PEDIATRIC HOSPITAL MEDICINE

MEDICINE

Textbook of Inpatient Management

SECOND EDITION

Edited By

...ald M. Perkin, M.D., M.A.

Professor & Chairman
Department of Pediatrics
The Brody School of Medicine
East Carolina University
Greenville, North Carolina

James D. Swift, M.D.

Medical Director
Sunrise Children's Hospital
Director of Critical Care and Hospitalist Program
Santa Barbara Cottage Children's Hospital
Santa Barbara, California
Riverside County Regional Medical Center
Riverside, California

Dale A. Newton, M.D.

Professor of Pediatrics
Senior Vice Chair for Operations
Clinical Professor of Medicine
Head, Division of General Pediatrics
Department of Pediatrics
The Brody School of Medicine
Greenville, North Carolina

Nick G. Anas, M.D.

Medical Director
Pediatric Intensive Care Unit
Children's Hospital of Orange County
Clinical Professor of Pediatrics
David Geffen School of Medicine at UCLA
Orange, California

Wolters Kluwer | Lippincott Williams & Wilkins
Health

Philadelphia · Baltimore · New York · London
Buenos Aires · Hong Kong · Sydney · Tokyo

Acquisitions Editor: Sonya Seigafuse
Managing Editor: Ryan Shaw
Marketing Manager: Kimberly Schonberger
Project Manager: Fran Gunning
Manufacturing Coordinator: Kathleen Brown
Design Coordinator: Stephen Druding
Compositor: International Typesetting and Composition

© 2008 by LIPPINCOTT WILLIAMS & WILKINS, a WOLTERS KLUWER business
530 Walnut Street
Philadelphia, PA 19106 USA
LWW.com

Printed in the USA

Library of Congress Cataloging-in-Publication Data
ISBN-13: 978-0-7817-7032-3
ISBN-10: 0-7817-7032-7

Pediatric hospital medicine : textbook of inpatient management / [edited by]
Ronald M. Perkin . . . [et al.]. -- 2nd ed.
    p. ; cm.
  Includes bibliographical references and index.
  ISBN-13: 978-0-7817-7032-3
  ISBN-10: 0-7817-7032-7
  1. Pediatrics. 2. Clinical medicine. 3. Teaching hospitals. I. Perkin, Ronald M.
  [DNLM: 1. Pediatrics--methods. 2. Clinical Medicine--methods. 3. Hospitals, Teaching.
WS 200 P37127 2008]
  RJ47.P367 2008
  618.92--dc22
                                                                    2007015408

Care has been taken to confirm the accuracy of the information presented and to describe
generally accepted practices. However, the authors, editors, and publisher are not responsible for errors or omissions or for any consequences from application of the information in
this book and make no warranty, expressed or implied, with respect to the currency, completeness, or accuracy of the contents of the publication. Application of the information in a
particular situation remains the professional responsibility of the practitioner.

The authors, editors, and publisher have exerted every effort to ensure that drug selection and dosage set forth in this text are in accordance with current recommendations and
practice at the time of publication. However, in view of ongoing research, changes in government regulations, and the constant flow of information relating to drug therapy and drug
reactions, the reader is urged to check the package insert for each drug for any change in
indications and dosage and for added warnings and precautions. This is particularly important when the recommended agent is a new or infrequently employed drug.

Some drugs and medical devices presented in the publication have Food and Drug
Administration (FDA) clearance for limited use in restricted research settings. It is the
responsibility of the health care provider to ascertain the FDA status of each drug or device
planned for use in their clinical practice.

To purchase additional copies of this book, call our customer service department at
(800) 638-3030 or fax orders to (301) 223-2320. International customers should call (301)
223-2300.

Visit Lippincott Williams & Wilkins on the Internet: at LWW.com. Lippincott Williams
& Wilkins customer service representatives are available from 8:30 am to 6 pm, EST.

10 9 8 7 6 5 4 3 2 1

DEDICATION

With appreciation for the support of our spouses,
Susan
Nancy
Emmie
Nancy

for the love of our children and grandchildren,
Nick, Matt, Jeff, Mitch, Benjamin, and Savannah
Allison and Chandler
Alan, Dan, David, Abby, and Kacy
Lauren, Nikki, Katie, and Stephen

and the education by and encouragement of our many teachers and mentors, but especially
Drs. Lewis Barness, James Hallock, and Dan Levin
Drs. Ronald Perkin and Nick Anas
Drs. Floyd Denny, Harvey Hamrick, and Ed Sumpter
Drs. Dan Levin, Charles Ginsburg, John Brooks, and John McBride

We also appreciate the encouragement and stimulation of our students, residents, and colleagues.

Special thanks is extended to
Barbara J. Heath
Nancy P. Leggett
April Andrews
Nicole Wagner
and
Ryan Shaw

Who helped us make revisions, meet deadlines, and tolerated our bad moods.

Again, we thank you all!
Ronald M. Perkin, MD, MA
James D. Swift, MD
Dale A. Newton, MD
Nick G. Anas, MD

Mary-Alice Abbott, M.D. Ph.D.
Associate Professor, Department of Pediatrics, Tufts University School of Medicine; Clinical Genetics, Bay State Medical Center, Springfield, Massachusetts

William T. Adamson, M.D.
Assistant Professor of Surgery, Division of Pediatric Surgery, Department of Surgery, University of North Carolina at Chapel Hill School of Medicine, Chapel Hill, North Carolina

Sana Al-Jundi, M.D.
Associate Clinical Professor, Department of Pediatrics, David Geffen School of Medicine at UCLA, Los Angeles, California Pediatric Intensive Care Attending Children Hospital of Orange County, Orange, California

Nick G. Anas, M.D.
Medical Director, Pediatric Intensive Care Unit, Children's Hospital of Orange County, Clinical Professor of Pediatrics, David Geffen School of Medicine at UCLA, Orange, California

Katherine Andreeff, M.D.
Pediatric Hospitalist, Pediatric Subspecialty Faculty, Children's Hospital of Orange County, Orange, California

Jeff Armstrong, M.D.
Pediatric Hospitalist, Hospitalist Division, Children's Hospital of Orange County, Orange, California

Pamela H. Arn, M.D.
Chief, Division of Genetics, Nemours Children's Clinic, Jacksonville, Florida

Antonio C. Arrieta, M.D.
Director, Pediatric Infectious Diseases, Children's Hospital of Orange County, Orange, California

Negar Ashouri

Stephen Ashwal, M.D.
Chief, Department of Pediatrics, Division of Neurology, Loma Linda University School of Medicine, Loma Linda, California

Howard I. Baron, M.D.
Associate Professor, Department of Pediatrics, University of Nevada School of Medicine; Vice Chief of Staff, Sunrise Hospital and Sunrise Children's Hospital; Pediatric Gastroenterology and Nutrition Associates, Las Vegas, Nevada

Sudipa Barr, M.D.
Section of Pediatric Endocrinology, Division of Pediatrics, Cleveland Clinic Children's Hospital, Cleveland Clinic Foundation, Cleveland, Ohio

Anjan S. Batra, M.D.
Assistant Professor, Division of Cardiology, Department of Pediatrics, University of California-Irvine; Director of Electrophysiology, Children's Hospital of Orange County, Orange, California

Cassie A. Billings, B.S. Pharm., Pharm.D.
Affiliate Instructor, Department of Pediatrics, The Brody School of Medicine, East Carolina University; Clinical Pharmacy Specialist—Pediatrics, Department of Pharmacy Services, University Health Systems of Eastern Carolina, Greenville, North Carolina

Sheryl Boon

Kristin Brown, M.S., RD
Pediatric Dietitian, Clinical Nutrition Services, The Children's Hospital, Denver, Colorado

Kristina K. Bryant, M.D.
Assistant Professor, Department of Pediatrics, Hospital Epidemiologist, Kosair Children's Hospital, Louisville, Kentucky

Melissa C. Brinn, M.D.
Clinical Assistant Professor, Department of Pediatrics, The Brody School of Medicine, East Carolina University; Active Medical Staff, Department of Pediatrics, Children's Hospital, University Health Systems of Eastern Carolina, Greenville, North Carolina

Nathan Andrew Brinn, M.D.
Clinical Assistant Professor, Department of Pediatrics; Medical Director, Adult and Pediatric Health Care; The Brody School of Medicine, East Carolina University; Active Medical Staff, Department of Pediatrics, Children's Hospital, University Health Systems of Eastern Carolina, Greenville, North Carolina

Stephen C. Boos, M.D.
Clinical Associate Professor of Pediatrics, University of Medicine and Dentistry of New Jersey, School of Osteopathic Medicine, NJ Cares Institute, Stratford, New Jersey; Medical Director, Treehouse Child Assessment Center, Rockville, Maryland

Tyrone G. Bristol, M.D., M.P.H.
Attending Pediatrician, Albany Medical Center Pediatric Group, Associate Professor of Pediatrics, Albany Medical College, Albany, New York

Ronald A. Bronicki, M.D.
Assistant Clinical Professor, Department of Pediatrics, Harbor-UCLA Medical Center, University of California Los Angeles School of Medicine; Clinical Director, Cardiac Intensive Care Unit, Children's Hospital of Orange County, Orange, California

Elaine S. Cabinum-Foeller, M.D.
Associate Professor of Pediatrics, Medical Director, TEDI BEAR: Children's Advocacy Center, Department of Pediatrics, The Brody School of Medicine, East Carolina University; Active Medical Staff, Department of Pediatrics, Children's Hospital, University Health Systems of Eastern Carolina, Greenville, North Carolina

James P. Cappon, M.D.
Medical Director of Quality and Patient Safety, and Pediatric Critical Care Medicine, Children's Hospital of Orange County; Clinical Assistant Professor of Pediatrics, Harbor-UCLA Medical Center, UCLA Geffen School of Medicine, and University of California, Irvine Medical Center, Orange, California

Teresa R. Carroll, R.N., M.S.N., P.N.P.
Pediatric Gastroenterology and Nutrition Associates, Las Vegas, Nevada

Ying T. Chang, M.D., M.P.H.
Professor and Head, Section of Endocrinology, Department of Pediatrics, The Brody School of Medicine, East Carolina University; Active Medical Staff, Department of Pediatrics, Children's Hospital, University Health Systems of Eastern Carolina, Greenville, North Carolina

Minakshi Chaudhari, M.D., M.S.
Pediatric Rheumatology, Children's Hospital of Orange County, Orange, California

Paul A. Checchia, M.D.
Chief, Pediatric Cardiac Critical Care Service, Co-Director, Pediatric Intensive Care Unit, St. Louis Children's Hospital; Assistant Professor of Pediatric Critical Care and Cardiology, Washington University School of Medicine, St. Louis, Missouri

Anthony Cherin, M.D.
Clinical Faculty, Pediatric Critical Care, Children's Hospital Orange County, Orange, California; Clinical Faculty, Pediatric Critical Care, University of California at Irvine, Irvine, California

Melinda C. Clark-Gambelunghe, M.D.
Assistant Professor, Department of Pediatrics, Albany Medical College, Albany, New York

William E. Cleve, M.T., M.P.H.
Public Health Epidemiologist, Infection Control Department, Pitt County Memorial Hospital, Greenville, North Carolina

Michael H. Cohen, J.D., M.B.A., M.F.A.
President, Institute for Integrative and Energy Medicine; Assistant Clinical Professor of Medicine, Harvard Medical School, Boston, Massachusetts

Paul P. Cook, M.D.
Associate Professor, Department of Medicine, The Brody School of Medicine, East Carolina University; Active Medical Staff, Department of Medicine, Pitt County Memorial Hospital, University Health Systems of Eastern Carolina, Greenville, North Carolina

David N. Collier, M.D., Ph.D.
Assistant Professor, Department of Pediatrics; Adjunct Assistant Professor, Department of Family Medicine and Department of Exercise and Sport Science, The Brody School of Medicine, East Carolina University: Active Medical Staff, Department of Pediatrics, Children's Hospital, University Health Systems of Eastern Carolina, Greenville, North Carolina

Joseph P. Cravero, M.D.
Professor of Anesthesia and Pediatrics, Dartmouth Hitchcock Medical Center, Dartmouth Medical School, Lebanon, New Hampshire

George W. Crowl, M.D.
Associate Clinical Professor, Department of Physical Medicine and Rehabilitation and Department of Pediatrics, The Brody School of Medicine, East Carolina University; Director of Pediatric Rehabilitation, Pitt County Memorial Hospital, Greenville, North Carolina

James J. Cummings, M.D.
Professor of Pediatrics and Adjunct Professor of Physiology, Department of Pediatrics, The Brody School of Medicine, East Carolina University; Active Medical Staff, Department of Pediatrics, Children's Hospital, University Health Systems of Eastern Carolina, Greenville, North Carolina

Coleen K. Cunningham, M.D.
Associate Professor, Department of Pediatrics, Division of Infectious Diseases, Duke University Medical Center, Durham, North Carolina

Charles W. Daeschner, III, M.D.
Professor, Department of Pediatrics, The Brody School of Medicine, East Carolina University; Active Medical Staff, Department of Pediatrics, Children's Hospital, University Health Systems of Eastern Carolina, Greenville, North Carolina

William A. B. Dalzell, M.D.
Assistant Clinical Professor of Pediatrics, Section of Infectious Diseases, The Brody School of Medicine, East Carolina University; Active Medical Staff, Children's Hospital, Department of Pediatrics, University Health Systems of Eastern Carolina, Greenville, North Carolina

Debra S. Demos, M.D.
Assistant Professor, Department of Pediatrics, Division of Child Neurology, Loma Linda University School of Medicine, Loma Linda, California

Carl V. Dezenberg, M.D.
Assistant Professor, Department of Pediatrics, University of Nevada School of Medicine, Pediatric Gastroenterology and Nutrition Associates, Las Vegas, Nevada

Sharron L. Docherty, Ph.D., C.P.N.P.(AC)
Assistant Professor, Pediatric Acute/Chronic Care Advanced Practice Specialty Director School of Nursing, Duke University; Pediatric Nurse Practitioner, Valvano Day Hospital, Pediatrics, Duke University Hospital, Durham, North Carolina

Joseph B. Domachowske, M.D.
Associate Professor, Department of Pediatrics, Division of Infectious Diseases, State University of New York (SUNY) Upstate Medical University, Syracuse, New York

David L. Eldridge, M.D.
Assistant Professor, Department of Pediatrics, The Brody School of Medicine, East Carolina University; Active Medical Staff, Department of Pediatrics, Children's Hospital, University Health Systems of Eastern Carolina, Greenville, North Carolina

Jeffrey P. Engel, M.D.
State Epidemiologist and Chief, Epidemiology Section, Division of Public Health, Department of Health and Human Services, Raleigh, North Carolina

Duncan M. Fagundus, M.D.
Staff Physician, Division of Rheumatology, Physicians East, Consultant Physician, Department of Pediatrics, Children's Hospital, University Health Systems of Eastern Carolina, Greenville, North Carolina

David L. Fairbrother, M.D., M.S.C.R.
Assistant Professor, Department of Pediatrics, Division of Pediatric Cardiology, The Brody School of Medicine, East Carolina University; Active Medical Staff, Department of Pediatrics, University Health Systems of Eastern Carolina, Greenville, North Carolina

Irma Fiordalisi, M.D.
Professor, Department of Pediatrics, The Brody School of Medicine, East Carolina University; Director, Pediatric Intensive Care Unit, Department of Pediatrics, Children's Hospital, University Health Systems of Eastern Carolina, Greenville, North Carolina

Anna Grattan Flik, M.D.
Assistant Professor of Pediatrics, Albany Medical College, Division of General Pediatrics, Albany Medical Center, Albany, New York

Emily Fontane, M.D.
Assistant Professor, Department of Emergency Medicine, The Brody School of Medicine, East Carolina University; Attending Physician, Department of Emergency Medicine, Pitt County Memorial Hospital, Greenville, North Carolina

Lori D. Frasier, M.D.
Professor of Pediatrics, University of Utah School of Medicine; Medical Director, Medical Assessment Program, Center for Safe and Healthy Families, Primary Children's Medical Center, Salt Lake City, Utah

Herbert E. Fuchs, M.D., Ph.D.
Associate Professor, Head of Pediatric Neurosurgical Services, Division of Neurosurgery, Department of Surgery, Duke University School of Medicine, Durham, North Carolina

Patricia S. Gerber, M.D.
Staff Physician, National Allergy, Asthma & Urticaria Centers of Charleston, Charleston, South Carolina

Gary Goodman, M.D.
Clinical Instructor of Pediatrics, UCLA School of Medicine; Director, PICU and Hospitalist Service, CHOC at Mission, Orange, California

David A. Gremse, M.D.
Professor and Chair, Department of Pediatrics, Section on Pediatric Gastroenterology, University of Nevada School of Medicine, Las Vegas, Nevada

David W. Hannon, M.D.
Professor, Department of Pediatrics, The Brody School of Medicine, East Carolina University; Active Medical Staff, Department of Pediatrics, Children's Hospital, University Health Systems of Eastern Carolina, Greenville, North Carolina

Glenn D. Harris, M.D.
Professor, Department of Pediatrics, Section of Endocrinology/Diabetology, The Brody School of Medicine, East Carolina University; Active Medical Staff, Department of Pediatrics, Children's Hospital, University Health Systems of Eastern Carolina, Greenville, North Carolina

Timothy H. Hartzog, M.D.
Pediatric Hospitalist, Assistant Professor of Pediatrics, Medical University of South Carolina, Charleston, South Carolina

David A. Hicks, M.D.
Pediatric Critical Care and Pulmonary Diseases, Director of the Cystic Fibrosis Care, Research and Teaching Center, Children's Hospital of Orange County, Orange, California; Clinical Instructor, University of California at Irvine, School of Medicine

Karin M. Hillenbrand, M.D.
Professor, Department of Pediatrics, The Brody School of Medicine, East Carolina University, Active Medical Staff, Department of Pediatrics, Children's Hospital, University Health Systems of Eastern Carolina, Greenville, North Carolina

Susan C. Hoffman, M.D.
Medical Director Pediatric Hospitalits, Pediatrix Medical Group; Medical Director Pediatric Unit, Sky Ridge Medical Center, Lone Tree, Colorado

Opal Jean Hood, M.D.
Associate Professor, Emeritius, Honorary Medical Staff, Department of Pediatrics, The Brody School of Medicine, East Carolina University; Active Medical Staff, Department of Pediatrics, Children's Hospital, University Health Systems of Eastern Carolina, Greenville, North Carolina

Patrician M. Hopkins, M.D.
Assistant Professor, Department of Pediatrics, Albany Medical College, Albany, New York

Thomas G. Irons, M.D.
Professor of Pediatrics, The Brody School of Medicine, East Carolina University, Greenville, North Carolina

Dina M. Iwai, M.D.
CHOC Clinical Attending Pediatric Critical Care, Board Certified, Orange, California

Katherine L. Jacoby, R.N., M.S.N., C.P.N.P.
Cardiovascular Nurse Practitioner, Children's Hospital of Orange County, Orange, California

Donald L. Janner, M.D.
Associate Professor, Department of Pediatrics, Division of Infectious Diseases, Loma Linda Children's Hospital, Loma Linda, California

Amy J. Jones, B.S., R.R.T.
Coordinator, Center for Children with Complex and Chronic Conditions, Children's Hospital, University Health Systems of Eastern Carolina, Greenville, North Carolina

Sue Joan Jue, M.D.
Associate Professor of Pediatrics, University Medical Group, Department of Pediatrics, Section of Infectious Diseases, Greenville Memorial Hospital, Greenville, South Carolina

Kathi J. Kemper, M.D., M.P.H.
Caryl J. Guth Chair for Holistic and Integrative Medicine, Professor, Pediatrics; Family and Community Medicine; and Public Health Sciences, Wake Forest University School of Medicine, Winston-Salem, North Carolina

Jean F. Kenny, M.D.
Professor Emeritus, Department of Pediatrics, Division of Infectious Diseases, The Brody School of Medicine, East Carolina University, Greenville, North Carolina

Loretta M. Kopelman, Ph.D.
Professor, Department of Medical Humanities, The Brody School of Medicine, East Carolina University, Greenville, North Carolina

James D. Korb, M.D.
Director, Academic Affairs; Director, Pediatric Residency Program, Children's Hospital of Orange County, Orange, California

Jason M. Knight, M.D.
Medical Director, Emergency Transport Services; Clinical Faculty, Pediatric Critical Care, Children's Hospital Orange County, Orange, California; Clinical Faculty, Pediatric Critical Care, University of California at Irvine, Santa Ana, California

Patricia A. Lange, M.D.
Assistant Professor of Surgery, Division of Pediatric Surgery, Department of Surgery, University of North Carolina at Chapel Hill School of Medicine, Chapel Hill, North Carolina

Pamela G. Larsen, Dr.P.H., D.N.Sc., F.N.P.
Clinical Faculty, Department of Pediatrics, Division of General Pediatrics, The Brody School of Medicine, East Carolina University, Greenville, North Carolina

Michael A. Levine, M.D.
Lerner Research Institute, Division of Pediatrics, Cleveland Clinic Children's Hospital, Cleveland Clinic Foundation, Cleveland, Ohio

Russell C. Libby, M.D.
Clinical Instructor, Department of Pediatrics, Virginia Commonwealth University School of Medicine; Chief, General Pediatrics, Inova Fairfax Hospital for Children, Falls Church, Virginia

Amy E. Lovejoy, M.D.
Director, Hemophilia and Thrombosis Treatment Center, Rady Children's Hospital; Assistant Clinical Professor, Department of Pediatrics, University of California, San Diego, California

Patricia V. Lowery, M.D.
Duke Endowment Fellow for the Masters in Public Health, East Carolina University; Fellow of Neonatology, Department of Pediatrics, The Brody School of Medicine, East Carolina University, Pitt County Memorial Hospital, Greenville, North Carolina

Paul S. Lubinsky, M.D.
Assistant Clinical Professor, Harbor-UCLA Medical Center, David Geffen School of Medicine at UCLA, Torrance, California; Associate Director PICU Children's Hospital Orange County, Orange, California

Judith A. Lucas, M.D.
Assistant Professor, Pediatrics, Albany Medical College, Albany, New York

Karen F. Lurito, M.D.
Clinical Assistant Professor, Section of Cardiology, Department of Pediatrics, The Brody School of Medicine, East Carolina University; Active Medical Staff, Department of Pediatrics, Children's Hospital, University Health Systems of Eastern Carolina, Greenville, North Carolina

Jennifer MacFarquhar, R.N., M.P.H., C.I.C.
Public Health Epidemiologist Program Director, North Carolina Statewide Program for Infection Control and Epidemiology, University of North Carolina, Chapel Hill, North Carolina

Scott S. MacGilvray, M.D.
Clinical Associate Professor of Pediatrics, Department of Pediatrics, The Brody School of Medicine, East Carolina University; Active Medical Staff, Department of Pediatrics, Children's Hospital, University Health Systems of Eastern Carolina, Greenville, North Carolina

Sharon A. Mangan, M.D.
Associate Clinical Professor, Department of Pediatrics, The Brody School of Medicine, East Carolina University, Greenville, North Carolina

Chalmer D. McClure, M.D., Ph.D.
Assistant Professor, Department of Pediatrics, Division of Child Neurology, Loma Linda University School of Medicine, Loma Linda, California

Mark S. McConnell, M.D.
Co-Medical Director, Pediatric Intensive Care Unit, St. Luke's Children's Hospital, Boise, Idaho

Troy McGuire, M.D.
Hospitalist, Director of Medical Informatics, Children's Hospital of Orange County, Orange, California

Donna M. Messenger
Director of Operations, Medical Management and Billing Network, Las Vegas, Nevada

David J. Michelson
Assistant Professor of Pediatrics, Division of Neurology, Loma Linda University School of Medicine, Loma Linda, California

Claude J. Migeon, M.D.
Professor, Department of Pediatrics, Pediatric Endocrinology, Johns Hopkins University, Baltimore, Maryland

Daniel P. Moore, M.D.
Professor and Chairman, Department of Physical Medicine and Rehabilitation; Professor, Department of Pediatrics, The Brody School of Medicine, East Carolina University, Active Medical Staff, Children's Hospital, University Health Systems of Eastern Carolina, Greenville, North Carolina

Dale A. Newton, M.D.
Professor of Pediatrics, Senior Vice Chair for Operations; Clinical Professor of Medicine, Head, Division of General Pediatrics, Department of Pediatrics, The Brody School of Medicine, Greenville, North Carolina; Active Medical Staff, Department of Pediatrics, Children's Hospital, University Health Systems of Eastern Carolina

Khanh P. Nguyen, M.D.
Clinical Assistant Professor, Department of Pediatrics, The Brody School of Medicine, East Carolina University; Active Medical Staff, Department of Pediatrics, Children's Hospital, University Health Systems of Eastern Carolina, Greenville, North Carolina

Jessica R. Nichols, M.D.
Fellow, Division of Pediatric Infectious Diseases, University of Arkansas for Medical Sciences, Little Rock, Arkansas

Bruce G. Nickerson, M.D.
Associate Clinical Professor, Department of Pediatrics, University of California-Irvine; Director, Pulmonary Medicine, Children's Hospital of Orange County, Orange, California

William E. Novotny, M.D.
Associate Professor, Department of Pediatrics, The Brody School of Medicine, East Carolina University, Active Medical Staff, Department of Pediatrics, Children's Hospital, University Health Systems of Eastern Carolina, Greenville, North Carolina

John M. Olsson, M.D.
Associate Professor, Department of Pediatrics, The Brody School of Medicine, East Carolina University; Active Medical Staff, Department of Pediatrics, Children's Hospital, University Health Systems of Eastern Carolina, Greenville, North Carolina

Gary M. Onady, M.D., Ph.D.
Associate Professor, Departments of Internal Medicine and Pediatrics, Wright State University; Division Head, Department of Internal Medicine, The Children's Medical Center, Dayton, Ohio

Sameer S. Pathare, M.D.
Pediatric Hospitalist, Hospitalist Division, Children's Hospital of Orange County, Orange, California

Jack M. Percelay, M.D., M.P.H.
New Jersey Pediatric Board Representative, Society of Hospital Medicine; Pediatric Hospitalist, St. Barnabas Medical Center, Livingston, New Jersey

Ronald M. Perkin, M.D., M.A.
Professor and Chairman, Department of Pediatrics, The Brody School of Medicine, East Carolina University; Chief of Pediatrics, Department of Pediatrics, Children's Hospital, University Health Systems of Eastern Carolina, Greenville, North Carolina

Laura E. Peter, M.D.
Resident, Department of Physical Medicine and Rehabilitation, The Brody School of Medicine, East Carolina University; Pitt Memorial Hospital, Greenville, North Carolina

J. Duncan Phillips, M.D.
Associate Professor of Surgery, Division of Pediatric Surgery, Department of Surgery, University of North Carolina at Chapel Hill School of Medicine, Chapel Hill, North Carolina

Curtis B. Pickert, M.D.
Medical Director, Pediatric Critical Care, Cottage Children's Hospital, Santa Barbara, California

David M. Polaner, M.D., F.A.A.P.
Associate Professor of Pediatric Anesthesiology, University of Colorado School of Medicine; Attending Anesthesiologist and Chief, Acute Pain Service, The Children's Hospital, Denver, Colorado

J. Rainer Poley, M.D.
Clinical Professor and Head, Section of Gastroenterology, Department of Pediatrics, The Brody School of Medicine, East Carolina University; Active Medical Staff, Department of Pediatrics, Children's Hospital, University Health Systems of Eastern Carolina, Greenville, North Carolina

Jenifer L. Powell, Ph.D.
Pediatric Psychologist, Department of Psychology, Pitt County Memorial Hospital, Greenville, North Carolina

Kathleen Vincent Previll, M.D.
Clinical Professor, Department of Pediatrics, The Brody School of Medicine, East Carolina University; Active Medical Staff, Department of Pediatrics, University Health Systems of Eastern Carolina, Greenville, North Carolina

Julia T. Raper, RN, MSN
Administrator, Children's Hospital, University Health Systems of Eastern Carolina, Greenville, North Carolina

Daniel A. Rauch, M.D.
Director, Pediatric Hospitalist Program, New York University of Medicine, New York

Christopher Rhee, M.D.
Assistant Professor, Department of Pediatrics, University of Nevada School of Medicine, Pediatric Gastroenterology and Nutrition Associates, Las Vegas, Nevada

Taryn R. Richardson, M.D.
Fellow, Division of Allergy and Immunology, Department of Pediatrics, University of North Carolina School of Medicine, Chapel Hill, North Carolina

Sarah M. Roddy, M.D.
Associate Professor, Departments of Pediatrics and Neurology, Loma Linda University School of Medicine, Loma Linda, California

Philip Rosenthal, M.D.
Professor of Pediatrics and Surgery, Departments of Pediatric Gastroenterology, Hepatology, Nutrition and Liver Transplant and Pediatrics, University of California, San Francisco, California

Joseph Rosenthal
Associate Professor, Director, Pediatric Bone Marrow Transplantation, City of Hope Medical Center, Duarte, California

Adam K. Rowden, D.O.
Director, Division of Toxicology, Department of Emergency
Medicine, Albert Einstein Medical Center, Philadelphia,
Pennsylvania

Michael E. Reichel, M.D., M.P.H.
Clinical Professor and Head, Section of Behavioral and
Developmental Pediatrics; Medical Director, Children's
Developmental Services Agency; Department of Pediatrics,
The Brody School of Medicine, East Carolina University;
Active Medical Staff, Department of Pediatrics, Children's
Hospital, University Health Systems of Eastern Carolina,
Greenville, North Carolina

Charlie J. Sang, Jr., M.D.
Associate Professor, Department of Pediatrics, Section of
Pediatric Cardiology, The Brody School of Medicine, East
Carolina University; Active Medical Staff, Department of
Pediatrics, University Health Systems of Eastern Carolina,
Greenville, North Carolina

Roytesa R. Savage, M.D.
Assistant Professor, Department of Pediatrics, The Brody
School of Medicine, East Carolina University; Active Medical
Staff, Department of Pediatrics, Children's Hospital,
University Health Systems of Eastern Carolina, Greenville,
North Carolina

Karen Russell Schmidt, M.D.
Visiting Associate Professor of Pediatrics, Children's Hospital
of Pittsburgh, University of Pittsburgh Medical Center,
Pittsburgh, Pennsylvania

Jennifer Schneiderman, M.D., M.S.
Assistant Professor of Pediatrics, Division of Hematology,
Oncology, and Stem Cell Transplant, Children's Memorial
Hospital, Feinberg School of Medicine, Northwestern
University, Chicago, Illinois

Carrin E. Schottler-Thal, M.D.
Department of Pediatrics, Division of General Pediatrics,
Albany Medical College, Albany, New York

Binita R. Shah, M.D.
Professor, Departments of Emergency Medicine and
Pediatrics, State University of New York (SUNY) Downstate
Medical Center; Director, Pediatric Emergency Medicine,
Department of Emergency Medicine, Kings County Hospital
Center, Brooklyn, New York

Samir S. Shah, M.D., M.S.C.E.
Assistant Professor of Pediatrics and Epidemiology,
University of Pennsylvania School of Medicine; Attending
Physician, Divisions of Infectious Diseases and General
Pediatrics, The Children's Hospital of Philadelphia,
Philadelphia, Pennsylvania

Robert R. Shelton, Psy.D.
Clinical Psychologist, Department of Psychology, Pitt County
Memorial Hospital, Greenville, North Carolina

Stanford Shu, M.D.
Assistant Professor, Department of Pediatrics, Division of
Child Neurology, Loma Linda University School of Medicine,
Loma Linda, California

Kristina L. Simeonsson, M.D.
Assistant Professor of Pediatrics and Family Medicine
(Masters of Public Health Program), The Brody School of
Medicine, East Carolina University, Greenville, North
Carolina; Active Medical Staff, Department of Pediatrics,
Children's Hospital, University Health Systems of Eastern
Carolina

Sara H. Sinal, M.D.
Professor of Pediatrics and Family and Community Medicine,
Department of Pediatrics of Wake Forest University School of
Medicine, Brenner Children's Hospital, Winston Salem,
North Carolina

Jasjit Singh, M.D.
Associate Director, Pediatric Infectious Diseases Children's
Hospital of Orange County Orange, California

Seema Singla, M.S., R.D., L.D.N., C.N.S.D.
Pediatric Nutrition Specialist, Private Practice, Greenville,
North Carolina

Mark A. Sperling, M.D.
Professor of Pediatrics, University of Pittsburgh School of
Medicine, Division of Endocrinology, Diabetes, and
Metabolism, Department of Pediatrics, Children's Hospital of
Pittsburgh, Pittsburgh, Pennsylvania

Betty S. Spivack, M.D.
Clinical Assistant Professor, Department of Pediatrics,
University of Louisville, Louisville, Kentucky

R. Dennis Steed, M.D.
Associate Professor of Pediatrics, Pediatric Cardiology, The
Brody School of Medicine, East Carolina University; Active
Medical Staff, Department of Pediatrics, University Health
Systems of Eastern Carolina, Greenville, North Carolina

Gerald L. Strope, M.D.
Clinical Professor and Head, Section of Pulmonology,
Department of Pediatrics, The Brody School of Medicine,
East Carolina University: Active Medical Staff, Department
of Pediatrics, Children's Hospital, University Health Systems
of Eastern Carolina, Greenville, North Carolina

James D. Swift, M.D.
Medical Director, Sunrise Children's Hospital, Las Vegas,
Nevada; Director, Department of Critical Care, Santa
Barbara Cottage Children's Hospital, Santa Barbara,
California and Riverside County Regional Medical Center,
Riverside, California

Gregg M. Talente, M.D., M.S.Ed.
Associate Professor, Departments of Internal Medicine and
Pediatrics, The Brody School of Medicine, East Carolina
University; Active Medical Staff, Department of Pediatrics,
Children's Hospital, University Health Systems of Eastern
Carolina, Greenville, North Carolina

Tina Q. Tan, M.D.
Associate Professor, Department of Pediatrics, Feinberg
School of Medicine, Northwestern University, and
Department of Pediatrics, Children's Memorial Hospital,
Chicago, Illinois

Jeffrey A. Towbin
Professor, Departments of Pediatrics (Cardiology) and
Molecular & Human Genetics, Baylor College of Medicine;
Chief of Pediatric Cardiology, Texas Children's Hospital,
Baylor College of Medicine, and Texas Heart Institute; Texas
Children's Foundation Chair in Pediatric Cardiac Research,
Houston, Texas

Debra A. Tristram, M.D.
Clinical Professor of Pediatrics, Section of Infectious
Diseases, The Brody School of Medicine, East Carolina
University; Active Medical Staff, Children's Hospital,
Department of Pediatrics, University Health Systems of
Eastern Carolina, Greenville, North Carolina

Dawn A. Tucker, R.N., M.S.N., C.P.N.P.
Cardiovascular Nurse Practitioner, Children's Hospital of
Orange County, Orange, California

Karen R. Underwood, M.D.
Assistant Professor, Department of Pediatrics, Division of
Critical Care Medicine, Washington University School of
Medicine, St. Louis, Missouri

Daniel vonAllmen, M.D.
Associate Professor of Surgery, Division of Pediatric Surgery,
Department of Surgery, University of North Carolina at
Chapel Hill School of Medicine, Chapel Hill, North
Carolina; Surgeon-in-Chief, North Carolina Children's
Hospital, Chapel Hill, North Carolina

Kelly M. Waicus, M.D.
Team Physician, UNC Sports Medicine, University of North
Carolina; Active Medical Staff, Department of Pediatrics,
UNC Hospitals, Chapel Hill, North Carolina

Carrie E. Waller, M.D., M.S.
Attending Pediatrician, Washington Pediatrics, Washington,
North Carolina

David O. Walterhouse, M.D.
Assistant Professor of Pediatrics, Division of Hematology,
Oncology, and Stem Cell Transplant, Children's Memorial
Hospital, Feinberg School of Medicine, Northwestern
University, Chicago, Illinois

Timothy M. Weiner, M.D.
Associate Professor of Surgery, Division of Pediatric Surgery,
Department of Surgery, University of North Carolina at
Chapel Hill School of Medicine, Chapel Hill, North Carolina

Robert C. Welliver, Sr., M.D.
Professor, Department of Pediatrics and Co-Director, Division
of Infectious Diseases, Women and Children's Hospital of
Buffalo, Buffalo, New York

Charles F. Willson, M.D.
Clinical Professor, Department of Pediatrics, The Brody
School of Medicine, Greenville, North Carolina; Active
Medical Staff, Department of Pediatrics, Children's Hospital,
University Health Systems of Eastern Carolina

Judy W. Wood, M.D.
Clinical Professor of Pediatrics, The Brody School of
Medicine, Greenville, North Carolina

Guy Young, M.D.
Director, Hemostasis and Thrombosis Center, Children's
Hospital; Associate Professor of Clinical Pediatrics,
University of Southern California Keck School of Medicine,
Los Angeles, California

Anchalee Yuengsrigul, M.D.
Assistant Professor of Pediatrics, Department of Pediatrics,
University of California Irvine; Pediatric Subspecialty Faculty,
Division of Pediatric Pulmonology, Department of Pediatrics,
Children's Hospital of Orange County, Orange, California

Joseph R. Zanga, M.D.
Jefferson-Pilot/Catherine and Max Ray Joyner, Distinguished
Professor in Primary Care; Assistant Dean for Generalist
Programs, Director, Office of Generalist Programs, Professor
of Pediatrics; The Brody School of Medicine at East Carolina
University, Active Medical Staff, Department of Pediatrics,
Children's Hospital, University Health Systems of Eastern
Carolina, Greenville, North Carolina

In 2003 we were honored to have the opportunity to bring *Pediatric Hospital Medicine* into publication with the help of the publishing company of Lippincott Williams & Wilkins. At that time this was the first textbook to specifically address the clinical information needed for providers of pediatric hospital care. Subsequent reviews were positive and in turn the textbook was well received by our colleagues. We are now honored to have the opportunity to produce a second edition with the assistance of the fine staff at Lippincott Williams & Wilkins (now a division of Wolters Kluwer).

The goals for this edition are to retain and refine those of the first edition. The content of the book focuses on the information needed to provide timely high-quality care on the general pediatric ward and in the newborn nursery. For issues related to the care of patients in the pediatric intensive care or neonatal intensive care units, we refer the reader to the excellent texts and resources specific to those patient care areas. The goals for this book do not include the attempt to achieve comprehensive depth, but rather to focus on the information necessary to quickly develop differential diagnoses and management plans for common clinical problems and presentations on the ward and newborn nursery. It is intended to be relatively concise and user friendly.

As a second edition, we hope that this book achieves these goals even better than the first edition. When appropriate, suggestions and corrections from readers and colleagues were included. The content has been edited in selected areas to be more useful and to better meet the above goals. Much of the material has been edited to reflect changes and advances based on recent journal publications. We also added an additional editor (thank you, Nick) and a number of new chapter authors who help make this book an even better clinical and educational resource.

The paradigm of care for hospitalized children continues to evolve. Pediatric hospitalists are increasing in number, especially in urban centers and large community hospitals. Yet in many locales, inpatient pediatric care continues to be provided by primary care community pediatricians, family physicians, and physician extenders. Regardless of the specifics of the community setting, practitioner training, or practice environment, we have attempted to make this book a useful resource by providing the information necessary to quickly provide high-quality medical care to infants and children.

Pediatric Hospital Medicine continues to have an extensive section on newborn nursery care. Such care overlaps with issues within the neonatal intensive care unit, but often there are issues of newborn care specific to the newborn nursery that need to be addressed. This textbook includes material that should provide information and guidance pertinent to the care of term and near-term infants in that clinical setting.

This edition also includes expanded material about the care of children with chronic medical conditions. Increasingly, hospitalized children are not otherwise healthy children with an acute medical illness, but are children with a chronic underlying disease process. In turn, these children have medical issues that are more complex, with hospital stays that are more frequent and often longer. The editors selected additional material for inclusion with the hope that it would assist the pediatric provider in meeting the needs of these children with improved pediatric care and quality of life, and by acknowledging the need for a different paradigm of care to achieve these goals and decrease the hospitalization rate (and attendant costs) for these children.

The editors appreciate the support of our readers and solicit additional input about this publication and suggestions for any future edition. Most importantly, we hope that your patients have good outcomes.

CONTENTS

SECTION IV ■ CARDIOVASCULAR

SECTION V ■ PULMONARY DISEASE

SECTION VI ■ NEUROLOGIC

SECTION VII ■ GASTROENTEROLOGY

Section Editor: James D. Swift

SECTION VIII ■ HEMATOLOGY–ONCOLOGY

Section Editor: Nick G. Anas

SECTION IX ■ RENAL

Section Editor: Nick G. Anas

SECTION X N VASCULITIS/ RHEUMATOLOGIC

Section Editor: Nick G. Anas

CHAPTER 1 ■ THE TRANSFORMATION OF CHILD HEALTH

RONALD M. PERKIN AND CHARLES F. WILLSON

A child is born, healthy and vigorous. A great-grandparent dies a peaceful death in her sleep. A recently married couple rejoices at a positive home pregnancy test. Proud parents watch as their child graduates from college and enters adulthood. A pediatrician sees a child in a busy office and reassures the parent that this viral illness will pass with minimal discomfort and inconvenience. These are the expected outcomes in the cycles of our daily lives, in an ideal world.

All too often, these positive expectations are not realized. Approximately 20% of children in America have a chronic, and in some cases disabling, condition (1). Children are born with handicapping genetic syndromes. Trauma, some accidental and some inflicted, too often leads to permanent injury and death. Children and sometimes their parents suffer daily from mental illnesses. Many deadly infectious diseases have been conquered through good public health practices and immunizations, but new infectious agents such as pandemic influenza, Severe Acute Respiratory Syndrome (SARS), Human Immunodeficiency Virus (HIV), and drug-resistant *Staphylococcus aureus* and *Enterobacter* threaten to fill our hospital wards with severely sick and dying children. The need for a well-planned, well-equipped, and superbly staffed children's hospital or pediatric ward in a local hospital remains as pressing today as it was 75 years ago as the specialty of pediatrics was being created.

When is hospital care needed for a child? The simple but correct answer is, when the level of care needed cannot be achieved in the child's home. To remove a child from the familiar, safe, and comfortable setting of her own home should never be taken lightly. Hospital care, no matter how well intentioned and planned, is always complex and dangerous. Mistakes and errors of commission and omission occur all too frequently, even in our nation's finest children's hospitals. Hospital care is stressful at best for the child and the family, and at worst may be psychologically damaging. The child's support system, her family, must be included in all activities within the hospital care plan and beyond.

From the moment of admission to the hospital, the planning for discharge begins. Who will assume the care at home? What strengths and resources does the family possess that can be leveraged in the future care to assure a complete or optimal recovery? What stresses and weaknesses are present that might foil even the most carefully developed care plan? Who is the referring physician, and can that practice truly function as a medical home for a child with a condition of that complexity? How can we make the transition from hospital care to outpatient care as safe and seamless as possible? Hospital care is not an end unto itself but rather a hopefully brief but intense interruption in the normal cycle of the life of a child, the family, and even the community.

To assure that hospital care will be available and affordable when needed requires that all health care professionals for children be involved in all aspects of the life of the child's community, state, region, and nation. Good health care policy leads to best outcomes for children and their families. The lack of good schools, safe streets, and job opportunities will foil the goals of maximizing the life potential of our children. A lack of pediatric specialty care, therapeutic services, and respite care will diminish the chances of achieving maximal outcomes, especially for our children with complex and chronic conditions.

Following the vision for a new health care system articulated by the report from the National Institute of Medicine, *Crossing the Quality Chasm* (2), pediatric inpatient care must be viewed as part of a continuous healing relationship, based in a competent medical home in the child's community. If a pediatric hospitalist is to assume the care of the child in the hospital, that hospitalist should take every opportunity to get to know the referring physicians and the communities from which his patients come. Information must be shared freely yet confidentially. Safety of care must be a priority, especially focusing on transitions from one unit to another or from inpatient to outpatient care. Waste in the form of unnecessary, defensive, or duplicative tests and procedures must be eliminated. In an era where some radiologic examinations at night are being interpreted by highly trained and skilled professionals in other countries during their waking hours, we truly have the resources of the world available to treat our patients no matter where our hospital is located. The phrase, "That test or procedure is not done at night or on weekends in our hospital" should not be uttered in our new system.

Finally, we must measure and track what we do. Gone are the days when a physician could point to a list of research grants and publications as a proxy to evaluating the quality of care being delivered. Research and publications remain extraordinarily important in advancing medical knowledge, but the care delivered and actual outcomes achieved must be recorded and celebrated within every health care setting for children (3). Harmful sentinel events must be reported, investigated, and remedied in an open and blameless culture of continuous improvement. When a parent calls to ask where her child should go for a particular procedure, we should have at our fingertips the outcome profiles of the hospitals caring for children in that state or region. Our care must be transparent to the public and to ourselves. If we don't measure our care, we are truly flying blind. Here's a snapshot of what we do know about the health care of the child in the United States.

TRENDS IN ACUTE AND CHRONIC ILLNESS

Acute Illness

There has been little change in the incidence of acute illness among U.S. children (4). Data from the National Health Interview Survey (NHIS), a cross-sectional annual survey of approximately 40,000 households containing some 30,000 to 40,000 children, were used to track trends in acute illnesses over the past four decades (5). The NHIS defines *acute illness* as any disease or injury that requires an activity restriction or medical attention for less than 3 months. Overall, there was only a modest reduction in acute illness among children, as the average annual rate fell from 3 to 2.4 per child. This modest overall reduction was attributable almost entirely to declines among school-age children and adolescents, while the rate for young children remained remarkably stable. Children younger than 5 years of age averaged the highest number of acute illnesses per year, with approximately 3.2; school-age children averaged 2.1; and adolescents were reported to have experienced an average of 1.7 acute illnesses per year.

Although acute illnesses among school-age children fell only modestly, the number of days children were in bed because of illness fell 41% between 1962 and 2000. This dramatic decline was associated with a concomitant fall in days absent from school. Although the reasons for this elasticity between illness and its impact on bed disability and school absence cannot be ascertained from this data source, they likely reflect major trends in maternal employment and widespread use of effective medications to control fever.

Chronic Illness

Trends in the prevalence of chronic illness among American children have been difficult to ascertain due to the variability in the definition and diagnosis of chronic illness over the past several decades (6).

Estimates of childhood chronic illness have varied from less than 5% to more than 30% (7). The lower estimates tend to include only those children with diagnoses associated with significant disability or the need for specialized services or equipment. The estimates that approach one-third of all children include all chronic conditions regardless of their impact on child well-being, including allergic conditions, serous otitis media, and acne.

Of greatest relevance to the issue of pediatric practice, however, are likely to be estimates of children with chronic disorders that require an elevated use of health services. This dual requirement—the presence of a chronic disorder and elevated service—has been used by the Maternal and Child Health Bureau as a basis for a consensus definition of a subset of children with chronic conditions: "children with special health care needs" (8). Several recent efforts to operationalize this definition suggest that somewhere between 15% and 20% of all American children could be considered to have a special health care need (6).

Some children are more profoundly affected by their chronic condition than others. One study estimated that approximately 0.7% of children were not able to conduct their expected, age-appropriate activity (e.g., play for preschoolers, school for school-age children); another 4% were limited in some form in conducting these major activities; and 1.8% were limited not in their expected major activity but in other activities. Therefore, a total of 6.5% of all American children were estimated to be limited, or disabled, by their chronic illness in some manner (9).

Not surprisingly, the 15% to 20% of children categorized as having special health care needs have elevated use of health services. They are more than 3 times as likely to be confined to bed due to illness, visit a physician 2.5 times as often, and average more than 5 times as many days in the hospital compared with children without such special health care needs. For the estimated 6.5% of children with a reported disabling chronic condition, their average number of contacts with physicians was more than triple the average for all children without a disabling condition. It was estimated that some 11.4% of children with a disabling condition were hospitalized in the year prior to the survey, while 2.8% of children without such conditions were hospitalized over the same period, accounting for an eightfold difference in days of hospitalization (6,9).

When comparisons over time have been conducted, large increases in the prevalence of chronic childhood illnesses have been observed (10). Large increases in the reported prevalence of asthma and of behavioral and developmental problems have accounted for the bulk of the rise in chronic conditions.

There has also been considerable concern that clinical innovation, while increasingly efficacious, has actually served to increase the number of children with serious chronic illness and disability. Of special interest has been the potential impact of clinical interventions late in pregnancy and during the neonatal period. These obstetrical and pediatric interventions have resulted in dramatic declines in neonatal mortality. However, the question remains as to whether these improvements in survival have been associated with significant growth in the prevalence of serious disabilities among surviving children (11).

In addition, low-birthweight (LBW) infants have 20.5% more physician visits than their heavier-birthweight peers during the first 5 years of life (12). This implies that LBW infants are growing into a subpopulation of children with a greater likelihood to return to children's hospitals for everything from inguinal hernia repair to respiratory infections, apnea, gastroesophageal reflux, and more acute specialty care later in life.

Advances in treatments for chronic illnesses that were uniformly fatal in the past have resulted in a new population of older children and young adults that rely on children's hospitals for their medical care. Children with cystic fibrosis, sickle-cell anemia, and congenital heart disease are living longer and returning to hospitals over extended periods of time.

The broader mental health needs of children have become more apparent in recent years and account for some of the rise in chronic illness in children (13).

Dramatic increases in childhood obesity have also received considerable recent attention. Although obesity does not usually result in the kinds of functional impact that underlie most definitions of major chronic illness, it can be associated with a variety of chronic problems such as type II diabetes, asthma, hypertension, and sleep apnea.

The rise in the prevalence of chronic disorders can also be observed in patterns of bed disability days: in 1982 approximately 13% of all bed disability days in children were attributable to chronic conditions; the comparable figure for 2000 was approximately 25% (4).

SEVERITY OF PEDIATRIC ILLNESS AND HOSPITALIZATION

Even at a time when the capabilities of outpatient management are growing rapidly, hospitalization remains among the best general indicators of the severity of illness in children.

Analysis of data from the National Hospital Discharge Survey (NHDS), an annual sampling of U.S. acute care hospitals, suggests significant reductions in hospitalization, with a 45% decline between 1962 and 2000 (4,14). However, the precise cause of these reductions is undoubtedly heterogeneous, and incentives for outpatient treatment, including those associated with managed care, are likely to have played an important role. The length of hospital stay for children fell slightly over this time period as well.

To assess the relative contributions of acute and chronic illness to changing hospitalization patterns, the NHDS data were analyzed using a categorical, diagnosis-based definition for chronic illness based on NHIS criteria. Injuries accounted for approximately 9% of childhood admissions in 2000. Noninjury admissions were separated into acute and chronic hospitalizations. Chronic conditions were defined using the NHIS categorical system for conditions lasting at least 3 months. Although changes in diagnostic capacity and coding over more than four decades make detailed temporal comparisons somewhat problematic, the scale of the shift toward chronic diseases seems to have been profound. Among all medical admissions (excluding injury-related causes) for children younger than age 17, approximately one-fourth were associated with a chronic diagnosis in 1962; by 2000 the figure had more than doubled to approximately 55%.

The precise reasons for this dramatic shift remain poorly defined. However, evidence suggests that hospitalization rates and lengths of stay for children with chronic illness have fallen more slowly than among children without a chronic disease (15). In 1962, approximately 4% of hospital bed days for children were accounted for by children who had had two or more admissions that year; by 2000 this figure had risen to approximately 25%.

Acute infectious diseases remain an important cause for health service use and spending. However, chronic illness, particularly asthma and mental disorders (which include developmental, learning, and psychiatric disorders), accounts for a large portion of child health spending. When spending for all causes is assessed, approximately 80% of all nontraumatic spending was attributable to chronic illness, a figure applicable to just 20% of all children (16).

TRENDS IN MORTALITY

U.S. mortality rates for children have fallen dramatically over the past several decades. This should be viewed as the most recent extension of a long-standing trend of declining mortality among all age groups in the United States. Mortality from injuries remains the leading cause of death among children, although major reductions have been made in virtually all injury categories. Of the 13,555 total childhood deaths that occurred in 2001, some 6,646 were the result of unintentional injuries, by far the largest contributor (4).

Chronic illness contributes strikingly to U.S. child mortality. Data from Washington State suggest that children with complex chronic conditions—a small subset of children with chronic conditions—account for more than half of all childhood deaths from medical causes, excluding the perinatal age group (17). Other data suggest that approximately one-quarter of all medical pediatric deaths occur among children with two or more complex chronic conditions (18). Analysis of the National Vital Statistics Death Files suggests that these trends have occurred nationally as well, with significant increases in the contribution of chronic disorders to noninjury mortality rate (4). In 2000, some 70% of noninjury deaths among children ages 1 to 4 years and more than 80% of deaths among all school-age children were the result of chronic causes.

IMPLICATIONS FOR PRACTICE

Hospitalization and death among children have increasingly been associated with chronic illness. At the same time, well children have a far smaller risk of experiencing a serious acute illness than ever before. The terms "well" and "chronically ill" are used cautiously here, because well children can experience a variety of health problems, and chronic illness can reflect a spectrum of severity. However, the primary focus here is on the risk of serious illness, one likely to require specialized services or result in hospitalization or death. From this perspective, the concentration of hospitalization and mortality in chronic causes suggests a growing separation of the service needs of generally well children from those of chronically ill children. This dichotomy in the challenges confronting the child health care system is likely to be expressed as growing pressures for the high-volume provision of an array of preventive interventions and general counseling for the majority of children and the increasingly complex management of children with serious chronic illnesses (4,19).

The central focus for addressing the health care needs of all children rests with the provision of primary care. Recommendations to improve the health of children with complex health needs have relied on special programs with strong primary care services that offer high continuity of care and increased competence in coordinating linkages with subspecialty services, community-based support services, and hospital-based care, sites commonly referred to as "medical homes" (20). However, recent surveys have documented that this model characterizes the care of only about half of children with special health care needs (21). Other studies of children with specific chronic disorders such as asthma, cystic fibrosis, and sickle-cell disease have also found major deficiencies in the quality and coordination of services (4). At the same time, high-quality well-child care will increasingly require improvements in the provision and documentation of a growing number of immunizations, standardized screening protocols, guidance regarding sudden infant death syndrome (SIDS) and injury prevention, and general counseling techniques.

The reimbursement patterns of Medicaid and State Children's Health Insurance Program (SCHIP) continue to generate major disincentives to the development of medical homes and other comprehensive approaches to the care of chronically ill children (22). Managed care efforts have generally not improved the provision of appropriate services for these children (23). The Supplemental Security Income (SSI) program, while providing important cash and Medicaid benefits for some of the most seriously affected children, does not make provisions for establishing systems of care. In addition, proposals to extend coverage for "basic care" to currently uninsured children by eliminating specialized benefits for chronically ill children can only exacerbate these financial disincentives. Similarly, impulses to move away from the relatively comprehensive, mandated-benefit provisions of Medicaid toward the far more flexible structure of SCHIP could, without purposeful protections, lead to the erosion of covered benefits for chronically ill children. The implementation of medical homes will need to become the organizing principle around which child health financing and care is restructured in the years to come.

The dramatic improvements in the survival of children with serious chronic illness has meant that almost half a million children with special health care needs now reach adulthood each year (24). However, there remains a serious gap in policies and services that support this critical transition. Discontinuities in eligibility criteria for Medicaid, SCHIP, and SSI and related programs can often leave adolescents and young adults with severe medical conditions lacking coordinated health care or support services.

The dichotomization of child health may also require changes in the organization and training of child health care personnel. Physicians, particularly pediatricians, will need to focus more directly on the comprehensive management of children with chronic disorders. Pediatric hospitalists will play a larger role as the complexity of hospitalized patients rises. These developments could provide a much stronger platform to organize integrated primary and specialty systems of care and better coordinate the increasingly blurred lines between inpatient and outpatient care. The blurred distinction between inpatient and outpatient care implies that high-quality hospitalist care will require deep expertise, with the outpatient management of complex pediatric patients and the providers and systems in place for their care upon discharge. Indeed, pediatricians based in hospitals and even in intensive care settings will increasingly be required to engage or even help institute integrated systems of inpatient and outpatient care. Pediatric departments will increasingly find that the best guarantee of efficient high-quality inpatient care is the development of integrated programs that transcend traditional inpatient/outpatient barriers and ensure that hospitalists and intensivists who may come to know many chronically ill children extremely well interact seamlessly with pediatricians responsible for the care of these children in community settings. From this perspective, the true promise of the movement toward hospitalists may lie in their capacity to practice and ultimately to teach a deep respect for the transitional nature of pediatric care in the years to come.

References

1. Kastner T, Committee on Children with Disabilities. Managed care and children with special healthcare needs. *Pediatrics* 2004;114:1693–1698.
2. Committee on Quality of Health Care in America, Institute of medicine. *Crossing the Quality Chasm: A New Health System for the 21st Century.* Washington, DC: National Academics Press, 2001.
3. Landrigan C, Conway P, Edwards S, et al. Pediatric hospitalists: a systematic review of the literature. *Pediatrics* 2006;117:1736–1744.
4. Wise PH. The transformation of child health in the United States. *Health Affairs* 2004;23:9–25.
5. National Center for Health Statistics. National Health Interview Survey (NHIS). 2001 NHIS survey description. www.cdc.gov/nchs/about/major/nhis/quest_data_related_doc.htm.
6. Newacheck PW, Strickland B, Shonkoff JP, et al. An epidemiologic profile of children with special health care needs. *Pediatrics* 1998;102:117–123.
7. Newacheck PW, Stoddard JJ. Prevalence and impact of multiple childhood chronic illnesses. *J Pediatr* 1994;124:40–48.
8. Westbrook LE, Silver EJ, Stein REK. Implications of estimates of disability in children: a comparison of definitional components. *Pediatrics* 1998;101:1025–1030.
9. Newacheck PW, Halfon N. Prevalence and impact of disabling chronic conditions in childhood. *Am J Public Health* 1998;88:610–617.
10. Newacheck PW, Budetti PP, Halfon N. Trends in activity-limiting chronic conditions among children. *Am J Public Health* 1986;76:178–184.
11. Schmidt B, Asztalos EV, Roberts RS, et al. Trial of indomethacin prophylaxis in preterms (TIPP) investigators. Impact of bronchopulmonary dysplasia, brain injury, and severe retinopathy on the outcome of extremely low-birth-weight infants at 18 months: results from the trial of indomethacin prophylaxis in preterms. *JAMA* 2003;289:1124–1129.
12. McClimon PJ, Hansen TN. Why are children's hospitals so busy? *J Pediatr* 2003;142:219–220.
13. Kellcher KJ, McInerny TK, Gardner WP, et al. Increased identification of psychosocial problems. *Pediatrics* 2000;105:1313–1321.
14. National Center for Health Statistics. Design and operation of the National Hospital Discharge Survey. *Vital Health Stat 1* 2000;39:1–12.
15. Neff JM, Valentine J, Park A, et al. Trends in pediatric hospitalizations of children in Washington State by insurance and chronic condition status, 1991–1998. *Arch Pediatr Adol Med* 2002;156:703–709.
16. Elixhauser A, Machlin SR, Zodet MW, et al. Health care for children and youth in the United States:2001 annual report on access, utilization, quality, and expenditures. *Amb Pediatr* 2002;2:419–437.
17. Feudtner C, Silveira MJ, Christakis DA. Where do children with complex chronic conditions die? Patterns in Washington State, 1980–1998. *Pediatrics* 2002;109:656–660.
18. Feudtner C, Christakis DA, Zimmerman FJ, et al. Characteristics of deaths occurring in children's hospitals: implications for supportive care services. *Pediatrics* 2002;109:887–893.
19. Cheng TL. Primary care pediatrics: 2004 and beyond. *Pediatrics* 2004;113:1802–1809.
20. Sia C, Tonniqes TF, Osterhas E, et al. History of the medical home concept. *Pediatrics* 2004;113: 1473–1478.
21. Strickland B, McPherson M, Weismann G, et al. Access to the medical home: results of the national survey of children with special health care needs. *Pediatrics* 2004;113:1485–1492.
22. Neff JM, Anderson G. Protecting children with chronic illness in a competitive marketplace. *JAMA* 1995;274:1866–1869.
23. Ferris TG, Perrin JM, Manqanello JA, et al. Switching to gatekeeping: Changes in expenditures and utilization for children. *Pediatrics* 2001;108:283–290.
24. Newacheck PW, Taylor WR. Childhood chronic illness: prevalence, severity, and impact. *Am J Public Health* 1994;82:364–371.

CHAPTER 2 ■ PEDIATRIC HOSPITALIST: PATIENT CARE, ADMINISTRATION, AND EDUCATION

TIMOTHY H. HARTZOG, JACK M. PERCELAY, AND DANIEL A. RAUCH

THE PEDIATRIC HOSPITALIST

The first description of a "hospitalist" comes from a 1996 *New England Journal of Medicine* article by Wachter and Goldman (1). Since that time, hospitalists have become one of the fastest growing specialties in pediatrics. Pediatric hospitalists programs have been started in academic and community hospitals across all regions of the country. There is no single definition of the roles and responsibilities for a pediatric hospitalist; however, the best working definition is a pediatrician who spends 25% of her time providing care in the hospital setting. The Society of Hospital Medicine (SHM) established the following definition: "Hospitalists are physicians whose primary professional focus is the general medical care of hospitalized patients. Their activities include patient care, teaching, research, and leadership related to Hospital Medicine" (2). Pediatric inpatients range from those with routine diseases to chronically and critically ill patients, and encounter a vast number of health care providers including nurses, pharmacists, respiratory therapists, social workers, discharge planners, pediatric subspecialists, non-pediatric subspecialists, radiologists, sedation subspecialists, and anesthesiologists.

Hospitals are highly complex organizations influenced by economic and non-economic factors that comprise the care of children, and without an advocate, children's care suffers. Optimizing care requires hospitalists to coordinate and lead the interdisciplinary team. Physicians often do not realize that ordering a lab or antibiotics can involve as many as 30 steps and 5 to 10 different providers in the process—a complex process that has great potential for errors. Hospitals are currently facing shortages of skilled ancillary services along with nurses and pharmacists. Hospitalists can reduce burnout and help retain talented people in the hospital by coordinating and leading the health care team. Hospitalists must lead by using skills in communication, collaboration, and financial/business management.

FORCES DRIVING THE DEVELOPMENT OF PEDIATRIC HOSPITAL PROGRAMS

One factor driving the development of hospitalists is the increasing demands on private practice outpatient pediatricians to see increasingly complex outpatients, in addition to the constant pressure to see more patients per hour while using fewer resources including lower reimbursement from health care companies. Only the sickest of patients are now admitted to the hospital, with the typical pediatrician only admitting 20 to 25 patients per year. Therefore, just the time required to drive to the hospital is lost productivity and many complicated patients require more than one visit per day. Also, parents in a typical pediatric office will not tolerate being left waiting as a pediatrician leaves to handle an inpatient crisis. From the hospital side, hospitals depend on physicians to volunteer time to serve on the many hospital committees, perform quality control, and improve patient safety. With the increasing demands on physicians, many physicians are unwilling and/or unable to serve on committees, leaving the hospitals at risk.

The traditional model of medicine is that one primary care provider handles all of an individual's health care needs including outpatient, inpatient, and rehabilitation needs. The theory was that a single provider knew the patient's entire medical history and family dynamics, and had a trusting relationship with the family. *New England Journal of Medicine* editorials feared that hospitalists would only disrupt patient care at the critical time of inpatient admission (3). However, other factors also pushed for the development of inpatient-only physicians. With increasingly complex illness in the hospital, many pediatricians have become uncomfortable with moderately to critically ill patients. Physicians not only cannot leave the office to check on patients whenever a significant event occurs, but there is no time for rounds, talking with families, and then rushing to the office to see numerous outpatients.

From the hospital perspective, hospitalists fill a void by allowing a small number of physicians to care for a large number of patients, making the implementation of care paths easier. Multiple studies also suggest that length of stay decreases by 10% to 15% with hospitalists, resulting in tremendous cost savings (4,5,6). Also, hospitalists serve on many of the needed committees and quality-improvement processes, filling a void left by private practice physicians.

STARTING A HOSPITALIST PROGRAM

The benefits of starting a pediatric hospitalist program are numerous, but the creation takes time and skill. Benefits of hospitalist programs include greater physician accessibility during hospital stays, and concentration on outpatients by primary care physicians. Hospitalists are often a recruiting tool for new primary care physicians, due to the lack of assigned call times or nighttime admissions, which leads to an improved lifestyle. For primary care physicians, the admission process is streamlined. The ER and nurses appreciate improved access to physicians (7).

The American Academy of Pediatrics (AAP) has compiled a list of recommended basic principles for hospitalist programs in their policy statement. These include the following.

1. All pediatric hospitalist programs should be based on voluntary referrals. Pediatricians and other qualified primary (or specialty) care physicians should always retain the option to admit and manage their own patients. They should also retain the privilege to accept and participate in unassigned patient admissions at their desire or discretion.
2. Each pediatric hospitalist program should be designed to meet the unique needs of the patients, families, and physicians in the community it serves.
3. Physicians serving as hospitalists should be board certified in pediatrics or have equivalent qualifications.
4. Pediatric hospitalist programs should include in their design provision for appropriate outpatient follow-up of patients on discharge.
5. Pediatric hospitalist programs should provide for timely and complete communication between the hospitalist and the physicians responsible for a patient's outpatient management, including the primary care physician and all involved subspecialists.
6. Pediatric hospitalist programs should include data-collection and outcome-assessment capabilities to monitor their performance and are encouraged to contribute to research studies involving the care of hospitalized children (8). (Reproduced with permission from *Pediatrics*, Vol. 115(4), Pages 1101–1102, Copyright © 2005 by the AAP.)

TYPES OF HOSPITALIST PROGRAMS

Each hospitalist program is unique due to geographic, economic, and hospital-specific factors. Therefore, many different types of hospitalist programs exist across the country. Few places have sufficient pediatric inpatient volume to justify starting a hospitalist program to only care for pediatric inpatients. Less than 25% of hospitalist programs make enough from professional billings to cover salary and benefit cost (9). Therefore, programs are looking to other avenues to increase revenues. Hospitalists may be involved in such varied areas as urgent care, emergency medicine, neonatal intensive care unit (NICU) coverage, pediatric intensive care unit (PICU) coverage, sedation services, and palliative care (see Table 2.1). Because of the varied responsibilities, there is not one standard description of the role of a hospitalist. Studies, regarding pediatric critical care outcome, have shown that a PICU covered by hospitalists at night with PICU as back-up showed improved outcome and significantly decreased length of stay for critically ill children (10,11,12). Although hospitalists should not practice critical care medicine independently of intensivists, there may be a joint management role for patients with immediate back-up of the intensivist.

In neonatal care units, hospitalists can fill an important role including covering deliveries, neonatal resuscitation, and night coverage for neonatologists (see Table 2.2) (13). Another successful service for many pediatric hospitalists is sedation services. These services are revenue generating and increase the efficiency and accessibility of radiology services. Sedation services require extra training in airway and sedation medications and defined protocols on which patients are safe for a hospitalist and which need referral to anesthesia (14).

TABLE 2.1

MOST COMMON PEDIATRIC DIAGNOSES FOR A PEDIATRIC HOSPITALIST PROGRAM

- Asthma (n = 515)
- Bronchiolitis (n = 282)
- Pneumonia (n = 219)
- Upper respiratory tract infection (n = 142)
- Sickle-cell disease (n = 130)
- Urinary tract infection (n = 128)
- Convulsions (n = 119)
- Viral infection (n = 113)
- Rotavirus gastroenteritis (n = 101)
- Other gastroenteritis/colitis (n = 91)
- 10 most frequent diagnoses (n = 1840)
- Remaining diagnoses (n = 1967)

Source: Dwight P, MacArthur C, Friedman JN, et al. Evaluation of a staff-only hospitalist system in a tertiary care, academic children's hospital. *Pediatrics* 2004;114:1545–1549.

There are two basic models of hospitalist programs: the 24/7 versus the traditional model. The 24/7 model requires a physician in-house at all times, covering floor issues, new admissions, emergency department consults, delivery, and the NICU. This schedule is designed around a shift model similar to that used by emergency medicine physicians. The shift model can be configured in a number of ways, but most include physicians doing daily rounds and checking out to the night call person. The advantage of this type of system includes having a physician present at any time during the hospital stay, especially for critical events. The disadvantages include adding full time employees (FTEs) with the night person without an increase in patient care revenue, and the fact that night call is tough on the family and the body.

The traditional model involves a physician who is responsible for daily rounds and admissions, but takes calls from home at night. The advantage includes fewer FTEs required to staff the program. However, there can be a longer response time for acute events at night.

TABLE 2.2

HOSPITALIST SKILLS IN THE NEONATAL INTENSIVE CARE UNIT

- Umbilical catherization
- Endotracheal intubation
- Arterial and venous blood draws
- Percutaneous venous and arterial line placement
- Lumbar puncture
- Thoracocentesis
- Exchange transfusion
- Suprapubic tap

PEDIATRIC HOSPITAL MEDICINE PROFESSIONAL ORGANIZATIONAL ACTIVITY

Current Status

The most important professional organizations for pediatric hospitalists are the American Academy of Pediatrics (AAP), the Ambulatory Pediatric Association (APA), and the Society of Hospital Medicine (SHM). These three organizations work together to represent the various interests and needs of pediatric hospital medicine and pediatric hospitalists. The AAP is the umbrella organization for all pediatricians. Within the AAP, the Section on Hospital Medicine (SOHM) focuses on clinical issues related to inpatient care from the perspectives of the pediatrician and the child and family. It is the largest group of pediatric hospitalists, with more than 500 members. The APA is the professional home for academic pediatricians. Its focus is research and teaching. The Hospital Medicine Special Interest Group (SIG) coordinates hospitalist activity within the APA. In contrast, SHM represents hospitalists and hospital medicine as a whole, adult and pediatric. Its membership consists primarily of internists. For the pediatrician, SHM offers valuable insights into logistic and systems issues involved in the care of hospitalized patients. Pediatric activity within SHM is coordinated through the SHM Pediatric Committee.

Although the focus of each organization is distinct, the AAP, APA and SHM have considerable overlapping interests in clinical care, logistics and systems of care, research, education, and advocacy. By creating shared entities and avoiding redundant and potentially competing programs, the three organizations have worked together to advance the field and thus the care of hospitalized children. These collaborative efforts are best exemplified through a shared LISTSERV, research network, and annual meeting.

The AAP Section on Hospital Medicine LISTSERV is open to all clinicians with an interest in general inpatient pediatrics. Although the LISTSERV is housed within the AAP, it is not restricted to AAP members. This open structure has created a large, dynamic, and often loquacious community. Neither the APA nor SHM has attempted to develop a competing LISTSERV, thereby ensuring maximum participation for all hospitalists and a simple, single vehicle to communicate with colleagues nationally and internationally.

The PRIS (Pediatric Research in the Inpatient Setting—pronounced "prize") network is the collaborative research network for pediatric hospitalists. The acronym and organizational structure were modified with the consent and encouragement of the AAP's very successful PROS (Pediatric Research in the Office Setting) network. PRIS is housed within the APA for purposes of grant allocation, but structurally PRIS is a joint project of all three organizations. Its bylaws specifically include representation from each organization on the PRIS steering committee. PRIS projects thus far have examined practice patterns among pediatric hospitalists and the use of evidence-based modalities (15). More than 50 sites are involved with PRIS. The network serves as both a vehicle to answer common inpatient problems and a means to develop pediatric hospitalist research skills.

The annual pediatric hospital medicine conference is the biggest success of the three organizations. In July 2005, the three organizations co-sponsored a 4-day pediatric hospital medicine conference in Denver that brought together more than 230 pediatric hospitalists. Based on the overwhelming success of this meeting, similar conferences will be presented annually beginning in 2007. The APA was the lead sponsor for the first meeting. This responsibility will rotate among the

TABLE 2.3	
ORGANIZATION WEBSITES	
American Academy of Pediatrics	www.aap.org
Ambulatory Pediatric Association	www.ambpeds.org
Society of Hospital Medicine	www.hospitalmedicine.org

AAP, APA, and SHM for future meetings, but all will share the same stand-alone, multiday structure with multiple networking opportunities. Together the AAP, APA and SHM have helped facilitate the growth of pediatric hospital medicine as a field, and contributed to the improved care of hospitalized children and their families while laying the groundwork for establishing hospital medicine as a distinct discipline within pediatrics. These organizations need the continued support of pediatric hospitalists to continue with their missions. In return, participation in these organizations offers opportunities for professional growth, personal satisfaction, and the privilege of contributing to and influencing the development of our field. More information about each organization and membership materials are available through the websites listed in Table 2.3 and in other recent publications (16).

Future Issues

Subspecialty Certification

One of the major issues facing pediatric hospital medicine is the question of certification and creation of a subspecialty. The authors believe that whatever precedents are established by adult hospitalists and the American Board of Internal Medicine will strongly influence any decisions made by the American Board of Pediatrics. As of this writing, the adult hospital medicine community is not seriously considering a distinct sub-board or subspecialty. Instead, internists would continue to complete a core residency, with the potential for emphasis on ambulatory medicine, hospital medicine, or subspecialty medicine. Initial board certification coming out of residency would be relatively unchanged, but maintenance of certification would be dramatically altered. After a several-year period with appropriate (documented) clinical experience, one would be eligible to recertify with special expertise in ambulatory and/or hospital medicine. Requirements to meet recertification would include demonstrated clinical proficiency based on a log of clinical activity and assessment of outcomes, a secure exam of cognitive knowledge, evidence of continued learning, and completion of relevant performance improvement activities.

The same such structure could readily be applied to pediatric hospital medicine. In fact, the pediatric core curriculum being developed by SHM forms the framework for the cognitive knowledge portion of certification. This document will identify the core clinical, procedural, and systems knowledge expected of a pediatric hospitalist. Details are listed in Table 2.4.

Performance improvement modules specific for pediatric hospital medicine will need to be developed for maintenance of certification. The AAP SOHM is interested in developing such a module for inpatient asthma management that would be similar in structure to an outpatient module already under development for office-based practitioners. Systems-based materials developed by SHM for adult hospitalist recertification addressing such issues as patient safety, communication with

TABLE 2.4

SOCIETY OF HOSPITAL MEDICINE CORE CURRICULUM

Proposed pediatric clinical topics (17)	Selected adult systems topics (18)
Acute abdomen	Care of vulnerable populations
Apparent life-threatening event (ALTE)	Communications
Asthma	Diagnostic decision-making
Bone and joint infection	Drug safety, pharmacoeconomics
Diabetes	Pharmacoepidemiology
Failure to thrive	Equitable allocation of resources
Febrile infant	Evidence-based medicine
Fluids/electrolytes/nutrition	Hospitalist as consultant
Gastroenteritis	Hospitalist as teacher
Jaundice	Information management
Kawasaki disease	Leadership
Lower respiratory infection	Management practices
Meningitis and encephalitis	Palliative care
Non-accidental trauma and neglect	Patient education
Pneumonia	Patient handoff
Seizure	Practice-based learning and improvement
Sickle-cell disease complications	Prevention of health care–associated infections and antimicrobial resistance
Soft-tissue infection	
Special technology needs patients	Professionalism and medical ethics
Toxic ingestion	Quality improvement
Upper respiratory infection	Risk management
Urinary tract infection	Team approach and multidisciplinary care
	Transitions of care

referring physicians, and coordination of care could easily be modified for pediatric hospitalists.

Academic Growth

Academic growth is another key factor required for the development of pediatric hospital medicine as a distinct discipline. Here the APA has taken the lead to highlight research in pediatric hospital medicine by offering plenary sessions on hospital medicine at its annual meetings and offering faculty development workshops. Works such as this textbook, the PRIS network, and individual contributions by individual hospitalists are the building blocks that support the academic foundation of the field. Each organization's peer-reviewed journal (*Pediatrics* for the AAP, *Ambulatory Pediatrics* for the APA, and *The Journal of Hospital Medicine* for SHM) welcomes submissions on pediatric hospital medicine topics. Comprehensive Web-based resources also need to be developed. Ideally, these resources will not be restricted to members of any particular organization, but will be freely available internationally through the Web to all persons caring for hospitalized children—physicians, nurses, and pharmacists, hospitalists, subspecialists, and primary-care physicians.

Other Issues

Clinical issues abound, both in the science and the art of medicine. Improved evidence-based pathways for pediatric inpatient care will continue to remain a focus. Much of this work will be done by subspecialists in their individual fields looking at pneumonia, asthma, gastroenteritis, and meningitis, for example. However, as pediatric hospital medicine matures as a discipline, these illnesses will become the domain of the hospitalist, with occasional consultation by the subspecialist. Systems issues are another area ripe for the hospitalist to tackle. Patient safety, computerized physician order entry, patient flow throughout the hospital, discharge planning, coordination of care, and medication reconciliation are all areas where the hospitalist plays a key role.

Financial Viability of Programs

Pediatric hospital medicine programs are not financially self-sufficient given the wide range of under- and un-reimbursed services these programs provide. The explosive growth of hospitalist programs indicates that those who take a global view of the value provided by hospital medicine programs are convinced that hospitalists are a wise investment. The challenge is documenting this value on an income and expense statement. Compared to adult programs, pediatric programs face particular financial challenges due to differences in reimbursement between Medicare and Medicaid, lower inpatient volumes with significant seasonal variation, and the appropriately time-consuming nature of dealing and communicating with two patients—the child and the family.

All three organizations are working to improve the financial landscape for pediatric hospital medicine. On the national political level, the AAP and APA lobby regularly for universal health care coverage for all children. More immediately relevant issues relate to the current CPT inpatient coding structure and reimbursement paradigms. For now, inpatient coding is likely to continue to be based on the model of the single daily visit. Although neonatology and pediatric critical care have developed global codes to reflect comprehensive care delivered over a 24-hour period, such changes are unlikely for (pediatric) hospitalists. This would fundamentally alter the compensation structure for all physicians, and any changes that involve Medicare are bound to move slowly.

On the other hand, Medicare's push for pay for performance is likely to have a strong impact on hospitalist reimbursement. Current Medicare proposals involve a differential of several percent in reimbursement for hospitals that report outcomes for quality indicators such as percent of patients with an MI who receive beta-blockers or percent of patients with pneumonia who get antibiotics within 4 hours of entry into the health care system. These small percentages turn into large amounts of absolute funds given the volume of services provided. SHM has been at the forefront in welcoming performance-based measurements and providing the resources to teach the hospital and hospitalist how to improve systems to drive better outcomes. Large private payers have similarly endorsed pay for performance. One can readily imagine similar inpatient pediatric performance measures being adopted, such as percent of patients with asthma discharged with an asthma care plan or influenza vaccine, or time to antibiotics for the febrile neonate.

Another financial issue related to pay for performance involves revising Stark regulations. Current Stark regulations prohibit nearly all incentives, including incentives not to provide harmful care. Hospitals and hospitalists must be allowed to structure contracts that align incentives and permit the hospital to provide financial support to a hospitalist group to deliver the quality services desired. Clearly, any new legislation must also include safeguards to prevent individuals and/or organizations from profiting by withholding appropriate and needed care.

Other professional and practice concerns facing hospitalists include determination of reasonable work expectations. Surveys by the AAP and SHM have been useful to provide comparison data on the average number of clinical hours a hospitalist works in a week or in a year, as well as compensation standards. Other related issues include determining appropriate patient loads and call schedules for the individual hospitalist. The most current information is generally available to dues-paying members on the particular organization's website.

HOSPITAL ADMINISTRATION

Hospitalists must work with hospital administration to develop and maintain pediatric inpatient services. Administrators are trained to maintain financial stability and legally protect the institution, but often do not understand the complete picture of the resources needed to return a healthy child to society. Likewise, physicians often believe, or act as if they believe, that the money just magically appears and do not understand the tremendous economic pressures hospital administrators are under to achieve a balanced budget and maintain current resources.

Health care is a very regulated industry, and must maintain compliance with all standards of the Joint Commission on Accreditation of Healthcare Organizations (JCAHO). Without this accreditation, hospitals will not get reimbursed by insurance companies. The JCAHO rules are complex and extremely detailed, requiring a tremendous amount of documentation. The JCAHO has developed new strategies for surveying

hospitals called "Shared Visions." Now the JCAHO will make unannounced visits, and will use a new method of tracers where one patient's care is traced from entrance to the facility until exit, with the JCAHO demanding that the hospital show safe and effective delivery of health care (19,20). In addition, any hospital that accepts Medicaid and Medicare must follow the rules of the Centers for Medicare and Medicaid Services (CMS) with another set of documentation.

Another layer of regulation is by the state facilities services that must inspect and approve health care facilities to ensure facility safety and strict engineering for all hospital construction, fire containment, and uninterrupted power supplies. Also, some states require a certificate of need (CON) to purchase equipment over a set amount. For example, in North Carolina, the state is divided into regions and each region has a set number of beds, magnetic resonance imaging (MRIs), surgery bed services, and so forth. When the state determines that a region needs more of a particular service, hospitals compete for the right to purchase or develop the desired service. Only the hospital with the "best" proposal is able to start the new service. High-profit-margin services such as surgery or cardiology are the most sought-after CONs (21).

Corporate compliance officers also have an incredibly tough role to ensure hospital legal compliance in ethics, finances, conflicts of interest, Health Insurance Portability and Accountability Act of 1996 (HIPAA), and Emergency Medical Treatment and Active Labour Act (EMTALA), as violations of these standards can lead to substantial fines and even jail time. Key laws for the hospitalist are the Stark regulations, which strictly prevent kickback; therefore, hospitalists cannot give bonuses or services to referring pediatricians based on the number and type of referrals.

Sometimes pediatricians think that administrators are able to dispense money without realizing the small profit margins a hospital has and that even minor imbalances can create peril. Many profitable hospitals run on 0.5% to 4% margins, which means that 96% to 99.5% of income is used in the daily operations, leaving little for new projects and expansion. Although the profit is in the millions of dollars, even small mismanagements and miscalculations can create deficits. The mantra for some health care administrators is "no margin, no mission." This statement seems very cold, but is true—without profit, no program or service is possible.

FINANCING A HOSPITALIST PROGRAM

Most hospitalist programs do not collect enough from professional billing to cover physician salaries. The reasons for this problem vary, from the relative underpayment for inpatient service, uncompensated committee work, and the fact that admissions between midnight and 8 AM do not increase daily revenue, but that time must be covered by physicians. One struggle for hospitalists is to convince the hospital to subsidize a program to meet salary demands with reasonable work hours. Pediatric hospitalists provide many services that are indirectly profitable for the hospital including decreased length of stay, service development, quality management, and activity on pharmacy and therapeutics committees (22,23) (see Table 2.5).

A downstream income source is increased referral to the hospital's emergency room because admissions are easier with hospitalists in-house. Hospitalist services allow for decreased time from the ER admission decision until the patient has orders and is physically out of the ER. ERs are overcrowded, and emptying beds reduces the demand for new, very expensive bed space. The same is true of decreased length of stay—if a hospitalist program is constantly rounding and discharging a

TABLE 2.5

HOSPITAL BUSINESS PLAN

Full-time hospitalist (FTE)	1	3	5
Salary per FTE	$120,000	$360,000	$600,000
Benefits per FTE	$42,000	$126,000	$210,000
Malpractice	$8,000	$24,000	$40,000
Support personnel per FTE	$12,000	$36,000	$60,000
Total cost of hospitalist	$182,000	$546,000	$910,000
BILLINGS/REVENUES			
Patient admissions	800	2,400	4,000
Revenue per admission	$180	$180	$180
Patient care revenue	$144,000	$432,000	$720,000
Straight financial deficit	−$38,000	−$114,000	−$190,000
INDIRECT INCOME SOURCES			
Committee work hours per year	25	75	125
Rate per hour ($58)	$1,450	$4,350	$7,250
Reduced costs ($200 per admission)	$160,000	$480,000	$800,000
Total advantage to hospital	$123,450	$370,350	$617,250

Note: Numbers are for example only

child when he is ready, not just at morning rounds, fewer beds can accommodate more patients.

Keys to a successful practice are communicating your needs to hospital administration. Physicians must approach administrators with respect and with numbers in hand. Statements such as "we need more people" are just too generic. Before approaching administration, obtain data from sources such as the Medical Group Management Association (MGMA) or the SHM. Useful data include encounters per year per hospitalist, average salaries, and other benchmarks. Know your current FTE workload. Allow time for administration to review the numbers and verify your claims. Make sure to request your needs before yearly budgets are started. Also, document nonclinical activities such as committee work, quality improvement projects, patient satisfaction, and decreased length of stay (LOS) when talking to administration. In addition, add measurable goals to your request (e.g., we will decrease patient time from the ER admission decision to arriving on the floor from 120 minutes to 60 minutes; we will increase coverage during peak admission time; we will provide on-demand sedation for radiology to prevent costly rescheduling while increasing the overall efficiency of radiology). Regardless of how the data are received, keep communication open and be willing to compromise (24,25).

IMPORTANCE OF EFFECTIVE COMMUNICATION WITH PHYSICIANS, PARENTS, AND PATIENTS

One of the objections to hospital medicine is the perception that continuity of care would be destroyed if outpatient split from inpatient medicine. The term "voltage drop" has been used to describe loss of information when transferring a patient to an inpatient setting (26). The problem is really just poor communication skills, not an inevitable part of hospital medicine. To counteract this problem, hospitalists must develop excellent communication skills when communicating with a wide variety

of physicians, nurses, and ancillary staff (27). Standardizing the process of communication with primary care providers at the time of admission, discharge, or significant inpatient change improves primary care provider satisfaction with hospitalist programs. Many programs have the dictated HP and dictated discharge summary sent to the primary care physician's office. Also, providing the patient with a short form describing the diagnosis, treatment, and discharge medicines will keep the family informed regarding what occurred during admission.

Communication with parents is crucial to satisfaction with hospitalist programs. Parents have a rush of emotions when children are admitted to the hospital, combined with sleep deprivation and financial concerns—hospital admission is a trying time for families. A technique used by one of the authors (THH) is to explain in 2 to 5 minutes the disease being treated, the treatment plans, when to expect lab results back, and the next time they will see a physician. For diseases such as Respiratory Syneytial Virus (RSV), gastroenteritis, asthma, and the febrile neonate, it is helpful to have a whiteboard talk for the parents that helps them to understand the admission.

An inevitable problem is dealing with angry and upset patients. Advice from Stephen Lazoritz, "Dealing with Angry Patients," (28) includes the following.

1. Listen and try to understand the patient's expectations, including what did not meet expectations.
2. Sit down—do not hover over the bed and do not sit on the bed.
3. Eliminate distractions—lower the television, turn the pager to vibrate, let the patient talk for at least a minute prior to interrupting.
4. Listen as long as possible before speaking.
5. Recapitulation or summarize what you heard to ensure understanding of the issues at hand.
6. Validate the emotion, but you do not have to validate the issues. Many times once a patient has had a chance to voice the concerns and feel that you have listened, she is satisfied.
7. If follow-up is needed, ensure that the patient receives any follow-up to questions raised. From the authors' experience, many issues resolve themselves with active listening and allowing the patient time to process all that has happened during the admission (28).

COMMUNICATION WITH STAFF

Communication with nursing and ancillary staff is important to the overall success of a hospitalist program. Nursing has a vital role in the delivery of health care, and effective communication enhances physician and nurse job satisfaction (29). The key is to explain the treatment plan to nurses, any unusual or complex orders, and ask if they have questions. Ensure that the nurses feel comfortable calling with questions or when they do not understand orders. Medical errors occur when nurses do not call physicians for questionable orders.

When communicating with staff, principal skills are respectful listening and not being argumentative. One style of physician communication that is harmful is the contentious style, where physicians argue about precise details and definitions while missing the overall point of the conversation. These behaviors both inhibit further communication and prevent dialogue. Additionally, the skill of "letting it pass" needs to be learned. This skill enables a person to develop judgment in recognizing when it is necessary to stop a conversation and insist on clarification because an important point is at issue, and when it is better to ignore a comment that one disagrees with because bringing the other person to one's exact way of thinking is not essential to one's goal (30,31).

Another key is respectful disagreement. Listen to nurses—they follow patients and know when the conditions change—so listen. Most of the time, staff makes, helpful suggestions and remind us when we forget things. Sometimes staff proposes a wrong course of action, and physicians need to listen and then explain why a different choice in treatment was made. Staff can contribute to a patient's care but only if physicians listen and attempt to elicit opinions. Other keys are to make eye contact when speaking, to smile, and when appropriate, to use humor. Never make fun of or belittle ideas and embarrass staff. Never use yelling to control people, as the cost on staff morale is too great. If dealing with chronic misbehavior, write down the details and quietly talk with either your medical director or nurse manager. Deal in fact and specifics—not in innuendo and hearsay. Ensure that you communicate the plan of care and explain when nurses need to call the physician. In particular, explain about patients who have unusual syndromes or conditions. Never ignore staff concerns about a worsening patient.

Another key to successful hospitalist programs is dealing with physicians who are disruptive. Disruptive physicians are physicians who use abusive language, physical intimidation, foul language, or sexual harassment when dealing with interpersonal conflict. Although only 3% to 5% of physicians regularly exhibit disruptive behavior, any occurrence must be handled with a steady fair hand, but with zero tolerance. Hospitals should have a policy about acceptable behavior, but if not, your group should have a defined plan to monitor members for recurrent patterns of behavior. When surveys are done, one of the significant reasons stated for nurses leaving the profession is disruptive physician behavior. Given an already stressful nursing shortage and an average cost of $47,000 to recruit and train a nurse, controlling disruptive behavior is necessary for successful growth (31,32).

STRATEGIES FOR HOSPITAL COMMITTEE WORK

Most physicians dislike meetings, but meetings are an unfortunate necessity of modern health care management. Hospitalists can be change leaders—developing quality improvement programs, protocols, and changes to rate-limiting processes, but to accomplish these admirable goals one must collaborate with nursing, social work, discharge planning, and hospital administration. The key is to understand that meetings are nothing more than academic attending rounds without the military stratification. In collaborative meetings, everybody's voice is equal and must be heard. If the hospitalists become effective change leaders, their value to the institution is invaluable, and allows for ongoing improvements, but change does not occur without time and effort.

During meetings when conflicts are present, seven key points are outlined in Marvel's "Push and Pull: Resolving Differences of Opinion During Meetings"(33).

1. Acknowledge differences of opinion with simple nonjudgmental statements. Be an advocate for your position by explaining your point without degrading the opinions of other people.
2. Inquire about the other person's position and opinions.
3. Affirm/validate that you understand the opposition's opinion. Genuinely try to understand other opinions.
4. Self-disclosure—when emotions begin to run high, acknowledge your own emotions to the group.
5. Summarize—provide a summary of both positions.
6. Interruption—use very sparingly.
7. Humor—a great tool.

Do not force immediate decisions on the group—instead, try to schedule a follow-up meeting prior to implementing the changes. Be careful to discuss only the issues and not criticize a person or make slanderous remarks. Do not belittle or disregard emotions.

Good meeting skills allow for members of the team to contribute to improvements. Ensure that all opinions can be heard and expressed. When someone voices an opinion, never belittle or immediately dismiss new ideas. Be aware of emotional attitudes, as sometimes after tragic events or bad outcomes people may be allowing emotions to overrule logic.

Early in your tenure as a hospitalist, deal with easy issues and build a consensus. Stress relationship building with all team members and ancillary staff. A trick of one of the authors (JP) was to individually meet with key leaders after grand rounds and ask if they needed help with any issues. In this way minor issues were often dealt with before they became larger issues. Sometimes the conversation is completely a social conversation, but as the issues get tougher, relationships are crucial to progress.

HOSPITALIST AS EDUCATION LEADER

The hospitalist has the opportunity to play a powerful role in medical education. This opportunity arises from the hospitalist's presence on the inpatient service and expertise in hospital processes. It also arises from the unique perspective of a hospitalist in the larger context of health care for children.

The classic venue for medical education on the inpatient service is attending rounds. Attending rounds can be educational as well as the method for directing care as the responsible physician in charge. The challenge for the hospitalist is to promote an educational environment. This is best accomplished by paying attention to the tenets of small group facilitating. A small group leader must set an agenda and be prepared. On day one, or sometimes even in advance, it is important to be clear about your expectations of various team members and to define everyone's role. The agenda is dependent on the learners' level and the role of the inpatient service in the larger curriculum for the student or resident.

The hospitalist should LEAD: L—leadership position stated, E—expectations clarified, A—assess learners, and D—develop a feedback plan. Dissatisfaction is often the result of ambiguous expectations. Preparation means being ready to do whatever it is you are going to do, whether it is to lecture, discuss patients, or go to the bedside. Being prepared does not mean that the attending physician must know all of the information or answers, but he or she should be equipped for the selected teaching format. The content of rounds can vary from person to person and day to day. Adult learning theory states that learners are best engaged when the learner sets the objectives, principles are stressed over facts, and the knowledge is readily applicable. Additionally, there must be a safe learning environment that is supportive and nonjudgmental. It is important for the hospitalist to be aware of her preferred teaching approach and remain open to other styles. Finally, it is vital to set aside some time for reflection and feedback about the teaching encounter. This may come as self-reflection or solicited feedback from the learners or an invited observer.

The content of attending rounds is where a hospitalist can make a real difference in the larger curriculum because of the specific expertise that the hospitalist brings to bear. Direct patient care includes not only relevant medical knowledge, but also clinical reasoning in management, issues in transition to outpatient care, and procedure skills. The hospitalist is a potent role model for the practice of evidence-based medicine in utilizing the medical literature and best-practice pathways. The Accreditation Council for Graduate Medical Education (ACGME) competencies may be addressed with discussions of resource utilization, cost containment and health care finances, cultural competencies, and ethical issues.

The true impact of the hospitalist on medical education comes when he takes advantage of the teaching opportunities present outside attending rounds. The most effective educational intervention is the direct observation of the learner. As an ongoing presence on the inpatient service, the hospitalist has the chance to observe learners doing admissions, physical exams, procedures, discussions with families, and interacting with other staff. Watching any of these events, even briefly, provides ample fodder for high-quality feedback. Making feedback a frequent occurrence allows easier feedback and helps to create a supportive educational environment. Besides direct observation, there are many other teaching points. The hospitalist should serve as a role model for interdisciplinary coordination between other physicians as well as the ancillary staff. As such, the hospitalist can coordinate total evaluation of the learner by incorporating evaluations by nurses and other staff. Chart review can be used to demonstrate proper documentation skills and attention to medicolegal issues. The hospitalist should be skilled in information technology and able to show how to use it to benefit patient care.

It should also be recognized that many learners spend the single largest portion of their time on the inpatient service. This means that the hospitalist should have a significant role in creating the overall curriculum and determining which aspects, in the context of that department/hospital/school, are best served by covering on the inpatient service.

Finally, the hospitalist must be able to share his understanding of the milieu in which hospitalized children exist. There needs to be an appreciation for the effect of access to care and effective preventative care on the hospitalization of a child. Community and societal priorities have an impact on services for children that affect admissions and discharges. Hospitalist may have a broader view of health trends because the sickest children are concentrated in the hospital and not in any single outpatient practice or clinic.

Good teaching skills and a full utilization of the hospitalist's expertise in inpatient care will combine to make any hospitalist a valuable educator.

Bibliography

Arond-Thomas M. Understanding emotional intelligence can help alter problem behavior. *Physician Executive* September/October 2004:36–39.

Baudendistel TE, Wachter RM. The evolution of the hospitalist movement in the USA. *Clin Med* 2002;2:327–330.

Calzada PJ. The impact of hospitalists: one system experiences major problems after hospitalists arrive. *Physician Executive* November/December 2002: 37–39.

Dichter JR. Teamwork and hospital medicine: a vision for the future. *Crit Care Nurs* 2003;23:8–11.

Hospitalist and case managers team up for better outcomes. *Hosp Case Management* 2004;12:81–84.

Keogh T, Martin W. Managing unmanageable physicians—leadership, stewardship and disruptive behavior. *Physician Executive* September/October 2004:18–22.

Landrigan CP, Muret-Wagstaff S, Chiang VW. Effect of a pediatric hospitalist system on house staff education and experience. *Arch Pediatr Adolesc Med* 2002;156:877–883.

Landrigan CP, Srivastava R, Muret-Wagstaff S, et al. Impact of a health maintenance organization hospitalist system in academic pediatrics. *Pediatrics* 2002;110:720–728.

Meyerson DE. Radical change, the quiet way. *Harvard Business Review* October 2001:92–100.

Shulman ST. What's a hospitalist? Benefits and obstacles should be weighed when trying to develop an individual model. *Pediatr Ann* 2003;32:777.

Srivastava R, Landrigan C, Gidwani P, et al. Pediatric hopitalists in Canada and the United States: a survey of pediatric academic department chairs. *Amb Pediatr* 2001;1:338–339.

Summers JA, Ginn D, Nunley D. The rotating hospitalist: a solution for an academic internal medicine practice. *South Med J* 2003;96:784–786.

Wachter RM. Hospitalists in the United States—mission accomplished or work in progress? *N Engl J Med* 2004;350:1935–1936.

Wachter RM. The evolution of the hospitalist model in the United States. *Med Clin North Am* 2002;86:687–706.

Wachter RM. Hospitals and hospitalists can reach across the "quality chasm" by restructuring inpatient care. *Cost & Quality* June 2001:21–22.

Weber DO. Poll results: doctors' disruptive behavior disturbs physician leaders. *Physician Executive* September/October 2004:6–14. http://www.jcaho.org/accredited+organizations/unannounced.htm Accessed Feb. 2, 2006.

References

1. Wachter RM, Goldman L. The emerging role of "hospitalists" in the American health care system. *N Engl J Med* 1996;335:514–517.
2. Society of Hospital Medicine. Definition of a Hospitalist. http://www.hospitalmedicine.org/Content/NavigationMenu/AboutSHM/Definitionofa Hospitalist/Definition_of_a_Hosp.htm. Accessed Feb. 20, 2006.
3. Epstein D. The role of "hospitalist" in the health care system. *N Engl J Med* 1997;336:444–446.
4. Dwight P, MacArthur C, Friedman JN, et al. Evaluation of a staff-only hospitalist system in a tertiary care, academic children's hospital. *Pediatrics* 2004;114:1545–1549.
5. Rogers JC. Pediatric hospitalist programs offer chance to improve quality and cost. *Health Care Strategic Management* March 2003:12–15.
6. Bellet PS, Whitaker RC. Evaluation of a pediatric hospitalist service: impact on length of stay and hospital charges. *Pediatrics* 2000;105:478–484.
7. Polk DH. Managing a pediatric hospitalist practice requires team approach. *Pediatr Ann* 2003;32:797–801.
8. Percelay J. Guiding principles for pediatric hospitalist programs. *Pediatrics* 2005;115:1101–1102.
9. Ward C, Reckewey K, Silbaugh B. Financial benchmarks for hospitalist programs. *Physician Executive* November/December 2002:43–47.
10. Ottolini MC, Pollack MM. Pediatric hospitalists improve critical care outcomes. *Crit Care Med* 2003;31:986–987.
11. Tenner PA, Dibrell H, Taylor RP. Improved survival with hospitalists in a pediatric intensive care unit. *Crit Care Med* 2003;31:847–852.
12. Swift JD. Integrating hospitalists into the pediatric intensive care unit. *Pediatr Ann* 2003;32:813–816.
13. Carlson DW, Fentzke KM, Dawson JG. Pediatric hospitalists fill varied roles in the care of newborns. *Pediatr Ann* 2003;32:802–810.
14. Carlson D. Hospitalist run sedation services. http://www.ambpeds.org/site/sp_int_groups/PHM2005/HospitalistRunSedationServices.ppt. Accessed Feb. 2, 2006.
15. Landrigan CP, Stucky ER, Chiang VW, et al. Variation in Inpatient Management of Common Pediatric Diseases: A Study From the Pediatric Research in Inpatient Settings, Platform Presentation at 2004 Pediatric Academic Societies' annual meeting, San Francisco, May 2004.
16. Rauch DA, Percelay JM, Zipes D. Introduction to pediatric hospital medicine. *Pediatr Clin North Am* 2005;52:963–977.
17. Cornell T, Rauch D, Amin A. A Pediatric Hospital Medicine Curriculum. Poster presentation at 2004 AAP NCE meeting, San Francisco, October 11, 2004.

18. Pistoria M, Amin A, Dressler D, et al. The core competencies in hospital medicine. *J Hosp Med* 2006;1: 82–95 (suppl 1).

19. The launch of shared visions—new pathways. *Joint Commission Perspectives* 2004;24:1–3.

20. DeLorenzo M. Shared visions—new pathways: what to expect at your next JCAHO survey. *Nurs Management* 2005;36:26–31.

21. Overview of CON process. North Carolina Division of Facility Services Certificate of Need Section 2005;Nov. 21.

22. Ward C, Reckewey K, Silbaugh B. Financial benchmarks for hospitalist programs. *Physician Executive* November/December 2002:43–47.

23. Nelson JR, Whitcomb WF. Organizing a hospitalist program: an overview of fundamental concepts. *Med Clin North Am* 2002;86:887–909.

24. Weymier RE. The hospital/physician divide: understanding the drivers of their relationships. *Physician Executive* May/June 2004:60–62.

25. Tarantino DP. Six steps to negotiating hospital stipends. *Physician Executive* May/June 2004:63–64.

26. Rauch DA, Percelay JM, Zipes D. Introduction to pediatric hospital medicine. *Pediatr Clin North Am* 2005;52:963–977.

27. Auerbach AD, Aronson MD, Davis RB. How physicians perceive hospitalist services after implementation. *Arch Intern Med.* 2003;163:2330–2336.

28. Lazoritz S. Dealing with angry patients. *Physician Executive* May/June 2004:28–31.

29. Sotile WM, Sotile MO. How to shape positive relationships in medical practices and hospitals. *Physician Executive* July/August 1999:57–60.

30. Rosenstein AH Nurse–physician relationships: impact on nurse satisfaction and retention. *AJN* 2002;102:26–34.

31. Coeling HVE, Cukr P. Communication styles that promote perceptions of collaboration, quality, and nurse satisfaction. *J Nurs Care Qual* 2000; 14:63–74.

32. Weber DO. For safety's sake disruptive behavior must be tamed. *Physician Executive* September/October 2004:16–17.

33. Marvel K, Gunn W, Brezinski KL. Push and pull: resolving differences of opinion during meetings. *Physician Executive* September/October 2004: 44–48.

CHAPTER 3A ■ ADVANCED-PRACTICE NURSES IN PEDIATRIC HOSPITAL CARE

SHARRON L. DOCHERTY

HISTORY OF ADVANCED-PRACTICE NURSING IN PEDIATRIC HOSPITAL CARE

The rise in the complexity, technology, and cost of pediatric hospital care over the past decade has created the need to bring together a collaborative health care team that can meet the multi-factorial needs of infants, children, adolescents, and their families (for the purposes of this chapter, the term "children" will be used to refer to infants, children, adolescents, and their families). This interdisciplinary team with diverse skills must be poised to offer a seamless, dynamic, efficient, and responsive model of care delivery to hospitalized children (1,2). The skills and competencies of the pediatric advanced-practice nurse (APN) are a good fit to play a unique yet critical role on this team.

Advanced-practice nursing is a broad label given to describe several diverse yet interconnected nursing roles. An APN is a registered nurse who has met advanced, graduate-level educational and clinical practice experience requirements (3). There are four broad groups of APNs in North America: the nurse anesthetist, nurse-midwife, clinical nurse specialist (CNS), and nurse practitioner (NP). For the purposes of this chapter the discussion will be confined to the roles of the CNS and NP as the key APNs who can contribute to the pediatric hospitalist team goal of delivering high-quality, safe, and cost-effective care in pediatric hospital settings.

Advanced-practice nurses have been contributing to the care of hospitalized children since the 1960s. The CNS role was the first to be developed in pediatric inpatient units after successful implementation of this role in the care of adult psychiatric patients (4). Historically, due to challenges in demonstrating the impact and cost-effectiveness of care outcomes, hospital administrators have been inconsistent in the value that they have placed on the CNS role. Thus the 1980s saw an increase in demand for the CNS role, followed by the health-care spending cutbacks of the 1990s and a resultant sharp decline in CNS numbers, only to be followed by the current rise in interest in the role after the year 2000 brought about in part by an increased focus on patient safety and efficient case management. Despite this instability, the positive effects of the CNS on the care of the pediatric patient and family, as well as the immeasurable contributions made to efficient pediatric unit management, was noted and laid the ground work for the introduction of other nurses with advanced education and practice experience to the pediatric hospital setting.

The birth of the pediatric NP role also occurred in the 1960s but was initially designed by Loretta Ford and Dr. Henry Silver to provide ambulatory care to poor children in rural Colorado (5,6). One of the key developments that helped to move the pediatric nurse practitioner (PNP) role into hospital settings was the success engendered by neonatal nurse practitioners (NNPs). In the late 1970s, a shortage of neonatologists, increasing complexity of care requirements, and a limitation in the amount of time pediatric residents could devote to neonatal intensive care, spurred the growth of the NNP role. The extremely positive clinical outcomes demonstrated by NNPs in the 1980s blazed the path for the nurse practitioner role in other areas of acute care (7–9). Beginning in the 1980s and extending into the 1990s, changes in the health care needs of acute and chronically ill adult and pediatric patients brought about the introduction of the acute-care nurse practitioner role into a variety of inpatient and outpatient hospital settings. The increasing acuity of illness requiring care in a highly technological environment, combined with a decreasing number of medical residents, brought about the need for a health care provider who could assist with the assessment, monitoring, and management of adults and children experiencing episodic and chronic health problems across the continuum of acute-care services (10). Again, the positive clinical outcomes demonstrated by acute-care nurse practitioners in the care of adult patients (11–13) provided even further evidence of the potential effectiveness of this role in the care of hospitalized children.

In pediatric inpatient settings, the PNP role, more accurately known as the acute-care pediatric nurse practitioner (AC-PNP—see Table 3.1), has expanded in response to the health and illness needs of children who are acutely ill and/or who have exacerbations of chronic health problems (14). Similar trends as reviewed above (positive clinical outcomes, economics of health care, alterations in medical resident work hour availability) are responsible for the exponential growth of the role in the care of children throughout the hospital, from the intensive care unit, through the emergency department and across a variety of specialty areas (15,16). In 1999, the American Academy of Pediatrics endorsed the PNP as a contributor to the improvement of the quality of care of hospitalized children (17). In a survey by the National Association of Children's Hospitals and Related Institutions (18), 88% of hospitals reported that they employed NPs in their hospital. Thus there is growing evidence and support for the role of the pediatric APN as a critical and essential component of the health care team in the acute-care setting (19,20).

TABLE 3.1

COMPARISON OF PEDIATRIC ADVANCED-PRACTICE ROLES

	Clinical nurse specialist	Pediatric nurse practitioner
Focus of Care	Indirect patient care to defined population of children	Direct patient care to individual children
Education	Master's degree in nursing—Specialization as a Clinical Nurse Specialist in Pediatrics	Master's degree in nursing—Specialization as a Pediatric Nurse Practitioner
National Board Certification	American Nurses Credentialing Center: Clinical Nurse Specialist in Pediatric Nursing	Three national exams available: 1. Pediatric Nursing Certification Board: Pediatric Nurse Practitioner in Acute Care 2. Pediatric Nursing Certification Board: Pediatric Nurse Practitioner in Primary Care 3. American Nurses Credentialing Center: Pediatric Nurse Practitioner in Primary Care

Post-Nominal Designation	After graduation:
	   CNS: Clinical Nurse Specialist
	After national certification:
	   CCNS: Certified Clinical Nurse Specialist
		After graduation:
		   PNP-AC: Pediatric Nurse Practitioner in Acute Care
		   PNP-PC: Pediatric Nurse Practitioner in Primary Care
		After national certification:
		   CPNP-AC: Certified Pediatric Nurse Practitioner in Acute Care
		   CPNP-PC: Certified Pediatric Nurse Practitioner in Primary Care

PEDIATRIC APN ROLE CONCEPTUALIZATIONS, COMPETENCIES, AND SCOPE OF PRACTICE

A conceptual model is a constructive way in which to view the key competencies, skills, and values held by a professional body. Several models are available that can assist in articulating the professional role, identity, and function of the pediatric advanced-practice nurse; however, the Strong Model of Advanced Practice was chosen for use here as it was developed within an acute-care setting (21). The Strong Model of Advanced Practice was developed in 1994 by a group of APNs and faculty members at Strong Memorial Hospital, University of Rochester Medical Center (21–23). According to this model five domains of practice (see Fig. 3.1) comprise the APN role:

- Direct comprehensive care: patient-focused activities including history-taking; physical assessment procedures; ordering, performing, and interpreting diagnostic tests; case management; prescribing medications and other therapies; and patient counseling.
- Support of systems: indirect patient care activities representative of professional contributions to optimal functioning of the clinical setting, immediate department, and broader institution (e.g., consultation, participation in strategic planning, quality-improvement initiatives, establishing and evaluating standards of practice).
- Education: formal and informal education of caregivers, students, patients, families, and the public.
- Research: activities that promote a culture of practice that places high value on evidence-based practice through scientific inquiry. These may include both the use and conduct of research.

- Publication and professional leadership: activities that demonstrate professional leadership both within and outside of the institution. These may include dissemination of knowledge about the role, involvement in professional organizations, influencing health and public policy, and publishing (21,23).

The Strong model also includes critical unifying threads, illustrated in Figure 3.1, as circular and continuous practice values that influence each domain. These threads are collaboration,

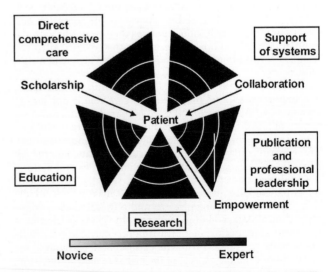

FIGURE 3.1. The Strong Model of Advanced Practice. (From Mick DJ, Ackerman MH. Advanced practice nursing role delineation in acute and critical care: application of the Strong model of advanced practice. *Heart Lung* 2000;29:210–221.)

scholarship, and empowerment (22), and they are the essential ties that bind together the five domains of practice.

APNs have the educational preparation and, at least, novice-level experience with all five domains of practice. Thus the most comprehensive and effectual position would allow for some level of functioning in all of the domains. The particular constellation in which the five domains of practice exist and are operationalized is unique to each role, practice setting, and individual APN position. As will be described, there are some generalities to the constellation that broadly characterize the CNS and PNP role, but beyond these broad categories, the manner in which the domains are operationalized is usually negotiated by the APN, supervising physician, and reporting department.

The Strong model is useful in demonstrating the key competencies, skills, and values of the pediatric APN, both the CNS and the AC-PNP. The distinction between these two roles lies in the proportionate amount of time, and thus focus, that the APN gives to each of the five domains of practice. In general, the pediatric CNS tends to spend proportionately more time focusing on support of systems, education, and consultation, and relatively less time on direct care. Historically, the pediatric CNS has focused her knowledge on the care required by a population of patients, and thus she functions very well as a resource for nurses, PNPs, and other care providers. The CNS is involved in establishing and evaluating standards of care within a unit, or for a particular patient population. Clinical nurse specialists are responsible for assessing and identifying the educational needs of the patient, family, unit, and community. They provide consultation to others on the unit, within the hospital, or in the community regarding needs of a particular population of patients. They are involved in initiating, participating in data collection, and implementing changes based upon research findings. Most pediatric clinical nurse specialists are employed by the institution under the department of nursing.

In contrast to the pediatric CNS, the AC-PNP tends to spend proportionately more time on direct patient care than on the other domains. In most states, the AC-PNP is employed and licensed to work in a collaborative relationship with a physician. The meaning of the term "collaboration" is highly variable and influenced by national, state, and local regulations (24). It can vary from mandated, on-site supervision to no required physician collaboration or supervision (see Fig. 3.2). Terms such as physician extender, midlevel provider, or physician substitute have been used interchangeably with the term NP (24). These terms may cause role confusion and tend to hold a negative connotation as they do not fit with the nonhierarchical, collaborative nature that is critical to the seamless functioning of the interdisciplinary pediatric hospitalist team.

Although most AC-PNPs practice in hospital-based units, it is important to note that the acute-care role is not setting specific (25). Acute-care PNPs are prepared to function in a variety of locations that provide direct patient care to children with complex and rapidly changing clinical conditions (26). These settings may include intensive care units, emergency departments, subacute inpatient areas, as well as ambulatory, rehabilitative, and specialty-based clinic settings. The scope of direct patient care given by the AC-PNP may include admitting patients, performing histories and physical exams, evaluating clinical data, rounding with the physician, developing a treatment plan, performing invasive procedures, and consulting with case managers to facilitate discharge planning. One of the more valuable aspects of the role is related to the coordination of patient care management when many consultants are involved in decision-making (27). Although most AC-PNPs have prescriptive privileges, the level of physician involvement varies from state to state (see Fig. 3.3).

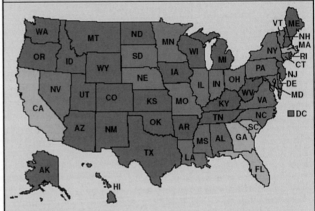

Summary of Advanced Practice Nurse (APN) Legislation: Legal Authority for Scope of Practice*

■ States with nurse practitioner** title protection; the board of nursing has sole authority in scope of practice, with no statutory or regulatory requirements for physician collaboration, direction, or supervision: AK, AR, AZ, CO, DC, HI, IA, ID, KS, KY, ME, MI, MT, ND, NH, NJ, NM, OK, OR, RI, TN, TX, UT, WA, WI, WV, WY

■ States with nurse practitioner** title protection; the board of nursing has sole authority in scope of practice, but scope of practice has a requirement for physician collaboration: CT, DE, IL, IN, LA, MD, MN, MO, NE†, NV, NY, OH, PA, VT

■ States with nurse practitioner** title protection; the board of nursing has sole authority in scope of practice, but scope of practice has a requirement for physician supervision: CA, FL, GA, MA, SC

■ States with nurse practitioner** title protection, but the scope of practice is authorized by the board of nursing and the board of medicine: AL, MS, NC, SD, VA

[Washington, D.C., is included as a state in this table.]

* This table provides a state-by-state summary of the degree of independence for all aspects of NP scope of practice, including diagnosing and treating (except prescribing). See Table: "Summary of APN Legislation: Prescriptive Authority" for a state-by-state analysis of NP prescriptive authority.
** This information may apply to other APNs (clinical nurse specialists, certified nurse midwives, and certified registered nurse anesthetists). See "Summary of Advanced Practice Nurse Poplulation" for details.
† State with APRN Board.

FIGURE 3.2. Legal authority for scope of practice. (From Phillips SJ. 18th Annual legislative update. *Nurse Practit* 2006;31:6–38.)

EDUCATIONAL PREPARATION

The development of nationally reviewed, credible, and stable educational programs has been a critical step in the continued development of the pediatric advanced-practice nursing role. Historically, there has been great variability in the level and type of educational programming required in order to be considered a "nurse specialist." From the 1960s through the 1980s, there was a general lack of agreement about the educational preparation and experience required in order to be considered an APN. In addition, there was great confusion regarding the titles being used (8). In 1965, the American Nurses Association (ANA) declared that only those nurses with a master's degree or higher in nursing could claim the title of CNS (4). Since the year 2000, all APNs entering the field must have a post-baccalaureate graduate degree. In a survey published by the American Academy of Nurse Practitioners as of 2004, 88% of NPs meet this criterion (28).

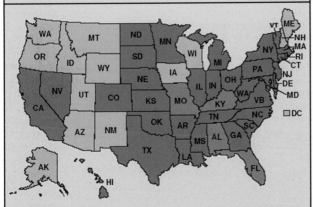

Summary of APN Legislation: Prescriptive Authority*

■ States where nurse practitioners** can prescribe (including controlled substances) independent of any required physician involvement in prescriptive authority: AK, AZ, DC, IA, ID, ME, MT, NH, NM, OR, UT†, WA, WI, WY

■ States where nurse practitioners** can prescribe (including controlled substances) with some degree of physician involvement or delegation of prescription writing: AR, CA, CO, CT, DE, GA‡, HI, IL, IN, KS, LA, MA, MD, MI, MN, MS, NC, ND, NE, NJ, NV, NY, OH, OK, PA, RI, SC†, SD, TN, TX, VA, VT, WV

■ States where nurse practitioners** can prescribe (excluding controlled substances) with some degree of physician involvement or delegation of prescription writing: AL, FL, KY, MO

All states: Nurse practitioners** may receive and/or dispense drug samples based on authorized scope of practice, rules and regulations, or statutes.

[Washington, D.C., is included as a state in this table.]

* This table provides a state-by-state analysis of NP prescriptive authority. For analysis of other aspects of the NP scope of practice (including diagnosing and treating), see Table: "Summary of APN Legislation: Legal Authority for Scope of Practice."
** The information may apply to other APNs (clinical nurse specialists, certified nurse midwives, and certified registered nurse anesthetists). See "Summary of Advanced Practice Nurse Population" for details.
† Schedule IV and/or V controlled substances only.
‡ Nurse practitioners do not have written prescribing or dispensing authority; the process falls under delegated medical authority.

FIGURE 3.3. Prescriptive authority. (From Phillips SJ. 18th Annual legislative update. *Nurse Practit* 2006;31:6–38.)

In 1995, the American Association of Colleges of Nursing (AACN) supported the merging of the CNS and NP roles in the curricula of graduate education, and published a document that functioned then and now as one of the primary guidelines for schools of nursing in the development of curricula. The Essentials of Master's Education for Advanced Practice Nursing (29) defines the essential elements of master's education for all APNs and acts as a standard for educational programming. According to this document, master's education (http://www.aacn.nche.edu/education/ mastessn.htm) for all APNs must include three components: a graduate nursing core, an advanced-practice nursing core, and specialty nursing content. The graduate core includes content required by all areas of practice (e.g., research, ethics, theory courses). The advanced-practice nursing core includes advanced health/physical assessment, advanced physiology and pathophysiology, and advanced pharmacology. Specialty curricula include content and clinical practice experiences that help students acquire the knowledge and skills essential to the specific advanced-practice role (4).

The Essentials document was a first critical step in helping to ensure that educational program offerings at the APN level across the United States met minimum standards. For nurse practitioner programming, a second key document assisted in establishing more specific standards. In 2002, The National Organization of Nurse Practitioner Faculties (NONPF) and the AACN partnered and published a set of standards for the preparation of nurse practitioners. This was titled "Nurse Practitioner Primary Care Competencies in Specialty Areas: Adult, Family, Gerontological, Pediatric, and Women's Health." This document described entry-level competencies of graduates prepared as adult, family, gerontological, pediatric, and women's health primary care nurse practitioners. These competencies set the national standard for guiding program development in the five different primary care focus areas, and provided the model for the 2004 publication of Acute Care Nurse Practitioner Competencies.

Despite the fact that less than half of practicing pediatric nurse practitioners are in primary care roles, with 56% reporting themselves as being employed outside of primary care practice (30), the majority of PNPs practicing today graduated from educational programs that specialized in primary care. This occurred in part because there was a paucity of educational programs specializing in the care of acutely ill children. Prior to 2002 there were fewer than six programs in the United States that specialized in the care of acutely ill children. The situation also arose because the PNP certification exam tested primary care competencies. Several national trends that have occurred over the past 5 years have rapidly changed this situation. As discussed earlier, positive clinical outcomes demonstrated by nurse practitioners in acute-care settings, changes in the economics of health care, and alterations in medical resident work hour availability, have combined to open many new employment opportunities for those nurses who wished to work in pediatric acute-care settings. Because of this new interest in this specialized role, in 2005 a national certification exam for AC-PNPs became available (26). These events have resulted in the rapid expansion in the number of AC-PNP educational programs. As of 2006, the number of AC-PNP educational programs had doubled.

Today, the AC-PNP who has graduated from a program that has been reviewed and recognized by the Pediatric Nursing Certification Board can expect to be prepared to function in a variety of settings to provide care to children with complex physiologic conditions and rapidly changing clinical conditions, including the recognition and management of emerging crises and organ dysfunction and failure (26). The short-term goal of care provided by the AC-PNP is stabilization of the child, minimizing complications, and providing physical and psychological care measures. The long-term goal of care is to restore maximal health potential through implementation of strategies to reduce health risks.

CERTIFICATION, LICENSING, AND CREDENTIALING

Certification, licensing, and credentialing of the pediatric APN are separate yet very interrelated processes that work together to protect the health, safety, and welfare of the public. Although the order varies widely from state to state, national certification is usually a prerequisite to state licensing as an APN, and both certification and licensing are a prerequisite for employment and thus credentialing.

The successful completion of a national certification examination attests to the achievement of specialty knowledge beyond basic nursing preparation. Table 3.1 lists role-specific national certification examinations. Medicare regulations stipulate the completion of a national certification examination as a requirement for NPs to obtain reimbursement (25).

Licensure to practice is a requirement for the PNP but not for the CNS. Nurse practitioners, in general, are independently licensed and authorized to provide care within state regulations and they are independently liable for their practice. Even in the states in which physician supervision is required (see Fig. 3.2), nurse practitioners retain the sole responsibly (and thus liability) for their license. Licensure is determined by individual states under the federal Constitution that provides standards to ensure basic levels of public safety (31). In most states, the board of nursing maintains authority over nurse practitioner licensing. However, in 11 states there is joint authority with the board of medicine (see Fig. 3.2). In most states, a PNP is licensed to work in collaboration with a physician (see Fig. 3.2). In these states, the PNP can provide only those services specifically articulated by state statute and in accordance with a written practice agreement with a licensed physician. In other states, NPs have been granted independent practice and prescribing authority.

Credentialing is the process through which an employer verifies that a practitioner has the required qualifications for the position into which he is being hired. It is critical that each institution develop a detailed credentialing process for AC-PNPs. This process is ideally undertaken jointly by the department of nursing and medicine. A separate but integrated part of credentialing is the delineation of clinical privileges that will be offered by the PNP. Both of these processes are mandated through the Joint Commission on Accreditation of Healthcare Organizations (32). In 2004, a survey of NP practice revealed that 92% of NPs maintained national certification and 39% held hospital privileges (28).

CLINICAL OUTCOMES: EFFECTIVE AND ECONOMICAL CARE PROVIDERS

The study and documentation of clinical outcomes of APN practice has been a critical component in the role advancements over the last several decades. The ability to be able to demonstrate the high-quality, cost-effective care that is characteristic of APN practice is essential (33). The vast majority of research in this area has used NPs providing care to adult populations in both primary care and acute-care settings.

Several researchers compared primary-care nurse practitioner practice outcomes with that of physicians and have demonstrated no significant differences in regard to process of care, resource use, and cost (34). Primary-care NPs have been found to contribute to patient safety, consumer satisfaction, and efficient and cost-effective delivery of health care (35).

Numerous studies have documented the positive clinical outcomes of acute-care nurse practitioners in providing safe, cost-effective care in a variety of adult hospital settings (12,14, 36–39). Christakis and colleagues were able to demonstrate that NP practice in an emergency department helped to improve continuity of care, which assisted in decreasing emergency room visits and related hospitalization (40). In a large study examining nurse practitioner and physician outcomes of care given to emergency department patients with minor injuries, no significant differences were found in the number of clinically important errors, in accuracy of examinations, and adequacy of treatment. In this study, NPs were found to be better at recording medical histories, and fewer patients seen by an NP had to seek unplanned follow-up advice about their injury (41). Several studies have also documented outcomes of care

provided in adult critical-care environments and found that NPs assisted in decreasing length of stay (42) and number of days on mechanical ventilation days (43). A study comparing outcomes in a subacute medical intensive-care unit of patients managed by either an acute-care nurse practitioner or a physician found that the care outcomes did not differ in terms of length of stay or duration of mechanical ventilation (44).

There are relatively fewer studies available describing APN outcomes with pediatric acute-care populations. Verger and colleagues provide an excellent review of research examining studies conducted on neonatal populations (45). Martin found positive parent and staff nurse satisfaction with pediatric nurse practitioners in an intensive-care unit (46). CNS practice in general has been studied and found to have improved compliance, decreased length of stay, and improved staff nurse clinical judgment skills (47–50). With the recent role advancements made by pediatric acute-care nurse practitioners and clinical nurse specialists, more research is needed to examine clinical outcome indicators.

CONCLUSIONS

Pediatric advanced-practice nurses are poised to make significant contributions to the care of hospitalized infants, children, adolescents, and their families. The opportunity to play a unique and critical role on an interdisciplinary team in providing safe, cost-efficient, and effective care is one that cannot be taken lightly.

References

1. Liguori R, Ricciardi R, Jones DC, et al. The 40-year-story of PNP caregiving—still being written. *Contemp Pediatr* 2005;22:56.
2. Mundinger M. Toward a quality workforce. *Pediatrics* 2003;112:416–418.
3. American Nurses Association. *Nursing's social policy statement.* 2nd ed. Washington, D.C.: ANA; 2003.
4. Dunphy LM, Youngkin EQ, Smith NK. Advanced practice nursing: Doing what had to be done. In: Joel LA, ed. *Advanced practice nursing: essentials for role development.* Philadelphia: F.A. Davis; 2004:3–30.
5. Ford LC, Silver HK. The expanded role of the nurse in child care. *Nurs Outlook* 1967;15:43–45.
6. Silver HK, Ford LC, Stearly SG. A program to increase health care for children: The pediatric nurse practitioner program. *Pediatrics* 1967;39: 756–768.
7. Bissinger RL, Allred CA, Arford PH, et al. A cost-effectiveness analysis of neonatal nurse practitioners. *Nurs Economics* 1997;15:92–99.
8. Keeling AW, Bigbee JL. The history of advanced practice nursing in the United States. In: Hamric AB, Spross JA, Hanson CM. eds. *Advanced practice nursing. An integrative approach.* St. Louis: Elsevier; 2005:4–45.
9. Mitchell-DiCenso A, Guyatt G, Marrin, M, et al. A controlled trial of nurse practitioners in neonatal intensive care. *Pediatrics* 1996;98:1143–1148.
10. Keane A, Richmond T, Kaiser L. Critical care nurse practitioners: evolution of the advanced practice nursing role. *Am J Crit Care* 1994;3:232–237.
11. Dahle KL, Smith JS, Ingersoll GL, et al. Impact of a nurse practitioner on the cost of managing inpatients with heart failure. *Am J Cardiol* 1998;82: 686–688, A-8.
12. Spisso J, O'Callaghan C, McKennan M, et al. Improved quality of care and reduction of house staff workload using trauma nurse practitioners. *J Trauma* 1990;30:660–663.
13. Weinberg RM, Liljestrand JS, Moore S. Inpatient management by a nurse practitioner: Effectiveness in a rehabilitation setting. *Arch Phys Med Rehabil* 1983;64:588–590.
14. Teicher S, Crawford K, Williams B, et al. Emerging role of the pediatric nurse practitioner in acute care. *Pediatr Nurs* 2001;27:387–390.
15. Christensen J, Akcasu N. The role of the pediatric nurse practitioner in the comprehensive management of pediatric oncology patients in the inpatient setting. *J Pediatr Oncol Nurs* 1999;16:58–67.
16. Verger JT, Marcoux KK, Madden MM, et al. Nurse practitioners in pediatric critical care. Results of a national survey. *AACN* 2005;16:396–408.
17. American Academy of Pediatrics Committee on Hospital Care 1997–1999. The role of the nurse practitioner and physician assistant in the care of hospitalized children. *Pediatrics* 1999;103:1050–1052.
18. Pitts J, Seimer B. The use of nurse practitioners in pediatric institutions. *J Pediatr Health Care* 1998;12:67–72.

19. Brilli RJ, Spevetz A, Branson RD, et al. Critical care delivery in the intensive care unit: defining clinical roles and the best practice model. *Crit Care Med* 2001;29:2007–2019.

20. Maloney AM, Volpe J. The inpatient advanced practice nursing roles in a Canadian pediatric oncology unit. *J Pediatr Oncol Nurs* 2005;22:254–257.

21. Mick DJ, Ackerman MH. Advanced practice nursing role delineation in acute and critical care: application of the Strong model of advanced practice. *Heart Lung* 2000;29:210–221.

22. Ackerman MH, Norsen L, Martin B, et al. Development of a model of advanced practice. *Am J Crit Care* 1996;5:68–73.

23. Spross JA, Lawson MJ. Conceptualizations of advanced practice nursing. In: Hamric AB, Spross JA, Hanson CM. eds. *Advanced practice nursing. An integrative approach.* St. Louis: Elsevier; 2005:47–84.

24. Todd BA, Resnick A, Stuhlemmer R, et al. Challenges of the 80-hour resident work rules: collaboration between surgeons and nonphysician practitioners. *Surg Clin North Am* 2004;84:1573–1586.

25. Hravnak M, Kleinpell RM, Magdic KS, et al. The acute care nurse practitioner. In: Hamric AB, Spross JA, Hanson CM, eds. *Advanced practice nursing. An integrative approach.* St. Louis: Elsevier; 2005:475–514.

26. Pediatric Nursing Certification Board. Definition of ACPNP. Available online at: http://www.pncb.org/ptistore/control/exams/ac/ac_ques

27. Wachter RM. An introduction to the hospitalist model. *Ann Inter Med* 1999;130:338–342.

28. American Academy of Nurse Practitioners. *U.S. nurse practitioner workforce 2004.* Retrieved March 20, 2006 from http://www.aanp.org 2004.

29. American Association of Colleges of Nursing. *Essentials of master's education for advanced practice nursing.* Washington, D.C.: AACN; 1996.

30. Jackson PL, Kennedy C, Sadler LS, et al. Professional practice of pediatric nurse practitioners: implications for education and training of PNPs. *J Pediatr Health Care* 2001;15:291–298.

31. Hanson CM. Understanding regulatory, legal, and credentialing requirements. In: Hamric AB, Spross JA, Hanson CM, eds. *Advanced practice nursing. An integrative approach.* St. Louis: Elsevier; 2005:782–808.

32. Magdic KS, Hravnak M. Credentialing for nurse practitioners. An update. *AACN Clin Issues* 2005;16:16–22.

33. Ingersoll G. Evaluation of the advanced practice nurse role in acute and specialty care. *Crit Care Nurs Clin North Am* 1997;7:25–33.

34. Mundinger MO, Keefe RL, Lenz ER, et al. Primary care outcomes in patients treated by nurse practitioners or physicians: a randomized trial. *JAMA* 2000;283:59–68.

35. Bryant R, Graham MC. Advanced practice nurses: a study of client satisfaction. *J Am Acad Nurs Pract* 2002;14:88–92.

36. Rudy EB, Davidson LJ, Daly B, et al. Care activities and outcomes of patients cared for by acute care nurse practitioners, physician assistants, and resident physicians: a comparison. *Am J Crit Care* 1998;7:267–281.

37. McMullen M, Alexander MK, Bourgeois A, et al. Evaluating a nurse practitioner service. *Dimensions Crit Care Nurs* September/October 2001;20:30–34.

38. Howie JN, Erickson M. Acute care nurse practitioners: creating and implementing a model of care for an inpatient general medical service. *Am J Crit Care* 2002;11:448–458.

39. Van Soeren M, Micevski V. Success indicators and barriers to acute nurse practitioner role implementation in four Ontario hospitals. *AACN Clin Issues* 2001;12:424–437.

40. Christakis DA, Mell L, Koepsell TD, et al. Association of lower continuity of care with greater risk of emergency department use and hospitalization in children. *Pediatrics* 2001;107:524–529.

41. Sakr M, Angus J, Perrin J, et al. Care of minor injuries by emergency nurse practitioners or junior doctors: a randomized controlled trial. *Lancet* 1999;354:1321–1326.

42. Russell D, VorderBruegge M, Burns SM. Effect of an outcomes-managed approach to care of neuroscience patients by acute care nurse practitioners. *Am J Crit Care* 2002;11:353–362.

43. Burns SM, Marshall M, Burns JE, et al. Design, testing, and results of an outcomes-managed approach to patients requiring prolonged mechanical ventilation. *Am J Crit Care* 1998;7:45–57.

44. Hoffman LA, Tasota FJ, Zull TG, et al. Outcomes of care managed by an acute care nurse practitioner/attending physician team in a sub acute medical intensive care unit. *Am J Crit Care* 2005;14:121–312.

45. Verger J, Trimarchi T, Barnsteiner JH. Challenges of advanced practice nursing in pediatric acute and critical care: education to practice. *Crit Care Nurs Clin North Am* 2002;14:315–326.

46. Martin SA. The pediatric critical care nurse practitioner: evolution and impact. *Pediatr Nurs* 1999;25:505–510.

47. Crimlisk J, Bernardo J, Blansfield J. Endotracheal intubation: a closer look at a preventable condition. *Clin Nurs Specialist* 1997;11:145–150.

48. Gurka A. Process and outcome of clinical nurse specialist consultation. *Dimensions Crit Care Nurs* 1991;10:169–175.

49. Lombness P. Differences in length of stay with care managed by clinical nurse specialists or physician assistants. *Clin Nurs Specialist* 1994;8:253–260.

50. Naylor M, Brooten D, Campbell R. Comprehensive discharge planning and home follow-up of hospitalized elders: a randomized control trail. *JAMA* 1999;281:613–620.

CHAPTER 3B ■ ROLE IMPLEMENTATION OF THE PEDIATRIC ACUTE-CARE NURSE PRACTITIONER

DAWN A. TUCKER AND KATHERINE L. JACOBY

Nurse practitioners play an integral role in care of the hospitalized child. There are more than 100,000 nurse practitioners (NPs) in the United States, with 90% of pediatric hospitals employing NPs (1,2). As changes and new challenges in health care have occurred, the role of the pediatric acute-care nurse practitioner (pediatric ACNP) has evolved to provide comprehensive care with the multidisciplinary care team that includes patients and families. These changes include an increase in complexity and chronicity of pediatric illnesses. Not only are patients presenting to acute-care settings with increasing complex medical conditions, but many patients and families are more knowledgeable consumers and realize they have choices regarding where they receive health care. The challenge in today's health care system is to be better service providers. Patients and families expect care that is coordinated including consistent communication with all members of the interdisciplinary team and the primary care physician. Integral to the patient and family experience is education

about health issues related to normal growth and development as well as the presenting acute problem. It is imperative to consider the nature and complexity of patient problems as they transition across the continuum of care from the hospital to the home.

These challenges are important factors to consider when developing the staffing composition of a hospitalist's practice. Pediatric ACNPs and hospitalists have an opportunity to work synergistically in the delivery and coordination of patient care. The successful introduction of pediatric ACNPs into a hospitalist's practice requires understanding of educational preparation, role delineation, and collaboration models, and recognition of opportunities for improved patient outcomes. Important questions are: What skill set and qualities does an ACNP bring to the practice? What value is added to the practice by using an ACNP? Why choose an ACNP versus adding part-time or moonlighting physicians or using residents?

EDUCATIONAL PREPARATION

The pediatric ACNP has advanced education and clinical training beyond the nursing education required for state licensure (3,4). Pediatric ACNPs are registered nurses with master's degrees in nursing who are prepared for advanced practice in pediatric acute care (5). Pediatric ACNPs receive education and training including didactic and mentored clinical experience in pediatric critical, acute, and chronic care settings. National certification is available for the pediatric ACNP through the Pediatric Nursing Certification Board (PNCB).

ROLE OF NURSE PRACTITIONERS IN THE ACUTE-CARE SETTING

The role of the pediatric ACNP is to provide continuous and comprehensive advanced nursing care to patients who are acutely and critically ill (6). Pediatric ACNPs practice in any setting in which patient care requires complex monitoring and therapies, high-intensity intervention, or continuous nursing vigilance. Practice settings are most often hospital based, including emergency room, acute-care inpatient units, and intensive-care units; however, the role may expand across the continuum of care to ambulatory care, urgent care, and rehabilitative care settings (7).

The scope of practice includes providing direct patient care management such as performing admission history and physical exams, conducting patient rounds, developing treatment plans, interpreting results of laboratory and diagnostic tests, prescribing medications, providing education, consulting, providing discharge planning, and performing procedures (7). The pediatric ACNP works collaboratively with the multidisciplinary care team to promote stabilization and restoration of health. She also builds rapport with patients and families while providing education and emotional support. The pediatric ACNP has a wonderful opportunity to be an educator to staff while providing direct patient-care services. The constant presence at the bedside ensures that practices are consistent among caregivers.

ACNPs are also utilized in pediatric subspecialties such as cardiac surgery. In this model, the pediatric ACNP will provide seamless specialized care continuously for patients as they move from high-acuity to lower-acuity inpatient care units, facilitate patients' movement through the health-care system, and plan for and implement discharge. The cardiac ACNP participates in daily rounds with the multidisciplinary team; they become the "spokesperson" for the cardiac surgeon. The cardiac ACNP is the link and complement between surgeons, residents, attending physicians, patients, families, and nursing staff. As an example, Table 3.2 illustrates a job description for a pediatric ACNP working in the hospital's division of cardiothoracic surgery.

COLLABORATION

The pediatric ACNP role is complementary to the pediatric hospitalist. Literature supports that pediatric ACNPs have the skill set and knowledge to manage highly acute and complex medical conditions (8). Although this knowledge is extremely valuable, the ability to provide continuity of care from hospital to home, patient and family education, interdisciplinary care coordination, initiating communication with the primary care pediatrician, discharge planning, and additional manpower are among the greatest advantages of adding a pediatric ACNP to the hospitalist team.

In collaboration, the ACNP and hospitalist can improve quality of care. A major impetus for the utilization of ACNPs in the hospital setting was the result of imposed limitations in residency work hours in the face of increasing patient care management needs. In hospital settings where medical residents and fellows are not available, NPs have been used successfully to improve the continuity of care delivered in critical care facilities (8–10). Also, the shortage of pediatric subspecialties has been addressed through the training of ACNPs to participate in the provision of subspecialty medicine. For example, ACNPs can function as specialists, complementing and augmenting the vital role of cardiologists, surgeons, and other specialty care physicians.

Pediatric ACNPs provide consistent care to patients from admission to discharge and across the multiple hospitalizations experienced by chronically ill children. Some hospitalist practices have manpower shortages. These practices may use "moonlighters" to supplement staffing needs. This type of structure poses particular concern regarding consistency of care delivery. Continuity of care is imperative particularly in tertiary-level hospitals that care for a disproportionate number of chronically ill children.

Patient satisfaction has been found to improve in a physician/NP team over a physician alone (11,12). They provide patients and families with skills to navigate transitions along the health care continuum. Results of collaborative practice are synergistic because the contributions of both health care professionals are optimized to a level that would not be achievable through independent practice.

While 85% to 88% of the pediatric ACNP's responsibilities are related to direct management of patient care, ACNPs are engaged in many activities that can be identified as systems support or indirect patient care activities (7). They are active members of multiple hospital committees. ACNPs are actively involved with research publication and education at the university level (7,13). They facilitate processes of change within the health care system to provide evidence-based, cost-effective care models and mentor innovative systems and resource use among the health care team. Pediatric ACNPs are leaders in coordination of multidisciplinary teams to develop or revise programs to enhance patient care. They are the line of communication between nursing, social services, dietary, interdisciplines, and attending hospitalist. This communication continues throughout the hospitalization into the outpatient setting. The NP is excellent in the discharge planning process. He provides seamless care throughout the continuum, resulting in optimal-quality safe care.

STANDARDIZED PROCEDURES

Performance of tasks involving invasive skills depends on job descriptions and collaborative practice agreements. Standardized procedures are legal mechanisms for pediatric ACNPs to perform functions that would otherwise be considered the practice of medicine. Pediatric ACNPs perform invasive procedures such as chest tube insertion, central and peripheral inserted catheterizations, and lumbar punctures. Table 3.3 provides a list of common standardized procedures performed by pediatric ACNPs. Although comprehensive, this is not a complete list of all procedures performed by pediatric ACNPs. NPs provide leadership in the development of standardized procedures, protocols, policies, and outcome measures.

TABLE 3.2

CARDIOVASCULAR NURSE PRACTITIONER JOB DESCRIPTION

SUMMARY

The Cardiovascular Nurse Practitioner functions in an Advanced Practice role as a clinical expert in the management of pediatric cardiac patients within a family-centered care environment. Practicing within developed Standardized Procedures and Process Protocols, the Cardiovascular Nurse Practitioner plans, implements, and evaluates the plan of care for pre- and postoperative cardiac patients. Management includes but is not limited to performing history and physical examination, ordering and interpreting appropriate diagnostic and laboratory tests, and furnishing of pharmacologic and nonpharmacologic therapies in a cost-efficient manner. The Cardiovascular Nurse Practitioner functions both as an independent practitioner and in collaboration with the multidisciplinary cardiac team. He/She provides consultation and education to patients, families, and members of the multidisciplinary teams.

ESSENTIAL DUTIES AND RESPONSIBILITIES

I. Clinical Practice (70%)
    A. Measures to Promote and Maintain Health
        1. Inpatient
            a) Provides appropriate care based on the physiological, emotional, and cognitive needs of infants, preschool children, and adolescents.
            b) Performs and documents comprehensive age appropriate history and physical examination.
            c) Implements, plans, and reevaluates daily plan of care in collaboration with the multidisciplinary team. Writes orders and progress notes daily to effectively communicate the designated plan of care.
            d) Performs diagnostic and therapeutic procedures according to standardized procedures.
            e) Orders appropriate laboratory and diagnostic studies as indicated with appropriate follow-up.
            f) Differentiates between normal and abnormal laboratory and radiographic results and intervenes appropriately.
            g) Orders treatment modalities within practice guidelines, and in collaboration with the physician.
            h) Facilitates discharge planning with multidisciplinary team as appropriate.
            i) Documents or dictates transfer and/or discharge summaries as indicated.
        2. Preoperative Clinic
            a) Obtains comprehensive health history and physical examination on all preoperative patients.
            b) Orders and interprets appropriate preoperative laboratory and radiographic studies and ensures appropriate follow-up.
            c) Communicates with surgeon and anesthesiologist regarding patient's status (illness), readiness for surgery, etc.
            d) Performs preoperative education to patient and family regarding surgery, medications, hospitalization, and anticipated discharge needs.
        3. Postoperative Clinic
            a) Performs physical examination.
            b) Reviews patient progress since discharge, ensuring follow-up appointments are in place.
            c) Initiates referrals based on identified needs to appropriate resources.
    B. Patient/Family Education and Resource
        1. Interacts with families to identify unmet psychosocial needs.
        2. Assesses and identifies learning needs of patient and family.
        3. Discusses patient progress and plan of care with family.
        4. Initiates and participates in family conferences as appropriate.
        5. Educates patient and family regarding disease process, postoperative course, and progress.
        6. Initiates appropriate referrals and educates patients and families regarding utilization.
    C. Coordination/Consultation
        1. Facilitates patient progression throughout surgical course: preoperative, hospitalization, and postoperative.
        2. Facilitates communication between patient/family and interdisciplinary team members; between patient/family and the community; and between members of the multidisciplinary team.
        3. Initiates consultations with appropriate interdisciplinary team members.
        4. Provides consultation and meets with health care team at frequent intervals to discuss patient progress and ensure continuity of care.
II. Professional Development/Leadership (15%)
    A. Viewed as a leader and resource to the interdisciplinary and multidisciplinary team
    B. Acts as a change agent in providing creative solutions to clinical and/or systems problems to impact patient care or service.
    C. Participates on hospital/departmental committees.
    D. Maintains a current knowledge base by active participation in professional organizations as well as attending applicable national conferences.
    E. Acts as a mentor for advanced practice nursing students and educators when possible.
    F. Participates in the development, updating, and implementation of standardized protocols and procedures for practice.
III. Research/Education (15%)
    A. Integrates current research into clinical practice, projects, and education.
    B. Develops and/or participates in and promotes research.
    C. Disseminates research and clinical finding through publications, presentations, seminars, etc.
    D. Assists with educational classes and provides mentorship for nursing and medical staff.
    E. Clinical resource for nursing staff, residents, fellows, and referring facilities.
    F. Participates in Quality Resource Management activities.
    G. Develops and/or participates in the development of patient and family educational materials.

TABLE 3.3

NURSE PRACTITIONER STANDARDIZED
PROCEDURES

1. Bone marrow biopsy
2. Central venous catheterization
3. Peripherally inserted venous catheterization
4. Umbilical vessel catheterization
5. Removal of intracardiac lines
6. Insertion of arterial lines
7. Needle aspiration of pneumothorax
8. Thoracentesis
9. Chest tube placement
10. Chest tube removal
11. Epicardial pacemaker wire removal
12. Lumbar puncture
13. Neonatal exchange transfusion
14. Oral endotracheal intubation
15. Skin punch biopsy
16. Suturing
17. Procedure sedation
18. Casting
19. Intrathecal infusion pump manipulation
20. Vagus nerve stimulator therapy
21. Ventricular reservoir tap

REIMBURSEMENT FOR SERVICES

Pediatric ACNPs can bill for their services. The Balanced Budget Act of 1997 with clarifications from the Health Care Financing Administration gives some structure to direct reimbursement for NPs (13). Pediatric ACNPs employed by physician practice plans are also eligible for reimbursement for their services. NPs working in the hospital often do not bill for services since they are salaried employees paid by the hospital, physician group, or a combination of both. In the combination practice agreement where salary of the ACNP is shared between the hospital and the physician practice, both the hospital and practice benefit financially because of cost sharing.

CHALLENGES AND BARRIERS TO THE ACNP ROLE

Lack of role clarity and expectations contribute to problems such as role conflict, role overload, and variable stakeholder acceptance of ACNP roles. Inexperience with ACNPs by those involved in introducing the roles can lead to misinterpretation, underuse of the role, and inconsistency among ACNPs. Insufficient administrative support and competing time demands associated with clinical practice and medical functions are frequently reported barriers to participating in education, research, and leadership activities.

ROLE COMPARISON OF ACNPS AND PHYSICIAN ASSISTANTS

ACNPs are different from physician assistants (PAs). The PA role is under the jurisdiction of physician licensure, which is supervisory rather than collaborative and does not allow for independent functions. A PA is registered by the state after 2 years of undergraduate education (which may or may not be in a health-related field) followed by nine to fifteen months of didactic and clinical education. ACNPs are master-prepared registered nurses. Although some of the care provided by PAs is similar to that provided by ACNPs, there are differences in philosophy, education, scope of practice, and patient approach (13). The ACNPs direct clinical practice competencies provide for the promotion and protection of health. A further differentiation is that the ACNP practice focuses on patient and family education, coordination of care, consultation, and research.

CONCLUSIONS

Opportunities for innovation and improved patient health care systems outcomes occur when the introduction of ACNP roles represent a complementary addition to the model of care rather than a transfer of role functions between care providers. The challenges for the future will focus on further demonstrating the value added of hiring an ACNP to the practice or team. Pediatric ACNPs practicing in collaboration with hospitalists in a collegial relationship will enhance evidence-based decision-making for patient management that leads to increased patient and family satisfaction and clinical outcomes. The continuity of care provided by the ACNP enhances the patient and family experience during a stressful hospitalization. Moreover, the transition to home and the plan for follow-up care are responsibilities well suited to the training and expectations of the ACNP.

Suggested Readings

Cowan MJ, Shapiro M, Hays RD, et al. The effect of a multidisciplinary hospitalist/ physician and advanced practice nurse collaboration on hospital costs. *J Nurs Admin* 2006;36:79–85.

Hickey J. Advanced practice nursing at the dawn of the 21st century: practice, education, and research. In: Hickey J, Ouimette R, Venegoni S, eds. *Advanced practice nursing: changing roles and clinical applications.* 2nd ed. Baltimore: Lippincott Williams & Wilkins; 2000:3–33.

Hravnak M, Kleinpell R, Magdic K, et al. The acute care nurse practitioner. In: Hamric A, Spross J, Hanson C, eds. *Advanced practice nursing: an integrative approach.* 3rd ed. St. Louis: Elsevier Saunders; 2005:475–514.

Meyer S, Meirs L. Cardiovascular surgeon and acute care nurse practitioner. *AACN Clin Issues* 2005;16:149–158.

National Panel for Acute Care Nurse Practitioner Competencies. *Acute care nurse practitioner competencies.* Washington, DC: National Organization of Nurse Practitioner Faculties; 2004.

References

1. Health Resources Services Administration. The registered nurse population: national sample survey of registered nurses. Washington, D.C.: United States Department of Health and Human Services; 2004.
2. Pitts J, Seimer B. The use of nurse practitioners in pediatric institutions. *J Pediatr Healthcare* 1998;12:67–72.
3. American Academy of Pediatrics. The role of the nurse practitioner and physician assistant in the care of hospitalized children. *Pediatrics* 1999; 103:1050–1052.

4. Kleinpell R, Perez D, McLaughlin R. Educational options for the acute care nurse practitioner practice. *J Am Acad Nurs Practitioners* 2005;17:460–471.
5. National Association of Pediatric Nurse Practitioners. Position statement: the acute care pediatric nurse practitioner. *J Pediatr Healthcare* 2005;19: 38A–39A.
6. ANA. Standards of clinical practice and scope of practice for the acute care nurse practitioner. Washington, D.C.: American Nurses Association; 1995.
7. Kleinpell R. Acute care nurse practitioner practice: results of a 5-year longitudinal study. *Am J Crit Care* 2005;14:211–220.
8. Hoffman LA, Tasota FJ, Zullo GT, et al. Outcomes of care managed by an acute care nurse practitioner/attending physician team in a subacute medical intensive care unit. *Am J Crit Care* 2005;12:121–128.
9. Carzoli RP, Martinez M, Cuevas LL, et al. Comparison of neonatal nurse practitioners, physician assistants, and residents in the neonatal intensive care unit. *Arch Pediatric Adolesc Med* 1994;148:1271–1276.
10. Karlowicz M, McMurray J. Comparison of neonatal nurse practitioners and pediatric residents care of extremely low birth weight infants. *Arch Pediatric Adoles Med* 2000;154:1123–1126.
11. Martin SA. The pediatric critical care nurse practitioner: evolution and impact. *Pediatr Nurse* 1999;25:505–510.
12. Molitor-Kirsch S, Thompson L, Milonovich L. The Changing face of critical care medicine: nurse practitioners in the pediatric intensive care unit. *AACN Clin Issues* 2005;16:172–177.
13. The Balanced Budget Act of 1997. 42 USC; 4511–4512:1997.

CHAPTER 4 ■ EVIDENCE-BASED MEDICINE AND CLINICAL DECISION-MAKING IN THE PRACTICE OF PEDIATRICS

GREGG M. TALENTE AND GARY M. ONADY

Evidence-based medicine (EBM) has been defined as the integration of best research evidence with clinical expertise and patient values (1). Evidence-based clinical decision-making should be applied at all times by physicians in pediatric hospital medicine—as with all areas of pediatrics. This model integrates clinical expertise, research evidence, and patient values to help physicians make the best decision for their patients.

Practitioners often misinterpret EBM as "cook-book medicine," and reject the principles outlined above to rely solely on their personal "experience" and "expertise." Practicing EBM, by definition, relies solidly on physician expertise. The additional misconception that EBM ignores the patient's wishes is also dispelled by the definition in which incorporating patient values is a core feature. The truth about EBM is that it simply calls for the physician to apply her expertise to the critical appraisal of pertinent literature regarding the clinical decisions she makes daily. In turn, the EBM process ensures that these decisions lead to the greatest benefit demanded by the patient with the least risk of harm.

This chapter provides EBM methods that can be applied in the everyday hospital practice of physicians and other providers taking care of children. The five EBM steps highlighted in this chapter consist of the following: (1) asking answerable clinical questions, (2) efficiently searching relevant literature, (3) critically evaluating the literature, (4) applying valid evidence to clinical decision-making, and (5) evaluating and improving the process.

STEP 1: ASKING ANSWERABLE CLINICAL QUESTIONS

The well-read physician who is familiar with the relevant data and the standard of care is able to make many clinical decisions without any additional review of the literature or other effort. However, all providers will find clinical situations where the correct course of action is not so clear. In these situations, a careful examination of the literature and how it pertains to the patient will be necessary. The first step in EBM is to formulate a clear and answerable question.

The most frequently recommended model for formulating a specifically focused clinical question is the PICO model (Table 4.1). This model provides the framework for a researchable clinical question. The following are the essential components of the question: (1) the presenting *Problem*; (2) the *Intervention* being considered; (3) *Comparison* intervention(s)

if they exist; and (4) the clinical *Outcome* relevant to the case (1). After these components are defined, a clear clinical question can be easily stated. This will be made clear by reviewing a simple example:

> A 1-year-old infant presents with cough, congestion, wheezing, and respiratory distress. The infant requires nasal cannula oxygen support for moderate hypoxia. A chest x-ray shows bilateral perihilar infiltrates, and the respiratory syncytial virus (RSV) antibody test is positive. The child was previously healthy and has no history of reactive airway disease. For this patient, will inhaled albuterol will be beneficial or prevent worsening of the condition?

Table 4.1 shows how the PICO format is used to define a clinical question for this example. Thus applied, the format defines the patient problem (RSV bronchiolitis), intervention, comparison, and outcome. This question addresses treatment, but the method can be used to clearly state questions that inform and address decisions regarding illness manifestations and etiologies, usefulness of clinical findings, most useful diagnostic test(s), and best methods for preventing illness.

STEP 2: EFFICIENTLY SEARCHING RELEVANT LITERATURE

Once the clinical question has been clearly stated, the second step is to find relevant literature to answer the question. The most commonly used tool for searching the medical literature is MEDLINE, a free Internet database provided by the U.S. National Library of Medicine. It is an "on your own" search engine consisting of scientific abstracts from more than 4,000 journals from 1966 to the present. Content area is indexed by subject (keywords), article type (e.g., review, randomized trial), patient age ranges, publication language, author name(s), publication date ranges, and journal names, with the ability to select limits within these fields. Free online search versions such as PubMed (*www.pubmed.gov*) provide economy and quick access from an office-based personal computer for both foreground and background questions. Background information is usually found in textbooks and review literature while foreground information is more specific, journal based, and subsequently constructed to answer the PICO question.

Searching for literature to address a specific clinical question involves entering a series of search terms and combining them to appropriately limit the number of articles returned by

TABLE 4.1

PICO ORDER TO THE ANSWERABLE
CLINICAL QUESTION

Patient or problem	A 1-year-old with RSV
Intervention	Inhaled albuterol
Comparison	Placebo and supportive care measures
Outcome	Prevention of pediatric intensive care unit (PICU) transfer
Clinical question	Does inhaled albuterol compared to placebo reduce the frequency of PICU admission in children with RSV bronchiolitis?

the search engine. The intent is to find those articles that are pertinent, and hopefully a manageable number. A physician practiced in searching the medical literature can easily locate articles that directly address a clearly stated clinical question in a short amount of time. Search terms are combined using AND, OR, and NOT depending on whether you want to limit (i.e., AND, NOT) or expand (i.e., OR) the search. The search terms can usually be defined directly from a clearly stated clinical question.

In the example above, the clinical question was "Does inhaled *albuterol* compared to placebo reduce the frequency of *PICU admission* in *children* with *RSV bronchiolitis*?" Words that can easily be used as search terms are italicized. A search to find relevant literature to answer this question would usually start with the disease of interest. Thus the first search term would be "RSV bronchiolitis." Next the search would continue with the patient type, "children." Combining these two terms with AND will get every article about children with RSV. Age range can also be used to set limits to a search rather than as a search term.

Other useful resources for finding "best evidence" include formatted publications and evidence-based medicine databases. Examples of formatted publications include *Clinical Evidence*, which addresses therapeutic questions; and *Best Evidence*, which provides a wider range of clinical inquiries including etiology [cohort studies], clinical findings [diagnostic tests], diagnosis [differential diagnosis], diagnostic testing [sensitivity AND specificity], therapeutics [randomized control trial], prognosis [prognosis], economics, and quality improvement. The bracketed terms represent clinical operators that when used in combination with the AND/OR/NOT terms further limit the search to the context of that specific content category. These are updated quarterly with relevant pediatric content and can be useful resources for finding evidence to address clinical questions. The *Cochrane Library* provides a collection of quarterly updated systematic reviews focusing on therapeutics and prevention. This resource saves time and effort because other authors have researched and digested similar clinical questions and provided informed reports.

Returning to the case example, to further narrow the search, continue with a search for articles about "albuterol" therapy or "therapy" in general and combine the searches again. Finally, because randomized control trials are the best form of evidence, limit the search to include only randomized studies. The "search sentence" converted into an answerable question appears as [*RSV bronchiolitis* AND *albuterol* AND *therapy* AND *randomized control trial*]. This will finally result in a very short list of articles to review, with one or more that will address the specific question.

STEP 3: CRITICALLY EVALUATING THE LITERATURE

With the literature search completed and evidence located, step 3 requires a critical evaluation of the collected evidence. At this point the most important lead question to ask is: "Does this information have relevance to the treatment of my individual patient?" Finding what appears to be a high-quality study does not mean that this information applies to the patient of interest. Clinical expertise again contributes here significantly. Once applicability has been confirmed, formal application of step 3 proceeds by evaluating the found evidence with the following three criteria: (1) evaluating basic study design to check validity, (2) analyzing results for use in patient care decisions, and (3) applying these results to the specific clinical problem.

Guides have been published that help physicians perform these critical reviews (2–10). This chapter will focus on evaluating articles about diagnostic tests and therapy choices because these are the studies that are usually most helpful in answering clinical questions. Other article types such as meta-analyses, prognosis articles, and review articles can be used to answer questions as well but will not be discussed here. Table 4.2 provides a summary of critical evaluation questions and Table 4.3 provides definitions that are important in understanding and appraising the literature.

Examples

Critical Evaluation of Diagnostic Testing Articles

Start by determining study validity. Review the methodology and ensure that good research methods were used. A simple way to look at this is to answer the following questions:

1. Was there an independent, blind comparison of the test with a reference (gold) standard of diagnosis?
2. Was the diagnostic test evaluated in an appropriate spectrum of patients like the patient of interest?
3. Was the reference standard applied regardless of the diagnostic test result?
4. Was the test validated in a second, independent group of patients?

Answers to these four questions cover most of the important issues in assessing validity, and address most of the ways in which bias enters a study of a diagnostic test.

Critical evaluation then focuses on measuring statistical impact of the results. Most studies report how many patients test positive and negative with the proposed testing compared to currently accepted testing or a reference test (gold standard) that determines who has or does not have a specific disease. Sensitivity, specificity, positive predictive value, and negative predictive value are then calculated for the test. Sometimes a study reports only sensitivity and specificity. Alternatively, the article may report likelihood ratios calculated from the sensitivity and specificity. Figure 4.1 shows how these different measures are calculated.

Sensitivity and specificity for a specific test are independent of disease prevalence. Therefore sensitivity and specificity can be applied to individual patients who have a pretest disease prevalence different from the study population. In contrast, positive and negative predictive values look at the probability of disease in a preselected study population and vary based on the prevalence of the disease in the population. Thus in assessing an article about a diagnostic test, all of these factors and the prevalence of the disease in the population to whom the patient belongs must be considered.

Likelihood ratios (LRs) provide a more useful tool for assessing the quality of a diagnostic test in that they allow the

TABLE 4.2

MEDICAL LITERATURE CRITICAL EVALUATION GUIDES

		Clinical manifestations	Differential diagnosis	Diagnostic testing	Therapy/Prevention	Prognosis	Cause/Harm/Etiology	Reviews
Study	**Validity**	▪ Explicit use of diagnostic criteria ▪ Independent diagnostic criteria ▪ Study mirrors whole patient population with disease ▪ Thorough and consistent patient evaluation	▪ Well-defined problem ▪ Thorough evaluation ▪ Prevalence mirrors target population ▪ Similarity of services by clinics used ▪ Inclusion-Exclusion avoids missed patients ▪ Consistent diagnostic workup	▪ Independent, blind comparison test with a reference standard ▪ Test evaluated on appropriate patient spectrum ▪ Reference test applied regardless of test result ▪ Validated 2nd group of independent patients	▪ Controls randomized ▪ Small groups at start ▪ No other treatments details ▪ Lost patients accounted ▪ Non-compliant patients accounted ▪ Care given out of study accounted	▪ Population represented ▪ Well-defined disease ▪ Long enough F/U ▪ Adverse outcome defined ▪ Outcome blinded ▪ Rx altering outcome	▪ Comparable subjects non-exposed/exposed ▪ Confounding variables accounted ▪ Temporal relation of exposure correct ▪ Sufficient F/U ▪ Adjusted prognosis	▪ Clear, focused question ▪ Defines patient, exposure, method ▪ Good inclusion criteria ▪ Good quality studies ▪ Outcome differences documented ▪ Homogeneity
Statistical Results		▪ % patients with each clinical finding listed ▪ All CIs on + side of 0	▪ CIs minimal overlap among diagnosis	▪ LR ability to modify pretest probability	▪ ARR is best measure ▪ CIs crossing 0 do not demonstrate benefit	▪ Survival curves (Kaplan-Meier) ▪ CIs precisely estimate likelihood	▪ RR if prospective ▪ OR if retrospective ▪ CI tells size of effect	▪ Detailed data ▪ OR/RR reported ▪ CI tells size of effect
Applicable		▪ Close patient match provides confidence ▪ Culture can effect expressed disorder ▪ Consider change of disease over time ▪ Treatment advances can change course	▪ Close patient match provides confidence ▪ Other diseases controlled/eliminated ▪ No new diseases arise ▪ Survival improves ▪ Public health measures control disease	▪ Testing reproducible ▪ Similar interpretations ▪ Similar severity and competing diseases ▪ Impacts treatment thresholds	▪ Patient meets inclusion ▪ Treatment improves important outcome ▪ Value and range of NNT/NNH ▪ Risk of adverse event if not treated	▪ Similar study patients ▪ Results lead to therapy selection ▪ Results reassure patient ▪ Bad results lead to end of life decision-making	▪ Similar study patients ▪ Treatment improves patient outcome ▪ Risk to patient if exposure continues ▪ Positive consequence if exposure reduced	▪ Study consistently applied to wide range of patients ▪ Studies not included are considered ▪ Benefits weighted against harm and cost

The key points regarding validity, study results, and applicability are outlined under each of the different types of clinical questions that may arise in the care of hospitalized pediatric patients. CI, confidence interval; F/U, follow-up; ARR, absolute risk reduction; RR, relative risk; OR, odds-ratio; NNT, number needed to treat; NNH, number needed to harm; LR, likelihood ratio.

TABLE 4.3

TERMINOLOGY KEY

Term	Definition
Sensitivity	The percentage of patients with a disease who will test positive on the diagnostic test being studied
Specificity	The percentage of patients without a disease who will test negative on the diagnostic test being studied
Positive predictive value (PPV)	The percentage of patients testing positive on the diagnostic test being studied who actually have the disease, or the likelihood a person testing positive has the disease
Negative predictive value (NPV)	The percentage of patients testing negative on the diagnostic test being studied who do not have the disease, or the likelihood a person testing negative does not have the disease
Pretest probability	The likelihood a patient has a condition before the test being considered is done. This is an estimated likelihood based on clinical presentation and other available data
Post-test probability	The likelihood a patient has a condition after the test in question has been performed. This is calculated using the pretest probability and the positive or negative likelihood ratio
Likelihood ratio	A mathematical ratio calculated from the sensitivity and specificity of a given diagnostic test that can be used along with pretest probability to calculate the post-test probability of a patient having the condition
Event rate	The percentage of individuals in either the test or control groups in whom the outcome of interest occurs.
Absolute risk reduction (ARR)	Difference in event rates or risk between patients in the control or placebo group and patients in intervention or test group. (The outcome occurs ARR% fewer times in treated patients compared to controls.)
Relative risk reduction (RRR)	The proportional reduction in events in treated compared to untreated or control subjects. (The outcome in treated patient is reduced by RRR%.)
Number needed to treat (NNT)	Number of patients who need to be treated to achieve one additional favorable outcome

clinician to apply the pretest likelihood of having a disease based on a reference population and the test's sensitivity and specificity values (which are used to calculate the likelihood ratio) to an individual patient. This in turn allows the clinician to calculate a post-test probability that the individual patient has the disease. Likelihood ratios provide straightforward clinical relevance as ratios very close to one do not change the pretest likelihood of disease—that is, any value multiplied by one results in the same value. Thus a test with a likelihood ratio close to 1 provides little useful information. Tests that result in a +LR between 5 and 10 are good, and >10 provide

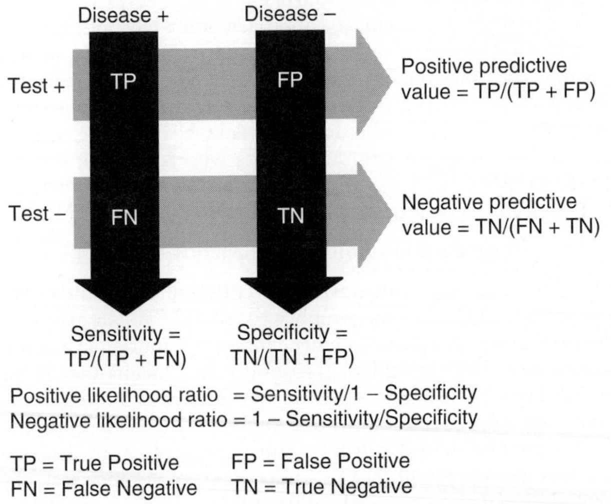

excellent tests toward advancing the post-test likelihood of disease. Tests with −LR between 0.2 and 0.5 are good, and tests <0.2 are also excellent tests.

Critical evaluation is completed by determining if study results are applicable to the patient. This evaluation can be omitted if the study was found not to be valid, or the results are not clinically applicable to the patient of interest. A final summary for appraising an article on diagnostic testing would be to ask the following questions:

1. Is the diagnostic test available, affordable, accurate, and precise in your setting?
2. Are the study subjects similar to your own patient?
3. Is the prevalence of the disease different for your patient than stated in the study, thus changing the predictive value of the test?
4. Would a positive or negative result on this test change the probability that your patient has the disease and change your management?
5. Would your patient be willing to have the test?
6. Would the consequences of the test help your patient?

In answering these questions the patient-centeredness of the EBM approach becomes evident.

Critical Evaluation of Therapy Articles

To ascertain study validity for therapy articles, start by reviewing the methodology and trying to determine whether good research methods were used. A simple way is to answer the following questions:

1. Was the assignment of patients to the treatment and control groups randomized?
2. Were the treatment and control groups similar at the start of the study?

FIGURE 4.1. Relationship of sensitivity, specificity, predictive values, and likelihoods.

TABLE 4.4

GRADING LEVELS OF EVIDENCE

Level of evidence	Type of study
Level I	Randomized controlled trial
Level II-1	Nonrandomized trial, well designed
Level II-2	Cohort, case-control, well designed
Level II-3	Uncontrolled, time series
Level III	Opinion, descriptive, case reports

3. Were all patients accounted for? Was follow-up complete? Were patients analyzed in the groups to which they were randomized?
4. Were patients, health workers, and researchers "blind" to treatment?
5. Were the groups treated equally?

Randomized trials serve as the strongest filter to eliminate bias and confounding variables; hence, they are the most trusted source of data and are preferred over other study types. Table 4.4 shows the various levels of evidence available in assessing treatments. The better the level of evidence, the more the results can be trusted as long as the study was well done and is otherwise valid.

After determining the level of the evidence and whether it is valid, an assessment is made of the statistical magnitude of the treatment effect. Randomized trials typically present results as a relative risk (RR), which is the ratio of risk for the therapeutic outcome of patients receiving the therapy compared to those not receiving the intervention of interest. Results are also frequently reported as relative risk reduction (RRR), representing the extent to which treatment reduces risk beyond the beneficial effect of the comparison intervention. The RRR can be misleading (see below). This calculation compares the difference between the event rate of the experimental group, the experimental event rate (EER), and the control event rate (CER; for the control group) divides this difference once again by the CER, or RRR = (CER−EER)/CER. A more "absolute" representation of response magnitude of therapeutic trials is the absolute risk reduction (ARR). This calculation simply reflects the difference between control and experimental results as ARR = CER − EER. Absolute risk reduction is sometimes not reported in published articles, but with the above equations can be easily applied. Why should a physician need both RRR and ARR numbers? When the control group rate is divided into the difference between the experimental and control groups, the magnitude of this effect becomes dependent on the size of control group response rate. Thus RRR can appear to have a greater effect than is really present. As an example, if the control group rate (CER) is 10% (0.10) and the experimental group rate (EER) is 5% (0.05), RRR is (0.1 − 0.05)/0.05 or 100%, whereas the ARR is only 5%. Which value has the most practical application to the treating clinician and to the patient?

A major discriminator in evaluating articles concerning therapeutics, prognosis, and harm is calculation of the numbers needed to treat (NNT) or harm (NNH). The concept behind NNT and NNH relates to answering the question, "How many patients do I need to medically manage with the desired intervention before one patient benefits (NNT) or is harmed (NNH) from that medical intervention?" This parameter is the reciprocal of the absolute risk reduction, or NNT = 1/ARR. Thus NNT makes the most conceptual sense toward communicating benefit to risk (or cost) before an intervention

is used. The NNT (or NNH) should be calculated in any study of a therapeutic intervention.

Some treatment studies look at outcomes of a particular intervention, for example, the effect of aerosolized epinephrine in croup on length of hospital stay. In such studies, the outcome variable presented is the difference between the two groups. These studies do not lend themselves to RRR, ARR, or NNT calculations. In such a study, the difference between the two groups is calculated as Y−X, and reported along with the 95% confidence intervals for that difference. The true finding or effect for similar patients under similar circumstances is likely to be within the 95% confidence interval. The narrower the 95% confidence interval (CI), the greater certainty of the difference presented. When the 95% CI includes zero, then it is possible that there is no difference in the outcomes between the test and control groups.

After reviewing the study results, the final step is to determine whether the study results are applicable to the patient of interest. Answer the following questions:

1. Are the patients in the study similar to my patient?
2. Were all clinically important outcomes considered?
3. Are the likely treatment benefits worth the potential harms and cost?
4. Is the therapy feasible in my community or practice?

The most valid study with the most impressive results is meaningless if it doesn't relate to your specific patient.

STEP 4: APPLYING VALID EVIDENCE TO CLINICAL DECISION-MAKING

Clinical expertise through identification of relevant clinical manifestations provides the essential database that sets the foundation for evidence-based decision-making. Traditional medicine utilizes a *possibilistic* approach to differential diagnosis that lists a potentially exhaustive list of diagnostic possibilities, which can in turn lead to exhaustive diagnostic strategies. Evidence-based decision-making applies a *probabilistic* approach that organizes a differential of diseases into one leading diagnosis and a few (typically <4) active alternatives that represent prognostic differentials with high likelihood of morbidity or mortality if left undiagnosed. Diagnostic testing is then judiciously chosen toward ruling in a working diagnosis by applying testing with high positive likelihood ratios (>5) or ruling out active alternatives with tests possessing low negative likelihood ratios (<0.5) (5).

The probabilistic diagnostic approach ultimately optimizes the post-test likelihood of disease for an individual patient, ideally reaching the point that crosses a treatment threshold. Treatment thresholds are derived from weighing the cost of bad outcomes in treating individuals who do not actually have disease, against the lost benefit of not treating patients who truly have disease. This analysis can be based on a cost-benefit analysis derived from prognostic data relevant to the working diagnosis (11):

$$\text{Treatment Threshold} = 1/([\text{Benefit/Cost}] + 1)$$

More serious diagnoses have low treatment thresholds, and less serious diagnoses have higher thresholds. As an example, the possibility of sepsis in a febrile infant without an infectious source has a 5% treatment threshold. This means that if the possibility of sepsis exceeds 5%, the infant needs to be covered with appropriate antibiotic therapy until a high-quality diagnostic test (blood culture) returns negative, thus decreasing this disease possibility to under 5%. By comparison, the probability of sinusitis needs to be at least 55% before electing to treat with an antibiotic course.

Many valuable outcomes are derived from isolated EBM applications, which can be directly utilized in making relevant medical decisions with the patient. For example, a weight-loss medication on the market achieves a 10% weight loss goal with a reported RRR = 0.56%. The clinician can easily calculate an ARR of 0.05; NNT = 1/0.05 = 20. Soiling is the major side effect of this medication, with an absolute risk increase (ARI) = 0.25; NNH = 1/0.25 = 4. Putting this into perspective, 20 patients need to be treated before one patient achieves a 10% weight-loss goal, while 5 will experience stool leakage. The patient (or patient's family) responsible for doing the laundry should easily reach an individualized medical decision when provided with this evidence-based perspective.

STEP 5: EVALUATING AND IMPROVING THE PROCESS

Providers taking care of children in the hospital setting who practice the application of EBM principles to their clinical questions will quickly realize the benefit this provides their patients. The steps in developing, researching, and answering a clinical question will take less and less time as practitioners hone their skills. The final step in applying an evidence-based model to the care of children involves asking and answering other types of questions using the same process. This chapter has focused on questions related to how to diagnose or treat individual patients. EBM can also be used to address other clinical questions (Table 4.2) or even systems-based issues that affect the care of all hospitalized children. The pediatric hospital care provider can use this model to determine best practices for the inpatient unit, for nursing procedures, or for almost any medically related decision he may need to make in an administrative role. The steps remain the same; the only difference is how the answer to the question is applied. In this case, it may be used to set policy on the inpatient ward.

CONCLUSION

The EBM approach prepares pediatric care providers to find the clinical evidence in the literature and apply this information to optimize the care of individual patients, and all of their patients. It relies on the expertise of the practicing physi-cian and his ability to appraise the evidence in direct relation to a specific patient. EBM provides clinicians with a set of tools to use when complex medical decisions need to be made to improve outcomes. Quality measures have become more important in our health care system, and EBM is a part of that process. Increasingly, third-party payers are imple-menting pay-for-performance programs that include meeting evidence-based standards for clinical practice. In such situa-tions, the pediatric hospital care provider should approach patient care based on the best available evidence. A solid understanding of how to interpret and assess the quality of published evidence has and will become more critical for suc-cessful practice.

References

1. Sackett DL, Richardson WS, Rosenberg WM, et al. *Evidence-based medicine: how to practice and teach EBM.* 2nd ed. London: Churchill Livingston; 2000:1.
2. Oxman AD, Cook DJ, Guyatt GH. Users' guides to the medical literature VI. How to use an overview. *JAMA* 1994;272:1367–1371.
3. Richardson WS, Wilson MC, Noyer VA, et al. Users' guides to the medical literature XXIV. How to use an article on the clinical manifestations of disease. *JAMA* 2000;284:869–875.
4. Richardson WS, Wilson MC, Guyatt GH, et al. Users' guides to the medical literature XV. How to use an article about disease probability for differential diagnosis. *JAMA* 1999;281:1214–1219.
5. Jaeschke R, Guyatt G, Sackett DL. Users' guides to the medical literature III. How to use an article about a diagnostic test A. Are the results of the study valid? *JAMA* 1994;271:389–391.
6. Jaeschke R, Guyatt G, Sackett DL. Users' guides to the medical literature III. How to use an article about a diagnostic test B. What are the results and will they help me in caring for my patients? *JAMA* 1994;271:703–707.
7. Guyatt GH, Sackett DL, Cook DJ. Users' guides to the medical literature II. How to use an article about therapy or prevention A. Are the results of the study valid? *JAMA* 1993;270:2598–2601.
8. Guyatt GH, Sackett DL, Cook DJ. Users' Guides to the medical literature II. How to use an article about therapy or prevention B. What were the results and will they help me in caring for my patients? *JAMA* 1994;271:59–63.
9. Levine ML, Walter S, Lee H, et al. Users' guides to the medical literature IV. How to use an article about harm. *JAMA* 1994;271:1615–1619.
10. Laupacis A, Wells G, Richardson WS, et al. Users' guides to the medical literature V. How to use an article about prognosis. *JAMA* 1994;272:234–237.
11. Pauker SG, Kassirer JP. Therapeutic decision making: a cost-benefit analysis. *N Engl J Med* 1975;293:229–334.

CHAPTER 5 ■ BILLING AND CODING

DONNA M. MESSENGER AND JAMES D. SWIFT

When health care providers hear "billing and coding," they automatically assume that the topic of conversation is payment for the services rendered in their respective area of expertise. At a minimum, billing and coding is only one aspect of physician or "practice revenue management." Physician billing, coding, and accounts receivable (A/R) management is one of the most complex revenue cycles in the business of medicine. The era when solely being a good physician guaranteed financial success has long since passed. In today's medical marketplace it is imperative that physicians understand the complex world of medical practice billing and A/R management. In this section we will cover the following components that comprise the medical practice revenue cycle:

> Documentation and coding
> Contracts
> Fee schedules
> Collection percentage
> A/R aging
> Payer mix
> Billing/collections

DOCUMENTATION AND CODING

Physicians are required to document pertinent facts and findings regarding a patient's health history including, but not limited to, past and present illnesses, test results, family history, examinations, medications, and vaccinations in the individual's medical record.

The medical record facilitates communication between physicians and other health care providers, as well as documenting services rendered for billing purposes. Medical records may also be viewed by risk management, insurance carriers, medical boards, and participants in legal proceedings.

Determining the correct level of service and documentation guidelines has been an ongoing controversy for many years. Requirements for the current level of service/documentation guidelines are determined by the Centers for Medicare and Medicaid Services (CMS), formerly known as HCFA (Health Care Financing Administration). These recommendations are contained in the 1995 or 1997 Documentation Guidelines, which providers can utilize based on the guideline year that the provider feels is more advantageous. The 1995 and 1997 Documentation Guidelines are templates for documenting the services provided, to support the correct evaluation and management (E/M) code assigned to a patient visit.

Documentation is absolutely critical. Medical record documentation must be clear and concise and must accurately reflect services performed. Auditors do not infer that services were performed; they strictly audit the chart note to ascertain whether the key elements were met. Failure to document properly can be construed as fraud and abuse, and lead to payment denials. Services not documented are reported by auditors as not having been performed. The method of chart documentation adopted—such as typed, handwritten, computer generated—is up to the physician or hospital. The medical record must reflect the date and the full name of the physician. Illegible signatures or initials are not sufficient. For time-sensitive codes, such as critical care, the total time must be stated in the medical record.

Current Procedural Terminology

Current procedural terminology (CPT) codes[1] developed by the American Medical Association (AMA) are numbers assigned for reporting medical services and procedures performed by physicians. Multiple codes are necessary because of the wide range of services provided, and the various methods and combinations of procedures performed. CPT codes are classified into the following categories:

> Evaluation and management (E/M) codes
> Anesthesia
> Surgery
> Radiology
> Pathology and laboratory
> Medicine

Evaluation and Management Codes

Evaluation and management (E/M) codes are the most commonly used codes and the most difficult to determine the correct level. E/M codes fall into several categories and subcategories. A few are listed below.

Category	Subcategory
Office/outpatient services	New/established patients
Hospital services	Initial/subsequent/ discharge
Critical care	Adult/pediatric/neonatal
Consultations	Hospital/office

There are seven components that comprise the level of E/M services: Office visits, consultations, hospital visits, critical care services, observation codes, and nursing facility care. These components can be divided into three key components:

> History
> Examination
> Medical decision-making

---

[1]CPT™—Current Procedural Terminology 2005 American Medical Association. All Rights Reserved.

Three contributory components:

Counseling
Coordination of care
Nature of presenting problems

One final component:

Time

The three key components are expanded further as shown in the following sections.

History. E/M services are based on four types of history: problem focused, expanded problem focused, detailed, and comprehensive.

Chief complaint
Statement describing reason for the visit
History of presenting Illness
Description of the patient's present illness
Location, quality, severity, timing, context, modifying factors, and associated signs/symptoms
Review of systems
An inventory of body systems, documented by a series of questions to identify signs/symptoms by positive responses and pertinent negatives.
Constitutional; eyes; ears, nose, mouth, and throat; cardiovascular; respiratory; gastrointestinal; genitourinary
Musculoskeletal; integumentary; neurologic; psychiatric
Endocrine; hematologic/lymphatic; allergic/immunologic
Past, family, and/or social history
A review of pertinent past, family, or social history
Prior medical history; age-appropriate immunizations
Age-appropriate feeding
Specific family diseases related to a chief complaint
Family history that may impact patient condition(s)
Living arrangements
Age dependent: sexual history or use of drugs/alcohol/ tobacco
Other relevant social factors

Examination. E/M services are based on four types of examinations: problem focused, expanded problem focused, detailed, and comprehensive.

Problem focused: A limited examination of the affected body area or organ.
Expanded problem focused: A limited examination of the affected body area or organ and any other symptomatic or related body area(s) or organ.
Detailed: An extended examination of the affected body area(s) or organ(s) and any other symptomatic or related body area(s) or organ system.
Comprehensive: A general multisystem examination or complete examination of a single organ system and other symptomatic or related body area(s) or organ system(s).

Documentation that notes "negative" or "normal" is sufficient documentation for normal findings related to unaffected areas. Simply documenting "abnormal" is not sufficient documentation. Abnormal findings and relevant negative findings from the examination should be described and well documented. A general multisystem examination must include documentation from eight or more of the twelve organ systems.

Medical Decision-Making. E/M services recognize four types of medical decision-making: straightforward, low complexity, moderate complexity, and high complexity. The number of possible diagnoses—the number of management options, the amount and complexity of data that must be obtained and reviewed, and the risk of complications/morbidity/mortality as well as co-morbidities associated with the patient's presenting problems—are measurements utilized when selecting the level of medical decision-making. Selection of the appropriate CPT and ICD-9 code is based on the documentation supported in the chart.

Time. Codes that are time sensitive, such as critical care and prolonged services, require that the actual time spent be documented in the medical record. When procedures are performed, the time spent on the procedure must be subtracted from the total encounter time.

Modifiers. Modifiers are two-digit codes reported in addition to the CPT code for further clarification of services performed. The lack of modifiers or the improper use can lead to payment delays or even denials. Commonly used modifiers include those described in the following sections.

Modifier 25: Significant, separately identifiable E/M service by the same physician on the same day of the procedure or other service

Example: A 4-year-old patient is admitted early in the morning for labored breathing, requiring O2 supplementation and nebulizer treatment. You perform a full admit workup. Within hours of the admission the patient's condition worsens and he is transported to the PICU. You spend an additional 45 minutes monitoring and treating.

This would be billed with both admit 99223 and 99291, providing the documentation in the medical record clearly reflects both services performed. These are two separately identifiable services. It would be incorrect to bill additional time (99292) for the time spent on the admit workup because the criteria for critical-care billing would not have been satisfied. The use of modifier 25 tells the insurance carrier that the critical care services were "significant and separate" from the admission. Carriers may require that two different diagnosis codes be used, one for the admission and one for the critical care. However, CPT guidelines do not require more than one diagnosis for two E/M codes.

Modifier 52/53: Reduced procedure discontinued. Physicians may elect to terminate a procedure if they feel that the well-being of the patient is in jeopardy.

Modifier 63: Procedure performed on neonates or infants less than 4 kg. This can only be added to some surgical procedures.

International Classification of Disease, Ninth Revision, Clinical Modification (ICD-9, CM)

ICD-9 CM codes are three-, four-, or five-digit numbers assigned to signs, symptoms, illnesses, disorders, and diseases, and are used to describe the medical necessity of the procedure or the encounter. An ICD-9 code is valid only when coded to the proper number of digits required. ICD-9 CM codes range from 001.0 to 999.9, V01.0 to V83.02, and E800.0 to E999.

When coding, always code to the highest level of certainty. If a definitive diagnosis is not immediately determined, code the presenting signs and symptoms. Be specific. Abdominal pain is not a valid diagnosis code. Indicate the location of the pain; upper right/left quadrant, lower right/left quadrant, or generalized.

Do not code; "rule out," "suspected," "probable," or "questionable." If you are ruling out meningitis, and have ordered a lumbar puncture, with a negative result, code the presenting signs and symptoms.

For billing purposes, four diagnosis codes are permitted per CPT code; many insurance carriers only consider the primary and secondary diagnosis codes. Medicare only considers the primary diagnosis code.

Chronic conditions can be coded as primary or secondary, depending on the reason for the encounter. If a patient with a chronic condition presents for a routine visit, code the chronic condition as primary. If that same patient presents with a complication to the chronic condition, or an unrelated illness that could become more severe because of the chronic condition, code the reason for the encounter as primary with the chronic condition as secondary.

Documentation in the medical record must match the billing record for diagnostic codes as well as procedural codes. Information sent to an insurance carrier for reimbursement needs to clearly indicate the reason for the encounter utilizing CPT and ICD-9 codes only.

Evaluation and Management CPT Codes may be assigned completely separate diagnosis codes than a procedure performed on the same day. Always assign the appropriate diagnosis code to the procedure being done. Codes begin with alpha prefix E or V.

V-Codes V01.0 to V83.02

V-codes generally designate reasons for encounters when:

1. A patient presents for services when she is not presently ill, such as a yearly physical.
2. A patient with a known disease presents for treatment related to the disease, such as renal dialysis.
3. When circumstances or problems are present that influence the patient's health status, such as shunt status.

E-Codes E800.0 to E999

E-codes are supplement diagnosis codes used to classify external causes of the injury, poisoning, or adverse effects. E-codes are never coded as primary; they are used only to help support the reason for the illness.

COLLECTION PERCENTAGE, A/R AGING, CONTRACTS/ CREDENTIALING, AND FEE SCHEDULE

These next four elements of the billing and collection cycle are all interrelated. The collection percentage is predicated on the established fee schedule and contractual reimbursement. Accounts receivable (A/R) aging is predicated on the timely filing of claims and the turnaround time of the reimbursement from the contracted insurance carriers.

Collection Percentage

There are two factors to review when looking at your collection percentage: net and gross collection percentage. Total net receipts divided by total charges equals net collection percentage. Total net receipts plus contractual adjustments divided by total charges equals gross collection percentage.

Contractual adjustments are the difference between the physician's fee schedule and the amount of reimbursement, based on the contract with the insurance carriers. Contractual adjustments do not take into consideration write-offs for bad debt.

If the charges are $655,233 and the net receipts are $368,629, then the monthly net collection percentage will be 56%. Based on the previous figures, the gross collection percentage is total net receipts, or $368,629, plus contractual adjustments, or $179,000 = $547,629. And then $547,629 divided by total charges, or $655,233 = 83%.

Lower collection rates do not necessarily indicate that a practice makes less money. Would you rather have 75% of $100,000 or 50% of $200,000? Payer mix, fee schedules, and contract rates all play an important part in determining if your collection percentage is acceptable or not.

Payer Mix

A graph similar to the one shown in Table 5.1 should be reviewed monthly and yearly. Track total charges, payments, adjustments, and percent of total A/R by carrier per month and per year. Tracking your A/R in this manner will provide you with:

1. Breakdown of carrier classifications (by contract). You will be able to see what your average collection percentage is by contract.
2. If you have a high concentration of Medicaid, which historically has the lowest reimbursement rate, your collection percentage is going to be lower than a practice with a relatively low Medicaid population.
3. Tracking reimbursement trends. If your contract with a carrier is 65% of your billed charges; any variances will be seen monthly and can be addressed. Is the carrier having financial difficulties, is it denying a greater percentage of your claims, and is your billing department not following up on outstanding claims?

Contract Rate

Since 1992, Medicare has reimbursed physician services under Section 1848 of the Social Security Act (the Act). The Act mandates payments under a fee schedule based upon national uniform relative value units (RVUs). Medicare's fee schedule, RBRVS (resource-based relative value scale), was established

TABLE 5.1					
	Charges	Payments	Contractual adjustments	Collection (%)	Total outstanding A/R (%)
Insurance A	$158,605	$75,945	$48,267	48%	23.5%
Insurance B	$269,842	$138,691	$90,653	51%	39.8%
Insurance C	$73,235	$23,496	$6,941	32%	19.5%

by combining a RVU (relative value unit) for each of these three components: physician work, practice expense, and malpractice expense. For each of these components there is a geographic practice cost index (GPCI) for each fee schedule area. The GPCIs reflect the relative cost of practice expense, malpractice insurance, and physician work in a geographical area compared to the national average for each component adjustment factor, and a national conversion factor (CF). Therefore Medicare's fee schedule equals:

$$\text{Payment} = [(\text{RVU work} \times \text{GPCI work}) \\ + (\text{RVU practice expense} \\ \times \text{GPCI practice expense}) \\ + (\text{RVU malpractice} \\ \times \text{GPCI malpractice}) \times \text{CF}]$$

Example

Let's look at 99291 (facility based).

Work RVU	3.99
Practice expense	1.28
Malpractice expense	.21
Total	5.48

Take the total RVU 5.48 and multiply that by the national conversion factor of $37.8975, giving $207.68. If Medicare did not take into consideration a geographical cost index, every physician across America would be paid $207.68 for facility-based critical-care services.

Medicaid and many Preferred Providers (PPOs) utilize Medicare's RBRVS when calculating reimbursement or fee schedules for physicians. Medicaid usually calculates reimbursement as a percent of Medicare's allowable. Other carriers establish their own proprietary fee schedule, usually based on some multiplier of the standard RVU. Whatever method a carrier utilizes it is imperative that you as a physician know what the reimbursement is before signing any contract.

How do you successfully negotiate or renegotiate a contract? Before going into negotiations with a carrier, do your homework and, as mentioned, know what percentages of your practice are comprised of patients from the different carriers. The more patient volume per carrier, the better position the practice is in to negotiate contracts that are more favorable to the practice.

Rate

Look at the reimbursement. If the reimbursement is not based on a percentage of RBRVS (Medicare), what is it based on? If it is based on the carrier's established fee schedule, possibly a proprietary unit value, provide them with a listing of your top 25 to 50 codes; request that they supply you with actual reimbursement per code. This will provide you with at a sampling of what your reimbursement will be.

If Based on RBRVS, What Year?

This may not seem like an important factor, but there are many carriers basing their reimbursement on previous years' RBRVS. The contract should read "current-year RBRVS," to indicate that the reimbursement is adjusted yearly. Also review the contract for stipulations on authorizations, timely filing of claims, and medical records. The majority of contracts currently in place were designed for the office-based practice, either primary care or specialist. Hospital-based physician groups need to fine tune carrier contracts to accommodate to today's evolving practices.

Fee Schedule

What is the best way for a practice to establish a fee schedule? There are many different methods for physicians to set their fee schedule, from: "That's the going rate" or "It's the most I am paid by my payers" to "I think my time is worth a set amount, so I will charge that set amount for the procedure." You might as well pull the numbers out of the sky.

The most effective method for establishing a fee schedule is as follows:

- Divide your procedure codes into categories: E/M, medicine, surgery, and so forth.
- List the RVU (relative value unit) per procedure code and total the value.
- List the base fee for each procedure (your current fee) and total the fees.
- Divide the total fees by the total RVUs to obtain the gross conversion factor, per category.
- Multiply the gross conversion factor by any RVU within a category to establish a benchmark fee for each procedure.
- Once the benchmark has been established, compare the results to your current fee schedule. Adjust up any procedures significantly lower than the benchmark; conversely adjust lower any procedures significantly higher.

A/R Aging

This is the number of days outstanding since the claim was submitted to the insurance carrier or patient sorted into the following aging categories (number of days): 0 to 30, 31 to 60, 61 to 90, 91 to 120, and over 120. Benchmark: The outstanding A/R should not be more than 90 days of charges.

BILLING AND COLLECTION

Effective billing and collections is a collaborative effort between the physician and the billing staff. Charge tickets, charge master, superbills, or whichever nomenclature is used represent the instrument physicians use to convey to the billing department the services provided, CPT code, the reason the service was provided, and the ICD-9 (diagnosis) codes. There are many variations of how a charge ticket looks, but the basic information that is needed is:

Patient name
Medical record number
Date of service
CPT
Diagnosis code
Consulting physician name, if applicable
Final disposition, if applicable, transferred off care, d/c to home, etc.

Charge tickets should be updated yearly. Each year, usually in July for ICD-9 and October for CPT, the AMA releases the following year's CPT and ICD-9 coding books. These should be carefully reviewed for new codes, deleted codes, and updated descriptions. To give you an example of yearly changes, in 2003 the AMA released new Pediatric Critical Care Service codes, 99293 and 99294, valid for children 31 days to 24 months, not location driven. In 2004, these codes changed to become valid for "inpatient" services only. In 2005, the age changed to 29 days through 24 months of age. The consequences of not reviewing the yearly changes to CPT codes are noncompliance and possible adverse effects to your A/R.

The billing staff should be diligent in all aspects of the billing collection process. Claims should be closely monitored for timely payment, correct reimbursement, and improper claim denials. There is no single benchmark that can serve as a standard indicator for judging the physician revenue cycle. Each piece of the pie must be reviewed, analyzed, and correlated with each component. The success of an individual practice depends on a good payer mix, good contract rates, a fee schedule that is not predicated on pulling numbers out of a hat, and good coding and documentation. A dedicated and diligent billing staff that will effectively follow up on the claims and get them paid can be the last piece of the puzzle. A successful practice may ultimately rely on the relationship of the physicians and their billing staff.

CHAPTER 6 ■ THE SAFETY OF INPATIENT PEDIATRICS: PREVENTING MEDICAL ERRORS AND INJURIES IN HOSPITALIZED CHILDREN

CURTIS B. PICKERT

In 1999, the Institute of Medicine (IOM) released a report on the morbidity and mortality resulting from medical errors occurring in hospitals within the United States (1). The report inferred that between 44,000 and 98,000 patients died each year as a result of medical mishaps of all types, while as many as 7,000 died specifically as a result of medication-related errors. An aggressive media response followed, and the matter of medical errors and patient safety received unprecedented national and worldwide attention. If accurate, the IOM report placed medical errors in hospitals as one of the ten leading causes of death in the United States. The reported numbers were the result of an extrapolation from other studies, and thus may not have quantified the magnitude of the problem precisely (2–4). However, the report left no doubt that medical errors constituted a significant problem of relevance to all health care providers in the United States and throughout the world.

Information from two large retrospective chart reviews of hospitalized patients suggests that adverse events occur in approximately 3% to 4% of hospitalizations, with between 6% and 13% of those events resulting in death (5–7). These figures potentially underestimate the global prevalence of the problem of medical errors, because retrospective analysis could not identify any unreported events. Also, the reports did not evaluate errors in the outpatient population. Total national costs from medical errors, including lost income and productivity, disability, and health care costs, have been estimated to be as high as $29 to $37 billion or more per year. Adverse drug events occurring after hospitalization, alone, may result in over $4 billion in hospital expenses, independent of related expenditures such as malpractice costs (8).

Though epidemiologic information is limited, children are potentially at higher risk of exposure because of the increased prevalence of medication errors in the pediatric population (9–12). Rates of hospital-reported medical errors in children range from 1.81 to 2.96 per 100 discharges, and there may be as many as 70,000 hospitalized children each year in the United States who experience an adverse event (13,14). Many, if not most, errors identified could have potentially been prevented (15).

Multiple factors contribute to this problem in hospitalized children, including failure to provide services demonstrated to be beneficial in the prevention of errors. Such services include ward-based clinical pharmacists, computerized physician order entry, and translation programs to overcome language barriers (16–21). Despite evidence of significant benefit, deficits in the provision of such services persist nationwide. Inadequate or failed communication between members of the health care team may result in significant errors in the pediatric inpatient setting. Additionally, many children still receive inpatient care from practitioners with limited pediatric training and expertise, often in nonspecialized environments. Thus, the matter of medical errors in children is of critical importance to the pediatric hospitalist or hospital-based pediatrician.

Medication-related errors warrant unique consideration because they are both prevalent and often preventable. These errors are of special relevance in children because of the significant variability of weight-based dosing in the pediatric population, and the clinical vulnerability of the infant and toddler. An area of particular concern is the use of verbal medication orders, either delivered in person or by telephone. Whenever possible, verbal or telephone medication orders should be given directly from the physician to the pharmacist, thus eliminating the role of additional practitioners and reducing the potential for misinterpretation of the order. There is currently widespread impetus to eliminate verbal orders from the practice of medicine, but in the interim there are specific types of preventable communication errors that have been identified. Many drug names are similar enough to be confused or interpreted in error, with the result being that knowledgeable and well-meaning practitioners, typically a doctor and a nurse or pharmacist, combine to deliver the wrong medication. The numerical element of dosing is also easily misunderstood when received verbally, such as a "15" sounding like "50," or a "2" sounding like "10." Absolute clarification of the quantity is necessary, such as stating "one five" for 15 or "five zero" for 50. A common order-writing practice that introduces risk is the use of inappropriate abbreviations. Drug names and doses should be written out completely and legibly. Abbreviations such as "mg" for milligram or "mcg" for microgram are easily confused, especially if the handwriting is not clearly legible. Abbreviating the frequency of medications with the terms "qid" or "qd," for four times a day, or daily, respectively, may also be misinterpreted, resulting in either inadequate or excessive drug administration. Writing "four times a day" or "daily" eliminates any potential misunderstanding of the intent. The appropriate placement of "leading" and "following" zeros, as in "5.0" or "0.5," is very important. Leading zeros, or those preceding a decimal point, are important to include. For example, ".5" is less apt to be interpreted as "5" if the leading zero is present ("0.5"). Following zeros, however, are a source of error and should not be used ("5.0" may be interpreted as "50," whereas "5" is unlikely to be misinterpreted). Finally, the problem of illegible practitioner handwriting remains a source of potential harm to patients. Though physicians are often stereotyped as having poor handwriting, the problem

35

extends to all care providers, including nurses, respiratory therapists, and pharmacists. Every member of the health care team has an obligation to write in a manner that is legible and easily understood.

Although attention to such practical preventive steps may reduce errors, more sophisticated interventions have been identified to effectively reduce medication-related adverse events in children. As previously stated, these measures include computerized physician order entry, the presence of specialized pharmacists and clinical pharmacologists in the inpatient setting, and individualization of drug therapy based on pharmacogenomics (22,23). Though not yet widely applied, computerized physician order entry can provide absolute legibility, direct communication, automated drug dosage and compatibility screening, surveillance for drug allergy or intolerance, and elimination of the need for human interpretation of medication orders. Further proliferation of the use of this technology is expected to have significant positive impact on the number and magnitude of medication-related errors. Alternatively, the implementation of very simple interventions, such as the use of preprinted prescription order sheets, has also been shown to reduce medication errors (24).

The 1999 IOM report called for a 50% reduction in the rate of medical errors within 5 years, but also noted that "health care is a decade or more behind other high-risk industries in its attention to ensuring basic safety." Other sectors of society, such as aviation and general industry, have implemented programs resulting in significantly greater progress in the reduction of errors. Characteristics of successful error reduction programs include intolerance of high error rates, confidentiality, error tracking mechanisms, root cause analysis, systems approaches that do not seek to find individual blame, creating organizational structure that enhances safety, and adequate resource allocation for error-reducing initiatives.

Though not a new problem, there is a new emphasis on identifying, understanding, and preventing errors in health care. There are, however, significant roadblocks to progress, including the nature of the U.S. health care system in general. This was addressed directly in the IOM statement: "The decentralized and fragmented nature of the health care delivery system (some would say 'non-system') also contributes to unsafe conditions for patients, and serves as an impediment to efforts to improve safety."

As a result, the federal government has recently become more involved in the matter. In February 2000, a bill was introduced in the 106th Congress entitled "The Medical Error Reduction Act of 2000" (25). This bill served to amend the Public Health Service Act in order to reduce accidental injury and death resulting from medical mistakes and to reduce medication-related errors. One year later, the U.S. Department of Health and Human Services released $50 million to fund research and projects to reduce medical errors (26). Throughout the private sector, there continues to be momentum for a comprehensive national solution, including mandatory reporting, increased utilization of medical information systems, and prevention programs.

In 2001, the IOM released a second comprehensive report entitled "Crossing the Quality Chasm: A New Health Care System for the 21st Century" (27). In that document, six aims for improvement were provided, including that care should be *safe, effective, patient-centered, timely, efficient, and equitable*. Furthermore, ten rules for redesign of the health care system were presented:

■ Care is based on continuous healing relationships.
■ Care is customized according to patient needs and values.
■ The patient is the source of control.
■ Knowledge is shared and information flows freely.
■ Decision-making is evidence based.
■ Safety is a system priority.
■ Transparency is necessary.
■ Needs are anticipated.
■ Waste is continuously decreased.
■ Cooperation among clinicians is a priority.

The report addressed critical issues necessary to accomplish a revamped, improved health care system, including the need to make available scientific evidence more useful and accessible, increasing use of information technology in health care, aligning payment and compensation with quality improvement, and preparing the health care workforce for change.

Also in 2001, the American Academy of Pediatrics established a policy statement on the matter, calling for patient safety guidelines, consideration of unique pediatric safety issues, increased research into the use of information technology for prevention of errors, and collaboration with pharmaceutical companies, the Agency for Healthcare Research and Quality, and other health care organizations to increase safety in children (28). Two years later, the AAP published an additional policy statement specifically regarding the prevention of medication errors, including a comprehensive list of recommendations for hospitals, prescribers, pharmacies and pharmacists, nurses, and parents (29).

One of the stated goals in the original IOM report was to "break the cycle of inaction." Research and common sense support that many medical errors can be prevented, and morbidity and mortality can be reduced. However, the matter of safely providing care to the hospitalized patient involves both individuals and systems. A critical element of the problem is contained within the title of the original IOM report: "To Err is Human." Diligent, conscientious care delivered by qualified practitioners must be applied in combination with the measures noted to assure the safest possible care of patients. Pediatric hospitalists are optimally positioned to be leaders in this endeavor.

References

1. Kohn LT, Corrigan JM, Donaldson M, eds. *To err is human: building a safer health system*. Washington, D.C.: Institute of Medicine, National Academy Press; 1999.
2. McDonald CJ, Weiner M, Hui SL. Deaths due to medical errors are exaggerated in Institute of Medicine report. *JAMA* 2000;284:93–95.
3. Leape LL. Institute of Medicine medical error figures are not exaggerated. *JAMA* 2000;284:95–97.
4. Brennan TA. The Institute of Medicine report on medical errors—could it do harm? *N Engl J Med* 2000;342:1123–1125.
5. Brennan TA, Leape LL, Laird LM, et al. Incidence of adverse events and negligence in hospitalized patients: results of the Harvard Medical Practice Study I. *N Engl J Med* 1991;324:370–376.
6. Thomas EJ, Studdert DM, Burstin HR, et al. Incidence and types of adverse events and negligent care in Utah and Colorado. *Med Care* 2000;38: 261–271.
7. Leape LL, Brennan TA, Laird N, et al. The nature of adverse events in hospitalized patients: results of the Harvard Medical Practice Study II. *N Engl J Med* 1991;324:377–384.
8. Bates DW, Spell N, Cullen DJ, et al. The costs of adverse drug events in hospitalized patients. *JAMA* 1997;277:307–311.
9. Kaushal R, Bates DW, Landrigan C, et al. Medication errors and adverse drug events in pediatric inpatients. *JAMA* 2001;285:2114–2120.
10. Lesar TS. Errors in the use of medication dosage equations. *Arch Pediatr Adolesc Med* 1998;152:340–344.
11. Agency for Healthcare Research and Quality. *Summary statement, summit: setting a research agenda for patient safety*. Elk Grove Village, IL: American Academy of Pediatrics; 2002. http://www.aap.org/advocacy/washing/patientsafety.htm.
12. Miller MR, Elixhauser A, Zhan C. Patient safety events during pediatric hospitalizations. *Pediatrics* 2003;111:1358 Elk Grove Village, IL: 1366.
13. Slonim AD, LaFleur BJ, Ahmed W, et al. Hospital-reported medical errors in children. *Pediatrics* 2003;111:617–621.
14. Woods D, Thomas E, Holl J, et al. Adverse events and preventable adverse events in children. *Pediatrics* 2005;115:155–160.

15. Sedman A, Harris M, Schulz K, et al. Relevance of the Agency for Healthcare Research and Quality patient safety indicators for children's hospitals. *Pediatrics* 2005;115:135–145.

16. Fortesque EB, Kaushal R, Landrigan CP, et al. Prioritizing strategies for preventing medication errors and adverse drug events in pediatric patients. *Pediatrics* 2003;111:722–729.

17. Simpson JH, Lynch R, Grant J, et al. Reducing medication errors in the neonatal intensive care unit. *Arch Dis Child Fetal Neonatal Ed* 2004;89: F480–F482.

18. King WJ, Paice N, Rangrej J, et al. The effect of computerized physician order entry on medication errors and adverse drug events in pediatric inpatients. *Pediatrics* 2003;112:506–509.

19. Potts AL, Barr FE, Gregory DF, et al. Computerized order entry and medication errors in a pediatric critical care unit. *Pediatrics* 2004;113:59–63.

20. Upperman JS, Staley P, Friend K, et al. The introduction of computerized physician order entry and change management in a tertiary pediatric hospital. *Pediatrics* 2005;116:e634–e642.

21. Cohen AL, Rivara F, Marcuse EK, et al. Are language barriers associated with serious medical events in hospitalized pediatric patients? *Pediatrics* 2005;116:575–579.

22. Bates DW, Leape LL, Cullen DJ, et al. Effect of computerized physician order entry and a team intervention on prevention of serious medication errors. *JAMA* 1998;280:1311–1316.

23. Phillips KA, Veenstra DL, Oren E, et al. Potential role of pharmacogenomics in reducing adverse drug reactions. *JAMA* 2001;286:2270–2279.

24. Kozer E, Scolnik D, MacPherson A, et al. Using a preprinted order sheet to reduce prescription errors in a pediatric emergency department: a randomized, controlled trial. *Pediatrics* 2005;116:1299–1302.

25. Medical Error Reduction Act of 2000 (S 2038). Introduced in the Senate of the United States, 106th Congress, February 8, 2000.

26. HHS announces $50 million investment to improve patient safety. Press release. Rockville, MD: Agency for Healthcare Research and Quality; Oct. 11, 2001. http://www.ahrq.gov/news/press/pr2001/patsafpr.htm.

27. Crossing the quality chasm: a new health system for the 21st century. Washington, D.C.: Institute of Medicine, National Academy Press; 2001.

28. National Initiative for Children's Health Care Quality Project Advisory Committee. Principles of patient safety in pediatrics (RE060027). *Pediatrics* 2001;107:1473–1475.

29. American Academy of Pediatrics. Policy statement: prevention of medication errors in the pediatric inpatient setting. *Pediatrics* 2003;112:431–436.

CHAPTER 7A ■ INTRODUCTION/GENERAL PRINCIPLES

LORETTA M. KOPELMAN

Moral principles offer general requirements that are intended to guide us in making practical choices, and several have become important focal points for discussions in medical ethics. The principle of *beneficence* instructs us to promote people's well-being and *nonmaleficence*, to avoid harming people. The principle of *distributive justice* directs us to promote a fair allocation of goods, benefits, and services among some group, whereas the principle of *social utility* guides us to promote the greatest good for the greatest number of people in a society. The principle of *autonomy* or *self-determination* prescribes that a person act to foster personal responsibility and plan her life to develop her abilities and opportunities to flourish.

It is a mistake to suppose that moral principles simply tell us what to do or require uniform action and conformity. First, because they are stated abstractly, they must be interpreted or specified. This is done by making practical moral judgments, leaving considerable room for interpretation and disagreement from person to person or from culture to culture, even among those who agree on the importance of these principles. Although none would seriously object to promoting justice, well-being, or self-development for children, we may easily disagree about the means to achieve those ends. For example,

in some parts of the world ritual burning of children and female genital cutting are considered important health practices. Many people from these regions would insist that they are promoting the well-being of children by engaging in these customs, and would be shocked to find that their actions are regarded as child abuse in other countries. This shows that agreement about principles is no guarantee that we will agree on a means to achieve them.

Second, because moral principles can conflict, they sometimes have to be ranked, and people may reasonably disagree about how to do this justifiably. For example, the duty to help a child may conflict with parental autonomy, and ranking one or the other as the greater duty may depend on the probability and magnitude of harm to be avoided. Third, even applications of the same principle can cause conflict. Beneficence requires doing what is best for one's patients, but if someone has many patients needing the same scarce resource, then a choice must be made among them, with the result that some will receive less than ideal treatment. The general agreement about the importance and meaning of moral principles, even across cultures, however, is an essential first step in deciding what is in fact best. Moral principles describe *prima facie* duties, prohibitions, obligations, values, virtues, rights, or permissions.

CHAPTER 7B ■ CONSENT OR PERMISSION FROM PARENTS OR GUARDIANS

LORETTA M. KOPELMAN

Parents or guardians usually have the authority to give consent or permission for children's health care or participation in research. Reasons for this social policy include, first, that parents in general have the greatest knowledge about, and interest in, the well-being of their own minor children. Another well-recognized reason why parents have legal authority to make these and many other decisions for their minor children is that parents or guardians must deal with the consequences of the choices made. Clinicians usually should try to respect the preferences of families' choices because of the importance families play in fostering children's well-being and shaping their values (1–3).

Parental consent, like other informed consent in a medical setting, must be adequately informed. That is, the parent giving consent must be provided with sufficient information to understand and authorize the treatment that has been recommended. Clinicians need to reveal all information they know or should know that would be regarded as important to parents in making their decisions. Those seeking consent, for example, should provide parents with information about the diagnosis and prognosis, so that they understand the disease process. Reasonable alternative treatment options should also be explained, along with their nature, duration, side effects, or potential harms or benefits. They also should be told the likely consequences of no treatment. Clinicians should then test for understanding of the information. Some ways to do this include asking them questions about what was discussed, or asking them to explain the material.

Clinicians are sometimes puzzled about how much information is enough for families. Two legal standards have emerged, although in practice they often come to the same thing. The older standard is the *professional community standard*, which requires that clinicians reveal what qualified medical practitioners in the same field would regard as appropriate to tell the parents under similar circumstances. The more recent *reasonable person standard* requires the clinician to reveal information that a reasonable person would consider material or important to reaching a decision about whether to consent.

The person who gives consent must have the capacity to make decisions. In the recent literature, the terms *competent* and *incompetent* are often reserved for legal contexts. Courts can make a determination about whether people are competent or not. The presumption is that adults are legally competent and minors are not. Minors, usually those younger than 18 years of age in most of the United States, are regarded as incompetent to make decisions about their own health care, especially if the decisions are momentous. The reality is that many adults lack decision-making capacity but have not been declared legally incompetent in the courts, and many legally incompetent minors have good decision-making capacity. In many jurisdictions, this is acknowledged by allowing minors to gain some legal rights, independent of parental permission, for medical care such as for sexually transmitted disease, substance abuse, contraception, or abortion. Legal doctrines of mature and emancipated minors also permit them to have more of a role in making decisions about their lives. Thus, the legal notion of competence and that of decision-making capacity should be distinguished.

For the purpose of health care, decision-making capacity concerns the individual's ability to understand information needed to make informed consent, evaluate this information in terms of stable personal values, and use and manipulate the information in a reasonable way (2,4,5). For important decisions, clinicians should assess how well people giving the consent can understand the information, deliberate, and make and defend choices; it also is important that they communicate

choices appropriately. These features should help clinicians decide if parents or older minors have the capacity to make important health care decisions.

Many authors favor a sliding scale (4) for determining if someone is capable of making medical decisions. That is, the lower the probability and magnitude of the risk of harm from the decision, the less clinicians need scrutinize the decision-making capacity of the person giving consent. But the greater the probability and risk of harm from the decision, the higher the level of scrutiny necessary to ascertain that the decision is rational. Reasoning by parents who refuse chemotherapy for a child with cancer, for example, needs to be very carefully assessed.

Consent, assent or permission also must be freely given, or voluntary. This means it must not be coerced or manipulated. The fact that the parents may be distraught does not make them legally incompetent or unable to give consent. If parents are not competent or are making an inappropriate decision, clinicians may have a legal and moral duty to seek a court order so the courts can authorize the needed intervention.

People's informed consent or permission, then, should have the following elements (6,7):

1. All information or material important to their decision has been disclosed to them.
2. They comprehend or understand the information that has been disclosed.
3. They voluntarily agree to participate.
4. They are competent to make a decision to participate.
5. They agree to the procedure, act, intervention, or research.

In some cases informed consent may be waived, as in medical emergencies, public health emergencies, or where parents cannot be reached.

Parents giving consent or permission should be guided by what is in the best interest of their child. Their decisions can be challenged, for example, if they endanger their child. The best interest of the child standard is one of four important standards for medical decision-making; the other three are self-determination, advance directive, and presumed consent. Although the best interest of the child standard is of special importance in pediatrics, each of the four standards has some role to play in making health care decisions for minors.

CHAPTER 7C ■ ASSENT AND SELF-DETERMINATION

LORETTA M. KOPELMAN

Self-determination as a standard for health care decision-making applies to competent adults and to many older or emancipated minors. This standard of self-determination presupposes that the person is autonomous or capable of self-determination, has informed understanding, and makes the choices voluntarily. It honors the basic moral principles just mentioned. It flows from the moral principle of autonomy or self-determination and honors people's liberty; it enables people to make choices about themselves, assess their own best interest, and develop their own capacities and life plans as they wish, as long as they do not harm others. This standard is

just or fair insofar as it extends the same liberty to others that most of us want for ourselves; most of us want to be free to make our own choices about how to determine our well-being and create opportunities. It is socially useful because most of us do better when we make our own life choices. Our successes and failures are lessons not only to ourselves but to others.

Although the law grants full competence to minors on the occasion of a specific birthday, this practical and useful legal practice fits poorly with medical decision-making. In medicine, it is more useful to view capacity as a matter of degree, and less like the "light-switch" concept found in the law.

In both law and medicine, young children are the paradigm of persons unable to make decisions for themselves. Infants are among the many incompetent and vulnerable of our citizens, but minors just before the age of majority are as competent as many adults. Although most young children lack the capacity, maturity, experience, or foresight to make important decisions for themselves, older adolescents may be entirely capable of making important choices for themselves and determining which of them promotes their well-being and opportunities. As children gain maturity, many, but of course not all, seek to understand important health care decisions being made about them, and older children may have serious views about their care.

In the United States, Canada, and northern European countries, empirical research about childhood understanding and needs has altered the practice of keeping children ignorant about serious conditions and even their imminent death (8). Studies showed that all people, including children, sense when family and clinicians are not being truthful, and feel isolated.

To acknowledge the child's emerging capacities, honor his point of view, and promote his well-being, clinicians seek the child's assent when possible, in addition to parental permission. Consequently, whenever possible, the assent or agreement of children even as young as 7 years of age should be gained; as minors become increasingly mature and competent, they should be accorded more self-determination. Children with life-threatening or chronic illnesses, for example, may want to participate in discussions and decisions about their care and find that this is a way to gain control and respect. Ignoring their desires to participate may cause pain, isolation, misunderstandings, and frustration. Some children, of course, do not want to participate, and their choices should be honored.

Assent is different from consent because the minor's preferences need not be honored in the same way as those of adults (9,10). Whether a minor's preference should be controlling may depend on the probability and magnitude of the harms involved and the irreversibility of the consequences. When children cannot enhance their own well-being and opportunities, then adults may have to override their decisions and not grant self-determination. The obligation to honor their wishes is not as binding as it would be for an adult. For example, children with cancer may strongly object to chemotherapy that causes their hair to fall out, saying they would "rather die first." Such responses cannot be controlling, although they should be the occasion for serious discussion and support.

In many parts of the world, however, adults who face serious illness or death are not privy to these conversations because family and clinicians believe that it is kinder to exclude them. Such cultural conflicts about how to apply the principles of beneficence and nonmaleficence have the potential to cause serious problems when people travel from one country to another seeking medical care. For example, older adolescents who have a serious illness may express the wish to clinicians to discuss their prognosis and options, while family members strongly object to telling them. Many clinicians find family members may change their minds when they see the social science evidence that children understand a good deal about their diseases and even imminent death and that excluding them increases their suffering. Some guardians, of course, remain adamant, and clinicians may have to choose between doing what they believe is best for the patients by informing them and honoring parental wishes. Other clinicians find that consultations with an ethics committee may help resolve such conflicts.

The recognition that older children can understand a great deal and be competent to participate in many decisions has been increasingly recognized in the scholarly literature and in social policy (11,12). As children grow older, they are increasingly able to discuss and participate in health decisions relating to them. Some adolescents have gained authority to make health care decisions independently of their parents. Depending on state law, they can get medical care such as contraceptives, contraceptive information and devices, abortions, and treatment for substance abuse without parental permission.

The ideal situation is to have shared decision-making and agreement among clinicians, family, and the child about what course to take. In the ordinary situation, however, parents or guardians have the authority to make decisions for children's medical care, unless they endanger them, just as they do for their religion and schooling. Children's assent, however, has been found to be increasingly important based on evidence that children with serious, chronic, or life-threatening illnesses understand a great deal and benefit from participating. In addition, the importance of their assent stems from understanding that they have the competence to make important contributions to these discussions.

CHAPTER 7D ■ ADVANCE DIRECTIVES

LORETTA M. KOPELMAN

Advance directives are used in framing health care decisions when the person has become incapacitated. They are statements made by the person who has decision-making capacity stating how decisions should be made when they are unable to make decisions. Adults and some older children may have such directives in order to extend their control over events. A competent adult may use a living will or power of attorney for health care to make their views about how decisions should be guided and who should make decisions for them. In rare cases, minors may decide they wish to make their views known.

For example, they may not want to be on a ventilator for an extended period if they lapse into a persistent vegetative state. Although such decisions are not as controlling as those of legally competent adults, they may be morally binding. Sometimes parents and children disagree about the sort of treatment that is appropriate at the end of life, with each making what the other regards as an inappropriate request. Whenever possible, however, clinicians should give the requests of the older minor serious consideration and seek a consensus among the family.

CHAPTER 7E ■ SUBSTITUTED JUDGMENT

LORETTA M. KOPELMAN

Substituted judgment is another rarely used standard for minors in making medical decisions because this standard applies to those who were once able to express their views, but left no advance directives. It instructs others to use their understanding of the person's views to select the option that they think the individual would have selected were she able to do so. Minors who are very sick may have expressed preferences that they hope will guide people, and such requests should receive great weight, if at all possible.

CHAPTER 7F ■ THE BEST INTEREST OF THE CHILD: STANDARD AND PARENTAL AND GUARDIAN'S CONSENT

LORETTA M. KOPELMAN

The best interest of the child standard is the most frequently used standard for medical decisions involving children or others who lack capacity to make their own medical decisions. According to the best interest standard, decisions for incompetent persons should be made by assessing the incompetent person's immediate and long-term interests and then deciding whether the benefits of the procedure or intervention outweigh the burdens (13–16). The burdens of enduring intense pain for a short time, for example, would be more than balanced by the benefits of a long and healthy life. The use of the best interest standard presupposes some agreement about how to assess, rank, and balance potential burdens and benefits (16,17). Controversies over the best interest standard sometimes are engendered because we disagree about how to rank potential harms and benefits. In general, however, parents have the legal authority to assess these potential harms and benefits for their minor children, although in some cases their choices should be challenged.

The best interest standard tends to be a conservative standard because it relies on agreement among people about what a reasonable individual would choose in the same or a similar situation. Without such agreement, the best interest standard is difficult to apply. However, it still may be used even where the parties cannot agree on a single best answer, if they can agree on a range of acceptable, albeit not ideal, responses for the incompetent person. Families may disagree with clinicians over whether life-sustaining treatment should be continued. Rather than insist that there is one best answer, it may be useful to consider what choices by the legal guardian are socially acceptable. Alternatively, the families and clinicians may agree on a plan (16). For example, they may agree on withdrawing life support if there is any further deterioration of the child's condition. These decisions are especially complicated because, in the case of younger children, the quality-of-life assessments must be based on the values of others, not the patient's values.

CHAPTER 7G ■ REFUSAL OF CARE

LORETTA M. KOPELMAN

Some older children refuse important interventions because they object to them or the results. Clinicians and parents may have a duty to override their wishes, although, as noted, their inappropriate requests should initiate support for the minor and discussions about why their wishes cannot be controlling.

Parents or guardians who place their children at serious risks, such as by refusing to permit a clinician to provide life-saving interventions to a child, may have their authority contested (18,19). Guardians have the authority to give consent because it is presumed they will promote the opportunities and well-being of their children. If, however, they harm or endanger their minor children, or do not take adequate means to prevent or minimize harms to them, clinicians should challenge parental authority. Guardians may lose custody of their children temporarily or permanently if they neglect, abuse, or exploit their children. Courts can order interventions if the child is assessed to be in danger in the parent's or guardian's care. It is not only health care professionals who have a responsibility to protect children from abuse and neglect, but also teachers, neighbors, and others in the community. Clinicians, however, often have special insights into how children are being treated, and hence special responsibilities to notify the authorities when parental acts or omissions endanger their minor children.

CHAPTER 7H ■ INAPPROPRIATE CARE REQUESTS

LORETTA M. KOPELMAN

Parents sometimes ask clinicians to provide treatments regarded as entirely unreasonable, such as herbal medicines for the treatment of cancer, antibiotics for viral illnesses, or highly invasive procedures for minor illnesses. In some cases, parents and others confuse their right to refuse treatment that they do not regard as beneficial with a belief they have a right to demand certain treatments. Clinicians have a duty to refuse such requests that may harm based on the moral principle of nonmaleficence. In addition, clinicians have a social duty to conserve resources and not provide costly, futile, or burdensome interventions. Simply put, futile treatments are not useful, or useful enough to justify the expense, potential harms, time, or energy (20). As a matter of professional integrity and personal morality, clinicians should refuse to provide costly, burdensome, or useless interventions. The question of when treatments are futile may of course be disputed among families or among clinicians.

Minors also sometimes make demands that are not appropriate. If an adolescent demands genetic testing for a late-onset illness such as Alzheimer disease, his preference should not prevail as it might for an adult because he may not have the maturity to consider his well-being and opportunities. Clinicians may have to override such inappropriate requests. They do not have a duty to provide medical interventions they regard to be wrong, ill-considered, or inappropriate. Most, but not all, requests for futile interventions may be the result of miscommunication. Some of these are embedded in social, ethnic, or religious differences. In some cases, families have unrealistic expectations, believe "everything must be done," or are "waiting for a miracle." Guilt and denial also may play a role in these irrational or unreasonable requests. Clinicians should show great sensitivity and patience in helping families come to terms with a diagnosis or prognosis.

In some cases, families have a general mistrust of the health care system, which seems vindicated by an unexpected and bleak prognosis. Their request for futile treatment may be an expression of this mistrust. It sometimes is helpful to include someone whom they trust and can help them understand, such as a minister or family member with a health care background. In rare cases, the disagreement is truly a value disagreement where family members may, for example, see maintaining someone in a persistent vegetative state as a positive value, whereas the clinicians do not. In these and other cases, doctors should maintain professional integrity and personal morality, but may find other clinicians willing to accept the families' decisions. Substantial literature exists on how to respond to such situations, when to override parental requests, and the dangers of using decisions about what treatments are futile as mechanisms for rationing health care. In general, however, for the practicing clinician, it is important to remember that most demands for futile interventions are likely to be the result of poor communication and inadequate understanding.

CHAPTER 7I ■ CONFIDENTIALITY

LORETTA M. KOPELMAN

The importance of confidentiality in medical practice has been acknowledged since ancient times. One reason for this is that respecting patients' confidentiality usually promotes the moral principle of beneficence or the patients' best interest. If patients are assured of confidentiality, they are more likely to be candid. Moreover, because privacy is what each of us wants for ourselves, then it is only just to extend it to others. In addition, it is fair to adopt this policy of respecting confidentiality because, in some sense, patients "own" the information about themselves, and confidentiality honors their privacy and rights to control this information. If some information about the individual is released, such as a genotype for a late-onset genetic disease, it has the potential to cause great harm through discrimination, labeling, or loss of self-esteem. The social utility of respecting patients' confidentiality also is acknowledged in policies allowing physicians to avoid testifying about patients' revelations to them in health care settings. Confidentiality may be important for minors as well as adults. Minors, for example, may seek medical care as a safe haven to express how they have been abused or exploited.

The clinician's duty to maintain confidentiality, however, is not absolute. The presumption in favor of confidentiality can be overruled if there is a greater duty at stake or if there is a recognized exception (21,22). For example, an exception to the duty to maintain confidentiality is to protect a third party, as in child abuse. If clinicians suspect that someone is abusing a child, they have a legal and moral duty to override confidentiality because a greater duty is at stake. In addition, there may be a duty to override confidentiality if there is a need to protect the patient from herself; there may be such a duty if the minor is suicidal. There also may be a duty to protect the community that is greater than the duty to maintain someone's confidentiality, such as a duty to report communicable diseases or gunshot wounds, regardless of whether the person wants them to be reported.

When trying to decide whether the duty to maintain confidentiality is the greater duty, certain features must be considered. The first is that in making the judgment about whether to overrule confidentiality, the clinician must consider the severity of the harm to be avoided and the probability of its occurrence. If there were a very small risk of a minor harm, the duty to maintain confidentiality would be secure. As the harm is greater and the likelihood higher, the duty to override confidentiality increases. Second, the most justifiable causes of overriding the duty of confidentiality for adults who are competent usually are to prevent harms, especially to third parties; this honors the principle of nonmaleficence. The duty to prevent harm usually is recognized as stronger than the duty of beneficence or providing benefits because our notions of what we think benefits competent adults may be wrong; acting on such views may be disrespectful of their autonomy. Clinicians

would have, for example, a strong duty to override a competent parent's confidentiality to prevent harm to a child who is endangered in the parent's care.

Respect for children's rights of confidentiality cannot be approached in the same way as for those of fully competent adults. Although children's wishes and values are important, the best interest standard of the child shapes decision-making for children and thus is the primary consideration. Yet older children may have rights to privacy independent of their parents. In some cases, clinicians may have a legal right to refuse to discuss with guardians intervention for the minor's substance abuse, sexually transmitted disease, abortion, or contraception. In addition, it may be in the best interest of children or adolescents who are abused, neglected, or exploited to be able to seek help without parental consent or involvement. Clinicians, of course, should explore the minor's reasons for not wishing to involve parents. Sometimes the child's concerns are not realistic, but in other cases the minor knows that parents would refuse to permit some interventions, such as allowing the provision of contraception. Because only one view can prevail where parents and minors disagree, it sometimes is morally and legally justifiable to respect the minor's preference not to involve his or her parents.

CHAPTER 7J ■ RESEARCH

LORETTA M. KOPELMAN

Participation in research can give children opportunities to gain access to programs or treatments that otherwise are unavailable to them, and most research is not dangerous. Research may benefit not only individual research subjects but also children as a group. Medical science cannot assess children's unique needs and reactions to interventions without systematic testing. Without good testing, physicians face a dilemma of prescribing untested interventions, thereby risking adverse reactions or undertreating children because they want to use only tested interventions.

The enormous social utility of conducting research with children, however, does not mask the fact that some children have been harmed by participation in research. This raises a serious moral and social issue about how to balance the values at stake. If we say the child's well-being must always take precedence such that if there is *any risk*, studies must be prohibited, then many important and relatively safe studies will be halted on the grounds that one cannot be certain there is no risk whatsoever. This policy is very problematic. To obtain information on normal growth and development, information must be collected from children's records that do not, strictly speaking, present any risk of harm to the children. Nonetheless, we cannot call this absolutely risk free. For example, a loss of privacy could cause great damage to the child through discrimination or loss of self-esteem. This application of the best interest of the child standard could harm children because it imposes too strict a standard.

One of the most difficult issues in medical ethics concerns when and under what circumstances children should be permitted to serve as research subjects when there is *no anticipated benefit* to them as research subjects. The problem is how does one promote children's well-being and help them develop their potential as self-determinant individuals by having the best therapies and interventions available for them, while

protecting them from being harmed in the research setting? When subjects are adults, they help solve this problem for themselves by the informed consent process, thus determining whether they want to be in research and the degree of risk that they are willing to assume to promote the common good. Different policy solutions about children's research should be assessed in terms of the principle of beneficence (will it promote their well-being?), and this raises the problem of how to justify research risk to children in studies that are unlikely to provide direct benefit to them.

Children cannot protect their own well-being, so if children are to be enrolled in research, others must give consent or permission for them. Many adults have this responsibility, not just the parents. In most institutional settings in which research is conducted, investigators, members of institutional review boards or ethics committees, and consultants have this duty as well as the parents. Together they must ensure that children are not abused, neglected, or exploited. Parental consent, then, is not sufficient because some guardians might make imprudent decisions about enrolling their children in studies. The intention may be to foster their child's well-being and prevent, remove, or minimize harms, yet the complexity of research programs usually also requires layers of approval from others. Moreover, competent adults have the right to volunteer themselves for high-risk studies to make a contribution to medical knowledge. Although this may be morally admirable, volunteering to put others in harm's way is not, and could conflict with the parent's role of protecting the well-being of children. Thus, parents cannot be permitted to decide to enroll children just as they would for themselves; additional regulatory protections are needed.

Even where parents, investigators, and institutional representatives agree that the child should be enrolled, they may have responsibilities to get the assent or agreement of the child to participate, especially if the study is not for the direct benefit of the child or if there is some risk. Children as young as 7 years of age are routinely consulted. Securing the agreement of the child and the consent of the parent, then, still is not sufficient to justify enrollment of children in research, and an elaborate set of federal regulations must be followed in almost all research involving children.

Until recently, the prevailing view regarding research was that studies should be done first on adults and only later on vulnerable groups such as children. They were excluded from many studies to protect them, but the consequences were that they could not obtain investigational new drugs or gain access to important studies. Thus, in attempting to protect children, these policies actually were harming children. The practice of excluding "vulnerable" groups such as pregnant women and children from investigations came under scrutiny when it seemed the policies sometimes were harming children or "protecting minors to death." Regulatory obstacles, for example, initially restricted how children with acquired immunodeficiency syndrome (AIDS) could be treated. In the early days of the epidemic, when zidovudine (AZT) was being tested, there were no other options. Yet a variety of state and federal laws forbade children from getting what appeared to be the only possible drug to help them on the grounds that it needed to be tested first on adults (23). Not only were the exclusions not a benefit and not a means of protecting these children, but it seemed frankly unfair.

It also became obvious that the restrictions to "protect" children sometimes were put in place for other reasons. Investigators prefer homogeneous subject populations to make it easier to hold down costs and analyze their findings. People of different ages react to interventions differently, so that the more subjects of different ages who are included in studies, the more people investigators have to enroll, and the more subjects, the higher the costs. Age is only one of many variables that can drive up costs. Thus, investigators often prefer similar subjects, and critics argue that they were often middle-aged white men. The difficulty is that the more one restricts the groups, the harder it is to generalize findings. Children react differently to drugs than adults. For example, chloramphenicol is an antibiotic commonly used among adults, yet it caused many deaths in neonates. In short, if studies are not done with children, the studies done on adults have uncertain benefits. Some pediatricians go so far as to say that evidence-based medicine does not yet exist in pediatrics. Only a small number of interventions in drugs used for treatment of diseases have been tested on children, according to the American Academy of Pediatrics, and most marketed drugs are unlabeled for pediatric populations (24); from 10% to 20% of research excludes pediatric populations without good reason.

Congress and the research community began addressing this problem, seeking a policy where unless there are good scientific or ethical reasons to do so, children should not be excluded from research. For example, researchers may show the topic is irrelevant to children's health or well-being, that the information already is available, that there are restrictions, that there are legal regulatory prohibitions against including them, or that the condition would be so rare in pediatric populations that it would be inappropriate to include them. Testing on pediatric populations should be done unless a case can be made that it would be unsafe, impractical, or otherwise unreasonable.

Thus, a narrow path runs between too many protections and too few protections for children (25). The two extremes are entirely unsatisfactory. One permits adults to consent for children just as they would for themselves, and the other would severely limit or even disallow studies on children. Because adults have different reactions to drugs, studies done with adults may be inapplicable to children. Drugs for childhood schizophrenia, diabetes, depression, infections, and respiratory distress need to be tested at some point on children themselves for safety and efficacy. Excluding vulnerable groups to protect their rights and welfare may have the opposite result. If good information about childhood disorders cannot be obtained for the pediatric population because of severe limiting of research, then it certainly does not promote their welfare, individually or collectively. Research rules, then, try to strike a balance between too much and too little protection of children, and they do this by trying to balance harms and benefits when assessing whether research should be approved.

CHAPTER 7K ■ RESEARCH REGULATION

LORETTA M. KOPELMAN

Many national and international research policies address the problem of when to permit studies with children as subjects in a similar way (26), including U.S. Federal Regulations (27) and the Council of International Organizations of Medical Science (CIOMS) (28). According to this approach, the goal is to "balance" the social utility of research with respect and protection for the child. This is done by allowing research that holds out direct benefit or does not place the child at unwarranted risk of harm, inconvenience, or discomfort. In this way, special protections are offered for children while important research is allowed to continue. It also requires informed consent from parents and, where possible, the assent of affirmative agreement to participate from the children.

The U.S. regulations are among the most elaborate, but similar to those in many other countries (26). The U.S. Federal Regulations distinguish four categories of research, and the greater the potential risk to children, the more rigorous the safeguards and the documentation of the probability and magnitude of benefits and harms, parental consent, and the child's assent required (28). The four categories of research are referred to by their nomenclature in the Code of Federal Regulations: 46.404, 46.405, 46.406, and 46.407.

46.404

Research with no greater than a minimal risk may be approved with institutional review board (IRB) approval, even if it does not hold out direct benefit to individual research subjects, as long as it makes adequate provisions for consent from at least one guardian and, when appropriate, the assent of the child subject. Because the risk is low, direct benefit does not have to be shown to individual research subjects. For example, gathering information about children's growth and development from their medical records may not benefit them directly, but may be of enormous benefit to children as a group. Watching children stack blocks or identify animals from sounds may not benefit children directly, but be very important for establishing normal growth and development. In some cases, IRBs, which have to approve studies as having no greater than a minimal risk, might determine that extra tests or procedures might be considered minimal risk as well. "Minimal risk" is understood as everyday risks such as those encountered in routine physical, dental, or psychological examinations. It is a widely used international research standard but defined differently in different countries (29).

46.405

Children are a distinctive group, and to test standard or new therapies for them, some members of the group have to be included. This second category of research allows IRBs to approve studies that have greater than minimal risk if they hold out direct benefit, and risks are justified because the intervention is at least as favorable for each subject as alternatives that are available. This category of research allows with IRB approval, parental consent, and the child's assent when appropriate, greater than a minimal risk if the risk can be justified by anticipated direct benefits to each subject that are at least as favorable to each subject as available alternatives. Children, of course, have many unique problems, and the results from studies with adults may be inapplicable to children. To test the safety and efficacy of drugs for premature infants, premature infants need to be subjects. Children with respiratory distress or infections need to be subjects in studies that evaluate the safety and efficacy of standard, innovative, or investigational drugs for children with these diseases.

46.406

This category of research allows local IRBs to approve studies that have a minor increase over minimal risk even if the study does not hold out the prospect of direct benefit to individual subjects. This requires that the children in the study have a condition or disorder, but there has been disagreement about what this permits (30,31). Consent from both parents is required if practicable, and the child's assent is needed if appropriate. To justify the higher level of risk, the study has to be similar to the children's actual or expected medical, dental, psychological, or educational experiences, as well as being likely to result in important information about the child's disorder and condition. "Minor increase over minimal risk" is undefined. Given the recent legal ruling, *Grimes v Kennedy Krieger Institute*, Kopelman has argued that it should mean a minimal risk for these children with a disorder or condition, but no more than a minor increase over minimal risk for otherwise healthy and normal children without conditions or disorders (31).

46.407

Local IRBs cannot approve non-beneficial studies having more than a minor increase over minimal risk for children, but they can seek approval for a study from the Secretary of the Department of Health and Human Services (DHHS). To gain approval, it must represent a reasonable opportunity to understand, prevent, or alleviate a serious problem affecting the health or welfare of children. The Secretary of DHHS can approve a study with more than a minor increase over minimal risk, but first must garner public comments, consult with a panel of experts about the study's value and ethics, and seek adequate provisions for parental consent, typically from both parents, and the child's assent. In the United States, this category also has been used to review studies that have become controversial (32).

CHAPTER 7L ■ CONCLUDING REMARKS

LORETTA M. KOPELMAN

Moral and social policy regarding children's health care is shaped by commitments to children that may be stated in terms of the principles of beneficence, self-determination or autonomy, nonmaleficence, justice, and social utility. Policies are better insofar as they promote these duties or ideals for children and worse if they do not.

Although all four standards of decision-making in health care are important for children (self-determination, advance directives, presumed consent, and the best interest standard), the best interest standard is used most frequently in pediatrics. Competent adults, including parents, clinicians, nurses, teachers, and others, have duties to ensure that children are protected and get good care. The primary responsibility for making decisions for children may fall to parents or guardians, but their decision can be challenged if they endanger their children or do not promote their well-being or opportunities to flourish. The ideal, of course, is that parents, the minor, clinicians, and other health care professionals agree about the best course of action for the minor.

References

1. Brock DW. What is the moral authority of family members to act as surrogates for incompetent patients? *Milbank Q* 1996;74:599–618.
2. Buchanan AE, Brock DW. *Deciding for others: the ethics of surrogate decision making.* Cambridge: Cambridge University Press; 1989.
3. Kopelman LM. Children/III: Health care and research. In: Reich WT, ed. *Encyclopedia of bioethics*, rev. ed. New York: Simon & Shuster Macmillan; 1995:357–368.
4. Kopelman LM. On the evaluative nature of competency and capacity judgments. *Int J Law Psychiatry* 1990;13:309–329.
5. U.S. President's Commission for the Study of Ethical Problems in Medicine and Biomedical Research. *Making health care decisions.* Washington, DC: Government Printing Office; 1982.
6. Beauchamp TL, Cook R, Fayerweather W. Ethical guidelines for epidemiologists. *J Clin Epidemiol* 1991:44(suppl):151S–169S.

7. Faden RR, Beauchamp TL, King NMP. *History and theory of informed consent*. New York: Oxford University Press; 1986.
8. Bluebond-Langner M. *The private worlds of dying children*. Princeton, NJ: Princeton University Press; 1978.
9. Kopelman LM. Children/III: health care and research. In: Reich WT, ed. *Encyclopedia of bioethics*. Rev ed. New York: Simon & Shuster Macmillan; 1995:357–368.
10. Holder A. *Legal issues in pediatrics and adolescent medicine*. 2nd ed. New Haven: Yale University Press; 1985.
11. President's Commission for the Study of Ethical Problems in Medicine and Biomedical Research. *Making health care decisions*. Washington, DC: Government Printing Office; 1982.
12. Faden RR, Beauchamp TL, King NMP. *History and theory of informed consent*. New York: Oxford University Press; 1986.
13. Buchanan AE, Brock DW. *Deciding for others: the ethics of surrogate decision making*. Cambridge: Cambridge University Press; 1989.
14. Kopelman LM. The best-interests standard as threshold, ideal, and standard of reasonableness. *J Med Philos* 1997;22:271–289.
15. Kopelman LM. Children as research subjects: a dilemma. *J Med Philos* 2000;25:745–768.
16. Kopelman LM. Rejecting the Baby Doe regulations and defending a "negative" analysis of the best-interests standard. *J Med Philos* 2005;30:331–352.
17. Kopelman LM. Are the 21-year-old Baby Doe rules misunderstood or mistaken? *Pediatrics* 2005;115:797–802.
18. Kopelman LM. Children/III: health care and research. In: Reich WT, ed. *Encyclopedia of bioethics*. Rev ed. New York: Simon & Shuster Macmillan; 1995:357–368.
19. Holder A. Legal issues in pediatrics and adolescent medicine. 2nd ed. New Haven: Yale University Press; 1985.
20. Kopelman LM. Conceptual and moral disputes about futile and useful treatments. *J Med Philos* 1995;20:109–121.
21. Faden RR, Beauchamp TL, King NMP. *History and theory of informed consent*. New York: Oxford University Press; 1986.
22. Beauchamp TL, Childress JF. The rule of confidentiality. In: *Principles of biomedical ethics*. New York: Oxford University Press; 1979:80–84.
23. Kopelman LM. How AIDS activists are changing research. In: Monagle JF, Thomasma DC, eds. *Health care ethics: critical issues*. Gaithersburg, MD: Aspen; 1994:199–209.
24. American Academic of Pediatrics, Committee on Drugs. Guidelines for the ethical conduct of studies to evaluate drugs and pediatric populations. *Pediatrics* 1995;95:286–294.
25. U.S. Federal Regulations, 45 CFR46 (1991).
26. Council for International Organizations of Medical Science (CIOMS). *International ethical guidelines for biomedical research involving human subjects*. Geneva: CIOMS; 1993.
27. Kopelman LM. Minimal risk as an international ethical standard in research. *J Med Philos* 2004;29:351–378.
28. Kopelman LM. What conditions justify risky nontherapeutic or "no benefit" pediatric studies: a sliding scale analysis. *J Law Med Ethics* 2004;32:749–758.
29. Kopelman LM. Pediatric, research regulations under legal scrutiny: Grimes narrows their interpretation. *J Law Med Ethics* 2002;30:38–49.
30. Kopelman LM., Murphy T. Ethical concerns about approval of risky pediatric studies. *Pediatrics* 2004;113:1783–1789.

CHAPTER 8 ■ ETHICS AND THE CHILD WITH A CHRONIC CONDITION

RONALD M. PERKIN

The course of a chronic condition is likely to include diagnosis and treatment; periods of recovery, exacerbations, stability, or instability; and in some cases, deterioration and death. These phases often are punctuated by recurring ethical questions, including the following: (1) defining what constitutes a life worth living, (2) recognizing the threshold for certainty in diagnosis and treatment, (3) choosing a decision-maker to decide about treatment or nontreatment, (4) determining the role of minors in making treatment decisions, (5) deciding whether to pursue experimental or innovative therapies, and (6) resolving conflicts. The range of chronic conditions in childhood and adolescence is paralleled by the range of values held by people with chronic conditions or caregivers of those with chronic conditions. Competing ethical obligations can create a set of problematic situations for children, families, and health care providers.

PRINCIPLES IN DECISION-MAKING

The ethical principles that guide medical decision-making in chronic care are similar to the principles used in other health care settings. Ethical theories and principles provide a foundation for ethical analysis and moral reasoning. Theories that focus on consequences (e.g., various utilitarian theories), motives (e.g., virtue theories), and duties (e.g., deontologic theories), guide the reasoning process. Ethical principles, such as beneficence (doing good), nonmaleficence (avoiding or minimizing harm), veracity (telling the truth), justice (ensuring fairness or equality), fidelity (keeping promises), and autonomy (deciding for oneself), commonly are applied to clinical situations.

Based on the principles of beneficence and nonmaleficence, health care professionals seek to promote the well-being of their patients and to reduce or alleviate harm. Choices among alternative treatments should benefit the infant or child and clearly outweigh the associated burdens and harms. Even though children are not autonomous of self-determining, respect for people still is required in decisions about their care because the lives of children have unique meaning. To treat children with respect is to acknowledge and value who they are outside of a medical context, rather than to treat them only according to how professional goals and values are advanced. Justice demands that individual patients be treated fairly and that decisions are not made based on subjective criteria such as race, age, sex, diagnosis, or socioeconomic status.

Autonomy implies the importance of the individual in making his or her own life decisions. This concept is accepted for adults, but vicarious decisions necessarily must be made for infants and children.

A triangle of understanding needs to be established among the child, family, and health care team. In children with chronic health care problems, this triadic relationship often is complex. Instead of one physician, there may be a health care team whose chief may change on a regular basis. Instead of two involved parents, there may be a single teenage mother, or the parents may already be separated or divorced, each accompanied by a new partner. The parents often are accompanied by a variety of family members with differing philosophies. The child is not yet autonomous but completely dependent on others for care, love, and decisions. In the setting of an acrimonious family, the ethical health care team must constantly think of what is best for the child.

Parental decision-making on behalf of children can provoke questions about parental rights versus the rights of children, parental rights versus the duty of the pediatric professional, and the interests of the decision-makers versus those of the state.

PARENTAL/FAMILY RIGHTS AND RESPONSIBILITIES

As a rule, the law protects the natural rights of parents to raise children free from unwarranted state interference, presuming that parents will act in the best interest of their children. Accordingly, parents are allowed considerable latitude for medical decisions on behalf of their children, even if the choices may not concur with the physician's recommendation. These rights are conditional on parental fulfillment of the duty to provide necessary care for minor children. Even more important than parental rights are parental responsibilities. If parents fail to provide their children with at least a minimum standard of medical care, the state may assert its interest in protecting the welfare of children by involving child protection statutes to override parental wishes.

Courts regularly uphold such interventions when parental refusals, even when genuinely motivated by strong family convictions, may be life-threatening. However, when the consequences for the child are grave but not life-threatening, states have differed in their willingness to intervene, reflecting the continuing struggle to balance the rights of individual children and family privacy. Many state child-protection statutes include exemptions for parents who seek nontraditional forms of treatment based on religious convictions. It must be emphasized that the central principal guiding decisions should be what protects the best interests of the child and not mere parental preference.

Despite the strong emphasis on patient self-determination and informed consent, the literature in medical ethics now includes persuasive arguments against the autonomy of even competent adult patients and in favor of including family members and their interests in decision-making. While this position is controversial, it deserves consideration.

As the severity of a child's disability and/or dependency upon medical technology increases, families often face difficult moral issues in attempting to understand the nature and the extent of their obligations to provide care. The extent of family caring indicates widespread recognition that families have a serious duty to provide care. On the other hand, families often are deeply perturbed by the inescapable need to set limits to this care. As the disabilities and dependencies of their children increase, many families face emotional and moral exhaustion. Trying to balance the demands of care against their own dwindling resources, they are caught between imperative duties and impossible demands.

Individual family members caring for loved ones regularly confront questions on their own identity and social roles. Parents caring for children dependent on technology naturally wish to maintain and foster an exclusively loving, nurturing, and comforting relationship with their child. Their natural role is to protect, to safeguard from harm, and to reassure. But these same parents, in their role as dispensers and maintainers of high-tech medical treatments, sometimes must inflict serious pain and suffering on their own children. In this second role, they must act more like doctors than parents, or more like technicians than nurturing mothers and fathers. Many may wonder whether their child who is dependent on a ventilator might be better off elsewhere, perhaps in a comfortable residential setting, where the child may focus his rage against others, and the family members may be better able to retain their identity as caring nurturers.

Faced with such challenges, family caregivers have a real stake in decisions affecting the focus and level of care for their children. Decisions about chronic care can seriously alter the lives of family caregivers, infringing on their independence, autonomy, and commitments to others. Depending on the extent and impact of family members' caregiving, their autonomous interests can move into the foreground of decision-making. This is not to suggest that chronic care requires a move from a model of patient as primary agent to one of family as primary agent. The ethical problem for chronic care becomes one of determining how the autonomy and interests of family members should counterbalance those of the child receiving care. When family members heavily share the challenges of care, decision-making becomes a horizontal, interactive process involving negotiation, mediation, compromise, and recognition of values. The traditional, patient-centered moral framework must give way to a new ethic for chronic care based on the notion of reasonable accommodation of competing legitimate interests.

In chronic care, family caregivers play crucial roles that have no parallel in acute care. These roles and their distinctive ethical challenges deserve fuller description and analysis. The following issues stand in the foreground: the basis of family obligation to provide direct care; the limits of this obligation; the relation between familial obligation and the wider societal obligation to provide home care; and the nature of autonomy and beneficence, as well as independence and paternalism, within family caregiving.

MALTREATMENT OF CHILDREN WITH DISABILITIES

The numbers of children surviving disabling medical conditions as a result of technological advances and children being recognized and identified as having disabilities are increasing.

The rates of child maltreatment have been found to be high in both the child population in general as well as in children who are blind, deaf, chronically ill, developmentally delayed, behaviorally or emotionally disordered, and multiply disabled.

Recent evidence revealed that children with disabilities were more likely to experience multiple episodes and multiple forms of abuse than their nondisabled peers. They are nearly four times more likely to be neglected, and physically abused and three times more likely to be sexually abused.

In general, the causes of abuse and neglect of children with disabilities are the same as those for all children; however, several elements may increase the risk of abuse for children with disabilities. Children with chronic illnesses or disabilities often place higher emotional, physical, economic, and social demands on their families. Parents with limited social and community support may be at especially high risk for maltreating children with disabilities because they may feel more overwhelmed and unable to cope with the care and supervision responsibilities that are required. Lack of respite or breaks in child care responsibilities can contribute to an increased risk of abuse and neglect.

The requirement of special health and educational needs can result in failure of the child to receive needed medications, adequate medical care, and appropriate educational placements, resulting in child neglect.

Parents or caregivers may feel increased stress because children with disabilities may not respond to traditional means of reinforcement, and children's behavioral characteristics (e.g., aggressiveness, noncompliance, and communication problems, which may appear as temper tantrums) may become frustrating. A behaviorally challenging child may further increase the likelihood of physical abuse. Parents of children with communication problems may resort to physical discipline because of frustration over what they perceive as intentional failure to respond to verbal guidance. It has been noted, however, that families who report higher stress levels may actually have greater insight into problems associated with caring for a disabled child, whereas parents with a history of neglect of a child may not experience the level of stress that a more involved parent may experience.

In regard to sexual abuse, infrequent contact of a child with disabilities with others may facilitate molestation, because there is decreased opportunity for the child to develop a trusting relationship with an individual to whom he or she may disclose the abuse. Also, children who have increased dependency on caregivers for their physical needs may be accustomed to having their bodies touched by adults on a regular basis. Children with disabilities who require multiple caregivers or providers may have contact with numerous individuals, thereby increasing the opportunity for abuse.

Children with disabilities are often perceived as easy targets, because their intellectual limitations may prevent them from being able to discern the experience as abuse. Impaired communication abilities may prevent them from disclosing abuse. Because some forms of therapy may be painful (e.g., injections or manipulation as part of physical therapy), the child may not be able to differentiate appropriate pain from inappropriate pain. Because children with disabilities are at increased risk for maltreatment, all health care providers should be vigilant in their assessment of these children.

DISCLOSURE

Many guidelines exist about the disclosure of a chronic illness to a child. In general, disclosure is geared to a child's level of cognitive development and psychosocial maturity. For most illnesses, young children receive simple explanations about the nature of their illness and what their responsibilities are in caring for themselves. The exact diagnosis and prognosis of the disease are less important in early discussions with young children. As children mature, they should be fully informed of the nature and consequences of their illness and encouraged to participate actively in their own medical care. Children with a variety of chronic diseases, including cancer, have exhibited better coping skills and fewer psychosocial problems when appropriately informed about the nature and consequences of their illness.

SELF-DETERMINATION

The commonly accepted concepts of parental consent and parental right to refuse consent raise serious ethical problems when they compete with the responsibilities of health care professionals to their minor patients who have the capacity to consent for their own medical treatment. Historically, the right of self-determination is recognized at the legal age of maturity, defined as 18 years. Many legislatures and courts have expanded minors' rights to consent to medical treatment. In most states a child may acquire status as an emancipated minor entitled to treatment as an adult through marriage, judicial decree, military service, parental consent, failure by the parents to meet legal responsibilities, living apart from and being financially independent of parents, and motherhood. In addition, statutory mature minor rules uphold the validity of consent given by minors if the treatment is appropriate and the minor is considered capable of comprehending the clinical circumstances and therapeutic options. As a child's powers to interpret and integrate life's experiences evolve from a characteristically concrete, shortsighted perspective to an appreciation of abstract, future-oriented concepts, concomitant expansion of decisional rights involving increasingly complex and risky alternatives may follow. Though it is well recognized that age alone is not an adequate gauge of maturity, some developmental psychologists suggest that most children older than 15 years of age have the ability to make their own medical decisions, and many between 11 and 15 years of age also have this capability. Courts have recognized the rights of minors approaching the age of 18 years to participate in decision-making, including choices involving life-and-death consequences.

STRESSORS ENCOUNTERED BY PARENTS OF CHILDREN WITH CHRONIC ILLNESS

The stressors experienced by parents of children who are chronically ill usually are multiple and ongoing. Although these stressors vary over time, they can be categorized as those that parents experience: (1) at the time of diagnosis, (2) during developmental transitions, (3) while meeting the ongoing health care needs of their child, and (4) as their child experiences illness exacerbations and hospitalizations.

Diagnosis

The diagnosis of a child's chronic illness is a stressful event for parents. Full comprehension of the diagnosis does not always occur simultaneously with the initial diagnosis. Uncertainty regarding the child's condition and his or her potential outcomes is a major stressor at the time of diagnosis. Parents experience the loss of the previously taken-for-granted world and fear the potential loss of their child, altered parenting roles, and role strain as stressors. Being unable to care for, protect, and parent their child is especially stressful.

Although disclosure of the diagnosis brings parents closure regarding the question of what is wrong with their child, it does not answer their questions of what they need to know about the illness and what their next steps are in caring for their child. Parents identify a high-technology environment at the time of diagnosis, such as a neonatal or pediatric intensive care unit, as an additional stressor.

Parental responses to the diagnosis of their child's chronic condition commonly include shock, disbelief, denial, and anger. Additional responses include despair, depression, frustration, and confusion.

Developmental Transitions

Children with chronic illnesses need to achieve the same developmental tasks as their healthy peers. However, because chronic illness may negatively affect the physical, cognitive, or emotional health of the child, accomplishment of these developmental tasks is challenging. Many parents experience recurrent or chronic sorrow as they watch their children struggle to achieve developmentally appropriate tasks, especially as they become acutely aware of differences and delays between their children and healthy peers.

Chronic sorrow is a coping mechanism that allows for periodic grieving. It is thought to be a recurrent phenomenon rather than a continuous process. The chronic sorrow model contends that parental reaction is one of functional adaptation rather than acceptance of the child's condition.

As normal healthy toddler and preschool children struggle with common developmental issues, children with chronic conditions also are challenged to develop autonomy, initiative, and mastery over their environment. Parents desire to promote their child's development, but simultaneously want to protect and assist their child with what they perceive she is unable to accomplish. Because they tend to view their child as fragile, vulnerable, and different, parents tend to engage in overprotective parenting.

The transition to school for a chronically ill child also is stressful for families. This may be the first time that parents realize the extent to which the child is different from peers in physical appearance, cognitive ability, and social skills. Children may face teasing, difficulties with establishing friendships, discrimination, and challenges performing many age-appropriate activities, which usually are painful for both the child and family alike.

When the child enters the school system, parents give up control of their child's health care management during the school day to teachers and other professionals (e.g., the school nurse). Relinquishing these caretaking activities may prove difficult, especially if the parents have assumed the sole care of their child to this point in time. Unfortunately, many teachers and school personnel have very little knowledge about childhood chronic illnesses, which is an added source of stress and concern for parents.

Ongoing Care (Chronic Burden of Care)

Many daily health care regimens are time consuming, rigorous, and unrelenting, which prove taxing to both parents and children. Parents report that seeing their children in physical or emotional pain and discomfort is heart-wrenching and frequently triggers overwhelming feelings of guilt and inadequacy. Balancing the competing demands from the child's chronic illness and the parent's personal and family daily responsibilities is challenging and exhausting. Parents of chronically ill children often experience role and marital strain as well as higher levels of psychological distress (e.g., depression and anxiety) than parents of healthy children.

The financial burden of ongoing care is another major stress for families and is an issue that is becoming more salient with increased health care control by insurance companies. Not only is health care expensive, but the costs related to housing and other lifestyle modifications, special equipment, and other services pose additional financial strains for families. Unfortunately, many of these costs are not reimbursed by health care insurance plans.

Exacerbations and Hospitalizations

Many chronic illnesses are fraught with exacerbations and deterioration in the child's functioning or quality of life, which tax parents' coping resources. These exacerbations frequently require hospitalization, increased services, and changes in family lifestyles. Hospitalizations create stress as they interrupt normal routines and place increased demands on parents who have to divide their time further between their normal responsibilities and their hospitalized child. The lack of control and sense of powerlessness many parents feel when their child is hospitalized may lead to controlling and overprotective behaviors by parents. Uncertainty and fear about the future is a constant worry for parents of children who are chronically ill.

ROLE OF HOME CARE

Home care is an exceptionally diverse endeavor covering a wide range of initiatives, from the care of those dependent on extremely complex technology to the continuing management of a person who needs assistance in the basic activities of daily life, such as feeding, ambulating, and personal hygiene.

Some children require a significant amount of daily care and much of that care has moved from hospitals into homes. Home care now includes the use of tracheostomy tubes, intravenous transfusions and infusions, peritoneal dialysis, and the long-term use of ventilators (see Section XV). The burden of care has shifted to the family, assisted to various degrees by home care nurses, therapists, and equipment companies. One distinctive ethical issue, broadly construed, of high-technology home care is the tendency to medicalize the home environment, subjecting the traditionally private sphere of home to the intrusions of medical personnel, timetables, and equipment.

Families often prefer home care because they believe it has benefits for the child and family and represents a safer, more normal environment than the hospital. In some cases, the life of the child may be prolonged, whereas in other cases, home is a more acceptable place to manage the final stages of a terminal illness. Home care provides many personal, social, and financial benefits, but it also presents the family with problems. The personal, social, structural, and financial barriers to successful home care can be overwhelming, and sources of support may be limited. Families with more resources often experience serious limitations in maintaining careers and preferred personal and family lifestyles. Some homes are not conducive to the successful provision of home care. The worst home is not necessarily better than the best medical institution. Children in these circumstances remain in institutions until alternatives can be found. The success of home care depends on the determination and resourcefulness of the family, and the quality of the support network that can be marshaled to assist them.

Fundamental ethical dilemmas arise when one set of problems (for the patient) is solved at the cost of creating a new set of problems (for the patient and caretakers). The relatively recent popularity of home care for patients who are chronically ill or dependent on technology has moved professionals into unfamiliar settings with great rapidity, often without time for contemplation of the significant changes in attitudes and priorities home care demands.

A main factor that has encouraged complex care in the home is the development of sophisticated medical technology. High-tech, safe equipment has permitted the introduction of a variety of treatments and mechanical supports in the home. However, the technology itself is largely responsible for the stress that families experience. The transition from hospital to home can be felt by patients and family members as a shift from technology overload to technological isolation. At home, some patients and their families can feel cut off from or even abandoned by the system of intensive medical supports present in the hospital. This lack of connection can be experienced by families as a profoundly alienating and isolating experience. Thrown back on their own resources and instincts, families must rely on impressions and guesswork rather than data. The ensuing magnification of uncertainty can be a source of great worry and anxiety.

The goal of a home health care program for infants, children, or adolescents with chronic conditions is the provision of comprehensive, cost-effective health care within a nurturing home environment that maximizes the capabilities of the individual and minimizes the effects of the disabilities.

Careful review of the patient's status and needs should be made by each professional participating in the patient's care. Each discipline should formulate goals and objectives for the patient. Eligibility for home health care should be based on a comprehensive analysis of the capabilities of the home health care program, whether the child's therapeutic needs can be met by home care, the potential benefits and risks, and the available resources. Families should not face excessive pressure to enroll their children in a home care program if such a move would be detrimental to the child or family.

Home care is mostly chronic care. It differs markedly from acute care, which focuses on short-term, cure-oriented treatment. Chronic care is ongoing, uncertain about prognosis, varied (even diffuse) in its modalities, and often directed at palliation and functional support rather than cure and return to normal function.

Because home care tends to be chronic in nature, it is not simply or even predominantly medical. Ethical problems arise, in less dramatic fashion, within the routines of daily life, and these dilemmas often are quite different from those encountered in the acute care setting. The home setting, the role of family as caregivers, the nonmedical dimensions of care, and the limited reimbursement system all create special problems that press ethical reflection beyond the standard acute care discussion.

Unfortunately, home care is relatively poor in status and resources; it often is ancillary and marginal. It functions with very little physician involvement, relies on nursing and social work supervision, and is heavily dependent on ancillary formal caregivers and a large but often "invisible" force of informal caregivers (mainly family members).

Decisions for or against long-term home care usually are made in the acute care setting. These decisions must be based on adequate and thorough information provided to patients and families. Once the information is provided and digested, a decision based on the collective best interests of patient and family should be sought. The decision must weigh the benefits and burden primarily for the patient, but also for the family members. Investigation and assessment of the family's ability to provide the environment as well as carry out the many duties required of patients who are dependent on technology must be conducted by clinicians experienced in chronic home care. One must search for the existence of psychological, social, or cultural barriers to effective care.

A number of issues related to the potential effects of having a child who is severely ill at home need to be explored with the family, including issues of privacy, physical burdens of care, role of the parents in coordinating care, and the social and financial aspects, including issues of confidentiality.

Placing complex life support systems in the home may create extraordinary challenges for parents and families. In the face of these challenges, one cannot simply judge parents acceptable if they provide recommended health care or neglectful if they do not. Professionals must be careful in deciding how vigorously to try to convince parents, explicitly or by implication, to assume obligations for such care.

The patient's general condition, including associated functional or cognitive disabilities and other medical problems, and ability to participate in social and academic activities, need to be weighed in the light of the natural history of the disease process to decide about benefits of long-term support. This judgment is fundamentally subjective, but it requires consideration by parents and caregivers. In this situation, informed consent must be seen as a dynamic process whereby both caregiver and patient/family benefit from each other's thinking, not as a finite moment in time. The home care process must allow decisions to be reviewed and revised and take into account the family's quality of life. Without a process to change decisions, families may resort to making their own decisions, such as implementing privately sanctioned do-not-resuscitate orders that are later explained as equipment failures or accidents. The home care movement must advocate a system of continuing assessment of the patient and family. High-tech home care contracts with the family should be renegotiable throughout the course of the patient's care.

Most home care patients receive formal (health care professionals) and informal (family) care and, therefore, the cooperation of family members is crucial to the success of care plans. A model for hospital discharge and home care planning should clarify relationships among physicians and establish mechanisms of accountability for all involved in caring for the child. It must be family centered, community based and include physician involvement at the tertiary and local levels. Roles and responsibilities should be established, to the extent possible, for the physician based in the tertiary care center and the community-based physician before hospital discharge. The community-based physician should be identified early in the planning process and should have the opportunity to supply input into the home care plan and to receive training, if needed, at the tertiary care center.

Providing care to these children can be frustrating and challenging for pediatricians serving this vulnerable and complex population. The frustrations generally fall into three categories: time, information, and coordination. First, high-quality primary care services for children with chronic conditions are time-consuming. As the managed care industry thrives, primary care physicians receive the same capitation rate for children with complicated problems as they do for other children. There is little financial incentive under most managed care plans to spend extra time on complex problems, and some insurers discourage primary care physicians from attracting children with high-cost health care needs into their practices.

Second, many primary care physicians feel inadequately informed about managing chronic illnesses and disabilities. Well-trained informal caregivers may be more knowledgeable about the management of the technology and even more expert in disease assessment for their unique patient than the primary pediatrician who joins the care team relatively late in the endeavor.

Finally, the child with chronic illness often requires extensive care coordination that involves the entire community. Communication between health care professionals can run the gamut from fair to inadequate. Sometimes there is no coordination at all; in other cases, children have multiple case managers who fail to communicate with one another.

Within communities, efforts should be made to develop effective and efficient chronic condition management programs. Pediatric practices can strengthen their services to children with special health care needs with a well-planned management approach that is part of the medical home model. This type of program earmarks specific children for extra services in the primary setting and improves access to office services, responsiveness to family needs, care coordination, ongoing education, and office efficiency and reimbursement.

The home environment is a secondary setting for formal providers and the primary setting for the family. This is a paradigm shift from the hospital, where formal caregivers were in control. In the home setting, parents are in the primary position of authority and, in the past, did not consult with others about how they functioned or the decisions they made about their child. In fact, to take the child with a disability home, they were required to become experts in their child's care and in most situations were lauded by the medical profession for their skills. This reversal of authority and narrowing, or even reversal, of the professional-parent expertise gap may cause conflict because it is a role foreign to the professional health care provider and parent. The role change is necessary in the home care environment, where the emphasis is on empowering parents to make critical decisions about their child's care, but it may be very uncomfortable for and even threatening to the physicians involved.

The autonomy and authority of formal caregivers can be muted by the home setting, the nature of the care provided, dependency on family caregivers, and tensions created by family supervision of care. Caregivers face sharp conflicts when patients and families, emboldened by these elements, press to control care in an unreasonable fashion. Even in less contentious situations, authority and control remain underlying problems.

The various tensions between caregivers, patients, and families require more than a strict ranking of autonomy and authority. The ethical equation becomes more complex, and it often is helpful to focus on goals of therapy rather than the ethical principles. The recognition of common, corresponding, or at least cohabitable goals often may be more productive than the determination of whose goal finally wins. In daily home care, autonomy is acutely protected by accommodation, the recognition of interdependence, mutuality, and the sharing of challenges.

Suggested Readings

American Academy of Pediatrics. Assessment of maltreatment of children with disabilities. *Pediatrics* 2001;108:508–511.

Melnyk BM, Feinstein NF, Moldenhouer Z, et al. Coping in parents of children who are chronically ill: strategies for assessment and intervention. *Pediatr Nurs* 2001;27:548–558.

Perkin RM, Orr R, DeLeon D. Ethical issues in pediatric home care. In: McConnell MS, ed. *Guidelines for pediatric home health care*. Elk Grove village, IL: American Academy of Pediatrics; 2002:431–462.

Ruston CH, Savage TA. Ethics and the child with a chronic condition. In: Jackson PL, Vessey JA, eds. *Primary care of the child with a chronic condition*. 3rd ed. St. Louis: Mosby; 2000:101–116.

CHAPTER 9A ■ PALLIATIVE CARE DEFINED

JULIA T. RAPER AND RONALD M. PERKIN

Palliative care is about quality of life. Pediatric palliative care is about "adding life to their days, not days to their life" (1). The World Health Organization revised its definition of palliative care in 2002 to say, "Palliative care is an approach which improves quality of life of patients and their families facing life-threatening illness, through the prevention and relief of suffering by means of early identification and impeccable assessment and treatment of pain and other problems, physical, psychosocial, and spiritual" (2).

Palliative care is:

■ Patient centered rather than disease focused.
■ Death accepting but also life enhancing.
■ A partnership between the patient and the caregivers.
■ Concerned with healing rather than curing.
■ Provided regardless of patient age or location.

"Palliative," derived from the Latin word *pallium*, means to cloak. In palliative care, symptoms are "cloaked" with treatments whose primary aim is to promote comfort. This extends far beyond physical symptom relief; it seeks to help patients achieve and maintain their maximum potential physically, psychologically, socially, and spiritually, however limited these have become as a result of disease progression. This helps the child and family come to terms with the impending death as fully and constructively as they can (Fig. 9.1).

When palliative care begins from the earliest recognition of a life-threatening condition, it can be concurrent with efforts to prolong life. As symptom control and supportive care increases, the child and family can be prepared for what to expect and participate in the decision-making. And as death begins, bereavement care can be initiated to a more prepared family. Recognize that the transition from active treatment of the underlying disease to provision of palliative care is gradual, with the latter assuming an increasing role as death becomes more of a certainty. It is not inconsistent for disease-specific treatment to continue in a predominantly palliative setting, especially if those treatments enhance symptom control.

Death is inherently solitary, and the process of dying should be inscribed with support and empathy for the comprehensive needs of young patients (3).

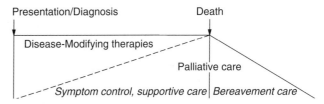

FIGURE 9.1. The relationship between disease-modifying therapy, supportive care, and palliative care.

CHAPTER 9B ■ UNIVERSAL PRINCIPLES OF PEDIATRIC PALLIATIVE CARE

JULIA T. RAPER AND RONALD M. PERKIN

1. The sole admission criterion for palliative care programs is that the child is not predicted to survive to become an adult. Prognosis for short-term survival should not be required, as it interferes with the provision of critical support from the time of diagnosis.
2. The unit of care is the child and the family. Family is defined as the persons who provide physical, psychological, spiritual, and social comfort to the child, regardless of genetic relationships.
3. Palliative/hospice services should be accessible to the children and their families in a setting that is desired and/or appropriate to their needs; whether home, inpatient hospice, hospital, or intensive-care unit. Research indicates that the home is generally considered the preferred

site of living until death, as bereavement outcome is enhanced for family members who otherwise may have limited access to the child.

4. Palliative care is not directed at foreshortening life. Symptom management is accomplished through means acceptable to the patient and the family.

5. Care provided focuses on the relief of physical, social, psychological, and existential or spiritual pain for the child and the family, whether they have chosen to continue with life-prolonging therapies or not.

6. Children and their families should have access to a team of caregivers, or at a minimum, a "key worker" whose care is seamless, that is, who cares for them where they prefer to be.

7. Care is designed to enhance the quality of life for the child and family; the child and family must be included in designing the priorities for care after being given as much information as is desired regarding the disease and treatment options.

8. The care team recognizes the individuality of each child and her family, and upholds their values, wishes, and beliefs unless unnecessary harm is at hand.

9. An interdisciplinary team with pediatric knowledge, generally including trained volunteers, social workers, nurses, physicians, and spiritual counselors, optimally delivers pediatric palliative care.

10. The palliative care team is available to the family 24 hours a day, 365 days a year.

11. The provision of respite, whether for a few hours or a few days at a time, is an essential service in palliative care.

12. Families should be able to refer themselves to a hospice/palliative care program.

13. Providing pediatric palliative care is difficult, though rewarding, work. Direct caregivers must be provided formal or informal psychosocial support and supervision.

14. Regardless of cause of death, supportive and bereavement care should be provided to all those who are affected by the child's death, for as long as they need it (4).

CHAPTER 9C ■ INTEGRATION

JULIA T. RAPER AND RONALD M. PERKIN

The death of a child is often described as one of the most difficult losses to bear. It is the responsibility of all those who care for children with life-limiting and life-threatening diseases and conditions to prevent unnecessary suffering. Palliative care for children is in the early stages of societal acceptance and is only beginning to receive its rightful place in the spectrum of health care services and medical education. The strongly held belief that "children are not supposed to die" creates societal barriers to facing this reality. Children require specialized approaches and services to meet their unique needs, and they require a combination of specialized caregivers in addition to their family. Family members, especially siblings, can have unique needs and concerns, too. Operating within a family-centered model of pediatric palliative care encourages families' participation in a mutually beneficial and supportive partnership, and facilitates seamless continuity in addressing children's and families' needs related to life-threatening conditions (5).

Clinically, palliative care should "alleviate and heal," with healing defined as not a cure, but the restoration of the patient's integrity (6). The assumption that palliative care cannot be offered until all curative options have been exhausted may interfere with early conversations about palliative issues, including limitations of burdensome interventions at the end of life. Health care providers, patients, and families may infer that discussions regarding accept natural death orders or comfort care equals "giving up the fight." Such inferences may inhibit individuals from voicing fears and concerns about the burdens of life-prolonging interventions and the dying process. Explaining usefulness of treatments and discussing the value of advance directives must be done with respect and empathy. It may be reassuring for the child and family to know that when therapies become burdensome or no longer provide comfort, they will be discontinued.

Integrating palliative care into the current model of acute care has multiple advantages:

1. Integration ensures that comprehensive supportive care is introduced earlier in the course of a severe disease or condition.

2. Palliative care principles benefit all patients regardless of prognosis, and introduction of these principles into the mainstream of therapy will benefit all pediatric patients and their families (through improved communication, respect for family and child values, and increased attention to the prevention and treatment of physical, social, emotional, and spiritual suffering of patients and families).

3. Integration ensures that grief and bereavement counseling is accessible to families during the entire course of the illness and after the child's death.

4. Integration provides the infrastructure for integrated medical care and facilitates a formal evaluation of the impact of emotional health and spirituality on disease and medical outcomes.

By integrating palliative care into the care of the severely injured or ill child, health care providers expand the range of appropriate care options. By providing a more comprehensive approach, health care providers ultimately provide relief of suffering and the provision of comfort and peace. The course of illness may be unpredictable, so the need for early integration of palliative care, including symptom management, attention to quality of life, and communication about the end of life with the child and family, should become the standard of care (7).

CHAPTER 9D ■ CHILDREN AND DEATH

JULIA T. RAPER AND RONALD M. PERKIN

Children who are dying know it (8). They are not dependent on information from parents or health care personnel. Experiencing loss of ambulation, energy, and enthusiasm; depression; unusual fatigue; and a keen awareness of the feelings and actions of those around them are some of the possible reasons a child would know he is dying. His understanding of death is based more on his personal experiences with his own diagnosis, course of disease and treatment, and the deaths of peers than on his age or intellectual development. This maturity reveals itself when terminally ill 3- or 4-year-olds demonstrate knowing more about illness and dying than healthy, unaffected 9- or 10-year-olds (9). Studies agree that by 7 years of age children can understand the death concepts of universality, irreversibility, no functionality, and causality (10). These concepts can be integrated with the child's developmental age and level (Table 9.1) (11,12).

Keep the following points in mind when considering children's understanding of death:

■ Providing emotional and psychological support for the dying child is as important as providing relief of physical symptoms.
■ Parents frequently have many questions about how much the child perceives of the terminal condition and how to be most supportive in allaying the child's fears and any misconceptions.
■ Parents are often struggling to meet the emotional needs of siblings.
■ The palliative care team can support the parents' efforts by providing education on a child's normal developmental understanding of death.

TABLE 9.1

CHILDREN'S CONCEPTS OF DEATH

Stage of development	Key concepts	Example	Practical implications
Infancy	Experience the world through sensory information Death is perceived as separation or abandonment Protest and despair from disruption in caretaking	Aware of tension, the unfamiliar, and separation	Comfort by sensory input (touch, rocking, sucking) and familiar people as well as transitional objects (toys)
Early verbal childhood (2–6 years)	See death as reversible or temporary Magical thinking that wishes can come true Death may be seen as punishment	Do not believe death could happen to them May equate death with sleep May believe they can cause death by their thoughts, such as wishing someone would go away	Provide concrete information about state of being; e.g., "A dead person no longer breathes or eats" Need to dispel concept of being responsible and therefore guilty because of thoughts
Middle childhood (7–12 years)	Personalize death Aware that death is final Earlier stage: understand causality by external causes Later stage: understand causality by internal causes	Aware that death can happen to them Believe that death is caused by an event, such as an accident Understand that death also can be caused by an illness	Child may request graphic details about death, including burial and decomposition May benefit from specifics about an illness
Adolescence (older than 12 years)	Appreciate universality of death but may feel distanced from it	May engage in risky behavior, stating "it can't happen to me" or "everyone dies anyway"	May have a need to speak about unrealized plans, such as schooling and marriage

Source: Modified from Frager G. Children's concepts of death. In: Joishy SK, ed. *Palliative medicine secrets.* Philadelphia: Hanley & Belfus; 1999: 170–171; and American Academy of Pediatrics, Committee on Psychosocial Aspects of Child and Family Health. The pediatrician and childhood bereavement. *Pediatrics* 2000;105:445–447.

CHAPTER 9E ■ END-OF-LIFE COMMUNICATION FOR CHILDREN

JULIA T. RAPER AND RONALD M. PERKIN

Patients continue to die following unnecessarily prolonged hospitalizations, sometimes without adequate relief of pain and symptoms. Children may be at greater risk for prolonged hospitalization and disease-specific interventions as families and professionals attempt to maximally prolong a child's life. Too often, however, the child's preferences about such treatments are not adequately addressed, documented, or followed. Effective communication is the key. Assuming that children and families prefer to avoid such a difficult topic should be questioned. According to a recent study, bereaved parents had no regrets about discussing death with their child (13).

One approach to improving competence in end-of-life communication is a six-stage protocol, originally promoted by Buckman for the communication of "bad news" (14). The protocol has been adapted into the American Medical Association-sponsored Education for Physicians on End-of-Life Care (EPEC) program. Von Gunten, Ferris, and Emanuel expand Buckman's communication system to a seven-step method (15). The seven steps address communication, decision-making, and the building of relationships:

Prepare the Patient, Caregivers, and Physician for Discussion of Important Information

1. Prepare for the discussion by confirming medical facts, creating a supportive physical environment, ensuring that there is adequate time, and arranging for the appropriate people to attend including, when possible, the child patient.
2. Establish what the patient and family know by using open-ended questions. Some parents may need to be counseled to be honest with their children.
3. Determine how the patient and family want the information to be delivered. This includes extent of information (in the United States, 90% of adult patients express a preference for full disclosure, regardless of the seriousness of the information) as well as methods of communication. It is important not to rely on assumptions about patient preferences based on the patient's chronological age and ethnic and cultural background. This step may be best accomplished early in the patient–provider relationship, long before the need to discuss sensitive information is anticipated.

Deliver Information

4. Use clear and unambiguous language, neither understating nor overstating the implications of the news. This conversation must be free of jargon and delivered in language the patient can understand, not in foreign medical terminology. Pace the delivery of information, giving many opportunities to ascertain the patient's reception of the information. Check for understanding.

Respond to Patients' Reaction and Planning

5. Respond to emotions. Stop if the patient or family seems overwhelmed. The extent to which the provider is prepared to respond to any emotional reaction with respect and support will be repaid with a stronger patient–provider relationship.

6. Discuss the goals of care, a critical component of good communication. A clear understanding of the patient's goals, and the family's goals, will inform the future course of treatment. The use of open-ended questions encourages patients to formulate their values and preferences regarding the goals of treatment. This step is often revisited in subsequent meetings when the patient and caregivers have had the opportunity to absorb the medical information and when response to therapy becomes clearer. The first six steps logically lead to the final step, establishing a plan.
7. Establish a plan. In view of the considerations and interactions noted above, the mutually elaborated goals of care (step 6) should be used to make a plan for the patient's care that is consistent with family and patient values and goals. This may at first be a short-term plan with certain goals of gaining stability and comfort and measuring the patient's health and response to any provided treatments, interventions, or comfort measures.

In discussions about the end-of-life phase, the child patient's and family's wishes and needs can be addressed in at least six different domains: patient goals; values of the family, caregiver, and patient; advance directives; accept natural death orders; plans for the relief of pain and symptoms; and attending to "unfinished business" (16). These domains may need special consideration in the case of pediatric patients, for whom legal recognition of advance directives and the processes whereby accept natural death or do-not-attempt-resuscitation orders can be obtained are special. Furthermore, children may require attention to particularly unique matters in addressing "unfinished business"—such as accomplishing unmet goals or leaving some kind of legacy. When the child patient, the parents, and the health care providers face the end of life together, these domains can be addressed in a logical and complete manner without resorting to uncomfortable, ill-timed, and artificial conversations. Improved communication will be accomplished by providing the patient and family with the freedom to clearly express their wishes to a health care provider and team who have the skills to listen.

A summary of some of the key points of this section is presented next.

END-OF-LIFE COMMUNICATION FOR CHILDREN (17)

■ One of the most difficult aspects of pediatric palliative care.
■ Majority of parents do want information and they want it from their physician.
■ Difficult conversations are more manageable if they are seen as a process.
■ Careful planning and consensus development. Remember cultural considerations.

Preferred Setting

■ Quiet.
■ Comfortable.
■ Convenient time.
■ Sufficient time.

- Private.
- Support person(s) for parent(s).
- Other members of health care team.
- Provide tissues.

Physician Obstacles

- Conflict with perceived role of curing, prolonging life, and improving health.
- Lack of education or formal training.
- Stress around the delivery of bad news.
- Sense of failure surrounding treatment efforts.
- Loss of relationship with the patient and the investment in their care.

Specific Fears Related to the Delivery of Bad News

- Fear of being blamed.
- Fear of how the child/family will react.
- Fear of expressing emotion or breaching "professional" conduct.
- Fear of not knowing the answers.

Value of Skilled Conversations

- Shift focus of care from cure or prolongation of life to skilled palliative care.
- Improved management of the child's pain and other symptoms.
- Decreased stress.

Talking with the Dying Child

- Most children with a life-threatening illness or condition have a greater understanding of what death means than do healthy children their own age.
- Terminally ill children are usually aware of their prognoses, even if they take great pains to hide that knowledge from the adults around them.
- Terminally ill children feel less isolated if they can communicate their concerns.
- Stay open and receptive when the child initiates a conversation.
- Recognize that many children communicate best through nonverbal means, such as artwork or music.
- Reassure continued love and physical closeness and minimization of pain.
- Respect the child's need to be alone.

Children's Understanding of Death

- Providing emotional and psychological support for the dying child is as important as providing relief of physical symptoms.
- Parents frequently have many questions about how much the child perceives of the terminal condition and how to be most supportive in allaying the child's fears and any misconceptions.
- Parents are often struggling to meet the emotional needs of siblings.
- Palliative care team can support the parents' efforts by providing education on a child's normal developmental understanding of death.

CHAPTER 9F ■ PEDIATRIC PALLIATIVE CARE IN UNIQUE POPULATIONS

JULIA T. RAPER AND RONALD M. PERKIN

Palliative care services are essential for all children, regardless of their age or location. This chapter will address the neonatal population, the intensive care arena, abused children, and the dying adolescent.

NEONATAL POPULATION

When parents lose an infant, they are losing more than a child. They are losing their hopes and dreams for the future. In the case of an infant who never was discharged home, the only memories that the parent has of that child are those that are created during pregnancy and during the hospitalization. The health care team must help the family focus on the positive aspects of the infant's life, no matter how short it was. Emotional support allows parents to express their feelings of loss and helplessness as well as to begin to adjust to life without their newborn (18). It is vital that we recognize the range of emotions that parents experience. Palliative care principles should be integrated into the care of newborns and their families but require addressing several considerations (Table 9.2).

There are many ways that members of the health care team can be supportive in anticipation of a neonatal death, whether it occurs in the delivery room or elsewhere, including talking to the family about what the death process may look like and assuring them that any symptoms, such as pain, will be meticulously treated. It is also helpful to encourage the family to name the infant and hold the infant, regardless of the presence of congenital malformations. Religious rituals such as baptism and pastoral counseling are often valued by families. The team should foster memories by providing photographs (especially in the parent's arms), footprints, and locks of hair. Helping parents plan for autopsy, organ donation, disposition of the body, and funeral arrangements promotes a sense of control in an otherwise uncontrolled situation. Families often appreciate help explaining the death to the infant's siblings (19). Child life specialists are a valuable resource trained to work with siblings. The physician can counsel the family about the cause of death and risk for future pregnancies and help answer the questions (spoken or unspoken).

Although the parents of a dying infant experience a variety of emotions ranging from denial to guilt, their primary fear is that their child will experience pain. It is inhumane to let

TABLE 9.2

CONSIDERATIONS FOR INTEGRATING PALLIATIVE CARE INTO THE NICU

- Determine how to identify those infants for whom palliative care should be considered.
- Identify and address barriers that might limit the provision of palliative care in the NICU (philosophical, physical environment, personal, or fiscal).
- Define what constitutes optional care for the newborn patient and the family.
- Design decision-making and advanced care planning to incorporate the family's values and preferences and mutually determine goals for minimizing suffering and achieving the infant's best interest.
- Determine an optional site of palliative or end-of-life care.
- Develop resources to meet family-centered care needs and to ensure excellent palliative care regardless of the site of care.

Source: Buchholz M, Karl HW, Pomietto M, et al. Pain scores in infants: A modified pain scale versus visual analogue. *J Pain Symptom Manage* 1998;15:117.

infants suffer from pain without appropriate intervention (Table 9.3). It is a challenge, however, to diagnose pain confidently in this vulnerable population.

Objective quantification of infant pain is generally based on recognizing the infant's responses to pain via physiologic changes (change in heart rate, blood pressure, or oxygen saturation) or behavioral responses (facial expressions, body movements, or cries) (Table 9.4). The body's response to pain results in increases in the release of cortisol and catecholamines and, unfortunately, the proposed clinical pain scales do not correlate well with increased concentrations of biochemical markers.

Regardless, regular use of pain and other symptom assessment tools will help caregivers gauge and manage pain in the newborn (20). Efforts to prevent, limit, or avoid painful stimuli should occur with nonpharmacologic interventions (swaddling, positioning, nonnutritive sucking or holding with skin-to-skin contact) or appropriate medications (Table 9.5).

INTENSIVE CARE ARENA

Palliative care is as applicable in the intensive care setting as it is in the home (4). Considering that the majority of children who die do so in hospitals, most often in neonatal and pediatric intensive care units (PICUs), it is imperative that the health care team and families "use extreme responsibility, extraordinary sensitivity, and heroic compassion" (21–24). Despite the initial apparent incongruence between the principles of palliative care and intensive care medicine, it is precisely because of the frequency of death in this setting that intensive care staff must be prepared to provide palliative care, including effective and compassionate communication, symptom prevention and control, and ethical decision-making.

Most children who die in a PICU do so after a decision has been made either to withhold or to withdraw life-extending therapies, including ventilators, antibiotics, intravenous fluids, and other potentially life-prolonging technologies (25–27). Understanding that the goal of withdrawing life-sustaining treatments is to remove unwanted treatments rather than to hasten death is essential in clarifying the distinction between active euthanasia (providing drugs or toxins that hasten death) and death that accompanies the withdrawal of life support. The steps clinicians take when they withdraw life support should parallel the steps they take when they perform a thoracentesis, lumbar puncture, or appendectomy. Withdrawing life-support measures is seldom an emergency decision, and time should be taken to resolve disagreements among the staff and with the family. Strategies to improve consensus include allaying fears of

TABLE 9.3

GENERAL PRINCIPLES FOR PREVENTION AND MANAGEMENT OF PAIN IN NEWBORNS

1. Pain in newborns is often unrecognized and undertreated. Neonates do feel pain. Compared with older age groups, newborns may experience a greater sensitivity to pain and are more susceptible to the long-term effects of painful stimulation.
2. If a procedure is painful in adults, it should be considered painful in newborns, even if they are preterm.
3. Adequate treatment of pain may be associated with decreased clinical complications and decreased mortality.
4. The appropriate use of environmental, behavioral, and pharmacological interventions can prevent, reduce, or eliminate neonatal pain in many clinical situations.
5. Sedation does not provide pain relief and may mask the neonate's response to pain.
6. Health care professionals have the responsibility for assessment, prevention, and management of pain in neonates.

Source: Adapted from Anand KJS and the International Evidence-Based Group for Neonatal Pain. Consensus statement for the prevention and management of pain in newborns. *Arch Pediatr Adolesc Med* 2001;155:113–120.

MODIFIED INFANT PAIN SCORE

Behavior	Behavior score[a]		
	0	1	2
Sleep during last hour	None	Five- to ten-minute naps	Less-than-ten-minute naps
Facial expression: brow bulge, open mouth, chin quiver, stretch mouth vertically, stretch mouth horizontally, nasolabial furrow, eye squeeze	Marked	Less marked	Calm
Quality of cry	Screaming, high pitched	Modulated; infant can be distracted	No cry
Spontaneous motor activity	Incessant agitation, thrashing	Moderate	Normal
Excitability and responsiveness	Tremulous, clonic movement, spontaneous Moro reflex	Excessive reaction to any stimulus	Quiet
Flexion of toes and fingers	Pronounced and constant	Less marked, intermittent	Absent
Sucking	Absent or disorganized	Three to four sucks, stops with crying	Strong, rhythmic; pacifies
Overall tone	Strong, hypertonic	Moderately hypertonic	Normal tone
Consolability	None after two minutes of comforting	Quiet after one minute of effort	Quiet within one minute
Sociability (eye contact) in response to face or smile	Absent	Difficult to obtain	Easy and prolonged

[a]Total score 0 (severe pain) to 20 (complete comfort).
Source: Adapted from Buchholz M, Karl HW, Pomietto M, et al. Pain scores in infants: A modified pain scale versus visual analogue. *J Pain Symptom Manage* 1998;15:117.

legal liability, encouraging face-to-face discussions between health care providers who disagree on the prognosis, eliciting the views of clinicians who are providing bedside care, and consulting with a senior clinician or ethics committee.

The following information provides a framework to guide clinical practice and proposes a protocol for the withdrawal of life-sustaining treatments.

Appropriate Setting and Monitoring

If the child is expected to live for several days following discontinuation of life-sustaining modalities, consideration of referral to hospice in the home setting should be made. If this is not possible, there are several options. One option is to transform the PICU into a suitable place to fulfill the new goals of terminal care (Table 9.6).

Another option is to transfer the patient from the PICU setting to a general pediatric unit, or preferably a palliative care room. As large a room as needed to accommodate the patient and his loved ones should be provided, if possible. University Health Systems of Eastern Carolina Children's Hospital is constructing a Pediatric Palliative Care room designed specifically for the function of palliative care. Input provided by patients, parents, physicians, nurses, the child life specialist, and hospital design and construction staff helped meet the following goals (28).

- The size is large enough (approximately 620 square feet) for family and friends to gather at the end of a special child's life.
- Respite areas are present; indoor family space can be divided from patient space, and outdoor seating areas are available.

- The aesthetic environment resembles a home environment, with natural and electrical light control and personalization areas for photos and trinkets.
- A queen-size bed promotes closeness between the child, family, pets, and friends.
- There is space for a crib for the infant patient.
- Window seating is large enough for a parent and child; suction and oxygen capability is in this area.
- A kitchen area is available for nourishment breaks.
- There is a technology station for communicating, electronic family diary entries, and diversion activities.
- The outer wall with numerous windows and a large doorway allows the patient, family, and friends to enjoy the healing landscape and changes in the weather.
- Privacy fencing allows for direct pet entry.
- A home-style bathroom is present with a large, multiple-jet shower for stress reduction.
- Closet areas are ample for patient/family storage and health care supply storage.

Once the location decision is made, the health care providers can begin the compassionate withdrawal of life-sustaining treatment. Implement the following guidelines to increase the comfort level of the patient, family, and health care team (Table 9.7).

Plan for Withdrawal

- Determine which life-support measures will be discontinued, in what order, and by whom.
- Redefine the goals of care in terms of patient comfort.

TABLE 9.5

MEDICATIONS FOR NEONATAL PALLIATIVE CARE

Drug	Category	Starting dose (per kg body weight)	Route and interval
Acetaminophen	Analgesic, antipyretic	24 mg load 10–15 mg 45–50 mg load 20–30 mg	PO once PO every 4–8 h PR once PR every 6 h
Chloral hydrate	Sedative, hypnotic	10–25 mg 25–75 mg	PO, PR every 6–8 h PO, PR single dose
EMLA (lidocaine-prilocaine 5%)—not to be used in neonates <37 weeks gestation	Topical anesthetic	A thin layer of cream	Topical, 1 hour before procedure; cover with occlusive dressing
Fentanyl	Opioid analgesic	0.5–4 µg 0.5–5 µg/kg/h	IV (or IM) every 2–4 h Continuous IV
Furosemide	Diuretic	1–2 mg	IV, PO, IM every 12 h
Glycopyrrolate	Anticholinergic drying agent	0.01 mg	IV, PO, IM every 4–8 h
Lorazepam	Benzodiazepine sedative, anxiolytic, anticonvulsant	0.05–0.1 mg	IV every 4–8 h
Methadone	Opioid analgesic	0.05–0.2 mg	IV, PO every 12–24 h
Metoclopramide	Antiemetic, promotility	0.03–0.1 mg	IV, PO, IM every 8 h
Midazolam	Benzodiazepine sedative, anxiolytic	0.05–0.15 mg 0.01–0.06 mg/kg/h 0.3–0.5 mg	IV, IM every 2–4 h Continuous IV PO
Morphine	Opioid analgesic, decreases dyspnea	0.05–0.2 mg 0.2–0.5 mg 0.1–0.2 mg/kg/h	IV, IM, every 2–4 h PO every 4–6 h IV continuous infusion
Naloxone	Opioid antagonist	0.1 mg 0.001 mg/kg/h	IV, IM, SC, per ET IV Infusion
Sucrose 12–25%	Analgesic	1–2 mL	PO

Source: Modified from Toce S, Leuthner SR, Dokken D, et al. The high-risk newborn. In Carter BS, Levetown M, eds. *Palliative care for infants, children, and adolescents.* Baltimore: Johns Hopkins University Press; 2004:247–272.
IV, intravenous; IM, intramuscular; PR, per rectum; SC, subcutaneous; ETT, endotracheal tube.

TABLE 9.6

SIMULATING A HOME ENVIRONMENT FOR DYING PATIENTS IN THE INTENSIVE CARE UNIT

Transportable aspect of a patient's home	Ways to provide this aspect in the intensive care unit
Privacy	Provide a private room. Close doors and curtains.
Ready access to family	Suspend restrictive visiting hours. Provide comfortable chairs, recliners, and cots for family members in patient's room.
Access to patient's own possessions and amenities	Allow family to bring in favorite music, clothes, religious icons, food, and pets.
Family serving as personal caregivers	When appropriate, allow family to assist with patient care.
Access to religious rituals and spiritual support	Provide religious and spiritual resources. Encourage religious and other family rituals at the bedside before and after death.

Source: Modified from Perkin RM, Swift JD, Raper JT. *Primer on pediatric palliative care.* Greenville, NC: University Printing and Graphics of East Carolina University Press; 2005.

TABLE 9.7

PROTOCOL FOR COMPASSIONATE TREATMENT WITHDRAWAL

When an informed decision has been made by patient/family/surrogate to withdraw supportive treatment with the expectation that the patient will die, discontinuing pressors or dialysis may sometimes lead to death. More commonly, it is stopping of the ventilator which is the final step. This step is sometimes uncomfortable, and often feared by the care team, but it needn't be. Discontinuation of ventilatory support may be done in one of three ways: extubation, rapid weaning (few hours), or slow weaning without reversal. Increasingly, intensivists and pulmonologists favor **extubation** as the more humane approach. Whichever method is used, the steps to be taken and your expectations should be thoroughly discussed with the family. Once this has been done and an agreeable time has been set, the following guidelines may increase family and staff comfort because they are designed to maximize patient comfort.

1. **Discontinue monitors.** All monitors (IVs, oximeters, pulse, pressure, respiration, etc.) should be disconnected from the patient and/or from their power source; it is difficult to be sure that all are off; someone who knows how they operate should be present to override the alarm of any that cannot be guaranteed off (e.g., some vent alarms).
2. **Free patient's hands.** Hands are for holding; anything that restricts access to hands should be removed (restraints, mitts, bedrails, IVs, etc.).
3. **Remove encumbering and disfiguring devices.** Anything that will get in the way of the family should be removed (e.g., warming blankets, IV poles, detached monitors, etc.); sheets, dressings, and supplies stained with blood or Betadine should be removed or covered; NG tubes should be removed before the family enters the room (they are gross); space should be made available for the family to be at the bedside.
4. **Invite family in.** Have tissues available in the room.
5. **The responsible physician should be present.** She should quietly stop the pressors (or ask the nurse to do so) and reduce the IV to TKO; IV access should be maintained.
6. **IV sedation should be already drawn up.** Valium, Ativan, or other sedation should be ready in case of distressing tachypnea; the family should have been made aware of agonal breathing, Cheyne-Stokes pattern, and so forth, but if the patient appears to be in respiratory distress, he should be further sedated.
7. **The vent is set to FiO2 of 21%.** The patient should be observed for signs of respiratory distress; if the scene is comfortable the ETT should be removed under a clean towel; a nurse should clean the patient's face with a damp washcloth; someone should be beside the vent to stop any alarm.
8. **Remain with the family.** Physician and nurse should remain in the room until death is declared; ask if the family wants some time alone with the body.

Source: Perkin RM, Swift JD, Raper JT. Primer on Pediatric Palliative care. Greenville, NC: University Printing and Graphics of East Carolina University; 2005.
IV, intravenous; NG, nasogastric; TKO, to keep vein open; ETT, endotracheal tube.

- The time course for withdrawal of life-sustaining treatments should equal the time to meet the child's needs for pain relief. Tapering treatments only delays death.
- Because the withdrawal of mechanical ventilation poses the greatest problems with ensuring comfort, all other life-support devices should be withdrawn before the ventilator.

Withdrawing Mechanical Ventilation (Table 9.8)

- Unless the patient specifically requests otherwise, analgesia and sedation should be provided before withdrawing mechanical ventilation support.
- Many clinicians prefer leaving the endotracheal tube in place during withdrawal of mechanical ventilation to prevent gasping and airway occlusion that may be uncomfortable for the patient and observers. It also facilitates suctioning in patients who are uncomfortable due to profuse secretions. Nevertheless, it may be appropriate to extubate the patient, particularly if the child can communicate or if prolonged survival off of life support is expected.
- It is very important to prepare the observers that agonal breathing is normal and part of dying.

Survival Despite Withdrawal of Life-Sustaining Treatment

- Patients may survive the withdrawal of life-sustaining treatments. Have a plan.
- Reassure the family that their child is comfortable and that the timing of death is out of the control of the clinical team.

- Consider transferring these patients out of the PICU to a more private area as long as the family has been prepared for the move.
- Be wary of revising plans and prognosis based on a perceived delay in the expected timing of death. These changes in plans can have a devastating effect on the family and the health care team.

ABUSED CHILDREN

Health care providers caring for a severely abused child who is supported with life-sustaining medical treatments face many difficult decisions. Concerns may include (1) how to proceed when the child apparently will survive with seriously disabling neurologic deficits or with continued reliance on medical support, or (2) conflict of interest when a decision to forgo treatment risks changing the legal charge faced by a perpetrator from assault to manslaughter or homicide.

Forgoing Life-Sustaining Therapy

Deciding to remove life-sustaining treatment for a critically ill child whose injuries are the result of abuse should be made using the same criteria as those used for any critically ill child (26). The primary considerations in forgoing treatment should be in the best interest of the child after carefully weighing the benefits and burdens of continued treatment. In cases of severe brain injury, decisions should not be based solely on a persistent vegetative state.

TABLE 9.8

METHODS OF WITHDRAWING VENTILATOR SUPPORT

Method	Positive aspects	Negative aspects
Prolonged terminal weaning	Allows titration of drugs to control dyspnea. Maintains airway for suctioning. Creates more "emotional distance" between ventilator withdrawal and patient's death.	May prolong the dying process. May mislead family to think that survival is still a goal of therapy. Interposes a machine between family and patient. Precludes any possibility of verbal communication.
Extubation	Allows patient to be free of unwanted technology. Is less likely to prolong the dying process.	Family may interpret noisy breathing caused by airway secretions or agonal breaths as discomfort. May cause dyspnea at time of extubation, especially if anticipatory sedation is not given.
Rapid terminal weaning	Maintains airway for suctioning. Is less likely to prolong the dying process.	Interposes machine between family and patient. Precludes any possibility of verbal communication.

Source: Faber-Langendoen K, Lanken PN. Dying patients in the intensive care unit: forgoing treatment, maintaining care. *Ann Intern Med* 2000;133:886–893.

Resolution of Conflict

The parent or guardian may be suspected or accused of the assault or may be protecting a friend or family member who is suspected or accused of the assault. If the physician suspects that a parent or guardian is not acting in a child's best interest, seek further review and consultation in hopes of resolving conflict. The complex legal issues may force the conflict into court (27). Sometimes the court will appoint a guardian *ad litem* for the purpose of protecting the abused child and for making medical decisions.

Prosecutors may not support a decision to forgo life-sustaining modalities out of concern that the case against the alleged abuser may be weakened. Furthermore, because the prosecutor may bring a charge of manslaughter or murder after the child's death, the prosecutor has an apparent conflict of interest in arguing before the court in favor of discontinuing certain treatments. It also may be difficult to find a judge who is willing to hear a request for appointing a guardian *ad litem* for medical decision-making, given the notoriety that such cases often bring. Finally, the application of pertinent child abuse laws varies from state to state, county to county, and judge to judge, making it difficult to predict with any certainty the outcome of such court proceedings. The American Academy of Pediatrics recommends the appointment of a guardian *ad litem* in all cases of child abuse requiring life-sustaining therapy in which a parent or guardian may have a conflict of interest (28).

Family Support

Decisions to forgo life-sustaining therapy should be based on complete and compassionate communication with the family. The American Academy of Pediatrics endorses a parent's participation in helping to make these determinations, even if one or both parents are suspected of causing the injury (27). Regardless of the cause, nature, and extent of a child's injuries and of the ongoing court proceedings, the parent or guardian should be treated with respect, compassion, and due consideration for privacy. Appropriate support for the parent should be offered, including a bereavement counselor, chaplain, or other persons identified by the parent as providing important psychological and spiritual support (29).

Tissue and Organ Donation

Although forgoing life support does not require the permission of the medical examiner or the district attorney, the medical examiner should be involved early and before the removal of life-support therapies in child abuse cases (27). There may be physical evidence, such as photographs of the injuries, that preferably would be obtained before the child's death.

Federal and state regulations require that the parent or guardian be given the option of tissue and organ donation. However, the permission of the medical examiner is absolutely necessary for tissue and organ procurement to take place, as valuable evidence may be altered or lost in the process (27). If tissue and organ donation are options, the physician should introduce the idea and then request that a person who is trained and comfortable in discussing tissue and organ donation describe the options and answer the family's questions. In addition, the medical examiner should be encouraged to attend the tissue and organ procurement to ensure that appropriate evidence is collected rather than routinely denying permission for procurement (27).

DYING ADOLESCENTS

Adolescents, especially those who are medically experienced, often demonstrate remarkable insight into their illnesses, prospects for survival, and preferences for how they wish to spend their remaining time. Research with adolescents suggests that experience with serious medical conditions, rather than chronological age, constitutes a more reliable indicator of decision-making capability (30,31). Experience suggests that the majority of terminally ill adolescents and their parents have established long-term relationships with their care providers and have acquired substantial medical experience through chronic illness. These facts are powerful adjuncts when facilitating a decisional role for a competent adolescent. When solicited in a sensitive and respectful way, many adolescents will share their feelings about impending death and their opinions concerning continued treatment and palliative care. These expressions of preference, when taken seriously by medical care providers and parents, are crucial. The American Academy of Pediatrics recommends that physicians respect the wishes of mature adolescents (32).

For younger adolescents who meet some but not all of the criteria for functional competence, they may be given a meaningful decisional role in which serious account is taken of their preferences while final authority rests with the responsible adult. The notion of assent rather than consent has been suggested for this population (33). This can be problematic when applied in practice. If the younger adolescent feels that she has veto power over a recommended care plan, care providers are forced to choose between honoring a poor decision not made competently and disregarding the child's stated wish, which violates the spirit of seeking assent in the first place.

CHAPTER 9G ■ SYMPTOMS IN DYING CHILDREN

JULIA T. RAPER AND RONALD M. PERKIN

Dying children are often highly symptomatic, and their symptom burden may increase with time, especially when the terminal phase is reached (34). This symptom burden consists of a matrix composed of physical, psychological, spiritual, and other factors. Although the entire matrix needs to be considered in the symptom assessment of the dying child, this chapter focuses on physical symptoms.

Physical symptoms may be caused by the underlying illness, side effects related to medical interventions and treatment, or causes unrelated to either the primary disease or its treatment. The assessment and diagnosis of symptoms is fundamental to the clinical care of dying children. Palliative therapeutics should generally only be implemented once the underlying causative mechanisms have been established, because therapies directed at the primary cause may ultimately have a more effective outcome for symptom management.

Attempts have been made to survey and describe the symptoms that occur in terminally ill adults (35). However, the recorded prevalence of symptoms may not actually represent the true prevalence of symptoms (36,37). Certain "core" symptoms (e.g., pain, dyspnea, constipation) are invariably elicited and/or recorded, while other "orphan" symptoms (e.g., dry mouth, sleep problems, itching) are less commonly elicited and/or recorded. Very little information is available about the symptoms occurring in dying children, especially those with nonmalignant disease (38).

Data on the prevalence of symptoms among dying children are gradually becoming available (38–42). Patients present with symptom complexes related to diagnosis and stage of disease as well as to therapeutic interventions. Symptoms change over time and in response to primary and palliative treatments, necessitating frequent reevaluation for symptom control.

The progress in symptom control in adults receiving palliative care does not have a parallel experience in children (34). This is due in part to the paucity of symptom measures in children, and explains the reliance of best practice in pediatric palliative care on the best evidence in adult palliative care.

Most of the validated symptom assessment tools in pediatrics have focused on two common symptoms: pain and nausea. In contrast to instruments measuring nausea and vomiting, instruments measuring pain in children have largely been validated predominantly in the noncancer setting. Few multidimensional symptom assessment scales exist for children. Systematic symptom assessment may be useful in assessing symptom burden as part of decision-making toward palliative care and in future epidemiologic studies of symptoms in dying children.

A retrospective study of 30 children at a children's hospice reported the signs and symptoms observed and recorded during the last month of life (38). Table 9.9 lists the symptoms that appear to have been most persistent during the last week of life. Similarly, Liben and Goldman (42) report the most common symptoms among 152 children dying the last month of life (Table 9.10).

TABLE 9.9

SYMPTOMS ASSOCIATED WITH CHILDHOOD TERMINAL ILLNESSES

Symptoms in final week	Percentage of children
Pain	71
Dyspnea	32
Oral symptoms	32
Excess secretions	25

Source: Hunt AM. A survey of signs, symptoms and symptom control in 30 terminally ill children. *Dev Med Child Neurol* 1990;32: 341–346.

TABLE 9.10

MOST COMMON SYMPTOMS AMONG 152 CHILDREN DURING THE LAST MONTH OF LIFE

Symptom	Percentage of children
Pain	92
Weakness	91
Weight loss	72
Anorexia	70
Decreased mobility	59
Nausea	59
Constipation	58
Vomiting	57
Sleepiness	52
Anxiety	46
Difficulty swallowing	44
Dyspnea	41

Source: Liben S, Goldman A. Home care for children with life-threatening illness. *Palliat Care* 1998;14:33–38.

TABLE 9.11

PREVALENCE OF SYMPTOMS IN 159 CHILDREN AGE 10–18 WITH CANCER

Symptom	Overall prevalence (%)
Lack of energy	49.7
Pain	49.1
Feeling drowsy	48.4
Nausea	44.7
Cough	40.9
Lack of appetite	39.6
Feeling sad	35.8
Feeling nervous	35.8
Worrying	35.4
Feeling irritable	34.6
Itching	32.7
Insomnia	30.8
Dry mouth	30.8
Hair loss	28.3
Vomiting	27.7
Weight loss	26.6
Dizziness	24.5
Numbness/tingling in hands/feet	22.0
Sweating	20.3
Lack of concentration	20.1
Diarrhea	20.1
Skin changes	20.1
Dyspnea	16.5
Change in the way food tastes	16.5
"I don't look like myself"	15.8
Mouth sores	13.9
Difficulty swallowing	12.6
Constipation	13.8
Swelling of arms/legs	12.0
Problems with urination	6.3

Source: Collins JJ, Byrnes ME, Dunkel I, et al. The Memorial Symptom Assessment Scale (MSAS): validation study in children aged 10–18. *J Palliat Symptom Manage* 2000;19:363–377.

Children aged 10 to 18 with cancer were surveyed at Memorial Sloan Kettering Hospital, New York, for symptom prevalence and distress (43). Symptom prevalence ranged from 49.7% for lack of energy to 6.3% percent for problems with urination (Table 9.11). Patients who had received chemotherapy had significantly more symptoms than patients who had not received chemotherapy for more than 4 months (11.6 ± 6.0 versus 5.2 ± 5.1), and those patients with solid tumors had significantly more symptoms than patients with leukemia, lymphoma, or central nervous system malignancies (9.9 ± 7.0 versus 6.8 ± 5.5 for leukemia, 6.8 ± 5.0 for lymphoma, or 8.0 ± 6.1 for CNS malignancies). The most common symptoms (prevalence > 35%) were lack of energy, pain, drowsiness, nausea, cough, lack of appetite, and psychological symptoms (feeling sad, feeling nervous, worrying, feeling irritable). Of the symptoms with prevalence rates higher than 35%, those that caused high distress in more than one-third of patients were feeling sad, pain, nausea, lack of appetite, and irritable. These data confirm a high prevalence of symptoms overall and the existence of subgroups with high distress associated with one or multiple symptoms. Systematic symptom assessment may be useful in future epidemiologic studies of symptoms and in clinical chemotherapeutic trials (33). Symptoms epidemiology may also provide a focus for future clinical trials related to symptom management in children with cancer.

A survey of symptom prevalence was performed in children aged 12 to 17 with cancer (44). Of the eight symptoms surveyed, the mean number of symptoms experienced by younger children was 1.9 (± 1.6). Symptom prevalence during the 48 hours prior to completion of the questionnaire is given in Table 9.12. More than half of the children who endorsed pain as a symptom rated their pain as a "medium amount" to "a lot." Although sadness was the least prevalent symptom, more than half of the patients who experienced it rated it as severe, frequent, and distressing. Tiredness and lack of appetite were less likely to be causes of high distress than pain, insomnia, itch, nausea, or worry (44).

The symptom burden of children dying in the hospital is high; ironically, the symptom burden may be reduced in the intensive care unit, where the most aggressive interventions are undertaken (45). A retrospective study examined symptom prevalence, characteristics, and distress of 30 children

TABLE 9.12

PREVALENCE OF SYMPTOMS IN CHILDREN AGE 7–12 WITH CANCER

Symptom	Overall prevalence (%)
Lethargy	35.6
Pain	32.4
Insomnia	31.1
Itch	25.0
Lack of appetite	22.3
Worry	20.1
Nausea	13.4
Sadness	10.1

Source: Collins JJ, Devine TB, Dick G, et al. The measurement of symptoms in young children with cancer: the validation of the Memorial Symptom Assessment Scale in children aged 7–12. *J Pain Symptom Manage* 2002;23:10–16.

dying in a children's hospital (45). Symptoms and their characteristics during the last day of life were determined from an interview of a nurse who cared for that child during the last day of life using a symptom assessment instrument. The dominant disease process was cancer, while the most likely location of death was intensive care. The mean duration of the "active phase of dying" was 25.2 hours and the major physiologic disturbances at this time were respiratory failure and encephalopathy. The mean (± SD) number of symptoms per patient was 11.1 ± 5.6 with significantly more ($p >$ 0.02) symptoms for children dying on the ward (14.3 ± 6.1) compared to children dying in the intensive care (9.5 ± 4.7). Six symptoms (lack of energy, drowsiness, skin changes, irritability, pain, and edema of the extremities) occurred with a high prevalence (affecting 50% or more of the children) in the last week of life. Symptoms in the last day of life—even if they occurred with a high prevalence, frequency ("a lot" to "almost always"), or severity ("moderate" to "very severe")—were in general not associated with a high level of distress ("quite a lot" to "almost always"). Lack of energy was the only symptom where over 30% percent of children with the symptom had a high level of distress ("quite a bit" to "very much"). The level of patient comfort as perceived from the medical notes indicated that the majority of children were "always comfortable" to "usually comfortable" in the last week (64%), day (76.6%), and hour (93.4%) of life.

CHAPTER 9H ■ TERMINAL SEDATION

JULIA T. RAPER AND RONALD M. PERKIN

Occasionally, a technique known as *terminal sedation* is necessary to control symptoms, most often pain, dyspnea, and intractable seizures (46,47). At least within the palliative care community, terminal sedation has become a generally accepted plan of care for adults in the case of otherwise uncontrollable symptoms, although somewhat more reluctantly so for children, who cannot always independently consent in advance. Although considered an "acceptable and justifiable form of euthanasia or physician-assisted suicide (PAS)" by some, others see those as erroneous and harmful concepts, and instead view terminal sedation as the extension of the tenet that, above all, the health care provider's duty is to relieve suffering (46). The intention is not to bring about the demise of the child (as in the case of PAS and euthanasia), but rather to control the symptom, even at risk of death (principle of double effect).

The term *terminal sedation* is being eschewed because of its ambiguous connotation, suggesting that inducing sedation is in fact a terminal event. The preferred term, now used by the National Hospice and Palliative Care Organization in its educational resource materials, is *total sedation*, suggesting complete relief of suffering (47). The indication for total sedation is to fulfill a patient's (or family's) expressed wish of being relieved of the perceived burden of consciousness in the presence of intractable suffering: physical, psychological, and spiritual (48).

Regardless of the philosophical underpinnings that lead to the practice, terminal sedation is widely regarded as the only humane solution to an otherwise uncontrollable and severely distressing problem. It is undertaken only when attempts at symptom control guided by consultation with a professional skilled in palliative care have failed and with the agreement of the child and family. Full explanations of the inability to reverse the underlying process must precede this decision.

Unfortunately, significant discomfort and uncertainty on the part of many critical care practitioners impede the availability of these therapeutic strategies. Clinicians fear being perceived as the proximate cause of death due to the administration of opioids, despite numerous well-known ethical opinions that the relief of symptoms is the primary obligation to the dying patient (46,47).

The child's medication history and the physician's preferences are the primary determinants guiding the choice of pharmacologic agent. The basic principles are the same whether opioids, benzodiazepines, barbiturates, neuroleptics, or others are used singly or in combination.

The usual approach is to increase the dose of the opioid for the child already being treated with opioids. In the circumstance of significant opioid tolerance and a very distressing symptom, however, sedation with opioids alone may be elusive, or unwanted side effects may be exacerbated with opioid escalation. This warrants the inclusion of a second agent, such as a neuroleptic, benzodiazepine, or barbiturate, while continuing opioid therapy. Meperidine, with its toxic metabolite normeperidine, should not be chosen as an opioid. The possible manifestations of neurotoxicity would be difficult for anyone attending the patient.

Table 9.13 refers to initial starting doses for several agents useful for sedation in this context. The reader is referred to Kenny and Frager for a more complete review (46).

The basic premises include frequent reassessment of the effect of the intervention, and remaining vigilant for breakthrough symptoms or adverse effects. Rapid titration to the end-point of comfort through sedation may be required for rapidly progressive symptoms, as sometimes witnessed in the imminently terminal phase. Each increment is based on an increase proportionate to the last dose given. For example, if 10 mg/h of hydromorphone has been inadequate in relieving dyspnea, a reasonable intervention would be to bolus with 10 to 20 mg and increase the basal dose by at least 50% to 15 mg; if distress continues, rebolus with 15 to 30 mg and increase the infusion to 22 mg/h and so on until comfort is achieved.

TABLE 9.13

PHARMACOLOGIC OPTIONS FOR TERMINAL SEDATION IN CHILDREN

Class of drug	Drug	Route (IV/SL/PR)[a]	Initial dose[b]	Initial frequency; titrate as needed
Opioid	Any of the opioids generally used for moderate to severe cancer pain can be used for terminal sedation. The dose is titrated to effect, with the end-point being sedation.			
Benzodiazepine	Lorazepam	SL IV/SC	0.02–0.05 mg/kg	Q6–8h
Initial dosing as for anxiolysis	Diazepam	PR/IV	0.1 mg/kg	
Beware of paradoxical reactions	Midazolam	V/SC	0.03 mg/kg	
Neuroleptics	Methotrimeprazine	IV/SC	0.1 mg/kg	Q8h
Potential extra-pyramidal effects	Chlorpromazine	PR IV/SC	0.5 mg/kg	
	Haloperidol	IV/SC	0.01 mg/kg	
Barbiturate	Pentobarbital	PR/IV	Load with 4 mg/kg then infusion/bolus	Continuous or Q12h
General anesthetic	Propofol	IV	Load with 0.5 mg/kg 1 mg/kg/h infusion	Infusion

[a]Oral route possible but not detailed here as generally precluded by terminal sedation.

[b] These are merely starting doses in the conservative range, as many patients will be receiving other centrally acting medications. Aggressive upward titration is anticipated. When treating infants younger than 6 months, starting doses are 0.25% to 0.33% of the usual initial dose.

Source: Kenny NP, Frager G. Refractory symptoms and terminal sedation of children: ethical issues and practical management. *J Palliat Care* 1996;12:30–45.

SL, sublingual; PR, per rectum; SC, subcutaneous; IV, intravenous.

CHAPTER 9I ■ COMPLEMENTARY THERAPIES

JULIA T. RAPER AND RONALD M. PERKIN

In recent decades, there has been increasing public use of complementary and alternative medicine (CAM). The incorporation of CAM into routine allopathic medical care has become known as *integrative medicine*, and challenges the health care profession to broaden the definition of healing (49). The National Center for Complementary and Alternative Medicine of the U.S. National Institutes of Health defines CAM as a broad range of activities and interventions that are outside standard allopathic medicine. These modalities (Table 9.14) are categorized into four areas (50). The following sections further explain the premise, potential benefits, and use of some of the complementary therapies (50–52).

LIFESTYLE THERAPIES

- Light and color
  - Premise: The use of visible and invisible light brings harmony to the energetic fields of the individual.
- Potential benefits include:
  - Metabolic alterations.
  - Thyroid stimulation.
  - Circadian rhythm development/maintenance.
- Examples of use:
  - Has been in use for many years in the neonatal population in the form of phototherapy to diminish the effects of bilirubin.
  - Treats Seasonal Affective Disorder caused by limited daylight exposure.
- Sound and music
  - Premise: Sound enters the body through the ear and stimulates the thalamus.
  - Includes various instruments such as voice, harps, drums, and tuning forks; various musical types such as classical, jazz, and nature sounds.
  - Potential benefits include (dependent on type of music and individual's preferences):
    - Phonic stimulation.
    - Sonic camouflage.

TABLE 9.14

COMPLEMENTARY THERAPIES

Modality	Examples
Lifestyle therapies	■ Light and color ■ Sound and music ■ Aromatherapy ■ Kangaroo care ■ Hospice practices ■ Prenatal and perinatal psychology
Biomechanical therapies	■ Massage ■ Reflexology ■ Osteopathy/craniosacral ■ Chiropractic care
Bioenergetic therapies	■ Acupuncture ■ Reiki ■ Energy work ■ Healing touch ■ Distant intentionality/prayer
Biochemical therapies	■ Homeopathy ■ Herbal medicine

Source: National Center for Complementary and Alternative Medicine, National Institutes of Health.

■ Decrease agitation.
■ Diminish presurgical and postsurgical stress.
■ Increase in appetite.
■ Examples of use:
  ■ Infants prefer the voice of their mother to any other auditory stimuli during the first few days of life.
  ■ Classical music eases and changes a baby's NICU stay.
■ Aromatherapy
  ■ Premise: Alters an individual's mood or behavior through the use of aromatic and essential oils distilled from herbs and flowers. Neurotransmitters in the brain are released involuntarily and immediately, which results in a calming, sedative, pain-reducing, stimulatory or euphoric effect depending on the oil.
  ■ Potential benefits include:
    ■ Relaxation.
    ■ Renewed energy.
    ■ Enhanced pleasure.
    ■ Soothing fatigued muscles.
    ■ Relief of headaches.
    ■ Increased creativity.
  ■ Examples of use:
    ■ Lavender alleviates insomnia and helps ICU patients cope with stress.
    ■ Jasmine increases efficiency and relieves stress.
    ■ Peppermint provides a stimulant effect.
    ■ Aromatherapy is beginning to be used to produce calming or stimulating effects similar to the use of Muzak.
■ Kangaroo care
  ■ Premise: The baby and parent benefit from skin-to-skin contact.
  ■ Potential benefits include:
    ■ Promotes parent–infant bonding and attachment.
    ■ Fewer apnea and bradycardia spells.
    ■ Improves flexion and tone.
    ■ Thermoregulatory control.
    ■ Decreases the disorganization of the infant's sleep states.

■ Examples of use:
  ■ Primarily in the NICU; neonate (usually wearing nothing except a diaper) is held on the bare chest of the mother or father.

BIOMECHANICAL THERAPY

■ Massage
  ■ Premise: Relieves muscle tensions while reducing stress and evoking calm feelings.
  ■ Numerous types: Friction, kneading, containment, vibration, and percussion.
  ■ Potential benefits include:
    ■ Reduces muscle soreness and stiffness.
    ■ Increases range of motion.
    ■ Improves lymph drainage.
    ■ Decreases edema.
    ■ With infants, encourages early coordination by assisting the myelination of nerves.
  ■ Examples of use:
    ■ Massaged infants experience weight gain and better-organized sleep states.
    ■ Hand or foot massage for relaxation for palliative care patients
■ Reflexology
  ■ Premise: Reflex zones exist in the feet and hands specific to all parts, organs, glands, and functions of the human body. By applying pressure to the reflex points, the blood flow is stimulated to the surrounding zone; the body produces endorphins; and the body eliminates waste materials.
  ■ Potential benefits include:
    ■ Improved circulation.
    ■ Alleviated pain.
    ■ Stress relief.
    ■ Energy balance.
  ■ Examples of use:
    ■ Relief of headaches.
    ■ Relief of earaches.
    ■ Increase blood flow to specific body areas.
■ Craniosacral therapy
  ■ Premise: Involves "listening with the fingers" to the body's subtle rhythms and patterns of inertia or congestion.
  ■ Potential benefits include:
    ■ Encourages and enhances the body's own self-healing and self-regulating capabilities
  ■ Examples of use:
    ■ Relief of neonatal sucking/swallowing/reflux caused by a compressed vagus nerve.
    ■ Relief of recurrent otitis media caused by a temporal lobe malalignment.
    ■ Relief of headaches caused by sphenoid issues.

BIOENERGETIC THERAPY

■ Acupuncture/acupressure
  ■ Premise: The healing energy known as Chi circulates through the body along specific pathways referred to as meridians; obstructions in the flow of this energy cause disease states.
  ■ Acupressure, as opposed to acupuncture, is more popular in the pediatric patient because it does not involve the use of needles. Acupressure involves the application of pressure to stimulate the body's healing energy from the acupuncture points along the 14 major energy meridians.
  ■ Potential benefits include:
    ■ Changes in brain activity.
    ■ Improvements in blood chemistry values.

TABLE 9.15

APPROACH TO CONSIDERING COMPLEMENTARY AND ALTERNATIVE MEDICINES IN PEDIATRIC PALLIATIVE CARE

- Consider each practice separately, based on the specific situation.
- Gather data on safety.
- Gather data on efficacy.
- Elicit beliefs and preferences of the patient and family.
- Present appropriate recommendations to patient and family.
  - If there is sufficient evidence of unacceptable risk and efficacy data are lacking, advise against the practice.
  - If risk is uncertain and efficacy data are lacking, advise accordingly (that is, that a medical recommendation cannot be made).
  - If efficacy data are sufficient, balance risk information in the usual risk–benefit analysis and advise accordingly.

- Increased immune responses.
- Increased endocrine responses.
- Examples of use:
  - Anesthesia.
  - Postoperative pain management.
  - Addiction recovery.
- Reiki
  - Premise: Energy is transferred from and through the hands of a trained practitioner to an individual.
  - Potential benefits include:
    - Restores balance.
    - Increases the body's healing process.
    - Provides relaxation.
    - Reduces stress levels.
    - Relieves pain.
    - Enhances the feeling of overall well-being.
  - Examples of use:
    - Assist infants recovering from acute infections.
    - Pain management.
    - Appetite stimulant.

Neuhouser and associates note that 66% of children with cancer use some form of CAM (53). Complementary and alternative medicine includes self-care practices such as relaxation, which can be performed by an individual without assistance, and acupuncture or other interventions that are generally performed by a licensed practitioner who has met credentialing requirements. Many "therapies" and dietary supplements (including herbal remedies) are unregulated. The degree of scientific evidence supporting some of these practices is extensive; for others, however, it is entirely absent. Factors influencing individuals' choices of CAM interventions are poorly understood. Specific cultural practices and the belief systems upon which they are based should therefore be fully appreciated by the professional health care team, especially in the pediatric setting. Health care professionals are further advised to approach patients and families in a respectful and organized way when discussing CAM interventions (49). Tolerance of harmless CAM practices, encouragement of helpful practices, and knowledge of harmful practices or therapies is critical to effective patient-centered care (Table 9.15).

BIOCHEMICAL THERAPIES

- Herbal medicine
  - Premise: Natural plants, plant extracts, or plant preparations work with the body instead of against a disease.
  - Potential benefits include (dependent on herb type):
    - Few adverse side effects when used appropriately.
    - Relief of pain.
    - Relief of inflammation.
    - Relief of cramps or spasms.
    - Facilitates sleep.
    - Balances hormone levels.
    - Soothes inflamed mucous membranes or digestive tissues.
    - Increases the immune system's ability to fight.
  - Examples of use:
    - 25% of current pharmaceuticals are derived directly from plants.
    - Digitalis for congestive heart failure.
    - Echinacea as an immune stimulant.
    - Ginger diminishes nausea.
    - Caffeine for apnea and bradycardia in neonates.
    - Aloe vera for skin protection or use with skin irritations/burns.
    - Tea tree oil for antifungal purposes.

These modalities have become increasingly popular, and consumers are spending large amounts of personal money on CAM.

References

1. American Academy of Pediatrics, Committee on Bioethics and Committee on Hospital Care. Palliative care for children. *Pediatrics* 2000;106:351–357.
2. Foley K. The past and future of palliative care. Improving end of life care: why has it been so difficult? *Hastings Center Rep* 2005;35(6):S42–S46.
3. Hartman RG. Dying young: cues from the courts. *Arch Pediatr Adolesc Med* 2004;158:615–619.
4. American Academy of Pediatrics, Committee on Bioethics and Committee on Hospital Care. Palliative care for children. *Pediatrics* 2000;106:351–357.
5. Gilmer MJ. Pediatric palliative care: a family-centered model for critical care. *Crit Care Nurs Clin North Am* 2002;14:207–214.
6. Kane JR, Barber RG, Jordan M, et al. Supportive/palliative care of children suffering from life-threatening and terminal illness. *Am J Hospice Palliat Care* 2000;17:165–172.
7. Mack JW, Wolfe J. Early integration of pediatric palliative care: for some children, palliative care starts at diagnosis. *Curr Opin Pediatr* 2006;18:10–14.
8. Martinson ID. Improving care of dying children. *West J Med* 1995;163:258–262.
9. Arrig T. Beyond pain: the existential suffering of children. *J Palliat Care* 1996;12:20–23.
10. Speece MW, Brent SB. The development of children's understanding of death. In: Corr CA, Corr DM, eds. *Handbook of childhood death and bereavement.* New York: Springer; 1996:29–50.
11. Frager G. Children's concepts of death. In: Joishy SK, ed. *Palliative medicine secrets.* Philadelphia: Hanley & Belfus; 1999:170–171.
12. American Academy of Pediatrics, Committee on Psychosocial Aspects of Child and Family Health. The Pediatrician and childhood bereavement. *Pediatrics* 2000;105:445–447.
13. Mack JW, Wolfe J. Early integration of pediatric palliative care: for some children, palliative care starts at diagnosis. *Curr Opin Pediatr* 2006;18:10–14.

14. Buckman R. *How to break bad news: a guide for health care professionals.* Baltimore: Johns Hopkins University Press; 1992.

15. Von Gunten GF, Ferris FD, Emanuel L. Ensuring competency in end-of-life care communication and relational skills. *JAMA* 2000;284:3051–3057.

16. Hays RM, Haynes G, Geyer JR, et al. Communication at the end of life. In: Carter BS, Levetown M, eds. *Palliative care for infants, children, and adolescents.* Baltimore: Johns Hopkins University Press; 2004:112–140.

17. Perkin RM, Swift JD, Raper JT. *Primer on pediatric palliative care.* Greenville, NC: University Printing and Graphics of East Carolina University Press; 2005.

18. Duhn LJ, Melves JM. A systematic integrative review of infant pain assessment tools. *Adv Neonatol Care* 2004;4:126–140.

19. American Academy of Pediatrics, Committee on Psychosocial Aspects of Child and Family Health. The pediatrician and childhood bereavement. *Pediatrics* 1992;89:516–518.

20. Buchholz M, Karl HW, Pomietton, et al. Pain scores in infants: A modified pain scale versus visual analogue. *J Pain Symptom Manage* 1998;15:117.

21. Levetown M. Pediatric care: The inpatient/ICU perspective. In: Ferrell BR, Coyle N, eds. *Textbook of palliative nursing.* Oxford: Oxford University Press; 2001:570–583.

22. Wanzer SG, Federman DD, Adelstein SJ, et al. The physician's responsibility toward hopelessly ill patients: A second look. *N Engl J Med* 1989;320:844–849.

23. Levetown M, Liber S, Audet M. Palliative care in the pediatric intensive care unit. In: Carter BS, Levetown M, eds. *Palliative care for infants, children, and adolescents.* Baltimore: Johns Hopkins University Press; 2004:273–291.

24. McCallum DE, Byrne P, Bruera E. How children die in hospitals. *J Pain Symptom Manage* 2000;20:417–423.

25. Garros D, Rosychuk RJ, Cox PN. Circumstances surrounding end of life in a pediatric intensive care unit. *Pediatrics* 2003;112:e371–e379.

26. Perkin RM, Swift JD, Raper JT. *Primer on pediatric palliative care.* Greenville, NC: University Printing and Graphics of East Carolina University Press; 2005.

27. American Academy of Pediatrics, Committee on Child Abuse and Neglect and Committee on Bioethics. Forgoing life-sustaining medical treatment in abused children. *Pediatrics* 2000;106:1151–1153.

28. DiScala C, Sege R, Li G, et al. Child abuse and unintentional injuries. *Arch Pediatr Adolesc Med* 2000;154:11–15.

29. American Academy of Pediatrics, Committee on Bioethics and Committee on Hospital Care. Palliative care for children. *Pediatrics* 2000;106:351–357.

30. Freyer DR. Care of the dying adolescent: Special considerations. *Pediatrics* 2004;113:381–388.

31. Maggiolini A, Grassi R, Adamsil L, et al. Self-image of adolescent survivors of long-term childhood leukemia. *J Pediatr Hematol Oncol* 2000;22: 417–421.

32. American Academy of Pediatrics, Committee on Bioethics. Guidelines on forgoing life-sustaining medical treatment. *Pediatrics* 1994;93:532–536.

33. American Academy of Pediatrics, Committee on Bioethics. Informed consent, parental permission, and assent in pediatric practice. *Pediatrics* 1995; 95:314–317.

34. Collins JJ. Intractable pain in children with terminal cancer. *J Palliat Care* 1996;12:29–34.

35. Potter J, Hami F, Bryan T, et al. Symptoms in 400 patients referred to palliative care services: prevalence and patterns. *Palliat Med* 2003;17:310–314.

36. Stromgren AS, Groenvold M, Pedersen L, et al. Does the medical record cover the symptoms experienced by cancer patients receiving palliative care? *J Pain Symptom Manage* 2001;21:189–196.

37. Shah S, Davies AN. Medical records versus patient self-rating. *J Pain Symptom Manage* 2001;22:805–806.

38. Hunt AM. A survey of signs, symptoms and symptom control in 30 terminally ill children. *Dev Med Child Neurol* 1990;32:341–346.

39. Hain RD, Patel N, Crabtree S, et al. Respiratory symptoms in children dying from malignant disease. *Palliat Med* 1995;9:201–206.

40. Mallinson J, Jones PD. A 7-year review of deaths on the general pediatric wards at John Hunter Children's Hospital. *J Pediatr Child Health* 2000;36:252–255.

41. Wolfe J, Grier HE, Klar N, et al. Symptoms and suffering at the end of life in children with cancer. *N Engl J Med* 2000;342:326–333.

42. Liben S, Goldman A. Home care for children with life-threatening illness. *Palliat Care* 1998;14:33–38.

43. Collins JJ, Byrnes ME, Dunkel I, et al. The Memorial Symptom Assessment Scale (MSAS): validation study in children aged 10–18. *J Palliat Symptom Manage* 2000;19:363–377.

44. Collins JJ, Devine TB, Dick G, et al. The measurement of symptoms in young children with cancer: the validation of the Memorial Symptom Assessment Scale in children aged 7–12. *J Pain Symptom Manage* 2002;23:10–16.

45. Drake R, Frost J, Collins JJ. The symptoms of dying children. *J Pain Symptom Manage* 2003;25:1–10.

46. Kenny NP, Frager G. Refractory symptoms and terminal sedation of children: ethical issues and practical management. *J Palliat Care* 1996;12:30–45.

47. Fine PG. Total sedation in end-of-life care: clinical considerations. *J Hospice Palliat Nurs* 2001;3:81–87.

48. Lo B, Rubenfeld G. Palliative sedation in dying patients. *JAMA* 2005; 294:1810–1816.

49. Hain R, Weinstein S, Oleske J, et al. Holistic management of symptoms. In: Carter BJ, Levetown M, eds. *Palliative care for infants, children and adolescents.* Baltimore: Johns Hopkins University Press; 2004.

50. Jones JE, Kassity N. Varieties of alternative experience: Complementary care in the neonatal intensive care unit. *Clin Obstet Gynecol* 2001;44: 750–768.

51. Dollemore D, Giuliucci M, Haigh J, et al. New choices in natural healing. In: Gottlieb B, Berg S, Fisher P, eds. *Palliative care for Infants, Children and Adolesents* Emmaus, PA: Rodale Press; 1995.

52. White L, Foster S. *The herbal drugstore: the best natural alternatives to over-the counter and prescription medicines.* Emmaus, PA: Rodale Press; 2000.

53. Neuhouser ML, Patterson RE, Schwartz SM, et al. Use of alternative medicine by children with cancer in Washington state. *Prev Med* 2001;33: 347–354.

CHAPTER 10 ■ COMPLEMENTARY THERAPIES IN PEDIATRICS—LEGAL PERSPECTIVES

KATHI J. KEMPER AND MICHAEL H. COHEN

Pediatric use of complementary medical therapies raises complex issues at the borderland of medicine, law, and public policy. This chapter will provide illustrative cases, definitions of essential terms, an overview of the epidemiology of complementary therapies use in pediatrics, an ethical framework for addressing the use of such therapies in the hospital setting, a discussion of legal issues, and additional resources about this topic for hospital-based physicians.

ILLUSTRATIVE CASES

1. Walking into an 8-year-old patient's room, you notice several bottles of herbs and dietary supplements on the bedside table. When you ask, the patient's mother tells you that her son has not been sleeping well in the hospital, and she has been giving him valerian, melatonin, and kava kava to help him sleep. She thinks they have helped. What should you do?

2. Despite his medications, a 12-year-old oncology patient has suffered moderately severe nausea and vomiting during this admission. Her father says he has looked on the Internet, and noticed that acupuncture might help. He wants to know if there is an acupuncturist on staff who can help. If not, can he hire one to come in and treat his daughter while she is hospitalized?

3. A 10-year-old with recurrent migraine headaches is hospitalized for treatment of a femur fracture sustained in a car accident. He practices guided imagery and uses biofeedback at home to help prevent headaches. He asks if he can bring in his biofeedback software to the hospital and whether there is someone who can help him with his guided imagery to help manage his pain with less medication.

4. Your neonatal intensive care unit wants to start a massage program, and asks you to advise them on the legal issues involved in hiring someone to provide services and teach parents how to give infant massage. What do you do?

5. Several nurses in the pediatric intensive care unit provide therapeutic touch to patients. There have been no patient complaints; in fact, patients seem to enjoy receiving this therapy. However, there are no written policies in your hospital about this therapy, and some of your physician colleagues have expressed concern about continuing to let the nurses do this. What do you do?

6. The parents of a hospitalized child with treatable leukemia announce that they want to take their child home, start a vegetable fast, see a shamanic healer, and fly to Mexico for a new nontoxic cancer cure. What do you do?

DEFINITIONS

The National Center for Complementary and Alternative Medicine at the National Institutes of Health (NIH) defines complementary and alternative medicine (CAM) as "a group of diverse medical and health care systems, practices, and products that are not presently considered to be part of conventional medicine." Specifically, complementary therapies are used *together with* conventional medicine, not in place of it. An example of a complementary therapy is using aromatherapy to help lessen a patient's discomfort following surgery. The last example above, in which a family decides to abandon effective conventional care in favor of an unproven alternative for a life-threatening condition, is *not* complementary or integrative medicine; it is a case of *alternative* medicine, where more communication, counseling and possibly even intervention by the courts, may be necessary. Integrative medicine combines mainstream medical therapies and complementary therapies for which there is some scientific evidence of safety and effectiveness.

EPIDEMIOLOGY

Use of complementary therapies is common among children as well as adults. Rates of use are often over 50% among children with chronic, recurrent, and incurable conditions such as asthma, allergies, cancer, cystic fibrosis, HIV infection, inflammatory bowel disease, and special health care needs. These are exactly the kinds of children who are frequently hospitalized. The parents of pediatric patients do not necessarily tell physicians that they are providing these therapies, nor do they necessarily stop providing them when their child is hospitalized.

In a national survey of 745 pediatricians, 87% reported being asked by a patient (or parent) about one or more CAM therapies (1). Most pediatricians (73%) agreed that "It is the role of pediatricians to provide patients/families with information about all potential treatment options for the patient's condition"; and 54% agreed that "Pediatricians should consider the use of all potential therapies, not just those of mainstream medicine, when treating patients." The movement toward multidisciplinary care in pediatrics also provides opportunities for pediatricians to collaborate with other clinicians such as massage therapists, naturopaths, chiropractors, acupuncturists, and others. Increasingly, hospitals are including such practitioners among their professional staff. Thus, physicians caring for hospitalized children need to ask and appropriately counsel patients about using these therapies in conjunction with ongoing care. Clinicians providing complementary therapies are licensed to provide care in many states, but licensure varies by discipline and state. For example, chiropractors are licensed in all 50 states, and services are often reimbursed by insurance; however, few chiropractors provide inpatient services. On the other hand, acupuncturists are licensed in over 40 states, and over one-third of pediatric pain treatment programs in teaching hospitals provide acupuncture; however, regulations about provision of Chinese herbal medicine are quite variable. Massage therapists are licensed by fewer states, and regulated by municipalities in others. As of 2007, only a minority of states license naturopathic physicians or homeopathic practitioners, but the status of these clinicians is rapidly changing. Furthermore, insurance reimbursement and hospital credentialing for complementary therapies also varies widely and is changing over time. This heterogeneity complicates the legal and ethical situation for clinicians incorporating complementary therapies in the hospital setting.

ETHICAL PRINCIPLES

Several other chapters in this text cover the principles of medical ethics. However, several principles bear repeating. First, good ethics start with good facts. Because patients and families may not raise the issue spontaneously, clinicians need to ask routinely about their use of complementary therapies. Asking tends to be most effective when (1) questions are asked in a routine way along with questions about medications and allergies, (2) questions are asked nonjudgmentally and respectfully, and (3) examples are provided. For example, a clinician caring for a child hospitalized with asthma may say, "I know that as parents, you want to do whatever you can to help your child be as healthy as possible. In addition to prescription medications, some families try special herbs, massage, prayer, acupuncture, avoiding certain foods and things like that. What have you tried, and how has that worked for your child?" When the parents respond that they have used complementary health products, ask them to bring them in so you can check the ingredient lists and manufacturer and make sure your records are complete and up to date.

Given the extent to which parents provide herbs and dietary supplements to their children, clinicians should (1) be aware of resources to identify potential drug interactions, toxicity, and adverse reactions; (2) be aware of potential benefits that may be associated with supplements; (3) inform patients that health problems from herbs and supplements can arise, from contamination, misidentification, and inaccurate labeling; and (4) caution families that expressing children's dosages for dietary supplements as a fraction of adult dosages is "strictly anecdotal" and may not truly be the optimal dose for the child.

Physicians also need to be aware of their institutions' policies about the use of home supply of medications, nonprescription products, herbs, dietary supplements, and devices. In a recent study, none of the states surveyed had laws concerning parental provision of complementary therapies to children (2). Hospital policies vary widely across different institutions and are changing over time. Once a physician knows that using certain products falls within institutional policies and guidelines, she may ethically advise the family about using complementary therapies using a simple 2 3 2 framework (Table 10.1).

TABLE 10.1

ETHICAL ADVICE ABOUT COMPLEMENTARY THERAPIES

		Effective	
		Yes	No/Unknown
Safe	Yes	Recommend	Tolerate
	No	Monitor	Avoid

Physicians should inquire whether the medical evidence (1) supports both safety and efficacy; (2) supports safety, but evidence regarding efficacy is inconclusive; (3) supports efficacy, but evidence regarding safety is inconclusive; or (4) indicates either serious risk or inefficacy. Within this framework, physicians can (1) recommend the CAM therapy; (2) allow patient use of the CAM therapy, but monitor efficacy; (3) allow patient use of the CAM therapy, but monitor safety; or (4) avoid and discourage use of the CAM therapy (3).

A key to this framework is continuing to monitor the patients closely, since most complementary therapies will fall in regions (2) and (3). Physicians must be aware that complementary therapies can shift regions as the medical evidence changes. For example, many herbal products once were considered safe (e.g., St. John's Wort) though of uncertain efficacy, whereas now evidence of both safety under certain conditions (e.g., St. John's Wort and indinavir) as well as efficacy is being questioned. Clinicians accordingly are responsible for monitoring the literature and framing decisions accordingly.

EFFICACY

Several studies have suggested potential efficacy for some CAM therapies in pediatrics (3), such as use of acupuncture for patients with chronic, severe pain (4); massage therapy to lower anxiety and stress hormones and improve the clinical course in infants and children with various medical conditions (5); and hypnosis, guided imagery, and biofeedback for pain (6).

SAFETY

On the other hand, complementary therapies may cause either direct or indirect harm. Direct harm includes direct toxic effects, poor nutrition, and interrupting or postponing beneficial therapies, while indirect harm can include an unwarranted financial and emotional burden. Case reports involving harm from use of CAM therapies include a chemical burn caused by topical vinegar application in a newborn infant (7); fatal hypermagnesemia in a child treated with megavitamin/megamineral therapy (7); multiple organ failure after ingestion of pennyroyal oil from herbal tea (8); lead encephalopathy due to herbal medicine and dietary supplements from developing countries, such as Ayurvedic remedies from India (9); quadriplegia after chiropractic manipulation in an infant with congenital torticollis (10); brucellosis from the treatment of a juvenile rheumatoid arthritis with intradermal injections of folk medicines (11); and one case of an infant developing botulism after being given home-grown chamomile tea (12). As the above suggests, most common side effects for CAM therapies are reported from herbs and other dietary supplements.

Other therapies such as massage, meditation, hypnosis, guided imagery, therapeutic touch, Reiki, prayer and homeopathy are extremely safe when they do not delay standard medical care.

If the CAM therapies selected are known to be unsafe or ineffective based on the medical literature, the physician should discourage them; if parents persist, and the child's life is thereby endangered, then reporting and state action may be appropriate. On the other hand, assuming that the clinical situation is not life-threatening, the complementary therapy will not delay imminently necessary medical care, and the therapy is not known to be unsafe or ineffective, then the pediatrician may continue to monitor the patient while the complementary therapy is provided. If the physician is uncomfortable with this role, rather than abandon the patient, the pediatrician may wish to find another physician who is able to supervise care.

PROFESSIONAL PRINCIPLES

Physicians may be concerned about the risk of being perceived as unprofessional in their conduct if they recommend or discuss complementary therapies. In some states, the definition of professional misconduct includes any clinical practice that departs from "acceptable and prevailing standards of care" (13). In response to narrow interpretations of this language, at least a dozen states enacted "medical freedom" statutes to protect physicians against the possibility of medical board discipline merely for recommending or delivering CAM therapies. In addition, a number of state medical boards have adopted regulations clarifying that incorporating CAM therapies by itself is not a sufficient departure from prevailing standards to warrant physician discipline (14).

Furthermore, the United States Federation of State Medical Boards (Federation) guidelines state that merely using complementary therapies does not constitute grounds for discipline. The guidelines, however, require that the selected complementary therapies are likely to provide "a favorable risk/benefit ratio compared to other treatments for the same condition"; be "based upon a reasonable expectation that it will result in a favorable patient outcome, including preventive practices"; and be based upon the expectation that a greater benefit than harm will result. Even if evidence of either safety or efficacy is inconclusive, risks to the practitioner and the patient are lessened if the patient continues to be monitored and the clinician is ready to intervene when necessary.

The authors have found no reported judicial decisions involving review of medical board discipline of a pediatrician under either the Federation guidelines or the applicable rules of a state medical board; nor have the authors learned about expulsion of any AAP member for using complementary therapies.

LEGAL PRINCIPLES

When advising patients concerning complementary therapies, physicians may also be concerned about legal risks such as malpractice. Malpractice is defined as unskillful practice that fails to conform to a standard of care in the profession, and thereby results in patient injury. It can be grounds for a civil lawsuit by an injured patient, and/or in professional discipline by the state medical board. New statutory language in several states clarifies that use of CAM therapies does not in itself constitute disciplinary grounds.

To minimize their risk and facilitate the provision of optimal comprehensive care, pediatricians should ask themselves several questions: (1) Are the parents abandoning effective care when the child's condition is serious or life-threatening? (2) Will use of the complementary therapy delay imminently necessary conventional treatment? (3) Is the complementary therapy known to be unsafe and/or ineffective? (4) Have the proper parties consented to the use of this therapy? (5) Is the

risk–benefit ratio of the proposed therapy acceptable to a reasonable, similarly situated clinician, and does the therapy have at least minority acceptance or support in the medical literature? (3).

RISKS WHEN REFERRING TO ANOTHER CLINICIAN

When making referrals, physicians should become familiar with the provider's credentials and (to the extent reasonably feasible) history of malpractice and professional discipline. If the treatment plan involves a therapy that is known to be unsafe and ineffective, referral is inadvisable, even if the therapist is licensed, has good credentials, and has no history of malpractice or professional disciplinary problems.

There are legal risks involved in referral to a CAM provider who turns out to be negligent. The general rule is that a physician is not liable for the negligence of the provider to whom a patient has been referred except when (1) the referral itself was negligent, because it caused harm by delaying necessary conventional treatment; (2) the referring provider knew or should have known that the CAM provider was "incompetent"; and (3) the physician had hired the CAM provider, or engaged in a highly coordinated "joint treatment" with that provider (15). As new models of "integrative" health care evolve, courts are increasingly likely to apply this "joint treatment" exception.

COULD USE OF COMPLEMENTARY THERAPIES BE CONSIDERED ABUSIVE OR NEGLECTFUL?

Because pediatricians are subject to the legal and ethical reporting requirements relating to child abuse and neglect, a pediatrician who accedes to parental demands for complementary therapies may feel caught between the impetus to please patients, the prospect of malpractice liability if the therapy fails, professional discipline for providing the requested therapy, and reporting of abuse and neglect by another pediatrician. Negotiating an evidence-based, family-centered outcome in such a charged context may be difficult. There have been few court cases concerning abuse and neglect involving complementary therapies. Generally, courts have been reluctant to overrule parental choice of treatment, except in life-threatening clinical situations when conventional care is imminently necessary (3).

In life-threatening clinical situations involving children, parents rejecting conventional care have faced prosecution for abuse and neglect (and/or child endangerment and homicide), and removal of the child from parental custody and transfer to a state authority such as the department of public welfare. In the most drastic cases, and upon clear and convincing evidence of neglect, courts have terminated parental rights and allowed adoption.

INFORMED CONSENT

As with other therapies, informed consent is required for treatment involving complementary therapies where informing the patient about such therapies will make a difference in the patient's choice of treatment. Parents or legal guardians typically are asked to provide informed permission for diagnosis and treatment of children, with the assent of the child whenever appropriate. In most states adolescents within a certain age range are considered mature minors who can consent to medical treatment.

Because the absence of adequate informed consent can be a basis for a malpractice claim, it is important to provide pediatric patients (and their families) with all information relevant to a treatment decision involving complementary therapies. Informed consent also can provide an opportunity to show sensitivity to and respect for the religious, cultural, or personal beliefs and practices of the family. Written informed consent to, and an assumption of risk regarding, complementary therapies may, in some states, provide a defense to malpractice, if the therapy is reasonably safe and effective and provided with careful clinical judgment (3).

A family-centered approach, using spiritual and psychological support, attention to the child's feelings, and concerns about the likely effects of treatment, is particularly appropriate to consideration of complementary therapies in the pediatric setting.

LIABILITIES AND RISKS FOR NOT ADVISING PATIENTS ABOUT COMPLEMENTARY THERAPEUTIC OPTIONS

The authors are not aware of legal cases involving suits by families against physicians who fail to offer or refer children for complementary therapies. It is possible that such cases might arise, as evidence about the efficacy of integrating complementary therapies grows and the standard of care shifts toward greater integration of these therapies in conventional hospital settings.

RESPONSES TO SPECIFIC THERAPIES IN CASES ABOVE

Physicians should ask all hospitalized patients about their use of herbs and dietary supplements, chart this information in the medical record, and check for known risks of side effects and interactions with the patients' medications. Do not ignore bottles of supplements sitting on bedside tables as in the first case described at the start of the chapter. Physicians should be familiar with their hospital's policy about use of home supply of nonformulary herbs and dietary supplements, and advise patients and families accordingly. These discussions should be documented in the medical record.

Physicians should also ask hospitalized patients about their use of other complementary therapies and therapists, and respond to families' questions such as the one about acupuncture services for children suffering from pain or nausea (Case 2). Generally, only therapists who have hospital privileges may provide care to patients during hospitalization. Increasing numbers of hospitals do have acupuncturists on staff and a credentialing policy in place. For those that do not have credentialed licensed acupuncturists, physicians may discuss with families the use of acupressure band devices including evidence of their effectiveness, safety, and potential contraindications to their use.

If the child's condition is not serious or life-threatening, the use of complementary therapies is unlikely to result in liability, unless the child is diverted from imminently necessary, conventional care and thereby injured. Thus, a time-limited trial of the proposed strategy may be appropriate. If the strategy involves referral to a licensed clinician, legal risk may be reduced if the steps suggested earlier are taken, and with the caveat that the referring pediatrician should continue monitoring the child and continue conventional treatment. The complementary provider should have hospital privileges to practice within the scope of his professional license in order to provide such services in the hospital setting.

Increasing numbers of hospitals also have psychologists or licensed professional counselors or pediatricians who can assist patients using guided imagery, as requested by the family of the 10-year-old with migraine headaches hospitalized with a femur fracture (Case 3). We are unaware of hospital policies limiting the use of devices such as computer-game–based biofeedback programs.

Increasingly, hospital nurseries are offering massage therapy for babies and massage classes for new parents (Case 4). It is important to ensure that those offering these therapies are properly credentialed and licensed to do so, and have undergone appropriate hospital training (e.g., covering HIPAA regulations and bloodborne pathogen control). Appropriately educating the existing staff through regular, experiential in-service training programs can help minimize the resistance to incorporating these therapies into routine care.

Many nursing schools offer classes in therapeutic touch and healing touch, and these practices are covered under nursing scope of practice (Case 5). Nurses and other hospital-based clinicians who provide these services should write and submit policy and procedure descriptions about them as they would with any other nursing procedure. As with massage services, health professionals who provide therapeutic touch, healing touch, or related biofield therapies should offer to demonstrate the techniques to physicians and other hospital-based health care professionals to familiarize them with the procedures, indications, and contraindications, and provide periodic in-service training to the nursing staff to better facilitate integrated care.

When parents of a hospitalized child with a treatable condition announce that they want to abandon effective care and instead seek alternatives (Case 6), physicians need to engage in a respectful dialogue, listening to the parents' needs, values, and perspectives; sharing in their concern for the child; and expressing their expert opinion on how the child's health needs can best be met. At times, it is helpful to bring in additional parties such as family friends, pastors, nurses, other health care providers, or the hospital ethics team to ensure that the discussions remain patient centered, respectful, and constructive. Respectful communication usually resolves these differences, and allows children to receive optimal care with agreement and collaboration among all those caring for them. If, however, after careful and thorough discussion, the parents insist on abandoning effective care for a life-threatening condition, legal intervention may be warranted.

SUMMARY

Use of complementary medical therapies is common and growing, even in hospital settings. Parents are providing these therapies to their children, and an increasing number of hospitals include complementary care providers on their medical staff. Clinicians should routinely ask about families' use of such therapies, be familiar with resources to answer common questions, and understand their own hospital policies regarding use of home supply of supplements as well as the availability of complementary therapists. Risks are minimized by understanding the effectiveness and safety of different therapies, and applying common-sense guidelines to recommending, tolerating, monitoring, or avoiding complementary therapies.

Resources for Pediatricians

Articles

Cohen MH, Hrbek A, Davis RB, et al. Emerging credentialing practices, malpractice liability policies, and guidelines governing complementary and alternative medical practices and dietary supplement recommendations. *Arch Intern Med* 2005;165:289–295.

Cohen MH, Kemper KJ. Complementary therapies in pediatrics: a legal perspective. *Pediatrics* 2005;115:774–780.

Cohen MH, Kemper KJ, Stevens L, et al. Pediatric use of complementary therapies: ethical and policy choices. *Pediatrics* 2005;116:568–575.

Committee on Children with Disabilities, American Academy of Pediatrics. Counseling families who choose complementary and alternative medicine for their child with chronic illness or disability. *Pediatrics* 2001;107:598–601.

Websites

Federation of State Medical Boards. Guidelines for physician use of complementary and alternative medical practice. Available at http://www.fsmb.org.

Institute of Medicine has convened a Committee on Use of Complementary and Alternative Therapies by the American Public. Available at http://www.iom.edu/cam.

National Institutes of Health, National Center for Complementary and Alternative Medicine. Available at http://nccam.nih.gov.

White House Commission on Complementary and Alternative Medicine Policy. Final report. Available at http://www.whccamp.org.

References

1. Kemper KJ, O'Connor KG. Pediatricians' recommendations for complementary and alternative medical (CAM) therapies. *Ambul Pediatr* 2004; 4:482–487.

2. Cohen MH, Hrbek A, Davis RB, et al. Emerging credentialing practices, malpractice liability policies, and guidelines governing complementary and alternative medical practices and dietary supplement recommendations: a descriptive study of 19 integrative health care centers in the United States. *Arch Intern Med* 2005; 165:289–295.

3. Cohen MH, Kemper KJ. Complementary therapies in pediatrics: a legal perspective. *Pediatrics* 2005;115:774–780.

4. Kemper K. Complementary and alternative medical therapies. In: Schechter NL, Berde CB, Yaster M, eds. *Pain in Infants, Children and Adolescents.* Lippincott, Williams and Wilkins; 2002:449–461.

5. Hernandez-Reif M, Field T, Krasnego J, et al. Children with cystic fibrosis benefit from massage therapy. *J Pediatr Psychol* 1999;24:175–181.

6. Jacobs J, Jiminez LM, Gloyd SS, et al. Treatment of acute childhood diarrhea with homeopathic medicine: a randomized clinical trial in Nicaragua. *Pediatrics* 1994;93:719–725.

7. Korkmaz A, Sahiner U, Yurdakok M. Chemical burn caused by topical vinegar application in a newborn infant. *Pediatr Dermatol* 2000;17:34–36.

8. McGuire JK, Kulkarni MS, Baden HP. Fatal hypermagnesemia in a child treated with megavitamin/megamineral therapy. *Pediatrics* 2000; 105:E18.

9. Coppes MJ, Anderson RA, Egler RM, et al. Alternative therapies for the treatment of childhood cancer. *N Engl J Med* 1998;339:846–847.

10. Yu EC, Yeung CY. Lead encephalopathy due to herbal medicine. *Chin Med J (Engl)* 1987;100:915–917.

11. Bose A, Vashistha K, O'Loughlin BJ. Azarcon por empacho—another cause of lead toxicity. *Pediatrics* 1983;72:106–108.

12. Montoya-Cabrera MA, Rubio-Rodriquez S, Velazquez-Gonzalez E, et al. Mercury poisoning caused by a homeopathic drug. *Gac Med Mex* 1991; 127:267–170.

13. Cohen MH. *Complementary and alternative medicine: legal boundaries and regulatory perspectives.* Baltimore: Johns Hopkins University Press; 1998.

14. Cohen MH. *Future medicine: ethical dilemmas, regulatory challenges, and therapeutic pathways to health and human healing in human transformation.* Ann Arbor: University of Michigan Press; 2003.

15. Cohen MH, Eisenberg DM. Potential physician malpractice liability associated with complementary and integrative medical therapies. *Ann Intern Med* 2002;136:596–603.

CHAPTER 11 ■ ABDOMINAL MASS

ROYTESA R. SAVAGE AND MELISSA C. BRINN

The discovery of an abdominal mass is concerning for both parents and practitioners. The differential diagnosis is long, but can often be focused with a careful history and physical exam. There are specific disease and nondisease processes that have typical patterns based on age, sex, and location of the mass in the abdomen. A careful evaluation of the pediatric patient with an abdominal mass can lead to a cost-effective, safe evaluation for the patient, followed by appropriate referrals and/or interventions.

The abdominal cavity houses the majority of the body's solid organs. Correspondingly, masses often originate in the intestines, kidneys, liver, and spleen. The stomach, pancreas, adrenal glands, gallbladder, and the female sex organs can also cause abdominal masses. Stool in the intestines can cause uncomfortable but very benign abdominal masses that can extend from the suprapubic area to past the umbilicus.

The history obtained from the child or caregiver will help to establish the signs and symptoms associated with the mass as well as how the mass was discovered and the known duration of existence. Weight loss, fever, pallor, pain, anorexia, and change in bowel or bladder habits are some important history questions. Often, the physical exam can localize the mass to a specific region in the abdomen. Size and consistency of the mass provide additional information, as do any other associated signs of illness. On exam, many masses can be outlined and marked on the skin or measured such that later growth in size or change in position can be detected.

DIFFERENTIAL DIAGNOSIS

The differential diagnosis can be narrowed by age—neonate, infant or child, or adolescent (Table 11.1). Furthermore, the location of the mass, such as flank, midabdomen, or suprapubic region, needs to be considered. Also, helpful in narrowing a differential diagnosis, are related systemic symptoms, localized tenderness or hepatosplenomegaly.

In the healthy term newborn, the most common causes of abdominal masses are renal in origin, including multicystic kidney dysplasia, polycystic kidney, or hydronephrosis. Many are diagnosed prenatally on ultrasound. In the preterm or sick infant, necrotizing enterocolitis can present with palpable loops of bowel, or present with a palpable kidney secondary to renal vein thrombosis complicating dehydration or placement of an umbilical vein catheter. In the newborn who has not passed stool, a palpable left colon can represent a distal obstruction by meconium. Less commonly a tumor of the liver including giant hemangiomas or other masses (e.g., neuroblastoma) can present in the newborn. Bladder distention can be a presenting sign of urinary tract obstruction, most commonly due to posterior urethral valves.

In infants, most abdominal masses are nonmalignant and are renal in origin. Renal vein thrombosis, multicystic kidney disease, and hydronephrosis are common etiologies. The most common cause of malignant abdominal mass is neuroblastoma in this age group. Wilms tumor, soft tissue sarcomas, germ cell tumors, and hepatoblastoma are other less common malignant tumors in this age group. Palpable stool can also present as an abdominal mass. Neuroblastoma is the most common extracranial solid tumor in childhood.

In children, Wilms tumor becomes a more common malignancy than neuroblastoma. Sarcoma and germ cell tumors are also common. More innocent masses such as palpable stool in the left lower quadrant are quite common and can usually be diagnosed with a good history and physical exam. Hepatoblastoma makes up 80% of the primary malignancies of the liver in children.

In adolescents, the range of possibilities increases to include pregnancy, ovarian torsion, and abscess. Wilms tumor and neuroblastoma are rare, but lymphoma, sarcoma, and germ cell tumors increase in frequency.

EVALUATION

The evaluation of the abdominal mass should always begin with a thorough history and physical exam. After a complete history and physical exam, further laboratory and imaging can help to diagnose the origin of the mass.

Laboratory investigation should begin with a complete blood cell count, which may show signs of anemia or a malignant process. Chemistries should be obtained to help determine electrolyte disturbances, ascertain renal function, and evaluate liver function. It is important to evaluate renal function before administering IV contrast material for radiologic studies. A urinalysis is also indicated. Other more specific lab testing (e.g., catecholamine or molecular markers) may be necessary, and selection is guided by the initial differential diagnosis. The type of radiologic studies ordered will depend on the most likely origin of the mass, based on physical exam, age, presentation of the child, and initial laboratory evaluation.

Abdominal X-Ray

Abdominal x-ray is a useful initial tool, especially if an abdominal ultrasound with an experienced ultrasonographer is not readily available. There are limitations specifically in evaluating the mass itself. The x-ray is very useful when constipation is high on the differential diagnosis, or to evaluate the neonate for enlarged bladder or signs of necrotizing enterocolitis. In the case of tumors, they may appear as stippled calcification on the radiograph, warranting further studies.

Abdominal Ultrasonography

Abdominal ultrasonography is usually an excellent initial evaluation for an abdominal mass. It does not usually require sedation, and avoids the radiation exposure of x-rays or CT

TABLE 11.1

DIFFERENTIAL DIAGNOSIS OF ABDOMINAL MASSES BY AGE

	Neonates	Infants and children	Adolescents
Genitourinary	Hydronephrosis[a] Renal vein thrombosis Polycystic kidney disease[a] Multicystic kidney disease[a] Bladder distention[a] Hydrocolpos Hematocolpos	Hydronephrosis Renal malformation Bladder distention[a]	Pregnancy[a] Bladder distention[a] Ovarian cyst Ovarian torsion Tuboovarian abscess Endometriosis Hydrometrocolpos
Tumors	Hepatoblastoma Hemangioma Teratoma Congenital mesoblastic nephroma[a]	Wilms tumor[a] Neuroblastoma[a] Rhabdomyosarcoma Hepatoblastoma Lymphoma	Lymphoma Ovarian tumors
Gastrointestinal	Storage diseases Choledochal cyst Bowel duplication Mesenteric cyst Volvulus Gallbladder hydrops	Feces[a] Pyloric stenosis Intussusception Choledochal cyst Duplication cyst Mesenteric cyst Pancreatic pseudocyst Abscess	Feces[a] Regional enteritis Abscess Pancreatic pseudocyst Choledochal cyst
Other	Adrenal hemorrhage Anterior meningocele		Parasitic infections Aortic aneurysm

[a]Common

scans. Ultrasonography can characterize a mass as solid or cystic, and may help determine the extent of the tumor. A child's fatty tissues usually also enhance the diagnostic detail of the exam. The pylorus can be visualized and sizes and consistencies of the other organs can be assessed. Quality can be limited by the experience and skills of the technician and/or supervising radiologist. Visualization of the mass can also be obscured by loops of air-filled bowel.

Barium Enema

Barium enema is the study of choice when intussusception or Hirshsprung disease is suspected. Barium enema may also be useful if extension of the mass (e.g., malignancy) into the gastrointestinal tract is a consideration. With the associated risk of perforation, prior to requesting a barium enema, consultation about appropriate imaging procedures should occur with the pediatric radiologist and the pediatric surgeon.

Computed Tomography (CT) or Magnetic Resonance Imaging (MRI)

CT and MRI have become essential in evaluation of abdominal masses. Such imaging often provides information about size, location, and consistency of the mass. A CT scan with and without IV contrast can help define the extent of the mass, but often is unable to determine if a tumor extends into the spinal canal. At times, CT scans that include the chest, abdomen, and pelvis are helpful in defining extension and infiltration when malignancy is felt to be likely. An MRI provides better soft tissue definition and may help in differentiating the mass from surrounding normal tissue and in visualization of spinal column involvement. MRI also adds information about other masses, metastases, or accompanying problems.

MANAGEMENT

Management is determined by the underlying disease process. For example, the common issue of constipation can be handled by the primary care physician, while other diagnoses (e.g., tumors) require consultation with other pediatric subspecialists. Occasionally, diagnosis cannot be made by noninvasive testing (e.g., gastric duplication), and the pediatric surgeon may need to be consulted to make a diagnosis.

PEARLS

- Wilms tumor is frequently discovered as a nontender abdominal mass by parents while bathing the child.
- Adolescents must have a careful sexual history taken. Their differential diagnosis list must include pregnancy and lymphadenopathy from sexually transmitted diseases.
- History and physical exam guide the initial evaluation process aided by laboratory work-up and imaging studies.
- Most abdominal masses in children should be considered a malignancy until proven otherwise.
- Abdominal masses are commonly an incidental finding.
- Infants commonly have a palpable abdominal mass, subsequently found to be a distended bladder.

Suggested Readings

Chandler JC, Gauderer MW. The neonate with an abdominal mass. *Pediatr Clin North Am* 2004;51:979–997.
Golden CB, Feusner JH. Malignant abdominal masses in children: quick guide to evaluation and diagnosis. *Pediatr Clin North Am* 2002;49:1369–1392.

CHAPTER 12 ■ APNEA

JUDITH A. LUCAS

Apnea is defined as a cessation of inspiratory gas flow for more than 20 seconds in an infant, or for a shorter period of time if there is associated cyanosis, pallor, or bradycardia. A careful history is often very helpful in determining the underlying cause of apnea. Apnea may in fact be the presenting symptom of a life-threatening condition. Therefore, the clinician must be familiar with the various causes of apnea in the infant and child, the initial diagnostic evaluation, and proper methods of stabilization and treatment.

TYPES OF APNEA

Apnea has been classified into three types depending on whether respiratory muscle effort is present.

Obstructive Apnea

In obstructive apnea, inspiratory effort is present. However, there is absent air flow due to obstruction of the upper airway. There is usually an anatomic cause, such as tonsillar and adenoidal hypertrophy, craniofacial abnormalities, micrognathia, or muscular hypotonia.

Central Apnea

In central apnea, respiratory effort is absent. There is often an underlying neurologic cause or severe systemic illness, such as sepsis.

Mixed Apnea

Apnea of prematurity is the most common type in an infant and is related to both central and obstructive causes. There are both immature brainstem regulation of respiration and inadequate mechanisms to maintain airway patency. The onset is usually gradual over the first week of life, with episodes increasing in frequency over time. A sudden increase in the number and severity of apneic episodes in a preterm infant suggests another etiology, such as infection or intracranial hemorrhage.

APNEA IN THE PRETERM INFANT

There are many different underlying causes for apnea in the premature infant. In *idiopathic apnea of prematurity*, there is no clear predisposing disease. The incidence varies inversely with gestational age. Generally, apnea develops between days 2 and 7 of life. Bradycardia may develop during prolonged apneic spells. Affected infants should be placed on apnea

monitors. For infants with mild or infrequent spells, cutaneous stimulation may be adequate therapy. For infants with more severe or frequent apneic spells, therapy with caffeine or theophylline may be necessary. Vital signs need to be closely monitored, and oxygenation maintained, especially with concomitant bradycardia. Treatment of anemia, either with transfusion or with erythropoietin, has been shown to be beneficial in reducing the severity and duration of apneic episodes. Some infants with severe episodes of apnea will require ventilatory support with nasal CPAP or even mechanical ventilation.

When infants reach the equivalent of 34 to 36 weeks of gestation, most will have resolved this disorder. Apnea of prematurity is not a risk factor for future development of sudden infant death syndrome. Any infant with apnea on the first day of life, after 2 weeks of age, or associated with clinical deterioration, likely has an underlying cause for apnea and should be evaluated. The list of possible causes is summarized in Table 12.1.

APNEA IN THE INFANT AND CHILD

Many infants are brought to medical attention for evaluation of an apparent life-threatening event (ALTE). The clinician must obtain a complete history regarding the prior health status of the child, and detailed information regarding the event and any resuscitation that has taken place. In approximately one-half of cases, an identifiable cause can be determined from history alone. A list of possible causes of apnea in the infant and child can be found in Table 12.2.

Evaluation

A careful, detailed history can be extremely helpful in elucidating the underlying cause of apnea. One must first review the child's prior health and developmental history. A report of antecedent fever, poor feeding, and decreased activity points to a possible infectious cause. Respiratory syncytial virus (RSV) has been known to cause apnea in small infants, and the apnea often precedes the febrile, catarrhal phase of the illness. Infants with pertussis are also prone to develop apnea, especially if they are incompletely immunized. Children with chronic upper respiratory infections are prone to develop tonsillar and adenoidal hypertrophy. Parents often report that their child snores loudly, struggles to breathe at night, and has breathing pauses during sleep. Due to disordered sleep/wake cycles, affected children may also develop nocturnal enuresis. There may also be excessive daytime somnolence, irritability, and declining school performance. It is important to note the physiologic effects of apnea, as listed below:

■ Decrease in arterial oxygen tension
■ Increase in carbon dioxide
■ Decrease in heart rate

TABLE 12.1

CAUSES OF APNEA IN THE PRETERM INFANT

Infection
Bacterial, viral, or fungal sepsis, meningitis, necrotizing enterocolitis (NEC)

Respiratory
Pneumonia, pneumothorax, atelectasis, respiratory distress syndrome, phrenic nerve paralysis, vocal cord paralysis, laryngotracheomalacia

Central Nervous System (CNS)
Intraventricular hemorrhage (IVH), asphyxia, seizures, medications (e.g., morphine), hydrocephalus, herniation, neuromuscular disorders

Gastrointestinal
Gastroesophageal reflux, esophagitis, NEC, intestinal perforation, passage of feeding tube

Cardiovascular
Patent ductus arteriosus, hypotension, hypertension, temperature instability, anemia, hypovolemia, hemorrhagic shock, heart failure, persistent pulmonary hypertension

Metabolic
Hypoglycemia, hypocalcemia, hypoxemia, hypernatremia, hyponatremia, acidosis

Idiopathic (Apnea of Prematurity)
Immature central regulation, abnormal response to hypoxia/hypercarbia, upper airway collapse

TABLE 12.2

CAUSES OF APNEA IN THE INFANT AND CHILD

Infection
Bacterial sepsis, meningitis, pertussis, respiratory syncytial virus (RSV), and other respiratory viruses

Respiratory
Airway abnormality, tonsillar and adenoidal hypertrophy, vascular ring, pulmonary sling, pneumonia, breath-holding spell, foreign body aspiration

Gastrointestinal
Gastroesophageal reflux, esophagitis, anaphylactic reaction to milk protein

Neurologic
Seizure disorder, meningitis, encephalitis, Chiari II malformation, vasovagal response, hydrocephalus, brain tumor

Cardiovascular
Arrhythmias, congestive heart failure, anaphylactic shock

Trauma/Abuse
Shaken baby syndrome, closed head injury, toxic ingestion, pediatric condition falsification

- Decrease in peripheral blood flow
- Increase in venous pressure and pulmonary arterial pressure
- Decrease in muscle tone

Chronic obstructive sleep apnea is particularly worrisome in young children due to the potential development of hypercarbia, pulmonary hypertension, and right-sided congestive heart failure. Breath-holding spells typically occur in young toddlers. The toddler is usually upset or frightened, and then holds his breath for a brief period of time. The child may become pale, cyanotic, or even lose consciousness briefly (see Chapter 13). Children with underlying airway abnormalities often have a history of stridor, cough, or an unusual-sounding cry. Sudden choking or coughing may indicate a possible foreign body aspiration (see Chapter 39a).

A feeding history is particularly important in any infant with apnea. Infants with GERD typically choke, cough, and spit up following feeds, especially if placed in the supine position. Irritability either during or after a feed suggests reflux esophagitis. Rarely, children with milk-protein allergy will present with apnea, pallor, or cyanosis with feeding.

A report of unusual movements associated with an apneic episode may indicate a possible seizure disorder. The child's developmental history should also be reviewed, looking for either a delay or loss of milestones. Review of growth data, especially a sudden increase in head circumference, may indicate developing hydrocephalus, subdural hematomas (seen in abuse), or even a brain tumor. Profound irritability, lethargy, and seizures raise the possibility of encephalitis. The type II Chiari brainstem malformation is characterized by progressive hydrocephalus and a myelomeningocele. Approximately 10% of type II malformations produce symptoms during infancy, including stridor, weak cry, and apnea, which may be relieved by shunting or decompression of the fourth ventricle.

A history of progressive dyspnea with feeds or exertion points to a possible cardiac abnormality. A family history of arrhythmia or sudden cardiac death suggests the possibility of a dysrhythmia. The child's heart rate and blood pressure need to be carefully monitored.

Apnea may be the presenting feature of several different forms of child abuse. First, the child who sustains a closed head injury as a result of being shaken may present with apnea related to seizure activity, diffuse axonal injury, or herniation. Alternatively, pediatric condition falsification (PCF; also Münchausen by Proxy, MBP) is a pattern of behavior in which a caretaker deliberately fabricates, exaggerates, or induces illness in a child to gain some form of personal gratification. A review of resuscitation efforts may indicate if in fact the infant experienced true physiologic changes. It is sometimes helpful to gather information from other household members and even EMS staff. In the setting of MBP, infants who "stop breathing" are at times intentionally smothered, drugged, or have had their noses occluded. A careful examination of the head and neck looking for signs of trauma is critical in these cases. The parent may also give a history of seeking medical care from multiple providers or emergency departments (see Chapter 139).

Diagnostic Testing and Management

First and foremost, the child's Airway, Breathing, and Circulation (ABCs) must be assessed and stabilized, while a prompt search for the underlying cause of apnea is undertaken. The underlying cause must be identified and treated promptly. Most infants and children who present with the sudden onset of apnea are admitted to the hospital for cardiopulmonary monitoring and further observation and management. This is also effective in reducing parental stress and anxiety. Any infant who is presumed to be septic should have a thorough sepsis evaluation and prompt administration of IV antibiotics. If the child appears unstable, or is having frequent or severe apneic episodes associated with bradycardia and/or hypoxemia, an intensive care setting may be appropriate. Nasopharyngeal specimens should be tested for RSV and/or

Bordetella pertussis. The child with possible RSV bronchiolitis should be monitored closely from a cardiorespiratory standpoint. The patient with presumed pertussis should be isolated, while empiric antibiotic therapy is initiated.

A chest radiograph may be helpful in ruling out pneumonia, air leak, or cardiac enlargement. A right-sided aortic arch is typically found with vascular rings. Posterior rib fractures may be present in cases of shaken baby syndrome. Air trapping may indicate an aspirated foreign body. An EKG can be helpful in looking for arrhythmias or evidence of right ventricular hypertrophy.

The following blood work may be helpful in managing the patient with apnea. A CBC can indicate possible infection or anemia. Serum electrolytes are usually obtained. An elevated serum bicarbonate may indicate chronic hypoventilation, whereas a decrease suggests acidosis that may have developed during the acute episode. Decreased serum sodium and calcium can lead to seizure activity. Arterial blood gas analysis provides an initial assessment of oxygenation and acid–base status.

If an airway abnormality is suspected, a fiberoptic bronchoscopy may be considered once the patient is stabilized. Lateral radiographs of the soft tissues of the neck can document tonsillar and adenoidal size. Consultation with an otorhinolaryngologist may be helpful in determining the need for tonsillectomy and adenoidectomy. Endoscopic evaluation of the esophagus and/or 24-hour esophageal pH monitoring with respiratory pattern recording may be helpful in defining GERD as the cause of apnea in a patient, although the relationship between these events remain controversial. Brain imaging and EEG monitoring may be appropriate in those patients with suspected hydrocephalus or seizures. With a thorough history and physical examination, close monitoring in the inpatient setting, and focused, appropriate diagnostic testing, most causes of apnea can be correctly diagnosed and treated.

Treatment

Therapy is directed at supporting the patient's cardiopulmonary status, while identifying and treating the underlying condition. If an infant appears ill, blood cultures are obtained and empiric IV antibiotics are promptly administered. Anticonvulsants are administered to patients with seizures. Anatomic lesions may need to be surgically corrected. Anti-reflux measures, such as small, frequent feeds, upright positioning after feeds,

medications, and occasionally surgery, are needed to treat the patient with GERD.

Occasionally, however, no clearly identifiable cause can be found. Many of these children undergo six-channel monitoring, measuring heart rate, blood pressure, oxygen saturation, esophageal pH, nasal air flow, and chest wall movement, over a 24-hour period. In some instances, even this testing fails to reveal a treatable cause for apnea. The role of *home monitoring* is controversial, as there has not been a clear benefit demonstrated in controlled clinical trials. The decision to monitor these children at home should be made in consultation with the family and primary care provider. Home monitoring may be considered for children with severe, recurrent, or frequent episodes, even though it has not been shown to improve long-term survival. Most parents and providers choose to discontinue home monitoring when the child has not triggered the alarm for several months, and the child's health status has generally improved.

PEARLS

■ A careful, detailed history of the actual apneic event, the child's previous health, and the resuscitation effort points to the underlying diagnosis in at least 50% of cases.
■ The child's <u>A</u>irway, <u>B</u>reathing and <u>C</u>irculation must be stabilized while the underlying cause of apnea is determined and appropriately treated.
■ The clinician must promptly consider a number of diagnostic possibilities, including infectious causes, seizures, GERD, airway abnormalities, and child abuse.
■ Home monitoring is seldom necessary or helpful in improving long-term outcome of these patients.

Suggested Readings

American Academy of Pediatrics policy statement: apnea, sudden infant death syndrome, and home monitoring. *Pediatrics* 2003;111:914–917.
Mitchell I, Brummitt J, DeForest J, et al. Apnea and factitious illness (Münchausen syndrome) by proxy. *Pediatrics* 1993;92:810–814.
Schechter, Michael S. Technical report: diagnosis and management of childhood obstructive sleep apnea syndrome. *Pediatrics* 2002;109:e69.

CHAPTER 13 ■ CYANOSIS

PATRICIA V. LOWERY AND GERALD L. STROPE

CYANOSIS AND HYPOXEMIA

Cyanosis is a physical sign manifest by dark blue coloration of the skin best seen in the mucous membranes and nail beds. Its presence may indicate hypoxemia, but its absence does not rule out hypoxemia. The discussion of cyanosis in this chapter is divided into five parts: (1) an overview, including differential diagnosis (Table 13.1); (2) pulmonary disease; (3) cyanotic heart disease; (4) methemoglobinemia; and (5) breath-holding spells.

Hypoxemia is subnormal oxygenation of arterial blood. It is detected by measuring arterial oxygen tension (partial pressure of oxygen, PaO_2 in mm Hg or torr). Normal newborns have a PaO_2 of approximately 50 mm Hg by 5 to 10 minutes after birth (see Section XIII, Chapter 106). Because it is common to make assumptions about PaO_2 based on pulse oximetry–measured saturation, or SaO_2 (percentage oxyhemoglobin), the relationship between PaO_2 and SaO_2 is important to understand. As Figure 13.1 shows, arterial oxygen saturation in-creases in an almost linear fashion when the partial pressure of oxygen increases from 10 to 50 mm Hg. Increases in oxygen tensions above 70 mm Hg, however, do not result in any significant rise in oxygen saturation.

Central cyanosis (at the highly vascularized lips and mucous membranes) correlates better with hypoxemia than *peripheral cyanosis* (in the extremities), and facilitates the assessment of cyanosis in darkly pigmented individuals. Slow movement of blood through the peripheral capillaries leads to increased oxygen extraction and localized cyanosis (acrocyanosis). Peripheral cyanosis therefore is a less reliable sign of hypoxemia than central cyanosis because peripheral cyanosis may occur even when arterial blood is well oxygenated (e.g., cold exposure, polycythemia). Two additional types of cyanosis should be remembered. Differential cyanosis may be seen in conditions with right-to-left shunting from the pulmonary artery to the descending aorta through the patent ductus arteriosus (PDA), with cyanosis of the lower half of the body and a pink (acyanotic) upper body. Reversed differential cyanosis, cyanosis of the upper body and a pink lower body, can occur with either transposition of the great arteries (TGA) or total anomalous pulmonary venous connection (TAPVC) and associated shunting through a patent ductus arteriosus (PDA). Both TGA and TAPVC are associated with a higher oxygen content in right ventricular blood, resulting in this unexpected distribution of cyanosis.

The presence of cyanosis is influenced by several factors, including the site of observation, pH, temperature, and concentrations of adult and fetal hemoglobins. Cyanosis appears when the absolute concentration of reduced hemoglobin (deoxyhemoglobin) in arterial blood is greater than 4 to 5 g/dL. Because this amount of reduced arterial hemoglobin (deoxyhemoglobin) is necessary to produce cyanosis, a low hemoglobin concentration (e.g., anemia with hemoglobin of 10 g/dL) requires an arterial saturation of 60% to produce approximately 4 g/dL of deoxyhemoglobin and cyanosis. The oxygen dissociation curve in Figure 13.1 shows that an oxygen saturation of 60% of adult hemoglobin corresponds to a PaO_2 of 32 mm Hg and represents severe hypoxemia. Fetal hemoglobin, given its higher affinity for oxygen, requires a lower PaO_2 than adult blood to be fully saturated but releases O_2 to the tissues less readily. Thus, the first sign of profound hypoxemia in an anemic infant may be bradycardia.

In contrast, a child who is polycythemic (e.g., total hemoglobin of 17 mg/dL) manifests cyanosis at a higher oxyhemoglobin saturation. This child, with a SaO_2 of 75% (25% deoxyhemoglobin), will have 4.25 g/dL of deoxyhemoglobin (25% of 17) and will likely appear cyanotic. As Figure 13.1 shows, an oxygen saturation of 75% of adult hemoglobin corresponds to a PaO_2 of 42 mm Hg. Thus, an anemic patient must be severely hypoxic before he/she will appear cyanotic, whereas a patient with polycythemia may appear cyanotic without as much hypoxia. In summary, hypoxemia may not correlate with the degree of cyanosis because this finding is dependent upon the absolute amount of deoxyhemoglobin.

The pH and temperature also influence whether cyanosis is present. The oxygen dissociation curve of hemoglobin shifts to the right in the presence of adult hemoglobin, acidosis, and increased temperature. If an infant is acidotic, febrile, or has more adult hemoglobin (e.g., post-transfusion), then at any given PaO_2 (any state of oxygenation) there is increased oxygen delivery to the tissues, less oxyhemoglobin, and more deoxyhemoglobin, such that cyanosis will occur more readily.

Pearls

- Cyanosis and hypoxemia are not synonymous.
- Both the hemoglobin level and oxyhemoglobin saturation must be known to understand why cyanosis is present or absent.
- Because a patient can be hypoxemic without cyanosis, to document hypoxemia, oxygen tension from an arterial blood gas (PaO_2) measurement is preferred to oxygen saturation (SaO_2).
- In an anemic infant, bradycardia may be the first sign of hypoxemia.

PULMONARY DISEASE

(See Chapters 35, 41, and 106 for further discussion of respiratory conditions.) Pulmonary conditions are by far the most common causes of cyanosis. Tachypnea is usually present, but this finding can occur with or without clinically apparent cyanosis. Major pulmonary causes of neonatal respiratory problems

TABLE 13.1

CAUSES OF CYANOSIS

A. Decreased availability of oxygen in inspired air
   1. Altitude
   2. Inhalation of nonphysiologic gas mixture

B. Alveolar hypoventilation
   1. Neurologic depression
      a. Trauma: cerebral hemorrhage or edema, birth trauma (e.g., phrenic nerve palsy)
      b. Drugs: maternal narcotic analgesia/anesthesia, narcotic withdrawal
      c. Infection
      d. Central hypoventilation: Ondine curse
   2. Airway obstruction
      a. Congenital: vocal cord paralysis, choanal atresia, laryngeal web, saccules, laryngoceles, subglottic stenosis, hemangiomas, craniofacial abnormalities
      b. Acquired: bronchiolitis, asthma, croup, pneumonia, chronic inflammation, epiglottitis
   3. Neuromuscular disease: Jeune thoracic dystrophy
   4. Restricted lung movement: pneumothorax, pulmonary interstitial emphysema, hypoplastic lung, diaphragmatic hernia, cystic adenomatoid malformation

C. Shunt
   1. Intracardiac: congenital heart disease (CHD-TGV, TAPVC, TOF, TA, tricuspid atresia, PS)
   2. Intrapulmonary: coarctation, bronchiectasis, persistent fetal circulation

D. Ventilation–perfusion mismatch ($\dot{V}°/\dot{Q}° <1$)
   1. Parenchymal disease: TTN, RDS, aspiration, pneumonia, pulmonary edema, hypoplasia
   2. Airway disease: asthma, cystic fibrosis, bronchiolitis
   3. Vascular disease: pulmonary embolus (thrombus, fat)

E. Major diffusion abnormalities
   1. Interstitial fibrosis
   2. Adult respiratory distress syndrome
   3. Oxygen toxicity
   4. Pulmonary edema

F. Abnormalities of hemoglobin and oxygen-carrying capacity
   1. Abnormal hemoglobin: anemia, methemoglobin, Hgb M, sulfhemoglobin, other mutant Hgb's
   2. Alterations in oxyhemoglobin affinity: pH, temperature, 2, 3-DPG levels
   3. Too much reduced hemoglobin: hyperviscosity, polycythemia

G. Poor tissue perfusion–low cardiac output: sepsis, hypovolemia, CHF

H. Causes of apparent (but not "real") cyanosis
   1. Vasomotor instability: mottling, acrocyanosis, Harlequin condition
   2. Bruising
   3. Vasoconstriction secondary to cold

I. Other conditions associated with cyanosis
   1. Hypoglycemia
   2. Hypocalcemia
   3. Hypothermia

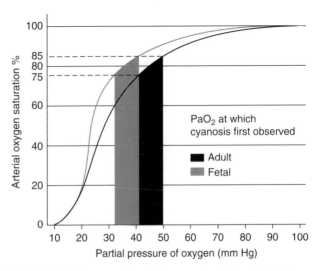

FIGURE 13.1. Oxygen dissociation curve for fetal and adult hemoglobin showing relationship of oxygen saturation (SaO_2) to oxygen (PaO_2). Note that under normal circumstances, cyanosis usually is observed at oxyhemoglobin saturations between 75% and 85%.

breathing, and tachypnea. Aspiration leads to overinflation, air leak disorders, atelectasis, and V/Q mismatches in addition to hypoxic pulmonary vasoconstriction. RDS or hyaline membrane disease (HMD) is caused primarily by surfactant deficiency, which leads to similar lung pathologies. Nonpulmonary causes of tachypnea include cardiac, infectious, neurologic, and metabolic disorders. The immediate goal in evaluating a cyanotic newborn is to differentiate between cardiac and noncardiac causes. Observation of the breathing pattern may assist in this process, as weak or irregular breathing is often associated with central nervous system pathology while vigorous or labored breathing is typically seen with cyanosis of cardiopulmonary origin. Cyanosis is generally an ominous finding of pulmonary pathology.

CYANOTIC CONGENITAL HEART DISEASE

Cyanosis from congenital heart disease (CHD; also see Chapter 29) may be classified into two basic categories: (1) lesions involving predominantly diminished pulmonary blood flow caused by *right-sided obstruction* with an intracardiac communication, or (2) lesions involving abnormal *intracardiac mixing*. For simplicity, all cyanotic CHD may be considered to occur by one of these two mechanisms.

The physical examination is helpful in differentiating the category of cyanotic CHD. Clues that the cyanosis may have a cardiac origin include deep cyanosis with minimal respiratory distress, a single second heart sound, a pathologic heart murmur, and/or extra heart sounds such as gallops or clicks. In the normal heart, the S_2 sound is split because the two semilunar valves close separately. In TAPVC, there is often an abnormally widely split S_2 because of severe RV volume overload. If the S_2 sounds single, it may indicate:

- An absent semilunar valve (e.g., pulmonary atresia) or aortic atresia (e.g., hypoplastic left heart syndrome, HLHS).
- Inaudible closure of a stenotic pulmonary valve (e.g., tetralogy of Fallot [TOF] or tricuspid atresia).
- Loud closure of the aortic valve (e.g., transposition of great arteries, where the aortic valve's anterior location allows it to obscure closure of the more distant pulmonary valve).

associated with cyanosis include transient tachypnea of the newborn (TTN), aspiration syndromes, and respiratory distress syndrome (RDS). In TTN, delayed resorption of lung fluid leads to reduced pulmonary compliance, increased work of

A diastolic murmur is always pathologic and is sometimes noted in the infant with persistent truncus arteriosus from truncal valve regurgitation during diastole. A gallop rhythm accompanies poor ventricular compliance and may occur in HLHS (also notable for poor peripheral pulses and perfusion). The long systolic murmur heard in TOF arises from the right ventricular outflow tract (RVOT) obstruction, not from the ventricular septal defect. Multiple systolic clicks are common in Ebstein anomaly of the tricuspid valve.

Pulse Oximetry

In evaluating the cyanotic infant or child, it is recommended that pulse oximetry be checked at two sites: preductally (usually the right arm) and postductally (either foot). If the child has cyanotic CHD, the preductal saturation should be low because blood leaving the heart is already desaturated. In contrast, if the infant has a normal heart structure but severe pulmonary artery hypertension with right-to-left shunting through the patent ductal artery, the preductal pulse oxygen saturation may be high but the postductal saturation may be low.

Hyperoxia Test

In patients with cyanotic heart disease, the systemic arterial PaO_2 is decreased because some deoxygenated blood never goes through the pulmonary circulation as a result of right-to-left shunting. So even if the inspiratory oxygen concentration (FIO_2) is increased to 100%, the infant will continue to be cyanotic. In patients with pulmonary disease, by contrast, the desaturated blood does go through the lungs, but there may be either inadequate ventilation (as with choanal atresia) or ventilation–perfusion mismatch (as with atelectasis). If sufficient ventilation is provided or occurs in a patient with a pulmonary etiology, increasing the FIO_2 to 100% should markedly increase both the PaO_2 and oxygen saturation.

As a rule, if an inspired oxygen concentration of 100% is provided for 15 minutes, then if the arterial PaO_2 on arterial blood gases increases to more than 150 mm Hg, the primary pathologic process is likely pulmonary. If the PaO_2 does not increase to this value, cardiac disease is more likely to be the cause (shunting implied). If it remains less than 100 mm Hg, the clinician should strongly suspect congenital cardiac disease. In infants with persistent pulmonary hypertension of the newborn (PPHN), a hyperoxia test may not be diagnostically helpful.

Chest Radiograph

Another basic diagnostic tool in evaluating the infant with possible cyanotic CHD is the chest radiograph. The clinician should look for heart size, pulmonary vascular markings, and heart configuration. Most cyanotic CHD is associated with cardiomegaly and can be divided for the purpose of broad differential diagnoses into diseases with increased pulmonary vascular markings and those with decreased pulmonary vascular markings.

If pulmonary vascularity is decreased, problems with the valves on the right side of the heart should be suspected. The right-sided obstructive lesions (TOF, pulmonary atresia, and critical pulmonary valve stenosis) involve the pulmonary valve. Other considerations include tricuspid atresia (absence of the tricuspid valve between the right atrium and right ventricle) and Ebstein anomaly (with an abnormal location of a leaky tricuspid valve). If the patient has increased pulmonary vascularity, the clinician should suspect cyanotic lesions with either mixing problems (TGA, persistent truncus arteriosus) or heart failure (HLHS, total anomalous pulmonary venous connection).

The contour of the heart on chest radiography may offer some clues. If the radiograph shows increased pulmonary vascular markings and cardiomegaly that looks like an egg on a string, TGA should be suspected. The mediastinum is narrow because of lack of thymus (CATCH 22 [cardiac defects, abnormal facies, thymic aplasia/hypoplasia, cleft palate, hypocalcemia], DiGeorge syndrome) and because the aorta is almost directly in front of the pulmonary artery rather than next to it. A "boot-shaped" heart caused by a small or absent pulmonary artery segment and associated with right ventricular hypertrophy should raise suspicion of TOF. A right aortic arch suggests truncus arteriosus if accompanied by increased pulmonary vascular markings, or TOF if accompanied by decreased pulmonary vascular markings. A normal-sized or small heart with pulmonary edema may occur with obstructed total anomalous pulmonary venous connection (TAPVC). A huge heart secondary to massive right atrial enlargement may be seen in severe Ebstein anomaly of the tricuspid valve.

Electrocardiogram

In newborns, the electrocardiogram (ECG) is much less useful in the assessment of suspected congenital heart disease. The QRS axis in the normal newborn is deviated to the right and can vary between +90° and +200°. If the axis is leftward (approximately −30°) with evidence of left ventricular hypertrophy, tricuspid atresia should be suspected. In older infants and children, the ECG has more utility. Other findings that can be considered suggestive include left ventricular hypertrophy with a QRS axis of 0° to +90°; suspect pulmonary atresia with an intact ventricular septum. If the QRS axis is +90° to +180° along with right ventricular hypertrophy, then consider TOF. In newborns, this latter finding is nonspecific because both right axis deviation and right ventricular hypertrophy are present normally.

If Ebstein anomaly is present, it may be accompanied by right atrial enlargement, right bundle-branch block, a long PR interval, or Wolff-Parkinson-White (WPW) type of pre-excitation. Interestingly, in HLHS the left-ventricular forces are found to be decreased in only one-third of affected infants.

With a careful clinical assessment, chest radiograph, and ECG, the clinician has enough information to begin to formulate the most likely cardiac etiologies for cyanosis. Immediate consultation with a pediatric cardiologist is indicated, so that guidance may be obtained for subsequent medical treatment and/or transfer to a tertiary care institution. Usually the definitive diagnosis is reached with the help of an echocardiogram in the hands of a pediatric cardiologist.

Medical Treatment

If definitive therapy is not available at the provider's institution, or if other delays in obtaining definitive pediatric cardiology consultation occur, prostaglandin E_1 (PGE_1) can be lifesaving. PGE_1 helps maintain patency of the ductal artery. Thus for cyanotic congenital heart defects that are "ductal-dependent," this intervention can be critical. An infusion of this medication may promote the following:

- Increased pulmonary blood flow in lesions with decreased flow, which is helpful for palliation and stabilization in ductal-dependent lesions with severe right-sided obstruction (TOF, critical pulmonary stenosis, pulmonary atresia, Ebstein anomaly, tricuspid atresia).
- Improved bidirectional mixing in TGA.
- Greater cardiac output in HLHS with maintenance of ductal artery patency.

Because of the issues involved and the risks to the infant, prior to beginning therapy with PGE₁, consultation with a pediatric cardiologist should occur, even if only by telephone. The dosage for PGE₁ is 0.03 to 2.0 µg/kg/min given as a continuous infusion, and the cardiac effects are seen within 2 to 3 minutes. If possible, a second intravenous (IV) site should be available to avoid interruption of the infusion if the initial site is lost. Side effects include apnea, hyperpyrexia, systemic hypotension, jitteriness/seizures, diarrhea, platelet inhibition, and, with chronic use, cortical proliferation of the long bones. Apnea is the most significant side effect, but is *not* an indication to stop the PGE₁ infusion, but rather to intubate and ventilate the infant. Of note, TAPVC typically worsens with administration of PGE₁.

Providing supplemental oxygen to cyanotic infants usually does not help in cyanotic CHD because of right-to-left shunting. In general, unless the patient is extremely hypoxic, it is best to maintain the child in room air to avoid oxygen's potential to enhance closure of the patent ductal artery, and to decrease pulmonary vascular resistance in patients with HLHS. Other supportive therapies include correcting acidosis and maintaining the hemoglobin at more than 13 g/dL to provide adequate oxygen-carrying capacity.

TOF spells (hypercyanotic "tet spells") may occur if systemic resistance falls and obstruction increases at the infundibulum (RVOT), as when a child with tetralogy of Fallot is placed in a warm bath or after vigorous physical activity (like crying). Treatment aims to increase peripheral resistance (systemic vascular resistance) and relieve RVOT obstruction. Knee-chest positioning or giving IV phenylephrine may increase systemic vascular resistance, thereby promoting more blood flow out the RVOT to the lungs. Propranolol may "relax" the infundibulum, decreasing right-sided obstruction and improving pulmonary blood flow. Morphine sulfate may both calm the patient (decrease activity) and act on the infundibulum. Fluid volume loading may expand intravascular volume and promote flow across the RVOT. Finally, transfusion with packed red blood cells may improve oxygen tissue delivery, but should be undertaken rarely because chronically cyanotic children often have secondary polycythemia.

Pearls

- A hyperoxia test is an important adjunct to the diagnosis of cyanotic CHD in the newborn period. On 100% FiO₂ with good ventilation, if the PaO₂ remains less than 150 mm Hg, suspect cyanotic CHD.
- Obstructed TAPVC is the cyanotic CHD most often mistaken for lung disease.
- Giving PGE₁ may help stabilize a patient with any type of cyanotic CHD.

METHEMOGLOBINEMIA

Methemoglobinemia (MHb) refers to the oxidation of ferrous iron (Fe^{2+}) to ferric iron (Fe^{3+}) in the hemoglobin molecule. This reaction impairs the ability of hemoglobin to transport oxygen, leading to tissue hypoxemia and, in severe cases, death. MHb most commonly results from exposure to an oxidizing chemical, but also may arise from genetic, dietary, or even idiopathic etiologies.

The most common cause of MHb is ingestion or skin exposure to an oxidizing agent. MHb is most common in children older than 6 months. Common agents are aniline, benzocaine, dapsone, phenazopyridine (Pyridium), nitrites, nitrates, and naphthalene (Table 13.2). Oxidizing agents can be divided into those that directly oxidize hemoglobin and those that

indirectly oxidize hemoglobin. Direct oxidizers react directly with hemoglobin to form MHb. Indirect oxidizers actually are powerful reducing agents that reduce oxygen to the free radical O_2, or water to H_2O_2, which in turn oxidizes hemoglobin to MHb.

Many drugs that produce MHb are not themselves the causative agents. Instead, these drugs are metabolized to an oxidative free radical. For example, aniline is metabolized by the cytochrome P450 system to a free radical phenylhydroxylamine, which, like nitrite, reacts with oxygen to form oxygen free radicals and then MHb. Because of the variability in metabolism among individuals, not every patient may experience MHb when exposed to such agents. This may explain why MHb does not develop in every child who ingests benzocaine. MHb develops only in those few who metabolize a significant amount of parent drug to the toxic metabolite. Poisoning is characterized by a latent period of several hours followed by nausea, vomiting, diarrhea, and then cyanosis (i.e., MHb), hemolysis, and renal failure. Some agents (e.g., nitrites) can be absorbed directly through the skin and from the gastrointestinal tract. Others (e.g., dapsone) are processed through the enterohepatic circulation and produce elevated MHb.

The second most common cause of MHb is idiopathic and related to systemic acidosis. MHb can be formed in some young infants (<6 months) when severe metabolic acidosis develops, most commonly as a result of diarrhea and dehydration. Several risk factors may predispose these infants to the development of MHb. Infants have quantitatively lower red blood cell levels of the protective enzyme, cytochrome-b_5 reductase (levels at birth = 50% to 60% of adult levels). Fetal hemoglobin also is more easily oxidized than adult hemoglobin. Finally, the higher intestinal pH of infants may promote the growth of gram-negative organisms that are able to convert dietary nitrates to nitrites, potent MHb inducers. The relative contribution to the formation of MHb from nitrites formed by intestinal gram-negative bacterial flora, the presence of fetal hemoglobin, lower MHb-reducing enzyme

TABLE 13.2

COMMON AGENTS THAT PRODUCE METHEMOGLOBINEMIA[a]

Acetanilid	Nitrates[b]
Alloxan	Nitric oxide
Aniline (dyes, ink)	Nitrites
Antipyrine	Nitroalkanes
Arsine	Nitrochlorobenzene
Benzene derivatives	Nitrofuran
Benzocaine	Nitroglycerin
Chlorates	Nitroprusside
Chlorobenzene	Paraquat/diquat
Chloroquine	Phenacetin
Dapsone	Phenazopyridine
Dinitrophenol	Phenol
Dinitrotoluene	Phenylhydrazine
Hydroxylamine	Phenytoin
Lidocaine	Prilocaine
Menadione	Primaquine
Methylene blue	Smoke inhalation
Metoclopramide	Sulfonamide antibiotics
Naphthalene	Trinitrotoluene

[a]Many chemicals may have oxidizing properties, and this list is not complete.
[b]Chemical and food sources.

levels during the first months of life, or formation of oxidative metabolites, remains unclear. In this clinical situation, no association with oxidant drugs has been established and the MHb resolves with time, suggesting that it is not inherited. Clusters of cases of infants with MHb have been reported, perhaps because of colonization with certain strains of gram-negative, nitrite-forming bacteria, such *Escherichia coli* or *Campylobacter jejuni*. However, a definite etiologic pathogen has not been identified in all such cases. In addition, some case reports implicate noninfectious diarrhea (e.g., cow's milk protein intolerance). There also are reports of infants with MHb and acidosis in the absence of diarrhea (e.g., renal tubular acidosis and vomiting). It may be that the common endpoint of metabolic acidosis is the greatest predisposing factor. There is evidence that endogenous MHb reduction is inhibited by an acidic pH and promoted by an alkaline pH. The exact cause is likely multifactorial.

A third cause of MHb is dietary and is related to well-water nitrates. This exposure deserves special consideration because it occurs in very young infants in whom toxic ingestions are extremely uncommon and often leads to delayed diagnosis and recurrent symptoms. Typically, affected patients are very young infants who live in rural areas where the water source is a well containing high levels of nitrates, possibly from fertilizer runoff. Intestinal bacterial flora convert the nitrates to nitrites, which are potent MHb-forming agents.

The fourth cause of MHb is genetic. These patients present at or very shortly after birth with cyanosis. Two different deficiencies may be present: cytochrome-b_5 reductase deficiency or cytochrome-b_5 deficiency. Both are transmitted in an autosomal recessive pattern. These subjects have moderately elevated MHb levels that usually are well tolerated. Hemoglobin M describes a group of abnormal hemoglobin molecules. This disorder is inherited in an autosomal dominant pattern. Presumably, the homozygous form is not compatible with life.

Regardless of etiology, the severity of symptoms depends on the MHb level (Table 13.3). Levels are reported as a percentage of total hemoglobin. Cyanosis caused by MHb becomes clinically apparent at an MHb level of 1.5 g/dL. In a normal person, this usually is approximately 15% of total hemoglobin. Levels above 70% may cause death. Because MHb usually is expressed as a percentage of total hemoglobin, levels may not correspond to symptoms in some patients. An anemic patient may have greater symptoms at a level of 20% than a nonanemic patient because the oxygen-carrying capacity is lower and more easily compromised. For example, a patient with an MHb level of 20% and total hemoglobin of 15 g/dL still has 12 g/dL of functioning hemoglobin, whereas a patient with an MHb level of 20% and total hemoglobin of 8 g/dL has only 6.4 g/dL of functioning hemoglobin. Anemia, acidosis, respiratory compromise, and cardiac disease may make patients more symptomatic than expected for a given MHb level.

Laboratory Diagnosis

When a patient presents with obvious cyanosis, an arterial blood gas analysis and pulse oximetry reading usually are performed. Unfortunately, results of these tests may be normal or near normal in a patient with significant MHb. Unless the clinician is familiar with the effect of MHb on these tests, the results may delay diagnosis.

Arterial Blood Gas Analysis

Arterial blood gas analyzers are based on electrochemistry. Voltage changes are determined with high-impedance electrodes to measure pH and PCO_2 and electrical current changes determined to measure PO_2. PO_2 refers to dissolved gas and not to oxygen molecules bound to hemoglobin. Subjects with MHb may have normal PO_2 levels despite life-threatening MHb.

Pulse Oximetry

The pulse oximeter detects significant levels of MHb as mild to moderate oxygen desaturation; unfortunately, it cannot be used to determine the actual percentage of MHb in the blood.

Co-oximetry

Co-oximetry is an accurate method of measuring MHb. A co-oximeter is also a simplified spectrophotometer, but unlike a pulse oximeter, it measures light absorbance at four different wavelengths. These wavelengths correspond to specific absorbance characteristics of deoxyhemoglobin, oxyhemoglobin, carboxyhemoglobin, and hemoglobin. A peak absorbance of light at 630 nm is used to characterize MHb.

TABLE 13.3

SYMPTOMS ASSOCIATED WITH METHEMOGLOBIN BLOOD CONCENTRATIONS

MHb Concentration (g/dL)	Total Hemoglobin[a] (%)	Symptoms[b]
<1.5	<10	None
1.5–3.0	10–20	Cyanotic skin discoloration
3.0–4.5	20–30	Anxiety, lightheadedness, headache, tachycardia
4.5–7.5	30–50	Fatigue, confusion, dizziness, tachypnea, increased tachycardia
7.5–10.5	50–70	Coma, seizures, arrhythmias, acidosis
>10.5	>70	Death

MHb, methemoglobin.
[a]Assumes hemoglobin = 15 g/dL. Patients with lower hemoglobin concentrations may experience more severe symptoms for a given percentage of MHb level.
[b]Patients with underlying cardiac, pulmonary, or hematologic disease may experience more severe symptoms for a given MHb concentration.

Bedside Tests

The primary diagnostic consideration in a patient with cyanosis is to differentiate deoxyhemoglobin from MHb. Blood containing high concentrations of MHb appears chocolate brown as opposed to the dark red/violet of deoxygenated blood. A simple bedside test is to place one or two drops of the patient's blood on white filter paper. The chocolate-brown appearance of MHb does not change with time; deoxyhemoglobin appears dark red/violet initially but brightens after exposure to atmospheric oxygen. Gently blowing supplemental oxygen onto the filter paper hastens the reaction with deoxyhemoglobin but does not affect MHb.

Treatment

Once recognized and confirmed, life-threatening MHb must be treated rapidly. However, not all patients require antidotal therapy, and many do well with only supportive care.

After an acute exposure to an oxidizing agent, the threshold for intervention is considered to be approximately 20% MHb in symptomatic patients and 30% in asymptomatic patients. Patients who are symptomatic or have significant concurrent problems that compromise oxygen delivery (e.g., heart disease, lung disease, carbon monoxide poisoning, or anemia) should be treated at levels between 10% and 30%.

The treatment of choice for severe acute MHb is methylene blue. Methylene blue is provided as a 1% solution (10 mg/mL). The dose is 1 to 2 mg/kg (0.2 mL/kg of a 1% solution) infused IV over 3 to 5 minutes. The dose may be repeated at 1 mg/kg if MHb does not resolve within 30 minutes. Methylene blue should reduce MHb levels significantly in less than an hour. Infants with MHb resulting from diarrhea and acidosis may improve with aggressive rehydration and bicarbonate to correct the acidosis. However, MHb levels greater than 20% should also be treated with methylene blue.

Complications of methylene blue treatment have been reported in two groups: patients with glucose-6-phosphate dehydrogenase (G6PD) deficiency and neonates. Patients with G6PD deficiency may develop a Heinz body hemolytic anemia from methylene blue. Paradoxically, methylene blue actually is an oxidant; the metabolic product leukomethylene blue is the reducing agent. Large doses of the drug (4 mg/kg) may result in proportionately higher levels of the oxidizing agent, methylene blue, rather than the reducing agent, leukomethylene blue. Thus methylene blue (1 to 2 mg/kg) may induce both hemolysis, and paradoxically, MHb in patients with G6PD deficiency. The perinatal administration of higher doses of methylene blue (4 mg/kg, amniotically) has been reported to induce hemolysis and MHb in non–G6PD-deficient infants.

BREATH-HOLDING SPELLS

Breath-holding spells occur in up to 5% of children and usually present between 6 and 18 months of age; there is often a family history. They are classified as either cyanotic (expiratory apnea) or pallid (pallid syncope). Cyanotic breath-holding spells usually start with anger or mild injury, which progresses to a breath-hold after a forced expiration. Cyanosis develops rapidly and may be followed by limpness and loss of consciousness. Some children posture but rarely have seizures. Anticonvulsant medications help control the seizure activity but have no effect on the occurrence of breath-holding spells.

Pallid breath-holding events occur less frequently than cyanotic breath-holding. They are most often triggered by minor trauma to the head or upper body. This trigger event may occur as long as 30 seconds prior to the breath-holding (apnea) and related pallor. Limpness develops and, if the event lasts more the a few seconds, is followed by generalized increased tone, and is sometimes accompanied by incontinence and mild clonus. The entire event may last less than a minute but may be followed by a period of confusion and sleepiness. These events are often misinterpreted as seizures.

There is no specific therapy for children with cyanotic breath-holding spells. Anticonvulsant medications may be effective for the rare associated seizures but have no effect on the breath-holding. Hence such medication is rarely indicated. Pallid breath-holding is associated with cardiac asystole followed by a period of brief brain hypoperfusion. In this setting, pallid breath-holding might be considered another form of autonomic dysregulation. If the asystole is prolonged (10 to 30 seconds), cardiology evaluation may be helpful for management.

Both types of breath-holding spells are thought to be benign paroxysmal involuntary events of childhood. Management should focus on behavioral issues associated with these events. There is some evidence that iron therapy may be helpful to decrease the number of the breath-holding spells. However, it is not effective in all children, and effectiveness is often not related to the hemoglobin level.

Suggested Readings

Anderson JE, Bluestone D. Breath holding spells: scary but not serious. *Contemp Pediatr* 2000;1:61.

Brousseau T, Sharieff GQ. Newborn emergencies: the first 30 days of life. *Pediatr Clin North Am* 2006;53:69–84.

Brown K. The infant with undiagnosed cardiac disease in the emergency department. *Clin Pediatr Emerg Med* 2005;6:200–206.

Crownover BK. Newborn respiratory problems: when the grunting and flaring won't go away. *Contemp Pediatr* 2004;21:57.

DeWolfe CC. Apparent life threatening event: a review. *Pediatr Clin North Am* 2005;52:1127–1146.

Greer FR, Shannon M. Infant methemoglobinemia: the role of dietary nitrate in food and water. *Pediatrics* 2005;116:784–786.

Hannon DW. Relief for the (missed) blue baby blues. *J Pediatr* 2003;142:231–233.

Langley JM, Bradley JS. Defining pneumonia in critically ill infants and children. *Pediatr Crit Care Med* 2005;6:S9–S513.

Sasidharan P. An approach to diagnosis and management of cyanosis and tachypnea in term infants. *Pediatr Clin North Am* 2004;51:999–1021.

Sharieff GQ. The pediatric ECG. *Emerg Med Clin North Am* 2006;24:195–208.

Woods WA, McCulloch MA. Cardiovascular emergencies in the pediatric patient. *Emerg Med Clin North Am* 2005;23:1233–1249.

Wright RO, Lewander WJ, Woolf AD. Methemoglobinemia: etiology, pharmacology, and clinical management. *Ann Emerg Med* 1999;34:646–656.

CHAPTER 14 ■ COMMON ELECTROLYTE PROBLEMS IN PEDIATRICS

RONALD M. PERKIN, WILLIAM E. NOVOTNY, AND PATRICIA M. HOPKINS

Electrolyte disorders are important sequelae of many diseases that result in pediatric hospitalization. Accurate identification of such abnormalities has significant potential impact on the treatment, outcome, and disposition of these patients.

SODIUM, OSMOLALITY, AND THE VOLUME OF BODY FLUIDS

Total body water, which is 55% to 72% of body mass, varies with sex, age, and fat content and is distributed between the intracellular and extracellular spaces. The extracellular fluid (ECF), which comprises approximately one-third of total body water, includes the intravascular plasma fluid and the extravascular interstitial fluid. Plasma ions include primarily sodium (Na^+), chloride (Cl^-), and bicarbonate (HCO_3^-), which are excluded from intracellular environments, and lesser amounts of potassium (K^+), magnesium, calcium, phosphates, sulfates, organic acids, and protein. Interstitial fluid, which surrounds the cells, has the same composition as plasma, but with less protein. The principal components of intracellular fluid (ICF) are K^+, proteins, magnesium, sulfates, and phosphates.

In the ECF, Na^+ and Cl^- constitute 90% or more of the effective solutes. Serum Na^+ concentration defines the relative amount of sodium and water in plasma; the maintenance of a normal Na^+ concentration thus contributes to regulation of the volume of body fluids. The size of the ECF and ICF compartments depends on the amount of water in each; the distribution of water depends on their osmolality. It is important to recognize that osmolality and tonicity are not identical. Osmolality is a measure of the number of solute particles per unit volume. Measured osmolality of a solution includes all particles, whether they are osmotically active or inactive. Sodium chloride or other impermeable solutes such as mannitol or glucose do not readily cross cell membranes to enter cells. They remain restricted to the ECF space and are thus "effective osmols" by obligating water to remain extracellular. Cell membranes are freely permeable to solutes such as urea, methanol, or ethanol. Although contributing to measured osmolality, these "ineffective osmols" do not obligate water to remain in the ECF space. Tonicity takes into account only osmotically active impermeable solutes and is the important physiologic parameter.

In a given patient, the osmolality may be calculated as follows, using the values of 2.8 and 18 to convert values of blood urea nitrogen (BUN) and glucose, respectively, to milliosmoles per liter (mOsm/L):

$$\text{Osmolality} = 2[Na^+ \text{ in mEq/L}] + [BUN \text{ in mg/dL}]/2.8 + [\text{glucose in mg/dL}]/18$$

Normal serum osmolality is maintained by kidney function, which dilutes or concentrates urine. This is accomplished by a variety of mechanisms involving glomerular filtration, arterial pressure, blood flow, the sympathetic nervous system, and hormones such as aldosterone, atrial natriuretic factor, and vasopressin. These systems converge to control water and electrolyte balance through glomerular ultrafiltration of the plasma followed by changes in the electrolyte content of this ultrafiltrate by tubular reabsorption and secretion. These mechanisms, together with thirst, control both plasma osmolality and plasma volume.

HYPONATREMIA

Hyponatremia usually is defined as a plasma sodium concentration ≤135 MEq/L (135 mmol/L). When assessing the child with hyponatremia, it is important to determine whether the low serum sodium is true or fictitious. It also is important to determine the patient's volume status (i.e., euvolemia, hypovolemia, or hypervolemia). This allows the basic distinction between hyponatremia caused by sodium loss, or hyponatremia caused by an increase in total body water resulting in a relative dilution of the ECF compartment. The serum sodium concentration usually cannot be used to estimate the patient's total body fluid status. Figure 14.1 summarizes the causes of hyponatremia.

Because serum sodium concentration is the main determinant of plasma osmolality, hyponatremia usually reflects hypoosmolality. Initially, the clinician must determine whether hyponatremia reflects true hypotonicity. There are two clinical circumstances in which hyponatremia may be present without hypotonicity. In the first situation, high levels of plasma lipids or proteins increase plasma volume, which decreases the percentage of plasma volume that is water. Because many clinical laboratories measure and report sodium concentrations in milliequivalents per liter of plasma (not in milliequivalents per liter of plasma water), the reported sodium concentration is artificially low. A clinical clue to such "pseudohyponatremia" is the presence of lipemic serum and a normal measured serum osmolality (because lipids or proteins have large molecular weights and therefore are minor components of overall plasma osmolality). In patients with nephrotic syndrome, a clinical rule of thumb is that an increase in triglycerides of 1 g/dL will decrease serum sodium concentrations by approximately 2 mEq/L. The second situation in which a patient may be hyponatremic, but not hypotonic, occurs when an osmotically active solute (e.g., glucose or mannitol) has been added to the extracellular space. Water drawn out of cells by such an osmotically active particle dilutes the serum sodium concentration despite isotonicity or even hypertonicity.

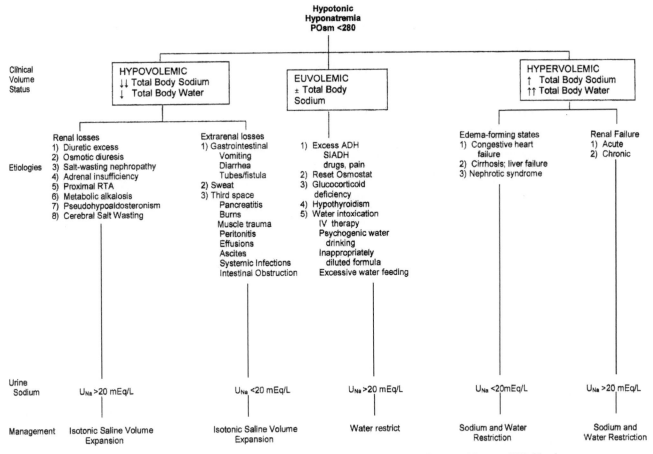

FIGURE 14.1. Diagnosis and treatment of true hyponatremia. (From Perkin RM, Novotny WE, Harris GD, et al. Common electrolyte problems in pediatric patients presenting to the ED. *Pediatr Emerg Med Rep* 2001;6:13–26, with permission.)

When hyperglycemia is present, a clinically useful method for bedside prediction of the serum sodium concentration once normoglycemia is achieved is that the serum sodium concentration is lowered by 1.6 mEq/L for each 100 mg/dL increase in glucose concentration. The presence of an osmotically active nonglucose solute in the extracellular space is readily identified by comparing the calculated osmolality with measured osmolality. If they differ by >10 mOsm/L, it can be inferred that some other solute (mannitol or glycerol) may be present.

The severity of signs and symptoms of hyponatremia depends on the rapidity of its development and the degree of decline in plasma osmolality. As the plasma osmolality decreases, an osmotic gradient across the blood–brain barrier develops that results in water movement into the brain. This cerebral overhydration is responsible for most of the symptoms seen in hyponatremia. In general, neurologic manifestations do not occur until the serum sodium concentration is <125 mEq/L. However, patients with preexisting neuropathologic processes may exhibit symptoms at higher serum sodium levels. Signs and symptoms may include headache, agitation, disorientation, lethargy, nausea, vomiting, muscular cramps, decreased deep tendon reflexes, seizures, coma, pseudobulbar palsies, and signs of cerebral herniation. The rapid development of hyponatremia (<24 hours) carries significant morbidity and mortality. Hyponatremia is a common cause of seizures in infants; it is the leading cause of afebrile seizures in this population. Hyponatremic seizures usually are generalized, with frequent progression to status epilepticus. Respiratory failure requiring intubation is not uncommon,

although most require mechanical ventilation for <24 hours. Correction of the underlying electrolyte disturbance is more effective than the use of anticonvulsants.

Hyponatremia occurs as a result of water retention, sodium loss, or both; therefore, the extracellular fluid volume may be low, normal, or high. History and physical exam findings may be of help in determining the overall volume status of the patient. An analysis of the urine sodium concentration may be of diagnostic aid in determining the etiology of the hyponatremia.

Hyponatremia with Hypovolemia

Fluid losses in these patients may have occurred by either renal or extrarenal routes. Most instances of hyponatremia presenting in the emergency department are caused by volume depletion resulting from an underlying disease; thus, appropriate fluid administration as well as treatment of the underlying disease usually is required to correct the hyponatremic state. Extrarenal losses most commonly occur through the gastrointestinal tract (vomiting or diarrhea), but may be secondary to other disorders such as burns, pancreatitis, or peritonitis. The normal kidney responds to these hypovolemic states by conserving sodium and water; thus, concentrated urine with a sodium concentration <20 mEq/L should be expected.

In hyponatremic, hypovolemic patients with urine sodium concentrations >20 mEq/L, the possibility of adrenal insufficiency exists, particularly if the serum potassium concentration is elevated. The most common cause in the infant and young child is the salt-losing form of congenital adrenal hyperplasia. Other causes include congenital adrenal hypoplasia, acute infection, hemorrhage into the adrenal glands, inadequate replacement of adrenocorticosteroids, and inappropriate tapering of steroids.

Hyponatremia is a well-recognized complication of traumatic brain injury and subarachnoid hemorrhage and is frequently ascribed to the syndrome of inappropriate antidiuretic hormone secretion (SIADH) or to cerebral salt wasting (CSW). Cerebral salt wasting, first described in 1950, is characterized by hyponatremia, diuresis, and natriuresis in the face of a contracted ECF, in contrast to SIADH, in which patients are euvolemic. The distinction is important because CSW is thought to be caused by excess secretion of natriuretic peptide and the treatment is saline replacement, whereas fluid restriction is appropriate treatment of SIADH. The treatment of hyponatremia in the volume-depleted patient should be directed toward expansion of the extracellular fluid volume with salt-containing solutions.

In addition to adequate water and salt, patients with adrenal insufficiency require efforts to correct hypoglycemia and hyperkalemia, and need replacement of deficient adrenal corticosteroids. If a patient presents with a salt-losing crisis, high doses of hydrocortisone (50 to 140 mg/m^2 per day in three to four divided doses) are required.

Acute symptomatic hyponatremia is a medical emergency for which the use of hypertonic saline may be required. Because of the dangers of congestive heart failure, osmotic demyelination syndrome, or cerebral hemorrhage, only enough hypertonic saline should be used to correct serum sodium to levels of 125 mEq/L. The amount of hypertonic saline needed can be calculated using the following formula:

$$\text{mEq Na}^+ = (0.6)\,(\text{body wt. in kg})\,(125 - [\text{Na}^+])$$

where [Na$^+$] = serum sodium concentration in milliequivalents per liter.

In the water-intoxicated patient, spontaneous water diuresis occurs so rapidly that treatment with hypertonic saline usually is unnecessary.

Neurologic complications as a result of overly rapid correction of hyponatremia have been reported in adults and older children. The syndrome of osmotic demyelination, or central pontine myelinolysis, is the result of neuronal dehydration. Hyponatremia-induced losses of intracellular potassium and amino acids shift the cells to a hypotonic state, predisposing them to acute dehydration when exposed to a normotonic or hypertonic solution aimed at rapidly correcting hyponatremia. Caution is required when contemplating rapid correction of acute symptomatic hyponatremia.

Euvolemic Hyponatremia

In patients with hyponatremia who have neither contraction of extracellular fluid volume nor expansion to the point of clinical edema, SIADH should be considered. Patients with SIADH have a concentrated urine in spite of the hyponatremia, and the urinary sodium concentration closely parallels the intake and usually is >20 mEq/L.

There are several factors that affect ADH secretion, the most important of which is plasma osmolality. Hyponatremia from SIADH occurs due to water retention secondary to a persistently elevated ADH level inappropriate to the stimuli that normally affect ADH secretion. SIADH is seen in a variety of clinical disorders, which can be subdivided into four categories: (1) increased hypothalamic production of ADH because of disease or the action of drugs, (2) ectopic production of ADH, (3) potentiation of ADH as an effect of drugs, and (4) exogenous administration of ADH. The diagnosis ultimately rests on the demonstration of an inappropriately high plasma concentration of arginine vasopressin when hyponatremia has appeared spontaneously or has been induced by increased water intake. In the absence of ADH levels, the following criteria can be used: (1) hyponatremia with corresponding plasma hypo-osmolality, (2) inappropriately elevated urine osmolality relative to plasma osmolality, (3) normal renal function, (4) normal adrenal and thyroid functions (particularly ruling out glucocorticoid deficiency and hypothyroidism), (5) high urine sodium excretion in the presence of normovolemia, (6) absence of clinical signs of hypovolemia and dehydration, (7) absence of edema-forming states or evidence of volume depletion, and (8) correction of hyponatremia and natriuresis by fluid restriction. SIADH commonly is seen in the presence of disorders that affect the central nervous system (CNS), in the presence of pulmonary diseases, and with use of certain drugs. Conditions associated with SIADH are listed in Table 14.1. As these conditions account for many of the diagnoses in hospitalized patients, judicious fluid and electrolyte management is important.

The management of SIADH can be considered under two headings: treatment of the hyponatremia and treatment of the disease process responsible for the syndrome. Because all the signs of uncomplicated SIADH result from excessive retention of water, they all respond to simple restriction of fluids. Reduction of fluid intake to the point where urinary and insensible losses induce a negative water balance leads to restoration of normal body fluid volume, a reduction in urinary sodium excretion, and an increase in serum sodium concentration. In some cases, the hyponatremia is so severe or has occurred so rapidly that signs of water intoxication (e.g., convulsions, coma) develop. In such instances a rapid form of treatment is preferred. The recommended treatment is hypertonic saline and furosemide. This combination causes a rise in serum sodium concentration and concurrent water diuresis. This treatment is reserved for emergency situations and should be followed by fluid restriction.

TABLE 14.1

CONDITIONS ASSOCIATED WITH SYNDROME OF INAPPROPRIATE SECRETION OF ANTIDIURETIC HORMONE

Central nervous system	Tumors
Meningitis	Lymphoma
Encephalitis	Ewing sarcoma
Head trauma	Thymoma
Brain tumors	Carcinomas
Brain abscess	Mesothelioma
Botulism	
Guillain–Barré syndrome	**Drugs**
Hypoxia (neonatal)	Antidiuretic hormone
Hydrocephalus	analogues
Rocky Mountain spotted	Chlorpropamide
fever	Vincristine
Cerebral thrombosis	Cyclophosphamide
or hemorrhage	Carbamazepine
Subarachnoid or subdural	Barbiturates
hemorrhage	Colchicine
Peripheral neuropathy	Haloperidol
Hypopituitarism	Amitriptyline
	Salicylates
Pulmonary	Indomethacin
Pneumonia	
Positive-pressure ventilation	**Miscellaneous**
Asthma	Idiopathic
Pneumothorax	Pain
Cystic fibrosis	Postoperative patients

In the presence of high vasopressin levels (appropriate or inappropriate), the imprudent administration of excessive fluid volumes can culminate in severe cerebral edema.

Hyponatremia with Hypervolemia (Dilutional Syndromes)

Hypervolemic hyponatremia occurs when net water retention exceeds that of sodium. Clinically, it may be seen with (1) edema-forming states such as congestive heart failure, cirrhosis, and nephrosis; and (2) acute or chronic renal failure. Under normal conditions, an increase in sodium intake results in sodium and water retention and an increase in intravascular volume. This increase in intravascular volume in turn results in an increase in renal perfusion and in subsequent activation of the afferent and efferent mechanisms controlling renal sodium excretion. The net effect is an increase in renal sodium excretion and water retention in an attempt to return the intravascular volume to normal.

These patients have an increase in total body sodium but disproportionately larger increases in total body water. Therapy should be directed at maximal improvement of the underlying disorder. Because total body sodium is already elevated, efforts to increase serum sodium through administration of saline result only in further expansion of extracellular fluid volume and may worsen the clinical status of the patient. Attempting to decrease total body water by severe restriction of fluid intake is the most appropriate therapy. The excess sodium needs to be treated concomitantly by sodium restriction and judicious use of diuretics.

HYPERNATREMIA

Hypernatremia, defined as a rise in the serum sodium concentration to a value ≥ 150 mmol/L, is a common electrolyte disorder. Because sodium is a functionally impermeable solute, it contributes to tonicity and induces the movement of water across cell membranes. Therefore, hypernatremia invariably denotes hypertonic hyperosmolality and always causes cellular dehydration, at least transiently. The resultant morbidity may be inconsequential, serious, or even life-threatening.

Hypernatremia represents a deficit of water in relation to the body's sodium stores, which can result from a net water loss or a hypertonic sodium gain (Table 14.2). Net water loss accounts for most cases of hypernatremia. It can occur in the absence of a sodium deficit (pure water loss) or in its presence (hypotonic fluid loss). Hypertonic sodium gain usually results from clinical interventions or accidental sodium loading. Intentional salt poisoning also has been described as a form of child abuse.

Because sustained hypernatremia can occur only when thirst or access to water is impaired, the groups at highest risk are patients with altered mental status, infants, and elderly patients. Hypernatremia in infants usually results from diarrhea, whereas in the other groups it usually is associated with infirmity or febrile illness.

Clinical signs and symptoms of hypernatremia with associated hypertonicity are directly related to cerebral cell dehydration resulting from water movement from the ICF to the ECF. Neurologic manifestations include varying degrees of depressed sensorium, ranging from lethargy to coma. Most patients exhibit marked irritability, a high-pitched cry, and seizure activity. Muscle tone may be normal or increased, and may be accompanied by hyperreflexia or twitching. Examination of the cerebrospinal fluid may show an elevated protein without pleocytosis. Some patients also may have hyperglycemia, hypercalcemia, hypokalemia, or metabolic acidosis. With extreme hypertonicity and resultant water movement from brain cells

<table>
<tr><td colspan="1">TABLE 14.2</td></tr>
<tr><td>CAUSES OF HYPERNATREMIA</td></tr>
</table>

Net water loss
  Pure water loss
    Unreplaced insensible losses (dermal and respiratory)
    Hypodipsia
    Neurogenic diabetes insipidus
      Posttraumatic
      Caused by tumors, cysts, histiocytosis, tuberculosis, sarcoidosis
      Idiopathic
      Caused by aneurysms, meningitis, encephalitis, Guillain–Barré syndrome
      Caused by ethanol ingestion (transient)
    Congenital nephrogenic diabetes insipidus
    Acquired nephrogenic diabetes insipidus
      Caused by renal disease (e.g., medullary cystic disease)
      Caused by hypercalcemia or hypokalemia
      Caused by drugs (lithium, demeclocycline, foscarnet, methoxyflurane, amphotericin B)
  Hypotonic fluid loss
    Renal causes
      Loop diuretics
      Osmotic diuresis (glucose, urea, mannitol)
      Postobstructive diuresis
      Polyuric phase of acute tubular necrosis
      Intrinsic renal disease
    Gastrointestinal causes
      Vomiting
      Nasogastric drainage
      Enterocutaneous fistula
      Diarrhea
      Use of osmotic cathartic agents (e.g., lactulose)
    Cutaneous cause
      Burns
      Excessive sweating
Hypertonic sodium gain
  Hypertonic sodium bicarbonate infusion
  Hypertonic feeding preparation
  Ingestion of sodium chloride
  Ingestion of sea water
  Hypertonic sodium chloride infusion
  Hypertonic dialysis
  Primary hyperaldosteronism
  Cushing syndrome

into the ECF, the entire brain can shrink away from the cranium and produce rupture of cerebral vessels. Consequently, focal intracerebral and subdural hemorrhages and/or venous thrombosis may occur.

Because the CNS is particularly vulnerable to hypertonicity, the brain cells adapt within hours by increasing intracellular osmolality with resultant movement of water back into the brain cells. Myoinositol, taurine, glycerylphosphorylcholine, and betaine are the organic osmolytes (formerly called *idiogenic osmoles*) responsible for normalizing brain water content. If hypertonicity develops rapidly, these intracellular osmoles or osmoprotective molecules may not be generated fast enough to prevent brain cell shrinkage. Therefore, the severity of clinical manifestations of hypernatremia and associated hypertonicity is related both to its degree and rate of development.

The mechanism of hypernatremia with normal volume status is excessive sodium intake. Most cases are iatrogenic, including the use of sodium bicarbonate or improperly diluted infant formula. Ultimately, even these disturbances result in a water deficit and hypovolemia because water is lost as the kidney attempts to excrete the salt load.

In clinical medicine, the most common cause of hypernatremia is a primary water deficit with a relative excess of sodium, resulting in hypernatremia with decreased volume status. Water and sodium loss may occur through the extrarenal route or the renal route (Table 14.2). Included in this category are patients with diabetes insipidus (DI). DI is characterized by complete or partial failure of ADH secretion (central DI) or decreased renal response to ADH (nephrogenic DI), resulting in excretion of hypotonic urine. Central DI may be idiopathic, but most patients have a history of head trauma, CNS infections, or tumors. Nephrogenic DI may be congenital or acquired, and results in hypernatremia usually associated with decreased water intake.

Hypernatremic dehydration also is well described in breast-fed newborns. The serum sodium concentration in these cases may be dramatically elevated and frequently is associated with complications. Some infants may present with the triad of fever, absence of overt signs of dehydration, and poor weight gain in the first week of life. In some of these earlier-presenting infants, serum bilirubin concentrations may be elevated. In these infants, the fever subsides quickly and the serum bilirubin concentrations fall rapidly within a few hours of rehydration. In general, the infants make an uneventful recovery without permanent neurologic sequelae. Fever, presumably secondary to dehydration, is a useful early warning sign. Such cases emphasize the importance of early and regular measurement of body weight in exclusively breast-fed infants. Hypervolemic hypernatremia results when sodium gain is greater than water intake. This may include administration of hypertonic saline or sodium bicarbonate. Hypernatremia with increased volume status also may be seen in patients with primary hyperaldosteronism or Cushing syndrome because of sodium retention.

Whenever possible, therapy of hypernatremic patients should be directed at the underlying disease process (e.g., administration of vasopressin analogues in DI). In the presence of shock or severe ECF volume contraction, restoration of the intravascular volume takes precedence over normalization of plasma osmolality. In this setting, isotonic saline solutions are the recommended fluid replacement to restore circulating blood volume.

The speed of correction of hypernatremia depends on the rate of its development and the accompanying clinical presentation. Correction of hypernatremia should be accomplished slowly, except in the setting of acute massive salt poisoning. Rapid lowering of serum sodium may result in water movement from the ECF into the brain cells, resulting in cerebral edema and possible herniation. When serum sodium acutely exceeds 175 mEq/L (as in salt poisoning), dialysis may be performed to lower serum sodium rapidly. Once serum sodium concentration is at 170 mEq/L, further reduction should be carried out over 48 hours, with the aim of lowering serum sodium no greater than 1 mEq/L/h.

A slower pace of correction is prudent in patients with hypernatremia of longer or unknown duration because the full dissipation of accumulated brain solutes occurs over a period of several days. In such patients, reducing the serum sodium concentration at a maximal rate of 0.5 mEq/L/h prevents cerebral edema and convulsions.

HYPERKALEMIA

Potassium is the major intracellular cation; only a very small fraction of total body potassium is in the intravascular space. Increased potassium concentration in serum is infrequent in pediatrics, but it can be life-threatening because of its effect on membrane potentials, particularly of heart muscle.

The serum potassium concentration is affected primarily by the kidney. Potassium is filtered by the glomerulus, then reabsorbed and secreted by the tubule. Processes that interfere with filtration or secretion (e.g., acute or chronic glomerulonephritis, interstitial nephritis) may cause hyperkalemia; processes that interfere with reabsorption may cause hypokalemia. The most common cause of an increased serum potassium is "pseudohyperkalemia" due to specimen hemolysis or to tissue hypoxia distal to the placement of a tourniquet. A repeat determination usually is sufficient to resolve whether hyperkalemia is present, but if an adequate specimen is difficult to obtain, electrocardiography (ECG) can be helpful. True hyperkalemia in children is associated most commonly with acute or chronic renal failure. Certain drugs used infrequently in pediatric practice can produce hyperkalemia: spironolactone, amiloride, triamterene, cyclosporin, and angiotensin-converting enzyme inhibitors (e.g., captopril, enalapril). Nonsteroidal anti-inflammatory drugs also are recognized as being capable of producing hyperkalemia, which is the result of chronic renal injury. Occasionally usual doses of nonsteroidal anti-inflammatory drugs given in the course of treatment of brief illness associated with poor fluid intake can result in renal failure and hyperkalemia.

Two clinical situations that physicians need to recognize are (1) the infant in the first weeks of life who vomits and has virilized genitalia (congenital adrenal hyperplasia) or normal genitalia (pseudohypoaldosteronism); and (2) a child of any age who has acute metabolic acidosis, including children with diabetic ketoacidosis.

Clinical signs of hyperkalemia usually are absent until the serum potassium is quite high, particularly when the accumulation of potassium has occurred gradually. At concentrations >7 mEq/L (usually >8.5 mEq/L), the patient may develop ascending muscle weakness to the point of flaccid paralysis. Cerebration and cranial nerve function are preserved. There usually are no clinical signs of altered cardiac function until concentrations exceed 9 or 10 mEq/L, when ventricular fibrillation or asystole may develop.

Changes in the waveform on ECG provide clues to the degree of hyperkalemia. The earliest changes are tall, peaked T-waves, with a normal or shortened QT interval and shortened PR interval; these are present at serum potassium concentrations of 5.5 to 6.5 mEq/L. As the serum potassium concentration rises, cardiac conduction is impaired. The QRS complex begins to widen and the PR interval lengthens at serum potassium concentrations of 6.5 to 7.5 mEq/L. With further increases in the serum potassium concentration, the P-waves become broad and of low amplitude, the QT interval is prolonged, and the ST segment is either elevated or depressed (7 to 8 mEq/L). When the serum potassium concentration exceeds 8 mEq/L, P-waves disappear; the QRS becomes markedly widened and may progress to a "sine wave" configuration, identifying the patient to be at risk of ventricular fibrillation or asystole.

Potential treatment (Table 14.3) includes (1) protecting the heart from the effects of hyperkalemia (e.g., calcium salt IV); (2) shifting potassium from the intravascular space to the intracellular space (e.g., sodium bicarbonate IV, insulin/glucose IV); and (3) eliminating potassium from the body (e.g., dialysis, ion exchange resins PO or PR).

An intravenous (IV) infusion of calcium ion acts rapidly but its effects last only approximately 1 hour (Table 14.3). Sodium bicarbonate or insulin/glucose causes potassium to move intracellularly. Sodium bicarbonate has no significant action on plasma potassium in the first 60 minutes after administration. Insulin binds to specific membrane receptors and through a second messenger stimulates the sodium–potassium adenosine triphosphatase (Na^+/K^+-ATPase) pump, resulting in intracellular uptake of potassium. This effect is independent

TABLE 14.3

EMERGENCY TREATMENT OF HYPERKALEMIA

Technique	Agent	Dose	Onset/Duration of action	Comment
Reversal of membrane effects	10% calcium gluconate	0.5 mL/kg	30–60 min	ECG monitor; discontinue if pulse rate <100
Movement of K into cells	Na bicarbonate, 7.5% (1 mEq = 1 mL)	2–3 mL/kg	30 min/1–4 h	May use in the absence of acidosis
	Glucose 50% plus insulin (regular)	1 unit for every 5–6 g glucose	Same	Monitor blood glucose
	Albuterol 0.5% solution	0.01–0.05 mL/kg (max 1 mL) aerosolized with 1–2 mL saline	15–30 min	Monitor heart rate
Enhanced excretion of K	Kayexalate	1 g/kg	Hours/variable	Can be given orally or by rectum; give with sorbitol (70%)

From Perkin RM, Novotny WE, Harris GD, et al. Common electrolyte problems in pediatric patients presenting to the ED. *Pediatr Emerg Med Rep* 2001;6:13–26, with permission.

of its hypoglycemic action. In children, a glucose load of 0.5 to 1 g/kg IV should be given over 15 to 30 minutes. This is because many children increase their endogenous insulin production with the administration of a glucose load. If blood glucose is elevated, insulin can be added starting at 0.05 U/kg IV or SC.

Beta$_2$-adrenergic agonists drive K^+ into cells by increasing Na^+/K^+-ATPase activity. They are effective in reducing the serum potassium concentration rapidly and can be delivered by aerosol. Studies have shown that in some patients albuterol can lower the K^+ by up to 1.5 mEq/L within 30 minutes.

Effects of calcium, insulin, bicarbonate, and β_2 agonists are transient. Therefore, these measures usually are followed by a cation exchange resin, diuretics, or dialysis to remove the excess K^+ from the body. Sodium polystyrene sulfonate resin (Kayexalate) is given at a dose of 1 g/kg in 20% sorbitol orally or in 70% sorbitol rectal installation. The latter must be retained for 20 to 30 minutes and can be repeated every 4 to 6 hours. In the gut, this resin takes up K^+ and, to lesser degrees, Ca^{2+} and Mg^{2+}, while it releases Na^+. Each gram of resin may bind 1 mEq of K^+ and release 1 to 2 mEq of Na^+. The major side effects are nausea, constipation, hypokalemia, and retention of Na^+ exchanged for K^+. Loop and thiazide diuretics increase urinary K^+ excretion by enhancing K^+ secretion in the distal nephron, but are not widely used because patients with impaired renal function are unlikely to respond. In acute or chronic renal failure, the aforementioned measures are used while preparations are made for dialysis. In stable patients with acute renal failure, hemodialysis is preferred to peritoneal dialysis because the rate of K^+ removal is faster (see Chapter 62).

HYPOKALEMIA

Hypokalemia is defined as a serum potassium level <3.5 mEq/L. As with hyperkalemia, nerves and muscles (including the heart) are most affected by hypokalemia, particularly if the patient has other preexisting disease, such as cardiovascular disease.

Both the total body stores of potassium and its distribution in the body are closely regulated by key hormones. The normal transcellular distribution of potassium (a high ratio of intracellular to extracellular potassium) is maintained by at least two hormonal signals that promote the entry of this cation into cells. Both insulin and β-adrenergic catecholamines increase cellular potassium uptake by stimulating cell membrane Na^+/K^+-ATPase. Administration of alkali causes a shift of potassium into cells, but the response is quite variable. In general, serum K^+ decreases by approximately 0.3 mEq/L for every 0.1 increase in pH above normal. In patients with end-stage renal disease, administration of bicarbonate has only a slight effect on the transcellular distribution of potassium.

It remains unclear whether aldosterone affects the transcellular distribution of potassium, but this hormone is clearly the major regulator of body stores of potassium through its effect on the excretion of potassium by the kidney.

Patients with hypokalemia often have no symptoms, particularly when the disorder is mild (K^+ = 3 to 3.5 mEq/L). With more severe hypokalemia, nonspecific symptoms, such as generalized weakness, lassitude, and constipation, are more common. When serum potassium decreases to <2.5 mEq/L, muscle necrosis can occur, and at serum concentrations of <2.0 mEq/L, an ascending paralysis can develop with eventual impairment of respiratory function. The likelihood of symptoms appears to correlate with the rapidity of the decrease in serum potassium. In patients without underlying heart disease, abnormalities in cardiac conduction are extremely unusual, even when the serum potassium concentration is <3.0 mEq/L. In patients with cardiac ischemia, heart failure, or left ventricular hypertrophy, however, even mild to moderate hypokalemia increases the likelihood of cardiac arrhythmias. Hypokalemia also notably increases the arrhythmogenic potential of digoxin. Thus, hypokalemia should be avoided or treated promptly in patients receiving digitalis derivatives.

Hypokalemia rarely is suspected on the basis of clinical presentation; the diagnosis is made by measurement of serum potassium. A low serum potassium concentration indicates disruption of normal homeostasis, with one very rare exception. In some patients with leukemia and markedly elevated white cell counts, potassium is taken up by the abnormal cells if the blood is left at room temperature for several hours prior to analysis. More commonly, hypokalemia in patients with leukemia is the result of renal potassium wasting.

Hypokalemia is suggested by changes in the ECG, including:

- U-waves
- T-wave flattening
- ST segment changes
- Arrhythmias (especially if the patient is taking digoxin)
- Pulseless electrical activity or asystole

Hypokalemia almost always is the result of potassium depletion induced by abnormal losses of potassium. More rarely, hypokalemia occurs because of an abrupt shift of potassium from the extracellular compartment into cells. In either case, drugs prescribed by physicians are the most common causes of hypokalemia. Thus, the first step in the management of hypokalemia is to review the patient's drug record.

In the absence of an inciting drug, hypokalemia can result from an acute shift of potassium from the extracellular compartment to cells, from inadequate intake, or from abnormal losses. Most commonly, hypokalemia is the result of either abnormal loss through the kidney induced by metabolic alkalosis or loss in the stool induced by diarrhea.

The various causes of hypokalemia are listed in Table 14.4. In some patients, more than one mechanism may be involved.

Hypokalemia is an almost invariable consequence of metabolic alkalosis. In the most common form of this disorder, induced by selective chloride depletion due to vomiting or nasogastric drainage, hypokalemia develops in parallel with the alkalosis as a result of increased renal potassium loss. In the chloride-sensitive form of metabolic alkalosis, the administration of chloride corrects the alkalosis and allows the repletion of body stores of potassium if potassium intake is adequate.

More rarely, metabolic alkalosis occurs independently of chloride depletion, as a result of systemic or intrarenal abnormalities that augment sodium reabsorption in the distal nephron. The most common of these abnormalities is *primary hyperaldosteronism*, a disorder often heralded by severe hypokalemia (K^+ <3 mEq/L). Hypokalemia also can develop in patients with Cushing syndrome, but it usually is milder than in patients with hyperaldosteronism.

Genetic abnormalities that influence the activity of renal ion transporters are rare causes of metabolic alkalosis and hypokalemia. Two of these disorders (Liddle syndrome and 11β-hydroxysteroid dehydrogenase deficiency) stimulate reabsorption of sodium by collecting duct cells and cause the *syndrome of apparent mineralocorticoid excess*, so named because this transport abnormality results in hypertension and hypokalemia, but serum aldosterone concentrations are low rather than high. In two other disorders, genetic mutations inactivate or impede the activity of chloride-associated sodium transporters in the loop of Henle (Bartter syndrome) and early distal tubule (Gitelman syndrome), causing metabolic alkalosis and hypokalemia without hypertension.

Magnesium depletion, induced either by dietary restriction or by abnormal loss, reduces the intracellular potassium concentration and causes renal potassium wasting. The depletion of intracellular potassium stores appears to be due to impairment of the activity of cell membrane NA^+/K^+-ATPase, but the mechanism by which magnesium depletion causes renal potassium loss is unclear. Magnesium depletion often coexists with potassium depletion as a result of drugs (e.g., diuretics and amphotericin B) or disease processes (e.g., hyperaldosteronism and diarrhea) that cause loss of both ions, making it difficult to assess whether the hypokalemia is caused by the hypomagnesemia or is an independent effect. Regardless of the cause, the ability to correct potassium deficiency is impaired when magnesium deficiency is present.

TABLE 14.4

CAUSES OF HYPOKALEMIA

Nutritional
  Poor intake of potassium-containing foods
  Parenteral fluids devoid of potassium

Transcellular shifts
  Metabolic or respiratory alkalosis
  Insulin or glucose therapy
  Elevated β-adrenergic activity; stress, β-agonist treatment
    for asthma
  Periodic paralysis—hypokalemic form
  Pseudohypokalemia
  Hypothermia

Gastrointestinal losses
  Diarrhea
  Vomiting
  Ureterosigmoidostomy
  Purgative abuse
  Intestinal fistulas
  Cystic fibrosis

Renal losses
  Polyuria
  Renal tubular damage
    Chronic interstitial nephritis
    Chronic pyelonephritis
    Nephrotoxins (e.g., chemotherapy, amphotericin,
      nonsteroidal anti-inflammatory agents)
  Excess mineralocorticoid effect
    Primary hyperaldosteronism
    Congenital adrenal hyperplasia
    Renin-secreting tumors
    Cushing syndrome
    Renovascular hypertension
    High-dose glucocorticoids
    Licorice ingestion
  Increased Na^+ delivery to the distal tubule
    Proximal tublopathy—proximal RTA, Fanconi syndrome
    Hypercalcemic states
    Diuretic therapy
    Distal RTA—type 1
  Nonreabsorbable anion
    Certain medications—penicillins
    Bicarbonate—nasogastral suction or vomiting, alkali
      therapy for RTA
    Ketones
  Primary renal tubular disorder—Bartter, Gitelman,
    and Liddle syndromes
  Magnesium depletion

RTA, renal tubular acidosis.

Principles of Potassium Replacement

Potassium replacement is the cornerstone of therapy for hypokalemia. Unfortunately, supplemental potassium administration also is the most common cause of severe hyperkalemia in patients who are hospitalized, and this risk must be kept in mind when one is initiating treatment. The risk is greatest with the administration of IV potassium, which should be avoided if possible. The treatment of hypokalemia includes minimizing further potassium loss and giving potassium replacement. Intravenous administration of potassium is indicated when arrhythmias are present or hypokalemia is severe (K^+ <2.5 mEq/L).

Acute potassium administration may be empirical in emergent conditions. When indicated, maximum IV K^+ replacement should be 0.3 to 1 mEq/kg/h (maximum, 40 mEq/h) with continuous ECG monitoring during infusion. Central or peripheral IV sites may be used. A more concentrated solution of potassium may be infused if a central line is used, but the catheter tip should not extend into the right atrium.

If cardiac arrest from hypokalemia is imminent (i.e., malignant ventricular arrhythmias), more rapid replacement of potassium is required. In the patient's chart, the clinician documents that rapid infusion is intentional in response to life-threatening hypokalemia. Once the patient is stabilized, the infusion is reduced to continue potassium replacement more gradually.

CALCIUM

Calcium is an essential ion for function of all cells in the body. It is the primary regulator of motion and regulates excitation–contraction coupling, neurotransmission, hormonal secretion, mitosis, ciliary motion, phagocytosis, and many other processes. These are all vital cell functions that are essential for cellular health.

In the serum, it consists of three fractions: (1) ionized or free calcium, accounting for approximately 50% of total calcium; (2) protein-bound calcium that is not filterable by the kidney, accounting for approximately 40%; and (3) calcium complexed to anions such as bicarbonate, citrate, sulfate, phosphate, and lactate, accounting for the remaining 10%. Ionized calcium is the physiologically active portion. In addition to serum protein concentration (principally albumin), pH also influences protein binding of calcium and thus the ionized calcium level. When available as a laboratory test, the ionized calcium level should be followed. Abnormalities in serum calcium concentration have profound effects on neurologic, gastrointestinal, and renal function. Maintenance of the normal serum calcium is a result of tightly regulated ion transport by the kidney, intestinal tract, and bone, mediated by calcemic hormones, especially parathyroid hormone (PTH) and 1,25-dihydroxyvitamin D [$1,25(OH)_2$ D]. Abnormalities in calcium transport that result in uncompensated influx into, or efflux from, the extracellular fluid result in hypercalcemia or hypocalcemia, respectively.

Hypocalcemia

Hypocalcemia usually is defined as an ionized calcium level <4 mg/dL (1 mmol/L). Hypocalcemia occurs when there is a net efflux of calcium from the ECF; calcium is lost from the ECF, often through renal mechanisms, in greater quantities than can be replaced by the intestinal transport or bone (Table 14.5). Falsely low levels of calcium due to hypoalbuminemia should be excluded by measuring ionized calcium.

In many cases, hypocalcemia is a result of an inability to mobilize calcium from the skeletal system. This is secondary to decreased secretion of PTH (hypoparathyroidism, hypomagnesemia), impaired synthesis of $1,25(OH)_2$ D (renal failure, vitamin D–dependent rickets), or inadequate responsiveness of target organs to PTH (pseudohypoparathyroidism, vitamin D deficiency, osteomalacia, renal failure, hypomagnesemia) or $1,25(OH)_2$ D (vitamin D–dependent type II rickets).

The manifestations of hypocalcemia may be ascribed to increased neuromuscular excitability and can range from numbness and tingling of lips, hands, and toes, to carpopedal spasms, irritability, laryngeal stridor, apnea, and generalized

TABLE 14.5
CAUSES OF HYPOCALCEMIA

True hypoparathyroidism
  Familial, with or without multiple endocrine abnormalities ("autoimmune")
  DiGeorge syndrome
  Postsurgical
  Idiopathic
  Magnesium deficiency

End-organ resistance to parathyroid hormone
  Primary vitamin D deficiency (dietary, sunlight)
  Secondary vitamin D deficiency
    Malabsorption (e.g., celiac disease, biliary atresia)
    Anticonvulsant therapy
    Chronic renal failure
  Primary vitamin D resistance (familial hypophosphatemic rickets, uncommonly)
  Secondary vitamin D resistance
    Fanconi syndromes (e.g., cystinosis, Lowe syndrome)
    Renal tubular acidosis
  Primary vitamin D dependence
    Type I (deficient I, α-hydroxylase)
    Type II [end-organ resistance to $1,25(OH)_2$ vitamin D]
  Magnesium deficiency

Miscellaneous causes
  Hypoproteinemia
  Hypernatremic dehydration with K^+ deficiency
  Postacidotic tetany
  Diuretic abuse
  Phosphate loading
  Critical illness

tonic-clonic seizures. Trousseau sign (contractions of the hand muscles induced by decreased blood flow to the extremity), and Chvostek sign (spasm of the facial muscles evoked by tapping the facial nerve anterior to the ear) may be present. Decreases in cardiac contractility and systemic vascular resistance result in hypotension. Cardiac manifestations also may consist of a prolonged QT interval, which may progress to ventricular fibrillation or heart block.

Severe, symptomatic hypocalcemia should be treated immediately. Calcium may be given IV as 10% calcium chloride (10 to 20 mg/kg/dose) or 10% calcium gluconate (50 to 100 mg/kg/dose) by slow infusion. The slow IV administration of calcium supplementation (10 to 15 minutes) and continuous ECG recording are critical to monitor for bradycardia or ventricular irritability. Intravenous access must be secure because calcium infiltration can result in phlebitis and tissue necrosis. Except in the setting of life-threatening hypocalcemia, calcium salts usually are best administered into a central vein. Multiple doses must be guided by frequent ionized calcium determinations.

Several general principles apply to the management of a hypocalcemic patient. The magnesium level should be checked and, if low, corrected. In a setting of sepsis or renal failure, metabolic acidosis may accompany hypocalcemia and calcium must be replaced before the acidosis is corrected to avoid worsening of hypocalcemia. Calcium and hydrogen ions compete for protein-binding sites, so an increase in pH with alkali therapy will increase the binding sites for calcium, leading to a rapid fall in ionized calcium, potentially resulting in cardiac arrest—unless the calcium is corrected first. Sodium bicarbonate and calcium salts must be infused in separate lines to avoid precipitation of calcium carbonate. Patients on digoxin should be monitored carefully because administration of calcium may potentiate digitalis toxicity and cause death. Intravenous calcium should be given cautiously in the presence of hyperphosphatemia; a total calcium × phosphate product of greater than 70 mg/dL may lead to soft tissue calcification. Similarly, aggressive replacement of phosphorus may precipitate tetany.

Hypercalcemia

In pediatrics, hypercalcemia is an uncommon occurrence. Hypercalcemia is defined as a measured total serum calcium concentration >11 mg/dL. This discussion excludes hypercalcemia in the newborn. The major causes of hypercalcemia in infants and children are outlined in Table 14.6. Hypercalcemia can result from increased calcium absorption from the gut or increased calcium resorption from bone. Hypercalcemia occasionally results from a massive increase in dietary calcium intake or a reduction in the renal excretion of calcium. In hyperparathyroidism, increased bone resorption of calcium results in hypercalcemia, and decreased renal reabsorption of phosphorus results in hypophosphatemia. Because PTH stimulates bone turnover, alkaline phosphatase is elevated. A serum PTH level that is inappropriately elevated for the concurrent serum calcium confirms the diagnosis. The vitamin D toxicity syndromes usually can be suspected from the history; hypercalcemia is the result of increased calcium absorption. If the intoxicating compound is conventional vitamin D, then hypercalcemia may be prolonged because of the storage of this compound in adipose tissue.

Symptoms of hypercalcemia may be attributed to its depressive effects on neuromuscular function. These include

anorexia, nausea, vomiting, lethargy, muscular weakness, confusion, and stupor. ECG changes (shortening of the QT interval) may be seen.

Treatment of a hypercalcemic crisis depends on the underlying cause, level of serum calcium, and severity of signs and symptoms. It always requires hospitalization in an intensive-care setting. The choice of therapy depends on whether the kidneys are functioning normally. The initial emergency treatment of symptomatic hypercalcemia is designed to enhance calcium excretion by saline infusion at a rate of twice maintenance followed by bolus injections of furosemide, 1 to 2 mg/kg every 6 to 8 hours. The subsequent amount and rate of saline to be administered depends on the state of hydration and presence or absence of hypertension or preexisting cardiac disease, but in an otherwise normal patient, saline flow rates of two to three times daily maintenance would be appropriate until the serum calcium returns to normal. In acute oliguric renal failure, peritoneal dialysis or hemodialysis against a low-calcium dialysate usually is effective.

For hypercalcemia that is poorly responsive to conventional treatment, treatment with bisphosphonates should be considered. Most pediatric experience is with pamidronate: a single dose of 0.5 to 1 mg/kg IV should normalize the serum calcium in 2 to 5 days. Hypersensitivity to the drug or its components is the only contraindication to IV administration. It should be used cautiously in renal insufficiency, and adequate hydration and urinary output should be ensured during treatment.

MAGNESIUM

Magnesium is the fourth most abundant cation in the body and the second most abundant intracellular electrolyte. Ninety-nine percent is found in the intracellular compartment, and the remaining 1% is in extracellular fluid. This important ion is a dependent co-factor in the function of more than 300 enzyme systems. It is an obligatory co-factor in reactions involving ATP, including maintenance of normal intracellular potassium by the Na^+/K^+-ATPase pump. It is essential to oxidative phosphorylation, protein synthesis, amino acid activation, and glucose use. Serum magnesium levels are regulated by the kidneys. The normal serum or plasma magnesium ranges from 1.7 to 2.2 mg/dL (0.75 to 0.95 mmol/L; 1.5 to 1.9 mEq/L).

The plasma magnesium concentration is composed of bound and unbound fractions in a manner that is similar to that of calcium; approximately 50% of the circulating magnesium is free (i.e., ionized). In critically ill patients, the total magnesium concentration may poorly reflect the physiologic (ionized) concentration; the latter can be measured with ion-selective electrodes. Particularly in pharmacologic concentrations, magnesium can inhibit calcium channels, which accounts for some of the potentially therapeutic effects of magnesium. Through inhibition of calcium channels and the subsequent reduction of intracellular calcium concentration, magnesium causes smooth muscle relaxation, which has been used in the treatment of acute severe asthma. In addition, the effects of magnesium on calcium channels, and perhaps other membrane effects, have been useful in the treatment of torsades de pointes ventricular tachycardia.

Hypomagnesemia

Magnesium deficiency is estimated to be present in 20% to 65% of critically ill patients and has been associated with increased mortality rates. Because magnesium deficiency is common and may lead to life-threatening complications, total

---

TABLE 14.6

CAUSES OF HYPERCALCEMIA

Increased intestinal absorption of calcium
  Hypervitaminosis D
  Hyperparathyroidism
  Postrenal transplantation
  Sarcoidosis
  Granulomatous diseases: tuberculosis; fungal infections
  Idiopathic hypercalcemia (William syndrome)
  Phosphate depletion
  Malignancy associated

Increased bone solubilization
  Hyperparathyroidism
  Malignancy
  Hyperthyroidism
  Immobilization

Increased renal tubular reabsorption of calcium
  Thiazide diuretics
  Familial benign hypocalciuric hypercalcemia

Miscellaneous
  Subcutaneous fat necrosis
  Vitamin A intoxication
  Recovery phase of acute tubular necrosis, especially after rhabdomyolysis or tissue necrosis
  Iatrogenic
  Hypophosphatasia
  Idiopathic hypercalcemia of infancy
  Milk–alkali syndrome
  Pheochromocytoma

TABLE 14.7

HYPOMAGNESEMIA

Cause of deficiency	Specific association
Gastrointestinal	Prolonged gastric/intestinal fluid losses Acute/chronic diarrhea and steatorrhea Protein-calorie malnutrition Prolonged parenteral nutrition without Mg
Renal loss	Osmotic diuresis (especially diabetes mellitus) Hypercalcemia
Renal diseases	Diuretic phase of acute tubular necrosis Postobstructive nephropathy Renal tubular defects Chronic pyelonephritis
Metabolic acidosis	Starvation Ketoacidosis Alcoholism
Endocrine	Hyperaldosteronism Hyperthyroidism Hypoparathyroidism/ hyperparathyroidism
Drugs	Diuretics Aminoglycosides Amphotericin B Cisplatin Cyclosporine Pentamidine Cardiac glycosides (possible)
Critical illness	

serum magnesium concentration has been viewed as the "fifth electrolyte" needed in every patient (in addition to sodium, potassium, chloride, and bicarbonate). The usual cause of hypomagnesemia is loss of magnesium from the gastrointestinal tract or the kidney (Table 14.7).

Most of the symptoms of moderate to severe hypomagnesemia are nonspecific, and symptomatic magnesium depletion usually is associated with additional ion abnormalities such as hypocalcemia, hypokalemia, and metabolic alkalosis.

Hypocalcemia is typically present in association with severe hypomagnesemia, and the degree seems to be related to the severity of the magnesium depletion, usually appearing at a serum Mg <1 mEq/L (0.5 mmol/L). Patients may present with evidence of neuromuscular hyperexcitability, with positive Chvostek and Trousseau signs or spontaneous carpopedal spasm. Most hypocalcemic/hypomagnesemic patients have a low or normal PTH concentration, suggesting impaired synthesis or secretion of PTH. Total body magnesium repletion leads to a rapid rise in plasma PTH.

Hypokalemia also is a frequent feature of magnesium deficiency (40% to 60% of cases). In magnesium deficiency, potassium secretion in the loop of Henle and the cortical collecting tubule increases. In this scenario, hypokalemia does not respond to potassium replacement alone and the magnesium deficit has to be corrected.

Magnesium depletion may produce acute ECG changes such as widening of the QRS complex and the appearance of peaked T-waves. In severe depletion, the PR interval is prolonged, with progressive widening of the QRS, T-wave inversion, and the appearance of U-waves. Hypomagnesemia has been implicated in severe ventricular arrhythmias, especially during myocardial ischemia and cardiopulmonary bypass procedures. There also is an association between hypomagnesemia and sensitivity to cardiac glycosides.

The use of IV magnesium should be considered for refractory arrhythmias, even in the presence of normal serum magnesium levels, particularly if the patient is on digoxin and diuretics. According to numerous case reports, magnesium sulfate has proven effective in treating a wide range of cardiac arrhythmias, especially ventricular arrhythmias, after conventional therapies have failed.

The choice of route of magnesium repletion varies with the severity of the clinical findings. An acute infusion of magnesium could decrease magnesium reabsorption in the loop of Henle, with most of the infused magnesium excreted in the urine. For this reason, oral replacement is preferred, especially in symptom-free patients. Oral magnesium replacement can be hampered by magnesium associated diarrhea.

Symptomatic magnesium deficiency should be treated parenterally. Magnesium sulfate can be supplemented at an IV dose of 25 to 50 mg/kg/dose (maximum single dose, 2 g) infused over 3 to 4 hours. Cardiorespiratory monitoring is required during IV administration of magnesium because hypotension, arrhythmias, and skeletal muscle weakness with respiratory failure have been reported (see Hypermagnesemia, below). Calcium should be readily available as an antidote. Concomitant hypocalcemia and hypokalemia should be corrected separately.

Hypermagnesemia

Hypermagnesemia is uncommon in pediatrics but, as in adults, usually is related to accidental overdose. This is particularly true in patients with impaired renal function. Magnesium-containing over-the-counter medications, particularly antacids and cathartics, may result in hypermagnesemia in infants and small children. Measurement of serum magnesium concentration is appropriate in the child with unexplained lethargy, hypotonia, respiratory depression, or hypotension. Pseudohypermagnesemia may be associated with hemolytic release of intracellular magnesium.

Manifestations of hypermagnesemia are based on this ion's affect on the CNS, cardiovascular system, and neuromuscular junction. CNS manifestations include drowsiness, confusion, lethargy, and coma. Effects on the cardiovascular system include hypotension and dysrhythmias. These effects are caused by the calcium channel–blocking properties of magnesium, which decreases entry of calcium into cells and enhances egress of calcium from cells. At the neuromuscular junction, magnesium sulfate decreases the amount of acetylcholine liberated, diminishes the sensitivity of the end-plate to acetylcholine, and depresses the excitability of the muscle membrane. This results in skeletal muscle weakness and respiratory distress. Clinical signs and symptoms correlate with plasma concentrations. ECG changes (prolongation of the PR interval, increased duration of the QRS complex, and increased height of the T-waves) are noted with concentrations of 6 to 12 mg/dL (5 to 10 mEq/L); deep tendon reflexes are lost when serum concentrations reach 12 mg/dL (10 mEq/L); respiratory paralysis and sinoatrial and atrioventricular block occur at 18 mg/dL (15 mEq/L); and cardiac arrest occurs at 30 mg/dL (25 mEq/L).

Management of hypermagnesemia is dictated by the cardiovascular, CNS, and neuromuscular changes that occur. Treatment consists of stopping the source of magnesium, respiratory and cardiovascular support, calcium, diuresis, and dialysis. Indications for dialysis include kidney failure, increasing magnesium levels despite diuresis, dysrhythmias, and persistent hemodynamic instability.

Suggested Readings

Adrogue HJ, Madias NE. Hypernatremia. *N Engl J Med* 2000;342:1493–1499.

Arieff AI, Kronlund BA. Fatal child abuse by forced water intoxication. *Pediatrics* 1999;103:1292–1295.

Bhalla P, Eaton FE, Coulter JGS, et al. Hyponatremic seizures and excessive intake of hypotonic fluids in young children. *BMJ* 1999;319:1554–1557.

Bushinsky DA, Monk RD. Calcium. *Lancet* 1998;352:306–311.

Gennari FJ. Hypokalemia. *N Engl J Med* 1998;339:451–458.

Harker HE, Majcher TA. Hypermagnesemia in a pediatric patient. *Anesth Analg* 2000;91:1160–1162.

Moritz ML, Ayus JC. Preventing neurologic complications from dysnatremias in children. *Pediatr Nephrol* 2005;20:1687–1700.

Ng PC, Chan HB, Fok TF, et al. Early onset of hypernatremic dehydration and fever in exclusively breast-fed infants. *J Paediatr Child Health* 1999;35: 585–587.

Perkin RM, Novotny WE, Harris GD, et al. Common electrolyte problems in pediatric patients presenting to the ED. *Pediatr Emerg Med Rep* 2001;6: 13–26.

Roberts KB. Hyperkalemia. *Pediatr Rev* 1996;17:106.

Schurman SJ, Shoemaker LR. Bartter and Gitelman syndromes. *Adv Pediatr* 2000;47:223–248.

CHAPTER 15 ■ FAILURE TO THRIVE

JOHN M. OLSSON

Failure to thrive (FTT) is a syndrome characterized by failure of physical growth and malnutrition resulting from organic disease, nonorganic factors, or a combination of the two. Failure of physical growth is established by plotting growth parameters on standard growth charts produced by the National Centers for Health Statistics (*www.cdc.gov/growthcharts*). In general, growth failure is defined by either a weight less than the fifth percentile for age, or reduction in weight gain such that plotted weight crosses two or more major percentile lines in 6 months' time.

It is important to consider a child's growth over time, ideally from the time of birth. Infants who are born prematurely should have their growth plotted on charts designed for premature infants. Alternatively, if one is using charts intended for term infants, growth parameters should be corrected for prematurity. Head circumference should be corrected until a chronologic age of 18 months, weight until a chronologic age of 24 months, and length until a chronologic age of 40 months. It also is important to identify the infant who is small for gestational age or has intrauterine growth retardation. Many of these infants, for uncertain reasons, do not "catch up" in their growth pattern and continue to be small for their chronologic age.

The clinician also must consider other normal growth patterns that may be confused with failure to thrive. These include infants and children with familial short stature, constitutional growth delay, and those who follow a changing growth curve related to genetic potential. Parental heights may suggest a diagnosis of familial short stature. Constitutional short stature is suggested by a family history of delayed puberty and a later growth spurt. Most infants who have changed their growth pattern because of genetic influences establish a new "growth channel" and do so by 13 months of age.

Traditionally, infants and children are thought to fail to thrive as a result of either organic or nonorganic processes. Unfortunately, this dichotomous approach often compels physicians to seek an obscure organic diagnosis and ignore the important nutritional context. Organic FTT is growth failure caused by a specific medical condition, whereas nonorganic FTT is growth failure without a diagnosable medical cause. Frequently, children fail to thrive because of coexisting organic and nonorganic reasons, often as a result of a mild, chronic medical condition that results in changes in temperament or feeding behavior.

The concept that is central to the issue of FTT or growth deficiency is inadequate nutrition. FTT may be viewed as a transactional model in which a combination of nonorganic and organic risk factors may cause malnutrition and growth failure (Fig. 15.1). Nonorganic risk factors that place a child at risk for inadequate nutrition include the temperament of the infant or child, the interaction between the infant and its caretakers or between the infant and the environment, the feeding behavior itself, and psychosocial stressors. Organic risk factors include minor congenital anomalies, prenatal or postnatal malnutrition, medically complicated prematurity, and other chronic medical conditions. FTT is identified in children of all socioeconomic backgrounds but is found more frequently in families living in poverty. It accounts for 3% to 5% of admissions to pediatric medical hospitals. Ten percent of children in rural outpatient populations and 10% of homeless children fail to thrive.

The differential diagnosis of FTT may be best divided into three categories: inadequate caloric intake, inadequate caloric absorption, and increased caloric requirements (Table 15.1). Inadequate caloric intake may result from poor appetite, difficulty with ingestion, improper formula preparation, lack of access to food, or loss of food by vomiting. Several other disease processes may interfere with the normal absorption of calories from the gastrointestinal tract. Finally, infants and children may have caloric needs above normal or they may have metabolic disorders that impair utilization of the energy absorbed.

CLINICAL FINDINGS

Evaluation and management of children who fail to thrive begins with a thorough history and physical examination (Fig. 15.2). Medical history should be comprehensive, with an emphasis on perinatal issues, recurrent health problems, family history of growth patterns, and a social history addressing family strengths and stressors. A nutritional history should include a detailed record of dietary intake, an assessment of parental feeding attitudes, a parental report of the infant's or child's feeding behaviors, and a description of the feeding environment. An assessment of dietary intake should reflect methods of feeding, breast-feeding patterns, formula preparation, volume consumed, and feeding techniques.

A careful and thorough physical examination should be performed and must include accurate measurements of weight, length, and head circumference (to age 3). Previous measurements should be obtained to appreciate the longitudinal pattern of growth. Dysmorphic features should be noted in an effort to identify any genetic syndrome associated with short stature. In addition, the clinician should note signs of malnutrition as well as of any medical condition requiring increased caloric expenditure.

Laboratory tests that help evaluate current nutritional status or complications of malnutrition should be measured. Prealbumin, protein, albumin, liver function tests, and hemoglobin/hematocrit may be useful as baseline values and for follow-up during nutritional therapy. In addition, standard electrolytes, bicarbonate, urinalysis, lead, and creatinine may be helpful in identifying the more frequent types of occult organic disease.

Extensive laboratory or radiologic studies to identify occult disease not suggested by the thorough history, physical

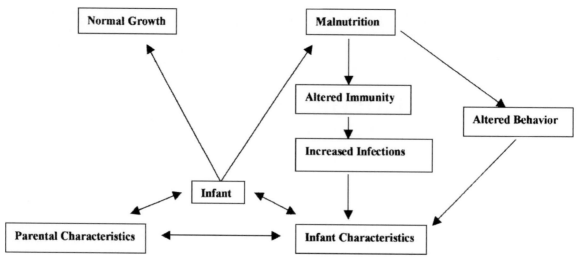

FIGURE 15.1. Transactional model of normal and abnormal growth.

examination, and basic laboratory results are not indicated as part of the initial evaluation. Sills, in a 1978 review of failure to thrive, found that of 2,607 laboratory tests performed in 185 patients, only 10 (0.4%) served to establish an organic diagnosis. In this study, organic etiologies were all suggested by history, physical examination, or a combination of the two.

TABLE 15.1

DIFFERENTIAL DIAGNOSIS OF FAILURE TO THRIVE

Inadequate caloric intake
- Lack of appetite (anemia, psychosocial problems, central nervous system disease)
- Difficulty with ingestion (craniofacial anomalies, cerebral palsy, feeding disorder)
- Lack of food (poor feeding technique, lack of sufficient food, excessive dilution of formula)
- Vomiting (gastroesophageal reflux, intestinal tract obstruction)

Inadequate caloric absorption
- Malabsorption (cystic fibrosis, food intolerance, celiac disease)
- Chronic diarrhea (parasitic infection, starvation)
- Hepatitis
- Hirschsprung disease

Increased caloric requirements
Increased use of calories

- Chronic/recurrent infection (tuberculosis, urinary tract infection, recurrent otitis media)
- Chronic pulmonary disease (bronchopulmonary dysplasia, recurrent pneumonia)
- Congenital heart disease (associated with congestive heart failure)
- Malignancy
- Toxin (lead)
- Metabolic (hyperthyroidism)

Ineffective caloric utilization

- Conditions associated with metabolic acidosis (inborn errors of metabolism)
- Renal tubular acidosis
- Chronic hypoxemia (cyanotic heart disease)

MANAGEMENT

In most FTT cases, once the pediatrician notes the change in growth pattern of the child, a nutritional assessment and treatment plan in the outpatient setting may be initiated. If the child continues to fail to gain weight appropriately, or if the child's weight falls below 60% of ideal body weight (severe malnutrition), the child should be admitted for further evaluation and treatment. Hospitalization has little impact on the diagnostic categorization of failure to thrive, but its controlled environment does facilitate a more accurate assessment of caloric intake and feeding behavior.

It is important to identify a multidisciplinary team for thorough evaluation and treatment of the child. It is essential to involve a nutritionist who is proficient in the nutritional needs of young and growing children. Individuals who are trained in social work and mental health issues also are important to evaluate the social and behavioral issues that invariably are present. The pediatrician performs the medical evaluation and should function as the leader of the inpatient team. Other health care professionals may include the child's primary nurse, occupational therapists, speech therapists, and child life specialists.

It also is helpful to observe the infant during feeding to assess the infant's oral motor function, parental feeding techniques, and infant or parental behaviors interfering with normal feeding. Important observers of oral motor function and feeding behavior may include nursing staff, speech therapists, occupational therapists, and pediatric nurse specialists/practitioners with expertise in this area.

Nutritional therapy is crucial in treating children who fail to thrive. Goals should include the achievement of ideal weight for height, correction of nutritional deficits with allowance for catch-up growth, restoration of normal body composition, and parental education in feeding and nutritional requirements.

Caloric needs of infants and children who fail to thrive are calculated based on their ideal body weight. Ideal body weight is the 50th percentile weight for the child's measured length. To provide for maintenance requirements and catch-up growth, these children usually require 150% of the usual maintenance calorie needs. This target caloric intake should be achieved over 5 to 7 days' time, not on the first day of treatment. Increasing the caloric density of formula and foods often is the mainstay of nutritional therapy, and details of how to do this are contained in a later chapter (Chapter 142). Hypercaloric feedings usually also are hyperosmolar and may

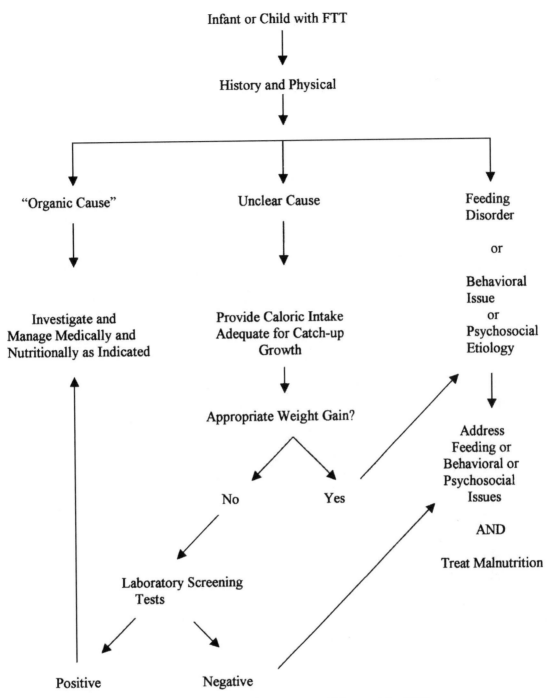

FIGURE 15.2. Diagnosis and management of failure to thrive (FTT).

not be tolerated by the child (i.e., osmotic diarrhea) if the feeding osmolality is advanced too quickly.

In addition, a multivitamin preparation with iron and zinc is recommended for all undernourished children. Catch-up growth may be reduced if the positive balance of these micronutrients is insufficient.

Behavioral interventions with the family may include emphasis on making mealtime a pleasant and social experience, limiting distractions while eating, allowing the child to choose how to eat and how much to eat, and providing positive reinforcement for appropriate feeding behaviors.

Psychosocial factors that contribute to FTT vary a great deal from family to family. It is necessary to identify the particular material and interpersonal stressors that bear on the

child and its family. This is best accomplished by conducting a detailed and sensitive interview, making home visits, and referral to appropriate community resources. For example, an intervention as simple as a referral to the WIC (Women, Infants, and Children) program may greatly improve access to food. Identifying a primary caregiver who is responsible for how well a child is fed may be important in households where, because of varied work schedules, several individuals share child care. There is no single form of treatment for all children; the pediatrician needs to develop a treatment plan that is unique for each family and child.

Although most children with FTT are not victims of physical abuse or medical neglect, it is vital to recognize the few cases where children are suffering from intentional withholding of food. Only in these instances of intentional food deprivation or in cases with evidence of associated physical or emotional abuse or neglect should a referral be made to child protective service agencies.

COURSE AND PROGNOSIS

In the same manner that weight is lost over a long period of time, weight gain and restoration of body composition take time. The purpose of hospitalization is to address nutritional, behavioral, and psychosocial issues pertaining to the FTT, and to develop a comprehensive plan to correct the problems identified. The child may be discharged to resume outpatient care once the home environment is thought to be safe and the family understands and demonstrates competence with the treatment plan.

Further evaluation is indicated only if the infant or child fails to gain weight on a diet meeting nutritional needs for catch-up growth along with improved or appropriate feeding technique. The history and physical examination should be reviewed and additional laboratory studies beyond the basic ones ordered as indicated.

There are very few longitudinal studies that have looked at the growth and developmental outcomes for infants and children who have failed to thrive. One 14-year follow-up study showed that a substantial number of children who had FTT in infancy had height ages and weight ages 1 or more years less than their chronologic ages compared with matched control subjects. Long-term growth is particularly compromised in situations where there are associated chronic medical conditions or when severe malnutrition was present in infancy. Likewise, many children who fail to thrive show developmental delays. During the preschool and school years, children hospitalized for FTT in infancy often continue to have depressed psychometric scores and high rates of school failure. In one 13-year follow-up study, former FTT children were significantly behind matched control children in language development, reading age, and verbal intelligence. It is crucial that these children have very close outpatient monitoring and intervention to address their growth and developmental needs.

PEARLS

- It is important to recognize four clinical conditions that meet the definition of FTT, but are actually physiologic: prematurity, familial short stature, constitutional growth delay, and small-for-gestational-age infants.
- Laboratory examinations rarely are helpful in identifying an organic cause of failure to thrive without an indication suggested by a thorough history and physical examination.
- Nutritional therapy must be based on a child's ideal body weight and should include an additional caloric need for catch-up growth and restoration of body composition.
- Because the prognosis for future growth and development is unclear, close follow-up of children with FTT for both growth and development is crucial.

Suggested Readings

Frank DA, Silva M, Needlman R. Failure to thrive: mystery, myth, and method. *Contemp Pediatr* 1993;10:114.

Gahagan S. Failure to thrive: a consequence of undernutrition. *Pediatr Rev* 2006;27:e1.

Maggioni A, Lifshitz F. Nutritional management of failure to thrive. *Pediatr Clin North Am* 1995;42:791.

Schwartz D. Failure to thrive: an old nemesis in the new millennium. *Pediatr Rev* 2000;21:257.

Sills RH. Failure to thrive: the role of clinical and laboratory evaluation. *Am J Dis Child* 1978;132:967.

CHAPTER 16 ■ DISORDERS OF TEMPERATURE: HYPER- AND HYPOTHERMIA

JOSEPH R. ZANGA

Throughout life the human organism experiences considerable variability in body temperature. These variations are caused by both intrinsic and extrinsic factors, and each may create realistic concern about the health and well-being of the organism. It is necessary for physicians and other health care professionals providing hospital care to determine whether a particular variation is meaningful.

Normal core body temperature, which is only approximated by our usual measurements, varies from 36°C to 37.8°C, and varies from individual to individual and at different ages and stages of life. In addition, each individual has a diurnal variation of 0.3°C to 0.5°C. The temperatures of infants and young children are particularly difficult to categorize, as their body temperature readily responds by rising with exercise, elevated ambient temperatures, and excessive clothing. The reverse of these is also true. We also must recognize that our operational standard of normal temperature (37°C) is not realized until sometime in mid-adolescence. As many as half of all toddlers will have a normal measured temperature approximating 37.8°C.

In this chapter we will consider both hyper- and hypothermia, although the former is more common in the inpatient environment.

DEFINITIONS

- Fever (hyperthermia, pyrexia): Temperature ≥38°C (100.4°F) rectal, ≥37.5°C oral.
- Fever without source (FWS): Fever of recent onset without clearly apparent source on history or physical examination (also called *fever without localizing signs*).
- Fever of unknown origin (FUO): Fever for more than 14 days with etiology unknown or unclear after careful history, physical examination, and often routine laboratory investigation.
- Hypothermia: Core temperature <35°C measured rectally.
- 37°C = 98.6°F; 38°C = 100.4°F; 39°C = 102.2°F; 40°C = 104°F.

FEVER

Health professionals have almost inadvertently encouraged parents and others to adopt the notion that fever of any sort is an intrinsic danger to the child and must be quickly and effectively treated. In doing this we have created a "disease" entity that has come to be known as *fever phobia*. This is unfortunate, as an elevation in temperature above the normal range occasioned by innocent outside influences rarely requires specific treatment, while an elevation caused by infections and certain other treatable disorders is merely a sign or symptom of the illness and not a treatable illness itself.

In most instances, parents and health care professionals should welcome fever as a marker of the disease, with its continuance alerting us to the ineffectiveness of our treatment. Fever may also be considered part of the treatment for the underlying disease. Recall that before the antibiotic era, artificially induced pyrexia was used to treat certain infections (e.g., syphilis). It is well known that fever hastens cytokine release, and improves chemotaxis and leukocyte phagocytosis of bacteria as well as bacterial killing in the white cells. It is rarely necessary to treat the fever itself, and we recommend that treatment be provided only when the child appears fatigued due to the increased metabolic demand of fever, or is unable to sleep or carry on other activities that would aid in the healing process. Naturally, a child with a history of seizures, particularly febrile seizures, or an unknown personal, but strong, family history of seizures of any sort should be treated with antipyretics. Unfortunately, because fever is often one of the first signs of illness, the first fever-induced seizure will be frightening to the parents, despite assurances that it will not harm the child.

Treatment

If it is decided that therapy for pyrexia should be instituted, it should be done thoughtfully and carefully. Of course, exogenous factors contributing to the elevation of temperature should be removed, or the child removed from them, and infections thought to be sources of the fever should be diagnosed and treated.

Medications used to treat fever are generally safe, but by no means benign. Because of *fever phobia* mentioned earlier, and because of the wide variety of well-advertised over-the-counter (OTC) medications that contain acetaminophen, parents often inadvertently use this drug in excessive quantities. Acetaminophen is a well-known hepatotoxic agent, and because families often don't carefully read OTC labels, poisoning may be insidious, which makes recognition, prevention of further damage, and treatment difficult.

The second most commonly used antipyretic, ibuprofen, is also safe when used singly and as directed, but it too appears in a variety of OTC preparations and is known to have some renal and gastric toxicity, the latter with as little as one dose.

With respect to treating fever, the best evidence-based recommendation would suggest choosing one of the above drugs, dosed maximally and on an appropriate schedule, as the safest approach. If thought to be required, acetaminophen may be given in a dose of 15 mg/kg every 4 to 6 hours, while ibuprofen is given at 10 mg/kg no more often than every 6 hours. Fevers that persist, regardless of use or nonuse of antipyretics, suggest that the underlying disease is not being adequately or appropriately treated, and are cause for concern in a hospital setting. Temperature, therefore should be taken on a regular schedule, charted and graphed for regular review by the patient care staff. Insistence on treating minor temperature elevations in the hospitalized child, presumably being appropriately treated for her underlying illness, is to be condemned. This is not only for reasons mentioned earlier, but also because some fever curves are helpful in diagnosing certain medical conditions.

In this regard, quotidian fevers are a hallmark of the febrile onset of juvenile idiopathic arthritis. These fevers start out at or below the child's normal temperature early in the day, climbing through the day to a single spike in the evening, before starting a decline to baseline or below by the next morning. Relapsing fever, one that waxes and wanes over a series of days, is suggestive of spirochetal illnesses such as *Borrelia*. These episodes present acutely with chills, back and leg pain, and at times, seizures. Paroxysms of fever, with elevations occurring approximately every 72 hours, are known as quartan fevers, and are suggestive of malaria. Many of these diseases and conditions are uncommon to unknown in North America, but with international travel now common, with travel times often shorter than the incubation period of some of these infections, they are useful to know and easy to spot on graphic displays of the patient's temperature. The unfortunate overuse of antipyretics often obscures these patterns, contributing to a delay in diagnosis.

Evaluation of the Febrile Child

The standard of care, and logic, require that the evaluation of a febrile child begin with the careful taking of a history from the parents (and the child, if possible), followed by a thorough examination. Vital signs are an essential part of this, with the rectal temperature still regarded as the gold standard. Blood pressure, pulse, and respiration should be recorded, with the latter especially important if pneumonia is part of the differential diagnosis. Pulse oxymetry is rarely if ever indicated. One or more laboratory tests may be suggested by the history and the occurrence of certain signs and symptoms. Among the more commonly ordered tests is a complete blood count, which is of little value alone in making a diagnosis, is generally unhelpful in deciding whether an illness has a bacterial or viral etiology, and rarely helps to categorize a child as moderately or severely ill. Band counts, especially a band to neutrophil ratio of >0.2, are regarded by some as suggestive of bacterial infection. Others, however, believe that the band count is so fraught with error as to be a useless test. For the young infant, a white count <5,000 or >15,000, with a concomitant erythrocyte sedimentation rate (ESR) >30, may be more indicative of serious bacterial infection. In some centers, the C-reaction protein (CRP) has replaced the ESR as the acute phase reactant of choice. Most investigators find that either is helpful, though the sedimentation rate is said to increase and decrease more rapidly than the CRP.

Diagnosis and Management

When the cause of the fever is known, the most common practice is observation or outpatient treatment. Fevers of unknown origin (FUO) and fevers without source (FWS), as well as fevers in children of certain ages (see below), often require hospitalization.

Age ≤ 28 Days

- Treatable etiologies (most common):
  - Group B streptococci
  - *Listeria monocytogenes*
  - *Escherichia coli* and other gram-negative rods
  - *Streptococcus pneumoniae*
  - Herpes simplex virus
- Sepsis workup (*all* patients):
  - Complete blood count (CBC) with differential
  - ESR (or CRP)
  - Blood culture
  - Urinalysis and urine culture: catheterized specimen or suprapubic aspiration (SPA)
  - Cerebrospinal fluid (CSF) culture: lumbar puncture
  - Chest radiography
- Hospitalization (*all* patients)
- Treatment (intravenous; the following dosages are for >7 days of age and >2 kg)
  - Ampicillin (50 mg/kg every 6 hours) *and* cefotaxime (50 mg/kg every 8 hours) *or* gentamicin (2.5 mg/kg every 8 hours).
  - Consider acyclovir (20 mg/kg every 8 hours), especially in first 2 weeks of age.

Age 29 to 90 Days

- Treatable common etiologies: The aforementioned neonatal organisms continue to be seen with decreasing frequency up to age 2 months. The usual childhood pathogens of *S. pneumoniae, Haemophilus influenzae, Neisseria meningitidis*, and *Salmonella* increase in frequency.

Low-risk infants in this age group can be managed safely at home. *All* elements of the "low risk" evaluation must be met to define the infant as low risk. The low-risk criteria are:

- History: Term birth (>37 weeks estimated gestational age). No history of:
  - Antibiotics perinatally or subsequently
  - Prolonged newborn hospitalization
  - Unexplained jaundice
  - Chronic underlying diseases
- Physical examination: Nontoxic and no focus for fever
- Laboratory
  - CBC: White blood cell count (WBC) between 5,000 and 15,000
  - ESR: <30
  - Urinalysis: Negative Gram stain; <10 WBC/high-power field (hpf; catheterized or SPA)
  - Chest radiography: Normal
  - CSF: <8 WBC/hpf, negative Gram stain, normal glucose and protein
  - If diarrhea: stool <5 WBC/hpf
  - Culture: blood, urine, CSF, stool (latter obtained if diarrheal stools positive for leukocytes, blood, or mucus)
- Social: Reliable caretakers with telephone, transportation, and willingness to bring infant for follow-up in 24 hours.

If the infant meets the preceding criteria, he can be discharged and reevaluated the following day (or sooner if interval worsening noted by parents). If *not* low risk, treatment for the infant includes:

- Hospitalization
- Ceftriaxone 50 to 100 mg/kg/day intravenously
- Vancomycin (15 mg/kg every 6 hours) if CSF studies suggest meningitis

Follow-up of low-risk infants: If blood, CSF, or urine cultures become positive (usually within 24 hours), and infant is still febrile, he should be immediately reevaluated, recultured, and hospitalized for intravenous antibiotics.

Age 91 Days to 3 Years

- Treatable common etiologies:
  - *S. pneumoniae*
  - *N. meningitidis*
  - *H. influenzae* type B
  - *E. coli*
  - *Klebsiella* and other gram-negative rods
  - *Salmonella*

The greatest risk of occult bacteremia has historically been between 6 and 24 months of age. Now that conjugated pneumococcal vaccine is widely used in this age group, the incidence of pneumococcal bacteremia has decreased.

Child >3 Years of Age

Children after age 3 years are more immunologically competent and better able to communicate information about their illness. The risk of occult bacteremia and serious bacterial infection is lower. Decisions about evaluation of children in this age group are based on clinical judgment. Laboratory investigation is suggested for fever >40°C, fever without source persisting >72 hours, or other symptoms suggesting serious infection.

Fever Without Source (FWS)

Previously published recommendations for evaluation of FWS were based on studies predating the implementation of universal pneumococcal vaccination. The following are commonly accepted diagnosis and treatment guidelines. *Toxic* infants and children should be admitted for evaluation and treatment. Nontoxic individuals in the 91 days to 3 years age group should be evaluated as follows:

- Threshold for laboratory evaluation: Children <39°C may be followed clinically if nontoxic and no focus for fever. The following evaluation should be considered for children ≥39°C or any significant FWS lasting more than 48 to 72 hours:
  - Urinalysis and culture (catheterized or SPA): Boys <6 months, girls <24 months
  - Stool culture: Diarrheal stool with 5 WBC/hpf, blood, or mucus
  - Chest radiography: Only if indicated by clinical findings (e.g., tachypnea, crackles)
- For infants and children >2 months after the third dose of conjugated pneumococcal vaccine (due at age 6 months), the following becomes optional:
  - CBC with differential
  - ESR or CRP
  - Blood culture (higher yield if WBC >15,000 or <5,000)
- Treatment options: The decision on whether to start empiric antibiotic therapy should be based on the clinical assessment, WBC and ESR/CRP, age of child, and immunization status (especially for *H. influenzae* and *S. Pneumoniae*).
  - Observation alone, and reevaluation in 24 hours
  - Ceftriaxone 50 mg/kg intramuscularly and reevaluation in 24 hours

Pearls

- Although an objective measurement of temperature is best, parents are among the most reliable observers of their children, and a report that the infant (or child) "felt warm" requires a careful evaluation.
- Infants under 3 months of age, historically febrile by rectal temperature measurement, will require a workup even if afebrile at the time of presentation. This is especially true for the neonate.
- Tympanic, skin, axillary, temporal artery, and most other alternative methods and sites for temperature taking are less reliable than rectal temperatures. Although teething may elevate temperature within the normal variability range, it does not cause fever, nor should ambient environmental temperatures absolve the health professional of responsibility for careful evaluation.
- Although the examination of the child is often easier when that child is not febrile, recent temperature elevations must be known. The child's response to antipyretic therapy does not aid in differentiating between bacterial and viral infections.

Diagnosis and Management of Heat Stroke

Although this condition is more commonly seen in the emergency department, children are sometimes severely enough affected that at least brief hospitalization is required for continued care and observation. Seizures, alterations of central nervous system function, and disseminated intravascular coagulopathy may occasionally be seen.

The typical patient is an older child or adolescent, particularly from the southern tier of states, engaged in late-spring or early-summer athletic competition or summer/autumn early-season sports practice. Individual susceptibility may play a role.

Diagnosis is made by history and physical findings including altered mental status, flushed, warm, usually dry skin, tachypnea, and tachycardia. Body temperature, measured rectally, is usually 40°C or more. Children with a genetically determined potential for malignant hyperthermia may be more susceptible to heat stroke, but this situation is rare and beyond the scope of this chapter.

Laboratory evaluation generally should include a metabolic panel as well as a prothrombin time and partial thromboplastin time.

Treatment in the hospital setting includes the use of cooling blankets and/or enhanced evaporative cooling using air circulation over dampened skin. Therapy also requires continuous measurement of approximate core body temperature, generally with a rectal probe. Some children with heat stroke require intensive care (pediatric intensive care unit, PICU) where esophageal thermometry is often used. Shivering resulting from too rapid cooling can be controlled with the use of intravenous benzodiazepines. There is no role for antipyretics in the treatment of heat stroke.

Fever of Unknown Origin (FUO)

An adult medicine patient is not labeled as having an FUO until 3 weeks have passed with temperatures >38.4°C. In pediatrics, the duration of fever necessary to label a child as having an FUO varies between experts from as short as 8 days to as long as 14. Fortunately, the majority of diseases presenting as FUO produce indolent infections with considerable morbidity but rare mortality. A small majority of FUOs are caused by infections, with viral diseases leading the list. Included, however, are such things as brucellosis, cat scratch disease, rickettsial infections, spirochetal infections, salmonellosis, tularemia, and tuberculosis. The etiologies can be localized (urinary tract infections, osteomyelitis, and occult abscesses, e.g., hepatic) or more disseminated, as with viral illnesses including HIV/AIDS.

Diagnosis is generally made by meticulous history and physical evaluation, with a high index of suspicion for the diseases previously mentioned. The laboratory evaluation should begin with the tests suggested for the workup of febrile illnesses as previously detailed, but should also include a careful examination of the peripheral blood smear, obtaining an HIV serology, and performance of tuberculin skin testing. Both aerobic and anaerobic blood cultures are often helpful, and the chest x-ray is more commonly part of the routine evaluation.

Noninfectious causes of fever should be considered and include connective tissue diseases, inflammatory bowel disease, and malignancies. Correspondingly, the diagnostic workup should also include an ESR and CRP, an antinuclear antibody test, and liver and renal (BUN and creatinine) function studies.

Therapy should be based on determination of the specific etiology; a "shotgun" approach should be avoided. Antipyretic therapy should also be avoided because, especially with FUO, a graphic representation of the fever curve is an important diagnostic parameter. Note that in as many as 25% of children with FUO, the child becomes afebrile without therapy and without an etiology for the fever being determined.

HYPOTHERMIA

Hypothermia is more commonly seen during the winter months in the northern tier of states. States with milder climates also occasionally report morbidity and mortality due to hypothermia even in warm-weather months. Hypothermia rarely occurs de novo, but usually is a part of accidental trauma related to exposure to ambient air or water temperatures lower than body temperature for an extended period of time. Younger children who survive hypothermic incidents usually have better outcomes than older children; who, in turn, do better than adults. Their general good health and the often rapid drop in core temperature allows for increased sparing of CNS function, even when hypoxia is a contributing problem.

The typical history is one of exposure or immersion. In the adolescent, such events often involve the prior use of alcohol or other drugs. As the body cools there is a progressive decline in CNS function, so that at core temperatures <35°C (mild hypothermia) there is confusion and disorientation, while tachycardia and tachypnea begin their decline to bradycardia and bradypnea. At core temperatures <32°C, unconsciousness often occurs along with atrial dysrhythmias. Core temperatures <28°C are considered severe hypothermia. At this level, the child is likely to have dilated pupils, ventricular arrhythmias progressing to fibrillation (poorly or not at all responsive to defibrillation), and asystole.

Diagnosis is based on history and the rectal or other core temperature. When hypothermia is suspected, special low-reading thermometers must be used.

Laboratory evaluation generally includes a determination of arterial blood gases, primarily to assess the degree of acidosis (usually lactic acidosis) from decreased tissue perfusion. Many experts recommend that the laboratory be informed of the patient's condition in order to correct for temperature. Others, however, recommend using uncorrected values to guide therapy.

An electrocardiogram is done to evaluate prolongation of the PR, QRS, and QT intervals, as well as T-wave inversions. Hyperglycemia (which resolves spontaneously as temperature rises) may be seen along with prolongation of the prothrombin time and partial thromboplastin time. Particularly with immersion hypothermia, electrolytes should also be measured. All laboratory parameters should be rechecked frequently during the rewarming process, as values can change rapidly. In the case of adolescents, screening tests for drugs of abuse should be sent, as their presence may make treatment more difficult.

Rewarming is the essential treatment for the hypothermic patient. The bradycardia, low cardiac output, and peripheral vasoconstriction make the evaluation of cardiac status, phlebotomy, and the administration of intravenous fluids difficult. Despite these challenges, because rapidly induced hypothermia

may protect the CNS, the current standard of care requires prolonged resuscitation (often for several hours) until the core (rectal) temperature approaches 35°C.

Whether in the field or ED, immediate management of the patient includes removal of wet clothing, drying of patient's skin, covering with dry blankets, administration of warm, humidified oxygen, and warm IV fluids. The efficacy of this latter recommendation has been challenged, because the length of tubing and the relatively slow drip rate required for children often results in IV fluids entering the child's circulation at room temperature (which is below the hypothermic state of the patient).

For patients who are only mildly hypothermic, *passive* external rewarming, which simply continues therapies begun in the ED, is usually sufficient. For the patient who is glycogen depleted, or known to have a chronic condition, *active* external rewarming might be necessary.

Active external rewarming is also used for moderately, and occasionally even severely hypothermic patients. It may require PICU admission for monitoring and involves the use of heating pads, radiant heat, forced warm air, or warm baths (40–41°C). A caution with this method is the potential for sudden vasodilatation and hypotension, which in turn may result in inadequate perfusion of the coronary vessels and ventricular fibrillation. Central warming prior to the warming of the extremities diminishes the likelihood of these problems. In addition to the very serious risk of arrhythmias with rewarming, thermal burns of poorly perfused skin may occur. Active external warming in a bath is also contraindicated when there are open wounds.

For the child who is severely hypothermic, aggressive active core rewarming is usually necessary. This may include gastrointestinal irrigation with warm fluids, warm saline lavage of plural and peritoneal cavities, hemodialysis, and cardiopulmonary bypass. These techniques, however, require PICU admission because of the need for considerable expertise and equipment. They also expose the patient to increased risk of infection, and efficacy is somewhat limited by splanchnic bed vasoconstriction with ineffective heat exchange.

Hypothermia in the Neonate

The neonate (to 28 days postdelivery) has an immature thermoregulatory system. Already noted is their often "febrile" response to environmental conditions. Often of more concern is that hypothermia in the newborn is often associated with sepsis or other serious illness. Newborns who are hypothermic should be aggressively evaluated for sepsis, warmed appropriately (overbed warmers or incubators are occasionally necessary), and treated in the hospital with antibiotics (see "Age ≤28 Days" earlier in the chapter) pending result of cultures of blood, urine, and cerebral spinal fluid.

Suggested Readings

Liu YP, Ni YH, Fang CC, et al. Fulminant hepatic failure due to chronic acetaminophen intoxication in an infant. *AJEM* 2005;23:94–95.

Newton DA. Fever. In: Perkin RM, Swift JD, Newton DA, eds. *Pediatric hospital medicine.* 1st ed. Philadelphia: Lippincott Williams & Wilkins; 2003: 134–137.

Pantell RH, Newman TB, Bernzweig J, et al. Management and outcomes and care of fever in early infancy. *JAMA* 2004;291:1203.

Watson WA, Litovitz TL, Klein-Schwartz, et al. 2004 annual report of the American Association of Poison Control Centers Toxic Exposure Surveillance System. *AJEM* 2005;23:589–666.

CHAPTER 17 ■ HYPOGLYCEMIA

MELINDA B. CLARK-GAMBELUNGHE

The metabolism of glucose is a complex physiologic process. Elaborate mechanisms are present to regulate serum glucose within a fairly narrow range and thus usually avoid hypoglycemia. Glucose is the preferred energy substrate for central nervous system (CNS) metabolism, so the brain is particularly vulnerable to the effects of hypoglycemia. The developing brain is especially vulnerable such that repetitive or sustained hypoglycemia in infants can result in permanent neurologic sequelae. Although the number, duration, or severity of episodes required to cause CNS damage is not well established, it is prudent to test any patient with symptoms suggestive of hypoglycemia and aggressively treat if the glucose value is ≤40 mg/dL.

Hypoglycemia in newborns can be most practically defined as a blood glucose level ≤40 mg/dL (2.2 mmol/L), although debate regarding this definition exists. The lower limit of acceptable glucose is higher (≤45 mg/dL) in a serum or plasma sample in older children. Symptoms of hypoglycemia can occur at any glucose level <60 mg/dL, and patients with symptoms attributable to hypoglycemia should be treated. Of special note, neonates often do not display "classic" signs and symptoms of hypoglycemia (for neonatal hypoglycemia, see Chapter 107). Therefore, even asymptomatic neonates with known risk factors for the development of hypoglycemia should be closely monitored.

Hypoglycemia results from the failure of one or more of the normal regulatory mechanisms involved in glucose homeostasis. Maintenance of normal plasma glucose levels requires the following factors:

■ Adequate intake of glucose or substrate for gluconeogenesis (protein and fat).
■ Normal functioning of the enzymes involved in glucose uptake, glycogenolysis, lipolysis, and gluconeogenesis.
■ A functional endocrine system to regulate these processes.

Following a meal, glucose is first utilized by peripheral tissues, but some is synthesized into glycogen by muscle and liver cells, and some converted into fatty acids for storage in fat cells. In the fasting state, the body must generate glucose from stored substrate via glycogen degradation and the conversion of muscle and fat into glucose. The liver has the largest reserve of available glycogen for glycogenolysis and is also the organ primarily responsible for gluconeogenesis. Gluconeogenesis is the process of de novo synthesis of glucose from noncarbohydrate sources including pyruvate, lactate, glycerol, and amino acids (primarily alanine). The lactate and amino acids are generated by proteolysis of muscle, while the glycerol and fatty acids result from hydrolysis of peripheral lipid stores. The fatty acids undergo beta-oxidation for energy metabolism and ketone production.

Glucose homeostasis is maintained by multiple hormones that have varying effects on plasma glucose. Insulin is the primary hormone responsible for lowering serum glucose, via promotion of peripheral tissue uptake of glucose and inhibition of gluconeogenesis and glycogenolysis. Multiple counterregulatory hormones elevate plasma glucose, including catecholamines, cortisol, glucagon, and growth hormone. Table 17.1 summarizes the major effects of these hormones.

ETIOLOGY

The causes of hypoglycemia in the pediatric patient vary by age and presentation. Normal neonates and young children are prone to hypoglycemia. This may develop within hours of beginning a fast. Children typically cannot maintain euglycemia for more than 24 hours of fasting. Several causes of hypoglycemia are issues only during the neonatal period. The causes of hypoglycemia that are transient and restricted to neonates are discussed in Chapter 107. However, many of the etiologies of hypoglycemia in infants and older children can also present in the neonatal period. For the sake of simplicity, all the causes of hypoglycemia are categorized together under the major metabolic or physiologic abnormality, followed by specific disease entities as examples. This classification is intended to facilitate a thoughtful, organized approach to evaluation. Hypoglycemia in an individual patient could potentially result from a combination of the factors described in the following sections.

Excess Insulin

The presence of insulin inhibits hepatic glycogenolysis and ketogenesis, so patients with excess insulin present with hypoglycemia, but no ketones. Excess insulin is most common and best characterized in the infant of a diabetic mother (see Chapter 107). Insulin overdose may be accidental (e.g., diabetic patients), iatrogenic, or intentional (e.g., Münchausen by proxy). Finally, persistent hyperinsulinemic hypoglycemia of infancy (PHHI) is common and has many possible causes, including:

■ Inherited forms of PHHI: A receptor or transporter defect inherited in an autosomal dominant, autosomal recessive, or sporadic manner.
■ Beckwith–Wiedemann syndrome (BWS): PHHI associated with macrosomia, macroglossia, hemihypertrophy, and omphalocele.
■ Pancreatic β-cell hyperplasia or islet-cell adenoma.

Inadequate Glucose Stores or Other Substrate

■ Ketotic hypoglycemia is the most common cause of hypoglycemia in childhood. A prolonged overnight fast (12 to 18 hours) or illness results in hypoglycemia due to the

TABLE 17.1

EFFECTS OF HORMONES ON GLUCOSE METABOLISM

	Activates gluconeogenesis	Activates glycogenolysis	Activates lipolysis	Limits muscle glucose uptake
Cortisol	X		X	X
Epinephrine	X	X	X	X
Glucagon	X	X	X	
Growth hormone			X	X

child's inadequate gluconeogenesis despite intact enzyme pathways. This is often related to reduced alanine levels (these patients are typically small with limited muscle mass). The clinical features of ketotic hypoglycemia include elevated ketones, due to fatty acid production for gluconeogenesis, accompanied by low insulin levels.

- Starvation and malabsorption also result in inadequate intake of glucose, protein, and fat.
- Small-for-gestational-age (SGA) and premature neonates are prone to hypoglycemia from insufficient substrate, as they often have inadequate glycogen stores and glucose intake.

Increased Metabolic Rate

Increased metabolic rate and glucose overutilization can result in hypoglycemia. Examples of this include sepsis, shock, burns, and polycythemia.

Disorders of Glycogenolysis

Patients with defects in glycogenolysis typically present with hypoglycemia onset 2 to 4 hours after a meal. It is important to note that *ketones will be present because lipolysis is unaffected.* Inadequate glycogenolysis to meet metabolic demands can result from:

- An enzymatic defect in the glycogen degradation pathway. These disorders are collectively termed the glycogen storage diseases (GSDs). Examples include glycogen synthetase deficiency (GSD type 0; rare) and glucose-6-phosphatase deficiency (GSD type I, von Gierke disease). The clinical features of GSD (types I, III, and VI) include hepatosplenomegaly (not found in type 0), growth and mental retardation, hypotonia, and lactic acidosis.
- Hepatic failure. Etiologies include viral hepatitis, toxins, Reye syndrome, and cirrhosis. Hypoglycemia occurs because the liver is the primary organ responsible for glycogenolysis (and gluconeogenesis).
- Insufficient hormones (catecholamines or glucagon) to stimulate glycogenolysis (see "Endocrine Imbalance" later in the chapter).

Disorders of Gluconeogenesis

The hypoglycemia from inadequate gluconeogenesis occurs 6 to 12 hours after a meal, so these disorders typically become evident during a prolonged fast, such as when an infant begins sleeping through the night. Failure to perform gluconeogenesis can result from:

- An enzymatic defect in the gluconeogenesis pathway, such as fructose 1,6-diphosphatase deficiency and phosphoenolpyru-

vate carboxykinase deficiency. The clinical features of these enzyme deficiencies include lactic acidosis, ketosis, failure to thrive, and hyperlipidemia.
- Substrate unavailability: Recall that glucose can be synthesized de novo from amino acids (primarily alanine), lactate, or free fatty acids. Therefore, a deficiency of these substrates will result in diminished gluconeogenesis. Amino acid depletion occurs in ketotic hypoglycemia (see above) and branched-chain amino aciduria (Maple syrup urine disease, MSUD). Fatty acid oxidation defects, of which medium-chain acyl-coenzyme-A dehydrogenase deficiency (MCADD) is the most common, cause hypoglycemia accompanied by low or no ketones, low serum carnitine (total and free), and increased serum free fatty acids.
- Insufficient hormones to stimulate gluconeogenesis (cortisol, epinephrine, glucagon), discussed in the next section.
- Toxin interference with gluconeogenesis (e.g., alcohol, salicylates).

Endocrine Imbalance

A decrease in the counterregulatory hormones that antagonize the effects of insulin will result in hypoglycemia. These hormones include cortisol, growth hormone (GH), glucagon, and epinephrine:

- Cortisol. A deficiency of cortisol is seen in primary adrenal insufficiency or ACTH deficiency from a pituitary or hypothalamic defect. Primary adrenal insufficiency etiologies include autoimmune conditions, (e.g., Addison disease), masses, and adrenal hemorrhage (Waterhouse–Friderichsen syndrome). Symptoms of cortisol deficiency include fatigue, weakness, weight loss, and nausea/vomiting, but severe deficiency presents as a "shock-like" state with low blood pressure. Characteristic skin hyperpigmentation is seen in Addison disease.
- Growth hormone (GH). An expected result of isolated GH deficiency is growth failure, but patients with panhypopituitarism will display the combined clinical effects of deficiencies of multiple hormones (ACTH, GH, TSH, and LH/FSH).
- Glucagon deficiency is very rare. Epinephrine deficiency is even more rare, and possibly nonexistent as an isolated cause of hypoglycemia.

Ingestion

Ingestion of a medication or toxin must always be considered in the differential diagnosis of hypoglycemia, especially in young children. Examples of ingestions that cause hypoglycemia include oral hypoglycemic agents (e.g., sulfonylureas), β-blockers (e.g., propranolol), salicylates, and alcohol.

Inborn Errors of Metabolism

Inborn errors of metabolism (IEM) include defects in the metabolism of carbohydrates, fatty acids, and amino/organic acids.

- Defects in carbohydrate metabolism include galactosemia (galactose-1-phosphate uridyl transferase deficiency) and hereditary fructose intolerance (fructosemia; fructose 1,6-bisphosphate aldolase deficiency). The clinical features of galactosemia and fructosemia are hypoglycemia, jaundice, hepatomegaly, vomiting, lethargy, and convulsions, which may occur within hours of ingestion of the offending agent.
- Fatty acid oxidation defects (MCADD, LCADD), discussed earlier.
- Amino acid and organic acid disorders (e.g., MSUD, propionic acidemia).

Other Important Clinical Considerations

- **Reactive hypoglycemia:** Postprandial hypoglycemia that occurs 1 to 3 hours after meals due to insulin oversecretion. Reactive hypoglycemia is most common in late-adolescent, overweight females.
- **CNS glucose transporter defect:** Serum glucose levels are normal, but the patient is unable to transport glucose into the CNS. Seizures are the presenting symptom and the diagnosis is made based on a low CSF glucose level.
- **Pseudohypoglycemia:** This is laboratory error due to an increased white-blood count (WBC) or red-blood count (RBC) with subsequent cell utilization of glucose in the sample. For example, this might occur in a patient with leukemia with a high WBC count when there is delay in the determination of glucose level.

PRESENTING SYMPTOMS AND SIGNS

Glucose is the preferred energy source for CNS function, accounting for 90% of cerebral metabolism. Therefore, a deficiency of glucose usually presents with neurologic signs and symptoms, including:

- Headache, irritability, confusion, difficulty concentrating, and visual changes.
- Ataxia, paresthesias, slurred speech, and seizures.
- Lethargy, somnolence, and coma.

The remaining signs and symptoms are due to the effects of the counterregulatory hormones discussed above and are primarily adrenergic effects:

- Tachycardia or palpitations.
- Tremor, shaking, and anxiety.
- Sweating, weakness, hunger, and nausea.

Neonatal hypoglycemia is often more subtle in presentation, but signs and symptoms include lethargy, decreased arousal, decreased tone, weak suck, poor feeding, jitteriness, tremor, seizures, apnea, and cyanosis.

DIAGNOSIS

History

A number of pertinent historical elements need to be carefully defined in the history. These include:

- Age of patient at onset of hypoglycemia, relevant birth history.
- Prior history of hypoglycemia, or episodes that could be accounted for by hypoglycemia, such as a history of unexplained behavior changes or seizures.
- Duration of fasting prior to symptom onset.
- Family history of hypoglycemia or unexplained "sudden infant death."
- Recent ingestion of new food (e.g., fructose).
- Possibility of medication ingestion.

Physical Exam

It is imperative to perform a complete physical exam, as physical findings may provide a hint to a diagnosis. Examples of possible exam findings (followed by the possible associated disease condition) are as follows: the presence of a cleft lip or palate (midline defect and pituitary insufficiency), microphallus (hypopituitarism), macrosomia (hyperinsulinism; e.g., BWS), hypotension or hyperpigmentation (Addison disease), growth failure (GH deficiency, IEM), visceromegaly (glycogen storage disease, BWS), and jaundice with hepatomegaly (galactosemia, fructosemia).

Laboratory Data

The initial diagnosis of hypoglycemia is typically made with a bedside glucometer. Although one must treat clinically based on this value, it is imperative to confirm the hypoglycemia with a serum level prior to the administration of glucose. Whenever possible, it is extremely important to *draw additional blood for diagnostic testing at the time the serum glucose is low,* that is, prior to glucose infusion. Many of the laboratory tests to confirm the etiology of hypoglycemia can only be interpreted in the presence of hypoglycemia.

Initial laboratory testing is directed at establishing a hormonal imbalance, confirming a suspected toxic ingestion, or providing indirect evidence of an enzymatic defect or inborn error of metabolism. The latter can be definitively established later (e.g., specific enzyme defects can be confirmed with a liver biopsy). Initial tests should include:

- Serum electrolytes (glucose, bicarbonate, anion gap), liver function tests, and an ammonia level.
- Serum lactate, ketones (especially β-hydroxybutyrate), free fatty acids, acylcarnitine profile, and total and free carnitine.
- Urine for ketones and reducing substances. It is important to note that the presence of a reducing substance in the urine *that is not glucose* implies hereditary fructose intolerance or galactosemia.
- Toxicology screen if the history or physical exam suggest ingestion. This should include screening for ethanol, sulfonylureas, and salicylates.
- Plasma amino acids and urine organic acids (e.g., MSUD).

Endocrine tests: Take caution to note that most *hormone measurements can only be interpreted when collected simultaneously with a plasma glucose sample.* Appropriate specific endocrine tests include serum insulin with C-peptide, cortisol, glucagon, GH, IGF-1, and IGFBP-1. In the normal state, insulin levels are depressed in the face of hypoglycemia. C-peptide is a marker of endogenous insulin production, so hypoglycemia with an elevated insulin level but a *low* C-peptide indicates exogenous insulin administration.

Additional testing should be considered if the above testing has not established a diagnosis. Considerations might include the following:

- Glucagon challenge.
- Elective fast. This can only be done safely after ruling out a fatty acid oxidation defect or carnitine metabolic defect by confirming normal plasma carnitine and acylcarnitine levels.
- Pancreatic imaging if PHHI has been established and there is suspicion of islet cell adenoma or hyperplasia.

MANAGEMENT

Start with assuring that an ABCs response is utilized if necessary for stabilization of the patient. Immediate attention should then be directed at correction of the hypoglycemia, the urgency obviously varying according to the severity of symptoms and level of hypoglycemia.

- Administer glucose. If the patient is awake and alert, oral glucose is the safest and easiest route (e.g., 20 mL/kg juice). If oral administration is not an option, administer glucose IV at a dose of 250 mg/kg of glucose (e.g., 2.5 mL/kg of 10% D10W or 1 mL/kg of D25W). An appropriate rate of glucose infusion should be calculated (usually 6 to 8 mg/kg/min) and then adjusted based on subsequent glucose values. A requirement of excessive rates of glucose infusion (>10 mg/kg/min) to maintain euglycemia suggests hyperinsulinemia. Consider glucocorticoids or GH for hypoglycemia unresponsive to glucose infusion.
- Glucagon can be administered if IV access is not readily available (0.02 to 0.03 mg/kg/dose IM/SQ for children up to max 1 mg/dose). Remember that glucagon is ineffective for hypoglycemia caused by defects in gluconeogenesis or glycogenolysis.
- Whole blood glucose should be monitored frequently (every 30 to 60 minutes) until the values have stabilized, and then every 2 to 4 hours.
- Ketotic hypoglycemia and some IEM (e.g., MCAD) can be managed long-term by avoidance of fasting via frequent feedings and supplying complex glucose polymers (e.g., uncooked cornstarch).
- PHHI long-term management includes diazoxide, octreotide, and possibly resection of an adenoma.

PEARLS

- Ketotic hypoglycemia is the most common cause of hypoglycemia in childhood. The hypoglycemia will be accompanied by a low insulin level and elevated ketones.
- Absence of ketones suggests hyperinsulinemia or a fatty acid oxidation defect.
- Defects in glycogenolysis usually present with hypoglycemia 2 to 4 hours after a meal. Ketones are present because lipolysis is unaffected.
- Defects in gluconeogenesis usually present with fasting hypoglycemia occurring 6 to 12 hours after a meal. Infants often present when they begin sleeping through the night.
- The presence of a reducing substance in the urine *that is not glucose* implies hereditary fructose intolerance or galactosemia.
- It is of paramount importance to draw blood for diagnostic testing at the time that the patient is hypoglycemic, prior to glucose infusion.
- Hormone measurements can *only* be interpreted when collected simultaneously with a plasma glucose sample.
- A requirement of excessive rates of glucose infusion (>10 mg/kg/min) to maintain euglycemia suggests hyperinsulinemia.

Suggested Readings

Losek JD. Hypoglycemia and the ABC'S (sugar) of pediatric resuscitation. *Ann Emerg Med* 2000;35:43–46.

Lteif AN, Schwenk WF. Hypoglycemia in infants and children. *Endocrinol Metab Clin North Am* 1999;28:619–646.

Stanley CA. Hyperinsulinism in infants and children. *Pediatr Clin North Am* 1997;44:363–374.

CHAPTER 18 ■ LYMPHADENOPATHY AND LYMPHADENITIS

DALE A. NEWTON, ROYTESA R. SAVAGE, AND TARYN R. RICHARDSON

LYMPHADENOPATHY

Introduction

The lymphatic system filters out and responds to antigenic material within the lymph nodes. The structure of a node is conducive to allowing contact between antigens and lymphocytes with subsequent antigen recognition. This in turn is followed by stimulation of the cellular and humoral immune response. This protective process is very important to the body's ability to recognize infection and respond appropriately. Regional lymph node enlargement commonly presents in children secondary to local infection. Local lymphadenopathy can have serious implications, but generalized lymphadenopathy is of even more concern because of its association with systemic diseases including malignancy.

Infants at birth rarely have palpable lymph nodes. After the newborn period, with subsequent childhood infections and immune system stimulation, a rapid increase in lymphoid tissue occurs. Children are more likely than adults to have palpable nodes. Normal lymph nodes usually are less than 1 cm in diameter; however, they tend to be larger in childhood (ages 2 to 10 years) than later in life. At puberty, the nodes begin to involute, a process that continues throughout life.

The presence of regional lymphadenopathy is common in children and adolescents, especially during the period of rapid lymphoid growth in late childhood. By far the most common etiology is viral infection, but parents are often anxious about enlarged lymph glands because of the possible association with malignancy. At times it can be difficult for the physician to determine whether a node is benign and deserving of observation, or malignant and requiring thorough investigation. Generalized lymphadenopathy is usually caused by systemic disease and results in more concern. The differential diagnosis remains broad with malignancy being only a lesser part. Reports of lymph node biopsy series vary between 10% and 30% malignancy. These reports are based on referred children and are quite different from the population seen in general pediatric practices. There are also a number of other subcutaneous lesions that can be confused with lymph nodes (e.g., lipomata, cysts, cervical ribs).

Regional adenopathy usually results from a local process and the differential diagnosis varies correspondingly. For example, occipital nodes are often secondary to scalp pathology such as tinea capitis, seborrhea, tick bites, or scalp folliculitis. Inguinal adenopathy is often secondary to sexually transmitted diseases or skin lesions on the distal lower extremities. Submaxillary lymphadenopathy can be caused by dental caries or a dental abscess. In a child with regional adenopathy, it is important that the examiner carefully examine the skin and other structures in the respective lymphatic drainage area for possible etiologies.

The specific node or group of nodes that are enlarged is significant. Cervical, axillary, and inguinal nodes are commonly palpable in children. Upper posterior cervical lymphadenopathy is rarely associated with significant diseases in children and inguinal lymphadenopathy in children is usually not associated with a specific etiology unless the nodes are very large (>3 cm). Conversely, supraclavicular, popliteal, abdominal, epitrochlear, and mediastinal nodes are most likely to represent significant underlying pathology.

Most children with lymphadenopathy can be evaluated as outpatients. Hospitalization may be necessary for evaluation (consultations and biopsies), treatment (some lymphadenitis or malignancies), or to allay parental anxiety.

Definitions

- *Lymphadenopathy* refers to a nontender lymph node greater than 10 mm with the following exceptions:
  - An epitrochlear node greater than 5 mm
  - An inguinal node greater than 15 mm
- *Generalized adenopathy* refers to enlarged lymph nodes in two or more noncontiguous lymph node regions (e.g., inguinal and cervical).
- *Lymphadenitis* refers to an inflamed node with heat and tenderness, which may subsequently suppurate.

Differential Diagnosis

Evaluation

The history should first focus on evidence of infection or malignancy. Fever and other systemic symptoms (night sweats, anorexia, and weight loss) may be found in both categories, but the time course and other features may suggest specific etiologies. A good review of symptoms will help to narrow your differential diagnosis. Other infectious etiologies should be investigated including contact with kittens or their fleas (cat-scratch disease), ticks, drugs, sexual activity (especially if high-risk), travel, and other infectious contacts (tuberculosis). Sometimes localizing symptoms are present with infectious or malignant diseases. See Tables 18.1 and 18.2.

During the physical examination, the patient should be completely examined with particular attention to skin, joints, liver, spleen, and tonsils. All sites of regional lymph nodes should be examined. Features that should be noted include location, size, tenderness, fixation, and consistency. All nodes should be noted (size limits as above), but in some locations, nodes can still be safely followed. For example, a 2-cm anterior

TABLE 18.1

CAUSES OF REGIONAL ADENOPATHY

Cervical (lymphatic drainage from face, neck, thyroid, mouth, pharynx, and esophagus)
  Viral infections ("reactive nodes")
    Usual upper respiratory pathogens
    Epstein-Barr B Virus (EBV)
    Cytomegalovirus (CMV)
    Rubella
    Rubeola
    Varicella
  Bacterial infections and cat-scratch disease (see Table 18.3)
  Toxoplasmosis
  Mycobacterial infections
    M. tuberculosis
    Atypical tuberculosis
  Fungal infections
    Aspergillosis
    Cryptococcosis
    Histoplasmosis
    Coccidioidomycosis
    Acinetobacter spp.
    Nocardiosis
  Kawasaki disease
  Malignancy
    Lymphoma
    Leukemia
    Neuroblastoma
    Thyroid tumors
    Langerhans histiocytosis
  Sarcoidosis
  Suppurative thyroiditis

Occipital (lymphatic drainage from scalp and upper neck)
  Dermatitis
    Seborrhea
    Eczema
    Infectious
    Impetigo
    Folliculitis
    Otitis externa
  Viral
    Rubella (postauricular)
    Roseola (suboccipital)
  Bites
    Ticks
    Mosquitoes
    Biting flies
    Lice

Preauricular (lymphatic drainage from ear, forehead, eye, and adjacent scalp)
  Viral: Adenovirus 3 and 8 (epidemic keratoconjunctivitis)
  Chronic eye infections
    Hordeolum (stye)
    Chalazion
    Chlamydial eye infection
  Bacterial
    Tularemia (with eye inoculation)
    Cat-scratch disease
    Otitis externa

Axillary (lymphatic drainage from arm, chest wall, and breast)
  Infection (local)
    Cat scratch disease
    Other bacteria, viral, fungal
  Inflammation: eczema or other chronic dermatitis
  Vaccination: BCG

Inguinal (lymphatic drainage from lower extremity, pelvic organs, genital area, buttocks, and lower abdominal wall)
  Infection (local)
    LGV
    Chancroid
    Rickettsial infections
    Fungal
    Impetigo
  Inflammation (local)
    Diaper dermatitis
    Monilial dermatitis
    Contact dermatitis
    Bug bites

Supraclavicular (nodes are not usually palpated in the supraclavicular area and should be considered abnormal if greater than 1–2 mm in size)
  Right: Thoracic diseases, especially malignancies
  Left: Abdominal processes, especially malignancies

Epitrochlear nodes (palpable nodes in this region are often pathologic in children)
  Infections of the hand or forearm
  Leukemia
  Lymphoma
  Atypical mycobacterial infections

cervical node is commonly palpated and can be followed in an otherwise well child. Tenderness is caused by infection or rapid increase in the size of the node causing tension within the node capsule. Fixation of nodes can occur by local invasion by a malignancy or the inflammatory response to some infections. Fixation can occur to deeper or more superficial structures or even to adjacent nodes ("matting"). Consistency is important with benign nodes having a characteristic texture. Hard nodes are found in some cancers. Rubbery, firm nodes can be found in lymphomas and some leukemias. Lymph nodes palpated in leukemia tend to be softer.

On careful examination of the skin, evidence of local infection or trauma may suggest the etiology of regional lymphadenopathy. A skin papule on the shoulder or a distal extremity may be found at the site of primary infection with cat-scratch disease. Careful examination of the abdomen should be performed with particular attention to detecting hepatomegaly and/or splenomegaly.

The utility of additional diagnostic tests usually depends on the specifics of the presentation and the most likely diagnosis. For a patient with localized adenopathy, observation for 2 to 4 weeks is appropriate if the risk of malignancy is felt to be low. If the enlarged node is cervical or tender, a therapeutic trial with an antibiotic is appropriate for possible lymphadenitis. Therapy should be with an antibiotic that covers most strains of *Staphylococcus* and *Streptococcus* such as first- and second-generation cephalosporins, dicloxacillin, or amoxicillin-clavulanate. If there is no response to antibiotics in the first 2 weeks, coverage may be broadened to include other pathogens such as atypical mycobacteria or anaerobes.

TABLE 18.2

GENERALIZED LYMPHADENOPATHY

Benign Lymphoidal Hyperplasia (nonspecific response to
  a number of viral infections)
Systemic infections
  Bacterial
    Salmonellosis
    Brucellosis
    Syphilis
    Leptospirosis
    Typhoid fever
    Streptococcal systemic infection
    Tuberculosis
  Viral
    EBV
    CMV
    HIV
    Enteroviruses
    Hepatitis A
    Rubella
    Rubeola
  Other
    Toxoplasmosis
    Histoplasmosis
    Malaria
    Mycoplasma
Connective tissue disorders
  Systemic lupus erythematosus
  Juvenile rheumatoid arthritis
Malignancies
  Leukemias
  Lymphomas
  Metastatic neuroblastoma
  Langerhans histiocytosis
Immunologic diseases
  Chronic granulomatous disease
  Serum sickness
  Autoimmune hemolytic anemia
  Angioimmunoblastic lymphadenopathy
  Dysgammaglobulinemia
Skin conditions
  Any chronic diffuse skin irritation/disease (eczema)
Drug reactions
  Allopurinol   Penicillin
  Atenolol   Phenytoin
  Captopril   Primidone
  Carbamazepine   Pyrimethamine
  Cephalosporins   Quinidine
  Gold   Sulfonamides
  Hydralazine   Sulindac
  Isoniazid   Antithyroid medications
Metabolic storage diseases
  Gaucher disease
  Niemann–Pick disease
  Tangier disease
Other
  Sarcoidosis
  Gianotti–Crosti syndrome
  Chediak–Higashi syndrome
  Hemophagocytic syndrome
  Hyperthyroidism
  Castleman disease
  Rosai–Dorfman disease
  Inflammatory pseudotumor
  Churg–Strauss syndrome

Ciprofloxacin is a good second-line choice if there are no contraindications. A 2- to 4-week delay in diagnosis is not crucial even if the patient is found later to have lymphoma or another malignancy. Assuring follow-up is crucial.

If findings suggest generalized lymphadenopathy, a chest radiograph can detect hilar adenopathy. The presence of supraclavicular adenopathy is specifically an indication for chest radiography. Oftentimes a CT scan is needed to fully evaluate hilar and abdominal nodes. These tests have also largely replaced lymphangiograms.

In the patient with generalized palpable nodes, a complete blood count is indicated. Other tests to consider include erythrocyte sedimentation rate (ESR) or C-reactive protein (CRP); PPD; serologies for EBV, CMV, cat-scratch fever, and toxoplasmosis; HIV antibody determination (PCR and viral load if acute infection suspected); serologic test for syphilis; and tests for collagen vascular disease (ANA) and sarcoid (angiotensin-converting enzyme).

If the diagnosis is unclear after the above evaluation, consideration should be given to a lymph-node biopsy. If other enlarged lymph nodes are available, biopsy of the axillary and inguinal nodes should be avoided. These nodes are more likely to be enlarged due to nonspecific regional processes, resulting in nondiagnostic biopsy results. These same sites also are closer to neurovascular structures, increasing surgical risk.

The biopsy can be performed in two very different ways: fine-needle aspiration (FNA) and open biopsy. FNA obviously has the advantages of less pain, cost, and sedation, but with the disadvantage of obtaining much less tissue. Because of the latter, the results are sometimes nondiagnostic or false negative. If malignancy is found, the sample is usually inadequate for necessary molecular studies. The open biopsy is more traumatic, but provides more information about the pathologic tissue and node architecture. It is the only acceptable option to rule out lymphoma or another malignancy. Even with an open biopsy, a biopsied node may sometimes be normal and an adjacent (unbiopsied) node abnormal, resulting in a false-negative interpretation. The diagnoses being considered, the involved nodes, and the skills of the available physicians should determine the biopsy technique.

Pearls

- Most adenopathy with rapid onset (≤7 days) is infectious in origin, usually of common viral or pyogenic bacterial causes.
- The etiologies of more indolent adenopathy (1 to 3 weeks) tend to be more varied and include cat-scratch disease (*Bartonella henselae*), EBV, CMV, and Kawasaki disease.
- Features on physical examination that suggest malignancy include firmness, nontenderness, coalescence into a mass of nodes (matting), and fixation to deeper structures or skin. Under age 8, leukemia is the most common associated malignancy. The first test should be a CBC with review of a peripheral smear. After age 8, suspicious nodes should be biopsied, because lymphoma is the most common malignancy.
- Lymph-node biopsy is indicated for children with unexplained fever, weight loss, night sweats, or the above nodal characteristics on exam.
- Even with biopsy (open or FNA), as many as 50% of children with enlarged nodes do not get a definitive diagnosis.
- Enlarged nodes may be very slow to resolve (month to years). This has no diagnostic significance.
- Many conditions can be confused with lymphadenopathy, including thyroglossal duct cyst, branchial cleft cyst, parotid or submandibular salivary gland hypertrophy, lipoma, and other benign lesions.
- Mediastinal adenopathy can be associated with malignancy. Bilateral hilar node enlargement can also be found with

mycoplasma pneumonitis, sarcoidosis, cystic fibrosis, and fungal infections. Unilateral node enlargement is more common with tuberculosis and rarely with viral and bacterial lung infections.

- Generalized lymphadenopathy is common with atopic eczema.

LYMPHADENITIS

Most children with lymphadenitis do not need hospitalization. Hospitalization is occasionally necessary because of the age of the child (very young), toxicity, associated lymphangitis or cellulitis, rapid progression of the infection, associated diseases (immunocompromised state), or for diagnostic evaluation. The involved nodes are usually warm, tender, and may have overlying erythema. The most common site for acute lymphadenitis is in the submandibular or cervical regions and is usually secondary to local spread of a bacterial infection from the pharynx, teeth and gums, or skin. Head and neck trauma can also result in lymphadenitis in this area. In addition to the local findings of inflammation, the patient with lymphadenitis usually has some systemic symptoms and an elevated white blood cell count.

Subacute and chronic lymphadenitis are less common than acute lymphadenitis. These are also more common in the cervical region, with the axillary, occipital, and inguinal regions progressively less common.

Differential Diagnosis

Evaluation

Needle aspiration of an infected node can often lead to identification (by stains and cultures) of the specific pathogen if bacterial or tuberculous. (Use an 18-gauge needle on a 20-mL syringe; can inject and reaspirate nonbacteriostatic saline if nothing is obtained on initial aspiration.) The node does not have to be fluctuant. There is a small risk of developing a persistent draining tract if the infection is caused by atypical mycobacteria. This is substantially greater if open drainage is performed. Warthin-Starry stain can be used to identify *Bartonella henselae*, but more often diagnosis is based on positive serology. If careful palpation of an involved node is unable to determine the presence of fluctuance, ultrasound evaluation can be helpful in the determination of abscess cavity formation. See Table 18.3.

Management

In the setting of an acute lymphangitis (usually pyogenic), initial intravenous therapy should be nafcillin 150 mg/kg/day divided Q4–6 H or ampicillin/sulbactam 100 to 200 mg/kg/day divided Q6H. If oral therapy is adequate, cephalexin 50 mg/kg/day divided Q6H has the advantages of palatability and efficacy. If the lymphadenitis is secondary to a dental infection, anaerobic coverage is necessary. Penicillin V is drug of choice (50 mg/kg/day divided Q6H) with clindamycin or erythromycin as alternatives for penicillin allergy.

If the time course and clinical presentation suggests a subacute or chronic infectious etiology, the specific therapy will depend on the most likely etiology. Cat-scratch disease is usually self-limited and benign, but total resolution may take months. Efficacy of antibiotic therapy is controversial, but azithromycin (10 mg/kg first day, then 5 mg/kg/day for 4 days) has been shown effective in one study. Aspiration may be needed for pain relief if suppuration occurs. Rarely is incision and drainage necessary.

Atypical tuberculosis is usually approached by total excision of infected nodes. Antituberculous medications have variable

TABLE 18.3

DIFFERENTIAL DIAGNOSIS OF LYMPHADENITIS

Acute lymphadenitis
Bacterial
β-hemolytic streptococci
Staphylococcus aureus
Anaerobic bacteria
Pasteurella multocida
Mycoplasma hominis
Chlamydia trachomatis (LGV)
Gram-negative bacilli
Others (see Table 18.2)
Viral
Herpes simplex
Enteroviral
EBV
Adenovirus
Varicella

Subacute or chronic lymphadenitis
Bacterial
Cat-scratch disease (*Bartonella henselae*)
Staphylococcus aureus
Atypical tuberculosis
Mycobacterium tuberculosis
Anaerobes
Syphilis
Tularemia
Brucellosis
Viral
EBV
CMV
Human immunodeficiency virus (HIV; acute)
HHV-6 (roseola subitum)
Other
Kawasaki disease
Chronic granulomatous disease
Sporotrichosis
Nocardiosis
Toxoplasmosis
Histoplasmosis
Tropical protozoan infections
BCG-itis
Kikuchi lymphadenitis

effectiveness in these strains, and sensitivity testing is necessary. Some strains respond to the quinolones and newer macrolides. *M. tuberculosis* is usually treated with a three-drug regimen as if treating disseminated infection. Actual dissemination is uncommon. Surgical drainage is usually not indicated although biopsy may be needed for diagnosis. A 5-TU PPD skin test usually results in >15 mm induration with *M. tuberculosis*, but 5 to 15 mm with the atypical mycobacteria. See Table 18.4.

Course and Prognosis

Resolution of acute lymphadenitis is usually rapid (1 to 7 days) with appropriate therapy. Subacute/chronic lymphadenitis resolves more slowly (over 1 to 3 weeks), and the course is often diagnosis dependent. Delay in diagnosis and therapy can result in a longer course, cellulitis, abscess formation, and even sinus tract formation (atypical tuberculosis). Infrequently, lymphadenitis will recur and should cause a careful search for an undiscovered etiology (e.g., foreign body, dental abscess).

TABLE 18.4

INDICATIONS FOR EARLY LYMPH NODE BIOPSY

Early lymph node biopsy should be considered in patients with the following clinical features:

- Systemic symptoms (fever >1 week, night sweats, weight loss >10%)
- Supraclavicular and lower neck nodes
- Fixed, nontender nodes in the absence of other symptoms
- Abnormal chest radiograph or CBC
- Lack of infectious symptoms
- Elevated ESR

Pearls

- Group B streptococcal "cellulitis-adenitis" is a variant of late-onset GBS disease in 1- to 2-month-old infants. Infants are febrile and irritable with tender submandibular or facial cellulitis/adenitis. Blood culture is often positive and otitis media is often a comorbidity.
- In cat-scratch disease, a papule can be found at site of initial infection in 60% of cases. Flea bites can also spread infection, sometimes explaining infection in the absence of known cat exposure. One-half of patients have lymphadenopathy without other symptoms; 15% progress to suppuration; 5% have

an atypical presentation including CNS involvement, FUO, or lesions in lung, liver, bone, or spleen.

- Adenitis related to *M. tuberculosis* rather than atypical organisms is more common in children over age 4, with known exposure to TB, in urban residence, with bilateral cervical or generalized lymphadenopathy, or with an abnormal chest radiograph.
- Nodular lymphadenitis is a distinctive form of lymphangitis with nodules along the lymphatics draining an area. A primary site of infection is usually present distally. Pathogens associated with this pattern include sporotrichosis, *Nocardia*, atypical tuberculosis, and tularemia.
- Acute mesenteric lymphadenitis is associated with fever, nausea, and abdominal pain. Because of associated abdominal findings on exam, this entity is frequently difficult to distinguish from appendicitis. It is usually associated with viral infections, but can be secondary to bacterial enteritis, especially *Yersinia*.

Suggested Readings

Kelly CS, Kelly RE. Lymphadenopathy in children. *Pediatr Clin North Am* 1998;45:875–888.
Leung AK, Robson WL. Childhood cervical lymphadenopathy. *J Pediatr Health Care* 2004;18:3–7.
McClain KL, Fletcher RH. Evaluation of peripheral lymphadenopathy in children, *UpToDate* Online 9.3.
Margileth AM. Sorting out the causes of lymphadenopathy. *Contemp Pediatr* 1995;12:23–40.
Peters TR, Edwards KM. Cervical lymphadenopathy and adenitis. *Pediatr Rev* 2000;21:399–405.

CHAPTER 19 ■ ORGANOMEGALY

DAVID L. ELDRIDGE AND DALE A. NEWTON

Organomegaly describes any organ that is pathologically enlarged. For the purposes of this chapter, the discussion will be restricted to enlargement of the liver and spleen. For discussion of other abdominal masses, see Chapter 11.

Palpation of an enlarged liver or spleen is very common in infancy. In older children, the margin of the liver or spleen is less commonly palpable. There is a broad range of diseases that can cause hepatosplenomegaly, and these vary greatly by age of presentation. Because there is much overlap in the pathologic states that can cause hepatomegaly and splenomegaly, the differential diagnosis of these two entities will be considered jointly (Table 19.1). Obviously, some of these entities may involve only the liver or the spleen.

HEPATOMEGALY

In newborns, the liver margin is commonly palpated 2 cm below the right costal margin. The liver margin is often not palpable in infants with intrauterine growth retardation. Conversely, the liver can be as much as 4 cm below the right costal margin in infants of diabetic mothers (IDM). In older infants and children, palpation alone should not be used as the sole criteria for hepatomegaly; other techniques, including percussion, can help define the upper margin of the liver and determine liver span.

At 2 months of age, the average liver span is approximately 5.5 cm, with a normal range of 3.5 to 7.2 cm. By age 5 years, the average span is 8.2 cm, with a normal range of 6.5 to 10 cm. There are also nomograms relating liver span to body surface area.

Diseases that cause hepatomegaly are quite varied and include vascular engorgement, cellular infiltrates, accumulation of storage products, inflammation, fatty infiltration, Kupffer cell hypertrophy, and tumors. This leads to the very broad differential diagnosis described in Table 19.1. The first step in evaluation beyond history and physical exam is usually the hepatic ultrasound to aid in the determination of size and consistency.

SPLENOMEGALY

The spleen is important to the fetus as a site of hematopoiesis. This function usually ceases in the third trimester. It remains important in filtration of particulate matter and abnormal cells from the circulation and in production of humoral factors that opsonize bacteria. The spleen is usually enlarged as a consequence of systemic or liver diseases and is rarely the site of primary disease.

The spleen is commonly palpable in preterm infants and in 30% of term infants. At 1 year of age, approximately 30% of children have palpable spleens. This decreases progressively to only 1% in normal adolescents. In some older children, the spleen tip is soft and barely palpable under the left rib margin. For many of these children, this represents visceroptosis (a lower position of the spleen) rather than true splenomegaly. Ultrasonography is the appropriate first test to confirm and evaluate splenomegaly.

Hypersplenism can complicate splenomegaly and represents the development of excessive splenic function. The latter notably results in splenic sequestration and subsequent deficiency of one or more blood cell lines (thrombocytopenia, leukopenia, and anemia) with normal or increased bone marrow production. The patient typically presents with pallor, fatigue, and splenomegaly. The most common cause of hypersplenism is portal vein hypertension, often secondary to thrombosis of the portal vein from processes such as umbilical vein catheterization, shock, dehydration, or omphalitis. Although uncommon in children, cirrhosis can also result in portal hypertension and hypersplenism. Other causes include storage diseases of the liver and malaria. Splenectomy cures hypersplenism, but the etiology usually determines whether this is appropriate therapy and whether other surgical procedures are indicated (e.g., vascular shunts).

PEARLS

- Isolated splenomegaly can be found with any of the causes of portal hypertension (e.g., cirrhosis from a number of causes, veno-occlusive disease, chronic congestive heart failure).
- Hepatic or splenic enlargement can be secondary to intraparenchymal hemorrhage from direct trauma.
- Pulmonary hyperinflation (acute or chronic) can cause apparent, but "pseudo" hepatosplenomegaly.
- Acute enlargement of the liver or spleen is a contraindication to sports participation. Chronic and/or stable hepatosplenomegaly needs individual assessment before permission to participate, especially in contact sports.
- A form of acute hypersplenism occurs in young children with sickle-cell disease. During these "splenic sequestration crises," the children present with sudden enlargement of the

TABLE 19.1

DIFFERENTIAL DIAGNOSIS OF HEPATOSPLENOMEGALY (BY AGE)

Newborn
Infection
  Bacterial infections
  TORCH infections
  Infectious hepatitis
  Syphilis
Hemolytic disease: Rh or ABO incompatibility
  (erythroblastosis fetalis)
Congestive heart failure: congenital heart disease
Liver disease
  Neonatal hepatitis
  Biliary atresia
  Inspissated bile syndrome
Metabolic
  Infant of diabetic mother
  Galactosemia
  Hyperparathyroidism
Miscellaneous
  Beckwith–Wiedemann syndrome
  Zellweger syndrome
  Hereditary spherocytosis
  G6PD deficiency
  Riedel lobe

Infant
Cystic fibrosis
Malnutrition
Malignancy
  Wilms tumor
  Neuroblastoma
  Hepatoma
  Hemangioma
  Histiocytosis
Metabolic
  Glycogen storage diseases
  Gaucher disease
  Mucopolysaccharidoses
  Galactosemia
Hemoglobinopathies
  β-thalassemia
  Sickle-cell disease
  Infantile pyknocytosis
Other
  Hyperalimentation
  Alpha-1-antitrypsin deficiency
  Klippel–Trenaunay–Weber syndrome

Younger child
Toxin/drug
  Acetaminophen
  Anticonvulsants
  Sulfonamides
Infection
  Viral hepatitis A, B, or C
  CMV
  EBV
  Enteroviruses
  HIV
  Visceral larva migrans
Malignancy
  Leukemia
  Lymphoma
  Metastatic tumors
  Hemangioendotheliomas

Histiocytosis
Hepatoblastoma
Other
  Benign hepatomegaly (secondary to non-hepatitis viral
    infection)
  Iron-deficiency anemia
  Hemolytic anemias
  Chediak–Higashi syndrome
  Chronic granulomatous disease
  Type I hyperlipoproteinemia
  Homocystinuria
  Polycystic disease of the liver
  Cystic fibrosis
  Cockayne syndrome

Older child/adolescent
Hepatitis
  Viral hepatitis A, B, or C
  CMV
  EBV
  HIV
  Enteroviruses
  Leptospirosis
Infections
  Rocky Mountain spotted fever
  Liver abscess
  Parasitic infections
  Brucellosis
  Malaria
  Babesiosis
  Tuberculosis
Toxin/drug
  Acetaminophen
  Anticonvulsants
  Sulfonamides
  Tetracyclines
  Oral contraceptives
  Corticosteroids
  Anabolic steroids
Collagen-vascular disease
  Juvenile rheumatoid arthritis
  Systemic lupus erythematosus
  Serum sickness
Malignancy
  Lymphoma
  Leukemia
Nutritional
  Starvation
  Hyperalimentation
Other
  Wilson disease
  Hemochromatosis
  Visceral larva migrans
  Inflammatory bowel disease
  Amyloidosis
  Reye syndrome
  Primary sclerosing cholangitis
  Hypervitaminosis A
  Constrictive pericarditis
  Diabetes mellitus (poorly controlled)
  Lipodystrophy
  Sarcoidosis
  Budd–Chiari syndrome

spleen and a large proportion of their circulating blood volume retained within the spleen. Clinical findings include pallor, dyspnea, left-sided abdominal pain, and tachycardia. Because this can rapidly progress to hypovolemic shock and death, recognition, fluid resuscitation, transfusion, and ultimately splenectomy are indicated.

Suggested Readings

Tunnessen WW. *Signs and Symptoms in Pediatrics.* 3rd ed. Philadelphia: Lippincott Williams & Wilkins; 1999.

Wolf AD, Lavine JE. Hepatomegaly in neonates and children. *Pediatr Rev* 2000;21:303–310.

CHAPTER 20A ■ ACUTE ABDOMINAL PAIN

KATHLEEN VINCENT PREVILL

Abdominal pain is a common pediatric symptom representing approximately 5% of all outpatient visits. Because of the many organ systems located in the abdomen, identifying the source of the pain requires astute clinical skill.

Acute abdominal pain has a defined beginning, hours or at most a few days before the examination, and must be accurately and immediately evaluated for surgical versus medical causes. Children may not be able to clearly describe their discomfort in the usual terms of character, quality, and timing. Often pain intensity can be quantified by having the patient rate the pain on a scale from 1 to 10. When assessing the intensity of pain in children less than 7 years of age, a picture scale depicting happy to anxious faces is helpful.

Children are frequently able to identify the location of abdominal pain. If the pain is visceral (i.e., intestinal, organ capsule), it typically is dull, mid-epigastric, and poorly localized. Once the intestinal wall is distended, vascular supply compromised, or lymphatics obstructed, the characteristic sharp pain of parietal peritoneum involvement begins and the pain becomes more localized.

Specific history should be taken concerning the association and onset of vomiting, diarrhea, fever, cough, constipation, urinary symptoms, trauma, rash, and anorexia. Male patients should be screened for scrotal or penile pain, and female patients should be evaluated for menarche, menstrual patterns, or vaginal discharge. Both male and female adolescents should be asked about sexual activity.

The pertinent past medical history includes information about prior surgical procedures, current mediations, and chronic illness such as sickle-cell anemia.

DIFFERENTIAL DIAGNOSIS

The most common causes of acute abdominal pain in children are viral gastroenteritis and mesenteric adenitis. Associated fever, vomiting, and diarrhea as well as sick contacts implicate these diagnoses. Acute appendicitis is the diagnosis of greatest concern because of its common occurrence and potential for appendiceal rupture. Appendicitis typically presents with acute pain that progressively worsens over 24 hours with vomiting following the onset of pain. In gastroenteritis, vomiting usually precedes abdominal pain or diarrhea. Classically the child with appendicitis is anorectic, lies very still, and has abdominal guarding and rebound pain. This diagnosis is more difficult in children younger than 3 years of age (Chapter 126B).

When children present with bilious emesis, conditions associated with bowel obstruction (e.g., midgut volvulus, perforated appendix) should be considered (Section XIV). In any age group, but especially in young children, urinary tract infections or stones may present without urinary frequency or dysuria; hence the diagnosis may become evident only from urinalysis or urine culture results (Chapter 80).

Constipation is common in children and can be a cause of intermittent severe pain or vague abdominal discomfort. The history of the child's defecation pattern is very important, but sometimes difficult to ascertain accurately in the toilet-trained young child. Encopresis is a form of severe constipation with soiling, and often is associated with pain (Chapter 52).

Adolescent girls present added diagnostic challenges, and evaluation of the genitourinary system with a pelvic examination is critical to diagnosing pregnancy, pelvic inflammatory disease, or other gynecologic causes of lower abdominal pain (Chapter 88). The clinician must respect the possibility that adolescent girls are as likely as young children to have the common causes of abdominal pain. The differential diagnosis of acute abdominal pain in the pediatric age group is similar to the differential for adults but does include some disorders specific to children, including Henoch Schönlein purpura and malrotation with volvulus (Table 20.1).

EVALUATION

Acute abdominal pain often causes discomfort relieved only by lying still with the legs flexed at the hips or assuming a semifetal position. Particular attention should be given to associated tachycardia, pallor, diaphoresis, or tachypnea. Among these, tachycardia is the most sensitive indicator of serious intra-abdominal disease.

The abdominal examination is done with care and sensitivity. The examiner looks for distention. Abdominal sounds are auscultated and their presence, pitch, and frequency described. High-pitched, infrequent sounds suggest paralytic ileus, whereas absent bowel sounds indicate obstruction.

The abdomen is palpated using gentle touch and warm hands. A child may wish to place her hand on top of the examiner's and thereby control the pressure exerted. The examiner describes any localized tenderness and further defines any mass by scratch percussion. Rebound pain may be quite painful and should not be repeatedly performed. When deciding to perform a rectal examination, the clinician must weigh the discomfort it may cause against the pertinent information the exam may reveal such as occult blood, pelvic masses, or anterior rectal wall tenderness. The child is asked to walk, hop, cough, straight-leg raise, or hyperextend the leg at the hip to ascertain peritoneal inflammation.

Pubertal patients should have a detailed genitourinary and pelvic examination as part of their evaluation.

MANAGEMENT

Any anorectic child with progressive pain or localized abdominal pain requires surgical consultation. The surgeon can help differentiate those conditions for which specific surgical intervention is

TABLE 20.1

ACUTE ABDOMINAL PAIN BY ORGAN SYSTEM

Esophagus/Stomach
- Esophagitis
- Peptic ulcer disease
- Gastroenteritis

Small Intestine
- Mesenteric adenitis
- Lymphoma
- Intussusception
- Midgut volvulus/malrotation
- Crohn's disease
- Incarcerated hernia

Large Intestine
- Appendicitis
- Intussusception
- Hirschprung disease
- Ulcerative colitis
- Constipation

Uterine
- Pelvic inflammatory disease
- Pregnancy
- Dysmenorrhea
- Endometriosis

Tubo-Ovarian
- Ovarian cyst
- Adnexal torsion
- Tubo-ovarian ischemia
- Ectopic pregnancy

Testes
- Torsion testes
- Trauma
- Torsion appendix testes

Liver/Gallbladder
- Hepatitis
- Hepatic tumor
- Cholecystitis/cholelithiasis

Kidney
- Pyelonephritis/cystitis
- Kidney stone
- Renal vein thrombosis

Adrenal
- Adrenal calcification
- Adrenal tumor

Spleen
- Ruptured capsule
- Infarcted spleen

Pancreas
- Pancreatitis
- Common bile duct stone

Omentum
- Peritonitis
- Omental hernia

Aorta/Arterial bed
- Vascular insufficiency
- Aortic dissection

Miscellaneous
- Referred pain from pneumonia and pleura
- Trauma
- Sickle cell crisis
- Henoch Schönlein purpura
- Strep pharyngitis

carefully measured output from the urinary and intestinal tracts are essential for management. Antibiotics with aerobic and anaerobic coverage are included in the preoperative management of appendicitis or any condition with potential bowel perforation. Many regimens are suggested, including meropenem or imipenem-cilastatin.

Screening laboratory tests include the complete blood count, urinalysis and culture, electrolytes, renal function tests, and pancreatic enzymes. If suggested by history or examination, screening liver functions, stool cultures, or stool analysis for parasites may be indicated.

Radiologic studies may help define the diagnosis. These should begin with an upright and supine plain radiograph to observe gas patterns, psoas sign, calcifications, feces, or free peritoneal air. Ultrasonography is a sensitive and specific tool for surgical disorders. The most definitive study is the abdominal computed tomography (CT) scan with contrast, although this study does expose children to added radiation.

PEARLS

- Intussusception is more common in boys between 3 months and 2 years of age. Most infants have severe episodes of pain and may have bloody stools.
- Peptic ulcer disease can occur in young children but is more common in adolescents. When suspected, a trial of a histamine-2 blocker is an appropriate first step before beginning a more invasive evaluation.
- Mesenteric adenitis can be caused by adenovirus, enterovirus, or *Yersinia*, or can be associated with streptococcal pharyngitis. Mesenteric adenitis commonly mimics appendicitis, and a collaborative pediatric and surgical approach is indicated.
- Any infant <3 months with a distended, painful abdomen requires immediate evaluation for sepsis, bowel perforation, or Hirschsprung disease. These are surgical emergencies (Section XIV).

indicated. The use of pain medications including narcotics is acceptable and does not obscure the ability to diagnosis an acute surgical condition (Chapter 134).

With any potential bowel obstruction, the stomach should be rested with nasogastric suction. Fluid resuscitation for deficits, normal saline to replace nasogastric losses, and replacement of

Suggested Readings

Ashcraft KW. Consultation with the specialist: acute abdominal pain. *PIR* 2000;21:363.

Green R, Bulloch B, Kabari A, et al. Early analgesia for children with acute abdominal pain. *Pediatrics* 2005;116:978–983.

Kharbanda AB, Taylor GA, Fishman SJ, et al. A clinical decision rule to identify children at low risk for appendicitis. *Pediatrics* 2005;116:709–716.

CHAPTER 20B ■ CHEST PAIN

DALE A. NEWTON AND DAVID W. HANNON

Chest pain is a common problem in the pediatric age group, especially in adolescents. One study noted that approximately one in four adolescents reported three or more episodes of chest pain in the previous year. Chest pain in a child often is a cause of significant anxiety, somewhat for the child and more so for the parent. Society associates chest pain with heart disease because of the prevalence of angina in adults and the highly publicized (although rare) cardiac deaths of several

famous athletes. Chest pain and the associated concerns often result in emergency department visits, urgent office visits, and frequently, pediatric cardiology consultations. About one-half of all children who complain of chest pain miss some school because of the complaint and more than two-thirds limit their physical activity. At times parents and even coaches will limit activity and sports participation until physician evaluation is completed.

Despite this level of concern caused by chest pain, cardiac etiologies are uncommon, accounting for approximately 5% of children presenting with chest pain. Most children and adolescents with cardiac etiologies of chest pain do not have life-threatening conditions.

When chest pain in children has an organic etiology, most often it is due to chest wall problems, reflux esophagitis, or pulmonary diagnoses, especially asthma, pneumonia, and chronic cough. The newly described orthostatic tachycardia syndrome also may be relatively common. Nonorganic chest pain commonly presents as a functional problem, sometimes with associated hyperventilation. Reported series vary greatly, but in approximately 25% of children with chest pain, no etiology can be found (i.e., idiopathic).

DIFFERENTIAL DIAGNOSIS

Evaluation

Most children with chest pain can be worked up in the outpatient setting (Table 20.2). A rare child or adolescent is admitted because of the severity of pain, patient or parental anxiety, or findings suggesting serious organic disease. A careful history of the pain should be obtained, including descriptions of the character, location, radiation, precipitating events, and relieving factors. Chronic recurrent pain is less likely to have a serious organic etiology. Other historical clues to the diagnosis may be such elements as pain associated with certain positions, movements, or eating, fever, pain awakening the child from sleep, history of chest trauma or asthma, or presence of sickle-cell anemia.

Of the lengthy differential diagnosis that follows, the diagnoses that may put the patient at greatest risk of death usually are related to the heart. To complete the cardiac investigation, it is important to pay careful attention to historical details such as a previous history of Kawasaki disease, chest pain or syncope during vigorous exercise, or concomitant autoimmune disease that could predispose to pericarditis (e.g., lupus or rheumatoid arthritis). Risk factors for coronary heart disease such as smoking, hyperlipidemia, hypertension, diabetes mellitus, and family history of premature cardiovascular disease should be elicited, although children and adolescents are unlikely to have atherosclerotic coronary artery disease. A rare exception is homozygous familial hypercholesterolemia. These children often have total cholesterol values exceeding 800 mg/dL and angina presenting in adolescence. A family history of hypertrophic cardiomyopathy or dilated cardiomyopathy mandates cardiac evaluation. Careful elicitation of a history of palpitations is appropriate because chest pain can be associated with arrhythmias. Palpitations also are characteristic of orthostatic-tachycardia syndrome.

Pulmonary etiologies should be investigated with questions about asthma, cough, or dyspnea. Some studies have suggested that undiagnosed exercise-induced asthma is a common cause of chest pain. Although pulmonary embolus is rare in adolescence, a history of leg problems suggesting deep venous thrombosis should be sought because of the potentially fatal outcome of pulmonary thromboembolism. Risk factors that increase the likelihood of pulmonary thromboembolism include prolonged travel, use of birth control pills, prolonged bed rest after surgery, and certain prothrombotic states. Pulmonary hypertension may present with chest pain, syncope, dyspnea, or effort intolerance. Pulmonary hypertension may be primary, or secondary to chronic airway obstruction (e.g., sleep apnea).

After the careful review of past medical history, family history, and social history, review of systems should be carefully performed. This should include a focus on findings suggesting chronic disease such as weight loss, fever, fatigue, night sweats, severe snoring, and malaise. Especially in adolescents, a careful history for situational stress or symptoms of depression should be obtained. Such a history often is associated with functional chest pain. A careful inquiry to patients about what they think is causing the pain often is enlightening, especially if there are stressors playing a role in psychogenic or physical etiologies. Eating disorders also should be considered because the self-induced vomiting associated with bulimia can result in chest pain due to esophagitis or esophageal mucosal tears.

The physical examination should include a careful review of the vital signs and equally careful observation of the patient, including emotional status. This is the examiner's opportunity to detect respiratory distress, cyanosis, tachypnea, murmurs, and rales. In the examination of the chest and heart, careful palpation of the chest and all chest structures is especially important. Chest wall tenderness is the finding most common in the pediatric age group that provides a ready explanation for musculoskeletal chest pain. This pain can be from costochondritis or secondary to trauma. The latter may be associated with other physical findings.

The examination of the lungs should focus on detecting wheezing, rales, and symmetric air movement. These findings may confirm asthma, pneumonia with pleurisy, or pneumothorax, respectively.

The cardiac examination may be negative in the setting of premature coronary artery disease or an aberrant coronary artery. With pericarditis, a pericardial friction rub may be heard. Decreased heart sounds and distended neck veins are present if tamponade occurs. With myocarditis, the findings are subtle, with clues such as tachycardia, third heart sound, and orthostatic blood pressure changes. Murmurs obviously can be associated with a number of valvular abnormalities. Severe aortic or pulmonic stenosis may cause chest pain. However, these are discovered only rarely in adolescents presenting with chest pain because a prior diagnosis of valvular cardiac disease almost always has been established. Severe coarctation of the aorta may present with chest pains in late adolescence and may be previously undiagnosed. Hypertension in the right arm should be present. Palpation of femoral pulses should be included in the physical examination of any adolescent.

A mid-systolic click with or without late systolic murmur suggests mitral valve prolapse. Several studies have concluded that mitral valve prolapse may not have a significantly greater incidence of chest pain than exists in a control population. Recent studies have suggested that symptoms of the so-called "mitral valve prolapse syndrome" may be more related to autonomic abnormality than to cardiac valvular abnormality. Some authors equate orthostatic tachycardia syndrome with the mitral valve prolapse syndrome, suggesting that a decreased preload to the heart during standing may result in an auscultatory click, but symptoms of palpitations and chest tightness may be related to autonomic dysfunction and orthostatic intolerance. The striking infrequency of chest pain complaints in adolescents with Marfan syndrome and true mitral valve prolapse (often with significant mitral valve regurgitation and myxomatous change) is consistent with the hypothesis that chest pain in most patients with mitral valve prolapse syndrome may not be cardiac but autonomic. Patients with true mitral valve prolapse may have an increased frequency of arrhythmia, but these are unlikely to be life-threatening in an adolescent population.

Chest pains in an adolescent with Marfan syndrome require consideration of acute, subacute, or even chronic aortic dissection. Therefore, the general physical examination should include attention to general appearance, especially skeletal (pectus excavatum, pectus carinatum, arm span, upper/lower body length ratio, narrow-arched palate,

TABLE 20.2

DIFFERENTIAL DIAGNOSIS OF PEDIATRIC CHEST PAIN

Idiopathic (common)

Musculoskeletal (common)
Trauma
  Contusion
  Muscle strain
  Rib separation or fracture
  Repetitive coughing
Inflammatory
  Costochondritis
  Juvenile idiopathic (rheumatoid) arthritis
  Juvenile ankylosing spondylitis
Idiopathic
  Slipping rib syndrome
  Xiphoid process syndrome
Malignancy: locally invasive (primary or metastatic)
Infectious: osteomyelitis

Pulmonary (common)
Infectious
  Pneumonia
  Pleurisy
  Pleurodynia
  Bronchitis/tracheitis
  Empyema
  Cystic fibrosis
Vascular
  Acute chest syndrome (sickle-cell disease)
  Pulmonary emboli
  Primary pulmonary hypertension
Malignancy: hilar or parenchymal tumor
Other
  Asthma
  Pneumothorax (spontaneous or secondary to underlying disease)
  Aspirated foreign body
  Systemic lupus erythematosus
  Precordial catch ("side stitch")

Neural (uncommon)
Neuritis: herpes zoster
Nerve root irritation
  Tumor
  Trauma
  Radiculitis

Gastrointestinal (common)
Peptic
  Esophagitis (peptic and eosinophilic)
  Peptic ulcer disease
Infectious
  Cholecystitis

Subphrenic abscess
Perihepatitis (Fitz–Hugh–Curtis syndrome)
Other
  Esophageal foreign body
  Cholelithiasis
  Esophageal spasm
  Caustic ingestion
  Candidal esophagitis
  Pancreatitis
  Esophageal tear

Cardiac (uncommon)
Ischemic
  Aberrant coronary artery
  Coronary artery aneurysm after Kawasaki disease
  Pulmonary hypertension
  Cocaine ingestion (or other sympathomimetic drugs)
  Premature atherosclerosis (familial hypercholesterolemia homozygote)
Pericardial
  Pericarditis
  Postpericardiotomy syndrome
  Pneumopericardium
Valvular
  Aortic stenosis
  Bacterial endocarditis
  Mitral valve prolapse syndrome
  Pulmonary stenosis
Other
  Dissecting aortic aneurysm (Marfan syndrome)
  Acute rheumatic fever
  Arrhythmias
  Hypertrophic cardiomyopathy (idiopathic hypertrophic subaortic stenosis/IHSS)
  Other cardiomyopathies
  Myocarditis

Other (common)
Breast
  Adolescent breast development
  Fibrocystic breast disease
  Mastitis
  Tumor
Renal: nephrolithiasis with colic
Psychological
  Functional (anxiety; often with hyperventilation)
  Conversion reaction (including globus hystericus)
  Depression
Malingering
Orthostatic tachycardia syndrome/orthostatic intolerance

arachnodactyly). The joints and skin also should be inspected for changes of Ehlers–Danlos syndrome, some forms of which are associated with aortic dissection. The vascular form of Ehlers–Danlos syndrome is more likely to occur in patients with thin, translucent-appearing skin. Patients with Ehlers–Danlos syndrome with lax, hypermobile joints were shown in one study to have an increased prevalence of orthostatic intolerance presenting as chronic fatigue, chest discomfort, palpitations, and syncope. Tall, thin adolescents with or without Marfan syndrome have an increased prevalence of spontaneous pneumothorax that may present as a nagging

unilateral chest pain of sudden onset but with duration of days to weeks.

Most children and adolescents presenting with chest pain do not need any additional evaluation other than a good history and physical examination. If history or physical examination suggests one of the more serious etiologies, appropriate diagnostic testing should be performed. However, in the absence of specific suggestive findings, testing should not be done just to reassure parents. Rather than decreasing anxiety, such testing often reinforces the thought that the doctors "can't find the problem" and thereby raises anxiety.

When indicated, tests to consider include the electrocardiogram (ECG), chest radiograph, pulse oximetry or arterial blood gas analysis, and drug screen. Cardiac enzymes are usually not indicated, but should be obtained if acute myocarditis is suggested by clinical or ECG findings. Associated symptoms such as recurrent palpitations, syncope, or presyncope may indicate need for an ECG looping event recorder. External leads are worn daily for a month or more and used to record a rhythm strip during a symptomatic event. This can later be transmitted by telephone to a receiving station for review. Twenty-four–hour ambulatory ECG (Holter monitoring) is less useful and has largely been replaced by prolonged event recorders. An echocardiogram may be considered for the patient with exertional chest pain, or exertional syncope or dizziness. This study should exclude aberrant origin of either coronary artery, coronary aneurysm from old Kawasaki disease, and cardiomyopathy. Pediatric cardiologists are more likely than internal medicine cardiologists to image specifically the coronary origins and courses. A treadmill test also may be useful in patients with exertional chest pain and can be used to diagnose exercise-induced asthma as well as look for exertional cardiac arrhythmia or ischemia. Thyroid function tests are indicated if clinical features suggest hyperthyroidism, or in the presence of an arrhythmia. If collagen vascular disease is suspected, complete blood count and erythrocyte sedimentation rate are indicated. An appropriate gastrointestinal workup may be indicated if the history suggests dyspepsia or gastroesophageal reflux. Esosinophilic esophagitis requires endoscopic biopsy for diagnosis, but is usually associated with both dysphagia and chest pain rather than isolated chest pain.

MANAGEMENT

Treatment is specific to the suspected etiology. Many children with chest pain need only reassurance and no specific medication. Children and adolescents with chest pain who are admitted to the hospital usually have features suggesting one of the more serious diagnoses. In addition to a workup directed by the history and examination, appropriate consultation may be needed with subspecialists in cardiology, gastroenterology, pulmonology, or psychiatry.

COURSE AND PROGNOSIS

If the initial evaluation is benign, rarely does long-term follow-up reveal a serious etiology. However, children with chest pain often have symptoms that persist for months and occasionally years. It is advisable to warn patients and parents about the natural history of recurrent chest pain and the concomitant frustration. This often helps families and children cope with the recurring problem without undue anxiety or unnecessary limitation of physical activities. They also need to be informed that long-term follow-up of children with chest pain shows that most (80%) eventually become pain free. When specific etiologies for chest pain are found, the prognosis becomes that of the underlying disease.

PEARLS

- A normal ECG often reassures parents and children. The clinician must remain aware that this does not rule out all cardiac etiologies. Echocardiography usually is not necessary or cost effective, but may be indicated for exercise-related chest pains.
- Pain in a dermatomal distribution may be herpes zoster (shingles). The neuritic pain may precede the characteristic rash by several days.
- A point of tenderness at a costochondral junction ("trigger point") often suggests costochondritis in the absence of a history of trauma. With a history of trauma, a similar trigger point may be a rib separation or fracture.
- A precordial "catch" is common in children (with exertion or at rest) and may be reproducible with certain movements. The pain (Texidor twinge) is sudden, sharp, does not refer elsewhere, and immediately remits.
- "Idiopathic" chest pain commonly is chronic. In long-term follow-up of these children and adolescents, severe diseases are not found.
- Patients with orthostatic-tachycardia syndrome complain of light-headed spells, headaches, and sensation of chest tightness with pounding and palpitations. These symptoms also may be seen in anxiety disorders. Both diagnoses need to be considered.
- In "slipping rib" syndrome, placing the examiner's fingers under the anterior rib margin of the 8th, 9th, or 10th ribs and pulling outward reproduces the sharp pain.
- Coxsackie virus can cause pleurodynia ("devil's grip"). This viral pleuritis presents with severe pleuritic chest pain, fever, and a pleural friction rub.

Suggested Readings

Cava JR, Sayger PL. Chest pain in children and adolescents. *Pediatr Clinic North Am* 2004;51:1553–1568.
Kocis KC. Chest pain in pediatrics. *Pediatr Clin North Am* 1999;46:189–203.
Robertson D. The epidemic of orthostatic tachycardia and orthostatic intolerance. *Am J Med Sci* 1999;317:75–77.

CHAPTER 20C ■ HEADACHE

TYRONE G. BRISTOL

Headache is a symptom commonly encountered in the child and adolescent population. Most headaches are mild and caretakers usually manage them at home with little or no assistance from a health care provider. According to Swaiman and Ashwal, the overall prevalence of headache increases quite strikingly from preschool age to adolescence. Headache prevalence by age 7 is 37% to 51%. At ages 7 to 15, it ranges from 57% to 82% (1). Headaches can be broadly classified as acute, chronic, and mixed; or alternatively, migrainous or non-migrainous. Migrainous headaches can be simple or complex with an aura. Non-migrainous headaches typically are due to stress and tension, or some other pathologic condition.

Children require hospitalization if their symptoms cannot be managed or if evaluation cannot be completed in the ambulatory setting. The consequences of a headache such as unmanageable pain, or nausea and vomiting with significant dehydration, may result in hospitalization for supportive care. Headaches associated with pathologic findings like increased intracranial pressure (ICP), meningismus, or neurologic deficits require the sophisticated medical resources of an inpatient setting where thorough assessment and management of potentially serious conditions can be completed.

DEFINITION

Headache generally refers to pain localized to areas above the neck including all parts of the cranium (intra- and extracranial) and upper neck muscles. Parents are often concerned that the headache is from malignant intracranial pathology or other significant organic processes. Fortunately, most headaches in children are benign, resolve with minimal treatment, and produce few sequelae. Although reassurance suffices for caretakers in most situations, the challenge for pediatric health care providers, especially those caring for the very young, preverbal child, is distinguishing benign headaches from the more ominous ones requiring hospitalization, in-depth evaluation, and complex management.

ETIOLOGY AND PATHOPHYSIOLOGY

The brain parenchyma and some of its supporting structures are insensitive to pain. However, via multiple mechanisms headaches can originate from many pain-sensitive structures in and around the cranium (Table 20.3). Externally, the facial, neck, and scalp muscles may cause pain from inflammation or prolonged contraction, (e.g., stress and tension). Trauma to bones, skin, and subcutaneous tissues of the face and skull cause localized headache. Headache may present due to referred pain from numerous structures including inflamed temporomandibular joints (TMJ), inflamed or infected mucous membranes and dental structures (gums and teeth), pharyngeal tissues (tonsils), ears (external auditory canal and middle ear), and paranasal sinuses. Idiopathic or psychogenic headaches have no obvious etiology despite a complete medical and psychological evaluation.

Intracranial inflammation and infection of meningeal tissue, increased ICP, and displacement or traction of the intracranial vessels and nerves from mass effect due to abscess, hemorrhage, hydrocephalus, and tumor are among the more serious pathologic causes of headaches. Vasospasm of intracranial arteries followed by vasodilation is reported in patients with migraine headaches, but the causal relationship

TABLE 20.3

PATHOPHYSIOLOGY

Increased ICP
Infection
Inflammation
Muscle contraction
Traction
Vasospasm

TABLE 20.4

ASSOCIATED SYMPTOMS

Aura	Mental status changes
Dental pain	Nausea
Emesis	Photophobia
Fatigue	Sinus pain
Fever	Somnolence
Irritability	Visual changes
Meningismus	Weight loss

between these vascular changes and the headaches continues to be debated. Although often attributed a causal role, refractive errors and strabismus do not usually cause headaches. With some eye disorders, pain in the globe may be noted and deserves evaluation, or frontal headache may occur after hours of close visual work. Pseudotumor cerebri is a more serious cause of headaches and may be associated with progressive visual loss.

CLINICAL PRESENTATION

A thorough history and physical examination is invaluable in determining the etiology of a headache. However, it may be more challenging in pediatrics due to the variable presentations (Table 20.4) in this age group and the inherent difficulty of gathering information, especially from the very young preverbal child or those with cognitive limitations. Patients may present with acute, chronic, and acute superimposed on chronic, diffuse, or localized headaches. They may be associated with an aura, photophobia, nausea, and vomiting. Concerning symptoms include focal or diffuse neurologic deficits, emesis during sleep or upon awakening, constitutional symptoms (fatigue, fever, lethargy, weight loss, somnolence), irritability, mental status changes, meningismus, and facial or paranasal sinus erythema, pain, and swelling. Headaches that awaken a child from sleep should also be considered a red flag for potentially serious diagnoses. Providers should suspect increased ICP if headaches are made worse by cough or Valsalva maneuvers. Dental diseases should be suspected if erythema, pain, and/or swelling are present around dental structures. Progressive visual loss and visual field defects raise the possibility of pseudotumor cerebri.

DIFFERENTIAL DIAGNOSIS

Pediatric practitioners are often faced with the difficult task of deciding which headaches are benign and require minimal intervention in the ambulatory setting versus the more malignant ones that require hospitalization, extensive evaluation, and more complex treatment. Fortunately, most of the diagnostic considerations for headaches in children are benign (Table 20.5) and beyond the scope of this text. The following discussion addresses the conditions that frequently require hospitalization.

Central nervous system (CNS) infections (abscess, encephalitis, meningitis) may present as a severe headache that requires urgent evaluation and treatment. Accompanying symptoms may include myalgias, dehydration, fatigue, fever, irritability, lethargy, nausea, rash, and/or vomiting. A history of ill contacts should be sought, and usually there is a negative history of trauma. Rather than meningismus, infants and young children

TABLE 20.5

DIFFERENTIAL DIAGNOSIS

Hemorrhage	Poor vision
Hypertension	Sinusitis
Infection	Stress/tension
Migraine	TMJ inflammation
Muscle strain	Trauma
Oral infections	Tumor
Pseudotumor cerebri	

TABLE 20.6

MIGRAINE VARIANTS

Abdominal	Benign paroxysmal vertigo
Acute confusional state	Cyclic vomiting
Alice-in-Wonderland	Hemiplegic
Basilar	Ophthalmoplegic
Benign paroxysmal torticollis	Retinal

more often present with nonspecific symptoms such as decreased oral intake, irritability or excessive somnolence. Meningeal signs (stiff neck, positive Brudzinski and Kernig signs) are commonly found in older children and teenagers. Patients may present with focal or generalized seizures and neurologic deficits. The presence of papilledema on examination suggests increased ICP (often associated with brain abscess) and may be a contraindication to lumbar puncture. In that setting, or if there are other signs and/or symptoms suggesting a mass lesion or increased intracranial pressure, computed tomography (CT) head imaging should be done. If there is no CT finding to provide a contraindication, prompt evaluation of cerebrospinal fluid (Gram stain, cell count, glucose and protein levels, culture or PCR for bacteria and virus) is appropriate. A complete blood count (CBC) may provide supporting evidence of infection, and a blood culture may later provide guidance for antibiotic therapy. Appropriate to the age and suspected disease process, broad-spectrum antibiotics against the most common pathogens should be initiated as soon as possible. Close observation in hospital with judicious fluid and electrolyte management, frequent vital signs, and serial exams, is necessary. Duration of treatment and prognosis depends on the pathogen isolated. Consultation with infectious disease colleagues is usually helpful in managing these patients.

Head trauma may result in significant headaches, either from concussive and postconcussive syndromes or the more alarming forms of CNS hemorrhage (subarachnoid, epidural, subdural, intraparenchymal). Although a history of trauma is usually present when causal, this is not the case when the CNS process is spontaneous such as stroke, rupture of an aneurysm, or hemorrhage from an arteriovenous malformation (AVM). Headache may initially be mild and localized but then progresses to severe and diffuse. When blood is in the subarachnoid space, the headache is usually accompanied by meningismus. Other signs and symptoms of a CNS mass lesion or increased ICP may be present. History and other signs of abuse and neglect should be sought if nonaccidental head trauma is suspected. CNS imaging should be conducted with haste and a LP may help confirm the diagnosis. Concussive syndromes are usually accompanied by negative imaging and supportive care is sufficient. CNS hemorrhage requires immediate consultation with pediatric intensive care and neurosurgical colleagues.

Migrainous headaches occur more frequently in children than previously suspected, and require a high index of suspicion when patients present to the emergency department or inpatient hospital setting. These are often chronic, nonprogressive, frontotemporal or unilateral headaches, which may have acute exacerbations due to triggers. Family history is usually positive, and if absent should suggest additional investigation. A history of motion sickness is very common in children with migraines. Triggers such as exercise, foods (chocolate, caffeine), menstruation, mild head trauma, and

stress are common. Migraines of the classic variety present more often in older adolescents. These unilateral throbbing headaches are often associated with motor, sensory, or visual aura, gastrointestinal (GI) symptoms, and photophobia. Patients will report that sleep relieves the headache. Younger children more frequently have "atypical" or common migraines. They are usually bilateral, steady, and lack the classic aura. These common migraines may also have GI symptoms, decreased oral intake, and irritability or malaise, leading to dehydration and hospitalization.

Migraine variants are common in young children and often difficult to recognize as such. Children with these variants may present with more complex signs and symptoms that obscure the associated headaches, and can even occur without a headache. These patients often have ED visits, and sometimes need hospitalization for further evaluation and management. Most of these migraine variants (Table 20.6) are considered diagnoses of exclusion in the pediatric population, requiring a search for other etiologies with assistance from appropriate subspecialists, often a neurologist. A few of these "complicated migraines" should be mentioned. *Basilar migraines* are headaches associated with cranial nerve dysfunction and ataxia, often leading to an extensive evaluation given the broad differential for this presentation. All of the neurologic symptoms usually resolve completely. *Hemiplegic and ophthalmoplegic migraines* present with unilateral neurologic deficits appropriate to those terms. Slow, complete resolution of symptoms is common. *Abdominal migraines* present with chronic, recurrent GI symptoms, including abdominal pain and persistent or cyclic vomiting. Photophobia is common and sleep relieves symptoms.

Brain tumor is a common concern of parents when their children develop headaches. In turn, health care providers often feel compelled to order imaging to "rule them out." Fortunately, malignancies are infrequently the cause of headaches and when they do occur, classic signs and symptoms suggestive of a CNS mass lesion accompany them. Negative family history of headaches and focal, progressive headaches awakening the child from sleep, or early morning headaches associated with nausea and vomiting, should prompt an investigation for brain tumor. There may be mental status changes and focal neurologic signs, especially suggestive of lesions in the posterior fossa, because these are very common in children. If initial CT is positive for mass lesion then magnetic resonance imaging (MRI) with contrast is indicated and consultation with a pediatric oncologist and neurosurgeon is warranted.

Pseudotumor cerebri should be suspected in patients presenting with acute or chronic headache associated with progressive visual loss, especially visual field deficits. Obesity is a risk factor for developing this disorder, and weight loss is an important part of management. Although the etiology is often idiopathic, a detailed history of medication use including lithium, tretinoin, tetracyclines, and endocrinopathies, should be taken. Excess ingestion of vitamin A and occlusion of CNS venous drainage are also possible etiologies. Visual acuity, visual field testing, and a thorough neurologic examination with special attention to the optic discs for papilledema should be done. CNS imaging is usually normal but should be performed prior to lumbar puncture. It is imperative to record opening pressure because an elevated pressure is diagnostic. Although this procedure can temporarily relieve symptoms, long-term management includes the use of acetazolamide, furosemide, weight loss if indicated, and consultation with a neurologist and ophthalmologist.

EVALUATION

The evaluation of headaches in the pediatric population should begin with a comprehensive history and physical examination (Table 20.7). The history should focus on when headaches were first noted, and the duration, location, and severity of symptoms. Situations, foods, medications, or other factors that exacerbate or relieve the headache should be elicited. Personal or family stressors, associated constitutional symptoms, and a family history of headache are also vital pieces of information helpful in solidifying a diagnosis. A history of dental or sinus symptoms and head trauma should be sought.

The physical examination of a pediatric headache patient should be complete, with special attention being paid to the following areas. Vital signs should include blood pressure, pulse, respiratory rate, temperature, and visual acuity. Palpation of the face, neck, and scalp for localized tenderness aids in the diagnosis of diseases related to these areas. An examination of the oral cavity for pharyngeal and dental abnormalities should be included. Fundoscopy and a test of visual fields should be performed. Special care should be taken to perform a complete neurologic examination, noting any mental status, motor, or sensory deficits.

The etiology of most headaches can be determined by a complete history and physical examination. Further diagnostic modalities (Table 20.8) should be guided by findings from the history and physical. An urgent CT scan is indicated for acute headaches associated with mental status changes, neurologic deficits, severe emesis, or trauma. It should also be done prior to lumbar puncture (LP) if increased intracranial pressure or mass lesion is suspected. Sinus disease causing severe headaches (more commonly facial pain) can also be diagnosed with CT. MRI of the brain is indicated to aid in the diagnosis of brain tumors or other intracranial pathology.

Lumbar puncture is needed if CNS infection, inflammation, or hemorrhage is suspected. Opening pressure should be recorded if pseudotumor cerebri is in the differential diagnosis. In this case, LP can be diagnostic and therapeutic. History and physical examination findings should guide the need for imaging and EEG. Blood chemistries, CBC, and blood culture are indicated to support the diagnosis of dehydration and infection if suspicion for these processes is high. Consultation

TABLE 20.8

EVALUATION

History
Vital signs
Visual acuity
Physical examination
CT/MRI
LP with opening pressure
Blood chemistries
Body fluid cultures
Consultants

with colleagues from Dental, Infectious Diseases, Neurology, and Ophthalmology may be necessary depending on symptomology and physical findings.

MANAGEMENT

Treating headaches (Table 20.9) and their complications in the hospital setting should focus on relief of symptoms and, if the etiology is unclear, further evaluation. Dehydration should be treated with the appropriate intravenous fluids until the patient is capable of tolerating oral fluids. Rarely, antiemetics are needed to control vomiting during an acute headache. Care should be taken because these medications can alter mental status and confuse subsequent neurologic examination. When fluids, rest, sleep, and removal of stressors do not control headache pain, the next element of management should be analgesics such as acetaminophen and nonsteroidal anti-inflammatory drugs (e.g., ibuprofen). Narcotics or other addictive drugs should be avoided during acute, severe headaches as much as possible.

Neurologic consultation is often necessary when patients are admitted to a hospital with complex headaches. Once an etiology for the headache is found, management should be focused on alleviating symptoms, treating the underlying cause, and preventing morbidity and mortality. The ultimate diagnosis will be migraines for most childhood headaches. Prompt treatment to relieve symptoms is imperative. Acutely, acetaminophen (15 mg/kg/dose every 4 to 6 hours) or ibuprofen (10 mg/kg/dose every 6 to 8 hours) should be administered. The triptans are now commonly used as abortive agents, especially in teenagers, but they have not been approved for use in young children. Sumatriptan has a rapid onset of action and short half-life. It can be administered by nasal, oral, or injection routes.

TABLE 20.7

HISTORY

Associated symptoms
Duration
Family history
Location
Severity
Triggers
What relieves
What worsens

TABLE 20.9

MANAGEMENT

Dehydration	Abortive/Analgesic Agents
■ IV/PO fluids	■ Acetaminophen
■ Correct electrolyte imbalance	■ Ibuprofen
	■ Triptans (IM, IN, PO)
Antiemetics	Prophylaxis
■ Promethazine	■ Amitriptyline/ nortriptyline
■ Prochlorperazine	■ Calcium channel blocker
■ Metoclopramide	■ Cyproheptadine
■ Diphenhydramine	■ Propanolol/atenolol
■ Ondansetron	■ Gabapentin/valproic acid/topiramate

Long-term treatment to prevent chronic migraine headaches should be accomplished first by avoiding triggers, then by using prophylactic medications. Cyproheptadine is very effective, especially in young children. Side effects include weight gain and somnolence. Other prophylactic options include beta-blockers, calcium channel blockers, tricyclic antidepressants, anticonvulsants, and acetazolamide (especially for perimenstrual headaches).

PROGNOSIS

The morbidity, mortality, and prognosis of headaches depend on their etiology. Non-migrainous headaches require prompt evaluation and management, and may require a team approach to care that includes appropriate subspecialists. Migrainous headaches have an excellent prognosis, especially in young children if rapidly recognized and optimally managed. Most outgrow their migraines. Aggressive treatment is necessary to prevent daily rebound headaches, especially in the adolescent age group. Avoidance of triggers and prophylactic use of medications is the best long-term therapy, but abortive treatment and supportive care in the hospital setting is sometimes necessary during acute exacerbations.

PEARLS

- A detailed history is usually the key element in the diagnosis of pediatric headache.
- A negative family history makes migraine headaches less likely.
- Neurologic deficits should prompt a search for serious pathology.
- Migraines are common but may present "atypically" in younger children.
- Avoid narcotics when treating acute headaches.

Suggested Readings

Fisher P. Help for headaches: a strategy for your busy practice. *Contemp Pediatr* 2005;22:34–41.
Fleisher G, Ludwig S, Henretig F (eds). *Textbook of pediatric emergency medicine.* 5th ed. Lippincott, Williams and Wilkins: Philadelphia; 2006:511–518.

Reference

1. Rother AD, Headaches. In: Swaiman KF, Ashwal S (eds). *Pediatric neurology: Principles and Practice.* 3rd ed. St. Louis, Mosby; 1999:747–758.

CHAPTER 20D ■ JOINT PAIN

KELLY M. WAICUS

A joint consists of a space encapsulated by synovial membrane and including articular cartilage. This articular capsule allows motion between two opposing bones. All joints are supported by soft tissues such as ligaments, tendons, and muscles. Trauma, infection, or inflammation to any of these structures leads to pain. *Arthralgia* refers to joint pain without associated erythema or swelling. When erythema and swelling are present, the joint has *arthritis*. This process may be acute, as in a septic joint infection, or chronic, as in juvenile idiopathic arthritis. Pain may also be referred to a joint from a pathologic process outside of the joint itself. Clinical evaluation involves astute clinical reasoning to differentiate the many causes of joint pain.

HISTORY

The history should include symptoms describing the pain including location, severity, duration, radiation, migration, and number of joints involved. Questions regarding timing of the pain may be helpful, such as whether the onset of pain was abrupt or gradual, intermittent versus persistent symptoms, and time of day when symptoms are worst. The pattern of pain may direct the evaluation. Inflammatory and rheumatologic conditions, such as juvenile idiopathic arthritis, are worse in the morning and at rest. The physician must ask about inciting injury, falls, or new/increased physical activity. Traumatic arthralgia or arthritis is made worse by exercise or prolonged use, as in overuse syndromes such as Little League elbow.

A thorough history should also include associated signs and symptoms. Inquiring about history of fever, periarticular redness, preceding viral or bacterial infection, pharyngitis, sexually transmitted disease (especially gonorrhea), skin infection, tick bite, rash, and recent immunizations or medications may prove particularly useful. Past medical history, family history, and a thorough review of systems should also be included.

The most common cause of joint pain in children is injury due to falls or sport-related activities. It is very important to differentiate these disorders from septic arthritis, which has the potential for rapid joint destruction if not treated appropriately, and from rheumatologic conditions, which may have other associated organ system involvement. The differential diagnosis of joint pain is reviewed in Table 20.10.

PHYSICAL EXAMINATION

A thorough physical exam including vital signs and height and weight percentiles is necessary. Poor growth may indicate the presence of chronic disease. The skin should be inspected for rashes, which may be seen in conditions such as acute rheumatic fever or other inflammatory diseases. The cardiac examination may reveal arrhythmia or murmur.

Examination of the involved joint should begin with observation of the child's spontaneous movements. Posture, gait, and use of the affected limb should be noted. The musculoskeletal examination should begin with the unaffected or lesser affected side. Both the affected and unaffected joints should be inspected for swelling, redness, and deformity.

TABLE 20.10

DIFFERENTIAL DIAGNOSIS OF JOINT PAIN

Inflammatory/Rheumatologic
    Juvenile idiopathic arthritis
    Acute rheumatic fever
    Lyme arthritis
    Postinfectious arthritis
        Streptococcal
        Rubella
        Hepatitis
        Parvovirus-B19
        Epstein-Barr virus
        Adenovirus
    Systemic lupus erythematosus
    Crohn disease
    Serum sickness
    Sarcoidosis
    Postdysenteric arthritis
        Shigella
        Salmonella
    Henoch–Schönlein purpura

Traumatic/Infectious/Nonrheumatologic
    Toxic synovitis
    Septic joint
    Osteomyelitis
    Leukemia
    Hemarthrosis
    Osteochondritis
    Hypermobility syndrome
    Overuse syndromes
    Ehlers–Danlos syndrome

Following observation, the examiner should proceed to palpating the affected ares for warmth, tenderness, and swelling. The dorsal surface of the examiner's fingers and hand may detect warmth more sensitively than the thicker palmar surfaces. Joint effusions may be ballotable, whereas swelling with a more doughy consistency may be a result of synovial thickening.

Finally, both active and passive range of motion should be evaluated. Weight bearing and motor strength may be helpful in assessing joint pain. Affected joints should be evaluated for both range of motion and strength. Severe pain may limit this portion of the exam. If there is a known history of trauma or obvious deformity, it is best to splint the extremity and obtain x-rays before manipulating the limb or joint. Once the painful joints are examined, all other joints should be evaluated for mobility and pain.

DIAGNOSTIC STUDIES

The history and physical examination should direct the laboratory evaluation. Any child suspected of having a septic joint requires urgent joint aspiration by a trained provider. Depending on the age of the patient and the joint involved, sedation or ultrasound guidance may be needed. Studies performed on aspirated synovial fluid should include cell count with differential, Gram stain, glucose, protein, and cultures (both aerobic and anaerobic). Polarized light microscopy is not usually indicated in children as acute crystal-induced arthritis (gout or pseudogout) does not usually affect this age group. Acid-fast staining for mycobacteria should be considered based on clinical presentation, especially in immunocompromised children. Blood cultures should also be obtained as septic joints usually result from hematogenous spread. Table 20.11 presents comparisons of joint fluid results.

Plain radiographs are most likely to be helpful when a single joint is involved. Joint radiographs can provide evidence of effusions and help diagnose fractures or chronic joint changes. Further radiologic studies such as CT scan or MRI are rarely needed in a child with joint pain. Bone scan may help differentiate septic arthritis from osteomyelitis when the clinical picture is unclear or when there is concern for bony involvement. Ultrasonography is a helpful technique for diagnostic evaluation of joints for effusions if the clinical examination is equivocal. This imaging modality may also be helpful for guidance in joint aspiration.

When joint pain exists in the absence of an obvious traumatic cause, blood work may be helpful. Recommended tests include complete blood count with differential, sedimentation rate, C-reactive protein, blood cultures, throat culture, and antistreptolysin-O titers. If the joint pain has been intermittent or chronic, Lyme titers, rheumatoid factor, ANA, and HLA-B27 typing should be considered.

Inflammatory joint effusions may be accompanied by an increase in serum acute-phase reactants. Erythrocyte sedimentation rate or C-reactive protein level can help evaluate systemic inflammation. The complete blood count may show an elevated white blood cell count (>15,000) if an infectious process is present or anemia in a chronic disease such as Crohn disease or systemic lupus erythematosus.

If acute rheumatic fever is suspected, recent streptococcal infection can be verified with throat culture and/or streptococcal serologies, including antistreptolysin-O or anti-DNase B titers. For juvenile idiopathic arthritis or postinflammatory

TABLE 20.11

JOINT FLUID INTERPRETATION

Etiology	Color/Clarity	WBC/mm^3	Percent PMNs
Normal	Clear/transparent	<200	<25
Noninflammatory	Yellow/transparent	200–2,000	<25
Traumatic effusions	Red/bloody	200–2,000	50–75 (fat globules indicate fracture)
Inflammatory effusions	Yellow/traslucent	2,000–10,000	>50
Septic effusions	Yellow to green/opaque	>100,000	>75 (Gram stain ± bacterial organisms)

PMNs, polymorphonuclear neutrophils.

arthritis, rheumatoid factor, antinuclear antibodies, Lyme serology, parvovirus B-19 serology, and complement levels (C3, C4, CH50) may be helpful.

MANAGEMENT

If the joint fluid studies are consistent with septic arthritis, antimicrobial therapy should be initiated immediately. Orthopedics should also be consulted immediately, as joint drainage may be necessary. For the hip and shoulder, this usually means open arthrotomy. There is controversy about open drainage in other joints versus repetitive needle aspiration. Factors to consider include the experience and opinion of the consulting orthopedic surgeon, age of the child, ease of aspiration, and viscosity of the infected joint fluid.

Bacterial etiologies of joint infections in children are most commonly *Staphylococcus aureus, Streptococcus pyogenes,* and *Streptococcus pneumoniae.* Empiric coverage pending culture results usually includes nafcillin or cefazolin. Vancomycin is added when β-lactam resistance is suspected, and ceftriaxone should be used when gonorrhea is likely (Chapter 86).

Supportive management of joint pain due to traumatic injuries such as sprains may be as simple as rest, ice, elevation, and nonsteroidal anti-inflammatory drugs (NSAIDs). Ibuprofen may be more effective than acetaminophen for joint pain. In general, aspirin should not be used in children younger than 16 years of age due to the associated risk of Reye syndrome. For acute rheumatic fever or juvenile idiopathic arthritis, aspirin remains a therapeutic option. This therapeutic decision will likely be determined by the pediatric rheumatologist involved.

Depending on the etiology of a child's joint pain, consultation with an orthopedic surgeon, sports medicine specialist, or rheumatologist may be indicated. For those rheumatologic conditions (e.g., juvenile idiopathic arthritis) associated with iritis, even if not clinically evident, ophthalmology consultation for slit-lamp examination is indicated due to the risk of progression to blindness if iritis is unrecognized or untreated (Chapter 69).

PEARLS

- If traumatic joint injury is present in the absence of an age-appropriate history, strongly consider child abuse in the differential diagnosis.
- Toxic synovitis (presumed viral etiology) of the hip is a common cause of acute or insidious unilateral hip pain without trauma, fever, or other findings of systemic disease. This is a diagnosis of exclusion, and resolves with bed rest.
- Legg–Calvé–Perthes disease is idiopathic ischemic necrosis of the proximal femoral epiphysis. Usually, this affects boys between 4 and 8 years of age, who present with limp and minimal/mild pain.
- Slipped capital femoral epiphysis is an idiopathic process occurring spontaneously in children (boys and African Americans more often affected) nearing skeletal maturity. Presentation is with limp, pain in the groin, thigh, or knee (referred), and the affected leg appears shortened and externally rotated.

Suggested Readings

Ansell BM. Rheumatic disease mimics in childhood. *Curr Opin Rheumatol* 2000;12:445–447.

Barness L. Extremities, joints, spine and muscles. In: Barness L (ed). *Manual of pediatric physical diagnosis* 6th ed. Chicago: Mosby-Year Book; 1991:139–156.

Denardo BA, Tucker LB, Miller LC, et al. Demography of a regional pediatric rheumatology patient population. *J Rheumatol* 1994;21:1553–1561.

CHAPTER 21 ■ PURPURA

ANNA GRATTAN FLIK

Purpura is the dermatologic lesion that results from the extravasation of red blood cells from the vasculature into the skin. Purpuric lesions are part of a spectrum of such lesions in a classification based on size: petechiae <2 mm, purpura 2 mm to 1 cm, and ecchymoses >1 cm. These lesions do not blanch with external pressure. Purpuric lesions are a manifestation of a hemostatic defect, either in platelets, plasma coagulation, or blood vessel integrity. Petechial lesions generally result from platelet disorders, ecchymosis from coagulation disorders, and palpable purpura from vascular abnormalities; however, overlap is common.

This section will focus on the approach to the older child (i.e., non-neonate) who presents with purpura per se, lesions between 2 mm and 1 cm. Although many of the etiologies for purpura are not serious, many are serious and potentially immediately life threatening. For this reason, any child presenting with purpura as part of the clinical illness deserves immediate and careful investigation.

ETIOLOGIES

As the etiologies for purpura are numerous and often representative of the underlying defect, it is useful to classify etiologies based on pathophysiology. See Tables 21.1 and 21.2.

INITIAL MANAGEMENT

As shown in Tables 21.1 and 21.2, purpura can be the result of many different disease processes ranging from relatively benign to life threatening. It is therefore important to approach the patient in a stepwise fashion, ruling in or out the most serious causes that may require immediate intervention.

Major considerations in the evaluations should include the following:

- Vital signs (temperature, blood pressure, pulse, capillary refill): Does the patient have signs of infection or sepsis? Such signs should cause consideration of meningococcemia or sepsis, with parenteral antibiotics initiated immediately.
- History: Is there any history of preceding illness, medication use, travel, exposure to animals, or ingestion of undercooked meat?
- Review of systems: Are any other organ system(s) affected?
- Physical exam: Are the purpuric lesions palpable? Are there signs suggesting viral/bacterial infection, malignancy, or hepatitis? Are other skin lesions also present? A thorough physical exam is essential in narrowing the differential diagnosis.
- Laboratory workup: Initial tests should include complete blood count with peripheral blood smear, liver function tests, electrolytes, blood urea nitrogen, creatinine, urinalysis, and erythrocyte sedimentation rate (ESR).
- Further tests: Consider skin biopsy. Consider further investigation for possible internal injuries if nonaccidental trauma remains a consideration.

Purpura is commonly seen both in the pediatric office and hospital settings. A framework by which to approach the child with purpura can lead to a swift and accurate diagnosis.

Suggested Readings

Drokt BA, Esterly NB. Purpura in infants and children. *J Am Acad Dermatol* 1997;37:673–705.

Behrman RE, Kliegman RM, Jenson HB, eds. *Nelson textbook of pediatrics.* 17th ed. Elsevier; 2004:826–827, 1670–1674.

Tunnessen W. *Signs and symptoms in pediatrics.* 3rd ed. Philadelphia: Lippincott Williams & Wilkins; Philadelphia 1999:790–801.

TABLE 21.1

ETIOLOGIES OF PURPURA IN CHILDREN

Platelet disorders	Vascular disorders	Coagulation disorders

THROMBOCYTOPENIAS
Decreased platelet production
 	
■ Neoplastic disorders (leukemia, lymphoma, neuroblastoma)
■ Aplastic anemia
■ Drugs (see Table 21.2)
■ AIDS
■ Fanconi anemia
 	
Increased platelet destruction
 	
■ Idiopathic thrombocytopenic purpura (ITP)
■ Systemic lupus erythematosis (SLE)
■ Hyperthyroidism
■ Acquired hemolytic anemia
■ Drugs (Table 21.2)
■ Disseminated intravascular coagulation (DIC)
   Sepsis
   Burns
   Severe trauma
   Snake and insect bites
■ Hemolytic uremic syndrome (HUS)
■ Wiskott–Aldrich syndrome
■ Sequestration
   Hypersplenism
   Sickle-cell anemia and other hemoglobinopathies
   Giant hemangioma
■ Glycogen storage diseases
 	
INFECTIONS (MAY CAUSE THROMBO-CYTOPENIA BY EITHER MECHANISM)
■ Viral
   Atypical measles
   Congenital rubella
   Cytomegalovirus (CMV)
   Enterovirus
   HIV
■ Bacterial
   Meningococcemia
   Gonococcemia
   Pneumococcal sepsis
   Haemophilus influenzae sepsis
   Pseudomonas aeruginosa sepsis
■ Rickettsial
   Rocky Mountain spotted fever
 	
THROMBOCYTOPATHIES
■ Drug-related
■ Uremia
■ Hereditary thrombocytopathies
	NORMAL VESSELS
	■ Mechanical causes:
	   Trauma
	     Accidental
	     Nonaccidental
	   Increased intravascular pressure
	     Cough
	     Vomiting
	     Straining
	   Suction (i.e., "hickey")
	   Factitious
	   Cupping, coin rubbing
	   Stasis
	
	VASCULITIS
	■ Drugs (see Table 21.2)
	■ Infection
	   Viral
	     Coxsackie A9, B3
	     Echoviruses 4,9
	     Atypical measles
	   Bacterial
	     Meningococcemia
	     Streptococcal pharyngitis
	     Septic emboli
	       SBE
	       Gonococcus
	   Rickettsial
	     Rocky Mountain spotted fever
	■ Immune-mediated
	   Henoch–Schönlein purpura
	   SLE
	   Wegener granulomatosis
	   Serum sickness
	   Other connective tissue disorders
	   Dysgammaglobulinemias
	
	INCREASED VASCULAR PERMEABILITY
	■ Scurvy
	■ Ehlers–Danlos syndrome
	■ Marfan syndrome
	■ Osteogenesis imperfecta
	■ Hereditary hemorrhagic telangiectasia
		■ von Willebrand disease
		■ Clotting factor deficiencies
		   Congenital
		     Hemophilias
		   Acquired
		     Acquired vitamin K deficiency
		       Cystic fibrosis
		       Diarrhea, chronic
		       Hepatitis
		       Biliary atresia
		       Celiac disease
		     Cyanotic congenital heart disease
		     Hepatorenal disease
		■ Protein C and S deficiencies
		■ Rat poison (warfarin) ingestion

TABLE 21.2

DRUGS THAT MAY CAUSE PURPURA IN CHILDREN

Mechanisms of drug-induced purpura may include vasculitis, abnormal platelet function, coagulopathies, or direct or immune-mediated thrombocytopenias.

ANALGESICS
- Aspirin
- Acetaminophen
- NSAIDs
- Codeine

ANTICONVULSANTS
- Barbiturates
- Carbamazepine
- Phenytoin
- Valproate

ANTI-INFLAMMATORY
- Corticosteroids

ANTICOAGULANTS
- Warfarin
- Heparin

CARDIOVASCULAR MEDICATION
- Digitalis
- Nitroglycerin
- Propranolol

DIURETICS
- Thiazides
- Furosemide
- Spironolactone

ANTIPSYCHOTICS/ANTIDEPRESSANTS
- Tricyclic antidepressants
- Phenothiazines

ANTIBIOTICS
- Penicillins
- Sulfonamides
- Nitrofurantoin
- Tetracyclines
- Erythromycin
- Cephalosporins
- Aminoglycosides

MISCELLANEOUS
- Chemotherapeutic agents
- Oral contraceptives
- Diphenhydramine
- Griseofulvin
- Dextroamphetamine
- Insulin
- Omeprazole

CHAPTER 22 ■ STRIDOR

PATRICIA V. LOWERY AND GERALD L. STROPE

Stridor, a respiratory noise of varying volume and pitch, is the result of increased velocity and turbulent air flow caused by partial laryngeal or tracheal obstruction. The word "stridor" is derived from the Latin *stridulus* meaning creaking, whistling, or grating. Stridor is most often somewhat musical, high-pitched, and monophonic and typically considered inspiratory. The degree of patient distress should dictate the approach to management of stridor of any cause, with priority given to the maintenance or emergent establishment of an airway for severe distress. Stridor is commonly mistaken as a wheeze.

When evaluating a patient with stridor, the clinician should note the phase of respiration in which stridor occurs. *Inspiratory stridor* is usually caused by extrathoracic obstruction in the supraglottic or glottic areas that produce inward collapse of loose structures as negative pressures are generated. Stridor occurring during *expiration* originates most often from obstruction below the level of the true vocal cords or below the thoracic inlet. *Biphasic stridor* usually suggests a severe fixed lesion at or below the level of the subglottic space. Depending on the location of the obstruction, stridor commonly varies with positioning of the patient, which may further assist with the differential diagnosis. Notably, stridor decreases when infants with laryngomalacia or anomalous artery compression of the airway are placed in the prone position. *Stertor*, or rattling, is due to obstruction of the structures in the supraglottic airway, that is, the nose, oral cavity, pharynx, and supraglottic larynx.

An appreciation of the anatomic and physiologic differences in the pediatric airway that underlie the pathophysiology of stridor is critical to thorough evaluation and management. Breathing should normally be effortless and quiet with air flowing from an area of greater to lesser pressure. On inspiration, the diaphragm, which plays a major role in the respiratory dynamics of infants and young children, descends, thereby creating an intrathoracic pressure that is less than atmospheric pressure such that air flows into the lungs. On expiration, the diaphragm relaxes and the elastic recoil of the lungs reverses this pressure gradient such that intrathoracic pressure is greater than atmospheric pressure and air flows out of the lungs. The small, funnel-shaped larynx of the infant is more anteriocephalad, lying at the level of C3-C4 and comprised of soft, elastic cartilage that is easily collapsed or compressed by abnormally altered airway pressures. The tongue, tonsils, and adenoids occupy a relatively larger portion of the oral cavity. The epiglottis is long, omega-shaped, and positioned close to the soft palate, thus rendering the young infant an obligate nose breather. The arytenoids are relatively large in proportion to the size of the larynx. The cricoid ring is the narrowest portion of the airway, averaging 3.5 to 5.0 mm in the full-term infant. According to Poiseuille's law, as the radius of the airway decreases by 1/2, the cross-sectional area decreases by 4-fold and the airway resistance increases by 16-fold assuming laminar airflow. Accordingly, a significant increase in resistance to airflow can occur with even a small decrease in the diameter of the infant airway.

Stridor thus results from increased velocity and turbulence of airflow caused by varying degrees of laryngeal or tracheal obstruction. Stridor is produced by narrowing or obstruction of the laryngeal opening or subglottic region with vibration of the soft tissues. The greater the airflow turbulence becomes, the worse the stridor, thus signifying a more significant obstruction. Dynamic compression of the trachea may occur because the tracheal rings of the infant and young child are more compliant. Further dynamic collapse of already compromised airways during expiration may produce an expiratory noise that can often be considered a monophonic wheeze.

When the clinical situation permits, the clinician should obtain a brief history seeking information regarding age, onset of symptoms, recent illnesses, associated fevers, ingestions, trauma, medications, cyanosis, allergies, previous airway manipulations, or pulmonary diseases. Observation of preferred posture, level of alertness and responsiveness, pattern of respirations, and presence of cyanosis should follow. Stridorous children should receive supplemental oxygen unless such intervention worsens agitation. In the setting of acute onset of stridor secondary to possible epiglottitis, definitive airway management should ensue with assembly of anesthesia, ENT, or pulmonary/critical care consultation. Bedside tracheotomy may be necessary if an attempt at endotracheal intubation is unsuccessful. If the presentation does not mandate emergent intervention, additional evaluation may include plain films of the neck and chest, fluoroscopy, barium swallow, bronchoscopy, MRI, and angiography when concern for vascular anomalies exists.

Conditions associated with stridor are generally classified as congenital or acquired (Table 22.1). They result from either intrinsic narrowing or extrinsic compression producing partial obstruction of the airway. These conditions can also be classified by the phase of respiration in which they occur.

INSPIRATORY STRIDOR

Congenital Conditions

The most common congenital cause of inspiratory stridor in infancy is *laryngomalacia*, caused by the prolapse of the aryepiglottic folds upon the glottis. The stridor has a somewhat high-pitched, fluttering quality, which may be appreciated from birth or during the first few weeks of life, worsens during the first 1 to 3 months on average, and usually resolves without intervention by 1 year of age. The stridorous sound may be transmitted throughout the chest on auscultation, but is best appreciated over the suprasternal notch/neck. Any stridor that does not improve over time, worsens, interferes with

131

TABLE 22.1

CAUSES OF STRIDOR

Congenital	Acquired
Laryngomalacia	Infections (e.g., epiglottitis)
Vocal cord paralysis	Trauma
Laryngeal webs	Foreign body
Laryngocele/saccular cysts	ingestion/aspiration
Laryngeal/tracheal clefts	Neoplasms
Tracheomalacia	Systemic disorders
Subglottic stenosis	Neurologic lesions
Trauma	Subglottic stenosis
Neurologic lesions/injury	Allergic
Metabolic disorders	
Vascular rings	
Tracheoesophageal fistulas	
Hemangiomas	
Craniofacial abnormalities	
Cystic hygroma	
Neoplasms	

feeding, or is complicated by obstructive sleep apnea should be referred to a pulmonologist or otolaryngologist for further evaluation. Approximately 10% to 15% of patients with severe laryngomalacia will have airway obstruction significant enough to result in tracheostomy or laser aryepiglottoplasty. The symptoms of laryngomalacia may be significantly worsened by co-existing gastroesophageal reflux disease (GERD).

Vocal cord paralysis (VCP), unilateral or bilateral, is the second most common cause of stridor in the infant. In the case of unilateral VCP, an adequate airway may exist unless the infant is agitated, which produces typical inspiratory stridor that does not change with positioning. Unilateral VCP occurs more often on the left side and may present several weeks after birth. In addition, the cry is somewhat breathy and weak. In comparison, the infant with bilateral VCP may have normal phonation/cry but, because the cords remain in the paramedian position, the airway obstruction may result in significant-enough stridor (sometimes biphasic) and distress during activity that a tracheostomy is necessary. Congenital central nervous system lesions or injuries, birth trauma, surgical injury, and cardiovascular anomalies are the most common causes of VCP. Infections and malignancies are also recognized causes. Iatrogenic causes include the administration of vincristine, surgical repair of cardiovascular and tracheoesophageal fistulas/atresias with secondary recurrent laryngeal nerve injury, and the placement of vagal nerve stimulators for treatment of medically refractory epilepsy. A genetic basis has also been suggested in bilateral VCP.

Papillomas of the vocal cords produce a croupy cough and stridor resulting from obstruction and perhaps altered vocal cord mobility. Optimally, fiber-optic visualization of the cords should occur without sedation to define the dynamics of movement.

Laryngotracheoesophageal cleft, although a rare cause of inspiratory stridor, must be considered during the evaluation because the associated recurrent aspiration can result in pneumonia and death. These infants have choking, coughing, and cyanosis in addition to stridor, often necessitating emergent airway management. Voice abnormalities are frequently noted. Gastrostomy feeding is often necessary pending definitive surgical correction or reconstruction. Clefts may be associated with other anomalies of the larynx, trachea, and esophagus such as congenital subglottic stenosis, esophageal atresias, and

tracheoesophageal fistulas. GERD and esophageal dysmotility disorders are also encountered.

Acquired Conditions

Acquired conditions that produce inspiratory stridor include infections, trauma (including iatrogenic causes, burns, and foreign body aspiration), systemic disorders, neurologic lesions, and neoplasms. As obstruction progresses with these conditions, expiratory stridor may also develop. Infectious considerations include *laryngotracheobronchitis (LTB)*, epiglottitis, retropharyngeal abscess, suppurative (bacterial) tracheitis, and diphtheria. LTB (croup), the most common infectious cause of stridor, presents with hoarseness, croupy or brassy cough, variable fever, and thin, often copious nasal secretions with progressive symptoms. Onset is usually gradual, most often in the winter in children 6 months to 3 years of age. In infants less than 6 months and children over 5 to 6 years of age, the diagnosis of LTB must be scrutinized. LTB is usually viral with parainfluenzae viruses, adenoviruses, and respiratory syncytial virus (RSV) most often the causative organisms, although a bacterial source may occasionally be seen (see below). LTB may also be of spasmodic (presumed allergic) origin; however, in these cases, there is usually little to no fever, no viral symptoms, and onset is sudden with rapid clearance of symptoms. Treatment of LTB includes humidification (with increasing evidence of lack of efficacy), assurance of good hydration, oxygen administration by hood or face mask, racemic epinephrine via nebulization, and steroids (dexamethasone 0.6 mg/kg). Cyanosis, progressive fatigue, and the use of racemic epinephrine at frequent intervals herald the need for intubation. The infant in moderate distress may warrant ICU observation and management.

Acute epiglottitis/supraglottitis (AE/S) occurs most typically in the 2- to 6-year-old with rapid onset of fever and typical signs of threatened airway obstruction (e.g., preferred sitting posture, open-mouthed with chin held forward in an effort to maintain airway patency, with drooling indicative of inability to handle secretions, muffled voice if any, extremely anxious, acutely ill/toxic). This constitutes a medical emergency where the only goal is rapid airway stabilization via brisk subspecialty consultation as noted above. No oral intake should be allowed. If the diagnosis is in question and the patient is stable, x-rays should be obtained only if a physician capable of definitive airway management accompanies the patient to radiology. When the diagnosis is considered, the more appropriate course of action is to proceed to the operating room or intensive care unit for direct visualization progressing to securing of the airway via endotracheal intubation or tracheotomy. AE/S occurs much less frequently since introduction of the Hib vaccine. Organisms associated with AE/S include *H. influenzae* type B and nontypable strains, *H. parainfluenzae*, *Streptococcus pneumoniae*, *Staphylococcus aureus*, and beta-hemolytic *Streptococcus* groups A, B, and C.

Retropharyngeal abscess occurs most commonly in children 2 to 4 years old. Symptoms relate to pressure and inflammation of the involved prevertebral/posterior pharyngeal space defined by fascia that fuses inferiorly at the level between T-1 and T-2. Thus, drooling, dysphagia, odynophagia, resistance to extension of the neck, and stridor are variably present. Swelling of one side of the posterior pharyngeal wall may be noted on visual inspection. Imaging with plain films is technically limited in young infants and children, as crying and swallowing may create problems with positioning and interpretation. CT, even with its own limitations, is the best imaging tool to identify abscesses and cellulitis in this space. Identification of complete rim enhancement indicates the presence of abscess. Antibiotic coverage should be directed at strep, staph, and oropharyngeal anaerobes. Surgical intervention is indicated when a large, hypodense area is discovered on CT or when the patient demonstrates poor response to a trial of antibiotic therapy.

Bacterial tracheitis is an infectious process that may present quite similarly to LTB and may complicate LTB. These children may initially have a clinical course compatible with LTB, but develop high fever, toxicity, and a leukocytosis. Soft-tissue x-rays of the trachea may demonstrate clouding due to the tenacious material in the airway. As this process progresses, bronchoscopy with removal of the thick secretions, and ventilatory support is often required. Broad-spectrum antibiotic coverage for staphlococcus, streptococcus, *Moraxella*, and *Haemophilus* is indicated.

BIPHASIC STRIDOR

Biphasic stridor indicates critical obstruction at any level or obstruction in the area below the glottis. Congenital laryngeal webs, subglottic hemangiomas, and congenital or acquired subglottic stenosis produce biphasic stridor.

Laryngeal webs, although quite uncommon, present with variable degrees of inspiratory stridor, recurrent croup, or high-degree obstruction with biphasic stridor. In the most severe cases, there is no stridor, because air movement is critically limited. Symptoms of laryngeal web are usually manifest at birth. Dysphonia is the most common presenting symptom followed by stridor. Thin webs may be excised or lasered endoscopically, while thick webs may require tracheostomy, multiple resections, and sometimes tracheal reconstruction.

Subglottic hemangiomas can manifest as hoarseness and stridor with potential for rapid progression to respiratory failure. Approximately 50% of these infants will have associated cutaneous hemangiomas. The symptoms are not usually present at birth but develop progressively over the following several weeks to months. The symptoms are notably worsened with crying as vascular engorgement increases the degree of obstruction. Initially stridor is inspiratory but with time becomes biphasic as the lesion enlarges. Of note, the clinical course is variable with periods of improvement or abatement of symptoms such that recurrent croup may be erroneously diagnosed. As many as 60% of infants with extensive hemangiomas involving the preauricular regions, chin, lower lip, and anterior neck (beard-like distribution) have symptomatic airway disease. The PHACE(S) syndrome consists of *p*osterior fossae malformations, *h*emangioma, *a*rterial anomalies, *c*oarctation of the aorta and other cardiac defects, *e*ye abnormalities, and occasionally *s*ternal defects. The hemangiomas are typically cervicofacial and plaque-like. These infants require close observation for respiratory distress. Tracheostomy and/or laser therapy are the most favorable treatment options for subglottic hemangiomas.

Subglottic stenosis may be congenital or acquired. The congenital form consists of two types. The more common type results from thickening of tissues in the subglottic area and/or of the true vocal cords, and presents with varying degrees of biphasic stridor—except in very mild cases when the stridor is largely inspiratory and noted only with physical activity or when worsened by URI. This type most often improves with growth of the larynx, and surgical intervention should be avoided if possible. Rarely, congenital subglottic stenosis results from a malformation of the cricoid cartilage. These infants manifest severe respiratory distress at birth and require tracheostomy. The timing of subsequent decannulation is determined by expectant airway growth.

EXPIRATORY STRIDOR

Expiratory stridor occurs with critical obstruction at any level or with conditions associated with narrowing of the intrathoracic portion of the trachea. The latter include complete tracheal rings, tracheomalacia (TM), tracheoesophageal fistulas (TEF), and vascular rings/slings. It is important to recognize that these abnormalities may coexist. *Tracheal rings* result from posterior fusion of the cartilage with absence of the membranous portion of the trachea involving a few rings or the entire trachea. *Tracheomalacia (TM)*, in contrast, results from poorly formed or weakened c-shaped tracheal rings, and occurs as a primary or secondary abnormality. Secondary TM is seen with localized areas of abnormal cartilage (e.g., TEF), in prolonged compression (e.g., vascular rings/slings), or in the premature infant who develops BPD. Diagnostic evaluation of these disorders begins with plain films of the chest and esophagram. Further anatomic definition may be achieved with CT, MRI, or bronchoscopy. Evaluation and definitive management of these disorders is optimized with pulmonary, cardiac, or surgical consultation at a tertiary care center.

PEARLS

- Any stridor that does not improve with time, recurs with uncertain explanation, interferes with feeding, or is biphasic warrants referral to a pediatric pulmonologist.
- The administration of corticosteroids for presumptive croup will temporarily shrink hemangiomas, further confusing the clinical picture.
- Bronchoscopy or advanced imaging (CT, MRI) are necessary for the definitive diagnosis of tracheomalacia.

Suggested Readings

Andrus JG, Shapshay SM. Contemporary management of laryngeal papilloma in adults and children. *Otolaryngol Clin North Am* 2006;39:135–158.

Boogaard R, Sjoerd HH, Pijnenburg MW, et al. Tracheomalacia and bronchomalacia in children: incidence and patient characteristics. *Chest* 2005; 128:3391–3397.

Carden KA, Boiselle PM, Waltz DA, et al. Tracheomalacia and tracheobronchomalacia in children and adults: an in-depth review. *Chest* 2005;127:984–1005.

Fitzgerald DA. The assessment and management of croup. *Paediatr Respir Rev* 2006;7:73–81.

Kaditis AG, Wald ER. Viral croup: current diagnosis and treatment. *Pediatr Infat Dis J* 1998;17:827–834.

Long FR. Imaging evolution of airway disorders in children. *Radiol Clin North Am* 2005;43:371–389.

Parikh, SR. Pediatric unilateral vocal fold immobility. *Otolaryngol Clin North Am* 2004;37:203–215.

Paul I. A young boy with stridor. *Pediatr Case Rev* 2003;3:141–149.

Rock MJ. Noisy breathing and stridor in infants. In: Dozor AJ, ed. *Primary pediatric pulmonogy*. Blackwell: A mes, Iowa; 2001:23–42.

Zuckerberg AL, Backofen JE, Othman NA, et al. Upper airway diseases. In: Rogers MC, Helfaer MA, eds. *Handbook of pediatric intensive care*. 3rd ed. Baltimore Williams & Wilkins; 1998:53–79.

CHAPTER 23 ■ VOMITING

PATRICIA V. LOWERY AND J. RAINER POLEY

Vomiting involves a complex sequence of events in response to noxious or adverse stimuli resulting in the retrograde expulsion of gastric contents. The delivery of messages from the gastrointestinal tract is mediated via neural afferents that are integrated in a series of nuclei such as the nucleus tractus solitarius, the reticular formation in the medulla, the area postrema at the dorsal end of the floor of the fourth ventricle, and a series of paraventricular nuclei. These nuclei also receive input from cardiorespiratory and neurohumoral centers that are recruited into the emetic response. It is doubtful that a single anatomic structure exists that represents a "vomiting center" to which all emetic impulses converge, and it is equally doubtful that a single structure exists from which all efferent impulses derive.

The differential diagnosis of vomiting in the infant, child, or adolescent may be extensive and merits a systems-based, methodical approach to assure identification of the occasional patient with a significant, potentially life-threatening diagnosis (Table 23.1). An age-related approach to diagnosis provides a reliable template for initial diagnostic considerations (Table 23.2). When faced with this very common presentation, the clinician should consider digestive versus nondigestive sources of vomiting including infectious diseases, central nervous system pathology, psychological etiologies, metabolic disorders (including varied delayed presentations of inborn errors of metabolism), renal disorders, ingestion of toxic agents, or adverse reactions to medications. The recognition of additional symptoms obtained via a detailed and focused history, physical findings, appropriately selected laboratory tests, and imaging studies (for selected indications) will guide the clinician in diagnosis.

Fundamentally, the presence of bile in the emesis suggests an obstruction distal to the second portion of the duodenum, demanding an aggressive evaluation; however, with nonobstructive conditions associated with persistent vomiting, reflux of duodenal contents into the stomach may result in bile-stained emesis. Bloody emesis warrants consideration of causes of gastrointestinal hemorrhage such as accidental or nonaccidental trauma, peptic or duodenal ulcer disease, caustic or foreign-body ingestion, or posterior nosebleeds. Children and adolescents with vomiting can usually be evaluated and managed as outpatients.

ETIOLOGIES OF VOMITING IN INFANTS

When confronted with vomiting in infants, the clinician must distinguish between different types of vomiting. First, vomiting due to gastroesophageal reflux is very common and is due to a constant or intermittent relaxation of the lower esophageal sphincter (LES). Emesis is not forceful or projectile. With increasing age and with assumption of a more upright position,

the frequency of emesis will gradually decrease. Treatment with medications is often not necessary, but may be useful in selected infants. Appropriate therapy may consist of the administration of either an H_2-receptor antagonist (e.g., ranitidine or cimetidine) or proton-pump inhibitor with or without a prokinetic agent such as metoclopramide or erythromycin ethyl succinate (EES).

Second, forceful emesis is often associated with nasal escape of gastric contents, causing parental concern. However, some emetic material escaping through the nose is simply because of ineffective closure of the velopalatial region, mainly owing to the rapid and forceful upward flow of gastric contents. It is of great interest that almost all infants with forceful emesis have hiccupped in utero during the middle to end of the third trimester. This hiccupping is mostly due to refluxed acidified gastric contents, which are retained in the stomach because of delayed gastric emptying, possibly due to antral dysmotility. After birth, these infants exhibit forceful vomiting, have very frequent hiccups, and are difficult to burp. In this situation, treatment with EES administered at a dose of 5 to 6 mg/kg/dose 4 times daily is usually quite helpful along with an H_2 blocker or a PPI such as lansoprazole at 1 mg/kg daily.

Third, projectile vomiting, gastric contents exiting from the mouth as if delivered by a garden hose without a nozzle, is almost always indicative of hypertrophic pyloric stenosis. Diagnosis is best made by ultrasonography. Non-emergent surgical intervention should follow initial therapy directed at the correction of fluid and electrolyte abnormalities.

Other diagnostic modalities for the evaluation of vomiting include an upper gastrointestinal contrast study or a nuclear gastric emptying/reflux scan. Aside from emesis due to the common situations of reflux or delayed gastric emptying, thought must be given to the possibility of various forms of intestinal obstruction such as malrotation, duodenal stenosis or atresia, and volvulus; all of these may be heralded by bilious emesis.

Fourth, vomiting accompanied by colicky abdominal pain suggests possible intussusception. The infant with intussusception may also present with mental status changes (usually some degree of obtundation) without gastrointestinal symptoms.

Finally, and very commonly, the vomiting infant who is thriving may be being overfed. Observation of the caretaker feeding the infant may reveal feeding, bonding, anatomic, or mechanical problems. An in-depth discussion of specific causes of vomiting seen in the newborn can be found in Chapter 109.

ETIOLOGIES OF VOMITING IN CHILDREN AND ADOLESCENTS

Vomiting in the child or adolescent is most often caused by *viral gastroenteritis*, which is most commonly due to infection with rotavirus. Other viruses such as astroviruses, enteric

TABLE 23.1

DIFFERENTIAL DIAGNOSIS OF EMESIS

Nonbilious
  Infectious
    Viral gastroenteritis
    Bacterial gastroenteritis
    Urinary tract infections
    Sepsis
    Meningitis
    Encephalitis
    Otitis media
    Pneumonia
    Hepatitis
    Streptococcal pharyngitis
    Pertussis
    Parasites
    Sinusitis
    Orbital cellulitis
    Labyrinthitis
    Helicobacter pylori infection
  Metabolic
    Inborn errors of metabolism
      Disorders of carbohydrate metabolism
        Galactosemia
        Hereditary fructose intolerance
      Peroxisomal disorders
      Fatty acid oxidation disorders
      Mitochondrial disorders
      Urea cycle defects
      Organic acidurias
      Aminoacidurias
      Mucopolysaccharidoses (communicating
        hydrocephalus)
    Adrenal insufficiency
    Adrenogenital syndromes
    Diabetic ketoacidosis
    Porphyrias
    Pheochromocytoma
    Renal tubular acidosis
    Hereditary angioedema
  Neurologic
    Hydrocephalus
    Intracranial bleeding
    Ventriculo-peritoneal/ventriculo-atrial shunt malfunction
    Kernicterus
    Migraine
    Space-occupying lesion
    Chiari malformation
    Pseudotumor cerebri
    Abdominal epilepsy
    Dysautonomias
  Gastrointestinal
    Obstructive
      Pyloric stenosis
      Proximal duodenal web/band
      Intussusception (early)
      Esophageal stricture
      Closed loop obstructions (internal hernia)
      Superior mesenteric artery syndrome
      Duodenal hematoma
      Adhesions/bands/vascular rings
      Annular pancreas
    Nonobstructive
      GERD (gastroesophageal reflux disease)
      Overfeeding
      Gastritis

  Peptic and duodenal ulcer
  Eosinophilic esophagitis
  Eosinophilic gastroenteritis
  Achalasia
  Esophageal dysmotility
  Cholelithiasis/cholecystitis
  Pancreatitis
  Inflammatory bowel disease
  Meckel diverticulum (with intussusception)
  Appendicitis
  Celiac disease (gluten-sensitive enteropathy)
  Hirschsprung disease
  Chronic intestinal pseudo-obstruction (myogenic and
    neurogenic)
  Constipation (severe)
  Gastroduodenal dysmotility disorders
Psychogenic
  Anxiety disorders
  Depression
  Secondary gain
  Rumination
  Münchausen or Münchausen-by-proxy
  Eating disorder (bulimia)
Urogenital
  Ureteropelvic junction (UPJ) obstruction
  Hydronephrosis
  Nephrolithiasis
  Pregnancy
  Pelvic inflammatory disease
  Hydrometrocolpos
  Ectopic pregnancy
  Endometriosis
Toxins/Medications
  Chemotherapy
  Food poisoning
    Bacterial toxins
    Solanine poisoning (green or sprouting potatoes)
    Scombroid poisoning
    Ciguatera fish poisoning
  Heavy metals (arsenic, mercury, lead, iron)
  Hydrocarbon ingestion
  Caustic ingestion
  Cholinergic poisoning (muscarinic and nicotinic)
    Organophosphates
    Carbamates
    Plants (mushrooms, tobacco)
    Black widow spider envenomation
    Nerve agents
  Acetaminophen (stage 1)
  Aspirin (gastric irritation)
  Ibuprofen
  Digoxin
  Theophylline
  Ethanol, methanol, ethylene glycol
  Calcium channel blockers
  Nerve agents
  Carbon monoxide
  Selective serotonin reuptake inhibitors (SSRIs;
    less common)
  Ipecac
Other
  Coughing
  Improper formula preparation
  Cow's milk or soy allergy

(continued)

TABLE 23.1

CONTINUED

Cyclic vomiting syndrome	Incarcerated inguinal hernia
Reye syndrome	Hirschsprung disease
Familial Mediterranean fever	Adhesions
Collagen vascular disorders	Necrotizing enterocolitis
Bilious	Appendicitis
Malrotation/volvulus	Duodenal hematoma
Intestinal atresia/stenosis	Ileus
Duplications	Biliary dyskinesia/sphincter of Oddi dysfunction
Choledocal cysts	Extrinsic mass lesion/compression
Intussusception	Annular pancreas

adenoviruses, caliciviruses, and noroviruses must be considered. Enteroviral infections are frequently associated with mild gastrointestinal symptoms, whereas emesis associated with CNS findings, lethargy, or a stiff neck should arouse suspicion of meningitis due to enterovirus. The diagnosis of viral gastroenteritis is often supported by seasonal and community prevalence information.

The empiric use of antiemetics in the outpatient management of the younger child should generally be avoided, as the literature does not support their use (or that of antidiarrheal agents). However, ondansetron (Zofran), a 5-hydroxy-tryptamine-3 antagonist used for chemotherapy-associated nausea, is now FDA approved for use in infants as young as 1 month of age. If a youngster fails attempted oral rehydration, hospitalization or a period of observation and therapy for dehydration may be necessary. Oral rehydration is very effective but is more labor intense for the caretaker and patient. However, it offers the advantage of safety and early progression to refeeding. The specific intravenous rehydration strategy is chosen based on degree and classification of dehydration after review of the serum electrolytes. Parenteral rehydration is necessary only for those children with severe dehydration, or those with moderate dehydration who do not tolerate attempts at oral rehydration. In the mildly to moderately dehydrated child, the AAP does not recommend routine electrolytes. Rather, in the child who presents with clinical findings of severe dehydration, altered mental status, or prolonged diarrhea with numerous stools,

the AAP recommends that electrolytes be obtained. Of note, bicarbonate levels have not been shown to correlate with the degree of dehydration.

Gastroesophageal reflux disease (GERD) results from the retrograde movement of gastric contents into the esophagus and is the most common cause of vomiting in children of all ages. An infant may present with a variety of problems related to GERD including apnea, stridor, and lower-airway disease accompanying choking, spitting, gagging, irritability, a pattern of frequent small feeds, or feeding aversion. In contrast, the preschool child is more likely to present with regurgitation, while the older child or adolescent may experience epigastric abdominal or substernal chest pain suggesting gastritis or esophagitis. GERD is known to potentially aggravate or perhaps cause asthma. Conversely, the increased respiratory effort of coughing and wheezing likely worsens GERD via intra-abdominal pressure–volume dynamics. GERD may be managed in most children with a trial of an H_2 blocker or PPI. For those children where the diagnosis remains uncertain, the 24-hour esophageal pH probe may be helpful in assessing the degree of GERD and/or adequacy of therapy in the patient not responding to treatment. Endoscopy with mucosal biopsy is performed to document the presence and severity of esophagitis or to establish an alternative diagnosis. Obesity, a national pediatric epidemic, also likely contributes to the development of GERD, although the underlying pathophysiology remains controversial.

TABLE 23.2

DIFFERENTIAL DIAGNOSIS OF EMESIS BY AGE AND RELATIVE INCIDENCE

Infant (0–12 mo)	Child (1–12 yr)	Adolescent (>12 yr)
GERD	Gastroenteritis	Gastroenteritis
Overfeeding	GERD	GERD
Gastroenteritis	Gastritis	Gastritis
GI obstruction	Systemic infection	Systemic infection
Systemic infection	Ingestion	Migraine
Increased ICP	GI obstruction	Medication
IEM	Celiac disease	Toxic ingestion
	Increased ICP	Pregnancy
	IBD	Celiac disease
		Acute abdomen (e.g., appendicitis)
		Eating disorders
		IBD
		Increased ICP

GERD, gastroesophageal reflux disease; GI, gastrointestinal; IBD, inflammatory bowel disease; ICP, intracranial pressure; IEM, inborn errors of metabolism.

Biliary colic may produce vomiting and abdominal pain in the older child or adolescent. *Diseases of the gallbladder* associated with vomiting include acute hydrops, acute acalculous cholecystitis, cholelithiasis, acute or chronic cholecystitis, and biliary dyskinesia. Conditions associated with cholelithiasis include prolonged parenteral nutrition, chronic liver disease, ileal resection, inflammatory bowel disease (Crohn disease), obesity, pregnancy, cystic fibrosis, treatment of childhood cancer, chronic hemolytic disease (e.g., sickle-cell anemia, the thalassemias, red blood cell enzyme abnormalities), and prolonged fasting or rapid weight reduction. The premature infant is particularly at risk for developing cholelithiasis after a complicated medical and surgical course in the neonatal intensive care unit. A plain film of the abdomen may reveal opaque calculi but cholesterol stones are radiolucent and will not be visualized. Therefore, ultrasound is the imaging method of choice for detection of gallstones or initial delineation of disease of the gallbladder. Patients with hemolytic disease are at risk for developing black-pigment cholelithiasis. In the pediatric population, obese adolescent females are most frequently affected with cholesterol stones. One theory of the development of cholesterol stones is the result of cholesterol in excess compared to the cholesterol-carrying capacity of bile micelles. This can result either from elevated bile levels of cholesterol and/or decreased levels of biliary amphiphiles (bile salts and phospholipids).

Hydrops of the gallbladder is defined as noncalculous, noninflammatory distention without accompanying bacterial infection or congenital anomalies of the biliary tree. Conditions associated with hydrops of the gallbladder include Kawasaki disease, streptococcal pharyngitis, staphylococcal infections, sickle cell crisis, typhoid fever, viral hepatitis, leptospirosis, sepsis, parasitic infections such as ascariasis and threadworm, and mesenteric adenitis. Other recognized conditions include Henoch–Schönlein purpura and necrotizing enterocolitis. Prolonged fasting and parenteral nutrition are also associated with hydrops of the gallbladder. Fever, vomiting, and jaundice may be typical findings. On ultrasound, there is appreciation of a distended, echo-free gallbladder without dilatation of the biliary tree.

Although uncommon, *biliary dyskinesia* or *sphincter of Oddi dysfunction (SOD)* or stenosis is hallmarked by intermittent biliary obstruction (which produces biliary pain even after cholecystectomy) or by abdominal pain secondary to pancreatitis. Hepatobiliary scintigraphy (HIDA) and fatty-meal ultrasonography may assist in predicting which patients will gain long-term benefit from sphincterotomy. However, the diagnosis of SOD is established most reliably via endoscopic retrograde cholangiopancreatography (ERCP). Gallbladder disease and SOD are also recognized in the etiology of pancreatitis in children and adolescents.

Acute pancreatitis is most often caused by trauma, viral illnesses, systemic diseases, congenital anomalies, biliary diseases, and genetic causes; in 25% of cases, the etiology remains unknown. Epigastric pain, vomiting, and fever are often accompanied by a quite uncomfortable patient assuming an antalgic position. The epigastric pain may radiate into the mid-back. The amylase and lipase levels are typically elevated, the former for only several days. The lipase level is more specific, as amylase may be increased in salivary gland pathology, systemic disease, and other intra-abdominal pathology (including biliary tract disease, appendicitis, obstruction, and perforation). Severe pancreatitis, infrequent in the pediatric population, is seen with the systemic inflammatory response syndrome (SIRS) with multiorgan failure. Prognostic systems such as the Ranson criteria and the APACHE-III(Acute Physiology and Chronic Health Evaluation) score should not be used in the pediatric patient. Ultrasonography, CT scan, ERCP, and magnetic resonance cholangiopancreatography (MRCP) are useful in the diagnosis and follow-up of the pediatric patient with suspected recurrent,

acute pancreatitis. Mutations of the CFTR (cystic fibrosis transmembrane regulator), SPINK 1 (serine protease inhibitor Kazal type-1), cationic trypsinogen (or R122) gene may underlie recurrent or chronic pancreatitis. Pancreatitis may also be caused by hypercalcemia and hyperlipidemia.

In addition, *eating disorders*, such as bulimia nervosa (BN), may present with pancreatitis. The *Diagnostic and Statistical Manual of Mental Disorders* (1994) provides the criteria for diagnosis of BN. Approximately 2% of female and 0.3% of male adolescents meet the criteria for either purging or nonpurging BN. Purging is achieved via self-induced or pharmacologically produced vomiting, enemas, and laxatives. Diuretic and diet pill abuse may also exist. Patients with BN may be of decreased, normal, or increased weight. It is estimated that as many as 30% of adolescents who are obese meet the definition of binge eating disorder (BED). Physical findings include tachycardia, bradycardia, and other dysrythmias; orthostatic blood pressure changes; erosion of dental enamel; irritation or calluses on the dorsum of the joints of fingers used to induce vomiting (Russell sign); enlargement of the parotid glands; and lanugo or hirsutism related to hyperandrogenism and polycystic ovary syndrome (PCOS). The proposed mechanism for the development of PCOS is via potentiation of the insulin response. Laboratory abnormalities often include a hypokalemic, hypochloremic metabolic alkalosis. Decreased magnesium, calcium, and phosphorus levels may be seen with cathartic abuse, and hepatic toxicity with ipecac abuse. Altered thyroid hormone levels are often found, and abnormal ECG findings including T-wave inversion or flattening, ST depression, supraventricular tachycardia, ventricular arrhythmias, and QT prolongation may be present and are usually related to the electrolyte problems described above. Peripheral edema in the absence of hypoproteinemia or CHF may be explained on the basis of SIADH (syndrome of inappropriate antidiuretic hormone). Menstrual irregularities, such as oligomenorrhea and amenorrhea, are common and render the patient at increased risk for osteopenia. Hospitalization may be required for these acute medical issues as well as for psychiatric intervention when deemed medically or psychiatrically necessary. However, outpatient management is preferred to avoid further stigmatization and expense.

Renal conditions that may produce vomiting and abdominal pain include urinary tract infections, nephrolithiasis, and UPJ (ureteropelvic junction) or other obstructions that may result in hydronephrosis. Flank pain and/or an associated abdominal mass are distinguishing features on physical exam. Acute and chronic renal failure may also produce vomiting. In the young child or infant, lower urinary tract infections typically produce vomiting usually accompanied by fever and often mistaken for gastroenteritis. Pyelonephritis typically produces vomiting with fever and flank pain, and the latter usually includes costovertebral angle tenderness on physical examination. Renal tubular acidosis may present later in infancy, childhood, or adolescence.

Cyclic vomiting syndrome (CVS), to a large degree, remains poorly understood. New concepts involving neuroendocrine pathways involving the gastrointestinal, nervous, and perhaps cardiovascular systems are emerging. Considered to be a migraine variant, no laboratory or radiographic marker exists to affirm this relationship. Recent evidence suggests that CVS, abdominal migraine, and migraine headaches may have autonomic dysfunction with a dominance of sympathetic tone over the parasympathetic cholinergic tone. There is a family history of migraines or syncope in the majority of these individuals. The cyclic vomiting pattern is one of a severe, recurring, discrete, episodic nature. Children may go weeks without emesis followed by periods of days of severe vomiting, often enough to result in dehydration requiring parenteral fluids. Symptoms are often more severe than with gastroenteritis, with which it is commonly mistaken. Other causes of emesis must be eliminated. Many of these patients will go on to develop typical migraines. Anti-migraine and anti-emetic therapy is reported as useful in these patients. Precipitating factors include psychological stress, illness, fatigue, sleep deprivation, diet, motion sickness, and menses. Knowledge of this disorder should avoid misdiagnosis as psychogenic in origin.

space-occupying lesions that produce increased intracranial pressure may otherwise be missed. Early morning or nocturnal vomiting is of particular concern.
- Hiccups occurring in utero are associated with forceful emesis in the infant, which often responds to a prokinetic agent other than metoclopramide.

PEARLS

- Celiac disease may present with unexplained vomiting, particularly when associated with type-1 diabetes mellitus.
- Recurrent vomiting not due to GERD may be caused by celiac disease, which has a 5% to 10% prevalence rate in Down syndrome and should be considered in the health supervision of these patients.
- Intracranial pathologies must be considered in the infant and child with vomiting because nonaccidental trauma or

Suggested Readings

Berhman RE, Kliegman RM, Jenson HB, eds. *Nelson textbook of pediatrics.* 17th ed. Philadelphia: Saunders; 2004.

Li BU, Misiewicz L. Cyclic vomiting syndrome: a brain-gut disorder. *Gastroenterol Clin North Am* 2003;32:997–1019.

MacDonald MG, Seshia MKM, Mullett MD, eds. Avery's neonatology, pathophysiology and management of the newborn. 6th ed. Philadelphia: Lippincott; 2005.

McCollough M, Sharieff GQ. Abdominal pain in children. *Pediatr Clin North Am* 2006;53:107–137.

CHAPTER 24 ■ WHEEZING

JESSICA R. NICHOLS AND KARIN M. HILLENBRAND

Wheezing is a high-pitched, continuous lung sound caused by turbulent airflow through narrowed airways. It results from obstruction of the airway at any level from the intrathoracic trachea to the bronchioles. Wheezing is primarily an expiratory sound because during expiration pleural pressure becomes more positive and results in increased collapse of the airways distal to the obstruction.

Wheezing is a common complaint for children of all ages, but it is particularly common in young children. Their risk is increased both by more compliant and easily collapsible airways, and because smaller-diameter airways are more easily obstructed by bronchospasm, mucosal edema, and secretions.

DIFFERENTIAL DIAGNOSIS

Asthma is the most common etiology for wheezing in childhood. The diagnosis of asthma might better be considered a syndrome with three distinct phenotypes than a specific disease entity. *Transient infant wheezers* have recurrent episodes of wheezing in the first 3 years of life but do not develop persistent asthma. *Nonatopic wheezers* develop airway dysfunction after a significant lower respiratory tract infection, and continue to wheeze after 3 years of age, though symptoms may lessen with age. *Atopic wheezers* have onset of wheezing occasionally before, or more commonly after, 3 years of age. They also typically manifest other symptoms of atopic disease, and often have a family history of asthma. Asthma is discussed in greater detail in Chapter 37.

Infection is also a common cause of wheezing at all ages. In infancy, bronchiolitis is the most common infectious illness with wheezing. Many viruses can cause bronchiolitis, including respiratory syncytial virus (RSV), parainfluenza, influenza, adenoviruses, and human metapneumovirus. In older children and adolescents, bronchitis is more likely to cause wheezing. Bronchitis is generally viral, although infection with atypical organisms such as *Mycoplasma pneumoniae* or *Chlamydia pneumoniae* must be considered as well. Pneumonia may present with wheezing, but is primarily an alveolar disease and more likely to present with rales than wheezing alone. Tuberculosis is an uncommon but reemerging cause of pulmonary disease in children and may also present as new-onset wheezing.

The differential diagnosis for wheezing is extensive (Table 24.1). An understanding of the many different causes can direct a reasonable approach to the evaluation and diagnosis of the wheezing child and to the initiation of appropriate treatment.

EVALUATION

History

Wheezing is most commonly a finding on physical examination and is frequently inaudible to parents. Parents who report hearing their child wheeze often mistake upper-airway congestion for true wheezing. Associated symptoms include cough that may be worsened by exercise, play, or at night; difficulty feeding; and limitation of normal activities. When medications have been tried in the past, the reported clinical response may help direct current therapy.

The age at onset may provide a clue to the etiology of wheezing. Wheezing since birth suggests an intrinsic airway anomaly like bronchomalacia. Wheezing in early infancy is also seen with cystic fibrosis and bronchopulmonary dysplasia, but is very uncommon in asthma. Foreign-body aspiration is suggested by the sudden onset of coughing and choking in a previously well toddler. Sudden onset may also be seen when wheezing is caused by hypersensitivity reactions; a detailed history of new exposures is needed to identify potential triggers.

Environmental irritants and allergens can precipitate wheezing in susceptible children. A history of exposure to environmental tobacco smoke, pet dander, cockroach antigen, molds, dusts, pollens, or chemical irritants should be investigated.

Additional historical clues that aid in diagnosis are found in Table 24.2.

Physical Examination

The physical examination of a wheezing child is important for determining the degree of distress, and may provide clues to the underlying diagnosis. Wheezing that is primarily expiratory is usually due to constriction of small airways, whereas biphasic wheezing can occur with narrowing of larger, central airways. Wheezing should be distinguished from stridor, which is a louder and harsher breath sound generally noted during inspiration and attributable to extrathoracic airway compression. Wheezing and stridor may occur concomitantly in conditions with extensive airway involvement such as laryngotracheobronchitis (croup) and tracheobronchomalacia. Wheezing associated with crackles suggests an interstitial component such as that found in infection, broncho-pulmonary dysplasia (BPD), or pulmonary edema with congestive heart failure.

Assessment of vital signs may provide clues both to the severity of illness and the underlying diagnosis. Fever suggests an infectious etiology. Tachypnea is common in wheezing patients; when severe, it can serve as an early warning of impending respiratory fatigue and failure. Persistent tachypnea is a sensitive indicator of pneumonia, and is also common with bronchiolitis and congestive heart failure. Pulse oximetry provides a noninvasive means of approximating oxygen saturation and may predict the need for hospitalization, but it can be inaccurate in children with cool extremities or poor perfusion.

The respiratory exam is clearly critical in the examination of wheezing children. There have been many attempts to develop a standardized score to assess the level of respiratory

TABLE 24.1

DIFFERENTIAL DIAGNOSIS OF WHEEZING IN CHILDREN

Common causes	Less common causes
Infancy	
Asthma	Cystic fibrosis
Virally mediated wheezing	Congenital vascular malformations
Bronchiolitis	Aberrant vessel
Aspiration: Gastroesophageal reflux disease (GERD)	Vascular ring
	Congenital lung malformations
Bronchopulmonary dysplasia (BPD)	Bronchogenic cyst
	Congenital lobar emphysema
	Bronchomalacia
	Congenital heart disease
	Congestive heart failure
	Cardiomegaly
	Aspiration: dysfunctional swallowing
Toddler/Child	
Asthma	Foreign body aspiration
Pneumonia/bronchitis	Hypersensitivity reactions
	Congenital heart disease
	Cystic fibrosis
	GERD
Adolescent	
Asthma	Mediastinal mass
Exercise-induced bronchospasm	Hypersensitivity reaction
Pneumonia/bronchitis	Drug use: tobacco, marijuana, inhalants
Vocal cord dysfunction	GERD
	Cystic fibrosis
	Cardiomegaly (with airway compression)
	Congenital heart disease
	Tuberculosis
Rare	
Immunodeficiency syndromes (including HIV)	Hemosiderosis
	Aspiration
Ciliary dyskinesia	Laryngeal cleft
Visceral larval migrans	Tracheoesophageal fistula: H-type (TEF)
Allergic bronchopulmonary aspergillosis	Pulmonary vasculitis/collagen vascular disease
Bronchial stenosis	
Alpha$_1$-antitrypsin deficiency	Fungal pulmonary infections

distress and direct management. These scores have been shown to correlate with length of hospital stay and can be followed to assess response to treatment. Although there is no currently agreed-upon scoring system, the following elements are commonly included: mental status, severity of wheezing, air entry, expiratory time, and overall work of breathing (including visible discomfort, retractions, accessory muscle use, and nasal flaring).

Evidence of increased work of breathing is generally assessed visually rather than through auscultation. Retractions, particularly intracostal, suprasternal, and subcostal, are frequently noted in children with wheezing. Nasal flaring is seen with worsening respiratory distress, as is the use of accessory muscles (e.g., sternocleidomastoid, abdominal muscles). Patients may also be obviously short of breath and have difficulty speaking normally. Decreased level of alertness or any altered mental status is a particularly concerning and often overlooked part of respiratory assessment. Decreased alertness may warn of worsening respiratory fatigue and potential hypercarbia.

Additional clues to specific diagnoses that can be found during the physical examination are included in Table 24.2.

Diagnostic Studies

Of the many diagnostic tools available, the routine use of chest radiography in the evaluation of a wheezing child has been one of the most controversial. Historically, routine chest radiographs have been recommended for all children wheezing for the first time. Evaluation of this practice in more recent years has shown that most wheezing children have normal radiographs, or have findings suggestive of asthma or bronchiolitis. Routine radiography exposes children to unnecessary radiation and adds significantly to cost, and findings rarely alter clinical management of these patients. Current data suggest that chest radiographs should be performed in a more select group of wheezing children. They should be considered in the following situations:

- Persistently asymmetric lung findings (decreased air movement, focal wheezing, crackles).
- Low oxygen saturation or PaO$_2$.
- History or examination findings that suggest an etiology other than bronchiolitis or asthma, such as lack of family history of atopy, lack of upper respiratory infection findings, and failure to respond to bronchodilators.

TABLE 24.2

CLUES TO DIAGNOSIS FROM THE HISTORY AND PHYSICAL EXAMINATION

Diagnosis	History	Physical examination
Asthma	Recurrent wheezing; viral or allergic trigger; family history of asthma or atopic disease	Atopic dermatitis; allergic rhinitis; increased anteroposterior (AP) chest diameter if severe
Bronchiolitis	Age <18 months; seasonal: fall and winter; fever, cough, congestion	Fever; rhinorrhea; nasal congestion; rales
Pneumonia/bronchitis	Fever; cough, often productive; history of neonatal conjunctivitis or maternal infection (*Chlamydia trachomatis*)	Fever; rales; tachypnea; conjunctivitis (*Chlamydia trachomatis*, adenovirus)
Gastroesophageal reflux disease	Feeding difficulties: choking, cough, emesis; irritability	Poor growth
Dysfunctional swallowing	Developmental disability; choking or cough during feeds	Neuromuscular weakness or spasticity; craniofacial abnormality
Foreign-body aspiration	Sudden-onset cough, choking; proximity of small food objects or toys	Persistent unilateral wheeze; localized decreased breath sounds; deviated trachea
Bronchopulmonary dysplasia	Prematurity; history of mechanical ventilation	Poor growth; rales
Congestive heart failure	Fatigue, especially with feeding	Poor growth; tachypnea; rales; displaced apical impulse; heart murmur; hepatomegaly
Cystic fibrosis	Chronic cough; positive family history; steatorrhea; recurrent sinopulmonary infection	Poor growth; nasal polyps; increased AP chest diameter; clubbing
Hypersensitivity	Sudden onset; exposure to food, drug, environmental trigger	Urticaria; angioedema
Mediastinal mass	Chest pain; progressively worsening cough; recurrent fever; malaise; weight loss; night sweats	Adenopathy; hepatosplenomegaly; pallor
Tuberculosis	Travel or other exposure risks; weight loss; recurrent fever	Adenopathy
Vascular malformation	Feeding difficulty; symptoms may increase with agitation	Poor growth; stridor
Immunodeficiency	Onset in infancy; serious infections; recurrent sinopulmonary disease (ciliary dyskinesia)	Poor growth; sinus, ear disease

Studies suggest that significant fever or tachypnea are also associated with an increased incidence of abnormal chest x-rays.

Suspected foreign bodies pose unique diagnostic challenges. Many aspirated foreign bodies are not radiopaque and may be easily missed on plain radiography. Atelectasis or localized air trapping may be subtle clues, but are frequently absent. Paired inspiratory and expiratory views may reveal asymmetric emptying of a lung segment, asymmetric diaphragm movements, or shift of the mediastinum away from the affected bronchus during expiration, but these images can be very difficult to obtain in young children. Fluoroscopy requires less patient cooperation and more consistently reveals clues to the presence of a foreign body.

Although pulse oximetry has largely replaced blood gas analysis for assessment of oxygenation, it does not provide information about ventilation. Blood gas analysis is necessary to assess for hypoventilation or inadequate gas exchange in patients with severe distress. Careful attention should be given to the PCO_2 measurement in a tachypneic child: a "normal" or rising value in this setting may portend impending respiratory failure.

Spirometric measurement of lung function is helpful to document the presence of obstruction and to assess the response to treatment. An increase in airway hyperreactivity during a methacholine challenge and improvement with bronchodilator therapy may be clues to asthma as the etiology of wheezing. Additional studies that might be useful for specific diagnoses are outlined in Table 24.3.

TREATMENT

Treatment of wheezing is directed primarily at the underlying disease process. In some cases, definitive therapy may be available. Examples include removal of foreign bodies, surgical repair of anomalous vasculature and other anatomic anomalies, and antimicrobial treatment targeted at specific infectious etiologies such as *Chlamydia* or tuberculosis. Therapeutic options exist for symptomatic relief of disorders for which no definitive treatment is available, such as asthma and bronchiolitis. Specific management recommendations for these disorders are provided in Chapters 37 and 78.

With any patient in acute distress, the first priority is stabilization of cardiorespiratory status. An initial focused history and physical can be performed while simultaneously initiating measures to maintain the airway and alleviate acute respiratory compromise. This is often accomplished by allowing an alert child to assume a position of comfort, and assisting with clearance of secretions, particularly in infants.

TABLE 24.3

DIAGNOSTIC TOOLS FOR THE WHEEZING CHILD

Diagnosis	Studies to consider
Asthma	Total eosinophil count; serum IgE; skin prick tests for allergen triggers
Bronchiolitis	Nasopharyngeal washing for viral culture, rapid antigen detection, PCR
GERD; dysfunctional swallow	pH probe; videofluoroscopic swallow study; endoscopy
Foreign-body aspiration	Fluoroscopy, bronchoscopy (may be therapeutic as well as diagnostic)
Cystic fibrosis	Sweat chloride analysis
Vascular malformation	Barium esophagram; bronchoscopy; MRI
Cardiac abnormalities	Echocardiography
Mediastinal mass	Chest radiograph; CT, MRI
Tracheoesophageal fistula	Barium esophagram; bronchoscopy; endoscopy
Immunodeficiency	Complete blood count; serum immunoglobulin levels; CH50 level; HIV test

CT, computed tomography; GERD, gastroesophageal reflux disease; HIV, human immunodeficiency virus; MRI, magnetic resonance imaging; PCR, polymerase chain reaction.

Providing humidified *supplemental oxygen* is beneficial for most wheezing children who require hospitalization, even if pulse oximetry is normal. Humidification decreases the risk of ongoing airway obstruction by dried secretions. It is important to work with the child and her parent to find the means of oxygen delivery that will be most comfortable and most easily tolerated. Many children are upset or anxious when forced to wear a face-mask; in turn, this anxiety causes increased respiratory distress and oxygen consumption. Oxygen delivery may be more successful with the parent holding the oxygen tubing or mask to blow near the patient's face, or by using a less constrictive method, like a face tent or hood.

Heliox is a mixture of inhaled helium and oxygen, which provides a lower-density oxygen source. This can be useful in patients with many causes of wheezing as it allows oxygen delivery despite elevated airway resistance and can decrease the work of breathing. Heliox is not universally available or considered first-line therapy, but can be useful in patients with severe symptoms who are difficult to oxygenate by traditional means. However, the percent of oxygen that can be delivered is limited, so heliox cannot be used if hypoxia is severe.

Beta-adrenergic agonists are very effective bronchodilators and are considered first-line therapy in most cases of acute wheezing. Use of these agents can provide both symptomatic relief and clues to the potential etiology of wheezing, because bronchodilators provide minimal relief in a patient with a fixed obstruction such as an airway foreign body or extrinsic compression. If the patient improves after administration of an inhaled beta-agonist, medication administration may be repeated every 20 to 30 minutes as needed.

Nebulized epinephrine has also been used in patients with acute wheezing, particularly children with bronchiolitis. Epinephrine is an alpha-adrenergic agent and potent vasoconstrictor that reduces airway edema and mucous production. For patients with suspected cardiac disease as an etiology for wheezing, both groups of inhaled bronchodilators should be avoided until the patient is further evaluated.

Parenteral alpha- and beta-adrenergic agents, including subcutaneous epinephrine or terbutaline, are primarily indicated for wheezing associated with a systemic allergic reaction, but not for other causes of wheezing.

Beta-agonist medications for wheezing are usually administered via a metered-dose inhaler (MDI) with a valved holding chamber (spacer) or via nebulization. Studies have demonstrated equal or superior efficacy, as well as decreased time of administration, with metered-dose inhalation. When a nebulizer is used for infants or young children, a face-mask is necessary to assure adequate delivery of medication. The efficacy of treatment is greatly reduced if the mask or tubing is held passively in front of the patient's face.

In patients with suspected bronchiolitis, the use of bronchodilators is controversial. Although some patients clearly improve with inhaled albuterol or epinephrine, clinical trials have not shown a statistically significant difference in symptoms or outcome with these therapies. It is reasonable to attempt treatment with either or both of these inhaled bronchodilators and assess for clinical improvement by examining the patient immediately before and after the therapy is administered. Inhaled bronchodilator medications should not be continued in those patients who fail to respond to an initial trial.

There is extensive data supporting the use of systemic steroids in the treatment of acute asthma exacerbations. The use of corticosteroids with other causes of acute wheezing is less beneficial. In particular, the use of systemic steroids in bronchiolitis remains controversial.

PEARLS

- Although the differential diagnosis for wheezing is extensive, asthma is the most common cause of wheezing throughout childhood. Infections are also commonly found in the wheezing child but are most typically viral and do not require antibiotic therapy.
- Wheezing may be a sign of significant respiratory distress. A careful assessment for other signs of distress, as well as frequent reassessment is essential.
- Treatment with a bronchodilator is an appropriate initial intervention for the wheezing child regardless of etiology. For children who do not respond to this initial trial, bronchodilators should not be continued.

Suggested Readings

Hillenbrand KH, Perkin RM. Wheezing in children younger than 3: differential diagnosis and initial approach to management. *Emerg Med Rep* 2003;8:83–97.

Pope JS, Koenig SM. Pulmonary disorders in the training room. *Clin Sports Med* 2005;24:541–564.

Taussig LM, Wright AL, Holberg CJ, et al. Tucson children's respiratory study: 1980 to present. *J Allergy Clin Immunol* 2003;111:661–675.

CHAPTER 25 ■ JAUNDICE

KATHLEEN VINCENT PREVILL AND JUDY W. WOOD

Other than physiologic jaundice of the newborn, jaundice in an infant or child is always abnormal and caused by a variety of disorders resulting from liver dysfunction. Jaundice is observed in the sclera at a serum bilirubin level above 1.5 to 3 mg/dL, and is visible in skin color beginning at approximately 5 to 6 mg/dL. When jaundice is observed, the clinician must proceed with an evaluation. This clinical evaluation should focus on four main categories of liver and biliary tract problems:

■ Obstructive jaundice
■ Infectious hepatitis
■ Drug-induced jaundice
■ Metabolic/genetic liver disorders

The evaluation also includes the basic elements of a careful history and physical examination. Infants and children with jaundice may have abdominal pain, lethargy, fever, nausea, vomiting, or weight loss. A history of medication use and dosage must be taken. It is helpful to know if the urine color is dark or the stools light. Changes in mental status may suggest serious hepatic derangement. The family history should be reviewed for liver disease or consanguinity.

On physical examination, the liver is palpated for size, texture, and tenderness, and percussed for liver span. A careful inspection of the infant or child should be performed for dysmorphologic features. The abdomen is evaluated for ascites, or increased venous markings suggesting portal hypertension. In addition to the degree of cutaneous jaundice, the skin should be inspected carefully for xanthomata that can be associated with some genetic causes of icterus.

DIFFERENTIAL DIAGNOSIS

Obstructive Jaundice

Biliary Atresia

The most common cause of obstructive jaundice in infants beyond 2 weeks of age is biliary atresia. Of unknown cause, it results from complete obliteration or discontinuation of the hepatic or common bile duct. Early and accurate diagnosis of biliary atresia is critical because the prognosis rests on performing surgical correction (portoenterostomy; Kasai procedure) before 3 months of age. Because the clinical presentation of neonatal hepatitis and biliary atresia is similar, they must be differentiated by screening tests for hepatitis and ultrasound examination of the liver. The ultrasound is extremely useful if a "triangular cord sign" is seen, for this predicts biliary atresia well. When biliary atresia seems likely, an intraoperative cholangiogram is appropriate to rule out choledochal cysts or cystic dilatation of the intra- or extrahepatic bile ducts. A percutaneous liver biopsy may also be indicated.

Cholelithiasis

Though uncommon in children, gallstones usually can be detected by ultrasound. Cholelithiasis is associated with prolonged total parental nutrition, cystic fibrosis, hemolytic disorders such as sickle-cell anemia, obesity, and after ileal resection.

Hepatic Masses

Approximately 5% of abdominal masses in children are found in the liver. These may be either primary malignances of the liver, metastatic malignancy (usually Wilms tumor or neuroblastoma), or benign lesions. At presentation, all may be associated with jaundice in addition to a palpable abdominal mass, pain, hepatomegaly, and abnormal liver enzymes.

Between 0.5% and 2% of pediatric malignancies are primary hepatic neoplasms. The most common is hepatoblastoma, which classically (>90% of patients) presents before age 3 with painless liver mass and elevated alpha-fetoprotein. Children with genetic conditions such as hemihypertrophy, Beckwith–Wiedemann syndrome, biliary atresia, and Wilms tumor are predisposed to develop hepatoblastoma.

Hepatocellular carcinoma, the second-most common primary pediatric liver malignancy, peaks at 12 to 14 years of age. Serum alpha-fetoprotein will be elevated in more than 80% of cases. Half of these cases are associated with preexisting liver disorders such as hepatitis B, alpha-1-antitrypsin deficiency, or a glycogen storage disease.

Infantile hemangioendothelioma is a benign cause of a palpable hepatic mass. The classical presentation is an infant less than 6 months of age with an abdominal mass and high-output cardiac failure. Half of these patients have an associated cutaneous hemangioma, and 3% have an elevated alpha-fetoprotein level.

Infectious Hepatitis

Infectious hepatitis is the first concern for the older child with jaundice (see Chapter 55). Hepatitis A, an RNA virus, is the most common cause, and is associated with fever, nausea, and fatigue. The child younger than 6 years may not experience jaundice and is the prime carrier of this disease in the population. Hepatitis A is spread by the fecal–oral route, is rarely associated with fulminant hepatic failure, and is not associated with chronic hepatitis. Vaccine prevention is recommended.

Hepatitis B, a DNA virus, is spread by sexual contact, IV drug abuse, or vertical transmission at birth. This infection may be asymptomatic, but can result in chronic hepatitis and hepatic carcinoma. Vaccine prevention is highly effective.

Hepatitis C is caused by an RNA flavivirus and now is the major cause of post-transfusion hepatitis. There are serologic antibody tests and a polymerase chain reaction test to prove hepatitis C virus infection. Infants may acquire hepatitis C by vertical transmission.

Hepatitis D may occur as a co-infection with hepatitis B and, when present, may lead to fulminant hepatitis.

Hepatitis E is found in Southeast and Central Asia, the Middle East, Africa, and Mexico. It is spread by the fecal–oral route and contaminated water. It frequently causes fulminant hepatitis.

Hepatitis G is transmitted by blood transfusion and sexual contact. It does not cause significant disease and is considered harmless.

Other viral causes of hepatitis include cytomegalovirus, Epstein–Barr, herpes simplex, HIV, and enteroviruses. Lymphoproliferative hepatic disease and fungal inflammatory liver masses may occur in the immunosuppressed patient. *Bartonella henselae* is the cause of an inflammatory liver mass in about 10% of patients with cat-scratch disease.

Drug-Induced Jaundice

Drugs may displace bilirubin from albumin-binding sites or create toxic metabolites injurious to the hepatocyte. The liver is the main metabolic site for drug detoxification, and those metabolites are sometimes toxic, as in acetaminophen poisoning. Children on chronic anticonvulsants, antibiotics, antineoplastic medications, or exposure to environmental toxins are susceptible to drug-induced jaundice. See Table 25.1.

TABLE 25.1

DRUGS CAUSING JAUNDICE

ANTIMICROBIALS
- Amoxicillin-clavulanic acid
- Erythromycin
- Sulfonamides
- Minocycline
- Isoniazid
- Ketoconazole
- Griseofulvin

ANTICONVULSANTS
- Valproic acid
- Phenytoin
- Phenobarbital
- Carbamazepine

ANESTHETICS
- Halothane

ANALGESICS
- Acetaminophen
- Aspirin

ANTINEOPLASTICS
- Methotrexate and most chemotherapy drugs

ANTIRETROVIRALS
- Nucleoside reverse transcriptase inhibitors

OTHERS
- Oral contraceptives
- Alcohol
- Herbicides/insecticides/organophosphates

Metabolic/Genetic Liver Disorders

Inherited liver disorders associated with jaundice are better understood by breaking them into unconjugated and conjugated categories.

Unconjugated Hyperbilirubinemia of Genetic Origin

Red-cell membrane disorders trigger hemolysis in the reticular endothelial system and the increased heme byproduct is not adequately conjugated and cleared in the liver. Although more common in the newborn period (see Chapter 108), there are several RBC membrane disorders and hemoglobinopathies that result in increased unconjugated bilirubin in older infants and children. These include sickle-cell disease, thalassemia, pyruvate kinase deficiency, spherocytosis, and G-6PD deficiency.

Other genetic based causes of unconjugated hyperbilirubinemia exist in those children who have extreme deficiency or absence of uridine diphosphate glucuronosyltransferase. These syndromes include Crigler–Najjar types 1 and 2, which result in severe neurotoxicity if not recognized and treated. A benign form of reduced glucuronosyltransferase is expressed in Gilbert syndrome, which is present in 5% to 8% of the population and is not associated with long-term disease.

Conjugated Hyperbilirubinemia of Genetic Origin

The primary examples in this category include Alagille syndrome, Wilson disease, alpha-1-antitrypsin disorder, cystic fibrosis, and autoimmune hepatitis. Rare causes include progressive familial intrahepatic cholestasis, Rotor syndrome, and Dubin–Johnson syndrome.

Alagille syndrome is an autosomal dominant disorder presenting with jaundice because of a paucity of interlobular bile ducts. Children have triangular facies, congenital heart defects, vertebral anomalies, short stature, and eye defects. There is a molecular genetic marker in the *JAGGED*-1 gene.

In Wilson disease there may be a conjugated hyperbilirubinemia early in the disease with neurologic symptoms developing later that may include tremor, dysarthria, or psychiatric symptoms. Once neurologic symptoms are present, the diagnostic finding of Kayser–Fleischer rings may be seen with slit-lamp examination of the cornea. Wilson disease is caused by a deficiency of ceruloplasmin that results in excessive toxic accumulation of copper in the liver, kidneys, and central nervous system. Copper excess in the liver causes an oxidative insult to the liver mitochondria.

Patients who are homozygous for alpha-1-antitrypsin (a protease inhibitor) deficiency develop liver disease that manifests as conjugated hyperbilirubinemia. They may progress to cirrhosis and portal hypertension.

Although patients with cystic fibrosis may develop cholestatic jaundice, their clinical presentation is recognized earlier because of the associated gastrointestinal and/or pulmonary disease. Approximately 25% to 65% of patients with cystic fibrosis develop liver dysfunction including cholestasis and cholelithiasis. They may progress to cirrhosis.

Autoimmune hepatitis is described as an immune-mediated chronic inflammatory condition of the liver. This process destroys hepatic parenchyma if not recognized and treated with immune suppression. A dysfunctional autoimmune regulator gene is responsible for two types of autoimmune hepatitis. The clinical presentation is of noninfectious hepatitis with increased IgG levels. Serologic tests are positive for smooth muscle antibody (SMA) and antinuclear antibody (ANA) in type 1, and liver-kidney microsomal antibody (LKM1) in type 2.

A rare cause of cholestatic jaundice is progressive familial intrahepatic cholestasis. This is related to defects in bile acid transport across the canalicular membrane. Many variants of this hereditary problem have been identified.

EVALUATION

Laboratory evaluation of the jaundiced infant or child begins with measurement of conjugated and unconjugated bilirubin. The normal total serum bilirubin rarely exceeds 1.2 mg/dL, and the conjugated form should be <30% of the total. Liver enzymes should be determined and include alanine aminotransferase (ALT), γ-glutamyl transpeptidase (GGT), and aspartate aminotransferase (AST). An elevated GGT level is more specific for cholestatic disorders and an elevated ALT is most specific for hepatocellular dysfunction. Additional laboratory measurements needed include alkaline phosphatase, prothrombin time (PT), partial thromboplastin time (PTT), glucose, ammonia, albumin, and alpha-fetoprotein level.

All patients suspected of having obstructive jaundice deserve an ultrasound of the liver and spleen early in the workup. Liver biopsy may be indicated.

Specific serologies for various viral hepatitis etiologies are performed when indicated. For indirect hyperbilirubinemia one must consider Coombs positive hemolytic conditions and red blood cell membrane disorders. Review of peripheral blood smears with the pathologist or hematologist should be considered part of the evaluation. Hemoglobin electrophoresis may be indicated.

Wilson disease, alpha-1-antitrypsin deficiency, autoimmune hepatitis, and cystic fibrosis have specific tests for diagnosis. When Wilson disease is suspected, a 24-hour urinary copper excretion, urinary amino acid screen, serum ceruloplasmin, and serum copper level should be measured. Ceruloplasmin levels below 20 mg/dL are typical of Wilson disease.

MANAGEMENT

Management is supportive with hydration and close surveillance of hepatic function until the specific cause of jaundice is diagnosed. Signs of hepatic failure (see Chapter 56), especially hypoglycemia, prolonged PT, and encephalopathy, require referring the child to a center with liver transplant capability. Several of the metabolic/genetic causes of jaundice have specific interventions. These can be identified with evidence-based literature searches as well as consultation with a genetic or pediatric gastrointestinal specialist.

PEARLS

■ Fulminant hepatic failure is recognized by a PT >25 seconds, hyperammonemia, acidosis, and mental status changes depicting encephalopathy. The child may need an immediate liver transplant.
■ The liver span is 5 cm at 6 months, 7 cm at 3 years, 8 to 10 cm at 10 years, and 9 to 12 cm in adolescence.
■ Chronic hepatic injury may be associated with hepatic vein thrombosis and veno-occlusive disease.
■ Website for parents of children with infectious diseases: *www.pkids.org.*
■ Crigler–Najjar website: *www.crigler-najjar.com.*

Suggested Readings

Bezerra JA, Balistreri WJ. Cholestatic syndromes of infancy and childhood. *Semin Gastrointest Dis* 2001;12:54–65.

Donnelly LF, Bisset GS. Unique imaging issues in pediatric liver disease. *Clin Liver Dis* 2002;6:227–245.

Gilbert-Barness E, Barness LA. *Clinical use of pediatric diagnostic tests.* Philadelphia, Lippincott, Williams and Wilkins; 2003:302–336.

Pashankar D, Schreiber RA. Jaundice in older children and adolescents. *PIR* 2001;22:219–226.

Pineiro-Carrero VM, Pineiio EO. Liver. *Pediatrics* 2004;113:1097–1106.

CHAPTER 26 ■ SHOCK

CARRIN E. SCHOTTLER-THAL

DEFINITION

In the pediatric population, the early recognition and treatment of shock improves clinical outcomes dramatically. Because of this, it is important that the primary care physician recognizes shock and starts treatment immediately. Shock can be defined as a physiologic state that results in the hypoperfusion and deoxygenation of vital organs and tissues. As a result of this hypoxia, there is a disruption in critical cellular processes, resulting in cell ion pump dysfunction, intracellular edema, dysregulation of intracellular pH, and eventual cell death.

PATHOPHYSIOLOGY

In the normal physiologic state, oxygen delivery is directly related to arterial oxygen concentration and cardiac output. Cardiac output is determined directly by (1) stroke volume (SV), which is the amount of blood ejected from the left ventricle; and (2) heart rate (CO = SV × HR). Stroke volume is directly determined by (1) preload, which is the end-diastolic fiber length; and (2) ionotropy, which is myocardial contractility. Stroke volume is indirectly related to afterload, which is resistance to blood ejection from the ventricle. Physiologically, when there is an increased demand for cardiac output, infants differ from adults and older children in terms of response. When faced with increased cardiac output demands, infants will generally increase heart rate, because myocardial contractility is weaker at this age. On the other hand, in older children and adults, an increased need for cardiac output will result in increases in stroke volume through increased venous return to heart (preload), decreased arterial resistance (afterload), and increased ionotropy. It is important to be aware of these age-related differences in regulatory mechanisms when trying to understand the differences in age groups according to how children might present in shock.

CLASSIFICATION

First of all, shock is classified into two stages: compensated (pre-shock) and decompensated shock. Compensated shock is defined as inadequate tissue perfusion with the maintenance of systolic blood pressure in the normal range. In compensated shock, the blood pressure is normal, but other indicators of shock such as lactic acidosis, oliguria, and altered level of consciousness are present. On the other hand, decompensated shock is described as the presence of these signs of tissue hypoperfusion *with* a decrease in systolic blood pressure.

Shock can also be classified in three separate categories based on the physiological cause of hypoperfusion: hypovolemic, distributive, and cardiogenic shock. Categorizing the different types of shock often oversimplifies the disease process in any one patient because components of all of three shock processes can occur in the same person. For example a person in hypovolemic shock can later demonstrate impaired cardiac function as a result of progressive cardiac tissue hypoperfusion.

Hypovolemic Shock

Hypovolemic shock is the most common cause of shock in the pediatric population and annually accounts for millions of deaths worldwide. Hypovolemic shock results from acute hypovolemia secondary to blood loss, fluid/electrolyte depletion, third-space fluid loss from capillary leak, and renal fluid losses. When found in the pediatric population, hypovolemic shock can usually be classified into two categories: fluid loss and hemorrhage. Physiologically, hypovolemic shock can be attributed to excessive decreases in preload.

Worldwide, the most common cause of hypovolemic shock is dehydration from diarrhea (1). With appropriate treatment, the mortality rate for hypovolemic shock is less than 10% in uncomplicated cases (2). Recovery from hypovolemic shock depends on the degree of dehydration, pre-existing hydration status, and rapid recognition and treatment. Hypovolemic shock is best distinguished from other types of shock by history and the absence of any signs of heart failure and sepsis. In the patient with hypovolemic shock, the clinical finding of "cold shock" helps diagnostically. The body compensates for hypovolemia with vasoconstriction and diversion of blood flow away from the skin, mesenteric, and renal circulations and results in cool, poorly perfused extremities.

Distributive Shock

Distributive shock is a result of an abnormal distribution of blood flow. It is the result of decreased systemic vascular resistance that, in turn, causes inadequate perfusion of vital organ systems. In this type of shock, cardiac output is maintained at high or normal levels. There are several notable etiologies for distributive shock, including sepsis, anaphylaxis, and central nervous system injury.

Septic shock is the most common type of distributive shock in the pediatric population, and is not infrequently found in hospitalized patients being treated for infection. It can be associated with any of a number of infectious etiologies, most commonly a bacterial infection and more rarely a rickettsial, viral, or fungal process. Patients with septic shock generally have fever, lethargy, and an identified infectious focus, and sometimes petechiae or purpura. Patients at higher risk for this type of shock include children with indwelling catheters, asplenia, immunodeficiency, surgical incisions, burns, malnutrition, or chronic antibiotic therapy (2).

Septic shock is often referred to as "warm shock." Early in this disease process the patient is febrile and tachycardic with warm flushed skin. Often in early septic shock, systemic arterial blood pressure is normal with normal or increased cardiac output. At this point, clinical recognition may be difficult, and the diagnosis requires a strong index of suspicion. The diagnosis of septic shock is a clinical one, and does not require the presence of a positive blood culture. Septic shock remains a major cause of death and improved survival depends on early recognition and treatment.

Anaphylactic shock, another form of distributive shock, results from an allergic, IgE-mediated response from exposure to an exogenous antigen. In a previously sensitized person, anaphylaxis occurs after exposure to an appropriate allergen, resulting in the rapid release of inflammatory mediators from mast cells and basophils. These inflammatory mediators markedly decrease systemic vascular resistance (SVR). This SVR decrease results in a redistribution of cardiac output so that some tissue beds become inadequately perfused (e.g., renal, splanchnic) and other organ systems (e.g., brain, heart) are preferentially perfused.

Neurogenic shock is caused by an acute (and usually severe) injury to the central nervous system. This injury results in a loss of sympathetic tone with a resulting decrease in blood pressure. Neurogenic shock results in a decrease in both systemic vascular resistance and preload with a concurrent low to normal cardiac output. Neurogenic shock then results in a maldistribution of blood flow such that the microcirculation receives an excessive amount of blood flow and other vital parts of the body receive little perfusion. Classic findings in neurogenic shock include hypotension without the expected compensatory tachycardia or vasoconstriction.

Cardiogenic Shock

Cardiogenic shock results directly from myocardial dysfunction, although it is important to note that any child with sustained shock will eventually develop some degree of cardiac dysfunction. Cardiogenic shock is manifested by decreased systolic function and subsequently decreased cardiac output. Intravascular volume is maintained, but is not adequately distributed because of the inadequate cardiac function. The body attempts to compensate with vasoconstriction and diversion of blood flow away from skin, mesenteric, and renal circulations; thus cardiogenic shock can also be termed "cold shock." Cardiogenic shock results from several different mechanisms including cardiomyopathies, arrhythmias, mechanical abnormalities, and obstruction. Compared to the pediatric population, cardiogenic shock is significantly more common in adults because of the high prevalence of ischemic heart disease.

Primary cardiomyopathies are conditions that affect the myocardium. Most cardiomyopathies are idiopathic in origin, but other causes include infectious, genetic, and infiltrative disorders. With a cardiomyopathy, the usual mechanism is the development of left ventricular dysfunction that over time leads to cardiogenic shock. A multitude of both atrial and ventricular *arrhythmias* can lead to cardiogenic shock. The most common reasons for arrhythmias in children include drug intoxication, structural lesions, and hypothermia. The rapid heart rates associated with both ventricular and atrial arrhythmias can result in decreased preload, decreased ventricular filling, and decreased stroke volume. Bradycardia and heart block can result in cardiogenic shock simply because of the substantial decrease in heart rate.

Congenital heart disease and other mechanical abnormalities of the heart are also significant causes of cardiogenic shock in children. In most children with congenital heart disease, cardiogenic shock generally follows heart failure. The exception is hypoplastic left heart syndrome, where heart failure generally follows cardiogenic shock. Other mechanical abnormalities of the heart including coarctation of the aorta and intracardiac tumors can also cause cardiogenic shock by introducing a high afterload and subsequently resulting in diminished heart function by pressure overload.

Obstructive disorders can result in cardiogenic shock by introducing an extracardiac barrier to normal cardiac function. Examples of these extracardiac barriers include constrictive pericarditis, cardiac tamponade, severe pulmonary hypertension, and pulmonary embolism.

SIGNS OF SHOCK

The assessment of five physical signs should be conducted and analyzed when a child is suspected of being in shock. These signs include blood pressure, skin changes (warmth and perfusion), urine output, mental status, and lactic acidosis.

Low blood pressure occurs in most patients in shock when in the decompensated state, but this is often a late finding in children. Hypotension can be defined as a systolic blood pressure less than 90 mmHg in adults, or less than the fifth percentile for age in children.

Skin changes vary according to the type of shock (see above). In hypovolemic and cardiogenic shock, the body compensates by diverting blood flow from the peripheral, mesenteric, and renal vessels and redirecting the blood flow to coronary and cerebral vessels, thus resulting in "cold shock." In distributive shock (i.e., septic, anaphylactic, and neurogenic) the dysregulated peripheral vasodilation results in a flushed appearance, otherwise known as "warm shock."

As a result of diverting blood flow away from the renal vessels, another sign of shock is a decrease in glomerular filtration with a subsequent *decrease in urine output.*

Because of a decrease in blood flow to the brain, *impaired mental status* is also a typical sign of shock. This impairment initially starts as an agitated state, progresses to confusion, and ultimately leads to obtundation.

Tissue hypoperfusion ultimately leads to *increased lactic acid production* and also decreased clearance of lactic acid by the liver, kidneys, and skeletal muscle. In turn, this results in progressive metabolic acidosis, increased lactic acid levels, and an increased anion gap.

HISTORY AND PHYSICAL EXAM

Although a history may be difficult to obtain from the child in shock, obtaining several key elements of history should be attempted. Past medical history and the patient's general condition can aid in determining an etiology for the presentation of shock. Other key elements of history include the child's activities prior to presentation, allergies, medications, potential ingestions, immunosuppressive conditions, hypercoagulable conditions, recent illnesses, and recent trauma.

Physical examination is crucial and should occur rapidly and thoroughly. Important physical exam findings to note include:

- General appearance: agitated, confused, obtunded.
- HEENT: scleral icterus, dry mucous membranes, pinpoint or fixed, dilated pupils, nystagmus, sunken or bulging fontanelle.
- Neck: meningeal signs, jugular venous distention, adenopathy.
- Lungs: tachypnea, shallow breathing, crackles, wheezes, stridor.
- Heart: irregular rhythm, tachycardia or bradycardia, heaves, murmurs, distant heart sounds, pericardial rub.
- Abdomen: distention, tenderness, peritoneal signs, absent or high-pitched bowel sounds, hepatosplenomegaly, ascites.
- Rectal: bright red blood, melena.

- Extremities: weak pulses, delayed capillary refill, cyanosis, edema, disparity of blood pressures or pulses between extremities.
- Neurologic: paresis, focal deficits, seizure activity.
- Skin: cold, clammy, warm, hyperemic, petechiae, purpura, urticaria, cellulitis, catheters, recent surgical sites.

LABORATORY VALUES

There are many laboratory values appropriate to assist in the identification of shock, its etiology, and subsequent management. Tests to strongly consider include complete blood count (CBC) and differential, basic chemistry tests, liver function tests, amylase, lipase, fibrinogen/fibrin split products, lactate level, cardiac enzymes, arterial blood gas, toxicology screen, chest x-ray, abdominal x-ray, ECG, and urinalysis.

MANAGEMENT

Any child in suspected shock should be treated quickly and in accordance with the principles taught in Pediatric Advanced Life Support (PALS). Therapy should ultimately minimize the patient's cardiopulmonary workload while maintaining adequate cardiac output, blood pressure, and gas exchange. Management may need to begin with immobilization of the cervical spine, and avoidance of extension and flexion of the neck. After immobilization, the airway should be secured, breathing maintained, circulation supported (ABCs), and vascular access obtained. With the initial ABCs, 100% oxygen should be administered, a cardiorespiratory monitor attached, and four-limb blood pressures obtained, followed by monitoring blood pressure and pulse oximetry. Laboratory evaluation (especially glucose and potassium levels) should be done as soon as the ABCs are achieved. Two large-bore IV lines are preferable, but an interosseous (IO) line should be considered in children where peripheral access is not successful. Any child with obvious rib trauma, decreased breath sounds, distended neck veins, or tracheal deviation requires immediate chest decompression via needle or chest tube thoracostomy.

Further management is guided by the assessment for the type of shock. Volume resuscitation should be initiated immediately, especially if the history and physical are indicative of hypovolemic shock. Isotonic saline bolus infusions of 20 mL/kg (over 20 minutes) should be administered followed by reassessment. Often multiple boluses are necessary. If the child has significant blood loss from hemorrhage, 10 to 15 mL/kg transfusions of packed red blood cells should be administered. Children in any type of shock should be transferred to an intensive-care unit as promptly as possible.

In cases where distributive shock is suspected, decreased preload impairs cardiac function significantly. In these cases, fluid resuscitation with 20 mL/kg of isotonic saline is also indicated. If septic shock is suspected, broad-spectrum antibiotics should be administered and blood cultures obtained. In patients where anaphylaxis is suspected, epinephrine (1:10,000; 0.1 mL/kg every 3 to 5 minutes) should be administered intravenously or intratracheally.

If the child is determined to be in cardiogenic shock, initial management with isotonic saline should be much more conservative. Only if it is felt necessary to assure adequate preload, saline can be given as a conservative bolus of 5 to 10 mL/kg. It is important to be conservative with fluids in cardiogenic shock because excessive elevations in preload can cause pulmonary edema. In cyanotic infants with any suspicion of a ductal-dependent cardiac lesion, PGE1 (prostaglandin E1) infusion should be administered, but with guidance from a pediatric intensive care unit or pediatric cardiologist. Again, arrangements for immediate transfer to a pediatric intensive care unit should follow to allow for a full cardiac evaluation and initiation of ionotropic support with dopamine, or epinephrine and dobutamine if appropriate.

PEARLS

- Early recognition improves clinical outcome.
- Shock results in hypoperfusion and deoxygenation.
- Shock can be classified into compensated and decompensated shock depending upon whether the child is able to maintain blood pressure.
- Shock can also be classified as hypovolemic (most common in children), distributive, and cardiogenic.
- Signs of shock include low blood pressure, skin changes, decreased urine output, mental status changes, and increased lactic acid production.
- Initial treatment of shock should be in accordance with principles taught in PALS, focusing on airway, breathing, and circulation.

Suggested Readings

Hazinski MF, ed. Recognition of respiratory failure and shock. In PALS provider manual. Dallas: American Heart Association; 2002: 23–42.

Krug SE. The acutely ill or injured child. In: Behrman R, Kliegman R, eds. *Nelson essentials of pediatrics*. 3rd ed. New York: Saunders; 1998: 93–128.

Pappas A. The infant in shock. In: Lieh-Lai M, Ling-McGeorge KA Asi-Bautista MC, et al. *Pediatric acute care*. 2nd ed. New York: Lippincott Williams & Wilkins; 2001:38–39.

Pomerantz W, Roback M. Definition, classification, and initial assessment of shock in children. *Up to Date*, September 13, 2005, http://www.utdol.com/application/topic.

References

1. Thomas NJ, Carcillo JA. Hypovolemic shock in pediatric patients. *New Horizons* 1998;6:120–129.
2. Witte MK, Hill JH, Blumer JL. Shock in the pediatric patient. *Adv Pediatr* 1987;34:139–173.

CHAPTER 27 ■ SYNCOPE

DAVID W. HANNON AND DAVID L. FAIRBROTHER

DEFINITIONS

- Syncope: Brief loss of consciousness due to inadequate cerebral perfusion with spontaneous resolution.
- Presyncope: Symptoms that may occur prior to a syncopal event. These symptoms include sensation of warmth, lightheaded or dizzy spells, visual gray out or black out, or transient nausea. It is common in patients with neurocardiogenic syncope. Presyncope may be confused with the aura of an epileptic seizure.
- Orthostatic intolerance: Recurrent episodes of presyncope with or without full vasovagal syncope, which may be combined with episodic sensation of racing heart, chest pain, tightness in the chest, or shortness of breath. These symptoms are now termed postural tachycardia syndrome or POTS (postural orthostatic tachycardia syndrome). A number of young patients with idiopathic ("noncardiac") chest pain or palpitation may have postural tachycardia syndrome. Chronic fatigue is also described in these patients, and headaches are also a common symptom.

PATHOPHYSIOLOGY

Syncope generally falls into one of three categories: Vasovagal, vasodepressor, and cardioinhibitory. Vasovagal syncope is the most common, and occurs while standing or sitting when venous pooling in the lower extremities results in inadequate preload to the hear, triggering excessive catecholamine discharge. A vigorously contracting "empty" heart stimulates the firing of afferent C-fibers within the myocardium, which results in reflex withdrawal of sympathetic tone and (in some cases) vagal parasympathetic discharge. Withdrawal of sympathetic tone when there is compromise of adequate preload to the heart may be sufficient to cause syncope (vasodepressor-type syncope). However, additional vagal stimulation (cardioinhibitory syncope) will result in syncope accompanied at the onset by a brief convulsion from cardiac asystole. This is often presaged by the vagally mediated symptoms of nausea, sweating, or abdominal cramping. Cerebral hypoperfusion may also occur due to potentially life-threatening arrhythmias.

DIFFERENTIAL DIAGNOSIS

- Vasovagal/neurocardiogenic syncope.
- Pallid infantile syncope and toddler syncope.
- Pulseless ventricular tachycardias: long QT syndromes, Brugada syndrome, arrhythmogenic right ventricular cardiomyopathy, catecholamine-dependent ventricular tachy-cardia, repaired congenital heart disease, especially repaired tetralogy of Fallot.
- Pulseless supraventricular tachycardias: atrial fibrillation with Wolff–Parkinson–White syndrome; atrial tachycardia with rapid ventricular response, after atrial repair of transposition of the great arteries or after Fontan-type operations for single-ventricle anatomy.
- Pulseless bradyarrhythmias: episodic heart block (usually) below the AV node is rare but seen in some forms of myocarditis, sarcoidosis, and in the subacute phase of Lyme disease.
- Anomalous coronary artery.
- Cardiomyopathy: hypertrophic, dilated, or restrictive cardiomyopaties.
- Obstruction to ventricular outflow: severe aortic stenosis; severe pulmonic stenosis.
- Primary pulmonary hypertension.
- Seizure disorders.
- Metabolic: hypoglycemia, drug or intoxicant ingestion.
- Conversion disorders and other forms of factitious syncope.

PEARLS IN DIAGNOSIS

- History is the most important diagnostic tool.
- Physical examination is normal in vasovagal/neurocardiogenic syncope and in almost all patients with serious syncopal arrhythmias.
- Syncope that occurs during a venipuncture or when seeing an injury, surgery, or blood is almost always vasovagal. Faints occurring with prolonged standing (wedding faints, stage faints, church faints) are usually vasovagal.
- A prodrome of nausea and sensation that the room is hot is frequent in vasovagal/neurocardiogenic syncope.
- "Hair-grooming syncope" is vasovagal syncope. This occurs in a girl having her hair groomed while standing.
- Syncope that occurs during intense exercise is a "red flag" for life-threatening cardiac etiologies such as hypertrophic cardiomyopathy, congenital coronary artery abnormalities (aberrant course of one coronary artery), or dangerous arrhythmias (e.g., arrhythmogenic right-ventricular cardiomyopathy, catecholamine-triggered ventricular tachycardia, long QT syndromes, and rare instances of atrial fibrillation with rapid ventricular response in Wolff–Parkinson–White syndrome).
- Syncope that occurs immediately after exercise while in the upright position is most likely to be vasovagal, but other exercise-triggered syncopal etiologies also may occur with this history.
- Many patients with orthostatic intolerance will report a history of poor fluid intake, concentrated urine, or excessive caffeine intake.
- Family history in patients with vasovagal syncope may be positive for medical fainters, orthostatic fainters, migraine

headaches, or individuals with various presyncopal symptoms.
■ Family history of sudden death, congenital deafness, or drowning increases the suspicion for LQTS.
■ Severe aortic and pulmonic stenosis are rare causes of syncope as they are usually previously diagnosed (by murmur on physical exam). Hypertrophic cardiomyopathy is more subtle and can be missed. A systolic murmur that intensifies when standing is usually abnormal and suggestive, as is LVH on ECG. Equally subtle, primary pulmonary hypertension may present with syncope. There is usually no murmur. A loud single second heart sound and RVH on electrocardiogram are present.
■ The likelihood of pathologic arrhythmia increases with a history of repaired (or unrepaired) congenital heart disease.

DIAGNOSTIC EVALUATION

Most cases of pediatric syncope are worked up in outpatient settings. Patients who are hospitalized for syncope may have atypical features suggesting causes other than common vasovagal fainting.

Electrocardiogram is requisite: careful measurement of corrected QT interval (corrected for heart rate as $QTc = QT/$ square root of RR interval) to look for evidence of long QT (QTc over 0.450 sec), careful inspection for evidence of pre-excitation (delta wave of Wolff–Parkinson–White syndrome), or evidence of precordial lead ST or T-wave abnormalities (Brugada syndrome and arrhythmogenic RV cardiomyopathy), or atrioventricular or intraventricular conduction abnormalities. Tilt table testing is sometimes employed to provoke syncope and help identify an etiology. The specificity and sensitivity of tilt table testing with or without pharmacologic provocation (e.g., isoproterenol) is not well established, especially in young patients. Sensitivity and specificity both may be low enough that uncertainty about the cause of syncope will remain unless tilt testing is combined with a careful history, family history, and physical exam. A tilt test is occasionally performed if there is concern that the symptoms may not be due to cerebral hypoperfusion (i.e., pseudoseizure) or to study heart rate, respiratory changes, and blood pressure changes prior to syncope to guide medication choice. Twenty-four-hour ambulatory ECG monitoring (Holter monitor) is often not helpful and is not considered requisite. A 30-day ECG event recorder (looping type recorder) is more helpful if symptoms occur relatively frequently (>1 episode/2 weeks) and the history is suggestive of an arrhythmia. This can document the cardiac rhythm at the time of a recurrence of symptoms. Minimally invasive implantable long-term looping ECG event recorders are available for patients with unclear diagnosis after 30-day external event recordings, especially if symptoms suggest dangerous arrhythmia.

Syncope with repaired significant congenital heart disease (e.g., repaired tetralogy of Fallot) may warrant invasive electrophysiologic study to provoke syncopal arrhythmia by cardiac pacing.

Cerebral CT imaging is unlikely to secure syncope diagnosis in pediatric patients with normal neurologic exam. Rarely, a Chiari I malformation of the brainstem presents as syncope or as autonomic dysfunction. This diagnosis may require MRI with attention to posterior fossa anatomy. Standard or ambulatory electroencephalography (EEG) may be diagnostic of seizure disorders. EEG is rarely necessary when syncope rather than a convulsion is the clinical presentation in a child or adolescent with a normal neurologic exam. A neurology consultation is indicated if the history suggests a seizure disorder or if neurologic examination is abnormal.

TREATMENT

Patients with vasovagal syncope (neurocardiogenic syncope) should be told to perform avoidance maneuvers at the onset of presyncopal symptoms. These can include crossing the legs and tensing the thigh/buttocks/abdominal musculature, squatting, or lying down. Onlookers should never raise the head if a vasovagal faint occurs, because this may cause a brief seizure from prolonged cardiac asystole and resultant cerebral hypoperfusion. In addition to avoidance maneuvers, other nonpharmacologic measures include increasing fluid intake and not avoiding salt in the diet. All drugs that have been used for neurocardiogenic syncope are not FDA approved for this use in children, and consultation is encouraged before using drugs in children with syncope. Beta-blocker therapy may decrease syncope in vasovagal/neurocardiogenic syncope and may be useful for symptoms of postural tachycardia syncope. Fludrocortisone (0.1 to 0.3 mg/day) has been used in multiple studies in adult and pediatric patients with vasovagal/neurocardiogenic syncope but is an off-label use. Salt retention, blood pressure increase, and hypokalemia may occur in some patients. No large-scale controlled trials of fludrocortisone are published. Midodrine has been used in studies of adult patients with neurocardiogenic syncope, especially vasodepressor response type. It has also been used in orthostatic intolerance syndromes. It is FDA approved for use in adults with orthostatic hypotension but not for children with orthostatic intolerance or syncope. Side effects may include occasional marked supine hypertension and paresthesias. Midodrine has a short half-life and should not be given later than midafternoon to avoid sleeping hypertension. Sertraline is an SSRI-type antidepressant that has been evaluated in several studies showing possible benefit in neurocardiogenic syncope. It is not FDA approved for this indication in any age group, however. Double-blind placebo-controlled studies have shown iron supplementation significantly improves symptoms in infants and toddlers with breath-holding spells or infantile syncope when iron deficiency coexists with breath-holding spells.

Pacemaker therapy is usually not needed for neurocardiogenic (vasovagal) syncope in adolescence even with documented asystole. However, recent controlled studies have shown benefit in adults with recurrent neurocardiogenic syncope using dual-chamber pacemakers with a special rate drop response that "rescues" the patient with a high-paced heart rate when marked bradycardia occurs. Some adolescents with severe recurrent vasovagal syncope may require this type of pacing therapy.

Long QT syndrome responds to treatment with beta-blocker medication in some patients. Adjunctive pacemaker therapy is indicated if there is bradycardia dependent severe QT prolongation. Some of these patients will require an implantable cardioverter/defibrillator (ICD). Syncope in patients with LQTS should be considered to be due to torsades de pointes until proven otherwise.

Patients with "repaired" congenital heart disease may benefit from radiofrequency ablation of arrhythmia sites, reoperation to improve abnormal hemodynamics (e.g., residual pulmonic stenosis or severe pulmonic regurgitation in tetralogy of Fallot), implantation of a pacemaker (for sick sinus syndrome, high-grade late AV block, or anti-tachycardia pacing), or implantation of an ICD for refractory ventricular tachycardia.

PEARLS

■ Vasovagal syncope often results in a period of asystole with secondary cerebral hypoperfusion. A brief grand malconvulsion may occur at the onset of a vasovagal syncopal episode due to cardiac asystole.

- Vasovagal syncope is often familial with an autosomal-dominant mode of inheritance and marked variation in expression.
- Some types of breath-holding spells (pallid infantile syncope) represent infantile/toddler variants of vasovagal syncope. Studies document that cardiac asystole precedes cessation of respiration, loss of consciousness, or brief epileptic activity as also occurs in cardioinhibitory forms of vasovagal syncope. Other family members may report breath-holding during childhood or may report typical adolescent or adult presentations of vasovagal syncope.
- Life-threatening arrhythmias such as torsades de pointes (polymorphic ventricular tachycardia in long QT syndrome) may also cause a brief grand malconvulsion at the onset of the syncopal spells because of cerebral hypoperfusion. There are multiple reports of misdiagnosis of long QT syndrome as epilepsy.
- Syncope that occurs during sleep (sudden awakening with seizure or faint) is seen in some forms of long QT syndrome and in the malignant recurrent ventricular tachycardia syndrome called Brugada syndrome.
- Loss of consciousness that persists for longer than 1 minute points toward a different etiology than common vasovagal syncope, such as malignant arrhythmia. Loss of consciousness that persists for longer than 10 minutes followed by spontaneous recovery may suggest conversion or factitious syncope. Factitious fainters can be surprisingly resistant to sternal rub or other noxious stimuli to try to awaken them.
- Rare patients can have both vasovagal syncope and, on other occasions, factitious or conversion-type syncope, suggesting learned secondary gain from the true or vasovagal faints.
- Significant fasting normally causes increased circulating catecholamines (counterregulatory hormonal response), which is detrimental in patients who have a vasovagal predilection. This may be misdiagnosed as a primary hypoglycemic disorder, which is comparatively rare in otherwise healthy adolescents. Documentation during or after syncope of hypoglycemia severe enough to cause loss of consciousness must be done with a finger-stick blood analysis to secure a diagnosis of true hypoglycemia.
- Many patients with neurocardiogenic syncope will at some point have frequent or severe-enough headaches to result in a diagnosis of migraine headaches. This is especially true of patients with orthostatic intolerance or postural orthostatic tachycardia syndrome.
- One report suggests a relationship between marked joint laxity (hypermobile joints) and symptoms of orthostatic intolerance and chronic fatigue.
- Some young adults with the diagnosis of "mitral valve prolapse syndrome" and minimally abnormal or normal cardiac examination findings may actually have orthostatic intolerance with related symptoms of chest pain, light-headedness, palpitations, and shortness of breath.
- Rare patients with true mitral valve prolapse ("myxomatous valve") can have serious ventricular arrhythmia and sudden deaths are reported. Ventricular arrhythmia should be excluded as a cause of syncope in patients with bona fide mitral valve prolapse and significantly abnormal echocardiographic valve function or anatomy.

Suggested Readings

Grubb BP. Neurocardiogenic syncope and related disorders of orthostatic intolerance. *Circulation* 2005;111:2997–3006 Available at http://circ.ahajournals.org/cgi/content/full/111/22/2997.

Hannon DW. Breath-holding spells: waiting to inhale, waiting for systole, or waiting for iron therapy? *J Pediatr* 1997;130:510–512.

Hannon DW, Knilans TK. Syncope in children and adolescents. *Curr Probl Pediatr* 1993;23:358–384.

Jacob B, Fernando C, Shannon J, et al. The neuropathic postural tachycardia syndrome. *N Engl J Med* 2000;343:1008–1014.

Rowe PC, Barron DF, Calkins H, et al. Orthostatic intolerance and chronic fatigue syndrome associated with Ehlers-Danlos syndrome. *J Pediatr* 1999;135:494–499.

Stewart JM. Chronic orthostatic intolerance and the postural tachycardia syndrome (POTS). *J Pediatr* 2004;145:725–730.

Strickberger SA, Benson DW, Biaggioni I, et al. AHA/ACCF Scientific Statement on the Evaluation of Syncope. *J Am Coll Cardiol* 2006;47:473–484.

Willis J. Syncope. *Pediatr Rev* 2000;21:201–203.

CHAPTER 28 ■ ARRHYTHMIA AND CARDIAC PACING

DAVID L. FAIRBROTHER, ANJAN S. BATRA, AND DAVID W. HANNON

NARROW-COMPLEX TACHYARRHYTHMIAS

Definitions

Supraventricular tachycardia (SVT) can be used to describe any narrow-complex tachycardia with a "supraventricular morphology." This broad category includes sinus tachycardia, reentry-type SVT, atrial tachycardia, atrial flutter, and atrial fibrillation (Table 28.1).

Sinus tachycardia may be appropriate or inappropriate and involves a tachycardia originating from the sinus node with a rapid rate.

Reentry-type SVT can be classified into *atrioventricular reentry tachycardia (AVRT)*, which involves a reentry circuit between the atrium and the ventricle; and *atrioventricular nodal tachycardia (AVNRT)*, which involves a reentry circuit between a slow and fast conducting pathway within the atrium. AVRT can be further classified into those with *Wolff–Parkinson–White syndrome (WPW syndrome)*, where the accessary pathway is capable of antegrade and retrograde impulse conduction; and those with a *concealed pathway*, where the accessary pathway is only capable of retograde impulse conduction. A subset of patients with AVRT may present with an incessant form of tachycardia called *permanent junctional reciprocating tachycardia*.

Ectopic atrial tachycardia is a supraventricular tachyarrhythmia arising from a focus in the right or left atrium. Two basic types occur. *Automatic atrial tachycardia* is produced by increased automaticity of such a focus. *Atrial reentry tachycardia* is caused by a local reentry of an electrical wavefront that includes only atrial tissue. Atrial reentry tachycardia is not synonymous with classic atrial flutter.

Atrial flutter is a rapid atrial tachycardia due to a macroreentry circuit within the atrium (right atrial reentry circuit).

Atrial fibrillation is a rapid atrial tachycardia secondary to enhanced automaticity from atrial musculature that extends into the pulmonary veins.

Junctional ectopic tachycardia (JET) refers to a narrow-complex tachycardia arising within the atrioventricular (AV) junction secondary to increased automaticity.

Clinical Presentations and History

Sinus tachycardia (ST) is common in infants. The highest average heart rates occur at 6 to 8 weeks of life and decline afterward. Under 6 months of age, sinus tachycardia rates of up to 220 beats/minute can be seen with fever, sepsis, extreme stress, high doses of β-agonist medication, and so on.

AVRT and AVNRT are the most common causes of sustained SVT in pediatrics. Greater than 90% of infant SVT may be attributed to AVRT, whereas AVNRT is usually rare in infancy and becomes more prevalent with increasing age. In a significant proportion of patients with AVRT, the accessory pathway may spontaneously resolve by the first year of life. In the neonate with SVT, heart rates are usually 250 to 280 beats/minute with narrow-complex QRS, and these patients are more likely to present with a sustained tachycardia. However, presentation in the delivery room or newborn nursery without significant symptoms is not unusual. Fetal SVT can cause intrauterine congestive heart failure with stillbirth or delivery of a hydropic infant. Sustained SVT in first months of life may present with history of irritability, poor feeding, and poor color. Congestive heart failure may be evident on examination with a gallop on auscultation, tachypnea, hepatomegaly, and poor pulses. SVT of several days duration is suggested by this presentation (Fig. 28.1).

The first episode of AVRT or AVNRT may occur in later childhood or adolescence. It presents with sensation of a racing heart, sometimes accompanied by chest pain or dyspnea. Often, the patient will describe the cessation of tachycardia as occuring with a single beat, rather than a gradual termination. Heart rates from 180 to 220 beats/minute are typical. Congestive heart failure is rare if medical care is sought early. Patients with permanent junctional reciprocating tachycardia present with an incessant tachycardia with a high risk for developing tachycardia-induced cardiomyopathy.

Atrial flutter is much less common than AVRT-type paroxysmal SVT (PSVT) in the neonate, but it is not rare. Atrial rates in newborns with atrial flutter are 400 to 480 beats/minute; however, this is always associated with 2:1 AV conduction (ventricular rate 200 to 240) or with variable AV conduction. Flutter waves at twice the ventricular rate are usually not apparent unless the electrocardiogram (ECG) is taken while higher degrees of AV block (3:1 or 4:1 conduction) are induced with vagal maneuvers or adenosine. Atrial flutter should be suspected in the neonate with "SVT" that is slower than usual (Fig. 28.2). This form of atrial flutter has a high likelihood of resolving spontaneously.

Adolescents and adults with repaired complex congenital heart disease involving multiple atrial suture lines may present with slow forms of "atrial flutter" (atrial rates of 200 to 280) with 1:1 or 2:1 atrioventricular conduction. Survivors of the Mustard and Senning operations (intra-atrial baffle) for transposition of the great arteries are now adults and often present with this type of SVT. Late survivors of the Fontan operation for single-ventricle hearts also may have extensive atrial scarring and suffer from atrial tachycardia or "slow flutter," with 1:1 atrioventricular conduction. A fixed heart rate of 100 to

TABLE 28.1

MOST LIKELY DIAGNOSIS FOR NARROW COMPLEX TACHYCARDIA OF DIFFERING RATES

Age	Rate (bpm)	Diagnosis
Newborn/ neonate	260–280	AV reentry type PSVT
	210–225	Atrial flutter with 2:1 AV conduction (atrial rate 420–450 bpm)
Young infant	180–210	Sinus tachycardia, especially if febrile or crying[a]
	180–220	Atrial tachycardia possible, less likely than sinus tachycardia[b]
	230–260	AV reentry type tachycardia[a]
Older child	120–170	Sinus tachycardia, atrial tachycardia also possible
	190–220	AV reentry or AV node reentry tachycardia[c]
	120–150	With irregular narrow QRS rate—atrial fibrillation

[a]Sinus tachycardia may occur with rates to 260 bpm in ages 2–6 mo. when there is fever and crying. Careful inspection of 12-lead electrocardiogram reveals normal axis P waves preceding each QRS with short to normal PR interval.
[b]P wave with abnormal axis and/or abnormally long PR interval is often seen with atrial tachycardia.
[c]Some cases of PSVT (AV reentry or even AV node reentry SVT) can have rates as slow as 170 bpm in adolescents.
SVT, supraventricular tachycardia; AV, atrioventricular; bpm, beats per minute; PSVT, paroxysmal SVT; QRS,

140 beats/minute in a patient with previous atrial repair of complex congenital heart disease should always be considered an atrial tachycardia rather than sinus tachycardia until proven otherwise. Such patients are at risk for "tachycardia-mediated cardiomyopathy." In incessant, "slower" supraventricular tachycardias, a severe but reversible dilated cardiomyopathy can develop as a response to chronically high heart rate. Patients may be unaware that heart rate is incessantly in the range required to cause this syndrome (above 140 beats/min). Atrial flutter with 2:1 AV block and chronic atrial or junctional tachycardia can cause tachycardia-mediated cardiomyopathy. This should not be confused with primary dilated cardiomyopathy. Restoration of normal sinus rates will result in return of normal cardiac function. Ebstein anomaly is frequently associated with WPW and AVRT.

Atrial fibrillation is rare in childhood. It is uncommon but well described during adolescence. The typical case of pediatric atrial fibrillation is an athletic child presenting with sustained atrial fibrillation and sensation of continuous but irregular palpitation. These cases of "lone atrial fibrillation" are not associated with discernible structural heart disease (Fig. 28.3). Atrial fibrillation with WPW is a distinct clinical entity. Although it is a rare presentation of WPW syndrome, its potential for disastrous outcome makes understanding this pathophysiology important. These patients most commonly develop AV reentry (typical PSVT) that then degenerates into atrial fibrillation or somehow triggers atrial fibrillation. Atrial fibrillatory impulses may then conduct to the ventricles at dangerously fast rates via conduction over both the normal AV node and the accessory pathway. Hypotension, syncope, collapse, and death may occur. Well-documented cases exist where sudden death (usually with exercise) was the *first* symptom in patients with previously discovered WPW as an incidental finding on ECG. This tragic arrhythmia can occur in adolescents with normal hearts (no structural disease or cardiomyopathy). The rare case reports of *sustained* atrial fibrillation with rapid ventricular response in infants with WPW have involved abnormal hearts (e.g., cardiomyopathy). It is arguable that sustained atrial fibrillation with dangerous ventricular rate is not a risk for infants with WPW and completely normal hearts apart from the accessory pathway (Fig. 28.4). Ectopic atrial tachycardia is associated with a high incidence of congestive heart failure because of its incessant nature. The natural history of ectopic atrial tachycardia is unpredictable but mandates an aggressive treatment approach.

Automatic junctional tachycardia with no other underlying cardiac pathology is a very rare rhythm in pediatrics and may present in infancy as congenital junctional ectopic tachycardia or in young adulthood. The patients are often quite symptomatic and, if untreated, may develop heart failure, particularly if their tachycardia is incessant. Junctional ectopic tachycardia in the immediate postoperative period after congenital heart surgery, however, is relatively common, presenting in up to 10% of such patients. This arrhythmia is usually transient and spontaneously resolves in the first 3 to 5 days. Treatment for hemodynamic instability associated with this rhythm may be necessary.

Premature atrial beats or *premature atrial contractions (PACs)* are very common in newborns. These usually present

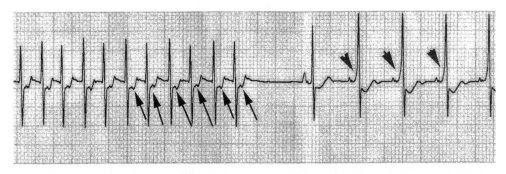

FIGURE 28.1. AV reentry tachycardia (common SVT) terminates with adenosine. Sinus rhythm after conversion shows Wolff–Parkinson–White syndrome with short PR and slurred initial QRS forces (delta wave). Delta wave is not present during SVT because the accessory pathway conducts only retrograde during SVT. Retrograde P-waves in SVT are indicated by arrows. Arrowheads show preexcitation (delta wave) during sinus rhythm.

ADENOSINE

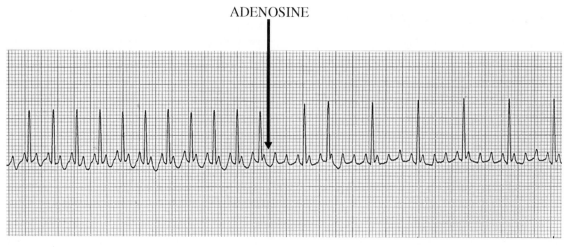

FIGURE 28.2. Atrial flutter in a neonate without structural heart disease. The ventricular rate of 220 beats/min is slow for typical SVT in the neonate. Atrial flutter waves at 440 beats/min are shown by arrowheads. There is 2:1 AV conduction.

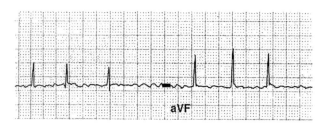

FIGURE 28.3. Atrial fibrillation in an athletic teen with sudden onset of palpitations related to irregular ventricular response to atrial fibrillation.

as irregular pauses in the heart rate, because the premature atrial beats often occur early enough that the AV node is refractory and does not allow conduction of the premature atrial complex to the ventricle. A subtle P-wave in the ST segment of the normal preceding QRS is present, but no QRS follows the premature P-wave (nonconducted PAC; Fig. 28.5).

Establishing a Diagnosis

For a summary of diagnoses, see Table 28.1. A full, 12-lead ECG should always be done. Diagnostic findings include narrow QRS morphology and abnormal heart rates, as described

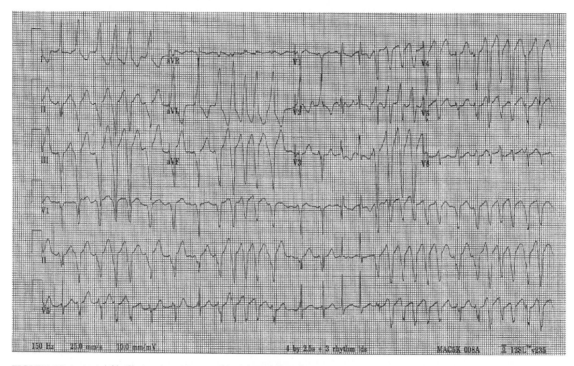

FIGURE 28.4. Atrial fibrillation in a 10-year-old with Wolff–Parkinson–White syndrome. The narrower QRS complexes are the result of conduction of atrial fibrillatory impulses over the AV node. Wide QRS complexes result from atrial impulses conducted over the accessory pathway.

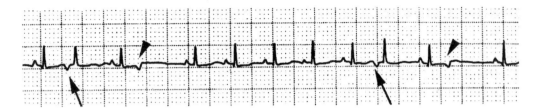

FIGURE 28.5. Premature atrial complexes in an asymptomatic neonate. Arrows indicate the premature P-waves that conduct with following QRS complexes. Arrowheads indicate two nonconducted premature atrial beats that result in pauses with no QRS.

above. Additional features that will narrow the diagnosis include:

■ Sinus tachycardia: There are upright P-waves in the inferior leads (II, III, AVF) and negative in AVR (normal P-axis), with a normal to short PR interval (less than 0.12 to 0.14 sec in the young child; Fig. 28.6). The presence of normal morphology P-waves preceding all QRS and gradual rate slowing as the stress or fever is treated distinguish very rapid sinus tachycardias from PSVT and other pathologic arrhythmias (Fig. 28.6).

■ AVRT: Careful review of ECG shows retrograde P-waves just after the QRS complex and within the ST segments due to reentry to the atrium over the accessory pathway. Inspection of the 12-lead ECG during sinus rhythm (after conversion) will in some cases show findings of WPW syndrome. The hallmark findings of WPW syndrome include a short PR interval and slurred initial QRS deflection ("delta wave"; Fig. 28.1).

■ AVNRT: No P-waves will be seen after the QRS (in the ST segment) or preceding the QRS. Electrophysiologic studies show the atrial activity to be nearly simultaneous with the QRS as reentry to the atrium occurs during impulse conduction to the ventricles over bundle branches.

■ Atrial flutter: During increased AV block (decreased AV conduction), the presence of very rapid atrial complexes ("flutter waves"), typically at twice the presenting SVT rate, will be appreciated. This is one reason that a "hard-copy" ECG should always be recorded during attempts to convert "SVT" with adenosine or vagal maneuvers, such as ice bag to face (Fig. 28.2). In pediatric patients, the atrial rate is usually 300 to 460 beats/minute. Normal AV conduction blockade results in a ventricular response (ventricular rate) of 150 to 230 beats/minute. A characteristic "sawtooth" pattern of the baseline may or may not be seen. AV node block with vagal maneuvers or adenosine can slow the ventricular response but not convert atrial flutter to sinus rhythm.

■ Atrial fibrillation: ECG findings of atrial fibrillation include absence of clearly discernable P-waves and an irregular ventricular rate.

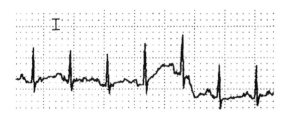

FIGURE 28.6. Sinus tachycardia in an infant with high fever and agitation at 230 beats/min. Sinus P-wave precedes each QRS. Normal P-wave axis with normal to short PR interval supports sinus tachycardia over atrial tachycardia. Treatment of fever slowed rate gradually.

■ Ectopic atrial tachycardia: P-waves precede each QRS, but the P-wave morphology or axis is abnormal because it does not arise from the sinus node. The PR may be slightly longer than would be expected with sinus tachycardia.

■ Junctional tachycardia: This is apparent as a narrow-complex tachycardia with the P-waves either not apparent when they occur simultaneously with the QRS complex or the P-waves dissociated from the QRS complex when the junctional rate is faster than the atrial rate.

For nonsustained SVT, 24-hour ambulatory ECG monitoring (Holter monitoring) is usually not helpful. Patients with episodic, nonsustained SVT are unlikely to oblige the physician with an episode during the 24-hour recording. Thirty-day ECG event recorders are helpful and can be diagnostic if the palpitation recurs within 30 days. These devices should replace Holter monitoring in the diagnostic workup of palpitations. Newer 30-day event loop recorders with the capability of auto-triggering a recording when the heart rate exceeds the programmed parameters may be helpful in smaller children unable to adequately communicate with the recorder to initiate a recording.

Pacing the heart (electrophysiologic studies) can provoke SVT in patients with electrical substrate for reentry (AVRT-type SVT, AVNRT-type SVT, atrial flutter, atrial reentry–type atrial tachycardia). It is possible to perform such pacing from a swallowed esophageal (atrial) pacing wire or via a transvenous pacing wire. The ability to induce and terminate SVT by pacing the heart may point toward a specific electrophysiologic mechanism.

Diagnostic Risk Stratification

Adolescents with WPW syndrome must be informed of the very small but real chance of sudden death due to extremely high ventricular rates from rapid AV conduction during an episode of atrial fibrillation. Some patients with WPW syndrome can be reassured that they have no risk of this rare catastrophe if the ventricular response to pacing-induced atrial fibrillation is clearly not life-threatening under conditions mimicking exercise-induced catecholamine stress (isoproterenol infusion). Provocative testing can be done as an outpatient procedure with a single, small, venous lead or with a transesophageal pacing wire. WPW patients also have a risk of sudden death that, in patients with structurally normal hearts, has been reported to be in the range of 0.09% to 0.6% per patient year follow-up.

Treatment

Acute Conversion of Sustained Supraventricular Tachycardia

Infants often convert to normal rhythm with application of ice bag to face as a vagal maneuver to block AV nodal conduction

TABLE 28.2

TREATMENT OF SUSTAINED COMMON SUPRAVENTRICULAR TACHYCARDIA

Age	Treatment
Neonate/Infant[a]	Five to 10 second application of large *ice/ice water bag to face* with continuous ECG recording.[b] Adenosine: 0.1–0.2 mg/kg *rapid* i.v. push (use "chaser" of 3–5 ml saline) with continuous ECG recording. Digoxin loading: 15 µg/kg i.v. as first dose (10 µg/kg in premature). See maintenance therapy for follow-up doses. If hemodynamically unstable, do *not* load with digoxin. *Synchronized DC electrical cardioversion* 0.5–1 J/kg. Give lidocaine one mg/kg i.v. pre-DC cardioversion if loaded with digoxin.
Older children	Vagal maneuvers (*carotid sinus massage/Valsalva maneuver*) with continuous ECG recording. Adenosine: 0.1–0.2 mg/kg rapid i.v. push with continuous ECG recording. Maximum single dose 12 mg. Diltiazem (i.v.): 0.25 mg/kg (maximum 20 mg) given over two minutes. Follow with continuous infusion 0.1–0.3 mg/kg/hour (maximum 15 mg/hour). Continuous monitoring required. Esmolol: 500 µg/kg i.v. over one minute, then 50 µg/kg/min. May need to rebolus and increase infusion rate in 50 µg/kg increments every five minutes to maximum of 300 µg/kg. Continuous monitoring for response effect required. Higher infusion rate may be needed in young children. Amiodarone: 5 mg/kg given slowly over 30 minutes as an infusion. Then 5 µg/kg/min. May increase to 10 µg/kg/min. For adult-sized patients, 150 mg over 10 minutes, then 360 mg over six hours, then 540 mg over 18 hours. Continuous ECG monitoring for sinus rate/AV block/QT prolongation needed.

ECG, electrocardiogram; DC, direct current; AV, atrioventricular
[a]i.v. Calcium channel blocking drugs (e.g., *verapamil/diltiazem*) *contraindicated* in neonate and infant.
[b]If ice/drug/DC electrical conversion to sinus is only transient, *ice or adenosine one hour after first digoxin loading dose will often produce sustained conversion.*

and interrupt the reentry circuit (Tables 28.2 and 28.3). Completely covering the face with a large plastic bag filled with crushed ice and water is more effective than ice alone. This can be safely done if the application is less than 6 to 7 seconds. Very brief (2 to 3 seconds) nasal airway compromise may be preferable to prolonged application (30 or more seconds) of an ineffective ice bag when attempts are made to keep the lower half of the infant's face uncovered. Rectal stimulation (e.g., with thermometer) or gagging can convert SVT by vagal stimulation. *Ocular compression is no longer recommended as a vagal maneuver.* Older children should not undergo ice application, although voluntary facial immersion in icewater has sometimes converted SVT. Carotid massage or Valsalva maneuver may cardiovert by vagal block of AV conduction. *Always* record a continuous-running ECG rhythm strip (preferably three leads at least) during these interventions.

Adenosine may also convert AVRT or AVNRT-types of paroxysmal SVT to sinus rhythm through AV node block. AV block will last seconds only. The dosage is 0.1 mg/kg rapid IV push with immediate saline push to flush the adenosine. A second dose of 0.2 mg/kg may be needed.

Atrial flutter will not convert to sinus rhythm with AV node blocking maneuvers or drugs. The ventricular rate may transiently slow, usually to one half the presenting rate as higher-grade AV block is induced. Recording an ECG during this time may establish the diagnosis of flutter. DC electrical cardioversion with 0.5 J/kg will usually establish sustained sinus rhythm. Atrial pacing via transesophageal pacing wire is an alternative.

In older children and adolescents, infusion of a calcium-channel blocker drug (e.g., diltiazem hydrochloride) or beta-blocker infusion (e.g., esmolol hydrochloride) can be used safely to block AV node conduction and convert PSVT to sinus rhythm or slow ventricular response rate in atrial flutter or atrial fibrillation. These should *not* be used in atrial fibril-

lation with WPW syndrome, where electrical cardioversion of this potentially life-threatening arrhythmia is usually the first-line treatment.

Maintenance Therapy

Digoxin may be effective in preventing recurrences of SVT in infants. Infants require 8 to 12 µg/kg (0.008 to 0.012 mg/kg) given daily or divided every 12 hours. Loading with 0.030 mg/kg (30 µ/kg) in divided doses over the first 24 hours can help establish a therapeutic effect earlier. Premature infants may require lower loading doses (0.020 to 0.025 mg/kg). Oral loading is usually effective. Intravenous loading may be needed in compromised infants, but may involve more risk of toxicity if the incorrect dose is given. Give one-half of the total dose followed by one-fourth 8 to 12 hours later and the final one-fourth 8 to 12 hours later.

Beta-blocker drugs are safe and effective maintenance drugs for most forms of SVT, including AVRT with WPW. In infants, propranolol is the best-studied beta-blocker. The usual dose is 1 to 4 mg/kg/day divided every 6 hours. It is available in oral liquid form. In older children, atenolol is the most studied and commonly used beta-blocker. A dose of 0.5 to 2 mg/kg/day divided every 12 hours is used.

Flecainide acetate, a class Ic agent, has been used in children with structurally normal hearts with refractory SVT. Use only with expert consultation due to the risk of sudden death if toxic levels occur related to excessive dose or other pharmacologic interactions.

Sotalol hydrochloride, a class III agent, has been effective in some cases of refractory SVT. It has been used in patients with structurally abnormal hearts. Sotalol hydrochloride–related bradycardia may rarely require concomitant pacemaker treatment. Sotalol hydrochloride should be used in pediatric patients only with expert consultation.

TABLE 28.3

SIDE EFFECTS/INTERACTIONS OF ANTIARRHYTHMIC DRUGS USED IN ACUTE SUPRAVENTRICULAR TACHYCARDIA

Drug	Side effects/interactions
Digoxin	Sinus bradycardia; AV block
Adenosine	Sinus bradycardia; AV block; premature ventricular beats (all transient) Atrial fibrillation (usually transient, but have DC cardioverter available if hemodynamic deterioration results—especially if WPW is present) Bronchospasm, dyspnea, chest pain, dizziness
Diltiazem hydrochloride	Hypotension; sinus bradycardia; AV block Do not use i.v. calcium channel blockers (e.g., diltiazem hydrochloride) in young infants Cautious use if concomitant beta blocker use (additive side effects) Headache, nausea may occur Increases levels of digoxin, beta blockers, fentanyl citrates benzodiazepines
Esmolol hydrochloride	Hypotension; sinus bradycardia; AV block; bronchospasm Increases digoxin level 10%–20%
Amiodarone hydrochloride (i.v.)	Hypotension; sinus bradycardia; AV block Availability of transthoracic external pacing desirable Longer term infusion may increase digoxin, warfarin sodium, calcium channel blockers, fentanyl citrate levels/effects Polymorphic ventricular tachycardia (torsade de pointes) is rare but may occur if coexisting hypokalemia present Adult respiratory distress syndrome reported in adults on high FiO_2 and i.v. amiodarone hydrochloride Hepatic enzyme elevation during high-dose amiodarone hydrochloride infusion Do not exceed two mg/ml concentration in drip unless central line

AV, atrioventricular; WPW, Wolff–Parkinson–White syndrome; FiO_2, inspired oxygen concentration.

Amiodarone hydrochloride, a class III agent, may be effective in refractory SVT with structurally abnormal hearts, but the risk of thyroid, pulmonary, skin, and eye complications mandate use with expert guidance in pediatric patients.

Radiofrequency catheter ablation can permanently treat refractory SVT in children with all forms of SVT except (possibly) atrial fibrillation. Concerns about scar formation in very small hearts limit its use in infants or toddlers. It is an excellent option for the adolescent with WPW and SVT where the potential for dangerous atrial fibrillation is a concern. Success rates for all pediatric arrhythmias reported by the Pediatric Radiofrequency Catheter Ablation Registry improved from 90% in the early era (1991 to 1995) to 95% in a more recent era (1996 to 1999). With the recent advent of electroanatomic and noncontact mapping techniques, higher success rates have been reported.

Among the possible complications of radiofrequency catheter ablation, atrioventricular block is probably the most worrisome. The highest risk of atrioventricular block occurs in ablating septal pathways adjacent to the normal conduction system. Recent studies have shown promising results in treating these high-risk pathways with cryoablation because of its potential for creating selective lesions that allow elimination of a juxta-AV nodal focus while preserving normal atrioventricular conduction.

Pearls and Important Concerns

- Calcium-channel blocking drugs (especially IV) *verapamil hydrochloride or diltiazem hydrochloride should not be given to infants under 1 year of age.* Hypotension and cardiovascular collapse may occur.

- Digoxin should *not* be used as maintenance therapy for SVT in patients with WPW found on ECG during sinus rhythm. Ventricular rate response to atrial fibrillation may be increased by digoxin. Some experts note that this risk may not apply to young infants with SVT and structurally normal hearts. Consultation should be obtained.
- If SVT immediately recurs after transient normalization of heart rate during vagal or adenosine conversion, consider the possibility that the SVT is atrial flutter and the transient "normal rhythm" was actually atrial flutter with a higher degree of AV block. Careful inspection of the ECG tracing taken during the "conversion" of SVT should show this and prevent unnecessary repetition of an ice-bag or adenosine.
- Reentry SVT may convert to normal sinus with an ice-bag or adenosine and then relapse. Multiple conversions are not indicated, effective, or usually necessary. Brief pauses in SVT will usually reestablish a more stable hemodynamic state in an infant. Intravenous digoxin can be given, and within several hours, spontaneous conversions and relapses will be seen prior to a final sustained conversion. In older children or adolescents, a long-lasting AV node blocking drug can be given, such as IV diltiazem hydrochloride. This can be titrated and given as an IV drip to control ventricular response.
- Repeated and prolonged applications of an ice-bag to the face will cause fatty necrosis of the cheeks ("popsicle panniculitis") several days afterward. The infant may be readmitted with misdiagnosis of facial cellulitis. No warmth is present, but a red mass in the buccal area that becomes violaceous and progressively more indurated over several days is seen.
- Adenosine may cause transient atrial fibrillation. WPW cannot be diagnosed during SVT. During PSVT, accessory pathway conduction is retrograde only; there is no anterograde

accessory pathway conduction. Therefore, no delta wave and short PR is apparent until sinus rhythm is established. If a patient has undiagnosed WPW and develops atrial fibrillation after IV adenosine, hypotension and collapse may occur. *Immediate direct current (DC) electrical cardioversion is required if this occurs.* Electrical cardioversion should be available bedside whenever adenosine is used.

WIDE-COMPLEX TACHYARRHYTHMIAS

Definitions

Wide-complex beats or rhythm is a more generalized term than *ventricular beat or rhythm*. Because normal QRS duration is shorter in younger children, QRS duration of 0.09 to 0.10 seconds in an infant is considered wide complex. In older children, QRS width above 0.10 seconds is an abnormally wide complex.

Premature ventricular beats (PVBs or PVCs) or ventricular ectopic beats arise from ventricular myocardium or from the specialized conduction tissues below the AV junction (fascicles) with abnormal QRS morphology and abnormally wide complexes.

Ventricular tachycardia (VT) can be defined as three or more ventricular ectopic beats in sequence. VT can be *sustained* or *nonsustained*, symptomatic or asymptomatic, and *monomorphic* (of one QRS morphology) or *polymorphic*.

Aberrancy is wide-complex QRS morphology of a supraventricular beat. This occurs when there is some conduction problem in the specialized conduction system (drug toxic state, rate-dependent aberrancy, or conduction over an abnormal pathway). Aberrantly conducted beats are not ventricular in origin but are of wide or abnormal morphology.

Clinical Presentations

Frequent PVCs occur in some asymptomatic children with no heart disease. These present with the incidental finding of premature beats on physical examination. These benign PVCs usually have one morphology (*unifocal PVCs*). They often suppress during exercise.

Accelerated ventricular rhythm occurs in children and infants with normal hearts and produces no symptoms. It is usually discovered incidentally when an ECG is done for other reasons. The wide-complex ventricular rhythm may sustain at rates just above the sinus rate when sinus rate is slow and disappears when the sinus rate exceeds the accelerated ventricular rhythm rate (Fig. 28.7). Neonatal forms of this rhythm usually resolve in weeks to months. Rapid hemodynamically unstable ventricular tachycardia is rare but can occur in children or adolescents with structurally normal hearts. Syncope during exercise may be due to *catecholamine-sensitive ventricular tachycardia*. Examples include the ventricular tachycardia of arrhythmogenic right ventricular cardiomyopathy and the polymorphic VT of the long QT syndromes.

Adolescents with repaired tetralogy of Fallot or other important congenital heart lesions may present with syncope or hypotension from rapid ventricular tachycardia.

Chronic, relatively slow ventricular tachycardia can result in a reversible dilated cardiomyopathy called *tachycardia-mediated cardiomyopathy*. This entity was discussed above in the section on supraventricular tachycardias and can also occur with chronic, incessant VT. In the case of incessant ventricular tachycardia with poor cardiac function, it is important to determine if the ventricular tachycardia has *caused* a dilated cardiomyopathy or is the *result of* a primary cardiomyopathy.

Types of Ventricular Tachycardia

Accelerated idioventricular rhythm (also called *nonparoxysmal ventricular tachycardia*) is characterized by ventricular rhythm with rates nearly the same as sinus node rate. It does not require treatment and does not produce symptoms (Fig. 28.7).

Nonsustained monomorphic VT is defined as three beats to 30 seconds of ventricular tachycardia with uniform-morphology wide QRS complexes (Fig. 28.8). *Sustained monomorphic VT* has greater than 30 seconds of ventricular tachycardia with uniform morphology wide QRS complexes.

Polymorphic VT has variable-morphology wide QRS complexes of ventricular origin. It may be sustained or nonsustained (Fig. 28.9).

Torsade de pointes is a polymorphic VT with "twisting of the points," in which QRS polarity is alternately positive then negative. It is often seen in situations where there is preceding long QT interval (Figs. 28.10 and 28.11).

Inducible VT can be monomorphic or polymorphic and sustained or nonsustained. Inducible ventricular tachycardias may be induced by pacing with a programmed electrical ventricular stimulation protocol during electrophysiologic catheter study (EP study).

Etiologies of Ventricular Tachycardia

Idiopathic types are often monomorphic but may be polymorphic. Brief monomorphic VT that suppresses during exercise, is asymptomatic, and is associated with no structural heart disease and normal resting ECG is the most likely VT to be benign.

VT secondary to dilated cardiomyopathy occurs with idiopathic dilated cardiomyopathy or with ischemic cardiomyopathy. In pediatric patients, ischemic dilated cardiomyopathy occurs with congenital anomalous left coronary artery and after Kawasaki disease with coronary aneurysm thrombosis or coronary stenosis.

VT also occurs in patients with hypertrophic cardiomyopathy (HCM). However, not all syncope in HCM is from VT; some can be bradyarrhythmic/neurocardiogenic. Nevertheless, syncope in these patients requires workup for ischemic and nonischemic VT.

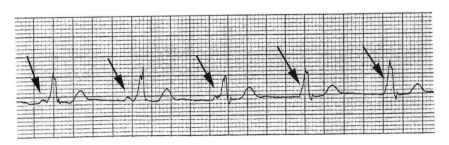

FIGURE 28.7. Accelerated idioventricular rhythm in an adolescent with no symptoms. P-waves (*arrowheads*) at 65–70 beats/min are gradually "lost" in the following wide QRS complexes with a ventricular rate that is slightly faster than the sinus rate. AV dissociation is not due to AV block but to the accelerated ventricular rhythm.

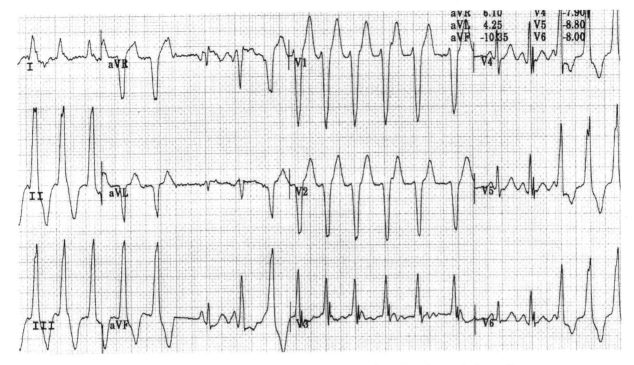

FIGURE 28.8. Monomorphic ventricular tachycardia arising from the right ventricular outflow tract. The morphology resembles sinus beats with left bundle branch block with an inferior QRS axis because of early activation of the superior right ventricle.

Congenital long QT syndromes and Brugada syndrome usually cause polymorphic VT or torsade de pointes. The presentation is often episodic syncope or even brief convulsions. A family history of epilepsy or sudden death may be present.

Drug-induced long QT syndromes can also cause polymorphic VT. Refer to Table 28.4 for a list of drugs associated with prolongation of QT interval.

Arrhythmogenic right ventricular cardiomyopathy (ARVC) or arrhythmogenic right ventricular dysplasia (ARVD) causes ventricular tachycardia arising from the dysplastic area of the right ventricular (RV) myocardium. VT in ARVD is often exercise related, may be monomorphic or polymorphic, and may cause syncope or sudden death in young individuals. It is often familial, but sporadic cases are common.

Idiopathic RV outflow tract VT is a monomorphic VT with left bundle-branch block morphology and positive QRS complexes in inferior leads (II, III, aVF), indicating a focus in the superior right ventricle. Some of these may represent forms of ARVD. Others represent a distinct entity, which can have a benign prognosis or cause syncope (Fig. 28.8).

Catecholamine-sensitive ventricular tachycardia or catecholamine-dependent ventricular tachycardia are terms applied to a polymorphic or "bidirectional" VT (two opposite polarity, wide QRS morphology complexes) that commonly presents as syncope, brief seizure, or sudden death during exercise. This VT can be accompanied by simultaneous JET or atrial tachycardia and is then called "double tachycardia" (Fig. 28.9).

VT in repaired congenital heart disease is most commonly seen in adolescents and young adults with repaired tetralogy of Fallot. It is usually characterized by inducible monomorphic VT with left-bundle branch block morphology and may cause exercise-related sudden death.

Belhassen ventricular tachycardia originates in the area of the left posterior fascicle of the specialized conduction system. Right bundle-branch block morphology with somewhat narrower QRS than other VTs is typical, usually with left axis deviation. Although it is not a type of SVT, this VT will often

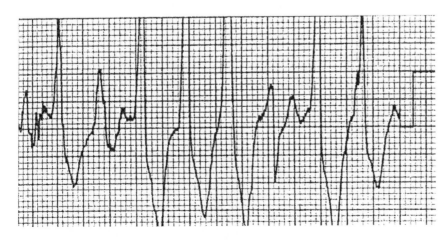

FIGURE 28.9. Exercise-induced, catecholamine-sensitive polymorphic ventricular tachycardia in a child who presented with syncope during intense exercise.

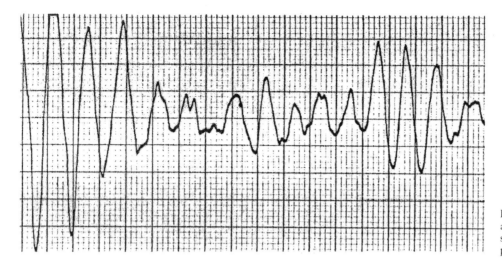

FIGURE 28.10. Torsade de pointes associated with congenital long QT syndromes and other causes of QT prolongation.

convert to sinus rhythm with calcium-channel blocker drugs. Other "fascicular" LV tachycardias may have similar ECG with variable axis.

PVCs or VT can occur in children with myocardial rhabdomyomas. These benign tumors are found in infants with tuberous sclerosis, although most do not result in arrhythmia. Benign LV or RV tumors can be diagnosed with echocardiography. A rare cause of incessant VT is myocardial histiocytic tumor. This may present as infantile sudden death or near sudden death.

Establishing a Diagnosis of a Wide-Complex Tachycardia

In a child, sustained wide-complex arrhythmia is probably ventricular tachycardia, but always consider severe hyperkalemia in the differential diagnosis of wide-complex tachycardia (see below). Other nonventricular, aberrant complex rhythms should also be considered. If sinus P-waves can be seen in the ECG that are unrelated to the wide QRS complexes and if the QRS rate is faster than the P-wave rate (AV dissociation), then ventricular tachycardia rather than aberrant conduction of SVT or sinus tachycardia is likely (Fig. 28.12).

During sinus rhythm, the ECG should be inspected for abnormal prolongation of the corrected QT interval to exclude long QT syndrome; other abnormalities in the QRS, ST, and T-complexes may provide clues to predilections toward ventricular tachyarrhythmia, such as ECG evidence of cardiomyopathy (Table 28.5).

Acute Treatment of Ventricular Tachycardia

Nonsustained ventricular tachycardia or accelerated ventricular rhythm may need no treatment (e.g., accelerated ventricular rhythm of the newborn). Benign premature ventricular beats require no treatment or activity restriction.

Severely symptomatic ventricular tachycardia with collapse should be treated with immediate DC cardioversion 1 to 2 J/kg

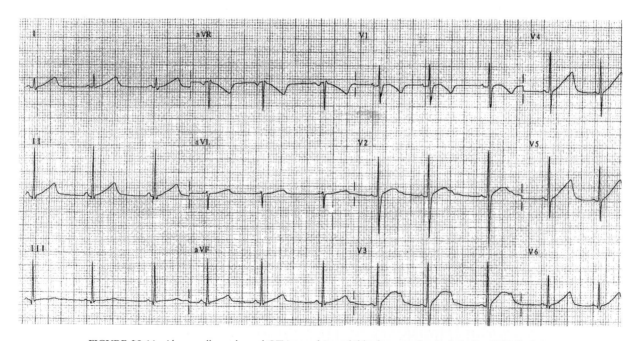

FIGURE 28.11. Abnormally prolonged QT interval in a child whose mother had similar ECG findings and who had seizures and syncopal spells due to torsade de pointes.

TABLE 28.4

DRUGS ASSOCIATED WITH PROLONGATION OF QT OR TORSADES[a]

Classification	Drug
Class Ia antiarrhythmic drugs	Quinidine, procainamide hydrochloride, disopyramide phosphate
Class Ic antiarrhythmic drugs	Flecainide acetate
Class III antiarrhythmic drugs	Sotalol hydrochloride, amiodarone hydrochloride, dofetilide
Antibiotics	Clarithromycin, erythromycin, sparfloxacin, levofloxacin, moxifloxacin hydrochloride
Other anti-infectives	Halofantrine, pentamidine
Antipsychotic agents	Haloperidol, chlorpromazine hydrochloride, thioridazine hydrochloride, pimozide, risperidone, quetiapine fumerate
Antireflux agents	Cisapride
Tricyclic antidepressants	Imipramine hydrochloride, desipramine hydrochloride, doxepin hydrochloride
SSRI antidepressants (association is not clear)	Fluoxetine hydrochloride, sertraline hydrochloride, paroxetine hydrochloride
Other antidepressants	Venlafaxine hydrochloride, ziprasidone
Antimigraine agents	Zolmitriptan, sumatriptan, naratriptan hydrochloride
Antiepileptics	Fosphenytoin sodium, felbamate
Antihypertensives	Isradipine, nicardipine, indapamide
Lipid lowering agents	Probucol
Immunosuppressives	Tacrolimus
Antinausea drugs	Dolasetron mesylate

[a]Prolongation of QT or torsade in FDA labeling. List may not be fully inclusive.
Note: Antifungal thiazole drugs: itraconazole, ketoconazole, fluconazole, etc. generally inhibit cytochrome P 450 3A4 and can increase levels of some drugs that cause prolonged QT (e.g., quetiapine fumerate, cisapride). Knowledge of drug metabolism/interactions is required to prevent drug-induced torsades.
Note: Hypokalemia may be an important contributing cause in some cases of drug-induced torsade de pointes. Electrolyte imbalance should be avoided when using any drug that prolongs QT interval.
SSRI, selective seratonin reuptake inhibitor.

(synchronized if ventricular tracking can be achieved). Repetitive episodes of severely symptomatic ventricular tachycardia may improve with lidocaine. Note that for adult patients, the 2001 Advanced Cardiac Life Support (ACLS) Guidelines of the American Heart Association now recommend IV amiodarone rather than lidocaine for severe ventricular tachycardia/ventricular fibrillation that is refractory to simple electrical cardioversion (Table 28.6).

Treatment of Chronic Ventricular Tachycardia

Beta-blocker drugs are occasionally very effective in some catecholamine-dependent ventricular arrhythmias that are serious enough to need treatment (long QT syndromes, catecholamine-dependent ventricular tachycardia).

Large clinical trials of antiarrhythmic drugs in adults with ischemic heart disease raised significant concerns that many antiarrhythmic drugs have excessive proarrhythmic potential. Mortality was higher with antiarrhythmic drug treatment than without for asymptomatic or minimally symptomatic ventricular ectopy and VT in patients with ischemic heart disease. This has led to significant increase in nonpharmacologic treatment of life-threatening arrhythmias with ICDs (implantable cardiac defibrillators). In children and adolescents, the roles and indications for ICDs, second- or third-tier antiarrhythmic drugs (e.g., sotalol hydrochloride, amiodarone hydrochloride), and catheter radiofrequency ablation

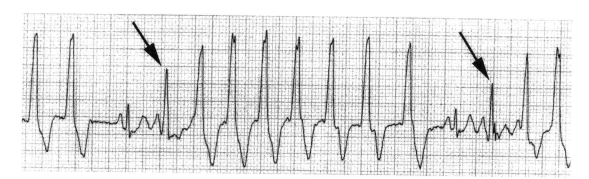

FIGURE 28.12. Fusion beats are indicated by arrows at initiation of brief runs of ventricular tachycardia. The intermediate-width QRS complexes represent partial depolarization of the ventricle from conduction of the sinus beat through the AV node and partial depolarization by the ventricular ectopic focus.

TABLE 28.5.

DIFFERENTIAL DIAGNOSIS OF WIDE QRS COMPLEX TACHYCARDIA

Rhythm	Diagnosis
Dissociation of P waves from wide QRS complexes	Ventricular tachycardia (VT) Junctional ectopic tachycardia (JET) with preexisting bundle branch block
One-to-one relationship of P waves with wide QRS complexes	Sinus tachycardia or with preexisting bundle branch block; normal P precedes QRS Sinus tachycardia with "toxic" intraventricular conduction delay (e.g., severe hyperkalemia, acute myocarditis); P precedes QRS, but often low amplitude SVT (AV reentry type) with preexisting bundle branch block; P follows QRS in ST segment[a] SVT (AV reentry type) with rate dependent aberrant intraventricular conduction; P follows QRS in ST segment VT with one-to-one ventriculoatrial retrograde conduction[a] Atrial ectopic tachycardia or atrial tachycardia with rate-dependent aberrant intraventricular conduction or with preexisting bundle branch block; P wave with abnormal P axis precedes wide QRS complexes
Wide QRS complex regular rate tachycardia with no visible P waves	VT with no visible P waves (dissociated or one-to-one retrograde conduction) SVT (AV node reentry type) with rate-dependent aberrant intraventricular conduction or with preexisting bundle branch block
Wide QRS complex irregular rate tachycardia with no visible P waves	Atrial fibrillation with Wolff–Parkinson–White syndrome Polymorphic ventricular tachycardias (e.g., congenital long QT syndromes, drug-induced long QT VT, severe CNS trauma/hemorrhage, myocarditis)

[a]If patient has had prior surgical repair of tetralogy of Fallot, and QRS morphology is left bundle branch block type, consider VT. If RBBB-type morphology, consider SVT with preexisting RBBB after tetralogy repair.

TABLE 28.6.

TREATMENT RECOMMENDATIONS FOR PULSELESS VENTRICULAR TACHYCARDIA/ VENTRICULAR FIBRILLATION

1) *DC electrical cardioversion/defibrillation*—two j/kg. Repeat twice at four j/kg if no response.
2) *Epinephrine i.v. (or i.o.)*—0.01 mg/kg (0.1 ml/kg of 1:10,000). Alternative of tracheal tube epinephrine 0.1 mg/kg (0.1 ml/kg of 1:1000).
3) *Repeat electrical defibrillation*—four j/kg within 30–60 sec.
4) *Amiodarone hydrochloride*—five mg/kg i.v./i.o. bolus; OR *Lidocaine*—one mg/kg i.v./i.o./tracheal bolus; OR *Magnesium*—25–50 mg/kg i.v./i.o. (if VT is polymorphic, torsades de pointes, or if hypomagnesemia present).
5) *Repeat electrical defibrillation*—four j/kg within 30–60 sec. of each medication. Continue pattern of CPR—drug—shock OR CPR—drug—shock—shock—shock.
6) *Do not use defibrillator or above antiarrhythmics if asystole is clearly documented* or pulseless bradyarrhythmia. Proceed with CPR—epinephrine.

If *ventricular tachycardia with pulse but poor perfusion*: Follow attempt at electrical cardioversion (one J/kg) with amiodarone hydrochloride five mg/kg i.v. over 30 min. OR procainamide hydrochloride 15 mg/kg i.v. over 30–60 min. OR lidocaine 1 mg/kg i.v. bolus.

of ventricular arrhythmia focus all continue to evolve and change.

ICD treatment may serve as a bridge to transplantation for pediatric patients awaiting orthotopic heart transplantation for dilated cardiomyopathy or for end-stage CHF with congenital heart disease. Hypertrophic cardiomyopathy with a strong family history of young sudden death has also been used as an indication to consider ICD treatment. Another indication for ICD implantation may be the adolescent or young adult with repaired tetralogy of Fallot who has episodic, sustained rapid ventricular tachycardia. Radiofrequency catheter ablation for ventricular tachycardia has been most successful with focal origin tachycardias without primary diffuse cardiomyopathy, including RV outflow tract tachycardia and Bellhassen tachycardia. When secondary cardiomyopathy is caused by one of these types of ventricular tachycardias, radiofrequency ablation by catheter can be very effective.

Pearls and Special Concerns

- *Severe hyperkalemia in children can cause wide QRS rhythm that is often confused with ventricular tachycardia.* Wide complexes are due to conduction delay in the myocardium secondary to loss of transmembrane potential, not due to primary ventricular arrhythmia. T-waves are *not* peaked at these potassium levels (K^+ of 9 to 11). DC cardioversion or antiarrhythmic drugs are of no value. Usual presentation is poor perfusion, shock, and distant heart tones from electromechanical dissociation. *A useful clue is that the wide-complex rhythm is at a rate that would not be fast enough to*

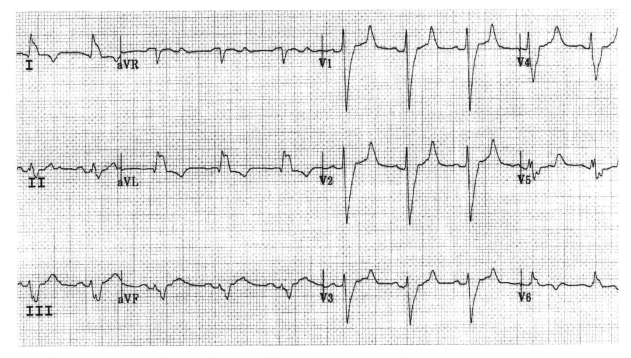

FIGURE 28.13. Hyperkalemia. Second-degree (2:1) AV block and extremely wide QRS complexes in a neonate with serum K$^+$ of 11 mEq/L. The sinus rate is 150 beats/minute with every other P-wave nonconducted because of the effect of hyperkalemia on AV conduction. QRS complexes are not of ventricular origin and are wide from the effects of hyperkalemia on the conduction system.

cause collapse if it were ventricular tachycardia (140 to 180 beats/minute). Intravenous calcium chloride or calcium gluconate will immediately narrow the QRS complexes, restore transmembrane potential, and reverse shock and collapse (Fig. 28.13).

■ Severe overdose of any tricyclic antidepressant (TCA) drug can result in an in-hospital cardiac arrest hours after admission for early symptoms of obtundation, seizures, or vomiting. The cardiac rhythm of TCA overdose is a pulseless, wide-complex rhythm that may not be responsive to DC cardioversion or any antiarrhythmic drug (the wide complex may not be due to ventricular arrhythmia but to myocardial conduction delay from cardiac toxicity). If cardioversion with and without lidocaine treatment has no effect, consider this possibility. Effective CPR has resulted in normal neurologic outcomes in TCA overdose, even when continued for periods of hours until the pulseless, wide-complex rhythm has resolved. Twelve to 24-hour use of extracorporeal-membrane oxygenation (ECMO) or ventricular assist devices (VADs) has also allowed for transition from prolonged CPR to cardiopulmonary bypass with good results.

BRADYARRHYTHMIAS

Definitions

AV block is abnormally decreased conduction from atria to ventricles through the normal AV node and/or bundle of His and specialized conduction tissues. *First-degree AV block* is an abnormally long PR with all P-waves conducted. *Second-degree AV block* is diagnosed when some but not all P-waves conducted. *Third-degree (complete) AV block* is present when no P-waves are conducted (Figs. 28.14 and 28.15).

Escape rhythm refers to an underlying rhythm that is unmasked by the failure of impulse initiation or conduction from above (e.g., junction escape rhythm unmasked by sinus bradycardia or junctional escape rhythm unmasked by lack of conduction of sinus P-waves to the ventricle in AV node block).

Sick sinus syndrome refers to abnormal sinus node function, usually bradycardic or sometimes with atrial tachyarrhythmias, occurring episodically in a patient with bradyarrhythmia.

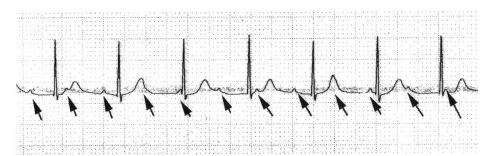

FIGURE 28.14. Congenital complete AV block in a neonate. Arrows indicate sinus P-waves at 165 beats/min. Escape rhythm is junctional (narrow complex) at 90 beats/min in this newborn. Some neonates have much slower junctional escape rates, necessitating pacemaker treatment.

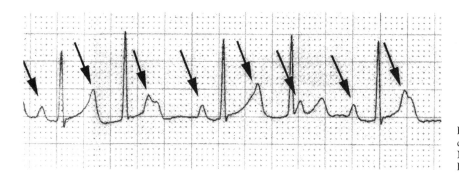

FIGURE 28.15. Wenckebach-type second-degree AV block. Arrows indicate P-waves. Note increasing PR interval with nonconducted P-wave after the conducted beats.

Clinical Presentation

AV block in an otherwise normal child is usually congenital. Congenital AV block may or may not cause complete (third-degree) AV block at birth. Presentation may be in infancy or even in late childhood or adolescence when an inappropriately slow heart rate is discovered. Exercise intolerance or syncope may occur if the (junctional) escape rhythm is too slow. Congenital AV block in the fetus may cause fetal demise or hydrops fetalis at birth (Fig. 28.14).

Childhood myocarditis may present as syncope or brief seizures due to cardiac arrest from paroxysmal complete AV block with no escape rhythm. Patients with congenital heart disease may develop paroxysmal complete AV block years after surgical repair and present with syncope or brief seizures (Figs. 28.16 and 28.17).

Sick sinus syndrome may be an early or late complication of atrial surgery for complex congenital heart disease (e.g., Fontan operation for single ventricle hearts or Mustard operation for transposition of the great vessels). Patients present with abnormally slow sinus rhythm or slow, nonsinus baseline rhythm (e.g., junctional rhythm). They may have episodes of a rapid atrial tachycardia type of SVT (so-called "brady-tachy syndrome"). Symptomatic palpitations may alternate with syncope or bradycardia-related fatigue.

Diagnosis

Complete heart block will result in a slow heart rate with cannon A-waves visible in the neck (atrium contracting during ventricular systole) and marked variation in intensity of the first heart sound. Both are due to AV dissociation with atrial rate faster than the junctional escape rhythm. ECG should show that the P-waves are unrelated to the QRS complexes and at a faster rate. QRS morphology should be narrow and normal with typical junctional escape rhythm found in congenital heart block (Fig. 28.14).

Sick sinus syndrome may be more obvious from inspection of a 24-hour ambulatory (Holter) ECG monitor. Thirty-day ECG event recorders may be needed to capture the bradycardia-related symptomatic event (syncope or presyncope) in an at-risk child/adolescent.

Treatment

Pacemaker therapy issues are listed in Tables 28.7A and B to 28.9.

Permanent pacemaker treatment is the mainstay for recurrent or permanent bradyarrhythmia. Its use depends on the rate and mechanism of the escape rhythm in AV block, or on the etiology of bradycardia and the bradycardia rate in other conditions.

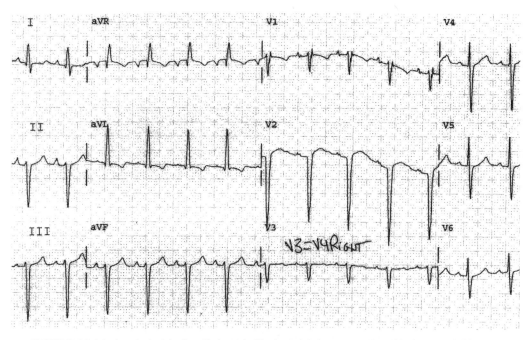

FIGURE 28.16. Atypical right bundle-branch block and left anterior hemiblock in a child with myocarditis. Left axis deviation suggests left anterior fascicle disease in addition to abnormal conduction in the right bundle. Increasing QRS duration in this child was followed by periods of complete AV block causing syncope.

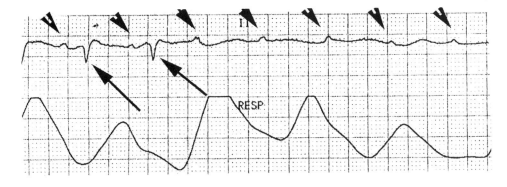

FIGURE 28.17. Prolonged asystole from paroxysmal complete AV block without escape rhythm causes a brief convulsion in the child illustrated in Fig. 28.16. Two conducted wide QRS complexes (*arrows*) are followed by nonconducted P-waves (*arrowheads*) with no escape rhythm.

TABLE 28.7A

RECOMMENDATIONS FOR PERMANENT PACING IN CHILDREN, ADOLESCENTS, AND PATIENTS WITH CONGENITAL HEART DISEASE

CLASS I
1. Advanced second- or third-degree AV block associated with symptomatic bradycardia, ventricular dysfunction, or low cardiac output.
2. Sinus node dysfunction with correlation of symptoms during age-inappropriate bradycardia. The definition of bradycardia varies with the patient's age and expected heart rate.
3. Postoperative advanced second- or third-degree AV block that is not expected to resolve or persists at least 7 days after cardiac surgery.
4. Congenital third-degree AV block with a wide QRS escape rhythm, complex ventricular ectopy, or ventricular dysfunction.
5. Congenital third-degree AV block in the infant with a ventricular rate less than 50 to 55 bpm or with congenital heart disease and a ventricular rate less than 70 bpm.
6. Sustained pause-dependent VT, with or without prolonged QT, in which the efficacy of pacing is thoroughly documented.

CLASS IIA
1. Bradycardia-tachycardia syndrome with the need for long-term antiarrhythmic treatment other than digitalis.
2. Congenital third-degree AV block beyond the first year of life with an average heart rate less than 50 bpm, abrupt pauses in ventricular rate that are two or three times the basic cycle length, or associated with symptoms due to chronotropic incompetence.
3. Long-QT syndrome with 2:1 AV or third-degree AV block.
4. Asymptomatic sinus bradycardia in the child with complex congenital heart disease with resting heart rate less than 40 bpm or pauses in ventricular rate more than 3 seconds.
5. Patients with congenital heart disease and impaired hemodynamics due to sinus bradycardia or loss of AV synchrony.

CLASS IIB
1. Transient postoperative third-degree AV block that reverts to sinus rhythm with residual bifascicular block.
2. Congenital third-degree AV block in the asymptomatic infant, child, adolescent, or young adult with an acceptable rate, narrow QRS complex, and normal ventricular function.
3. Asymptomatic sinus bradycardia in the adolescent with congenital heart disease with resting heart rate less than 40 bpm or pauses in ventricular rate more than 3 seconds.
4. Neuromuscular diseases with any degree of AV block (including first-degree AV block), with or without symptoms, because there may be unpredictable progression of AV conduction disease.

CLASS III
1. Transient postoperative AV block with return of normal AV conduction.
2. Asymptomatic postoperative bifascicular block with or without first-degree AV block.
3. Asymptomatic type I second-degree AV block.
4. Asymptomatic sinus bradycardia in the adolescent with longest RR interval less than 3 seconds and minimum heart rate more than 40 bpm.

TABLE 28.7B

DEFINITIONS OF CLASSIFICATIONS OF EVIDENCE FOR RECOMMEDATIONS TO IMPLANT PACEMAKERS

Class I: Conditions for which there is evidence and/or general agreement that a given procedure or treatment is useful and effective.

Class II: Conditions for which there is conflicting evidence and/or a divergence of opinion about the usefulness/efficacy of a procedure or treatment.
  IIa: Weight of evidence/opinion is in favor of usefulness/efficacy.
  IIb: Usefulness/efficacy is less well established by evidence/opinion.

Class III: Conditions for which there is evidence and/or general agreement that the procedure/treatment is not useful/effective and in some cases may be harmful.

TABLE 28.8

PACEMAKERS IN CHILDREN: TECHNICAL CONCEPTS

Technical aspect	Concept or common indications
Epicardial leads (transthoracic)	Newborns/infants with congenital heart block (inadequate SVC size)
	Patients with right to left intracardiac shunting (systemic embolism concerns)
	Complex congenital heart disease with no SVC route to desired atrium or ventricle
Endocardial leads (transvenous)	Lower lead thresholds may allow lower pacemaker current output and longer generator life
	Lead failure rates are lower than for epicardial leads
	Bipolar sensing capability from single ventricular lead or atrial lead is less sensitive to inappropriate sensing of muscle or other far field artifact when unipolar sensing is used with epicardial single leads
VVI pacing mode—(V)entricular pacing, (V)entricular sensing, (I)nhibition of ventricular pacing	Single chamber demand pacing of ventricle only
	Usually used for small infant with congenital AV block (requires only patients one lead)
	Lack of atrial contribution to cardiac output (AV dissociation)
AAI pacing mode—(A)trial pacing, (A)trial sensing, (I)nhibition of atrial pacing	Single chamber demand pacing of atrium only
	Requires normal AV node function
	Usually for sick sinus syndrome
	May help prevent atrial flutter or atrial tachycardia in patient with otherwise extreme sinus bradycardia (tachy-brady syndrome)
DDD pacing mode—(D)ual chamber pacing, (D)ual chamber sensing, (D)ual function with inhibition of pacing of either chamber and ventricular pacing triggered by sensing native atrial activity	Can track atrial rate and pace ventricle with appropriate AV delay in with complete AV block (most physiologic type of pacing)
Mode switching	Algorithm that detects high atrial rate is likely due to SVT and not exercise-induced sinus tachycardia
	DDD pacing reverts to VVI pacing at a preprogrammed rate to avoid rapid ventricular rate in response to the atrial arrhythmia
Rate responsive pacemakers—VVIR, AAIR, DDDR	"R" refers to "rate response" mode; piezoelectric or accelerometer activity sensor within the generator allows pacing at a rate appropriate to patient's level of exercise
	Usually required only in older children with inappropriately low atrial rates during exercise

SVC, superior vena cava.

TABLE 28.9

PACEMAKERS: PRECAUTIONS IN HOSPITAL OR AFTER DISCHARGE

Procedure or activity	Risk and precautions
Magnetic resonance imaging	MRI magnetic and radiofrequency fields can result in unpredictable reprogramming of pacemaker; rarely could be life-threatening MRI generally considered contraindicated in pacemaker patients
Electrocautery during surgical procedures	Improper use could damage pacemaker Improper use rarely can cause myocardial damage During proper use, temporary inhibition of pacing may occur Reprogram to VOO mode (ventricular pacing without inhibition enabled) during the surgery to avoid inhibition of pacing in patients who are pacemaker dependent Place ground contact plate where current will not travel though pacemaker or leads Do not use electrocautery closer than 15 cm from pacing system
Electrical cardioversion/defibrillation	Place paddles or pads for electrical cardioversion so that current will not pass through the generator External programmer available to interrogate/reprogram pacemaker after cardioversion (not essential when lifesaving defibrillation urgently required)
Radiotherapy	May damage some pacemakers if high doses are directed at the pulse generator Consultation with pacemaker engineer and limitation of direct radiation to pacemaker Diagnostic radiation not a risk
Diagnostic radiation-cellular phones	Cellular phones in normal use proximity, no significant risk Diagnostic ultrasound, not a significant risk
Diagnostic ultrasound contact sports	Contact sports prescribed to prevent lead fracture/damage

Pacemakers may become necessary in some patients with sick sinus syndrome when antiarrhythmic drugs are used to treat the tachyarrhythmia. This is especially a concern with structural heart disease, such as repaired complex congenital heart disease.

Sudden symptomatic bradyarrhythmia may respond to isoproterenol hydrochloride (0.01 to 0.10 µg/kg/min) while preparing for transvenous pacing. Noninvasive transthoracic pacing can be performed in children, but is a very temporary solution because of the significant discomfort associated with this form of ventricular pacing. Temporary transvenous pacing is the most effective (and comfortable) support in patients who will require permanent pacing with serious bradyarrhythmia. Temporary pacemaker output should be set above the "capture threshold," with a 2:1 safety margin (i.e., at twice the minimum pulse width or amplitude that reliably paces).

Sensing thresholds should be tested if the underlying non-paced rhythm may increase to the point that pacing will not be necessary and would compete with the patient's rhythm. The sensing function is set so that the native rhythm is reliably sensed. See Table 28.10 for Pacemaker Pacing modes.

Pearls

- Infants with congenital heart block are often said to have neonatal lupus syndrome. Conduction system damage is due to transplacental transfer of maternal antibodies during the pregnancy of the SS-A and SS-B type. In fact, the majority of mothers of such infants do not have clinical systemic lupus erythematosus (SLE), but may have or later develop a more subtle autoimmune disorder with clinical features more like Sjögren syndrome than SLE.

TABLE 28.10

PACEMAKER PACING MODES

Chamber paced (1st letter)	Chamber sensed (2nd letter)	Response to sensed beat (3rd letter)	Programmability rate modulated (4th letter)	Antitachycardia functions (5th letter)
V	V	T	R	P
A	A	I	O	O
D	D	D	C	S
O	O	O		D

V, ventricle; A, atrium; D, dual; O, none; T, trigger; I, inhibit; R, rate modulation; C, communicating; P, pacing (antiarrhythmia); S, shock.

Suggested Readings

Ammirati F, Colivicchi F, Santini M, et al. Permanent cardiac pacing versus medical treatment for the prevention of recurrent vasovagal syncope: a multicenter, randomized controlled trial. *Circulation* 2001;104:52–57.

Batra AS, Balaji S, Sahn D. Management of pediatric tachyarrhythmias in 2005: is ablation salvation? *JACC Rev* 2005:14;69–71.

Blomstrom-Lundqvist C, Scheinman MM, et al. ACC/AHA/ESC guidelines for the management of patients with supraventricular arrhythmias—executive summary. *J Am Coll Cardiol* 2003;42:1493–1521.

Case CL. Diagnosis and treatment of pediatric arrhythmias. *Pediatr Clin North Am* 1999;46:347–354.

Dunnigan A, Benson DW, Benditt DG. Atrial flutter in infancy: diagnosis, clinical features, and treatment. *Pediatrics* 1985;75:725–729.

Jaeggi ET, Hamilton RM, Silverman ED, et al. Outcome of children with fetal, neonatal, or childhood diagnosis of isolated congenital atrioventricular block. *J Am Coll Cardiol* 2002;39:130.

Kanter JR. Pediatric electrophysiology. *Curr Opin Cardiol* 1993;8:119–127. Review.

Kirsh JA, Gross GJ, O'Connor S, Hamilton RM. Transcatheter cryoablation of tachyarrhythmias in children: initial experience from an international registry. *J Am Coll Cardiol* 2005;45:133–136.

Kugler JD, Danford DA. Management of infants, children, and adolescents with paroxysmal supraventricular tachycardia. *J Pediatr* 1996;129: 324–338.

Kugler J, Danford D, Deal B, et al. Radiofrequency catheter ablation for tachyarrhythmias in children and adolescents. *N Engl J Med* 1994;330:1481–1487.

Schwartz PJ, Moss AJ, Vincent GM, et al. Diagnostic criteria for the long QT syndrome: an update. *Circulation* 1993;88:782.

Yabek SM. Ventricular arrhythmias in children with an apparently normal heart. *J Pediatr* 1991;119:1.

CHAPTER 29 ■ CONGENITAL HEART DISEASE

DAVID W. HANNON AND R. DENNIS STEED

Children with congenital heart disease require admission to a hospital more frequently than healthy children. They can be more susceptible to complications from common childhood illnesses. One such example is respiratory compromise in a child with respiratory syncytial virus (RSV) infection and a large left-to-right shunt from an unrepaired ventricular septal defect or patent ductus arteriosus. Another example is worsening cyanosis in a child with single ventricle who had a bidirectional Glenn shunt with dehydration from a gastrointestinal virus. Furthermore, treatments for common childhood illnesses requiring hospitalization are more likely to cause complications in children with heart disease. Intravenous fluids must be carefully managed to prevent fluid overload and pulmonary edema in children with congestive heart failure. Children with cyanotic congenital heart disease must have special care taken to ensure that air or clots cannot be introduced through intravenous lines because of the possibility of systemic embolism when right-to-left shunting of blood exists.

Other pitfalls exist for the hospitalized child with congenital heart disease. The signs and symptoms of decompensated cardiac status in children with previously diagnosed congenital heart disease may be confused with those of an unrelated childhood illness. An example is the presentation of severe heart failure as vomiting and anorexia. Some children with previously undiagnosed congenital heart disease may also be hospitalized with complications of the cardiac defect that are confused with another serious illness. The exemplar is the 1-month-old with a critical coarctation of the aorta diagnosed as having septic shock rather than congenital heart disease with profound cardiogenic shock.

Finally, children who are convalescing from surgical repair of congenital heart disease may not only be more susceptible to noncardiac illness but may have important complications of cardiac surgery that suggest noncardiac illness. An important example is the frequent presentation of cardiac tamponade from postpericardiotomy syndrome as abdominal pain and vomiting rather than the expected chest pain usually suggestive of pericarditis.

To avoid such problems the hospital physician needs to be familiar with the basic types of congenital heart diseases, the hemodynamic perturbations that they cause, and the signs and symptoms of those perturbations.

LESIONS CAUSING LEFT-TO-RIGHT SHUNTING

Ventricular Septal Defect and Patent Ductus Arteriosus

Ventricular septal defect (VSD) and patent ductus arteriosus (PDA) result in a volume overload of the left ventricle (LV).

The right ventricle (RV) is not volume overloaded with VSD because preload to the ventricle is a diastolic event and the shunting of blood from LV to the RV takes place during systole when the ventricles are emptying. The excess blood flow to the pulmonary vascular bed in patients with either VSD or PDA must return to the left atrium and then to the LV during diastolic filling. As pulmonary vascular resistance falls in the first weeks and months of life, the amount of excess pulmonary blood flow and excess left ventricular diastolic preload increase (Fig. 29.1). Enlargement of the LV may be apparent on physical exam as a left ventricular heave on precordial palpation. In addition to the expected holosystolic murmur of the shunting of blood through the VSD, or continuous murmur of shunting of blood through the PDA, the excess return to the LV may cause a low-pitched diastolic murmur or so-called "diastolic rumble." Signs and symptoms of "congestive heart failure" are related not to poor systolic contraction of the ventricle but to the pulmonary overcirculation and the diastolic LV overload. These infants often have tachypnea due to pulmonary overcirculation. Sinus tachycardia and sweating are seen due to increased plasma catecholamines. Increased caloric expenditure from the increased volume work of the LV and tachypnea can cause failure to thrive. This symptoms complex can mimic pulmonary disease or be complicated by common pulmonary infections. Fluid retention is promoted by activation of the renin-angiotensin-aldosterone cascade and worsens pulmonary symptoms.

Atrial Septal Defect

Atrial septal defect (ASD) results in volume overload of the RV (Fig. 29.2). The left-to-right shunt of oxygenated blood across the atrial defect results in pulmonary overcirculation, often to the same degree as with a significant VSD but almost never with the same degree of symptoms. This presumably is due to less activation of the neurohumoral cascade of "congestive heart failure" by right-ventricular volume overload than with left-ventricular volume overload. To some extent the absence of any excess pressure increase in the pulmonary vascular bed also mitigates symptoms from the left-to-right shunt. During the first year of life, many infants have small to moderate-sized defects in the secundum atrial septum that are not of any consequence. No untoward consequence occurs from lack of diagnosis of these defects in the young infant. The physical findings of significant ASD in older infants and children are right ventricular lift on precordial palpation, ejection murmur over the pulmonary artery (often subtle), and fixed splitting of the second heart sound due to the constant volume overload of the RV. Endocarditis prophylaxis is not required when procedures that produce bacteremia are performed in patients with isolated secundum ASD. Closure of secundum ASD by surgery or catheter occlusion devices is recommended in children but not

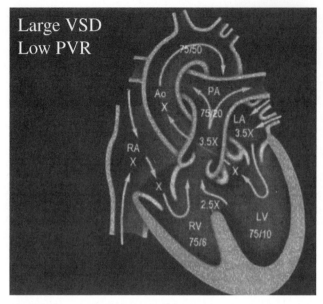

FIGURE 29.1. Large ventricular septal defect (VSD) and low pulmonary vascular resistance (PVR).

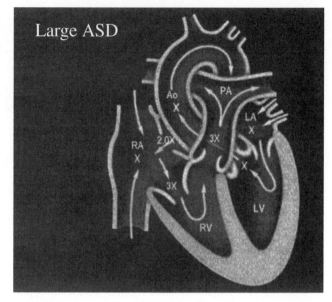

FIGURE 29.2. Large atrial septal defect (ASD).

in young infants. This approach ensures the best chance for good right ventricular function in late adult life but allows for the significant chance that moderate-sized defects found in young infants will close spontaneously.

Atrioventricular Septal Defect

Atrioventricular septal defect (AVSD) is sometimes called endocardial cushion defect or atrioventricular canal defect. In complete atrioventricular (AV) septal defects, the normal separation of the mitral and tricuspid components of the AV valve tissue does not occur, and there is a defect in the atrial septal above this common AV valve and a defect in the ventricular septal defect below it. Partial AV septal defects or ostium primum atrial septal defects have no shunting of blood at the ventricular level and are functionally similar to secundum atrial septal defect, with the important exception that there is often regurgitation of the left AV valve through a "cleft" mitral valve. A blowing systolic murmur that begins with S1 may be heard at the apex and left axilla. In children with complete AV septal defects, signs of a large left-to-right shunt at the ventricular level predominate. However, the large atrial shunt and the presence of pulmonary hypertension from the very large VSD often result in biventricular overload. Symptoms of "congestive heart failure" occur unless there is persistence of marked elevation of pulmonary arterial resistance that can impede the degree of left-to-right shunt. Most children with isolated complete AV septal defect have Down syndrome.

Management

Symptomatic VSD and PDA should be closed. Surgical closure of VSD can be safely performed at any age, but a trial of medical management is sometimes given if there is evidence the defect may decrease in size over time. PDA is closed surgically in small symptomatic infants. In older infants and children, closure of PDA is most commonly performed with coil or occluder device embolization in the catheterization lab. Medical treatment of "congestive heart failure" (CHF) from large left-to-right shunts usually includes diuretics to alleviate pulmonary and systemic venous congestion, digoxin, and sometimes angiotensin-converting enzyme inhibitors

(ACE inhibitors). The role of digoxin has been questioned, as poor contractile function of the enlarged left ventricle is only rarely present. However, digoxin may confer some benefits related to its vagotonic effects. Sympathetic excess is an important part of the pathophysiology of the symptoms of CHF in these infants. Spironolactone, a potassium-sparing diuretic, may also blunt sympathetic excess as it inhibits cardiac extraction of aldosterone. Attention to maximizing caloric intake is a crucial component in managing these infants. Some require nasogastric feeding while awaiting surgical treatment (Table 29.1).

Pearls

- Children with Down syndrome have a high incidence of AVSD, VSD, and ASD. Large ventricular defects especially with AVSD may not be associated with any significant systolic murmur. Elevated pulmonary vascular resistance may prevent left-to-right shunt to the degree that symptoms and murmur are absent. The second heart sound should be abnormally loud. If untreated, such defects ultimately produce irreversible pulmonary hypertension, cyanosis, and premature death. All children with Down syndrome should have cardiologic evaluation.
- Neonates with Down syndrome have an excessive incidence of primary pulmonary hypertension of the neonate (PPHN) and are over-represented in larger series of infants who require extracorporeal membrane oxygen support (ECMO). This occurs independently of traditional risk factors for PPHN such as sepsis, birth asphyxia, or meconium aspiration. Neonatal cyanosis in any infant with Down syndrome suggests the possibility of dangerous pulmonary hypertension even if the first day of life is uneventful. This complication occurs with and without ventricular and atrial septal defects and is not due to the ventricular defect but to the excessive vasoconstriction in the pulmonary vascular bed.
- CHF in the first 2 weeks of life in an infant with VSD should suggest possibility of a secondary lesion, especially coarctation of aorta.
- A superior axis in the limb leads of the electrocardiogram (ECG) suggests an AV septal defect in an infant with exam suggesting VSD or ASD.

TABLE 29.1

DRUGS USED FOR CONGESTIVE HEART FAILURE IN INFANTS WITH CONGENITAL HEART DISEASE

Drug and dose	Mechanism	Side effects	Important interactions/ Special concerns
Digoxin 8–12 μg/kg/day (PO)	Inotropy. Vagotonic effect may decrease sympathetic excess symptoms.	Nausea and vomiting. Poor feeding. Rare with trough levels less than 2 to 2.5 ng/dL. CHF may improve with low therapeutic level.	Use with caution or do not use in WPW syndrome or with AV block. Toxicity with impaired renal function. Spironolactone or ibuprofen may raise digoxin level.
Furosemide 1–3 mg/kg/day (PO or IV)	Loop diuretic. Treats pulmonary edema and systemic venous congestion.	Potassium wasting. Metabolic alkalosis. Young infants susceptible to hyponatremia and hypocalcemia.	Hypokalemia may potentiate digoxin toxicity. Ototoxicity in high doses with renal insufficiency/ aminoglycoside use.
Hydrochlorothiazide 1–3 mg/kg/day PO (divided b.i.d.)	Proximal tubule diuretic. Same indications as furosemide. Generally less potent but also less sodium, potassium, and calcium wasting.	Hyperuricemia.	
Captopril 0.2–3 mg/kg/day PO (divided q 6 to 8 hr)	Angiotension-converting enzyme inhibitor. Decreases systemic vascular resistance. Increases serum bradykinin.	Hyperkalemia is rare. "Captopril cough" is rare in infants. Hypotension with excessive dose. Renal dysfunction with excessive dose.	Begin at lower dose range and titrate to upper range.
Enalapril 0.1–0.5 mg/kg/day PO	Same as captopril. Single daily dose more convenient in older infants. Potassium sparing diuretic.	Same as captopril.	Same as with captopril. May be more difficult to titrate dose renal function in neonates.
Spironolactone 1–2 mg/kg/ day PO	Aldosterone inhibitor.	Hyperkalemia especially if used with ACE inhibitors.	Contraindicated in acute renal failure.
Alprostadil (PGE₁) 0.05–0.15 μ/kg/min IV	Establishes patency of ductus arteriosus.	Apnea, vasodilatation.	

ACE, angiotensin-converting enzyme; CHF, congenital heart failure; WPW, Wolff–Parkinson–White; AV, atrioventricular.

LESIONS CAUSING OBSTRUCTION TO VENTRICULAR OUTFLOW

Pulmonic Stenosis

All outflow obstructive lesions produce a pressure overload on one of the ventricles. Compensatory hypertrophy of the ventricular wall normalizes wall stress. Therefore, signs or symptoms of decompensation are only associated with long-standing or severe obstruction to outflow. Pulmonic stenosis only rarely causes symptoms in childhood. The exception is critical pulmonary valve stenosis in the neonate, which can result in cyanosis secondary to right-to-left shunt at the level of the normal neonatal atrial defect (patent foramen ovale). Even significant pulmonary valve stenosis in an older infant is not a cyanotic condition. Findings are a harsh ejection murmur at the left sternal edge and a pulmonic ejection click at the onset of the murmur produced in the dilated main pulmonary artery (post-stenotic dilation). There are few issues of importance regarding the hospitalized child with pulmonic stenosis other than a need for endocarditis prophylaxis for appropriate procedures.

Aortic Stenosis, Discrete Subaortic Stenosis, and Supravalvular Aortic Stenosis

Aortic stenosis can vary in severity from trivial (bicuspid aortic valve) to critical aortic stenosis of the neonate. The only concern in children with bicuspid aortic valve or asymptomatic aortic stenosis is the need for endocarditis prophylaxis during bacteremic procedures.

Critical aortic stenosis often presents at birth or soon after as profound congestive heart failure, often with shock and metabolic acidosis. The classic harsh ejection murmur of aortic stenosis that radiates to the carotids may be absent due to very poor left ventricular output. Closure of the ductus arteriosus results in a virtual absence of flow to the systemic vascular bed. Occasionally, severe aortic stenosis is asymptomatic in the neonate but presents with more subtle signs of congestive heart failure due to pulmonary venous congestion from the elevated end-diastolic pressure in the failing left ventricle. Tachypnea, sweating, and gallop rhythm are ominous prognostic signs, much more so than when they occur in infants with simple left-to-right shunt. Myocardial ischemia may be apparent on ECG.

The older child with unoperated aortic stenosis is unlikely to present special needs when hospitalized with noncardiac problems unless endocarditis is present and missed. It should always be included in the differential diagnosis of fever, malaise, weight loss, or other compatible signs and symptoms. If high-dose sympathomimetic medications (e.g., continuous nebulizer treatments) are used to treat severe asthma in a child with moderate or moderately severe aortic stenosis, ECG monitoring is important. Myocardial ischemia can occur in this setting from myocardial oxygen supply and demand imbalance.

Discrete subaortic stenosis produces a murmur that more closely mimics the systolic harsh murmur of a VSD than the ejection murmur of aortic stenosis. Although not truly S1 coincident nor holosystolic, it sounds "longer" than aortic stenosis and there is no ejection click. Supravalvular aortic stenosis is also not associated with any ejection click as there is no post-stenotic dilatation of the aortic root. Children with these forms of LV outflow tract obstruction will almost always present with abnormal murmurs rather than with symptoms.

Coarctation of Aorta

Critical neonatal coarctation of the aorta is associated with ductal-dependent systemic blood flow provided by the RV. Most often these infants present to a hospital at 2 to 6 weeks of life with a history of feeding and respiratory difficulties as the ductus arteriosus closes. The clinical exam suggests neonatal sepsis with gray mottled skin color and poor perfusion, tachypnea, and poor pulses. A murmur may not be apparent and hepatomegaly and gallop rhythm may be more detectable after fluid resuscitation. Oximetry may not reveal significant desaturation. Cardiomegaly is usually present on a chest radiograph.

Older children with coarctation usually have no symptoms but may have hypertension incidentally detected (especially if measured in the right arm). Femoral pulses can be present in the older child with coarctation due to flow through collateral vessels, and foot pulses may seem almost normal. However, palpation of femoral arterial pulse simultaneously with right brachial pulses will reveal the delay in femoral pulse and the relative decrease in amplitude.

A small number of infants will have noncritical but severe coarctation and present in the first 6 months of life with symptoms of congestive heart failure but without the picture of shock seen in the young infant with critical coarctation.

Management

Most infants with critical pulmonic valve stenosis will undergo urgent balloon dilation of the pulmonic valve in the catheterization lab. The infant with critical coarctation or critical aortic stenosis in cardiogenic shock requires stabilization by establishing patency of the ductus arteriosus to allow the RV to provide systemic blood flow below the aortic obstruction. Alprostadil (prostaglandin E1 infusion) can often accomplish this, but inotropic support with dopamine or dobutamine is often needed. This is followed by judicious use of diuretics to establish urine output and relieve pulmonary edema. Ventilator support is usually needed, but attempts to maintain minimal FiO_2 (often 21%) are important. High inspired FiO_2 acts as a pulmonary vasodilator and can "steal" systemic circulation to the pulmonary vascular bed. Treatment

for sepsis is often initiated in these infants before the diagnosis of cardiogenic shock is made. Continuation of antibiotic treatment may be advisable pending culture results, as these infants have an increased incidence of concomitant gram-negative sepsis, perhaps secondary to poor perfusion of the bowel.

The older infant with severe coarctation or aortic stenosis with congestive heart failure without shock requires surgical or catheter treatment. Surgical correction is the most common approach used for infants with coarctation. Catheter dilation has a more established record in the treatment of infants with severe aortic valve stenosis. Aortic valvotomy by catheter dilation or by surgery is palliative and will be followed by more definitive operation in the older child. In most cases the Ross operation is performed, in which the patient's native pulmonic valve is autotransplanted into the aortic position. A composite homograft pulmonic valve is used to replace the normal native pulmonic valve that has been placed in the aortic position. This approach seems to afford the best chance for long-term correction of aortic valve disease without the need for warfarin anticoagulation mandated by the use of mechanical valve prosthetics.

Pearls

- Bicuspid aortic valve is relatively common but difficult to diagnose. The diagnosis is suggested by an aortic ejection click often most easily heard at the cardiac apex. It mimics a "split S1," which is unlikely to be heard in that location as only mitral valve closure is apparent at the apex or lateral to it.
- If supravalvular aortic stenosis is discovered in an infant or young child, careful examination for the features of William syndrome should be performed. William syndrome is commonly missed in affected children until they are in the preschool age group. Deletion on chromosome 7 may be found in such children and in children with supravalvular stenosis who do not have William syndrome (familial supravalvular aortic stenosis).
- An infant with shock and severe CHF from critical coarctation may not have an obvious difference in the upper extremity and lower extremity pulse strength or blood pressures until successful fluid and inotropic resuscitation improves cardiac output.
- Infusion of alprostadil (prostaglandin E1) can reopen the ductus arteriosus and be life-saving in critical coarctation of the aorta even past 1 month of age. These infants often have profound metabolic acidosis with pH values less than 7.0. However, cerebral perfusion usually has not been critically deprived, and full recovery often follows successful resuscitation and surgery.

LESIONS CAUSING VALVULAR REGURGITATION

Aortic Valve Regurgitation and Mitral Valve Regurgitation

The left heart regurgitant lesions are most important regurgitant pathologic conditions. Both produce a volume overload on the LV even though mitral regurgitation is obviously a systolic event. The reason that the overload is volume type (diastolic) in mitral regurgitation is that the regurgitated blood volume must return to the left ventricle along with normal pulmonary venous return with each diastolic filling. Therefore, severe mitral valve regurgitation not only produces a holosystolic regurgitant murmur, but also a low-pitched diastolic filling murmur.

That aortic regurgitation creates left ventricular volume overload with LV dilatation that is more intuitively obvious because it is a diastolic phenomenon. Aortic valve regurgitation is usually caused by congenital abnormality (bicuspid aortic valve), but is seen after rheumatic fever as well. The characteristic physical finding is a decrescendo diastolic murmur, blowing in character and of fairly high pitch. Fairly severe aortic regurgitation may be tolerated without symptoms, but surgery is required if either left ventricular dysfunction or severe ventricular enlargement develops. The Ross operation is increasingly the procedure of choice, even in small children and infants.

Mitral valve regurgitation also is well tolerated until severe. The backward regurgitation into the lower pressure left atrium allows for a lower afterload on the enlarging left ventricle than if it were contracting against aortic resistance alone. This preserves systolic function but with the risk that decompensation can be sudden once the volume overload becomes too severe. Surgery should be performed prior to development of frank CHF. Newer surgical techniques allow for mitral valve repair rather than replacement in many instances. As with aortic valve regurgitation, the cause may be congenital or rheumatic. Management of significant but asymptomatic mitral or aortic valve regurgitation intends to prevent or delay the need for surgical intervention. There may be some utility of systemic afterload reduction with ACE inhibitors and other drugs to accomplish this, but the benefit of this type of therapy in the absence of ventricular dysfunction remains an unanswered question, especially in the setting of mitral valve regurgitation. When there is diminished ventricular systolic performance, the value of ACE inhibition and other CHF drug therapy is well established as helpful prior to surgical treatment.

CYANOTIC CONGENITAL HEART DISEASE

Cyanotic congenital heart lesions may be divided into those with biventricular anatomy, all of which are surgically repairable; and those with single ventricle type anatomy, all of which are only amenable to surgical palliation. All of these conditions require endocarditis prophylaxis at the time of bacteremic procedures regardless of prior surgical repair. Successfully repaired biventricular cyanotic congenital heart lesions become free from the risk of systemic embolization of venous thrombi or intravenously introduced air. Patients with univentricular cyanotic congenital heart disease require precautions to minimize this risk when receiving intravenous fluids in the hospital even if prior surgical "repair" has been performed.

Another way to characterize cyanotic congenital heart disease is whether there is a common mixing chamber for the combined systemic and pulmonary venous returns or whether there is abnormal pulmonary blood flow. Typical examples of the former physiology include double-inlet single ventricle, tricuspid atresia, and hypoplastic left heart. Examples of abnormally restricted pulmonary blood flow include tetralogy of Fallot with or without pulmonary valve atresia. Combinations of the two types exist. Transposition of the great arteries can be thought of as a special case of abnormal pulmonary blood flow because there is abnormal flow of the pulmonary venous blood back to the lungs. However, it is fundamentally different from other forms of cyanotic congenital heart disease because there is no restriction to pulmonary blood flow and the circulations are separated and not mixed.

The differential diagnosis of the cyanotic infant is not limited to congenital heart lesions and is discussed at length elsewhere in this text (Chapter 13).

Biventricular Types of Cyanotic Congenital Heart Disease

Tetralogy of Fallot

The combination of large subaortic VSD and right ventricular outflow tract obstruction may be associated with no visible cyanosis or even excessive pulmonary blood flow early in life, but eventually is replaced by cyanosis as obstruction to pulmonary blood flow progresses. On physical exam, the infant with tetralogy of Fallot usually has a long harsh systolic murmur created by flow through the obstructed right ventricular outflow tract. Prior to repair, infants with tetralogy of Fallot may be acyanotic or cyanotic depending upon the severity of chronic obstruction.

Hypercyanotic Spells

Hypercyanotic spells can occur in any patient with tetralogy of Fallot whether acyanotic or cyanotic. These spells present with the sudden development of profound cyanosis and a marked diminution in the loudness of the systolic murmur of flow through the pulmonary outflow tract. The infant is usually tachypneic with deep rapid inspirations and may also be obtunded. During these "hypercyanotic spells" there is hyperdynamic systolic contraction of the right ventricular infundibulum with increased right-to-left shunt and, more importantly, markedly decreased pulmonary blood flow. Oxygen, sedation, and knee-chest position are helpful. The knee-chest position transiently increases the preload to the RV as well as the aortic afterload, both of which increase pulmonary blood flow through the RV outflow tract. An intravenous volume push can often reverse a hypercyanotic spell, but afterload increase with phenylephrine drip may be needed to maintain good oxygen saturation as hypercyanotic spells are often relapsing once they occur (Table 29.2).

Tetralogy of Fallot Repair

Tetralogy of Fallot repair involves patch closure of the VSD with surgical relief of RV outflow obstruction, often with a patch across the pulmonary valve annulus to enlarge the outflow and main pulmonary artery. Some hemodynamic abnormality is present in all repaired tetralogy patients, either residual pulmonary stenosis with increased right-ventricular pressure load or residual pulmonary valve incompetence with increased right-ventricular volume load. Ventricular ectopy arising from the abnormal RV is common, but life-threatening rapid ventricular tachycardia is relatively rare. However, syncope should be considered a potentially serious symptom in repaired tetralogy for this reason. Most repaired tetralogy patients are allowed to participate in vigorous sports.

Transposition of the Great Arteries

Transposition causes severe cyanosis in the neonate. There is usually no murmur and the chest radiograph shows normal or increased pulmonary blood flow. Surgical correction is now performed in the first weeks of life with outstanding long-term prognosis. During surgical repair, the coronary arteries must be switched along with the great arteries. Problems with the coronary anastamoses can cause myocardial ischemia, but this is a rare complication. Far more common is mild obstruction in the pulmonary artery near the anastamotic site, which often causes a systolic murmur in these children. Most children with transposition of the great arteries who have undergone repair by arterial switch are allowed to play competitive sports.

Prior to the mid-1980s, arterial switch repair for transposition was not commonly performed. Redirecting the pulmonary venous and systemic venous returns by means of

TREATMENT OF HYPERCYANOTIC SPELLS IN INFANTS WITH TETRALOGY OF FALLOT

Intervention	Effect/Mechanism of action
Calming infant	Decreases catecholamine-induced tachycardia, which promotes improved RV filling (preload and size); decreases inotropy and infundibular hypercontractility.
Knee chest or fetal positioning	Increases RV filling; increases aortic/systemic afterload.
Oxygen administration	Increases pO_2 of pulmonary venous return.
Sedation (e.g., IV morphine 0.05–0.2 mg/kg)	Decreases catecholamine-induced tachycardia and inotropy.
IV volume push (15 mL/kg normal saline IV or IO)	Increases RV preload, decreases catecholamines, increases BP.
Phenylephrine drip (0.4–3.0 μg/kg/min). May give 5 μg IV slow push if response to drip not immediate	Increases aortic/systemic afterload without increasing inotropy or chronotropy; diminishes right-to-left shunt; may diminish RV hypercontractility via acute afterload increase.
Sodium bicarbonate 1 meq/kg IV	Treatment of metabolic acidosis. Often not needed if volume and phenylephrine rapidly normalize pulmonary blood flow.
Propranolol HCL (0.05–0.1 mg/kg IV) slow push over 10 minutes	Decreases tachycardia and RV hypercontractility. Often not needed if volume and phenylephrine rapidly normalize pulmonary blood flow. Risk of IV propranolol is hypotension.

atrial baffles was used to correct the cyanosis of children with transposition—many of whom now are young adults. The Mustard and Senning operations used for this type of repair involved extensive atrial suture lines and are associated with the late occurrence of atrial flutter and other atrial arrhythmias. Unlike patients who have had arterial switch repair, the Mustard and Senning patients depend upon the RV as the systemic ventricle. Congestive heart failure can occur if right ventricular failure with or without significant tricuspid regurgitation develops. Some adolescents may be seen with this type of transposition repair but most patients with this anatomy are now adults.

Total Anomalous Pulmonary Venous Return

Total anomalous pulmonary venous return (TAPVR) may be obstructed (most often when the pulmonary veins drain to an infradiaphragmatic site) or unobstructed (most typically when return is supracardiac to the innominate vein). Obstructed types present in the first day or two of life with severe pulmonary edema or with pulmonary hypertension and severe cyanosis. Unobstructed total anomalous pulmonary venous return often is not diagnosed until the infant is older and displays tachypea and signs of heart failure and pulmonary overcirculation. Wide fixed splitting of the second heart sound is often quite striking in these children due to the profound right ventricular volume overload from the anomalous pulmonary venous return. A patent foramen is found in all noncritically ill infants with TAPVR, which allows mixed cyanotic and oxygenated blood return to be delivered to the systemic circulation. Re-anastomosis of the pulmonary venous confluence with the left atrium with closure of the atrial septal defect is associated with normal late cardiac function, although some patients will develop episodic atrial arrhythmia such as atrial flutter years after surgical repair.

Truncus Arteriosus

Truncus arteriosus is anatomically similar to tetralogy of Fallot except that the pulmonary arteries arise from the ascending aortic trunk or truncus. As in tetralogy of Fallot, this arterial trunk overrides the large VSD. Mixing of oxygenated and deoxygenated venous returns occurs in the proximal truncus. Unrestricted pulmonary blood flow usually minimizes cyanosis. Presentation with excessive pulmonary blood flow and symptoms reminiscent of a large VSD is usual. The aortic or "truncal" valve may have two, three, or four valve cusps. Significant truncal valve stenosis or regurgitation complicates neonatal repair. On physical exam there is an LV heave, aortic ejection click, and a systolic murmur of exuberant pulmonary blood flow. There will be a diastolic decrescendo murmur if truncal valve insufficiency is present. The operation is in many respects similar to the repair of cases of tetralogy of Fallot when a conduit from RV to pulmonary artery is required. There is an association of truncus arteriosus with interrupted aortic arch. This combination is associated with deletion on chromosome 22 (DiGeorge and related syndromes).

Univentricular (Single Ventricle) Types of Cyanotic Congenital Heart Disease

All such hearts have two ventricles but usually one ventricle is hypoplastic, or abnormalities of AV valve alignment preclude successful partitioning of the heart into two functioning ventricles. Typical congenital lesions in this class include:

- Tricuspid atresia
- Pulmonary atresia with intact ventricular septum and hypoplastic right heart
- Double-inlet LV
- Hypoplastic left heart syndrome
- Heterotaxy syndromes

With all of these diagnoses there is mixing of both venous returns. The degree to which these patients have either cyanosis or heart failure in early life often relates to whether there is restriction to pulmonary blood flow or restriction of systemic blood flow. A Fontan-type operation, with its unique physiology and complications, is required for these patients.

Fontan physiology implies total connection of the systemic venous return (usually superior and inferior vena cavae) directly to the pulmonary arteries. The absence of a separate ventricle to pump desaturated blood to the lungs is compensated for by the diastolic suction of the single ventricle as it receives blood from the lungs to pump to the systemic circulation. This offers a reasonable palliation long term for most single-ventricle patients.

The physiologic transformation to this circulatory pattern from one in which both systemic and pulmonary venous returns go to the single ventricle to the Fontan physiology is usually accomplished in two stages. A bidirectional Glenn anastomosis routes the superior vena cava(ae) to the pulmonary arteries and is performed at 4 to 8 months of life. Routing the inferior caval flow to the pulmonary arteries after the first year of life completes the Fontan physiology. While awaiting the Fontan operation, patients with bidirectional Glenn shunts typically have arterial oxygen saturations in the low to mid-80s. Even after the Fontan operation, most single-ventricle patients do not have completely normal arterial oxygen saturation because there may be fenestrations in the IVC to PA connection left to decompress abdominal systemic central venous pressure (CVP).

Elevated CVP after either bidirectional Glenn shunting or Fontan operation may result in facial or extremity edema, and serous or chylous pleural and pericardial effusions. Ascites and protein-losing enteropathy from lymphatic congestion in the intestines may occur after Fontan operation if there is elevated CVP in the inferior cava. Respiratory distress, unexpectedly low oximetry, or abdominal complaints in the weeks to months after these two operations always should prompt imaging studies to rule out these complications.

A number of patients with single-ventricle palliation by Fontan operation have continued needs for anticongestive medications. All require the use of antiembolic "bubble filters" on IV lines when in hospital. Many are at risk for venous thrombosis and/or thromboembolism. Finally, the incidence of atrial tachyarrhythmias is significant in these patients early and late after surgery.

Pearls

- The "hyperoxia test" may be useful to exclude cyanotic congenital heart disease in the neonate with low pulse oximetry. However, pulse oximetry is not used during the hyperoxia test. Right radial arterial blood gas to obtain paO_2 values while breathing 100% FiO_2 in a head hood may be as low as 50 Torr while the oxygen saturation measured by pulse oximetry is in the upper 90s. Therefore, "normalization" of the pulse oximetry reading on high FiO_2 in no way excludes cyanotic congenital heart disease. An arterial pO_2 greater than 150 Torr while in 100% FiO_2 is needed to reliably exclude all cyanotic heart disease.
- The Norwood I operation for hypoplastic left heart syndrome uses the main pulmonary artery to provide systemic blood flow to the transverse and descending aorta. Pulmonary blood flow comes from an aortopulmonary shunt. Attempts to normalize oxygen saturation with supplemental oxygen risk "stealing" blood flow from the systemic circulation to the pulmonary circulation. Oxygen is not contraindicated when these infants are admitted to the hospital with pneumonia or respiratory distress. However, a goal of oximetry saturation values in the 80% to 85% range rather than above 90% should be specified to avoid pulmonary overcirculation.
- Midline stomach or liver or abnormal relationship of the cardiac situs to abdominal situs is suggestive of heterotaxy syndromes. Most have complex congenital cardiac lesions but some have less complex lesions. Bilateral right atrial appendages are associated with asplenia and bilateral left atrial appendages with polysplenia. Diminished splenic function may occur with both conditions that will require continuous antibiotic prophylaxis against pneumococcal

infection as well as pneumococcal vaccination. Problems with abdominal and cardiac situs mismatch and persistent sinus bradycardia suggests polysplenia syndrome because of absence of the normal right atrial sinus node. Howell–Jolly bodies on the peripheral blood smear indicate asplenia. The most reliable and inexpensive test to diagnose absent splenic function is quantitation of pitted red blood cells with a Nomarsky optics microscope.

- Irradiated red blood cells should be used if transfusion is required in the infant with lesions with a significant chance of deletion of chromosome 22 at the 22q11 locus. This deletion is often associated with features of DiGeorge syndrome with thymic aplasia. Lack of thymic T-cell function is a risk for the development of graft-versus-host disease if viable leukocytes are transfused into a susceptible patient. Traditionally this precaution was observed in infants with "aortic arch abnormality" because of the high association of the chromosome 22q11 deletion with interrupted aortic arch and with lesions associated with right aortic arch, especially tetralogy of Fallot. The recent demonstration of significant associations of this deletion with subaortic VSD, with right aortic arch and aberrant left subclavian artery and with other lesions widens the spectrum of patients in whom the chromosome 22 deletion precautions might apply. Low serum calcium can also be a significant problem for these infants due to parathyroid dysfunction and should be monitored in all sick neonates with compatible cardiac lesions. It is now clear that the 22q11 deletion may be found in more children with congenital heart disease than formerly appreciated. However, it is also apparent that not all infants with this deletion have impaired T-cell function or parathyroid dysfunction. Also, many that have such dysfunction may recover normal function later in infancy.
- Cyanotic congenital heart disease places patients at increased risk for neurologic problems. There is an excess incidence of infantile and childhood stroke and also of brain abscess. The latter may present as a focal seizure without significant fever. Brain abscess occurs presumably from septic embolism from the venous system allowed by the right-to-left intracardiac shunt. The risk for stroke increases when there is chronic cyanosis or polycythemia (erythrocytosis) with significant iron deficiency. In this situation, red blood cell microcytosis from iron deficiency during increased red cell production is associated with abnormal red cell deformability and abnormal rheologic properties of the blood that contribute to the risk for stroke. Therefore, adequate iron intake is important in infants with cyanotic congenital heart disease even if they do not have low hemoglobin values for a normal infant.
- "Reverse differential cyanosis" usually indicates that the infant has transposition of the great arteries. The oxygen saturation by oximetry is consistently lower in the preductal right hand than in the postductal foot in many of these infants because increased pulmonary resistance and an open ductus combine with the transposed circulations to result in highly oxygenated blood to flow out into the aorta from the hypertensive but highly saturated main pulmonary artery. Reverse differential cyanosis can also occur if there is supracardiac total anomalous pulmonary venous return with highly oxygenated superior caval venous return to the right ventricle and thence to the pulmonary artery and out the duct to the lower body. This model also assumes some pulmonary hypertension is present.
- Infradiaphragmatic (obstructed) total anomalous pulmonary venous return may be suggested by a return of red blood when an umbilical venous catheter is placed in a cyanotic infant. If the infant is receiving 100% FiO_2, the umbilical venous catheter pO_2 may be greater than 250 Torr even though the umbilical arterial pO_2 will be quite low. This

TABLE 29.3

CARDIAC CONDITIONS FOR WHICH ENDOCARDITIS PROPHYLAXIS IS OR IS NOT RECOMMENDED

Cardiac conditions for which antibiotic prophylaxis is recommended	Cardiac conditions for which antibiotic prophylaxis is not recommended
Prosthetic cardiac valves (includes homograft or bioprosthetic valves)[a]	Isolated secundum atrial septal defect
Cyanotic congenital heart disease preoperative or postrepair[a]	Surgically repaired atrial septal defect, ventricular septal defect, or PDA with no residual defect (6 or more months postoperative)
Cyanotic congenital heart disease palliated (e.g., aortopulmonary shunts)[a]	Mitral valve prolapse without valvar regurgitation
History of prior bacterial endocarditis[a]	Functional or innocent heart murmurs
Acyanotic congenital heart disease, unrepaired	Previous Kawasaki disease with no valvar regurgitation
Acyanotic congenital heart disease, repaired (except repaired VSD, PDA, ASD)	Previous rheumatic fever with no valvar regurgitation
Hypertrophic cardiomyopathy	Cardiac pacemakers (transvenous or epicardial) with no structural or congenital heart disease
Dilated cardiomyopathy with abnormal mitral valve regurgitation	
Mitral valve prolapse with mitral valve regurgitation	

[a]Higher risk category of lesions.
Adapted from American Heart Association Scientific Publications online at http://216.185.112.5/presenter.jhtml?identifier=1729.

occurs because of anomalous return of the pulmonary venous blood to the liver via the infradiaphragmatic channel. This sign is not always present if the obstructed pulmonary venous drainage does not communicate with the hepatic venous and ductus venosus confluence. Furthermore, it must be ascertained that the umbilical venous catheter has not passed into the heart and into the left atrium via the foramen ovale. Extremely high pO_2 values in an umbilical venous catheter in the left atrium suggests transposition of the great arteries in a severely cyanotic neonate.

Congenital Heart Disease: Bacterial Endocarditis

Antibiotic prophylaxis prior to procedures that can cause bacteremia is recommended for most congenital cardiac defects.

Isolated secundum atrial septal defect is the exception. Ostium primum–type atrial septal defects do have significant risk for endocarditis because of the associated mitral valve regurgitation. American Heart Association guidelines are available online and are summarized in Tables 29.3 and 29.4.

Bacterial endocarditis should be considered as a possibility in any febrile child with known congenital heart disease. The threshold for obtaining more than one blood culture prior to initiation of antibiotics should be low. If fever does not promptly resolve with antibiotic treatment or if a single blood culture becomes positive, having obtained two or more blood cultures prior to antibiotic may be very helpful in excluding or diagnosing bacterial endocarditis. In addition to fever, the signs of bacterial endocarditis may include weight loss, malaise, and signs of peripheral embolization or immune complex deposition such as petechial skin rash, splinter hemorrhages, Janeway lesions, splenomegaly, and microscopic hematuria.

TABLE 29.4

PROCEDURES FOR WHICH ENDOCARDITIS PROPHYLAXIS IS OR IS NOT RECOMMENDED

Antibiotic prophylaxis recommended	Antibiotic prophylaxis not recommended
Dental extractions	Fluoride treatments
Routine professional dental cleaning	Orthodontic appliance adjustment
Periodontal preocedures such as scaling, probing	Shedding of primary teeth
Dental implant of avulsed tooth	Restorative dentistry (filling cavities)
Initial placement of orthodontic bands	Endotracheal intubation
Tonsillectomy and/or adenoidectomy	Tympanostomy tube insertion
Bronchoscopy with rigid bronchoscope	Bronchoscopy with flexible bronchoscope with or without biopsy
Surgical operations involving respiratory or intestinal mucosa	Endoscopy including transesophageal echocardiography
Urethral dilation	Circumcision
Cystoscopy	Cardiac catheterization
	Vaginal delivery (optional for high risk patients)
	Urethral catheterization if uninfected
	Insertion of intrauterine devices if uninfected

Adapted from American Heart Association Scientific Publications online at http://216.185.112.5/presenter.jhtml?identifier=1729.

Postpericardiotomy Syndrome

Postpericardiotomy syndrome can occur after virtually any congenital heart surgery and causes a sterile reactive pericarditis with pericardial effusion. Operations performed via left thoracotomy such as coarctation repair do not present this risk, but even closed-heart procedures such as pulmonary artery banding have been followed by reactive pericardial effusions. Postpericardiotomy syndrome can cause cardiac tamponade. A discussion is presented elsewhere on the general features of pericarditis and tamponade. However, it bears emphasizing that in young children, symptoms of abdominal discomfort, anorexia, and vomiting are far more common signs of pericardial tamponade than symptoms of chest pain. With tragic results, physicians may misinterpret this symptom complex as a sign of viral gastroenteritis in children who are convalescing from heart surgery. In this setting, immediate evaluation with chest radiograph or echocardiography is mandatory unless physical exam is *completely* negative for all signs of large pericardial effusion. These include tachycardia, poor color, pulsus paradoxus, distant heart tones, and jugular venous distention. Postpericardiotomy syndrome with serious pericardial effusion can occur up to 2 months after heart surgery. Reversal of recovery of appetite and energy during convalescence should prompt consideration of this diagnosis.

If pericardial effusion is diagnosed before tamponade occurs, pericardiocentesis may be avoided by treatment with anti-inflammatory drugs. Some debate exists about the optimal regimen. Some experts add diuretics to improve any component of fluid retention that is contributing beyond the inflammatory response. Concerns have been raised that steroid treatment of postpericardiotomy syndrome may be associated with increased frequency of relapses, but it is possible that this apparent association is related to reserving use of steroids to cases where response to nonsteroidal anti-inflammatory medications has failed. Caution should be used in children who are on high doses of diuretic and angiotensin-converting enzyme inhibitor drugs when nonsteroidal anti-inflammatory drugs are added. Renal function must be monitored.

Pericardial effusion after bidirectional Glenn anastomosis or Fontan operation in patients with single ventricle can occur from excessive systemic venous pressure and is analogous to and often seen with pleural effusions in these patients. These problems are not inflammatory and usually do not respond to treatment for postpericardiotomy syndrome.

Respiratory Syncytial Virus

Respiratory syncytial virus (RSV) can cause prolonged hospitalization and respiratory failure in infants with congenital heart diseases. Those with symptoms of CHF, large left-to-right shunts, and cyanosis are most at risk. Palivizumab, a monoclonal anti-RSV antibody, has been shown to decrease admission rates and length of hospital stay in infants born prematurely, those with chronic lung disease, and in infants with serious congenital heart disease. Current recommendations are for RSV prophylaxis in infants under 12 months of age who are receiving medication to control CHF, infants with moderate to severe pulmonary hypertension, and infants with cyanotic congenital heart disease.

Pulmonary Hypertension in Congenital Heart Disease

Pulmonary hypertension in patients with congenital heart disease is usually thought of as a complication of unrepaired ventricular septal defect (Eisenmenger syndrome). However, there is a growing appreciation that unusual patients with appropriately repaired congenital heart disease may present years later with pulmonary hypertension, occasionally severe. Symptoms that may suggest this entity include syncope, dyspnea, chest pain, and effort intolerance. Presenting signs are auscultation of a loud pulmonic closure sound and right ventricular hypertrophy on ECG. Diagnosis is confirmed by echocardiography or cardiac catheterization. Obstructive sleep apnea as a contributing cause must be excluded and, if found, treated. Rare children and adolescents with successfully repaired congenital heart disease will require long-term treatment with pulmonary vasodilators such as bosentan or sildenafil.

Suggested Readings

Dajani AS, Taubert KA, Wilson W, et al. Prevention of bacterial endocarditis. Recommendations by the American Heart Association. *JAMA* 1997;277:1794–1801.

Doroshow RW. The adolescent with simple or corrected congenital heart disease. *Adolesc Med* 2001;12:1–22.

Grifka RG. Cyanotic congenital heart disease with increased pulmonary blood flow. *Pediatr Clin North Am* 1999;46:405–425.

Lee C, Mason LJ. Pediatric cardiac emergencies. *Anesthesiol Clin North Am* 2001;19:287–308.

Ohye RG, Bove EL. Advances in congenital heart surgery. *Curr Opin Pediatr* 2001;13:473–481.

Pillo-Blocka F, Adatia I, Sharieff W, et al. Rapid advancement to more concentrated formula in infants after surgery for congenital heart disease reduces duration of hospital stay: a randomized clinical trial. *J Pediatr* 2004;145:761–766.

Waldman JD, Wernly JA. Cyanotic congenital heart disease with decreased pulmonary blood flow in children. *Pediatr Clin North Am* 1999;46:385–404.

Woods WA, Schutte DA, McCulloch MA. Care of children who have had surgery for congenital heart disease. *Am J Emerg Med* 2003;21:318–327.

CHAPTER 30 ■ CARDIOMYOPATHY

JEFFREY A. TOWBIN AND CHARLIE J. SANG, JR.

Cardiomyopathy is any structural and/or functional abnormality of the ventricular myocardium that is not associated with disease of the coronary arteries, high blood pressure, valvular or congenital heart disease, or pulmonary vascular disease. Incidence estimates have ranged from 8 cases per 100,000 to 17.2 cases per 100,000 among all age groups. Recently, the Pediatric Cardiomyopathy Registry (PCMR) showed that the youngest of children (i.e., <1 year of age) have the highest incidence of 8.34 per 100,000 compared to an incidence of 0.70 per 100,000 in the 1- to 18-year-old age group.

ETIOLOGY

Cardiomyopathies have been divided into two categories. Primary cardiomyopathies are heart muscle diseases of unknown cause. With the advent of molecular biology, and of other etiologic diagnostic methods, idiopathic disease is likely to be lessened. Genetic findings have enabled clinicians to understand the underlying basis of these disorders, which includes problems of cytoarchitecture and metabolism.

Secondary cardiomyopathies are heart muscle diseases of known cause or associated with disorders of other systems. Systemic diseases, which may result in cardiomyopathies, are infections, metabolic conditions, general system diseases, heredofamilial conditions, and sensitivity and toxic reactions. Table 30.1 provides a detailed list of associated systemic diseases. Diagnosis and treatment of the systemic disease may result in the resolution of the cardiomyopathy. The following discussion will pertain to primary cardiomyopathies.

TYPES OF CARDIOMYOPATHY

Dilated cardiomyopathy (DCM) is the most prevalent form of heart muscle disorder and accounts for approximately 50% of cases. Typically the left ventricle (rarely both ventricles) is enlarged with thinning of the interventricular septum and free wall. Contractility is diminished in these patients and heart failure is common. Autosomal dominant forms of DCM are the most common inherited forms, although X-linked, autosomal recessive, and mitochondrial (maternal) transmission also occurs.

Hypertrophic cardiomyopathy (HCM) involves hypertrophy of the interventricular septum and/or left ventricular free wall and accounts for 35% of cases of heart muscle disease. Family history of other affected relatives in an autosomal dominant pattern may be seen in 50% of patients. Diastolic dysfunction with abnormal relaxation of the left ventricle (stiff ventricle that requires higher filling pressures), left ventricular outflow tract obstruction, ventricular arrhythmias, and sudden death are some of the problems seen in these patients. Left ventricular systolic function is hypercontractile in the majority of patients.

Restrictive cardiomyopathy (RCM) is the least prevalent form of cardiomyopathy, accounting for fewer than 5% of cases. There is diffuse fibrosis and rigidity of the myocardium resulting in poor diastolic relaxation, normal systolic function, and dilation of the atria. The patients have symptoms related to pulmonary congestion with right-sided heart failure, atrial arrhythmias, and syncope. Sudden death is common.

Left ventricular noncompaction (LVNC) is probably the third-most common form of cardiomyopathy, appearing to account for about 15% of cases in childhood. It is characterized by prominent trabeculations in the apex, and the free wall of the left ventricle may be dilated and/or hypertrophic or normal in size and thickness, while systolic function may be normal, depressed, or hypercontractile. The clinical presentation depends on whether the left ventricle has a hypertrophic or dilated cardiomyopathy-like physiology.

Finally, an uncommon form of cardiomyopathy in childhood, arrhythmogenic right ventricular dysplasia/cardiomyopathy (ARVD/C), presents with ventricular tachycardia of left bundle branch morphology, and is characterized by a dilated right ventricle with fibrofatty replacement. Right ventricle failure may occur.

PRESENTATION

Patients with dilated cardiomyopathy present with signs of congestive failure: tachycardia, tachypnea, diaphoresis, poor feeding, or decreased exercise tolerance with shortness of breath. Other symptoms include palpitations (ventricular arrhythmias), syncope, or abdominal pain/nausea. Physical examination is characterized by tachycardia, tachypnea, and normal to low blood pressure with narrow pulse pressure. The skin may be cool and pale. Breath sounds may be diminished with occasional rales. The cardiac examination demonstrates a diffuse, displaced apex, muffled heart sounds, and a gallop rhythm. A murmur of mitral insufficiency may or may not be present. The liver is enlarged, peripheral pulses are weak, and capillary refill is delayed in children with heart failure.

Patients with hypertrophic cardiomyopathy may present with signs and symptoms of congestive heart failure (CHF) when diagnosed at less than 1 year of age. Children with HCM are commonly asymptomatic, particularly when diagnosed after 1 year of age. Fewer than 70% of children with hypertrophic cardiomyopathy are diagnosed correctly on initial presentation by clinical findings alone. Children with HCM are prone to present with sudden death, particularly when associated with exercise. Physical examination may demonstrate an abnormal carotid upstroke. S3 or S4 gallops may be heard in 50% of patients. A systolic ejection murmur may be present in 40% of patients, particularly those with left ventricular outflow tract obstruction.

TABLE 30.1

SECONDARY CARDIOMYOPATHIES

INFECTIONS
Viral
  Coxsackie B
  Echo
  Mumps
  Rubella
  Rubeola
Bacterial
  Diphtheria
  Meningococcal
  Pneumococcal
  Gonococcal
Fungal
  Candidiasis
  Aspergillosis
Protozoal
  American trypanosomiasis (Chagas disease)
  Toxoplasmosis
Rickettsial
  Rocky Mountain spotted fever
Spirochetal
  Lyme disease

METABOLIC CONDITIONS
Endocrine
  Thyrotoxicosis
  Hypothyroidism
  Diabetes mellitus
    Infant of diabetic mother
    Diabetic cardiomyopathy
  Hypoglycemia
  Pheochromocytoma/neuroblastoma
    Catecholamine cardiomyopathy
Familial storage disease
  Glycogen storage disease
    Pompe disease (type II)
    Cori disease (type III)
    Andersen disease (type IV)
    McArdle disease (type V)
    Hers disease (type VI)
  Mucopolysaccharidoses
    Hurlers syndrome
    Hunters syndrome
    Sanfillipo syndrome
    Morquio syndrome
    Scheie syndrome
    Maroteaux–Lamy syndrome
  Sphingolipidoses
    Niemann–Pick disease
    Farber disease
    Fabry disease
    Gaucher disease
    Tay–Sachs disease
    Sandhoff disease
    G_{ml} gangliosidosis
    Refsum disease

Nutritional deficiency
  Protein: kwashiorkor
  Thiamine: bereberi
  Vitamine E and selenium (Keshan disease)
  Phosphate
Others
  Carnitine deficiency
    Primary
    Secondary: diphtheritic cardiomyopathy
  B-ketothiolase deficiency
  Hypertaurinuria

GENERAL SYSTEM DISEASES
Connective tissue disorders
  Systemic lupus
  Juvenile rheumatoid arthritis
  Polyarteritis nodosa
  Kawasaki disease
  Pseudoxanthoma elasticum
Infiltrations and granulomas
  Leukemia
  Sarcoidosis (not in children)
  Amyloidosis (not in children)
Others
  Hemolytic-uremic syndrome
  Mitochondrial cytopathy
  Reye syndrome
  Peripartum cardiomyopathy
  Osteogenesis imperfecta
  Noonan syndrome

HEREDOFAMILIAL CONDITIONS
Muscular dystrophies and myopathies
  Juvenile progressive (Duchenne)
  Myotonic dystrophy (Steinert)
  Limb-girdle (Erb)
  Juvenile progressive spinal muscular atrophy
    (Kugelberg–Welander)
  Chronic progressive external ophthalmoplegia (Kearns)
  Nemaline myopathy
  Myotubular myopathy
Neuromuscular disorders
  Friedreich ataxia
  Multiple lentiginosis

SENSITIVITY AND TOXIC REACTIONS
Sulphonamides
Penicillin
Anthracyclines
Iron (hemachromatosis)
Chloramphenicol

TACHYARRHYTHMIAS
Supraventricular tachycardia
Atrial flutter
Ventricular tachycardia

Reprinted with permission from *The science and practice of pediatric cardiology*. Philadelphia: Lippincott Williams & Wilkins; 1990:1618.

Restrictive cardiomyopathy is rare in children. In adults, the most common symptom is dyspnea followed by chest pain. Physical examination demonstrates a nonspecific systolic ejection murmur or a holosystolic murmur at the apex, S3 and S4 gallops, jugular venous distension, ascites, and pedal edema. In childhood, the most common presentation is sudden death. Hepatomegaly is typically seen in children with RCM and pulmonary hypertension is common. Children with LV noncompaction present with features typical of either DCM or HCM, although many will be asymptomatic. Children with ARVD are most commonly diagnosed after presenting with arrhythmias and/or syncope. In a small subgroup, right heart failure is the presenting feature.

LABORATORY DATA

Initial workup for patients with cardiomyopathy is based on history and clinical findings to find secondary causes. A complete blood count, erythrocyte sedimentation rate, C-reactive protein, and cultures (bacterial, viral, and fungal) of blood, nasopharyngeal, rectal, and urine are obtained to evaluate infectious causes. Electrolytes, calcium, magnesium, phosphorous, urine organic acids, urinalysis, and acylcarnitine levels are used to evaluate metabolic causes. Liver and renal function tests are obtained to look for other organ involvement and to determine dosing of medications that are metabolized by these organs. Thyroid function tests and skin and/or muscle biopsy are obtained based on clinical suspicion. In addition, B-type natriuretic peptide (BNP) is valuable to investigate heart failure, while creatine kinase measurements may be useful if suspecting ischemic (elevated CK-MB) or systemic disease (elevated CK-MM). Chest x-ray, electrocardiogram, and echocardiogram are obtained to differentiate the type of cardiomyopathy. Cardiac catheterization may be needed for diagnostic endomyocardial biopsy as well as for transplantation evaluation.

The chest x-ray in patients with dilated cardiomyopathy commonly demonstrates enlargement of the left atrium and left ventricle. Pulmonary venous congestion or pulmonary edema may be present. Left-sided atelectasis may be the result of compression of the left mainstem bronchus by an enlarged left atrium. The electrocardiogram typically shows sinus tachycardia with abnormal ST segments. Left atrial and left ventricular enlargement may be present, along with ventricular arrhythmias. The echocardiogram shows enlargement of the left atrium and left ventricle with diminished ventricular systolic function. Mitral insufficiency is frequently present even if a mitral insufficiency murmur is not detected. Intracardiac thrombus in the apex of the left ventricle is not a rare finding. In some cases, a pericardial effusion is noted. Cardiac catheterization can be used as a diagnostic tool if no etiology for the cardiomyopathy can be found. One must identify the origins of the coronary arteries if not adequately seen by echocardiography to diagnose anomalous origin of the left coronary artery from the pulmonary artery. Endomyocardial biopsy samples can be used to diagnose myocarditis or storage diseases. Polymerase chain reaction (PCR) has been used to detect viral RNA in endomyocardial biopsies to confirm cases of myocarditis because other viral studies have typically not been conclusive. Sixty-seven to ninety-five percent of patients with hypertrophic cardiomyopathy have cardiomegaly with normal pulmonary vascular markings on chest x-ray. The electrocardiogram may present with nonspecific ST segment changes and T-wave abnormalities as well as biventricular hypertrophy in infants and left ventricular hypertrophy in children. Atrial and/or ventricular arrhythmias may be seen as well. In some cases, pre-excitation is noted.

Echocardiography demonstrates asymmetric septal hypertrophy or concentric left ventricular hypertrophy. Left ventricular outflow tract obstruction secondary to systolic anterior motion of the mitral valve as well as ventricular systolic and diastolic function can be assessed, along with evidence of mitral insufficiency. Cardiac catheterization with endomyocardial biopsy may aid in a pathologic diagnosis, although cardiac biopsy is rarely needed.

Patients with restrictive cardiomyopathy have cardiomegaly on chest x-ray with dilated atria, but in most cases the cardiac silhouette is not enlarged. The electrocardiogram may demonstrate nonspecific ST–T-wave changes, small QRS voltages, first-degree AV block, or atrial fibrillation. Atrial enlargement, with or without ventricular hypertrophy, is standard. The echocardiogram classically demonstrates significant atrial (usually biatrial) enlargement with normal (or occasionally decreased) ventricular volumes. Ventricular function is normal or increased. Mitral insufficiency and cardiac thrombi are common.

In LVNC, the chest x-ray is usually normal unless it presents as a dilated cardiomyopathy form of LVNC. The electrocardiogram demonstrates severe voltage increase in one-third of cases with or without pre-excitation. The classic echocardiogram demonstrates apical trabeculation of the LV and usually free wall trabeculations are visualized. Arrhythmogenic RV dysplasia/cardiomyopathy may be associated with an enlarged RV with or without RV outflow tract outpouching on chest x-ray. The electrocardiogram may show classical epsilon waves but this is rare. More typically, right ventricular hypertrophy, inverted T-waves and ST elevation in leads V_1 or V_2 are seen. Ventricular tachycardia with left bundle–branch morphology is also classically described. The echocardiogram can demonstrate RV dilation and dysfunction with RV outflow outpouches. Cardiac catheterization and angiography is consistent with hemodynamic abnormalities consistent with RV failure and angiograms show a thin-walled RV with depressed function and aneurysms of the RV apex and outflow tract A biopsy in the "triangle of dysplasia" will show fibrofatty replacement in this portion of the RV.

TREATMENT

Treatment of CHF is the initial therapy for patients with dilated cardiomyopathy and heart failure. Digitalis and diuretics (furosemide) were previously first line outpatient medications but currently afterload reducing agents (captopril, enalapril, or lisinopril) with beta bockers (carvedilol or metoprolol) are the first line drugs. Patients with severe heart failure and respiratory failure require intubation and mechanical ventilation. Intravenous therapy in the past has focused on inotropy and, therefore, high-dose epinephrine was used as standard therapy. Today, these drugs have come into disfavor due to poor outcomes, and therapy with dopamine, dobutamine, milrinone, and nesiritide have a role in these patients. Arrhythmias should be vigorously treated. Steroids and immunosuppressive agents are still controversial and have not been proven to be effective in controlled studies. L-carnitine and other vitamins (coenzyme Q10, thiamine, riboflavin) have been used with varying effectiveness. Those with very low ejection fraction or shortening fraction, or syncope or resuscitated sudden death, should be considered for ICD. Anticoagulation is needed in patients who develop intracardiac thrombi or those with very poor function. For patients refractory to medical management, ventricular-assist devices and an extracorporeal membrane oxygenator (ECMO) are used as a bridge to cardiac transplantation.

Beta-blockers (propranolol and atenolol) and calcium-channel blockers (verapamil and nifedipine) have been the preferred drugs to treat patients with hypertrophic cardiomyopathy for many years. The mode of action is to reduce heart rate as well as decrease contractility and wall stress. Beta-blockers have been reported by some to have somewhat limited effect on ventricular arrhythmias, whereas calcium-channel blockers have more effect. However, limited studies have been reported in children. Treatment of arrhythmias with amiodarone has improved survival rates. If severe bradycardia is induced with these medications, pacemaker support is recommended. Methods to reduce left-ventricular outflow-tract obstruction have included surgical myotomy–myectomy and mitral valve replacement. Dual-chamber (DDD) pacing and injection of septal perforators of the left anterior descending coronary artery with ethanol to relieve left-ventricular outflow-tract obstruction continue to be evaluated. Those children with high risk (extreme hypertrophy, syncope, resuscitated sudden death, or multiple familial sudden deaths) should be considered for ICD implant.

No specific therapy for patients with restrictive cardiomyopathy has been universally embraced. Therapies used for hypertrophic cardiomyopathy have also been used for patients with restrictive cardiomyopathy, but with very poor outcome. Heart transplantation is the only treatment proven effective to date. Those with syncope should be considered for ICD. LV noncompaction cases are treated based on their mode of presentation (i.e., DCM versus HCM). In ARVD/C, however, ICD treatment is becoming common.

PEARLS

If a patient presents with tachycardia and hypotension, do not simply provide fluid resuscitation (decreased heart rate and increased blood pressure), but instead evaluate the heart size by chest x-ray at presentation to diagnose dilated cardiomyopathy.

Monitor patients with dilated cardiomyopathy for arrhythmias and cardiac output while instituting medical therapy. Inotropic agents can induce arrhythmias. Anti-arrhythmics can decrease cardiac function, but are usually safe unless severe ventricular dysfunction exists. Consider use of ICD in high-risk patients. The underlying etiology of the cardiomyopathy may

influence treatment and outcome and, therefore, should be thoroughly sought.

Inotropic agents and diuretics may increase left-ventricular outflow-tract obstruction in patients with hypertrophic cardiomyopathy by increasing contractility and decreasing ventricular filling pressures.

Children with LVNC have an "undulating phenotype"; that is, they can change from one form to another (i.e., DCM-like to HCM-like, or vice versa) and therefore need close monitoring.

Bibliography

Franz WM, Muller OJ, Katus HA. Cardiomyopathies: from genetics to the prospect of treatment. *Lancet* 2001;358:1627–1637.

Friedman RA, Duff DF, Schowengerdt KO, et al. Myocarditis. In: Feigin RD, Cherry JD, eds. *Textbook of pediatric infectious diseases.* 4th ed. Philadelphia: Saunders; 1998:349–371.

Helton E, Darragh R, Francis P, et al. Metabolic aspects of myocardial disease and a role for L-carnitine in the treatment of childhood cardiomyopathy. *Pediatrics* 2000;105:1260–1270.

Lipshultz SE, Sleeper LA, Towbin JA, et al. The incidence of pediatric cardiomypathy in two regions of the United States. *N Engl J Med* 2003;348: 1703–1705.

Pignatelli RH, McMahon CJ, Dreyer WJ, et al. Clinical characterization of left ventricular noncompaction in children: a relatively common form of cardiomyopathy. *Circulation* 2003;108:2672–2678.

Towbin JA. Cardiomyopathy and heart transplantation in children. *Curr Opin Cardiol* 2002;17:274–279.

Towbin JA. Pediatric myocardial disease. *Pediatr Clin North Am* 1999: 46(2):289–312.

CHAPTER 31 ■ PERICARDITIS

KAREN F. LURITO AND CHARLIE J. SANG, JR.

Pericarditis is an inflammatory reaction of the pericardium to injury—infectious or noninfectious. The incidence is one case per 850 hospital admissions. In children less than 2 years of age, 90% of cases are purulent pericarditis.

The pericardium is a double-layered sac that surrounds the cardiac chambers and extends to the great vessels and systemic/pulmonary veins. The pericardium prevents overdistension of the heart, protects from infection and adhesions, maintains the heart in a fixed position in the chest, and regulates the stroke volumes of the two ventricles.

ETIOLOGY

Pericarditis may result from idiopathic, infectious, and noninfectious causes (Table 31.1). Typically, when infection is the etiology, there is a primary site of infection with hematogenous or direct spread to the pericardium. In most cases, treatment of the primary cause will result in resolution of pericarditis. Upper airway obstruction producing cor pulmonale has also been associated with pericardial effusions. A common noninfectious cause, postpericardiotomy syndrome, will be discussed in further detail.

PATHOPHYSIOLOGY

Infectious pericarditis begins with fibrin deposition adjacent to the great vessels that causes the pericardium to lose its smoothness and translucency. The intruding agent spreads via direct extension from the lung/pleura or the bloodstream. Fluid accumulates in the pericardial space, increasing intrapericardial pressure. The rate of accumulation determines presentation of symptoms. A slow accumulation allows accommodation of large volumes due to gradual expansion of the pericardium. The venous, atrial, and ventricular pressures of the heart rise equally. The resultant decrease in venous return due to cardiac compression results in decreased cardiac output. Reflex tachycardia and peripheral vasoconstriction are activated to maintain cardiac output. Pulsus paradoxus, a greater than 10-mm mercury drop in systolic pressure during inspiration, occurs because of decreased inflow to the cardiac chambers. Kussmaul sign is a paradoxical rise in jugular venous pressure during inspiration due to the tense pericardial sac limiting blood return to the right atrium from diastolic compression.

PRESENTATION

The most common symptoms are fever, tachypnea, and tachycardia. Chest and abdominal pain may be seen in 15% to 80% of patients. Upper respiratory tract symptoms may be present 10 to 14 days prior to presentation in patients with

viral pericarditis. Signs and symptoms consistent with other systemic causes may be present.

The physical examination may demonstrate jugular venous distension with hepatosplenomegaly. Heart tones are muffled. A pericardial friction rub is typically present but may be absent if there is sufficient pericardial fluid to prevent apposition of the pericardium. A pericardial rub is a high-frequency murmur with a scratchy quality. Rubs are best heard in the leaning forward or kneeling position with the diaphragm of the stethoscope pressed against the chest to amplify the opposing visceral and parietal pericardium. Decreased peripheral pulses and poor capillary refill may be present in early cardiac tamponade.

LABORATORY DATA

Recommended baseline studies include a complete blood count, erythrocyte sedimentation rate, C-reactive protein, and cultures of blood, nasopharyngeal, rectal, and urine to evaluate for bacterial and viral causes. Tests to confirm other systemic diseases should be obtained if history and physical examination are suggestive. These include blood urea nitrogen and serum creatinine levels, urinalysis, thyroid-stimulating hormone levels, antinuclear-antibodies, HIV serology, and tuberculin skin test if indicated. Cardiac muscle enzymes may be elevated if there is associated muscle damage due to involvement of the myocardium in cases of myopericarditis. Pericardiocentesis and analysis of the pericardial fluid is indicated in patients with moderate to large pericardial fluid collection presenting in tamponade, in patients suspected of bacterial or neoplastic pericarditis, and in patents with chronic pericarditis refractory to treatment.

Chest radiograph may demonstrate increased cardiothoracic ratio without increased pulmonary vascular markings if the pericardial fluid collection is gradual in subacute pericarditis. The cardiothoracic silhouette may be normal in cases of rapid accumulation of pericardial fluid, or in acute pericarditis without substantial fluid collection. Electrocardiogram initially demonstrates ST segment elevation with PR segment depression. As recovery ensues, the ST segments return to normal with development of T-wave inversion (Spodick stages).

Echocardiography is indicated in all patients with suspected or presumed pericarditis, (class I recommendation from the 2003 task force of the American College of Cardiology and the American Heart Association). The echocardiogram may demonstrate abnormal fluid space in the pericardial sac, or echogenic pericardium without significant fluid collection. Cardiac tamponade is present when diastolic collapse of the right atrium and right ventricle is demonstrated, and there is abnormal respiratory variation in the mitral inflow Doppler peak velocity.

TABLE 31.1

CAUSES OF PERICARDITIS

Type	Cause
IDIOPATHIC	
Benign	
Recurrent	
INFECTIOUS	
Purulent	Bacterial: *Staphylococcus aureus*, *Haemophilus influenzae*, streptococci, *Neisseria meningitidis*, *Streptococcus pneumoniae*, anaerobes, *Francisella tularensis*, *Salmonella*, enteric bacilli, *Pseudomonas*, *Listeria*, *Neisseria gonorrhoeae*, *Actinomyces*, nocardiosis
	Tuberculosis
	Fungal: histoplasmosis, coccidioidomycosis, aspergillosis, candidia sis, blastomycosis, cryptococcosis
Viral	Coxsackie viruses B
	Other: influenza A and B, mumps, echoviruses, adenoviruses, infectious mononucleosis, hepatitis, measles, cytomegalovirus
Other	Rickettsial: typhus, Q fever
	Mycoplasmal: *Mycoplasma pneumoniae*
	Parasitic: *Entamoeba histolytica*, *Echinococcus*
	Spirochetal: syphilis, leptospirosis
	Chlamydial: psitticosis
	Protozoal: toxoplasmosis
NONINFECTIOUS	
	Postpericardiotomy syndrome
	Rheumatic fever
	Connective tissue disorders: juvenile rheumatoid arthritis, systemic lupus erythematosus, dermatomyositis, periarteritis nodosa
	Trauma: blunt or penetrating
	Metabolic: uremia, myxedema
	Hypersensitivity: serum sickness, pulmonary infiltrates with eosinophilia, Stevens–Johnson syndrome, drugs (hydralazine, procainamide, chemotherapy)
	Neoplasm: leukemia, metastatic
	Postirradiation

From Feigin RD, Cherry JD, eds. *Textbook of pediatric infectious diseases.* 4th ed. Philadelphia: Saunders; 1998:339, with permission.

TREATMENT

Patients who present with cardiac tamponade and hemodynamic instability require emergent pericardiocentesis and management in an intensive care unit. Draining the pericardial fluid using a large-bore needle, angiocath, or pigtail catheter placed under echocardiogram guidance may be life-saving.

Patients presenting with risk factors for complications and adverse sequelea require inpatient care. These include patients with high fever (>100.4°F), subacute onset, immunocompromised state, history of anticoagulant therapy or trauma, or failure to respond to nonsteroidal anti-inflammatory therapy.

If purulent pericarditis is diagnosed, surgical drainage with a pericardial drainage tube may be required because the viscous fluid will not drain from smaller tubes. Based on culture results, intravenous antibiotic therapy for 3 to 4 weeks is required. The most common organisms are *Staphylococcus aureus* and *Haemophilus influenzae*.

Idiopathic and viral pericarditis may resolve spontaneously over 3 to 4 weeks. Anti-inflammatory therapy with aspirin (80 to 100 mg/kg/day divided into four doses), ibuprofen (5 to 10 mg/kg/dose given every 6 to 8 hours) or prednisone (2 mg/kg/day) has been recommended in cases where the pericardial fluid continues to accumulate. In their 2004 published guidelines, the European Society of Cardiology gave a class I recommendation for the use of nonsteroidal anti-inflammatory agents in acute pericarditis.

Treatment of underlying noninfectious causes typically results in resolution of pericardial fluid. Patients with hypothyroidism, renal failure, and systemic lupus erythematosus have dramatic recoveries. Rare cases that are recurrent and unresponsive to routine medical management have required surgical pericardial windows for long-term drainage.

Colchicine has been used in adults for the treatment of recurrent and refractory pericarditis. The European Society of Cardiology in their 2004 guidelines published the results of an open-label sudy, the COPE trial, a prospective randomized trial evaluating 120 adult patients with a first episode of acute pericarditis. The results supported the use of colchicine (0.5 to 1 mg/kg/day) alone or in addition to an NSAID for the treatment of acute pericarditis. Their guidelines also recommended the use of corticosteroids in patients refractory to NSAID and colchicine therapy, and in patients with known systemic autoimmune disorders. Several observational studies have also suggested that corticosteroid use early in acute pericarditis is associated with recurrent refractory pericarditis and should therefore be limited to patients who are nonresponders to NSAIDs and patients with autoimmune diseases.

PROGNOSIS

Purulent pericarditis has a high mortality rate. One late sequelae of purulent pericarditis is constrictive pericarditis. A thick, fibrotic, and occasionally calcific pericardium develops and restricts diastolic function. Surgical resection of the pericardium is the therapy of choice when constrictive pericarditis occurs.

The recurrence rate for viral pericarditis is 15% to 30%. Patients may have associated viral myocarditis that requires therapy after the pericarditis has resolved.

POSTPERICARDIOTOMY SYNDROME

Postpericardiotomy syndrome is the most common postoperative inflammatory syndrome. This syndrome occurs in patients who have undergone heart surgery during which the pericardium has been insulted. Although the inflammatory response is attributed to extensive trauma to the pericardium, epicardium, and myocardium, cases have been reported with atrial septal defect closure and patent ductus arteriosus ligation and division. An autoimmune response with the production of antisarcolemmal and antifibrillary antibodies is felt to be the etiology.

These patients develop a fever 1 to 2 weeks postoperatively with malaise, decreased appetite, irritability, vomiting, and nonspecific chest and abdominal pain. Physical findings are tachycardia, pericardial rub, and hepatomegaly. Cardiac tamponade is rare. A left-sided pleural effusion may be present. A complete blood count may show a left shift, and the erythrocyte sedimentation rate and C-reactive protein may be elevated. Chest radiograph will demonstrate enlargement of the cardiac silhouette and possible left pleural effusion. The echocardiogram will demonstrate pericardial fluid collection of varying size with echogenic pericardium heralding pericardial inflammation.

Anti-inflammatory therapy with aspirin, ibuprofen, indomethacin, or prednisone typically aids in resolving the pericarditis and eliminating the pericardial fluid. Frequent follow-up is required to document resolution of the fluid collection. Pericardiocentesis or surgical drainage/window has been required in cases that are not responsive to medical management.

PEARLS

■ Diuretics given to patients with pericardial fluid may make them hemodynamically unstable by decreasing filling pressures, resulting in cardiac tamponade physiology.

■ Complications of pericardiocentesis include laceration of coronary arteries and perforation of the heart. If the patient does not improve during the procedure, reevaluate that the needle or catheter is in the pericardial space and not the ventricular cavity. Typically, pericardial fluid will not clot and the hematocrit of the fluid is less than the venous blood. Patients may require volume resuscitation while extracting pericardial fluid to improve preload.

Suggested Readings

Clapp SK. Postoperative inflammatory syndromes. In: Garson A, Bricker JT, McNamara DG, eds. *The science and practice of pediatric cardiology.* Philadelphia: Lea & Febiger; 1990:1600–1604.

Maisch B, Severovic PM, Ristic AD, et al. Guidelines on the diagnosis and management of pericardial diseases executive summary. The task force on the diagnosis and management of pericardial diseases of the European Society of Cardiology. *Eur Heart J* 2004;25:587.

Pinsky WW, Friedman RA. Pericarditis. In: Garson A, Bricker JT, McNamara DG, eds. *The science and practice of pediatric cardiology.* Philadelphia: Lea & Febiger; 1990:1590–1599.

Pinsky WW, Friedman RA, Jubelirer DP, et al. Infectious pericarditis. In: eds. *Textbook of pediatric infectious diseases.* 4th ed. Philadelphia: Saunders; 1998:339–348.

Spodixk, DH. Pericardial disease. In: Braunwald E, Zipes D, Libby P, eds. *Heart disease. A textbook of cardiovascular medicine.* New York: Saunders; 2001:1823–1876.

CHAPTER 32 ■ MYOCARDITIS

KAREN R. UNDERWOOD AND PAUL A. CHECCHIA

Cardiac inflammation is difficult to diagnose and even if diagnosed, can we then treat it effectively?
— Jean Baptiste Senang, physician to Louis XV, 1773

Myocarditis is defined as an inflammation of the myocardium. The etiologies are varied, but are usually considered viral when using the term (see Table 32.1). Inflammatory and infiltrative diseases of the heart such as Kawasaki disease and sarcoidosis are usually considered as separate disorders, although there may be inflammatory cardiac changes. Myocarditis affects both children and adults, can be acute or more insidious in its onset, and can be life threatening or life shortening. This review will concentrate on the incidence, presenting features, available approaches to the diagnosis, and treatment options of myocarditis in children. An important distinction must be made regarding the separation of diagnostic versus prognostic examination, and between the more general diagnosis of severe heart failure or shock versus the specific diagnosis of myocarditis.

INCIDENCE

The incidence of myocarditis has been reported to be approximately 0.1% to 0.6% in the general pediatric population (1). A difficulty in measuring the incidence of myocarditis, especially in a pediatric population, is the variability of existing diagnostic protocols. Also, there is considerable clinical and histologic overlap with the diagnosis of dilated cardiomyopathy. Finally, compared with studies of adults, there is relatively little data examining myocarditis in pediatric populations to define potential age-related differences in the pathophysiology and presentation of myocarditis. This is an important fact because more than half of all cases of myocarditis in children present within the first year of life.

CLINICAL PRESENTATION

Common presenting features of myocarditis in children are those of sudden onset of cardiac insufficiency or failure. However, myocarditis can present in a more insidious fashion such as failure to thrive or with acute catastrophic symptoms such as life-threatening dysrhythmias, cardiogenic shock, or sudden death. The clinical features of the presentation of myocarditis vary depending on age.

DIAGNOSIS

The diagnosis of myocarditis requires a high index of suspicion, attention to historical clues, and thorough physical exam. Regardless of etiology, the diagnosis of myocarditis is based on clinical findings, echocardiographic evaluation, and endomyocardial biopsy sampling. There are, however, limitations to the use of each of these examinations, including sampling errors related to heterogeneity of disease, the invasiveness of the procedure, and inability of the pathologic examination of tissue to reflect the physiologic effect of circulating mediators. A simple, highly sensitive, and specific test that could accurately detect myocyte injury during the course of myocarditis, etiologic agent, and response to therapy would be clinically valuable. Unfortunately, no sensitive or specific clinical or laboratory clues to the diagnosis of acute myocarditis have been found.

The diagnosis of myocarditis starts with ruling out other causes of myocardial dysfunction. Structural cardiac lesions, in particular left-sided outflow obstruction and anomalous coronary artery, can cause congestive heart failure, and must be ruled out by echocardiography. The signs and symptoms of pericarditis, especially with pericardial tamponade, may resemble those of acute myocarditis; significant pericardial effusion is easily diagnosed with an echocardiogram. Incessant or chronic arrhythmia such as supraventricular tachycardia and the permanent form of junctional reciprocating tachycardia may cause significant myocardial dysfunction mimicking myocarditis, but should be detected by electrocardiography. Arrhythmia as a presenting sign of myocarditis is discussed below. Systemic hypertension can present with congestive heart failure. Inherited metabolic causes of myocardial dysfunction may be more difficult to rule out, although a positive family history, long-standing failure to thrive, other abnormalities on physical exam (e.g., hypotonia), and characteristic electrocardiographic (ECG) changes when present (e.g., for glycogen storage disease of the heart) may suggest the need for detailed investigation along those lines.

Having ruled out other causes of myocardial dysfunction, there are multiple tests which may lend support to the diagnosis of myocarditis, and/or offer important information relevant to the therapy provided.

ECG Findings

Electrocardiographic findings in patients with acute myocarditis are highly variable. The most typical findings are (1) sinus tachycardia; (2) low-voltage QRS in standard (total voltage <5 mm) and precordial leads, and low-amplitude q-waves in the lateral precordial leads; and (3) flattening or inversion of T-waves in the standard or L precordial leads.

Marked elevation of ST segments on electrocardiogram (ECG) may be a striking finding. Several studies in adults have documented symptoms, cardiac enzyme changes, and ECG findings including ST elevation that suggested myocardial infarction, but occurred in patients with normal coronary arteries and histologic evidence of myocarditis (2).

Arrhythmia is not uncommon in myocarditis, including supraventricular tachycardia, atrial ectopic tachycardia, ventricular premature beats, ventricular tachycardia, and ventricular

TABLE 32.1

VIRAL CAUSES OF MYOCARDITIS

Enteroviruses (coxsackie B)
Adenovirus
Influenza
Parvovirus B19
Epstein–Barr virus
Varicella-zoster
Herpes simplex
Human immunodeficiency virus
Cytomegalovirus

fibrillation. Several studies have described children and adolescents with ventricular tachycardia or frequent ventricular ectopy who had biopsy findings of myocarditis without obvious myocardial dysfunction (3). Variable degrees of atrioventricular block, including complete heart block, have also been well documented.

Chest Radiograph

The cardiac silhouette is generally enlarged with acute myocarditis, but may be normal in size and configuration. Pulmonary edema may be present in variable degree. Pleural effusion and interstitial infiltrates may also be observed.

Echocardiography

The most characteristic echocardiographic appearance is that of enlarged ventricular end-systolic and diastolic dimensions, as well as reduced shortening and ejection fractions; atrioventricular valve regurgitation, especially mitral regurgitation, is also common. However, multiple studies of adults with clinically and/or histologically established myocarditis have described regional wall-motion abnormalities, without global dysfunction or ventricular dilation, and in whom ischemic causes for such abnormalities has been excluded (4). There appears to be little published data regarding regional wall-motion abnormalities in children. Transiently increased ventricular wall thickness has also been observed.

Other cardiac ultrasound findings include pulmonary arterial hypertension secondary to increased left atrial pressure, and ventricular thrombi. Evidence of restrictive ventricular physiology and dystrophic calcification is rarely observed.

Serum Markers of Myocardial Injury

Creatine Kinase-MB

There is limited data on the use of CK-MB in the diagnosis of myocarditis in children. Data on the utility of CK-MB in myocarditis mainly examines its sensitivity and specificity in comparison to cardiac troponin measurements. One pediatric study showed that CK-MB, as well as cardiac troponin-T, were significantly higher for myocarditis than for dilated cardiomyopathy or congestive heart failure from excessive left-to-right shunting (5).

Cardiac Troponin

Several investigators have demonstrated elevation of cardiac troponin measurements in patients with suspected myocarditis (6). Some suggest a greater sensitivity and specificity of troponin measurements in comparison to CK-MB. These investigations

have utilized both troponin-I and troponin-T measurements with equivalent findings. However, some studies have suffered from their lack of consistency in their comparison to histologic findings obtained by biopsy.

In one pediatric-specific study, a serum cardiac troponin-T (cTnT) level of 0.052 ng/mL was shown to be an appropriate cutoff point for distinguishing acute myocarditis diagnosed by endomyocardial biopsy from dilated cardiomyopathy or from congestive heart failure from large ventricular septal defect (7). The role of troponin in the timing of biopsy and its role in the management of immunosuppressive regimes have not been well studied. Timing endomyocardial biopsy coincident with a high troponin might improve the yield of finding active inflammatory infiltrate.

Endomyocardial Biopsy

Endomyocardial biopsy remains the standard for diagnosing myocarditis, despite its known limitations, including sampling error, procedural complications, variability of pathologic interpretation, and low negative predictive value. The standard histologic criteria for establishing the diagnosis of myocarditis, the Dallas Criteria, were established in an adult population (8). Although studies have applied these criteria to pediatric populations, modifications based on age groups have not been found. Several pediatric-specific studies have found that endomyocardial biopsy was helpful but not universally diagnostic (9,10).

Recent advances in molecular biology techniques are increasing its sensitivity and overall utility. It is now possible to routinely use polymerase chain reaction and ribonucleic acid hybridization to provide rapid, reliable, and specific detection of viral genetic material in biopsy samples. Viral genome has been detected in the majority of biopsy samples in patients with myocarditis but is rarely present in controls (11).

MRI

Several noninvasive strategies are emerging as adjunctive diagnostic tests. Antimyosin scintigraphy, contrast-enhanced cardiovascular magnetic resonance imaging (CMR), and echocardiographic digital image processing may each be useful for the noninvasive localization and assessment of the extent of inflammation in patients with presumed myocarditis.

Investigators have evaluated the role of CMR in the diagnosis of acute myocarditis in both pediatric and adult populations. Several methods have been studied, including contrast enhancement and noncontrast T2-weighted imaging (12,13).

Diagnosis: Summary

The diagnosis of myocarditis must be based on a synthesis of the patient's clinical history, physical examination, imaging studies, and laboratory tests; no single diagnostic modality can suffice. Clinical history, physical exam, and imaging—especially echocardiography—are important for ruling out non-myocarditis etiologies that may present in the same way as myocarditis. Electrocardiography may help confirm the diagnosis of myocarditis. Classically this includes low voltages in the limb and precordial ECG leads and flattening of T-waves. In other cases of proven myocarditis, the ECG findings may be more confusing, as in the patient with marked ST segment elevation falsely suggesting myocardial infarction or in cases with incessant or frequent arrhythmia as a manifestation of myocarditis rather than a primary arrhythmia causing ventricular dysfunction. Chest x-ray findings are highly variable and nonspecific. Echocardiographic assessment of ventricular dimensions and systolic function is an essential part of the evaluation because myocardial dysfunction is the most common mode of presentation of myocarditis in children.

CK-MB, troponin-I, and troponin-T have all been found to be elevated with myocarditis; probably the best data to date regards elevation of troponin-I. Endomyocardial biopsy, looking for histologic evidence of inflammation, has served as the "gold standard" for diagnosis, although it is clearly positive for myocarditis in only a relatively small fraction of patients for whom there is a strong clinical index of suspicion for the disease. Searching for the presence of viral genome in myocardial samples appears to considerably increase the sensitivity of endomyocardial biopsy.

Advanced imaging modalities, such as antimyosin scintigraphy and contrast-enhanced cardiovascular magnetic resonance imaging (CMR), may allow noninvasive imaging and study of myocardial biology and take on more important diagnostic and prognostic roles (14).

TREATMENT

Immunotherapies

Varying successes are reported with immunotherapies early in the course of treatment of myocarditis. These have included intravenous immune globulin as well as immunosuppressive agents such as prednisone, methylprednisolone, azathioprine, and OKT3.

Because the early form of myocarditis is thought to be due to an inflammatory response usually secondary to a viral pathogen, immune globulin could potentially enhance viral clearance if it contains neutralizing antibodies to the virus. Likewise, immune globulin may help to reduce the inflammatory response triggered by proinflammatory cytokine release. There are no randomized controlled studies proving efficacy of immune globulin in this situation, although some reports suggest possible benefits (15,16). In one pediatric study, 21 children presenting with presumed myocarditis were treated with an intravenous gamma globulin infusion of 2 g/kg over 24 hours after presentation. Twenty-five historical untreated patients were used as the control group. Improvement in the left ventricular shortening fraction favored the treated group and differences at the 3- to 6-month follow-up and 6- to 12-month intervals were significantly different from the historical controls. The 12-month survival trended favorably for the treated patients; the observed differences were not statistically significant. Age less than 2 years along with biopsy status showed significantly better outcome than historical controls (15).

Other immunosuppressive therapies may act to suppress cell-mediated inflammatory reactions within the myocardium during the subacute phase of myocarditis. Because an autoimmune reaction may play a role in chronic myocarditis, immunosuppression may help to reduce this reaction. There is preliminary data suggesting a beneficial effect from multiple immunosuppressive agents, and this is an area that needs to be explored in a multicenter, randomized controlled study (17,18).

Supportive Care

In fulminant myocarditis, aggressive treatment and hemodynamic monitoring may be necessary in a critical care setting. Mechanical ventilation with the initiation of inotropic support, afterload reduction, anticoagulation, and diuresis are often required with severely depressed function as detailed in other chapters within this text. Other mainstays of therapy include beta-blockers and calcium-channel blockers.

Mechanical Circulatory Support and Heart Transplantation

For those patients with continued depressed cardiac function despite aggressive management with mechanical ventilation, inotropic support and afterload reduction, cardiopulmonary support may be a reasonable option. It appears that these patients develop aggressive myocyte injury from the initial impact of the viral infection, and medical treatment does not seem to alter the unrelenting fulminant course. Extracorporeal support has been used as a life-saving maneuver while the myocardium recovers or as a bridge to heart transplantation. In one study, eight pediatric patients with biopsy-proven myocarditis were supported on extracorporeal membrane oxygenation (ECMO). Five of these patients were successfully separated, of whom three had restoration of normal cardiac function, one had residual myocardial dysfunction, and one died of fungal sepsis. One patient died while on support, and two additional patients underwent cardiac transplantation (19).

Summary: Therapy

Despite a common practice of immune globulin administration, the pediatric literature is void of randomized controlled studies to render a definitive opinion regarding the use of immune globulin in the management of myocarditis. No Class I studies exist in the pediatric literature addressing this treatment and no meaningful meta-analysis of available studies exists. Data does suggest that benefit may exist and this warrants further investigation. Further, the available studies do not reveal a risk of immune globulin treatment in this patient population.

Likewise, there is a lack of evidence-based data to conclude whether the use of other immunosuppressive therapies (steroids, and immunosuppressives) benefits the pediatric myocarditis patient. Preliminary data suggest a beneficial effect particularly from multiple immunosuppressive agent use, and this needs to be explored in a multicenter, randomized controlled study. Data in the adult myocarditis patient suggests that a favorable clinical response to immunosuppressive treatments may be predicted by the presence of cardiac antibodies and absence of viral genome by PCR in the myocardium. Such screening should be incorporated in the study design of future pediatric treatment studies.

References

1. Wheeler DS, Kooy NW. A formidable challenge: the diagnosis and treatment of viral myocarditis in children. *Crit Care Clin* Jul 2003;19:365–391.
2. Angelini A, Calzolari V, Calabrese F, et al. Myocarditis mimicking acute myocardial infarction: role of endomyocardial biopsy in the differential diagnosis. *Heart* 2000;84:245–250.
3. Friedman RA, Kearney DL, Moak JP, et al. Persistence of ventricular arrhythmia after resolution of occult myocarditis in children and young adults. *J Am Coll Cardiol* 1994;24:780–783.
4. Shirani J, Ilercil A, Chandra M, et al. Cardiovascular imaging in clinical and experimental acute infectious myocarditis. *Frontiers in Bioscience* 2003;8: e323–e336.
5. Soongswang J, Durongpisitkul K, Ratanarapee S, et al. Cardiac troponin T: its role in the diagnosis of clinically suspected acute myocarditis and chronic dilated cardiomyopathy in children. *Pediatr Cardiol* 2002;23:531–535.
6. Lauer B, Niederau C, Kuhl U, et al. Cardiac troponin T in patients with clinically suspected myocarditis. *J Am Coll Cardiol* 1997;30:1354–1359.
7. Soongswang J, Durongpisitkul K, Nana A, et al. Cardiac troponin T: a marker in the diagnosis of acute myocarditis in children. *Pediatr Cardiol* 2005;26:45–49.
8. Aretz HT, Billingham ME, Edwards WD, et al. Myocarditis. A histopathologic definition and classification. *Am J Cardiovasc Pathol* 1987;1:3–14.
9. Schmaltz AA, Apitz J, Hort W, et al. Endomyocardial biopsy in infants and children: experience in 60 patients. *Pediatr Cardiol* 1990;11:15–21.
10. Chandra RS. The role of endomyocardial biopsy in the diagnosis of cardiac disorders in infants and children. *Am J Cardiovasc Pathol* 1987;1:157–172.

11. Martin AB, Webber S, Fricker FJ, et al. Acute myocarditis. Rapid diagnosis by PCR in children. *Circulation* 1994;90:330–339.

12. Gagliardi MG, Bevilacqua M, Di Renzi P, et al. Usefulness of magnetic resonance imaging for diagnosis of acute myocarditis in infants and children, and comparison with endomyocardial biopsy. *Am J Cardiol* 1991;68: 1089–1091.

13. Abdel-Aty H, Boye P, Zagrosek A, et al. Diagnostic performance of cardiovascular magnetic resonance in patients with suspected acute myocarditis: comparison of different approaches. *J Am Coll Cardiol* 2005;45:1815–1822.

14. Mahrholdt H, Goedecke C, Wagner A, et al. Cardiovascular magnetic resonance assessment of human myocarditis: a comparison to histology and molecular pathology. *Circulation* 2004;109:1250–1258.

15. Drucker NA, Colan SD, Lewis AB, et al. Gamma-globulin treatment of acute myocarditis in the pediatric population. *Circulation* 1994;89:252–257.

16. English RF, Janosky JE, Ettedgui JA, et al. Outcomes for children with acute myocarditis. *Cardiol Young* 2004;14:488–493.

17. Gagliardi MG, Bevilacqua M, Bassano C, et al. Long term follow up of children with myocarditis treated by immunosuppression and of children with dilated cardiomyopathy. *Heart* 2004;90:1167–1171.

18. Kleinert S, Weintraub RG, Wilkinson JL, et al. Myocarditis in children with dilated cardiomyopathy: incidence and outcome after dual therapy immunosuppression. *J Heart Lung Transplant* 1997;16:1248–1254.

19. Lee KJ, McCrindle BW, Bohn DJ, et al. Clinical outcomes of acute myocarditis in childhood. *Heart* 1999;82:226–233.

CHAPTER 33 ■ ENDOCARDITIS

KAREN F. LURITO AND DEBRA A. TRISTRAM

Infective endocarditis results when microorganisms (bacteria or fungi) adhere to the endocardial surface of the heart, usually on the heart valves. Infection begins on abnormal endocardium at the sites of congenital defects or damage by previous surgery, disease, or trauma. Infective endocarditis can be classified as either acute or subacute based on the progression of untreated disease. Acute endocarditis has a much more fulminant course, with high fever, systemic toxicity, and rapid death in untreated conditions. Subacute bacterial endocarditis (SBE) follows a more indolent course, 6 weeks to several months, with intermittent low-grade fever, vague systemic complaints, and various forms of embolic phenomenon.

In children, the most common bacteria causing endocarditis are streptococci, especially the viridans streptococci. Staphylococci are the next most common bacterial pathogens, with *Staphylococcus aureus* more common than coagulase-negative staphylococcal species. Staphylococci predominate among causes of endocarditis after cardiac surgery. Occasionally, gram-negative enteric bacteria are found in endocarditis. These organisms tend to be associated with prior surgery or the presence of indwelling vascular catheters. In children, nutritionally deficient streptococci and fastidious gram-negative coccobacilli in the HACEK group (*Haemophilus aphrophilus*, and *Actinobacillus*, *Cardiobacterium*, *Eikenella*, and *Kingella* species) are unusual causes of endocarditis. Fungal endocarditis may be encountered, and seems to cluster among sick neonates. Indwelling catheters, prolonged antibiotic courses, and prior bowel surgery may predispose to the development of transient fungemia and subsequent fungal endocarditis. Approximately 5% to 10% of cases of endocarditis have sterile blood cultures, most commonly in circumstances where antibiotics have been given before obtaining the blood cultures.

Since the early 1990s, the incidence of infective endocarditis in children has increased, possibly because of the improved survival of children with complex congenital heart disease. Mortality rates for endocarditis have fallen and are close to 10% or less. Prosthetic valves and valve conduit repairs in children with complex heart disease are predisposing factors to the development of endocarditis (Table 33.1). The incidence of prosthetic valve endocarditis varies from approximately 2% to 4% after surgery. Aortic and mitral valves are infected most often. Native valve endocarditis results from the bacterial seeding on heart valves or endocardium disrupted by turbulent blood flow. Transient bacteremia occurs during dental and other procedures that disrupt the integrity of the mucosal surface. The microorganisms in the blood are then deposited on the platelet–fibrin thrombi present at the site of turbulence. Although most episodes of native valve endocarditis occur in children with abnormal cardiac structure due to congenital heart disease, an increasing number of children with normal cardiac structure have been reported with endocarditis. Risk factors in normal children include indwelling vascular catheters (especially where the tip is in the right side

of the heart), prolonged parenteral nutrition, and acquired immunodeficiency states (patients on chemotherapy and renal transplant recipients).

Prosthetic valve endocarditis is divided into early and late disease in relationship to the surgical intervention. Early endocarditis (within 2 months of surgery) results from bacterial contamination at the time of surgery or in the immediate postoperative period. Perioperative poor nutrition and impaired host defenses may contribute to the bacteria's ability to adhere and proliferate. Late-onset endocarditis occurs outside of the 2-month postoperative period, when the operative site and valves/conduits have been reepithelialized. Risk factors for late-onset endocarditis closely parallel those for native valve endocarditis.

The differential diagnosis of endocarditis depends on the duration of symptoms. If the onset of endocarditis is insidious, prolonged or intermittent fever in conjunction with muscle aches or arthralgias may suggest a viral illness (e.g., Epstein–Barr virus) or a collagen vascular disorder (e.g., juvenile rheumatoid arthritis). With sudden onset of endocarditis, fever and toxic appearance suggest septicemia or other acute cardiac inflammatory disease such as pericarditis or myocarditis. Patients with embolic disease may have unrecognized cardiac disease, particularly if they have only a single site of peripheral embolization such as a lung or brain abscess.

CLINICAL FINDINGS

The clinical presentation usually allows infective endocarditis to be classified as subacute or acute. SBE generally manifests with a prodrome of several weeks to months consisting of general malaise and low-grade fever. In contrast, acute endocarditis has a short prodrome and a sepsis-like presentation. There may be considerable overlap between acute disease and SBE. The most common symptoms of endocarditis in children are fever, malaise, and worsening cardiac function. Because of the subtle nature of SBE symptoms, there can be a delay in diagnosis of weeks to months. Endocarditis should be suspected in any child with a history of congenital heart disease who presents with an unexplained, fatiguing illness and fever. There may be a history of limited improvement after empiric oral antibiotics are given.

The classic physical findings in endocarditis are fever, new or changing heart murmur(s), and the presence of embolic phenomena. Fever is a nearly universal finding and probably can be used to date the onset of disease. Occasionally, a patient with subacute bacterial endocarditis does not have fever, particularly if he has received antibiotics for another reason. Splenic enlargement is a relatively common feature and may be found in up to 75% of children with endocarditis. Embolic phenomena such as petechiae or vasculitis, especially involving the mucous membranes, may be present. Splinter hemorrhages

TABLE 33.1

CARDIAC CONDITIONS ASSOCIATED WITH ENDOCARDITIS

High risk	Moderate risk	Minimal or no risk
Prosthetic cardiac valves not listed in high- or minimal-risk	Other congenital cardiac malformations categories	Isolated secundum atrial septal defect
Previous bacterial endocarditis	Acquired valvular disease	Surgical repair of atrial septal defect, ventricular septal defect or patent ductus arteriosus (without residua and more than 6 months postoperative)
Complex cyanotic congenital heart disease	Hypertrophic cardiomyopathy	Mitral valve prolapse without regurgitation
Surgically constructed systemic–pulmonary shunts and conduits	MVP with valvular regurgitation or thickened leaflets	Physiologic, functional, or innocent murmurs Previous Kawasaki disease without valvular dysfunction Previous rheumatic disease without valvular dysfunction Electrical cardiac devices (e.g., pacemakers, defibrillators)

may be seen in the nailbeds of fingers and toes and appear as dark linear streaks from microemboli and increased capillary fragility. Osler nodes, the small, painful, purplish lesions found in the pulp of fingers and toes, or Janeway lesions, the painless hemorrhagic macular plaques on the palms and soles, occasionally may be found. A careful examination of the retina may reveal Roth spots, small hemorrhagic retinal lesions with a pale center that usually are found near the optic discs. All of these features are not common findings in patients with endocarditis, but still should be sought carefully on physical examination.

Laboratory tests should be performed to support the diagnosis of infective endocarditis. Usually, three blood cultures performed at separate times are obtained before the institution of antibiotics if the patient is otherwise stable. The total peripheral white blood cell count usually is elevated and anemia often is present. Inflammatory indicators such as erythrocyte sedimentation rate or C-reactive protein are almost always elevated. A positive serum rheumatoid factor and hematuria may be present in 25% to 50% of patients. A low serum complement, particularly with long-standing infective endocarditis, may be found in a small number of individuals.

The echocardiogram can visualize endocardial vegetations and lesions as small as 2 mm. Early in the course of infective endocarditis, valve leaflet thickening can be seen. Serial echocardiographic examination demonstrates the development of irregularly shaped lesions on the valve leaflets, the chordee, or the base of the valves. Doppler flow can demonstrate new regurgitation or turbulence as the vegetations change over time. Transesophageal echocardiography increases the sensitivity for imaging vegetations and should be performed in cases where initial transthoracic echocardiography is negative and endocarditis is strongly suspected.

The diagnosis of endocarditis is straightforward in a patient with positive blood cultures, known cardiac disease, and a new vegetation. It is far more difficult in situations where there may be culture-negative disease with new vegetations or positive blood cultures without evidence of cardiac lesions. The set of diagnostic criteria proposed by Von Reyn may be helpful in such cases. *Modifications of the Duke Criteria have been proposed specifically to improve diagnosis of pediatric endocarditis*

and are available online in the article by Tissieres and associates cited in the Suggested Readings. Consultation with a pediatric cardiologist also can be a valuable resource in such cases.

MANAGEMENT

The antibiotic treatment of infective endocarditis depends on the microorganism responsible for infection. Suggested regimens for antibiotic therapy are outlined in Table 33.2.

Surgery plays an important role in some cases of infective endocarditis. The indications for surgery include (1) persistently positive blood cultures despite appropriate antibiotics, (2) abscesses of the valve annulus or the myocardium, (3) two or more serious embolic events during treatment, (4) rupture of the valve leaflet or chordee with subsequent acute valvular insufficiency and intractable cardiac failure, (5) progressive cardiac failure that cannot be controlled by medical management (usually due to mitral or aortic valve insufficiency), and (6) fungal or coagulase-negative staphylococcal endocarditis. In most cases, the decision to remove an infected prosthetic device depends on the response to antimicrobial therapy and the organism involved. It may not be necessary if the patient responds rapidly to medical treatment, but it is definitely necessary if the clinical response is poor, blood cultures continue to be positive, cardiac status deteriorates, or clinical relapse occurs after completion of the antibiotic regimen. For coagulase-negative staphylococci and for fungi, the likelihood of true sterilization is extremely low even with an apparent rapid response to medical therapy. In these instances, the foreign material (valves, conduits) should be removed promptly if at all possible.

As many as 20% of children who present with endocarditis have recently undergone a procedure associated with a high risk of bacteremia (e.g., dental cleaning). Antibiotic prophylaxis is recommended and has been shown to be useful in patients with cardiac defects who need procedures that are associated with a high risk of bacteremia. For more specific recommendations on the cardiac defects and surgical procedures requiring prophylaxis, and the appropriate antibiotic

TABLE 33.2

ANTIBIOTICS FOR BACTERIAL ENDOCARDITIS

Bacteria	Antibiotic choice, dose, and duration
Viridans streptococci	Penicillin G 200,000–300,000 U/kg/day IV div q4–6h × 4 weeks; *or* Ceftriaxone 100 mg/kg/day q24h × 4 weeks *and* penicillin G 200,000–300,000 U/kg/day IV div q4–6h × 2 weeks *or* Ceftriaxone 100 mg/kg/day q24h × 2 weeks *and* gentamicin 3 mg/kg/day IM, IV div q8h × 2 weeks *or* Vancomycin 40 mg/kg/day IV div q6h
(For nutritionally variant viridan streptococci)	Penicillin G 300,000 U/kg/day IV div q4–6h × 4–6 weeks *and* gentamicin 3 mg/kg/day IM, IV div q8h × 4–6 weeks *or* Vancomycin 40 mg/kg/day IV div q6h
Enterococci	Ampicillin 300 mg/kg/day IV, IM div q6h × 30 days *and* gentamicin 6–7.5 mg/kg/day IM, IV div q8h *or* Penicillin G 250,000 U/kg/day IV div q8h q4–6h *and* streptomycin 30 mg/kg/day IM div q12h × 30 days
Staphylococcus aureus	Nafcillin or oxacillin 200 mg/kg/day IV div q6h × 6 weeks
Staphylococcus epidermidis (for methicillin-resistant staphylococci)	Vancomycin 40 mg/kg/day IV div q6h; consider adding rifampin or aminoglycoside for synergy
Other bacteria and fungi	Consult with infectious disease or cardiology for treatment options

div, divided; IM, intramuscular; IV, intravenous.

regimen, readers may see the tables in Chapter 29, or are referred to the references at the end of this chapter.

COURSE AND PROGNOSIS

Most of the survivors of infective endocarditis remain hemodynamically stable at long-term follow-up. Cure rates for endocarditis caused by viridans streptococci are nearly 100%. The cure rate for *S. aureus* endocarditis is less than for streptococci, but still is close to 75%. Fungal endocarditis has the worst prognosis, with a cure rate of only approximately 50% even in the face of valve replacement. Those features associated with a poor prognosis include the presence of prosthetic material, especially artificial heart valves; very young infants; and giant vegetations.

PEARLS

- Serum rheumatoid factor is very often positive in subacute or chronic endocarditis owing to immune complex deposition.
- When present, microscopic hematuria may be associated with red cell casts in the urine and with low serum complement levels.
- Secundum atrial septal defect is not a risk for endocarditis prophylaxis *before or after* surgical closure. However, a primum atrial septal defect is really a kind of endocardial cushion defect and always requires SBE prophylaxis before and after operative repair because the mitral valve is abnormally formed and is associated with SBE risk.

Suggested Readings

Baddour LM, Wilson WR, Bayer AS, et al. AHA scientific statement. Infective endocarditis. Diagnosis, antimicrobial therapy, and management of complications: a statement for healthcare professionals from the Committee on Rheumatic Fever, Endocarditis, and Kawasaki Disease, Council on Cardiovascular Disease in the Young, and the Councils on Clinical Cardiology, Stroke, and Cardiovascular Surgery and Anesthesia, American Heart Association—executive summary: endorsed by the Infectious Diseases Society of America. *Circulation* 2005;111:3167–3184. Available at *http://circ.ahajournals.org/ cgi/content/full/111/23/e394*.

Bayer AS, Bolger AF, Taubert KA, et al. Diagnosis and management of infective endocarditis and its complications. *Echocardiogr Circ* 1998;98:2936–2948.

Brook MM. Pediatric bacteria endocarditis treatment and prophylaxis. *Pediatr Clin North Am* 1999;46:275–287.

Dajani, AS, Taubert KA, Wilson W, et al. Prevention of bacterial endocarditis. American Heart Association. *Circulation* 1997;96:358–366. Available at: *http://circ.ahajournals.org/cgi/content/full/96/1/358* or *http://www.american-heart.org/presenter.jhtml?identifier=3004539*

Dajani AS, Taubert KA, Wilson W, et al. Prevention of bacterial endocarditis: recommendations by the American Heart Association. *JAMA* 1997;272:794–1801 and *Circulation* 1997;96:358–366.

Ferrieri P, Gewitz MH, Gerber MA, et al. Committee on Rheumatic Fever, Endocarditis, and Kawasaki Disease of the American Heart Association Council on Cardiovascular Disease in the Young. Unique features of infective endocarditis in childhood. *Circulation* 2002;105:2115–2127. Available at *http://circ.ahajournals.org/cgi/content/full/105/17/2115*.

Hoyer A, Silberbach M. Infective endocarditis. *Pediatr Rev* 2005;26:388–393. Available at *http://pedsinreview.aappublications.org/cgi/content/full/26/11/394*.

Millar BC, Jugo J, Moore JE. Fungal endocarditis in neonates and children. *Pediatr Cardiol* 2005;26:517–536. Review.

Tissieres P, Gervaix A, Beghetti M, et al. Value and limitations of the von Reyn, Duke and modified Duke criteria for the diagnosis of infective endocarditis in children. *Pediatrics* 2003;112:e467–e471. Available at *http:// pediatrics.aappublications.org/cgi/content/full/112/6/e467*.

Von Reyn CF, Levy BS, Arbeit RD, et al. Infective endocarditis: an analysis based on strict case definitions. *Ann Intern Med* 1981;94:505.

CHAPTER 34 ■ SHOCK STATES

RONALD A. BRONICKI

Definition and Classification of Shock

Shock results from inadequate oxygen delivery and/or impaired utilization leading to tissue hypoxia, cellular dysfunction, and cellular necrosis. Shock is not necessarily a problem of blood volume, cardiac output, or blood pressure, but it is always a problem of inadequate tissue oxygenation. Delivery of oxygen depends upon the integrated function of three organ systems: the lungs for oxygenation, the blood for oxygen-carrying capacity, and the circulatory system for perfusion. Accordingly, tissue hypoxia or shock results from one or more of the following mechanisms: *hypoxic hypoxia* occurs when the partial pressure of oxygen in blood is reduced, and *anemic hypoxia* results from a reduction in oxygen-carrying capacity; in either case, oxygen content is severely reduced; *stagnant hypoxia* results from low cardiac output; and *histotoxic hypoxia* results from impaired cellular utilization of oxygen.

Cellular Respiration and Oxygen Consumption

Cells generate energy in the form of adenosine triphosphate (ATP) in order to maintain cellular integrity and function. Oxidative phosphorylation is the primary means by which cells generate ATP, a process that consumes oxygen. As cellular oxygen tension decreases, oxygen consumption and oxidative ATP synthesis decrease, and ATP is increasingly produced by anaerobic glycolysis. Anaerobic metabolism is far less efficient at generating ATP than is oxidative phosphorylation, and produces lactic acid as a byproduct. As cellular oxygen tension decreases further, anaerobic metabolism is incapable of generating sufficient ATP to maintain cellular function, and ultimately cellular viability is lost. Thus, a continuous delivery of oxygen is needed to sustain normal cellular function.

Physiology and Pathophysiology of Tissue Oxygenation

The relationship between oxygen delivery (DO_2) and oxygen consumption (VO_2) is reflected in the Fick equation: $VO_2 = DO_2 \times$ oxygen extraction (Fig. 34.1). Oxygen consumption varies in accordance with cellular activity. Oxygen delivery is the product of oxygen content (hemoglobin concentration $\times$ arterial O_2 saturation + dissolved O_2) and cardiac output. Cardiac output is the product of heart rate (HR) and stroke volume (SV), where SV is affected by ventricular preload, myocardial function, and afterload. Because oxygen is poorly soluble in water, the amount of oxygen normally dissolved in blood is negligible. Oxygen extraction is the difference between arterial oxygen content and venous oxygen content and is equal to VO_2/DO_2, an important ratio that reflects the balance between oxygen requirements and oxygen delivery (i.e., *oxygen transport balance*).

Oxygen consumption is maintained constant as DO_2 decreases by progressive increases in oxygen extraction (Fig. 34.2). However, below a given DO_2, oxygen extraction continues to increase but not enough to maintain a constant VO_2, and anaerobic metabolism ensues. This represents the critical DO_2, and the corresponding percent oxygen extraction represents the critical oxygen extraction ratio. From studies in animals and humans, the critical DO_2 is between 8 and 10 mL/min/kg (a decrease in DO_2 of greater than 50% from normal), and is the same whether the decrease in DO_2 results from a reduction in oxygen content or cardiac output (CO). The corresponding critical oxygen extraction ratio is approximately 50% (1,2). The critical DO_2 varies with changes in VO_2; however, the critical oxygen extraction ratio remains unchanged (Fig. 34.3).

A further appreciation of the relationship between VO_2, DO_2, and oxygen extraction can be obtained by observing the compensatory responses that attempt to maintain oxygen transport balance as VO_2 increases, or oxygen content and cardiac output decrease (Table 34.1). If VO_2 increases, as with exercise, the initial compensatory mechanism for maintaining adequate DO_2 is an increase in CO. If this compensation is inadequate, oxygen extraction increases as well. Similarly, if oxygen content decreases, as with hypoxemia or anemia, CO increases to maintain DO_2. If the circulatory response is inadequate, oxygen extraction increases. Finally, regardless of the lesion, when CO is limited, the sole acute compensatory mechanism to maintain DO_2 is an increase in oxygen extraction. Thus, as long as oxygen extraction is not significantly elevated, DO_2 is adequate and VO_2 is maintained. The exception to this occurs when shock is due to impaired utilization of oxygen or histotoxic hypoxia.

Monitoring oxygen extraction is the most sensitive indicator of tissue oxygenation because it reflects the balance between oxygen requirements and oxygen delivery (VO_2/DO_2) or *oxygen transport balance* (Table 34.2). Oxygen extraction is readily assessed by calculating the oxygen extraction ratio (OER). The OER is derived from the Fick equation: OER = $SaO_2 - SmvO_2/SaO_2$, where SaO_2 is the arterial oxygen saturation and $SmvO_2$ the mixed venous oxygen saturation. The mixed venous saturation is obtained from the pulmonary artery and represents the weighted average of venous return from all viscera. The normal SaO_2 is 100% and $SmvO_2$ is 75% for an OER of 25%. The OER is independent of the hemoglobin concentration and accounts for arterial hypoxemia when calculating the percent oxygen extraction. For example, if the SaO_2 is 90% and the $SmvO_2$ 67%, the OER is normal. In this instance, the $SmvO_2$ is depressed because of arterial hypoxemia and not because of diminished DO_2.

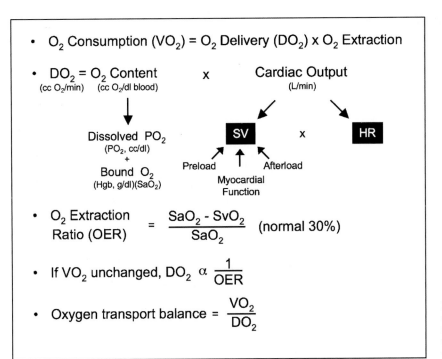

- O_2 Consumption (VO_2) = O_2 Delivery (DO_2) x O_2 Extraction

- DO_2 = O_2 Content   x   Cardiac Output
  (cc O_2/min) (cc O_2/dl blood)   (L/min)

  Dissolved PO_2 SV   x   HR
  (PO_2, cc/dl)

  Preload   Afterload
  +
  Bound O_2 Myocardial
  (Hgb, g/dl)(SaO_2)   Function

- O_2 Extraction Ratio (OER) $= \dfrac{SaO_2 - SvO_2}{SaO_2}$ (normal 30%)

- If VO_2 unchanged, $DO_2 \propto \dfrac{1}{OER}$

- Oxygen transport balance $= \dfrac{VO_2}{DO_2}$

FIGURE 34.1. The Fick equation, determinants of DO_2, oxygen extraction ratio, and oxygen transport balance. SaO_2, arterial oxygen saturation; SvO_2, mixed venous oxygen; SV, stroke volume; HR, heart rate;

Compensatory Mechanisms to Maintain Tissue Oxygenation

Blood flow and therefore DO_2 is distributed in order to match the metabolic demands of various organs. As DO_2 decreases and/or VO_2 increases, three separate but interrelated processes attempt to preserve adequate tissue oxygenation: CO is augmented, blood flow is redistributed between organs, and microcirculatory changes enhance tissue extraction of oxygen.

As DO_2 becomes inadequate, cardiopulmonary receptors, arterial baroreceptors, and chemoreceptors are stimulated. This leads to activation of neurohormonal systems and an increase in circulating levels of catecholamines, angiotensin II, aldosterone, and vasopressin; direct sympathetic stimulation of the myocardium also occurs. These vasoactive substances cause venoconstriction, thereby reducing venous capacitance, and stimulate fluid retention, both of which serve to increase ventricular preload; additionally, they increase heart rate, enhance myocardial function, and increase arterial vascular tone. The net result is an increase in CO, DO_2, and arterial pressure.

FIGURE 34.2. The relationship between oxygen delivery (DO_2), oxygen consumption (VO_2), and oxygen extraction (OE). Initially, as $DO_2 \downarrow$, VO_2 remains constant due to an $\uparrow$ in OE (i.e., VO_2 is independent of DO_2). As $DO_2 \downarrow$ further, OE $\uparrow$ but not enough to maintain a constant VO_2 (i.e., VO_2 becomes dependent on DO_2). The critical DO_2 represents the commencement of anaerobic metabolism.

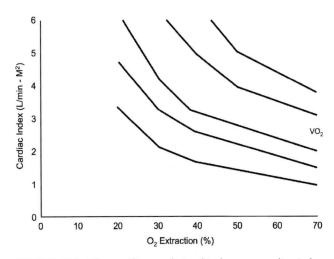

FIGURE 34.3. The curvilinear relationship between cardiac index and oxygen extraction as oxygen consumption (VO_2) varies.

TABLE 34.1

COMPENSATORY RESPONSES TO CHANGES IN OXYGEN DELIVERY (DO_2) AND OXYGEN CONSUMPTION (VO_2)

Hypoxic or Anemic Hypoxia
$CaO_2 \downarrow \rightarrow CO \uparrow \rightarrow DO_2$ and VO_2 maintained
$CaO_2 \downarrow \downarrow \rightarrow CO \uparrow + OER \uparrow \rightarrow VO_2$ maintained

Stagnant Hypoxia
$CO \downarrow \rightarrow OER \uparrow \rightarrow VO_2$ maintained
$CO \downarrow \downarrow \rightarrow OER \uparrow \uparrow \rightarrow VO_2 \downarrow$

Histotoxic Hypoxia
$VO_2 \downarrow \rightarrow CO + DO_2 \uparrow \rightarrow OER \downarrow \downarrow$

Increased Metabolism
$VO_2 \uparrow \rightarrow CO \uparrow \rightarrow DO_2 \uparrow$, O_2 requirements met
$VO_2 \uparrow \uparrow \rightarrow CO \uparrow + OER \uparrow \rightarrow DO_2 \uparrow$, O_2 requirements met

DO_2, oxygen delivery; VO_2, oxygen consumption; OER, oxygen extraction ratio; CO, cardiac output; CaO_2, arterial oxygen content.

The redistribution of blood flow between organs represents an additional mechanism by which to optimize DO_2. Less vital organs, such as the mesentery and dermis, and organs with considerable flow reserve, such as the kidneys, experience an increase in vascular resistance and therefore a reduction in perfusion. Vital organs such as the brain, myocardium, and diaphragm do not experience an increase in vascular resistance and perfusion increases. This represents an important compensatory mechanism, as these vital organs have high resting oxygen extraction, necessitating a relatively large percentage of CO under normal conditions, and an increase in flow as oxygen requirements increase.

Finally, although there may be alterations in vascular resistance that reduce blood flow, all organs are capable of microcirculatory adjustments that oppose systemic vasoconstriction and allow for an increase in oxygen extraction; these compensatory changes attempt to maintain a constant VO_2 when DO_2 is limited. Metabolism-linked (i.e., autoregulatory) mechanisms mediate a redistribution of microcirculatory blood flow leading to capillary recruitment. The local accumulation of adenosine, a byproduct of ATP utilization, and a decrease in tissue oxygen tension, for example, have

TABLE 34.2

RELATIONSHIP BETWEEN OXYGEN EXTRACTION AND THE DEVELOPMENT OF SHOCK AND MULTIORGAN SYSTEM FAILURE

Oxygen Extraction Ratio

30%	Normal	$VO_2 \uparrow$
30–40%	Increased	and/or
40–50%	Impending Shock	$DO_2 \downarrow$
>50–60%	Shock	

$\downarrow$ Multi-Organ System Failure $\downarrow$ Lactic Acidosis
Death

VO_2, oxygen consumption; DO_2, oxygen delivery.

been shown to mediate these changes. The recruitment of additional capillary networks improves oxygen extraction by several mechanisms. The distance for oxygen diffusion decreases, and the capillary surface area available for gas exchange, increases. In addition, the cross-sectional area of the individual vessel and of the vascular bed increases; because the linear velocity of blood is inversely related to the cross-sectional area, RBC velocity decreases and its transit time increases, increasing oxygen diffusion times. Finally, the oxyhemoglobin dissociation curve is shifted to the right secondary to tissue acidosis and an increase in red blood cell 2,3-DPG levels; this shift represents a decrease in the affinity of oxygen for hemoglobin, thus enhancing oxygen release in the periphery. In sum, cardiovascular function and the balance between systemic and local vascular changes determine tissue oxygenation.

CLINICAL RECOGNITION AND ASSESSMENT OF SHOCK

The evaluation of shock requires a thorough understanding of the pathophysiology of tissue hypoxia. Serial physical exams and an accurate interpretation of hemodynamic and laboratory data are essential for a timely diagnosis, as it is much more advantageous to *implement anticipatory rather than resuscitative strategies*. There are, however, important limitations of the clinical evaluation that merit discussion.

Physical Exam

It is important to consider the limitations of the physical exam when assessing critically ill patients. For example, some shock states are characterized by an elevated CO and good perfusion exam. Nonetheless, oxygen delivery or utilization is inadequate. Furthermore, the clinical impression of experienced physicians is frequently discordant with objective data (3,4). In a study of pediatric intensive care patients, estimations of CO correlated poorly to measured values, irrespective of the observer's level of experience, confirming conclusions from studies in adult patients.

Metabolic Acidosis

The hallmark of shock is metabolic acidosis resulting from the accumulation of lactic acid. An elevated lactate level is highly specific for shock. However, a normal lactate level does not exclude the presence of marginal or inadequate perfusion and tissue oxygenation. First, tissue clearance of lactate is highly efficient. A majority of lactate is reutilized during gluconeogenesis in the liver and kidneys or is metabolized in the Krebs cycle. More importantly, oxygen extraction increases significantly as CO and DO_2 decrease. It is not until DO_2 is less than 50% of normal before VO_2 decreases and anaerobic metabolism commences (Table 34.2).

The presence of metabolic acidosis and a base deficit are nonspecific findings and correlate poorly with an elevated lactate level. The first step in interpreting metabolic acidosis is to determine if it is an anion gap or non-anion gap acidosis. The anion gap is the difference between "unmeasured" cations and anions and is readily calculated from serum electrolytes: $Na^+ - (Cl^- + HCO_3^-)$. The concentration of total cations in the serum must equal the concentration of total anions. The normal gap is approximately 10 ± 2 mEq/L. An elevated anion gap result from either decreased unmeasured cations (K^+, Ca^{2+}, Mg^{2+}) or increased unmeasured anions. An anion gap resulting from an increase in unmeasured anions occurs primarily from lactic acidosis (shock states), ketoacidosis (diabetic ketoacidosis), or from accumulation of renally excreted organic and inorganic anions (uremia). The hydrogen ion from the acid converts bicarbonate to carbonic acid, which is then converted to CO_2 and eliminated by the lungs. As the bicarbonate anion is titrated away, metabolic acidosis is created; in addition, the retention of the unmeasured anion restores the law of electroneutrality and generates an anion gap. Lactic acidosis may even occur in the absence of acidemia if metabolic alkalosis was present prior to the onset of anaerobic metabolism; however, the anion gap will be elevated. Other causes of lactic acidosis include inborn errors of metabolism. Non-anion gap acidosis primarily results from either intestinal or renal losses of bicarbonate, in which case the chloride ion is retained, or from hyperchloremia, as seen with large saline infusions, which produces metabolic acidosis by increasing free hydrogen ions. In each case, the anion gap remains normal (5).

Blood Pressure

Blood pressure correlates poorly with CO. Because blood pressure is the product of CO and SVR, any decrease in output is offset by an increase in SVR. This is exemplified in patients with hypovolemic shock who require >30% reduction in intravascular volume and a decrease in CO before blood pressure begins to drop.

Mixed Venous Oxygen Saturations

The most accurate assessment of tissue oxygenation is mixed venous oxygen saturation, which allows for calculation of an OER and therefore an assessment of oxygen transport balance (Table 34.2). The true mixed venous saturation is obtained from a pulmonary artery catheter, which allows for the measurement of mixed venous oxygen saturation, CO, and DO_2. A venous oxygen saturation obtained from a central venous line located in the right atrium or superior vena cava is an acceptable alternative. The normal OER is 33% and 25% for a sample obtained from the superior vena cava and right atrium, respectively. A sample obtained from the inferior cava is unreliable due to vascular streaming.

Cerebral Oximetry

Cerebral oximetry provides an additional means by which to monitor oxygen transport balance. A relatively new technology, cerebral oximetry, has been used intraoperatively to monitor cerebral oxygen delivery during cardiac surgery, and is increasingly being used in the postoperative setting. Cerebral oximetry is similar to pulse oximetry in that they both utilize near-infrared spectroscopy (NIRS) to determine oxygen saturations. Cerebral oximetry, however, monitors the nonpulsatile signal component reflecting tissue circulation. Because the cerebral microcirculation contains arteries, capillaries, and venous components, the cerebral saturation represents a weighted average, with approximately 80% of the signal originating from venules. The FDA-approved cerebral oximeter (INVOS; Somanetics, Troy, MI) closely tracks changes in jugular and superior vena cava saturations and, in contrast to venous saturations, provides continuous, noninvasive data (6,7).

GENERAL THERAPEUTIC CONSIDERATIONS

All types of shock have varying degrees of multiorgan system involvement, including hypoxic respiratory failure, renal failure, liver dysfunction, and a consumptive coagulopathy.

Positive pressure ventilation improves gas exchange and oxygen transport balance. Hemodialysis is often indicated, as is replacement of clotting factors and platelets. Serum electrolytes should be closely monitored, ensuring adequate calcium and glucose metabolism.

Infant Cardiopulmonary Function

Infants have considerably less cardiopulmonary reserve than do children and adults, an important consideration when managing critically ill infants. The myocardium of an infant has less contractile reserve and is less compliant than that of a child and adult. The cardiomyocyte possesses relatively few, poorly organized contractile proteins, and a majority of the myocyte is composed of noncontractile elements. Furthermore, the cardiomyocyte has reduced intracellular stores of calcium and the sarcoplasmic reticulum is less organized (8,9). Thus, the immature myocardium is less responsive to fluid and inotropes, and more susceptible to increases in afterload. As a result, increases in CO result primarily from an increase in heart rate, rather than from an increase in SV.

The functional residual capacity (FRC) is the lung volume at end-expiration and is set passively by the balance between the inward recoil of lung and outward recoil of the chest wall. Because the infant has a relatively high chest wall to lung compliance ratio, the end-expiratory lung volume is reduced, which predisposes the infant to atelectasis and hypoxemia. Furthermore, the infant is less able to defend tidal volume when faced with an increased respiratory load (10). The highly compliant chest wall is at a mechanical disadvantage and a significant portion of the energy generated by the respiratory pump is wasted in distorting the rib cage (retractions), rather than in exchanging tidal volume. Finally, the infant diaphragm has less contractile reserve because it contains few fatigue-resistant type muscle fibers and immature sarcoplasmic reticulum, and it is inefficient as storing energy. Respiratory pump function improves over the first several months of life, primarily because of chest wall ossification and improved respiratory muscle performance.

These limitations of infant cardiopulmonary function are compounded by the fact that infants have a much higher VO_2 per unit mass necessitating a relatively greater CO and minute ventilation. In addition, the hemoglobin of an infant is comprised mostly of fetal hemoglobin, which has a much greater affinity for oxygen, thus impairing its release in the periphery. Thus, the propensity for the critically ill infant to develop respiratory failure is great and is due to a precarious interplay between oxygen transport balance for the respiratory pump, respiratory load, and respiratory pump function.

Mechanical Ventilation

Although the primary role of mechanical ventilation is to improve gas exchange, it has beneficial effects on oxygen transport balance. By unloading the respiratory apparatus and by increasing intrathoracic pressure, mechanical ventilation improves global and myocardial oxygen transport balance.

Under normal conditions, the diaphragm consumes less than 3% of global VO_2 and receives less than 5% of CO. However, with an increase respiratory load, diaphragmatic VO_2 may increase to values over 50% of the total VO_2. In order to meet these increased oxygen demands, diaphragmatic blood flow must increase. When diaphragmatic oxygen transport balance is inadequate, either because of excessive oxygen requirements or limited DO_2, respiratory pump failure ensues (11). Thus, when global $D\overline{O}_2$ becomes limited, diaphragmatic blood flow is protected to an equal or even greater extent than is cerebral and myocardial blood flow. In a dog model of cardiogenic shock in which CO was decreased by 70%, respiratory muscle blood flow increased to 21% of CO during spontaneous respiration. However, during mechanical ventilation, respiratory muscle blood flow decreased to 3% of CO and blood flow to the liver, kidneys, and brain increased significantly (12).

In addition to releasing substantial quantities of oxygen for use by other organs, mechanical ventilation directly increases SV and CO in the setting of ventricular dysfunction. By increasing intrathoracic pressure, positive pressure ventilation decreases ventricular transmural pressure and therefore ventricular afterload. This leads to improved ventricular emptying. However, as intrathoracic pressure increases, the pressure gradient for venous return decreases (see "Cardiovascular Physiology and Cardiopulmonary Interaction" under "Stagnant Hypoxia" later in the chapter). Thus, the net effect of positive pressure ventilation on CO depends on where the ventricle resides on the pressure–volume curve. If ventricular preload is maintained, CO increases as well (13). At the same time, myocardial oxygen requirements decrease. As the respiratory apparatus is unloaded, global oxygen VO_2 decreases, leading to reduced CO requirements and myocardial work. Finally, myocardial oxygen requirements decrease as ventricular afterload decreases. As a result of these changes, global and myocardial oxygen transport balance improves substantially (14,15).

HYPOXIC HYPOXIA

Etiology and Pathophysiology

Hypoxic hypoxia results from a marked reduction in arterial oxygen tension (PaO_2). This results from a decrease in the inspired concentration of oxygen (e.g., high altitude); from hypoventilation (e.g., apnea); from ventilation–perfusion mismatch and intrapulmonary shunting (e.g., acute respiratory distress syndrome); and from cyanotic congenital heart lesions. Hypoxemia stimulates peripheral chemoreceptors, leading to hyperventilation and an increase in catecholamine release. Cardiac output increases to maintain adequate DO_2 and constant VO_2; with severe hypoxemia, oxygen extraction increases as well. Chronic hypoxemia stimulates erythropoiesis and the concentration of hemoglobin increases; as a result of the increase in oxygen-carrying capacity, DO_2 returns to normal, and CO decreases, although it remains elevated above normal. Chemoreceptor sensitivity to hypoxemia wanes and hyperventilation abates.

Therapy

With acute hypoxemia, therapies are directed at improving oxygenation and oxygen transport balance. The critical PaO_2 and PvO_2 in animals with isolated hypoxemia are 25 to 30 mm Hg and 15 to 20 mm Hg, respectively. When severe hypoxemia is accompanied by anemia or when CO is limited, the critical PO_2 increases. The "optimal" hematocrit is in the range of 40% to 45% (16). As the hematocrit rises, the oxygen-carrying capacity of blood increases; however, the attendant increase in blood viscosity, SVR, and resistance to venous return cause DO_2 to decrease as the hematocrit exceeds 45% to 50%. Finally, the circulatory response to hypoxemia requires adequate ventricular preload and function.

ANEMIC HYPOXIA

Etiology and Pathophysiology

Anemic hypoxia occurs when the oxygen-carrying capacity of blood is severely reduced. This results from a decrease in red blood cell and hemoglobin production, hemolytic processes,

and from dyshemoglobinemias (e.g., methemoglobinemia). Anemia stimulates aortic chemoreceptors, leading to an increase in catecholamine release and CO. The most important determinant of the cardiovascular response is volume status. In contrast to hemorrhagic anemia, where CO is low and SVR is high, normovolemic anemia is characterized by an increase in CO. This results primarily from changes in ventricular loading conditions. As viscosity decreases, the resistance to venous return and SVR decrease, which leads to an increase in ventricular preload and SV (16). Increases in heart rate and contractility also contribute to elevating CO, albeit to a lesser extent. An additional compensatory response is an increase in red blood cell 2,3-DPG levels, which shifts the oxyhemoglobin dissociation curve to the right, thus enhancing oxygen release in the periphery. The degree to which oxygen extraction increases depends on the severity of the anemia, the adequacy of the circulatory response, and oxygen requirements. With isolated normovolemic anemia, the critical hematocrit is approximately 10% to 15%. The substantial increase in CO causes myocardial VO_2 to increase significantly. At the critical hematocrit, myocardial oxygen delivery becomes inadequate to support any further increase in myocardial performance and CO. In other words, myocardial oxygen transport balance becomes the rate-limiting factor (1).

Therapy

Clinical efforts are directed at identifying and treating the underlying process responsible for the anemia, and at maintaining adequate oxygen transport balance. Red blood cells are transfused carefully so as to avoid precipitating congestive heart failure.

Dyshemoglobinemias

Dyshemoglobinemias such as methemoglobinemia (met-Hgb) and carboxyhemoglobinemia (CO-Hgb) represent unique types of anemia, both in terms of their clinical evaluation and treatment. Methemoglobinemia occurs primarily with use of certain medications and in infants with gastrointestinal infections and sepsis. Several endogenous reduction systems maintain the iron moiety of hemoglobin in the reduced state. However, under conditions of oxidative stress, iron is oxidized to form met-Hgb, which is unable to carry oxygen. In addition, the nonoxidized hemoglobin subunits bind oxygen more tightly, thereby impairing the release of oxygen in the periphery. Some degree of hemolysis also occurs in met-Hgb.

Methemoglobinemia presents with a variety of symptoms. Cyanosis is invariably present despite supplemental oxygen. Pulse oximetry saturations usually range from 85% to 90%, while arterial blood gas analysis reveals an elevated PO_2 and an arterial saturation of 100%, for a saturation gap of 15%. When a blood gas is obtained, the arterial blood appears dark or chocolate-colored in the syringe. This clinical picture should prompt further investigation. The oxygen saturation obtained from an arterial blood gas is inaccurate because it is calculated from the PaO_2. Co-oximetry is required to determine the presence of dyshemoglobinemias. Routine pulse oximeters measure light absorbance at only two wavelengths of light. Because dyshemoglobinemias have absorption characteristics in the same region of the spectrum as oxyhemoglobin and deoxyhemoglobin, dyshemoglobinemias cause significant inaccuracies in pulse oximetry readings. Co-oximetry uses spectrophotometry to measure light absorbance at four different wavelengths. These wavelengths correspond to specific absorbance characteristics of deoxygenated hemoglobin, oxygenated hemoglobin, met-Hgb, and CO-Hgb. Levels are reported as a percentage of total hemoglobin. Symptoms do not necessarily correspond with met-Hgb levels and depend on the other determinants of DO_2, such as hemoglobin concentration, intravascular volume, and myocardial performance. Met-Hgb is treated with methylene blue, which reduces the iron moiety, thus restoring the oxygen carrying capacity of hemoglobin.

Carboxyhemoglobinemia (CO-Hgb) results from the inhalation of carbon monoxide. There are several mechanisms by which carbon monoxide interferes with tissue oxygenation. Carbon monoxide competes with oxygen for binding to hemoglobin. The affinity of hemoglobin for carbon monoxide is 200 to 250 times as great as its affinity for oxygen, and the binding of carbon monoxide to hemoglobin causes a leftward shift of the oxyhemoglobin dissociation curve, impairing the release of oxygen in the periphery. Carbon monoxide also interferes with tissue oxygenation by binding to cytochrome-c oxidase of the respiratory chain, thereby interfering with cellular respiration. Thus, it causes anemic hypoxia and histotoxic hypoxia. Similar to met-Hgb, pulse oximetry cannot distinguish CO-Hgb from oxyhemoglobin, producing a low oxygen saturation relative to the PaO_2. Co-oximetry is required to measure CO-Hgb and oxyhemoglobin levels. The mainstay of therapy for carbon monoxide poisoning is provision of maximal supplemental oxygen, which displaces it from hemoglobin.

STAGNANT HYPOXIA

Inadequate perfusion results from one or more of the following: hypovolemia; ventricular failure; obstructive lesions, which depress CO despite adequate ventricular preload and function; and distributive lesions, where vasomotor dysfunction leads to the maldistribution of blood flow. A thorough understanding of cardiovascular physiology is essential to a discussion of the pathophysiology of low CO states, as well as the circulatory response in other types of tissue hypoxia. Cardiac physiology will be reviewed according to the determinants of CO: preload, myocardial function, afterload, and heart rate. In addition, the effects that changes in intrathoracic pressure have on cardiovascular function (i.e., cardiopulmonary interaction) will be discussed.

Cardiovascular Physiology and Cardiopulmonary Interaction

Preload

Preload is the load on a muscle before contraction has started. In isolated muscle strips, the length to which a muscle is stretched before activation determines the force generated with stimulation. In the intact circulation, this phenomenon is referred to as the length dependence of cardiac contractility, and results from an increase in myofilament sensitivity to the prevailing cytosolic calcium concentration. The effects of changes in preload can be further appreciated by reviewing the observations made by Frank and Starling. Frank demonstrated that if the heart was not allowed to eject, increasing preload increases the pressure-generating capabilities of the ventricle ("afterload reserve"). Starling demonstrated that SV increases in proportion to increases in preload ("preload reserve"). With normal ventricular function, volume loading produces elevated end-diastolic volume (EDV) and SV, and end-systolic volume remains the same. The actual measure of ventricular preload is EDV. The relationship between EDV and SV is linear within physiologic limits (Fig. 34.4). However, EDV is not readily assessable clinically. Instead, ventricular preload is inferred from the central venous pressure (CVP), where the relationship between end-diastolic pressure (EDP) and EDV is curvilinear (Fig. 34.4). The response to changes in preload depends on myocardial function and where the ventricle resides on the

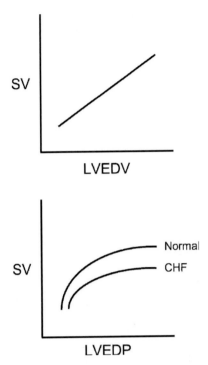

FIGURE 34.4. The relationship of stroke volume (SV) to left ventricular end-diastolic volume (LVEDV) (*top*) and left ventricular end-diastolic pressure (LVEDP) (*bottom*). As LVEDV increases, SV increases within physiologic limits. As LVEDP increases, SV increases to a point due to the compliance of the heart. As ventricular function decreases, increases in LVEDP have less of an effect on SV.

pressure–volume curve (Fig. 34.4). When the ventricular filling pressure is reduced, large volume infusions significantly augment SV and have little effect on ventricular pressure. Conversely, when filling pressures are elevated, volume loading has little effect on SV but filling pressures increase significantly. Finally, when ventricular filling pressures are low, further reductions in preload will lead to a decrease in SV.

There are important limitations to using CVP as a surrogate for ventricular preload. As stated, the relationship between ventricular pressure and volume is curvilinear. However, the position and shape of the curve change as ventricular compliance changes. Compliance is equal to the change in volume divided by the change in pressure. When ventricular compliance is decreased, a given filling pressure is associated with a reduced ventricular volume. Ventricular compliance is altered by diseases of the myocardium and pericardium and by changes in intrathoracic pressure (ITP). Ventricular hypertrophy and ischemia are the most common causes of reduced ventricular compliance, and positive pressure ventilation (PPV) decreases ventricular compliance by increasing juxtacardiac pressure. Another potential pitfall is using the CVP or right atrial pressure (RAP) as an indicator of LV preload. If the function of right and left ventricles is discordant or pulmonary vascular disease is present, the RAP may not accurately reflect LV conditions. This is a particularly common finding in congenital heart disease.

Determinants of Ventricular Filling

RV filling or preload is determined by venous return, ventricular compliance, and the diastolic transmural pressure (Tmp) for the RV (Table 34.3). *Venous return* is proportional to the pressure gradient between extrathoracic venous structures (i.e., mean systemic pressure, MSP) and intrathoracic venous

TABLE 34.3

DETERMINANTS OF VENOUS RETURN

- Venous Return = $\dfrac{\text{Mean Systemic Pressure} - \text{Right Atrial Pressure}}{\text{Resistance to Venous Return}}$

- Mean Systemic Pressure = $\dfrac{\text{Intravascular Volume}}{\text{Intravascular Capacitance}}$

- Right atrial pressure is affected by:
  - Cardiovascular function
  - Pericardial disease
  - Intrathoracic pressure

structures (i.e., RAP), and is inversely related to the resistance to venous return (17,18).

MSP is equal to the ratio of intravascular volume to vascular capacitance, where a great majority of intravascular volume and vascular capacitance reside with the venous circulation (17,18). Thus, therapies or conditions that affect venous capacitance affect the MSP and therefore venous return. Similarly, a great majority of resistance to venous return resides with the venous circulation. Resistance to venous return is significantly affected only with marked changes in viscosity (16–18).

RAP is affected by cardiovascular function, pericardial disease, and changes in ITP. Heart failure raises RAP and impedes venous return. *Changes in ITP affect the gradient for venous return.* Positive-pressure ventilation increases ITP and RAP, thereby decreasing the gradient for venous return. The degree to which PPV increases RAP depends on the magnitude of positive pressure, parenchymal lung compliance, and the degree to which airway pressure is transmitted to the cardiac fossa. As RAP increases, adrenergic-induced venoconstriction increases the intravascular volume to capacitance ratio in an attempt to maintain the pressure gradient for venous return. Without this circulatory response, a rise of 1 mm Hg in RAP would decrease venous return by 15%, and a rise of 3.5 mm Hg in RAP would decrease venous return by half. In contrast to PPV, spontaneous respiration, by virtue of decreasing ITP and RAP, enhances venous return.

Finally, in addition to the gradient for venous return, *ventricular compliance,* the *diastolic ventricular Tmp,* and the *duration of ventricular diastole,* determine ventricular filling (Fig. 34.5) (19). The diastolic Tmp is equal to ventricular diastolic pressure minus ITP. If ventricular filling pressures and compliance are equal between two ventricles, the ventricle exposed to negative ITP will fill to a greater extent. Similarly, if filling pressures and the Tmp gradients are the same, the more compliant ventricle will fill to a greater extent.

Myocardial Function

The assessment of myocardial performance has traditionally focused on LV systolic function. However, the importance of diastolic or lusitropic function has gained increasing recognition. Similarly, the focus has shifted to include assessment of RV performance as well. Evaluation of biventricular diastolic and systolic function is essential in managing critically ill patients, particularly in the setting of congenital heart disease.

Systolic function or contractility is the intrinsic ability of heart muscle to shorten and generate force independently of changes in loading conditions. With an increase in contractile function, the rate of tension development, and the velocity and extent of fiber shortening increase. Systolic dysfunction is characterized by an elevated ventricular filling pressure and volume

with decreased ejection fraction and SV. In contrast to the LV, the highly compliant, thin-walled RV is designed to pump blood into a low-resistance, high-capacitance pulmonary circulation, while maintaining a low atrial pressure to optimize venous return. In fact, a significant portion of RV-developed pressure and volume outflow depends on LV contraction, a phenomenon known as *systolic ventricular interdependence* (20). As a result, the RV is less capable of maintaining SV when afterload is increased.

Diastolic function is the ability of the ventricle to receive blood under low pressure. Diastolic function is determined by

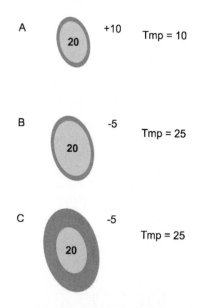

Determinants of Ventricular Filling:
Ventricular Compliance, Ventricular Filling Pressure and Intrathoracic Pressure

Tmp = ventricular transmural pressure
Tmp = intracavitary - extracavitary pressure

FIGURE 34.5. The relationship of ventricular filling pressure (EDP), ventricular compliance, and intrathoracic pressure (ITP) to ventricular filling. The EDP is 20 for each ventricle. **A.** The ITP is +10 (positive pressure ventilation). **B.** The ITP is −5 (spontaneous breathing). **C.** Ventricular compliance is reduced. *Ventricle A vs. B.* Ventricular compliance is the same; however, because ventricle B has a greater Tmp, it fills to a greater extent. *Ventricle B vs. C.* The Tmp is the same; however, because ventricle B is more compliant, it fills to a greater extent.

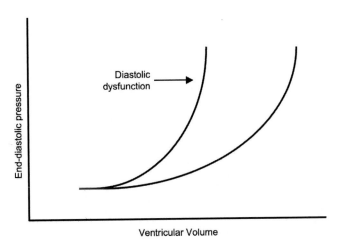

FIGURE 34.6. Ventricular compliance curve. In the normally compliant ventricle, as ventricular volume increases, end-diastolic pressure increases slightly. With diastolic dysfunction, modest increases in ventricular volume produce significant elevations in end-diastolic pressure.

TABLE 34.4

DETERMINANTS OF VENTRICULAR AFTERLOAD

- Ventricular Wall Stress

$$\text{Stress} = \frac{\text{Tmp} \times r}{2t}$$

- Tmp = transmural pressure
- r = radius of the chamber
- t = thickness of the chamber wall

- Tmp = intracavitary minus extracavitary pressure
- Intracavitary pressure is peak LV pressure or aortic systolic pressure
- Extracavitary pressure is intrathoracic pressure

- Vascular Impedance
  - According to Poiseuille's Law:

$$\text{Resistance} \, \alpha \, \frac{\text{viscosity}}{\text{radius}^4}$$

- Radius or cross-sectional area of the arteriolar bed

the process of active relaxation and by the passive elastic properties of the heart. Ventricular relaxation is an energy-dependent process involving the dissociation of calcium from myofilaments, the reuptake of calcium from the cytosol by the sarcoplasmic reticulum, and the uncoupling of actin-myosin cross-bridges. The passive elastic properties of the heart are influenced by the composition of the cardiac interstitium and the myocytes themselves. Diastolic dysfunction refers to an abnormality of diastolic distensibility, filling, or relaxation of the ventricle. As a result, the curve for ventricular diastolic pressure in relation to volume is shifted upward and to the left (Fig. 34.6), ventricular compliance is reduced, the time course of filling is altered, and the diastolic pressure is elevated. In marked contrast to systolic dysfunction, chamber volumes are reduced, the ejection fraction is normal, and SV is maintained. The most common cause of impaired relaxation is ischemic heart disease, and abnormal passive elastic properties most commonly result from conditions that produce ventricular hypertrophy, such as obstructive lesions and hypertension.

Afterload

Afterload is a major determinant of both CO and myocardial oxygen transport balance. In the intact ventricle, afterload is the force opposing ventricular contraction and emptying. The two principal vascular determinants of afterload are systolic wall stress and vascular impedance (Table 34.4).

For a spherical chamber such as the LV, stress or the force per unit of cross-sectional area of myocardium is defined by La Place's law. *Left ventricular systolic wall stress* is proportional to the Tmp and the radius of the chamber, and is inversely related to chamber thickness. The systolic Tmp is equal to peak LV cavitary pressure or aortic systolic pressure minus ITP. As aortic systolic pressure increases, left ventricular Tmp and afterload increase. *Changes in ITP* also affect the Tmp. PPV increases ITP and thus decreases the Tmp and ventricular afterload. Spontaneous respiration has the opposite effect. When negative ITP is exaggerated as with respiratory disease, the Tmp and ventricular afterload are *significantly* elevated. As ventricular preload or EDV decrease, or as the myocardium thickens or hypertrophies, ventricular wall stress decreases. Ventricular hypertrophy represents a major compensatory mechanism to maintain SV and to reduce wall stress when ventricular volume or pressure is chronically elevated. According to Poiseuille's law, *vascular impedance* or resistance

is proportional to viscosity and inversely related to the radius of the vessel. Thus, vasoactive agents that cause systemic vasodilation reduce afterload by increasing the cross-sectional area of the arteriolar bed.

The importance of afterload in patients with ventricular dysfunction resides with its effects on SV, CO, and myocardial oxygen demands. With increases in afterload, both the rate and extent of myofiber shortening decrease. In the intact circulation, if myocardial function is normal and afterload is increased, a compensatory increase in EDV maintains SV even though the ejection fraction is decreased. However, when ventricular function is depressed, increases in afterload lead to a decrease in SV and CO despite significant increases in ventricular volume and pressure (Fig. 34.7). Finally, afterload is one of the major determinants of myocardial oxygen demands.

Heart Rate

Heart rate is an important determinant of CO, especially in the neonate, where recruitable SV is limited. In addition, as heart rate increases, the force of ventricular contraction increases. This phenomenon is known as the force–frequency relationship. The increase in inotropy is due to an increase in cytosolic calcium availability, which results from reduced calcium sequestration by the sarcoplasmic reticulum during a shortened diastole. In the failing myocardium, the force–frequency relationship is depressed and in some patients it may become negative. Excessive heart rates may also limit ventricular filling and coronary perfusion, both of which occur during diastole. Finally, optimal cardiac performance requires synchronized activation of myofibers. The sequence of electrical activation is an important determinant of both right and left ventricular output.

Myocardial Oxygen Transport Balance

Inadequate myocardial oxygen transport balance impairs diastolic and systolic function, and if severe, leads to myocyte necrosis. Thus an understanding of the determinants of myocardial oxygen transport balance is essential and provides a rationale for implementing various therapies.

Because baseline myocardial oxygen extraction is high, increases in oxygen demands are met primarily by an increase in myocardial oxygen delivery. This is especially concerning in

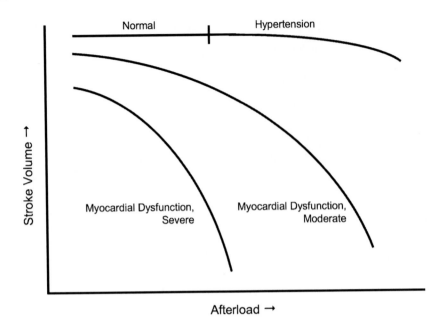

FIGURE 34.7. Relation of LV stroke volume to afterload in normal and diseased hearts. If cardiac function is normal, a rise in resistance results in hypertension because cardiac output remains fairly constant. When myocardial function is severly depressed, stroke volume and resistance are inversely related.

the setting of heart failure, where myocardial oxygen consumption is elevated while CO and coronary blood flow are limited. The primary determinant of myocardial oxygen demand is ventricular wall stress (Table 34.4). Therefore, myocardial oxygen requirements increase as intraventricular pressure and volume increase. Inotropic stimulation and heart rate elevations significantly increase myocardial oxygen consumption. Coronary perfusion of the systemic ventricle occurs predominantly during diastole when intramyocardial and intraventricular pressures are much lower. Coronary blood flow is linked to the metabolic requirements of the myocardium (i.e., autoregulatory mechanism). As myocardial oxygen demands increase, myocardial biochemical changes (e.g., oxygen tension) modulate coronary vascular tone, allowing for a commensurate increase in coronary blood flow. When the compensatory increase in coronary blood flow is unable to meet the metabolic requirements of the myocardium (i.e., maximum coronary vasodilation has occurred), coronary flow reserve has been exhausted. At this point, coronary perfusion is the product of the pressure gradient between aortic diastolic and ventricular diastolic pressures.

HYPOVOLEMIC SHOCK

Etiology and Pathophysiology

Hypovolemic shock is the most common cause of shock in pediatric patients and results from a variety of etiologies (Table 34.5). Gastroenteritis may produce significant fluid and electrolyte losses. Hemorrhagic lesions can rapidly progress to shock due to the combination of hypovolemia and anemia. Regardless of the etiology, intravascular volume is severely reduced, leading to a decrease in MSP, venous return, ventricular preload, and consequently SV and CO. Neurohormonal activation leads to an increase in heart rate and SVR, which compensates for low CO. Blood pressure is maintained until greater than 30% of intravascular volume is depleted.

Clinical Assessment

The findings on physical exam are proportionate to the degree of intravascular volume depletion and include cool extremities, poor peripheral pulses, prolonged capillary refill, dry mucus

membranes, tachycardia, and tachypnea. Placement of a bladder catheter yields minimal urine. A decreasing respiratory rate or irregular breathing signals impending cardiopulmonary failure. Hypotension and altered mental status are late findings, as are the presence of an anion gap metabolic acidosis and elevated lactate level. Hypovolemia complicated by anemia and no obvious source of bleeding requires a thorough investigation for occult bleeding.

Treatment

Effective resuscitation of hypovolemic shock begins with intravascular access. Peripheral venous access should be attempted concurrently with other attempts at vascular access, including placement of an intraosseous needle and central venous catheter. Isotonic fluids such as 0.9% normal saline, lactated Ringer, or colloid solutions should be administered as rapidly as possible. Securing the airway and providing ventilatory support are prudent. However, the medications used for

TABLE 34.5
COMMON CAUSES OF HYPOVOLEMIC SHOCK

I. Fluid and Electrolyte Losses
  ■ Vomiting
  ■ Diarrhea
  ■ Excessive sweating

II. Hemorrhage
  ■ Traumatic
    ■ Hepatic rupture
    ■ Splenic rupture
    ■ Intracranial
      ■ Especially in neonates
    ■ Fractures
    ■ Major vessel injury
  ■ Gastrointestinal

III. Vascular Leak Syndrome
  ■ Sepsis/SIRC
  ■ Burns
  ■ Peritonitis

intubation and the attendant increase in intrathoracic pressure will decrease venous return and may precipitate circulatory collapse. Hypovolemic shock should respond dramatically to fluid resuscitation. The perfusion exam and heart rate should promptly improve and urine output should increase. Once intravascular volume has been restored, the underlying etiology, serum electrolytes, and ongoing losses dictate fluid therapy. Failure to make progress with fluid therapy should prompt further investigation for complicating factors.

CARDIOGENIC SHOCK

Etiology and Pathophysiology

Heart failure results from a variety of etiologies (Table 34.6) and several pathophysiologic processes. Although heart failure is most often due to a decrease in myocardial performance, in some cases it is caused by conditions in which the normal heart is suddenly presented with a load that exceeds its capacity (e.g., malignant hypertension). In either case, systolic or diastolic failure, or both, leads to low CO and shock.

Immune-mediated myocardial damage is a common cause of acute and chronic heart failure. Myocardial injury from myocarditis results from viral cytotoxicity and more importantly from the host inflammatory response to infection. Because of the insidious nature of *myocarditis*, most cases are probably unrecognized. The clinical presentation and causes of myocarditis are discussed in a separate chapter in this text. *Kawasaki disease* is an acute, self-limited panvasculitis of unknown etiology that occurs predominantly in infants and young children. The pathogenesis of Kawasaki disease is unclear; however, most hypotheses focus on an immunologic response that is triggered by any of several different microbial agents. Myocardial function in Kawasaki disease is often depressed secondary to myocarditis and occasionally patients present with low CO and shock.

Another mechanism of myocardial injury is *ischemia* resulting from inadequate coronary perfusion. An *anomalous left coronary artery from the pulmonary artery (ALCAPA)* is a congenital lesion that most often presents with severe heart failure in infancy. As pulmonary vascular resistance (PVR) decreases over the first several weeks of life, the perfusion pressure across the distribution of the left coronary artery decreases, and ischemia ensues. Other *congenital heart lesions require a patent ductus arteriosus* for pulmonary perfusion, systemic perfusion, or to enhance intercirculatory mixing. These patients often present with shock during the first several days of life as the ductus arteriosus begins to close. Finally, other *shock states* may cause myocardial ischemia leading to ventricular failure.

Tachydysrhythmias can lead to shock. High heart rates shorten diastole, thereby compromising ventricular filling. Cardiac output and coronary perfusion are further compromised when atrioventricular synchrony is lost. The attendant increase in myocardial oxygen consumption coupled with marginal coronary perfusion leads to inadequate myocardial oxygen transport balance and the development of heart failure.

Systolic Heart Failure

Systolic heart failure is characterized by decreased SV and CO despite elevated ventricular volumes and pressure. Several adaptive mechanisms attempt to maintain CO, arterial pressure, and perfusion of vital organs. Neurohormonal activation is a compensatory response to low CO. Adrenergic activation and parasympathetic system withdrawal lead to stimulation of myocardial contractility, tachycardia, and generalized systemic vasoconstriction. In addition to catecholamine-mediated increases in SVR, activation of the renin–angiotensin–aldosterone system (RAAS), the augmented release of vasopressin, endothelial production of endothelin, and decreased basal production of endothelial-derived nitric oxide, contribute to further elevations in SVR. Activation of neurohormonal systems also leads to an increase in sodium and water retention, which serves to increase preload. An increase in ventricular preload augments ventricular performance, thereby maintaining SV and CO (preload reserve). Atrial natriuretic peptide (ANP) and brain natriuretic peptide (BNP) are released in response to increases in wall stress. Natriuretic peptides act as counterregulatory hormones, producing vasodilation, increased sodium and water excretion, and inhibition of the sympathetic nervous system. When the ventricle is chronically exposed to an increase in volume or pressure, it undergoes hypertrophy in order to decrease myocardial wall stress and to preserve function. These compensatory mechanisms maintain cardiac performance. Over time, however, mechanical, neurohormonal, and possibly genetic factors produce molecular and cellular events that worsen ventricular function, increase ventricular wall stress, and promote further pathologic remodeling. This cycle ultimately leads to the loss of myocytes and the development of heart failure.

Left Ventricular Systolic Failure

Left ventricular failure is characterized by a significantly elevated EDV and EDP. The increase in ventricular volume often produces mitral regurgitation, which further increases ventricular wall stress while decreasing SV and CO. At the same time, an elevated ventricular EDP decreases the coronary

---

TABLE 34.6

CAUSES OF CARDIAC FAILURE

I. Arrhythmias
  - Supraventricular tachycardia
  - Ventricular tachycardia

II. Infectious/Immunologic Disorders
  - Myocarditis: viral, bacterial
  - Kawasaki disease
  - Acute rheumatic fever
  - Polyarteritis nodosa

III. Ischemia
  - Shock states
  - ALCAPA

IV. Congenital and Structural Heart Disease

V. Metabolic Disorders
  - Hypoglycemia
  - Hypocalcemia
  - Glycogen storage disease
  - Carnitine deficiency
  - Mitochondrial disorders

VI. Neuromuscular Diseases
  - Duchenne muscular dystrophy
  - Friedreich's ataxia

VII. Cardiomyopathy
  - Dilated
  - Restrictive
  - Hypertrophic

perfusion gradient and coronary flow reserve. In addition, increased ventricular pressures are transmitted to the pulmonary circulation. This elevates the pulmonary vascular hydrostatic pressure, producing pulmonary edema. With severe elevations in pulmonary vascular pressures, ultrastructural microvascular changes increase vascular permeability, contributing further to the formation of pulmonary edema. Finally, pulmonary hypertension leads to pulmonary endothelial dysfunction. As a result, the pulmonary endothelium releases endothelin, a vasoconstrictive peptide, and basal production of nitric oxide is decreased, leading to further increases in PVR and worsening pulmonary hypertension.

Right Ventricular Systolic Failure

Right ventricular failure is characterized by an elevated EDV and EDP. Marked RV dilation is often accompanied by tricuspid regurgitation. Right ventricular failure adversely affects left ventricular filling and therefore SV and CO by three mechanisms (20). First, pulmonary venous return is diminished. Second, right ventricular diastolic hypertension decreases the transeptal pressure gradient. As a result, the ventricular septum occupies a more neutral position between the two ventricles during diastole. This decreases left ventricular cavitary volume and therefore compliance, leading to reduced ventricular filling. This phenomenon is known as *diastolic ventricular interdependence*. Finally, as a result of *systolic ventricular interdependence*, right ventricular-dependent reductions in left ventricular filling diminish the magnitude of left ventricular systolic pressure, decreasing left ventricular assistance to right ventricular pressure and flow. Finally, right ventricular failure causes central venous hypertension, which impedes lymphatic drainage, producing pleural effusions and interstitial pulmonary edema.

Pulmonary Hypertension

Pulmonary hypertension is a common cause of RV failure. Interactions between the pulmonary vascular endothelium and smooth muscle cell determine the functional features of the pulmonary circulation in disease. Over time, vascular remodeling and endothelial dysfunction lead to pulmonary hypertension. Vascular remodeling occurs in progressive stages, which ultimately results in luminal occlusion. Endothelial injury results in the release of the vasoconstrictive peptide endothelin and decreased basal production of the vasodilator nitric oxide.

Neonatal pulmonary vascular disease can be due to several pathophysiologic processes. Pulmonary hypoplasia occurs with congenital diaphragmatic hernia, for example, and leads to a decrease in the cross-sectional area of the pulmonary circulation; excessive in utero muscularization of peripheral pulmonary arteries results from intrauterine hypoxia and stress; and postnatal failure of the pulmonary vasculature to dilate results from perinatal stress. Congenital heart lesions that have a large, nonrestrictive ventricular septal defect or aortopulmonary communication cause pulmonary hypertension by virtue of complete transmission of systemic pressure to the pulmonary circulation during systole. Over time, however, PVR increases, resulting in bidirectional shunting. Another cause of pulmonary hypertension is lesions that produce pulmonary venous hypertension, such as LV failure, mitral stenosis, and total anomalous pulmonary venous return.

Effects of Mechanical Ventilation on PVR

Pulmonary vascular resistance is lowest at FRC. Resistance increases as the end-expiratory lung volume decreases below FRC. As lung volume decreases, radial traction provided by the pulmonary interstitium decreases, leading to a decrease in the cross-sectional area of extra-alveolar vessels. Furthermore, as end-expiratory lung volume decreases, the propensity to develop atelectasis increases. This reduces alveolar oxygen tension, leading to compensatory hypoxic pulmonary vasoconstriction. Conversely, as lung volume increases above FRC, interalveolar vessels are compressed, increasing PVR.

Ventricular Diastolic Failure

Ventricular diastolic failure occurs when the ventricular chamber is unable to accept an adequate volume of blood to maintain an appropriate SV. Systolic function is often normal. Left ventricular diastolic failure leads to pulmonary hypertension, pulmonary edema, and low CO. Right ventricular diastolic failure leads to systemic venous congestion and impaired left ventricular filling. The latter results from ventricular interdependence and diminished pulmonary venous return.

Clinical Assessment

The clinical assessment of cardiogenic shock begins with a history, physical exam, and review of laboratory data. Patients with low CO require an emergent echocardiogram to evaluate cardiac anatomy and function, including indices of systolic and diastolic function. The most common measurements of systolic performance are the shortening fraction and ejection fraction for the LV. Assessment of RV function is difficult due to its geometrical shape. The findings on physical exam depend on the severity of heart failure, which ventricle is affected, whether diastolic or systolic failure is present, and the rapidity with which the disease is evolving. The characteristic findings on exam include cool extremities, prolonged capillary refill, poor peripheral pulses, tachycardia, and hepatomegaly. A chest radiograph demonstrates cardiomegaly and pulmonary edema. Central venous access is essential, and it allows for monitoring of mixed venous oxygen saturations and ventricular filling pressures. Cerebral oximetry is a surrogate for mixed venous oximetry, providing continuous, noninvasive data.

Therapy

As with other types of shock, addressing the determinants of oxygen transport balance provides a rationale for implementing therapies. Mechanical ventilatory support coupled with adequate sedation significantly decrease global oxygen demands and should be considered first-line treatment for circulatory failure and shock. Increasing DO_2 involves manipulating the determinants of oxygen content and CO.

The rationale for selecting vasoactive agents to treat heart failure is based on their effects on myocardial oxygen transport balance, whether diastolic or systolic failure is present, and whether pulmonary or systemic vascular resistance is elevated. In general, therapies are directed at optimizing ventricular preload and afterload, and providing inotropic support. There are several vasoactive agents to choose from with varying pharmacokinetic and pharmacodynamic properties (Table 34.7). Vasoactive agents that decrease ventricular preload, either by increasing venous capacitance or decreasing intravascular volume, reduce ventricular diastolic pressure and volume without appreciable effects on SV and CO. In contrast, vasoactive agents that reduce SVR increase SV and CO but have minimal effects on LV filling pressures. Combined venoarterial dilators significantly reduce LV diastolic volume and pressure while increasing SV and CO (21). The net effect is a marked improvement in myocardial oxygen transport balance. The benefits of afterload reduction therapy require an adequate, albeit elevated, ventricular filling pressure; otherwise reducing SVR may lead to an inadequate compensatory increase in SV, precipitating hypotension. Inotropic agents increase SV and CO while

TABLE 34.7

VASOACTIVE AGENTS HEMODYNAMIC EFFECTS

	Ventricular loading conditions				Ventricular function				
	Venous capacitance	LVFP	SVR	PVR	Inotropic properties	Lusitropic properties	HR	CO	Dose (μg/kg/min)
Milrinone	↑	↓	↓	↓	+	+	+/−	↑	0.25–0.75
Nesiritide	↑	↓	↓	↓	−	+	−	↑	0.01–0.03
Nitroprusside	↑	↓	↓	↓	−	+	+/−	↑	0.1–5.0
Nitroglycerin	↑	↓	+/−	+/−	−	+	+/−	+/−	0.1–5.0
Vasopressin	↓↓	−	↑↑↑	+/−	−	−	↓	−	0.0003–0.002
Catecholamines									
Dopamine	−	−	−	−	+	−	↑	↑	<10
	↓	−	↑	+/−	+		↑	↑	>10
Dubutaine	−	↓	↓	−	+	−	↑	↑	2–20
Epinephrine	−	−	↓	↓	++	−	↑	↑	<0.1
	↓↓	−	↑↑	↑	+++	−	↑↑	↑↑	>0.1–0.2
Norepinephrine	↓↓	−	↑↑↑	↑	+	−	↑	+/−	0.01–1.0
Isoproterenol	↑	↓	↓	↓	+++	−	↑↑	↑↑	0.01–1.0

SVR, systemic vascular resistance; PVR, pulmonary vascular resistance; LVFP, left ventricular filling pressure; CO, cardiac output; HR, heart rate.

reducing ventricular filling pressures. However, inotropic stimulation and the attendant increase in heart rate that accompanies most inotropic agents, significantly increase myocardial oxygen consumption. Finally, several vasoactive agents improve diastolic function by improving myocardial oxygen transport balance, and by their direct effects on the myocardium. There are several therapies available to treat pulmonary hypertension. Alkalosis and alveolar hyperoxia decrease PVR. Several vasoactive agents decrease pulmonary and systemic vascular resistance (Table 34.7). In contrast to these nonselective intravenous vasodilators, inhaled nitric oxide selectively vasodilates the pulmonary vasculature.

Mechanical circulatory support should be implemented if cardiac output and oxygen delivery remain inadequate despite escalating medical therapy. The decision to proceed to mechanic circulatory support is based in part on the etiology of heart failure and clinical progression. Optimal timing for mechanical assistance is subjective but critical in order to minimize organ damage. Similar thoughts should be directed at potential surgical intervention.

Catecholamines

The hemodynamic effects of catecholamines are dose dependent, and are mediated by a variety of adrenergic receptors that use the cAMP-dependent signaling cascade. As intracellular cAMP increases, intracellular calcium metabolism and cellular function are altered. Activation of β-2 receptors leads to vascular smooth muscle relaxation and vasodilation, while activation of cardiomyocyte β-1 receptors leads to enhanced contractility and, to a lesser extent, increased heart rate. Activation of α-1 receptors leads to vascular smooth muscle contraction and vasoconstriction. β-adrenergic receptors experience agonist-mediated receptor desensitization in which an attenuated physiologic response to beta agonists occurs with prolonged exposure to elevated levels of endogenous and exogenous catecholamines. In heart failure, circulating and myocardial norepinephrine and epinephrine levels are chronically elevated and acute tolerance may develop to catecholamine therapy. Catecholamines are primarily metabolized by two enzyme systems: catechol O-methyltransferase and monoamine oxidase. All catecholamines have a very short half-life, allowing for easy titration.

All catecholamines increase myocardial oxygen demands as a result of their chronotropic and inotropic effects. If myocardial oxygen delivery does not increase to the same extent as demand, myocardial ischemia may ensue. This is a particular concern when using epinephrine and isoproterenol. Tachydysrhythmias result from stimulation of β-1 receptors. The agents most commonly associated with induction of dysrhythmias are isoproterenol and epinephrine and, to a lesser extent, dopamine and dobutamine. Finally catecholamines with alpha-agonist activity, such as epinephrine, norepinephrine, and dopamine, should be administered through a central venous line to avoid the risk of extravasation and resulting tissue necrosis.

Dopamine. Dopamine is the immediate precursor of norepinephrine in the endogenous catecholamine biosynthesis pathway. Approximately half of the dopamine-induced response results from dopamine-induced release of norepinephrine from sympathetic nerve terminals. Dopamine directly stimulates α, β, and dopaminergic receptors.

Dopamine is primarily used in the treatment of oliguria, septic shock, and ventricular dysfunction. Dopamine in low doses (<3–5 μg/kg/min) stimulates renal vascular dopaminergic receptors, increasing renal blood flow and the glomerular filtration rate. Moderate doses (<10 μg/kg/min) have chronotropic and inotropic effects. In adults with congestive heart failure, dopamine significantly increases CO by increasing SV and, to a lesser extent, heart rate. Left ventricular filling pressures either remain unchanged or increase (22). Data in children are limited but demonstrate similar results (23). At high doses (>10 μg/kg/min) alpha-adrenergic effects predominate and SVR begins to increase. The effects of dopamine on PVR and pulmonary artery pressure are conflicting.

Dobutamine. Dobutamine is a synthetic catecholamine that provides inotropic support. In adults with ventricular dysfunction, dobutamine significantly increases CO by increasing SV and, to a lesser extent, by increasing heart rate and reducing SVR. In contrast to dopamine, dobutamine consistently decreases ventricular filling pressures (22). Data in children are limited but demonstrate similar results (24).

Epinephrine. Epinephrine is an endogenous catecholamine formed from norepinephrine through N-methylation. It is largely produced by the adrenal medulla in response to stress. Epinephrine is used frequently in the management of severe septic and cardiogenic shock, and during cardiopulmonary resuscitation. In low doses (<0.1 µg/kg/min), epinephrine provides significant inotropic and chronotropic support. Additionally, it stimulates β-2 receptors, causing a reduction in SVR, PVR, and diastolic blood pressure. At high doses, activation of α-1 receptors leads to vasoconstriction of venous capacitance and arterial resistance vessels, which may compromise renal and mesenteric blood flow.

Norepinephrine. Norepinephrine is the neurotransmitter of the sympathetic nervous system. It is released from terminal nerve endings and acts locally. Norepinephrine primarily causes vasoconstriction of venous capacitance and arterial resistance vessels by activating α-1 receptors, while providing minor inotropic support. The primary use for norepinephrine is to restore an adequate perfusion pressure in the setting of vasodilatory shock. As with epinephrine, significant increases in SVR may compromise renal and mesenteric blood flow.

Isoproterenol. Isoproterenol is a synthetic catecholamine. It is a potent, nonspecific β-agonist that provides significant inotropic and chronotropic support as well as reductions in SVR and PVR. Isoproterenol is associated with significant tachycardia and the propensity to develop tachydysrhythmias. It also increases myocardial oxygen demands, while a shortened diastole and diastolic hypotension compromise coronary perfusion. For these reasons, isoproterenol is primarily used to treat bradycardia.

Non-Catecholamine Vasoactive Agents

Milrinone. Milrinone does not act via adrenergic receptors but rather through selective inhibition of phospodiesterase III. This leads to a reduction of cAMP degradation, causing vasodilation of venous capacitance and pulmonary and systemic arterial resistance vessels. It also provides modest inotropic support with little effect on heart rate. Milrinone improves diastolic function by improving myocardial oxygen transport balance or by having a direct effect on the myocardium. Half-life is age-dependent and ranges from <1 hour in children to >3 hours in infants. Milrinone is predominantly cleared via renal excretion; therefore, dosing must be adjusted in patients with renal insufficiency. In children with acute ventricular dysfunction, the combined inotropic and afterload-reducing properties of milrinone produce a significant increase in CO and reduction in ventricular filling pressures (25).

Vasopressin. Vasopressin is a hormone that is essential for osmotic and cardiovascular homeostasis. In addition to its antidiuretic effect, physiologic levels of vasopressin are required for normal vascular tone. Vasopressin interacts with vasopressin-specific receptors located on vascular smooth muscle and renal tubular cells. Vasopressin constricts systemic arterial and venous capacitance vessels in a dose-dependent fashion. Based on these properties, vasopressin has utility in cardiac arrest and vasodilatory shock. Vasopressin has been demonstrated to significantly increase blood pressure, allowing for the reduction of catecholamine therapy in adult and pediatric patients with catecholamine-resistant vasodilatory shock (26, 27). While CO and DO$_2$ remain unchanged, SV increases significantly despite increases in afterload. It is unclear whether vasopressin provides inotropic support because of its effects on preload, heart rate, and coronary perfusion.

Nesiritide. Nesiritide is the human recombinant form of BNP. Nesiritide produces dose-dependent dilation of systemic and pulmonary arterial resistance and venous capacitance vessels by stimulating natriuretic receptors present on the surface of vascular smooth muscle cells. Nesiritide also affects vasomotor tone by inhibiting both the RAAS and the release of endothelin, and it reduces sympathetic tone by suppressing sympathetic outflow from the central nervous system and postganglionic sympathetic nerve endings. Nesiritide also improves diastolic function by stimulating natriuretic peptide receptors on cardiomyocytes, leading to an increase in cGMP levels. Nesiritide causes a dose-dependent natriuresis and diuresis by reducing sodium reabsorption in the proximal and distal tubules, and by inhibiting adrenal cortical production of aldosterone. Nesiritide has a half-life of 15 minutes, allowing for easy titration. It is cleared by binding to natriuretic peptide receptor C, at which time it is internalized and degraded. Additionally, circulating natriuretic peptides are inactivated by neutral endopeptidases. The primary indication for nesiritide is in the acute management of congestive heart failure (CHF). Because nesiritide decreases afterload and increases venous capacitance, CO is increased while ventricular filling pressures are reduced. The evaluation of nesiritide in pediatric patients has been limited to small, retrospective analysis.

Nitroprusside. Nitroprusside (NTP) spontaneously releases nitric oxide, which activates the soluble form of guanylate cyclase, producing increased levels of cGMP. NTP causes dose-dependent dilation of systemic and pulmonary arterial resistance and venous capacitance vessels. NTP decomposes nonenzymatically in the blood, releasing cyanide, which undergoes transulfuration to form thiocyanite. Thiocyanite is excreted by the kidneys and has a half-life of 3 days in patients with normal renal function. While thiocyanite is not vasoactive, it does accumulate in the setting of renal failure and may cause neurotoxicity. When thiosulfate stores are depleted, cyanide toxicity ensues. Prevention of cyanide toxicity is thus dependent on the availability of sulfur. Cyanide toxicity is rare, however, when low-dose infusion rates (<3 µg/kg/min) are used for a short period of time (<3 days). The primary adverse event resulting from the use of NTP is hypotension. One advantage of NTP is its short half-life of 2 minutes, which allows for easy titration. NTP is effective in the acute management of CHF. Because NTP decreases afterload and increases venous capacitance, CO is increased while ventricular filling pressures are reduced. As with other therapies that increase myocardial cGMP levels, NTP appears to improve diastolic function.

Nitroglycerin. Nitroglycerin (NTG) undergoes biotransformation to yield nitric oxide. NTG produces dose-dependent dilation of systemic and pulmonary arterial and venous capacitance vessels. NTG is hydrolyzed by hepatic glutathione-organic nitrate reductase into inorganic nitrite and denitrated metabolites. These metabolic byproducts have little if any vasoactivity. NTG has a short half-life of 2 minutes, allowing for easy titration. In contrast to NTP, tolerance develops rapidly to NTG and may result from impaired biotransformation. Adverse events with intravenous NTG are similar to other vasoactive agents. Hypotension results from inadequate ventricular filling pressures. Intravenous NTG is primarily used in the acute management of CHF. In low to modest doses (<3 µg/kg/min), NTG mainly increases venous capacitance thus ventricular filling pressures are reduced without significant changes in CO (28). In higher doses, NTG reduces SVR and PVR, and CO increases (29). Finally, as with other therapies that increase myocardial cGMP levels, NTG improves diastolic function.

DISTRIBUTIVE SHOCK

Distributive shock is characterized by vasomotor dysfunction leading to the maldistribution of blood flow. A marked reduction in vasomotor tone causes a significant increase in venous capacitance and reduction in SVR. This leads to a state of relative hypovolemia and hypotension. Distributive shock is seen with anaphylaxis, spinal cord injuries, cortisol-deficient states, and septic shock. Anaphylaxis is characterized by the release of inflammatory mediators, which cause vasodilation and increased vascular permeability. Spinal shock occurs with cord trans-section above T1, which causes total loss of sympathetic cardiovascular tone. Finally, cortisol is required to maintain vasomotor tone and vascular responsiveness to endogenous catecholamines.

SEPTIC SHOCK

Etiology and Pathophysiology

Septic shock results from the direct effects of the invading microorganism and its toxins, and from the patient's inflammatory response to infection. The current definition of sepsis is a systemic inflammatory response resulting from suspected or proven infection (30). A systemic inflammatory response syndrome (SIRS) is present when at least two of the following criteria are present: hypo- or hyperthermia ($>38.5°C$ or $<36.0°C$), tachycardia or bradycardia, tachypnea, and leukocytosis or leukopenia. Septic shock is characterized by sepsis and cardiovascular dysfunction (30). The latter is defined by hypotension ($<$5th percentile for age), the need for vasoactive medications to maintain blood pressure, metabolic/lactic acidosis, and poor perfusion despite administration of >40 mL/kg of isotonic intravenous fluid in the first hour.

The invading microorganism, as well as released structural components and exotoxins, activate several plasma protein systems and blood cells to release inflammatory mediators. Complement, the contact system, and the coagulation/fibrinolytic systems are activated, as well as endothelial cells, platelets, neutrophils, lymphocytes, and macrophages. The release of inflammatory mediator sets into motion a series of events that culminate in tissue injury. During this process, the endothelium is damaged. This increases microvascular permeability, which leads to interstitial edema, and the endothelium is converted to a procoagulant state. In addition, several inflammatory mediators such as bradykinin, histamine, and prostaglandins cause functional changes in the microvasculature, which further increases vascular permeability, contributing to edema formation.

Myocardial dysfunction develops in virtually all patients with septic shock. Serum from patients with septic shock was shown to depress myocardial function. Subsequent experiments demonstrated that TNF-α and interleukin-1 individually and synergistically, in addition to other mediators, are myocardial depressants (31). The characteristic pattern of cardiac performance during septic shock is one of reduced LV and RV ejection fractions, increased end-diastolic and end-systolic volumes of both ventricles, and normal SV. As compared to normal subjects, adults with septic shock usually have normal or increased coronary blood flow. Nonetheless, inadequate coronary perfusion and impaired utilization of oxygen may contribute to myocardial dysfunction in some instances. In addition, the myocardium is less responsive to adrenergic stimulation during septic shock due to adrenergic receptor desensitization.

In addition to myocardial dysfunction, some degree of vasomotor dysfunction is present in septic shock. Vasodilation of venous capacitance and arterial resistance vessels leads to reduced venous return and hypotension. With fluid resuscitation, CO normalizes and, despite significantly elevated levels of endogenous vasoconstrictors such as catecholamines, angiotensin II, and endothelin, SVR remains low and hypotension persists. This is the hemodynamic profile of *vasodilatory shock*. In some instances, patients remain hypotensive despite vasopressor therapy. There are several mechanisms thought to be responsible for the failure of vascular smooth muscle cells to constrict to endogenous and exogenous vasoconstrictors (32). Inflammatory mediators such as bradykinin and histamine are potent vasodilators. In addition, plasma levels of vasopressin are low. Normally, vasopressin plays a minor role in arterial pressure regulation, but it plays a major role in the defense of blood pressure during hypotension. During the initial phase of septic shock, vasopressin levels are markedly elevated. However, as shock worsens, vasopressin levels become low. Correction of inappropriately low plasma vasopressin levels to those found in acute hypotension significantly increase arterial pressure (26,27). The mechanism responsible for the low levels is unknown, but it may result from depleted neurohypophyseal stores after profound and sustained stimulation of vasopressin release early in shock.

An additional mechanism responsible for vascular failure involves modulation of ATP-sensitive potassium channels. Vasoconstrictors such as angiotensin II and norepinephrine bind to and activate receptors on vascular smooth muscle cells, which ultimately leads to an increase in the concentration of calcium in the cytosol and vascular smooth muscle cell constriction. This increase results from the release of calcium from intracellular stores and from the entry of extracellular calcium into the cell through voltage-gated calcium channels. However, under conditions of increased tissue metabolism or tissue hypoxia, when the cellular concentration of hydrogen ion and lactate are elevated, potassium channels become activated. This causes potassium to exit the cell, the plasma membrane becomes hyperpolarized, and inactivation of the voltage-gated calcium channels prevents an increase in the cytoplasmic calcium concentration in response to vasoconstrictors. Finally, increased synthesis of the vasodilator nitric oxide contributes to the hypotension and resistance to vasopressors that occur in vasodilatory shock. The mechanisms responsible for increased expression of inducible nitric oxide synthase remains unclear. Nitric oxide also activates calcium-sensitive potassium channels in the plasma membrane of vascular smooth muscle cell, contributing to vasopressor resistance. Thus, septic shock is characterized by altered ventricular preload, myocardial function, and afterload. As a result, there are a variety of hemodynamic states on presentation, which may vary over time. These include low CO/high SVR and high CO/low SVR states. Unlike adults, death from septic shock in children is most commonly associated with progressive cardiac failure, not vascular failure.

Shock results from either inadequate oxygen delivery or impaired utilization. The latter reflects impairment of oxidative metabolism, the pathophysiology of which remains unclear. Oxygen consumption wanes despite seemingly adequate oxygen delivery, and oxygen extraction is not increased. Furthermore, increasing oxygen delivery does not lead to an increase in aerobic metabolism, based on *direct measurements* of oxygen consumption (33,34). In addition to cardiovascular failure, multiorgan dysfunction and failure occurs and is due to either tissue hypoxia or inflammatory-mediated damage. Both the intrinsic and extrinsic coagulation pathways and endothelium are activated. This produces disseminated intravascular coagulation and the consumption of clotting factors, antithrombotic factors, and platelets, leading to a thrombotic and hemorrhagic state.

Clinical Assessment

Septic shock presents with a wide spectrum of clinical findings. Patients may present with brady- or tachycardia, hypo- or hyperthermia, tachypnea, and leukocytosis or leukopenia. On exam, the earliest indicator may be an isolated altered mental status. A few petechial lesions on presentation may rapidly progress to extensive hemorrhagic lesions, or purpura fulminans. Patients present anywhere along a spectrum ranging from hyperdynamic or "warm shock" to nonhyperdynamic or "cold shock." The former is characterized by bounding pulses and warm extremities with an instantaneous capillary refill; the latter is characterized by weak pulses and cool extremities. Similarly, various degrees of organ system involvement are present. Permeability pulmonary edema, or acute respiratory distress syndrome, pre-renal or renal azotemia, impaired liver function, and a coagulopathy often accompany cardiovascular instability.

Treatment

As with other shock states, the determinants of oxygen transport balance should be addressed. All children with septic shock require volume resuscitation. It is not uncommon to administer more than 100 to 150 mL/kg of isotonic fluid over the first few hours. There are no convincing data demonstrating a benefit of colloid over crystalloid during resuscitation. While attempts are made at generating and maintaining an adequate ventricular filling pressure, inotropic support should be provided. The patient's hemodynamic profile, the rapidity with which the disease is progressing, and the pharmacokinetic and pharmacodynamic properties of the various vasoactive agents (Table 34.7) should dictate additional therapies. Patients at risk for cortisol deficiency should receive corticosteroids. A history of recent glucocorticoid therapy, central nervous system disease, and patients with purpura fulminans (at risk for adrenal hemorrhage and Waterhouse–Friderichsen syndrome) should receive therapy. In addition, there is increasing evidence that preterm and stressed term neonates are at risk for a relative adrenal insufficiency due to an immature hypothalamic–pituitary–adrenal axis (35). In addition, corticosteroids prevent adrenergic receptor desensitization and they induce expression of additional receptors. Additional therapies are directed at treating organ system failure and include hemodialysis, administration of clotting factors and platelets, and provision of adequate nutritional support. Antibiotics should be started without delay, and surgical debridement, if indicated, should be performed emergently. Nosocomial sepsis requires broad-spectrum antibiotics. If a toxin-producing organism is suspected, clindamycin should be used in conjunction with appropriate antibiotics. Finally, granulocyte-macrophage colony-stimulating factor has been shown to improve survival in newborns with neutropenic septic shock.

OBSTRUCTIVE SHOCK

Obstructive shock is characterized by low CO despite normal intravascular volume and myocardial function. The most common causes are cardiac tamponade, tension pneumothorax, and excessive ventricular afterload due to obstructive congenital heart lesions, pulmonary hypertension, or malignant hypertension. Cardiac tamponade results from the accumulation of liquid in the pericardial space, which leads to a significant increase in intrapericardial pressure and reduction in RV diastolic Tmp. This leads to a marked reduction in venous return and RV filling. Isotonic fluid administration may be indicated to increase ventricular filling and preserve CO until emergent fluid removal can be accomplished by pericardiocentesis. A tension pneumothorax causes progressive ipsilateral lung collapse, a shift of the mediastinum, and obstruction of venous return. Therapy requires an emergent thoracentesis. Pulmonary hypertension and malignant hypertension are due to a variety of etiologies and pathophysiologic processes. In this instance, the normal heart is presented with a load that exceeds its capacity, producing heart failure. The myocardial response is determined by the rapidity with which the lesion evolved, and

therefore the time allotted for ventricular hypertrophy to develop, the magnitude of afterload, and intravascular volume status. Once afterload reserve is exhausted, SV and CO decrease. Obstructive congenital heart disease is a common cause of shock in infants. *Ductal-dependent lesions* manifest during the first 2 weeks of life as the ductus arteriosus is closing. Ductal patency allows for pulmonary perfusion with right-sided lesions, such as critical pulmonary stenosis, and for systemic perfusion with left-sided lesions, such as critical aortic stenosis and hypoplastic left heart syndrome. Effective resuscitation begins with a high index of suspicion and requires the prompt institution of a continuous infusion of prostaglandin E_1.

HISTOTOXIC HYPOXIA

Histotoxic hypoxia is characterized by impaired cellular utilization of oxygen. It most commonly occurs in the stetting of septic shock, but cyanide and carbon monoxide toxicity also inhibit oxidative phosphorylation. Despite a normal or elevated CO and DO_2, lactate levels are elevated and the OER is decreased. Reports of normal levels of tissue oxygenation in patients with septic shock and lactic acidosis and of the inability to increase VO_2 in the face of increased DO_2 support the presence of impaired oxygen utilization. A number of possible mechanisms may be responsible for deranged cellular energy metabolism (36). Carbon monoxide and cyanide bind to cytochrome oxidase, inhibiting mitochondrial respiration and the generation of ATP. Cyanide and carbon monoxide are products of combustion in many fires, and toxicity should be suspected in all victims of smoke inhalation.

CONCLUSION

A thorough understanding of the pathophysiology of shock is necessary for managing critically ill patients. Shock is not necessarily a problem of cardiac output and arterial pressure, but it is always a problem of inadequate tissue oxygenation. Viewing shock as an imbalance between oxygen delivery and oxygen utilization allows for a comprehensive understanding of all shock states, and provides a rationale for diagnosing and treating shock states.

References

1. Cain SM. Oxygen delivery and uptake in dogs during anemic and hypoxic hypoxia. *J Appl Physiol* 1977;42:228–234.
2. Van Der Linden P, Gilbert E, Paques P, et al. Influence of hematocrit on tissue oxygen extraction capabilities during acute hemorrhage. *Am J Physiol* 1993;264:H1942–H1947.
3. Tibby SM, Hatherill, Marsh MJ, et al. Clinicians' abilities to estimate cardiac index in ventilated children and infants. *Arch Dis Child* 1997;77:516–518.
4. Connors AF, McCaffree DR, Gray BA. Evaluation of right heart catheterization in the critically ill patient without acute myocardial infarction. *NEJM* 1983;308:263–267.
5. Scheingraber S, Rehm M, Sehmisch C, et al. Rapid saline infusion produces hyperchloremic acidosis in patients undergoing gynecologic surgery. *Anesthesiology* 1999;90:1265–1270.
6. Daubeney P, Pilkington SN, Janke E, et al Cerebral oxygenation measured by near infrared spectroscopy: comparison with jugular bulb oximetry. *Ann Thorac Surg* 1996;61:930–934.
7. Tortoriello TA, Stayer SA, Mott AR, et al. A noninvasive estimation of mixed venous oxygen saturation using near-infrared spectroscopy by cerebral oximetry in pediatric cardiac surgery patients. *Pediatr Anesth* 2005;15:495–503.
8. Legato MJ. Cellular mechanisms of normal growth in the mammalian heart: I. Qualitative and quantitative features of ventricular architecture in the dog from birth to five months of age. *Circ Res* 1979;44:250–262.
9. Marijianowski MH, Van Der Loos CM, Mohrschladt MF, et al. The neonatal heart has a relatively high content of total collagen and type I collagen, a condition that may explain the less compliant state. *J Am Coll Cardiol* 1994;23:1204.

10. Nichols DG. Respiratory muscle performance in infants and children. *J Pediatr* 1991;118:493–502.
11. Vassilakopoulos T, Zakynthinos S, Roussos C. Muscle function. In: Marini JJ, Slutsky AS, eds. *Physiological basis of ventilatory support*. New York: Marcel Dekker; 1998:103–152.
12. Viires N, Sillye G, Aubier M, et al. Regional blood flow distribution in dog during induced hypotension and low cardiac output. *J Clin Invest* 1983;72:935–947.
13. Pinsky MR, Marquez J, Martin D, et al. Ventricular assist by cardiac cycle-specific increases in intrathoracic pressure. *Chest* 1987;91:709.
14. Rasanen J, Nikki P, Heikkila J. Acute myocardial infarction complicated by respiratory failure. The effect of mechanical ventilation. *Chest* 1984;85:21.
15. Rasanen J, Vaisanen IT, Heikkila J, et al. Acute myocardial infarction complicated by left ventricular dysfunction and respiratory failure. *Chest* 1985;87:158.
16. Guyton AC, Jones CE, Coleman TG. Effects on cardiac output of alterations in peripheral resistance—especially the effects of anemia and polycythemia. In: Guyton AC, Jones CE, Coleman TG, eds. *Circulatory physiology: cardiac output and its regulation*. Philadelphia: Saunders; 1973:394–411.
17. Guyton AC, Jones CE, Coleman TG. Mean circulatory pressure, mean systemic pressure, and mean pulmonary pressure and their effect on venous return. In: Guyton AC, Jones CE, Coleman TG, eds. *Circulatory physiology: cardiac output and its regulation*. Philadelphia: Saunders; 1973:205–221.
18. Guyton AC, Jones CE, Coleman TG. Effect of peripheral resistance and capacitance on venous return. In: Guyton AC, Jones CE, Coleman TG, eds. *Circulatory physiology: cardiac output and its regulation*. Philadelphia: Saunders; 1973:222–236.
19. Wiedemann HP, Matthay MA, Matthay RA. Cardiovascular-pulmonary monitoring in the intensive care unit (part 1). *Chest* 1984;85:537–549.
20. Santamore WP, Gray L. Significant left ventricular contributions to right ventricular systolic function. *Chest* 1995;107:1134–1145.
21. Artman M, Graham TP Jr. Guidelines for vasodilator therapy of congestive heart failure in infants and children. *Am Heart J* 1987;113:994–1005.
22. Leier CV, Heban PT, Huss P, et al. Comparative systemic and regional hemodynamic effects of dopamine and dobutamine in patients with cardiomyopathic heart failure. *Circulation* 1978;58:466–475.
23. Driscoll DJ, Gillette PC, Deuff DF, et al. The hemodynamic effect of dopamine in children. *J Thorac Cardiovasc Surg* 1979;78:765–768.
24. Perkin RM, Levin DL, Webb R, et al. Dobutamine: a hemodynamic evaluation in children with shock. *J Pediatr* 1982;100:977–983.
25. Chang AC, Atz AM, Wernovsky G, et al. Milrinone: systemic and pulmonary hemodynamic effects in neonates after cardiac surgery. *Crit Care Med* 1995;23:1907–1914.
26. Rosenzweig EB, Starc TJ, Chen JM, et al. Intravenous arginine-vasopressin in children with vasodilatory shock after cardiac surgery. *Circulation* 1999;100 (suppl II):182–186.
27. Dunser MW, Mayr AJ, Ulmer H, et al. Intravenous vasopressin in advanced Vasodilatory shock. *Circulation* 2003;107:2313–2319.
28. Miller RR, Vismara LA, Williams DO, et al. Pharmacological mechanisms for left ventricular unloading in clinical congestive heart failure. *Circ Res* 1976;39:127–133.
29. Ilbawi MN, Idriss FS, DeLeon SY, et al. Hemodynamic effects of intravenous nitroglycerin in pediatric patients after heart surgery. *Circulation* 1985;72 (suppl II):101–107.
30. Goldstein B, Giroir B, Randolph A, et al. International pediatric sepsis consensus conference: definitions for sepsis and organ dysfunction in pediatrics. *Pediatr Crit Care Med* 2005;6:2–8.
31. Parrillo JE. Pathogenetic mechanisms of septic shock. *NEJM* 1993;328:1471–1477.
32. Landry DW, Oliver JA. The pathogenesis of vasodilatory shock. *NEJM* 2001;345:588–595.
33. Ronco JJ, Fenwick JC, Wiggs BR, et al. Oxygen consumption is independent of increases in oxygen delivery by dobutamine in septic patients who have normal or increased plasma lactate. *Am Rev Respir Dis* 1993;147:25–31.
34. Phang PT, Cunninghan KF, Ronco JJ, et al. Mathematical coupling explains dependence of oxygen consumption on oxygen delivery in ARDS. *Am J Respir Crit Care Med* 1994;150:318.
35. Sasidharan P. Role of corticosteroids in neonatal blood pressure homeostasis. *Clin Perinatol* 1998;25:723–740.
36. Creery D, Fraser DD. Tissue dysoxia is sepsis: Getting to know the mitochondrion. *Crit Care Med* 2002;30:483–484.

CHAPTER 35 ■ SIGNS AND SYMPTOMS OF PEDIATRIC PULMONARY DISEASE

DINA M. IWAI

HISTORY

Obtaining a thorough history is an essential factor in the proper identification, diagnosis, and treatment of respiratory disease in children. Attention must be paid to not only medical history, but also to environmental, psychosocial, and family information that may be pertinent.

The history begins with the chief complaint or reason for referral. If the child is old enough, it is important to allow her to participate in the discussion. The child can often provide details that may be overlooked by a parent. In addition, parents frequently misuse terms such as *wheeze* to describe any form of noisy breathing. For this reason, the hospitalist should try to understand and clarify a parent's terminology in order to avoid misdiagnosis.

The description of the chief complaint should include duration and chronology of symptoms. Each symptom should be characterized by timing (time of day and relation to respiratory cycle), aggravating and relieving factors, type of onset (sudden or gradual), and associated features. The age of onset is also key as symptoms beginning shortly after birth may be related to an underlying congenital abnormality.

An arbitrary time-frame should be assigned in the evaluation of duration of symptoms as follows: acute (less than 3 weeks), subacute (>3 weeks and <3 months), and chronic (>3 months). It is essential to distinguish chronic or persistent symptoms from those that are recurrent with a period of wellness or good health in between.

Cough

One of the most common and earliest signs of respiratory disease is cough. Cough can be characterized by its nature (dry or productive), its quality (staccato, barking, or brassy), its timing (nocturnal, intermittent, or constant), its triggering factors (cold, exertion, positioning), its alleviating factors (response to bronchodilator therapy or antibiotics, change in position), and its associated symptoms (e.g., wheezing or vomiting).

Cough associated with sputum production is always considered significant in a child. It may be difficult to document sputum production in younger children or infants who frequently swallow rather than expectorate their sputum. If possible, it is important to establish the character of the sputum including volume, odor, color, and the presence of blood.

The timing and associated factors of the cough often lend insight into determining the underlying diagnosis. For example, in infants, cough associated with feedings may be due to gastroesophageal reflux, tracheoesophageal fistula, or swallow incoordination. A cough associated with recurrent wheezing is suggestive of airway obstruction such as occurs in asthma.

Noisy Breathing

"Noisy breathing" generally describes one of the following signs: snoring, stridor, wheezing, or grunting. Although frequently noisy breathing is assumed indicative of a pulmonary problem, it is important to remember that noisy breathing can also indicate a problem in the nose, nasopharynx, or upper airway. Noisy breathing during sleep or snoring may be a sign of obstructive sleep apnea.

Chest Pain

Chest pain, especially in adolescents, is not an uncommon complaint and may be caused by respiratory or other inciting factors. Organic chest pain can arise from a variety of anatomic structures such as chest wall, myocardium, pericardium, pleura, and esophagus. Pleural pain is generally localized to the involved area and is augmented with respirations. Diaphragmatic pleural irritation can result in referred pain to the abdomen or neck.

Dyspnea

Dyspnea is labored or difficult breathing. It is frequently associated with a subjective sensation of breathlessness.

PHYSICAL EXAMINATION

The physical examination of infants and children should begin with observation even before a formal examination is initiated. It is important to make observations before approaching or touching the child, which often invokes anxiety. The examination is best accomplished in the position in which the child feels most comfortable such as sitting in the parent's lap. The order of the physical examination should leave the most uncomfortable aspects of the examination for the end. A comprehensive examination includes the following four components: (1) inspection, (2) palpation, (3) auscultation, and (4) percussion.

Inspection

A large amount of information can be gained from simple observation. First, observe the child's *respiratory rate*, which varies with age, activity, state of wakefulness, and anxiety. It is important to remember that nonrespiratory factors such as anxiety, acid–base status, fever, anemia, metabolic disorders, and nervous system disturbances can also affect respiratory rate. Although determining a child's respiratory rate may be difficult in the examination setting, the examiner should count the respiratory rate for a full minute while the child is as calm as possible. *Tachypnea*, an abnormally high respiratory rate, can be due to respiratory diseases in patients with decreased compliance or an increase in upper airway resistance or non-respiratory disorders such as metabolic acidosis or fever. *Bradypnea*, an abnormally low respiratory rate, can indicate central nervous system depression or metabolic alkalosis.

Once the respiratory rate has been determined, the next focus of attention is on the rhythm of respirations. Variations in the rhythm of respirations occur in children and are especially prominent in infants and younger children. Children younger than 3 months of age commonly have pauses in their respiratory pattern of less than 10 seconds. *Periodic breathing* is a respiratory pattern in which three or more of these pauses occur with less than 20 seconds of breathing between pauses. *Apnea* is the cessation of breathing for more than 15 seconds, and is classified as central or obstructive. Central apnea occurs when there is no air flow and no apparent effort. In obstructive apnea there is vigorous effort with no resultant air flow.

Other common variations in respiratory rhythm include Kussmaul breathing and Cheyne–Stokes breathing. *Kussmaul breathing* is a pattern of deep, slow, regular respirations with a prolonged expiratory phase that is seen in ketoacidosis. *Cheyne–Stokes breathing* consists of a cyclical variation in rate and increasing and decreasing depths of tidal volume which become slower until breathing stops for several seconds before speeding up to a peak and then slowing again. This pattern occurs when the sensitivity of the respiratory centers in the brain is impaired, such as in children with increased intracranial pressure.

While observing a child's respirations, it is important to note the shape of the thorax. In general, infants' chests are more rounded than in older children due to the more horizontal position of the ribs. Abnormalities such as pectus excavatum (indrawing of the sternum or funnel chest) and pectus carinatum (bowing out of the sternum or pigeon chest) can be readily observed. Although these abnormalities may be isolated findings, pectus carinatum may be indicative of a chronic cardiorespiratory problem. A barrel-shaped chest with increased anteroposterior diameter is usually the result of chronic air trapping such as occurs in disease in the small airways that results in air trapping. Marked scoliosis may alter the thoracic cavity in such a way that impedes normal pulmonary function. Newborns and young infants have an excessively compliant chest wall; as a result, respiratory distress is characterized by collapse of the chest wall on inspiration, thus limiting the generation of tidal volume.

After assessing the rate and rhythm of respirations, the effort of respirations must be assessed. Objective signs of increased respiratory effort include chest wall retractions, use of accessory muscles, paradoxical respiratory movements, nasal flaring, head bobbing, grunting, orthopnea, and increased pulsus paradoxus.

When assessing respiratory effort, it is important to remember that breathing occurs as a result of complex coordination of the respiratory center, nervous system, and muscles of respiration. The dome-shaped diaphragm is the main muscle of respiration. Contraction of the diaphragm results in an outward movement of the ribcage and displacement downward of the abdominal compartment. As disturbances in normal respiratory mechanics occur, use of accessory muscles such as the intercostals muscles, scalene muscles, and sternocleidomastoid muscles can be observed. Use of these accessory muscles results in observed retractions. Retractions are due to a difference in intrathoracic and atmospheric pressure that results from airway obstruction or decreased lung compliance. Subcostal retractions generally occur when the lungs become hyperinflated and cause flattening of the diaphragm. In order to create sufficient negative intrathoracic pressure and allow inspiration to occur, the accessory muscles move the chest outward

and the sternum begins to shift anteriorly. When paradoxical use of respiratory muscles is observed (i.e., abdominal muscle movement opposite chest wall movement), respiratory failure and ultimately apnea is impending and action must be taken to assist with respirations.

In addition to thoracic inspection, there are key extrathoracic areas that should also be examined. The nasal cavity and oropharynx should be assessed for any abnormalities. Findings such as allergic shiners (dark discoloration of the lower eyelids that occurs due to venous stasis), Dennie line (an accentuated line below the margin of the lower eyelid), or an allergic salute (a wiping or rubbing of the nose with a transverse or upward movement of the hand) may indicate an allergic component to respiratory problems. The fingers should also be inspected for any evidence of clubbing (proliferation of the nail bed tissue that raises the nail base), which may be subtle and can be a result of a variety of respiratory, cardiac, and gastrointestinal disorders.

Palpation

Position of the trachea is important for the evaluation of possible mediastinal shift. The tracheal position in the suprasternal notch can be assessed by extending the neck slightly with the head in a midline neutral position and using two fingers in the older child, and one finger in the younger child. Although slight tracheal deviation to the right is normal, the trachea may be shifted when there are differences in intrathoracic pressure or volume between the two sides of the thorax. Depending on the location and nature of the abnormality, such as pneumothorax or collapsed alveoli, the mediastinum can be pushed or pulled to one side.

In addition to assessing the position of the trachea, palpation is used to identify the presence of *pulsus paradoxus*. Pulsus paradoxus describes the fluctuation in arterial pressure that occurs with respiration. As a result of changes in right ventricular preload and left ventricular afterload, arterial pressure normally falls with inspiration and rises in expiration. When a higher than normal increase in negative intrathoracic pressure occurs during inspiration, such as in airway obstruction, the difference in arterial pressures between inspiration and expiration becomes exaggerated. In order to assess for pulsus paradoxus, a blood pressure cuff and a stethoscope are used. The highest pressure at which any systolic sound is heard is recorded. The pressure is then lowered until all systolic sounds are heard. The difference is normally less than 10 mm Hg. Bronchial obstruction such as occurs in asthma may result in values greater than 20 mm Hg. If significant airway obstruction is present, variations in the amplitude of the continuous waveform of a pulse oximeter may be appreciated as an indication of pulsus paradoxus.

Auscultation

Although important information can be gathered from other aspects of the physical exam, auscultation is the key component in the assessment and diagnosis of pulmonary disease. Attention must be paid to the location, timing, and quality of the breath sounds. In general it is recommended that the diaphragm of the stethoscope be used, because lung sounds tend to be higher in pitch than heart sounds.

Location

When determining the origin of the location of the breath sounds one must recall the anatomy of the lungs. It is necessary to listen to each lobe of the lung and to compare both sides of the chest. One must determine whether the breath sounds are normal, increased, or decreased. The sounds that are appreciated are created by flow through the airways. Larger airways such as the trachea produce more turbulent flow and result in more audible sounds than the smaller distal airways. When the diaphragm of the stethoscope is placed over the trachea, "tubular" sounds louder during expiration than inspiration can be heard; these are referred to as *tracheal breath sounds*. When the stethoscope is placed in the left axilla, the softer, lower-pitched sounds of the distal airways can be heard. These sounds are louder in inspiration than in expiration and are referred to as *vesicular breath sounds*. A third type of breath sound, known *as bronchovesicular breath sounds*, can be appreciated by placing the diaphragm below the center of the right clavicle. The breath sounds heard in this location are equal in inspiration and expiration and are more turbulent in quality than vesicular breath sounds. The final type of breath sounds that can be encountered are *bronchial breath sounds*. These breath sounds are slightly louder in expiration than inspiration and are rather harsh, although less pronounced than with tracheal breath sounds.

Timing

When performing auscultation, it is important to listen to at least two cycles of respirations. There are three phases of the respiratory cycle that should be appreciated: (1) inspiration, (2) expiration, and (3) pause. It may not always be clear when the expiratory phase ends and the pause begins. In general, a normal inspiratory-to-expiratory (I:E) ratio is 1:2 or 1:3.

Specific Sounds

There are a variety of different adventitious or "extra" sounds that can be appreciated and that have been described. Although differentiating the various types of adventitious sounds can be challenging, experience can lead to identification of the more common types of sounds that frequently occur in pulmonary disease. It is always important not only to identify these sounds but to appreciate the timing, loudness, pitch, and location of these extra sounds.

Crackles/Rales. Crackles are described as popping or crackling, nonmusical sounds that are heard more frequently in inspiration but occasionally may be heard during expiration. Crackles are a result of air passages or alveoli opening up or by air bubbling through fluid. When crackles are low in pitch and heard early in the respiratory cycle, they are referred to as *coarse crackles*. Coarse crackles are an indication of fluid in the larger airways. When a significant amount of fluid is present in the larger airways, coarse crackles may also be heard during expiration. *Fine crackles* occur later in inspiration, are higher in pitch, and are a sign of fluid in the smaller airways.

Wheezes. Wheezes are prolonged, musical sounds produced by air flowing across an obstruction such as a narrowed airway. Depending on the caliber of the narrowed airway, wheezes may be high pitched or low pitched and may occur in inspiration or expiration. Widespread obstruction such as in asthma leads to wheezing that is polyphonic in nature. Fixed obstruction of a large airway such as with a foreign body leads to monophonic wheezing. During inspiration, airways are normally tethered open, and therefore airway narrowing may be reduced and a wheeze may disappear. As expiration begins and airways return to their resting caliber, narrowing increases and wheezes will return. Therefore wheezing that occurs during both inspiration and expiration (i.e., biphasic wheezing) is an indication of more significantly narrowed airways than that of wheezing that occurs solely during expiration.

Tubular Breath Sounds. Tubular breath sounds that are louder during expiration than inspiration are abnormal when they are heard in the peripheral areas, where only vesicular sounds should occur. When these sounds are appreciated in the periphery, they are an indication of consolidated lung such as occurs in pneumonia.

Absent or Muffled Breath Sounds. Absent or muffled breath sounds are inaudible or reduced in loudness. They may represent a reduction in airflow to a portion of the lung (such as in atelectasis), air or fluid around the lung (pneumothorax or pleural effusion), or an increase in chest wall thickness.

Stridor. Although stridor is frequently confused with a wheeze, stridor is a harsh, vibratory sound of a single pitch. Stridor occurs as a result of oscillations of a narrowed large extrapulmonary airway. As with a wheeze, depending on the cause, stridor may take place during inspiration or expiration. In general, inspiratory stridor results from an extrathoracic obstruction while expiratory stridor is caused by an intrathoracic narrowing.

Friction Rub. A friction rub is described as a harsh, grating sound that can occur during inspiration and expiration. The sound produced is a result of friction between the two layers of the pleura, which results in vibrations of the chest wall and the pulmonary parenchyma.

Snoring. Snoring is a rough, hoarse noise that occurs from the vibration of tissues in the oropharynx. Snoring may be present in both inspiration and expiration. It may be heard intermittently during sleep in normal children, but chronic snoring can be indicative of underlying pathology if associated with other signs and symptoms of obstructive sleep apnea.

Grunting. Grunting is a low-pitched, expiratory sound caused by partial closure of the glottis. Grunting occurs in an attempt to maintain end-expiratory pressures in order to hold the airways open, and is typically observed in patients with parenchymal lung disease characterized by a loss of lung volume.

Percussion

Chest percussion can be used in order to detect dull, flat, or hyper-resonant areas. By tapping the terminal phalanx of the third finger placed on the chest, vibrations through the tissues are produced. Vibrations that are not dampened will be resonant or tympanitic, whereas rapid attenuation of the vibrations will lead to a flat or dull note. Dullness to percussion may indicate an area of consolidation, while a hyperinflated area may produce hyper-resonance. By comparing symmetric chest sites, slight differences may be detected.

CONCLUSION

When evaluating a child with suspected pulmonary disease it is essential to begin with a detailed history. One must characterize symptoms based on timing, aggravating and relieving factors, onset, and associated features. Once a complete history is obtained, a thorough physical examination including inspection, palpation, auscultation, and percussion is performed. Although evaluation of pediatric pulmonary disease can be challenging, a patient and detailed approach often leads to proper diagnosis.

Suggested Readings

Chang AB, Glomb WB. Guidelines for evaluating chronic cough in pediatrics: ACCP evidence-based clinical practical guidelines. *Chest* 2006;129:260S–283S.

Epstein SK. An overview of respiratory muscle function. *Clin Chest Med* 1994; 15:619–636.

Hartert TV, Wheeler AP, Sheller JR. Use of pulse oximetry to recognize severity of airflow obstruction in obstructive airway disease: correlation with pulsus paradoxus. *Chest* 1999;115:475–481.

Hilman BC. Clinical assessment of pulmonary disease in infants and children. In: Hilman BC. *Pediatric respiratory disease: diagnosis and treatment.* Philadelphia: Saunders; 1993:57–67.

Hughes DM. Evaluating the child's respiratory system. In: Goldbloom RB. *Pediatric clinical skills.* 2nd ed. New York: Churchill Livingstone; 1997: 171–191.

CHAPTER 36 ■ PULMONARY FUNCTION TESTING

BRUCE NICKERSON

Pulmonary function tests (PFTs) are often underutilized in pediatrics. PFTs can quantify the degree of disease and disability. They can elucidate the response to therapy. Improvement or worsening in the natural course of respiratory disease can be tracked by PFTs. Physicians can better understand the physiology of a patient's illness by judicious use of the pulmonary function lab. Sometimes organic disease problems can be ruled out and proper focus placed on psychological factors. PFTs provide a classification of lung functions by physiologic impairment (Table 36.1).

The technician in a Pediatric Pulmonary Function Lab is the crucial ingredient to obtaining useful, reproducible, valid results. The tech should be skilled in relating to children of different ages, degrees of disability, and those with medical or neurologic illness. Helping the child to be in a comfortable, cooperative state is essential for obtaining good pulmonary functions. Sometimes, the child must revisit the Pulmonary Function Lab several times to get valid results. It is crucial that the child have a good experience in the lab even if the results are suboptimal. This will ensure that on future visits, the child is less anxious and more confident and able to do a better job. Often it is beneficial if the parent is in the room with the child. However, sometimes the parent–child interaction is not helpful and it is better if the technician relates one-on-one with the child without the parent in the room. Many tests that are limited by cooperation or effort can generate values that at least put a floor on the pulmonary function. Over time these values will increase as the child becomes more comfortable, cooperative, and skilled in performing the tests.

Spirometry is the most widely employed measure of pulmonary function. Spirometry generates a forced vital capacity, forced expiratory volume in one second, and forced expiratory flow between 25% and 75% of vital capacity. These three values have good standard normals for children over 5 years of age and are well validated and correlate with other indices of health and disease and response to therapy. A wide range of other flow rates at specific lung volumes, (e.g., peak expiratory flow, forced expiratory time) are less reproducible or well standardized. PFT labs all report forced vital capacity, FEV_1, and FEF_{25-75}, and sometimes include other parameters (Fig. 36.1).

A valid forced expiratory maneuver requires a good inspiration, and a rapid, forceful expiration for long enough for flow to get back to baseline. Often young children stop their forced expiratory maneuver early (sometimes before 1 second). This produces an incomplete curve and falsely elevated values of FEF_{25-75} and low values of forced vital capacity. If the forced expiratory time is greater than 1 second, it does not affect FEV_1. It is important that spirometry is taken as the best of three curves with the highest sum of forced vital capacity

and FEV_1 by American Thoracic Society standards. Most children by age 4 to 6 can produce reproducible spirometry.

It is important to look at the shape of the curve. Sudden falls in expiratory flow with a rapid re-upswing can indicate coughing. Scalloping may be seen in obstructive disease such as asthma or cystic fibrosis (Fig. 36.2) A sawtooth inspiratory flow at a low value can be seen in vocal cord dysfunction.

Often spirometry is done before and after bronchodilators. Generally, an increase in forced expiratory volume in 1 second, more than 10% to 15%, and an increase in FEF_{25-75} of 15% to 25%, are taken as valid indicators of improvement with bronchodilators. Of course, a child with reactive airways when tested on a day when there is no bronchospasm will have normal pulmonary function without a significant response to bronchodilators. This test can also be used to check the child's technique using a metered dose inhaler and spacer, and this opportunity should not be lost.

Many clinicians use home peak expiratory flow meters for children with asthma. This allows the family to quantitate the airway function on a daily or several times a day basis. Generally, the best of three peak expiratory flows is taken and recorded. Patients are encouraged to keep a diary with recordings of the numbers or graph to establish a good baseline. A 20% fall in peak flow is taken as an indicator for increased therapy, and a 50% fall warrants consulting a physician.

For children with neuromuscular disease, maximal inspiratory and expiratory pressures can be measured. Particularly in transient illnesses such as botulism or Guillain–Barré syndrome, these may change from day to day. When maximum inspiratory and expiratory pressures are first measured, there is a significant learning effect, so the patient should try at least ten times to generate a true maximum. The literature citing these tests is flawed by studies with low values, as investigators did not ask the children to truly learn how to perform the tests. Normal values for maximum inspiratory and expiratory pressure are usually greater than 100 cm H_2O. Patients with pressures near 20 cm H_2O are near respiratory failure and may require endotracheal intubation and mechanical ventilatory support.

Exercise is increasingly used for children. A variety of tests have been used. A simple 6-minute walk can quantify a child's ability to exercise. Adding recordings of heart rate and oxygen saturation can demonstrate oxygen desaturation such as in those with pulmonary hypertension. This test has been used in adults and in some children to quantify response to therapy in the treatment of pulmonary hypertension.

Exercise-induced bronchospasm occurs in most children with asthma. This can be a phenomenon difficult to demonstrate in a lab. The reason is that the stimulants for exercise-induced bronchospasm are cooling and drying of the airways at about

TABLE 36.1

LUNG FUNCTION AND PHYSIOLOGIC IMPAIRMENT

OBSTRUCTIVE LUNG DISORDERS	RESTRICTIVE LUNG DISORDERS
Reduced FEV_1, FEV_{25-75}, PEFR	Symmetric reduction in lung volumes
Increased RV/TLC	FVC decreased
Increased RV and decreased VC	TLC decreased
FEV_1/FVC reflects a disproportionate reduction in flow of FEV_1 to FVC	FEV_1/FVC normal
Increased airway resistance	

FEV_1, forced expiratory volume in 1 sec; FEV_{25-75}, forced expiratory volume at 25–75% vital capacity; PEFR, peak expiratory flow rate; RV, residual volume; TLC, total lung capacity; VC, vital capacity; FVC, forced vital capacity.

the fifth generation. Thus, the exercise should be performed in a laboratory with cool air and a low humidity. Often hospitals are kept at a relative humidity of 75% with a room temperature around 20°C, and the patient may not have exercise-induced bronchospasm even with adequate exercise in the circumstances. The exercise should be vigorous enough to obtain a heart rate approximately 80% of predicted rate, and have a sudden start, 5 to 10 minutes, of vigorous exercise, and a sudden stop. Spirometry is done before and at 3- to 5-minute intervals after the exercise. Typically, after exercise-induced bronchospasm, spirometry values will fall shortly after exercise. A bronchodilator can be given after 15 minutes to see if there is reversibility with bronchodilators.

A maximum exercise stress test can be used to better quantify a child's exercise capacity. A good level of maximum exercise requires adequate cardiac and circulatory function, adequate maximum voluntary ventilation, adequate oxygen-carrying capacity (i.e., hemoglobin), and adequate muscle conditioning.

ASTHMA

Children with asthma often have home peak flow meters. Many have an action plan with a sequence of responses when their peak flow falls below 80% of their previous best, and to start steroids and call the physician when it falls below 50%. Once patients are hospitalized, their progress can be followed using pulmonary function. During an acute episode of bronchospasm, there may be significant scalloping of the expiratory portion of the flow-volume loop. Vital

capacity, FEV_1, and FEF_{25-75} may be markedly diminished. It may take several weeks before spirometry returns to normal. In addition, nearly all children with asthma have exercise-induced bronchospasm. Thus, the significant fall in FEV_1 and FEF_{25-75} may occur after exercise. Even normal children following a respiratory infection will demonstrate exercise-induced bronchospasm for as long as 2 months after a significant infection.

VOCAL CORD DYSFUNCTION

Sometimes children believed to have a diagnosis of asthma will demonstrate a normal expiratory flow-volume loop. This should suggest the possibility of vocal cord dysfunction. A careful look with a good inspiratory effort should be made. Typically, patients with vocal cord dysfunction will have a relatively normal expiratory flow-volume loop or a truncated peak flow and lower FEV_1 but without the scalloping typically seen on the expiratory side. On the inspiratory side, there will be a sawtooth or jagged inspiratory flow as the vocal cords vibrate in the inspiratory column. Typically, inspiratory flows will be limited to the 1 to 2 L/sec range rather than being in the normal 4 to 6 L/sec range.

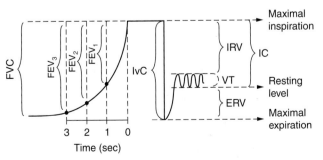

FIGURE 36.1. Lung volumes and capacities measured by spirometry. (IVC, inspiratory vital capacity; FVC, forced vital capacity; FEV_1, FEV_2, FEV_3, forced expiratory volumes in the first, second, and third seconds, respectively.)

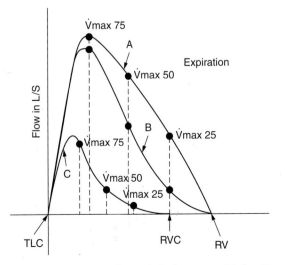

FIGURE 36.2. Note middle flow-volume loop (curve B) that demonstrates "scalloping" typical of obstructive lung disease.

CHEMOTHERAPY

Patients undergoing chemotherapy may experience toxicity from the chemotherapeutic agents. Often this will first manifest as a problem in diffusion capacity. The lab will make appropriate corrections for alveolar volume and hemoglobin. With increasing levels of toxicity, the vital capacity and total lung capacity may also be decreased, followed by a decrease in flow rates with a restrictive pattern. Recognizing this early can be life-saving by limiting the dose of chemotherapy to avoid lung toxicity.

RHEUMATOID DISEASES

Patients with a variety of rheumatologic syndromes may experience pulmonary function abnormalities. Patients with juvenile rheumatoid arthritis, systemic lupus erythematosus, and scleroderma in particular may manifest lung disease. They may have restrictive defects with a decrease in total lung capacity and forced vital capacity. They may have pulmonary vascular disease with evidence for pulmonary hypertension and a reduction in diffusion capacity. They may have decreased exercise tolerance above that caused by their disease.

PULMONARY HYPERTENSION

The advent of a number of new therapies for pulmonary hypertension has generated new interest in this often fatal syndrome. Because these drugs have been studied mainly in adults, there are few studies or protocols available for children. Nevertheless, it is important to evaluate on an ongoing basis the degree of lung disease, vascular disease, and response to therapy. Adult clinicians have used a 6-minute run/walk test to quantify the degree of disability and response to therapy. Children with pulmonary hypertension may also have oxygen desaturation during exercise or during a 6-minute walk. Recognition of oxygen desaturation with exercise can be very helpful in writing an appropriate exercise prescription for children with pulmonary hypertension.

CONGENITAL HEART DISEASE

Many children with congenital heart disease may also have pulmonary disease. The pulmonary function laboratory can be used to help distinguish and guide treatment. After cardiac surgery, patients may have unilateral vocal cord paralysis from damage to the recurrent laryngeal nerve. Others may have paralysis of a hemidiaphragm. Still others may require prolonged mechanical ventilation and have chronic inflammation of their lungs and residual airway reactivity secondary to pneumonitis, pulmonary edema, barotraumas, and hyperoxygen therapy. Vocal cord dysfunction can be demonstrated by limitation of inspiratory flows on the inspiratory side of the flow-volume loop. A paralyzed diaphragm will manifest as a decreased forced vital capacity and decreased total lung capacity and residual volume (i.e., a restrictive pattern). Chronic lung disease following mechanical ventilation may have an obstructive pattern with a positive response to bronchodilators. In addition, these patients may suffer from bouts of atelectasis or from tracheomalacia or bronchomalacia. Atelectasis is manifested in the pulmonary function lab as decreased lung volumes and a restricted pattern. Bronchomalacia or tracheomalacia demonstrates decreased flow rates and an obstructive pattern.

CHEST PAIN

Chest pain in the pediatric population is often due to pulmonary or chest wall problems and seldom due to cardiac lesions. Patients with asthma often have chest pain due to hyperinflation of the lungs and consequent distortion of the costochondral junctions. This can be demonstrated as an obstructive pattern on spirometry with a positive response to bronchodilators. They may also demonstrate significantly elevated lung volumes. An exercise study may demonstrate exercise-induced bronchospasm and relief of the pain with a bronchodilator.

Patients with neuromuscular weakness often have a decreased vital capacity and restrictive pattern. Maximal inspiratory pressures and maximal expiratory pressure are significantly decreased. These pressures can also give a quantitative measure of the effectiveness of cough.

SICKLE-CELL DISEASE

Patients with sickle-cell anemia often have a decrease in their pulmonary function. They may experience poor lung growth due to vascular disease. They may have decreased pulmonary function due to pain during acute chest syndrome. Many also have asthma. Some may develop chronic lung disease. Lung disease is one of the more common causes of death in patients with sickle-cell anemia.

THALASSEMIA

Patients with thalassemia may develop restrictive disease from iron overload in the pulmonary parenchyma. Serial pulmonary functions may reveal this over time.

PECTUS EXCAVATUM

Children with pectus excavatum often want the appearance of their chest wall improved. Most have normal pulmonary function. However, a few have impairment in pulmonary function with decreased lung volumes. The hospitalist should also look for evidence of upper airway obstruction with a decrease in inspiratory flows, which can cause a secondary problem with pectus excavatum. Some have asthma, which may be untreated because their symptoms are blamed on the chest wall deformity. Therefore, a response to bronchodilators may be very helpful diagnostically. Often chest surgeons want to know the pulmonary function and presence or absence of significant abnormality prior to surgical correction.

KYPHOSCOLIOSIS

Kyphoscoliosis commonly results in pulmonary function defects. The defects may show a mixed obstructive and restrictive pattern, as some areas of the lungs are compressed and restricted while others are overstretched and give an obstructive appearance. Pulmonary functions are helpful in the preoperative evaluation as they indicate the degree of pulmonary reserve these patients have. Particularly, patients with severe defects or secondary scoliosis due to neuromuscular weakness may have profoundly reduced vital capacity, FEV_1, and maximal inspiratory and expiratory pressures. Some of these patients are at high risk for respiratory failure following surgery. Thus the preoperative pulmonary function values can help in assessing their risk for these complications and provide the family, surgeons, and intensivists adequate preparation.

Pulmonary functions may be helpful in quantifying the degree of physiologic abnormality in other chest wall deformities. They may also be helpful in delineating progression of the disease and for optimal timing of surgery. Often, the surgeon must gauge a balance between minimizing the severity of the progressing defect while maximizing height growth. Thus, the progression of pulmonary functions may aid in this judgment.

In summary, the Pulmonary Function Laboratory can be quite useful in evaluating and following children with a wide variety of pulmonary and other lung diseases and their response to therapy. The hospitalist should develop a working relationship with a pediatric pulmonologist who can consult on pertinent clinical matters and can provide recommendations for the use and interpretation of PFTs.

CHAPTER 37 ■ ASTHMA

SUE HOFFMAN AND MARK BANKS

Asthma (reactive airways disease, RAD) is the most prevalent chronic disease in childhood. It affects approximately 6.2 million children under the age of 18 years. Asthma is the most frequent admitting diagnosis in hospitalized children. A male predominance is seen, with 10% to 15% of boys affected as compared to 7% to 10% of girls. The prevalence and mortality of this condition have been increasing over the past three decades although the reasons for this are unknown. Those children most severely affected have the onset of wheezing during the first year of life and also have a strong family history of asthma and atopy (particularly atopic dermatitis). Exposure to second-hand smoke plays a significant role. Approximately 30% of children with asthma will develop symptoms during the first year of life, while 80% to 90% experience first symptoms by the age of 5 years.

Asthma has a wide range of severity, and can be characterized by:

1. Reversible airways obstruction
2. Airway inflammation
3. Airway hyper-responsiveness to stimuli

The most severe form of asthma is that of status asthmaticus. This condition is defined as significant respiratory distress despite administration of beta-2 agonists and corticosteroids. Every child with asthma, regardless how mild, is at risk for an acute exacerbation. Pediatric hospitalists are responsible for both the management of an acute exacerbation of asthma and the coordination of outpatient management.

PATHOPHYSIOLOGY

Asthma is a chronic inflammatory disorder characterized by reversible airways obstruction. The disease is characterized by an exaggerated inflammatory response to environmental stimuli. The stimuli are foreign antigens, referred to as allergens when they trigger an allergic response. Atopy is the tendency for the body to react to these seemingly harmless proteins as if they were infectious agents. Allergens include dust mites, fungi, pollen, cigarette smoke, and animal dander. Although all atopy does not manifest as asthma, atopic pediatric patients are more at risk for developing this disease. Nonallergic triggers for asthma include exercise, cold air, atmospheric pollutants, and infectious agents. The resulting physiologic insult is the same regardless of the etiology.

Multiple physiologic changes contribute to the airway abnormalities seen in asthmatic patients. Smooth muscle surrounding the airways demonstrates an exaggerated bronchoconstriction and contributes to airway obstruction. Although this response is protective when undertaken to defend against infection, asthmatic patients demonstrate this airway constriction to an inappropriate degree and to inappropriate stimuli. Goblet cells generate excessive mucus that is thicker than normal and

can become inspissated. Mucus plugs contribute to airway obstruction, air trapping, and lung hyperinflation. Airway inflammation and mucosal lining edema also are also components of asthma. Inflammatory mediators can stimulate the parasympathetic nervous system and cause a release of acetylcholine. Acetylcholine can bind to muscarinic receptors along the airway and contribute to bronchoconstriction. The airways in an asthmatic patient are infiltrated with eosinophils and mononuclear cells. There is also epithelial cell destruction, goblet cell hyperplasia, collagen deposition beneath the basement membrane, vasodilatation, and vascular leak leading to bronchial wall edema (see Figs. 37.1 and 37.2).

The degree of inflammation in asthma is due to a complex set of interactions between inflammatory cells, inflammatory mediators, and resident cells along the airway. Allergen-induced bronchoconstriction results from an IgE-stimulated release of inflammatory mediators including histamine, leukotrienes, prostaglandins, and other cytokines (Fig. 37.3). Mast cells play an important role in these allergen-induced responses. In atopic patients, allergen exposure generates a specific IgE-antibody sensitization. Allergen-specific IgE then becomes bound to cells such as mast cells. Upon re-exposure, allergens can bind to surface-IgE on the mast cell. This allows for cross-linking of the surface-bound IgE and the subsequent release of inflammatory mediators. This is an immediate hypersensitivity response. There can be a symptom recurrence 4 to 12 hours later in the case of significant exposure to allergen. This is referred to as the late asthma response. The late response is mediated by activated lymphocytes and eosinophils. Eosinophils also play a large role in both allergic and nonallergic asthma. The degree to which they are present within the bronchial airway and bronchial secretions correlates with the severity of the disease. Eosinophils are mobile and present themselves in large numbers to the bronchial airways in asthmatic patients. Once present, they can become activated and contribute to the inflammatory response.

Chronic asthma is associated with airway remodeling. This refers to a process of subepithelial collagen deposition, myofibroblast accumulation, smooth muscle hypertrophy, goblet cell hyperplasia, vascular neogenesis, and epithelial disruption. This remodeling and subsequent airway fibrosis may cause a fixed airflow obstruction that is not reversible with medication (Fig. 37.4).

The airway obstruction characteristic of asthma increases resistance to expiratory airflow. This causes air trapping, lung hyperinflation, and increased work of breathing. Some alveoli become atelectatic and others become hyperinflated. This causes ventilation–perfusion (V/Q) mismatch. Air trapping increases intrapleural and alveolar pressures, which compromises pulmonary blood flow and causes decreased perfusion to some alveoli. This imbalance in perfusion and ventilation of the alveoli leads to V/Q mismatch. Hypoxemia is the result. Hypoxemia stimulates the respiratory centers, resulting in the

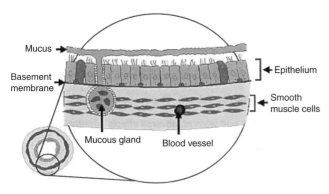

FIGURE 37.1. Histologic findings of a normal airway.

respiratory alkalosis characteristic of an early asthma attack. If the airway obstruction persists and worsens, further alveoli will become compromised and carbon dioxide retention may result. As the lungs and thorax become increasingly hyperinflated, the muscles of respiration become fatigued, and hypercapnic respiratory failure is the result.

TRIGGERS

Identifying and avoiding the triggers that can provoke asthma symptoms is essential in preventing asthma exacerbations. The most frequently described triggers are described in the following sections.

Inhalant Allergens

- Animal dander or saliva
- House dust mites
- Cockroaches
- Indoor mold or mildew
- Outdoor allergens (trees, grass, weed pollen, flowering plants)

Medications and Foods

- Aspirin and nonsteroidal anti-inflammatories
- Sulfite containing foods (shrimp, dried fruit, potatoes, beer, wine)
- Nonselective beta-blockers

Irritants

- Cigarette smoke, ashes, fireplace smoke
- Aerosol sprays, cleaning supplies

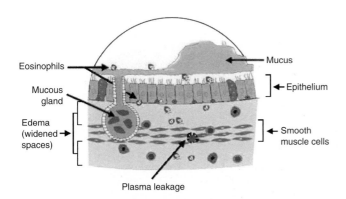

FIGURE 37.2. Histologic findings of an inflamed airway.

Cell-derived mediators

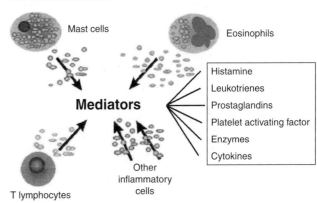

FIGURE 37.3. Inflammatory cells and mediators.

- Perfumes
- Car exhaust, gas fumes
- Air pollution, weather conditions (e.g., cold air)
- Shower steam

Infections

- Rhinovirus: Significant contributor to exacerbations in children with reactive airways, but does not appear to contribute to the development of the disorder.
- Respiratory syncytial virus (RSV): Common cause of wheezing in the first 2 years of life. RSV can contribute to the development of asthma (some studies cite up to 56% of those affected in the first 2 years of life), but generally in conjunction with other risk factors such as maternal smoking, family history of atopy/asthma, and elevated IgE levels.
- Metapneumovirus (in the *Paramyxoviridae* family, to which RSV also belongs): A newly recognized human pathogen that can lead to upper and lower respiratory infection and wheezing in young children.
- Influenza, parainfluenza, and adenovirus are other viruses associated with the provocation of asthma symptoms but not in the development of the disorder.
- Ear infections, sinus infections, and pneumonia can lead to exacerbations of asthma as they cause airway inflammation and increased mucous production.

Other Triggers

- Gastroesophageal reflux
- Exercise
- Emotions

Reviewing these with the child (when appropriate) and family, and eliminating or decreasing those involved, can produce a decrease in the child's symptoms and reduce the frequency of exacerbations.

DEFINITIONS OF ASTHMA BASED ON SEVERITY

Definitions based on severity of symptoms have emerged that also direct the course of therapy for the asthmatic (Table 37.1). These can help standardize management, which can facilitate

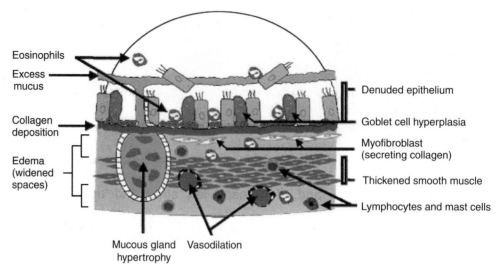

FIGURE 37.4. Processes in airway remodeling.

improved outpatient compliance by both the patient and primary care physician. The use of long-acting beta-2 agonists as well as inhaled steroids is dictated by the severity of the child's asthma symptoms (Table 37.2).

TEACH: All should be made aware of the basic facts of asthma including proper inhaler/spacer/nebulizer use, peak expiratory flow rate (PEFR) to guide therapy, medication roles, use of an action plan, rescue plan, and environmental controls.

THERAPY should be stepped up or down as symptoms dictate. Therapy should be reviewed every 1 to 6 months.

GOAL is to gain quick control and then taper off treatment as possible.

PHYSICAL EXAM

Asthma is a clinical diagnosis. Children with acute asthma can have a variety of presentations, ranging from minimally abnormal to anxious and air-hungry. The physical exam can deliver clues to the severity of the presentation (Table 37.3).

Children having an asthma attack can be pale or they can be cyanotic. They may be diaphoretic and tripoding in an effort to breathe or they may be wheezing "happily." It is the patient's effort to breathe that is the most important clinical marker. Children having an asthma attack are working harder than normal to breathe. The increased respiratory work can

TABLE 37.1

DEFINITIONS OF ASTHMA SEVERITY

	Symptoms	Nocturnal symptoms	PEFR
Step 4 Severe Persistent	Constant symptoms. Limits physical activity. Frequent exacerbations.	Frequent symptoms affecting quality of sleep	PEFR <60% predicted
Step 3 Moderate Persistent	Daily symptoms. Requires daily use of short-acting beta-2 agonists. Exacerbations affect physical activity. Exacerbations >2×/week and persist for days.	Sleep disturbing >1×/week	PEFR 60–80% predicted
Step 2 Mild Persistent	Symptoms occur >2×/week but <1×/day. May affect activity.	>2×/month	PEFR >80% predicted
Step 1 Mild Inflammatory	Symptoms <2×/week. Asymptomatic with normal PEFR between exacerbations. Exacerbations are brief.	< or = 2×/month	PEFR >80% predicted

PEFR, peak expiratory flow rate.

TABLE 37.2

CHRONIC THERAPY BASED ON SEVERITY

Step	Long-term daily therapy	Rescue
Step 4 Severe persistent	1. High-dose inhaled steroids *and* 2. Long-acting inhaled beta-2 agonists[a] *and if required* 3. Short- or long-term oral steroids Consider theophylline	Short-acting beta-2 agonist
Step 3 Moderate persistent	1. Low- to medium-dose inhaled steroids *and* 2. Long-acting beta-2 agonist[a] Alternative 1. Medium- or low-dose inhaled steroids *with* 2. A leukotriene modifier Consider theophylline	Short-acting beta-2 agonist

Step 2 Mild persistent	1. Low-dose inhaled steroid
	Alternative
	    Leukotriene modifier,
	    Chromolyn,
	    Nedocromil,
		Short-acting beta-2 agonist

Step 1 Mild inflammatory	No daily medications	Short-acting beta-2 agonist

[a]Evidence of cardiovascular side effects and severe asthma exacerbations can be seen if used without inhaled steroid.

manifest as retractions (intercostal, subcostal, sternocleido-mastoid), audible wheezing, and severe dyspnea. The respiratory rate is generally greater than 30 breaths/min, although this will vary with age. Tachycardia with a heart rate greater than 120 beats/min is also characteristic, particularly if the patient has been receiving beta-2 agonists. The patient's temperature may be normal or elevated if the asthma trigger is infectious. Blood pressure is usually within age-adjusted norms. Signs of hypovolemia such as dry mucus membranes are often present as tachypnea leads to increased insensible losses. Patients with an acute asthma attack are hypoxemic and they may have symptoms such as irritability or a change

TABLE 37.3

SIGNS OF ASTHMA EXACERBATIONS

	Mental status	Respiratory status	Skin color	PEFR	Retractions
Mild exacerbation	Alert/appropriately responsive	Mild dyspnea. Mild increase in RR. Easily speaks in sentences.	Pink, well perfused	70–90% of child's best level	None
Moderate exacerbation	Alert/appropriate	Increasing dyspnea. Elevated RR for age. Speaks in broken sentences/phrases. Complaints of wheeze, shortness of breath, chest tightness.	Normal to pale	50–70% of child's best	Slight to moderate retractions (subcostal/intercostal)
Severe exacerbation	Irritable to drowsy and confused	Extreme dyspnea. Either significantly elevated or decreased RR with laboring. Difficulty speaking. Severe complaints of wheeze, air hunger, chest tightness.	Poor color, pale to cyanotic	Less than 50% of child's best	Severe subcostal, intercostal, and supraclavicular

PEFR, peak expiratory flow rate; RR, respiratory rate.

TABLE 37.4

DETERMINING THE NEED FOR HOSPITALIZATION[a]

	Status	Disposition
Good	1. PEFR >70% predicted or patient's baseline 2. O_2 sat >95% on RA 3. Clearing breath sounds, resolution of retractions, normalization of vital signs	Home with good follow-up
Incomplete	1. PEFR 40–70% of predicted/baseline 2. Improving but not optimal physical signs 3. O_2 sat 91–95% on RA	Continued treatment in observation unit or on pediatric floor
Poor	1. PEFR <40% predicted/baseline 2. O_2 sat <91% on RA 3. Lack of improvement in clinical signs of airflow obstruction	Prompt hospitalization to the pediatric floor or PICU dependent on severity

[a]Generally determined after 2 to 6 hours of observation/therapy in ED or office.
PEFR, peak expiratory flow rate; PICU, pediatric intensive care unit; RA,

in personality. Although pallor is commonly seen, overt cyanosis is a late finding and should raise concern.

Wheezing is the symptom most associated with asthma. However, the degree of wheezing does not correlate with the severity of the disease. Inspiratory wheezes suggest an extrathoracic process that may be severe asthma or a foreign body. Wheezing is not, however, pathognemonic of asthma. Wheezing can also be caused by bronchiolitis, tracheomalacia, congenital heart disease with pulmonary edema, or vocal cord dysfunction. A high index of suspicion is warranted for these other possibilities in the absence of a history of asthma. Cough is often the initial, and sometimes the only, symptom of an asthma attack. Older children may have increased sputum production. Rales may also be appreciated. Rales result from the reopening of collapsed alveoli associated with mucus plugging and airway obstruction. Rales may also be the result of pulmonary edema. Young children with viral pneumonia may present with rales as well as wheezing. Pulmonary infections are the most common precipitants of RAD in young children. It is not uncommon for children to have elements of both pneumonia and RAD upon presentation. Asymmetric breath sounds can be from atelectasis, pneumothorax, or a foreign body. A silent chest is the most concerning sign of all. This suggests severe hyperinflation, air trapping, and an inability to generate sufficient expiratory airflow.

EVALUATION

Asthma is primarily a clinical diagnosis; therefore, additional tests are rarely required. Indications for obtaining a chest radiograph during an asthma exacerbation include:

- Physical symptoms of an extra-alveolar air leak
- Chest pain
- Fever >38.5°C
- Rales
- Lack of response to conventional therapy

At this point the differential of wheezing must be widened and further evaluation undertaken based upon symptoms and CXR results. Arterial blood gases are rarely required, as oxygenation can be monitored via pulse oximetry and venous blood gases can be used to follow trends in PCO_2 and pH if necessary. PEFR correlates well with the FEV_1 but is much

more easily obtained, although it is effort dependent and unable to be obtained in young children.

DETERMINING THE NEED FOR HOSPITALIZATION

The pediatric hospitalist is often asked to aid in the decision of whether to hospitalize a child with asthma. Table 37.4 describes the patients with the lowest to highest likelihood for admission based on PEFR, oxygen saturation, and clinical signs in response to therapy. Those in the "Good" category generally can be discharged home; the children with an incomplete response to therapy require prolonged observation. Poor responders require hospitalization.

Being familiar with the risk factors for fatal asthma is also extremely important to the pediatric hospitalist (Table 37.5). In particular, multiple recent ED visits (3 or more in the preceding 12 months), low oxygen saturations (<90% at sea level), longer asthma duration, and high serum IgE levels are all significant risk factors in children. Another study found that only 39% of children who died from asthma had potentially preventable triggers. Ultimately, it remains difficult to

TABLE 37.5

RISK FACTORS FOR FATAL ASTHMA

1. History of multiple visits to the emergency room (>3) within the past year
2. Significant hypoxemia on room air (<90% oxygen saturation at sea level)
3. Elevated serum IgE
4. Previous ICU admission
5. Poor compliance
6. Failure to perceive symptom severity
7. Lack of parental education
8. Severe atopy
9. Longer duration of asthma
10. Inner-city residence

determine who is at risk for death; even children with mild asthma are at risk for an acute life-threatening attack.

TREATMENT

Treatment for asthma exacerbations (Table 37.6) must be approached in a stepwise process dependent upon the severity (Fig. 37.5). Medications and frequency of delivery require adjustment during the acute period and as the child improves.

Humidified oxygen is an indicated for any hospitalized child with asthma. Oxygen increases the partial pressure of arterial oxygen, decreases work of breathing, and has bronchodilatory properties. Until the child clearly is resolving the exacerbation, oxygen must be applied regardless of the oxygen saturation. Dehydration must also be assessed and fluid replacement is recommended to regain euvolemia if the child is unable to maintain adequate oral intake. Over-hydration is not recommended as it can lead to pulmonary edema.

Systemic steroids, if not begun in the ED or office, should be administered as soon as possible in an acute exacerbation. Although there is no clinically significant difference in efficacy based on the route of administration, the parenteral route is suggested with severe asthma. It has been shown that administration of steroids early in the course of the exacerbation can lessen the severity and decrease the need for hospitalization primarily by decreasing the airway inflammation. Oral prednisone or prednisolone should be administered at a dose of 2 mg/kg/day divided twice a day or once a day. Methylprednisolone IV should be used for a significant exacerbation and especially when IV hydration is required at a dose of 0.5 to 1 mg/kg every 6 hours. Hydrocortisone can also be used, although not as commonly, at a dose of 2 to 4 mg/kg IV every 6 hours. Higher doses do not appear to generate added benefit. Steroids administered for more than 5 days should be tapered due to the risk of adrenal suppression. Inhaled steroids do not have a role in acute asthma management.

Nebulized albuterol, a beta-2 agonist, in a dose of 2.5 to 5 mg/kg/dose (administration should be oxygen-driven), is administered initially every 2 to 4 hours dependent on severity and weaned when possible as the exacerbation abates. Reassessment is required frequently. If the child is extremely tight with significant work of breathing, hourly or continuous albuterol nebulization may be required. Dosing for continuous nebulization is 10 to 25 mg/hr (Fig. 37.6). Diastolic hypotension is the most common and important hemodynamic side effect of continuous beta-2 agonist therapy; this may require fluid support. Tachycardia, increased QT interval, arrhythmia, and hypertension have been reported, but the incidence is rare. Hypokalemia can be seen with frequent or continuous albuterol therapy and should be monitored. Albuterol also reverses hypoxic pulmonary vasoconstriction and therefore its administration often results in a decrease in the child's arterial oxygen saturations. Whether hourly or continuous albuterol nebulization can be done on the pediatric unit is institution dependent; however, children requiring this intensity of therapy must have a physician present as deterioration may occur rapidly. If this level of treatment is required for 2 or more hours without significant improvement, or if during this time the child deteriorates with increasing oxygen requirement, increasing work of breathing, or decreasing PEFR, transfer to a pediatric intensive-care unit must be instituted.

If a child fails high-dose nebulized albuterol, subcutaneous terbutaline (0.005 to 0.01 mg/kg SC every 15 to 30 minutes × 2 as required) or epinephrine (0.01 mg/kg of the 1:1000 concentration every 15 to 30 minutes × 2 as required) should be administered. These are beta agonists that are very rapid acting in this form and do not require respiratory effort to deposit the medication in the area required. Terbutaline is often preferred to epinephrine as it has fewer adverse side effects such as nausea, vomiting, muscle tremor, and tachycardia with the same level of bronchodilatation. Also it can be helpful to determine how well the child will respond to terbutaline

TABLE 37.6

MEDICATIONS IN ASTHMA EXACERBATIONS

Drug	Dosage	Route	Frequency
Prednisone/ prednisolone	2 mg/kg/day	Oral	Q day or divided BID
Methylprednisolone	0.5–1 mg/kg	IV	Q 6 hr
Hydrocortisone	2–4 mg/kg	IV	Q 6 hr
Intermittent albuterol	2.5–5 mg/kg	Nebulized	Q 1–4 hr
Continuous albuterol	10–25 mg/hr	Nebulized	Continuous
Terbutaline	0.005–0.01 mg/kg 0.1–10 µg/kg/min	SQ IV	Q 15–30 min × 2 Continuous drip
Epinephrine 1:1000 concentration	0.01 mg/kg	SQ	Q 15–30 min × 2
Ipratropium bromide	250 g/kg if <30 kg 500 µg/kg if >0 kg	Nebulized	Every 4–6 hr
Magnesium	25–75 mg/kg	IV	Q 6 hr
Aminophylline	1–6 mg/kg load Then 0.7–1.2 mg/kg/hr infusion	IV	Continuous drip

Asthma severity score			
RR score (from table below)			
Room air O$_2$ saturation: > 90% = 1 85–90% = 2 < 85% = 3			
Auscultation: Normal breathing or end-exp. wheeze = 1 Expiratory wheeze = 2 Insp. & exp. wheeze ± ↓ breath sounds = 3			
Retractions: None/mild intercostal = 1 Intercostal + substernal = 2 Intercostal + substernal + supraclavicular = 3			
Shortness of breath: speaks in: sentences, coos, babbles = 1 Phrases, short cries = 2 Words, grunts = 3			
Total asthma severity score 5–7 mild 8–11 moderate 12–15 severe			
RN/RT initials			
Comments			

Respiratory rate score for asthma severity

Age	1 point	2 points	3 points
≤ 3 yo	≤ 34	35–39	≥ 40
4–5 yo	≤ 30	31–35	≥ 36
6–12 yo	≤ 26	27–30	≥ 31
> 12 yo	≤ 23	24–27	≥ 28

FIGURE 37.5. Asthma severity score.

should the child's status continue to decline and ICU management becomes necessary, as IV terbutaline (at a dose of 0.1 to 10 μg/kg/min) would become the next step. Long-acting beta agonists such as salmeterol have no place in the acute setting.

The benefits of other adjunctive therapy such as ipratropium bromide or IV magnesium remain unclear. Ipratropium (250 μg nebulized × 3) in the emergency department literature appears to enhance the effect of albuterol, improving symptoms and reducing need for hospitalization in the acute (ED) setting. Its benefit in the inpatient setting remains uncertain. If used, it should only be continued for the first 24 hours at a dose of 250 to 500 μg every 4 to 6 hours. Magnesium is another agent with uncertain benefits in the inpatient setting. There are studies that demonstrate improvement in symptoms with its usage in the ED, as magnesium sulfate promotes smooth muscle relaxation. It is given at a dose of 25 to 75 mg/kg. Usage on the inpatient pediatric unit is again likely to be institution dependent and its efficacy is unclear. If used, it requires careful administration and a physician immediately available for evaluation and intervention.

Aminophylline remains a treatment option for the acute severe asthmatic, although it is infrequently used in most institutions. It is recommended to load the patient with 1 to 6 mg/kg and run a continuous infusion at 0.7 to 1.2 mg/kg/hr. The recommended therapeutic level is 10 to 20 μg/mL; however, toxicity is seen even at these levels, with severe and even life-threatening toxicity at levels of 35 μg/mL. Therefore, care must be exercised if this medication is added to the treatment regime.

PEFRs should be followed as an objective measure of the child's status. However, this is effort dependent and likely not reliable in children less than 6 years of age. Incentive spirometry or flutter valves can be helpful in decreasing associated atelectasis although there is no literature to support this. Antibiotics do not play a role in the treatment of acute asthma unless a pneumonia, sinusitis, or other bacterial process is present.

The role of Heliox in the treatment of status asthmaticus is uncertain at this time. Lack of response to usual therapy requires further evaluation for other precipitants such as gastroesophageal reflux, sinus infections, viral infections, or pneumonias. Foreign bodies must also be considered in the appropriate settings (younger age group, developmentally disabled).

PICU CONSIDERATIONS

Every child with an acute severe asthma attack requires cardiopulmonary monitoring. Increasing oxygen requirement along with worsening asthma symptoms should prompt transfer to a PICU unless the child rapidly improves with usual therapy. The decision to intubate an asthmatic patient should be considered carefully. Positive pressure ventilation increases the risk of barotrauma and circulatory collapse. The belief that respiratory acidosis dictates the need for intubation needs to be reconsidered in the light of the more aggressive beta-2 agonist therapy that is currently recommended. Typically fewer than 1% of the children admitted for asthma need to be intubated. Indeed, some studies have found better outcomes in pediatric centers that are less likely to intubate patients with status asthmaticus. It is the patient's work of breathing that dictates the need for intubation. If you observe

Addressograph above

CHOC

**Continuous nebulized
albuterol order form**

Wt:_____kg   Ht:_____cm   Allergies: _____

◆   **Start continuous albuterol for inhalation.** Pharmacy to prepare an albuterol solution to deliver the
dose specified below:

Rate of delivery (expressed in mg/hr)	Continuous albuterol nebulized solution prepared	
	Not mechanically ventilated via *heart*® nebulizer	**Mechanically ventilated or nasal CPAP** via *mini-heart*® nebulizer
5	125 mg/500 mL NS	125 mg/200 mL NS
10 (Recommended start < 20 kg)	250 mg/500 mL NS	250 mg/200 mL NS
15 (Recommended start >/= 20 kg)	375 mg/500 mL NS	375 mg/200 mL NS
20	500 mg/500 mL NS	500 mg/200 mL NS
25	625 mg/500 mL NS	625 mg/200 mL NS
	Flow rate at 10 liters/min (which nebulizes 20 mL/hr)	**Flow rate at 2 liters/min** (which nebulizes 20 mL/hr)

◆   **Aerosolize albuterol at _____ mg/hr** (must specify, refer to dosing guide above)

◆   **Method of delivery** (must specify)

   ❑   Tent

   ❑   Mask

   ❑   Tracheostomy **(not mechanically ventilated)**

   ❑   Tracheostomy or endotracheal tube **(mechanically ventilated)**

   ❑   Nasal CPAP

◆   **If heart rate is persistently greater than _____ beats/min**, notify physician.

◆   **If needed, re-order before the current albuterol solution is completed.**

Date/Time:_____   MD: _____   Date/Time:_____   RN:_____
Form 99906 (Rev. 06/03) p:preprint/albuterolform0603

FIGURE 37.6. Childrens Hospital of Orange County (CHOC) method for utilizing continuous albuterol in status asthmaticus.

a patient become exhausted after a prolonged period of increased effort, then intubation may be required. Absolute indications for intubation include cardiopulmonary arrest, severe refractory hypoxia, and rapid sudden deterioration in mental status.

Intubating an asthmatic raises specific considerations given the conditions' unique pathophysiology. Following preoxygenation and nasogastric decompression, the patient should receive sedation, atropine, and neuromuscular blockade. Ketamine has a bronchodilatory effect and can be considered

Sample Action Plan for Children Ages 5 and Older

Doctor: _____ Date: _____ Consistent personal best peak flow: _____ Type of peak flow meter: _____

Green zone (Stable)

This is when you:
- Have no symptoms
- Can do daily activities without difficulty
- Sleep undisturbed by your breathing

Calculated peak flow: _____ to _____
(80 percent to 100 percent of personal best)

☐ Take daily long-term control medications:

_____ _____ puffs _____ time(s)/day.
_____ _____ puffs _____ time(s)/day.
_____ _____ puffs _____ time(s)/day.

☐ Take quick-relief medications:

_____ _____ puffs
up to _____ time(s)/day as needed.

☐ 15 to 30 minutes before exercise,
take _____ puffs of _____ if needed.

☐ Get annual flu vaccination.

Yellow zone (Caution)

Consider additional treatment if you experience:
- Increased difficulty breathing
- Sleep disturbed by asthma symptoms
- Frequent, tight coughing
- Wheezing
- Difficulty doing daily activities
- Other _____

Calculated peak flow: _____ to _____
(50 percent to 80 percent of personal best)

☐ Take quick-relief medications:

_____ _____ puffs
up to _____ time(s)/day as needed.

☐ Increase: _____ to _____
_____ puffs _____ time(s)/day.

☐ Continue: _____

☐ Add: _____

If treatment doesn't provide relief within
_____ hours or if symptoms suddenly worsen:

☐ Add prednisone _____ for _____ days.

☐ Call _____

Red zone (Alert)

Severe signs and symptoms requiring immediate medical care:
- Prolonged shortness of breath that medication relieves only briefly or doesn't relieve
- Trouble walking or talking
- Inability to do daily activities because of breathing trouble

Calculated peak flow: _____ to _____
(Less than 50 percent of personal best)

Seek emergency care or call 911.

☐ **Call your doctor.**

☐ Take quick-relief medications:
_____

up to _____ times.

☐ Add or increase prednisone: _____

☐ Continue other **green** and/or **yellow** zone medication(s).

Special instructions: _____

Triggers

☐ Infections
☐ Exercise
☐ Household pets
☐ Pollen
☐ Dust mites
☐ Mold
☐ Smoke/pollution
☐ Workplace
☐ Weather/temperature
☐ Household products

☐ Emotions
☐ Foods: _____

☐ Strong odors and sprays
☐ Medications: _____

☐ Other allergies: _____

Notes: _____

Contacts

Primary doctor: _____
  Phone: _____
Asthma specialist: _____
  Phone: _____
Hospital phone: _____
  Address: _____
Ambulance: _____ Taxi: _____
Pharmacy name: _____
  Phone: _____

Find this article at www.MayoClinic.com/invoke.cfm?id=hq000273

FIGURE 37.7. Home Action Plan for management of childhood asthma.

DANGEROUS ABBREVIATIONS – DO NOT USE

U or u	Q.D.	MS	µg	A.S.	Zero after decimal point	No zero before decimal point
IU	Q.O.D.	MSO₄	T.I.W.	A.D.		
		MgSO₄		A.U.		

Do not use these abbreviations, acronyms and symbols in any form (upper or lower case, with or without periods after the letters).

ANOTHER BRAND OF DRUG IDENTICAL IN FORM AND CONTENT MAY BE DISPENSED UNLESS CHECKED. ✓

PEDIATRIC STATUS ASTHMATICUS PHYSICIAN'S ORDERS

☑ **CHECK ALL THAT APPLY**   **PAGE 1 OF 2**

Medication Allergies (include nature of reaction if known):

Other Allergies (include nature of reaction if known):

☐ Admit to the pediatric ward   ☐ Admit to the PICU

☐ Inpatient status   ☐ Observation status

Other diagnoses:

Admitting MD:

Condition:

☐ Vital Signs q 4 hours

☐ Vital Signs:

☐ Activity:

☐ Nursing; per routine

☐ Strict I/Os

☐ Other for nursing:

☐ Regular age-appropriate diet

☐ Other diet:

☐ Labs to be drawn on arrival:

☐ Pulmonary Consult to be called, Dr._____

☐ Confirm patient height and weight as needed, start continuous pulse oximetry, start O₂ to maintain saturation > 92%

Isolation Precautions:

☐ Standard

☐ Contact

☐ Droplet

☐ Other:

☐ Initiate Telemetry for moderate–severe exacerbations

Begin treatment as follows:

☐ Mild Exacerbation (PASS 5-7, Peak Flow > 80% predicted) start albuterol (0.5% sol) nebulizer treatment based on weight

☐ < 30 kg, 2.5 mg Albuterol every _____ hours   ☐ > 30kg, 5 mg Albuterol every _____ hours

Select a steroid to administer:

☐ Prednisolone_____ mg PO (1-2 mg/kg, max 80 mg)

☐ Prednisone_____ mg PO (1-2 mg/kg, max 80 mg)

☐ Methylprednisolone _____ mg IV (1-2 mg/kg)

☐ Dexamethasone _____ mg (0.6 mg/kg, max 10 mg) ☐ PO ☐ IV ☐ IM, then _____ mg

(0.5-2 mg/kg/day divided q 6 hours) every _____ hr

Signature: **Date:**   **Time:**

FIGURE 37.8. Sample protocol for admitting a child with an asthma exacerbation.

for sedation in this setting, although the benefits remain controversial. The most experienced physician should handle the airway given the risk of complications. These include hypotension, severe oxygen desaturation, pneumothorax, and cardiac arrest. The majority of complications occur in the immediate postintubation period. Dynamic hyperinflation can contribute to both barotrauma as well as hypotension. Initially, slow hand-delivered breaths must be delivered. Remember to allow for long, prolonged expiratory times to facilitate airway emptying. It is prudent to place greater emphasis on "primary confirmation" for endotracheal tube placement. Primary confirmation includes looking for chest rise, water vapor in the

---

DANGEROUS ABBREVIATIONS – DO NOT USE

U or u	Q.D.	MS	µg	A.S.	Zero after decimal point	No zero before decimal point
IU	Q.O.D.	MSO₄	T.I.W.	A.D.	(1.0) ⊘	(.X) ⊘
		MgSO₄		A.U.		

Do not use these abbreviations, acronyms and symbols in any form (upper or lower case, with or without periods after the letters).

ANOTHER BRAND OF DRUG IDENTICAL IN FORM AND CONTENT MAY BE DISPENSED UNLESS CHECKED. | ✓

PEDIATRIC STATUS ASTHMATICUS PHYSICIAN'S ORDERS

☑ **CHECK ALL THAT APPLY**   **PAGE 2 OF 2**

☐ Moderate or Severe Exacerbation (PASS 8 or greater, Peak Flow < 80% predicted)

    ☐ Three consecutive nebulized treatments given q 20 minutes to include:

        ☐ For patients < 30 kg, 2.5 mg Abuterol and 250 mcg Ipratroprium (Atrovent)

        ☐ For patients > 30 kg or severe, 5 mg Albuterol and 500 mcg Atrovent

    ☐ Initiate continuous nebulizer treatment q 1 hr for persistent symptoms to include:

        ☐ Albuterol _____ mg (10-20 based on weight and severity)

        ☐ Atrovent (500 mcg)

Additional Orders:

☐ Magnesium Sulfate____ mg IV given over 20 min (25-75 mg/ kg, max 2.5 gm)

☐ Terbutaline ____ mcg bolus dose ☐ SQ ☐ IV (2-10 mcg/ kg, max 300 mcg)

☐ Terbutaline ____ mcg IV continuous infusion (begin 0.1 mcg/kg/min, increase by 0.1 mcg/kg/min q 30 min as needed for

    persistent symptoms, max 6 mcg/kg/min)

☐ IVF: _____ type, _____mL bolus over 1 hr (20 mL/kg)

☐ IVF: _____ type, _____ mL/hr continuous infusion (4 mL/kg first 10 kg, 2 mL/kg additional for

    second 10 kg, 1 mL/kg additional over 20 kg to max 125 mL/hr)

☐ CXR

☐ Antibiotics: _____ type, _____ mg, ☐ PO, ☐ IV, ☐ IM

☐ Acetaminophen (Tylenol) _____ mg (15 mg/kg), every _____ hours ☐ PO, ☐ PR, ☐ PRN _____

☐ Ibuprofen (Motrin): _____ mg (10 mg/kg), every _____ hours ☐ PO ☐ PRN _____

Other:

_____

_____

_____

_____

_____

_____

_____

_____

☐ Initiate Pediatric Asthma Protocol with Respiratory Therapy in _____ Zone,

    albuterol dose_____ (mg) Q _____ hr, atrovent dose (if any) _____ (mcg).

Signature: _____   **Date:** _____ **Time:** _____

FIGURE 37.8. *Continued*

---

endotrachial tube, breath sounds in both lung fields, and a lack of breath sounds over the abdomen. Volume loading with crystalloid will increase preload and can improve cardiac output. If the patient becomes hypotensive with intubation, IV crystalloids should be administered until blood pressure improves.

Mechanical Ventilation

When mechanical ventilation is initiated you should not aim to restore normocapnia, as this can unnecessarily increase the risk for barotrauma. Rather, aim to keep pH >7.1 and peak inspiratory pressure <40 mm H_2O. Permissive hypercapnia is well tolerated by children in this setting as long as oxygenation is adequate. Respiratory rates should be lower than age-adjusted norms and the I/E ratio 1:3 or greater. Continued neuromuscular blockade is sometimes required to prevent patient–ventilator dyssynchrony. Given the risk of subsequent myopathy due to the combination of muscle relaxants and corticosteroids, every effort should be made to discontinue paralysis as soon as possible. Pressure control ventilation (PCV) may be useful in this setting given the concern for ventilation-induced lung injury (VILI). PCV can ensure that peak pressures never exceed 40 mm H_2O. Volume control can be utilized but tidal volumes should be kept low normal (6 to 8 cc/kg) to keep the peak pressure acceptable. Given the degree of mucus plugging and air trapping, it is the plateau pressure that more likely reflects the pressure that is being delivered to the lower airways. Peak end expiratory pressure (PEEP) should be kept at 4 to 6 cm H_2O to promote small-volume patency at end-expiration. When patients have an adequate spontaneous respiratory effort they may be more comfortable in a pressure support (PS) mode. Patients who require mechanical ventilation need to be in an intensive-care unit. Numerous studies have demonstrated improved outcomes for critically ill patients when cared for in a PICU.

QUALITY MEASURES FOR ASTHMA

The way we practice medicine in the United States is undergoing a remarkable transformation, and the care of hospitalized children with asthma is being closely examined. The 1999 publication of *To Err is Human* opened our eyes to how unsafe the practice of medicine can be. Groups like the Institute for Healthcare Improvement (IHI) have helped to galvanize a unified response toward making patient safety our first priority. The Department of Health and Human Services now publishes a webpage (www.hospitalcompare.hhs.gov) with information on how hospitals are complying with basic practices designed to improve health care delivery. As yet, there is little such data available within pediatrics. However, accreditation bodies like the Joint Commission on the Accreditation of Healthcare Organizations (JCAHO) have taken note. The 2007 National Patient Safety Goals and implementation expectations are now available online at www.jointcommission.org. Some of these initiatives are just as applicable to pediatrics as they are to adult medicine. They include measures such as "encourage patients' active involvement in their own care as a patient safety strategy." As the Joint Commission accredits 15,000 hospitals in the United States, these initiatives will affect us all.

In order to address the lack of hospital performance measures relevant to pediatric medicine, the Joint Commission has started an industry-wide initiative called the Pediatric Data Quality Systems. Although this initiative is currently limited to 26 pilot programs, the quality measures they cover will likely move to national implementation rapidly. They include the following: Use of relievers (beta-2 agonists) for inpatient asthma, use of systemic corticosteroids for inpatient asthma, and a home management plan of care given to patient/caregiver (Fig. 37.7). Interestingly, a recent literature review found that such an asthma management plan did not prevent subsequent ED visits or unscheduled doctor visits. Other studies offer contradictory results. However, what is different about these initiatives is that when implemented, the Joint Commission will be looking for data as to how well hospitals are complying with the measures. Accreditation may be linked to hospital compliance. Hospitals and practitioners alike need to begin altering their health care practice to deliver these quality measures. Although most of us already ensure that our patients receive

beta agonists and steroids with an acute asthma attack, perhaps we are not aware of what education, if any, our patients are given before being discharged home. Practitioners need to define these expectations clearly and ensure they are delivered systematically. Furthermore, the hospital needs a record of the patient education that the Joint Commission can access easily during a site visit.

Other initiatives that are rapidly gaining acceptance are patient care "bundles." Bundles are brief guidelines that are designed to standardize the care of specific medical presentations. When implemented faithfully, bundles can improve the efficacy and safety of patient care. An example would be a Ventilator Bundle that would be utilized for patients in respiratory failure on the mechanical ventilator. Another more involved example is the asthma protocol (Fig. 37.8). Such guidelines can ensure that each patient receives standard-of-care treatment regardless of the circumstances of their admission. The importance of patient safety dictates that we deliver "best-practice" medicine, even if it has yet to be clearly defined in pediatrics, or set into motion.

Suggested Reading

1. Foroughi S, Thyagarajan A, Stone KD. Advances in pediatric asthma and atopic dermatitis. *Curr Opin Pediatr* 2005;17:658–663.
2. UpToDate. NAEPP expert panel report II (1997). 3. Pathogenesis and definition. www.uptodate.com.
3. Dinwiddie R. Diagnosis and management of paediatric respiratory disease. New York: Churchill Livingstone; 1997.
4. MerckMedicus Modules. Asthma—pathophysiology; function and structure of the respiratory system. 2006.
5. Tillie-Leblond I, Gosset P, Tonnel AB. Inflammatory events in severe acute asthma. *Allergy* 2005;60:23–29.
6. Fireman P. Understanding asthma pathophysiology. *Allergy Asthma Proc* 2003;24:79–83.
7. Strunk RC, Bloomberg GR. Omalizumab for asthma. *N Engl J Med* 2006; 354:2689–2695.
8. Apter AJ, Szefler SJ. Advances in adult and pediatric asthma. *J Allergy Clin Immunol* 2006;117:512–518.
9. McCance KL, Huether SE. Pathophysiology; the biological basis for disease in adults and children. Elsevier Mosby; 2006.
10. UpToDate. Acute severe asthma in children: assessment and prevention. 2006. www.uptodate.com.
11. Higgins JC. The crashing asthmatic. *Am Fam Physician* 2003;67:997–1004.
12. Werner HA. Status asthmaticus in children. *Chest* 2001;119:1913–1925.
13. Belessis Y, Dixon S, Thomsen A, et al. Risk factors for an intensive care unit admission in children with asthma. *Pediatr Pulmonol* 2004;37:201–209.
14. Russell G. Pediatric respiratory mortality: past triumphs, future challenges. *Thorax* 2005;60:985–986.
15. McFadden ER, Warren EL. Observations on asthma mortality. *Ann Intern Med* 1997;127:142–147.
16. Gorelick MH, Stevens MW, Schultz TR. Performance of a novel clinical score, the pediatric asthma severity score (PASS), in the evaluation of acute asthma. *Acad Emerg Med* 2004;11:10–18.
17. UpToDate. Pharmacologic therapy of acute severe asthma in children. 2006.
18. Streetman DD, Bhatt-Mehta V, Johnson CE. Management of acute severe asthma in children. *Ann Pharmacother* 2002;36:1249–1260.
19. Carroll CL, Schramm CM. Protocol-based titration of intravenous terbutaline decreases length of stay in pediatric static asthmaticus. *Pediatr Pulmonol* 2006;41:350–356.
20. Salpeter SR, Buckley NS, Ormiston TM, et al. Meta-analysis: effect of long-acting beta-agonists on severe asthma exacerbations and asthma-related deaths. *Ann Intern Med* 2006;144(12):904–912.
21. Smith M, Ighal S, Elliot TM, et al. Corticosteroids for hospitalized children with acute asthma. *Cochrane Database Syst Rev* 2003;CD002886.
22. Blitz M, Blitz S, Beasely R, et al. Inhaled magnesium sulfate in the treatment of acute asthma. *Cochrane Database Syst Rev* 2005;3:CD003898.
23. Wheeler DS, Jacobs BR, Kenreigh CA. Theophylline versus terbutaline in treating critically ill children with status asthmaticus: a prospective, randomized, controlled trial. *Pediatr Crit Care Med* 2005;6:142–147.
24. Rodrigo G, Pollack C, Rodrigo C, et al. Heliox for non-intubated acute asthma patients. *Cochrane Database Syst Rev* 2003;4:CD002884.
25. Roberts JS, Bratton SL, Brogan TV. Acute severe asthma: differences in therapies and outcomes among pediatric intensive care units. *Crit Care Med* 2002;30:581–585.
26. Dennis R, Solarte I, Fitzgerald MJ. Asthma; interventions. Clinical evidence: respiratory disorders. *BMJ* 2006. www.clinicalevidence.com.

27. Allen JY, Macias CG. The efficacy of ketamine in pediatric emergency department patients who present with acute severe asthma. *Ann Emerg Med* 2005;46:43–50.

28. Joint Commission on Accreditation of Healthcare Organizations. Performance measurement initiatives: children's asthma candidate core measure set. 2006.

29. Joint Commission on Accreditation of Healthcare Organizations. National patient safety goals: 2007 hospital/critical access hospital national patient safety goals. 2006.

30. Haby MM, Waters E, Robertson CF, et al. Interventions for educating children who have attended the emergency room for asthma. *Cochrane Database Syst Rev* 2001;1:CD001290.

31. Banasiak NC, Meadows-Oliver M. Inpatient asthma pathways for the pediatric patient: an integrative review of the literature. *Pediatr Nurs* 2004;30:447–450.

32. Shelledy DC, McCormick SR, LeGrand TS, et al. The effect of a pediatric asthma management program provided by respiratory therapists on patient outcomes and cost. *Heart Lung* 2005;34:423–432.

CHAPTER 38A ■ CHRONIC PULMONARY DISEASE: CYSTIC FIBROSIS

DAVID A. HICKS

CARE OF THE HOSPITALIZED CYSTIC FIBROSIS PATIENT

The medical care of cystic fibrosis (CF) patients is now very complex and labor intensive. As in most chronic, unremitting, slowly progressive disorders, such care is best provided at a CF center specifically set up to care for that disorder. The United States Cystic Fibrosis Foundation has 120 recognized centers that care for CF patients.

With the advent of Diagnosis Related Groups (DRGs), Health Maintenance Organizations (HMOs), better home health companies, inhaled and oral forms of therapy, and the patient's desire for a more normal life, hospitalizations are now less frequent and shorter. Nonetheless, a period of time in the hospital can allow for more education or re-education, and multiple consultations and procedures.

As everyone's time is precious, the benefits of hospitalizing the CF patient should be maximized. As approximately 90% of the care of CF patients is outpatient, each hospitalization should have goals that are set and met. The care team (including patient and family) should all be knowledgeable and aware of the reasons for admission and the treatment plans and goals.

Physiology

It is beyond the scope of this chapter to discuss the details of the genetics, physiology, pathophysiology, diagnosis, and differential diagnosis of CF. The reader is referred to the Suggested Readings at the end of the chapter.

The improved survival of CF patients is due to basic science and clinical care teams working together. The CF gene has been present in humans for hundreds if not thousands of years. It is an autosomal recessive genetic disease. It is the most common lethal genetic disease of the Caucasian race. One in twenty of the Caucasian population is a carrier. Birth rates for the disease are as follows: 1/2,000 to 1/3,500 white, 1/18,000 to 1/20,000 black, 1/90,000 Asian. Rates in other societies and cultures are not clearly defined.

Research over the Past 20 years has given us insight into the pathophysiology of CF, but the exact cellular mechanism of disease is still elusive. The CF gene is known to be located on the long arm of chromosome 7. There are nearly 2,000 distinct mutations. The most common (80%) occur at the 508 position (F508). At that position, a 3-base pair deletion results in the deletion of phenylalanine.

The CF gene encodes for a protein called CFTR (cystic fibrosis transmembrane conductance regulator). This protein is part of a family of ATP-binding cassette proteins. The CFTR is located in the apical membranes of the airways and glandular epithelium. The protein acts as a chloride channel, and proper function of the chloride channel is necessary for the airway surface fluid to have the correct ionic and water content. Disruptions in the ionic and water content lead to abnormalities in airway fluid physiology. Ion abnormalities in the sweat glands result in high chloride concentrations (the basis of the sweat test). Abnormalities in the airway surface fluid lead to thickened mucus, which is difficult for cilia to move and in which bacteria become entrapped, leading to chronic infection. The highly viscous airway fluid also contains a multitude of inflammatory cells, particularly netrophils. These inflammatory cells produce a myriad of inflammatory mediators and chemicals. The combination of entrapped bacteria, inflammatory cells, and mediators contributes to the chronic damage. Inflammation and chronic bronchitis can be found even in children less than 1 year of age. Bronchiectasis soon occurs and leads to continued tissue destruction and respiratory failure.

This same protein malfunction occurring in glandular epithelium leads to mucus obstruction in other organ systems: in the pancreatic ducts, leading to fibrosis and loss of exocrine function; in the hepatic bile canaliculi, leading to hepatitis; in the vas deferens, leading to azospermia.

Initial Evaluation

Once hospitalization is recommended, the entire CF support team should be notified (nutrition, physical therapy, psychology, social services, respiratory therapy, clinical nurse specialists, and MD consultants as needed). The first hospitalization is always the most difficult. Many families see this as the beginning of the end. All team members should be positive and encouraging. A patient with a chronic, unremitting disease that has frequent exacerbations is approached differently from a healthy normal child with a single disease who is expected to return to full health.

A complete history is important. What events led to the hospitalizations? How often are they seen in clinic? What medications are being taken? Are they taken correctly? Any medication side effects or complications? What respiratory programs are being used? How often is chest physical therapy being done? Which method? A detailed evaluation of the nutritional program is very important. Psychosocial and school questions are important.

The system review should be complete. Central nervous system: headache, sinus pain/pressure, eye pain, numbness, tingling. Respiratory: shortness of breath (sob); dyspnea on exertion (doe); hemoptysis; sputum production; sputum type—quality, color; night cough; post-tussive emesis; chest pain. Gastrointestinal: quality and number of stools, foul smelling, fatty-oily, abdominal pain, food types, gastroesophageal reflux (ger) symptomology. Menses and reproductive systems should be evaluated.

The diagnosis of cystic fibrosis is based on the results of either a sweat chloride test or DNA analysis. CF should be suspected if the child presents with meconium ileus, "salty" skin when kissed, chronic cough, wheezing, chest x-ray evidence of chronic infiltrates with lung hyperinflation, fat malabsorption, failure to thrive, digital clubbing, or a positive family history. For more detailed information, the Cystic Fibrosis Foundation can be contacted through their website: www.cff.org.

Physical Exam

The physical exam should have complete vital signs including oxygen saturation, SaO_2, and FiO_2 with flow rate, body weight, and BMI (body mass index). It is necessary to compare these data points with previous points and graph them. The HEENT exam should include evaluation for nasal polyps, and sinus or teeth pain. The chest exam: AP diameter, retractions, dullness, resonance, crackles (when in the inspiratory cycle, location, scattered, diffuse, wet, dry, bubbly), cough (dry, productive,) wheeze, stridor. The heart: splitting of S2, loudness of P2, perfusion, cyanosis. Abdomen: distension, pain, masses, span of liver and spleen. Extremities: muscle mass, subcutaneous tissue, hydration, salt crystals on the skin, clubbing (grade 1 minimal to 4 maximal), cyanosis. The neurologic-psychological exam is also important.

Laboratory Exam

The lab exam may depend upon what has been done in the clinic or emergency room. Prior to admission, all patients should have a CBC, complete metabolic panel, a sputum or throat culture, a chest radiograph, and (if old enough) a pulmonary function test (PFT). PFTs can usually be done on children as young as 6 to 7 years old.

Other tests may be appropriate, such as quantitative IGE (looking for *Aspergillus*); prealbumin (nutritional screen), prothrombin time (vitamin K function). The microbiologic lab must be able to isolate *Pseudomonas aeruginosa* (mucoid and nonmucoid), *Burkholderia cepacia*, *Aspergillus*, and non-*Mycobacterium* tuberculosis organisms from the sputum of CF patients. Sputum or throat specimens should be marked "CF" patient so the lab knows what to do.

Lab evaluation of the nutritional status can also include vitamins A, D, E, and K levels. They are done at least yearly or in a malnourished patient.

Evaluations of the endocrine function of the pancreas are now being done yearly on adolescents. The best evaluation is the 3-hour oral glucose tolerance test (OGTT). Other tests can include hemoglobin A1C, fasting blood sugar (FBS), and 2-hour postprandial (PP) glucose test. Special radiographic studies can be helpful: sinus CT scans with coronal views (headache, sinusitis); high-resolution CT scans of the lungs (usually without contrast) and abdominal series (for patients with abdominal pain). Lung CT scans are becoming a useful tool in following the status of the lung disease.

Complaints of abdominal pain can lead to gallbladder evaluation, barium studies, and CT evaluations of the abdomen. Gastroesophageal reflux, peptic ulcer disease, and pancreatitis are reasonably common. Amylase and lipase can be helpful in abdominal pain. Probably the most common etiology of abdominal pain is DIOS (distal intestinal obstruction syndrome—so-called meconium ileus equivalent). DIOS is evaluated with standard radiographs: CT scans or, rarely, contrast enema studies.

Antibiotic Therapy

Although there are many reasons for admission to hospital, the most common is for antibiotic therapy. With the advent of home health services, HMOs, and DRGs, hospital stays are often much shorter. Then there is the so-called "2 week cleanout."

The usual length of IV antibiotic therapy is 2 weeks; that said, an antibiotic course of 3 or 4 weeks is occasionally necessary. The length of therapy depends on the patient's response: exam, improved PFTs, vital signs, weight, and oxygen requirements. Most patients are now treated with 1 to 3 days in hospital and then finish IV therapy as outpatients.

The choice of antibiotics depends upon the pathogenic organism. In the first several years of life, *H. influenzae*, *Staphylococcus aureus*, and *E. coli* are often found. As the disease progresses, *Pseudomonas aerugenosa* (mucoid and nonmucoid) becomes predominant. The mucoid variety is rarely seen in other diseases. The sputum culture, cough-throat culture is the most important guide. The CF cough-throat culture is obtained by getting the younger CF patient to cough and then quickly doing a throat swab. It is important to notify the lab to look for CF pathogens not just beta-strep. By 6 or 7 years of age, expectorated sputum can usually be obtained. In patients with serious changes on the chest film, who cannot expectorate sputum and in whom the organism is not known or who are not responding to therapy, flexible bronchoscopy should be considered as a means for obtaining an adequate sample for culture.

Individuals with only staph or *H. influenzae* can often be treated with single-drug therapy—a semisynthetic penicillin or cephalosporin. Once *Pseudomonas* or other gram-negative organisms are found, then at a minimum double-drug therapy is needed. Most often a semisynthetic penicillin or cephalosporin and an aminoglycoside are used. It is important to use drugs from different classes to lessen the emergence of resistance. The doses should be the highest possible for that particular agent and patient. It takes high concentrations of drugs to overcome barriers found in the lungs of CF patients. Typical doses for ceftazidime can be 180 to 200 mg/kg divided q8 hours. Cefepime can be used q12 hours; however, for serious infections q8-hour dosing can be helpful. Semisynthetic penicillins such as piperacillin (up to 400 mg/kg divided q4–6 hr) and ticarcillin (300–400 mg/kg divided q4–6 hr) are often used. The dose of antibiotics such as Timentin or Zosyn is based upon the penicillin component. Many seriously ill patients may benefit from continuous infusions of antibiotics. CF patients usually require aminoglycoside doses of 10 to 15 mg/kg/day. Recently many centers have been using a single daily dose of aminoglycosides. The dose is usually between 10 and 12 mg/kg. Drug levels are drawn at 12 hours postdose. The desired level is less than 2. Using a traditional 8- to 12-hourly schedule, the desired trough is less than 2 and the peak between 8 and 10. While on aminoglycoside therapy it is important to monitor kidney function (BUN, creatinine). Years of therapy can have a negative cumulative effect on kidney function and then creatinine clearance becomes important. Periodic evaluation of hearing and vestibular function is necessary. Other organisms such as *B. cepacia*, *Staphylococcus. maltophilia*, *Aspergillus* and non-MTB, require specific therapy often guided by infectious disease specialists.

For highly resistant organisms, the CF Foundation can guide someone to special centers to do antibiotic synergy studies to determine which two or three antibiotics may work better together. Aerosolized antibiotics can achieve high concentrations in the larger airways and areas of better ventilation/airflow. These antibiotics (aminoglycosides, colymycin, and astreonam) are generally reserved for chronic/recurrent outpatient therapy.

Patients suffering from advanced complications of CF lung disease may benefit from combined intravenous and aerosolized antimicrobial therapy.

Quinalone antibiotics are among the most frequently used outpatient drugs. The bioavailability of this group and its antimicrobial patterns are the main factors leading to a reduction in IV therapy. This class of antibiotics is often used for inpatient therapy for patients with multiresistant organisms. Ciprofloxacin is used in a dose of 20 to 60 mg/kg divided q8 hours IV or oral. Levoquin can be given q24 hours: 250 µg for a child, 500 mg for an adolescent, or 750 mg for an adult.

Methacillin-resistant *S. aureus* (MRSA) is often found. This organism is best treated with Zyvox. Vancomycin has been the standard in the past. The newer antibiotics are better clinically and have much fewer side effects.

Azithromycin has recently been found to have a positive effect in CF patients. This is presumably due to an anti-inflammatory effect. The CF Foundation has recommended its routine use in CF patients age 5 and above. The drug is given by mouth Monday, Wednesday, and Friday. The dose is 250 mg for weight less than 40 kg and 500 mg for those weighing more than 40 kg. The drug should be continued when on IV antibiotics.

The pediatric pharmacist and infectious disease specialist can be very helpful in guiding antimicrobial therapy.

Chest Physiotherapy

Chest physiotherapy (PT) is a vital part of the CF patient's daily existence. Chest PT should continue in the hospital. The only real contraindication is active hemoptysis. The hospitalist must be careful to distinguish between chronic, small-volume bleeding and active, large-volume bleeding. Large, active bleeding deserves chest rest until the hemorrhage has subsided; then gentle chest PT resumes, advancing to vigorous PT as the bleeding stops. Routine chest PT is given q4 to 6 hours. Chest PT can be accomplished by various means: hand percussion, hand-held chest machine percussion, chest wall percussion by high-frequency chest wall vibrator, hand-held mouthpiece airway vibrators (acapella, flutter valve), intrapulmonary percussive ventilation (IPV), and special breathing techniques (Huff coughing). Chest PT is best accompanied by a comprehensive program of inhaled agents to relieve bronchoconstriction if present, mucolytics, steroids, and antibiotics. Hospitalization is useful to teach and to re-enforce such daily therapy.

Mucolytic therapy can be very useful. Recombinant human DNase (Pulmozyme) has supplanted the use of n-acetylcystine. This newer agent rapidly destroys any DNA that it comes in contact with in the airway. DNA from bacteria and the patient's own cells are a significant cause for the very tenacious CF sputum. The dose of DNase is 2.5 mg aerosolized once a day. Studies did not demonstrate a positive effect when used BID. However, many CF centers do increase the use of DNase to BID during acute exacerbations.

Reactive airways are a common complaint for many CF patients. However, airway obstruction in some CF patients actually worsen with a bronchodilator. Airway stability is maintained by cartilaginous support and muscle tone. If the cartilage is destroyed by bronchiectasis, then the airway patency may depend on muscle tone. If these muscles are relaxed with a bronchodilator, airway collapse can occur upon expiration. The patient worsens. PFTs can help guide the clinician in such cases. It is important for the CF patient's family, with the help of the CF team, to decide which form of chest PT works best for that patient and then to do it frequently.

Recent data has supported the use of 7% saline as an inhalation agent to lessen the viscosity of the airway secretions. The mechanism of action may simply be that of hydration to the airway mucus. Many patients who have not been sputum producers now seem to be able to cough up mucus. The dose is 4 mL inhaled several times per day. Once again, the patient must help design the respiratory program that works for her.

Nutritional Support

The typical CF patient has a variety of nutritional issues. The primary pancreatic defect results in the loss of pancreatic enzymes. Foodstuffs are not properly digested and are lost to the patient. Eighty-five percent to ninety percent of patients with the most common defect (deltaF508) are pancreatic insufficient. This means they require oral pancreatic enzyme supplementation. There are various enzyme preparations on the market. The dosage is determined by calculating units of amylase (in the capsules) per kilogram of body weight per meal. Adjustments of more or less enzymes are based on clinical response, including oil-grease fats in the stool, and quality, quantity, and frequency of bowel movements. A small dose would be 500 to 1,000 U/kg/meal; medium dose 1,000 to 2,000 U/kg/meal; and high dose over 2,500 U/kg/meal. The CF Foundation and its centers do not recommend generic enzymes.

The hospital dietary service should have available high-calorie, high-quality food for the CF patient. Frequent snacks of similar quality should be offered. A low-fat diet is no longer appropriate. A high-quality normal diet is required.

Calorie needs for CF patients are higher than in normal individuals, often 150% of normal during times of health and 200% or more during exacerbation. Getting the CF patient to eat properly is one of the biggest challenges for the CF care team (including the family). Chronic infections (with abundant inflammatory mediators) often lead to anorexia.

Nutritional failure, as evidenced by the growth chart and BMI, will hasten lung destruction. Patients with advanced lung disease need aggressive intervention. This intervention can be short-term hyperalimentation, nasogastric tube feedings, and gastric tube placement. Night-time intralipid supplementation is often used during hospitalization. The amount of lipids is about 2 g/kg body weight, delivered over 8 to 10 hours. Most patients with nutritional failure will require some nutritional support. Many oral, high-calorie supplements are available. The biggest problem is getting the patients and families to follow through on frequent supplementation. After a failed oral program, patients with nutritional failure will require tube feedings. Such tubes are self-placed (or parental placed) nasogastric tubes, surgical or percutaneous gastric tubes, or jejunal tubes. It is critical to provide enzymes for whatever nutritional support program the patient is on. Enzymatic support is usually in the range 2,000 to 4,000 units of lipase per 120 mL full-strength formula.

Antacids or proton pump inhibitors are frequently used to allow the enzyme products to function more efficiently. Adding these medications is usually the first step to improve nutrition.

SPECIFIC COMPLICATIONS— SPECIAL CONSIDERATIONS

Headache

The most frequent cause of headache in the patient with CF is sinus disease. Most patients with CF will have abnormal sinus CT scans. However, not all of these will have disease serious enough to warrant endoscopic sinus surgery. Frequent headaches, associated with sinus problems, may often lead to surgery. Antibiotics will help to lessen the bacterial load prior to surgery. Nasal steroids can help to lessen obstruction to the ostia, and inflammation in the mucosa, and help to relieve sinonasal congestion. Other causes for headaches can include brain abscesses and medication side effects.

Chest Pain

Chest pain is a very common complaint, often leading to the abuse of analgesics and narcotics. The most common cause is pleurisy secondary to underlying pneumonia. Treatment is antibiotics for infection and analgesics for pain. Short-term narcotics can be very useful. It is important to keep the narcotic use limited to several days as other treatments begin to have their effect. This will help prevent abuse. It is our opinion that any narcotics should be given slowly or even by infusion rather than push. This also may help to lessen abuse. We prefer narcotics other than demerol. Demerol is very effective but can be very addictive.

All patients with chest pain should have a chest x-ray to determine if a pneumothorax is present. Sudden onset of chest pain, with or without dyspnea or shortness of breath, is a usual sign of a pneumothroax. Other frequent causes of chest pain are gastroesophageal reflux, rib fractures (osteoporosis and cough), and muscle spasms (from cough).

Pneumothorax

Pneumothorax is a common cause of chest pain and respiratory distress. The most common etiology is from rupture of surface blebs. These are disruptions—emphysematous changes in the periphery of the lung that have direct communication with an airway. These airways are dilated and bronchiectatic. A moderate to large pneumothorax must be treated with a chest tube. It is important to re-expand the lung so that proper airway drainage can occur. The longer the lung stays down, the more secretions are retained, which can worsen the underlying lung damage. Antibiotics are recommended. Small leaks of 10% to 15% can often be observed. Frequent clinical exams and radiographs are needed to monitor resolution. During observation and treatment, chest physiotherapy is usually withheld to aid healing. The high intrathoracic pressure changes with coughing can prolong the air leaking. Most air leaks will resolve when the visceral and parietal pleura adhere. Installation of pleural irritating agents can be useful in resistant recurrent leaks.

Gastroesophageal Issues

Gastroesophageal reflux is very common. Overexpansion of the lungs, a flattened diaphragm, and high intra-abdominal pressure (with cough) are part of the causative factors. Treatment with antacids or proton-pump inhibitors is usually successful. Reglan may or may not be helpful. Persistent complaints should lead to investigations to determine if the medications have failed or if a hiatal hernia is present. Such problems can be surgically addressed.

Pancreatitis

Pancreatitis can be a recurring problem. Standard therapy is usually successful for this problem. A search for pancreatic duct blockage may be necessary in difficult or persistent cases.

Peptic Ulcer Disease

Peptic ulcer disease is also common. Standard therapy is again usually successful. Patients with CF have numerous stresses in their life and take multiple medications that can potentiate abdominal complaints.

Psychosocial Issues

Psychosocial issues are a real problem, and these should be addressed in a complete program to solve the abdominal complaints.

Distal Intestinal Obstruction Syndrome

Distal intestinal obstruction syndrome (DIOS) is a frequent and in some patients recurring complication. Prevention centers around proper enzymatic support and hydration. Once obstruction occurs, treatment can be as simple as a Fleets enema or Gastro-Grafin enema if the site of obstruction is the large intestine. For ileal obstruction, polyethylene glycol (Colyte) is often used. Colyte intestinal lavage is accomplished by ingesting (PO or nasogastric tube) large volumes of 2 to 6 L, 150 to 500 mL/hr, until rectal effluent runs clear. If the site of obstruction is the terminal ileum, often a Gastro-Grafin enema can help if the material is able to reflux into the terminal ileum. Abdominal films are needed to help localize the site of the obstruction. Symptoms of obstipation, constipation, change in stool pattern, abdominal pain, and vomiting are common. Go-Lyte (or similar) is the primary treatment for ileal obstruction. Oral intake or nasogastric instillation is required. GI consultation can be helpful in difficult cases. Recurrent cases can be treated at home with proper patient–family instruction.

Failure to Thrive

Failure to thrive can be a medical emergency in patients with CF. If intensive OPD nutritional support has failed, admission to hospital becomes necessary. As in any chronic illness, etiologies can be varied and complex—psychosocial, medical, surgical, abuse, or neglect. All causes need to be considered, eliminated, and/or treated. Lengthy hospitalizations can be required. These patients often need temporary nasogastric feeds. Hyperalimentation should be reserved for those not able to take full enteral support. Permanent g-tubes are often necessary.

Hemoptysis

Hemoptysis can be frightening and even life threatening. It is a very common complaint in patients with advanced bronchiectasis-bronchitis. The most frequent cause is superficial mucosal erosions caused by the chronic infections. This bleeding is small, dark, and streaking, associated with venous or low-pressure bleeding. The most troublesome, worrisome, and frightening is arterial bleeding. This is high-pressure bleeding from dilated tortuous bronchial arteries or other collateral arteries (internal mammary, intercostal, or subclavian). This bleeding is commonly large, bright red, not associated with exacerbations, often brought on by activity or a change in position. It is often felt as a gurgling "sound-feeling" in the chest. Treatment is bed rest, no chest therapy, antibiotics, type and cross-match, and hydration. One should look for treatable causes such as liver dysfunction, vitamin K deficiency (protime), clotting abnormalities (PTT, bleeding time), or medication side effects (thrombopathy secondary to penicillin or aspirin). Extra doses of vitamin K can be considered, 2.5 μg for a child, 5 μg for an adolescent or adult. Most often such bleeding will subside and stop. If the bleeding is continuous, recurrent, large volume, and requiring transfusion, consideration should be made for bronchial artery embolization. Such procedures should be done by experienced radiologists.

Mechanical Ventilation

Ventilator support is often needed after surgical procedures. Preparation before surgery is key to speedy recovery. Critical attention must be paid to pulmonary function. Several days (or more) of antibiotics, vigorous pulmonary toilet, and nutritional support will aid in faster recovery and extubation. Such support is mandatory while on mechanical ventilation. Endotracheal lavage with saline, normal or 7%, along with mechanical percussion, vibrating the chest, will aid in mucus removal. Aerosolized or even direct instillation of Pulmozyme may be very helpful. Pulmozyme is usually given BID for acute or serious problems; short-term more frequent use (QID) may help in very serious exacerbation or critically ill ventilated patients. Bronchoscopic lavage is quite helpful in removing mucus. Light sedation is best, as the patient's own cough is helpful in pulmonary toilet. Paralyzation of a CF patient can lead to more retention of mucus, purulent secretions, and a longer course on the ventilator.

CF patients can often be successfully weaned from endotracheal support with the use of facemask or nasal bi-pap. The distending pressure should not be too high, so as to reduce the possibility of pneumothorax. Provision should be made to continue vigorous chest PT and aerosol therapy. Permissive hypercapnia is often necessary for patients with advanced lung disease.

Terminal or end-stage patients should avoid endotracheal ventilation. Heavy sedation is necessary for comfort and this further compromises lung failure. Endotracheal support during the final stages of lung failure would mean little or no communication with loved ones. Bi-pap in these circumstances can be life prolonging, while avoiding heavy sedation and maintaining some pulmonary toilet. Mechanical ventilation is often necessary if the patient and/or family is not prepared for death. Good communication between the team and family can avoid this often-futile therapy. Endotracheal ventilation is not a bridge to transplant. However, bi-pap is considered such a bridge. Bi-pap can allow a patient on a transplant list sufficient time until a donor can be found.

If a terminal or end-stage patient or family asks for endotracheal ventilation, it is reasonable to advise that such therapy is often futile and will be offered only for a limited time, such as a week or even a few weeks. If no improvement is seen, then the ventilator should be withdrawn. Such decisions are difficult but needed to avoid unnecessary suffering.

Suggested Readings

Boucher RC. New concepts in the pathogenesis of cystic fibrosis lung disease. *Eur Respir J* 2004;23:146–158.

Bush A, Alton EW, Davies JC, et al. eds. *Cystic fibrosis in the 21st century, progress in respiratory research*. Vol. 34. Karger; 2006.

Chernick V, Boat T. Kendig's disorders of the respiratory tract in children. 6th ed. Philadelphia: Saunders; 1998.

Cystic Fibrosis Foundation, Bethesda, MD 20814, www.cff.org.

Davis P, ed. Cystic fibrosis. In: *Lung biology in health and disease*. Vol. 64. Marcel Dekker; 1993.

De Rose V. Mechanisms and markers of airway inflammation in cystic fibrosis. *Eur Respir J* 2002;19:333–340.

Doershuk C, ed. *Cystic fibrosis in the 20th century*. New York, AM Publishing; 2001.

Donaldson S, et al. Mucus clearance and lung function in cystic fibrosis with hypertonic saline. *N Engl J Med* 2006;354:241–249.

Elkins M, Robinson M, Rose B, et al. A controlled trial of long-term inhaled hypertronic saline in patients with cystic fibrosis. *N Engl J Med* 2006; 354:229–240.

Haddad G, Abman S, Chernick V, eds. *Basic mechanisms of pediatric respiratory disease*. 2nd ed. New York, B. C. Decker; 2002.

Orenstein D, Stern R, eds. Treatment of the hospitalized cystic fibrosis patient. In: Lung biology in health and disease. Vol. 109. New York, Marcel Dekker; 1998.

Ramsey BW, Pepe M, Quan J, et al. Intermittent administration of inhaled tobramycin in patients with cystic fibrosis. *N Engl J Med* 1999;340:23–30.

Rowe S, Miller S, Sorscher E. Cystic fibrosis. *N Engl J Med* 2005;352: 1992–2001.

Taussig Z, Landau L, eds. *Pediatric respiratory medicine*. St. Louis: Mosby; 1999.

CHAPTER 38B ■ CHRONIC PULMONARY DISEASE: BRONCHOPULMONARY DYSPLASIA

GARY GOODMAN

Chronic lung disease (CLD) is an all-inclusive term for persistent pulmonary dysfunction in childhood. The most recognized form of chronic lung disease is bronchopulmonary dysplasia (BPD), first described by Northway in 1967 in prematurely born infants with clinical symptoms of respiratory distress, a persistent oxygen requirement, and classic radiologic changes (see Fig. 38.1). Bronchopulmonary dysplasia is the final, common pathway of neonatal lung injury. The original form of BPD originated in a presurfactant era when immature lungs were exposed to excesses of pressure, volume, and oxygen, while being mechanically ventilated, and produced severe lung dysfunction that was often debilitating and fatal. Fortunately, the rates of severe bronchopulmonary dysplasia have steadily declined (from 9.7% in 1994 to 3.7% in 2002 in infants less than 33 weeks gestational age), although a "new" BPD has emerged. This "new" BPD occurs in infants born more prematurely (at 25 to 26 weeks gestational age and weighing less than 1 kg) and in term infants with residual lung disease after surviving advanced therapy for such disorders as neonatal pneumonia, meconium aspiration syndrome, diaphragmatic hernia, and persis-

tent pulmonary hypertension of the newborn (Fig. 38.2). The most recent National Institutes of Health consensus definition of BPD comprises infants with the need for supplemental oxygen beyond 28 days chronologic age with or without the need for ongoing assisted ventilation and radiologic changes on chest x-ray. Many infants will also require diuretic therapy and aerosolized bronchodilators. Under the broader heading of chronic lung disease are infants with congenital heart disease complicated by pulmonary disfunction, acquired airway abnormalities, neuromuscular disease with respiratory insufficiency or chronic respiratory failure, and even previously healthy infants with lung sequelae of acute infection, most notably respiratory syncytial virus (RSV) and adenovirus (Table 38.1).

PATHOPHYSIOLOGY

Regardless of the etiology, lung disease extending beyond the period of acute lung illness is a complex condition affecting many areas of the lung. CLD can affect the airway: both upper

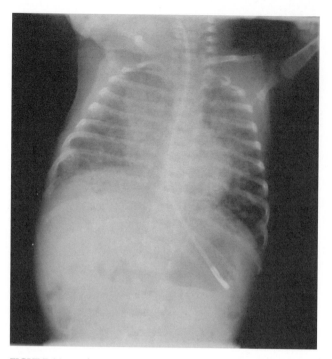

FIGURE 38.1. Chest x-ray with BPD.

and small airways, the lung parenchyma, and the pulmonary vascular bed. The physiologic consequences are altered gas exchange as well as abnormal lung mechanics. Clinical manifestations include chronic respiratory symptoms (tachypnea, increased work of breathing, and cough), airflow limitation (wheezing and prolonged expiratory phase), gas trapping (hyperinflation), and exercise intolerance. The most severely affected infants will not thrive despite comprehensive medical management and are candidates for long-term mechanical ventilation. Sleep is an especially vulnerable time period when occult hypoxemia can occur secondary to lung volume loss and hypoventilation. Secondary lung insults, especially gastroesophageal reflux and intercurrent infection, can exacerbate the pulmonary symptoms and require immediate intervention. Infants with chronic lung disease are also at unique risk for seasonal respiratory virus infections that exacerbate the underlying lung disease thereby worsening gas exchange and often promoting pulmonary hypertension.

EVALUATION AND TREATMENT

The cornerstone of therapy for CLD is supplemental oxygen. Hypoxemia contributes to acute respiratory dysfunction and growth failure, and is probably the primary risk factor for the development of pulmonary hypertension. Hypoxemia also has adverse effects on developmental outcomes in premature infants. Supplemental oxygen is a safe and effective treatment of infants with established chronic lung disease who are not at risk of further progression of retinopathy of prematurity. Oxygen saturation (SaO_2) below 92% should be avoided, with 94% to 96% the goal of therapy. Improvement in respiratory stability has been documented in otherwise healthy premature infants receiving supplemental oxygen during sleep, as evidenced by a decrease in apnea, periodic breathing, and bradycardia, without adverse effects on alveolar ventilation.

The infant or child with chronic lung disease may require hospitalization for primary exacerbation of their lung disease or with a secondary illness. Admission criteria are listed in Table 38.2. Support of the respiratory system is a priority. First, it is necessary to monitor the adequacy of gas exchange with noninvasive pulse oximetry and with blood gases when appropriate. For the patient with impending respiratory failure (increasing oxygen requirements, rising $PaCO_2$, or increased work of breathing), transfer to the pediatric intensive-care unit is indicated. Other diagnostic tests that may be helpful include a chest x-ray (with comparison, when possible, with previous films), rapid respiratory viral testing, and a

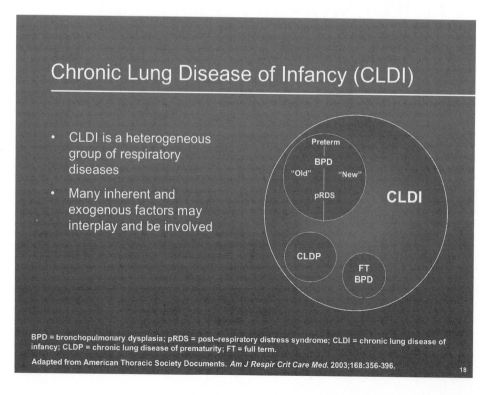

FIGURE 38.2. Chronic lung disease of infancy (CLDI).

TABLE 38.1

ETIOLOGIES OF CHRONIC LUNG DISEASE

NEONATAL PERIOD
Prematurity with surfactant deficiency (classic BPD)
Pulmonary hypoplasia
Term
  Neonatal pneumonia
  Meconium aspiration syndrome
  Congenital diaphragmatic hernia
  Tracheoesophageal fistula
  Persistent pulmonary hypertension of the newborn
  Congenital anomalies (e.g., cystic adenomatoid
    malformation)

INFANTS
Airway abnormalities
  Vocal cord dysfunction
  Subglottic stenosis
  Tracheomalacia, bronchomalacia
Congenital heart disease
Neuromuscular disease
Viral infections (RSV, adenovirus)

basic chemistry panel to assess electrolytes (important for patients on diuretics) and bicarbonate (to demonstrate primary or compensatory metabolic alkalosis).

For children with chronic lung disease admitted to the hospital for nonpulmonary conditions, close respiratory monitoring remains important. Fluid therapy should be adjusted to the patient's needs with accurate recording of intake and output. Continuation of home medications and respiratory care is necessary, and isolation to prevent nosocomial respiratory infection is mandatory. Often, infants with chronic lung disease will be admitted to the hospital for extended monitoring after even minor elective surgical procedures as they have a higher incidence of anesthetic complications including apnea and sensitivity to narcotic analgesics.

Bronchospasm and pulmonary edema formation are two of the most common clinical consequences of BPD, particularly with intercurrent infections such as RSV disease. With respect to bronchospasm, albuterol is the most commonly used bronchodilator (beta-2 agonist). Lev-albuterol (Xopenex) is sometimes used when patients have excessive tachycardia or irritability with albuterol, but its benefit is controversial. Alternately, reducing the dose of albuterol may also decrease the frequency of adverse reactions. Aerosolized ipratropium bromide (Atrovent) may also be used in conjunction with a beta-2 agonist. Diuretic

TABLE 38.2

ADMISSION AND DISCHARGE CRITERIA

Admission criteria	Discharge criteria
Increased respiratory rate	Stable respiratory exam
Increased respiratory effort	Stable oxygen requirement
Increasing oxygen requirements	Stable blood gases
Feeding difficulties	Stable ventilator settings
Respiratory acidosis	Steady weight gain
Failure to thrive	
Unstable ventilator settings	
"Spells" (desaturations, bradycardia, blue spells)	

therapy for pulmonary edema often includes lasix (which has diuretic properties and also directly improves pulmonary compliance) in combination with aldactazide to conserve potassium. It is important to monitor the serum bicarbonate level to avoid metabolic alkalosis, which accentuates respiratory insufficiency. Supplemental potassium can further help maintain a normal serum bicarbonate level. The benefit of corticosteroids in chronic lung disease exacerbations is variable, but both inhaled and systemic steroids (Solu-Medrol 1 mg/kg q6° or prednisone 1 mg/kg q12 hr) are often used to decrease airway inflammation and bronchial hyperreactivity. Other important aspects of care include nutritional support and treatment of gastroesophageal reflux when present. Caloric intake can be increased by concentrating infant formula to 22, 24, 27 or 30 calories/ounce as tolerated. Aspiration can also contribute to exacerbations of chronic lung disease. Study of such infants with barium swallow/upper gastrointestinal series and pH probe can be diagnostic and can indicate the need for antireflux therapy or gastrostomy tube placement if there is an aspiration risk present or inability to attain a sufficient caloric intake.

The most serious complication of chronic lung disease is pulmonary hypertension, which can be insidious and life threatening. Cardiovascular monitoring of infants with chronic lung disease begins with pulse oximetry, especially during feedings, sleep, and when sitting in the infant carrier/car seat. Routine monitoring of blood pressure and serial electrocardiograms may also demonstrate signs of pulmonary hypertension (systemic hypertension and right-ventricular hypertrophy). Echocardiography can further demonstrate right-ventricular hypertrophy, estimate pulmonary artery pressures, and show rightward displacement of the intraventricular septum. The gold standard for measuring pulmonary artery pressures, however, is cardiac catheterization, which can further rule out anatomic cardiac disease, pulmonary vein stenosis or occlusion, and the presence of a left-to-right shunt (patent ductus arteriosus, patent foramen ovale, atrial septal defect, and bronchial collaterals), which can exacerbate pulmonary hypertension. Pulmonary artery catheterization can be both a diagnostic as well as a therapeutic intervention. After measuring baseline pulmonary artery pressures, a variety of therapies can be tested including supplemental oxygen, inhaled nitric oxide, and epoprostenol (Prostacylin). Novel vasodilators for pulmonary hypertension include oral sildenafil and bosentan (an endothelin-1 receptor antagonist). Finally, infants with severe chronic lung disease who do not thrive with conventional medical therapy may also be candidates for long-term mechanical ventilation. The patient will require tracheostomy. A number of portable, battery-operated ventilators are currently available. Our lung center has had good results with the Pulmonetic LTV1000. Home ventilation is an imposing responsibility for families and requires complex, multidisciplinary planning that includes provision of home nursing care (see Chapter 131D).

Discharge criteria for children admitted with BPD are listed in Table 38.2.

Suggested Readings

Abman SH. Monitoring cardiovascular function in infants with chronic lung disease of prematurity. *Arch Dis Child Fetal Neonatal Ed* 2002;87: F15–F18.

Kotecha S and Allen J. Oxygen therapy for infants with chronic lung disease. *Arch Dis Child Fetal Neonatal Ed* 2002;87:F11–F14.

Smith VC, Zupancic JAF, McCormick MC, et al. Rehospitalization in the first year of life among infants with bronchopulmonary dysplasia. *J Pediatr* 2004; 144:799–803.

Smith VC, Zupancic JAF, McCormick MC, et al. Trends in severe bronchopulmonary dysplasia rates between 1994 and 2002. *J Pediatr* 2005;146: 469–473.

Allen J, Zwardling R, Ehrenkranz R, et al. Statement on the care of the child with chronic lung disease of infancy and childhood. *Am J Respir Crit Care Med* 2003;168:356–396.

CHAPTER 39A ■ FOREIGN BODY ASPIRATION

JASON M. KNIGHT

Foreign body aspiration is a common pediatric problem and a leading cause of accidental death in children under 5 years of age. Children between the ages of 1 and 4 years explore their environment, which often includes introducing objects into their mouths. It follows that nearly all foreign body aspirations occur in this age group.

The most commonly aspirated objects are food materials such as peanuts, seeds (sunflower and watermelon), nuts, and beans. Some inert objects that are easily aspirated into the child's airway include small toys, buttons, toy parts, lids of ballpoint pens, and straight pins (1).

CLINICAL PRESENTATION

Laryngeal impaction (complete obstruction of the trachea at the level of the glottis) is life threatening and tragic outcomes are not unusual (2). These children usually exhibit some degree of choking followed by acute respiratory arrest that may be unmanageable even by the trained provider. Respiratory arrest eventually progresses to asphyxia and cardiac arrest. If adequate circulation is restored, the majority of these patients suffer eventual brain death or severe neurologic insult due to their severe asphyxial injury.

Children with foreign body aspiration often present with nonspecific signs and symptoms of pulmonary disease such as cough, wheezing, respiratory distress, decreased breath sounds, and fever. Any history of "penetration syndrome," defined as the sudden onset of choking and intractable cough with or without vomiting (3), requires the hospitalist to rule out foreign body aspiration.

A foreign body can be found at any site in the airway, from the nose to the lung parenchyma. Before 15 years of age, there is no anatomic difference in the angle formed by each main bronchus, and therefore foreign bodies may not lodge preferentially in the right main bronchus in children (2).

After the foreign body passes the vocal cords into the trachea and bronchi, the symptoms often cease immediately. Unless the aspiration was witnessed and severe in nature, the patient will usually enter an asymptomatic period of days to years until a suspecting parent or physician considers the diagnosis or the child develops a complication from the chronic presence of the foreign body. Karakoc and Karadag (4) found that patients who aspirated organic foreign bodies had an abnormal physical exam 92% of the time versus 26% who aspirated inorganic foreign bodies. The risk of long-term complications increased with increasing elapsed time from aspiration to diagnosis; complications were as high as 60% in children who were diagnosed 30 days after foreign body aspiration, with bronchiectasis being the most common (4).

Therefore, the hospitalist must remember to consider the diagnosis of foreign body aspiration in any child, especially those less than 4 years of age, when symptoms include "unexplained" or prolonged cough, wheezing, and fever. One investigator found that 20% of all children were treated for other disease for over a month before undergoing bronchoscopy and foreign body removal.

STUDIES AND WORKUP

A management algorithm for children with suspected foreign body aspiration can be found in Table 39.1. The first study to be obtained when considering the diagnosis of foreign body aspiration is the plain radiograph of the chest, including inspiratory and expiratory films. Unfortunately, most foreign bodies are radiolucent and cannot be identified on radiographs. Multiple studies have shown that radiographs are neither sensitive nor specific to make the diagnosis of foreign body aspiration. In one series, 80% of children with laryngotracheal foreign bodies had normal x-ray findings while 68% of the children with bronchial foreign bodies had positive x-ray findings. The most common findings included obstructive emphysema, inspiratory shift of the mediastinal shadow, pneumonia, and atelectasis (5).

If the clinician is suspecting foreign body aspiration in the face of inconclusive radiographs, there are other imaging modalities available. Fluoroscopic exam occasionally aids the examiner when there is asymmetric, inadequate emptying of one lung or inspiratory–expiratory mediastinal shift indicating a unilateral bronchial obstruction (5). Computed tomography (CT) virtual bronchoscopy is a noninvasive technique that provides an internal view of the trachea and major bronchi by three-dimensional reconstruction (6). This modality may be useful when the history and preceding studies are unconvincing and the physician is unwilling to subject the patient to bronchoscopy. The disadvantages of CT virtual bronchoscopy include false-positive findings (retained secretions and artifacts); inability to show the morphology, vascularity, or color of the mucosa; and inability to detect endoluminal lesions smaller than 2 to 3 mm (6).

MANAGEMENT AND THERAPY

Bronchoscopy is the mainstay of foreign body removal and in most cases treatment is complete once the foreign body is removed. Some centers advocate the use of flexible bronchoscopy for foreign body removal in children. These groups have bronchoscopists who are trained in rigid bronchoscopy and they also have rigid bronchoscopy equipment available at the time of all flexible bronchoscopic foreign body removal (7).

TABLE 39.1

MANAGEMENT ALGORITHM FOR CHILDREN WITH SUSPECTED
FOREIGN BODY ASPIRATION

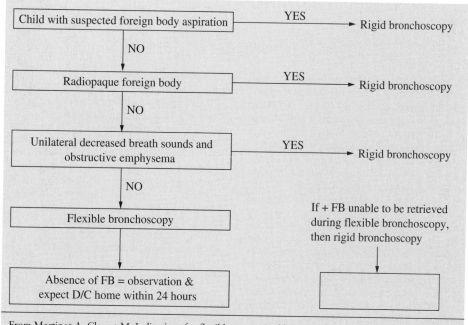

From Martinot A, Closset M. Indications for flexible versus rigid bronchoscopy in children with suspected foreign-body aspiration. *Am J Respir Crit Care Med* 1997;155:1676–1679.

The "gold standard" remains rigid brochoscopy due to the ability to fully control the airway, provide adequate oxygenation and ventilation and utilize all instruments that may be necessary for foreign body removal. Despite being relatively "safe," there is a small risk of morbidity and mortality with bronchoscopy. Complications include major airway injury, pneumothorax, and failure to extract the foreign body on the first attempt necessitating a second or third rebronchoscopy. Secondary complications may include deterioration of the patient's respiratory status post-bronchoscopy, occasionally requiring tracheostomy (8). There have been deaths associated with rigid bronchoscopy, which are most often related to asphyxia and cardiac arrest during the actual procedure (9). "Delayed" death can be caused by brain death secondary to severe, prolonged hypoxia or severe, irreversible respiratory failure.

OUTCOME

Outcome following aspiration of a foreign body is determined by the material or object aspirated, location in the tracheobronchial tree, length of time the object remains in the airway prior to removal, and the resultant complications. The longer the object has been present, the more likely the child will develop significant complications including pneumonia, obstructive emphysema, lung abscess, or bronchiectasis requiring surgical intervention and possibly lobectomy.

Despite foreign body removal, a number of patients will have persistent respiratory symptoms such as cough and wheezing. Nearly all of these patients respond positively to inhaled corticosteroids and bronchodilators. Those patients who failed to respond to intensive medical treatment, usually including antibiotics, underwent surgical treatment of their bronchiectasis and made a complete recovery (4).

PEARLS

- Foreign body aspiration is more common in children between the ages of 1 and 4 years.
- Food materials are most frequently aspirated.
- Physical examination and studies have low diagnostic sensitivity and specificity.
- A high degree of suspicion is enough to proceed with bronchoscopy.
- Delay in removal of a foreign body can lead to severe bronchial sequelae.

References

1. Friedman EM. Tracheobronchial foreign bodies. *Otolaryngol Clin North Am* 2000;33:179–185.
2. Lima JA, Fischer GB. Foreign body aspiration in children. *Pediatr Resp Rev* 2002;3:303–307.
3. Baharloo F, Veyckemans F. Tracheobronchial foreign bodies. Presentation and management in children and adults. *Chest* 1999;115:1357–1362.
4. Karakoc F, Karadag B. Foreign body aspiration: what is the outcome? *Pediatr Pulmonol* 2002;34:30–36.
5. Mu L, Sun D. Radiological diagnosis of aspirated foreign bodies in children: review of 343 cases. *J Laryngol Otolaryngol* 1990;104:778–782.
6. Haliloglu M, Ciftci AO. CT virtual bronchoscopy in the evaluation of children with suspected foreign body aspiration. *Europ J Radiol* 2003;48:188–192.
7. Swanson KL, Prakash UB. Flexible bronchoscopic management of airway foreign bodies in children. *Chest* 2002;121:1695–1700.
8. Sersar SI, Rizk WH. Inhaled foreign bodies: presentation, management and value of history and plain chest radiography in delayed presentation. *Otolaryngol Head Neck Surg* 2006;134:92–99.
9. Ciftci AO, Bingol-Kologlu MB. Bronchoscopy for evaluation of foreign body aspiration in children. *J Pediatr Surg* 2003;38:1170–1176.

CHAPTER 39B ■ FOREIGN BODY INGESTION

SAMEER S. PATHARE

Foreign body ingestion is a very common pediatric problem. Most ingestions occur in children under the age of 4 years. The majority of ingested foreign bodies (up to 80% to 90%) are harmless and pass spontaneously without complication. When patients are symptomatic, most foreign bodies are lodged in the esophagus. Foreign body ingestion can lead to partial obstruction or even complete obstruction of the airway. Airway obstruction is most common when the foreign body is in the mid- to distal esophagus. Symptoms include dysphagia, increased salivation, emesis, odynophagia, and chest pain.

Materials that lodge in the esophagus are divided into food bolus impactions and true foreign bodies. The food bolus impactions account for 34% to 60% of ingestions. True esophageal foreign bodies in children are most commonly smooth, blunt objects that lodge in the proximal esophagus. In children, up to 66% of true foreign bodies are coins. Other possibilities include small toys, toy parts, button batteries, and sharp objects. Button batteries should be removed promptly if lodged, due to the risk of erosion and esophageal perforation. Sharp objects include toothpicks, safety pins, glass, bones, and tacks, which have a 15% to 35% risk of perforation (1).

Most true foreign bodies are radiopaque and can be identified on plain films. A contrast esophagram can also be performed if a radiolucent foreign body is suspected. Flexible endoscopy is the mainstay of foreign body removal. Other possible removal techniques include balloon catheter removal and rigid esophagoscopy, which requires general anesthesia. Balloon catheter removal should be reserved for smooth objects that have been lodged for only a few hours. Rigid esophagoscopy may be necessary for prolonged foreign bodies. Observation without intervention may also be an option.

COIN INGESTION

Over 92,000 coin ingestions were reported to poison centers in 2003. Conners (2) studied management of coin ingestions and noted that once coins are in the stomach, they generally pass in children with normal anatomy. Coins spontaneously pass in 27% of patients. It is noteworthy that two-thirds of spontaneous passage occurs in the first 8 hours. Children with asymptomatic esophageal coins are far likelier to pass the coins into the stomach than those patients who have symptoms. Also, asymptomatic esophageal coins are more likely to be in the lower esophagus. Upper esophageal coins passed in only 8% of cases. Middle or distal esophageal coins passed 47% of the time. Spontaneous passage is far more likely in older patients. Prompt removal prevents complications such as esophageal perforation, esophageal stricture, and respiratory distress. However, most agree that an 8- to 16-hour period of observation is appropriate in the asymptomatic child. If the coin is in the stomach, then observation and follow-up radiographs can be done to determine passage.

Positioning of a coin can reveal the location on the AP films. The flat aspect of the coin can easily be visualized on an AP film. Esophageal coins typically have this appearance. A coin in the trachea generally has the slit-like appearance on AP views due to the tracheal cartilage that is incomplete posteriorly.

TREATMENT

Therapeutic intervention in foreign body ingestion depends on the type of foreign body, location in the gastrointestinal tract, time since ingestion, presence of symptoms, and clinical findings. The majority of foreign body ingestions can be successfully treated with observation and close follow-up (3). If removal is indicated, then a flexible endoscopic removal is currently the method of choice at our institution by an appropriately trained gastroenterologist. If rigid esophagoscopy is indicated, due to duration of symptoms or distress, then an otorhinolaryngologist may be preferred.

References

1. Duncan M, Wong R. Esophageal emergencies: things that will wake you from a sound sleep. *Gastroenterol Clin North Am* 2003;32:1035–1052.
2. Conners G. Management of asymptomatic coin ingestion. *Pediatrics* 2005;116;752–753.
3. Bendig DW. Removal of blunt esophageal foreign bodies by flexible endoscopy without general anesthesia. *Am J Dis Child* 1986;140:789–790.

Suggested Readings

Rotta A, Wiryawan B. Respiratory emergencies in children. *Respiratory Care.* 2003;48(3);248–260.
Waltzman M, Baskin, Wypij D, et al. A randomized clinical trial of the management of esophageal coins in children. *Pediatrics.* 2005;116;614–619.

CHAPTER 40 ■ PLEURAL EFFUSIONS

TONY CHERIN

The pleural space is a small, potential space between the visceral pleura that covers the lungs and the parietal pleura that lines the inside of the chest cavity. This space usually contains less than a single milliliter of a low-protein, acellular, sterile fluid. The pleural fluid acts as a lubricant to prevent the lungs from abrading against the ribcage with each breath.

Pleural fluid is formed continuously, usually at an extremely low rate. The hydrostatic pressure in the capillaries that supply both visceral and parietal pleura is normally greater than the oncotic pressure within the plasma, resulting in the filtration, or production, of pleural fluid. Venous and lymphatic vessels reabsorb pleural fluid, and are assisted in this endeavor by movements of the chest wall and diaphragm. Under normal physiologic conditions, the capacity for reabsorbing pleural fluid is several times higher than the rate of pleural fluid production. Various disease states can result in elevated capillary hydrostatic pressure, decreased plasma oncotic pressure, altered capillary membrane permeability, or impedance of lymphatic/venous drainage. Any of these changes will lead to excessive production of pleural fluid. When the capacity for reabsorption is overcome, a pleural effusion is the result. This is usually defined as at least 10 to 20 milliliters of fluid in the pleural space.

Pleural effusions can be classified as either transudates or exudates based on the number of cells and amounts of protein, glucose, and LDH that they contain. However, the utility of determining transudate versus exudate has been debated of late. Perhaps more notable is that the vast majority of effusions in children are parapneumonic effusions, caused by infectious agents. Congenital heart disease and malignancy are the second and third most common causes, respectively.

FREQUENCY

There are approximately 1 million cases of pleural effusion in the United States each year, but numbers vary widely by age and disease process. The Children's Hospital of Orange County is a 230-bed tertiary care facility that serves an estimated pediatric population of 800,000. In 2005, the hospital treated 152 cases of pleural effusions.

MORTALITY AND MORBIDITY

A frankly purulent pleural effusion, also termed an empyema, can have a prolonged, complicated course. If untreated, pleural-cutaneous fistulae may result, leading in frank pus erupting from the chest wall (empyema necessitatis). Large effusions that are treated with antibiotics alone, without surgical drainage or intervention, may result in a layer of proteinaceous debris also known as a pleural peel. This peel may take months to resolve and may impair lung function. Historically, the mortality rate for children with empyema was extremely high. Current antibiotic and surgical strategies have reduced the mortality rate to less than 10% in children under a year of age. Malignant effusions and those associated with congenital heart lesions have variable mortality/morbidity rates, depending on the underlying process.

ETIOLOGY

In the past, *Staphyloccocus aureus* and *Haemophilus influenzae* (type B) were the causative organisms for most cases of parapneumonic effusions. In the modern, post-HIB vaccine era, the three most common bacterial pathogens causing clinically significant effusions are *Streptococcus pneumoniae*, *Staphylococcus aureus*, and *Streptococcus pyogenes* (group A strep, GAS). The incidence of community-acquired, methicillin-resistant *Staphylococcus aureus* (MRSA) and cephalosporin-resistant *Streptococcus pneumoniae* continues to rise in most locales, and should be considered when making decisions regarding antibiotic coverage.

Other bacterial pathogens include non-typeable *H. influenzae*, *Klebsiella pneumoniae*, and anaerobes (particularly in cases of aspiration pneumonia). In the immunosuppressed child, *Pseudomonas aeruginosa* should be considered, although it infrequently causes effusions.

There are many nonbacterial infectious agents that can cause pleural effusions. Viruses, especially adenovirus, and *Mycoplasma pneumoniae* may in fact cause more effusions than the various bacterial pathogens. However, these effusions are usually small and transient, and rarely clinically significant. *Legionella pneumoniae*, although rarely seen in children, may also cause effusions and should be considered during regional outbreaks. Mycobacterium tuberculosis should always be considered as a potential cause for a newly discovered effusion, as up to 10% of pediatric pulmonary tuberculosis cases include effusions.

Pleural effusions are often associated with congenital heart disease, and are frequently chylothoraces. A chylothorax is a pleural effusion consisting of lymphatic fluid, comprised of lymphocytes and triglycerides. A chylothorax is usually the result of trauma to the thoracic duct, the largest lymphatic vessel in the body. The surgical cases most frequently implicated in thoracic duct trauma are aortic coarctation repair, ductus arteriosus ligation, and central shunt placement.

Chylothoraces may also occur spontaneously when the central venous pressure is high, preventing drainage of lymphatic fluid from the thoracic duct into the left subclavian vein, or from the right lymphatic duct into the right subclavian vein. This situation may arise with subclavian venous obstruction, thrombosis, or after the Fontan repair for single-ventricle physiology. Nonchylous effusions are occasionally seen with obstructive congenital heart lesions that lead to right ventricular failure, and hence increased central venous pressure.

Less frequent causes of pleural effusions in children include trauma, congestive heart failure, hypoalbuminemia, nephrotic syndrome, cirrhosis, pulmonary embolism, juvenile rheumatoid arthritis, systemic lupus erythematosis, pancreatitis, and sarcoidosis. Occasionally, a centrally placed venous catheter may migrate into the pleural space, leading to an infusion of IV fluids.

HISTORY AND PHYSICAL EXAM

The history given by patients and family members can be quite variable and is usually nonspecific. Patients often have antecedent upper respiratory symptoms. Presenting symptoms can include fever, cough, shortness of breath, chest pain, loss of appetite, nausea, vomiting, abdominal pain, and other generalized complaints. Small effusions may be entirely asymptomatic. Large effusions may lead to respiratory distress or respiratory failure. Often, the patient has been diagnosed clinically or radiographically with a lower respiratory tract infection but has not improved, or has actually deteriorated despite empiric antibiotic therapy.

As with the history, the physical exam can be surprisingly nonspecific and nonsensitive. Depending on the size of the effusion, the underlying cause, and the age/size/cooperation of the patient, the presence of an effusion may escape detection by even the most experienced and suspicious examiner. Larger effusions often lead to nonspecific findings such as tachypnea, anxiety, low oxygen saturation, and decreased air exchange on the affected side. A pleural rub, described as the sound of two pieces of dry leather rubbing against one another, is rarely detected. If present, a rub will be heard early in the disease process, and will disappear as the effusion grows in size. Very large effusions can cause absent breath sounds, dullness to percussion, decreased vocal/tactile fremitus, and voice egophony over the affected side.

WORKUP

Although a chest radiograph should be obtained whenever a pleural effusion is suspected, often a pleural effusion is detected by chance on a routine anterior–posterior chest film. A small effusion leads to the loss of the costophrenic angle on both AP and lateral views. As the effusion increases, a lateral fluid line may extend from the scapula to the diaphragm. On a right-sided effusion, fluid may be seen in the transverse fissure. A larger effusion will obscure the hemidiaphragm on the affected side. A very large effusion or an effusion overlying consolidated or atelectatic lung may result in complete opacification of the affected side.

A moderate to large effusion, or any effusion with clinically significant symptoms, should then be followed up with a lateral decubitus film with the affected side down. Gravity-dependent layering out of the fluid collection on the lateral decubitus film is a reliable indicator that fluid is free flowing. When the practitioner suspects a large effusion to be more than 2 to 3 days old, the lateral decubitus film can be foregone in favor of an ultrasound study of the chest. This is recommended for the purpose of determining whether the effusion is free flowing versus organized, with loculations and debris. Findings on ultrasound are often useful in guiding choice of surgical therapeutic options.

Although a CT scan is the definitive study for determining size and quality of an effusion, it is not often needed, especially in uncomplicated cases. CT scanning is reserved for patients with large, complex effusions, or for those in whom there is suspicion of marked parenchymal lung disease or an intrathoracic mass underlying the effusion.

As with any lower respiratory tract infection, a routine CBC with manual differential and blood culture should be obtained. The WBC and band count may be low, normal, or high, and the blood culture only occasionally yields a causative organism. The CRP and ESR can be followed for trending in response to therapy but should not be used to differentiate bacterial from nonbacterial causes. A complete metabolic panel, including renal and hepatic function screens, total protein, albumin, and LDH should be obtained. Mycoplasma serologies are warranted in school-aged children, and viral screens are uniformly indicated. A PPD should be placed on any patient with an unexplained effusion, particularly in areas where TB is prevalent. When considering less frequent causes, ANA, RF, complement, amylase, and lipase levels may be diagnostic.

Pleural fluid, if obtained, should be sent for routine Gram stain and culture, cell count and differential, and cytology. LDH, pH, protein, glucose, and triglyceride levels should be obtained for comparison with serum values to determine transudates versus exudates. Transudates typically have an effusion/serum LDH ratio of less than 0.6 g/dL, pH greater than 7.45, and protein less than 3 g/dL. Transudates may be parapneumonic but are more often associated with the rarer causes of effusions. Exudates are more common in pediatric patients, and usually have an effusion/serum LDH ratio of greater than 0.6, pH less than 7.2, protein greater than 3 g/dL, and effusion/serum glucose ratio of less than 0.5. A chylothorax will demonstrate a high triglyceride level and a predominance of lymphocytes. Acid-fast bacillus stain and culture should be considered.

TREATMENT

Due to the predominance of infectious etiologies, patients with a pleural effusion should be treated with antibiotics to cover lower respiratory tract pathogens while the initial workup is underway. In patients with very small effusions, no lung consolidation, and high suspicion for viral infection, antibiotics may be withheld while more data are obtained and clinical progression is observed.

All children with moderate or large effusions and/or consolidations should receive empiric coverage for staphylococcus, pneumococcus, and GAS. An initial combination of nafcillin and ceftriaxone provides excellent coverage, although the hospitalist may consider substituting vancomycin or linezolid for nafcillin, depending on regional incidence of community-acquired MRSA. Ceftriaxone has been found to provide high enough levels in both lung parenchyma and infected pleural effusions to overcome resistant strains of *Streptococcus pneumoniae*. In school-aged children, empiric mycoplasma coverage with azithromycin or erythromycin should be initiated pending serologic studies.

Clindamycin should be used in cases of suspected toxin producing staph or GAS infections. The use of clindamycin or other anaerobic coverage is also needed for suspected aspiration events, which may occasionally lead to effusions. In the immunosuppressed child, coverage of pseudomonas aeruginosa should be initiated immediately, using ceftazidime, cefipime, or piperacillin/sulbactam, pending workup.

The drainage of pleural effusions has long been the subject of considerable debate. As mentioned previously, small effusions can be managed conservatively, but moderate to large effusions may develop into long, complicated illnesses if not drained. Many approaches have been tried, tested, and touted, including serial needle thoracentesis, placement of intrapleural "pigtail" drainage catheters, bedside thoracotomy and chest tube placement, video-assisted thoracoscopic surgery (VATS), and open thoracotomy with debridement and chest tube placement. For thick empyemata, instilling streptokinase, urokinase, or TPA into obstructed chest tubes and "pigtails" has been tried with varying success.

When considering these options, the hospitalist should recall the tenet of *primum non nocere* (first do no harm). Do not, however, allow this attitude to lead to familiarity with another Latin phrase: *nolo contendere* (I do not wish to contend). The patient with a clinically significant pleural effusion should have it drained for diagnostic and/or therapeutic purposes.

In freely flowing effusions, as determined by lateral decubitus film or ultrasound, needle thoracentesis may suffice. A patient with purulent appearing pleural fluid on thoracentesis, or with a large free-flowing effusion, should have a bedside thoracotomy and chest tube placement, with conscious sedation at a minimum. A patient with a thick, organized, loculated effusion, as determined by ultrasound or CT scan, should proceed to early VATS for drainage and decortication if necessary. In complex effusions, early VATS has been shown to significantly decrease length of hospitalization. Rarely, patients with protracted disease, large pneumatoceles, or necrotic lung parenchyma will require open thoracotomy for surgical resection.

Children with chylothorax should be put on a low-fat diet, with enteral nutrition containing medium-chain triglycerides (MCT). Failing this strategy, persistent chylothorax may be treated with octreotide infusions, thoracic duct ligation, and/or pleural-peritoneal shunts. However, the success rate with each of these treatment strategies is variable. Long-term complications of persistent chylothorax include malnutrition, alteration of immune function, and occasionally chronic lung disease. Follow-up with a pulmonologist after recovery is recommended.

CHAPTER 41 ■ RESPIRATORY FAILURE

PAUL LUBINSKY AND JAMES P. CAPPON

Respiratory failure is the inability to maintain adequate gas exchange, due to inadequate alveolar ventilation and/or inadequate arterial oxygenation. The respiratory system includes the upper and lower airways; lungs (parenchyma and gas exchanging units); respiratory muscles and thoracic cage (respiratory muscles, ribs, spine, and pleura); and the central nervous system (CNS) and peripheral nervous system (PNS). The cardiovascular and respiratory systems are interdependent, and failure of one will compromise the other. Respiratory failure may be secondary to abnormalities in any of these components. Airway diseases are characterized by luminal obstruction and increased resistance. Diseases of the lungs manifest with decreased compliance and reduction of functional residual capacity (FRC). Respiratory pump failure may be acute (due to conditions such as spinal cord injury, Guillain–Barré syndrome, or infant botulism) or chronic (due to neuromuscular diseases, including the muscular dystrophies, myasthenia gravis, and deformities of the thoracic cage). Abnormalities of the central and peripheral nervous system include central apnea due to brain pathology or pharmacologic agents, phrenic nerve palsy, and metabolic derangements. One of the primary concerns with any CNS pathology is control and protection of the airway, and respiratory drive. Disease processes that may lead to respiratory failure are listed below.

DIFFERENTIAL DIAGNOSIS

I. Upper airway obstruction
  A. Choanal atresia
  B. Adenotonsillar hypertrophy
  C. Retropharyngeal abscess
  D. Laryngomalacia
  E. Angioneurotic edema
  F. Epiglottitis
  G. Vocal cord abnormalities
  H. Hemangioma
  I. Congenital syndromes, associations (e.g., Treacher–Collins, Pierre–Robin)
  J. Subglottic stenosis
  K. Croup (laryngotracheobronchitis)
  L. Tracheitis
  M. Foreign body inhalation
  N. External airway compression (e.g., neck mass, vascular ring)
II. Lower airway disease
  A. Foreign body
  B. Asthma/reactive airway diseases
  C. Bronchiolitis
  D. Bronchomalacia
  E. Bronchial compression
III. Pulmonary disease
  A. Viral pneumonitis
  B. Bacterial pneumonia
  C. Atypical pneumonia
  D. Opportunistic infections
  E. Aspiration/chemical pneumonitis
  F. Acute respiratory distress syndrome (ARDS)
  G. Vasculitic disease
  H. Cardiogenic pulmonary edema (left ventricular failure)
  I. Congenital pulmonary malformations (e.g., congenital adenomatoid malformation)
  J. Pulmonary fibrosis
  K. Pulmonary contusion
IV. Extrapulmonary restriction
  A. Pleural effusion, hemothorax, chylothorax
  B. Pneumothorax
  C. Thoracic cage deformity (e.g., kyphoscoliosis)
  D. Abdominal distension
V. Neuromuscular etiologies
  A. Altered mental status (e.g., acute encephalopathies, electrolyte/metabolic derangements, seizures, toxins, medications)
  B. Impaired secretion handling, lack of airway patency, and/or loss of airway reflexes
  C. Abnormal respiratory drive
  D. Muscular dystrophy
  E. Infant botulism
  F. Guillain–Barré syndrome
  G. Spinal muscular atrophy
  H. Transverse myelitis
  I. Myasthenia gravis
  J. Spinal cord trauma
  K. Prolonged paralysis, (following use of neuromuscular blocking agents)
VI. Diaphragmatic muscle fatigue
VII. Cardiovascular failure
  A. Pulmonary edema
    1. Cardiogenic pulmonary edema, (left ventricular failure)
    2. Fluid overload
  B. Inadequate oxygen delivery to respiratory muscles

The circulatory and respiratory systems are interdependent and failure of one will impact the other. Inadequate oxygen delivery in shock states will lead to compromise of respiratory muscle function. Pulmonary edema, which occurs in many primary cardiac diseases, is characterized by reduced lung compliance and hypoxemia. Interstitial edema may produce elevations in airway resistance (e.g., cardiac asthma). Elevated transpulmonary pressures will compromise left ventricular function.

CLINICAL FINDINGS

The differential diagnosis for respiratory failure is extensive, and a well-focused *clinical history* is essential. The history must include the nature and time course of the symptoms, medications (particularly those associated with respiratory depression), and concurrent symptoms (including fever, emesis, or neurologic changes). In addition to a complete history, the review must include (1) previous respiratory events, (2) medications for the present and prior respiratory events, (3) family history, (4) history of cardiovascular or neurologic disorders, (5) exposure to ill contacts, (6) recent travel, and (7) possibility of foreign body inhalation. It is often useful to ask about participation in school physical education programs to determine if there is unrecognized chronic respiratory insufficiency.

On physical examination, information on respiratory status can be rapidly obtained from close observation of the patient and review of vital signs. Mental status as a gauge of systemic oxygenation is important, as a patient with impending respiratory failure may be either agitated or lethargic. Diaphoresis is a sign of systemic stress and increased release of endogenous catecholamines. Although an infant is unable to position itself, an older child will assume the position of maximal comfort. With upper airway obstruction, the patient characteristically assumes the sniffing position and may drool due to the inability to swallow secretions. A patient in severe respiratory distress may position himself in the tripod position, sitting upright and leaning forward to maximize use of accessory muscles. A patient with congestive heart failure will avoid lying flat. Dyspnea when speaking or inability to suck a bottle indicate severe respiratory distress.

Increased work of breathing is manifest by nasal flaring, grunting, head bobbing, and chest wall retractions. Pulsus paradoxus is a sign of respiratory distress, sufficient to impair cardiac function. The presence of pulsus paradoxus is suggested by a reduction in the amplitude of the pulse oximetry wave form on inspiration. (When a patient has an arterial line in place, the reduction in blood pressure on inspiration can be quantified, as it can be with the use of a blood pressure cuff.) Diaphragmatic fatigue is manifested by abnormal respiratory patterns: paradoxical movement of the abdomen, respiratory alternans, or apnea. The physical assessment can then proceed with careful auscultation of the chest. A thorough assessment of other organ system involvement is necessary due to the diverse causes of respiratory failure.

The most common *laboratory measures of gas exchange* are pulse oximetry and a blood gas analysis, which may be of arterial (ABG), venous (VBG), or capillary (CBG) samples. Pulse oximetry is indicated in any patient with respiratory distress; with few exceptions, it is a very reliable measure of arterial oxygen saturation (SaO_2). Hypoxemia is a low arterial oxygen tension (PaO_2) while hypoxia is a low tissue oxygen level (reduced oxygen delivery).

The causes of hypoxemia may be derived from the alveolar gas equation based on Dalton's law:

Total pressure of gas in the alveolus
= The sum of the partial pressures of all of the individual gasses

The Alveolar Gas Equation, therefore, states:

$$PAO_2 = FiO_2(P_{atm} - P_{H_2O}) - PaCO_2/R$$

where PAO_2 = alveolar oxygen tension (mm Hg), PaO_2 = arterial oxygen tension (mm Hg), FiO_2 = fraction of inspired oxygen (0.21 for room air, 1.0 for 100% oxygen), P_{atm} = atmospheric pressure (760 mm Hg at sea level), P_{H_2O} = partial pressure of water at 37°C (47 mm Hg), $PaCO_2$ = arterial carbon dioxide tension (in mm Hg), and R = respiratory quotient (the ratio of CO_2 production to O_2 consumption, usually estimated to be 0.8). (Partial pressure of nitrogen is the same in the air and blood is dropped from both sides of the equation. The dissolved oxygen is inconsequential at atmospheric pressure and is "ignored.")

For example, in room air at sea level

$$\begin{aligned} PAO_2 &= 0.21(760 - 47) - 40/0.8 \\ &= (0.21 \times 713) - 50 \\ &= 150 - 50 \\ &= 100 \text{ mm Hg [normal A-a gradient} \\ &\quad \text{(intrinsic shunt) is } 5-10 \text{ mm Hg]} \end{aligned}$$

The A-a gradient is determined using the Alveolar Gas Equation to calculate the alveolar PAO_2 and then subtract the measured PaO_2. $AaDO_2 = PAO_2 - PaO_2$. In general terms, the wider the $AaDO_2$, the worse the physiologic derangement.

With cellular defects such as cyanide poisoning, there may be adequate delivery of oxygen but failure of cellular respiration. The etiology, pathophysiology, and initial treatment of hypoxemia are presented in Table 41.1.

PULSE OXIMETRY

Correct interpretation of pulse oximetry requires that the detected heart rate correlates with the patient's pulse rate. In clinical states with poor perfusion, an accurate reading may be difficult to obtain. Pulse oximetry assumes that there are only two forms of hemoglobin in the blood, oxyhemoglobin and deoxyhemoglobin, and is unreliable in states of carboxyhemoglobinemia or methemoglobinemia. In these conditions, the pulse oximeter will provide a falsely elevated reading of the percentage of oxygenated blood, as the oximeter does not detect carboxyhemoglobin or methemoglobin. Direct measurement of the oxygen saturation in the blood gas laboratory will therefore be necessary, to document abnormal hemoglobin moieties. In patients with cyanotic heart disease, an arterial saturation of 70% to 80% may be present, but oximeters are less accurate in this range. Pulse oximetry is nonetheless used in these patients, but the clinician must be aware that obtained values have less precision in this range.

INTERPRETATION OF ABGS

ABG analysis provides important information on ventilation, oxygenation, and acid–base status.

The pH is the primary determinant of acid–base status.

pH >7.40 $\Rightarrow$ alkalosis
$\Rightarrow$ due to $\uparrow$ serum bicarbonate (metabolic) or $\downarrow$ $PaCO_2$ (respiratory)

pH <7.40 $\Rightarrow$ acidosis
$\Rightarrow$ due to $\downarrow$ serum bicarbonate (metabolic) or $\uparrow$ $PaCO_2$ (respiratory)

(Compensatory adjustments in bicarbonate or $PaCO_2$ occur in response to the primary physiologic derangement.)

Elevated $PaCO_2$ (>45 mm Hg) $\Rightarrow$ Hypoventilation
$\Rightarrow$ Determine etiology

Normal $PaCO_2$ (35–45 mm Hg) $\Rightarrow$ Appropriate minute ventilation

Reduced $PaCO_2$ (<35 mm Hg)
$\Rightarrow$ Hyperventilation (usually secondary to increased respiratory drive as a result of hypoxemia or metabolic acidosis)

Normal PaO_2 $\Rightarrow$ Normoxia
Reduced PaO_2 $\Rightarrow$ Hypoxemia $\Rightarrow$ Administer 100% O_2

No increase in PaO_2 is indicative of intracardiac or intrapulmonary shunt. Improved oxygenation is indicative of low V/Q matching.

TABLE 41.1

ETIOLOGY, PATHOPHYSIOLOGY, AND INITIAL TREATMENT OF HYPOXEMIA

Etiology	Pathophysiology	Treatment
Alveolar hypoventilation	Alveolar CO_2 displaces O_2 No ↑ in A-aDO_2	Open airway Increase minute ventilation
Low V/Q	Reduced gas exchange (e.g., pneumonia syndromes)	Oxygen
Intrapulmonary shunt (V/Q = 0)	No gas exchange by perfused alveoli (e.g., ARDS)	PEEP
Dead space (V/Q = ∞)	No perfusion of ventilated alveoli Pulmonary hypertension Excessive PEEP Shock states Pulmonary embolus	Pulmonary vasodilation Consider nitric oxide Decrease PEEP Augment cardiac output Thrombolysis/anticoagulation
Intracardiac shunting	Bypasses pulmonary circuit	Surgical correction
Diffusion disturbances	Slows gas exchange	Diuretics, steroids
Low PvO_2	Low cardiac output states, SVO_2 <65%	Inotropes to improve cardiac output Decrease utilization
High altitude	Decreased barometric pressure	Increase FiO_2
Despite adequate arterial oxygen level, (PaO_2) may have inadequate arterial oxygen content and oxygen delivery (DO_2) resulting in tissue hypoxia:		
Anemia	Decreased DO_2	Transfuse
Carbon monoxide poisoning	Decreased DO_2	100% oxygen, consider hyperbaric therapy
Methemoglobinemia	Decreased DO_2	2 mL/kg methylene blue IV

ARDS, acute respiratory distress syndrome; PEEP, positive end-expiratory pressure; V/Q, ventilation-perfusion.

In patients with acute lung diseases associated with carbon dioxide retention, a measured arterial carbon dioxide concentration ($PaCO_2$) greater than 50 mm Hg indicates inadequate ventilation and frequently the need for escalation of support (e.g., mechanical ventilation). For patients with chronic respiratory insufficiency, a $PaCO_2$ of 60 mm Hg may be acceptable and the practitioner must evaluate pH and bicarbonate levels to determine if there is an acute rise in $PaCO_2$. A 5-mm Hg increase in $PaCO_2$ will result in an approximately 0.05 decrease in the pH, and vice versa.

Conversely, in severe asthma, minute ventilation is initially increased, resulting in a $PaCO_2$ that is lower than normal. A normal $PaCO_2$ during an acute asthma episode indicates significant disease with evidence of respiratory fatigue. An ABG may also be useful to identify when tachypnea results from severe metabolic acidosis with respiratory compensation. Arterial oxygen concentration (PaO_2) is used to calculate the alveolar-arterial oxygen gradient (A-a gradient), which provides an assessment of the severity of injury. The normal value for an A-a gradient in children without lung disease or intracardiac shunt is approximately 10 mm Hg. A similar calculation to define the severity of hypoxemia is the ratio of PaO_2/FiO_2 (P/F ratio). Acute lung injury (ALI) and acute respiratory distress syndrome (ARDS) are defined by the P/F ratio.

ALI: PaO_2/FiO_2 <300 (e.g., PaO_2 <150 on FiO_2 >0.5)
ARDS: PaO_2/FiO_2 <200 (e.g., PaO_2 <100 on FiO_2 >0.5)

Another commonly calculated measure of respiratory insufficiency is the oxygenation index (OI)

$$OI = MAP \times FiO_2/\text{Postductal } PaO_2$$

where MAP = mean airway pressure. (An advantage of this equation is the inclusion of the MAP required to achieve the level of oxygenation.)

A measured PaO_2 is required to calculate the A-a gradient, P/F ratio, and OI. However, a capillary blood gas sample from a warmed, well-perfused extremity will provide accurate measurements of pH and $PaCO_2$ while the oximeter provides a reliable measurement of oxygenation. When available, a central venous blood gas measurement provides an alternate to measurement of arterial blood gas, with accurate estimations of arterial pH and CO_2. (This should preferably be a mixed venous sample from a pulmonary artery catheter; however, a central venous sample provides an acceptable surrogate recognizing that right atrial sampling is more accurate than the superior vena cava, which is more accurate than inferior vena cava.) In general terms, the venous pH is estimated to be .05 lower than the arterial, and the vCO_2 approximately 5 mm Hg higher than the arterial pH and CO_2. The venous saturation (SvO_2) provides additional information regarding the adequacy of oxygen delivery and extraction. In addition to blood gas analysis, most patients should have an electrolyte panel and complete blood count along with other laboratory investigations as indicated to aid the diagnostic evaluation. In addition to the pulse oximeter, near infrared spectroscopy (NIRS) is a new monitoring technique that will provide a valuable assessment of cerebral and somatic oxygen delivery. NIRS will approximate and trend the SvO_2.

The continuous measurement of the end-tidal CO_2 ($P_{ET}CO_2$), capnography, provides a noninvasive means of assessing the adequacy of either minute ventilation and/or pulmonary perfusion, comparing $PaCO_2$ to $P_{ET}CO_2$. Increased gradients between $PaCO_2$ and $P_{ET}CO_2$ correlate with increased physiologic dead space (e.g., decreased right ventricular output or increased pulmonary vascular resistance).

RADIOLOGY

A chest roentgenogram (CXR) is essential in the evaluation of respiratory failure. The chest radiograph can identify diffuse or focal airspace disease, pulmonary edema, pleural effusions, pneumothoraces, mediastinal abnormalities, or cardiomegaly. Skeletal and bony structures must always be evaluated. Soft-tissue neck radiographs are useful to evaluate upper airway compromise with disease processes like croup or retropharyngeal abscesses. Computed tomography (CT) scans of the chest have become an integral modality in the evaluation of many cases of respiratory failure and have significantly enhanced the understanding of the pathophysiology of many intrathoracic disease processes.

OTHER TESTS

Additional laboratory evaluation will depend on the differential diagnosis and frequently includes a complete blood count, often with C reactive protein (CRP) and a viral respiratory panel (enzyme immunoassay or direct fluorescent antibody). In addition, a basic metabolic panel (BMP) or comprehensive metabolic panel (CMP) may be indicated. More specific laboratory evaluation should be tailored to the differential diagnosis.

INITIAL SUPPORT

In the acutely ill patient, the hospitalist must first assess airway, breathing, and circulation to determine whether a patient requires emergent intervention as outlined by the Pediatric Advance Life Support (PALS) guidelines. A patent airway must be maintained or established, and supplemental oxygen should be administered to any patient in respiratory distress as the assessment is initiated. As a general guideline, all patients with respiratory distress should have stable intravenous access to facilitate administration of fluids and medications. Vascular access will also facilitate further interventions such as invasive and noninvasive ventilation, and cardiopulmonary resuscitation (CPR) should the patient's clinical status deteriorate. Patients with moderate to severe respiratory distress should be made nothing by mouth (NPO) to decrease the risk of emesis and aspiration. For patients with documented or suspected bacterial infectious processes, appropriate antibiotics should be administered.

In many cases, the management of respiratory distress in pediatric patients requires only noninvasive support with supplemental oxygen. Supplemental oxygen should be provided to maintain oxygen saturations greater than 92% (in patients with cyanotic heart disease, lower oxygen saturations may be acceptable). Common oxygen delivery systems include nasal cannula, simple face masks, and masks with reservoir bags. Nasal cannulae are capable of delivering between 22% and 40% oxygen, with the higher oxygen delivery in young patients with small minute ventilation. Flow rates are routinely set at 2 L/min initially and should not exceed 4 L/min. Simple face masks can deliver up to 60% oxygen and are designed for flow rates of 4 to 8 L/min. A minimum flow rate of 4 L/min should be maintained to avoid rebreathing exhaled CO_2. A reservoir bag can be attached to a simple face mask to increase the delivery of oxygen. The partial rebreather mask can deliver up to 80% oxygen, and a nonrebreather mask can deliver close to 100% inspired oxygen when the mask fits snugly. When using partial rebreather and nonrebreather masks, it is important to ensure high gas flow from the oxygen

source (15 L/min) to meet inspiratory demand and wash out exhaled carbon dioxide.

Another method of noninvasive support that may be useful is the use of Heliox, a blend of helium and oxygen. Helium is less dense than nitrogen and decreases turbulence through narrowed airways, allowing more laminar flow of gas. Heliox is used primarily for upper airway obstruction (e.g., croup, foreign body inhalation, postextubation stridor); it may also be considered in asthma. For optimal clinical effects, a helium concentration of at least 60% is required. Therefore helium-oxygen gas mixtures are limited to patients who can tolerate an FiO_2 <0.4. It is recommended that only commercially available tanks are used to deliver helium–oxygen mixtures to prevent circumstances where hypoxic gas mixtures are administered. Noninvasive ventilatory support (NIV), which includes nasal continuous positive airway pressure (CPAP) and bilevel positive airway pressure (BIPAP), has been demonstrated to be of benefit in certain clinical situations. These devices should be used by individuals experienced in their use as well as endotracheal intubation, as the patient's respiratory status may continue to deteriorate and their cardiopulmonary reserve to tolerate intubation, following a failed trial of NIV, may be limited.

Intubation and mechanical ventilation are indicated for patients in respiratory failure who are unable to maintain adequate ventilation and oxygenation despite less invasive means. Indications for mechanical ventilation in the treatment of respiratory failure are listed below.

INDICATIONS FOR ENDOTRACHEAL INTUBATION

- Apnea.
- Severe upper airway obstruction.
- Alveolar hypoventilation.
- Uncompensated respiratory acidosis with a $PaCO_2$ greater than 60 mm Hg.
  Some patients with chronic respiratory failure may have a compensated respiratory acidosis with a $PaCO_2$ >60 mm Hg but do not require mechanical ventilatory assistance, while patients with asthma may demonstrate signs of respiratory failure with much lower $PaCO_2$.
- Hypoxemia unresponsive to supplemental oxygen.
  Cyanosis with FiO_2 greater than or equal to 0.6 in the absence of cyanotic heart disease.
  PaO_2 less than 70 mm Hg with FiO_2 greater than 0.6.
  Alveolar-arterial oxygen gradient greater than 300 mm Hg with $FiO_2 = 1.0$
  P/F <300.
- Other clinical indices of severely impaired systemic oxygenation.

RELATIVE INDICATIONS FOR ENDOTRACHEAL INTUBATION

- Secure control of ventilatory pattern and function
- Shock states (SvO_2 <65 mm Hg)
- Decrease metabolic cost of breathing
- Chronic respiratory failure
- Deteriorating mental status
- Glasgow Coma Scale less than 8
- Intracranial hypertension
- Prolonged transport
- Procedures requiring sedation for an extended time, (e.g., MRI)

There is no absolute degree of hypercapnea or hypoxemia that necessitates mechanical ventilatory assistance and NIV is frequently becoming a first-line choice when airway control and ventilatory drive are maintained. Tracheal intubation is indicated when NIV is not feasible or is inadequate, but rarely is necessary when the $PaCO_2$ is less than 55 mm Hg and oxygen saturations can be maintained greater than 90%. The most common exceptions to this rule are status asthmaticus, where there is a clear benefit to maintaining spontaneous respiration, and chronic lung disease with chronic CO_2 retention. In patients with increased intracranial pressure, endotracheal intubation is indicated to control the airway and to prevent an increase in $PaCO_2$, as hypoventilation increases cerebral blood flow and accelerates intracranial hypertension. Relative indications for intubation include increased work of breathing with evidence of fatigue and altered mental status, the need to sedate for a critical procedure while ensuring adequate airway protection, or a prolonged transport.

Details of airway management and tracheal intubation are presented in Chapter 148. It is important to emphasize that all appropriate equipment must be at the bedside before proceeding with tracheal intubation. Sedation, with loss of endogenous catecholamines, and positive-pressure ventilation, which increases intrathoracic pressure and decreases preload, may cause an acute fall in cardiac output, especially in situations of volume depletion or ventricular dysfunction. Therefore, isotonic fluids should be readily available during intubation. Following placement of the endotracheal tube (ETT), correct placement and position must be confirmed. The use of a colorimetric CO_2 detector or $ETCO_2$ monitoring, to confirm tracheal intubation, is now standard of care.

Once the child has been intubated and placed on the ventilator, the clinician should reassess for adequacy of ventilation, noting chest expansion, quality of air movement, and symmetry of the breath sounds. Unequal breath sounds may result from endotracheal tube malposition, pneumothorax, pleural effusion, or severe atelectasis. A chest radiograph should be performed immediately to confirm appropriate tube position. Oxygenation should be continuously monitored by pulse oximetry, and a blood gas should be obtained. With severely elevated $PaCO_2$ due to lung disease, it is not expected to normalize the $PaCO_2$ immediately after intubation. Elevated but improving $PaCO_2$ can be tolerated as long as the pH is greater than 7.25. In situations with increased ICP or suspected pulmonary hypertension, the clinicians should achieve a $PaCO_2$ in the range of 33 to 37 mm Hg.

Whether utilizing a self-inflating or anaesthesia bag a manometer should be available to monitor delivered airway pressures, in addition to assessing chest rise and listening to breath sounds. It may initially be necessary to transiently occlude the pop-off valve on the self-inflating bag or utilize a PEEP valve in patients with poor compliance and/or loss of lung volume.

INITIAL VENTILATOR SETTINGS

Initial ventilator settings depend on the age of the patient and the severity of the lung disease. Basic ventilator parameters, to provide adequate alveolar ventilation and maintain oxygenation, until the patient can be transported to a pediatric intensive care unit, are outlined below.

Provision of Adequate Alveolar Ventilation

Rate (breaths/min) based on physiologic norm for age:

- Newborn: ~30 breaths/min
- 1 year old: 20 to 25 breaths/min
- 1 to 8 years: ~20 breaths/min
- Greater than 8 years: ~16 breaths/min

Tidal volume: adequate to move chest and generate good breath sounds:

- 6 mL/kg measured at endotracheal tube

The peak inspiratory pressure (PIP) should be monitored and maintained <35 cm H_2O.

Inspiratory time (Inspiratory/Expiratory ratio):

- The I:E ratio is generally 1:2.
- Obstructive diseases require prolonged expiratory time and lower rate (I:E $\Rightarrow$ 1:3 to 4).
  This can be determined by evaluating ventilator graphics or listening with a stethoscope to ensure that exhalation ends before the next breath is delivered.

Immediately assess for signs of adequate ventilation. Adjust synchronized intermittent mandatory ventilation (SIMV) rate and/or tidal volume to maintain $PaCO_2$ between 35 and 50 mm Hg.

Maintenance of Adequate Oxygenation

- FiO_2: 1.0 initially and wean as tolerated for SaO_2 >92%.
- Positive end-expiratory pressure (PEEP): 5 cm H_2O (check CXR for lung expansion).
- Immediately assess for signs of adequate oxygenation (e.g., color, pulse oximetry) and circulatory depression (e.g., hypotension, diminished peripheral pulses).
- Poor lung compliance and oxygenation may require higher PEEP.

The goal is FiO_2 <0.6, with expansion to approximately 9 ribs on anteroposterior chest x-ray. The hospitalist may choose either volume control or pressure control ventilation. The team caring for the patient must be familiar with whichever mode is chosen, and the patient on mechanical ventilation must be constantly monitored for changes in ETT air leak, pulmonary compliance, and displacement of the ETT. The parameters may require modification in several scenarios. In small infants, where the compliance of the ventilator tubing is high relative to the compliance of the lungs, tidal volumes as high as 15 mL/kg measured at the ventilator may be necessary to adequately ventilate the patient. The stomach should always be decompressed particularly following bag valve mask ventilation. In patients with poorly compliant lungs and difficulty with oxygenation, the PIP may exceed 30 cm H_2O, and a higher PEEP of 7 to 15 cm H_2O may be indicated. Patients with respiratory failure due to status asthmaticus require a lower respiratory rate and prolonged expiratory time (I:E ratio 1:2 to 1:4) to prevent further air trapping and CO_2 retention. FiO_2 should initially be set at 100%, but can be weaned to maintain saturations of 92% to 96% (or 80% in patients with cyanotic heart disease).

While stabilizing the patient with respiratory failure, the hospitalist should be arranging transport to a pediatric intensive care unit. Several important steps are necessary to prepare the patient for a safe transport. The endotracheal tube position should be adjusted as indicated by chest radiograph, and the patient should be sedated to help ensure stability of the airway during transport. The importance of securing the endotracheal tube properly with benzoin and strong adhesive tape or other device with which the team is familiar, cannot be overemphasized. Due to the potential detrimental effects of sedation and positive airway pressure on cardiac output, the cardiovascular system should be reassessed and stabilized. Monitoring during transport, even within the same institution, should include continuous electrocardiogram monitoring, continuous pulse oximetry, and intermittent blood pressure monitoring.

ADJUNCTIVE THERAPIES

High-Frequency Oscillatory Ventilation

High-frequency oscillatory ventilation (HFOV) is an alternative technique for providing mechanical ventilatory assistance that is being utilized more frequently in the ICU setting. HFOV is initiated with the goal of reducing tidal flow of ventilatory gasses while safely applying high mean airway pressures, thus minimizing alveolar distending pressures and maintaining FRC. When transitioning conventional mechanical ventilation to HFOV, the MAP is usually set approximately 5cm H_2O higher. Sufficient amplitude is provided to achieve visible movement of the chest wall (refered to as "wiggle"), and the initial oscillatory frequency in the pediatric population is usually 5 to 8 Hz. In order to increase ventilation (increase CO_2 removal), the frequency is decreased and the amplitude increased. Decreasing the frequency allows an increased tidal excursion of the piston producing an increase in the bulk flow of gas, while increasing the amplitude drives the piston a greater distance producing an increase in the bulk flow of gas. To increase oxygenation the FiO_2 or MAP are increased. Adequacy of the applied MAP is determined by evaluating lung expansion on an AP CXR with a goal of approximatley 9 ribs. There are no randomized, controlled studies to date mandating the use of either conventional ventilation or HFOV; however, many practitioners favor the use of HFOV when ventilating stiff, noncompliant lungs or in the presence of an air leak (e.g., pneumothorax or pneumomediastinum).

Nitric Oxide

Inhaled nitric oxide (NO) reduces pulmonary vascular resistance when the pulmonary vascular bed is reactive. It is a gaseous agent delivered with the ventilatory gases to ventilated lung units, where it induces vasodilation of the pulmonary vasculature associated with those ventilated lung units. NO induces cyclic GMP formation as it crosses the alveolar capillary membrane. NO is then rapidly deactivated upon contact with hemoglobin, minimizing systemic effects. Although it has been demonstrated to be efficacious in neonates and select cardiac patients with pulmonary hypertension, and does improve oxygenation in some patients with acute respiratory failure, NO has not been demonstrated to improve outcome with respect to ventilator-free days or survival beyond the neonatal period.

Prone Positioning

Prone positioning has been advocated to optimize V/Q matching and has been shown to improve oxygenation, without significant adverse effects. Prone positioning has not been shown to improve outcome with respect to ventilator-free days or survival in randomized, controlled trials in adult and pediatric populations.

Surfactant

Surfactant is an excellent therapeutic modality in neonates with surfactant deficiency, but the dose and indications for the use of surfactant preparations in respiratory failure beyond the neonatal period are under study and have not yet been determined.

Extracorporeal Life Support

Extracorporeal life support (ECLS) is an extreme method of cardiopulmonary support that enables CO_2 removal and oxygenation of blood outside the body by means of a membrane oxygenator (i.e., artificial lung). The therapeutic intent is to minimize ventilator-induced lung injury (VILI) while optimizing oxygen delivery and CO_2 removal. With improving survival statistics for patients with ARDS (now greater than 80% in some instances), the use of ECLS is declining. ECLS remains a rescue technique for patients failing to demonstrate an adequate response to mechanical ventilatory support alone. ECLS is initiated to allow partial bypass of the "pulmonary circuit" and enable "lung rest." Definitive criteria for initiating ECLS are not well established. In general terms, ECLS is initiated when, in the opinion of the managing physician, the patient is likely to succumb without ECLS. It is, however, well established that if ECLS is indicated, the earlier it is instituted, the more favorable the outcome, by reducing VILI. Veno-venous ECLS is favored by many practitioners, but if there is any cardiac dysfunction then veno-arterial ECLS is instituted. There remains an approximately 50% survival rate for pediatric patients with acute hypoxemic respiratory failure who require ECLS.

PEARLS

- Establishment of a patent airway and administration of supplemental oxygen are immediate priorities in the management of respiratory distress with the addition of ventilatory assistance in the event of respiratory failure.
- Pulse oximetry monitoring must be instituted.
- Observation of the patient is the most accurate determinant of the degree of respiratory disease.
- The patient's response to oxygen is a determinant of the amount of intrapulmonary shunting and therefore the severity of lung disease.
- Respiratory distress and failure are initially clinical diagnoses and initial therapy should not be delayed while awaiting laboratory confirmation.
- Respiratory muscle fatigue is common in children and may be manifested by abnormal respiratory patterns.
- Gastric distention may precipitate respiratory failure in an infant by compromising diaphragmatic excursion, and gastric distention predisposes to regurgitation and aspiration of gastric contents.
- SvO_2 is an excellent marker of oxygen utilization and demand.
- Hypoxemia and hypercarbia may have different etiologies. Acute hypercarbia requires intervention, although the presence of chronic hypercarbia may mitigate against assisted ventilation.
- There are multiple causes of, and treatments for, hypoxemia.
- Knowledge of the technical details of oxygen supplementation is essential.
- Effective bag mask ventilation is preferable to unsuccessful and repeated attempts at endotracheal intubation.
- A measured pulsus paradoxus of 15 mm Hg (palpable by the examiner) is associated with an $FEV_1 < 40\%$ of predicted, while a pulsus paradoxus of 20 mm Hg is associated with an $FEV_1 < 20\%$ of predicted, in patients with acute severe asthma.

Suggested Readings

Acute Respiratory Distress Syndrome Network. Ventilation with lower tidal volumes as compared with traditional tidal volumes for acute lung injury and the acute respiratory distress syndrome. *N Engl J Med* 2000;342: 1301–1308.

Brower RG, Lanken PN, MacIntyre N, et al. National Heart, Lung, and Blood Institute ARDS clinical trials network. Higher versus lower positive end-expiratory pressures in patients with the acute respiratory distress syndrome. *N Engl J Med* 2004;351:327–336.

Steinhorn DM, Green TP. The treatment of acute respiratory failure in children: a historical examination of landmark advances. *J Pediatr* 2001;139:604–608.

CHAPTER 42 ■ SLEEP-DISORDERED BREATHING

ANCHALEE YUENGSRIGUL

Sleep plays a major role in children's well-being. The maturation of the sleep–wake system exerts significant influences on the psychosocial and neurobehavioral functioning of the child. Furthermore, endocrine and metabolic physiology in humans is strongly influenced by sleep and wakefulness states. For example, growth hormone secretion is pulsatile and episodic, and there is a consistent relationship between growth hormone secretion and slow-wave sleep. Thus, the early identification and treatment of childhood sleep disorders is essential for the child's well-being. Sleep-disordered breathing has been associated with various physiologic and neurobehavioral dysfunctions including sleep fragmentation and disorganization of sleep stages and cycles, behavioral problems and neurocognitive impairment, failure to thrive, and cor pulmonale.

Normal Respiration During Sleep

Sleep induces changes in the physiology of breathing and control of the respiratory system. Ventilation during sleep is decreased compared to the awake state. There is a decrease in tidal volume and respiratory rate, which results in a decline in minute ventilation. In addition, a sleep-related decrease in upper-airway tone results in a marked increase in upper-airway resistance. Finally, hypoxic and hypercapnic ventilatory drives decrease during sleep, especially during rapid-eye movement sleep. Normal children experience an increase in the partial pressure of carbon dioxide and a decrease in arterial oxyhemoglobin saturation during sleep. These effects are exaggerated and may result in significant ventilatory and gas exchange abnormalities in children with underlying pulmonary or upper airway problems such as adenotonsillar hypertrophy, obesity, craniofacial anomalies, chronic obstructive lung disease, and neuromuscular disorders (1).

Upper Airway

The pharyngeal airway behaves like a collapsible tube. The maintenance of a patent pharyngeal airway requires a variety of upper airway muscles to generate enough force to overcome the collapsing tendency of the inspiratory negative intrapharyngeal pressure produced by the diaphragm. Both anatomic and neural factors determine the collapsibility of the pharynx and the size of the upper airway. In children, the lymphoid tissue of the upper airway increases from birth until approximately 12 years of age. Simultaneously, there is gradual growth in the size of the skeletal boundaries of the upper airway. Thus, between 2 and 8 years of age, the tonsils and adenoid are the largest in relation to the underlying airway, resulting in a relatively narrow upper airway (2).

Arousal

Arousal is the important defense mechanism for sleep-breathing disorders. Hypercapnia and increased upper airway resistance are potent stimuli for arousal. Hypoxemia is the less potent stimulus for arousal, especially in infants and young children. Children have a higher arousal threshold and fewer spontaneous arousals than adults (2).

CLASSIFICATION OF APNEA

Sleep apnea is the cessation of breathing during sleep. These episodes result in hypoxemia and sleep disruption. Apnea can be classified as obstructive, central, or mixed.

- Central apnea is defined as pauses in respiration without ventilatory effort, which is caused by a reduction of neural impulses from the central nervous system to the muscles of respiration.
- Obstructive apnea is the cessation of breathing during sleep from obstruction of the upper airway despite ventilatory effort.
- Mixed apneas usually begin with a central respiratory pause followed by obstructive apnea from increasing breathing efforts against an obstructed airway.

Central Apnea

Central apnea is an absence of both airflow at the nose and mouth and movements of the chest wall and abdomen. Central apnea without physiologic consequence is found in both normal infants and children. Central apneas of short duration (less than 10 seconds) are common in neonates and occur more often during rapid-eye movement (REM) than non-rapid eye movement (NREM) sleep. In addition, other physiologic apneas such as movement-associated apnea and sigh-preceded central apneas are common in children of all ages. In general, these episodes last less than 20 seconds. Central apneas have been considered significant if they last longer than 20 seconds or if they are associated with oxygen desaturation, bradycardia, or arousal.

Periodic Breathing and Sighs

Periodic breathing is the alternation between breathing periods and 5- to 10-second apnea. It is defined as three episodes of apnea lasting longer than 3 seconds, separated by continued respiration of 20 seconds or less. It occurs in waking and all sleep stages but more commonly in REM sleep. Periodic breathing is more frequent in preterm infants, varies across studies in full-term infants, and decreases during the first year of life.

Many factors can increase periodic breathing in neonates and infants, including hypoxia, hyperthermia, and sleep deprivation.

Sighs are large (more than twice baseline tidal volume) augmented breaths that are necessary to reopen airways and recruit underventilated zones. Sighs are initiated by an inspiration-augmenting reflex arising in vagal afferents, probably from rapidly adapting pulmonary mechanoreceptors. This vagally mediated stimulus triggers an end-inspiratory reinforcement gasp that is superimposed near the peak of an apparently normal breath. Sighs are more frequent on the first days of life in preterm compared to term infants and in REM compared to quiet sleep. There is no strong association between sighs and apnea, with apnea being equally distributed either before or after a sigh. Decrease in lung volume during REM sleep and the relative hypoxemia of this sleep state plays a role in triggering sighs.

Obstructive Apnea

Obstructive apnea is defined as cessation of airflow at the nose and mouth in the presence of continued respiratory effort lasting longer than two respiratory cycle times, usually but not always associated with hypoxemia.

Mixed Apnea

Mixed apneas begin with a central respiratory pause followed by increasing breathing efforts against an obstructed airway. Mixed apneas share the same pathophysiology and clinical significance as obstructive apneas.

Hypopnea

Hypopneas occur when airflow decreases significantly but does not stop altogether. It is defined as a 50% or greater decrease in the amplitude of the nasal/oral airflow signal, often accompanied by hypoxemia or arousal. It can be classified into obstructive and nonobstructive subtypes. In obstructive hypopnea, there is a reduction in airflow without a reduction in effort. In contrast with nonobstructive hypopnea, there is a reduction in both airflow and respiratory effort by 50%.

Normal Data

Apnea

Central apneas are common in infants and children, particularly during REM sleep. In general, these episodes are less than 20 seconds in length. However, some normal physiologic central apnea of longer than 20-second duration is commonly observed after sighs or movement. Central apneas are considered significant if they last longer than 20 seconds, or are associated with desaturation, bradycardia, or arousal. However, these central apnea episodes are considered clinically significant if they occur frequently or there are associated gas-exchange abnormalities. In contrast to central apneas, obstructive apneas of any length are rare in normal children (2). In a multicenter study of 1,053 healthy infants with polygraphic recordings, the incidence of obstructive apnea index was in the range of 0 to 4.2/hour (3). A study of 50 normal children aged 1 to 18 years found that only 18% had even a single obstructive apnea during the night, and all obstructions were 10 seconds or less in duration. The mean obstructive apnea index was 0.1 ± 0.5/hour (4). There are no normative data for hypopneas in children. The only study evaluating hypopneas did not publish the hypopnea data separately, but found a total respiratory disturbance index (apneas and hypopneas) of 1.1/hour (5).

Gas Exchange

Infants and healthy children have baseline pulse oximetry values (SpO_2) between 95% and 100%. Brief desaturations frequently occur in association with central apnea or periodic breathing in normal infants. Hourly transient desaturations to less than 80% occurring in conjunction with short central apneas are seen in 80% of the 1- to 2-month-old infants. In healthy children 2 to 16 years of age, the frequency of transient desaturation is much lower than in infants, and decreases with advancing age. During sleep, normal children and adolescents rarely show more than an 8% drop in SpO_2, more than four desaturation episodes per hour, or an SpO_2 nadir below 90% (1).

During sleep, there is relative hypercapnia compared with wakefulness. Transcutaneous CO_2 tension (PCO_2) increases 1 to 3 mm Hg from wakefulness to sleep. Baseline PCO_2 values during sleep are generally between 36 and 42 mm Hg in newborns and infants (6). In 50 normal children ranging in age from 1.1 to 17.4 years, the mean maximal end-tidal CO_2 tension ($EtCO_2$) value during sleep was 46 ± 4 mm Hg (range, 38 to 53). Normal children have shown an increase in $EtCO_2$ values of 4 to 10 mm Hg during sleep (4).

ABNORMAL BREATHING DURING SLEEP

The clinical problems of sleep apnea and sleep-disordered breathing include a number of different disorders, either resulting from different pathophysiologic mechanisms or representing different points along a continuous spectrum:

- Snoring
- Obstructive sleep apnea syndrome (OSAS)
- Chronic pulmonary disease and sleep
  - Obstructive lung disease
  - Restrictive lung disease: pulmonary and chest wall
  - Restrictive lung disease: ventilatory muscle weakness
- Syndromes affecting respiratory control during sleep
  - Idiopathic congenital central hypoventilation syndrome
  - Myelomeningocele with Arnold–Chiari malformation
  - Prader–Willi syndrome
  - Obesity hypoventilation syndrome

Snoring

Snoring is loud upper airway breathing sounds in sleep, which is caused by vibration of the soft palate and indicates upper-airway narrowing during sleep. Snoring is a cardinal symptom of obstructive sleep and breathing disorders; as such, it can be a marker of obstructive sleep apnea. Habitual snoring in children is a common phenomenon. It occurs in 3% to 12% of preschool-aged children (7,8). It is possible that a certain amount of pharyngeal narrowing during sleep is unimportant, as it does not produce significant sleep fragmentation or sleep apnea. However, in a subpopulation of snorers, there are symptoms that it seems reasonable to ascribe to sleep fragmentation. Most of this association seems to be due to snoring and sleep disturbance, without frank sleep apnea.

It is possible, however, that habitual snoring, even in the absence of clear-cut OSAS, places children at risk. Recent studies demonstrated that snoring without overt OSAS may be associated with neurocognitive abnormalities. Ferreira and associates (9) demonstrated in a population-based cross-sectional study of 988 Portuguese children that habitual snorers were twice as likely as nonsnorers to have an abnormal score on the Children's Behavioral Questionnaire. Blunden and co-workers (10) compared 16 children referred for adenotonsillectomy or snoring to a control group and found impaired selective and sustained attention scores only in the children who snored. They also reported that the snoring children had significantly lower average IQ scores.

Obstructive Sleep Apnea Syndrome

Obstructive sleep apnea syndrome (OSAS) in children is a disorder of breathing during sleep characterized by partial upper airway obstruction and/or intermittent complete obstruction that disrupts ventilation and sleep quality. It is associated with symptoms including snoring, sleep difficulties, and/or daytime neurobehavioral problems. Complications may include growth abnormalities, neurologic disorders, and cor pulmonale, especially in severe cases. Adenotonsillar hypertrophy is the most common cause of OSAS in normal children between the ages of 2 and 6. Children with craniofacial anomalies and/or neurologic disorders affecting upper-airway configuration and collapsibility during sleep may present at any time from early infancy through childhood.

Prevalence

The prevalence of childhood OSAS is estimated to be around 2%, whereas habitual snoring is more common and is estimated to occur in 3% to 12% of preschool-aged children. OSAS occurs in children of all ages, including neonates. The peak age of OSAS is reported to be between 2 and 6 years, paralleling the developmental peak of adenotonsillar hyperplasia. Children with other underlying conditions affecting the structure of the upper airway, such as craniofacial anomalies, may present with symptoms of obstruction early in the neonatal period, while a later onset of symptoms may be found in obese children, associated with excessive weight gain or growth of the tonsils and adenoids.

Pathophysiology

Obstructive sleep apnea syndrome (OSAS) is characterized by recurrent closure of the pharyngeal airway during sleep. Its pathophysiology remains poorly understood. Although OSAS is related to adenotonsillar hypertrophy in children, this is not likely the sole cause of sleep-disordered breathing in this age group. The upper airway is a collapsible structure, the patency of which is dictated by a combination of passive mechanical properties and active neural mechanisms. Sleep produces changes in airway physiology, which in association with abnormal anatomy, lead to sleep-disordered breathing events and the syndrome of obstructive sleep apnea. Additional interactions between abnormal anatomy and normal or pathologic variables, including ventilatory, neurologic, and other factors, contribute to further compromise an inherently vulnerable upper airway.

Children with OSAS appear to have a deficit in arousal mechanisms. Studies have shown that these patients have elevated arousal thresholds in response to hypercapnia and increased upper airway resistance. Children with OSAS often do not have EEG arousals following obstructive apneas, and sleep architecture is preserved. Although apnea-related EEG arousals are less common in children than adults, subcortical arousals such as movement or autonomic changes occur frequently. These factors may contribute to neurobehavioral and autonomic complications (2).

Risk Factors

Although most cases of OSAS in children are secondary to enlarged tonsils and adenoids, many other medical conditions may lead to OSAS including patients with craniofacial and neurologic disorders affecting upper airway anatomy and patency during sleep (Table 42.1). Children who are neurologically impaired are at additional risk for developing OSAS due to multiple factors including muscular hypotonia, abnormal control of ventilation, and poor arousal mechanisms.

Adenotonsillar Hypertrophy. Adenotonsillar hypertrophy is the leading cause of OSAS in children. The peak prevalence of childhood OSAS occurs at 2 to 6 years, which is the age when the tonsils and adenoid are the largest in relation to the underlying airway size. Although enlarged tonsils and adenoids are clearly an important risk factor in children, a number of studies have shown that there is no absolute correlation between the size of the tonsils and adenoids and the presence of OSAS. The etiology of OSAS is likely multifactorial, involving a combination of the structural characteristics and neuromotor control of the child's upper airway during sleep.

Craniofacial Anomalies. OSAS occurs frequently in children with craniofacial anomalies with midfacial hypoplasia, micro- or retrognathia, or macroglossia, such as Crouzon syndrome, Pfeiffer syndrome, Treacher–Collins syndrome, Goldenhar syndrome, and Pierre Robin sequence. These anomalies lead to a decrease in the size of the nasopharynx, oropharynx, or hypopharynx, and can predispose to upper airway collapse during sleep. Some children with severe craniofacial anomalies require tracheostomies soon after birth because of fixed upper airway narrowing. However, less severely affected individuals may develop upper airway obstruction only during sleep, suggesting that there must be some combination of structural and dynamic factors for OSAS to occur. In some patients with craniofacial anomalies, OSAS begins or recurs during early childhood, in conjunction with adenotonsillar hypertrophy.

Obesity. Obesity has been increasingly recognized as a risk factor for the development of OSAS in the pediatric population. In a large epidemiologic study (11) of 399 children and adolescents aged 2 to 18 years, obesity was the strongest predictor of sleep-disordered breathing, with an odds ratio of 4.59. Several factors may contribute to OSAS in this group. Upper airway narrowing may result from deposition of adipose tissue within the muscles and soft tissues surrounding the upper airway and result in narrowing of the upper airway and increased pharyngeal resistance. In addition, obese subjects have been shown to have decreased chest wall compliance and displacement of the diaphragm resulting in restrictive lung defect in the supine position. This may result in decreased lung volumes and oxygen reserves during sleep, and may increase the severity of OSAS in this group.

Sign and Symptoms

The most common complaints of parents with children with OSAS are snoring and difficulty breathing during sleep. Increased respiratory efforts described as retractions, vigorous breathing, gasping, and grunting are often described by the parents. Airflow and ventilation disruptions due to airway obstruction during sleep cause significant gas exchange abnormalities with hypoxemia and hypercapnia. Restless sleep and unusual sleep positions (prone, neck extension, propped up on pillows) are well-observed phenomena in childhood OSAS. Other abnormal behavior during sleep such as night sweats and nocturnal enuresis are variable findings in children with OSAS. Furthermore, abnormal daytime behavior including hyperactivity and aggressiveness have been observed in 31% to 42% of children with OSAS (12). In contrast to adults, excessive daytime sleepiness is not a common complaint in children with OSAS, and is rarely the main presenting symptom in children. In the most severe cases, these nocturnal disturbances have been associated with

TABLE 42.1

PREDISPOSING FACTORS AND CONDITIONS FOR CHILDHOOD
OBSTRUCTIVE SLEEP APNEA SYNDROME

Craniofacial syndromes
- Midfacial hypoplasia
  Apert syndrome
  Crouzon syndrome
  Pfeiffer syndrome
  Treacher–Collins syndrome
- Macroglossia/glossoptosis
  Down syndrome
  Beckwith–Wiedeman syndrome
  Pierre Robin sequence
- Others
  Achondroplasia
  Hallerman–Streiff syndrome
  Klippel–Feil syndrome
  Goldenhar syndrome
  Marfan syndrome

Nasal obstruction
- Adenoid hypertrophy
- Nasal stenosis/hypoplasia
- Choanal atresia
- Septal deviation

Oropharyngeal obstruction
- Tonsil hypertrophy
- Macroglossia
- Micrognathia
- Retrognathia

Laryngeal obstruction
- Laryngeal web
- Laryngeal papilloma/other tumors
- Laryngeal web
- Subglottic stenosis
- Laryngomalacia
- Laryngeal hemangioma
- Vocal cord paralysis
- Previous airway surgery/scar/stenosis
- Laryngomalacia
- Airway papillomatosis
- Subglottic stenosis

Neurologic disorders
- Cerebral palsy
- Myasthenia gravis
- Möbius syndrome
- Arnold–Chiari malformation

Miscellaneous disorders
- Obesity
- Prader–Willi syndrome
- Hypothyroidism
- Mucopolysaccharidosis
- Sickle-cell disease
- Face and neck burns
- Gastroesophageal reflux disease

Modified from Arens, R. Obstructive sleep apnea in childhood: clinical features. In: Loughlin GM, Carroll JL, Marcus CL, eds. *Sleep and breathing in children. Lung biology in health and disease.* New York: Dekker; 2000:578.

daytime hypersomnolence, failure to thrive, and right heart failure.

Physical Examination

Most of the children with OSAS have a normal physical examination while awake. However, various physical findings suggest the underlying conditions associated with OSAS.

- Mouth breathing, hyponasal voice can indicate nasopharyngeal obstruction such as adenoidal hypertrophy.
- Nasal cavity: mucosal or turbinate swelling, septal deformity, and intranasal masses.
- Pharynx: small naso-oropharyngeal cavity, narrow cross-sectional area in patients with high-arched and elongated soft palate, large tongue, tonsilar hypertrophy, or reposition of the mandible.
- Craniofacial anomalies: midface hypoplasia, retrognathia, and micrognathia.
- Chest deformities: pectus excavatum can be present in some children with long-standing OSAS as the consequence of prolonged periods of ribcage paradox.
- Growth pattern: mildly diminished height and weight and in severe cases, failure to thrive have been described as the consequence of OSAS. Obesity, on the other hand, is associated with increased incidence of OSAS.
- Cardiovascular examination: evidence of systemic and pulmonary hypertension. Systemic hypertension, especially diastolic hypertension, has been reported to be associated with OSAS in children (13).
- Neurologic examination: focus on developmental status, muscle tone and strength, and cranial nerve functions.

Sequelae

The clinical consequences of OSAS are a direct result of a combination of sleep and breathing disorders. The repetitive arousals from sleep needed to reestablish collapsed upper airway patency lead to sleep fragmentation and poor sleep quality, which further exerts significant influences on the psychosocial and neurobehavioral functioning of the child. In addition, the apneic and hypopnic episodes represent periods of asphyxia that can result in hypoxemia, hypercapnia, and profound hemodynamic disturbances.

Cognitive and Behavioral Abnormalities. Neurologic and behavioral symptoms are commonly seen in children with sleep-disordered breathing. Cross-sectional studies suggest a nearly threefold increase in behavior problems, and neurocognitive abnormalities in children with sleep-disordered breathing include attention disorders, memory and learning disabilities, school failure, developmental delay, hyperactivity, aggressiveness, and withdrawn behavior. Improvement in academic and school performance has been demonstrated following successful treatment of obstructive sleep apnea syndrome, suggesting a link between abnormal breathing during sleep and these neurocognitive problems (14).

Growth. Early reports of children with OSAS described children with failure to thrive. Even though overt failure to thrive is uncommon these days because of early recognition and treatment, children with OSAS often have poor growth. This appears to be due to increased work of breathing associated with upper airway obstruction and increased airway resistance (15) and disruption of nocturnal growth hormone secretion caused by poor sleep quality and sleep fragmentation (16).

Improved growth has been demonstrated after treatment of childhood OSAS with adenotonsillectomy.

Cardiovascular Complications. Severe untreated OSAS can lead to cardiovascular complication including systemic and pulmonary hypertension, cor pulmonale, and heart failure. These appear to be reversible after adenotonsillectomy or after specific treatment of the OSAS. Systemic hypertension is a known complication of adult OSAS, and elevated diastolic blood pressure has been found in children with OSAS. The degree of blood pressure dysregulation correlates with the severity of the OSAS. Increased blood pressure variability and systemic hypertension during sleep have been shown to be associated with end-organ damage and an increased risk for cardiovascular diseases (17). Pulmonary hypertension results from the recurrent severe nocturnal hypoxemia, hypercarbia, and acidosis that occur during hypoventilation or apnea. OSAS in children can result in cardiac remodeling and hypertrophy of both the right and left ventricles. A study of 27 children with OSAS using radionuclide to evaluate ventricular function showed significantly abnormal right heart function. There was a decreased right ventricular ejection fraction in 37% of these children and abnormal wall motion in 67%. All of the 11 patients who had a repeat evaluation after adenotonsillectomy showed improvement (18). Cor pulmonale is readily reversible by treatment of OSAS, but perioperative precautions are required in these high-risk patients.

Diagnosis

Symptoms. OSAS can cause a variety of daytime and nighttime symptoms in children. A sleep history screening for snoring should be part of routine health care visits. Snoring and difficulty breathing during sleep are the most common complaints of parents of children with OSAS. In addition, parents often report nighttime sweating, restless sleep, and sleeping in unusual positions. Daytime symptoms associated with OSAS include mouth breathing, nasal obstruction, and hyponasal speech. Excessive daytime sleepiness and morning headache are less common in children with OSAS. Problems with learning and behavior also have been reported repeatedly in case series of children with OSAS.

Physical Examination. Physical examination of the child with OSAS is highly variable. Signs and symptoms of upper airway obstruction should be evaluated including nasal obstruction, adenotonsillar hypertrophy, micrognathia and retrognathia, midfacial hypoplasia, large tongue, and high-arched and elongated palate. Evidence of complications of OSAS may be present. These include systemic hypertension, an increased pulmonic component of the second heart sound indicating pulmonary hypertension, and poor growth. Obesity, on the other hand, with increasing incidence in children, is a risk factor for developing OSAS. Chest and respiratory examination are usually normal, although pectus excavatum has been reported in some patients secondary to prolonged periods of ribcage paradox.

Diagnostic Evaluation. *Overnight Polysomnography.* The gold standard for diagnosis of OSAS is overnight polysomnography (PSG) performed in a sleep lab. Polysomnography simultaneously records multiple physiologic variables including sleep state, respiration, cardiac rhythm, muscle activity, gas exchange, and snoring. It is the only diagnostic technique shown to quantify the ventilatory and sleep abnormalities associated with sleep-disordered breathing. It can distinguish primary snoring from OSAS. It can objectively determine the severity of OSAS and related gas exchange and sleep disturbances. It appears that the severity of PSG abnormality is an important predictor of complications in the immediate postoperative period after adenotonsillectomy. Polysomnography can be performed in children of any age, and should be scored and interpreted using age-appropriate criteria as outlined in the American Thoracic Society consensus statement on pediatric polysomnography (19).

Normative respiratory data during sleep are far more controversial (Table 42.2). Although a number of studies are available, they are based on relatively small sample sizes, and do not necessarily address the ages at which childhood OSAS is most prevalent. On the basis of normative data, an obstructive apnea index of 1 is often chosen as the upper limit of normal. However, although an apnea index of 1 is statistically significant, it is not known what level is clinically significant. Sleep-disordered breathing in childhood consists of a spectrum of disease, ranging from primary snoring to upper airway resistance syndrome, obstructive hypoventilation, and obstructive sleep apnea. Parameters for defining these conditions have not been established. Furthermore, few normative data are available for some of the important factors required in establishing these diagnoses, such as hypopneas, degree of paradoxical inward ribcage movement during inspiration, and esophageal pressure swings.

Alternatives to Polysomnography. History and physical examination are poor at predicting OSAS. Videotape and

TABLE 42.2

POLYSOMNOGRAPHIC VALUES AND RECOMMENDED NORMAL VALUES

	Mean ± SD	Range	Recommended normal values	Children classified as abnormal (%)
Apnea index (number/hr)	0.1 ± 0.5	0–3.1	≤1	2
Maximum PETCO$_2$ (mm Hg)	46 ± 4	38–53	≤53	0
Minimum PETCO$_2$ (mm Hg)	38 ± 3	28–44	NA	NA
Δ PETCO$_2$ (mm Hg)	7 ± 3	2–11	≤13	0
Duration of PETCO$_2$ >45 mm Hg (%TST)	6.9 ± 19.1	0–90.5	≤60	6
Maximum SaO$_2$ (%)	100 ± 1	98–100	NA	NA
Minimum SaO$_2$ (%)	96 ± 2	89–98	≥92	4
Desaturation >4%/hr TST (number)	0.3 ± 0.7	0–4.4	≤1.4	2
Δ SaO$_2$ (%)	4 ± 2	0–11	≤8	4

NA, not applicable.
Modified from Marcus CL, Omlin KJ, Basinki DJ, et al. Normal polysomnographic values for children and adolescents. *Am Rev Respir Dis* 1992; 146:1235–1239.

audiotape recoding have been helpful in predicting OSAS when positive and can be used as screening studies, but unfortunately do not rule out the diagnosis of OSAS when negative. Overnight oximetry can be useful if it shows a pattern of cyclic desaturation. A study that compared overnight oximetry with simultaneous polysomnography in a group of children with suspected OSAS demonstrated high positive predictive value but low negative predictive value (20).

In summary, other studies such as videotaping, nocturnal pulse oximetry, and daytime nap polysomnography tend to be helpful if results are positive but have a poor predictive value if results are negative. Thus, children with negative study results should undergo a more comprehensive evaluation.

Treatment

Tonsillectomy and Adenoidectomy. Adenotonsillectomy remains the first-line treatment of OSAS in otherwise healthy children. Adenotonsillar hyperplasia plays a key role in the compromise of airway patency during sleep, and removal of tonsils and adenoids cures OSAS in most children. Although obese children may have less satisfactory results, many will be adequately treated with adenotonsillectomy, and it is generally the first-line therapy for these patients. Potential complications of adenotonsillectomy include anesthetic complications, postoperative problems such as pain and poor oral intake, and hemorrhage. In addition, patients with OSAS may develop respiratory complications, such as worsening of OSAS or pulmonary edema, in the immediate postoperative period. Death attributable to respiratory complications in the immediate postoperative period has been reported in patients with severe OSAS. Identified risk factors are young age, failure to thrive, cor pulmonale, presence of neuromotor disease, craniofacial abnormalities, history of prematurity, recent respiratory infection, obesity, and severe OSAS on polysomnography. High-risk patients should be hospitalized overnight after surgery and monitored continuously with pulse oximetry (21).

Predictors of Postoperative Complications. Tonsillectomy and adenoidectomy (T&A) is the standard first-line treatment for childhood OSAS, resulting in a cure in the majority of patients. However, children with OSAS are at greater postoperative risk for respiratory compromise than children undergoing T&A for other indications. Postoperative respiratory complications include transient worsening of OSAS secondary to postoperative edema and increased secretions; respiratory depression from anesthetic agents, narcotics, and the use of oxygen in children with a blunted hypoxic ventilatory drive; and the occurrence of postobstructive pulmonary edema. Risk factors for postoperative respiratory complications in children with OSAS undergoing adenotonsillectomy include age younger than 3 years, severe OSAS on polysomnography, cardiac complications of OSAS (e.g., right ventricular hypertrophy), failure to thrive, obesity, prematurity, recent respiratory infection, craniofacial anomalies, and neuromuscular disorders (22). High-risk patients should be monitored as inpatients postoperatively.

Continuous Positive Airway Pressure (CPAP). Continuous positive airway pressure (CPAP) and bilevel positive airway pressure (BiPAP) are the alternative treatment for childhood with persistent OSAS after adenotonsillectomy or for children with contraindications for surgery. CPAP delivers pressurized air via a mask interface to stent the upper airway and increase functional residual capacity in the lungs. The pressure requirement varies among individuals; thus, CPAP must be titrated in the sleep laboratory before prescribing the device, and it must be periodically readjusted as indicated. Children may develop central apneas or hypoventilation at higher pressure levels. This can be treated by placing the patient on bilevel ventilation with a backup rate. Complications of CPAP or BiPAP usually are minor and include eye irritation, conjunctivitis, and skin ulcera-

tion from poor mask fit. Nasal symptoms such as congestion or rhinorrhea also are common, and can be relieved by nasal steroids or humidification. Other uncommon complications are midfacial depression and nasal deformities from prolonged use of the device. CPAP and BiPAP are generally well tolerated in older children. However, young children or older children with learning or behavioral problems may require behavioral or desensitization techniques. CPAP is a long-term therapy and requires frequent clinician assessment of adherence and efficacy and monitoring of possible potential complications.

Other Treatment Modalities. Some patients, especially those with underlying craniofacial malformations, cerebral palsy, and hypotonia of the upper airway muscle, may continue to have significant obstructive apnea despite adenotonsillectomy. In these selected cases, a uvulopalatopharyngoplasty, a tongue reduction, or a craniofacial reconstruction has been used, with varying success. Some specific cases with severe obstruction may require tracheostomy to bypass the upper airway obstruction if these surgeries cannot provide the relief of the obstruction. Oral appliances have been the effective treatment for some adults with mild OSAS (22). However, this is not recommended in children due to concern about interference with facial bone development and configuration.

Weight loss should be implemented in obese patients. Some studies reported transient benefit of intranasal corticosteroids for nasal and nasopharyngeal obstruction (23). Supplemental oxygen has been used as a temporary treatment of hypoxemia in some patients. However, oxygen therapy does not prevent sleep-related upper airway obstruction, sleep fragmentation, and increased work of breathing. Furthermore, it may worsen hypoventilation and hypercapnia. If oxygen therapy is to be used in children with OSAS, it should be evaluated during continuous PCO_2 monitoring to assess its effect on hypoventilation (24).

Follow-Up of Patients Undergoing Surgical Treatment for OSAS

All patients should have clinical follow-up for reassessment of symptoms and signs associated with OSAS after initial treatment. Although T&A is helpful in relieving OSAS in patients with adenotonsillar hypertrophy, children with severe disease may not be completely cured by surgery. Patients who continued with symptoms, who have severe OSAS, or who are obese require objective reevaluation to determine whether additional therapy, such as CPAP, is required.

Prognosis

The long-term prognosis and the natural history of childhood OSAS is unknown. It is possible that children at risk for OSAS have underlying factors such as a small pharyngeal airway or decreased upper airway neuromuscular tone. These may predispose to the recurrence of OSAS during adulthood if they acquire additional risk factors, such as androgen secretion at puberty and weight gain. A study by Guilleminault and associates (26) has demonstrated a 13% recurrence rate in adolescents who had been successfully treated for childhood OSAS. This suggests that children with OSAS, despite treatment, may be at a higher risk for the development of adult OSAS.

Chronic Pulmonary Disease and Sleep

Ventilation during sleep is decreased compared to the awake state. Normal children experience an increase in the partial pressure of carbon dioxide and a decrease in arterial oxyhemoglobin saturation during sleep. These effects are exaggerated and may result in significant ventilatory and gas exchange abnormalities in children with lung disease and a limited pulmonary reserve, such as in obstructive lung disease, bronchopulmonary dysplasia, asthma, and cystic fibrosis; restrictive lung disease from pulmonary and chest wall abnormalities; and ventilatory muscle weakness.

Obstructive Lung Disease

Patients with obstructive lung disease have little functional reserve, and are more likely to desaturate, especially during REM sleep, as the result of sleep-related intercostal muscle hypotonia and increased ventilation–perfusion mismatch. Thus, patients with adequate oxygenation during wakefulness may desaturate during sleep, especially during REM sleep. Other physiologic factors that will exacerbate sleep-disordered breathing in children with chronic lung disease include bronchoconstriction, reduced mucociliary clearance, and decreased cough during sleep. Pediatric patients with bronchopulmonary dysplasia, asthma, and cystic fibrosis have been shown to have prolonged episodes of hypoxemia during sleep, despite the presence of adequate oxygenation while awake.

Bronchopulmonary dysplasia (BPD). In infants with BPD, the combination of abnormal pulmonary mechanics and REM-related loss of inspiratory muscle activity results in ribcage paradox and hypoxemia. These episodes are not always predicted by blood gas measurements when awake and may not be detected by monitoring oxyhemoglobin during daytime naps, direct observation, or by recording techniques with delayed response time, such as transcutaneous PO_2 monitoring. Oxygen saturation during feeding and sleep should be measured for an extended period in infants and children with BPD who are on oxygen or recently been weaned to room air when awake if unusual conditions develop such as polycythemia, cor pulmonale, failure to thrive, disturbed sleep patterns, or apnea and bradycardia during sleep (20,25).

Studies have shown that maintaining SaO_2 above 92% in infants with resolving BPD was associated with better growth. In the most severe cases, oxygen supplementation alone may not be sufficient to maintain health. Nocturnal ventilatory support may be necessary and can be managed at home. A full polysomnography study can be of assistance in deciding when to discontinue the ventilatory support.

Cystic Fibrosis. Episodes of desaturation unrelated to apnea have been observed in some patients with cystic fibrosis. The mechanisms underlying O_2 desaturation during sleep in cystic fibrosis patients include alterations in ventilation–perfusion matching, decrease in the tonic activity of intercostal and diaphragmatic muscles in REM sleep stage, decrease in end-expiratory lung volume, and decreases in tidal volume and minute ventilation. Patients with cystic fibrosis who have an awake $PaO_2 < 70$ mm Hg or an equivalent SaO_2 (<95%) during a period of disease stability are at risk for worsening hypoxemia during sleep and should have continuous determination of SaO_2 during nocturnal sleep. This study should be performed during a period of disease stability in order to determine the extent and severity of sleep-associated hypoxemia and confirm the adequacy of prescribed supplemental oxygen. Patients with cystic fibrosis who develop polycythemia, cor pulmonale unexplained by awake blood gas or SaO_2 measurements, or who complain of headaches upon awakening, excessive daytime sleepiness, or disturbed sleep patterns, should also undergo continuous documentation of SaO_2 for at least 8 hours overnight during sleep. Patients with cystic fibrosis receiving supplemental oxygen may require PSG to rule out OSAS, if there is a history of snoring, desaturation episodes during sleep, cor pulmonale, polycythemia or disturbed sleep. Polysomnography should also be considered for assessing the potential adverse effects of supplemental oxygen during sleep in patients with advanced lung disease who are hypercapnic when awake.

Asthma. Many patients with asthma experience nocturnal symptoms. The contributing factors to exacerbations of asthma at night include circadian changes in ventilation, airway responsiveness and inflammation, mucociliary clearance, ventilatory responses to hypercapnia and hypoxia, and hormone levels. The circadian variation in airway caliber seen in normal children is amplified in patients with asthma and may produce as much as a 50% decrease in peak flow rate. Patients with asthma, including those suboptimally controlled, tend to have small changes in SaO_2 during sleep (26). Asthmatic children who have nocturnal symptoms should have a thorough clinical investigation including an assessment of the environment and the appropriateness of nocturnal therapy to identify factors that may contribute to these symptoms. PSG with esophageal pH monitoring should be considered if there is concern about the presence of gastroesophageal reflux during sleep as a trigger for nocturnal symptoms. PSG may be abnormal in children with poorly controlled nocturnal asthma who exhibit disturbed sleep, morning headaches, or cor pulmonale (20,25).

Restrictive Lung Disease: Pulmonary and Chest Wall

Kyphoscoliosis. Children with severe kyphoscoliosis may have significant sleep-related breathing problems. Failure of alveolar multiplication and enlargement play a major role in respiratory abnormalities in congenital kyphoscoliosis. Respiration is more vulnerable during sleep due to decreased ventilatory responses to hypoxia and hypercapnia, reduced chest wall compliance, and abnormal configuration of the diaphragm and diminished diaphragmatic contraction. These problems are compounded by reduced tone in the upper airway muscles during REM sleep. Patients with severe kyphoscoliosis cannot increase ventilatory activity because of a combination of mechanical and chest deformity, airway distortion, and depressed ventilatory drive. Nocturnal hypoventilation generally precedes respiratory failure diagnosed by conventional blood gas analysis during wakefulness and may be detected even when waking blood gases are normal. The best indicators are the level and severity of the scoliosis, forced vital capacity, resting arterial PCO_2 during the day and night, and presence or absence of muscular weakness.

Patients with scoliosis frequently have severe nocturnal hypoxemia, obstructive apnea, and hypoventilation. The greatest oxygen desaturation occurs in most patients during REM sleep. Sleep related breathing disorder may be recognized by clinical features, such as early morning headaches caused by carbon dioxide retention, daytime sleepiness caused by sleep deprivation because of repeated apnea-induced arousals, or restlessness during sleep caused by movement or arousal. PSG is useful in analyzing the severity of nocturnal oxygen desaturation, hypoventilation, and sleep derangements in children with kyphoscoliosis. Short-term ventilation has been associated with a marked improvement in clinical signs of respiratory failure in kyphoscoliosis. Children have been provided with noninvasive ventilatory support at night using negative-pressure ventilators, nasal bilevel ventilatory support, or nasal intermittent positive-pressure ventilation. For many patients, ventilatory support is usually only needed at night to improve quality of life and prognosis (27).

Achondroplasia. Achondroplasia is an autosomal-dominant skeletal dysplasia from defective endochondral ossification resulting in small stature with disproportionate shortening of the proximal limbs, short flared ribs, megalencephaly with a short cranial base, small foramen magnum, and midface hypoplasia. These patients are at risk for several types of respiratory complications. Their abnormal ribcage results in restrictive lung disease with low functional residual capacity that may cause airway closure, atelectasis, hypoxemia, and alveolar hypoventilation. The abnormal skull base, and stenosis of the foramen magnum with resultant brainstem compression, can result in spinal cord compression and central apnea or vocal cord paralysis that may produce sudden unexpected death. Patients with achondroplasia are at high risk for sleep-disordered breathing. A study of 88 children with achondroplasia found that 48% had sleep-disordered breathing and 44% had at least one episode of desaturation to <90%. However, in this study many of the patients had isolated hypoxemia, and 7 patients required supplemental oxygen. This was not a population-based study, and many of these patients had additional lung disease. However, their hypoxemia appeared out of proportion to the degree of lung disease, suggesting a restrictive component (28). All patients with achondroplasia warrant a thorough pulmonary evaluation including chest roentgenograms and overnight polysomnography, including measurement of exhaled CO_2 to evaluate central and obstructive apnea and hypoventilation. Electrocardiography and an echocardiogram may be needed to evaluate right heart strain from hypoxemia. Pulmonary function testing is helpful in patients old enough to cooperate. Although there appears to be no relationship between foramen magnum stenosis and sleep-disordered breathing, patients with respiratory problems not caused by OSA, restrictive pulmonary disease, or other primary pulmonary system disorders should undergo brainstem imaging studies to evaluate the brainstem because they may benefit from cervical cord decompression. Adenotonsillectomy was less effective and nasal CPAP may be the best treatment for OSA in patients with achondroplasia (29,30).

Restrictive Lung Disease: Ventilatory Muscle Weakness

Neuromuscular Disease. Children and young adults with a variety of pediatric neuromuscular disorders are at risk of developing both central and obstructive apnea/hypoventilation during sleep. These disorders include Duchenne muscular dystrophy (DMD), myotonic dystrophy, spinal muscle atrophy, diaphragmatic paralysis, cerebral palsy, poliomyelitis, and congenital muscle diseases. Abnormal breathing during sleep in these disorders is often not predicted by pulmonary function testing, arterial blood gases, or the degree of muscle involvement when awake.

Patients with muscular dystrophies demonstrate increasing weakness with age, and if left untreated, usually die of either respiratory or cardiac failure as adolescents or young adults. Respiratory muscle weakness, apneas and hypopneas, and abnormalities of breathing pattern and ventilatory drive may all contribute to nocturnal desaturation and sleep disruption, even before daytime ventilatory failure ensues. The most common form of sleep-disordered breathing in patients with respiratory muscle weakness is hypoventilation due to reduced tidal volume, particularly during REM sleep. In addition, they have a high incidence of obstructive apnea, presumably due to upper airway muscle weakness. Polysomnography, including either end-tidal or transcutaneous CO_2 monitoring, is indicated in evaluating children with neuromuscular disease who demonstrate impaired respiratory muscle function evidenced by a forced vital capacity <40%, a peak inspiratory pressure <15 cm H_2O, pharyngeal dysfunction (snoring or swallowing abnormalities), cor pulmonale, morning headaches, personality or behavioral changes, failure to thrive, or developmental delay disproportionate to the degree of neurologic impairment or the typical course of the disease.

Treatment

Oxygen Therapy

Supportive therapy is essential in patients with chronic lung disease and nocturnal hypoxemia. Medical management should be maximized with bronchodilators and anti-inflammatory agents, and nutrition should be optimized. Airway clearance with chest physical therapy and other modalities to enhance coughing and secretion clearance is useful in patients with ventilatory muscle weakness. Adequate oxygenation is necessary for neurocognitive development, cardiac function, and optimal growth.

Correction of sleep-related hypoxemia has been demonstrated to improve growth in infants with BPD. Supplemental oxygen is recommended to maintain SaO_2 >93% in infants with chronic lung disease in order to optimize health.

Supplemental oxygen is used frequently in patients with cystic fibrosis, particularly in patients with severe disease and a PaO_2 <60 mm Hg during wakefulness. The long-term consequences of brief episodes of oxygen desaturation during sleep are unknown. Nocturnal oxygen supplementation may improve the quality of life during the day by improving cognitive function. Oxygen therapy has been shown to be safe, with no excessive CO_2 retention, in most patients who are free from hypercapnia during the daytime. However, in some patients, carbon dioxide retention to this degree can have a clinically significant effect Importantly, there is currently no evidence that the improvements in nocturnal oxygen saturation with supplemental oxygen use are accompanied by changes in sleep quality, daytime function, or survival (31).

Noninvasive Positive-Pressure Ventilation

The use of noninvasive positive-pressure ventilation (NIPPV) for both acute and chronic respiratory failure in children has been increasing rapidly in recent years. NIPPV is being used frequently in children with advanced cystic fibrosis, either as supportive therapy or as a bridge to transplantation. Studies over months to years of use have shown an improvement in oxygenation, ventilation, and vital capacity, as well as subjective symptomatic improvement. NIPPV has also been used successfully to treat respiratory failure secondary to kyphoscoliosis in adults. NIPPV via nasal mask has been used widely in children and adolescents with ventilatory muscle weakness, including Duchenne muscular dystrophy and spinal muscular atrophy (2).

NIPPV improves survival and quality of life in patients with neuromuscular diseases. Positive-pressure breathing corrects obstructive sleep apnea, improves hypoventilation, and assists diaphragm failure in neuromuscular disease. The upper airway is supported, preventing obstructive apneas or hypopneas, and leading to a greater improvement in both oxygenation and sleep architecture (32). Daytime arterial blood gases improve with long-term nocturnal ventilation, and are associated with an increased ventilatory response to carbon dioxide (33). Supplemental oxygen via a mask is recommended when positive air pressure therapy is insufficient to overcome SpO_2 <90%. Bilevel positive airway ventilation is tolerated better by patients who have weak chest walls and diaphragm and who cannot overcome expiratory forces. Supplemental oxygen via nasal cannula may be sufficient in some cases to correct REM sleep-related desaturation. Tracheostomy may be indicated in some patients with advanced restrictive lung disease and severe chest-wall and diaphragmatic muscle weakness, but the dependence and complications that it causes have to be weighed against the benefits. Ethical considerations of prolongation of life versus improvement of quality of life may have to be addressed in patients who have terminal neuromuscular disease. Young children tolerate nasal ventilation poorly, and other therapeutic measures may have to be considered, including temporal use of tracheostomy (34).

Syndromes Affecting Respiratory Control During Sleep

There are multiple neurologic disorders of respiratory control that will affect breathing, especially during sleep and in some cases while awake.

- Idiopathic congenital central hypoventilation syndrome
- Myelomeningocele with Arnold–Chiari malformation

- Prader–Willi syndrome
- Obesity hypoventilation syndrome

Idiopathic Congenital Central Hypoventilation Syndrome

Idiopathic congenital central hypoventilation syndrome (CCHS) is a rare disorder with approximately 160 to 180 living children worldwide (35). It is defined as the disorder of autonomic control of breathing since birth of unknown etiology. Patients have the characteristic of hypoventilation with shallow breathing most severely affected while asleep, especially during quiet sleep. The severity of this disorder can range from mild hypoventilation during sleep with adequate awake ventilation to the severe degrees with hypoventilation both awake and asleep. Patients have nearly absent respiratory response to hypoxia and hypercapnia and no respiratory discomfort during CO_2 inhalation.

The cause or causes of CCHS are unknown. There is an association between CCHS and Hirschsprung disease, a condition characterized by abnormalities of the cholinergic innervations of the gastrointestinal tract. The estimated incidence of Hirschsprung disease among patients with CCHS ranges from 10% to 50% (36). These associations suggest that autonomic neuropathy, particularly of the parasympathetic system, is important in CCHS. In addition, recent studies have demonstrated abnormalities of the gene encoding the transcription factor Phox 2b, a transcription factor belonging to signaling pathways known to be essential for early autonomic nervous system development. Approximately 90% of patients with CCHS have heterozygous mutations in the Phox 2b gene. These findings are consistent with an autosomal-dominant pattern of inheritance for CCHS (37–39).

Patients with CCHS require nocturnal ventilatory support and some patients require support both awake and asleep. Several ventilatory support options are available. These include positive-pressure ventilation via tracheostomy, noninvasive positive-pressure ventilation, negative-pressure ventilation, and diaphragmatic pacers. Supplemental oxygen alone is inadequate treatment. Early diagnosis and adequate ventilatory support are key to management for optimal neurodevelopment and good quality of life.

Myelomeningocele with Arnold–Chiari Malformation

Arnold–Chiari malformations (ACMs) are congenital or acquired herniations of the cerebellum through the foramen magnum. The primary anatomic abnormality is caudal displacement of the cerebellum through the foramen magnum, resulting in brainstem compression. Type 1 is characterized by caudal displacement of the brainstem occasionally with herniation of the cerebellar tonsils through the foramen magnum. It is usually not accompanied by myelomeningocele. Type 2 includes cerebellar vermis herniation, in association with myelomeningocele, hydrocephalus, and displacement of the fourth ventricle below the foramen magnum (40).

Sleep-disordered breathing has been recognized with ACM, especially with ACM type 2, including obstructive sleep apnea, central apnea, and hypoventilation. Abnormal vocal cord motility and the resultant obstructive apnea in infants with myelomeningocele is a major manifestation of abnormal ventilation. In addition, infants with myelomeningocele, hydrocephalus, and ACM have abnormalities in their ventilatory pattern during sleep. High clinical suspicion for sleep-disordered breathing in ACM, early investigation, and early treatment may improve the clinical outcome. Management includes surgical treatment of hydrocephalus and brainstem decompression and evaluation for proper treatment of sleep-disordered breathing. Brainstem decompression may improve sleep-disordered breathing in ACM, but significant numbers of patients continue to have sleep-disordered breathing after decompression surgery.

Patients with signs of upper airway obstruction or obstructive sleep apnea should undergo laryngoscopy to evaluate vocal cord function. Tracheostomy is usually required if vocal cord paralysis is present. Some infants and children with myelomeningocele and ACM develop inadequate ventilation during sleep or during both sleep and wakefulness. This central hypoventilation syndrome requires chronic ventilatory support. Infants and children with myelomeningocele with severe neurologic damage, who also require assisted ventilation, have a poor prognosis because of progressive neurologic deterioration (41).

Prader–Willi Syndrome

Prader–Willi syndrome (PWS) is a multisystemic disorder characterized by neonatal hypotonia, dysmorphic facies, obesity, hyperphagia, hypogonadism, mental retardation, behavioral disorders, and sleep disorders. The prevalence of this disorder is estimated at 1 per 10,000 to 1 per 25,000 live births. PWS is a sporadic genetic mutation. Approximately 70% of affected people acquire PWS from a sporadic microdeletion of the long arm of chromosome 15 at q11q13, and 20% inherit both copies of chromosome from their mother (42).

Patients with PWS often exhibit sleep-disordered breathing. This is characterized by snoring, obstructive sleep apnea, restless movements during sleep, hypoventilation, hypoxia, excessive daytime sleepiness, and abnormalities of sleep architecture (43). Various studies have demonstated disorder of ventilatory control in patients with PWS. Rebreathing ventilatory responses to hypercapnia are depressed in obese PWS patients but not in nonobese patients. Ventilatory responses to hypoxia are depressed in both obese and nonobese PWS patients, suggesting a primary disorder of ventilatory control from peripheral chemoreceptor dysfunction. In addition, hypothalamic dysfunction in this syndrome may contribute to the ventilatory control abnormality seen in these patients (42).

Patients with PWS generally exhibit behavior disorders. Although neurobehavioral abnormalities are assumed to be of genetic origin, it is possible that sleep-disordered breathing and sleep hypoxemia also contribute to these symptoms. Polysomnographic studies in PWS demonstrate that the majority of PWS patients exhibit obstructive sleep apnea syndrome. Age-adjusted body mass index was associated with more severe hypoxemia during sleep and more sleep disruption. Increasing severity of obstructive sleep apnea (OSA) or sleep disturbance was associated with daytime inactivity/sleepiness, autistic-related behavior, and impulsiveness (44).

Hypothalamic dysfunction appears to underlie many of the features of PWS, including short stature, hypogonadism, and the defective regulation of energy balance. Growth hormone deficiency and blunted growth hormone secretion have been demonstrated in PWS (45). Many studies have investigated the effect of GH administration on body size and body composition in children with PWS.

Many studies have demonstrated growth hormone–induced alterations in body composition, decreased body fat, increased lean body mass, and increased linear growth in children with PWS. Many of these children appear to have growth hormone deficiency. Dosages used have varied in different studies. Higher doses may be necessary to sustain improvements in body composition (46).

There have been reports of fatalities associated with the use of exogenous growth hormone treatment in children with PWS. The deaths were associated with respiratory problems and/or were unexpected. The patients had one or more of the following risk factors: severe obesity, sleep apnea, or respiratory infection. Whether the deaths were directly related to the use of growth hormone therapy is unknown. Children with PWS appear to have an increased risk of sudden unexpected death independent of growth hormone therapy (47,48). However, growth hormone therapy may exacerbate an underlying condition in a subset of patients with PWS. Growth hormome and insulin growth factor-I have been proposed to lead to increased lymphoid tissue growth in some cases. Tonsillar and adenoidal hypertrophy could contribute to sleep apnea. Patients with PWS should be evaluated for signs of upper airway obstruction and sleep apnea before initiation of treatment with growth hormone. Growth hormone is contraindicated in PWS patients who are severely obese or have severe respiratory impairment. If, during treatment with growth hormone, patients show signs of upper airway obstruction and/or new-onset sleep apnea, growth hormone treatment should be interrupted (49).

Obesity Hypoventilation Syndrome

Obesity, particularly morbid obesity, is associated with a wide range of respiratory disturbances. Obesity leads to alterations of respiratory mechanics, airflow resistance, breathing pattern, and respiratory drive; impaired gas exchange; impaired exercise capacity; and sleep-disordered breathing from obstructive sleep apnea and alveolar hypoventilation. Obesity leads to reductions in lung, chest wall, and total respiratory system compliance. Obesity hypoventilation syndrome (OHS) is commonly defined as a combination of severe obesity and awake arterial hypercapnia ($PaCO_2$ >45 mm Hg) in the absence of other known causes of hypoventilation. Patients may present with symptoms such as excessive daytime sleepiness, fatigue, or morning headaches, similar to symptoms seen in obstructive sleep apnea-hypopnea syndrome. However, patients with OHS have daytime hypercapnia and hypoxemia, which is associated with pulmonary hypertension and right-sided congestive heart failure. This syndrome results in substantial morbidity and probable early mortality if left untreated (49). An abnormality in respiratory control has been suggested by the demonstration that patients with OHS have decreased respiratory responsiveness to both hypoxemia and hypercapnia. The syndrome may result from complex interactions among impaired respiratory mechanics, abnormal central ventilatory control, possible sleep-disordered breathing, and neurohormonal disturbances. OHS has been demonstrated in children with morbid obesity. These children with severe obesity hypoventilation syndrome often have severe obstructive sleep apnea, hypoxia, hypercapnia both awake and asleep, hypersomnolence, and cor pulmonale similar to adults with OHS.

Treatment of OHS in children includes the treatment of obstructive sleep apnea and weight loss. Adenotonsillectomy remains the initial therapeutic procedure for obstructive sleep apnea. These patients have increased risk of postoperative complications, including worsening of OSAS or pulmonary edema, apnea, and hypoventilation due to abnormal breathing control from chronic prolonged hypoxemia and hypercapnia. Ventilatory support with CPAP or bilevel positive-airway pressure may be required postoperatively in some patients. Some patients will require therapy in addition to tonsillectomy and adenoidectomy. In severely affected patients, a tracheostomy may be required to relieve the upper airway obstruction. Supplemental oxygen can be used as interim therapy while awaiting more definitive treatment. Hypercapnic patients should be carefully monitored with end-tidal PCO_2 during the introduction of supplemental oxygen to be sure that hypoventilation does not worsen (42).

References

1. Rosen CL. Maturation of breathing during sleep: infant through aldolescents. In: Loughlin GM, Carroll JL, Marcus CL, eds. *Sleep and breathing in Children. Lung biology in health and disease.* New York: Dekker; 2000: 181–196.

2. Marcus CL. Sleep-disordered breathing in children. *Am J Respir Crit Care Med* 2001;164:16–30.
3. Kahn A, Franco P, Kato I, et al. Breathing during sleep in infancy. In: Loughlin GM, Marcus CL, Carroll JL, eds. Sleep and breathing in children—a developmental approach. New York: Dekker; 2000:405–422.
4. Marcus CL, Omlin KJ, Basinki DJ, et al. Normal polysomnographic values for children and adolescents. *Am Rev Respir Dis* 1992;146:1235–1239.
5. Acebo C, Millman RP, Rosenberg C, et al. Sleep, breathing, and cephalometrics in older children and young adults. *Chest* 1996;109:664–672.
6. Hoppenbrouwers T, Hodgman JE, Arakawa K, et al. Transcutaneous oxygen and carbon dioxide during the first half year of life in premature and normal term infants. *Pediatr Res* 1992;31:73–79.
7. Ali NJ, Pitson DJ, Stradling JR. Snoring, sleep disturbance, and behaviour in 4–5 year olds. *Arch Dis Child* 1993;68:360–366.
8. Gislason T, Benediktsdottir B. Snoring, apneic episodes, and nocturnal hypoxemia among children 6 months to 6 years old. *Chest* 1995;107: 963–966.
9. Ferreira AM, Clemente V, Gozal D, et al. Snoring in Portuguese primary school children. *Pediatrics* 2000;106:e64. Available at: http://www.pediatrics.org/cgi/content/full/106/5/e64.
10. Blunden S, Lushington K, Kennedy D, et al. Behavior and neurocognitive performance in children aged 5–10 years who snore compared to controls. *J Clin Exp Neuropsychol* 2000;22:554–568.
11. Redline S, Tishler PV, Schluchter M, et al. Risk factors for sleep-disordered breathing in children: associations with obesity, race, and respiratory problems. *Am J Respir Crit Care Med* 1999;159:1527–1532.
12. Guilleminault C, Korobkin R, Winkel R. A review of 50 children with obstructive sleep apnea syndrome. *Lung* 1981;159:275–287.
13. Guilleminault C, Winkle R, Korobkin R, et al. Children and nocturnal snoring: evaluation of the effects of sleep related respiratory resistive load and daytime functioning. *Eur J Pediatr* 1982;139:165–171.
14. Marcus CL, Greene MG, Carroll JL. Blood pressure in children with obstructive sleep apnea. *Am J Respir Crit Care Med* 1998;157:1098–1103.
15. Gozal D. Sleep-disordered breathing and school performance in children. *Pediatrics* 1998;102:616–620.
16. Marcus CL, Carroll JL, Koerner CB, et al. Determinants of growth in children with the obstructive sleep apnea syndrome. *J Pediatr* 1994;125:556–562.
17. Nieminen P, Lopponen T, Tolonen U, et al. Growth and biochemical markers of growth in children with snoring and obstructive sleep apnea. *Pediatrics* 2002;109:1–6.
18. Amin RS, Carroll JL, Jeffries JL, et al. Twenty-four-hour ambulatory blood pressure in children with sleep-disordered breathing. *Am J Respir Crit Care Med* 2004;169:950–956.
19. Tal A, Leiberman A, Margulis G, et al. Ventricular dysfunction in children with obstructive sleep apnea: radionuclide assessment. *Pediatr Pulmonol* 1988;4:139–143.
20. American Thoracic Society. Standards and indications for cardiopulmonary sleep studies in children. *Am J Respir Crit Care Med* 1996;153:866–878.
21. Brouillette RT, Morielli A, Leimanis A, et al. Nocturnal pulse oximetry as an abbreviated testing modality for pediatric obstructive sleep apnea. *Pediatrics* 2000;105:405–412.
22. American Academy of Pediatrics: Section on Pediatric Pulmonary and subcommittee on obstructive sleep apena syndrome. Clinical practice guideline: diagnosis and management of childhood obstructive sleep apnea syndrome. *Pediatrics* 2002;109:704–712.
23. Ferguson KA. The role of oral appliance therapy in the treatment of obstructive sleep apnea. *Clin Chest Med* 24;2003:355–364.
24. Brouillette RT, Manoukian JJ, Ducharme FM, et al. Efficacy of fluticasone nasal spray for pediatric obstructive sleep apnea. *J Pediatr* 2001;138: 838–844.
25. Brouillette RT, Waters K. Oxygen therapy for pediatric obstructive sleep apnea syndrome: how safe? How effective? *Am J Respir Crit Care Med* 1996;153:1–2.
26. Guilleminault C, Partinen M, Praud JP, et al. Morphometric facial changes and obstructive sleep apnea in adolescents. *J Pediatr* 1989;114:997–999.
27. Smith TF; Hudgel DW. Arterial oxygen desaturation during sleep in children with asthma and its relation to airway obstruction and ventilatory drive. *Pediatrics* 1980;66:746–751.
28. Bandla H, Splaingard M. Sleep problems in children with common medical disorders. *Pediatr Clin North Am* 2004;51:203–227.
29. Mogayzel PJ, Carroll JL, Loughlin GM, et al. Sleep-disordered breathing in children with achondroplasia. *J Pediatr* 1998;132:667–671.
30. Zucconi M, Weber G, Castronovo V, et al. Sleep and upper airway obstruction in children with achondroplasia. *J Pediatr* 1996;129:743–749.
31. Waters KA, Everett F, Sillence DO, et al. Treatment of obstructive sleep apnea in achondroplasia: evaluation of sleep, breathing, and somatosensory-evoked potentials. *Am J Med Genet* 1995;59:460–466.
32. Milross MA, Piper AJ, Dobbin CJ, et al. Sleep disordered breathing in cystic fibrosis. *Sleep Med Rev* 2004;8:295–308.
33. Barbe F, Quera-Salva MA, de Lattre J, et al. Long-term effects of nasal intermittent positive-pressure ventilation on pulmonary function and sleep architecture in patients with neuromuscular diseases. *Chest* 1996;110: 1179–1183.
34. Annane D, Quera-Salva MA, Lofaso F, et al. Mechanisms underlying effects of nocturnal ventilation on daytime blood gases in neuromuscular diseases. *Eur Respir J* 1999;13:157–162.

35. Culebras A. Sleep and neuromuscular disorders. *Neurol Clin* 2005;23: 1209–1223.

36. American Thoracic Society. Idiopathic congenital central hypoventilation syndrome: diagnosis and management. *Am J Respir Crit Care Med* 1999; 160:368–373.

37. Trang H, Dehan M, Beaufils F, et al. The French Congenital Central Hypoventilation Syndrome Registry: general data, phenotype, and genotype. *Chest* 2005;127:72–79.

38. Gaultier C, Amiel J, Dauger S, et al. Genetics and early disturbances of breathing control. *Pediatr Res* 2004;55:729–733.

39. Weese-Mayer DE, Berry-Kravis EM, Zhou L, et al. Idiopathic congenital central hypoventilation syndrome: analysis of genes pertinent to early autonomic nervous system embryologic development and identification of mutations in PHOX2b. *Am J Med Genet* 2003;123A:267–278.

40. Gaultier C, Trang HA, Dauger S, et al. Pediatric disorders with autonomic dysfunction: what role for PHOX2B? *Pediatr Res* 2005;58:1–6.

41. Zolty P, Sanders MH, Pollack IF. Chiari malformation and sleep-disordered breathing: a review of diagnostic and management issues. *Sleep* 2000; 23:1–7.

42. Keens TG, Ward SL. Syndromes affecting respiratory control during sleep In: Loughlin GM, Carroll JL, Marcus CL, eds. *Sleep and breathing in children. Lung biology in health and disease.* New York: Dekker; 2000: 525–548.

43. Mascari MJ, Gottlieb W, Rogan PK, et al. The frequency of uniparental disomy in Prader-Willi syndrome: implications for molecular diagnosis. *N Engl J Med* 1992;326:1599–1607.

44. Cassidy SB, McKillop J, Morgan W. Sleep disorders in Prader-Willi syndrome. *Dysmorphol Clin Genet* 1990;4:13–17.

45. O'Donoghue FJ, Camfferman D, Kennedy JD, et al. Sleep-disordered breathing in Prader-Willi syndrome and its association with neurobehavioral abnormalities. *J Pediatr* 2005;147:823–829.

46. Angulo M, Castro-Magana M, Mazur B, et al. Growth hormone secretion and effects of growth hormone therapy on growth velocity and weight gain in children with Prader-Willi syndrome. *J Pediatr Endocrinol Metab* 1996;9: 393–400.

47. Wilson TA, Rose SR, Cohen P, et al. Update of guidelines for the use of growth hormone in children: the Lawson Wilkins Pediatric Endocrinology Society drug and therapeutics committee. *J Pediatr* 2003;143:415–421.

48. Nagai T, Obata K, Tonoki H, et al. Cause of sudden, unexpected death of Prader-Willi syndrome patients with or without growth hormone treatment. *Am J Med Genet A* 2005;136:45–48.

49. Schrander-Stumpel CT, Curfs LM, Sastrowijoto P, et al. Prader-Willi syndrome: causes of death in an international series of 27 cases. *Am J Med Genet A* 2004;124:333–338.

50. Olson AL, Zwillich C. The obesity hypoventilation syndrome. *Am J Med* 2005;118:948–956.

CHAPTER 43 ■ NEURODIAGNOSTIC STUDIES

STANFORD SHU

DIAGNOSTIC REASONING IN NEUROLOGY

The analysis and interpretation of the history and physical examination may be adequate for diagnosis. Special diagnostic studies then only corroborate the clinical impression. However, often the disease process is narrowed down to one of several possibilities. When this occurs, one then resorts to the ancillary tests discussed in this chapter. The aim of the clinician is to arrive at a final diagnosis by careful analysis of the data with the least number of laboratory procedures.

SPINAL FLUID EXAMINATION

Cerebrospinal fluid (CSF) has several functions including acting as a buffer against trauma and as a means to return various substrates back to the venous circulation.

Most of the CSF is secreted by the choroid plexus via a carbonic anhydrase–dependent mechanism. Some CSF is from water and other substances passively diffusing from meningeal vessels and the ependyma. The rate of CSF formation varies from 25 mL/day in a neonate to 750 mL/day in an adult. Total CSF volume ranges from 50 mL in a neonate to 150 mL in an adult. The CSF volume changes completely five times per day. Normal CSF pressure ranges from 90 to 120 mm H_2O in a neonate to 60 to 180 mm H_2O in a young child to 120 to 200 mm H_2O in a teenager or adult.

CSF secreted in the lateral ventricles passes through the foramina of Munro into the third ventricle and subsequently through the aqueduct of Sylvius into the fourth ventricle. CSF leaves the ventricular system either through the lateral foramina of Luschka or the midline foramen of Magendie to either flow upward over the cerebellar hemispheres or downward to the spinal cord. CSF is primarily reabsorbed through the arachnoid villi and to a limited extent by blood vessels and the lymphatic system.

A lumbar puncture for evaluation of the CSF is indicated when there is suspicion for infectious, demyelinating, or autoimmune processes. Increased intracranial pressure or a coagulopathy are contraindications to a lumbar puncture. Severe increased intracranial pressure may be manifested by papilledema, lack of venous pulsations over the optic disc, a bulging anterior fontanel, effacement of the cortical sulci, or tonsillar herniation on a neuroimaging study. Therefore, a neuroimaging study is always recommended prior to a lumbar puncture in a patient with a closed fontanel.

Local anesthesia with either lidocaine or EMLA cream should be placed in an area that is not infected. Common puncture sites are between L3 and L4, L4 and L5, and L5 and S1. A 20- or 22-guage needle with a stylet that is 2.5 to 5 cm long is used after the skin is sterilized. The needle is inserted in the midline with the bevel of the needle angled horizontally so that it passes vertically between the fibers of the dura mater. The needle is then advanced slowly until the ligamentum flavum and dura mater are pierced with a "popping" sensation. The stylet is then removed and the opening pressure is measured. If no fluid appears, the needle should then be rotated 90°. If this is still not effective, then withdraw the needle and select another interspace. Opening pressure is measured with the child in a relaxed lateral decubitus position. If the child is sitting, the opening pressure is then measured from the point where the foramen magnum is located. Approximately 5 mL of fluid should be collected in 4 tubes with 1 to 2 mL per tube. Cells from the CSF are calculated from tubes 1 and 3. Neonates have 7.5 ± 9 white blood cells/mm^3. Children up to 1 year of age may still have up to 10 cells/mm^3. Eight white blood cells/mm^3 is the upper limit up to 4 years of age. In older children and adults, the upper limit is 5 cells/mm^3. Excessive red cells indicate either hemorrhage or traumatic puncture. Fewer red cells in tube 3 as compared to tube 1 suggest a traumatic puncture. The ratio of 1 white blood cell for every 750 red blood cells after a traumatic puncture does not reliably differentiate white blood cells due to CSF pleocytosis from an inflammatory or reactive process.

Fluid from tube 1 may also be used to evaluate microorganisms visually through a Gram stain (bacteria), India ink (cryptococcus), or acid-fast stain (tuberculosis). Bacterial and viral cultures require at least 0.5 mL of fluid each. Approximately 20% of patients with signs of bacterial meningitis may have no evidence of pleocytosis in the CSF but have a positive culture. Counterimmunoelectrophoresis (CIE) can distinguish among the encapulated organisms, but has low sensitivity and high false-negative results. Latex agglutination is more sensitive than CIE. PCR amplification for *Streptococcus pneumoniae*, *Haemophilus influenzae*, herpes simplex, enterovirus, and cytomegalovirus are very accurate. The presence of CSF lactate or C-reactive protein studies for bacterial meningitis are nonspecific.

Glucose enters the CSF via a carrier-mediated transport system and is approximately two-thirds of serum glucose. Low glucose can be caused by increased metabolism of glucose or decreased entry of glucose into the CSF (Table 43.1).

Total CSF protein content is relatively high at birth with a mean of 80 mg/dL and decreases to adult levels by 10 years of age. Total CSF protein content is lowest in the ventricles and highest at the lumbar region (Table 43.2). Froin syndrome is caused by an obstruction of CSF flow due to a mass lesion causing a lumbar CSF protein content greater than 500 mg/dL.

TABLE 43.1

ETIOLOGY OF CSF HYPOGLYCEMIA

INCREASED GLUCOSE METABOLISM
Infection
Subarachnoid hemorrhage
Carcinomatous meningitis
Chemical meningitis

DECREASED GLUCOSE TRANSPORT
Glucose transporter defect

TABLE 43.2

TOTAL CSF PROTEIN CONTENT

Anatomic area	Protein (mg/dL)
Ventricles	<5
Cisterna magna	10–25
Lumbar region	15–45

Electrophoresis and immunoelectrophoresis of the CSF protein allow for identification of individual proteins that are helpful in diagnosing various CNS processes (Table 43.3). The changes in immunoglobulins are expressed as percentage of total protein, percentage of albumin, or ratios of CSF IgG/serum IgG to CSF albumin/serum albumin.

Neurometabolic studies from the CSF are helpful in identifying mitochondrial disorders (lactate/pyruvate) and other metabolic disorders (quantitative amino acids for alanine, glycine, creatine kinase, aspartate, acetylcholine, and phospholipids).

Cerebrospinal rhinorrhea may be caused by a dural tear and/or bone fracture. A rapid, but unreliable, test is a glucose level >5 mg/dL on glucose oxidase paper. Immunoelectrophoresis of 0.5 mL of nasal secretions for beta$_2$-transferrin, a protein that is specific for human CSF, is the most accurate test to determine if a patient has CSF rhinorrhea.

NEUROIMAGING

Neuroimaging studies continue to make rapid advances in our ability to noninvasively evaluate the central nervous system. Ultrasound, computed tomography (CT), and magnetic resonance imaging (MRI) are the most commonly used studies. Myelography, angiography, single-photon emission tomography (SPECT), positron-emission tomography (PET), and xenon-computed tomography are used only in specific circumstances.

The advantages of ultrasound include portability, speed, and multiplanar imaging. The primary disadvantage is poor resolution. The ultrasound image is produced by nonionizing pulses at 3.5 to 10 MHz sent by a transducer. The ultrasound waves are then reflected at different amplitudes depending on the density of the tissues they encounter. The reflected wave is shown as a dot with a brightness that depends upon the strength and location of the reflected signal. Duplex Doppler

sonography displays color-coded information about vascular flow direction and velocity. It is used for evaluation of cardiac and vascular blood flow as well as CSF flow. B-mode scanning produces several images per second, allowing for real-time sonography of echogenic (bright) structures such as choroid plexus, hemorrhage, tumors, and cerebritis as well as sonolucent structures such as cysts and CSF.

CT has been available since the 1970s and MRI since the 1980s, and they are now the mainstays for neuroimaging. Headache is a common disorder in which one must consider if neuroimaging is indicated and what type of imaging is the best. We will use the approach to headache to introduce us to these two neuroimaging modalities.

If a patient has an acute onset of the "first" or "worst" headache, or the neurologic examination is abnormal with stiff neck, nausea, vomiting, or focal deficits, then a neuroimaging study is always recommended. If the examination is normal, then the decision to image is on a case-by-case basis (Table 43.4). Once the decision is made to perform a neuroimaging study, the next question is to decide whether CT or MRI is the study of choice and whether contrast is required.

As outlined in Table 43.5, the head CT is helpful in the acutely ill patient with acute severe headache or altered sensorium, because it can quickly identify large hemorrhages, bone fractures, or increased intracranial pressure. The primary drawbacks to CT are the radiation and the risk for acute nephritis from the iodinated contrast.

Head MRI has many advantages over CT, including the lack of radiation, higher resolution, and the ability to perform special sequences: the susceptibility-weighted image (SWI) sequence can detect acute hemorrhage, magnetic resonance angiography (MRA) can detect vascular disease, diffusion weighted MRI (dwRMI) can detect ischemia, magnetic resonance spectroscopy (MRS) can detect biochemical changes in the brain, diffusion tensor (dt) studies can evaluate white matter tracts, and functional MRI (fMRI) can localize areas of brain activity during cognition or while performing specific tasks.

Contrast is helpful whenever there is a concern about a possible breakdown in the blood–brain barrier such as in tumor, abscess, or an infectious process. The iodinated contrast used in CT carries a small risk for acute nephritis due to

TABLE 43.3

CSF PROTEIN IMMUNOELECTROPHORESIS

Immunoglobulins	Myelin-basic/ antimyelin-basic protein	Myelin-associated glycoprotein (MAG)
Autoimmune	Demyelination	Autoimmune
Infection	White matter injury	Infection
Inflammatory processes		Tumor
Oligoclonal bands		
Tumor		

TABLE 43.4

NEUROIMAGING IN HEADACHES

Symptoms	Neuroimaging
Abnormal neurologic examination	Yes
"First" or "worst" headache	Yes
Normal neurologic examination with neurologic symptoms	Yes/No
Headache worsened by Valsalva	Yes/No
Headache that awakens patient from Sleep	Yes/No
Progressively worsening headache	Yes/No
Migraine	Yes/No
Tension	Yes/No

Lewis D, Ashwal S, Dahl G, et al. Practice parameter: Evaluation of children and adolescents with recurrent headache. Report of the quality standards subcommittee of the American Academy of Neurology and the Practice Committee of the Child Neurology Society. *Neurology* 2002;54:490–498.

hypertonicity and chemical toxicity. The contrast used in MRI has little toxicity.

There are three methods of angiography of the brain, each with its own advantages and disadvantages. Magnetic resonance angiography (MRA) is the safest method of angiography but it has the lowest resolution (2.5 mm) and is subject to flow artifact, which may underestimate the extent of the vascular lesion. MRA has low sensitivity for dural malformations. CT angiography has excellent resolution but carries the risk of radiation and interference from bone. Conventional angiography has the best resolution but has a 0.5% (children) to 2% (elderly) risk of contrast-induced vasospasm causing stroke.

Perfusion studies evaluating the rate of blood flow to brain tissues in acute stroke can be done with both CT and MRI.

Positron emission tomography (PET), single-photon emission computed tomography, and xenon computed tomography use radioactive tracers to provide information about cerebral function. These studies are helpful for evaluating the metabolism of a specific area and can distinguish between tumor and ischemia as well as evaluate for functional changes related to learning disabilities.

NEUROPHYSIOLOGY

Neurophysiology is the study of neurochemical changes in the nervous system related to pathologic states, and includes electroencephalography (EEG), evoked potentials, and electromyography.

Electroencephalography measures the voltage differences between two electrodes on the scalp. The electrodes are placed on the skull according to the International 10–20 System of electrode placement in which each electrode is spaced either 10% or 20% of the total distance between pairs of skull landmarks. The voltage represents the normal oscillatory and spontaneous electrical patterns of the brain. The background oscillatory patterns are regulated by the inferior olive, thalamus, and hippocampus. Spontaneous electrical activity represents the summation of the excitatory postsynaptic potentials and the inhibitory postsynaptic potentials for a set of neurons.

The EEG allows the neurologist to evaluate and characterize seizure activity and overall function of the brain (Table 43.6). The background of the EEG detects abnormalities in organization, symmetry, and suppression, which allows for evaluation of brain function or recent activity (Table 43.7). Abnormal spontaneous electrical activity is usually excitatory, but can be inhibitory. Abnormal focal waveforms such as spikes and sharp waves indicate focal areas of epileptiform activity arising from the cortex. The spike and wave waveform indicates generalized epileptiform activity arising from the thalamus or brainstem reticular activating system.

Magnetoencephalography is a method in which EEG and MRI are combined to allow detailed localization of seizures.

TABLE 43.5

HEAD MRI VERSUS HEAD CT

	Head MRI	Head CT
Radiation	No	Yes
Contrast-induced nephritis	No	Yes
Speed	10–30 min	1–15 min
Bone	Poor	Good
Increased intracranial pressure	Good	Good
Large hemorrhage	Good (SWI sequence)	Good
Petechial hemorrhages	Good (SWI sequence)	Poor
Abscesses	Good	Fair
Tumor	Good	Fair
White matter injury	Good	Fair
Congenital malformation	Good	Fair
Stroke/ischemia detection	20 min (dwMRI)	12–24 hr
Vasculitis/aneurysm/AVM	Good (MRA)	Good (CT angiogram)
Biochemical changes	Good (MRS)	Not available
Blood flow	Good (Perfusion MRI)	Good (Perfusion MRI)
Brain activity	Good (fMRI)	Not available

dwMRI, diffusion-weighted MRI; fMRI, functional MRI; MRA, magnetic resonance angiography; MRS, magnetic resonance spectroscopy; SWI, susceptibility-weighted imaging.

TABLE 43.6

INDICATIONS FOR EEG

Routine	Video EEG telemetry

Characterization of seizures
Brain death
State of consciousness—coma vs.
  nonconvulsive status epilepticus
	Management of seizures
	Management of status epilepticus
	Seizure vs. pseudoseizure
	Seizure localization for epilepsy
	  surgery

TABLE 43.7

EEG BACKGROUND

	Organization	Symmetry	Suppression
PHYSIOLOGIC PROCESS	Maturity Sleep/wake cycle Encephalopathy	Mass lesions Postictal Slowing	Mass lesion Skull defect Encephalopathy

TABLE 43.8

EVOKED POTENTIALS

Type	Indications
Brainstem auditory evoked potentials (BAER)	Integrity of the auditory system Hearing loss, demyelination, brainstem tumor or prognosis
Visual evoked reponse (VER)	Integrity of the visual system Prechiasmal vs. retrochiasmal lesions
Electroretinograms (ERG)	Photoreceptors of the retina
Somatosensory evoked potentials (SEP)	Integrity of the dorsal columns and medial lemniscal system of the spinal cord and brainstem Neurodegenerative diagnosis or prognosis

TABLE 43.9

BRAINSTEM AUDITORY EVOKED POTENTIALS

Waveform	Anatomic structure	Delayed latency between waveforms—lesion location
I	Acoustic nerve	Delayed I-III: Medulla-pons
II	Cochlear nucleus and trapezoid body	Delayed III-V: Pons-midbrain
III	Superior olive	Delayed I-V: Medulla-mibrain
IV	Lateral lemniscus	
V	Inferior coliculus	
VI	Medial geniculate body of the thalamus	
VII	Auditory radiations	

Evoked potentials evaluate conduction and neuronal processing of information through the central nervous system from an environmental stimulus (Table 43.8). Each evoked potential is represented by a sequence of waves. The amplitude and latency of each wave represent conduction and processing of information. A decreased amplitude or a delayed latency of a waveform signify a lesion or injury to a site distal to the structure represented by the waveform (Table 43.9).

Electromyography (EMG) and nerve conduction studies (NCS) are the most helpful tools for evaluating the peripheral nervous system—anterior horn cell, peripheral nerve, neuromuscular junction, and muscle. The NCS consist of recording and stimulating electrodes that allow the neurologist to study the conduction velocity of each nerve, the motor and sensory amplitudes, and the pattern of neuromuscular involvement.

The EMG localizes lesions to either nerve or muscle as well as evaluating for denervation, anterior horn cell dysfunction, and pseudoweakness.

Suggested Readings

Barkovich AJ. *Pediatric neuroimaging.* 4th ed. Philadelphia: Lippincott Williams & Wilkins; 2005.

Daly DD, Pedley TA. *Current practice of clinical electroencephalography.* 2nd ed. New York: Raven; 1990.

Fishman RA, *Cerebrospinal fluid in diseases of the nervous system.* 2nd ed. Philadelphia: Saunders; 1992.

Misulis KE. *Essentials of clinical neurophysiology.* 2nd ed. Boston: Butterworth-Heinemann; 1997.

Misulis KE. *Spehlman's evoked potential primer.* 3rd ed. New York: Butterworth-Heinemann; 2001.

CHAPTER 44 ■ SEIZURES

SARAH M. RODDY

Seizures are caused by abnormal discharges of neurons and may have a wide variety of clinical manifestations. A seizure should be considered a symptom of systemic or central nervous system dysfunction. Management consists not only of controlling seizures, but also of diagnosing any potentially treatable underlying condition. Acute conditions associated with seizures include metabolic disturbances, fever, meningitis, encephalitis, and toxic encephalopathy. The terms *seizure disorder* and *epilepsy* are synonymous and are applied to the condition in which there is a tendency for recurrent, unprovoked seizures.

CLASSIFICATION OF SEIZURES

Classification of seizures has provided a means to study seizures that have similar pathophysiology and is important for treatment decisions. Electroencephalography (EEG) monitoring has aided in the current classification, which is based on characterization of seizure onset and progression. Seizures are either partial or generalized. Epilepsy syndromes have also been defined in terms of a cluster of signs and symptoms including age of onset, severity, diurnal or nocturnal occurrence, clinical course, associated neurologic dysfunction, inheritance, and EEG findings. Febrile seizures, which can be generalized or focal, are considered separately, as are pseudoseizures.

Generalized Seizures

Generalized seizures result from simultaneous involvement of both cerebral hemispheres from the onset of the seizure. Types of generalized seizures include absence, myoclonic, atonic, and generalized tonic/clonic.

Absence seizures are generalized, nonconvulsive seizures characterized by interruption of activity, staring, and unresponsiveness; they usually last between 5 and 15 seconds. The episode starts abruptly, without warning, and ends abruptly with resumption of the child's preictal activity. The child may be unaware that the episode occurred. At times, unresponsiveness is accompanied by eyelid fluttering, upward rotation of the eyes, and occasionally, by mild clonic movements or automatisms, such as lip smacking, grimacing, or swallowing. Seizures may occur over 100 times/day and may interfere with learning ability. The age of onset is generally between 4 and 8 years of age; rarely does it occur before 3 years or after 15 years. Girls are affected more commonly than boys. The classic finding on the EEG in patients who have absence seizures is bilaterally synchronous 3-Hz spike-and-wave discharges. Hyperventilation may be used to precipitate the electrical discharges and a clinical seizure.

Myoclonic seizures are characterized by brief, sudden muscle contractions that may involve only part of the body or may be generalized. They may occur in clusters, especially during the period of falling asleep or shortly after awakening. There may be no alteration in consciousness associated with the jerks.

Atonic, or astatic, seizures have also been termed drop attacks. They are characterized by a sudden decrease in muscle tone, which may result in head nodding or mild flexing of the legs. More significant decreases in muscle tone may cause the patient to slump to the floor. There is usually no detectable alteration in consciousness with these seizures.

Generalized tonic-clonic seizures are also known as grand mal seizures and consist of motor manifestations and loss of consciousness. The tonic phase is characterized by a sustained contraction of muscles; as a result, the patient falls to the ground, usually in opisthotonus. There is usually extensor posturing with tonic contraction of the diaphragm and intercostal muscles. This halts respirations, which, in turn, produces cyanosis. The tonic phase lasts less than 1 minute and is followed by the clonic phase, which consists of bilateral and rhythmic jerking. The jerks may be accompanied by expiratory grunts produced by diaphragmatic contractions against a closed glottis. The frequency of the clonic jerks decreases as the seizure progresses, although the intensity actually may increase. The tongue may be bitten, and bowel and bladder incontinence may occur. The clonic activity usually stops after several minutes. The seizure may be followed by vomiting, confusion, and lethargy, with gradual recovery of consciousness over a period of minutes to hours. Generalized tonic-clonic seizures may be primary generalized or secondary generalized. Primary generalized seizures usually are idiopathic or genetic in origin and are associated with bilaterally synchronous electrical discharges on EEG. Secondary generalized seizures begin as partial seizures but may generalize so rapidly that any suggestion of focal origin is lacking. The EEG may demonstrate a focal discharge that may spread to both hemispheres or may show only bilateral synchronous discharges. History that is helpful in determining that a seizure is secondary generalized is the presence of an aura, head or eye deviation, or focal clonic movement at the onset of the seizure. Neurologic examination may reveal subtle focal signs, such as a mild hemiparesis or visual field defect.

Generalized Epilepsy Syndromes

Infantile spasms are a unique form of epilepsy, with onset during the first year of life. The seizures are characterized by a sudden contraction of neck, trunk, and extremity muscles. The spasms may be flexor, extensor, or mixed flexor-extensor and last only a few seconds each, but they often occur in clusters of up to 100 individual spasms. A typical episode is characterized by dropping of the head with abduction of the shoulders and flexion of the lower extremities. The infant may cry during or after the spasm. Pallor, flushing, grimacing, laughter, and nystagmus are observed during some episodes. Episodes are common on awaking from sleep, during drowsiness, and with feedings, but are rare during sleep. The peak age of infantile spasm onset is between 3 and 7 months, with boys more likely to be affected than girls. Infantile spasms are usually divided into symptomatic and cryptogenic groups based on the presence of a predisposing etiologic factor. Included among symptomatic infantile spasms are infants who have abnormal neurologic development before the onset of spasms. Causes include structural abnormalities of the brain, hypoxic-ischemic insults, central nervous system infections or hemorrhages, and inborn errors of metabolism. Children who have tuberous sclerosis account for up to 25% of patients who have infantile spasms. The cryptogenic group includes those patients in whom no etiologic factor can be found. Infants in this group tend to be older at the onset of infantile spasms compared with infants in the symptomatic group. The EEG pattern associated with infantile spasms is known as *hypsarrhythmia* and is characterized by high-voltage slow waves with irregularly interspersed multifocal spike and sharp waves. Hypsarrhythmia may precede the onset of clinical manifestations, or it may occur later or not at all. Over time, the hypsarrhythmia usually evolves into other focal or generalized abnormalities; in some cases, the EEG may normalize. The prognosis for infants who have infantile spasms remains grave. The average mortality is approximately 20%, with aspiration pneumonia being a common cause of death. Approximately 80% of survivors are mentally retarded. The spasms usually remit by a few years of age, but 55% to 60% of patients subsequently develop other forms of seizures. The prognosis is more favorable for those infants whose neurologic development had been normal before the onset of the spasms.

Lennox–Gastaut syndrome is a severe epileptic encephalopathy characterized by a variety of primary generalized seizures. Tonic seizures cause sudden, sustained contraction of the muscle groups, at times causing the patient to fall. Atypical absence seizures consist of a brief period of staring and immobility. The onset and recovery of atypical absence seizures are less abrupt than those of typical absence seizures. The episodes may be associated with mild tonic motor manifestations, automatisms, or loss of postural tone. Atonic seizures occur and may be preceded by myoclonic jerks. Tonic-clonic seizures and partial seizures also may occur in patients who have Lennox–Gastaut syndrome. The majority of these patients begin to have seizures between 3 and 5 years of age, with boys affected slightly more often than girls. Many patients have neurologic deficits before the onset of Lennox–Gastaut syndrome, including mental retardation and cerebral palsy, which may be related to hypoxic encephalopathy or other insults to the brain. Patients may have a history of infantile spasms. The EEG typically shows an irregular, high-voltage, slow (2.5 Hz or slower) spike-wave pattern. The discharges are bilaterally synchronous. The treatment of the seizures associated with Lennox–Gastaut syndrome is disappointing. Generally, the goal of treatment is to achieve reasonable seizure control with as few medications as possible to minimize adverse effects. Sometimes the seizures typical of Lennox–Gastaut syndrome occur in otherwise normal preschool-age children, associated with normal background and fast polyspike-and-wave changes on EEG. These children have a much better prognosis for seizure control and cognitive development.

Juvenile myoclonic epilepsy is a primary, generalized epilepsy with an age of onset of 12 to 18 years. It represents 7% of all epilepsy and is characterized by myoclonic jerks that mainly affect the upper extremities and less commonly the lower extremities. The jerks usually occur shortly after awakening, and patients may complain of clumsiness or difficulty holding objects early in the morning. Approximately 80% of patients have generalized tonic-clonic seizures, and 25% have absence seizures in addition to myoclonic seizures. Myoclonic jerks almost always precede the onset of generalized tonic-clonic seizures by months to years. A teenager who has generalized tonic-clonic seizures should be questioned carefully regarding myoclonic jerks. Both the myoclonic jerks and the tonic-clonic seizures may be precipitated by sleep deprivation, stress, alcohol, and hormonal changes. Patients remain neurologically normal. The ictal EEG typically shows generalized, symmetrical polyspike and waves at 4 to 6 Hz. In some patients, photic stimulation precipitates the electrical discharges. The recommended treatment for juvenile myoclonic epilepsy is valproate sodium. There is a high rate of seizure recurrence among patients who discontinue treatment. Juvenile myoclonic epilepsy is therefore considered a life-long condition that requires continuous treatment.

Partial Seizures

Partial seizures are caused by seizure discharges that begin in one hemisphere. They are divided into simple partial seizures, in which consciousness is preserved; and complex partial seizures, in which consciousness is impaired. Partial seizures of either type may progress to become secondarily generalized.

Simple partial seizures are characterized by seizure activity restricted to one side of the body, with preserved consciousness. The symptoms may be motor, sensory, or cognitive, depending on the location of the neuronal discharge. Motor seizures may be restricted to part of the body, such as the face or a limb, or they may spread to involve the entire side. If the seizure discharge spreads to structures involved in consciousness, the seizure will become a complex partial seizure. The seizure activity also may spread to the opposite side of the brain, causing a generalized seizure. A partial seizure may be followed by a Todd paralysis, a weakness of the limbs involved in the seizure. Partial sensory seizures are most often manifested by paresthesias lasting less than 1 to 2 minutes. Seizure discharges from one occipital lobe may cause visual symptoms, such as scintillating colored spots or scotomata in the visual field contralateral to the discharge. Seizures with more complex visual hallucinations often progress to complex partial seizures with diminished consciousness. Auditory seizures are manifested by hearing noises and, less commonly, by elaborate but usually nonverbal auditory hallucinations, such as music. Although simple partial seizures are caused by focal epileptiform discharges, a focal structural lesion may not be found in 30% to 50% of patients. Causes associated with these seizures include prenatal and perinatal insults, central nervous system malformations, and metabolic disturbances such as hypocalcemia, hypoglycemia, and inborn errors of metabolism.

Complex partial seizures are seizures that originate in a limited area of one cerebral hemisphere and result in impaired consciousness. A complex partial seizure may begin as a simple partial seizure that progresses to impairment of consciousness. The initial portion of a seizure that occurs before consciousness is lost is referred to as the aura. The aura may consist of any of a wide variety of symptoms, depending on the location of cortical discharges. There may be auditory, olfactory, or visual illusions or hallucinations. Affective symptoms, such as fear or other unpleasant feelings, can occur. Anger or rage is extremely rare as a seizure manifestation but may occur during postictal confusion if the patient is restrained. Deja vu, the feeling that an experience has occurred before, and jamais vu, the feeling that a previously experienced sensation is unfamiliar and strange, have been described. Young children have difficulty describing deja vu and may say only that there was a "funny feeling" that occurred in the head or stomach. Staring and automatisms, which are involuntary coordinated motor activity, occur when there is clouding of consciousness. Automatisms include simple phenomena, such as chewing, lip smacking, swallowing, and hissing; and more complicated activities, such as picking at clothes, searching, or ambulating.

Automatisms usually are followed by postictal amnesia. The child may become tired and go to sleep. Complex partial seizures must be distinguished from absence seizures, which are also characterized by staring and unresponsiveness. Episodes of absence seizures have an abrupt onset and termination, compared with complex partial seizures, which have a more gradual onset and termination. Absence seizures last less than 30 seconds and are not associated with postictal confusion. Automatisms can occur if absence episodes are prolonged, but they often are just a continuation of motor activity present before the onset of seizure. The most frequent EEG finding in complex partial seizures is an anterior temporal lobe spike discharge, although some patients will have spike discharges from other areas. Interictal EEGs are often normal. Repeating the EEG increases the likelihood of demonstrating the abnormal discharge. Causes of complex partial seizures include perinatal insults, head trauma, encephalitis, and possibly status epilepticus, all of which may be associated with scarring of the temporal lobe. Indolent tumors, such as hamartomas and low-grade gliomas, can also cause complex partial seizures and are found in approximately 20% of persons who have intractable partial seizures.

Partial Epilepsy Syndromes

Benign partial epilepsy of childhood also is known as rolandic epilepsy, sylvian seizures, and centrotemporal epilepsy. This epilepsy syndrome is a common type of partial motor epilepsy in childhood. The onset is usually between 5 and 8 years of age, and boys are more often affected than girls. Genetic factors play a role in the etiology. The seizures typically occur during sleep, although patients occasionally may have an episode during wakefulness. Episodes are characterized by the child awakening with one side of the face twitching. The oropharyngeal muscles are also often involved, causing the child to make unintelligible gurgling sounds. The ipsilateral upper extremity may be involved, but only rarely is the lower extremity involved. In rare cases, a seizure episode will become generalized. Consciousness is often retained during the seizure, although the child may not be able to speak. Most seizure episodes last less than 2 minutes. The frequency of seizures is low—25% of patients have a single seizure episode and 50% have fewer than five episodes. The typical EEG findings are midtemporal or centrotemporal spike discharges that are usually unilateral, often very frequent, and present in light sleep. Neuroradiologic studies show no abnormalities to correlate with the EEG focus. If a child has infrequent episodes, no treatment may be needed. The seizure episodes remit when the child is around 9 to 12 years of age, but no later than 17 years. Remission is long lasting, and no developmental or neurologic impairment is associated with these episodes.

Epilepsia partialis continua is a rare type of seizure in which twitching is continuous and limited to one side of the body. The twitching frequently involves only a few muscles and occurs most often in the hand or foot. Consciousness is preserved, but the seizure activity might weaken the extremity involved. Seizure activity may persist for hours to months. Focal encephalitis and tumor have been associated with this type of seizure. Medical treatment of epilepsia partialis continua generally is unsuccessful.

Febrile Seizures

Febrile seizures are seizures that occur in young children who have fever but no evidence of intracranial infection or acute neurologic illness. Simple febrile seizures are generalized tonic-clonic convulsions that last less than 15 minutes and do not recur within 24 hours. Complex febrile seizures are less common and are focal or prolonged beyond 15 minutes or recur within 24 hours. Febrile seizures occur in children between 3 months and 5 years of age; the median age of occurrence is 18 to 22 months. Approximately 2% to 5% of children will experience a febrile convulsion, and boys are more susceptible than girls. Familial clustering of febrile seizures suggests that genetic factors play a role in the etiology. A febrile seizure may be the first sign that a child is ill. It is not known whether the seizure activity is triggered by the rapid rise of fever or the actual height of the temperature. Febrile seizures can be triggered by any illness that causes fever, most frequently by otitis media and upper respiratory tract infections. There is a high rate of febrile seizures with roseola, salmonellosis, and shigellosis possibly related to a direct effect they have on the central nervous system or to a neurotoxin they produce. One-third of children who have a febrile seizure will have another one with another febrile illness, and the younger the child at the time of the first episode, the greater the risk of recurrence. Approximately 50% of recurrences occur within 6 months of the initial seizure, and 75% occur within 1 year.

Usually seizure activity has stopped by the time the child is evaluated. However, if the seizure continues, lorazepam or diazepam should be administered. The temperature should be brought down using rectal antipyretics, removing blankets and clothing, and sponging. Once seizure activity is controlled, evaluation is directed toward finding the cause of the fever. If the child is under 1 year of age or has not rapidly returned to normal, a lumbar puncture should be strongly considered to evaluate for meningitis. EEG is generally not helpful in the evaluation of children who have febrile seizures and is not predictive of febrile seizures or the development of epilepsy.

Treatment of febrile seizures includes family education that addresses the benign nature of the seizures, the use of antipyretics, and first aid for seizures. Administration of oral diazepam (0.33 mg/kg body weight every 8 hours during febrile illness) reduces the risk of recurrent febrile seizures. Administration of phenobarbital at the onset of a febrile illness, however, does not prevent seizure activity because therapeutic blood levels are not achieved soon enough. Prophylactic treatment with anticonvulsant agents should be considered if neurologic development is abnormal, it is a complex febrile seizure, or the child is under 1 year of age. Administration of phenobarbital in doses that achieve blood levels greater than 15 mg/mL *reduces* the recurrence of febrile seizures. Valproate sodium also appears to be effective in prophylaxis; phenytoin sodium and carbamazepine do not prevent recurrences. The adverse effects of anticonvulsant therapy must be weighed against the possible benefits. There is no evidence that prophylactic treatment reduces the risk of subsequent epilepsy, which is less than 5% in children who have febrile seizures. Factors associated with subsequent development of afebrile, partial seizures include focal seizures, prolonged seizures, and repeated episodes of seizures with the same febrile illness. Factors associated with development of afebrile, generalized seizures include more than three febrile seizures, a family history of afebrile seizures, and age over 3 years at the time of the first febrile seizure.

Pseudoseizures

Pseudoseizures are uncommon but must be recognized if inappropriate treatment is to be prevented. They differ from true epileptic seizures in several respects. The movements are usually not clonic but may be quivering or random thrashing movements. There is usually no incontinence, injury, or tongue biting associated with pseudoseizures. Episodes may be dramatic, with screaming and shouting. Episodes may also vary greatly in the same patient. Usually there is no postictal period. Pseudoseizures can occur in early childhood but are more frequent in adolescence, especially in girls. Pseudoseizures are most likely to occur in children who have true epileptic

TABLE 44.1

COMMON ANTIEPILEPTIC MEDICATIONS

Drug	Indications	Half-life (hours)	Dose (mg/kg/d)	Therapeutic levels (mcg/ml)	Adverse effects
Carbamazepine	Partial, secondary generalized	3–23 (18–55 initially)	5–25	5–10 (monotherapy 4–12)	Allergic rashes, nausea, diplopia, blurry vision, dizziness, hypersensitivity, hepatitis, aplastic anemia
Phenytoin	Partial, secondary generalized, primary generalized	7–42 (nonlinear kinetics)	5–7	10–20 (occasionally lower)	Rashes, hirsutism, gingival hyperplasia, coarse features, psychomotor slowing, neuropathy, folate deficiency myelosuppression, drug-induced lupus
Valproic acid	Primary generalized, absence, myoclonic, akinetic, febrile, infantile spasms, some partial	7–16	10–30 20–50 (infants and in polytherapy)	50–100 (150 if tolerated)	Nausea, tremor, weight gain, hair loss, thrombocytopenia, hepatic failure, pancreatitis
Phenobarbital	Neonatal, febrile, partial, secondary generalized, primary generalized, akinetic	36–120	3–5 (<25 kg) 2–3 (25–50 kg) 1–2 (>50 kg)	10–40	Sedation, inattention, hyperactivity, irritability, cognitive impairment, rare hypersensitivity reactions
Ethosuximide	Absence, myoclonic, akinetic	15–68	15–40	40–100	Nausea, abdominal discomfort, hiccups, drowsiness, behavioral problems, dystonias, myelosuppression, drug-induced lupus
Clonazepam	Absence, primary generalized, infantile spasms	20–36	0.01–0.2	0.01–0.07	Sedation, hyperactivity, inattention, aggressiveness, tolerance, ataxia, withdrawal seizures
Felbamate	Partial (in patients >12 yr), Lennox–Gastaut syndrome	20 (in monotherapy)	15–45 (maximum of 3,600 mg)	*	Anorexia, weight loss, nausea, insomnia, headache, fatigue, aplastic anemia
Gabapentin	Partial, with or without secondary generalized seizures	5–7	Total daily dosage 900–1,800 mg	*	Somnolence, dizziness, ataxia, fatigue
Lamotrigine	Partial, primary generalized, absence, atypical absence, atonic, and myoclonic	7–45	5–15 without valproic acid, 1–5 with valproic acid	*	Somnolence, rash, vomiting
Topiramate	Partial, primary generalized, tonic, atonic, atypical absence	20–30	1–9	*	Somnolence, anorexia, fatigue, difficulty with concentration, nervousness
Tiagabine hydrochloride	Partial	3–9	0.25–1.5 (maximum of 56 mg)	*	Dizziness, somnolence, headache, depression
Oxcarbazepine	Partial	8–11	10–30		Somnolence, diplopia, nausea, vomiting, rash, hyponatremia
Levetiracetam	Partial, photosensitive epilepsy, generalized	6–8	20–40	*	Ataxia, asthenia
Zonisamide	Partial, generalized, absence, myoclonic, infantile spasms	27–60	1.5–15 (usual 4–8)		Somnolence, dizziness, drowsiness, ataxia, confusion, anorexia

*Therapeutic levels have not been established. Partial, secondary generalized.

seizures. A detailed history and observation of an episode often is all that is needed to diagnose pseudoseizures; EEG monitoring can be used in patients in whom the distinction cannot be made clinically. Once the diagnosis is established, treatment is directed toward the psychosocial issues involved.

APPROACH TO AN INITIAL SEIZURE

The first step in treating a child who has an initial seizure is making the correct diagnosis. The risk of recurrence is important when deciding whether to initiate antiepileptic therapy. Some types of seizures, such as absence, myoclonic, akinetic, and infantile spasms, have a recurrence rate of virtually 100% and usually have recurred by the time the child is seen by the physician. These types of seizures require treatment. However, children who have a generalized tonic-clonic or partial seizure have a recurrence risk of about 40%. Factors that increase the risk of recurrence include a partial complex seizure, an abnormal neurologic examination, and focal epileptiform abnormalities on the EEG. The best prognosis is in those children who have a generalized seizure, a normal neurologic examination, and a nonepileptiform EEG. Many patients who have a single seizure should be observed for recurrence but should not be started on antiepileptic medication. Over 50% of the recurrences occur within 6 months, and up to 90% within 1 year. If a second seizure occurs, initiation of antiepileptic medication should be considered because approximately 80% of children who have a second seizure will have more seizures.

DIAGNOSTIC PROCEDURES

- Laboratory tests usually performed at the time of the initial seizure include measurement of serum electrolytes, calcium, magnesium, and blood glucose. In some cases, the history or examination may indicate that a more extensive laboratory evaluation is required.
- EEG, which measures the physiologic function of the brain, changes throughout childhood, reflecting brain maturation. The EEG is important in the evaluation of a child who has seizures, because it helps to define the seizure type. An epileptiform EEG may support the diagnosis of epilepsy, but a normal tracing does not exclude the diagnosis. Other abnormalities, such as slowing and background disorganization, are much less specific. Repeat tracings increase the likelihood of detecting epileptiform discharges in patients with seizures. Hyperventilation, photic stimulation, and sleep should be used when obtaining EEG recordings. Video EEG monitoring is useful in correlating clinical symptoms with electrical seizure activity and may be useful when clinical manifestations are atypical. Although the EEG provides electrophysiologic evidence to support the diagnosis of epilepsy, EEG abnormalities must be interpreted in view of the clinical symptomatology. Some individuals have epileptiform discharges and other EEG abnormalities without ever experiencing a clinical seizure; treatment is not indicated for such individuals.
- Neuroimaging studies can be helpful. CT and, preferably, MRI should be considered. CT and MRI detect structural abnormalities; MRI is more sensitive than CT in the detection of low-grade tumors, changes in myelination, and heterotopic gray matter. However, neuroimaging studies are not warranted in every child who has epilepsy; MRI should be performed in children who have focal neurologic abnormalities on examination or have intractable epilepsy.
- Lumbar puncture is rarely helpful and is not routinely indicated. The cerebrospinal fluid should be examined in patients in whom meningitis or encephalitis is suspected.

TREATMENT WITH ANTIEPILEPTIC MEDICATION

Once the child has had recurrent seizures and antiepileptic medication is indicated, the physician is faced with the decision of which medication to prescribe. Diagnosing seizure type correctly is the critical first step in treatment, because some seizure disorders respond to certain medications. In choosing among potentially effective antiepileptic agents, the drug that has the least adverse effects should be selected. The medication is started at a dosage that will result in a low therapeutic blood level. The dosage should be increased until seizures are controlled or adverse effects become intolerable. If the initial medication is not fully effective, a second medication may be added. Consideration should be given to discontinuing the first medication if seizures are fully controlled with the second medication. It is important to use monotherapy if possible, because polytherapy often does not improve seizure control but may dramatically increase toxicity. The efficacy of an antiepileptic medication should be evaluated only after five half-lives have elapsed, because this is the period of time required for the medication to reach a steady state. Table 44.1 outlines commonly used antiepileptic medications and their properties.

Suggested Readings

Annegers JF, Hauser WA, Shirts SB, et al. Factors prognostic of unprovoked seizures after febrile convulsions. *N Engl J Med* 1987;316:493.

Arzimanoglou A, Guerrini R, Aicardi J. *Aicardi's epilepsy in children*. Philadelphia: Lippincott Williams & Wilkins; 2004.

Baumann RJ, Duffner PK. Treatment of children with simple febrile seizures: the AAP practice parameter. *Pediatr Neurol* 2000;23:11.

Berg AT, Shinnar S. The risk of seizure recurrence following a first unprovoked seizure: a meta-analysis. *Neurology* 1991;41:965.

Camfield PR, Camfield C. Pediatric epilepsy: an overview. In: Swaiman K, Ashwal S, eds. *Pediatric neurology: principles and practice*. St. Louis: Mosby; 1999:629–633.

Commission on Classification and Terminology of the International League Against Epilepsy. Proposal for revised clinical and electroencephalographic classification of epileptic seizures. *Epilepsia* 1981;22:489.

Crumrine PK. Antiepileptic drug selection in pediatric epilepsy. *J Child Neurol* 2002;17(suppl 2):2S2.

Genton P, Dravet C. Lennox-Gastaut syndrome and other childhood epileptic encephalopathies. In: Engel J, Pedley TA, eds. *Epilepsy: a comprehensive textbook*. Philadelphia: Lippincott-Raven; 1997:2355–2366.

Guerrini R. Epilepsy in children. *Lancet* 2006;367:499.

Hirtz D, Ashwal S, Berg A, et al. Practice parameter: evaluating a first nonfebrile seizure in children. *Neurology* 2000;55:616.

Janz D. Juvenile myoclonic epilepsy. In: Dem M, Gran L, eds. *Comprehensive epileptology*. New York: Raven Press; 1990:171–185.

Pellock JM, Dodson WE, Bourgeois BFD, et al., eds. *Pediatric epilepsy diagnosis and treatment*. New York: Demos; 2001.

Rosman NP, Colton T, Labazzo J, et al. A controlled trial of diazepam administered during febrile illness to prevent recurrence of febrile seizure. *N Engl J Med* 1993;329:72.

Shinnar S, Berg AT, Moshe SL, et al. The risk of seizure recurrence after a first unprovoked afebrile seizure in childhood: an extended follow-up. *Pediatrics* 1996;98:216.

CHAPTER 45 ■ STATUS EPILEPTICUS

SARAH M. RODDY

The most widely accepted criterion for diagnosis of status epilepticus is any seizure that continues for 30 minutes, or intermittent seizures lasting for 30 minutes or longer in which the person does not regain consciousness between the episodes. The incidence of status epilepticus in patients who have epilepsy is as high as 16%. Its relative frequency, based on age, is highest in younger age groups. Infants and children also are much more likely than adults to have status epilepticus as the manifestation of their first seizure. Up to 70% of children with epilepsy beginning before the age of 1 year will experience status epilepticus.

ETIOLOGY

- Idiopathic in approximately 15% of cases.
- Fever present in 20% to 25% of cases.
- Acute symptomatic status epilepticus accounts for another 25% of cases and is an expression of an acute encephalopathy or brain injury. Causes in this group include meningitis, electrolyte disturbance, drug ingestion, and poor compliance with antiepileptic medication.
- Remote symptomatic status epilepticus occurs in patients with a prior history of central nervous system insult known to be associated with increased risk of seizure. This group accounts for another 30% of the cases of status epilepticus in children, and the majority have cerebral palsy or mental retardation.
- The etiology of status epilepticus in a small percentage of cases is a progressive encephalopathy. Included in this category are neurodegenerative diseases and neurocutaneous syndromes.

CLASSIFICATION

Status epilepticus can be classified in terms of the type of seizure.

- Generalized convulsive status epilepticus is the most common form and is an easily recognized type of seizure in children. The seizure activity is usually tonic-clonic or clonic, or less often, tonic or myoclonic.
- Simple partial status epilepticus or epilepsia partialis continua with prolonged seizure activity restricted to one side of the body without loss of consciousness.
- Nonconvulsive status epilepticus manifests as a confused, drowsy state in which the patient moves in slow motion. This condition results from continuing or repetitive absence seizures or partial complex seizures.

MANAGEMENT

Nonconvulsive status epilepticus and epilepsia partialis continua require prompt treatment, but there is less urgency because these seizures do not alter the body's homeostatic

mechanisms to the degree that convulsive status epilepticus does. Convulsive status epilepticus is considered a medical emergency because it is life-threatening and sometimes followed by neurologic sequelae. The longer convulsive status epilepticus continues, the more resistant it is to therapy and the greater the incidence of mortality and morbidity.

The objectives of treating convulsive status epilepticus are to:

- Maintain vital functions
- Identify and correct any precipitating factors
- Control seizure activity

A plan for management is outlined in Table 45.1. Because neurologic sequelae of status epilepticus can result from complicating factors, such as hypoxia, hypotension, and acidosis, attention should be given immediately to the respiratory and cardiovascular status of the child. If the patient is febrile, reducing body temperature is extremely urgent because of the synergism of fever and status epilepticus in producing brain damage.

EVALUATION

- History should be obtained from an accompanying family member and should include any history of previous seizures, chronic and recent medication use, intercurrent illness, head trauma, and details of the onset of status epilepticus.
- On physical examination, fever, any evidence of head trauma, increased intracranial pressure, and infection should be noted.
- Laboratory testing should include the tests in Table 45.1. A urine toxicology screen is helpful in determining if the seizures were precipitated by drug ingestion. Computed tomography (CT) scanning may be required to rule out an intracranial lesion if the etiology of status epilepticus remains obscure.

If the history or physical examination suggests a central nervous system infection, antibiotics should be administered immediately and a lumbar puncture performed as soon as seizure activity has been controlled. Once seizure activity is controlled, management should be directed toward preventing recurrence of seizures, including maintenance anticonvulsant therapy. The appropriate duration of therapy after an initial episode of idiopathic status epilepticus is not clear.

PROGNOSIS

Neurologic sequelae from status epilepticus include intellectual impairment and motor dysfunction. Over the past 20 years, morbidity and mortality from status epilepticus have declined, probably because of better access to medical care, more aggressive treatment, and the availability of benzodiazepines. In children with idiopathic or febrile status epilepticus, less

TABLE 45.1

PROTOCOL FOR TREATMENT OF STATUS EPILEPTICUS

- Assess cardiovascular function by making sure the airway is clear and the patient is breathing. Provide oxygen or respiratory support as necessary. Temperature should be monitored and fever treated aggressively.
- Establish an IV line and obtain blood samples for electrolytes, blood urea nitrogen, calcium, a complete blood count, and anticonvulsant medication levels. A blood dextrostix test should be performed immediately, and if the glucose is under 60 mg, then 1 to 2 mL/kg of D25W should be administered.
- One member of the emergency team should obtain a history while another does a physical examination.
- Administer anticonvulsant drugs in the following order until seizure activity is controlled.
- Initial therapy.
  Lorazepam should be the initial anticonvulsant administered IV at a dose of 0.1 mg/kg (maximum 4 mg) over 2 min; a dose of 0.05 to 0.1 mg/kg may be repeated every 5 min if necessary up to a maximum of 0.5 mg/kg, but not more than 10 mg.
  If lorazepam is not available, diazepam should be administered IV at a dose of 0.1 to 0.2 mg/kg (maximum 10 mg) by "pushing" half the dose over 1 min and the remainder at 1 mg/min. A dose of 0.1 mg/kg may be repeated in 5 min if necessary. Because of diazepam's short duration of anticonvulsant effect, another anticonvulsant, such as phenytoin, must be administered immediately. If the patient is known to be receiving phenytoin on a chronic basis, it should be administered as the initial anticonvulsant (see above).
- If status epilepticus continues, administer phenytoin or fosphenytoin sodium, which is a water-soluble prodrug of phenytoin with a more neutral pH value. The dose for both drugs is 15 to 20 mg/kg up to a total dosage of 1,000 mg. Phenytoin must be given IV, but fosphenytoin sodium can be given IM if IV access is not available. A quarter of the dose may be administered during the first 2 min and then at a rate of 1 to 2 mg/kg/min (maximum rate of 50 mg/min) for phenytoin and 3 mg/kg/min (maximum rate of 150 mg/min) for fosphenytoin sodium. If the patient is known to be receiving phenytoin chronically, 5 to 8 mg/kg of phenytoin may be administered as the initial anticonvulsant. Monitor the heart rate, and slow the rate of phenytoin infusion if bradycardia occurs. If seizure activity continues despite a full loading dose of phenytoin, correct for presumed acidosis with a modest dose of sodium bicarbonate.
- If status epilepticus continues, administer phenobarbital, 15 to 20 mg/kg IV up to a total dosage of 800 mg. Administer phenobarbital over 15 min, monitoring respirations and blood pressure, especially if the patient has been given a benzodiazepine.
- If seizure activity still persists, consult a neurologist to determine the need for other anticonvulsants, general anesthesia, or induction of pentobarbital sodium, diazepam, or midazolam hydrochloride coma. Electroencephalography monitoring is required to determine if there is ongoing electrical seizure activity, especially if paralytic agents are given.

than 5% develop new neurologic dysfunction. Mortality in children from status epilepticus currently does not exceed 6%. Death attributable to status epilepticus is rare, with most resulting from the illness that precipitated the seizure.

Suggested Readings

Berg AT, Shinnar S, Testa FM, et al. Status epilepticus after the initial diagnosis of epilepsy in children. *Neurology* 2004;63:1027.

Gross-Tsur V, Shinnar S. Convulsive status epilepticus in children. *Epilepsia* 1993;34(suppl 1):S12.

Hauser WA. Status epilepticus: epidemiologic considerations. *Neurology* 1990;40(suppl 2):9.

Maegaki Y. Risk factors for fatality and neurological sequelae after status epilepticus in children. *Neuropediatrics* 2005;36:186.

Maytal J, Shinnar S, Moshe SL, et al. Low morbidity and mortality of status epilepticus in children. *Pediatrics* 1989;83:323.

Shinnar S, Pellock JM, Moshe SL, et al. In whom does status epilepticus occur: age-related differences in children. *Epilepsia* 1997;38:907.

Shinnar S, Berg AT, Moshe SL, et al. The risk of seizure recurrence after a first unprovoked afebrile seizure in childhood: an extended follow-up. *Pediatrics* 1996;98:216.

Shinnar S, Maytal J, Kraynott L, et al. Recurrent status epilepticus in children. *Ann Neurol* 1992;31:598.

vanEsch A, Ramlal IR, VanSteensel-Mall HA, et al. Outcome after febrile status epilepticus. *Dev Med Child Neurol* 1996;38:19.

CHAPTER 46 ■ CHILDHOOD CEREBROVASCULAR DISEASE

CHALMER D. MCCLURE

Strokes occur in all age groups. In adults, strokes are unfortunately common events that are readily recognized because of the acute stereotypical physical changes. Strokes are less commonly recognized in children because of overlapping disease presentation and variable physical findings.

The two primary forms of stroke in both adults and children are ischemia and hemorrhagic, but the causes are different. The more common etiologies in adults include atherosclerosis, hypertension, and diabetes mellitus. In children, acute ischemic infarcts occur slightly more frequently than hemorrhagic infarcts, and are sequelae from sickle-cell disease, congenital heart disease, infections, and dehydration. Hemorrhagic strokes most often result from vascular malformation leakage. Cerebral sinus venous thrombosis (CSVT) is another prominent cause of childhood strokes, and occurs approximately one-third as often as ischemic strokes. Unlike adult stroke research, few prospective studies have been performed in children. In the past, treatment of strokes in children has been largely anecdotal, being extrapolated from adult stroke research. Over the past 5 years, several retrospective and prospective pediatric studies have been undertaken to determine etiologies and benefits of specific treatment.

ACUTE STROKE ETIOLOGIES

Ischemic Stroke

Sickle-cell disease is the single most common cause of ischemic stroke, yet these children have a known predisposition and often already receive prophylaxis by routine transfusions. If an acute infarct occurs, these children typically receive exchange transfusion in addition to aggressive hydration. In this chapter, the focus will instead be on identifying the multitude of other risk factors for acute arterial ischemic stroke.

In acute arterial ischemic strokes, large and small arterial thrombotic occlusions develop not only in the cerebral vasculature but also systemically. Irregular endothelial lining and/or intimal disruptions lead to flow turbulence and deposition of prothrombotic agents, which in turn, form enlarging clots. Homocystenuria and Williams syndrome lack appropriate endothelial cohesion, allowing for platelet aggregation and clot formation. Pregnancy, deficiencies of antithrombin III, low proteins C and S, presence of factor V Leiden and anticardiolipin antibodies, are prothrombotic states in which clots readily form at any endothelial disruption. Red blood cell deformation or proliferation, as seen in sickle-cell disease, thrombocytosis, and leukemias, mechanically disrupts the endothelium, leading to diminished blood flow and increased clot formation. Vasculitis arises from autoimmune-mediated deposition of immune complexes on endothelial cell membranes and is seen in systemic lupus erythematosus (SLE), rheumatoid arthritis, Takayasu arteritis, and dermatomyositis. Postinfectious vasculopathies are sequelae to varicella and herpes encephalitis, involving immune complex activation of viral infected cells. Spontaneous vessel occlusion and compensatory neovascularization is present in Moyamoya disease.

Carotid stenosis is common in adults with hypertensive disease due to underlying hypercholesterolemia/hyperlipidemia. Its occurrence in children is relatively uncommon; however, familial hyperlipidemia puts children at risk for hypertensive disease and its sequelae. Carotid dissection, from neck trauma, reduces cerebral blood flow and results in large territory ischemia. Often, the first presentation of carotid dissection is acute unilateral blindness.

Emboli to the central nervous system (CNS) most often originate from the heart, although trauma may release fat and air emboli, which may bypass the lungs by means of a patent foramen ovale (PFO). Cardiac shunting with right-to-left flow allows an embolus to bypass the lungs and travel to medium-sized vessels of both the anterior and posterior cerebral circulation. Complex congenital heart diseases in childhood predispose to intracardiac turbulence and thrombus formation (e.g., transposition of the great vessels, tetrology of Fallot, and pulmonary artery stenosis). A thrombus may enlarge in areas of stagnation and turbulence surrounding an abnormal vessel, later embolizing to the CNS. Left atrial fibrillation may lead to thrombus formation, which in turn may also embolize to the CNS. Valvular vegetations from bacterial endocarditis frequently "shower" the cerebrum with emboli in wide distribution and of varying age.

Embolization to the anterior cerebral circulation (areas supplied by the common carotid) presents clinically as headache, focal deficits, confusion, and/or focal seizures. Involvement of the posterior circulation (areas supplied by the vertebral/basilar system) clinically presents as obtundation with blood pressure instability and respiratory distress.

The mechanism of cerebral ischemia, whether initiated by thrombosis or embolism, involves diminished blood flow in the area distal to the occlusion. This brings about diminished oxygen and glucose supply to an increasingly hypoxemic/hypoglycemic brain parenchyma. If clinical symptoms are transient, that is, lasting less than 24 hours, then only a small area of necrosis may be present. If, however, symptoms persist for longer than 24 hours, extensive cellular necrosis and apoptosis have occurred. The surrounding ischemic parenchyma (penumbra) has potential recovery with minimal persisting deficits, if blood flow is restored in a timely manner. Still, the penumbra and areas of hypoxic injury are at risk for reperfusion hemorrhage because of blood–brain barrier breakdown and vessel wall disruption.

Cerebral Sinus Venous Thrombosis

Sinus occlusion may occur in any part of the cerebral venous drainage system. Although the superior sagittal sinus is the site most often involved, the inferior sagittal, transverse, and sigmoidal sinuses are sites of thrombosis. Prothrombotic states are the most common etiologies of CSVT. In neonates and young children, bacterial sepsis, polycythemia, and dehydration initiate a prothrombotic sequence by enhancing stagnation in the low-pressure venous system. Direct extension of a mastoiditis, particularly in older children and adolescents, by erosion through the adjacent bone to the transverse sinus, promotes a thrombophlebitis. With this, sufficient irritation to the sinus endothelial lining promotes clot formation. In cancer patients of all ages, L-asparaginase is notoriously prothrombotic and is associated with an increased incidence of CSVT formation.

Because cerebral veins do not have valves, CSVT produces backpressure leading to cerebral venous congestion, which in turn brings about vasogenic edema as arterial blood continues to pour into the slowly draining capillaries and veins. Cerebral venous congestion is usually bilateral, with generalized symptoms suggestive of bihemispheric involvement. These symptoms include altered level of consciousness, bilateral weakness, and generalized seizures. Occasionally, independent focal seizures represent asymmetrical venous congestion. In addition, sluggish venous drainage leads to poor CSF circulation, reabsorption, and the cascade of ventriculomegaly, communicating hydrocephalus, and increased intracranial pressure.

Hemorrhagic Stroke

Hemorrhagic strokes may involve either brain parenchyma or extra-axial fluid spaces. They are often the result of trauma, catastrophic vessel rupture, or bleeding diathesis.

Hemorrhages in brain parenchyma can originate from either arterial or venous structural anomalies (e.g., arteriovenous malformations, venous angiomas, and telangectasias). Cavernous angiomas rarely bleed. Pathologically, the differences between these malformations are readily identifiable, but may be difficult to discern clinically or by conventional neuroimaging. Angiography gives better characterization of these anomalies, thereby directing more appropriate interventions.

Vascular malformations have inherent structural instabilities, and are prone to leakage and rupture. Often located at junctions of small or medium-sized branches of major cerebral arteries, they are susceptible to undampened arterial pressure surges. Additionally, a multilumen malformation pools blood and reduces blood flow. In those areas where the vessel musculature is thin or absent, a small distention may evolve into an aneurysm. The aneurysm may then rupture under the stress of elevated arterial pressure. Symptoms associated with bleeding reflect location within the CNS (e.g., seizures, headaches, and focal motor deficits).

The CNS is susceptible to other causes of intraparenchymal bleeding. Both drug-induced and hypertensive bleeds have predisposition to the basal ganglia. Cardiac infections and valvular vegetations release emboli to both the anterior and posterior circulation. Thromboembolic events cause mechanochemical disruption of the blood–brain barrier, leading to transudative movement of blood components and other large molecules into the brain parenchyma. Blood in extravascular/extracellular spaces irritates neuronal membranes and causes local injury with edema. This promotes mass effect, midline shift, increased intracranial pressure, herniation, and possibly death. If no progression occurs, and once the thromboembolus resolves, reperfusion bleeding may also occur. If the bleeding remains localized to the basal ganglion, with minimal mass effect, sequelae may be limited to extrapyramidal symptoms.

Vasculopathies such as sickle-cell disease, Moyamoya disease, and Ehlers–Danlos syndrome (type IV) demonstrate specific pathologies leading to disrupted blood flow, neovascularization, and vessel fragility. Disseminated intravascular coagulation (DIC), associated with overwhelming sepsis, leads to multiorgan hemorrhages, including the CNS.

Other Hemorrhages

Subarachnoid hemorrhage most often results from aneurysmal rupture, usually originating from the circle of Willis. Extravasation of blood into the subarachnoid space interferes with CSF reabsorption, and subsequently increases intracranial pressure. Blood in itself is sufficiently irritating to cause vasospasm and secondary ischemia. Sentinel headaches herald slow or brief aneurysmal leaks, and portend later significant bleeding. An explosive headache, photophobia, and meningismus, followed by alteration of consciousness and/or coma, characterizes an acute subarachnoid hemorrhage. In neonates, a small amount of subarachnoid bleeding may be present following a normal vaginal delivery, but is usually asymptomatic.

Subdural and epidural hemorrhages in children stem from accidental cranial injury, nonaccidental trauma, and rarely from ruptured bridging veins. A transverse fracture of the temporal bone and rupture of the underlying middle meningeal artery is most often associated with an epidural hematoma. In this instance, blood collecting outside the dura mater (between the calvarium and periosteum) produces an expansive mass effect, which in turn rapidly leads to coma and death. A subdural hemorrhage dissects along the potential space between dura mater and arachnoid. Nonpenetrating trauma and the accompanying shearing forces can tear bridging veins that span the dura. Rarely, as in glutaric academia, an atrophic brain pulls away from the calvarium and dura stretching bridging veins. The veins may either spontaneously rupture or be sheared by mild transverse forces leading to extra-axial bleeding. Symptoms of extraparenchymal hemorrhaging include acute loss of consciousness, or in the case of a chronic bleed, unexplained emesis from increasing intracranial pressure (ICP), confusion, bizarre behavior, and eventual loss of consciousness.

INTERVENTIONS

First and foremost in treatment of childhood stroke is a thorough neurologic examination. This is the prerequisite for accurate anatomic localization and identification of the stroke type. It will then guide the practitioner to further investigation and treatment (Table 46.1). For example, if the child is febrile with a headache, then one should look for an infective source; if the child has a history of a focal seizure with severe headache leading to obtundation, then one should be concerned about causes of increased intracranial pressure.

Head imaging is the next step in investigating stroke etiologies. Often a head CT is the first neuroimaging performed in the emergency department, and it can be helpful in identifying intraparenchymal/extraparenchymal bleeding and midline shift. In CSVT, a head CT accurately demonstrates a thrombosis in 60% of cases, but has a high false-positive rate. Head CT poorly localizes acute ischemic infarcts because hypodense changes only become identifiable approximately 48 hours after the event. Rather, a head MRI with and without contrast, and diffusion-weighted imaging (DWI), are better at identifying acute ischemic changes (Fig. 46.1). Adding in susceptibility-weighted imaging (SWI) can also help identify old hemorrhagic changes. Magnetic resonance venography

TABLE 46.1

RECOMMENDED STUDIES IN SUSPECTED STROKE PATIENTS

IMMEDIATE STUDIES	RATIONALE
CBC	Anemia, leukocytosis/leukopenia, thrombocytosis
Chemistry profile	Hypocalcemia, acidosis, alkalosis, hypoglycemia
Thyroid function: TSH, T3, free T4	Hypo/hyperthyroidism
ESR	Systemic inflammatory reaction
SERUM	**ABNORMAL WHEN**
Lupus anticoagulant	Present
Factor V Leiden	Present
Lysophosphatidic acid	Elevated (LPA)
Methylenetetrahydrofolate reductase	Homozygous (MTHFR)
Antithrombin III	Low
Antiphospholipid/anticardiolipin abs	Present
Homocysteine	Elevated
Lipoprotein A	Elevated
Prothrombin gene mutation	Present (PT 2021A)
Proteins C&S	Low
Urine organic acids	Specific organic acids abnormal
URINE	
Homocysteine	Elevated
OTHER METABOLIC STUDIES	
Lactate/pyruvate	Elevated/low
Mitochondrial DNA panels I & II	Mutation present (MELAS)
CDG transferrin	Present
CSF STUDIES AND SERUM EQUIVALENTS	
Xanthochromia	Present, subarachnoid hemorrhage
Herpes IgG &IgM	Present
Varicella IgG & IgM	Present
Mycoplasma IgG & IgM	Present
EBV IgG & IgM	Present
CMV IgG & IgM	Present
IMAGING	**ABNORMAL FINDINGS**
MRI with DWI	T2 lengthening
MRA/MRV	Beading/low-flow system
Echocardiogram	PFO, LA thrombus (preferably TEE)
IF NECESSARY	
Conventional angiogram	Vessel stenosis
Carotid Doppler	Carotid dissection, turbulence
Transcranial Doppler	Diminished flow
ECG (12 lead)	Arrhythmia
EEG	Focal slowing, epileptogenic potentials

(MRV) is more accurate than CT, with fewer false-positive results, by demonstrating diminished venous sinus blood flow (Fig. 46.2).

In children with suspected vasculitis or postinfectious vasculopathies, magnetic resonance angiography (MRA) is quickly becoming the investigative tool of choice. Angiography, while still the gold standard for visualization of the affected area, has a greater risk of morbidity and mortality than MRA.

An echocardiogram is helpful for structural evaluation of the heart, occasionally revealing right-to-left shunting or other congenital malformations. The transesophageal echocardiogram (TEE) allows better visualization of the left atrium and aortic valve, so that they may be evaluated for thrombi and vegetations, respectively. Doppler flow studies demonstrate the presence or absence of a common carotid stenosis and/or dissection.

Evaluation of CNS bleeding, as in other CNS processes, is accomplished by a systematic approach: an accurate history, clinically confirmed deficits, neuroimaging, and lumbar puncture. Details about the head trauma, no matter how insignificant, can help direct more detailed examination; focal weakness, vision loss, or cranial nerve deficit can guide choice

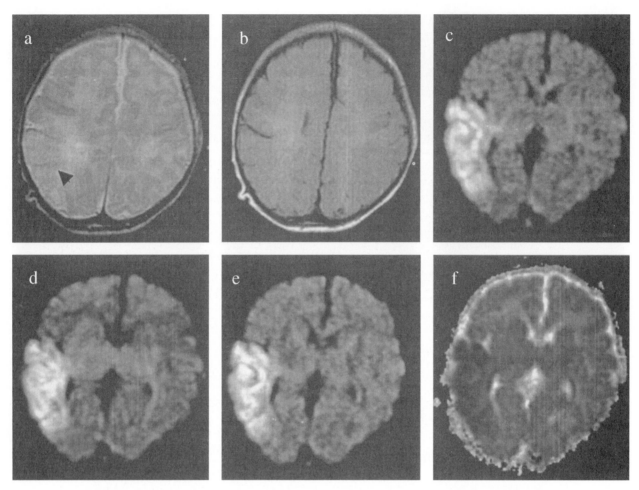

FIGURE 46.1. Right middle cerebral artery ischemic infarct in a 6-day-old infant: T-2 (**a**) and T-1 (**b**) weighted images and diffusion-weighted images (**c–f**). (Images courtesy of LLUMC Department of Radiology.)

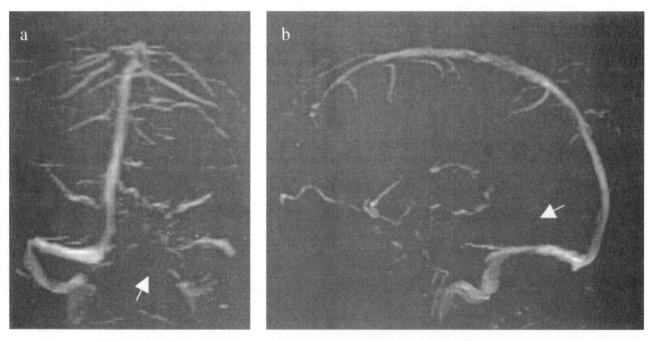

FIGURE 46.2. Magnetic resonance venography (MRV) demonstrating absent left transverse (**a**) and straight sinuses (**b**). (Images courtesy of LLUMC Department of Radiology.)

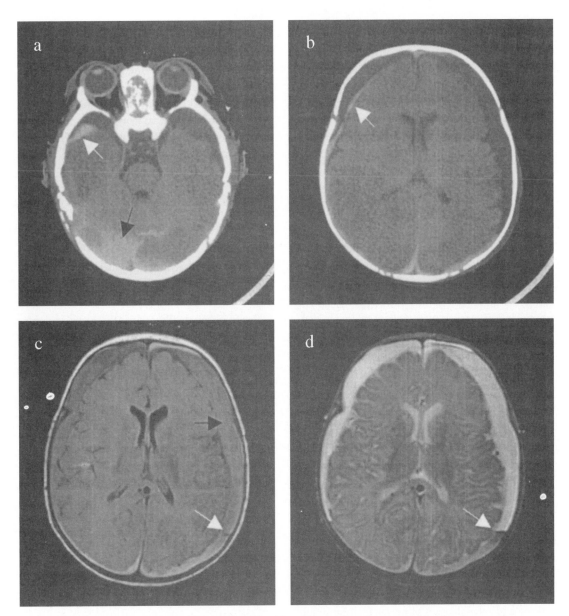

FIGURE 46.3. Four-month-old girl with subdural hematomas of varying age resulting from nonaccidental trauma. Head CT (**a & b**) demonstrates an acute subdural hematoma (*white arrows*) and possible subarachnoid hemorrhage along tentorium (*black arrow*). FLAIR and T-2 weighted head MRIs (**c & d**) exhibit dependent fluid/fluid level of acute blood products and resolving hematoma (*white arrows*). Faint demarcation of hematomas with varying age present (*black arrow*). (Images courtesy of LLUMC Department of Radiology.)

of imaging. A head CT readily demonstrates acute intra-parenchymal, subdural, and subarachnoid hemorrhaging based on location and shape (Fig. 46.3). A subdural hemorrhage appears as cerebral concavity, whereas a subarachnoid bleed displaces the brain as it follows contours of the gyri and sulci. The lumbar puncture in the presence of a subarachnoid hemorrhage shows xanthochromia and a nonclearing bloody CSF. An epidural hemorrhage has the appearance of an expanse of blood between brain and skull limited only by the periosteum of the affected bone.

Initial treatment for ischemic and hemorrhagic infarcts remains primarily supportive: adequate hydration, mild hypertension (to ensure blood flow to the affected area), mild sedation, and use of a stool softener to avoid straining are still recommended. Attention must be paid to "the clock," as maximum CNS edema occurs at 72 hours. Should the child have a

deteriorating level of consciousness, care must be paid to clinical signs of impending herniation. Mannitol, used to increase serum osmolarity, is still an effective means of reducing edema. Use of hyperventilation to reduce cerebral blood flow is controversial. An intracranial pressure (ICP) monitoring device is sometimes placed.

Other interventions for intraparenchymal bleeding involve avoiding blood pressure surges, removing risk factors for further bleeding, and avoiding anticoagulation. As with subdural and epidural hemorrhages, if an intraparenchymal bleed causes mass effect and increased ICP, it may require draining. Aneurysms are "clipped"; vascular malformations can be resected, embolized (by either chemical sclerosing or coil insertion), or radiologically sclerosed (proton beam or gamma knife). Because rebleeding may occur, close monitoring for alteration of clinical signs is imperative.

Thrombolytic therapy in children was initially extrapolated from adult stroke studies, but greater experience with childhood stroke has led to specific recommendations. Recognition of childhood ischemic stroke is often delayed and outside the 6-hour window for acute IV thrombolytic administration. Only in rare cases has interarterial TPA been used, and most of these have been associated with emboli being dislodged during cardiac catheterization. Unfractionated heparin was previously the mainstay of thromboembolic stroke treatment in adults; it activates antithrombin III to prevent extension of old clots or formation of new ones. The disadvantage of unfractionated heparin is the potential for cerebral hemorrhage. Consequently, with less risk of promoting cerebral bleeding, low-molecular weight heparin (LMWH) has become the acute anticoagulant of choice. As the majority of childhood thromboembolic events resolve without persistent clinical deficit, the use of any type of heparin in children is limited to those with increased risk for clot extension or recurrent emboli.

Treatment of CSVT depends upon the etiology of the thrombosis. If, for example, either bacterial meningitis with sepsis or dehydration is present, then IV antibiotics and fluid hydration should be initiated. Use of thrombolytic agents in children with meningitis/sepsis is almost universally avoided, as it may release a shower of septic emboli, further spreading infectious material. If thrombophlebitis is associated with erosive mastoiditis, surgical drainage of the mastoid and debridement of the thrombophlebitis should be done. When no clear infectious etiology is present, LMWH may be considered to prevent further clot extension. The risk to benefit ratio of thrombolytic therapy remains controversial, because thrombus in childhood CSVT often recannulizes without direct intervention.

Current guidelines from the United Kingdom and *Chest*, on evidence-based treatment for CSVT, cardioembolic stroke, or stroke resulting from arterial dissection, recommend warfarin or LMWH for 3 to 6 months. The guidelines offer different recommendations for treatment of ischemic strokes—one recommends LMWH for 5 to 7 days followed by aspirin at 1 to 5 mg/kg/day for 3 to 6 months, and the other recommends the aspirin only for the same duration. If possible, daily factor Xa levels are drawn to monitor the effectiveness of the LMWH.

Soon after hospitalization, rehabilitation should be initiated, so that long-term recovery can begin in a timely and effective way. Important to this recovery is the inclusion of the physical medicine and rehabilitation physicians, physical and occupational therapists, as well as speech therapists. Do not forget to contact the case manager early so that they can begin working with the family and insurance for maintaining these therapies in the outpatient setting.

RECURRENCE

The risk of stroke recurrence is dependent on etiology. Acute arterial ischemic stroke has estimated recurrences of between 6% and 30% in the first 6 months following the initial event, with congenital heart diseases and procoagulable states having the greatest incidence. Although the stroke mortality rate is 0.6/100,000 for children between 1 and 15 years of age, for children under 12 months of age the rate is higher. Hemorrhagic stroke recurrence is greatest within the first year following the initial event, but the mortality rate is higher than that of ischemic stroke, at between 7% and 54%. Most of the children who die, do so while still hospitalized from the initial event. For CSVT, no recurrence rates are available, but most of these children have recannualization of the thrombus without further extension.

Specific genetically associated procoagulable states and congenital heart diseases have higher risks of recurrence than does dehydration or infection. Table 46.1 lists recommended laboratory studies associated with prothrombotic states that should be checked in children who do not have a clear stroke etiology. Knowing the etiology allows the practitioner to appropriately treat the underlying disorder and give informed guidance to the patient and family.

Suggested Readings

deVeber G. In pursuit of evidence-based treatments for paediatric stroke: UK and *Chest* guidelines. *Lancet Neurol* 2005;4:432–436.

deVeber G, Roach ES, Riela AR, et al. Stroke in children: recognition, treatment, and future directions. *Semin Pediatr Neurol* 2000;7:309–317.

Garcia JH, Pantoni L. Strokes in childhood. *Semin Pediatr Neurol* 1995;2: 180–191.

Lynch JK, Han CJ. Pediatric stroke: what do we know and what do we need to know? *Semin Neurol* 2005;245:410–423.

Lynch JK, Han CJ, Nee LE, et al. Prothrombotic factors in children with stroke or porencephaly. *Pediatrics* 2005;116:447–453.

Sebire G, Tabarki B, Saunders DE, et al. Cerebral venous sinus thrombosis in children: risk factors, presentation, diagnosis, and outcome. *Brain* 2005; 128:477–489.

CHAPTER 47 ■ FLOPPY INFANT

DEBRA S. DEMOS

Hypotonia in infants may result from disturbance in cerebral function, spinal cord injury, anterior horn cell dysfunction, metabolic derangement, muscle structural abnormality, or chromosomal abnormality. The physical examination helps direct appropriate laboratory investigations to confirm or refute etiologies. Depending on the origin, hypotonia may herald numerous sequelae including failure to thrive, respiratory distress, and death.

ETIOLOGIES

Central Nervous System

Hypotonia resulting from cerebral dysfunction has many origins including hypoxic-ischemic encephalopathy (HIE). In the perinatal period, lack of blood flow and oxygen to the brain promotes neuronal cell death by necrosis or apoptosis. This occurs in cerebral gray matter and spinal cord and if sustained can involve white matter. Injury to the gray matter is associated with an encephalopathy and extrapyramidal symptoms while white matter injury initially manifests as weakness, diminished tone, and hyporeflexia.

Affected infants later progress to hypertonicity, hyperreflexia, and abnormal reflexes. Lesions of the cerebellar vermis exhibit abnormal tone in postural and antigravity muscle groups. Dandy–Walker malformation, vermian hypoplasia, Joubert syndrome, and the muscle-eye-brain variant of Walker–Warburg disease may all exhibit diminished axial strength and tone.

Anterior horn cell infections leading to hypotonia are primarily due to enteroviruses (coxsackie, echovirus, poliomyelitis). Infants usually have a predisposing gastroenteritis or recent polio immunization. Although the wild-type poliovirus has almost been eradicated in the United States, immunocompromised children can develop symptoms of progressive weakness following immunization. Neurologic symptoms among the enteroviruses may be clinically indistinguishable—that is, progressive generalized weakness and respiratory compromise. Coxsackie virus and echovirus may cause aseptic meningitis in late summer or early autumn. Poliovirus can be isolated from stool, but cerebral spinal fluid (CSF) is required to detect coxsackievirus and echovirus by polymerase chain reaction (PCR). CSF also exhibits a predominantly lymphocytic pleocytosis. Treatment is primarily supportive.

With the increased prevalence of cesarean sections, neonatal spinal cord injury is relatively infrequent. Injury does still occur after difficult vaginal deliveries (dystocia, macrosomy, or breech presentation) where twisting of the head or body (MacRoberts maneuver) is performed to free the child from the birth canal. Injuries are most often to the cervical or thoracic cord, and hypotonia results from spinal shock (hemorrhage and edema). Infants with high cervical lesions usually do not survive.

Spinal muscular atrophy (SMA I-III) is a disorder of the anterior horn cell. SMA is caused by a deletion of the survivor motor neuron gene (SMN) located on chromosome 5 and is characterized by a loss of anterior horn motor neurons, and results in progressive muscle weakness. Electromyography (EMG) and nerve conduction velocities (NCV) confirm the diagnosis of SMA, and muscle biopsy reveals a characteristic "checkerboard" pattern of type II muscle fiber atrophy. Blood DNA analysis for gene mutation may be diagnostic and eliminate the need for EMG and NCV.

The spectrum of this disease is divided by age of presentation. Type I disease (Werdnig–Hoffman) presents by age 6 months and is characterized by generalized weakness, respiratory distress, and poor suck and swallow with progression to respiratory failure by 12 to 18 months and death by 2 years of age. Type II disease, with onset between 6 and 18 months of age, also has extremity weakness, skeletal deformities, and respiratory failure and death in many patients. Symptoms associated with type III SMA (Kugelberg–Welander) include occasional respiratory difficulties and progressive proximal muscle weakness presenting after age 18 months or older; most children survive to adulthood.

Peripheral Nervous System

Disorders of the peripheral nervous system in children include axonal, demyelinating, or hypomyelinating neuropathies. Hereditary motor-sensory neuropathy I (HMSN-I, Charcot–Marie–Tooth I) may present in infancy. More commonly HMSN-3 (Dejerine–Sottas disease) presents with generalized hypotonia in the neonatal period or in infancy. HMSN-I is usually a demyelinating disorder, whereas HMSN-III is associated with hypomyeliantion. HMSN-III is characterized by initial distal weakness with eventual proximal weakness, areflexia, diminished sensation, chorea, and nystagmus. Mutation on the PMP22 gene occurs in both HMSN-I and HMSN-III. Sural nerve biopsy characteristically reveals an "onion bulb" formation consistent with cyclic demyelination and remyelination. HMSN-I becomes problematic in adolescence and has similar characteristics of distal extremity weakness and pes cavus.

HMSN-II is associated with axonal degeneration, is most readily seen in older children, and has similar findings to

The author would like to thank Dr. Chalmer McClure and Dr. Stanford Shu for allowing the use of "The Floppy Infant" from the first edition of this book.

type I with initial muscle wasting of the distal extremity muscles, pes cavus, unsteady gait, and sensory losses. Diagnosis is by family history and abnormalities on electromyographic testing.

Children with familial dysautonomia (Riley–Day syndrome) often have hypotonia, temperature and blood pressure instability, meconium aspiration at birth, and absent suck. An abnormal intradermal histamine challenge with an absent axon-flare response suggests the diagnosis, and further genetic testing can be done to confirm the diagnosis.

Demyelinating diseases resulting from autoimmune injury to the myelin sheath include acute inflammatory demyelinating polyneuropathy (AIDP/Guillain–Barré syndrome) and chronic inflammatory demyelinating polyneuropathy (CIDP). Guillain-Barré syndrome most often arises in older children, but has been diagnosed in several 9- to 12-month-old children. CSF protein is elevated approximately 2 weeks after initial URI symptoms; oligoclonal banding may be present. Although AIDP is most often described as an ascending weakness with sensory changes and areflexia, the clinical presentation may be variable and include cranial nerves. High-dose steroids (total 2 g/kg), intravenous immunoglobulin, and plasmaphoresis are used to treat severely affected patients. CIDP has similar findings as AIDP, but either progresses beyond 2 months or chronically relapses. Treatment is also similar to that for AIDP.

Neuromuscular Junction

Neuromuscular junction abnormalities may be intermittent or chronic in presentation. Infantile botulism is a neuromuscular junction disease of infectious origin and is usually self-limited. Infantile myasthenia gravis is usually transient but congenital myasthenia gravis has chronic symptoms.

Infantile botulism is caused by the gram-positive obligate anaerobe *Clostridium botulinum* and typically presents with generalized weakness, constipation, and diminished suck. If not recognized and treated, respiratory failure occurs as the toxin affects the neuromuscular junction of diaphragmatic muscles. It is spread by dust, but honey and corn syrup have also been implicated. The disease presents within the first year of life, and 95% of cases occur by 6 months of age. This is consistent with the lack of immune factors such as secretory IgA and lactoferrin in younger infants. Botulinum toxin binds to proteins in the synaptic vesicles, and inhibits acetylcholine (ACh) release from active zones of the presynaptic bouton.

EMG can be used to screen for botulism and stool cultures may grow *Clostridium*, which can then demonstrate the presence of either toxin type A or type B. Infantile botulism requires supportive care (parenteral nutrition and ventilator support) and treatment with human-derived botulinum immune globulin (HBIG). Antibiotics are avoided as lysis of the *C. botulinum* releases more of the intracellular neurotoxin into the gut, exacerbating the illness. Recovery time varies from 4 weeks to 1 year depending upon the strain of toxin released; treatment with HBIG reduces severity and improves recovery time.

Myasthenia gravis can present in the neonatal period transiently as the result of transplacental transfer of maternal antibodies during pregnancy, as an expression of genetic transmission in familial disease, or de novo as in congenital disease.

Transitory neonatal myasthenia gravis occurs in approximately 10% of births to mothers with myasthenia during pregnancy. Affected infants are alert but have a poor suck, weak cry, and generalized weakness. Measuring serum antibody titers and maternal history establish the diagnosis. Treatment includes symptomatic support and daily administration of pyridostigmine in moderate or severely affected cases. Duration of symptoms can range from 1 week to 2 months.

Infants with congenital myasthenic syndrome (CMS) also have weakness and feeding and respiratory difficulties. Subcategories of CMS reflect structural and functional abnormalities. Presynaptic defects include inadequate ACh resynthesis and packaging or reduced synaptic vesicle number. Synaptic defects involve endplate acetylcholinesterase deficiency, while postsynaptic defects entail diminished ACh receptor number, reduced synaptic fold surface area, impaired receptor function, or slow channel syndrome (prolonged receptor open time). Most entities have autosomal recessive inheritance although some occur de novo.

Interpretation of the Tensilon (pyridostigmine) test performed on these infants is difficult and highly subjective because the subject rarely cooperates. Substitution of neostigmine prolongs the effect, increasing the chance of a demonstrable clinical change. Repetitive electrical stimulation of selected nerves demonstrates approximately a 10% decremental response with resolution following a period of rest. Before attempting to define the CMS subtypes, efforts should be made to determine whether autoimmune forms of myasthenia are present by obtaining serum titers of ACh receptor and cross-reacting anti-striatal muscle antibodies and chest CT to evaluate for the presence of a mediastinal mass. Thymectomy has no effect on the course or duration of CMS and should not be performed. Pyridostigmine inhibits acetylcholinesterase action, allowing for longer action of ACh at the postsynaptic receptor site. Its effect is variable in CMS but still used to ameliorate symptoms. Pyridostigmine is not helpful in slow channel syndrome. Some antibiotics (aminoglycosides, erythromycin, sulfonamides), anesthetics (lidocaine), anticonvulsants (phenytoin), and iodinated contrast may worsen symptoms of myasthenia gravis.

Muscle Disease

Myotonic dystrophy is an autosomal dominantly transmitted disease with triplet (CTG) expansion of the protein kinase gene on chromosome 19q13.3. The incidence of myotonic dystrophy is estimated at 1 in 8,000 live births. Affected children are without symptoms until the CTG repeat number is greater than 800. If maternally inherited, there is expansion in the number of repeats (>1,500) with symptom onset in the neonatal period with generalized hypotonia, weakness, facial diplegia, respiratory distress, and arthrogryposis. Ventilatory support is usually required but the majority of infants are eventually weaned. Weakness and hypotonia improve and many children have long-lasting problems associated with global developmental delay. Congenital and childhood myotonic dystrophy may have some transient respiratory involvement. As these children mature, weakness and hypotonia give way to "stiffness" as voluntarily contracted muscles are unable to relax (myotonia). Percussion of the thenar eminence or other large muscle group can elicit myotonia. Typical facies also become apparent: high hairline, temporal wasting, "fish mouth" appearance, and dull affect. Associated cardiac arrhythmias and endocrine dysfunction may occur. The EMG/NCV reveals a characteristic "divebomber" sound. Antiepileptic drugs ameliorate muscle "stiffness," and older children respond to the antiarrhythmic drug mexiletene.

The spectrum of congenital muscular dystrophy includes subsets of absent or partially functioning merosin. Merosin is

TABLE 47.1

INITIAL LABORATORY INVESTIGATION OF HYPOTONIC INFANT

Diagnostic study	Disease
TORCH: toxoplasmosis, syphilis, rubella, cytomegalovirus, herpes titers/PCR	Infection
Chromosomes and subtelomeric chromosomes	Trisomy and other large genetic defects
Head MRI	Congenital brain malformations
Urine organic acids	Organic acidurias, mitochondrial disease
Arterial lactate, plasma pyruvate	Ratio >20:1 suggests mitochondrial disease
Serum ammonia	Defects in urea cycle and protein metabolism
Creatine Kinase (CK)	Screen for myopathy and congenital muscular dystrophy
Specific studies if indicated	
Spinal cord neuroimaging	Trauma
Acylcarnitine profile	Fatty acid oxidation defects
Total and free carnitine	Carnitine deficiency
Very-long-chain fatty acid (VLCFA), phytanic acid, pipecolic acid, plasmalogen	Zellweger syndrome, neonatal adrenoleukodystrophy, Refsum disease (HSMN IV)
DNA for mitochondrial deletions and mutations	Mitochondrial disorders—MELAS, MERRF, Leigh syndrome
DNA for myotonic dystrophy trinucleotide repeats	Myotonic dystrophy
DNA analysis for gene mutation	Spinal muscular atrophy (SMA)
FISH for chromosome 15 deletion	Prader–Willi syndrome, Angelman syndrome
Histamine skin challenge	Familial dysautonomia (Riley–Day syndrome)
Muscle biopsy	Myopathies (such as congenital, mitochondrial and beta oxidation) and storage diseases (such as acid maltase deficiency—Pompe disease)
Ophthalmology evaluation	Ophthalmologic abnormalities (e.g., retinal pigmentary abnormalities, cataracts, hemorrhage)
Additional metabolic and genetic testing as appropriate	

a protein partially embedded in the basement membrane surrounding muscle fibers that interacts with actin and dystrophin to produce movement. Although variable in presentation, congenital muscular dystrophy has proximal greater than distal muscle weakness and depressed deep tendon reflexes. Congenital muscular dystrophy is diagnosed following immunohistochemistry of biopsied muscle.

Unlike the merosin dependent congenital muscular dystrophies, the Fukuyama type has a CNS migrational abnormality in addition to the muscle component. Proximal greater than distal muscle involvement is noted, as is absent deep tendon reflexes. Affected children have severe motor and cognitive delays. Seizures may also be present. Muscle biopsy demonstrates a disrupted basement membrane and extremely variable fiber size.

Duchenne and Becker muscular dystrophies are part of a phenotypic continuum of dystrophin gene expression (Xp21). Deletion of DNA base pairs causes frame shifts in transcription leading to stop codons and no product or partial functional protein. The protein dystrophin attaches F-actin to merosin by way of sarcolemmal-bound glycoprotein. Without dystrophin, interaction between actin and merosin is greatly reduced, resulting in muscle weakness. Duchenne muscular dystrophy has absent or poorly functioning dystrophin resulting in significant clinical symptoms. Occasionally, severely affected boys present during infancy. The milder Becker muscular dystrophy has a more functional form of dystrophin, exhibiting less debilitating symptoms and later onset. In both, creatine kinase is markedly elevated; in Duchenne muscular dystrophy it is usually greater than 10,000 units.

The term *congenital myopathy* includes a host of extremely rare diseases of muscle pathology. Among these disorders, central core, nemaline, centronuclear, and congenital fiber-type disproportion are well-established entities. As a group, affected infants are the archetypal "floppy infant." Treatment is primarily supportive. Diagnosis requires muscle biopsy including light and electron microscopic studies and enzymatic staining. These diseases are severe in the infantile form and often lethal.

Central core disease gains its name from the histologic appearance of fused myotubules in the center of type 1 muscle fibers. It has an autosomal dominant inheritance with incomplete penetrance isolated to chromosome 19. Associated malignant hyperthermia becomes apparent following general anesthesia. Nemaline (rod) myopathy exhibits characteristic myogranules located eccentrically beneath the sarcolemma, best seen with trichrome staining of fresh frozen muscle. It has autosomal dominant (chromosome 1) and autosomal recessive (chromosome 2) transmission. Centrally located nuclei in myofibers are the hallmark of centronuclear myopathy. The neonatal/infantile form is an X-linked trait (Xq28), with additional clinical features of extraocular muscle weakness. Although numerous myopathies eventually show fiber-type prevalence with age, some investigators describe a congenital fiber-type disproportion with predominance of type 2 fibers in infancy. Still others describe a type 1 myofiber predominance. Differences are demonstrated by enzymatic muscle staining.

Metabolic Myopathies

Abnormalities of glycogen metabolism and deficiency of glycolytic enzymes give rise to several disorders including acid maltase disease (Pompe disease) as well as phosphorylase and phosphofructokinase deficiencies. Muscle storage of excess substrate has the clinical consequence of weakness and pain.

Infants with acid maltase deficiency are hypotonic and weak, and because of abnormal storage of glycogen, hepatomegaly,

TABLE 47.2

DIFFERENTIAL DIAGNOSIS OF LOWER MOTOR NEURON DISEASES

Anatomic location	Disease
Anterior horn cell	Spinal muscular atrophy
	Poliomyelitis
	Neurogenic arthrogryposis
Peripheral nerve	Congenital hypomyelinating neuropathy
	Giant axonal neuropathy
	Hereditary sensory-motor neuropathies
	Metachromatic leukodystrophy
	Neonatal adrenoleukodystrophy
	Neuroaxonal dystrophy
Neuromuscular junction	Congenital myasthenia gravis
	Transient neonatal myasthenia gravis
	Infantile botulism
Muscle	Fiber-type disproportion myopathies
	Central-core disease
	Congenital fiber-type disproportion
	Myotubular (centronuclear)
	Nemaline rod
	Metabolic myopathies
	Acid maltase deficiency (Pompe disease)
	Cytochrome-c-oxidase deficiency
	Phosphofructokinase deficiency
	Phosphorylase deficiency (McArdle disease)
	Muscular dystrophies
	Bethlem limb-girdle myopathy
	Cerebro-oculo-muscular syndrome
	Congenital muscular dystrophy (merosin + or −)
	Congenital myotonic dystrophy
	Fukuyama type

cardiomegaly, and macroglosia are common. Muscle biopsy demonstrates periodic acid Shiff (PAS) positive staining of glycogen vacuoles. Although a high-protein, low-carbohydrate diet has been helpful in some patients, it has not generally been proven to be effective. Most infants succumb to progressive cardiac failure.

A multitude of enzymatic defects are lumped together under the heading of *mitochondrial encephalomyelopathies*. These include deficiencies of enzymes from the Krebs cycle through electron transport chain, carnitine transport, and beta-oxidation. Prominent among these are Kearns–Sayre and Leigh syndromes; myoclonic epilepsy and ragged red fibers (MERRF); mitochondrial encephalopathy with lactic acidosis and stroke-like episodes (MELAS); and decreased carnitine content or transport across mitochondrial membranes. MERRF and MELAS become apparent in older children. Kearns–Sayre disease can be present at birth, usually with a progressive cardiac conduction defect, external ophthalmoplegia, weakness, and ataxia. This form is associated with complex I NADH-coenzyme Q reductase deficiency.

Infants with Leigh syndrome (subacute necrotizing encephalomyelopathy) are severely hypotonic, have poor spontaneous muscle movement, display abnormal eye movement, and are susceptible to respiratory distress. Magnetic resonance imaging (MRI) reveals periqueductal gray matter destruction, which extends from the hypothalamus to the brainstem tectum but does not include the mammilary bodies. Serum lactic acidosis can be detected, as well as enzyme abnormalities traced to pyruvate dehydrogenase and cytochrome c oxidase (complex IV) functioning. Dietary supplementation of thi-

amine has improved functioning in some patients; limiting carbohydrate intake is helpful in others.

Cerebrohepatorenal syndrome (Zellweger syndrome) and neonatal adrenoleukodystrophy are peroxisomal diseases with defective oxidation leading to accumulation of very-long-chain fatty acids (VLCFAs). Neonates have severe hypotonia, dysmorphic features, cerebral dysgensis, seizures, arthrogryposis, retinal abnormalities, and hepatomegaly. Diagnosis is further suggested by measuring serum VLCFA and performing a liver biopsy.

EVALUATION

When initially assessing the floppy infant, consider first that most causes are not neuromuscular in origin. Therefore, one must evaluate for sepsis, meningitis, electrolyte imbalances, dehydration, and other systemic illnesses that cause hypotonia (Table 47.1). Following this, establish involvement of either upper or lower motor neurons, or both. Lower motor neuron disease presents with hyporeflexia, muscle atrophy, and fasciculations; while upper motor neuron involvement usually demonstrates hyperreflexia and hypertonicity. When lower motor neuron deficits are suspected, the differential diagnosis is extensive (Table 47.2), and many of the tests listed in Table 47.3 will be necessary. Treatment for most of the neuromuscular disorders remains supportive. However, as many of these conditions are genetic in origin, it is likely that in the future new therapies will be available.

TABLE 47.3

EVALUATION OF LOWER MOTOR NEURON DISEASE

Test	Function
Serum creatine kinase	Reflects skeletal or cardiac muscle injury. If normal, then it is unlikely that there is a myopathy.
Electromyography and nerve conduction studies	Localizes lesion to a specific portion of the peripheral nervous system.
Tensilon test	Edrophonium chloride (Tensilon) 0.15–0.20 mg/kg to rule out disorder of neuromuscular transmission. If there is no adverse reaction 30–60 seconds after the first 10% of the dose is given, then the remainder is given.
Muscle biopsy	Human skeletal muscle can be divided into two types based on the intensity of reaction to myosin ATPase at pH 9.4. Type I and II fibers are generally equal in number and randomly distributed throughout the fascicle. Type I fibers (tonic) react weakly to ATPase. Type II fibers (phasic) react intensely to ATPase.
Nerve biopsy	Rarely needed.

Suggested Readings

Bodensteiner J. Congenital myopathies. *Neurol Clin* 1966;6:499–518.
Crawford TO. Clinical evaluation of the floppy infant. *Pediatr Ann* 1992;21: 348–354.
Johnston H. The floppy infant revisited. *BrainDev* 2003;52:155–158.

Miller VS, Delgado M, Iannoaccone ST. Neonatal hypotonia. *Semin Neurol* 1993;13:73–83.
Paro-Panjan D, Neubauer D. Congenital Hypotonia: is there an algorithm? *J Child Neurol* 2004;19:439–442.
Prasad A, Prasad C. The floppy infant: contribution of genetic and metabolic disorders. *Brain Dev* 2003;25:457–476.
Tein I. Neonatal metabolic myopathies. *Semin Perinatol* 1999;23:125–151.

CHAPTER 48 ■ THE COMATOSE CHILD

STEPHEN ASHWAL

Evaluation of the comatose child in the hospital setting must be viewed as a medical and surgical emergency. Fortunately, the near universal ability to obtain neuroimaging, toxicology screening, and other "routine" laboratory studies has made the ability to diagnose and treat children easier and has resulted in improved outcomes. It remains important to understand the different types of altered states of consciousness, to recognize important features of the examination that aid in the evaluation of the patient, and to have a readily available differential diagnosis to methodically pursue.

DEFINITIONS

Consciousness is the spontaneously occurring state of awareness of self and environment. Consciousness has two dimensions: wakefulness and awareness (1). Normal consciousness requires arousal, an independent, autonomic-vegetative brain function subserved by ascending stimuli, emanating from pontine tegmentum, posterior hypothalamus, and thalamus, which activate mechanisms inducing wakefulness. Cerebral cortical neurons and their reciprocal projections to and from the major subcortical nuclei subserve awareness. Awareness requires wakefulness, but wakefulness can be present without awareness.

Confusion is the state of impaired ability to think and reason clearly at a developmentally and intellectually appropriate level. Confused children have persistent difficulty with orientation, simple cognitive processing, and acquisition of new memory. Normal suggestibility and anxiety in younger children may be misleading when assessing confusion.

Impairment of Consciousness with Activated Mental State

Several conditions can be considered in this category. *Hallucinations* are perceptions of sensory input that are not present. *Illusions* are misinterpretations of actual sensory stimuli. *Delusions* are incorrect thoughts or beliefs that do not change when challenged by contradictory evidence or logical reason. *Delirium* refers to an activated mental state, which may include disorientation, irritability, fearful responses, and sensory misperception. Visual hallucinations, when present, are more common than auditory hallucinations and the patient may experience delusional thought or illusions. Delirium is usually due to diffuse nervous system disease; the most common causes in children include intoxication, infection, fever, metabolic disorders, and epilepsy.

Impairment of Consciousness with Reduced Mental State

Obtundation is a condition in which there is mild to moderate reduction in alertness with decreased interest in the environment and slower-than-normal reactivity to stimulation. Obtunded patients appear abnormally drowsy and often sleep when left alone. *Stupor* is a state of unresponsiveness with little or no spontaneous movement resembling deep sleep from which the patient can only be aroused by vigorous and repeated stimulation. Communication is absent or minimal. The best-aroused level of consciousness is still quite abnormal, and without continuous stimulation, the patient returns to the pre-stimulation state.

Coma is a state of deep, unarousable, sustained pathologic unconsciousness with the eyes closed resulting from dysfunction of the ascending reticular activating system either in the brainstem or both cerebral hemispheres (1). Coma usually requires the period of unconsciousness to persist for at least 1 hour to distinguish coma from syncope, concussion, or other states of transient unconsciousness. The term *unconsciousness* implies global or total unawareness and applies equally to patients in either coma or a vegetative state. Patients in coma are unconscious because they lack both wakefulness and awareness. In contrast, patients in a vegetative state are unconscious because, although they have retained wakefulness, they lack awareness. The depth of coma may be further specified by assessment of brainstem reflexes, breathing pattern, change of pulse or respiratory rate to stimulation, or stimulus-induced nonspecific movement.

Table 48.1 lists several of the major neurologic conditions that the clinician must be aware of and capable of differentiating from coma (1,2). Differentiating features of these conditions from coma are described in the following sections.

Vegetative State

The vegetative state can be described as a condition of complete unawareness of the self and the environment accompanied by sleep–wake cycles with either complete or partial preservation of hypothalamic and brainstem autonomic functions. Criteria to diagnose the vegetative state have been recommended for adults and children by the Multi-Society Task Force on PVS (Table 48.2). Children in a vegetative state lack evidence of self-awareness or recognition of external stimuli. Rather than being in a state of "eyes-closed" coma they remain unconscious but have irregular periods of wakefulness alternating with periods of sleeping. Vegetative patients have inconsistent head- and eye-turning movements to sounds and inconsistent nonpurposeful trunk and limb movements. Perhaps of most importance and most easy to objectively examine is the fact that they do not have evidence of sustained visual fixation nor do they demonstrate sustained visual tracking.

The clinical course of evolution to a vegetative state after an acute injury usually begins with eyes-closed coma for several days to weeks followed by the appearance of sleep–wake cycles (3). Other responses such as decorticate and decerebrate

TABLE 48.1

SEVERE DISORDERS OF CONSCIOUSNESS AND RELATED CONDITIONS

Condition	Self-awareness	Pain and suffering	Sleep–wake cycles	Motor function	Respiratory function	Outcome
Coma	Absent	No	Absent	No purposeful movement	Variably depressed	Evolves to PVS, death, or recovery, in 2 to 4 wk
Vegetative state	Absent	No	Intact	No purposeful movement	Normal to variably depressed	Depends on etiology
Minimally conscious state	Very limited	Yes	Intact	Severe limitation of movement	Variably depressed	Recovery unknown
Akinetic mutism	Limited	Yes	Intact	Moderate limitation of movement	Normal to variably depressed	Recovery unlikely or limited
Locked-in syndrome	Present	Yes	Intact	Quadriplegia; pseudobulbar palsy; eye movements preserved	Normal to variably depressed	Recovery unlikely; remain quadriplegic
Brain death	Absent	No	Absent	None or only reflex spinal movements	Absent	None

Based in part on Multi-Society Task Force on PVS. Medical aspects of the persistent vegetative state. *N Engl J Med* 1994;330:1499,1572; and Giacino J, Ashwal S, Childs N. The minimally conscious state: definition and diagnostic criteria. Report of the Aspen Work Group. *Neurology* 2002;58:349–353.

posturing, roving eye movements, and eye blinking appear earlier than sleep–wake cycles.

Diagnosis of the vegetative state is made clinically. There are no confirmatory laboratory tests. However, absence of somatosensory evoked responses to median nerve stimulation has been associated with the vegetative state in several studies (4). Neuroimaging usually demonstrates diffuse or multifocal cerebral disease involving the gray and white matter. In patients with traumatic and nontraumatic brain injury, serial imaging studies usually demonstrate progressive atrophy. It is important to correctly identify children who are in a vegetative state because of the implications for continued care, family expectations, and the need for rehabilitation. Children in a vegetative state have been reported to have considerably shorter than normal life expectancy (3).

Minimally Conscious State

The term *minimally conscious state* (MCS) has been proposed to describe patients who were in coma or a vegetative state and who are beginning to show minimal signs of awareness (5). The minimally conscious state has been defined as a condition of severely altered consciousness in which the person demonstrates minimal but definite behavioral evidence of self or environmental awareness (2). Patients in an MCS are able to (1) follow simple commands, (2) show some ability to manipulate objects, (3) have gestural or verbal "yes"/"no" responses, (4) have intelligible verbalizations, and (5) have stereotypical movements (e.g., blinking, smiling) that occur in a meaningful relationship to the eliciting stimulus and are not attributable to reflexive activity. Based on limited literature of this disorder in adults (6), it is possible that children in a minimally conscious state, depending on the etiology of the insult, may have a better potential for neurologic recovery and a longer life expectancy than those children who remain vegetative.

Locked-In Syndrome

In locked-in syndrome, patients retain consciousness and cognition but are unable to move or communicate because of severe paralysis of the voluntary motor system (7). This condition is due to diseases involving the descending corticospinal and corticobulbar pathways at or below the pons or to severe involvement of the peripheral nervous system. By definition,

TABLE 48.2

CRITERIA FOR DIAGNOSIS OF THE VEGETATIVE STATE

1. No evidence of awareness of themselves or their environment; they are incapable of interacting with others.
2. No evidence of sustained, reproducible, purposeful, or voluntary behavioral responses to visual, auditory, tactile, or noxious stimuli.
3. No evidence of language comprehension or expression.
4. Intermittent wakefulness manifested by the presence of sleep–wake cycles.
5. Sufficiently preserved hypothalamic and brainstem autonomic functions to survive if given medical and nursing care.
6. Bowel and bladder incontinence.
7. Variably preserved cranial nerve (pupillary, oculocephalic, corneal, vestibulo-ocular, gag, and spinal reflexes).

From Multi-Society Task Force on PVS. Medical aspects of the persistent vegetative state. *N Engl J Med* 1994;330:1499,1572.

patients in locked-in syndrome are conscious and differ from those in a coma or vegetative state, although this may be difficult to determine. The locked-in syndrome is quite rare in children (8). Some patients with this condition can establish limited communication using eye movements.

Akinetic Mutism

Akinetic mutism is a rare condition consisting of pathologically slowed or nearly absent bodily movement accompanied by a similar loss of speech (7). The original description of this condition in 1941 was in an adolescent with symptoms of intermittent depressed states of consciousness secondary to a craniopharyngioma (8). Since then, akinetic mutism has been seen with bacterial and viral CNS infections, other tumors of the nervous system, hydrocephalus, and occasionally as a postoperative phenomena. Wakefulness and self-awareness are usually preserved in most patients but the level of mental function is reduced. The condition characteristically accompanies gradually developing or subacute, bilateral damage to the paramedian mesencephalon, basal diencephalon, or inferior frontal lobes. The long-term outlook for children with akinetic mutism is unknown because few patients with this disorder have been reported. It is most likely related to the etiology and severity of the associated disease.

Brain Death

Brain death describes the permanent absence of all brain functions, including those of the brainstem. Brain dead patients are irreversibly comatose, apneic, and have absent brainstem reflexes including the loss of all cranial nerve functions. The appearance of brain death can be imitated by deep anesthesia, sedative overdose, or severe hypothermia. Patients who are brain dead differ from patients who are in a coma, as these latter patients usually have preserved brainstem functions and some degree of respiratory drive. Guidelines for the diagnosis of brain death in infants and children are well established and reviewed in a different section of this book.

CONSCIOUSNESS RATING SCALES

Several rating scales have been developed to assess patients with acute brain injury (Table 48.3). The best known and most widely used is the Glasgow Coma Scale (GCS), which yields a score of 3 to 15 based on best response to stimuli in three categories: eye opening, verbal response, and motor response (Table 48.3) (9). In its original form, the GCS was not developmentally suitable for assessment in newborns, infants, and younger children, and a variety of alternate scales have been proposed (8).

The Pediatric Coma Scale (Table 48.4) makes minor changes in the verbal scale of the GCS and redefines the "best" score based on developmental and age-appropriate norms (10). It has the advantage of prospective evaluation and interrater reliability and the disadvantage of different maximum scores based on age, thus making outcome prediction and comparison difficult to study using the GCS.

The Children's Coma Scale (Table 48.5) redefines certain criteria and the "maximum" score and changes the "eye opening" category to "ocular response" (11). This scoring system

---

TABLE 48.3

GLASGOW COMA SCALE (GCS) SCORE AND MODIFICATION FOR CHILDREN

Sign	GCS	GCS-MC	Score
EYE OPENING	Spontaneous	Spontaneous	4
	To command	To sound	3
	To pain	To pain	2
	None	None	1
VERBAL RESPONSE	Oriented	Age appropriate-verbalization	5
	Confused, disoriented	Cries but consolable, irritable, uncooperative, aware of environment	4
	Inappropriate words	Irritable, persistent cries, inconsistently consolable	3
	Incomprehensible sounds	Inconsolable crying, unaware of environment	2
	None	None	1
MOTOR RESPONSE	Obeys commands	Obeys commands, spontaneous movement	6
	Localizes pain	Localizes pain	5
	Withdraws	Withdraws	4
	Abnormal flexion to pain	Abnormal flexion to pain	3
	Abnormal extension to pain	Abnormal extension to pain	2
	None	None	1
BEST TOTAL SCORE			15

Glasgow Coma Scale (GCS) from Teasdale G, Jennett B. Assessment of coma and impaired consciousness. A practical scale. *Lancet* 1974;2:81. Glasgow Coma Scale Modified for Children (GCS-MC) from Hahn YS, Chyung C, Barthel MJ, et al. Head injuries in children under 36 months of age. *Childs Nerv Syst* 1988;4:34.

TABLE 48.4

PEDIATRIC COMA SCALE

Response	Score
EYE OPENING	
Spontaneous	4
To speech	3
To pain	2
None	1
BEST VERBAL RESPONSE	
Oriented	5
Words	4
Vocal sounds	3
Cries	2
None	1
BEST MOTOR RESPONSE	
Obeys commands	5
Localizes pain	4
Flexion to pain	3
Extension to pain	2
None	1
NORMAL AGGREGATE SCORE	
Birth to 6 months	9
>6 to 12 months	11
>1 to 2 years	12
>2 to 5 years	12
>5 years	14

From Reilly PL, Simpson DA, Sprod R, et al. Assessing the conscious level in infants and young children: a pediatric version of the Glasgow Coma Scale. *Childs Nerv Syst* 1988;4:30.

TABLE 48.5

CHILDREN'S COMA SCALE

Sign	Score
OCULAR RESPONSE	
Pursuit	4
Extraocular movement intact; pupils react appropriately	3
Fixed pupils or extraocular; movement impaired	2
Fixed pupils and extraocular; movement paralyzed	1
VERBAL RESPONSE	
Cries	3
Spontaneous respiration	2
Apneic	1
MOTOR RESPONSE	
Flexes and extends	4
Withdraws from painful stimuli	3
Hypertonic	2
Flaccid	1
BEST TOTAL SCORE	11

From Raimondi AJ, Hirschauer J. Head injury in the infant and toddler. Coma scoring and outcome scale. *Childs Brain* 1984;11:12.

includes pupillary reflexes, extraocular movements, and apnea in its categories and is different from the GCS and requires different training and forms to be used.

The Glasgow Coma Scale Modified for Children (GCS-MC) maintains the same categories as the GCS and the same maximum and minimum scores while allowing developmental and age-appropriate scoring (12,13). It does, however, equate spontaneous movement with following commands to achieve 6 points in the best motor response category, to allow inclusion of infants and young children (Table 48.3). The GCS-MC allows best direct comparison to the GCS for scoring of consciousness impairment and assessment of outcome.

These different scoring systems are useful to objectively quantify the continuum from consciousness to coma and allow serial reassessments with good interrater reliability. The scores also allow a relatively large amount of information to be conveyed quickly and concisely with minimum need to remember cumbersome definitions or write long descriptions. However, these scoring systems do not take into account all-important brainstem reflexes (e.g., pupillary, corneal, oculocephalic, and oculovestibular reflexes), and these should also be performed as part of the initial and ongoing assessment of these patients.

EVALUATION OF THE COMATOSE CHILD

Table 48.6 provides a classification of the causes of coma that can occur in children. It is important to evaluate the evolution of symptoms to determine if there is a need for immediate life support treatment and to try to identify the cause of coma and institute specific therapy.

Clinical Evaluation

Immediate Life Support

The ABCs (airway, breathing, circulation) of basic life support must be evaluated and managed emergently. Early airway control is essential to prevent further brain injury from hypoxia and hypercarbia. Additionally, it is essential to assess adequacy of perfusion, as children in shock may appear stable initially but then rapidly deteriorate. Glucose, the essential substrate for brain energy metabolism, must be provided via an intravenous line. Because unobserved or unreported trauma may have occurred, it is important to consider the possibility of a cervical fracture or other injury while implementing immediate life-support measures.

Identification of Cause

The history and physical examination are the basis for identifying the cause of coma. Time constraints and evaluation of symptoms will often require rapid transition to ordering diagnostic tests.

History. Coma may present as the progression of a known underlying illness, unpredictable consequence or complication of a known disease, or totally unexpected event or illness. An accurate history of the events and circumstances prior to the onset of symptoms and basic information concerning past medical history and medications may be invaluable in determining the cause of coma and quickly lead to the most appropriate diagnostic testing and treatment (7,8,14).

Sudden onset of coma in an otherwise normal and awake child suggests convulsions or intracranial hemorrhage. Coma preceded by sleepiness or unsteadiness suggests ingestion of a drug or toxin in an otherwise well child. Fever is typical when

TABLE 48.6

ETIOLOGIES OF IMPAIRED CONSCIOUSNESS AND COMA

Structural—Intrinsic	Metabolic—Toxic

A. TRAUMA
Concussion
Cerebral contusion
Epidural hematoma
Subdural hematoma/effusion
Intracerebral hematoma
Diffuse axonal injury
 	
B. NEOPLASMS
 	
C. VASCULAR DISEASE
Cerebral infarction
  Thrombosis
  Embolism
Cerebral hemorrhage
  Arteriovenous malformation
  Aneurysm
  Other acquired congenital vascular
    wall weakness
Vasculitis
Congenital abnormality of vascular
  supply
Trauma to carotid or vertebral arteries
  in the neck
 	
D. FOCAL INFECTION
Cerebritis
Empyema (subdural or epidural)
Abscess
 	
E. HYDROCEPHALUS
	A. HYPOXIA—ISCHEMIA
	Shock
	Cardiac or pulmonary failure
	Near drowning
	Carbon monoxide poisoning
	Strangulation
	
	B. METABOLIC DISORDERS
	Hypoglycemia
	With acidosis
	  Diabetic ketoacidosis
	  Organic acidemias
	  Amino acidemias
	With hyperammonemia
	  Hepatic encephalopathy
	  Reye syndrome
	  Urea cycle disorders
	  Valproic acid encephalopathy
	  Disorder of fatty acid metabolism
	Uremia
	Fluid and electrolyte imbalance
	  dehydration, hyponatremia, calcium
	  and magnesium imbalance
	Endocrine disorders (thyroid disorders,
	  hypoparathyroidism, adrenal
	  insufficiency)
	Hypertensive encephalopathy
	Vitamin deficiency (thiamin, pyridoxine,
	  niacin)
	Mitochondrial disorders
	
	C. EXOGENOUS TOXINS AND POISONS
	Narcotics, neuroleptics, antidepressants,
	  MAO inhibitors, anticonvulsants,
	  stimulants
	Over-the-counter drugs: acetaminophen
	Biological toxins (mushroom poisoning,
	  jimsonweed intoxication)
	Industrial toxins (organophosphates,
	  heavy metals, cyanide, volatile
	  hydrocarbons)
	Substance abuse (alcohol, cocaine,
	  heroin, amphetamine)
	Poisoning in Münchausen by proxy
	
	D. INFECTIONS
	Bacterial
	Viral
	Rickettsial
	Acute disseminated encephalomyelitis
	
	E. PAROXYSMAL DISORDERS
	Epilepsy
	Migraine

coma is due to an infectious process, but may not be present when shock is present or if the ambient temperature is low. The history of headache may suggest elevated intracranial pressure due to hydrocephalus or neoplasm but may also be seen in migraine syndromes with alteration of consciousness. When traumatic brain injury has occurred, coma may exist from the moment of impact or may be preceded by a lucid interval. The presence of a period of consciousness followed by coma warrants immediate CT of the head to assess for an expanding intracranial mass lesion such as an epidural hematoma. A history of fever or recent illness suggests an acute infectious etiology, but should also lead to considerations of complications from infectious disease such as acute disseminated encephalomyelitis, Reye syndrome, or mitochondrial disorders. Children with diabetes may have coma due to hypoglycemia or ketoacidosis. Children with congenital heart disease may be susceptible to brain abscess or infarction. Intermittent episodes of coma should suggest ingestion, drug overdose, inborn errors of metabolism, or Münchausen syndrome by proxy. A history of the use of an unvented kerosene stove or heater should suggest carbon monoxide poisoning.

General Physical Examination. The general physical examination begins with assessment of the vital signs: temperature, heart rate, respiration, and blood pressure. Fever usually suggests infection but infrequently can be caused by an abnormality of the central control mechanisms that regulate body temperature. Fever with coma suggests sepsis, pneumonia, meningitis, encephalitis, intracranial abscess, or emphysema. Very high fever and dry skin may be due to heat stroke or antihistamine ingestion. In children, hypothermia is most often seen with drug intoxication, especially if the ambient temperature is cold. Rapid heart rate suggests hypovolemic shock, secondary effects of fever, heart failure or a tachydysrhythmia such as paroxysmal atrial tachycardia (supraventricular tachycardia may be the better rhythm to note, as it is the most common pathologic tachydysrhythmia in children). An abnormally low heart rate may reflect myocardial injury, the late effect of hypoxemia, or increased intracranial pressure. Rapid respiration suggests a primary abnormality of oxygenation as seen in pneumonia, asthma, or pulmonary embolus; or acidosis as in diabetic ketoacidosis and uremia. Brainstem lesions may cause central neurogenic hyperventilation. Slow, irregular, or periodic breathing patterns may indicate toxic ingestion or increased intracranial pressure. Hypotension is seen in shock, sepsis, certain drug ingestions, myocardial injury or failure, and adrenal insufficiency. Hypertension may be a primary cause of unresponsiveness as in hypertensive encephalopathy, but may also be a compensatory mechanism to assure brain perfusion in children with increased intracranial pressure or stroke.

Inspection of the head, scalp, and skin can be most helpful. Cyanosis suggests poor oxygenation, jaundice is seen in liver failure, extreme pallor may be seen in anemia and shock, and a cherry-red color suggests carbon monoxide poisoning. The presence of a cephalohematoma, boggy or swollen areas of the scalp, or head bruises, suggest cranial trauma. Bleeding or clear fluid leaking from the nose or ears suggests a basilar skull fracture. Certain types of burns and multiple bruises of characteristic shape and location or varied age may suggest child abuse. Various rashes may be seen with infectious causes of coma such as meningococcemia or rickettsial disease. The presence of neurocutaneous lesions such as the depigmented areas of tuberous sclerosis suggests seizures or intracranial mass as the cause of coma. Generalized increased pigmentation may be seen in Addison disease or adrenoleukodystrophy.

The odor of exhaled breath can be characteristic in alcohol intoxication, diabetic ketoacidosis (sweet or fruity), uremia (urine-like), and hepatic coma (musty).

The cardiovascular exam may suggest congenital heart disease or endocarditis, both sources of intracranial abscess dissemination. Abdominal discoloration or rigidity may suggest intra-abdominal bleeding as a source of shock.

Neurologic Examination. Examination of the optic fundi, pupillary size and reactivity, eye movement control, corneal reflexes, motor responses, body posture, and the presence or absence of meningeal signs, gives important information about the potential causes and localization of brain dysfunction in the comatose patient (8,14).

Funduscopic examination offers important clues to the etiology of coma including papilledema as an indicator of raised intracranial pressure and retinal hemorrhages in occult trauma.

In acute increased intracranial pressure, there may not have been time for papilledema to develop at the time of presentation in the emergency department. Pupil size and reactivity are also important to assess. Pupillary reactivity can be elicited by shining a light on the eye or by opening and closing the eyelid. The afferent limb of the pupillary light reflex is through the optic nerve and the efferent limb is through the parasympathetic fibers, which travel with the oculomotor nerve. In the presence of normal visual acuity and absence of corneal clouding, an abnormality of the pupillary light reflex suggests midbrain dysfunction. With unilateral loss of visual acuity, the opposite pupil may dilate when the light is moved from the unaffected to the affected side. This is due to a defect in the afferent limb of the reflex arc on the affected side.

Many metabolic disorders and drug ingestions produce symmetrically small pupils that retain some reactivity to light. Severe hypoxic-ischemic injury produces symmetric dilated pupils, which may not respond to light. Structural or mass lesions of the cerebral hemispheres typically do not produce pupillary abnormalities unless herniation occurs. For example, herniation of the temporal lobe over the tentorium with compression of the parasympathetic fibers traveling with the oculomotor nerve will produce unilateral pupillary dilation due to unopposed sympathetic innervation. Hypothalamic lesions produce small pupils by interrupting sympathetic fibers at the point of origin. Structural lesions in the pons may disrupt sympathetic fibers descending from the hypothalamus. In either case, unopposed parasympathetic tone will produce small or "pinpoint" pupils that may mimic those seen in metabolic disorders or toxin or drug ingestions. Midbrain injuries may interrupt both sympathetic and parasympathetic pupillary innervations producing midposition unresponsive pupils.

The oculomotor (cranial nerve III), trochlear (cranial nerve IV), and abducens (cranial nerve VI) nuclei in the midbrain and pons control extraocular movements. Conjugate gaze is coordinated by the yoking together of these cranial nerve nucleii via the medial longitudinal fasciculus (MLF). Supranuclear control of conjugate gaze resides in the two primary cerebral gaze centers found in the frontal lobes and parieto-occipital areas. The frontal gaze center produces rapid or saccadic eye movement contralateral to the side stimulated, while the more posterior center produces smooth pursuit or tracking movements ipsilateral to the side stimulated. Unilateral stimulation of the frontal gaze center produces conjugate eye deviation to the opposite side and can be produced by seizure activity or other unilateral irritating stimuli. Unilateral injury, destruction, or metabolic exhaustion of the frontal gaze center produces conjugate deviation toward the affected side (the patient is said to look toward the lesion). This yoked system also has important input from the vestibular system, the cerebellum, and proprioceptive pathways from neck muscles. These pathways are the basis for the doll's-eye (oculocephalic) and caloric (oculovestibular) responses.

The oculocephalic maneuver is performed by moving the head side to side or vertically, and should only be performed when there is certainty that there is no cervical spine injury or abnormality. A positive oculocephalic response consists of conjugate deviation of the eyes in the direction opposite head movement. Absence of a positive oculocephalic response may be seen in structural abnormalities of the brainstem, where it may be asymmetrical; and in metabolic-toxic encephalopathies, where it is almost always symmetrical. A common cause of an abnormal oculocephalic response is sedation routinely used for procedures, tests, or critical care support.

Caloric or oculovestibular responses are obtained by irrigating one or both external ear canals with warm and cold water and should only be performed when the external canal can be visualized and the tympanic membrane is intact. The usual protocol for unconscious patients involves cold-water irrigation with the head elevated 30 degrees from the horizontal, which induces convection currents in the endolymphatic fluid of the labyrinth. The resulting vestibular nucleii stimulation affects the ipsilateral paramedian pontine reticular formation–abducens nuclear complex, and through the MLF also the contralateral oculomotor and trochlear nucleii. In awake patients, cold-water irrigation produces a lateral nystagmus with the quick phase away from the stimulated ear. Warm water stimulation has the opposite effect. This gives rise to the mnemonic COWS (cold—opposite; warm—same). In the unconscious patient, however, the quick phase is lost, and slow tonic deviation is noted toward the irrigated ear. An intact oculovestibular response suggests functional connections from the vestibular system in the medulla to the ocular cranial nerve nuclei in the mesencephalon and pons connected by the MLF. Unilateral or asymmetric caloric responses suggest a brainstem structural abnormality while bilateral absence can be seen in metabolic as well as structural abnormalities. The oculocephalic response is an objective measure of lower brainstem integrity and an important addition to the neurologic exam when other medullary-controlled activities such as respiration are abnormal or controlled by mechanical ventilation. Caloric stimulation of the noncomatose patient may provoke nausea and vomiting and care should be exercised to avoid the possibility of aspiration.

The corneal reflex consists of closure of the eyelid elicited by gently touching the cornea with suitable stimuli such as sterile gauze or cotton. The afferent or sensory limb of this reflex involves the first division of the trigeminal nerve (cranial nerve V), and the efferent or motor limb is via the facial nerve (cranial nerve VII). A normal response to unilateral corneal stimulation is bilateral blinking due to pontine interconnections. An absent response suggests abnormal afferent or trigeminal input or bilateral pontine involvement. A contralateral blink response suggests intact sensory input via the fifth cranial nerve, whereas an abnormal motor limb response on the ipsilateral side is more consistent with an ipsilateral structural abnormality. Metabolic lesions typically produce bilateral loss of response. Absence of the corneal reflex must be interpreted with caution in the presence of conjunctival edema, injury, or with the use of sedative or paralytic agents that are commonly used in the intensive-care unit setting. Care should again be taken when eliciting this reflex to avoid corneal abrasion or perforation.

Passive resistance to neck flexion suggests meningeal irritation, tonsillar herniation, or craniocervical trauma. Patients with acute subarachnoid hemorrhage may not develop signs of meningeal irritation for several hours.

Observation of spontaneous movement and motor responses to stimulation are important clues in the assessment of coma and localization of the level of injury or lesion. Asymmetric involvement is a hallmark of structural abnormality. Unilateral cortical or subcortical structural lesions may cause contralateral weakness. Bilateral absence of movement or tone (flaccidity) occurs in metabolic-toxic encephalopathies such as drug intoxications and in disruption of brainstem–cortical interconnections above the pontomedullary junction. Flaccidity due to spinal cord injuries or neuromuscular paralysis is not associated with coma unless other injuries exist.

Posturing may occur spontaneously or in response to stimulation. "Decorticate" posturing involves flexion of the upper extremities and extension of the lower extremities and usually involves cortical or subcortical abnormalities with preservation of brainstem function. "Decerebrate" posturing involves extension of all extremities with internal rotation and may be seen with metabolic-toxic disorders or midbrain compression. Decorticate and decerebrate posturing do not have the same exquisite localizing value in clinical medicine as they do in experimentally lesioned animals. It is generally believed, however, that decerebrate posturing is "worse" than decorticate posturing, and that asymmetry of posturing is more likely seen in patients with structural than with metabolic-toxic disorders. Herniation syndromes should always be considered when posturing is present. The importance of recognizing herniation syndromes lies in the opportunity for early intervention.

Uncal herniation is the medial displacement of the uncus of the temporal lobe over the free lateral edge of the tentorium, usually associated with an asymmetric supratentorial mass or edema. Because of direct pressure on the oculomotor nerve, the most reliable early indicator of uncal herniation is ipsilateral oculomotor dysfunction with ipsilateral pupillary dilation and sluggish reactivity to light due to parasympathetic dysfunction. Parasympathetic fibers are peripherally located along the oculomotor nerve and therefore first affected. As herniation continues, the ipsilateral pupil becomes more widely dilated and subsequently loses all reactivity to light. Partial ophthalmoplegia is present and ipsilateral hemiparesis may ensue due to compression of the contralateral cerebral peduncle. Without appropriate treatment, more generalized brainstem ischemia ensues with catastrophic results.

Infratentorial herniation can occur when mass lesions in the posterior fossa produce upward herniation of brainstem structures through the tentorial notch, frequently resulting in ischemia and death. Typically, however, posterior fossa mass lesions are discovered well before this occurs because of disturbances in lower cranial nerve or cerebellar function, headache, or other symptoms due to obstructive hydrocephalus. Herniation of infratentorial structures has become quite rare since the introduction of computed tomography.

Transtentorial herniation can occur when there is a generalized increase in intracranial pressure with gradual downward displacement of the diencephalon (thalamus and hypothalamus) through the tentorium cerebelli that produces progressive compression and ischemia of the brainstem. The relatively slow evolution of this syndrome allows identification of a series of clinical stages that may blend together (7). In the diencephalic stage, patients do not follow instructions but will localize to noxious stimuli and have small reactive pupils and preserved oculocephalic and oculovestibular reflexes. Respiration may be regular with yawns or sighs or Cheyne–Stokes respiration may appear. Cheyne–Stokes respirations consist of a cyclical gradual build-up and decrease in the volume of air inhaled with each breath. Increased rigidity or decorticate posturing may appear. In the midbrain–upper pontine stage, patients have decerebrate rigidity or no movement, midposition pupils that may be irregular in shape and show no reactivity, and abnormal or absent oculocephalic and oculovestibular reflexes. Patients usually hyperventilate, although Cheyne–Stokes respiration may still be noted. In the lower pontine–medullary stage, there is no spontaneous motor activity or activity in response to stimuli, midposition fixed pupils, absent oculocephalic and oculovestibular reflexes, and shallow and rapid or slow and irregular (ataxic) respirations. The lower extremities may withdraw to plantar stimulation. Finally, in the medullary stage, there is generalized flaccid tone, absence of pupillary reflexes and ocular movements, further slowing and irregularity of respiration, and ultimately death.

Diagnostic Testing
Laboratory Tests Including Lumbar Puncture

All patients with significant impairment of consciousness or coma should have immediate blood glucose determination by Chemstrip or Dextrostix and blood drawn for a chemistry profile and complete blood count. The blood chemistry profile should minimally include glucose, sodium, potassium, BUN, calcium, magnesium, and ammonia. Hypoglycemia, derangements of osmolality (hyponatremia, hypernatremia), and ketoacidosis are important causes of mental status change in children. Uremia with encephalopathy may be seen in patients with acute renal failure with evolution over hours to days. It may also be the presenting feature in the hemolytic–uremic syndrome. Disorders of calcium metabolism may impair consciousness as well as cause peripheral symptoms. Abnormalities of calcium or magnesium may precipitate unexpected seizures, especially in infants and young children. Hyperammonemia may alter consciousness, particularly in conjunction with hepatotoxicity due to valproic acid or other agents, Reye syndrome, inborn errors of metabolism, or other disorders. A complete blood count will assist in determining the presence of infection, anemia, or toxin exposure such as lead poisoning.

A urine specimen should be sent for toxicology screening (see Chapter 146). Toxic ingestions are best identified by history and by the recognition of specific clinical syndromes (toxidromes), but it is known that children are more likely than adults to present with unfamiliar or atypical clinical features. Some laboratory tests can provide rapid results and are commonly ordered as a batch, including standard urine tests for common drugs of abuse (barbiturates, benzodiazepines, opioids, amphetamines, cocaine metabolites, phencyclidine, and marijuana metabolites) and serum tests for acetaminophen, salicylates, ethanol, sympathomimetic amines, and tricyclic antidepressants. Broader drug screens, such as thin-layer chromatography and ultraviolet spectroscopy, can detect less common causes of intoxication, but may take days for results to become available.

Arterial blood gas determination is often necessary, as is pulse oximetry to evaluate for hypercapnea or hypoxemia as a cause of altered mental status. Methemoglobin and carboxyhemoglobin levels may need to be specifically requested. When infection is suspected, blood and urine cultures should be obtained.

Additional blood and urine studies, which may be worth obtaining when the patient is first seen but which are not usually immediately available, include urine and blood specimens for amino and organic acid disorders, thyroid function studies, plasma cortisol, free fatty acid and carnitine levels, and urine testing for disorders of porphyrin metabolism.

Lumbar puncture (LP) should be performed when there is a suggestion of infection of the central nervous system with or without fever. Depending on the clinical findings and evaluation, computed tomography (CT) may need to be performed prior to the LP to minimize potential morbidity. Measuring the opening CSF pressure should be performed if increased intracraniol pressure (ICP) is suspected, as in some children neuroimaging may not reflect increased ICP (Reye syndrome, metabolic encephalopathies, or pseudotumor cerebri). Caution must however be used in such situations as in some patients relatively low increases in ICP may precipitate herniation.

Neuroimaging

When medically stable, all patients in coma, and most if not all patients with impairment of consciousness of undetermined etiology, should have a CT performed as rapidly as possible. In children with closed head injury (CHI), CT or preferably magnetic resonance imaging (MRI) may be critical in identifying the specific cause of impaired loss of consciousness (15). MRI is also invaluable in identifying evidence of herpes simplex encephalitis or an acute demyelinating process such as acute disseminated encephalomyelitis (ADEM).

CT is most suited to the critically ill patient because it can be done quickly. CT is able to detect pathology in need of immediate surgical intervention, including hydrocephalus, her-

niation, and mass lesions due to infection, neoplasia, hemorrhage, and edema. MRI provides greater stuctural detail and may be uniquely able to show early evidence of infection, infarction, diffuse axonal injury, petechial hemorrhage, sinovenous thrombosis, and demyelination. Some special MRI techniques, such as proton spectroscopy, also offer valuable information regarding prognosis in patients with anoxic or traumatic coma. MRI is therefore preferred, but may need to be delayed until a child is stable enough to endure the long procedure. Some form of neuroimaging should be considered prior to lumbar puncture given the increased risk of herniation.

Additional neuroimaging studies may be suggested by the initial CT or MRI, such as magnetic resonance angiography or conventional angiography for cases of suspected vascular malformation, vasculitis, or venous thrombosis. Repeat scanning, usually with CT, is often undertaken on an emergent basis in patients with acute clinical deterioration, and can demonstrate worsening edema, hemorrhage, herniation, and hydrocephalus. Patients without a surgically remediable lesion on initial 24- or 48-hour CT scans do not appear to benefit from continued routine imaging. There is currently no role for the routine use of functional MRI, positron emission tomography, or single-photon emission tomography in the evaluation of comatose patients.

Electrophysiologic Tests

An electroencephalogram (EEG) should be among the tests performed routinely in patients with coma of unknown etiology, and is often the only means of recognizing nonconvulsive status epilepticus (NCSE), especially in patients who are paralyzed. NCSE can be seen in as many as 20% to 30% of children with status epilepticus. The EEG is useful in the serial reassessment and evaluation of patients in status epilepticus or persistent coma as well as those requiring pharmacologic paralysis or sedation. Periodic epileptiform discharges (PEDs) have been associated with NCSE. In patients without epilepsy, PEDs are suggestive of underlying brain injury and, when lateralized (PLEDs), are suggestive of herpes encephalitis or infarction. Multifocal or generalized periodic discharges can also be seen with metabolic and infectious causes of widespread cerebral dysfunction and are characteristic of subacute sclerosing panencephalitis. Non-epileptiform features of the EEG, such as slowing or asymmetry, are largely nonspecific, but can sometimes provide diagnostic or prognostic information. Continuous EEG is useful to assess and titrate the depth of sedation in patients placed under anesthesia for control of status epilepticus or increased ICP.

Other electodiagnostic tests, such as somatosensory, auditory, and visual evoked potentials, are sometimes used in comatose patients for assessment of prognosis but do not have a well-defined diagnostic utility. Nerve conduction and needle electromyographic studies also have no place in the routine evaluation of coma, although they are essential for diagnosing the locked-in syndrome caused by peripheral nervous system disorders, and are generally useful in the evaluation of paralysis in critically ill patients.

TREATMENT

Treatment of the child with impaired consciousness or coma requires attention to certain basic principles while diagnostic tests are obtained and therapy is initiated. Specific treatments of many individual causes of disordered consciousness are reviewed in other sections of this book. The principles of management are similar in the majority of patients and are outlined in Table 48.7.

TABLE 48.7

TREATMENT GOALS FOR PATIENTS WITH IMPAIRED
CONSCIOUSNESS AND COMA

- Assure oxygenation and ventilation
- Maintain circulation
- Give glucose
- Consider specific antidote
- Reduce increased intracranial pressure
- Stop seizures
- Treat infection
- Correct acid–base and electrolyte imbalance
- Adjust body temperature
- Manage agitation

Assure Oxygenation

Maintenance of an adequate airway remains one of the most important principles in the management of children with altered states of consciousness and coma to prevent secondary brain injury. When necessary, an artificial airway should be established and artificial ventilation provided early, with even the slightest suspicion of inadequate ventilation or oxygenation as well as depression or loss of protective airway reflexes, even if this necessitates use of sedative or paralytic agents. It is important to ensure that cervical spine injuries are not worsened in the process of managing a patient's respiratory problems.

Maintain Circulation

The second important principle in the management of these patients is to maintain cardiovascular function. Inadequate cardiac output can severely alter mental status, especially with sepsis. Intravascular access is critical and should be provided by an appropriate intravenous line or intraosseus access. Fluid resuscitation should be prompt with early institution of inotropic agents when necessary.

Administer Glucose

Glucose is the essential source of ATP for cerebral energy metabolism. Once the initial glucose level is ascertained, glucose administration is recommended if the results show an abnormally low level. All other therapies are superfluous when oxygen and essential metabolic substrates (e.g., glucose) are not delivered to neurons and toxic metabolites are not removed.

Consider Specific Antidotes

Naloxone is available for treatment when an opiate overdose is suspected. Although opiate overdosage is rare in children, the risks of naloxone are minimal and administration should always be considered. Physostigmine may reverse central nervous system and cardiac effects of anticholinergic agents. However, physostigmine may cause nonspecific central nervous system stimulation or seizures. Flumazenil, a benzodiazepine receptor antagonist, may be valuable in such patients.

Reduce Increased Intracranial Pressure

Increased intracranial pressure (ICP) may exist for a variety of structural, metabolic, or toxic reasons. It is essential to identify surgically treatable causes of elevated ICP quickly to allow appropriate intervention. Head CT should be performed in all children with coma due to closed head injuries and in all children in whom the cause of coma is not immediately apparent or in whom the onset was not observed or is unknown.

When a surgically treatable lesion does not cause increased intracranial pressure, a variety of therapeutic interventions can be considered. Fluid administration can be limited to half or two-thirds of maintenance provided that cardiovascular function is maintained. Fluid restriction as a treatment for increased intracranial pressure should only be used when cerebral perfusion is deemed adequate. Isotonic fluid use is essential to minimize exacerbation of cerebral edema. Often-overlooked methods to control increased ICP by facilitating jugular venous drainage include positioning of the head at 30 degrees above the horizontal, keeping the head midline, and avoiding excessively restrictive cervical collars for children with suspected cervical spine injuries. Sedation can also be helpful. Hyperventilation via mechanical ventilation may be valuable in the short term, but may contribute to poorer long-term prognosis. Hyperventilation may reduce cerebral blood flow and potentially worsen outcome in certain forms of CNS injuries. Agents that reduce intracranial volume, such as mannitol, can be beneficial. Hypertonic saline, 3% to 21%, is now frequently used as an osmotically active agent that decreases brain cellular edema and helps lower and control elevated ICP with the added benefit of improved hemodynamics due to its volume-expansion properties. With hypertonic saline there also is no concomitant loss of intravascular volume, and there may be associated beneficial anti-inflammatory effects. Administration of corticosteroids (e.g., high-dose methylprednisone or dexamethasone) may be useful, especially when intracranial pressure is related to peritumoral edema.

Stop Seizures

Treatment of status epilepticus and other seizure emergencies is discussed elsewhere. It is always important to consider seizures even when there are no obvious outward seizure manifestations. EEG is essential in identifying subclinical nonconvulsive status epilepticus or other forms of seizure activity.

Treat Infection

Underlying infectious process should be treated, provided specific treatment is available. Usually the diagnosis of infectious diseases that involve the central nervous system requires lumbar puncture. When there is concern about elevated ICP, it may be appropriate to start antibiotic therapy for meningitis or antiviral therapy for encephalitis prior to lumbar puncture. In certain clinical situations, treatment can be initiated and the lumbar puncture deferred.

Correct Acid–Base and Electrolyte Imbalance

Electrolyte imbalance seen after CNS insults is often mediated by inappropriate antidiuretic hormone secretion. Inappropriate administration of fluids may worsen this situation. More commonly, hyponatremia, hypernatremia, hypocalcemia, or hypomagnesemia may occur in conjunction with systemic illness and be the cause of coma. Metabolic or respiratory acidosis or alkalosis should also be identified and corrected.

Adjust Body Temperature

Usually normal body temperature is best for recovery and prevention of acidosis. Patients with fever should have appropriate antipyretic agents administered with active cooling if necessary. The use of prolonged hypothermia is generally no longer considered a potential treatment for coma, although brief periods of mild hypothermia may be cerebroprotective.

Manage Agitation

It is particularly important to prevent agitation because of the problems it may present in the critical care management of patients with altered consciousness or coma. Agitation may increase ICP and make it difficult to control respiration with mechanical ventilation. The decision to sedate, however, may make serial neurologic examination to measure change in a patient's status difficult. In these circumstances, additional serial neurodiagnostic tests such as EEG may be valuable.

PROGNOSIS

A commonly used and widely accepted measurement of outcome following severe CHI is the Glasgow Outcome Scale (GOS), originally used in adults after closed head injury, and now commonly used for many types of injuries. The GOS has five broad outcome categories: (1) death, (2) persistent vegetative state (PVS), (3) severe disability (conscious but disabled), (4) moderate disability (disabled but independent), and (5) good recovery (16). A modified form of the GOS for children, the Pediatric Cerebral Performance Category Scale (PCPCS), was published by Fiser in 1992 (17). This six-point outcome scoring system was validated in 1,469 pediatric patients suffering acute CNS injuries. The score includes the following outcomes: (1) normal: able to perform all age-appropriate activities; (2) mild disability: conscious, alert and able to interact at an age-appropriate level but may have a mild neurologic deficit; (3) moderate disability: conscious, sufficient cerebral function for most age-appropriate independent activities; (4) severe disability: conscious, dependent on others for daily support because of impaired brain function; (5) persistent vegetative state (PVS); and (6) death.

Other scoring systems include the Disability Rating Scale (DRS), and the Functional Independence Measure (FIM) and its pediatric counterpart, the WeeFIM. The DRS consists of eight items divided into four categories: (1) arousability and awareness (best eye opening, verbal and motor response); (2) cognitive ability for self-care activities (feeding, toileting, and grooming); (3) physical dependence on others; and (4) psychosocial adaptability for work or school (8). The DRS is a more sensitive measure of improvement during inpatient rehabilitation than the GOS. The Functional Independence Measure (FIM) and its pediatric counterpart, the WeeFIM, further refine outcome assessment using 6 items and 18 categories. The WeeFIM items and categories are (1) self-care (eating, grooming, bathing, dressing upper body, dressing lower body, toileting); (2) sphincter control (bladder and bowel); (3) mobility: transfer (chair or wheelchair, toilet, tub/shower); (4) locomotion (walking, wheelchair, crawling, stairs); (5) communication (auditory and/or visual comprehen-sion and verbal and/or nonverbal expression); and (6) social cognition (social interaction, problem-solving, memory). The WeeFIM has good interrater reliability and allows serial assessment throughout the pediatric age range. Other standardized measures used to assess intellectual, cognitive, language, and behavioral development in children without injury are useful in evaluating and assessing outcomes in children following severe CHI. In children old enough and cooperative enough, neuropsychological testing is the most sensitive and specific way to measure and monitor change in these domains. Valuable reviews of these issues are available (8). A detailed discussion of the outcomes after different types of pediatric brain injuries is beyond the scope of this chapter and the reader is referred to other sources (8,17).

References

1. The Multi-Society Task Force on PVS. Medical aspects of the persistent vegetative state. *N Engl J Med* 1994;330:1499,1572.
2. Giacino J, Ashwal S, Childs N. The minimally conscious state: definition and diagnostic criteria. Report of the Aspen Work Group. *Neurology* 2002;58:349–353.
3. Ashwal S. The persistent vegetative state in infancy and childhood. In: Frank Y, ed. *Pediatric behavioral neurology*. New York: CRC Press; 1996:113.
4. Beca J, Cox PN, Taylor MJ, et al. Somatosensory evoked potentials for prediction of outcome in acute severe brain injury. *J Pediatr* 1995;126:44.
5. Ashwal S, Cranford R. The minimally conscious state in children. *Semin Pediatr Neurol* 2002;9:19–34.
6. Giacino JT, Kalmar K. The vegetative and minimally conscious states: a comparison of clinical features and functional outcome. *J Head Trauma Rehabil* 1997;12:36.
7. Plum F, Posner JB. *The diagnosis of stupor and coma*. 3rd ed., revised. Philadelphia: FA Davis: 1982.
8. Taylor D, Ashwal S. Impairment of consciousness and coma. In: Swaiman KF, Ashwal S, eds. *Pediatric neurology: principles and practice*. St. Louis: Mosby; 2006:1377–1400.
9. Teasdale G, Jennett B. Assessment of coma and impaired consciousness. A practical scale. *Lancet* 1974;2:81.
10. Reilly PL, Simpson DA, Sprod R, et al. Assessing the conscious level in infants and young children: a pediatric version of the Glasgow Coma Scale. *Childs Nerv Syst* 1988;4:30.
11. Raimondi AJ, Hirschauer J. Head injury in the infant and toddler. Coma scoring and outcome scale. *Childs Brain* 1984;11:12.
12. Hahn YS, Chyung C, Barthel MJ, et al. Head injuries in children under 36 months of age. *Childs Nerv Syst* 1988;4:34.
13. Rubenstein JS. Initial management of coma and altered consciousness in the pediatric patient. *Pediatr Rev* 1984;15:204.
14. Cohen BH, Andrefsky JC. Altered states of consciousness. In: Maria BL, ed. *Current management in child neurology*, 2nd ed. New York: Decker; 2002: 470–480.
15. Ashwal S, Holshouser BA. New neuroimaging techniques and their potential role in patients with acute brain injury. *J Head Trauma Rehabil* 1997;12:13.
16. Jennett B, Bond M. Assessment of outcome after severe brain damage, a practical scale. *Lancet* 1975;1:480.
17. Fiser DH. Assessing the outcome of pediatric intensive care. *J Pediatr* 1992;121:68.

CHAPTER 49A ■ INFLAMMATORY NEUROPATHIES: GUILLAIN–BARRÉ SYNDROME

DAVID J. MICHELSON

In the context of immune activation against illness and vaccination, inappropriate direction of the immune system against self-antigens in the nervous system can precipitate acute neurologic dysfunction, inflammation, demyelination, and permanent injury. The process may involve one or more areas of the central nervous system (CNS), including the optic nerves, brain, cerebellum, and spinal cord, or may predominantly affect one or more components of the peripheral nervous system, including motor, sensory, and autonomic nerves. Presentations can range across a wide spectrum of extent and severity, influenced by multiple environmental and host factors. The most common clinical syndromes are further described in this chapter.

DEFINITION

Patients with Guillain–Barré syndrome (GBS) have acute immune-mediated inflammation of the spinal roots and peripheral nerves that causes motor, sensory, and autonomic nerve dysfunction. The best-known clinical presentation is that in which weakness and sensory changes begin symmetrically in the lower legs and progress in an ascending fashion over several days to weeks to involve the hands and arms, the muscles of respiration, and the cranial nerves. Many variants with more selective motor, sensory, cranial, or autonomic nerve involvement have been characterized. Diagnosis of GBS is one of exclusion, based on the presence of supportive clinical, laboratory, radiographic, and neurophysiologic findings. Immunomodulation, as with intravenous immunoglobulin (IVIG) or plasma exchange (PE), has been shown to be of benefit in the speed but not the extent of recovery.

EPIDEMIOLOGY

Estimates of the childhood incidence of GBS in developed countries range from 0.5 to 1.5 per 100,000 children, with a high percentage of cases seen in children less than 3 years of age, making it the most common cause of acute flaccid paralysis among such children in the post-polio era. A prodromal illness within 2 to 4 weeks of the onset of symptoms is reported in 50% to 70% of cases. A great number of infections have been associated with GBS, with the most common being Epstein–Barr virus, cytomegalovirus, *Mycoplasma pneumoniae*, and *Campylobacter jejuni*. Autoimmunity toward peripheral nerve antigens may be induced in these circumstances by molecular mimicry or by nonspecific superantigen activation. The most common antibodies, directed against

various components of the myelin sheath, lead to cellular infiltrates around endoneurial vessels, vesicular myelin degeneration, and impaired nerve conduction. Some infectious agents are known to induce less common antibodies and clinical variants of GBS. Antibodies toward the GM1 gangliosides of the peripheral nerve axons are associated with infection with certain *Campylobacter jejuni* strains and antibodies against the GQ1b glycolipids of cranial nerve axons are associated with cytomegalovirus infection.

CLINICAL FEATURES

The majority of cases of GBS have a history of rapidly ascending weakness that manifests initially as difficulty walking or refusal to bear weight. In 15% to 20% of cases, the weakness begins proximally and may present with initial difficulty climbing stairs or rising from a chair. In up to half of children, however, lower-extremity pain and dysesthesias are the first noticeable symptoms. This discomfort can, in some cases, be accompanied by headache, vomiting, and meningismus or by significant irritability. Apparent gait ataxia is usually due to loss of strength and proprioception, rather than cerebellar involvement. However, cerebellar ataxia, external ophthalmoplegia, and areflexia without limb weakness are features that are characteristic of the Miller–Fisher variant of GBS. Cranial nerve involvement is eventually seen in up to 45% of pediatric GBS, although internal ophthalmoplegia with loss of pupillary reactivity to light is so rare as to suggest a reconsideration of alternative causes of paralysis. Respiratory muscle weakness typically evolves gradually as weakness ascends to involve the upper arms, but acute respiratory failure has rarely been the initial presenting symptom of GBS. Sensory loss can be found in 40% of cases but a transverse sensory level should suggest a myelopathy and the need for further investigation. Autonomic dysfunction, seen in 25% of cases, can manifest as blood pressure instability, arrhythmia, and altered bladder and gastrointestinal function. Urinary and rectal sphincter dysfunction is rarely prominent in GBS and should prompt reconsideration of possible spinal pathology. Diagnostic criteria for typical GBS, proposed by Ashbury and Cornblath, are listed in Table 49.1.

TESTING

The diagnosis of GBS is often made on a clinical basis but can be supported by cerebrospinal fluid (CSF) analysis and electrophysiologic studies. The CSF commonly shows

TABLE 49.1
SUGGESTED DIAGNOSTIC CRITERIA FOR GUILLAIN–BARRÉ SYNDROME
SUPPORTIVE CLINICAL FEATURES Development of essentially symmetric limb weakness Loss or decrease in deep tendon reflexes within 1 week of onset Progression of weakness over several days to 4 weeks Paresthesias of the hands and feet
SUPPORTIVE LABORATORY FEATURES Greater than 45 mg/dL of protein in the CSF within 3 weeks of onset Neurophysiologic evidence of polyneuropathy in at least two limbs
UNSUPPORTIVE FEATURES Prominent and persistent asymmetry of weakness Abrupt onset of weakness without progression Identifiable sensory level Severe and persistent bladder or bowel dysfunction Greater than 50 nucleated cells/mm^3 in the CSF
Adapted from Asbury AK, Cornblath DR. Assessment of current diagnostic criteria for Guillain–Barré syndrome. *Ann Neurol* 1990;27: S21–S24.

cytoalbuminologic dissociation, elevation of CSF protein without corresponding CSF pleocytosis. This is due to inflammatory demyelination of the spinal nerve roots, disrupting the blood–CSF barrier. A slight elevation (10 to 50 cells/mm^3) in nucleated cells can be seen in typical GBS, but higher degrees of inflammation suggest meningoencephalitis or myelitis. Nerve conduction studies show slowed nerve conduction, conduction block, and dispersion of motor responses due to demyelination, and decreased amplitudes of motor and sensory responses due to axon loss. Electrophysiologic criteria that are predictive of poor outcome in adults with GBS are much less predictive in children. Spinal imaging should be performed urgently in children with symptoms suggestive of spinal cord compression such as back pain, a transverse sensory level, or prominent sphincter dysfunction. Enhancement of the cauda equina and lumbar nerve roots can be seen in patients with GBS who undergo spinal magnetic resonance imaging (MRI), but this finding is not diagnostic.

TREATMENT

Children with even mild initial symptoms of GBS can progress rapidly to respiratory failure. Patients should be admitted and have their vital capacity and negative inspiratory force monitored closely so that interventions to ensure adequate ventilation can be anticipated. Intubation and mechanical ventilation is required by approximately 15% to 20% of children with GBS and is generally considered necessary when the vital capacity falls below 12 to 15 mL/kg, the negative inspiratory force falls below -25 mm H_2O, the arterial pO$_2$ falls below 70 to 80 mm Hg, or when there is rapid progression, poor handling of secretions, dysphagia, or significant fatigue. Patients also require close monitoring for autonomic instability, which can cause tachy- and bradyarrhythmias, hypotension and hypertension, ileus, and urinary retention. Nonsteroidal anti-inflammatory agents and treatments for neuropathic pain can be employed for the management of pain but may be inadequate in the first few weeks of the illness. Corticosteroids can sometimes provide effective pain relief in such cases, but opiate analgesia may prove necessary, even though they may cause respiratory depression. Supportive measures should include maintenance of adequate nutrition and hydration, provision of regular physical therapy and skin care, and treatment of any consequences of immobility, such as hypercalcemia, pressure sores, and constipation.

Immune modulation should be considered for any child presenting with rapid progression of symptoms, loss of ambulation, dysphagia, or respiratory compromise. Intravenous immunoglobulin (IVIG) and plasma exchange (PLEX) are both associated with faster recovery in retrospective studies of adults and children, but neither appears to affect long-term outcome. IVIG at a total dose of 2 g/kg over 2 to 5 days is generally well tolerated and, because it is easier to administer than PLEX, is considered the treatment of choice. PLEX with a total 250 mL/kg volume exchange divided over 4 to 6 sessions on an alternate-day schedule is also generally well tolerated in patients weighing more than 10 kg.

OUTCOME

Clinical recovery from GBS is somewhat better in children than in adults, with more than 90% of patients making a full recovery and most of those with a persistent deficit being able to walk independently with only minor weakness of ankle dorsiflexion. Children with GBS have a low mortality rate, around 1% to 2%, but many of the deaths from respiratory failure and arrhythmias may be preventable with earlier diagnosis, closer monitoring, and earlier anticipation of complications.

CHAPTER 49B ■ INFLAMMATORY NEUROPATHIES: TRANSVERSE MYELITIS

DAVID J. MICHELSON

DEFINITION

In acute transverse myelitis (ATM), inflammation of the spinal cord gives rise to motor, sensory, and autonomic deficits. ATM is preceded by infection or vaccination in at least two-thirds of children, but the same clinical picture can also result from mass lesions causing spinal cord compression (tumor, empyema), vascular disorders causing spinal cord infarction (embolism,

TABLE 49.2

SUGGESTED DIAGNOSTIC CRITERIA FOR IDIOPATHIC ACUTE
TRANSVERSE MYELITIS

INCLUSION CRITERIA
Development of bilateral signs and symptoms of spinal cord dysfunction
Clearly defined sensory level
Evidence of inflammation on spinal cord neuroimaging[a]
Evidence of inflammation on cerebral spinal fluid (CSF) analysis[a]
Progression to nadir between 4 hours and 21 days after symptom onset

EXCLUSION CRITERIA
History of previous spinal irradiation within the past 10 years
Clinical deficits with clear spinal artery distribution
Abnormal surface flow voids on spinal cord neuroimaging
Extra-axial cord compression on neuroimaging
Findings suggestive of multiple sclerosis on cranial neuroimaging
History of clinically apparent optic neuritis
Serologic or clinical evidence of connective tissue disease
Central nervous system (CNS) manifestations of syphilis, Lyme disease, HIV, mycoplasma,
or other infection

[a]Required for a diagnosis of definite idiopathic ATM but not for possible idiopathic ATM.
Adapted from Transverse Myelitis Consortium Group. Proposed diagnostic criteria and nosology of acute
transverse myelitis. *Neurology* 2002;59:499–505.

watershed infarction, arteriovenous malformation), systemic inflammatory disorders associated with vasculitis (systemic lupus erythematosis, Sjögren syndrome, Behçet syndrome), and demyelinating disorders with greater involvement of the central nervous system (CNS) such as acute disseminated encephalomyelitis (ADEM), neuromyelitis optica (NMO), and multiple sclerosis (MS). Diagnostic criteria that have recently been put forward for idiopathic ATM are listed in Table 49.2.

EPIDEMIOLOGY

Estimates put the annual incidence of ATM at 1 to 4 per million per year. There is a bimodal age distribution, with peaks between 10 and 19 years and between 30 and 39 years, such that about one-third of cases occur in children. There is no clear racial, gender, familial, or seasonal variation.

CLINICAL FEATURES

Presenting features may initially be limited to neck or back pain, headache, and/or fever, but progressive neurologic deficits develop over several hours to weeks. Weakness is often initially asymmetric but becomes symmetric with further progression. At their nadir, 50% of patients have complete paraplegia and at least some weakness of the upper extremities. Flaccid weakness may be seen initially, due to spinal shock, but deep tendon reflexes of the extremities can eventually be normal, increased, or decreased depending on whether the anterior horn cells involved in the reflex are above, below, or within the area of spinal cord inflammation, respectively. Respiratory compromise is uncommon but can occur when there is cervical spinal involvement. Sensory disturbances, including a transverse band of dysesthesia or upper limit of numbness that can help to define clinically the upper boundary of spinal inflammation, occur in 80% to 90% of patients. Autonomic disturbances are nearly universal and can include urinary urgency, bowel or bladder incontinence, and difficult or incomplete bowel or bladder evacuation. GBS and ATM are equally important considerations in patients who present with rapidly progressive flaccid weakness and sensory loss.

The clinical and laboratory features that help to distinguish between GBS and ATM are presented in Table 49.3.

TESTING

Inflammatory myelitis can be difficult to differentiate from other causes of spinal cord injury. The patient history will usually identify prior neurologic illness, spinal cord irradiation, or spinal trauma. The first priority of diagnostic testing in patients with progressive spinal cord dysfunction should be expedited neuroimaging to exclude cord compression that would require urgent neurosurgical evaluation. MRI with gadolinium is ideal, as it will show the spinal cord itself, but computed tomography (CT) with myelography, which requires injection of iodinated contrast into the cerebral spinal fluid (CSF), is an acceptable alternative for excluding compressive lesions in patients who cannot tolerate MRI. Spinal CT without myelography is not sensitive enough.

Once compressive myelopathy has been excluded, the remaining diagnoses are either inflammatory or noninflammatory. MRI with gadolinium will show evidence of spinal cord inflammation in 40% to 50% of patients with ATM. Lesions in idiopathic ATM tend to appear as central cord edema involving most of the cross-sectional area of the cord, extending over 3 to 4 vertebral segments, with ring-like contrast enhancement. In contrast, the myelitis associated with multiple sclerosis tends to show edema that is more eccentric, extends over a shorter segment of the cord, involves a smaller cross-sectional area, and shows more central enhancement.

Lumbar puncture should be the next test performed to look for evidence of inflammation. CSF pleocytosis, oligoclonal bands, and/or an elevated IgG index are present in 20% to 30% of patients with ATM. About one-third of patients with suspected ATM lack initial evidence of inflammation on either MRI or CSF analysis and can only be given a diagnosis of possible ATM. Repeat imaging and CSF testing can be considered after 2 to 7 days in these patients.

Patients with a clearly inflammatory myelitis still must be differentiated into idiopathic, parainfectious, and disease-associated groups. Infectious and parainfectious myelitis should

TABLE 49.3

DIFFERENTIATING ACUTE TRANSVERSE MYELITIS (ATM) AND GUILLAIN–BARRÉ SYNDROME (GBS)

	GBS	ATM
Motor	Quadriparesis without a gradient or paraparesis without arm involvement	Ascending weakness, with legs more affected than arms initially
Sensory	Transverse sensory level, usually without arm involvement	Ascending dysesthesia, with legs more affected than arms initially, and no sensory level
Autonomic	Early and prominent bladder and bowel dysfunction, rare cardiovascular instability in severe cases with involvement above T6	Late and transient bladder and bowel dysfunction, common cardiovascular instability in moderate to severe cases
Cranial nerves	No involvement	Possible involvement of CN for facial and ocular control
Spinal MRI with contrast	Focal area of edema within the cord, with or without contrast enhancement	Normal or mild contrast enhancement of spinal nerve roots
Cerebrospinal fluid	Mild to moderate pleocytosis and protein elevation, with increased IgG index	Mild to moderate protein elevation, normal to mildly elevated cell count, and normal IgG index
Electrophysiology	Evidence of polyneuropathy on NCS, suggestive of demyelination and/or axon loss	No evidence of peripheral neuropathy on NCS studies and signs of spinal cord dysfunction on SSEP

CN, NCS, nerve conduction study; SSEP, somatosensory evoked potential.
Adapted from Krishnan C, Kaplin AI, Deshpande DM, et al. Transverse myelitis: pathogenesis, diagnosis, and treatment. *Front Biosci* 2004;9:1483–1499.

be considered more likely in patients presenting with fever, meningismus, rash, concurrent pneumonia or other systemic infection, recurrent genital infection, adenopathy, radicular pain (with or without a vesicular skin eruption) suggestive of zoster radiculopathy, an immunocompromised state, or residence in an area endemic for parasites. Testing for infectious agents in the CSF may include Gram, India ink, and acid-fast stains; bacterial, viral, mycobacterial, and fungal cultures; PCR testing for HSV-1, HSV-2, HHV-6, VZV, CMV, EBV, enteroviruses, and HIV; titers for antibodies against HSV, VZV, HTLV-1, and *Borrelia burgdorferi*; and VDRL. Serologic tests may include titers for antibodies to HSV, VZV, HTLV-1, *B. burgdorferi*, hepatitis A, B, and C, *Mycoplasma*, and parasites. Plain chest radiography is also recommended.

Myelitis associated with an underlying systemic autoimmune disease is more likely in patients who present with or have a history of rashes, oral or genital ulcers, adenopathy, livedo reticularis, serositis, photosensitivity, inflammatory arthritis, erythema nodosum, xerostomia, keratitis, conjunctivitis, contractures or thickening of skin, blood dyscrasia, Raynaud phenomenon, or arterial or venous thrombosis. Testing for suspected inflammatory disorders may include a plain chest radiograph or chest CT, serum ACE and complement levels, serum titers for ANA, antiphospholipid antibodies, and autoantibodies against ds-DNA, SS-A (Ro), SS-B (La), Sm (Smith), and RNP; urinalysis with microscopic analysis for hematuria; lip or salivary gland biopsy; and Schirmer test to quantify lacrimation.

The final goal of immediate testing in patients with myelitis is to define the extent of CNS involvement. MRI of the brain with gadolinium should be done looking for acute inflammation, which would suggest a diagnosis of ADEM, or signs of past demyelination and scarring in the typically periventricular pattern of MS. A patient whose brain MRI suggests demyelination has an 83% chance of being diagnosed with MS within 10 years, compared with 11% of patients with a normal brain MRI. An abnormal visual evoked potential (VEP) consistent with

demyelination of the optic nerves may suggest the diagnosis of NMO and an increased risk of recurrent symptoms. However, in the absence of a clinically recognized episode of optic neuritis, the implications of an abnormal VEP are unknown. Checking serum titers for the NMO-specific IgG antibody, which binds to an aquaporin channel, may be of greater prognostic value. Prospective studies should determine whether either test is beneficial in patients presenting with ATM.

Patients without signs of inflammation may suffer from cord ischemia or from a toxic or hereditary myelopathy. Spinal cord ischemia should be considered in patients whose symptoms develop abruptly or progress over fewer than 4 hours. Causes of ischemia include arterial or venous occlusion, watershed injury from hypotension, vascular steal from an arteriovenous malformation, radiation necrosis, epidural lipomatosis, and fibrocartilaginous embolism from a disrupted nucleus pulposus. Anterior spinal artery occlusion spares the posterior columns clinically and on neuroimaging. Abnormal flow voids on the surface of the spinal cord suggest the possibility of cord ischemia due to an arteriovenous malformation.

Further tests that may inform prognosis include CSF analysis for 14-3-3 protein levels and somatosensory evoked potentials. Bladder sphincter dysfunction is not always suggested by the history but should always be investigated through ultrasonography for postvoid residuals in the acute phase of illness and by urodynamic studies in the recovery period.

TREATMENT

Several small, open-label studies have found that patients given a 3- to 5-day course of high-dose IV methylprednisolone (IVMP) had higher rates of independent ambulation at 1 month and 1 year than was seen in historical controls that were treated with oral prednisone alone. Other small studies, including one with a prospective design, have failed to find a clear benefit to the use of IV steroids. Recognizing that more research is needed

TABLE 49.4

TABLE 49.4

SYMPTOM-BASED SUPPORTIVE CARE FOR ACUTE TRANSVERSE MYELITIS

Symptom	Management
Weakness and immobility	PT, OT, splinting, and orthoses as needed, daily weight bearing
Spasticity	PT, baclofen, tizanidine, diazepam, botulinum toxin injection
Pain and dysesthesia	PT, gabapentin, carbamazepine, nortriptyline, tramadol, TENS
Urinary retention	Clean intermittent bladder catheterization, anticholinergics for bladder spasticity, antiadrenergics for sphincter dyssynergia, cranberry extract or vitamin C for urine acidification
Constipation	High-fiber diet, increased fluids, stool softeners, laxatives, and enemas as needed for regularity
Depression	Psychiatric counseling, antidepressants
Fatigue	Amantadine, methylphenidate, modafinil, coenzyme Q10

PT, physical therapy; OT, occupational therapy; TENS, transelectrical nerve stimulation.
Adapted from Krishnan C, Kaplin AI, Deshpande DM, et al. Transverse myelitis: pathogenesis, diagnosis, and treatment. *Front Biosci* 2004;9:1483–1499.

to establish the role for this and other immunomodulatory treatments, the current practice is to treat ATM with 15 to 20 mg/kg of IVMP for 3 to 5 days before assessing the clinical and radiographic response. If significant improvement is perceived, IVMP therapy can be continued for another week. If improvement is not appreciable, alternatives to consider include IVIG, PLEX, and pulse cyclophosphamide. Suggestions for early supportive care and rehabilitation are outlined in Table 49.4.

OUTCOME

Clinical symptoms should stop progressing within 2 to 3 weeks, and most patients reach their nadir within 10 days. Complete recovery can be expected in approximately one-third of patients, with another third having minimal sequelae and another third experiencing more significant persistent impairment of motor or sphincter function. Prognosis is less favorable in patients who present with more severe and more rapid onset of symptoms and is more favorable in patients who begin to show improvement in the first week of recovery or regain independent walking within the first month. A high CSF 14-3-3 protein level and an abnormal SSEP also predict more permanent motor impairment and incontinence. Improvement in sensory and motor impairments usually begins within the first 2 months, with most of the eventual improvement seen within the first 6 months, but slowly incremental improvement may be seen as late as 2 years.

Recurrent ATM has been reported to occur in 10% to 25% of historical cases, but most of these patients had ATM as an initial presentation of MS, NMO, or systemic collagen-vascular disease. As such, a higher recurrence rate was associated with an abnormal brain MRI, a history of clinically apparent optic neuritis, or the presence of high serum titers of one or more autoantibodies. Even so, some laboratory findings in patients with idiopathic ATM are associated with later recurrence, including oligoclonal bands of IgG in the CSF and multiple distinct lesions on spinal MRI.

CHAPTER 49C ■ ACUTE DISSEMINATED ENCEPHALOMYELITIS

DAVID J. MICHELSON

DEFINITION

As the name implies, acute disseminated encephalomyelitis (ADEM) is typically a single, acute episode of demyelination that can simultaneously affect multiple areas of the CNS, including the optic nerves, brain, brainstem, and spinal cord. Like GBS and ATM, it most often develops 1 to 4 weeks after a systemic illness or vaccination and is believed to be triggered by the collateral activation of an immune response directed against self-antigens in myelin.

EPIDEMIOLOGY

The estimated incidence of ADEM is 1 to 3 per 100,000 persons per year. Although most of those who are affected are young children and adolescents, cases have been reported in infants and in adults as well. Most studies find no clear gender predominance, although some suggest a slight male predominance; or seasonal variation, although some report a higher incidence in winter and spring. A variety of infections and vaccinations have been associated with ADEM, particularly measles virus, rubella

TABLE 49.5

DIFFERENCES BETWEEN ADEM AND CHILDHOOD MS

Characteristic	ADEM	Childhood MS
Median age	6.5 years	143 years
Female:male ratio	Roughly 1:1	2:1
Presentation	Preceding infection or vaccination Headaches, fever, lethargy Multiple neurologic deficits Altered mental status	Isolated neurologic deficit
CSF	Lymphocytic pleocytosis and protein elevation common Oligoclonal bands in 0–29%	Lymphocytic pleocytosis and protein elevation less common Oligoclonal bands in 40–95%
MRI	Extensive, confluent and poorly defined lesions Bilateral lesions of the deep gray matter (basal ganglia, thalami) Absence of evidence of prior episodes of demyelination	Areas of T1 hypointense "black holes" within the subcortical white matter Well-defined, ovoid periventricular lesions of T2 hyperintensity with a long axis perpendicular to the corpus callosum (Dawson fingers)
Follow-up MRI	No change or resolution of prior lesions	Evolution of new lesions, which may be clinically silent

Adapted from Menge T, Hemmer B, Nessler S, et al. Acute disseminated encephalomyelitis: an update. *Arch Neurol* 2005;62:1673–1680.

virus, Epstein–Barr virus, cytomegalovirus, herpes simplex virus, and *Mycoplasma*. In most modern series, however, the majority of cases present after nonspecific symptoms of a respiratory or gastrointestinal illness that is never attributed to a specific pathogen.

CLINICAL FEATURES

Neurologic deficits attributable to the brain and brainstem develop acutely or subacutely over hours or days, often in association with more constitutional signs of inflammation and increased intracranial pressure such as fever, lethargy, headache, nausea, vomiting, and meningismus. Brainstem and cerebellar symptoms are common, including ataxia, vertigo, diplopia, dysphagia, and encephalopathy, which can range from obtundation to agitation. Clinical optic neuritis, usually bilateral, or transverse myelitis, usually complete, may be present in association with other impairments. Fulminant ADEM, more likely to affect children under 2 to 3 years of age, can progress quickly to coma and signs of impending central or uncal herniation from malignant cerebral edema.

TESTING

MRI of the brain and spinal cord is the study of choice for the evaluation of patients with suspected demyelinating disease. There are no findings that are specific to ADEM, but several patterns are recognized, including extensive, confluent subcortical white matter involvement and bilateral deep gray matter involvement. In some instances, particularly those with eventual isolated appearance of abnormalities in the deep gray matter, the initial MRI is normal, even when neurologic deficits are maximal. Hemorrhages may occur in the most severe, fulminant cases, often referred to as acute hemorrhagic encephalomyelitis (AHEM). There should not be radiologic evidence of past episodes of demyelination on the initial MRI nor evolution of new lesions on follow-up MRI done at least

6 months later, two findings that are commonly seen in patients with MS. Well-defined, ovoid periventricular lesions whose long axis is perpendicular to the corpus callosum are also more commonly seen in multiple sclerosis (MS). Table 49.5 reviews the clinical and radiologic distinctions between ADEM and childhood MS.

Consideration of a possible intracranial infection should lead to a lumbar puncture for CSF analysis. ADEM will often be associated with a mild to moderate lymphocytic pleocytosis with a corresponding elevation in CSF protein. The presence of intrathecal IgG synthesis and of oligoclonal bands does not exclude the diagnosis of ADEM, although they are more commonly seen in MS, especially after multiple relapses. The range of CSF tests ordered for the exclusion of viral, bacterial, mycobacterial, fungal, and parasitic infection should be informed by the clinical, travel, and exposure history. CSF with intense pleocytosis, neutrophilia, eosinophilia, or low glucose should also prompt a more extensive investigation for infection.

Demyelination or vasculitic ischemia associated with systemic autoimmune or inflammatory diseases should be excluded, as discussed previously for ATM, in patients with an atypical presentation of ADEM or a suggestive history. Diffusion-weighted MRI should be able to distinguish areas of ischemia from areas of demyelination, identifying patients who should be referred for angiography. Magnetic resonance and CT angiography have a low sensitivity for small to medium-sized vessel vasculitis and conventional angiography should be considered the gold standard.

Brain tumors and degenerative diseases such as mitochondrial encephalopathy (e.g., MELAS) or adrenoleukodystrophy can have a very similar appearance on MRI but are distinguished from ADEM by their more insidiously progressive and chronic clinical course. When patients present with neuroimaging showing intense perilesional vasogenic edema and mass effect, suggesting an aggressive tumor or infection, biopsy may be unavoidable. MR proton spectroscopy, if available, may show a pattern of metabolite changes, such as an isolated increase in the choline/creatine ratio, which is most consistent with demyelination and helps to avoid more invasive testing. The pathologic findings in ADEM are perivascular cuffs of macrophages and T-cells, patches of demyelination, and late gliosis; but these are nonspecific changes.

TREATMENT

Immunosuppressive in immunomodulatory therapies are here again used on an empirical basis, without the benefit of prospective research data. High-dose IV MP is the most commonly given therapy, with most retrospective studies seeing faster recovery and reduced complications in comparison to untreated historical controls. A taper of oral steroids over 2 to 6 weeks is often prescribed in conjunction, although again there is only sparse data to suggest that this may reduce the incidence of recurrence. There are multiple case reports of benefit from intravenous immunoglobin (IVIG), (PLEX), or cytotoxic immunosuppresants in patients who did not initially respond well to other therapies.

OUTCOME

Recent case series report excellent recovery in up to 90% of children with ADEM, and there is surprisingly little predictive value to the severity of the neurologic deficits at presentation or nadir. Many of the children with a near-complete recovery have only mild visuospacial processing deficits that manifest as difficulty in school. Mortality from ADEM was as high as 25% in reports predating widespread use of the measles vaccine in developed countries. Measles-associated ADEM is more often associated with hemorrhagic lesions and with a high morbidity, with as many as 35% surviving with severe and persistent neurologic disability.

Some patients will undergo an early relapse of their initial symptoms, with flare-up of the previously involved areas of the CNS on repeat neuroimaging within 4 weeks of initial presentation. This can occur as steroid therapy, tapered or stopped. In some series with long-term follow-up, up to 35% of patients undergo one or more distinct recurrences, with new neurologic deficits and areas of demyelination developing more than 1 month after the resolution of a prior episode. These patients with recurrent ADEM may be diagnosed with multiphasic disseminated encephalomyelitis (MDEM) or with MS, depending on the way in which recurrences present.

There are currently no absolute differences in the clinical, laboratory, or radiographic characteristics of ADEM, MDEM, and cases eventually diagnosed as clinically definite MS. Late follow-up neuroimaging, looking for the development of new asymptomatic lesions 3 to 6 months after initial diagnosis, may be particularly useful in the identification of patients at the highest risk for progression and relapse. There is ongoing debate as to whether ADEM and MS are distinct disorders or coexist on a spectrum of autoimmune demyelination.

Suggested Readings

Defresne P, Hollenberg H, Husson B, et al. Acute transverse myelitis in children: clinical course and prognostic factors. *J Child Neurol* 2003;18:401.

Garg RK. Acute disseminated encephalomyelitis. *Postgrad Med J* 2003;79: 11–17.

Krishnan C, Kaplin AI, Deshpande DM, et al. Transverse myelitis: pathogenesis, diagnosis, and treatment. *Front Biosci* 2004;9:1483–1499.

Menge T, Hemmer B, Nessler S, et al. Acute disseminated encephalomyelitis: an update. *Arch Neurol* 2005;62:1673–1680.

Ryan MM. Guillain-Barré syndrome in childhood. *J Paediatr Child Health* 2005;41:237–241.

CHAPTER 50 ■ GENERAL OVERVIEW AND MISCELLANEOUS DISEASES

HOWARD I. BARON

A pediatrician who spends her time providing care exclusively for hospitalized patients is a relatively new concept over the past decade. For those who have chosen this as an area of expertise, it is important to have a fundamental knowledge of gastrointestinal (GI) disorders, as a sizeable portion of all hospitalized children will require some attention to a disturbance of the GI tract. This may appear either as a primary reason for the admission, or as a secondary problem arising during the hospital stay. It is with this in mind that we have compiled the next several chapters, aimed mostly at common GI disorders in hospitalized children. Although a great deal of care for each of these problems is provided in the outpatient setting, children with these GI disturbances have specific diagnostic and therapeutic challenges when they are admitted to a hospital, and the hospitalist is often called on to make a diagnosis, render appropriate treatment, and discharge the patient in as expeditious a fashion as possible. Adherence to the general principle that *history is everything* in pediatric gastroenterology will usually allow the hospitalist to accomplish her goals.

Although a large percentage of admissions to a hospital setting will have identifiable GI pathology, a substantial portion of children and adolescents presenting with various GI complaints will not have a disease identifiable on physical exam, laboratory testing, or imaging. These patients are often the most frustrating, consume the most time for the practitioner, and take up as many or more hospital bed days as those with identifiable disease. Given the limitations on space in a textbook such as this, a brief discussion of the functional GI disorders of childhood seems most appropriate within this general overview chapter.

CHRONIC ABDOMINAL PAIN

Children with chronic abdominal pain account for 5% of all outpatient visits in the pediatric age group. Up to one-third of all children have this complaint, yet less than 10% of these children will have an identifiable organic etiology for their pain. These issues can have great impact on the functioning of the entire family, often causing work absence for the parents, excessive school absence for the child, and feelings of helplessness for the entire family unit.

Chronic abdominal pain is defined as at least 3 episodes occurring within a 3-month time-span that interferes with normal activity. It is slightly more common in girls than in boys, and usually occurs between the ages of 5 and 12 years. There is an increased incidence of recurrent abdominal pain in the families of these children.

The evaluation of a child with chronic abdominal complaints—or for that matter, any problem at all—starts with a comprehensive history. This should start with an interview of the child, as long as he is of the developmental stage in which he can respond to questions with verbal answers. Once exhausting the information available from the child, the parent or caretaker is interviewed. This allows the child to become part of the process, rather than feeling like an excluded object, and generally ensures that you will be able to interview the parent without as much interruption when the child has been asked to speak first.

Two major questions that help separate functional gastrointestinal complaints from disease-based problems are:

1. Does the pain wake you up out of sleep in the middle of the night?
2. Can you point with one finger to the spot that hurts?

As a general rule, children who spontaneously wake up out of deep sleep with abdominal symptoms have an organic basis for their complaint, while children with functional pain may have trouble falling asleep, but generally sleep soundly without interruption once they do. Similarly, children who cannot identify a specific site of pain, or who point exclusively to the periumbilical region when asked to identify a spot, will usually have a functional basis for their complaint. Those who can identify a specific quadrant or radiation pattern of their pain will more commonly have an underlying disease process.

In addition to the above, establishing a pattern of the pain occurrence is most helpful in deciding on an etiology. Questions that help establish specific patterns, are listed below:

Does the child wake up in the morning with pain?
Does the pain feel worse or better with eating? If worse, how soon after eating does it occur, and how long does it last?
Are there any foods that make the pain better or worsen it?
Is there any associated dysphasia/odynophagia (difficulty/pain with swallowing)?
Is there any nausea or vomiting?
What time does the child go to bed/fall asleep/wake up in the morning?
What is the pattern/consistency/completeness of evacuation of bowel movements?
Does the pain occur only on certain days of the week?
Does the child stay home from school or is there early school dismissal because of the pain?
What is the location/character/intensity/duration of the pain?
Have any medications been tried, and what is the success of each of these? (Be sure to ask about complementary/alternative treatments being offered as well as conventional medications.)

TABLE 50.1

ROUTINE LABORATORY EVALUATION FOR CHRONIC ABDOMINAL PAIN

- Urinalysis
- Complete blood count (CBC)
- Erythrocyte sedimentation rate (ESR)
- Comprehensive metabolic panel (electrolytes, blood urea nitrogen, creatinine, glucose, liver function tests)
- Amylase, lipase
- Fecal occult blood, white blood cells, ova and parasites

TABLE 50.3

DIFFERENTIAL DIAGNOSIS OF ORGANIC DISORDERS

- Chronic constipation
- Lactose intolerance
- Infectious (parasitic)
- Acid-peptic disorders
- Inflammatory bowel disease
- Celiac sprue
- Cystic fibrosis
- Hepatobiliary disorders
- Extraintestinal (e.g., urinary tract, gynecologic)

Is there any relationship between other prescribed/nonprescribed medications or treatments and the onset of the pain?

Have there been any changes in the child's life recently, including family deaths, loss of a close friend or pet, moves, separation/divorce, school location or performance changes?

What thoughts or fears do the parents or child have about the potential cause of the pain?

Any history of recent travel, pets, or a family history of GI disorders?

This set of questions will narrow down the differential diagnosis, and usually help identify the likelihood that laboratory testing or imaging studies will uncover an organic etiology for the pain.

The physical exam in children with chronic abdominal complaints is also critical in helping separate functional from disease-related pain. The exam focuses on establishing not only growth parameters upon admission, but if possible, a trend of growth over the preceding months or years that may signal an organic disorder of the digestive tract. For example, a child presenting at the 50th percentile for weight and height may not appear concerning, but if he had been following the 90th percentile for weight until his symptoms started a few months earlier, this could point the practitioner to a more extensive evaluation for malabsorption, especially if additional symptoms are suggestive.

The physical exam, although comprehensive, also should focus on the abdomen, with careful palpation for masses, hernias, and organomegaly. Careful note should be taken of fever, rash, oral lesions, arthropathy, and a rectal exam with perianal inspection, and fecal occult blood testing should be performed whenever possible. It is important to recognize that school-aged children are usually independent when using the restroom, and parents do not usually have an accurate sense of their defecation patterns or completeness. Even the child herself may not pay close attention to her own defecation pattern and stool appearance, so answers to questions on this topic need to be interpreted within this context.

Routine laboratory evaluation for children with chronic abdominal pain includes the tests listed in Table 50.1. A urinalysis helps diagnose infections or may uncover primary renal disease or calculi. A complete blood count (CBC) and differential may be helpful in identifying features of a chronic disease, such as a microcytic anemia, or even a blood-born malignancy presenting with GI complaints. An erythrocyte sedimentation rate (ESR) can help determine if an acute inflammatory process is present, although it is not specific for GI luminal disease. A comprehensive chemistry panel, including tests of liver function, electrolyte balance, renal function, and pancreatic enzymes, may help uncover a process in any of the visceral organs. Fecal occult blood testing, along with a fresh specimen for white blood cells, may suggest an intraluminal inflammatory process, and intestinal parasites are protean causes of abdominal pain in this age group.

Radiologic imaging is often indicated, and it is important to tailor the imaging toward the suspected cause of the pain. For example, contrast radiography such as upper GI and small bowel follow-through x-rays can be helpful in diagnosing structural problems such as intestinal malrotation, pyloric stenosis, or bowel obstruction. However, contrast studies are not useful in quantifying disorders of GI tract function, such as gastroesophageal reflux, delayed gastric emptying, or disorders of the solid viscera such as the liver or spleen. Similarly, computed tomography (CT) can be quite helpful in identifying extraluminal disease such as an abscess, ruptured appendicitis, and pancreatic pseudocysts. However, it may miss gallbladder sludge or stones, or even pancreatic disease if the amount of oral contrast is insufficient to separate intraluminal from extraluminal contents. A listing of commonly ordered imaging modalities can be found in Table 50.2.

A list of a typical differential diagnosis with fairly broad categories is listed in Table 50.3. Note that these are commonly found *organic* causes of abdominal pain.

FUNCTIONAL ABDOMINAL DISORDERS IN CHILDHOOD

When faced with a difficult set of GI symptoms in a child or adolescent who is hospitalized, the clinician frequently orders a battery of diagnostic tests. When these tests do not yield a diagnosis, the hospitalist may presume that the child is suffering from symptoms that are emotionally based. Although in some instances, this may be true, it is very important to understand that functional abdominal pain is *REAL* pain, and that the child is rarely suffering from a psychiatric illness or malingering.

Functional abdominal complaints usually *do* have a physiologic basis, and are related to maladaptive coping with the symptom(s). Failed diagnosis and inappropriate treatment can

TABLE 50.2

RADIOLOGIC EVALUATION OF ABDOMINAL PAIN

- Plain abdominal film
- Upper GI and small bowel follow-through
- Abdominal ultrasound
- More specific (when indicated):
  Abdominal/pelvic CT scan with contrast
  Nuclear medicine studies (gastric emptying, HIDA scan)

TABLE 50.4

CHILDHOOD FUNCTIONAL
GASTROINTESTINAL DISORDERS

- Vomiting
  - Infant regurgitation syndrome
  - Infant rumination syndrome
  - Cyclic vomiting syndrome
- Abdominal pain
  - Functional dyspepsia
    - Ulcer-like dyspepsia
    - Dysmotility-like dyspepsia
    - Unspecified (nonspecific) dyspepsia
  - Irritable bowel syndrome
  - Functional abdominal pain
  - Abdominal migraine
  - Aerophagia
- Functional diarrhea
- Disorders of defecation
  - Infant dyschezia
  - Functional constipation
  - Functional fecal retention
  - Functional nonretentive fecal soiling

result in needless physical and emotional suffering on the part of the patient and family. It is for this reason that hospital-based physicians need to familiarize themselves with the specific criteria for each of the functional gastrointestinal disorders, outlined by the ROME II criteria. Understanding that functional disorders of the GI tract have specific patterns will help prevent unnecessary testing or anxiety, and may reassure patients and families, allowing for more expedient care and shorter hospital stays.

The ROME II criteria separate functional GI disorders in childhood into four categories: vomiting, abdominal pain, functional diarrhea, and disorders of defecation (Table 50.4). Although a more exhaustive discussion of each disorder can be found in Drossman and associates (1), several of these are useful to outline for the pediatric hospitalist who will be called upon to evaluate and treat children with these problems on a regular basis.

Cyclic Vomiting Syndrome

Cyclic vomiting syndrome (CVS) consists of recurrent, distinct episodes of nausea and vomiting lasting hours to several days, separated by symptom-free intervals. Attacks may occur in very regular intervals or more sporadically. Accompanying symptoms may include pallor, weakness, increased salivation, abdominal pain, intolerance to noise/light/odors, headache, diarrhea, fever, tachycardia, hypertension, skin blotchiness, and leukocytosis. Up to 80% of patients can identify specific triggers for their episodes. Among these are anxiety, excitement, exhaustion, asthma, and infections.

Onset may occur anytime from infancy to midlife, but most commonly from ages 2 to 7 years. Males and females are equally affected. Migraine, motion sickness, and functional bowel disorders of other types are more prevalent in patients with CVS. The majority of patients with this disorder have been characterized as competitive, high-achieving, perfectionist, strong-willed, moralistic, caring, and enthusiastic. Depression and anxiety are common in part because of the unpredictable nature of the disorder.

The diagnostic criteria for CVS include:

- A history of 3 or more periods of intense, acute nausea and unremitting vomiting lasting hours to days, with intervening symptom-free intervals lasting weeks to months.

- There is no metabolic, GI, or CNS structural or biochemical disease identifiable.

The differential diagnosis of CVS is broad, and includes brainstem tumors, obstructive uropathy, acid-peptic disease with pyloric outlet obstruction, recurrent pancreatitis, intermittent small bowel obstruction, chronic intestinal pseudo-obstruction, pheochromocytoma, adrenal insufficiency, diabetes mellitus, and several of the chronic organic acidemias, as well as porphyria.

The disorder is thought to be related to the activation of the emetic reflex centrally. This consists of a pre-ejection phase accompanied by autonomic activation (pallor, headache, nausea, drooling) followed by an ejection phase with retching and vomiting. Intense autonomic discharge and release of ACTH, vasopressin, norepinephrine, and prostaglandin-E2 have been described in these patients. Although many of these mechanisms overlap in patients with abdominal migraines, the most distressing symptom in CVS is the vomiting, while with abdominal migraines, it is pain.

Although there is no single approved treatment for CVS, many patients who can identify triggers for their episodes can successfully avoid repeated attacks. Prophylactic treatments have included cyproheptadine, amitriptylene, erythromycin, phenobarbital, and propranolol, and have been met with varying rates of success.

Aborting episodes is often possible if the patient has a recognizable prodrome. Orally administered medications such as ondansetron, histamine-2 receptor antagonists, proton-pump inhibitors, and lorazepam have been used individually or in combination if the profound nausea and vomiting has not yet set in. Our group has often arranged home health care for intravenous administration of anti-emetics, intravenous fluids, and antacids once a pattern has been established and other disease processes have been comfortably ruled out, thus avoiding costly recurrent emergency room visits or hospitalizations. These regimens are continued until the patient has stopped vomiting and is able to tolerate liquids reliably without vomiting.

Functional Dyspepsia

Dyspepsia is generally defined as persistent or recurrent pain or discomfort centered in the upper abdomen. Organic disorders can cause dyspepsia, such as gastroesophageal reflux, *Helicobacter pylori*-associated gastritis, or Crohn disease. However, functional dyspepsia (FD) is by far more common, with prevalence in adolescents of 10%. FD has two distinct presentations, one ulcer-like and the other dysmotility-like, with some overlap between the two. Patients with the ulcer-like variety suffer predominantly from pain, often relieved by food and by inhibiting gastric acid secretion. In dysmotility-like dyspepsia, the patient complains more of early satiety, nausea, bloating, postprandial fullness, and retching or vomiting rather than pain.

The diagnostic criteria for FD are dependent on the child being mature enough to provide an accurate pain history, and includes at least 12 weeks (not necessarily consecutive) in the preceding 12 months of:

- Persistent or recurrent pain or discomfort present in the upper abdomen (above the umbilicus).
- No evidence of organic disease (including at upper endoscopy) that is likely to explain the symptoms.
- No evidence that dyspepsia is exclusively relieved by defecation or associated with the onset of a change in stool frequency or form (i.e., not irritable bowel).

The differential diagnosis for FD is also broad, and includes GI mucosal diseases (esophagitis, gastritis, duodenitis, and ulcer disease and disorders of the liver, gallbladder, or pancreas. Medications such as the nonsteroidal anti-inflammatory agents are to be avoided in these patients, and certain triggers in the diet, such as caffeine or spicy/fatty foods may also exacerbate the condition.

Although some children diagnosed with FD have demonstrated disorders of antroduodenal motility and electrogastrography, there have been no uniform studies demonstrating similar patterns in all children who meet these criteria for FD.

The treatment for FD is by no means uniform. Reassurance after a thorough diagnostic evaluation may be all that is required. However, many patients with ulcer-like FD respond to typical acid suppressors, while dymotility-like FD sufferers often respond to smaller, more frequent meals, low-fat diets, and occasionally, prokinetic agents such as metoclopramide, cisapride, or erythromycin. Antinausea medications are occasionally helpful as well (phenothiazines, serotonin agonists). Symptomatic relief is the goal in these patients, and no controlled trial exists for medications for FD in children.

Irritable Bowel Syndrome

Irritable bowel syndrome (IBS) is an often-misused term. It is important to recognize the criteria set forth by Rome II for this disorder. Specifically, these patients have abdominal pain that is associated with defecation or a change in bowel habit, and often have features of disordered defecation. IBS is one of the most common causes of recurrent abdominal pain in children, and it is estimated that 6% to 14% of adolescents will have some features of this disorder.

The diagnostic criteria for IBS includes at least 12 weeks, which need not be consecutive, in the preceding 12 months of continuous or recurrent symptoms of:

- Abdominal pain or discomfort that has two out of three features:
  - Relieved with defecation
  - Onset associated with a change in frequency of stool
  - Onset associated with a change in form (appearance) of stool
- There are no structural or metabolic abnormalities to explain the symptoms

Typical symptoms that support the diagnosis of IBS include abnormal stool frequency, defined as greater than 3 per day or less than 3 per week; abnormal stool form (lumpy/hard or loose/watery); abnormal stool passage (straining, urgency, or sensation of incomplete evacuation); passage of mucus; and bloating or feeling of abdominal distention.

Although the criteria for IBS generally provide enough guidance to make the diagnosis after a thorough history and physical exam, overlapping issues can be elicited in the history, such as relationship of dairy ingestion to the symptoms (lactose intolerance); overindulgence in nonabsorbable sugars (sorbitol, inositol) frequently found in dietetic foods, gums, and candies; and adequacy of dietary fiber intake in children with constipation-predominant symptoms. It is true that in adult studies, there have been motility and sensory abnormalities identified in IBS patients, but no data have been collected in children supporting a specific physiologic mechanism for IBS.

Treatment for IBS includes reassurance and suppression or elimination of symptoms. Presence or severity of the pain (as in all functional GI disorders of childhood) should not be disputed. Focus on the link between the brain and enteric nervous systems, addressing how outside influences such as stress or anxiety can play a role in exacerbating symptoms. Often, a clinician who develops a therapeutic alliance with the patient and family can introduce a therapist (psychologist, psychiatrist, counselor) into the treatment plan as an adjunctive way to make the patient regain normal function more rapidly. This is much less threatening and less anxiety provoking than simply throwing one's hands up and declaring that "we did all the tests and they were all normal, so it must be a mental illness."

Medications play a role in IBS treatment. Tricyclic antidepressants such as migraine and amitriptyline in low dose have been used for chronic visceral pain with much success. Amitriptyline has greater sedative and anticholinergic effects, and thus may be a better choice for patients with diarrhea-predominant (IBS-D) symptoms, or for those with disturbed sleep at night. Imipramine, however, may be a better choice for constipation-predominant (IBS-C) symptoms, as at low doses it rarely exacerbates the constipation. Antispasmodics with primarily anticholinergic effects, including dicyclomine, hyoscine, mebeverine, and octylonium, have some usefulness, but no controlled trials exist in children to measure efficacy. Increased dietary fiber (recommended daily intake = age in years + 5 grams) may act both as a stool softener (in patients with IBS-C) as well as adding form to otherwise formless stools (in patients with IBS-D). Finally, a wide array of laxative products may be recommended for patients with IBS-C, although we favor the nonstimulant osmotic agents such as polyethylene glycol (PEG-3350) preparations or lactulose syrup, or for diapered children over 1 year of age, mineral oil.

Functional Abdominal Pain

Children with recurrent abdominal pain that does not fall into the IBS or FD categories may be classified as having functional abdominal pain (FAP). In this case, there is no temporal association of the pain, which is usually periumbilical, with eating, defecation, menses, or exercise. It may be episodic or continuous, and affects the daily function of the child. It may affect school attendance and is often associated with unrecognized learning problems, especially in children from families with high achievement expectations.

The diagnostic criteria for FAP include at least 12 weeks of:

- Continuous or nearly continuous abdominal pain in a school-aged child or adolescent
- No or only occasional relationship of the pain with physiologic events (e.g., eating, menses, or defecation)
- Some loss of daily functioning
- The pain is not feigned (e.g., malingering)
- Insufficient criteria for other functional gastrointestinal disorders that would explain the abdominal pain

In these children, the pain is the predominant complaint, but other symptoms such as weakness, headache, fatigue, and nausea (without vomiting), may be present. The physical exam and laboratory evaluation are generally all normal, and specific physiologic features for this entity have yet to be defined in children. There is often a history of anxiety, depression, separation anxiety, school phobia, maternal–child enmeshment, and sleep disturbance.

Treatment requires a therapeutic alliance with the family, which may find it difficult to understand how a physiologic symptom can occur in the absence of a disease process. In fact, each negative test may serve to heighten anxiety that something is being missed, leading to further consultations, testing, and even more anxiety on the part of the patient and family. The child and family must be educated as to how sensitive nerves send pain signals to the brain, and that the way to treat the problem is to decrease these signals. Continued availability needs to be promised to the family to guide it through this transition toward functionality, and to respond if/when the pain changes character in any way. Providing something for the patient and family to do actively, such as increasing exercise, keeping a pain diary, and use of tricyclic antidepressants at bedtime to facilitate sleep while using nonsedating serotonin-reuptake inhibitors during the day, may be effective. Incorporation of a psychologist/therapist to help the child regain function is usually accepted once the patient and family have an understanding of the problem, and are comfortable that the clinician does not think the pain is "all in the head."

Abdominal Migraine

Abdominal migraine is characterized by the acute onset of midline abdominal pain that is noncolicky, incapacitating, and can last for hours. It is often associated with pallor and anorexia. A family history of migraines, increased susceptibility to motion sickness, prodromal changes of mood and activity, and other migraine-like symptoms (photophobia, phonophobia, headache, vomiting, sleepiness) is usually reported. The patients are usually well between attacks, and have a stereotypical presentation with their episodes. The onset of abdominal migraines may be part of the clinical expression of migraine, and affects about 2% of all children. It starts usually between 2 and 7 years of age, and girls outnumber boys 2 to 1.

The diagnostic criteria for abdominal migraine are:

- In the preceding 12 months, 3 or more paroxysmal episodes of intense, acute midline abdominal pain lasting 2 hours to several days, with intervening symptom-free intervals lasting weeks to months.
- Evidence of metabolic, GI, and CNS structural or biochemical diseases is absent.
- Two of the following features:
  - Headache during episodes
  - Photophobia during episodes
  - Family history of migraine
  - Headache confined to one side only
  - An aura or warning period consisting of visual symptoms (e.g., blurred or restricted vision), sensory symptoms (e.g., numbness or tingling), or motor symptoms (e.g., slurred speech, inability to speak, paralysis).

All organic causes of intermittent severe abdominal pain should be considered. A favorable response to medications used for prophylaxis of migraine headaches supports the diagnosis of abdominal migraine. No physiologic mechanism or psychological features have been established for this disorder. No treatment regimen has been proven effective, although some patients with migraine headaches and cyclic vomiting syndrome derive benefit from prophylaxis using cyproheptadine, and this agent might be useful in abdominal migraine prevention as well.

In summary, functional gastrointestinal disorders in childhood take up a significant amount of the pediatric hospitalist's time and attention. An understanding of these disorders and a consistent approach to evaluation and treatment will help minimize unnecessary intervention, and expedite the transition to outpatient care. Future validation of these criteria will be addressed in the soon-to-be-published ROME III criteria, and clinical trials measuring symptom change as the primary outcome measure will help us learn which interventions improve outcome in childhood functional gastrointestinal disorders.

Reference

1. Drossman DA, Corazziari E, Talley NJ, et al., eds. *ROME II: the functional gastrointestinal disorders.* 2nd ed. Lawrence, Kansas: Allen Press; 2000.

Suggested Reading

Walker WA, Goulet O, Kleinman RE, et al., eds. *Pediatric gastrointestinal disease: pathophysiology, diagnosis, and management.* 4th ed. Hamilton, Ontario: Decker; 2004.

CHAPTER 51 ■ ACUTE GASTROINTESTINAL BLEEDING

DAVID A. GREMSE

The presence of blood in vomitus or in bowel movements is an alarming symptom that prompts evaluation by the physician. The optimum management of gastrointestinal (GI) bleeding begins with a determination of the hemodynamic status to identify those patients with potentially life-threatening conditions, followed by a diagnostic evaluation to ascertain the etiology. Immediate intervention is required for those patients with significant gastrointestinal blood loss, while minimal evaluation and reassurance may be all that is needed for children with minor causes of bleeding. In some patients, the source of bleeding cannot be found even after an extensive evaluation.

Gastrointestinal hemorrhage can present as hematemesis, hematochezia, or melena. Hematemesis is the vomiting of blood and indicates bleeding proximal to the ligament of Treitz (1). Hematemesis may include either bright red blood or "coffee grounds," which are produced when hemoglobin is denatured by gastric acid (2). Hematochezia is the presence of bright red blood in the stool that usually occurs when the source of blood is in the ileum or colon (3). The blood may precede or be mixed in the stool when the source of bleeding is the intestinal mucosa. Massive upper GI bleeding can have a laxative-like effect to decrease the time available to denaturation of the blood, so passage of bright red blood per rectum can occur (4). In contrast, streaks of bright red blood on the stool suggest that the source of blood is the anal canal or rectal vault.

PATHOPHYSIOLOGY

The gastrointestinal tract is supplied by a rich vasculature, which can lead to massive blood loss with some of the causes of GI hemorrhage. Bleeding can occur from any part of the digestive tract via arterial bleeding, venous oozing, or arteriovenous malformations.

Acid-peptic diseases are one of the more common etiologies for GI hemorrhage. Ulceration of the GI mucosa that results in bleeding occurs when there is an imbalance between "aggressive factors" such as acid, pepsin, and bile acids (5) and "defensive factors" that include the mucus–bicarbonate layer and prostaglandins (6). The maxim "no acid, no ulcer" is the basis for treatment of peptic ulcers. As the term "acid-peptic disease" implies, the presence of both acid and pepsin combine to produce breaks in the upper GI mucosa (7). The inactive proenzyme pepsinogen becomes the active compound pepsin in acid milieu, so decreasing gastric acidity not only reduces the noxious effect of acid itself, but also decreases the amount of pepsin in the stomach. The mucus layer overlying the upper GI epithelium is impermeable to pepsin, but this agent is constantly eroding this barrier. Once pepsin comes into contact with the epithelial cell membrane it can exert its proteolytic effects.

The gastroduodenal epithelium produces a mucus layer that acts as a barrier to hydrogen ions and pepsin. Bicarbonate secretion is increased by prostaglandins and calcium, but is inhibited by alcohol, nonsteroidal anti-inflammatory drugs (NSAIDs), norepinephrine, and bile acids. In addition to their beneficial effect on local bicarbonate secretion by GI epithelium, prostaglandins also have direct cytoprotective effects. NSAID-associated gastritis results from a combination of a direct cytotoxic effect and the inhibition of prostaglandin synthesis.

Once clinically significant GI blood losses occur, the resulting hypoperfusion induces several compensatory responses. Hypovolemia causes decreased venous return to the heart, resulting in decreases in preload and cardiac output. However, blood pressure is initially maintained through increased systemic vascular resistance. Blood flow is diverted from the peripheral and splanchnic circulation to the central circulation. In addition, an "autotransfusion" from the extracellular and intracellular compartments can reach up to 15 mL/kg/hr in adults. Once 30% to 35% of the blood volume has been lost, irreversible shock can occur.

Children without underlying cardiovascular conditions are capable of compensating well initially and may have stable blood pressure and good color while mild tachycardia may be the only sign of hypovolemia. Treatment at this stage is most effective to prevent potential complications. This is especially important in young infants and children in whom clinical findings are not as prominent and hemodynamic and circulatory reserves are limited.

CLINICAL PRESENTATION

In the patient with clinically significant GI hemorrhage, obtaining pertinent history and physical findings must be coordinated with stabilization of the patient and initial management. The clinical setting dictates whether the history and physical examination should be brief or detailed.

When a patient presents with a history of passage of material that suggests upper or lower GI bleeding, it is important to confirm whether the material is actually blood. Substances that can be mistaken for blood include the red food dye seen in drinks or foods such as beets. The ingestion of bismuth or iron supplements can produce black stools. The presence of blood in the stool can be tested by biochemical analysis using guaiac. Commercially, the Hemoccult kit uses a guaiac-impregnated card to which the stool specimen is applied followed by the addition of two drops of hydrogen peroxide on the reverse side. The peroxidase activity of hemoglobin, if blood is present, leads to oxidation of the reagent, resulting in a blue discoloration. Because this reaction is less reliable in acidic fluids, the testing of gastric fluid should be done with Gastroccult cards (8).

Prior to performing an extensive evaluation to determine the source of GI hemorrhage, it is important to ensure that the patient is hemodynamically stable (9). Vital signs should include assessment of orthostatic changes of the heart rate and blood pressure. Tachycardia may be present, and orthostatic changes are not observed when the blood loss is less than 10%. The presence of orthostatic changes in blood pressure or heart rate indicates that the blood loss exceeds 10%. Tachycardia at rest and hypotension occur when the loss reaches 30% of blood volume.

If signs of clinically significant blood loss are present, volume resuscitation should be the first priority. One or two large-bore intravenous lines should be placed and isotonic fluid of normal saline or lactated Ringer solution given, followed by packed red blood cells. Patients who receive significant fluid resuscitation need to be monitored in a hospital setting. Patients without orthostatic changes, anemia, or ongoing blood loss can be observed for a period of time and then considered for outpatient follow-up. Moderately ill patients with tachycardia, tachypnea, delayed capillary refill, and orthostatic hypotension should be hospitalized, preferably in an intensive care unit, for monitoring as well as for potential interventional treatments. All newborns with significant GI bleeding, regardless of other findings, should be admitted for observation. Severely ill patients with the above findings plus obtundation and decreased urine output should all be admitted to the intensive-care unit. A transfusion requirement that equals or exceeds the calculated blood volume prior to surgical intervention, a coagulation disorder, or other systemic disease are associated with a poor prognosis (9).

Once the patient is stabilized, the focus can shift to determining the location of the bleeding. When hematemesis is the presenting symptom, the source is proximal to the ligament of Treitz. In contrast, streaks of blood on the stool indicates a distal colon source. However, hematochezia or melena can occur when the location of bleeding is either from an upper or lower source. For example, melena or maroon-colored stool can arise from an upper GI or right colon source, depending on the intestinal transit time. The passage of melanotic stool in adults or older adolescents indicates blood loss of at least 200 mL (10). Placement of a nasogastric tube can aid in localizing the bleeding site, but is not always specific. For instance, the nasogastric aspirate may be clear in patients with a duodenal ulcer without any gastric reflux of blood through the pylorus back into the stomach.

CLINICAL CONDITIONS

Upper Gastrointestinal Bleeding

Although there are many conditions that cause GI hemorrhage that can occur in any age group, the most likely diagnoses vary in infants, children, and adolescents (Table 51.1). For patients with upper GI bleeding, the diagnoses of duodenal ulcer, gastric ulcer, esophagitis, gastritis, and esophageal varices account for the majority of cases (1,2).

There are causes of GI bleeding that are unique to newborns. For example, swallowed maternal blood has been reported to explain 30% of GI bleeding in newborns (11). An Apt–Downy test, which distinguishes fetal from maternal hemoglobin, is useful in this setting to determine whether any further diagnostic evaluation is indicated. Another cause of bleeding that occurs early in infancy is hemorrhagic disease of the newborn. It is important to verify that vitamin K was administered at the time of delivery. Other risk factors for vitamin K deficiency include maternal medication that can cross the placenta and interfere with production of vitamin K–dependent factors. These medications include warfarin, phenytoin, and promethazine. On examination, petechiae and edema may appear from trauma during delivery, but progressive petechiae and ecchymoses suggest a platelet defect.

Upper GI mucosal disease leading to gastritis or stress ulcers can develop in newborns with conditions such as perinatal asphyxia or sepsis. Although these can be associated with significant blood loss, most are self-limited, and the neonate's ultimate prognosis depends more on the underlying disease. Blood-streaked emesis from erosive esophagitis occurs less commonly in young infants. When erosive esophagitis is seen in the first few months of life, it is often associated with

TABLE 51.1

DIFFERENTIAL DIAGNOSIS OF PEDIATRIC GASTROINTESTINAL BLEEDING

Infants	Children	Adolescents
MORE COMMON		
Infectious colitis	Infectious colitis	Infectious colitis
Allergic colitis	Anal fissure	Inflammatory bowel disease
Intussusception	Juvenile polyps	Peptic ulcer disease
Anal fissure	Intussusception	Gastritis
Lymphoid hyperplasia	Peptic ulcer disease	Mallory–Weiss syndrome
Swallowed maternal blood	Gastritis	Prolapse gastropathy
	Erosive esophagitis	
	Mallory–Weiss syndrome	
	Prolapse gastropathy	
LESS COMMON		
Malrotation with midgut	Esophageal varices	Hemorrhoids
Volvulus	Meckel diverticulum	Esophageal varices
Necrotizing enterocolitis	Lymphonodular hyperplasia	Esophagitis
Meckel diverticulum	Henoch–Schönlein purpura	Angiodysplasia
Hemorrhagic disease of	Foreign body	Graft-verus-host disease
the newborn	Angiodysplasia	

milk protein allergy rather than reflux esophagitis. Gastric outlet obstruction can lead to hematemesis in patients of any age. Coffee ground emesis can follow weeks of projectile non-bilious vomiting and poor weight gain in infants with pyloric stenosis.

In immunocompromised hosts, opportunistic infections can lead to GI bleeding. Infectious esophagitis can be caused by fungal pathogens such as *Candida albicans* or viral agents that include herpes simplex virus or cytomegalovirus. Infections with any of these pathogens can cause ulcerative lesions of the esophagus that may present as hematemesis with associated dysphagia (12). Risk factors for these infections include primary immunodeficiencies or secondary immune suppression owing to chemotherapeutic or immunosuppressive drugs. Other medications, including antibiotics or inhaled steroids, have been reported as risk factors for either candidal or herpetic esophagitis in nonimmunocompromised pediatric patients.

Retching injuries such as Mallory–Weiss syndrome or prolapse gastropathy are common causes of hematemesis in previously healthy children with an acute onset of vomiting. Mallory–Weiss syndrome is a mucosal laceration at the gastroesophageal junction that occurs after forceful or prolonged vomiting (13). On the other hand, prolapse gastropathy is a broad area of erosion in the gastric fundus near the gastroesophageal junction (Fig. 51.1) caused when the diaphragm descends during vomiting and the affected portion of the stomach protrudes through the diaphragmatic hiatus (14). The history for either of these conditions typically involves patients with no prior significant GI symptoms, who have several episodes or days of nonbloody vomiting followed by a sudden onset of hematemesis. With either condition, antisecretory therapy is commonly prescribed until mucosal healing occurs, and the prognosis is good (15). Even though retching injuries are the most common traumatic injuries around the gastroesophageal junction, other traumatic causes of upper GI bleeding include foreign bodies ingestion or ulceration of the stomach due to gastrostomy tubes.

The acid-peptic diseases that can cause hematemesis include erosive esophagitis, gastritis, and peptic ulcers (1,2). Erosive

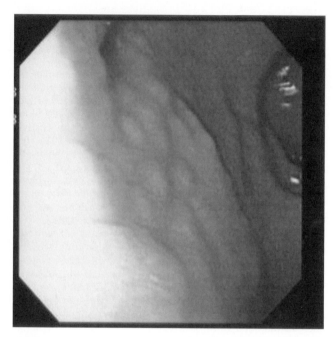

FIGURE 51.2. Nodularity in the mucosa of the gastric antrum in a patient with *Helicobacter pylori* infection.

esophagitis is a complication of chronic gastroesophageal reflux disease (16). Patients with gastroesophageal reflux disease who are neurologically impaired are at higher risk for the development of this complication. Esophageal erosions may not be apparent on upper GI series radiographs and thus may require upper endoscopy for diagnosis (16).

Gastritis and peptic ulcer disease are categorized as primary and secondary, depending on the underlying cause of mucosal inflammation (17). Factors contributing to secondary gastritis or peptic ulcers include stress from surgery, shock, major trauma, burns, or sepsis; drugs such as NSAIDs or steroids; or infection with *Helicobacter pylori* (Fig. 51.2). Risk factors for upper GI bleeding in pediatric intensive-care unit patients include respiratory failure, coagulopathy, or PRISM score ≥10 (9). Primary gastritis is a chronic inflammatory process that is often associated with duodenal ulcers. Symptoms of primary or secondary acid-peptic disease include recurrent epigastric pain, nocturnal pain that either awakens a child from sleep or is increased upon awakening, postprandial pain, and vomiting (18). Diagnosis is made endoscopically in most cases, and treatment includes the use of either histamine-2 receptor antagonists such as cimetidine, ranitidine, famotidine, or nizatidine; or proton-pump inhibitors such as omeprazole or lansoprazole. In the case of *H. pylori* infection, a combination of a proton-pump inhibitor with antibiotics such as amoxicillin, and metronidazole, or clarithromycin is used.

One of the most serious complications of portal hypertension is the development of esophageal varices. GI bleeding associated with esophageal varices can result in massive losses. The portal hypertension that causes esophageal varices can originate from an intrahepatic or extrahepatic source. Intrahepatic portal hypertension is usually associated cirrhosis from chronic liver conditions such as biliary atresia, congenital hepatic fibrosis, cystic fibrosis, autoimmune hepatitis, alpha-1-antitrypsin deficiency, or parenteral nutrition–associated liver disease. Extrahepatic portal hypertension in many cases is associated with portal vein thrombosis. The past medical history may indicate that an umbilical vein catheterization was performed in the neonatal period, or reveal a previous episode of severe dehydration. Patients with bleeding from esophageal varices

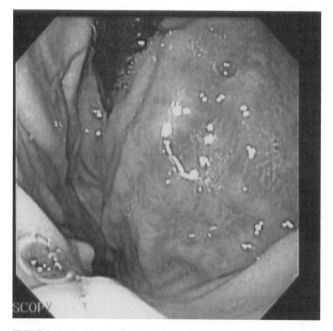

FIGURE 51.1. Hemorrhagic region of prolapse gastropathy in the gastric cardia near the gastroesophageal junction.

may have a sudden onset of hematemesis or melena, pallor, and fatigue without any warning. Other findings of portal hypertension such as splenomegaly, ascites, or caput medusa may be seen upon physical examination. Diagnosis is made by endoscopy, and treatment can include the use of octreotide, esophageal variceal sclerotherapy, or band ligation. In some severe cases of extrahepatic portal hypertension, surgical shunting may be necessary, whereas placement of a transjugular portosystemic shunt may temporarily alleviate intrahepatic portal hypertension pending liver transplantation.

Lower Gastrointestinal Bleeding

The more common conditions found in the age-related differential diagnosis of lower intestinal bleeding are listed in Table 51.1. In infancy, causes of lower intestinal bleeding that may require surgery include conditions that result in mucosal ischemia such as malrotation with midgut volvulus or intussusception and conditions that lead to ulceration of ectopic gastric mucosa such as Meckel diverticulum or bleeding from a duplication cyst. Eighty percent of patients with intestinal malrotation present with midgut volvulus in the first month of life, and 90% are symptomatic in infancy. Symptoms of midgut volvulus are poor feeding, bilious emesis, abdominal distention, and sometimes melena. Midgut volvulus is a surgical emergency because the vascular compromise can lead to intestinal ischemia and bowel necrosis. In preparation for surgery, a nasogastric tube should be placed and intravenous fluid replacement should be given. Intussusception typically occurs in children less than 3 years of age, but is unusual in the first 3 months of life. The usual history is that of a previously well child with paroxysmal, severe abdominal pain with progressive lethargy between pain episodes. The colicky pain may recur for hours, with the child eventually passing stools mixed with blood and mucus ("currant-jelly" stools), usually after symptoms have been present > 12 hours. A sausage-shaped mass may be palpated in the right lower quadrant. Radiographic contrast enema using air, water-soluble, or barium contrast may be diagnostic and therapeutic. Exploratory laparotomy for surgical reduction of the intussusception is needed if contrast radiography is not successful. As with any intestinal obstruction, a nasogastric tube and intravenous fluid resuscitation should be started prior to radiographic or surgical reduction.

Ulceration of ectopic gastric mucosa can lead to massive intestinal bleeding. Ectopic gastric mucosa can be found in Meckel diverticulum or intestinal duplication cysts. Meckel diverticulum is the result of incomplete obliteration of the omphalomesenteric duct and is located on the antimesenteric border of the distal small intestine within 100 cm of the ileocecal valve. Intestinal duplications can be cystic or tubular and can occur anywhere from the mouth to anus, but are most common in the small bowel. Duplications can enlarge to obstruct the adjacent bowel, or lead to volvulus or intussusception. Duplications with ectopic gastric mucosa can ulcerate and hemorrhage or perforate. The most common presentation of Meckel diverticulum or ulcerated ectopic gastric mucosa from intestinal duplication is painless rectal bleeding that varies from melena, to maroon-colored, to bright red depending on the volume and intestinal transit time. Diagnosis is made by technetium pertechnetate scan (Meckel scan) and treatment is surgical resection. Antisecretory therapy with H_2-receptor antagonists or proton-pump inhibitors can assist in the management of bleeding prior to surgery and can increase the sensitivity of the Meckel scan.

Less serious causes of lower intestinal bleeding in infants include anal fissures and allergic colitis. Anal fissure typically occur when passage of hard and large feces stretch and tear the perianal skin usually in the midline, either anteriorly or posteriorly. Anal fissures are usually self-limiting and heal unless the underlying cause such as constipation persists. The presence of anal outlet bleeding is suggested by a description or direct observation of a few streaks of bright red blood on the outside of a hard stool.

Allergic colitis due to cow's milk and/or soy protein intolerance typically occurs within the first 2 months of life (19). It also can be seen in exclusively breast-fed infants and presents with passage of stools containing blood and mucus along with irritability. Signs of infection such as fever are not present, although in some cases associated symptoms of vomiting and failure to thrive may occur. The estimated incidence of allergic enteropathy is 0.3% to 7.5% (20). Laboratory evaluation may be normal, but mild anemia, leukocytosis, eosinophilia, and thrombocytosis may be detected. More severe cases may lead to hypoalbuminemia due to protein-losing enteropathy. In atypical cases, flexible sigmoidoscopy can be used to confirm the diagnosis. Endoscopic findings include superficial erosions or lymphonodular hyperplasia in the rectosigmoid mucosa (20). Classically, biopsies demonstrate an eosinophilic infiltrate in the lamina propria or an eosinophilic cryptitis. Initial treatment is a trial of a casein-hydrolysate formula. The gross blood in the stool typically resolves within 72 hours, but guaiac-positive stool may continue for up to 2 weeks. Recurrence of symptoms appear if the offending milk protein is reintroduced into the diet. Soy formulas are not recommended because a high percentage of infants with cow's milk protein intolerance will also become sensitized to soy proteins (21). If symptoms persist with a casein-hydrolysate formula, an amino acid–based formula is required.

Inflammatory conditions of the bowel mucosa can occur in necrotizing enterocolitis or Hirschsprung enterocolitis and lead to lower intestinal bleeding in infancy. Necrotizing enterocolitis is usually seen in premature infants, but can rarely develop in full-term infants. Symptoms progress from abdominal distention, vomiting, lethargy, and poor feeding, to passage of grossly bloody or guaiac positive stools and signs of shock. Abdominal radiographs may show dilated loops of bowel, intramural thickening, air–fluid levels, or pneumatosis intestinalis, which is the classic finding of the disease (22).

Hirschsprung disease occurs in 1 in 5,000 live births and is caused by the failure of craniocaudal migration of ganglion cells during the fifth through twelfth weeks of embryonic development. Affected infants fail to pass meconium in the first 24 hours of life and usually do not have bowel movements without stimulation by enema, suppository, rectal thermometer, or digital stimulation, which can cause rapid expulsion of stool. Signs of Hirschsprung enterocolitis include abdominal distention, explosive watery to bloody stools, and fever, and may progress to hypovolemic shock (23).

The most common causes of hematochezia in the preschool- and school-aged child are nonsurgical and include infectious colitis, juvenile polyps, and inflammatory bowel disease. The most common bacterial pathogens associated with infectious colitis are *Salmonella* species, *Shigella* species, *Campylobacter jejuni*, and enteroinvasive and enterohemorrhagic *Escherichia coli*. In the patient who has a history of antibiotic usage or hospitalization, pseudomembranous colitis due to *Clostridium difficile* infection can produce bloody diarrhea (24). In certain parts of the world, amoebic colitis due to *Entamoeba histolytica* should be considered. The presence of blood in the stools is uncommon in viral gastroenteritis.

Juvenile polyps are a common cause of painless rectal bleeding from the ages of 2 to 6 years (Fig. 51.3). In most cases, the bleeding is slight, with streaks of fresh blood on the outside of the stool. However, occasionally a patient can autoamputate a polyp and have significant bleeding. The passed polyp may be mistaken for a "clot" within the bloody rectal discharge. Abdominal pain may be associated with traction on the polyp or the polyp may protrude from the rectum through the anus.

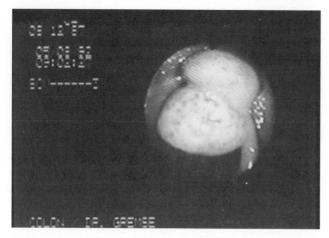

FIGURE 51.3. Pedunculated juvenile polyp in the sigmoid colon of a patient with painless rectal bleeding. (photo by David A. Gremse)

Juvenile polyps are benign inflammatory polyps and differ from the adenomatous polyps that are associated with familial polyposis syndromes. Juvenile polyps can be diagnosed and treated by pancolonoscopy with polypectomy using electrocauterization.

Multisystem diseases such as hemolytic–uremic syndrome and Henoch–Schönlein purpura can be distinguished from other causes of rectal bleeding by the associated features of these syndromes. Hemolytic–uremic syndrome, characterized by hemolytic anemia, thrombocytopenia, and uremia, can begin with bloody diarrhea in the prodrome (27). The features of Henoch–Schönlein purpura (HSP) include an urticarial or purpuric rash, arthralgias or arthritis, hematuria, and abdominal pain. The colicky abdominal pain in HSP can be associated with melena or bloody diarrhea and can lead to intussusception. The bloody stools may precede the development of the purpuric rash in HSP, making it more difficult to establish an early diagnosis. If endoscopy is performed to evaluate the source of GI bleeding in these patients, coalescing purpuric mucosal lesions from submucosal edema and hemorrhage are suggestive of HSP (25).

The peak age of onset of pediatric inflammatory bowel disease occurs in the second decade of life (26). The clinical features of IBD can be divided into two broad categories, those of small intestinal and colonic symptoms. Small bowel symptoms of IBD include cramping postprandial abdominal pain, growth failure, and malabsorptive type of diarrhea. In contrast, bloody, mucusy diarrhea is the classic colonic symptom of IBD that occurs in ulcerative colitis or in Crohn disease with colonic mucosal involvement. Extraintestinal manifestations of IBD, including perianal disease, skin lesions such as pyoderma gangrenosum or erythema nodosum, oral aphthous ulcers, arthritis, or sclerosing cholangitis, when present in combination with the GI manifestations, distinguish IBD from other causes of lower GI bleeding. Characteristic findings on colonoscopy with biopsies confirm the diagnosis.

DIAGNOSTIC EVALUATION

Establishing an accurate diagnosis aids in planning the specific management of the pediatric patient with GI hemorrhage. Confirmatory tests for blood (Hemoccult or Gastroccult) should be performed prior to scheduling any invasive procedures.

A history of hematemesis or blood in the nasogastric aspirate indicates a bleeding source proximal to the ligament of Treitz. If blood clears from the nasogastric tube, so that the upper GI mucosa can be thoroughly examined, the bleeding site can usually be identified by esophagogastroduodenoscopy (EGD). Even if the nasogastric aspirate is negative for blood, EGD is also the first diagnostic test recommended in patients with melena to rule out a duodenal lesion (28).

In patients with massive upper gastrointestinal bleeding, a nasogastric tube should be placed for gastric decompression and to clear as much blood from the stomach as possible to facilitate diagnostic evaluation. After the patient is stabilized, then EGD can be performed to determine the diagnosis.

Most cases of lower GI bleeding in children are not life threatening, so a planned approach can be employed to establish the diagnosis. The presence of mucus in the stool and detection of fecal leukocytes suggests an inflammatory or infectious etiology. Stool specimens should be collected in this clinical setting for culture, ova and parasite examination, and *Clostridium difficile* toxin to exclude infectious colitis. If an infectious etiology is not found, a colonoscopy is scheduled to evaluate for the source of bleeding. In a patient with maroon-colored stool whose EGD is negative and in whom the colonoscopy reveals melanotic stool in the lumen with normal underlying colonic mucosa, a Meckel scan is the next step. If all of the above tests are not diagnostic, angiography should be considered if the estimated rate of bleeding is at least 0.5 mL per minute (29). If the rate of bleeding is too slow to be detected by angiography, a ^{99m}Tc-labeled red-cell scan can help to localize the area of bleeding (30). Alternatively, in pediatric patients old enough to use the device, capsule endoscopy is a useful diagnostic imaging technique to identify lesions in the small intestinal that cannot be visualized by EGD or colonoscopy with ileoscopy (31).

MANAGEMENT

The initial management of the child with GI hemorrhage centers around the question of whether hypovolemic shock is present or imminent. The initial goals for stabilization are to correct or prevent hypovolemia and to restore hemoglobin levels to maintain adequate tissue oxygenation (2). One or two large-bore IV catheters should be placed depending on the clinical situation. If the bleeding is significant, central line access should be considered. After intravenous access is established, an initial isotonic fluid bolus of 20 mL/kg body weight should be given rapidly, with further boluses as needed to achieve acceptable vital signs and tissue perfusion. If 50 to 70 mL/kg is required over 6 hours, central venous access should be established if that has not already been done in the course of management.

Placement of a nasogastric tube is helpful as an initial assessment to identify an upper GI source of bleeding and to monitor ongoing losses. Historically, iced saline lavage through the nasogastric tube was used in the management of upper GI bleeding. However, animal studies have shown that iced saline lavage may have deleterious effects including a prolongation of the bleeding time with cooling (32) and an increased susceptibility to stress ulcers resulting from decreased gastric blood flow and a shift of the hemoglobin–oxygen dissociation curve to the left with cooling (33).

Antisecretory therapy with H-2 receptor antagonists or proton-pump inhibitors are indicated in the management of patients with upper GI bleeding or suspected Meckel diverticulum. Cytoprotective agents such as sucralfate also have a role in management. GI bleeding can be managed in most pediatric patients with supportive care. However, GI hemorrhage that does not respond to conservative management may require infusion therapy, therapeutic endoscopy, or surgical management. Octreotide has been proposed as a treatment for upper GI bleeding due to its pharmacologic effects of inhibiting gastric secretion, decreasing splanchnic blood flow. It is more effective in variceal hemorrhage, but its use has also been reported in nonvariceal upper GI bleeding. The recommended dose is a 1 to 2 µg/kg bolus, followed by a constant infusion of 1 to 2 µg/kg/hr (34).

Possible therapeutic interventions during upper GI endoscopy vary depending on the cause of bleeding. In patients with bleeding esophageal varices, sclerotherapy (35) or band ligation (36,37) are effective acute interventions. Sclerotherapy is also useful in the treatment of other vascular lesions such as Dieulafoy lesions (38) or rectal vascular lesions (39). Management of actively bleeding mucosal lesions includes thermal coagulation (40), electrocoagulation, or argon plasma coagulation (41). The use of these endoscopic techniques is restricted to patients who are actively bleeding or who are at high risk of rebleeding (42).

There are many causes of GI hemorrhage, and in pediatric patients with significant bleeding a team approach including the pediatric gastroenterologist, pediatric surgeon, and radiologist, may be needed for optimum management of the diagnosis and treatment. Endoscopy is not required in every child with a GI hemorrhage. Children with a history that suggests an acute self-limited illness who are not anemic and are hemodynamically stable can be monitored for further evidence of bleeding. Patients who have experienced a major GI bleed or those who rebleed usually require endoscopy as part of their evaluation. When lesions are actively bleeding or in situations where bleeding is likely, hemostasis can be achieved by a variety of endoscopic techniques. Surgery is indicated for certain causes of intestinal bleeding in children such as Meckel diverticulum or duplication cyst, but should also be considered for the child with persistent or recurrent bleeding with continued blood transfusion requirements for lesions not accessible by endoscopy or when therapeutic endoscopy is unsuccessful.

References

1. Fox V. Upper gastrointestinal bleeding. *Int Semin Pediatr Gastroenterol Nutr* 1999;8:1–9.
2. Cox K, Ament ME. Upper gastrointestinal bleeding in children and adolescents. *Pediatrics* 1979;63:408–413.
3. Murphy M. Lower gastrointestinal bleeding in infancy, childhood, and adolescence. *Int Semin Pediatr Gastroenterol Nutr* 1999;8:9–15.
4. Mezoff A, Preud'Homme D. How serious is that GI bleed? *Contemp Pediatr* 1994;11:60–92.
5. Drumm B, Rhoads JM, Stringer D, et al. Peptic ulcer disease in children: etiology, clinical findings and clinical course. *Pediatrics* 1988;92:410–414.
6. Cheung LY, Ashley SW. Gastric blood flow and mucosal defense mechanisms. *Clin Invest Med* 1987;10:201–208.
7. Venables CW. Mucus, pepsin, and peptic ulcer. *Gut* 1986;27:233–238.
8. Rosenthal P, Thompson J, Singh M. Detection of occult blood in gastric juice. *J Clin Gastroenterol* 1984;6:119–121.
9. Chaïbou M, Tucci M, Dugas MA, et al. Clinically significant upper gastrointestinal bleeding acquired in a pediatric intensive care unit: a prospective study. *Pediatrics* 1998;102:933–938.
10. Schnaffer J. Acute gastrointestinal bleeding. *Med Clin North Am* 1986;70:1055–1066.
11. Sherman NJ, Clatworthy HW. Gastrointestinal bleeding in neonates: a study of 94 cases. *Surgery* 1967;62:614–619.
12. Rahhal RM, Ramkumar DP, Pashankar D. Simultaneous herpetic and candidal esophagitis in an immunocompetent teenager. *J Pediatr Gastroenterol Nutr* 2005;40:371–373.
13. Yu PP, White D, Iannuccilli EA. The Mallory-Weiss syndrome in the pediatric population: rare condition in children should be considered in the presence of hematemesis. *R I Med* 1982;65:73–74.
14. Pohl JF, Melin-Aldana H, Rudolph C. Prolapse gastropathy in the pediatric patient. *J Pediatr Gastroenterol Nutr* 2000;30:458–460.
15. Bishop PR, Nowicki MJ, Parker PH. Vomiting-induced hematemesis in children: Mallory-Weiss tear or prolapse gastropathy? *J Pediatr Gastroenterol Nutr* 2000;30:436–441.
16. Gremse DA. Gastroesophageal reflux disease in children: an overview of pathophysiology, diagnosis, and treatment. *J Pediatr Gastroenterol Nutr* 2002;35:S297–S299.
17. Dohil R, Hassall E, Jevon G, et al. Gastritis and Gastropathy of Childhood. *J Pediatr Gastroenterol Nutr* 1999;29:378–394.
18. Gremse DA, Shakoor S. Symptoms of acid-peptic disease in children. *South Med J* 1993;86:997–1000.
19. Chong SK, Blackshaw AJ, Morson BC, et al. Prospective study of colitis in infancy and early childhood. *J Pediatr Gastroenterol Nutr* 1986;5:352–358.
20. Xanthakos SA, Schwimmer JB, Melin-Aldana H, et al. Prevalence and outcome of allergic colitis in healthy infants with rectal bleeding: a prospective cohort study. *J Pediatr Gastroenterol Nutr* 2005;41:16–22.
21. Halpin TC, Byrne WJ, Ament ME. Colitis, persistent diarrhea, and protein intolerance. *J Pediatr* 1977;91:404–407.
22. Klingman RM, Fanaroff AA. Necrotizing enterocolitis. *N Engl J Med* 1984;3340:1093–1103.
23. Bill AH, Chapman ND. The enterocolitis of Hirschsprung's disease—its natural history and treatment. *Am J Surg* 1962;103:70–74.
24. Gremse DA, Dean PC, Farquhar DS. Cefixime and antibiotic-associated colitis. *Pediatr Infect Dis J* 1994;13:331–333.
25. Tomomosa T, Has JY, Itoh K, et al. Endoscopic findings in pediatric patients with Henoch-Schönlein purpura and gastrointestinal symptoms. *J Pediatr Gastroenterol Nutr* 1987;6:725–729.
26. Marx G, Seidman EG. Inflammatory bowel disease in pediatric patients. *Curr Opin Gastroenterol* 1999;15:322–325.
27. Lieberman E. Hemolytic uremic syndrome. *J Pediatr* 1972;80:1–16.
28. Tedesco FJ, Goldstein PD, Gleason WA, et al. Upper gastrointestinal endoscopy in the pediatric patient. *Gastroenterology* 1976;70:492–494.
29. Afshani E, Berger PE. Gastrointestinal tract angiography in infants and children. *J Pediatr Gastroenterol Nutr* 5:173–186.
30. Alavi A, Ring EJ. Localization of gastrointestinal bleeding: superiority of 99mTc-sulfur colloid compared with angiography. *AJR* 1981;137:741–748.
31. Guilhon de Araujo Sant'anna AM, Dubois J, Miron MC, et al. Wireless capsule endoscopy for obscure small-bowel disorders: final results of the first pediatric controlled trial. *Clin Gastroenterol Hepatol* 2005;3:264–270.
32. Waterman NG, Walker JL. The effect of gastric cooling on hemostasis. *Surg Gynecol Obstet* 1973;137:80–82.
33. Menguy R, Masters YF. Influence of cold on stress ulceration and on gastric mucosal blood flow and energy metabolism. *Ann Surg* 1981;194:29–34.
34. Eroglu Y, Emerick KM, Whitingon PF, et al. Octreotide therapy for control of acute gastrointestinal bleeding in children. *J Pediatr Gastroenterol Nutr* 2004;38:41–47.
35. Yachha SK, Sharma BC, Kumar M, et al. Endoscopic sclerotherapy for esophageal varices in children with extrahepatic portal venous obstruction: a follow-up study. *J Pediatr Gastroenterol Nutr* 1997;24:49–52.
36. McKiernan PJ, Beath SV, Davison SM. A prospective study of endoscopic esophageal variceal ligation using a multiband ligator. *J Pediatr Gastroenterol Nutr* 2002;34:207–211.
37. Fox VL, Carr-Locke DL, Connors PJ, et al. Endoscopic ligation of esophageal varices in children. *J Pediatr Gastroenterol Nutr* 1995;20:202–208.
38. Stockwell JA, Werner HA, Marsano LS. Dieulafoy's lesion in an infant: a rare cause of massive gastrointestinal bleeding. *J Pediatr Gastroenterol Nutr* 2000;31:68–70.
39. Keljo DJ, Yakes WF, Andersen JM, et al. Recognition and treatment of venous malformations of the rectum. *J Pediatr Gastroenterol Nutr* 1996;23:442–446.
40. Wyllie R, Kay MH. Therapeutic intervention for non variceal gastrointestinal hemorrhage. *J Pediatr Gastroenterol Nutr* 1996;22:123–133.
41. Johanns W, Luis W, Janssen J, et al. Argon plasma coagulation (APC) in gastroenterology: experimental and clinical experiences. *Eur J Gastroenterol Hepatol* 1997;9:581–587.
42. Swain CP, Storey DW, Brown SG, et al. Nature of the bleeding vessel in recurrently bleeding gastric ulcers. *Gastroenterology* 1986;90:595–608.

CHAPTER 52 ■ CONSTIPATION AND ENCOPRESIS

TERESA R. CARROLL

Constipation is both a symptom and a diagnosis universally defined as an abnormal defecation pattern including hard, difficult-to-pass, painful, and infrequent bowel movements. This is a common functional problem in childhood affecting more than 60% of healthy children. Boys outnumber girls fo310ur to one.

In childhood, the normal expected defecation pattern can vary by age. During the newborn period, diet plays an important role in what would be accepted as a normal bowel pattern. Breastfed infants vary greatly, with a normal range of a bowel movement after every feeding to once every 7 to 10 days. Infants who are formula fed can average 1 to 4 stools per day. Toddlers and school-aged children can have defecation patterns that range from 3 times per week up to 3 times per day.

The key to these widely varied bowel patterns being normal is that there are no complications. Common complications include painful defecation, bleeding from traumatic defecation, early satiety and anorexia, abdominal pain, and encopresis. Encopresis is the overflow soiling of stool around a fecal impaction in the rectum. Of all these complications, encopresis can be the most problematic for the child due to the social consequences of incontinence.

Constipation and its complications can account for approximately 3% of outpatient visits to the pediatrician and as many as 25% of visits to the pediatric gastroenterologist. Even though there are organic causes of constipation, most of the cases of constipation in infants and children are functional, and most of these are the result of function fecal retention. The pediatric hospitalist needs to be able to differentiate between organic disease and functional constipation, perform the evaluation of functional constipation and encopresis, and be familiar with the treatment in both the inpatient and outpatient settings.

ORGANIC VERSUS FUNCTIONAL

Most cases of constipation during childhood are not based on organic disease. Table 52.1 lists the more common organic causes of constipation. The most important information needed to differentiate between organic and functional constipation is the patient's history. Having a detailed comprehensive history will alert the provider to red flags warranting further evaluation for an organic cause. Defecation patterns need to be assessed starting at birth with passage of meconium stools. Normal passage is in the first 24 hours of life, and the possibility of organic disease increases with a history of delayed meconium passage beyond 48 hours of age. The onset of defecation difficulties may be recalled by the parents as occurring since birth, indicating that a normal bowel pattern was never established. Bowel movement frequency should be assessed in relationship to the

infant's diet or the child's age. Stool size and consistency is also important to discuss, as small-caliber, ribbon-like or mucoid stools may indicate organic disease. Poor response to stool softeners or laxatives may also be part of the history. Symptoms of vomiting, feeding difficulties, and poor growth can be part of the history for both organic and functional constipation. Painful defecation, bleeding during stool passage, and retentive behaviors (e.g., stiffening up, grunting, rocking back and forth, applying pressure to the perineum) are more indicative of functional constipation.

Functional constipation in infants most often starts during a time of dietary change, such as weaning from breast milk, adding solid foods, and transitioning off formula. Another common time of onset associated with diet is when children transition from being passive feeders to self-feeding, thus potentially decreasing their intake of vegetables and fruits.

Toddlers can develop constipation from withholding behaviors during toilet training. Another common age of onset associated with withholding behaviors is with the school-aged child, around 6 to 7 years of age. In toilet-trained children this can be difficult information to obtain, as the parents generally cannot monitor this closely once the child is independently using the bathroom. Stool consistency is most often hard with associated discomfort during defecation. Size is also important, as withholding behaviors result in rectal stretching and the passage of large-caliber stools that may obstruct a commode.

EVALUATION

A thorough physical examination should follow a detailed history. The first assessment should be of the infant's or child's growth pattern. Growth can be affected in both functional constipation and organic disease, but in functional constipation it is often episodic, whereas with organic disease failure to thrive is chronic. This is due to the chronic obstructive nature of the underlying organic disease that results in discomfort and limited oral intake. The abdominal assessment, looking at contour of the abdomen and palpation of masses or excessive stool levels, should be carefully performed. Checking anal position on infants should be included, using the anogenital index, which can be estimated as follows: in boys, the position of the anal opening should measure about halfway between the base of the scrotum and the tip of the sacrum, and in girls the position of the anal opening should measure about one-third the distance between the base of the vaginal fourchette and the tip of the sacrum. The anal opening should be inspected because fissures or lesions may contribute to discomfort and withholding behaviors. A rectal exam, although unpleasant, needs to be completed. In patients with a history of encopresis it is important to assess for fecal impaction. The presence or absence of stool and

TABLE 52.1

ORGANIC DISEASE RELATED TO CONSTIPATION

- Anal stenosis
- Anterior ectopic anus
- Intestinal pseudo-obstruction
- Congenital aganglionosis (Hirschsprung disease)
- Segmental dilatation of the colon
- Atonic dilated colon
- Hypothyroidism
- Lesions of the lower spinal cord

the caliber of the rectum is also important in differentiating between organic and functional constipation. For example, in a child with retentive functional constipation, the rectum can be dilated with packed or scybalous stool. Conversely, in the child with Hirschsprung disease, stool retention is proximal to the aganglionic segment, and the rectum may be empty and narrow.

Red flags in the history or abnormal exam findings may warrant further diagnostic evaluations. A barium enema will assess the anatomy of the colon when a structural abnormality is suspected, as with Hirschsprung disease or anorectal malformation. This should be completed unprepped so that the transition zone may be visualized. Abnormal colonic stool volume is not always noted on exam, and a plain abdominal x-ray can be of assistance. A lateral view should be ordered if spinal abnormalities are suspected.

Anorectal manometry is also available to further assess both organic and functional disorders. Water-perfused catheters with balloon inflation are used to assess the rectal sensation threshold, which increases in the presence of functional fecal retention. This is due to chronic stretching of the rectum with impacted stool resulting in an increase in rectal compliance. Neuromuscular function is also assessed with balloon inflation. In healthy patients, the rectoanal inhibitory reflex (the reflex relaxation of the involuntary internal anal sphincter) can be seen as the internal sphincter pressure drops in response to the balloon inflation and rectal distension. This is absent in patients with Hirschsprung disease. Electromyography tracing is useful in assessing pelvic floor function. Pelvic floor dyssynergia is a common finding in children with functional constipation. The child may paradoxically squeeze the external sphincter and voluntary pelvic floor muscles tighter while attempting to bear down (Valsalva). This abnormality may be amenable to biofeedback therapy, allowing the child to learn to relax the voluntary muscles of defecation while attempting to evacuate.

TREATMENT

Chronic constipation is treated in three phases. The first phase is the most important to the future success of the treatment. This is the cleanout phase, which involves aggressive bowel cleansing at home or in the hospital setting. The second phase is long-term maintenance with daily stool softeners, behavior modification, and dietary changes. The final phase includes weaning of medications and focusing on management with diet and a bathroom schedule.

Outpatient

Cleanout Phase

For most patients, the bowel cleanout phase can be completed comfortably at home. If the child is impacted, the first goal is disimpaction. This can be done with daily phosphate enemas.

Some children respond better to mineral oil enemas because they provide extra lubrication. Milk-and-molasses enemas can be made at home by combining equal parts of both products and administering once a day with a commercially available enema kit. However, all of these techniques carry some reported risk of fluid shifts and acute dehydration. Parents need to be cautioned about this, especially if use is expected to be prolonged.

Once disimpaction is achieved, the bowel cleanout can start. One of the most common and effective products used is oral magnesium citrate, with a dose of 1 ounce per year of age up to 10 ounces per day, given once a day for at least 3 consecutive days. The product can be mixed with juice and ice to make it more palatable for the child. Family education should be provided about the product in that it needs to be given over less than 2 hours, and possible side effects can include vomiting, abdominal pain, weakness, and blurry vision.

Additional cleanout options for home treatment are available. Toddlers can be placed on mineral oil 15 mL per year of age per dose, 3 to 4 doses per day for 3 to 4 days. Oral phosphosoda is helpful in children resistant to the magnesium citrate. Recommendations are 1 to 3 ounces mixed in a minimum of 6 to 8 ounces of any beverage once a day for 3 consecutive days. Fluid intake needs to be increased significantly if this agent is used. Polyethylene glycol (PEG 3350) solutions can also be used. Commercially available bowel prep kits containing this product can be given once a day for 3 days. PEG 3350 oral is also available in powder form, and this can be given 17 g in 8 oz of any beverage 3 to 4 times per day for 3 to 4 consecutive days. A nightly stimulant, such as senna or bisacodyl, can be given in conjunction with the PEG treatments. Side effects of stimulant use include abdominal cramps. Long-term use of stimulants can lead to tachyphylaxis, melanosis coli, and colonic inertia.

An abdominal x-ray can be ordered after the disimpaction and cleanout process is completed to ensure proper evacuation. This cleanout process can be repeated on a weekly basis as long as the child is making progress and is not having any complications. If no progress is made after several attempts at home, or if the child is having complications from the treatment, then inpatient treatment is recommended.

Maintenance Phase

Once cleanout is achieved, long-term maintenance is started. This phase includes the use of a daily stool softener for several months. Treatment options are based on the child's history and age. For children less than 1 year of age, osmotic agents such as lactulose or PEG 3350 can be used safely. Toddlers over 1 year of age who are still in diapers and do not have neurologic impairment often benefit from daily doses of mineral oil. This can be easily mixed into age-appropriate foods such as yogurt, pudding, pureed or creamed foods, and pastas. For older children who are out of diapers, treatment with PEG 3350 is preferred. The volume of mineral oil necessary may be prohibitive or messy, with oil leakage into undergarments; and higher doses of osmotic agents can cause excess gas and discomfort. Dosage recommendations are listed in Table 52.2.

If the child is unable to make appropriate progress during the maintenance phase and compliance with the prescribed regimen is good, testing for neuromuscular dysfunction is

TABLE 52.2

DRUG AND DOSAGE OF DAILY STOOL SOFTENERS

Lactulose	1 mL/kg/dose 1 or 2 times per day
Mineral oil	15 mL/year of age 1 or 2 times per day
PEG 3350	0.74–1.0 g/kg/dose 1 to 3 times per day

TABLE 52.3

HIGH-RISK POPULATIONS FOR CHRONIC
CONSTIPATION

- History of ADD, ADHD
- Autism
- Neurologic deficits, CP
- Developmental delays
- Obesity
- Frequent surgeries (opiate pain medications)

CP, cerebral palsy; ADD, attention deficit disorder; ADHD, attention
deficit hyperactivity disorder.

TABLE 52.4

SAMPLE ORDERS FOR PEG BOWEL CLEANOUT

- Admit to pediatric floor for NG bowel cleanout.
- KUB now and repeat in 24 hr.
- Place #10-14F NG tube with topical lidocaine (if not
  allergic).
- Start PEG solution via NG tube at 5 mL/kg/hr; if tolerated,
  after 4 hr increase rate to a maximum of 240 mL/hr until 3
  to 4 L are infused and rectal effluent is clear.
- If patient vomits, stop infusion and restart in 30 min after
  careful reassessment.
- If patient is impacted, start soapsuds enemas every 4 hr
  until clear.
- Clear liquid diet during NG bowel cleanout.
- IVF of D5 $\frac{1}{2}$ NS with 20 mEq KCl/L at fluid maintenance
  rate (unless cardiac, pulmonary, or renal status precludes
  this).
- Reglan 0.2 mg/kg/dose IV every 8 hr during bowel
  cleanout.
- Benadryl 1–2 mg/kg/dose IV every 8 hr during bowel
  cleanout.
- Call MD for abnormal vitals signs or persistent vomiting.

IV, intravenous; IVF, intravenous fluid; KUB, x-ray designed to look at
Kidneys Ureters and Bladder. NG, nasogastric; NS, . . . ; PEG, polyethylene glycol.

warranted. This is accomplished through anorectal manometry testing. Children with chronic fecal retention often have
elevated resting sphincter pressures and an elevated conscious
rectal threshold. In some cases, pelvic floor dyssynergia is
noted, which may be treated with biofeedback therapy.

Weaning Phase

Once the child has completed several months of stable maintenance treatment, the final phase can begin. This must start
with a risk assessment, which includes the child's medical
history, psychosocial status, behavioral changes, and dietary
changes. Table 52.3 provides a list of risk factors that warrant continued chronic treatment without a weaning phase
due to a high rate of relapse.

Inpatient

When outpatient treatments fail, children can be admitted for
a more aggressive approach. If disimpaction was unsuccessful
at home, the child can be seen in an acute care facility for
hypertonic enemas. If this is successful, the child can be sent
home for continued oral cleanout treatments.

Some children fail both disimpaction and oral cleanout
attempts at home, and continue to experience complications
such as abdominal pain and encopresis. For these children,
admission to a pediatric hospital should be arranged for both
disimpaction and a bowel cleanout. Disimpaction may be
achieved with hypertonic (e.g., soapsuds) enemas. The bowel
cleanout is completed by placing a nasogastric tube and infusing a commercial PEG solution. Table 52.4 lists orders that
can be used for a PEG cleanout.

Although rare, some children fail treatment because the
impacted stool is too large to pass without significant
trauma. These children can be manually disimpacted under
sedation.

FOLLOW-UP AND PATIENT EDUCATION

Successful long-term treatment depends on the caregiver's
understanding of the problem including the need for continued follow-up with the pediatrician or GI specialist. In the
outpatient clinic, the family's education should be completed
in steps that follow the three phases of treatment.

Education at presentation should start with the basic function of the colon and pathophysiology of functional constipation. If encopresis is also present, a simple diagram of how
overflow soiling occurs is often helpful. An overview of the
three-phase treatment at this time also helps the family under-

stand the chronic nature of the problem, and it stresses the
importance of close follow-up. The cleanout phase is then
reviewed for outpatient or inpatient protocol.

During the maintenance phase, the frequency of follow-up
visits planned for each patient is based upon the patient's history, progress, and social environment. At each visit, the family is reminded of the three phases of treatment, and assessment is made as to how the child is currently progressing.
Each visit should also review the importance of bowel retrain-
ing with frequent toilet sitting or the dietary changes needed
to increase daily fiber intake. The clinician should provide the
family with a list of age-appropriate foods that are high in
fiber, and reinforce the importance of daily treatment with
prescribed medications.

When the child is ready to start the last phase of treatment
including laxative weaning, assessment of the family's understanding of the problem is critical. The clinician should review
the phases that were completed and the behavioral changes that
have occurred. Weaning instructions should be written clearly
in a stepwise approach. A short list of complications should be
included for the family to monitor. The importance of continued follow-up as a means to prevent relapse or complications
should be discussed. It should be stressed that there is a high
rate of relapse of functional constipation due to the permanent
increase in rectal compliance, which does not change even after
many months of normalizing stool frequency.

Suggested Readings

Hay WW Jr., Hayward AR, Levin MJ, et al. *Current pediatric diagnosis and
treatment.* 15th ed New York: McGraw-Hill; 2001:561–562.
North American Society for Pediatric Gastroenterology and Nutrition. Consti-
pation in infants and children: evaluation and treatment. A medical position
statement of the North American Society for Pediatric Gastroenterology and
Nutrition. Available at www.NASPGN.com.
Taketomo CK, Hodding JH, Kraus DM. *Pediatric dosage handbook.* 8th ed.
Hudson, New York: Lexi-Comp; 2001.
Walker WA, Durie PR, Hamilton JR, et al. *Pediatric gastrointestinal disease.* Vol 1.
Philadelphia: Decker; 1991:90–108, 818–827.

CHAPTER 53 ■ GASTROESOPHAGEAL REFLUX DISEASE

CHRISTOPHER RHEE

Gastroesophageal reflux (GER) is one of the most common gastrointestinal problems encountered in children. GER is defined as retrograde passage of gastric contents into the esophagus. Gastroesophageal reflux disease (GERD) refers to reflux that produces symptoms or complications that can produce a wide variety of symptoms that vary in severity from physiologic regurgitation to a life-threatening disorder.

PATHOPHYSIOLOGY

The pathophysiology of GERD requires noxious substances (such as acid, digestive enzymes, and bile acids) in refluxed gastric contents to come in contact with the esophagus, resulting in damage to the epithelium. Although GERD is usually a multifactorial disorder, one of the primary mechanisms of GERD in infants and children is believed to involve increased reflux episodes due to transient relaxations of the lower esophageal sphincter (LES), which is the principal barrier to reflux. Transient LES relaxations (TLESRs) are abrupt decreases in sphincter pressure unrelated to swallowing and usually of a longer duration than the typical relaxations triggered by the normal esophageal peristaltic mechanism. Other causes of increased reflux episodes include pathology such as a hiatal hernia or gastric factors such as decreased gastric compliance, large meals, delayed gastric emptying, and increased intra-abdominal pressure. Additional mechanisms that may contribute to GERD include poor esophageal clearance of the refluxate, a defective esophageal mucosal barrier, and increased noxiousness of the refluxate.

CLINICAL MANIFESTATIONS

GER can be a normal physiologic process in healthy children and adults. It is common, particularly during the first year of life, with recurrent vomiting occurring in 50% of infants in the first 3 months of life and with a peak prevalence of approximately 67% by 4 months of age. A small minority of infants and children go on to develop problems suggestive of GERD. GER, in addition to pathologic infant reflux, typically resolves in the majority of infants by 1 to 2 years of age. Reflux disease tends to persist in older children and adults, 50% of whom have a chronic, relapsing course.

Although the classic symptoms of heartburn and regurgitation are the most common complaints in adolescents and adults, the presentation in younger children and infants may be more variable (Table 53.1). In infants with GERD, symptoms can include dysphagia (difficulty swallowing), odynophagia (painful swallowing), anorexia, irritability, arching of the back during feedings, hematemesis, and failure to thrive.

GERD can cause apparent life-threatening events (ALTEs) in infants, and is associated with chronic respiratory disorders such as reactive airway disease, recurrent stridor, chronic cough, and recurrent pneumonia. In children, complications associated with GERD include recurrent vomiting, regurgitation, hematemesis, dysphagia, and odynophagia, as well as respiratory symptoms such as reactive airway disease, stridor, hoarseness, and chronic cough. Older children and adolescents are more likely to exhibit the same symptoms seen in adults with GERD, such as chronic heartburn and regurgitation. Although rare, esophageal pain causing stereotypical, repetitive arching and stretching movements can be mistaken for atypical seizures or dystonia (Sandifer syndrome).

Erosive esophagitis is a potential complication seen with GERD and can present not only as pain, but also with chronic blood loss associated with anemia, hematemesis, hypoproteinemia, or melena. If the inflammation is left untreated, chronic esophagitis can ultimately result in an esophageal stricture, or Barrett esophagus, which is the replacement of the normal stratified squamous epithelium of the esophageal mucosa with metaplastic columnar epithelium that is potentially malignant.

GERD is commonly seen in neurologically impaired children, with approximately one-third of children with severe psychomotor retardation estimated to have significant GERD as a result of diffuse gastrointestinal dysmotility. Although recurrent aspiration pneumonia from GER is uncommon in most children, patients in this group are particularly at risk due to increased risk of GERD, impaired protective reflexes of the airway, and discoordinated swallow reflexes.

DIAGNOSTIC APPROACH AND TESTING

In most cases of infants with vomiting and in older children with regurgitation and heartburn, a history and physical examination are sufficient to make a reliable diagnosis of GER or to recognize complications or warning signs suggestive of GERD. For infants, it is especially important to obtain a good feeding history in order to identify the possiblity of overfeeding, formula intolerance, and signs or symptoms suggestive of complications from GER.

Because the symptoms of GERD in children vary, the differential diagnosis is broad and can include an anatomic, metabolic, infectious, neurologic, cardiac, or respiratory etiology (Table 53.2). During the history and physical examination of an infant with recurrent vomiting, a number of warning signals can suggest a diagnosis other than GER and perhaps a more serious condition. These signs include bilious

TABLE 53.1

COMPLICATIONS OF GASTROESOPHAGEAL DISEASE

SYMPTOMS

Recurrent vomiting
Failure to thrive
Irritability in infants
Regurgitation
Heartburn or chest pain
Hematemesis
Dysphagia or feeding refusal
Apnea or apparent life-threatening event (ALTE)
Wheezing or stridor
Hoarseness
Persistent cough
Posturing (Sandifer syndrome)

FINDINGS

Esophagitis
Esophageal stricture
Barrett esophagus
Laryngitis
Hypoproteinemia
Anemia

Adapted from Rudolph CD, Mazur LJ, Liptak GS, et al. Guidelines for evaluation and treatment of gastroesophageal reflux in infants and children. *J Pediatr Gastroenterol Nutr* 2001;32(suppl 2):S1–S31.

vomiting, bulging fontanelle, macrocephaly/microcephaly, abdominal tenderness, severe abdominal distention, FTT, hepatosplenomegaly, seizures, and lethargy.

Although several tests are available for evaluating the child with suspected GERD, the diagnostic approach depends on the presenting signs or symptoms of the individual patient. In most cases of uncomplicated GER in infants, diagnostic tests are not needed.

The *24-hour esophageal pH monitoring (pH probe study)* is the most sensitive test for diagnosis of GER. The test is performed by placing a catheter with a microelectrode that measures pH in the distal esophageal lumen for a duration of 24 hours. An episode of acid reflux usually is defined as an esophageal pH <4, for a duration greater than 15 to 20 seconds. Interpretation of the pH probe study generally includes the total number of reflux episodes, the average duration of episodes, and the percentage of the total time for the entire study that the esophageal pH is <4, which is called the *reflux index* (RI). Because the RI is determined by the frequency and duration of the episodes of acid reflux, the reflux index indicates the cumulative amount of acid exposure in the esophagus and is therefore considered the most valid measure of GER. Because asymptomatic reflux episodes can occur in infants and adults in varying degrees as a normal physiologic process, age-dependent normal values for esophageal acid exposure have been established. Based on several studies, it is recommended that the upper limit of normal of the RI can be defined as up to 12% during the first year of life and up to 6% thereafter. The pH probe study also takes into account other parameters that can reflect problems with esophageal clearance

TABLE 53.2

DIFFERENTIAL DIAGNOSIS OF GERD SYMPTOMS

Vomiting

Gastrointestinal obstruction	Pyloric stenosis, malrotation, antral/duodenal web, foreign body
Gastrointestinal disorders	Achalasia, hiatal hernia, gastroparesis, peptic ulcer disease, food allergy, gastroenteritis, pancreatitis, gallstones, eosinophilic esophagitis
Neurologic	Hydrocephalus, intracranial mass or hemorrhage
Infectious	Meningitis, urinary tract infection, otitis media, sinusitis, hepatitis
Metabolic	Galactosemia, hereditary fructose intolerance, urea cycle defects, amino and organic acidemias, congenital adrenal hyperplasia
Renal	Obstructive uropathy, renal insufficiency
Toxic	Lead, iron, vitamin A or D, medications (ipecac, digoxin, theophylline, etc.)

Epigastric pain

Gastrointestinal	Peptic ulcer disease, inflammatory bowel disease
Musculoskeletal	Costochondritis
Infectious	Candida or herpetic esophagitis

Respiratory symptoms

Reactive airway disease/asthma, pneumonia, bronchiolitis, foreign body, laryngomalacia, tracheoesophageal fistula, vascular ring, cardiac disease

Neurologic symptoms

Seizures, movement disorders, metabolic disorders

of the refluxate. Such parameters include the number of reflux episodes greater than 5 minutes, the duration of the longest episode, and the mean duration of reflux during sleep.

Aside from quantifying the presence of an abnormal amount of reflux, esophageal pH monitoring can also be helpful in assessing whether a temporal relationship exists between symptoms and actual episodes of acid reflux. Furthermore, in patients who do not appear to be responding to acid-suppression therapy, a pH probe study performed while on treatment may be useful in determining whether the therapy is effectively blocking acid production.

A pH probe study should be used only in selected clinical situations. It most likely is not needed in infants with simple regurgitation, patients with classic symptoms of GERD in whom the diagnosis is not in doubt, or those already documented with reflux esophagitis by endoscopy. There are limitations to pH monitoring studies. Episodes of reflux that are too brief to register on the recorder may still cause respiratory complications such as ALTE, cough, or aspiration pneumonia. Conversely, some studies have shown significant reflux and apnea can also coexist without being related. Therefore, evaluation of infants with apnea or an ALTE remains controversial.

Esophageal pH monitoring may be useful if the apnea occurs frequently enough that it is likely to be detected during the study. In these situations, esophageal pH monitoring with polysomnography, which is the simultaneous monitoring of respiratory function through chest wall movement, nasal air flow, oxygen saturation of the blood, and heart rate, can be of added value in documenting the true association of reflux episodes with the apneic events. Another major drawback to the pH probe study is that it does not detect non-acid reflux episodes. This can be a diagnostic problem, especially in infants who often have inadequate acid production in addition to the buffering effects of the formula. Therefore, acidification of the formula or administration of acidic liquids, such as apple juice, is routinely used during the pH probe study for infants. With recent advances, multiple intraluminal impendance monitoring along with simultaneous pH monitoring has allowed the capablility of detecting both non-acid and acidic reflux. Impedance is the resistance to the flow of current between two points, which is lower between electrodes immersed in liquid. Using this principle, a catheter with several pairs of electrodes becomes capable of measuring impedance continuously at multiple sites along the length of the esophagus. A sudden decrease in impedance suggests that liquid (or refluxate) surrounds the electrode pair. By observing the movement of impedance changes up or down a linear array of several pairs of electrodes, one can determine the direction of fluid flow and differentiate a swallow from a retrograde reflux event irrespective of the acidity. A conventional pH electrode remains at the distal tip of the impedance catheter, allowing the clinician to see whether the fluid moving up or down the esophagus is acid or non-acid. Current limitations include time-consuming interpretation, and normal values in pediatric age groups which have yet to be defined.

The *upper gastrointestinal (UGI) series* is most useful in children with recurrent vomiting for detecting anatomic abnormalities (congenital or acquired) such as pyloric stenosis, malrotation, web, or hiatal hernia. It can also be helpful in detecting complications of GERD such as an esophageal stricture. However, it is insensitive for detecting erosions or superficial mucosal changes. Furthermore, the UGI series is neither sensitive nor specific for the diagnosis of GER. The brief duration of the study not only results in frequent false-negative results, but the frequent occurrence of physiologic or non-pathologic reflux results in false-positive tests. Evaluation starting with at least an upper GI study is warranted in those infants with a delayed presentation of persistent vomiting after 6 months age or in children who continue to have significant GER beyond 18 to 24 months of age.

Endoscopy with biopsy allows direct visualization and biopsy of the esophageal mucosa in order to assess the presence and severity of reflux esophagitis as well as to exclude other etiologies such as eosinophilic or infectious esophagitis. Upper endoscopy also may identify a hiatal hernia or web, in addition to other complications of GERD including esophageal strictures or Barrett esophagus.

Gastric scintigraphy can sometimes be used to demonstrate gastroesophageal reflux, aspiration, and possibly delayed gastric emptying, which may be an exacerbating factor in children with GERD. The technique involves feeding the patient a technetium-99m sulfur colloid-labeled meal and scanning postprandial images up to 24 hours after administering the feeding. Unlike esophageal pH monitoring, scintigraphy can demonstrate non-acid reflux. However, a lack of standardized techniques and absence of age-specific normative data limit the value of this test. Because aspiration episodes with GER can occur intermittently, a negative test result does not definitively exclude the diagnosis.

In children with concerns of aspiration, additional studies that may be helpful are barium swallow studies to look for actual aspiration with swallowing and a bronchoscopy with bronchoalveolar lavage for lipid-laden macrophages. A large lipid content in alveolar macrophages is a marker for chronic aspiration. However, this finding does not differentiate between aspiration associated with GER from aspiration that may occur upon swallowing. Routine performance of *esophageal manometry* is not helpful in diagnosis and management of pediatric GERD.

MANAGEMENT

Conservative Measures

Treatment options vary from conservative measures such as lifestyle modifications to pharmacologic or surgical therapies. Initial treatment options for infants with GERD can include alterations in formula volume and composition in addition to sleep positioning. For those infants with symptoms of GERD, the possibility of overfeeding should be initially addressed. Alterations to the feeding schedule by administering smaller volumes at more frequent feedings can be used to minimize gastric distention and the risk of GER. Thickening of the formula can also help reduce GER. Although a formula with added rice starch is commercially available, rice cereal can also be manually added to thicken a formula by using 1 to 3 teaspoons per ounce of formula. There is also evidence to support the trial use of a hypoallergenic formula for the subset of infants who may respond if they have vomiting due to cow's milk protein allergy. In older children, dietary modification includes avoidance of caffeine, chocolate, and spicy or acidic foods that may provoke symptoms. Other lifestyle changes include avoidance of alcohol, cessation of smoking, and weight loss in obese patients.

In hospitalized patients who are more acutely or chronically ill, other options to reduce reflux episodes include changing the formula to a higher caloric concentration so that a lower volume of feedings may be required. The administration of the feedings through a nasogastric tube or gastrostomy tube more slowly or even continuously may be necessary to minimize GER. For patients with persistent vomiting or significantly delayed gastric emptying, bypassing the stomach and administering transpyloric tube feedings may be an alternative as well.

Although it has been demonstrated during pH monitoring that infants have less GER with prone positioning, it is generally not recommended due to the fact that its potential benefits are outweighed by the increased risk of sudden infant death syndrome (SIDS). General reflux precautions include keeping an infant upright for 20 to 30 minutes after meals, elevation of the head of the bed while supine, or left side positioning.

Pharmacotherapy

Pharmacologic treatment of GERD primarily consists of acid suppression and prokinetic agents. Prokinetic agents are used to improve esophageal clearance and gastric emptying as well as raising the LES tonic pressure. Acid-suppression therapy is used to reduce the exposure of the esophagus or respiratory tract to acidic refluxate, thereby alleviating symptoms as well as promoting mucosal healing. At times, therapy is complemented with the use of surface agents such as sucralfate, which adheres to the mucosal lining and further protects it, making it particularly useful in children with erosive esophagitis.

Metoclopramide, a dopamine antagonist, is one of the more commonly used prokinetic agents in the treatment of GERD due to the fact it increases LES pressure and enhances esophageal peristalsis and gastric emptying. Unfortunately, the use of this medication can be limited due to its frequent incidence of adverse central nervous system (CNS) effects. Other alternative medications include erythromycin and bethanecol. Erythromycin, which is a motilin receptor agonist, increases LES pressure and accelerates gastric emptying at smaller doses than those required for antimicrobial purposes. Bethanechol is a cholinergic agonist, directly stimulating smooth muscle and enhancing contractions throughout the gastrointestinal tract, improving esophageal clearance, and increasing LES pressure. It has had mixed clinical results and its use is frequently limited by the occurrence of side effects due to its cholinergic activity. Despite the physiologic effects of these prokinetic agents, results from several studies looking at the clinical efficacy of these medications, including metoclopramide, have shown to be equivocal or inconsistent. The only prokinetic medication proven to reduce esophageal acid exposure in children was cisapride, a mixed serotonergic agonist. However, due to concerns about the potential for cardiac arrhythmias in patients while taking this medication, it is no longer available in the United States.

Acid suppression therapy can reduce symptoms caused by acid-induced esophagitis and promote mucosal healing. Histamine-2 receptor antagonists (H$_2$ RAs) and proton-pump inhibitors (PPIs) suppress stomach acid secretion through different mechanisms on the parietal cell. H$_2$ RAs have traditionally been used as first-line therapy in blocking acid secretion. Because PPIs directly inhibit the proton pump, they are more effective in suppressing acid production and are therefore used in patients who are refractory to treatment with H$_2$ RAs. Although data are limited in infants and children, omeprazole and lansoprazole have been studied the most extensively in case series and have proven to be effective in the treatment of reflux esophagitis. Therefore, these two medications are currently the only PPIs with an approved label for use in children. For lansoprazole, the recommended dosage in children 1 to 11 years of age is 15 mg once a day for children weighing less than or equal to 30 kg, and 30 mg a day for those patients weighing more than 30 kg. The dosage recommendation for omeprazole is 1 mg/kg/day once a day or divided twice a day for children 2 to 16 years of age, with a maximum dose of 20 mg once a day.

Surgical Therapy

In cases where symptoms of GERD are refractory to pharmacotherapy or considered life-threatening, surgical therapy can be considered. The Nissen fundoplication, which involves wrapping the gastric fundus around the distal esophagus, is the most popular of the many surgical procedures that have been used. A gastric scintigraphy study performed before fundoplication can be helpful in identifying children, particularly those with neurologic impairment, who would benefit from a concomitant procedure to facilitate gastric emptying. The majority of pediatric series have demonstrated a reduction or the complete relief of symptoms in greater than 90% of children following antireflux surgery. Common complications of fundoplication surgery include breakdown of the wrap, dumping syndrome, gas bloat syndrome, small bowel obstruction from adhesions, and esophageal obstruction. Experience with laparoscopic fundoplication in children have shown that the results and complication rates of this procedure are similar to those with the more traditional open laparotomy approach.

COURSE AND PROGNOSIS

Most cases of GER in infants present as regurgitation or vomiting and resolve by 1 to 2 years of age without requiring extensive diagnostic evaluation or pharmacotherapy. However, the presenting symptoms can vary. In patients with suspected complications or severe symptoms, appropriate diagnostic testing should be performed to help determine the best treatment. Acid suppression therapy and the use of a prokinetic agent are the main pharmacologic treatment options. Surgery should be considered only when maximal medical management has failed.

Suggested Readings

Orenstein SR. Gastroesophageal reflux. In: Wyllie R, Hyams JS, eds. *Pediatric gastrointestinal disease*. 2nd ed. Philadelphia: Saunders; 1999:164–187.

Rudolph CD, Mazur LJ, Liptak GS, et al. Guidelines for evaluation and treatment of gastroesophageal reflux in infants and children: recommendations of the North American Society for Pediatric Gastroenterology and Nutrition. *J Pediatr Gastroenterol Nutr* 2001;32(suppl 2):S1–S31.

Suwandhi E, Ton MN, Schwarz SM. Gastroesophageal reflux in infancy and childhood. *Pediatr Ann* 2006;35:259–266.

CHAPTER 54 ■ INFLAMMATORY BOWEL DISEASE

HOWARD I. BARON

Inflammatory bowel disease (IBD) is a fairly common problem in children who may be seen by a pediatric hospitalist. It is characterized by chronic inflammation of various portions of the gastro-intestinal (GI) tract, leading to symptoms such as abdominal pain, diarrhea, growth failure, and GI bleeding. However, it commonly includes extraintestinal manifestations such as arthropathy, dermatologic conditions, ophthalmologic findings, and various signs of malnutrition.

The etiology of IBD is thought to be multifactorial. Recent discovery of specific gene loci linked to patients with these disorders has renewed enthusiasm for a genetic basis of these disorders. However, it is recognized that the genetics of IBD are not simply Mendelian in pattern, but likely derive from a host of gene loci on multiple chromosomes, thus allowing for additional factors such as environment (including infections) and immune dysregulation to play roles in the etiopathogenesis.

IBD is generally divided into two distinct clinical entities: Crohn disease (CD) and ulcerative colitis (UC). Although there are often histopathologic differences between the two, they are differentiated mostly by their location within the GI tract. CD traditionally appears anywhere within the GI tract, from mouth to perianal disease, while UC is by definition limited to the colon. Over 40% of newly diagnosed children with CD will have terminal ileal involvement, with colonic disease being a close second, often in combination with ileal inflammation. Ten to twenty-five percent of children will present with some perianal finding, such as fissures, fistulae, or skin tags. Less classic presentations occur with proximal GI disease, and patients may at first be suspected as having acid-peptic disorders such as gastroesophageal reflux disease, gastritis, or ulcers of the stomach or duodenum. Some children with CD have only extraintestinal manifestations upon presentation, such as growth failure, iritis, arthritis, aphthous stomatitis, or delayed onset of puberty. Children and adolescents with UC tend to have a more protean presentation, with rectal bleeding, diarrhea, and crampy abdominal pain.

PRESENTING FEATURES

Because the common presenting symptoms of IBD are individually nonspecific, it commonly takes a median of 14 months for a child with IBD to attain a correct diagnosis, and during that time, severe manifestations of malnutrition can occur. It also makes the differential diagnosis of IBD quite broad (Table 54.1).

Presenting symptoms of IBD typically include diarrhea, abdominal pain, weight loss, and bleeding (usually rectal). However, less common presentations can occur; for example, up to 10% of children and adolescents with new-onset IBD will complain of constipation. Hospital presentation may appear as an acute gastrointestinal illness, but on further questioning, there is usually a prolonged history of symptoms, including abdominal pain complaints, alteration in bowel habits, fatigue, weakness, pallor, and frequent absence from school or activities. Occasionally, a more fulminant presentation can occur, with severe, rapid onset of focal abdominal pain mimicking appendicitis or other acute abdominal crisis, and a small percentage of patients with IBD are first diagnosed intraoperatively by a surgeon, who may find a thickened, narrowed loop of small intestine, serosal changes such as creeping fat, or overt perforation of transmural CD with abscess formation or a fistula linking a loop of inflamed bowel to another adjacent structure. Obstructive symptoms, such as bilious vomiting, may signal intraluminal disease that has caused complete blockage of the small bowel, requiring immediate surgical attention. As such, it is important when evaluating a child with possible IBD to differentiate the acutely ill from the chronically ill, allowing rapid assessment when needed, and allaying further anxiety when not needed.

HISTORICAL CLUES

In taking a history of a patient with potential IBD, there are several clues to uncover. The following is a list of questions that may help the clinician include or discard IBD as a possibility:

How long have the symptoms been present?
Is there diarrhea, urgency (tenesmus), night-time wakening to defecate, or visible blood or mucus in the stool?
Is there abdominal pain? If so, where?
Is the pain associated with meals?
Has there been weight loss, or a plateau in linear growth?
Has there been appropriate pubertal maturation (e.g., consistent with when the parents had onset of menarche or pubertal changes)?
Are there episodes of nausea, vomiting, regurgitation?
Are there mouth ulcers, joint pains or swelling, skin rash, fevers?
Any known exposures to others with similar illness?
Have there been any new medications associated with the onset of the symptoms?
Is there a family history of IBD, autoimmune disorders, or other associated GI illnesses?

PHYSICAL EXAM

Once the history is taken, the physical exam can uncover a number of signs of IBD. Special attention to weight, height, and velocity of growth pattern is needed, because these disorders often manifest with growth and nutritional deficiencies. Signs of specific vitamin and trace element deficiencies are important

TABLE 54.1

DIFFERENTIAL DIAGNOSIS OF INFLAMMATORY
BOWEL DISEASE

Bacterial infections (*Salmonella, Shigella, Campylobacter, Yersinia, Eschericia coli, Clostridium difficile*, tuberculosis, *Aeromonas*)
Viral infections (HIV, cytomegalovirus, herpes simplex, rotavirus, adenovirus, Norwalk virus)
Parasitic infections (*Entamoeba histolytica, Giardiasis, Cryptosporidium, Strongyloides stercoralis, Isospora belli*)
Allergic enterocolitis
Henoch–Schönlein purpura
Hemolytic-uremic syndrome
Ischemic colitis
Hirschsprung enterocolitis
Necrotizing enterocolitis
Graft-versus-host disease
Radiation/chemotherapy-induced colitis
Behçet syndrome
Constipation with encopresis, anal fissure
Meckel diverticulum
Enteric duplication cyst
Lactose intolerance/disaccharidase deficiency
Postinfectious enteropathy
Intussusception
Polyposis
Hemorrhoids
Neoplasms of the GI tract
Celiac sprue
Cystic fibrosis/pancreatic insufficiency
Anorexia nervosa/eating disorders
Nephropathy/cardiopathy
Non-GI malignancy
Mesenteric adenitis
Appendicitis
Bowel obstruction
Irritable bowel syndrome
Diabetes mellitus
Hyper/hypothyroidism
Hyper/hypoparathyroidism

TABLE 54.2

LABORATORY ASSESSMENT OF INFLAMMATORY
BOWEL DISEASE

Complete blood count with differential and red cell indices
Comprehensive chemistry panel (AST, ALT, alkaline phosphatase, bilirubin total and direct, sodium, potassium, chloride, bicarbonate, BUN, creatinine, glucose, albumin, globulin, total protein, amylase, lipase, calcium, magnesium, phosphorous)
Erythrocyte sedimentation rate (ESR)
C-reactive protein (CRP)
Fecal leukocytes, red blood cells, bacterial culture, *Clostridium difficile* toxins, ova and parasites, alpha-1-antitrypsin, lactoferrin, *Rotavirus* antigen (when indicated), *Cryptosporidium* prep (when indicated)
In selected patients: zinc level, vitamin B$_{12}$ level, folic acid, iron studies, inflammatory bowel disease serologic markers (pANCA, pASCA)

to note; these include skin rash, hair loss, thinning or depigmentation, cheilosis, buccal lesions, pallor, and nail-bed pitting. Abdominal palpation for masses, organomegaly, and perianal inspection are mandatory. Intrarectal digital exam should focus on the presence of a fluctuant mass or gross blood, but may be quite uncomfortable in patients with active proctitis.

LABORATORY EVALUATION

The laboratory evaluation of a patient with possible IBD is crucial to making the diagnosis, yet there is not one specific laboratory result that is pathognomonic of IBD. Table 54.2 lists the typical laboratory assessment, and it should be noted that even after all of the lab results have been analyzed, the diagnosis may still be in question. Acute-phase reactants, such as erythrocyte sedimentation rate (ESR) and C-reactive protein (CRP), are sensitive markers of acute inflammation, but are nonspecific, and may also be less accurate in patients with chronic nutritional deficiencies, including hypoproteinemia. Liver assessment is important but also nonspecific. It can uncover mild abnormalities in the transaminase levels in CD, or help identify the 10%

to 15% of patient with UC who also have sclerosing cholangitis, an autoimmune disease of the biliary tract that may be even more devastating to the patient than UC itself. A complete blood count and peripheral smear often uncover the microcytic anemia of iron deficiency, resulting from either chronic GI blood loss, poor intake of iron in the diet, or malabsorption of enteral iron. Macrocytic anemia can be seen in IBD patients with a history of terminal ileal resection or chronic disease, due to poor absorption of vitamin B$_{12}$, or rarely in patients with proximal small bowel disease who malabsorb folic acid. Lipase may be useful to check, because a small percentage of CD patients may manifest pancreatitis due to CD, or possibly due to medications commonly used for the treatment of IBD. Stool samples looking for common bacterial pathogens in patients with a clinical history of potential exposure, and fecal leukocyte testing, are necessary to heighten the suspicion of IBD and to eliminate common acute causes of enterocolitis in previously healthy individuals. Ova and parasite testing is useful in this regard as well. A spot test for fecal alpha-1-antitrypsin will uncover a protein-losing enteropathy, and in the differential diagnosis of these disorders, IBD is most common. Recently, there has been increased enthusiasm for stool lactoferrin analysis as a sensitive marker of inflammation.

In the past several years, there has been a large body of work on specific antibodies commonly recovered from patients with IBD. Perinuclear anti-saccharomyces cervasiae antibody (pASCA) and perinuclear anti-neutrophil cytoplasmic antibody (pANCA) have been enthusiastically adopted as potential screening labs for suspected cases of IBD, as well as to help differentiate CD from UC when only colonic involvement is found, and when the histopathology is nonspecific. However, these antibodies have a low sensitivity (50%–65%) and do not replace clinical acumen when making the diagnosis of IBD. They are statistically about as sensitive as the acute phase reactants, although further identification of additional antibodies commonly found in IBD patients, when used in combination with these initial two, are increasing the sensitivity of these assays, and should prove more useful in the future when clinical scenarios are confusing.

IMAGING

Imaging studies can be useful, if often nonspecific in evaluation of IBD. Fluoroscopic evaluation with upper GI series and small bowel follow-through has been the gold standard for many years in the evaluation of suspected small bowel CD. Characteristic findings of separation of edematous bowel loops, coin-stacking appearance of prominent valvulae conniventes, and string-like narrowed areas of inflammation as well as fistula detection can be seen in these patients. Barium enema evaluation of the colon and terminal ileum may reveal absence of haustral markings, narrowed areas of luminal inflammation, or fistula formation connecting other abdominal or pelvic structures. However, its use is limited when active colitis is suspected, because endoscopic evaluation is more sensitive and yields tissue for histologic examination. Computed tomography (CT) scanning is often performed in the acute care setting when a patient presents with acute or severe abdominal pain, and is most helpful when intraluminal contrast is ingested, so that luminal contents can be differentiated from extraluminal processes. CT scans are often read as showing mural thickening of an area of intestine, such as terminal ileum, colon, or even more proximal small intestine. Although a more chronic history coupled with isolated mural thickening of the ileum may raise suspicion of IBD, these radiographic findings are nonspecific, and can be seen in acute infectious illnesses as well as in IBD. Again, they need to be interpreted within the clinical context of the history and exam.

Recently, video capsule endoscopy has allowed examination of the small bowel lumen in previously endoscopically unreachable areas. Lesions that may be more subtle and not apparent on contrast radiography can be seen with this modality, although the quality of the study interpretation is somewhat user-dependent; the more experience we attain with this method of imaging, the more precise it will become as a tool to find previously occult small bowel disease. Its weakness at present is the inability to obtain tissue samples for diagnostic accuracy, as well as the size of the recording capsule, which at present precludes its use in children less than 4 years old.

ENDOSCOPIC FINDINGS

Endoscopy has been the gold standard method for diagnosis of IBD for more than 30 years in pediatrics. Esophagogastroduodenoscopy can examine the upper digestive tract lumen up to the ligament of Treitz, while colonoscopy can evaluate the entire colon and terminal ileum. Gross endoscopic findings of IBD include loss of vascular markings, friability, ulceration, edematous folds, luminal narrowing, pesudopolyp formation, and active bleeding. CD typically has a patchy distribution, manifesting skipped areas between actively inflamed areas, while UC is characteristically more contiguous, and limited to the colon. Occasionally, acute ileal findings can be seen with UC ("backwash ileitis"), but this is usually easily distinguishable from CD on histologic examination of ileal biopsies. UC often starts with proctitis only, or "left-sided" disease involving the rectum to the splenic flexure but sparing the rest of the more proximal colon. Pancolitis is also common in UC, but rectal sparing or exclusively right-sided inflammation is usually more prevalent in CD.

Histologic findings on biopsies obtained at endoscopy may overlap between CD and UC. The pathognomonic finding of noncaseating granulomas is seen in fewer than 30% of patients with CD, and transmural inflammation, typical of CD only, is found less often when endoscopic examination is undertaken earlier in the course of the disease. Crypt abscesses can be found in either CD or UC, and the population of white blood cells in the lamina propria may overlap in either disorder. More often than not, the diagnosis of CD versus UC is made based on the distribution of disease, as well as the clinical presentation, rather than the histologic findings alone.

MANAGEMENT

Management of IBD can be divided between acute inpatient settings and outpatient chronic care. In patients with active UC, hospital admission is required for hydration, control of bleeding, nutrition support if bowel rest is indicated, pain control, and management of any acute abdominal processes. Often, transfusion of packed red blood cells is required if the blood loss is acute and the patient is suffering any cardiorespiratory compromise. In contrast, patients admitted with a chronic microcytic anemia but no acute blood loss or cardiorespiratory distress can be managed with iron replacement therapy. In either UC or CD, bowel rest is useful to stop the accelerated diarrhea and dehydration these patients often experience; and in some cases, it can also assist in curbing the active bleeding. Depending on the condition of the patient at presentation, a decision to initiate nutritional support can be made shortly after initial stabilization, especially if bowel rest is expected to be employed more than 72 hours. Often, a central venous catheter is placed (either peripherally inserted, or directly into a central vein) to allow higher concentrations of dextrose and electrolytes to be infused. Older, larger adolescents can sometimes be supported with peripheral access only, as they may tolerate larger volumes of fluid, thereby removing the need for increasing dextrose concentrations. Close monitoring of vital signs, fever trends, stool volume, blood loss, and fluid balance is necessary in these cases. Because underlying infections may not be apparent at the moment of presentation, careful assessment of the need for intravenous antibiotic coverage should be made upon presentation and repeatedly throughout the hospitalization.

Corticosteroids given intravenously are the mainstay in controlling an acute exacerbation of either CD or UC. The dose ranges from 1 to 2 mg/kg/day, and can be divided into 2 to 4 doses per 24 hours. When symptoms diminish (i.e., cessation of bleeding grossly, reduced diarrhea and abdominal pain), the corticosteroids are converted to oral form and given in doses ranging from 1 to 2 mg/kg/day divided twice daily, with a maximum daily dose of 60 mg. Generally, after a 10-to 14-day quiescent period at this dose, a tapering schedule is given to the patient, with the intent that maintenance therapy with agents having fewer potential side effects will be used during and after the taper. Studies have shown that there is a reduction in disease exacerbation rates and less adrenal insufficiency with a gradual taper off corticosteroids, than with a rapid removal of these agents.

Several maintenance treatments are used, depending on the location and severity of disease in UC. Five-aceltylsalicylate (5-ASA) products are typically used for mild to moderate disease as first-line therapy, and can be given orally or rectally through enemas or suppositories for patients with primarily left-sided or rectal disease. Several forms are available, including sulfasalazine, olsalazine, mesalamine, and balsalazide. They differ in their site of release in the GI tract. Their ability to block prostaglandin production in the colon is thought to be their main mechanism of action. Antibiotics such as metronidazole or ciprofloxacin are often used adjunctively for patients with solely colonic disease or the perianal disease often seen in patients with CD, while immunomodulatory agents such as 6-mercaptopurine, azathioprine, cyclosporine, and tacrolimus are used when patients either do not respond to 5-ASA products or present with more severe disease initially, or in the case of CD, with disease outside of the colon. Cyclosporine and tacrolimus are usually reserved for rescue of patients who do not respond to bowel rest and IV corticosteroids, but because of the need to monitor levels in the serum, and due to the relatively high rates of nephrotoxicity and neurotoxicity, they are not agents used as long-term therapy. Recently in adults, there has been recognition that infliximab, an antitumor necrosis factor

(TNF) bioengineered monoclonal antibody, has some benefit in refractory UC, whereas it was approved for refractory CD in 1998. Ultimately, the toxicities of each of these agents has to be measured against the effectiveness and ultimate cure of patients with UC, who may opt instead for surgical colectomy. In patients with CD, who cumulatively have only a 10% chance of curing their disease surgically, the risk–benefit ratio may favor the potentially more toxic medications.

NUTRITIONAL THERAPY

As stated, patients with either UC or CD may benefit from a short course of bowel rest and potential nutritional support. In general, enteral nutritional support is preferred due to its lower risk of hepatotoxicity, as well as the inherent risk of central venous catheter complications such as thrombosis, infection, and dislodgement. Contraindications to enteral nutritional support include high-grade bowel obstruction, high-output enteric fistulae, or lack of tolerance of nasogastric (NG) tube placement. Studies have shown that, especially in children, nutritional therapy as first-line treatment in CD can be as effective as corticosteroid treatment, and often support with an elemental formula via oral or NG route is employed. This is not as effective for colonic CD or for UC, and the lack of palatability of these formulas, or the resistance to NG or gastrostomy placement, precludes their effective use.

Parents often ask what foods should be avoided, and there is no controlled data to support the cessation of any particular food group in patients with CD or UC. In general, we recommend that any patient with active colitis symptoms reduce fiber intake and observe a low-residue diet until the symptoms (bleeding, diarrhea) remit. Caffeine-free diets are recommended because of the alteration in GI blood flow seen in patients with caffeine intake. At least one study in adults indicated a higher incidence of lactose maldigestion in patients with UC compared to a control group, but no data exist that supports the complete removal of dairy products from the diet in IBD. In general, a diet replete with enough calories and protein is recommended when the patient transitions to outpatient care.

SURGICAL TREATMENT

As indicated, in patients with UC, surgical colectomy is curative. However, the patient may still be at risk of suffering some of the extraintestinal manifestations of the disease. Indications for colectomy in UC include refractory symptoms despite maximal medical therapy and bowel rest, including refractory pain or bleeding, as well as development of toxic megacolon. Surgery may also be indicated in marginally controlled disease when the side effects of medications are unacceptable, such as those seen when there is a recurrent need for corticosteroids. The custom for patients with UC undergoing surgery is first to create a temporary ileostomy, and then to create a J-pouch (neorectum) in second-stage surgery, and finally takedown of the diverting ileostomy. Patients undergoing this surgery successfully will be able to maintain continence and eat a normal diet, but will generally have more frequent bowel movements that will be softer in texture. Bouts of "pouchitis" or inflammation in the newly created neorectum are usually responsive to oral antibiotics such as metronidazole or ciprofloxacin.

In patients with CD, the indications for surgical intervention generally cannot promise a cure, such that surgery is often a last resort. Indications for surgery in CD include obstruction due to stricture formation, high-grade fistula, perforation with abscess formation, and relief of symptoms unresponsive to medical management. In some instances, primary reanastomosis is not feasible or advisable, and a temporary ostomy is created. In certain instances, a permanent stoma may be preferable to the potential need for more surgery when attempting to restore bowel continuity. Because of the potential for transmural inflammation in CD, the risk of perforation/fistula formation is higher, and adjacent structures may be compromised when this occurs. Perianal fistulae may erode into organs involved with reproduction, and there is some risk of sterility because of this complication. Fistulization to the skin surface, urinary tract, other loops of bowel, or even distant sites has commonly been reported. Although an attempt at medical therapy for fistulizing disease is often useful (using agents such as infliximab or 6-mercaptopurine), many patients require surgical intervention to combat chronic symptoms.

LONG-TERM FOLLOW-UP

Although the hospitalist is not usually in a position to manage patients with IBD long term, it is important to have an understanding of the importance of patient and family education at the outset, in order to effect better compliance and outcome in the ambulatory setting. Our group offers an extensive primer packet made of materials from the Crohn's and Colitis Foundation of America (CCFA) to all of our patients with newly diagnosed IBD. A website for the lay public can be accessed through www.CCFA.org. Dietician consultation in the inpatient setting is offered, and the physician performs extensive teaching about the disease and treatment as well as long-term outcome. Occasionally, mental health referral is useful for some children and especially adolescents who are more prone to depression and noncompliance with treatment. In essence, treatment of the whole patient rather than just the patient's intestinal tract is the best approach.

Although there is no specific cure for IBD, parents and children with this disease are counseled that there will be periods of remission and exacerbation, and strict adherence to medical regimens and follow-up are stressed. Support groups, or even an "IBD buddy," can allay the feelings of loneliness and body image concerns common to developing children and adolescents, and clinicians can make a huge impact on the long-term prognosis by providing some of these means of support for their patients.

In summary, IBD is a chronic condition that often begins during childhood. Although there is no known cure, advances in medical and surgical therapy have allowed patients with these diseases to live healthier, more productive lives. A basic understanding of the presenting symptoms, initial management, and long-term care of these patients is important for the practicing hospitalist.

Suggested Readings

Kleinman RE, ed. *Pediatric nutrition handbook.* 4th ed. American Academy of Pediatrics. Elk Grove Village, Illinois; 2004.
Walker WA, Goulet O, Kleinman RE, et al, eds. *Pediatric gastrointestinal disease: pathophysiology, diagnosis, and management.* 4th ed. Hamilton, Ontario: Decker; 2004.

CHAPTER 55 ■ HEPATITIS

CARL V. DEZENBERG

LIVER

Situated just below the right lung and diaphragm, the liver's right and left lobes receive blood from the hepatic artery and the portal vein, with total liver blood flow accounting for 20% to 25% of the cardiac output. The hepatic artery supplies 20% to 33% of the total blood flow through the liver with oxygen-rich blood, whereas the portal vein brings nutrient-rich blood from the intestines (1). In addition to its important roles in carbohydrate metabolism and protein and cholesterol synthesis, the liver forms bile, allowing excretion of bilirubin, steroids, cholesterol, and other compounds, including bile acids, which aid in the absorption of fat and fat-soluble vitamins (A, D, E, and K).

PATHOPHYSIOLOGY

Hepatitis is caused by any inflammatory process within the liver. Although direct cytopathic injury frequently occurs, immune reactions, such as from autoimmune diseases or hepatitis B infection, can also result in hepatocellular injury. As with glycogen storage diseases, obesity, and alpha-1 antitrypsin deficiency, accumulation of material may also result in injury, whereas inborn errors of metabolism can result in elevated metabolites that are toxic to the liver. Ischemia and toxins, including hyperalimentation, may cause damage as well. More common within neonates and infants, giant cell transformation can occur as a nonspecific response to injury. At any age, these insults commonly affect bile formation and excretion, such that cholestasis develops.

ETIOLOGY

Hepatitis in children is commonly caused by infectious agents (Table 55.2), but as seen in Table 55.1, other categories include drugs/toxins (Table 55.3), autoimmune disorders, metabolic diseases (Table 55.4), neoplasms, ischemia, and biliary disease. Graft-versus host disease, veno-occlusive disease, TPN cholestasis, passive congestion from cardiac disease, and steatohepatitis are also considered under appropriate circumstances. Of the many viral causes, children are now routinely vaccinated against hepatitis A, hepatitis B, and varicella. Although primary immunodeficiencies rarely affect the liver, secondary infections and malnutrition frequently do.

CLINICAL PRESENTATION

Many cases of hepatitis go undiagnosed because there may be few to no clinical symptoms, lack of localized symptoms or jaundice to suspect it, or a presentation with flu-like or acute gastroenteritis symptoms, resulting in symptomatic treatment only; while the less common presentation with jaundice and dark urine is more obvious. Even so, the etiology often is not readily apparent. A wide range of symptoms are possible, including malaise, anorexia, nausea, vomiting, fever, myalgias, arthralgias, abdominal pain, and diarrhea. There may be a rash or recent respiratory symptoms. With chronic disease or a neoplastic process, there may only be organomegaly or a mass on exam. An initial presentation with variceal bleeding can occur with portal hypertension, or epistaxis with a coagulopathy or thrombocytopenia.

DIAGNOSIS

Although it is difficult to directly measure liver health, certain lab findings are helpful. Elevations of alanine aminotransferase (ALT) and aspartate aminotransferase (AST) are suggestive of liver cell injury, especially if the ALT elevation is higher than the AST elevation. These enzymes can also be from other organs such as muscle, in which case a creatine phosphokinase (CPK) level may help to differentiate. Increased alkaline phosphatase and gammaglutamyltranspeptidase (GGT) are more indicative of intrahepatic and/or extrahepatic biliary system disease. Elevated bilirubin levels are seen with inflammatory, obstructive, or other disease states that interfere with its uptake, conjugation, or excretion, and in turn this cholestasis can result in fat-soluble vitamin deficiencies. Protein synthesis can be looked at by measuring various proteins, such as albumin and prealbumin. A prothrombin time can be elevated because of poor synthesis or vitamin K deficiency. This can usually be differentiated based on response to vitamin K supplementation. Ammonia levels can become elevated if the liver's ability to convert it to urea is reduced.

Specific etiologies are initially suspected based on the patient's age, history, physical examination, family history, and initial laboratory testing. Questioning should include specific medications, supplements, and herbs taken, as well as a detailed past medical history. As appropriate, travel history, sick contacts, developmental milestones, and vaccination records should be reviewed as well.

Radiologic imaging is very helpful to assess for focal lesions, including choledochal cysts, abscesses, tumors, and choledocholithiasis. Ultrasonography, which is noninvasive, readily available, and less expensive than other methods, is generally sufficient for initial evaluation, and it can even include Doppler flows to evaluate the vessels. Specific abnormalities may then need to be further defined through CT or MRI imaging. A liver biopsy is usually not required for diagnosis, but at times, especially with chronic disease, it is instrumental in evaluating liver health or establishing the diagnosis.

TABLE 55.1

CAUSES OF HEPATITIS IN CHILDREN

INFECTIONS (SEE TABLE 55.2)

DRUGS/TOXINS (SEE TABLE 55.3)

METABOLIC DISORDERS (SEE TABLE 55.4)

NEOPLASMS
Leukemia, lymphoma
Hepatoblastoma
Hepatocellular carcinoma
Metastatic (neuroblastoma, Wilms tumor)

AUTOIMMUNE/COLLAGEN VASCULAR DISEASE
Autoimmune hepatitis (types 1–3)
Sclerosing cholangitis (± association with inflammatory
bowel disease)
Systemic lupus erythematosus
Juvenile rheumatoid arthritis

BILIARY DISEASE
Biliary atresia
Paucity of interlobular bile ducts (Alagille syndrome versus
nonsyndromic)
Ductal plate malformations (congenital hepatic fibrosis with
autosomal recessive polycystic kidney disease, Caroli
disease)
Choledochal cyst
Choledocholithiasis

ENDOCRINE DISORDERS
Hyperthyroidism (cholestasis with hypothyroidism)
Cushing syndrome (cholestasis with adrenal insufficiency)
Diabetes mellitus (including Mauriac syndrome)
Hypopituitarism (possibly from Septo-optic dysplasia)

OTHER
Neonatal hepatitis
Ischemia
Hemoglobinopathies
Lymphohistiocytic disorders
Porphyrias

TABLE 55.2

INFECTIOUS CAUSES OF HEPATITIS IN CHILDREN

VIRAL
Hepatitis A, B, C, D (requires B), E, and G
Epstein–Barr virus
Cytomegalovirus
Herpes simplex virus
Varicella-zoster virus
Enteroviruses (Coxsackie)
Adenovirus
Parvovirus (Fifth disease)
Rubella
Human immunodeficiency virus (HIV)

BACTERIAL
Neonatal: E. coli, *Streptococcus*, *Staphylococcus*, *Listeria*
Multiple gram-positive and gram-negative organisms
Mycobacterium tuberculosis
Toxic shock syndrome (staphylococci, streptococci)
Cat scratch disease (*Bartonella henselae*)
Rickettsial infections (spotted fevers, Q fever)
Lyme disease (*Borrelia burgdorferi*)
Syphilis, brucellosis, leptospirosis
Perihepatitis (Fitz–Hugh–Curtis syndrome): *Chlamydia*,
Neisseria

FUNGAL
Candida
Coccidiomycosis
Cryptococcosis
Aspergillosis
Histoplasmosis
Trichosporon cutaneum

PARASITIC
Amebiasis
Schistosomiasis
Toxoplasmosis
Ascariasis
Alveolar echinococcus (*Echinococcus multilocularis*)
Visceral larva migrans (*Toxocara*)
Visceral leishmaniasis
Hepatic capillariasis
Liver flukes (*Clonorchis*, *Opisthorchis*)
Malaria

Aside from serologic testing for possible infectious causes, screening may be indicated for alpha-1 antitrypsin deficiency with protease inhibitor phenotype determination, Wilson disease with a ceruloplasmin level and urinary copper measurement, hemochromatosis with ferritin and transferrin saturation levels, tyrosinemia with urinary succinylacetone, or even cystic fibrosis with a sweat chloride test. The presence of reducing substances in the urine of an infant on a lactose-containing diet suggests galactossemia. Patterns of acidosis, hypoglycemia, and hyperammonemia may suggest specific inborn errors of metabolism, while hypergammaglobulinemia should prompt more specific autoimmune testing.

TREATMENT

Although most children can be treated as outpatients, hospitalization is sometimes required, particularly if there is dehydration with the inability to maintain and tolerate appropriate oral intakes, or there is a coagulopathy, encephalopathy, gastrointestinal bleeding, or concern for possible progression toward fulminant failure. Also, concomitant disease may prompt admission for closer monitoring. Liver failure with acidosis, severe coagulopathy, or encephalopathy should prompt referral to a liver transplantation center once stabilized as best as possible. Maintenance of appropriate hydration and blood sugars, as well as close monitoring of vital signs and laboratory values, is necessary for the hospitalized patient, but overexpansion may affect portal pressures and affect bleeding. Unless there is bleeding, coagulopathies can initially be treated with vitamin K. Severe coagulopathy or active bleeding should be treated with fresh frozen plasma and possibly recombinant factor VIIa (2). Pharmacologic treatment, such as with octreotide, may be as helpful as endoscopic procedures (3). Platelet counts should be kept over 25,000. An

TABLE 55.3

DRUG AND TOXIN CAUSES OF HEPATITIS

ANTIPYRETICS, ANTI-INFLAMMATORY DRUGS
Acetaminophen
Salicylates
Ibuprofen
Indomethacin

ANTIMICROBIALS
Isoniazid, rifampin
Ketoconazole
Erythromycin
Sulfonamides
Tetracyclines
Nitrofurantoin
Penicillins

ANTICONVULSANTS
Valproic acid
Phenytoin
Carbamazepine
Phenobarbital

ANESTHETICS
Halogenated inhalation agents (halothane, sevoflurane, desflurane)
Chloroform

ANTINEOPLASTIC/IMMUNOSUPPRESSIVE
6-mercaptopurine, azathioprine
L-asparaginase
Cytosine arabinoside
Nitrosureas (carmustine, lomustine, streptozocin)
Metal salts (carboplatin, cisplatin)

OTHER
Steroids (estrogens/contraceptives, anabolic steroids)
Methyldopa
Hypervitaminosis A
H_2-receptor antagonists (ranitidine, cimetidine)
Oral hypoglycemic agents
Environmental/industrial (pesticides, aromatic compounds)
Mushrooms (*Amanita, Gyromitra, Galerina*)
Illegal (alcohol, cocaine, amphetamines)

TABLE 55.4

METABOLIC CAUSES OF HEPATITIS

Alpha-1 antitrypsin deficiency
Cystic fibrosis
Iron storage disorders
　Neonatal hemochromatosis
　Hemochromatosis
Copper storage disorders
　Wilson disease
　Indian childhood cirrhosis
Tyrosinemia
Inborn errors of carbohydrate metabolism
　Galactosemia
　Disorders of fructose metabolism
　Glycogen storage disease
Inborn errors of fatty acid oxidation
Inborn errors of bile acid metabolism, peroxisomal disorders
Mitochondrial hepatopathies (Leigh syndrome, MELAS, Alpers disease, etc.)
Lysosomal storage diseases
　Mucopolysaccharidoses (Hurler syndrome, Hunter syndrome, Sanfilippo disease, etc.)
　Sphingolipidoses (Gaucher disease, Niemann–Pick disease, Farber disease, etc.)
　Lipidoses (Wolman disease, cholesterol ester storage disease)
　Mucolipidoses, glycoproteinoses
Porphyria

or immunosuppression, or possibly liver transplantation. It can affect growth and development and necessitate parenteral nutritional support. Liver failure, cirrhosis, portal hypertension, variceal bleeding, and even hepatocellular carcinoma can develop. Among other variables, prognosis is dependent upon the underlying etiology, liver status at time of diagnosis, and response to therapy.

References

1. Lautt WW, Greenway CV. Conceptual review of the hepatic vascular bed. *Hepatology* 1987;7:952–963.
2. Ramsey G. Treating coagulopathy in liver disease with plasma infusions or recombinant factor VIIa: an evidence-based review. *Best Pract Res Clin Haematol* 2006;19:113–126.
3. Yan BM, Lee SS. Emergency management of bleeding esophageal varices: drugs, bands or sleep? *Can J Gastroenterol* 2006;20:165–170.
4. Martindale RG. Contemporary strategies for the prevention of stress-related mucosal bleeding. *Am J Health Syst Pharm* 2005;62:S11–17.

H_2-receptor antagonist or proton-pump inhibitor can reduce the risk of bleeding from gastritis or stress ulceration (4). Ascites may prompt fluid and sodium restrictions and possibly diuretic therapy. Other specific treatments are directed by the underlying etiology of the hepatitis.

COMPLICATIONS

Acute hepatitis can range from an asymptomatic self-limited illness to fulminant hepatic failure and death. Chronic hepatitis (>6 months) may require long-term anti-infective therapy

Suggested Reading

Suchy FJ, Sokol RJ, Balistreri WF, eds. Liver disease in children. 2nd ed. Philadelphia: Lippincott, Williams & Wilkins; 2001.

CHAPTER 56 ■ ACUTE LIVER FAILURE

CHRISTOPHER RHEE

Acute liver failure is defined as severe liver injury and necrosis, resulting in severe impairment of liver function as manifested by jaundice, hepatic encephalopathy, and coagulopathy. Acute liver failure is commonly referred to fulminant hepatic failure (FHF) when hepatic encephalopathy occurs in less than 8 weeks after the onset of the jaundice and in the absence of any pre-existing liver disease. In children, it is a rare but often fatal disorder due to complications from cerebral edema, bleeding, sepsis, or renal failure. Liver transplantation remains the only effective treatment for those patients who do not spontaneously recover.

ETIOLOGY

Acute liver failure in children can be due to a variety of causes (Table 56.1) including infectious hepatitis, toxin- or drug-induced injury, metabolic disorders, and ischemia. In contrast to the adult population, the cause of liver failure in children is often the result of a suspected infection with a yet-to-be-identified non-A-G (or non-A, non-B [NANB]) hepatitis virus that can account for as many as 50% of cases. In these patients, there is generally an absence of markers for known viral agents, along with lack of exposure to drugs or toxins, negative markers for autoimmune disease, and no evidence of infection with nonviral agents capable of causing hepatitis. A high fatality rate is characteristic of FHF due to non-A-G hepatitis.

The causes of acute liver failure in children are often age-dependent. The differential diagnosis in early infancy particularly includes infectious etiologies as well as metabolic disorders. Viral etiologies include Epstein–Barr virus, cytomegalovirus, herpes virus, echovirus, adenovirus, and hepatitis B, while inborn errors of metabolism presenting as acute liver failure in the infant can include hereditary fructose intolerance, galactosemia, hereditary tyrosinemia, neonatal hemochromatosis, urea cycle disorders, and mitochondrial fatty acid oxidation defects. In infants, a previous hypoglycemic event, developmental delay, or history of seizures may suggest a metabolic disorder. In older children, the more common viral etiologies include hepatitis A, B, and non-A-G; EBV; parvovirus; and varicella zoster virus. History of any blood transfusions, immunization status to hepatitis A and B, and travel should be looked into. In regards to evaluation, viral serologies along with hepatitis serologies should be obtained for anti-hepatitis A virus IgM, hepatitis B surface antigen, anti-hepatitis B core IgM, and anti-hepatitis C virus. Although hepatitis C itself is a very unusual etiology of acute liver failure, it has been suggested that coinfection with hepatitis B virus can produce severe hepatitis.

Although patients with autoimmune hepatitis and Wilson disease have pre-existing liver disease and frequently chronic liver disease, these disorders can also present acutely with liver failure. Although serum ceruloplasmin levels classically are decreased in Wilson disease, a normal serum ceruloplasmin does not rule out Wilson disease, and a 24-hour urinary copper analysis or eventual liver biopsy for copper quantitation may be necessary. If autoimmune hepatitis is suspected, autoimmune markers, including antinuclear antibody, anti-smooth muscle antibody, anti-liver-kidney microsomal antibody, and anti-mitochondrial antibody should be obtained. A reversal in the albumin/globulin serum protein ratio or markedly increased IgG also may be suggestive of autoimmune disease.

Ischemic injury and perfusion defects may be the result of veno-occlusive disease, congenital heart disease, cardiac surgery, myocarditis, or severe asphyxia. Drug-induced liver toxicity can be dose-related, as seen with acetaminophen; or may represent an idiosyncratic reaction most commonly seen with anti-seizure medications (valproic acid, phenytoin), antituberculous drugs (isoniazid), and halothane. The most common cause of drug-related liver failure in adolescents is intentional acetaminophen overdose. An accurate acetaminophen history should be obtained with the amount and interval of doses. At times, parents have accidentally used acetaminophen children's elixir instead of the infant drops, resulting in a significant overdose. A history of ingestion, whether accidental or intentional, and use of herbal medications or recreational drugs should be considered. If suggestive, a toxicology screen and aspirin level should be obtained in addition to an acetaminophen level.

Other causes of acute liver failure in children include toxins such as ingestion of the *Amanita phalloides* mushroom. Rarely, primary malignancy or malignant infiltration (hepatoblastoma, leukemia, lymphoma, hemophagocytic lymphohistiocytosis) may result in liver failure.

CLINICAL MANIFESTATIONS

Abnormal Liver Tests

Clinically, the initial symptoms may be nonspecific, such as malaise, nausea, vomiting, and abdominal pain followed by jaundice. On physical examination, patients with FHF have rapidly progressing jaundice with marked elevated bilirubin levels of both the total and direct component. The liver can be normal in size or enlarged. Splenomegaly does not necessarily accompany FHF. Serum aminotransferases (aspartate [AST] and alanine aminotransferase [ALT]) are usually strikingly elevated, particularly with acetaminophen overdose. However, the degree of elevation in the liver transaminases is not necessarily predictive of outcome in patients with liver failure. Decreasing or lower transaminase values with increasing bilirubin levels may be suggestive of ongoing liver deterioration rather than improvement.

Electrolyte Changes and Renal Failure

Acute liver failure is associated with a hyperdynamic circulation that involves high cardiac output and a decrease in systemic

TABLE 56.1

CAUSES OF FULMINANT HEPATIC FAILURE
IN CHILDREN

Infectious	Hepatitis A, hepatitis B (with or without hepatitis C or D superinfection or co-infection), hepatitis E, non-A-G hepatitis, cytomegalovirus, Epstein–Barr virus, varicella-zoster virus, adenovirus, echovirus, herpes, parvovirus, sepsis
Drugs/toxins	Acetaminophen, valproate, phenytoin, isoniazid, rifampin, propylthiouracil, halothane, carbon tetrachloride, *Amanita phalloides*
Metabolic	Galactosemia, tyrosinemia, hereditary fructose intolerance, neonatal hemochromatosis, urea cycle disorders, mitochondrial fatty oxidation defects, Wilson disease
Ischemia	Congenital heart disease, myocarditis, pericardial tamponade, cardiac surgery, severe asphyxia, Budd–Chiari syndrome/hepatic vein thrombosis, veno-occlusive disease
Miscellaneous	Autoimmune hepatitis, acute fatty liver of pregancy, malignancies (hemophago-cytic lymphohistiocytosis, leukemia, lymphoma, hepatoblastoma)

vascular resistance and mean arterial pressure. Vasodilation may trigger activation of neurohumoral factors that results in extracellular fluid volume expansion and decreased water excretion. These patients typically have marked renal vasoconstriction despite systemic vasodilation that frequently results in functional renal failure, or hepatorenal syndrome. Its features include sodium retention (low urine sodium concentration), normal urinary sediment, and reduced urinary output. Although patients may go on to require hemodialysis or hemofiltration support, renal function generally recovers after successful liver transplantation. The renin–angiotensin–aldosterone pathway is stimulated with increased plasma renin activity and hyperaldosteronism, which results in hyponatremia due to excessive fluid retention despite sodium retention as well. Aside from serum

sodium disturbances, hypokalemia, hypocalcemia, and hypomagnesemia can also be seen.

Hypoglycemia

Hypoglycemia is due to the depletion of hepatic glycogen stores in addition to ineffective gluconeogenesis as a result of extensive injury and necrosis of the liver. Other contributing factors include increased insulin levels due to decreased catabolism by the liver as well as abnormal glucagon levels.

Coagulopathy

The liver is responsible for the synthesis of clotting factors I (fibrinogen), II (prothrombin), V, VII, IX, and X. During liver failure, there is impaired production of these clotting factors, in addition to impaired post-translational modification of vitamin K–dependent factors (II, VII, IX, and X). Therefore, a prolonged prothrombin time is one of the simplest clinical measures of hepatic dysfunction. Other contributing causes of coagulopathy include possible thrombocytopenia and disseminated intravascular coagulation. Therefore, clinically significant coagulopathy and hemorhage frequently complicate acute liver failure in children.

Hepatic Encephalopathy and Cerebral Edema

Manifestations of hepatic encephalopathy can vary from mild confusion or somnolence to coma; hepatic encephalopathy is graded from I to IV (Table 56.2). A worsened prognosis from acute liver failure has been shown to correlate with the degree of encephalopathy. Hepatic encephalopathy is not the same as cerebral edema. Although the pathophysiology of hepatic encephalopathy is poorly understood, it is generally accepted that it involves the accumulation of neurotoxic substances such as ammonia and agents that may possibly activate the gamma-aminobutyric acid (GABA) inhibitory neurotransmitter pathway. However, the serum ammonia level does not correlate with the development of or the degree of hepatic encephalopathy.

Cerebral edema is a major cause of mortality in patients with acute liver failure. Cerebral edema leads to intracranial hypertension, ischemic brain damage, and subsequent cerebral herniation, which is rapidly fatal. Signs suggestive of cerebral edema include pupillary changes and increased muscle tone. Papilledema is rare. Although cerebral edema can be visualized on CT scan, it is not sensitive for following increased

TABLE 56.2

CLINICAL STAGES OF HEPATIC ENCEPHALOPATHY

Stage	Clinical	Asterixis/Reflexes	Neurologic signs	Electroencephalographic changes
I	Confused, forgetfulness, mood changes, altered sleep–wake cycle	None/normal	Tremor, apraxia, impaired handwriting	Normal or minimal changes
II	Drowsy, inappropriate behavior, disorientation	Present/hyperreflexic	Dysarthria, ataxia	Abnormal, generalized slowing
III	Stuporous, obeys simple commands	Present/hyperreflexic, positive Babinski sign	Muscle rigidity	Abnormal, generalized slowing
IV	Comatose, arouses with painful stimuli (IVa), or no response (IVb)	Absent	Decerebrate or decorticate posturing	Abnormal, very slow delta activity

Adapted from Whitington PF, Soriano HE, Alonso EM. Fulminant hepatic failure in children. In: Suchy F, Sokol R, Balistreri W, eds. *Liver disease in children*. 2nd ed. Philadelphia: Lippincott Williams & Wilkins, 2001: 63–88.

intracranial pressures since these changes are late-findings. Dysfunction of the blood–brain barrier and impaired regulation of cellular osmolarity have been suggested as possible mechanisms for the development of cerebral edema.

MANAGEMENT

Management of liver failure is primarily supportive and focuses on the prevention and treatment of complications until spontaneous recovery or eventual liver transplantation. Survival has shown to be improved in those patients undergoing earlier rather than late transfer to a transplant center.

Management should be in an intensive-care unit setting. Venous access is mandatory. An arterial line should be considered if the child's condition is deteriorating and blood gas analysis is necessary for monitoring with intubation and mechanical ventilatory support. A urinary catheter should be placed to monitor fluid status and renal function. A nasogastric tube may be required to monitor for gastric bleeding and for administration of medications. Acid suppression with histamine-2 blockers or proton pump inhibitors is indicated as prophylaxis for the increased risk of stress ulcers and gastrointestinal bleeding. N-acetylcysteine should be administered to any patient suspected of toxic acetaminophen ingestion. Although most effective within 12 hours of ingestion, it has demonstrated beneficial effects up to 36 hours after the initial overdose.

Although a liver biopsy can sometimes provide a clue in establishing the cause of acute liver failure, this is infrequently the case. More commonly, the biopsy demonstrates diffuse and massive necrosis. In the presence of significant coagulopathy, a transjugular liver biopsy may be a safer alternative to a percutaneous biopsy if necessary. An abdominal ultrasound with Doppler study of the hepatic vessels can be useful to evaluate anatomic or vascular etiologies.

Patients with acute liver failure are at risk for complications including electrolyte and acid–base disturbances, hypoglycemia, and renal failure. Although these patients are frequently hyponatremic, fluid and sodium restriction (to 1.0 mEq/kg/day) are required because of fluid retention along with sodium overload. Frequent serum glucose monitoring is essential because patients are at risk of hypoglycemia and generally require increased dextrose concentrations of 10% to 20% in intravenous fluids.

In children with liver failure, the management of coagulopathy and hemorrhage represents a major part of the care due to the fact that they are frequent complications. The prothrombin time, which reflects the vitamin K–dependent clotting factors synthesized by the liver, often is the most useful laboratory parameter to follow serially in order to monitor the synthetic function of the liver. If the prothrombin time is prolonged, a trial of intravenous vitamin K daily for 3 consecutive days can be administered. Improvement in the prothrombin time suggests viable hepatocytes capable of synthesizing clotting factors and possibly potential for regeneration and recovery, whereas no improvement or a continued prolongation of the prothrombin time is a poor prognostic indicator. Along with the prothrombin time, fibrinogen levels should also be followed closely. In patients with severe prolongation of the prothrombin time or with active bleeding, administration of fresh frozen plasma and/or cryoprecipitate is required. In general, mild coagulopathy does not require treatment and aggressive use of fresh frozen plasma in attempts to fully correct the coagulation parameters within the normal range should be avoided. The judicious use of fresh frozen plasma and clotting factors is required in these patients to avoid the risk of fluid overload.

Due to the risk of hepatic encephalopathy and cerebral edema, frequent neurologic assessments should be performed. It is generally believed that ammonia, mainly of gut origin, accumulates in patients with liver failure and contributes to the development of hepatic encephalopathy. Therefore, therapy is aimed at reducing ammonia production and accumulation. In order to minimize ammonia production, protein intake should be limited. However, in order to maintain nitrogen balance and prevent muscle catabolism, a minimum of 0.8 to 1.0 g/kg of protein should be administered parenterally. Oral or rectal administration of antibiotics such as neomycin reduce ammonia absorption by reducing urease-producing bacteria that are responsible for ammonia production in the gut. Unfortunately, with chronic administration of neomycin, there is the potential for some absorption of this drug, leading to ototoxicity and nephrotoxicity, which may outweigh the possible benefits. Lactulose (β-galactosidofructose), a nonabsorbable disaccharide, can be also given orally or rectally, to reduce ammonia absorption due to its cathartic effects, as well as acidifying colonic contents to trap ammonia (NH_3) by conversion to NH_4^+, thereby promoting ammonia excretion. Specimens for serum ammonia levels should be sent immediately to the laboratory on ice in order to avoid falsely elevated levels. In general, sedating drugs, and especially benzodiazepines, are avoided not only because they are predominantly metabolized by the liver, but also since their administration may confound the mental status examination.

Because cerebral edema is a major cause of mortality and carries a poor prognosis, preventive measures are vital. Intracranial pressure (ICP) should be lower than 25 mm Hg to decrease the risk of herniation, while the cerebral perfusion pressure (CPP), should be maintained higher than 40 to 50 mm Hg to reduce the chances of ischemic brain injury. The CPP is defined as mean arterial pressure (MAP) minus the ICP. Because changes from cerebral edema on CT of the brain are late findings, intracranial pressure monitoring may be needed. Methods to reduce ICP include elective intubation with hyperventilation, mannitol infusion, and sodium and fluid restriction.

COURSE AND PROGNOSIS

Although acute liver failure is uncommon in children, it is associated with significant morbidity and mortality. Generally, spontaneous recovery is unusual, especially in children with FHF of unknown etiology. An exception to this generalization is acetaminophen overdose in children who undergo timely treatment. In those patients whose liver failure progresses, liver transplantation remains the only definitive cure, and intensive-care support and early referral to a transplantation center is crucial in improving survival outcome. Advances in transplantation through the use of living-related donors and split-liver transplants have helped alleviate the ongoing predicament of the shortage of donor organs and have helped reduce waiting times and pretransplant morbidity in pediatric liver transplant candidates. With the combination of improved immunosuppressive modalities and surgical techniques, pediatric 1-year survival rates have approached 90% in many large centers. The use of bioartificial liver support and hepatocyte transplantation in order to provide temporary hepatic support may hold promise in the future, but currently remain in experimental stages.

Suggested Readings

Lee WM. Acute liver failure. *N Engl J Med* 1993;329:1862–1872.

Hoofnagle JH, Carithers Jr. RL, Shapiro C, et al. Fulminant hepatic failure: summary of a workshop. *Hepatology* 1995;21:240–252.

Whitington PF, Soriano HE, Alonso EM. Fulminant hepatic failure in children. In: Suchy F, Sokol R, Balistreri W, eds. *Liver disease in children*. 2nd ed. Philadelphia: Lippincott Williams & Wilkins, 2001:63–88.

CHAPTER 57 ■ PANCREATITIS

CARL V. DEZENBERG

PANCREAS

The pancreas is formed from ventral and dorsal endodermal buds originating from the duodenum. Through growth and fusion of these buds, each originally with its own ductal system, the resulting pancreas typically drains through the ventral bud's duct of Wirsung into the major Vaterian papilla following regression of the dorsal bud's duct of Santorini and minor papilla. The ductal cells produce bicarbonate-rich fluid to neutralize stomach acid as it enters the duodenum, acinar cells synthesize and store digestive enzymes to aid digestion, and islet cells are responsible for hormone production. The endocrine portion accounts for about 2% of the cell mass, whereas the exocrine portion makes up the majority of the organ. Digestion of starch and proteins is aided by pancreatic amylase and proteases, whereas pancreatic lipase and colipase with bile acids help with the luminal digestion of triglycerides. The splenic artery provides most of the blood supply with a common blood supply between the pancreatic head and the duodenum via superior and inferior pancreaticoduodenal arteries. The pancreas is almost entirely extraperitoneal.

PATHOPHYSIOLOGY

Premature proenzyme activation or acinar cell injury, whether directly or via the canalicular, lymphatic, or vascular systems, can result in activation of the digestive enzymes. This may spontaneously resolve or continue as autodigestion with edema, hemorrhage, parenchymal and fat necrosis, and an inflammatory infiltrate. Pancreatitis is divided into acute and chronic, noting that recurrent bouts of acute pancreatitis can lead to chronic pancreatitis with its irreversible changes and possible endocrine and exocrine dysfunction.

ETIOLOGY

As opposed to adults, in whom gallstones and alcohol abuse are common causes of pancreatitis, common causes in children are more diverse, as listed in Table 57.1. Children are likely to have a systemic infection (Table 57.2), a drug exposure (Table 57.3), trauma, anatomic malformations of the pancreaticobiliary system, choledocholithiasis, or an idiopathic cause (1,2). Even a single exposure to a drug, such as propofol for sedation (3), may result in acute pancreatitis. Less likely etiologies include metabolic disorders, vasculitis, Crohn disease, and familial pancreatitis.

CLINICAL PRESENTATION

Over 90% of patients have abdominal pain, typically in the mid-epigastrium, but possibly in the right or left upper quadrant, diffusely, or even the lower abdomen. There may be extension to the back. Nausea, vomiting, and anorexia are common, whereas diarrhea and dyspnea are less so. Depending on the etiology and severity, there may be fevers, jaundice, abdominal distention, upper GI bleeding, anemia, or shock. Physical exam may reveal a bluish discoloration of the umbilicus (Cullen sign) or flanks (Grey–Turner sign).

DIAGNOSIS

In addition to the history and physical exam, laboratory testing and radiologic imaging aid in diagnosing pancreatitis. Although normal levels can be seen, elevation of amylase and/or lipase in the presence of abdominal pain supports this diagnosis. The pancreatic proteases trypsin, chymotrypsin, and elastase have not yet found favor in the diagnosis of pancreatitis (4). Serum amylase peaks in the first 24 to 48 hours and returns to normal in 3 to 5 days, whereas lipase may remain elevated for up to 2 weeks. Because of the rapid clearance of amylase, levels are sometimes normal in acute pancreatitis and frequently normal in chronic pancreatitis. It is also important to keep in mind other possible causes of hyperamylasemia, including intestinal obstruction or perforation, peritonitis, appendicitis, salivary gland inflammation, decreased clearance in renal failure, macroamylasemia, acidosis (including diabetic ketoacidosis), eating disorders (anorexia nervosa, bulimia), ovarian cysts, ectopic pregnancy, salpingitis, and various infections such as Epstein–Barr virus (EBV), mumps, or Human immunodeficiency virus (HIV).

Initial radiographic imaging usually includes ultrasonography or CT scan. In relatively uncomplicated pancreatitis, an ultrasound is preferred because of cost, ease of performing, lack of radiation exposure, and avoidance of the need for contrast; although CT imaging has its place for severe or complicated courses, or if ultrasonography is technically poor. Magnetic resonance cholangiopancreatography (MRCP) can help define ductal anatomy, such as pancreas divisum, in cases of recurrent pancreatitis, whereas endoscopic retrograde cholangiopancreatography (ERCP) should be reserved for some instances of gallstone pancreatitis or for recurrent pancreatitis in which either a structural abnormality is suspected or manometric studies indicated.

TREATMENT

Treatment depends on the severity of the attack, etiology, and associated complications, but the mainstays of therapy are

TABLE 57.1

CAUSES OF PANCREATITIS IN CHILDREN

SYSTEMIC INFECTION (SEE TABLE 57.2)

DRUGS (SEE TABLE 57.3)

TRAUMA
Blunt abdominal trauma (bicycle handlebar, child abuse)
Iatrogenic (ERCP, surgery)

ANATOMIC MALFORMATIONS
Pancreas divisum
Choledochal cyst

CHOLEDOCHOLITHIASIS

METABOLIC DISORDERS
Hyperlipoproteinemia types I, IV, V
Diabetes mellitus
Hyperparathyroidism
Aminoacidurias
Glycogen storage disease type I

VASCULITIS
Kawasaki disease
Henoch–Schönlein purpura
Systemic lupus erythematosis

OTHER
Cystic fibrosis
Crohn disease
Reye syndrome
Familial
Hypertensive sphincter of Oddi
Ischemia
Postirradiation
Scorpion of Trinidad bite

TABLE 57.2

INFECTIOUS CAUSES OF PANCREATITIS IN CHILDREN

BACTERIA
Mycoplasma
Salmonella, typhoid fever
Escherichia coli associated with hemolytic-uremic syndrome
Campylobacter
Yersinia
Legionella
Mycobacterium
Leptospira
Brucella

VIRUSES
Mumps
Coxsackie
Cytomegalovirus
Parainfluenza
Enterovirus
Human immunodeficiency virus
Influenza A and B
Epstein–Barr virus
Varicella
Hepatitis A and B
Rubeola
Rubella

FUNGAL
Aspergillus
Candida
Cryptococcus
Pneumocystis pneumonia

PARASITES
Malaria
Cryptosporidium
Ascariasis with ductal obstruction
Clonorchis with ductal obstruction

pancreatic rest, volume expansion/intravenous hydration, pain control, and close monitoring of cardiovascular and respiratory status. Also, close monitoring of hematocrit, glucose, and calcium are important. Because morphine can produce ampullary spasm, meperidine is generally preferred for pain control if narcotics are required. Nasogastric tube decompression with gastric acid aspiration, or acid suppression therapy, may reduce pancreatic exocrine secretion by reducing secretin levels, but both H_2-receptor antagonists and proton-pump inhibitors have been associated with pancreatitis in and of themselves. Further, clear benefits from H_2-receptor antagonists, as well as octreotide and protease inhibitors, have yet to be established (5), although somatostatin may be effective in the prevention of post-ERCP pancreatitis (6) and octreotide can reduce exocrine function after pancreatic surgery or help with treating pseudocysts (7).

Nutritional support should not be overlooked, especially if unable to initiate oral feeds within 5 to 7 days. It has been established that transpyloric feeds, or even gastric feeds with a low-fat elemental formula, are as safe and well tolerated as parenteral hyperalimentation. Enteral feeds may actually be preferred, considering the cost benefit, lack of potential central line complications, and fewer problems with hyperglycemia (8,9). Limiting fat in the diet to less than 20% of the total calories helps to minimize pancreatic stimulation, and

should be routinely taught to patients following an acute episode or with chronic pancreatitis. Also, in the presence of exocrine insufficiency in chronic pancreatitis, enzyme replacement therapy, fat-soluble vitamins, and possibly antioxidants should be considered, especially if testing reveals a deficiency (10). Prophylactic antibiotics should be considered in necrotic pancreatitis, especially considering the morbidity and mortality associated with infectious complications (11). Management of pseudocysts ranges from simple observation for regression to external, endoscopic, or surgical drainage, depending on the size, location, and associated complications, such as hemorhage or infection.

COMPLICATIONS

Risk factors for increased morbidity and mortality in children include age under 7 years and weight under 23 kg, as well as an initial white count over $18.5 \times 10^3/mm^3$ and LDH over 2,000 IU/L (12). Infected necrotic tissue and multisystem organ failure are associated with a higher risk of mortality. Acute pancreatitis may result in acidosis, hyperglycemia,

TABLE 57.3

DRUGS ASSOCIATED WITH PANCREATITIS

ANTICONVULSANTS
Valproic acid
Phenytoin

DIURETICS
Chlorothiazides
Furosemide
Ethacrynic acid

IMMUNOSUPPRESSIVES
Azathioprine, 6-mercaptopurine
L-asparaginase
Steroids

ANTIMICROBIALS
Sulfonamides
Tetracycline
Metronidazole
Pentamidine
Erythromycin
Rifampin
Nitrofurantoin

ACID SUPPRESSION
H_2-receptor antagonists
Proton-pump inhibitors

OTHER
Iatrogenic hypercalcemia
Acetaminophen overdose
Methanol, ethanol
Propofol
Estrogens
Organophosphates
Amphetamines
Heroin

hypocalcemia, hyperlipidemia, and hyperkalemia. Circulatory failure may occur from fluid losses, bleeding, or pericarditis, whereas respiratory failure can occur with large pleural effusions, acute respiratory distress syndrome (ARDS), disseminated intravascular coagulation (DIC), or aspiration. Renal failure can occur secondary to hypovolemic shock, DIC, or vascular thrombosis. Other complications include ileus, stress ulcers, bile duct strictures or rupture, portal vein thrombosis, abscesses, fluid collections, and pseudocysts.

References

1. Werlin SL, Kugathasan S, Frautschy BC. Pancreatitis in children. *J pediatr gastroenterol nutr* 2003;37:591–595.
2. Benifla M, Weizman Z. Acute pancreatitis in childhood: analysis of literature data. *J Clin Gastroenterol* 2003;37:169–172.
3. Gottschling S, Larsen R, Meyer S, et al. Acute pancreatitis induced by short-term propofol administration. *Paediatr Anaesth* 2005;15:1006–1008.
4. Goldberg DM. Proteases in the evaluation of pancreatic function and pancreatic disease. *Clin Chim Acta* 2000;291:201–221.
5. Kohsaki T, Nishimori I, Onishi S. Treatment of acute pancreatitis with protease inhibitor, H2 receptor antagonist and somatostatin analogue. *Nippon Rinsho* 2004;62:2057–2062.
6. Hoogerwerf WA. Pharmacological management of pancreatitis. *Curr Opin Pharmacol* 2005;5:578–582.
7. Mulligan C, Howell C, Hatley R, et al. Conservative management of pediatric pancreatic pseudocyst using octreotide acetate. *Am Surg* 1995;61:206–209.
8. Pandol SJ. Acute pancreatitis. *Curr Opin Gastroenterol* 2005;21:538–543.
9. Takeda K, Takada T, Kawvada Y, et al. JPN guidelines for the management of acute pancreatitis: medical management of acute pancreatitis. *J Hepatobiliary Pancreat Surg* 2006;13:42–47.
10. Scolapio JS, Malhi-Chowla N, Ukleja A. Nutrition supplementation in patients with acute and chronic pancreatitis. *Gastroenterol Clin North Am* 1999;28:695–707.
11. Moyshenyat I, Mandell E, Tenner S. Antibiotic prophylaxis of pancreatic infection in patients with necrotizing pancreatitis: rationale, evidence, and recommendations. *Curr Gastroenterol Rep* 2006;8:121–126.
12. DeBanto JR, Goday PS, Pedroso MR, et al. Acute pancreatitis in children. *Am J Gastroenterol* 2002;97:1726–1731.

Suggested Reading

Walker WA, Goulet O, Kleinm RA, et al. eds. *Pediatric gastrointestinal disease.* 4th ed. Hamilton, Ontario: Decker; 2004: Chapters 6 and 64.

CHAPTER 58 ■ ANEMIAS

JOSEPH ROSENTHAL

DEFINITION OF ANEMIA

Anemia is defined as a pathologic deficiency in oxygen-carrying capacity by red blood cells (RBCs). The function of RBCs is to deliver oxygen from the lungs to the tissues and carbon dioxide from the tissues to the lungs. This is accomplished using hemoglobin, a tetramer protein composed of heme and globin. The ability to transport oxygen and carbon dioxide is impaired in anemia. Anemia is characterized by a reduction in the number of circulating RBCs, the amount of hemoglobin, or the volume of packed red blood cells (hematocrit). Acute anemia denotes a precipitous drop in the RBC population due to acute hemorrhage, hemolysis, or abrupt interruption of normal RBC production.

The rate of reduction of RBCs is critical: an acute reduction in hemoglobin from normal levels to a level <8 g/dL will result in symptomatic patients (shock), while gradual and slow drop of hemoglobin to levels of 3 to 5 g/dL may be well tolerated by children with chronic anemia as a result of successful compensatory mechanisms.

INITIAL APPROACH TO THE ANEMIC CHILD

Because the normal range for hemoglobin (Hb) and hematocrit (Hct) vary with age and sex (Table 58.1), it is important to make sure a child is truly anemic before embarking on an extensive and/or expensive evaluation. The first step in evaluating the anemic child is to compare the patient's hemoglobin and hematocrit with normal values for children of the same age and sex. Spurious Hb or Hct results can occur due to sampling or laboratory errors. Venous samples are preferred and more accurately reflect the patient's Hb status. When capillary samples are obtained, it is important that the extremity is warm and that a free flow of blood is obtained. To ensure accurate results, an adequate volume of blood should be obtained to avoid excessive dilution by the anticoagulant. Analysis of the hemoglobin concentration is preferred as it is determined by direct spectrophotometry.

In defining anemia, the clinician should also consider the patient's utilization of oxygen and the accompanying cardiovascular compensation. Individuals with a clinical reason to have an elevated hemoglobin may actually be hemoglobin-deficient with values in the low normal range. For example, children with cyanotic congenital heart disease, respiratory insufficiency, or a hemoglobinopathy that alters oxygen affinity can be functionally anemic with normal hemoglobin levels. Anemia can be classified either by red blood cell indices (Table 58.2) or by the physiologic disturbance responsible for the anemia (Table 58.3). Once it is determined that a child is anemic, the next step is to evaluate the red cell indices. Of

these, the mean corpuscular volume (MCV) is the most useful. It is the only red cell index directly measured by the electronic counter and enables the classification of anemia by red blood cell size as microcytic, normocytic, or macrocytic. Although this classification is arbitrary and categories are not mutually exclusive, it provides a useful starting point for directing further evaluation (Table 58.2). The mean corpuscular hemoglobin (MCH) and mean corpuscular hemoglobin concentration (MCHC) are calculated values and generally less diagnostic. The MCH usually parallels the MCV. Both the MCV and MCH have small measurement errors and biological variation. The MCHC is a measure of cellular hydration status. It remains relatively constant throughout development and in most clinical settings. A high MCHC (>35 g/dL) is characteristic of spherocytosis, while a low value is most commonly associated with iron deficiency. The red cell volume distribution width (RDW) reflects the variability in cell size and can be used as a measure of anisocytosis. The use of RDW and the total RBC count aid in further differentiating between specific etiologies of anemia.

Microscopic examination of the peripheral blood smear can also aid in further focusing the differential. The clinician should assess the size, color, and shape of the red cells. The normal red blood cell is about the size of the nucleus of a small lymphocyte. On a well-stained blood smear the area of central pallor is seen in spherocytosis. Polychromasia with large cells is indicative of reticulocytosis. Distinctive abnormalities in shape are suggestive of red cell membrane disorders (e.g., spherocytosis, stomatocytosis, or elliptocytosis) or hemoglobinopathies (e.g., sickle-cell disease, thalassemia). Presence of inclusions such as basophilic stippling (i.e., thalassemia, lead poisoning) should be noted. Nucleated red blood cells are never normal, except in the newborn, and are indicative of a stressed marrow.

A normal erythrocyte lives approximately 120 days and then is removed from the circulation as it passes through the reticuloendothelial system. Under normal steady-state conditions, this daily loss of RBCs is balanced by effective erythropoiesis. Anemia results whenever the homeostatic balance between cell production and loss is disrupted. Because anemia is a sign of disease and not a final diagnosis, the goal of diagnostic evaluation of the anemic infant or child is to determine the cause of perturbed erythrocyte homeostasis.

In Table 58.3, the major childhood anemias are classified according to physiologic disturbance. Distinguishing between these causes can be daunting, but often is facilitated by a reticulocyte count. Most commonly, anemia is an incidental finding during routine screening of an otherwise well child, or an unanticipated observation during the evaluation of an acute or chronically ill child.

A detailed history (Table 58.4) and a careful physical examination are helpful in further defining the cause of anemia. In addition to the patient's history, a maternal history should be

TABLE 58.1

NORMAL HEMATOLOGIC VALUES BY AGE

Age (y)	Hemoglobin (g/dL)		Hematocrit (%)	
	Mean	Lower Limit	Mean	Lower Limit
0.5–0.9	12.5	11.0	37	33
2–4	12.5	11.0	38	34
5–7	13.0	11.5	39	35
8–11	13.5	12.0	40	36
12–14				
Female	13.5	12.0	41	36
Male	14.0	12.5	43	37
15–17				
Female	14.0	12.0	41	36
Male	15.0	13.0	46	38
18–49				
Female	14.0	12.0	42	37
Male	16.0	14.0	47	40

Hermiston ML, Mantza WL. A practical approach to the evaluation of the anemic child. *Pediatr Clin North Am* 2002;49(5):877–91.

included in evaluation of anemic infants (up to 6 months of age). Because many anemias have a hereditary basis, it is essential to include a thorough family history in the evaluation of any anemic child.

In obtaining the history, the relative frequency of the various causes of anemia with age should be considered. For example, iron deficiency anemia is the most common anemia of childhood. However, iron deficiency is never responsible for anemia in healthy term infants prior to 6 months of age. In the absence of blood loss, the term neonate is born with adequate iron stores for the first 6 months of life. The premature infant has lower total iron stores and can become anemic from nutritional iron deficiency at a younger age. More likely causes of anemia in the neonatal period include recent blood loss, isoimmunization, congenital infection, or the initial manifestation of a congenital hemolytic anemia. β-chain hemoglobinopathies such as sickle-cell disease or

β-thalassemia are generally not apparent until 3 to 6 months of age, when synthesis of the β-globin chain increases, whereas α-chain hemoglobinopathies are evident during fetal life and at birth. Iron-deficiency anemia is unusual in school-age children unless ongoing blood loss, malabsorption, or a very poor diet is concomitant.

Although relying on physical examination alone to diagnoses anemia has often been unreliable, the physical examination can provide several clues to the etiology of anemia. Tachycardia suggests an acute process with poor compensation necessitating prompt intervention (Section IV). A normal heart rate suggests a more chronic process. Jaundice points to a hemolytic process. Splenomegaly may be seen with inherited hemolytic anemia, malignancy, acute infection, or hypersplenism secondary to portal hypertension. The presence of petechiae indicates multiple cell lineages (i.e., platelets) are involved.

TABLE 58.2

CLASSIFICATION OF ANEMIA BASED ON RED CELL MCV AND RDW

MCV low (Microcytic)		MCV normal (Normocytic)		MCV high (Macrocytic)	
RDW normal	RDW high	RDW normal	RDW high	RDW normal	RDW high
Thalassemia trait	Iron deficiency	Normal	Mixed deficiency	Aplastic anemia	Folate deficiency
	C-β thalassemia	Chronic disease	Early iron or folate deficiency	Preleukemia	B₁₂ deficiency
Chronic disease	Hemoglobin H	Sickle/Hb C trait	Hemoglobinopathy		Immune hemolysis
	Fragmentation	Hereditary spherocytosis	Myelofibrosis		Cold agglutinins
		Transfusion Chemotherapy CLL, CML	Sideroblastic anemia		
		Hemorrhage			

Walters MC, Ableson HT. Interpretation of the complete blood count. *Pediatr Clin North Am* 1996;43:599–622. CLL, chronic lymphocytic leukemia; CML, chronic myelogenous leukemia; Hb, hemoglobin; MCV, mean corpuscular volume; RDW, red cell distribution width; S, sickle.

TABLE 58.3

CLASSIFICATION OF ANEMIA BY PHYSIOLOGIC MECHANISM

I. BLOOD LOSS
  A. *Acquired life-threatening blood loss*
    Traumatic injuries
    Massive upper and lower GI hemorrhage
    Ruptured ectopic pregnancy in an adolescent female
    Acute anemia due to disseminated intravascular coagulation
    Bleeding due to heparin induced thrombocytopenia
    Bleeding due to thrombocytopenia secondary to azotemia (renal failure)
  B. *Inherited syndromes of blood loss*
    Blood loss due to congenital bleeding disorders
    1. von Willebrand disease
    2. Hemophilia A (classic hemophilia)
    3. Hemophilia B (Christmas disease)
  C. *Blood loss due to acquired platelet disorders*
    Idiopathic thrombocytopenic purpura (ITP)
    Platelet function disorders, inherited or acquired such as in uremia

II. IMPAIRED PRODUCTION OF RED BLOOD CELLS
  A. *Deficiency as a cause of anemia*
    Iron
    Folate
    Vitamin B_{12}

Vitamin C
Vitamin B_6
Malnutrition
Anemia of chronic disease
  B. *Marrow failure*
    1. Inherited
      Pure red cell aplasia Blackfan–Diamond anemia
      Fanconi anemia
      Dyskeratosis congenita
      Pearson syndrome
    2. Acquired
      Severe aplastic anemia
      Erythroblastopenia of childhood
      Chemotherapy-induced anemia

III. EXCESSIVE DESTRUCTION OF RED BLOOD CELLS—HEMOLYSIS
  D. *Inherited*
    Membrane defects: spherocytosis, elliptocytosis
    Enzymatic defects: G6PD deficiency
    Qualitative globin defects: sickle cell syndromes
    Quantitative globin defects: thalassemia syndromes
  E. *Acquired*
    Autoimmune hemolytic anemia
    Secondary to auto immune systemic disorder

TABLE 58.4

IMPORTANT FEATURES IN THE HISTORY OF THE ANEMIC CHILD

1. Maternal history (for infant <6 months old)
   a. Pregnancy/delivery complications
   b. Drug ingestion
   c. Pica, nonfood-product ingestion
   d. Anemic during pregnancy

2. Family history
   a. Ethnicity
   b. Anemia
   c. Jaundice
   d. Splenomegaly
   e. Gallstone
   f. Bleeding disorders
   g. Cancer
   h. Transfusions

3. Patient history
   a. Hyperbilirubinemia
   b. Prematurity
   c. Diet history
      Type/quality of milk
      Ingestion of nonfood items
   d. Medications
   e. Activity level
   f. Acute or recent infection
   g. Evidence of chronic infection/disease
   h. Evidence of endocrinopathy
   i. Evidence of liver disease
   j. Easy bruising/blood loss

HEMOLYTIC ANEMIAS

Sickle-Cell Anemia

Sickle-cell anemia is an inherited disorder present in about 1 in 500 African Americans and to a lesser extent in other ethnic groups. The presence of Hgb S in sickle-cell disease and trait is detected by the characteristic pattern on Hgb electrophoresis. Hgb S polymerizes to form rigid, nondeformable, sickle-shaped RBCs that are trapped in the reticuloendothelial (RE) system. The deformed cells also occlude capillary beds throughout the body, causing tissue anoxic injury, organ dysfunction, and severe pain. These vaso-occlusive events (painful crises) represent the most frequently encountered acute complication in patients with sickle-cell disease. In addition, splenic sequestration, increased risk for sepsis, and marrow hypoplastic episodes are potential complications (discussed below).

The anemia of sickle-cell disease (SCD) is typically a chronic, compensated hemolytic anemia with an appropriate reticulocytosis. The average lifespan of red cells of affected individuals is 7 to 20 days (normal, 100 to 120 days). Clinically, this manifests as varying degrees of anemia with a brisk compensatory reticulocytosis, tachycardia, a hyperdynamic flow murmur, scleral icterus, mild jaundice, hyperbilirubinemia, and elevated LDH levels. Characteristic findings on blood smear include sickle shapes, target cells, polychromasia, anisopoikilocytosis, and thrombocytosis.

There are two conditions in which an acute decline in hemoglobin concentration can develop in patients with SCD: splenic sequestration crisis and aplastic crisis. These are true hematologic emergencies associated with appreciable morbidity and mortality.

Acute splenic sequestration is a life-threatening emergency that can occur without warning in children with SCD.

Vaso-occlusion within the spleen and splenic pooling of red cells and plasma can result in an abrupt decline in hemoglobin concentrations and blood volume. The spleen may enlarge dramatically within several hours. This condition typically affects infants and young children with SCD whose spleens have not yet undergone autoinfarction and fibrosis. Splenic sequestration may be the initial symptom in as many as 20% of children with SCD, and one-third of children will have acute splenic sequestration before 2 years of age. Children with Hb SC and Hb S-beta thalassemia are at continued risk for splenic sequestration throughout childhood because of the lower incidence of splenic scarring and atrophy associated with these SCD hemoglobin variants. There is a 10% to 15% mortality rate from splenic sequestration if not recognized rapidly and managed effectively. There is also a 50% recurrence rate in survivors; hence splenectomy is recommended after the first episode of splenic sequestration.

Clinically, patients with splenic sequestration present with pallor, marked tachycardia, splenomegaly, abdominal distention, irritability, and hypovolemic shock. Laboratory findings include profound anemia with a brisk reticulocytosis. Occasionally, platelets are also trapped in the spleen, resulting in mild thrombocytopenia.

Treatment is directed primarily toward restoration of circulating blood volume to maintain adequate tissue perfusion. Emergent transfusion of packed RBCs is indicated for severe anemia (Hb <4–5 g/dL) or cardiovascular compromise. Cefotaxime or cefuroxime should be given to febrile patients for presumptive treatment of bacterial sepsis. Patients with sequestration crisis should be hospitalized in a monitored setting. Serial blood counts are followed to determine the need for additional red cell transfusions. As splenic sequestration abates, previously sequestered red cells return to the circulation. Blood volume and hemoglobin level may rise above post-transfusion levels.

Transient aplastic crisis (TAC) results from the transient arrest of red cell production in patients with hemolytic anemia. As a consequence of rapid hemolysis and shortened RBC survival in patients with SCD, a dramatic decline in hemoglobin occurs over a short period of time, often within several days.

Parvovirus B19 is the infective agent most often associated with TAC, and is the causative agent of erythema infectiosum ("fifth" disease), a benign, self-limited illness associated with a characteristic facial rash. Parvovirus B19 may affect proliferating RBC progenitors in the bone marrow with marrow suppression typically lasting from 2 to 14 days. More than 60% of children with SCD have serologic evidence of parvovirus B19 infection by the age of 15 years. Recurrent infection with parvovirus is rare. TAC also has been associated with *Streptococcus pneumoniae*, *Salmonella*, and Epstein–Barr virus infections.

Clinically, patients with TAC present with pallor, fatigue, and tachycardia. In contrast to acute sequestration crisis, splenomegaly is absent. Laboratory findings include marked anemia and severe reticulocytopenia. Red cell transfusions are indicated to ameliorate symptoms of severe anemia while waiting for the eventual recovery of native red cell production.

When severe anemia has developed over several days, patients may be at risk for volume overload if the volume is corrected too quickly. Therefore, correction of anemia with slow packed RBC transfusion, at 4 to 5 mL/kg over 4 hours, is recommended, and administration of furosemide should be considered. Serial CBC and reticulocyte counts should be monitored. Recovery from TAC initially is heralded by the appearance of reticulocytes in the blood smear and ultimately by return to baseline levels of anemia.

Acute painful episodes (APEs) are the most frequent complications in children with SCD, and were formerly referred to as painful vaso-occlusive crises. Fever, infection, dehydration, exposure to cold, stress, menses, alcohol consumption, and nocturnal hypoxemia are typical precipitating factors leading to APE. Acute painful episodes account for nearly 90% of all SCD patient visits to the ED and nearly 70% of SCD hospital admissions. There is much variability in the frequency and severity of APE experienced by patients with SCD.

In children and adolescents, the most common anatomic sites for APE are the vertebrae, ribs, and long extremity bones. Pain generally is diffuse and may be accompanied by low-grade fever and mild swelling of the affected areas. Children often experience pain in the same sites with repeated episodes, although this is not always the case. Although far less common than APE, osteomyelitis must be included in the differential diagnosis. Nonaccidental injury and trauma are additional considerations.

Dactylitis (hand-foot syndrome) is painful swelling of the hands or feet arising from infarction of the metacarpal or metatarsal bones. This presentation is often the first sign of disease in young infants with SCD and is seen rarely after age 4. Typically, the infant will refuse to grasp an object placed in the affected hand or to bear weight on his feet. Erythema and low-grade fever may be present. Other than soft-tissue swelling, there is no radiologic evidence that can identify an acute episode of dactylitis. Recurrent dactylitis can lead to a mottled appearance of bones on x-ray and possibly to shortening of the affected metacarpal, metatarsal, or phalangeal bones. Treatment of dactylitis consists of hydration and administration of analgesic agents, anti-inflammatory medications, and hot packs. Febrile patients should receive antibiotics after blood cultures are obtained.

Chest or back pain is a particularly worrisome symptom in patients with SCD. Painful rib infarctions can lead to splinting, atelectasis, and hypoventilation, which can generate a worsening cycle of infarction, hypoxemia, and progressive sickling. Clinical presentation, in addition to pain, may include tachypnea, labored breathing, diminished or absent breath sounds, and hypoxia. Continuous pulse oximetry should be instituted with maintenance of oxygen saturation levels ≥92%. A chest x-ray is indicated in any patient with hypoxia, respiratory distress, abnormal or diminished breath sounds, fever, cough, or worsening symptoms. Although adequate pain control should be provided, dosing of opioid analgesia must be monitored carefully to avoid hypoventilation. The differential diagnosis of chest or back pain includes acute chest syndrome, pulmonary infarction, and pneumonia.

Abdominal pain is especially problematic in patients with SCD and is thought to arise from ischemia of the mesenteric circulation. Tissue ischemia and hypoxia can lead to progressive sickling and infarction of various organs and tissues, particularly the liver and spleen. Hepatic infarction typically presents with right upper quadrant tenderness, jaundice, scleral icterus, nausea, and vomiting. Liver dysfunction and hepatomegaly can occur as a result of intrahepatic sickling, transfusion-acquired infection, hemosiderosis, and autoimmune hepatitis. Analgesia and hydration are the mainstays of treatment. Asymptomatic, pigmented gallstones have been identified in children as young as 3 years and occur in about 70% of patients with SCD.

Acute splenic enlargement with sequestration crisis can present with abdominal pain (see above). In most children, splenic infarction occurs with time. Gradually, the child develops splenic hypofunction that ultimately leads to a functional asplenic state.

The clinician must remember that in addition to abdominal complications specific to SCD, the differential diagnosis of abdominal pain includes more commonly occurring disorders (e.g., acute appendicitis, gastroenteritis, constipation). Further evaluation (especially radiology) should be considered in patients who have an atypical presentation of an APE, but many usual laboratory tests have limited utility. The level of several acute-phase reactants (e.g., C-reactive protein, fibrinogen, LDH, interleukin-1, tumor necrosis factor, and serum viscosity) changes during acute painful episodes, but the clinical relevance of these tests is not clear.

Management of acute painful episodes in a child should start with oxygen administration to maintain arterial oxygen saturation levels >92%. Intravenous hydration should be provided when necessary to avoid the development of dehydration with potential worsening of the painful crisis.

The use of pain medications for the management of painful crisis in patients with SCD is complex. Wide variation in treatment regimens exist among practicing physicians, and the subjective interpretation of pain is influenced by the patient's clinical condition, psychological state, and prior experience with pain control. Patients and their families typically begin medical intervention at home prior to the patient's visit to the ED or office. Treatment generally includes oral hydration and administration of analgesic agents, heat packs, and rest.

An accepted approach to pain management in the acute setting is titration of the analgesic until adequate pain control is achieved. The goal is to diminish the patient's pain symptoms as quickly as possible, usually by providing repeated doses of analgesic agents administered at frequent intervals. This approach requires careful and continuous monitoring, particularly in patients who are at risk for the development of acute chest syndrome.

Acetaminophen with codeine or ibuprofen should be given for mild to moderate pain, and are usually taken prior to arrival in the ED or office. Subsequently, these patients should receive more potent analgesic agents. Because of its low abuse potential, ketorolac may be useful and is approved for use in children older than 16 years old or weighing more than 50 kg. Ibuprofen and ketorolac should not be used in combination because of their additive side effects. Contraindications to ketorolac or ibuprofen include gastritis, peptic ulcer disease, coagulopathy, and renal impairment.

Morphine sulfate (MS) is among the most frequently prescribed opioid analgesic agents for patients with SCD. The recommended starting dose is 0.1 to 0.15 mg/kg/dose, although many patients require higher doses to achieve pain relief. Additional doses of 0.05 to 0.1 mg/kg/dose can be given at intervals of 15 to 30 minutes, as needed, to achieve adequate pain control. Meperidine and hydromorphone can be substituted in patients who report adverse reactions to MS. Repeated doses of meperidine should be avoided because of the reported risk of seizures. Patient-controlled analgesia (PCA), using devices designed to administer opioids on demand, has been effective in allowing patients to participate directly in their pain management. Children as young as 6 years can be instructed in the use of this method of opioid administration.

Febrile episodes are potentially serious in any patient with SCD. Susceptibility to bacterial infections is increased as the result of impaired splenic function (asplenia) leading to inadequate clearance of bacteria from the circulation (e.g., *Streptococcus pneumoniae, Haemophilus influenzae,* and *Mycoplasma pneumoniae*). The presence of Howell–Jolly bodies (nuclear remnants in the red cells) on blood smear confirms the absence of the spleen. Thus, febrile children with SCD should be evaluated immediately (i.e., physical examination, CBC, differential, reticulocyte count, blood culture, and appropriate radiographic studies) and treated with appropriate antibiotics. Children ≥3 years of age with a normal physical examination, CBC, and chest x-ray can be discharged home after one dose of parenteral antibiotic (e.g., ceftriaxone) and with careful observation and follow-up. Immunization with a polyvalent pneumococcal polysaccharide vaccine in infancy (3 doses by 6 months), at 2 years of age, and every 5 years thereafter substantially reduces the risk of pneumococcal sepsis. Daily amoxicillin prophylaxis should be considered for children less than 5 years of age.

Acute chest syndrome (ACS) is a serious, rapidly progressive condition that is the leading cause of death from SCD. The low-pressure, slow flow rate in the relatively hypoxic environment of the pulmonary circuit is an ideal environment for the polymerization of sickle hemoglobin. Bacterial pneumonia, pulmonary infarction with thrombosis, and fat embolism from bone marrow infarction are the principal causes of ACS. Pulmonary infection is common in children with ACS. Although *S. pneumoniae* and *H. influenzae* are the most common organisms, mycoplasma and chlamydia are being seen more frequently. Thromboembolic phenomena secondary to fat and bone marrow embolism have been well described as a cause of microvascular pulmonary infarction.

Typically, patients with ACS present with back, chest, or rib pain; tachypnea; difficulty breathing; and cough. Fever and hypoxia may be present. Lung sounds may be deceptively clear, but the patient is often in extreme distress. A chest radiograph is essential and may show evidence of uni- or multilobar infiltrates, an elevated hemidiaphragm, and/or pleural effusions. Laboratory findings typically include leukocytosis, a declining hemoglobin concentration, thrombocytosis or thrombocytopenia, and elevated LDH and bilirubin levels.

Intravenous antibiotic agents are indicated in the presence of pneumonic infiltrates because it is not possible to distinguish infection from infarction. Antibiotic agents should treat both community-acquired bacterial and atypical pulmonary pathogens. Cefotaxime or cefuroxime plus azithromycin or erythromycin are recommended. Opioid analgesia should be administered judiciously to patients with ACS to avoid potential respiratory depression, the development of pulmonary edema, and further hypoxemia.

Type and cross-match for packed RBCs should be obtained at the time of initial blood drawing. Administered blood should be sickle-negative, leukocyte-depleted, and matched for RBC minor-antigen phenotypes to reduce red cell antibody formation. Such transfusions improve oxygenation and should be considered early in the course of treatment with ACS. Exchange transfusion is indicated in refractory cases or in the presence of progressive pulmonary infiltrates. Unstable patients with ACS can deteriorate rapidly and should be monitored closely in an intensive-care setting.

Inhaled nitric oxide is currently under investigation as a potential therapy for ACS. It is believed to downregulate the expression of vascular cell adhesion molecule-1 (VCAM-1), which may play a role in red cell adhesion to endothelium exposed to hypoxic conditions. Although anecdotal reports exist, there is currently insufficient evidence to support the use of nitric oxide in the treatment of ACS.

Neurologic complications such as cerebral infarction and hemorrhage are common in the child with SCD. Ten percent to twelve percent of children with sickle-cell anemia suffer a symptomatic stroke in childhood, and an additional 20% have evidence of an asymptomatic cerebral infarction on brain MRI. In the child with a symptomatic stroke, the rapid institution of transfusions often can reverse motor deficits that otherwise become life-long. Children with asymptomatic cerebral infarction on MRI also have been shown to have significant neuropsychological deficits.

Most strokes in children are the result of infarction, but intracranial hemorrhage also occurs, and increases in frequency in older children. The vessels of the anterior portion of the circle of Willis show progressive narrowing with eventual occlusion, collateral vessel development, and, often, progression to moyamoya. It is not known why children with SCD develop these lesions, particularly so early in life, but the altered rheology of the sickle red cell and the abnormal adherence of the sickle red cell to the endothelium likely contribute to endothelial injury in these vessels.

In the child who presents with an apparent cerebrovascular accident, exchange transfusions should be emergently undertaken. Initiation of this therapy should not be delayed pending further radiologic studies such as brain MRI. Exchange transfusion is undertaken to reduce the level of circulating hemoglobin S to less than 30%. After transfusion, children often have remarkable recovery from motor deficits; however, these children remain high risk for developing seizures. Once the patient has been stabilized, further radiologic confirmation of the nature of the cerebrovascular accident can be obtained. Usually a CT scan is obtained first, as this is generally more readily available and can show the presence of hemorrhage that may require immediate attention. Conversely, early CT scanning may completely miss the presence of a cerebral infarction and may appear normal. To detect a cerebral infarction, an MRI is definitive with immediate evidence of infarction. However, an MRI early in the course may miss the presence of bleeding. After a stroke, the affected child needs to be maintained on a chronic, monthly transfusion regimen to maintain the hemoglobin S level at less than 30%, and thereby decrease the risk of another stroke. Without transfusion therapy, a recurrent stroke occurs in 70% to 90% of patients and may be fatal.

In the absence of focal neurologic findings, the pediatric provider should be alert to some of the more subtle signs of an asymptomatic cerebral infarction. Changes in behavior or school performance can be subtle signs of an otherwise asymptomatic neurologic injury. In these cases, MRI and MRA scanning should be considered to rule out undetected cerebral infarction. Patients with asymptomatic cerebral infarction are at higher risk for developing symptomatic strokes, and MRA scanning may detect the stenosis of the circle of Willis vessels that predisposes to a clinically apparent stroke.

Because of the lifelong morbidity associated with strokes, there have been many efforts to identify which patients are at high risk for stroke. Natural history studies have demonstrated that the risk factors associated with stroke are different from those associated with other manifestations of SCD, suggesting a different pathophysiology. The risk factors identified to date include a history of transient ischemic attacks, seizures, low baseline hemoglobin level, elevated white blood cell count, systolic hypertension, and recent or remote history of ACS. Transcranial Doppler (TCD) ultrasound is a valuable tool in identifying SCD patients at high risk for stroke. Stenosis in the circle of Willis vessels results in an increased velocity across these vessels detectable with TCD. Although TCD is a valuable tool for the screening of sickle-cell patients, adequate training in the performance and interpretation of this test is critical.

Renal and genitourinary complications occur commonly with SCD, and manifest in a variety of problems including priapism, hematuria, enuresis, and renal failure. Enuresis is a common complaint from families with children with SCD. Unlike in other children, enuresis in the child with SCD is caused by nocturnal polyuria related to their kidneys' inability to concentrate urine. Because enuresis is the result of a renal problem, it can be particularly difficult to treat.

Hematuria is found on screening urinalysis fairly commonly in children with SCD. It is usually intermittent but is particularly concerning if found in association with proteinuria or hypertension. Proteinuria is a common finding in adults with SCD but can begin in childhood or the teenage years. Proteinuria is a harbinger of progressive renal injury and should be aggressively treated. Angiotensin-converting enzyme inhibitors (e.g., enalapril) have been shown to be effective in reducing proteinuria in these children.

Papillary necrosis also is seen in children with SCD, and manifests with the acute-onset of bloody or red-appearing urine. Treatment for papillary necrosis involves aggressive intravenous hydration and monitoring of hemoglobin level. Hematuria usually resolves with aggressive hydration, although bleeding can be prolonged. Frank renal dysfunction, as reflected by elevated creatinine, is uncommon in children with SCD, but glomerulomegaly and focal segmental glomerulosclerosis can begin as early as the second decade of life.

Priapism is common in pediatric patients with SCD and generally manifests in one of two ways. Young, prepubertal children often present with "stuttering" priapism consisting of short-lived episodes of penile erection, mild penile tenderness, and spontaneous resolution. Adequate hydration and treatment of any underlying infection are important, but more aggressive means are rarely needed because it usually resolves on its own. More concerning is the severe, painful priapism that develops in pubescent or older teens. Early recognition and treatment are critical, and priapism should be treated as a medical emergency. Initial management should consist of aggressive hydration and adequate pain relief. Priapism can be severe enough to obstruct the urinary stream, so urinary obstruction and urinary tract infection need to be quickly ruled out. Pain management usually requires the use of parenteral narcotics.

A variety of therapies have been reported to be of benefit in priapism, including oral alpha-agonists, alkalization of the blood, and direct injection of alpha-agonists into the corpora cavernosa. Rapid resolution of priapism can be achieved in most patients with aspiration and injection of alpha-agonists into the corpora cavernosum. When performed appropriately, this is a safe and rapidly effective procedure. Rarely do patients require repeated aspiration and injections for an acute event. After resolution, oral pseudoephedrine and antiandrogen therapies have been reported to be effective in preventing recurrences. Unfortunately, even with rapid treatment and resolution, a significant portion of young men with priapism develop fibrosis and impotence.

Avascular necrosis (AVN) of the femoral and humeral heads is a common complication of SCD and results in substantial physical disability. Although AVN of the humeral head is most common, this joint is not weight-bearing, and so disability is less frequent than with AVN of the hip. By 35 years of age, AVN of the femoral head develops in more than 50% of patients with SCD. Femoral head AVN can present in many ways, including reports of pain in the knee, thigh, or hip, or simply painless limitation of movement at the hip. A careful examination of hip flexion, extension, and rotation reveals pain or decreased range of motion, especially with internal rotation of the hip. AVN of the head is frequently bilateral but severity may vary between hips.

Therapy for avascular necrosis is largely supportive, with bed rest, NSAIDs, and limitation of movement during the acute painful episode. Transfusion therapy does not seem to delay progression of AVN.

Osteomyelitis is a bacterial infection of cortical bone and occurs more readily in children with SCD. Salmonella species, distinctly uncommon in healthy children, is the most common infecting organism, followed by *Escherichia coli* and other gram-negative bacteria. *Staphylococcus* accounts for only about one-quarter of all cases of osteomyelitis in SCD. Children typically present with fever, pain, tenderness, and localized swelling of the hand, foot, over a joint, or on the shaft of an extremity. There may be overlying cellulitis. The differential diagnosis of osteomyelitis includes APE and septic arthritis. Limitation of movement is generally more pronounced with septic arthritis. Unremitting pain, despite adequate analgesia, should heighten one's suspicion for osteomyelitis.

Orthopedic consultation should be sought to obtain a bone aspirate or biopsy for culture. Initial radiographs may be negative because several days to a week may be required to develop radiologic evidence of infection. Blood cultures and an erythrocyte sedimentation rate (ESR) measurement should be obtained. The ESR, typically very low in children with SCD, will be markedly elevated in children with osteomyelitis. Radionuclide bone imaging may be useful to localize the site of involvement. An important caveat: Patients with SCD frequently have abnormal bone scan findings due to previous bone infarctions. Areas of increased radionuclide uptake, which reflect healing bone, can make interpretation difficult.

Antibiotic therapy should be directed against both *Salmonella* and *Staphylococcus* species. Nafcillin or oxacillin plus ceftazidime are recommended. Vancomycin or clindamycin plus ceftazidime can be substituted in penicillin-allergic patients. Treatment may take as long as 6 weeks for complete resolution of the bone infection.

Acute cholecystitis and *cholelithiasis* are common in patients with SCD. Because of ongoing hemolysis, patients have chronically elevated bilirubin that leads to the formation of bilirubin stones and sludge. Stones can develop early in life, and any child who presents with right upper quadrant pain should be evaluated for the presence of cholelithiasis. The presence of biliary sludge does not mandate the removal of the gallbladder, as many patients do not progress rapidly to stone formation. If gallbladder stones are documented, the patient should be treated symptomatically with hydration and pain medications until the symptoms have resolved. Subsequently, the patient can be readmitted for elective cholecystectomy, as removal of the gallbladder during acute events should be avoided. After the gallbladder is removed, patients may still form stones that lodge in the common bile duct. Common bile duct stones often cause biliary obstruction and result in severe right upper quadrant pain and extreme hyperbilirubinemia. Patients with a common bile duct stone generally require more invasive measures such an endoscopic retrograde cholangiopancreatography (ERCP).

Thalassemia Syndromes

The thalassemia syndromes are characterized by decreased production of globin (alpha or beta) chains. Patients with thalassemia major (homozygous for beta thalassemia) develop severe anemia that requires transfusion from the first year of life.

Alpha thalassemia is the most common of the thalassemia syndromes. It results from the deficient or absent production of alpha-globin synthesis. Normally, alpha-globin chains bind with beta-globin chains to form the tetramer αα/ββ in hemoglobin A. The imbalance of alpha- and beta-globin chains creates the pathology in thalassemia. The clinical problems vary widely and the level of severity depends on the degree of alpha-chain deletion.

Beta-thalassemia syndromes are a group of hereditary disorders characterized by a defective synthesis of beta-globin chains. Beta-thalassemia major is the homozygous state, and beta-thalassemia trait (i.e., thalassemia minor) causes mild to moderate microcytic anemia.

A family history of anemia or the presence of microcytosis and mild anemia in a patient from the Mediterranean region should alert the pediatrician to the possibility of a beta-thalassemia trait. Similar findings in patients from Southeast Asia suggest alpha-thalassemia trait, beta-thalassemia trait, or a hemoglobin E syndrome. The blood hemoglobin concentration usually is low-normal with few or no associated symptoms, but chronic fatigue and pallor may be present. The family's name may not suggest the relevant ethnicity if, for example, the mother has taken the father's last name. It is particularly important to explore both the maternal and paternal family history for anemia because the potential for beta-thalassemia major or E-beta-thalassemia in future children is one of the primary reasons for establishing a diagnosis of beta-thalassemia trait or hemoglobin E in a patient. Aside from mild pallor, little is found on physical examination, and there is no enlargement of the liver or spleen in beta-thalassemia trait. Organomegaly suggests a more severe form of thalassemia.

No specific treatment is required for patients with beta-thalassemia minor. Patients, and in case of minors, their caretakers, need to be informed that the condition is hereditary and that physicians may misdiagnose the disorder as an iron-deficiency anemia. Some patients with beta-thalassemia trait may develop concurrent iron deficiency and severe anemia; they may require transfusional support if not responsive to iron repletion modalities.

Treatment for patients with thalassemia major includes chronic transfusion therapy, iron chelation, splenectomy, and allogeneic hematopoietic transplantation. The goal of long-term hypertransfusional support is to maintain the patient's Hb at 10 to 12 g/dL, thus improving the patient's sense of well-being while simultaneously suppressing enhanced erythropoiesis. This strategy not only treats symptoms of anemia, but also suppresses endogenous erythropoiesis so that extramedullary hematopoiesis and skeletal changes are suppressed. However, this regimen is frequently associated with manifestations of transfusion-related iron overload even with regular chelation therapy with deferoxamine. Lower target levels of hemoglobin are used to allow more effective prevention of iron loading, with higher likelihood of spontaneous pubertal development and without allowing excessive erythropoiesis.

Glucose-6-Phosphate Dehydrogenase Deficiency

Glucose-6-phosphate dehydrogenase (G6PD) deficiency is an X-linked trait common in the African-American population, having an incidence of about 10%. The ability of RBC to detoxify oxidants depends on the activity of G6PD. G6PD catalyzes the reduction of nicotinamide adenine dinucleotide phosphate (NADP) to NADPH in the hexosemonophosphate shunt. NADPH converts glutathione disulfide (GSSG) to reduced glutathione (GSH). GSH, in return, inactivates hydrogen peroxide (H_2O_2) and protects protein sulfhydryl groups from oxidation. In the absence of G6PD, the red cell membrane and hemoglobin can be damaged by oxidant exposure, leading to rapid hemolysis. Avoidance of oxidants (Table 58.5) and careful observation during stress (e.g., infection and surgery) are necessary. Patients with severe pallor or abdominal pain need immediate evaluation. RBC transfusion is sometimes necessary during episodes of severe hemolysis.

Hereditary Spherocytosis

Hereditary spherocytosis (HS) is the most common hemolytic anemia characterized by the presence of spherocytes (small ball-shaped cells instead of the normal biconcaved erythrocytes) and increased erythrocyte osmotic fragility. The disease is usually inherited in an autosomal dominant pattern but recessive variants occur. The primary defect is in the erythrocyte membrane cytoskeleton, a network of proteins underlying the lipid bilayer, including spectrin, actin, ankyrin, band 3 (AEI, the RBC anion exchange protein), and proteins 4.1 and 4.2.

Clinically, HS is characterized by the presence of spherocytes in peripheral smears with varying degrees of hemolysis and splenomegaly. There is increased fragility of the red cell membrane, leading to the vesiculation of the membrane, loss of membrane surface area, and trapping and destruction of the red cells in the spleen. The diagnosis of HS is suggested by asymptomatic splenomegaly. Splenectomy ameliorates the degree of hemolysis and is indicated in severely affected patients, but the intrinsic abnormality of the red cells remains after the procedure.

HS has a wide spectrum of clinical presentation, ranging from an asymptomatic condition that may be diagnosed in adulthood to a fulminant hemolytic anemia detected in early childhood. The morphologic hallmark of HS, the microspherocyte, is caused by loss of membrane surface area, so that the affected cells have a smaller ratio of cell surface area to cell volume compared to normal RBC. As a result, RBC survival is shortened and there is increased osmotic fragility in vitro. The

TABLE 58.5

AGENTS PRECIPITATING HEMOLYSIS
IN G6PD DEFICIENCY

MEDICATIONS
- Antibacterial
  Sulfonamides
  Trimethoprim–sulfamethoxazole
  Nalidixic acid
  Chloramphenicol
  Nitrofurantoin
- Antimalarials
  Primaquine
  Pamaquine
  Chloroquine
  Quinacrine
- Other medications
  Phenacetin
  Vitamin K analogs
  Methylene blue
  Probenecid
  Acetylsalicylic acid

CHEMICALS
- Phenylhydrazine
- Benzene
- Naphthalene

FOODS
- Fava beans in susceptible patients

Modified from Segal GB, Hirsh MG, Feig SA, et al. *Pediatr Rev* 2002;23:117.

major complications are aplastic or megaloblastic crisis, hemolytic crisis, cholecystitis, and severe neonatal hemolysis.

Hemolysis can begin in the first 24 hours of life, causing early neonatal jaundice. Hypoplastic episodes are also common following viral infection. RBC transfusion is sometimes necessary during episodes of acute hemolysis or prolonged hypoplasia. Splenectomy is necessary if the Hb concentration is persistently below 10 g/dL and the reticulocyte count above 10%. Splenectomy is usually deferred until after 5 years of age to minimize the risk of postsplenectomy sepsis.

Autoimmune Hemolytic Anemia

This group of acquired hemolytic anemias may be life threatening. The disorder is seen in association with autoimmune diseases (e.g., lupus, certain types of hematologic malignancies) or it may be drug induced. In about 50% of cases, there is no identifiable etiology.

This disease manifests itself with sudden pallor and fatigue, often following a viral illness. Because of the rapid onset, jaundice, hyperbilirubinemia, and reticulocytosis might not be present initially. The laboratory findings reveal a rapidly falling Hb, increased bilirubin metabolites in the urine, positive Coombs tests, and abundant spherocytes on the smear. The direct Coombs test confirms the diagnosis (the presence of antibodies or complements C3 and C4 on the RBC). The antibody specificity is detected by the indirect Coombs test. Hemolysis occurs with either IgG or IgM antibodies. IgG antibodies react at 37°C and do not agglutinate RBC in vitro, and thus are termed *warm* or *incomplete* antibodies. In contrast, IgM antibodies cause in

vitro agglutination at less than or equal to 20°C; thus they are termed *cold* or *complete* antibodies. The antibody-coated RBCs are destroyed primarily in the reticuloendothelial system; intravascular hemolysis is rare. The treatment involves hospitalization, careful observation, high-dose steroids, and if necessary, RBC transfusion using the most compatible blood.

Hemolytic-Uremic Syndrome (HUS) and Thrombotic Thrombocytopenic Purpura (TTP)

These syndromes are characterized by microangiopathic hemolytic anemia, thrombocytopenia, and renal failure (HUS) or central nervous system abnormalities (TTP). HUS and TTP represent different presentations of a similar disease mechanism. Endothelial cell injury appears to be the primary event in the pathogenesis of both disorders. The endothelial damage triggers a cascade of events that results in microvascular thrombi that occlude arterioles and capillaries. The platelet aggregation results in a consumptive thrombocytopenia. The epithelial damage that initiates this cascade often results from toxins released by bacteria, viruses, or chemical agents.

In TTP, the hyaline microthrombi occur throughout the microcirculation, and microvascular thromboses may be found in the brain, skin, intestines, skeletal muscle, pancreas, spleen, adrenals, and heart. In contrast, in HUS the damage is limited to the renal vasculature. In children, HUS often follows an infectious disease, usually diarrhea (90%) and less often an upper respiratory infection (10%). The most common cause of HUS is a toxin produced by *E. coli* serotype O157:H7. Additional agents include *Shigella, Salmonella, Yersinia,* and *Campylobacter* species. The Shiga and Shiga-like toxins, produced by some strains of *Shigella dysenteriae* and *E. coli* O157:H7, respectively, have been associated with approximately 70% of cases of HUS in children. In patients with organ or marrow transplants, HUS may be precipitated by immunosuppressive therapy with calcineurin inhibitors (tacrolimus or cyclosporine).

HUS presents in children usually after an acute diarrheal illness. The GI prodrome occurs a few days to a few weeks before the onset of HUS. Risk factors include eating rare hamburgers, visits to a petting zoo, or even a nursing home visit to a relative with diarrhea. The clinical picture can suggest a GI bleed, as opposed to toxic gastroenteritis, because the stool may be grossly bloody. The finding of grossly bloody stools in children is a strong predictor of *E. coli* disease, yet fever is often absent. Decreased urine output and even anuria may occur with HUS. Decreased platelet function secondary to uremia may lead to bleeding (typically with a BUN <80 mg/dL). TTP presents with neurologic symptoms, such as transient ischemic attacks, stroke, or seizures.

The hallmarks of HUS or TTP are thrombocytopenia, mild to severe anemia, and the presence of schistocytes (fragmented, deformed, irregular, or helmet-shaped RBCs) in the peripheral smear. These cells are the result of fragmentation of RBCs that occurs as the RBCs traverse vessels partially occluded by platelet and hyaline microthrombi. The peripheral smear may also contain giant platelets. This is a reflection of the reduced platelet survival time resulting from the peripheral platelet consumption and destruction. The reticulocyte count is elevated. A moderate leukocytosis may be present, but rarely more than 20,000/mm³.

Initial treatment should focus on supportive management, treatment of blood pressure elevation, blood transfusions, and hospitalization for adequate renal replacement therapy as needed.

BONE MARROW FAILURE/DECREASED RBC PRODUCTION

Aplastic anemia is a group of acquired and inherited disorders characterized by single lineage or multilineage deficient hematopoietic stem cells, hypocellular bone marrow, and peripheral blood cytopenias. The incidence of aplastic anemia in the United States is approximately 2 to 3 cases per million per year. These figures exclude patients in whom suppression of the bone marrow develops secondary to exposure to irradiation, chemotherapy, or other drugs. Normal blood formation requires replication and differentiation of hematopoietic stem cells in a microenvironment that includes stromal cells, lymphocytes, and growth factors. Hematopoietic stem cell numbers are markedly decreased in patients with aplastic anemia.

Residual stem cells appear to be qualitatively deficient as well. These deficits may persist even in patients whose peripheral blood cell counts return to normal. Different possible mechanisms are defects in stromal cell growth and impaired production of cytokines. However, these defects are usually mild and occur in a minority of affected individuals. The high cure rate after bone marrow transplants for aplastic anemia suggests normal marrow stromal cells in these patients. Hematopoietic stem cells from patients with aplastic anemia grow poorly when plated on stromal cells from normal individuals, whereas stromal cells from patients with aplastic anemia effectively support growth of hematopoietic stem cells from normal individuals. A variety of clinical and experimental data suggests that aplastic anemia is an immune-mediated disease. This includes (1) failure, in many cases, of marrow from an identical twin to correct aplastic anemia unless preceded by immune suppression; (2) autologous marrow recovery after rejection of an allogeneic marrow transplant; (3) improvement of hematopoiesis after immunosuppressive treatments (e.g., antilymphocyte globulin, cyclosporine, cyclophosphamide); (4) suppression of normal hematopoiesis by lymphocytes from patients with aplastic anemia; and (5) activated cytotoxic lymphocytes in blood and bone marrow that suppress hematopoiesis by production of gamma-interferon or tumor necrosis factor.

Inherited Marrow Failure Syndromes

Ten percent to twenty percent of all cases of aplastic anemia are secondary to the large group of congenital syndromes associated with anemia or pancytopenia. The pathogenesis of most forms of *inherited aplastic anemia* is not known. However, the poor response of most of these patients to immunosuppressive therapy suggests that nonimmunologic mechanisms may be operative. The most common syndromes are described next.

Fanconi anemia (FA) is inherited in an autosomal recessive fashion. It occurs in all racial and ethnic groups and is classically diagnosed between 2 and 15 years of age. The defective gene is responsible for impaired ability to repair DNA damage. This results in marrow failure, resulting in pancytopenia. There is also increased risk for malignancies, specifically leukemia; liver tumors; cancers of the mouth, tongue, and throat (head and neck malignancies); cancers of the female genitals (particularly labial and cervical cancer); cancer of the esophagus and intestines; and brain tumors. Neutropenia predisposes the patient with FA to infections, while the lack of platelets and red blood cells may result in bleeding and fatigue (anemia), respectively. Major findings on physical examination include:

- Café au lait spots (brown birthmarks)
- Short stature
- Abnormal thumbs, often including abnormal radii in the forearm
- Abnormal male development, infertility
- Small head
- Small eyes
- Abnormal kidneys

Dyskeratosis congenital (DC) is characterized by abnormal shapes to fingernails and toenails, a lacy rash on the face and chest, and white patches in the mouth. It is more prevalent in males (75% of all DC patients). Marrow failure occurs in about half of DC patients. The age of onset varies from early childhood to the seventh decade of life, in part because the findings on physical examination become more obvious with age. Two genes have been identified, an X-linked gene, DKC1, and an autosomal-dominant gene designated DKC2, hTR, or hTERC. The pattern of marrow failure varies from a single-lineage failure (anemia, thrombocytopenia, or leukopenia) to pancytopenia. There is an increased risk for malignancy with this syndrome, including malignancies of the tongue, mouth, and throat (head and neck); cancer of the esophagus, stomach, colon, and rectum (gastrointestinal); and leukemia.

Diamond–Blackfan anemia (DBA) is found in patients with a single-lineage failure of red cell production. All other blood cell lineages are intact. Physical abnormalities, involving mostly malformations of the thumbs are present in about 25% of DBA patients. Most patients are diagnosed with severe anemia within the first year of life. A mutation in the DBA gene is found in 25% of the patients; however, failure to identify this mutation in a patient does not exclude the diagnosis of DBA. There appear to be at least two other genes that can cause DBA. Currently, the diagnosis of DBA is based on clinical findings after exclusion of other known causes of pure red cell aplasia. Males and females are affected equally.

Pearson syndrome is a rare, multisystem, mitochondrial abnormality characterized by refractory sideroblastic anemia, pancytopenia, defective oxidative phosphorylation, exocrine pancreatic insufficiency, and variable hepatic, renal, and endocrine failure. It is diagnosed in infancy and leads to death in infancy or early childhood due to infection or metabolic crisis. In survivors of the refractory anemia, Kearns–Sayre syndrome (KSS), a mitochondrial defect, may occur. KSS is characterized by progressive external ophthalmoplegia and weakness of skeletal muscle.

Typically, the first defining feature of Pearson syndrome is marrow failure. A macrocytic sideroblastic anemia occurs with characteristic vacuolation of hematopoietic precursors. The anemia is refractory, and patients may be transfusion dependent. Neutropenia and thrombocytopenia also may be present. Other defining features of Pearson syndrome include exocrine pancreatic dysfunction and persistent lactic acidemia. Hepatic involvement may cause increases in transaminases, hyperbilirubinemia, hyperlipidemia, and steatosis. Renal failure may present with tubulopathy. The endocrine pancreas usually remains functional; however, a few patients develop diabetes mellitus. Splenic atrophy and impaired cardiac function have also been reported.

Acquired Marrow Failure Syndromes

Transient erythroblastopenia of childhood (TEC) is a slowly developing anemia of early childhood characterized by gradual onset of pallor. As the name suggests, all patients with TEC recover completely with no sequelae. The etiology of transient erythroblastopenia of TEC remains unknown, although an association with viral infections has been proposed. Several investigators found an association with parvovirus B19 (HPV) infection. Erythroid colony suppression has been suggested as the mechanism for the disorder. TEC is not caused by the lack of erythropoietin. Bone marrow from patients with TEC exhibits an absence of red cell precursors. The median age at diagnosis in patients with TEC is 18 to 26 months; however, the disorder may occur in infants younger than 6 months and in children as old as age 10 years. In contrast, Diamond–Blackfan anemia usually presents in the first year of life. The male to female ratio is 1.4 to 1.

Chemotherapy-induced anemia (CIA) is a common side effect caused by chemotherapy, affecting between 20% and 60% of cancer patients. The anemia is multifactorial but is sustained in part by the relative deficiency in endogenous erythropoietin associated with chronic disease. Prior to the 1990s, blood transfusions were the only means through which practitioners could manage anemia.

Diagnosis and Management of Aplastic Anemia

The clinical presentations of patients with aplastic anemia are related to symptoms of pancytopenia due to marrow failure. Complaints related to anemia or bleeding are most likely to be the presenting symptoms, though fever or infections are also often noted at presentation. Anemia may manifest as pallor, headache, palpitations, dyspnea, fatigue, or foot swelling. Thrombocytopenia may result in mucosal and gingival bleeding, or petechiae or ecchymoses. Neutropenia may manifest as overt infections, recurrent infections, or mouth and pharyngeal ulcerations.

With regard to environmental agents, the time course of aplastic anemia and exposure to the offending agent varies greatly, and only rarely is an environmental etiology identified. A detailed history should include recent exposure to solvent agents, radiation, environmental, travel, and infectious disease. An association between hepatitis virus infection and aplastic anemia has been documented.

In the absence of obvious phenotypic features, the presentation of a patient with an inherited marrow-failure syndrome is subtle, and a thorough family history may first suggest the condition.

Pallor and tachycardia from anemia, petechiae, or ecchymoses from thrombocytopenia or fever secondary to neutropenia are frequent findings at presentation. A small subset of patients may present with jaundice secondary to hepatitis. The presence of café au lait spots, microcephaly, microphthalmos, hypogonadism, mental retardation, and skeletal anomalies (particularly of the hand and thumb) should raise suspicion for Fanconi anemia or Pearson syndrome. The oral pharynx, hands, and nail beds should carefully be examined for clues of dyskeratosis congenita.

Determination of CBC and review of peripheral smears are the most important initial tests. Typically, a decrease in platelets, RBCs, granulocytes, monocytes, and reticulocytes is found. Commonly, mild macrocytosis is observed. The severity of aplastic anemia is determined by the degree of cytopenias. The corrected reticulocyte count is uniformly low in aplastic anemia. In patients with TEC, CBC results demonstrate a normochromic normocytic anemia and normal red cell morphology on the peripheral smear. Mean corpuscular volume (MCV) usually is within the reference range; however, MCV may be elevated if the patient has begun to recover and has reticulocytosis.

The peripheral blood smear is often helpful in distinguishing aplasia from leukemia or myelodysplastic syndromes. The presence of teardrop poikilocytes (an increased number of abnormally shaped red blood cells) and leucoerythroblastic changes suggest an infiltrative process. Leukemia may present with blasts on the peripheral smear.

Bone-marrow aspiration and biopsy are useful to assess cellularity, both qualitatively and quantitatively. Histologic findings with aplastic marrow include hypocellular bone marrow with fatty replacement and relatively increased non-hematopoietic elements, such as plasma cells and mast cells. Aspiration samples alone may appear hypocellular because of technical reasons (e.g., dilution with peripheral blood), or they may appear hypercellular because of areas of focal residual hematopoiesis. By comparison, core-biopsy better reveals cellularity. Evaluation of the marrow is also critical to exclude a leukemic process or myelodysplasia.

Patients with aplastic anemia may require transfusion support until the diagnosis is established and until specific therapy can be instituted. For patients in whom bone marrow transplant (BMT) may be indicated, transfusions should be used judiciously because minimally transfused subjects achieve superior therapeutic outcomes. Limiting or avoiding transfusions from family members may reduce alloimmunization against non-HLA tissue antigens found in family donors. With current standard practices in transfusion medicine, all blood products should undergo leukocyte reduction for prevention of alloimmunization and minimizing risks for transfer of cytomegalovirus infection. They should also be irradiated to prevent third-party graft-versus-host disease in BMT candidates. Judicious use of blood products is essential, and transfusion in conditions that are not life threatening should be performed in consultation with a physician experienced in the management of aplastic anemia.

The risk for serious bleeding secondary to thrombocytopenia in patients with aplastic anemia requires close observation of platelet counts. No standard parameters for transfusion have been established. In most cases active mucosal bleeding or widespread petechiae or ecchymoses will constitute an indication for platelet transfusion. An asymptomatic platelet count of less that 10,000/mm^3 will be considered an indication for platelet transfusion in most centers.

Infections are a major cause of morbidity and mortality in patients with aplastic anemia. Risk factors include prolonged neutropenia and the indwelling catheters used for specific therapy. For fever and neutropenia, broad-spectrum empirical antimicrobial therapy should be started with gram-negative rod and gram-positive cocci coverage based on local microbial sensitivities. Addition of antifungal therapy should be considered for fever persisting for more than 72 to 96 hours after initiation of antibiotic therapy. Cytokine support with granulocyte-colony-stimulating factor (G-CSF) or granulocyte-macrophage-colony-stimulating factor (GM-CSF) may be considered in refractory infections, though it should be weighed against cost and efficacy.

In patients with idiopathic aplastic anemia the standard of care is an allogeneic BMT if an HLA-identical related donor is available. If a donor is not available, a course of immunosuppressive therapy is indicated. Hematopoietic stem cell transplantation from an alternate source (e.g., unrelated matched marrow donor or an unrelated matched or partially matched cord blood) should usually be considered.

Due to the transient nature of TEC, no specific therapy with curative intent is indicated. Supportive care, mostly packed red cell transfusions, may be indicated in severe symptomatic TEC. Conditions in which transfusion may be necessary include hemodynamic instability, exercise tolerance, or altered mental status. Refractory TEC also may be associated with failure to thrive and may require packed RBC transfusion.

Pediatric oncology patients with CIA are treated according to preset guidelines. Hemoglobin levels or hematocrit levels below 8 g/dL or <25%, respectively, are commonly treated with packed RBC transfusions. Treatment with synthetic erythropoietic agents has entered the clinical arena in adult patients with CIA. Current efforts have become focused on providing optimal use of these agents by developing an understanding of CIA and the implications of preventing or appropriately managing CIA. Several clinical trails have demonstrated that appropriate treatment with erythropoietic agents greatly reduces the need for blood transfusions and the associated complications in patients undergoing chemotherapy. The use in pediatric patients with CIA remains under investigation.

Selected Readings

Beutler E. G6PD deficiency. *Blood* 1994;84:3613–3636.

Brodsky R. Acquired severe aplastic anemia in children: is there a standard of care? *Pediatr Blood Cancer* 2004;43:711–712.

Brodsky RA, Jones RJ. Aplastic anemia. *Lancet* 2005;365:1647–1656.

Buchanan GR, DeBaun MR, Quinn CT, et al. Sickle cell disease. The Educational Program of the American Society of Hematology (ASH) Annual meeting 2004;35–47.

Fixler J, Stles L. Sickle cell disease. *Pediatr Clin North Am* 2002;49:1193–1210.

Guardiola P, Socie G, Li X, et al. Acute graft-versus-host disease inpatients with Fanconi anemia or acquired aplastic anemia undergoing bone marrow transplantation from HLA-identical sibling donors: risk factors and influence on outcome. *Blood* 2004;103:73–77.

Hermiston ML, Mentzar WC. A practical approach to the evaluation of the anemic child. *Pediatr Clin North Am* 2002;49:877–891.

McSherry KJ, Baron BJ, Skavik KL. Emergency management of children with sickle cell anemia. *Pediatr Emerg Med Rep* 2005;10:129–140.

Sadowitz PO, Amanullah S, Soud A. Hematologic emergencies in the pediatric emergency room. *Emerg Med Clin North Am* 2002;20:177–198.

Tse WT, Lux SE. Red blood cell membrane disorders. *Br J Haematol* 1999;104:2–13.

Walters MC, Ableson HT. Interpretation of the complete blood count. *Pediatr Clin North Am* 1996;43:599–622.

CHAPTER 59 ■ COAGULATION AND THROMBOTIC DISORDERS

AMY E. LOVEJOY AND GUY YOUNG

OVERVIEW OF HEMOSTASIS

Hemostasis is the result of a dynamic interplay between pro-coagulant and anticoagulant forces. When blood vessel injury occurs, an immediate response of plasma and cellular components must occur in order to minimize bleeding and begin tissue repair; however, this process must be confined to the area of injury such that pathologic thrombosis does not occur. Initiation of coagulation is often described in three phases—the vascular phase, the platelet phase, and the plasma phase—all of which occur simultaneously.

The vascular phase is mediated by the release of local vasoactive agents and results in vasoconstriction at the site of injury. An intact endothelial cell lining promotes the fluidity of blood by secreting substances such as prostaglandin-I2, which inhibits blood coagulation and platelet aggregation and promotes fibrinolysis. Once blood vessel injury occurs, the underlying subendothelium is exposed and procoagulant proteins such as tissue factor and come into contact with blood. Platelets then bind through von Willebrand factor (VWF) to the subendothelium, which initiates the second phase of coagulation. Once platelets are bound to the subendothelium, platelets are activated and bind fibrinogen and VWF, leading to platelet aggregation, which forms the platelet plug. The initiation of the plasma phase occurs on the platelet surface with expression of tissue factor from the subendothelium. Tissue factor binds activated factor VIIa (FVIIa), which then activates FX and FIX. Factor X then converts a small amount of prothrombin to thrombin. This relatively small amount of thrombin leads to the activation of FVIII, which in the presence of the now-activated FIX leads to the conversion of a large amount of FX. Thrombin also leads to the activation of FVa, which catalyzes the conversion by FXa of a large amount of prothrombin to thrombin, resulting in the thrombin burst, which is the key step on formation of a stable clot. Thrombin then catalyzes fibrinogen conversion to fibrin, which is then cross-linked by factor XIII and made resistant to fibrinolysis by thrombin-activatable fibrinolysis inhibitor (TAFI) and a stable clot is formed. The first part of this chapter will discuss disorders of clot formation that result in bleeding diatheses.

Once clot formation occurs, anticoagulant forces must be activated to confine the clot to the site of injury. Dissolution of the clot over time helps promote wound healing. The second half of the chapter will discuss disorders of thrombosis, which can occur if the procoagulant forces overwhelm the fibrinolytic system and result in pathologic clot formation.

APPROACH TO THE BLEEDING PATIENT

Patients with bleeding may have abnormalities at any step in the hemostatic process including the endothelium, platelet, and plasma clotting factors. The history and physical exam are important for guiding the diagnostic workup. A history of bleeding should include the site(s) of bleeding, duration and age at onset, as well as elucidating a history of bleeding when the hemostatic system is challenged (e.g., by surgery or menstruation). Family history of bleeding should be reviewed, as many bleeding disorders are inherited. Physical examination findings suggestive of a bleeding disorder include bruising that is in unusual locations or out of proportion to sustained trauma, petechiae, or any visible bleeding. The usual laboratory tests performed initially include a complete blood count and screening coagulation assays including a prothrombin time (PT) and activated partial thromboplastin time (aPTT). A basic workup is shown in Table 59.1. The specific tests should be based on the initial laboratory findings and continued review of the history and physical findings. Platelet function assays such as the platelet function analyzer-100 (PFA-100) and platelet aggregation studies and testing for von Willebrand disease may be undertaken if the history is suggestive of von Willebrand disease or platelet dysfunction (e.g., mucocutaneous bleeding). Well-appearing children with long-standing bleeding symptoms may be more likely to have congenital bleeding disorders whereas ill-appearing or acute bleeding may be secondary to an acquired bleeding condition.

COMMON COAGULATION DISORDERS

Hemophilia

Background

Hemophilia results from congenital or acquired deficiency of clotting proteins, termed *factors*, though the term *hemophilia* most often refers to deficiencies of FVIII (hemophilia A) and FIX (hemophilia B). Because FVIII and FIX deficiency are X-linked, the vast majority of patients are male. Neonates often present with excessive bleeding after heel sticks, circumcision, or excessive bleeding associated with birth trauma. Older children present with easy bruising, hematomas with mild trauma, oropharyngeal bleeding, joint and muscle bleeding with or without trauma, and rarely, intracranial hemorrhage.

TABLE 59.1

BASIC BLEEDING DISORDER WORKUP

FIRST-LINE TESTING
CBC with platelet count PT, aPTT, fibrinogen,
1:1 mix PT, aPTT if prolonged
Specific factor assays if PT or PTT prolonged
von Willebrand testing (vWF:ag, vWF:Rco, FVIII
activity and vWF multimers)

SECOND-LINE TESTING
Thrombin Time
Factor XIII activity
Platelet function analyzer 100
Platelet aggregation

PT, protime; aPTT, activated partial thromboplastin time;
VWF:Ag, von Willebrand factor antigen, VWF:Rco,
ristocetin cofactor activity.

Hemophilia can be mild, moderate or severe depending on the plasma level of clotting factor. Patients with mild hemophilia A or B have 5% to 30% of clotting factor activity and usually only bleed excessively after trauma or surgery. Moderate hemophilia patients have 1% to 5% of FVIII or FIX activity and can have excessive bleeding after minor trauma or minor surgery. Patients with severe hemophilia have essentially no measurable level of FVIII or FIX and have spontaneous bleeding into their joints and muscles or excessive bleeding after minor trauma or surgery. Recurrent bleeding into joints, a hallmark of severe hemophilia, can result in progressive arthropathy, potentially leading to significant disability.

Diagnosis

Fetal testing can be done if the mother is a known carrier but is not universally available and generally not indicated as persons with hemophilia can lead relatively normal and productive lives with currently available treatment. Neonatal testing is indicated if the mother is a known carrier and can be done utilizing a specimen from cord blood immediately after delivery. If there is no family history, patients suspected of having hemophilia can be

identified initially by demonstrating an abnormal aPTT (activated parial thromboplastin time) and the diagnosis can be confirmed by a FVIII or FIX assay. Once hemophilia is diagnosed (or suspected), a referral to a federally designated hemophilia treatment center (HTC) should be made, as patients treated at HTCs have been shown to have less morbidity and mortality (1).

Treatment

Prior to the development of clotting factor concentrates in the 1970s, patients with hemophilia often developed debilitating and crippling joint disease. With the advent of factor replacement therapy, joint bleeding (as well as other bleeding) was more effectively treated and the complications of acute and chronic joint bleeding lessened. Tragically, many hemophilia patients became infected with HIV and hepatitis as a result of contaminated blood products in the late 1970s and 1980s. Since 1985 for HIV and 1992 for hepatitis C, screening of blood products as well as various viral inactivation methods of factor replacement products have lead to safer clotting concentrates with no known cases of transmission of HIV since 1985 and hepatitis C since 1992. Purified plasma concentrates are still utilized for treatment, especially in developing countries, as these products are much less expensive than recombinant factors (2). Currently, recombinant factor concentrates are available for deficiencies of both FVIII and FIX and are considered the standard of care in the United States (3). Mild FVIII deficiency patients can sometimes be managed with desmopressin (DDAVP), which causes release of VWF from the endothelium and thus raises FVIII levels. Current acute management for factor replacement for different types of bleeding is shown in Table 59.2, but should be modified according to the severity of bleeding and the individual response to therapy under the guidance of a pediatric hematologist. Adjunctive therapies such as aminocaproic acid and topical hemostatic agents (topical thrombin and fibrin sealants) should be considered for the management of bleeding episodes, especially mucus membrane bleeding.

The development of neutralizing antibodies directed against factor VIII or factor IX is a serious complication of hemophilia. These neutralizing antibodies are termed *inhibitors*, and can occur in up to 30% of severe FVIII patients, but are much lower in FIX-deficient patients. Inhibitors are categorized as low or high titer and low or high responding inhibitors (4). The management of acute bleeding in patients with

TABLE 59.2

REPLACEMENT FOR FACTORS VIII AND IX DEFICIENCY

Product	Dose	Indication
FACTOR VIII DEFICIENCY		
Recombinant FVIII	50 U/kg daily or twice daily	Severe bleeding, including joint bleeds, intracranial hemorrhage and large musculoskeletal bleeds
	30 U/kg daily	Mild to moderate bleeding, oropharyngeal bleeding, epistaxis, small muscle bleeds
FACTOR IX DEFICIENCY		
Recombinant FIX	130 U/kg daily	Severe bleeding as above
	65 U/kg daily	Mild to moderate bleeding as above
Plasma-derived FIX	100 U/kg	Severe bleeding
	50 U/kg	Mild to moderate bleeding

inhibitors depends on their inhibitor titer and on whether they are a low or high responder (a high responder will develop a rapid rise in inhibitor titer upon exposure to factor). For patients with low titer, low responding inhibitors, factor replacement with FVIII or FIX concentrates is usually effective although higher doses are required in order to overcome the inhibitor. For patients with high titer inhibitors, factor replacement is ineffective, as the antibody quickly removes the factor from circulation, and the bypassing agents are the treatment of choice. Bypassing agents such as recombinant FVIIa and activated prothrombin complex concentrates or porcine FVIII (for FVIII deficiency) are used for acute bleeding symptoms and should be managed by a pediatric hematologist familiar with hemophilia (5,6). Immune tolerance therapy should also be instituted in patients with inhibitors and is directed at eradicating inhibitors with daily exposure over weeks to years of FVIII or FIX concentrate.

von Willebrand Disease

von Willebrand disease (vWD) is an autosomally inherited congenital bleeding disorder caused by a deficiency (type 1), dysfunction (type 2), or absence (type 3) of von Willebrand factor. It is the most common bleeding disorder, present in 1% of the population. von Willebrand factor (vWF) has two main functions: (1) it binds factor VIII in plasma and protects it from degradation, and (2) it mediates platelet/endothelial cell interactions and promotes the formation of a platelet plug (7). Deficiency of vWF results in mucocutaneous bleeding with easy bruising, epistaxis, menorrhagia, and prolonged bleeding from dental extractions, trauma, or surgery.

Subtypes of vWD are listed in Table 59.3. Type 1 vWD is the most common form and results from mild to moderate quantitative deficiency of vWF. Type 2 is subdivided into four types, 2A, 2B, 2M and 2N, which all result from qualitative defects of vWF. Type 3 von Willebrand patients have a complete deficiency of vWF and have bleeding similar to patients with severe hemophilia. Platelet type vWD results from a mutation in platelet glycoprotein receptor GP1b and has symptoms similar to type 2 vWD. Acquired von Willebrand syndrome can also occur and has been associated with malignancy, autoimmune disorders, and rarely, the use of valproic acid (8).

Diagnosis

Diagnostic tests for vWD should include factor VIII activity, VWF:Rco (ristocetin cofactor activity or von Willebrand activity), vWF antigen, and vWF multimers. An assay to determine vWF binding to collagen is also available at specialty laboratories and can assist in making the diagnosis, especially in patients in whom the ristocetin cofactor activity is normal. The bleeding time has been used in the past but is not specific for vWD. The aPTT can be prolonged but may be normal in vWD. Table 59.3 shows the levels of the diagnostic tests in the different sub-types of von Willebrand disease.

Treatment

Treatment is dependent on the site of bleeding as well as the particular subtype, as shown in Table 59.3. Desmopressin (DDAVP) can be effective in type 1 and occasionally type 2A vWD and results in the release of stored vWF from the endothelium. The individual response to DDAVP varies, and some patients do not respond with increased levels of vWF activity. Prior to using DDAVP, a patient should have a stimulation test assessing their responsiveness. Pasturized, purified plasma-derived von Willebrand factor concentrates are also available for patients with type 1 vWD who either do not respond to DDAVP or for patients with types 2 and 3 vWD. Adjunctive agents as described for hemophilia should also be considered.

Patients with platelet type vWD require platelet transfusions for significant bleeding. Consultation with a hematologist for the diagnosis and ongoing management of vWD is suggested.

Platelet Disorders

Platelets play an important role in hemostasis by binding to the subendothelium when injury occurs and aggregating to form a platelet plug. In addition, coagulation factors are activated on the surface of platelets, and factor V and other proteins are released from platelet granules to assist with clot formation. Mucocutaneous bleeding is the hallmark of platelet dysfunction, although any type of bleeding can occur. Problems with platelet number or platelet function can both lead to bleeding.

Inherited platelet disorders are not uncommon, and multiple defects of platelet structure and function have been characterized. The best-characterized platelet disorders are listed in Table 59.4. Inherited disorders can present with thrombocytopenia (Wiskott–Aldrich syndrome, X-linked thrombocytopenias, macrothrombocytopenias) or with a normal platelet count but defective platelet function (Bernard–Soulier syndrome, Glanzmann thrombasthenia). A full discussion of congenital platelet disorders is outside the scope of this chapter and the reader is directed to the references provided (9,10).

Acquired platelet disorders are common and usually manifest as thrombocytopenia. The pathophysiology for acquired thrombocytopenia can be divided into (1) decreased production, (2) increased destruction, and (3) platelet sequestration. An overview of different disorders is listed in Table 59.5.

Idiopathic Thrombocytopenic Purpura

Idiopathic thrombocytopenic purpura (ITP) is a common autoimmune disorder with an estimated incidence of 1 in 10,000 children per year. ITP is caused by autoantibodies against platelet antigens. Serious and life-threatening bleeding complications such as intracranial hemorrhage are fortunately exceedingly rare despite the fact that the platelet count is often less than 10×10^9/L (11). Most patients with ITP undergo spontaneously resolution usually within a year of diagnosis (12). Chronic ITP, defined as ITP that lasts more than 6 months, can lead to life-long thrombocytopenia, although significant bleeding complications even in these patients is not common. The peak age of diagnosis is at 2 to 5 years of age but can occur in infants, older children, adolescents, and adults as well.

Diagnosis

The most common clinical manifestation is a healthy-appearing child with numerous bruises and petechiae or with mucous membrane bleeding. Platelet counts are usually less than 10×10^9/L and antiplatelet antibodies can often be identified in patient sera although the poor sensitivity and specificity of this test precludes its use as a diagnostic test. Triggers for autoantibody production include recent immunizations, viral infections, and medications, but no underlying causative agent is identified in most cases. Exclusion of other causes of thrombocytopenia such as malignancy, hypersplenism, drug-induced thrombocytopenia, other autoimmune disorders such as systemic lupus erythematosus, and infections such as parvovirus, human immunodeficiency virus, and Epstein–Barr virus infections, is important because ITP is a clinical diagnosis. Bone marrow aspiration to exclude leukemia is not usually necessary; however, it should be considered if the white blood cell count or hemogolobin is abnormal or if other symptoms, signs, or laboratory tests suggestive of leukemia are present. Furthermore, it is critical not to begin corticosteroid therapy for ITP therapy without consultation with a pediatric hematologist/oncologist, as steroids can partially treat leukemia.

TABLE 59.3

VON WILLEBRAND DISEASE SUBTYPES, TESTING, AND TREATMENT

	Freq (%)	Defect	VWF:Ag	VWF:RCo	F VIII	Plts	Multimers	Usual Treatment
Type I	80	Mild to moderate decrease in plasma VWF	Low	Low	Low/normal	Normal	Reduced amount of all multimers	DDAVP
2A	10	Lack of high- and intermediate-molecular-weight multimers	Low	Low	Low/normal	Normal	Absence of high- and intermediate-molecular-weight multimers	DDAVP or FVIII:vWF concentrates
2B	5	Reduced high-molecular-weight multimers due to gain of function mutation causing HMW multimers to be attached to platelets	Normal/low	low/very low	Normal	Normal/low	Reduced high-molecular-weight multimers	FVIII:vWF concentrates, no DDAVP
2M	1–2	VWF protein with abnormal GP1b binding	Normal	Low	Low/normal	Normal	Normal	FVIII:vWF concentrates
2N	1–2	VWF protein with abnormal binding to FVIII	Low/normal	Low/normal	Low/very low	Normal	Normal	FVIII:vWF concentrates
3	1–3	Complete absence of VWF	Absent	Absent	Absent	Normal	Absent	FVIII:vWF concentrates, no DDAVP
Platelet type vWD	1–3	Gain of function mutation causing reduced HMW multimers due to mutation on GP1B on platelets	Normal	Absent	Normal	Low	Reduced high-molecular-weight multimers	Platelet transfusions

AD, autosomal dominant; AR, autosomal recessive; VWF:ag, von Willebrand Factor antigen; VWF:RCo, von Willebrand Factor ristocetin cofactor; Plts, platelets; DDAVP, desmopressin.

TABLE 59.4

DISORDERS OF PLATELET FUNCTION

Disease	Genetics	Defect	Severity	Primary treatment	Hallmarks of disease
Bernard–Soulier syndrome	AR	Deficiency in platelet glycoprotein 1b	Mild to severe	Platelets	Defect of platelet aggregation. Giant platelets on blood smear. Purpura, mucocutaneous bleeding.
Glanzmann thrombasthenia	AR	Deficiency in platelet glycoprotein IIbIIIa	Severe	DDAVP, platelets, r FVIIa	Defect of platelet aggregation. Severe mucocutaneous bleeding.
Gray platelet syndrome	Unknown	Absent platelet alpha granules	Mild	DDAVP	Gray platelets on light microscopy.
Storage pool release defects Delta storage pool diseases	Variable	Impaired secondary wave of aggregation	Variable	DDAVP, platelets	
Wiskott–Aldrich syndrome	XLR	WASp gene absent	Moderate to severe	Steroids, platelets	Thrombocytopenia, eczema and recurrent infections.
Hermansky–Pudlak syndrome	AR	Absent platelet dense granules	Mild	DDAVP, platelets	Nystagmus, oculocutaneous albinism.
Chediak–Higashi syndrome	AR	Abnormal platelet granules	Mild to moderate	DDAVP, platelets	Partial albinism, immune dysfunction impaired leukocyte chemotaxis.

AR, autosomal recessive; XLR, X-linked recessive; WASp, Wiskott–Aldrich syndrome protein; DDAVP, desmopressin.

Treatment

The decision to treat ITP is controversial because this disorder is usually benign and self-limited; however, in many cases, treatment of severe thrombocytopenia, especially in active children, is suggested to minimize the danger of rare, devastating life-threatening intracranial hemorrhage (13). The agents used as the first line of treatment include intravenous immunoglobulin, steroids, and anti-D immunoglobulin (in Rh+ individuals). Platelet transfusions are only given in life-threatening hemorrhages such as ICH, as their effectiveness is greatly reduced due to the presence of antiplatelet antibodies. Splenectomy is utilized in either the acute management of a life-threatening bleeding episode or for management of severe, chronic ITP.

Rare Coagulation Factor Deficiencies

Deficiencies of other clotting factors are rare and include deficiencies of fibrinogen, prothombin, FV, FVII, FX, FXI, and FXIII. These rare deficiencies can result in a large continuum of clinical presentation from mild to moderate bleeding to severe, life-threatening bleeding. Factor XII deficiency does not result in bleeding complications and may even predispose to thrombosis. Treatment of these rare coagulation factor deficiencies consists of fresh frozen plasma, cryoprecipitate, or more specific factor concentrates where available. Current treatment options for these rare disorders are listed in Table 59.6.

APPROACH TO THE HYPERCOAGULABLE PATIENT

The incidence of thromboembolic disease is becoming more common due to advances in the management of critically ill children and children with congenital heart disease and cancer. The overall rate of thrombosis in children is much lower than adults with a rate of 0.07 per 10,000 patients with the highest rate observed in infants and adolescents (14). Spontaneous thrombosis rarely occurs in children and most cases of thrombosis can be linked to multiple genetic and/or acquired risk factors. The majority of children with congenital thrombophilia who develop clots have a recently acquired risk factor that triggered thrombus formation. Thromboembolic disease can occur in both the venous and arterial systems. Signs and symptoms of clot formation are dependent upon the anatomic location of the clot (Tables 59.7 and 59.8).

Diagnosis

Symptoms of venous thrombosis are secondary to poor venous return and manifest as pain and swelling distal to the occluded vein. This can occur in any extremity or in the head and neck with occlusion of the superior vena cava (SVC) causing superior vena cava syndrome. Headaches, emesis, and signs of increased intracranial pressure occur in cerebral sinus thrombosis. Venous thrombosis in the abdominal veins presents with pain and swelling of the affected organ, occasionally leading to organ dysfunction. See Table 59.7 for specific symptoms associated with different areas of venous thrombosis. Pulmonary embolism also occurs when venous thrombi travel to the lungs, which may result in hypoxia secondary to ventilation–perfusion mismatching and is one of the more severe complications of venous thromboembolism.

Arterial thrombosis is rare but must be recognized to prevent ischemia of the downstream tissue. Arterial thrombosis usually occurs in association with arterial injury or malformation. Neonates with umbilical artery catheters, children with vascular malformations (e.g., anatomic narrowing of the vessels), children with congenital heart disease who undergo cardiac catheterization, and children who have inadvertent arterial punctures are at highest risk for arterial thrombosis. Symptoms are associated with decreased perfusion, which in

TABLE 59.5

ACQUIRED PLATELET DISORDERS

INCREASED PLATELET DESTRUCTION
Immune thrombocytopenia
  Acute and chronic ITP
  Cyclic thrombocytopenia
  Systemic lupus erythematosus
  Evans syndrome
  Antiphospholipid antibody syndrome
  Drug-induced immune thrombocytopenia
    Chlorothiazides, estrogens, ethanol, tolbutamine
  Neonatal alloimmune and autoimmune thrombocytopenia
Nonimmune thrombocytopenia
  Thrombocytopenia of infection
    Bacterial, viral, protozoal, and fungal
  Thrombotic microangiopathic disorders
    Hemolytic-uremic syndrome
    Thrombotic thrombocytopenic purpura
    Bone marrow transplant–associated microangiopathy
  Congenital heart disease
  Type 2B vWD or platelet type vWD
  Disseminated intravascular coagulation (DIC)
  Heparin induced thrombocytopenia (HIT)
  Kasabach–Merritt syndrome

PLATELET SEQUESTRATION
Hypersplenism
Hypothermia
Burns

IMPAIRED PLATELET PRODUCTION
Aplastic anemia
Myelodysplastic syndrome
Idiopathic
Radiation and drug-induced
Marrow infiltration
Osteopetrosis
Viral infections (EBV, HIV, hepatitis)
Nutritional deficiencies (folate, B_{12}, iron deficiencies)
Anorexia nervosa
Giant platelet disorders
Malignancy-associated thrombocytopenia

the extremities will initially manifest as a cool, pale limb with a faint pulse that transitions to a purple and then black limb as the ischemia worsens and pulses diminish. Symptoms of thrombosis in the arteries of the chest and abdomen are more subtle and are listed in Table 59.8. Arterial thromboemboli in the brain or stroke is covered elsewhere.

A high index of suspicion is needed to diagnoses venous and arterial thrombosis. Quick reestablishment of blood flow is a priority to prevent post-thrombotic syndrome in venous thrombosis and to reduce ischemic tissue damage in arterial thrombosis. Laboratory testing should include a complete blood count (CBC), PT, aPTT, and fibrinogen level. Laboratory testing should also include the D-dimer, which if elevated is suspicious for thrombosis but can also be elevated in infection, inflammation, and disseminated intravascular coagulation. In addition, a negative D-dimer does not rule out thrombosis. Diagnostic imaging is required to establish or exclude the presence of thrombosis when there is a clinical suspicion. Multiple imaging methods are available for diagnosis of thrombosis. Angiography and venography are generally thought to be the gold standard for arterial and venous thrombosis, respectively. These modali-

ties are invasive and require interventional radiology techniques, which limits their usefulness. Noninvasive color-flow compression Doppler ultrasound (duplex scanning) is usually the first-line test and is sensitive for lower-extremity and abdominal DVTs and aortic and abdominal arterial clots; however, this method has poor sensitivity in the upper venous system. Diagnosis of thrombosis in the upper venous system requires either venography or more recently, MRV/MRA and CT angiography. It should be noted that MRV/MRA and CT angiography have not undergone sufficient study in the pediatric population to evaluate their sensitivity.

Treatment

In the acute phase, treatment is directed at reestablishing blood flow to prevent the ischemic complication in arterial thrombosis and post-thrombotic syndrome in venous thrombosis. Patients with severe or unresolved DVT can develop post-thrombotic syndrome, which consists of a clinical constellation of pain, swelling, and skin changes with visible collateral vessels, hyperpigmentation, or ulcers that can occur months to years after the initial clot (15). The incidence of PTS may be related to clot persistence, so acute treatment of thrombosis is important (16). Arterial flow must also be reestablished quickly in the case of arterial thrombus to prevent damage secondary to ischemia. Long-term treatment is directed at preventing thrombus extension, thus allowing the fibrinolytic system to resolve the thrombi and permitting the endothelium to heal. Treatment options for the management of thrombosis include thrombolysis, either with systemic or catheter-directed tissue plasminogen activator (t-PA), streptokinase, or urokinase; or by thrombectomy by interventional radiology or vascular surgery. Current anticoagulants used in children include the heparin-like agents, vitamin K antagonists, and occasionally, direct thrombin inhibitors. Aspirin and other antiplatelet agents may be considered in treatment and prevention of arterial thromboembolism. Treatment of any underlying acquired risk factor is also essential in clot resolution.

No large-scale prospective studies in pediatrics exist for determining the proper therapy. Treatment guidelines have been published to help guide treatment; however, the data are extrapolated from the adult data and the few uncontrolled or case series studies done in children (17). A pediatric hematologist with experience in treating thromboembolic disease should be consulted for patients with thromboembolic disease.

The initial management of thrombosis is dependent upon the severity of the symptoms. Severe symptoms such as SVC syndrome or pulmonary embolism should be managed with thrombolytic therapy as long as there are no contraindications to thrombolysis such as active bleeding, CNS ischemia/hemorrhage/seizures within 10 days, or surgery or other invasive procedure within 7 days. The majority of uncomplicated DVT can be treated with anticoagulation, which prevents clot extension and allows clot resorption; however, the need for quick resolution of arterial thrombi to prevent severe complications may necessitate thrombolysis despite the risk of bleeding (18).

The most common anticoagulants used in children are heparin, low-molecular-weight (LMW) heparin, and warfarin. Standard dosing of anticoagulants in children is not established and varies with the age of the child, volume of distribution, and concurrent medications and medical conditions.

Heparin and LMW heparin bind to antithrombin (AT), potentiating its ability to reduce thrombin generation. Unfractionated heparin is given by continuous infusion and requires frequent monitoring with the aPTT due to its unpredictable pharmacokinetics. Infants and younger children as well as patients with nephrotic syndrome have a relative AT deficiency, so monitoring and maintaining therapeutic anticoagulation can be difficult. LMW heparin preferentially inhibits

TABLE 59.6

RARE COAGULATION FACTOR DEFICIENCIES

Disorder	Laboratory abnormalities	Severity	Hemostatic factor level	Treatment	Hallmarks of disease
Factor II deficiency	Prolonged PT and aPTT, normal TT, low prothrombin activity	Mild to severe	20–35% normal levels	PCC/FFP	Associated with post-traumatic hemorrage and mucocutaneous bleeding, ICH
Factor V deficiency	Prolonged PT and aPTT, low factor V activity	Mild to moderate	25% normal	FFP/platelets	ICH in neonates
Factor X deficiency	Prolonged PT and aPTT, low factor X activity	Mild to moderate	15–20% normal	FFP/PCC	Autosomal recessive, mucocutanous and post-traumatic bleeding, ICH
Factor VII deficiency	Prolonged PT, normal aPTT, low FVII activity	Mild to severe	10% normal, 15–25% for surgery	Recombinant FVIIa,	Autosomal recessive, variable bleeding from severe to mild, potential for ICH
Factor XI deficiency	Prolonged aPTT, normal PT, low factor XI	Mild	>30% minor surgery, >45% for major surgery	FFP, FXI concentrates where available	Autosomal recessive, high incidence seen in Jewish persons of Ashkenazi descent, mucocutaneous bleeding but rare joint bleeding
Factor XIII deficiency	Normal PT, aPTT and TT, abnormal factor XIII activity	Severe	10% normal	Cryoprecipitate, FFP, factor XIII concentrates where available	Delayed seperation of umbilical stump, ICH, poor wound healing, miscarriage
Hypofibrinogenemia and afibrinogenemia	Prolonged TT and reptilase time, decreased or absent fibrinogen	Moderate to severe	80 mg/dL	Cryoprecipitate, fibrinogen concentrates where available	Moderate to severe bleeding, similar to hemophilia, can use cryoprecipitate as prophylaxis to prevent severe bleeding
Dysfibrinogenemia	Prolonged TT and reptilase time, low activity of fibrinogen on functional assays	Mild to moderate	80 mg/dL	Cryoprecipitate, fibrinogen concentrates where available	Associated with mild bleeding or can be asymptomatic, some forms predispose to thrombosis

PT, prothrombin time; aPTT, activated partial thromboplastin time; TT, thrombin time; PCC, prothrombin complex concentrates; FFP, fresh frozen plasma; ICH, intracranial hemorrhage.

TABLE 59.7

SYMPTOMS OF DEEP VENOUS THROMBOSIS BASED ON ANATOMIC SITE

Site	Pain	Swelling	Potential organ damage
Extremity	Limb pain	Limb swelling	Postthrombotic syndrome
Superior vena cava	Headache/neck pain	Head and neck swelling	Rare neurologic symptoms
Splenic vein	Left upper quadrant pain	Splenomegaly	Hypersplenism
Portal vein	Abdominal pain	Ascites	None
Renal vein	Flank pain, hematuria	Enlarged kidney	Renal dysfunction
Hepatic vein	Right upper quadrant pain	Hepatomegaly	Hepatic dysfunction
Mesenteric vein	Abdominal pain	None	Ileus
Pulmonary artery	Chest pain, cough, respiratory distress	None	Hypoxemia, respiratory failure
Cerebral sinus	Headache	None	Neurologic symptoms/seizures

FXa (more than thrombin) and is given via a subcutaneous injection every 12 hours. LMW heparin is monitored via the anti-FXa assay, as it does not affect the aPTT. Therapeutic anti-Xa levels for the treatment of DVT are between 0.5 and 1.0 antifactor Xa units. The pharmacokinetics of LMW heparin are more predictable than heparin, but the need for twice-daily injections and the inability to quickly reverse its anticoagulant effect can be problematic. The heparin-like agents may lead to heparin-induced thrombocytopenia, a serious complication of therapy, and long-term use is associated with the development of osteopenia. Warfarin is an oral agent that inhibits vitamin K epoxide, an essential enzyme required for the synthesis of the coagulation factors II, VII, IX, and X. Although warfarin is administered orally, its pharmacokinetics are unpredictable, especially in small children and infants, resulting in the need for frequent laboratory monitoring with the international normalized ratio (INR), a mathematical manipulation of the PT. Generally, the therapeutic range for the management of DVT is an INR level between 2 and 3, although it is higher (2.5 to 3.5) for mechanical valve patients. Many medications as well as dietary changes with fluctuating levels of vitamin K can significantly affect the INR. Antiplatelet agents such as aspirin are used in congenital heart disease and arterial thrombosis; however, they are not routinely used for venous thromboembolism as venous clots tend to be more fibrin-based.

Optimal doses and duration are not known for children and multicenter collaborative trials are being organized to determine the best dosing and duration of anticoagulation. It is suggested to consult a pediatric hematologist/oncologist with expertise in thromboembolic disease to assist in developing a treatment plan. If one is not available, refer to the previously published guidelines until such a consultation can be performed (19).

RISK FACTORS FOR ARTERIAL AND VENOUS THROMBOEMBOLISM

Acquired Risk Factors

The most frequent acquired risk factor is the presence of a central vascular catheter (CVC). Other acquired risk factors

TABLE 59.8

SYMPTOMS OF ARTERIAL THROMBOSIS BASED ON ANATOMIC SITE

Site	Signs of decreased perfusion	Potential organ damage
Peripheral artery	Color change, decreased pulses, decreased temperature, skin and limb ischemia	Skin necrosis, gangrene, loss of extremity, limb length discrepancy
Renal artery	Hypertension	Renal failure
Hepatic artery	Elevated transaminases	Liver failure
Aorta	Usually asymptomatic, discrepant upper and lower exteremity blood pressures, skin and bilateral limb ischemia	Usually none, but can see renal failure or limb abnormalities above if large occlusion

TABLE 59.9

INHERITED AND ACQUIRED DISORDERS OF THROMBOSIS/FIBRINOLYSIS

Inherited disorders	Acquired risk factors
Antithrombin deficiency	Central venous catheter
Protein C deficiency	Surgery/trauma/immobilization
Protein S deficiency	Sepsis
Factor V Leiden/activated protein C resistance	Pregnancy
Prothrombin G20210A	Smoking
Hyperhomocystenemia	Obesity
Dysfibrinogenemia	Medications including estrogen and oral contraceptives, L-asparaginase
Plasminogen deficiency	Congenital heart disease including artificial heart valves
Elevation in FVIII levels	Systemic diseases
Elevated lipoprotein (a)	Inflammatory diseases and vasculidites
Platelet glycoprotein polymorphisms, PAI-1 polymorphisms	Diabetes
Reduced levels of tissue plasminogen activator (t-PA)	Renal disease (nephrotic syndrome)
	Congenital heart disease including artificial heart valves
	Sickle-cell anemia
	Hypercholesterolemia
	Hypertension

for thrombosis in children include infection, surgery, trauma, malignancy, inflammatory diseases, autoimmune disease diabetes, renal disease, congenital heart disease, and sickle-cell anemia. Inflammation also may play a role in thrombus formation as generation of thrombin activates proteins important in the inflammatory cascade leading to activation of endothelial cells and platelets.

The presence of antiphospholipid antibodies such as lupus anticoagulants, anti-beta 2 glycoprotein I antibodies, and anticardiolipin antibodies is a risk factor for thrombosis that can be assessed via laboratory testing. Lupus anticoagulants are found in a high proportion of children with thrombosis and have been associated with pulmonary embolism (20). Thrombosis occurring in the presence of antiphospholipid antibodies is termed the antiphospholipid antibody syndrome (APLAS), and may be primary or secondary to another autoimmune disease. This condition is associated with a high rate of recurrent thrombosis and may lead to the need for life-long anticoagulation. Lupus anticoagulants can also be found transiently during an infection or even in asymptomatic children during routine preoperative laboratory testing. The significance of transient, asymptomatic LA is unclear, and laboratory assays cannot discriminate a prothrombotic LA from a transient LA, necessitating follow-up testing of positive results.

Genetic Risk Factors

Hereditary thrombophilia, defined as a genetic predisposition to the development of thrombosis, should be suspected in children with idiopathic thrombosis, for those with recurrent or severe life-threatening thrombosis, or in children with a strong family history of venous thrombosis. A list of the known thrombophilia disorders is shown in Table 59.9.

The most common thrombophilia in the Caucasian population is a mutation in factor V termed factor V Leiden. This change in the factor V protein slows down degradation of FV by activated protein C. Heterozygotes have a fivefold to tenfold

increased risk of thrombosis, whereas homozygotes have an eighty-fold increased risk of thrombosis in their lifetime (21). In general, thrombotic complications in homozygous FV Leiden occur in teenagers and young adults. Children who carry the factor V Leiden mutation are generally asymptomatic; however, prospective studies of children in whom thrombotic events have occurred have been found to have a high odds ratio for the presence of factor V Leiden. Children who carry multiple genetic risk factors are likely at higher risk for the development of thrombosis; however, studies supporting this notion have not been performed.

The need for treatment or prophylaxis against recurrent thrombosis is dependent upon the severity of the underlying disorder and the presence of acquired risk factors. Families with hereditary thrombophilia should be counseled regarding the signs and symptoms of thrombosis as well as avoiding smoking, dehydration, prolonged immobility, and estrogen-containing medications that may trigger clot formation.

References

1. Baker JR, Crudder SO, Riske B, et al. A model for a regional system of care to promote the health and well-being of people with rare chronic genetic disorders. *Am J Public Health* 2005;95:1910–1916.
2. Josephson CD, Abshire TC. Clinical uses of plasma and plasma fractions: plasma-derived products for hemophilias A and B, and for von Willebrand disease. *Best Pract Res Clin Haematol* 2006;19:35–49.
3. Kessler CM. New perspectives in hemophilia treatment. *Hematology (Am Soc Hematol Educ Program)* 2005;429–435.
4. Lusher JM. Hemophilia treatment. Factor VIII inhibitors with recombinant products: prospective clinical trials. *Haematologica* 2000;85:2–5.
5. Young G. New approaches in the management of inhibitor patients. *Acta Haematol* 2006;115:172–179.
6. Lusher JM. Inhibitors in young boys with haemophilia. *Baillieres Best Pract Res Clin Haematol* 2000;13:457–468.
7. Lanzkowsky P. *Manual of pediatric hematology and oncology.* 4th ed. New York: Elsevier Academic Press; 2005.
8. Federici AB, Mannucci PM. Diagnosis and management of acquired von Willebrand syndrome. *Clin Adv Hematol Oncol* 2003;1:169–175.

9. Hayward CP, Rao AK, Cattaneo M. Congenital platelet disorders: overview of their mechanisms, diagnostic evaluation and treatment. *Haemophilia* 2006;12(suppl 3):128–136.

10. Nathan D, Orkin S, Ginsburg D, et al. *Hematology of infancy and childhood.* 6th ed. Philadelphia: Saunders; 2003.

11. Di Paola JA, Buchanan GR. Immune thrombocytopenic purpura. *Pediatr Clin North Am* 2002;49:911–928.

12. Nugent DJ. Childhood immune thrombocytopenic purpura. *Blood Rev* 2002;16:27–29.

13. Tarantino MD. The treatment of immune thrombocytopenic purpura in children. *Curr Hematol Rep* 2006;5:89–94.

14. Journeycake JM, Manco-Johnson MJ. Thrombosis during infancy and childhood: what we know and what we do not know. *Hematol Oncol Clin North Am* 2004;18:1315.

15. Manco-Johnson MJ. How I treat venous thrombosis in children. *Blood* 2006;107:21–29.

16. Franzeck UK, Schalch I, Bollinger A. On the relationship between changes in the deep veins evaluated by duplex sonography and the postthrombotic syndrome 12 years after deep vein thrombosis. *Thromb Haemost* 1997; 77:1109–1112.

17. Monagle P, Chan A, Massicotte P, et al. Antithrombotic therapy in children: the seventh ACCP conference on antithrombotic and thrombolytic therapy. *Chest* 2004;126:645S–687S.

18. Young G. Diagnosis and treatment of thrombosis in children: general principles. *Pediatr Blood Cancer* 2006;46:540–546.

19. Monagle P, Chan A, Massicotte P, et al. Antithrombotic therapy in children: the seventh ACCP conference on antithrombotic and thrombolytic therapy. *Chest* 2004;126:645S–687S.

20. Manco-Johnson MJ. Antiphospholipid antibodies in children. *Semin Thromb Hemost* 1998;24:591–598.

21. Lanzkowsky P. *Manual of pediatric hematology and oncology.* 4th ed. New York: Elsevier Academic Press; 2005.

CHAPTER 60 ■ HEMATOLOGIC AND ONCOLOGIC EMERGENCIES

JENNIFER SCHNEIDERMAN AND DAVID O. WALTERHOUSE

Children with hematologic or oncologic conditions can present with pathology affecting virtually any organ system. The first presentation of a child with cancer to a physician can be very dramatic, as illustrated by a mediastinal mass that compresses the airways or with neurologic abnormalities caused by spinal cord compression, or more commonly relatively subtle requiring astute diagnostic skills by the pediatrician or emergency room physician. Once a diagnosis has been established an oncologist, and perhaps a surgeon, a radiation oncologist, and a nurse practitioner, will care for every pediatric patient with cancer for the duration of their cancer therapy, as well as for several years thereafter. Hematologic disorders of childhood range from chronic inherited conditions, such as sickle-cell disease or hemophilia, to acute acquired abnormalities, such as iron deficiency anemia or idiopathic thrombocytopenic purpura. Severe life-threatening complications of sickle-cell disease and hemophilia need to be recognized and treated appropriately, and identifying the patient presenting with autoimmune hemolytic anemia may be life-saving.

Most large centers have established teams that care for patients with sickle-cell disease and hemophilia that involve hematologists, nurse practitioners, physical therapists, dentists, and pain specialists. Fortunately, the prognosis for children with oncologic and hematologic problems has dramatically improved since the late 1970s as a result of many factors, including cooperative group clinical trials, for which the field of pediatric oncology has served as a model; neonatal screening for disorders such as sickle-cell disease to facilitate early recognition and immediate treatment for signs or symptoms related to the disease; immunization and antibiotic prophylaxis programs; and the development of new treatment strategies, including recombinant clotting factor concentrates that remove the risk of transmitting infection, and novel anticancer agents some of which are directed at molecular targets found specifically in cancer cells. It is essential that a pediatric hematologist/oncologist be consulted early in the management of these complex patients, whether at the time of diagnosis or during their course of highly specialized treatment. In this chapter, we will review the approach to managing some of the most common and critical emergencies found in pediatric hematology and oncology patients.

HEMATOLOGIC EMERGENCIES

Sickle-Cell Disease

Fever

Patients with sickle-cell disease are at 200 to 400 times higher risk for overwhelming infection with *Pneumococcus* due to functional asplenia than the general population. The introduction of prophylactic penicillin in children with all types of sickle-cell disease (SS, SC, Sβ-thalassemia) in combination with immunization against *Pneumococcus* has reduced the incidence of infection with encapsulated organisms by approximately 80% (1). Patients with sickle-cell disease who develop fever (temperature 101.5°F/38.5°C or greater) must be promptly evaluated by a health care provider. Those who appear "toxic," have an infiltrate on chest x-ray, or are under 15 to 18 months of age should be admitted to the hospital for empiric antibiotics and close observation. Older, nontoxic appearing children may be managed as outpatients with empiric antibiotic coverage.

Initial evaluation should include a blood culture, complete blood count (CBC), and chest x-ray. These tests should be repeated on subsequent days as clinically indicated. Particular infectious agents to consider in the early phase of therapy include *Streptococcus pneumoniae* and *Haemophilus influenzae* (though *Haemophilus* infections are exceedingly rare in this era of vaccinations). Patients with pulmonary complaints such as cough, shortness of breath, or chest pain require close monitoring of oxygen saturation and respiratory rate. The pattern of hypoxemia, infiltrate, and chest pain, which often occurs in the setting of fever, defines acute chest syndrome (ACS); in addition to antibiotics, red cell transfusion or exchange is indicated for these patients. Those with an infiltrate on chest x-ray may have antibiotic therapy broadened to include coverage for *Mycoplasma pneumoniae*, as this infection is commonly found in children with ACS (2).

It is common for children with acute bone pain due to vaso-occlusion to develop fever. Therefore, it can be very difficult to distinguish an uncomplicated painful crisis from osteomyelitis or septic arthritis, as similar symptoms (fever, pain, decreased range of motion, and swelling) are often present. Radiographic imaging is confusing in these children, as changes on plain film, CT, bone scan, and MRI are similar during episodes of ischemia and osteomyelitis. If osteomyelitis is suspected, cultures of the blood and bone should be performed, and antibiotic coverage broadened to cover *Salmonella* and *Staphylococcus aureus*.

Patients who become afebrile with negative blood cultures may be discharged following 36 to 48 hours of parenteral antibiotics. Those with documented bacteremia should remain in the hospital until appropriate information regarding bacterial susceptibility is available and should be treated for at least 7 days from the first negative culture.

Acute Chest Syndrome

Acute chest syndrome (ACS) is characterized by hypoxemia, a new infiltrate on chest x-ray, and chest pain, and is usually accompanied by fever (though fever is not a necessary component of the diagnosis). Children with homozygous sickle-cell disease (Hgb SS) are at the highest risk for ACS, followed by Hgb SC and Hgb Sβ-thalassemia. ACS is most likely due to pulmonary infarction, and may occur in the setting of pulmonary fat embolization from distant bone marrow infarction or infection/pneumonia (viral or bacterial). The most common pathogens isolated from sputum and bronchoscopy samples in the setting of ACS include *Chlamydia, Mycoplasma, Staphylococcus aureus, Streptococcus pneumoniae, Haemophilus influenzae,* and viruses (2,3). Patients with vaso-occlusive crisis of the chest wall are at risk for developing ACS due to shallow breathing and "splinting," leading to tissue hypoxia, increased sickling of red cells, and pulmonary ischemia. Therefore, patients admitted with acute pain episodes must receive medications to provide adequate pain control (with care not to blunt respiratory drive) along with close monitoring for subtle signs of ACS such as gradually increasing tachypnea or decreasing oxygen saturations. In addition, time out of bed and frequent use of incentive spirometry help to promote better pulmonary function.

If at any time the development of ACS is suspected, a chest x-ray should be obtained to evaluate for new infiltrates. Oxygenation status should be monitored by pulse oximetry or serial arterial blood gasses to determine the alveolar–arterial gradient. Patients with worsening respiratory status (increasing oxygen requirements, respiratory distress, or worsening alveolar–arterial gradient) should be in an intensive-care setting for close monitoring. Transfusion with packed red blood cells (PRBCs) to raise the hemoglobin no higher than 10 g/dL is indicated. Erythrocytapheresis (exchange transfusion) should be considered in any patient with severe, rapidly progressing ACS (or in those who already have a hemoglobin of 10 g/dL) to reduce the Hgb S percentage to less than 30%. Blood cultures should be obtained, and empiric antibiotics started to cover the previously mentioned pathogens (for example, a second-generation cephalosporin plus a macrolide). A complete course of antibiotics sufficient to treat pneumonia should be prescribed. A trial of bronchodilator therapy should be considered, as approximately 20% of patients with ACS have been found to clinically improve (2).

Stroke

Patients with sickle-cell disease who develop neurologic abnormalities (for example, altered mental status, seizure, facial palsy; or abnormal speech, strength or gait) must be evaluated for stroke. In contrast to stroke in adult patients without sickle-cell disease, stroke in children with sickle-cell disease is usually (but not always) ischemic. Immediately following evaluation and stabilization, a noncontrast CT scan should be obtained to rule out hemorrhage. An early ischemic event, which is more likely in children with SS, may not be evident on initial imaging; therefore magnetic resonance imaging (MRI) should be obtained in every patient with sickle-cell disease and neurologic abnormality once able. The current standard of care for patients with sickle-cell disease in whom a stroke is suspected based on clinical evaluation includes intravenous hydration and erythrocytapheresis to relieve vascular occlusion caused by sickled cells. The goal for erythrocytapheresis is to reduce the percentage of sickle hemoglobin to 30% or less. PRBC transfusion is an acceptable adjunct when exchange transfusion therapy will be significantly delayed. If simple transfusion is used as bridging therapy, the hemoglobin should not be raised to greater than 10 g/dL, as this carries the risk of increasing viscosity, thereby potentially worsening parenchymal ischemia. Given that the pathophysiology of stroke in patients with sickle-cell disease differs from that of the adult non–sickle-cell population, therapy with tissue plasminogen activator is not indicated. Patients who have experienced one stroke are at risk for subsequent strokes and are therefore treated with long-term chronic transfusion therapy.

Splenic Sequestration

Splenic sequestration occurs most often in children with homozygous sickle-cell disease between the ages of 6 months and 5 years. Acute splenic sequestration is characterized by rapidly falling hemoglobin, associated with an increase in peripheral blood reticulocytes, thrombocytopenia, and abdominal pain due to an enlarging spleen. Patients are at risk for hypovolemic shock, and therefore should be admitted to the hospital for serial CBCs and physical exams (including frequent assessment of vital signs and spleen size). Children with prior episodes of sequestration are more likely to have subsequent episodes. Treatment with boluses of normal saline and PRBC transfusion may be necessary; however, care must be taken to avoid overtransfusion as sudden mobilization of trapped blood from the spleen may occur. Splenectomy should be considered in those with recurrent, severe episodes.

Hemophilia

Although the majority of children with hemophilia can be treated as outpatients for bleeding into joints and muscles with a single 20% to 40% factor correction (20 units/kg for factor VIII and 40 units/kg for factor IX deficiency provide a 40% correction; see Table 60.1); others may require 50% to 100% factor correction (50 units/kg for factor VIII and 100 units/kg for factor IX deficiency provide a 100% correction) and admission to the hospital in order to maintain therapeutic levels for several days for head trauma, intracranial hemorrhage, large retroperitoneal bleeds, compartment syndrome, or pain control. Patients requiring surgery should be corrected to 100% prior to the procedure. Depending on the "invasiveness" of the procedure, therapeutic levels should be maintained for 7 to 10 days. In general, patients with suspected intracranial bleeds should be treated with the appropriate factor concentrate *before* a CT scan is performed to prevent rapid intracranial expansion of blood. Doses to replete the deficient factor to levels of 50% to 100% should be given.

When determining the dose, factor should not be wasted—whole vials should be used, with the dose "rounded up" to the next appropriate vial. If factor is not available immediately, fresh frozen plasma may be administered (20 mL/kg IV), but will raise levels to only 20% to 30%. Patients with an inhibitor (neutralizing antibody against factor VIII or IX) require therapy with bypass agents such as activated recombinant factor VII (90 to 100 µg/kg) or activated prothrombin complex concentrate (50 to 75 units/kg).

If the child has an intracranial hemorrhage or other life-threatening bleed, it may be preferable to treat with continuous rather than intermittent bolus factor replacement for several days in an intensive-care setting, thereby avoiding subtherapeutic factor level troughs that may occur when using bolus treatments. Daily monitoring of plasma factor levels will ensure that adequate levels are maintained. It is important to monitor the patient's hemoglobin closely for significant reduction, as red cell transfusions may be required in this setting. An orthopedic surgeon should be consulted when there is a concern for compartment syndrome.

Autoimmune Hemolytic Anemia

Autoimmune hemolytic anemia (AIHA) is a potentially life-threatening acquired disorder in which autoantibodies bind to the surface of erythrocytes, leading to premature red cell destruction. AIHA is a heterogeneous disorder, which is strongly influenced by the antibody isotype (IgG versus IgM), its ability to bind complement (C3), and its thermal reactivity (37°C versus 4°C). It can arise de novo without evidence of

TABLE 60.1

BLEEDING EPISODES

	Factor VIII deficiency[a]	Factor IX deficiency[a]
MINOR BLEEDING EPISODES		
Mucocutaneous[b]		
Apply pressure		
Topical thrombin		
Antifibrinolytic agents		
Soft tissue[c]	20	30–40
Joint bleeds		
Mild[d]	20	30–40
Severe[e]	40	40–60
Fractures/lacerations[f]	40	60–80
MAJOR BLEEDING EPISODES		
Head/neck trauma[g]	50 (Immediate)	100 (Immediate)
Compartment syndrome	50 (Immediate)	100 (Immediate)
GI bleed	50 (Immediate)	100 (Immediate)
Prior to surgery	50 (Immediate)	100 (Immediate)
Ileopsoas bleed	40–50	80–100

[a]Use patient's usual product.
[b]If profuse or refractory, may use "minor" factor replacement.
[c]If significant pain or dysfunction.
[d]Treated early, minimal pain/swelling.
[e]Bleed into target joint, severe pain/swelling.
[f]Followed by prophylaxis until cast removed.
[g]Give factor PRIOR to CT scan without contrast.

concurrent systemic disease (primary), or it may accompany systemic autoimmune diseases (systemic lupus erythematosus), malignancy (Hodgkin disease), immunodeficiency, or infection (viral, *Mycoplasma*). Primary AIHA can be classified based on antibody isotype and thermal reactivity into warm AIHA (IgG that is reactive at 37°C), paroxysmal cold hemoglobinuria (IgG that is reactive at 4°C), and cold agglutinin disease (IgM that is reactive at 4°C).

Children with AIHA will present with pallor and fatigue, with or without splenomegaly, jaundice, tea-colored urine, and abdominal pain. A CBC and reticulocyte count should be performed, along with a direct antiglobulin test (DAT or Coombs), type-and-screen, urinalysis, and total and direct bilirubin. Microspherocytes, polychromasia, and occasional schistocytes can be observed on peripheral blood smear. Children usually present with a compensated anemia that may be severe (Hgb <5 g/dL). If the DAT is positive when performed at 37°C (agglutination of the red blood cells is seen), the blood will be tested further to distinguish IgG from complement on the red cell surface. The presence of IgG and complement indicates that a warm autoantibody is present that has the ability to bind complement. The presence of complement alone suggests the presence of a cold antibody that is not seen when tested at room temperature (IgM autoantibody). The DAT can be performed at 4°C in order to detect the presence and amount of cold antibodies.

Therapy for AIHA is determined by the severity of anemia at presentation and the antibody isotype. Children with an initial hemoglobin over 9 g/dL can be observed with serial blood tests to estimate the rapidity of hemolysis. Patients who present with hemoglobin less than 5 g/dL should be admitted to an intensive-care unit for close observation, as hemolysis may be rapid, particularly with warm AIHA. Those with warm AIHA who show rapid hemolysis or those whose hemoglobin is less than 5 g/dL should receive corticosteroids as soon as possible.

Plasmapheresis, exchange transfusion, or intravenous immune globulin may also be helpful in "quieting" the hemolysis if corticosteroids are not effective. Depending on the rapidity of hemolysis, the approach to patients who present with a hemoglobin between 5 g/dL and 9 g/dL may resemble that used for either extreme, but erring on the side of caution. For those with cold agglutinin disease, it is important to avoid cold. Corticosteroids are generally not effective in this setting, but there may be a role for plasmapheresis. Transfusion with "least incompatible" blood should be considered if the child is symptomatic, though PRBC transfusion may exacerbate hemolysis, leading to hemoglobinuria and renal failure. If necessary, transfusions should be started slowly, with frequent monitoring of hemoglobin and urine for free hemoglobin to ensure that accelerated hemolysis is recognized promptly if present. Intravenous fluids (without potassium) should be administered to preserve kidney function, with care to avoid overhydration and dilution of very low hemoglobin with subsequent reduction of oxygen delivering capacity. Hemoglobin levels must be followed closely to evaluate efficacy of therapy.

ONCOLOGIC EMERGENCIES

Tumor Lysis Syndrome

Tumor lysis syndrome consists of hyperuricemia, hyperphosphatemia, hyperkalemia, and hypocalcemia in a patient presenting with leukemia or lymphoma, especially those with a very high white blood cell count, Burkitt leukemia/lymphoma, or T-cell leukemia/lymphoma. Tumor lysis can occur prior to the onset of therapy due to spontaneous blast cell breakdown, but more typically occurs after initiating therapy. Tumor lysis syndrome has rarely been reported in children with other solid tumors. In order to prevent acute renal failure, it is essential that tumor lysis be treated aggressively. A patient with suspected tumor lysis syndrome should have the following laboratory studies performed at the time of presentation: CBC with manual differential, and chemistry panel (to include potassium, creatinine, calcium, phosphorus, and uric acid).

Therapy for tumor lysis syndrome includes IV hydration at 2 or more times maintenance ($\sim$3,000 mL/m^2/day), urinary alkalinization, and allopurinol to decrease the formation of uric acid. Potassium should *not* be included in the IV fluid. Hydration fluids should include 30 to 40 mEq/L of NaHCO$_3$ to maintain urine pH from 7 to 7.5 in order to facilitate excretion of uric acid and phosphate. Efforts should be made, however, to keep the urine pH below 8, as this promotes formation of calcium-phosphate stones. If phosphorus levels are rising rapidly, amphogel can be added to aid in its excretion.

Depending on the severity of the metabolic abnormalities, kidney function, uric acid, calcium, phosphorus, and potassium should be assessed every 6 to 8 hours. Frequency can be altered when therapy is started (every 4 hours if necessary), and when laboratory values have stabilized (daily). Dialysis is indicated in patients with refractory fluid overload, hyperkalemia, acidosis, or hyperphosphatemia. A pediatric nephrologist should be consulted early in the patient's course to facilitate dialysis if necessary.

Rasburicase is a recombinant urate-oxidase enzyme that directly breaks down uric acid (in contrast to allopurinol, which inhibits its formation). It has been shown to be effective in controlling uric acid levels in children and adults with hyperuricemia due to tumor lysis syndrome. Children receiving rasburicase have demonstrated rapid declines in serum uric acid levels, accompanied by a more rapid normalization of kidney function (4). Patients with hyperleukocytosis and/or impaired renal function should receive rasburicase instead of allopurinol to treat hyperuricemia (0.2 mg/kg IV daily until stable). Those who are treated with rasburicase do not require alkalinization of their urine (but still should receive aggressive hydration *without* potassium).

Hypercalcemia

Children presenting with malignancy are at risk for hypercalcemia, although this is a rare complication in pediatrics. Hypercalcemia is defined as serum calcium of 12 mg/dL or greater, and is most common in leukemia and lymphoma, but has been reported in rhabdomyosarcoma, neuroblastoma, and Ewing sarcoma. High serum levels of calcium may be due to inadequate renal excretion, increased bone resorption caused by osteoclast activation, or the production of a hormone by tumor cells that causes parathyroid hormone (PTH)-like effects. Signs and symptoms include nausea, vomiting, lethargy, and cardiac arrhythmia. Very high levels of calcium (>20 mg/dL) can lead to stupor, coma, and death, if untreated. First-line therapy includes "forced diuresis" with IV fluids plus furosemide, which blocks calcium resorption in the kidney. Bone resorption can be reduced with bisphosphonates, which inhibit osteoclast activity. Clinical trials in adults and children have shown that pamidronate (0.5 to 1 mg/kg IV as initial dose, repeated if necessary) effectively reduces serum calcium levels in cancer patients with hypercalcemia (5).

Hyperleukocytosis

Hyperleukocytosis is defined as a white blood cell count of greater than 100,000/μL, and occurs at presentation in approximately 10% of children with acute lymphocytic leukemia (ALL), 20% with acute nonlymphocytic leukemia (ANLL), and in the majority with chronic myelogenous leukemia (CML) presenting in chronic phase. Therapy for patients with hyperleukocytosis depends on the underlying disease. These children should be evaluated immediately with the assistance of a pediatric oncologist to make the best possible determination of the most likely diagnosis before any therapy (including hydration and PRBC transfusion) is undertaken. Patients with hyperleukocytosis are at risk for "sludging" of cells within the microvasculature due to the formation of blast cell aggregates and thrombi. These can lead to hypoxemia and end-organ damage. Organs at particular risk include the brain, kidneys, and lungs. Symptoms and signs may include (but are not limited to) cranial nerve abnormalities (visual changes, facial palsy, or headache), elevated blood urea nitrogen (BUN) and creatinine, reduced urine output, tachypnea, and hypoxia. In addition, hyperleukocytosis can cause hemorrhage (especially in the CNS). Myeloblasts are larger and "stickier" than lymphoblasts; therefore children with ANLL are at a higher risk for sludging, thrombi, and hemorrhage than are those with ALL, whereas children with ALL are at greater risk for the metabolic abnormalities associated with tumor cell lysis.

The management of all patients with hyperleukocytosis starts with hydration. Intravenous fluids that do not contain potassium should be started immediately. Platelets may be transfused to keep the count above 20,000 to 30,000/μL to avoid hemorrhage. Fresh frozen plasma and vitamin K should be administered if the patient has a coagulopathy. The hemoglobin level found on a CBC in a patient with hyperleukocytosis may be spuriously high (due to machine confusion between blasts and other cells); obtaining a spun hematocrit on the patient's initial samples can give a better indication of the degree of anemia. PRBC transfusion should be avoided if possible, as red blood cells will increase stasis and may contribute further to microvascular thrombosis. Once definitive cytotoxic therapy is initiated and the white blood cell count falls, PRBCs can be administered more safely (keep hemoglobin <10 g/dL). Patients presenting with a very high white blood cell count and an elevated uric acid should receive recombinant urate oxidase (rasburicase) to prevent hyperuricemia.

Performing leukopheresis to reduce the burden of leukemic cells in patients with hyperleukocytosis is controversial. Clinical trials comparing treatment with leukopheresis versus aggressive supportive care have not been performed. Whether leukopheresis reduces the symptoms or risks associated with hyperleukocytosis is not known (6,7), but it carries certain risks. For example, anticoagulation (within the machine circuit) is required, and may further increase the risk of bleeding and thrombocytopenia. In addition it may be difficult to establish adequate IV/central line access in small children to perform the procedure. However, leukopheresis may be considered in children with a peripheral white blood cell count greater than 300,000/μL in ALL and CML, and greater than 200,000/μL in AML (or in those with symptoms of stasis). Initiation of appropriate cytotoxic therapy is the most effective way to reduce the peripheral white blood cell count.

Anterior Mediastinal Mass/Superior Vena Cava Syndrome

Depending on location, the following diagnoses are most often associated with anterior mediastinal masses: T-cell leukemia/lymphoma, Hodgkin disease, and germ cell tumor. Signs and symptoms are secondary to compromise of venous return and/or bronchial/tracheal compression by the mass, and may progress rapidly. They include stridor, hoarseness, wheezing, cough, dyspnea, orthopnea, and swelling of the face, neck, and arms. The child may not be able to tolerate positioning for procedures (lumbar puncture, central line placement, or bone marrow) and should be allowed to maintain the physical position most comfortable for him to optimize respiratory status, frequently sitting up and leaning forward.

Performing biopsies under anesthesia of any kind (conscious sedation, general anesthesia) places these patients at significant risk for respiratory and cardiovascular arrest. A chest radiograph should be performed prior to the administration of sedating medication in children being evaluated for possible malignancy to evaluate for a mediastinal mass. A chest CT may be performed with the patient prone if there is significant distress while supine. A definitive diagnosis should be made using the least invasive modality possible. Although it is always desirable to obtain tissue for diagnosis prior to starting therapy, this may not be possible if signs of respiratory distress are severe or progressive. If it is impossible to obtain a definitive diagnosis prior to therapy, a biopsy can be performed at the earliest timepoint when the child is no longer in distress. Empiric therapy may consist of steroids and/or radiation therapy, and should be determined with the guidance of a pediatric oncologist. The administration of Heliox mixtures may be useful as a way to improve breathing by increasing airflow while definitive therapy is being instituted.

Spinal Cord Compression

Patients newly diagnosed with neuroblastoma, lymphoma, metastatic medulloblastoma, and sarcomas may present with spinal cord compression. Signs and symptoms include localized back pain, sensory loss, weakness, or change in bowel and/or bladder function, but may be difficult to establish in young patients. Spinal cord compression may also occur at the time of relapse and should be considered whenever a cancer patient complains of back pain. In the short term, a plain radiograph may show destruction of vertebral bodies and a CT scan may show extension of tumor into the spinal canal. Ultimately, an MRI is necessary to define the extent and severity of the compression.

Management of spinal cord compression varies according to diagnosis and for some diagnoses remains controversial. In the setting of cord compression, it is important to use the entire clinical picture, including history (age and duration of complaints), physical examination (searching for lymphadenopathy and masses, as well as a complete neurologic exam), blood counts (looking for abnormalities suggestive of leukemia), and chemistries (looking for metabolic abnormalities associated with tumor lysis syndrome) to rapidly establish a differential diagnosis and guide diagnostic procedures. For leukemia/lymphoma, a diagnosis may be established by bone marrow aspiration. Otherwise tissue biopsy will be necessary. Once diagnostic samples are obtained, combinations of dexamethasone, radiation therapy, laminectomy, and chemotherapy have been utilized to treat spinal cord compression. Dexamethasone (1 to 2 mg/kg/day) will help reduce edema caused by inflammation that can be associated with any tumor.

The decision to use surgery, radiation therapy, or initiate definitive chemotherapy as a definitive means to relieve spinal cord compression should be made with the involvement of specialists in each of these areas. A rapid response to dexamethasone (1 to 2 mg/kg/day) together with definitive chemotherapy is most likely with non-Hodgkin lymphomas. For other tumors, surgical decompression or radiation therapy (for tumors known to be sensitive to radiation) have been used historically for symptomatic patients. More recently, studies conducted in patients with neuroblastoma have revealed that when managed in a timely fashion, the majority of patients with partial neurologic deficits will recover neurologic function with either medical (chemotherapy) or surgical management (8,9). It is important to recognize that there are serious postsurgical sequelae; therefore neurosurgical intervention may be best reserved for children with rapidly progressive neurologic symptoms.

Infection/Fever in the Neutropenic Patient

Fever in the neutropenic patient should always be considered an emergency. Severity of neutropenia can be stratified according to the absolute neutrophil count (ANC). An ANC <500 is considered severe neutropenia, 500 to 1,000 moderate, and 1,000 to 1,500 mild. The ANC is calculated by multiplying the total white blood cell count by the percentage of bands and neutrophils present on peripheral blood smear. Children with fever (>38.5°C once or 38°C twice in 24 hours) and an ANC <500 (or those with an ANC <1,000 in whom a drop can be predicted) are generally admitted to the hospital for empiric IV antibiotics and close observation. All lumens of central lines must be cultured daily while febrile. Urinalysis, urine culture, and wound and stool cultures should be performed as clinically indicated. A chest radiograph should be performed in any neutropenic child with respiratory signs or symptoms to rule out pneumonia. Shock in the neutropenic patient is managed with aggressive IV hydration, correction of coagulopathy, and inotropic support as necessary.

Careful physical exam with particular attention to central line sites, the peri-rectal area, and mouth is essential. It is important to note that examination of the peri-rectal area does *not* involve a penetrating rectal exam (which could cause mucosal damage and seeding of bacteria), simply a visual exam with gentle palpation to assess for tenderness. The typical signs of infection (large areas of erythema or pus) may not be present in severely neutropenic children, so the examiner must look for subtle erythema and tenderness. Patients with typhlitis, or neutropenic enterocolitis, will present with abdominal pain, fever, and diarrhea, and may mimic acute appendicitis.

Empiric antibiotic therapy should be started as soon as possible. *Staphylococcus, Streptococcus, Enterococcus, Enterobacteriaceae, Pseudomonas aeruginosa,* and anaerobes are the most prevalent causes of bacterial infections in neutropenic patients. In the well-appearing febrile child, monotherapy with a fourth-generation cephalosporin (such as ceftazadime) or carbapenem (such as meropenem) may be employed. Those with physical evidence of a localized skin or central line infection, or those receiving chemotherapy leading to severe mucositis, may receive vancomycin as well to improve coverage of gram-positive bacteria. Additional gram-negative coverage can be given if a peri-rectal abscess or neutropenic entercolitis (typhlitis) is suspected. Children who are hypotensive or "toxic" appearing may be empirically started on a combination of antibiotics including a fourth-generation cephalosporin or carbapenem, vancomycin, along with additional gram-negative coverage such as tobramycin. Antifungal therapy should be considered in patients who remain febrile with *negative* cultures despite appropriate antibiotics. Viral etiologies of fever (influenza, parainfluenza, respiratory syncytial virus, cytomegalovirus, Epstein–Barr virus, and adenovirus) must not be overlooked in patients with persistent fever and negative cultures.

Neutropenic patients with respiratory distress should be evaluated first with a history and physical examination, with particular attention to recent therapy, respiratory rate, effort, breath sounds, and pulse oximetry while on room air. Arterial or venous blood gas measurements should be performed in children requiring supplemental oxygen to accurately and completely assess respiratory status. In the setting of neutropenia, infectious causes of respiratory distress are most common; however, complications caused by tumors and cancer therapy (including chemotherapy and radiation therapy) must be considered. A chest radiograph is usually sufficient initially; however, a chest CT is usually performed as well to more fully examine the pattern and extent of infiltrates, in order to provide additional clues to the etiology and to help direct therapy. The approach to obtaining culture material to identify the offending organism varies among institutions. The yield of flexible bronchoscopy and bronchoalveolar lavage (BAL) is determined by the cause of infection (specific in the diagnosis of *Pneumocystis carinii*, less so with fungi and bacteria), the location of the infection (more difficult with peripheral infiltrates), and the experience of the physician performing the procedure. In a series of 58 children with primary immunodeficiencies and various types of cancer (some following stem cell transplantation) undergoing BAL, a specific organism was isolated in 53% of patients, and probable infection (defined as the presence of purulent secretions without isolation of a particular organism) was documented in another 21% (10). Open-lung biopsies should be considered in patients with respiratory distress and infiltrates in whom a definitive diagnosis has not been established by other means.

Respiratory Emergencies

Patients undergoing therapy for oncologic disorders may present with a myriad of respiratory emergencies depending on their specific diagnosis and recent therapy. Potential respiratory emergencies at diagnosis include the presence of a mediastinal mass (T-cell lymphoma); large chest wall mass (sarcomas); metastatic tumor (Wilms tumor or sarcomas); pneumothorax (osteosarcoma); pleural effusion, which may accompany any of the above; and infections. Certain chemotherapeutic agents are associated with acute and subacute pulmonary sequelae. For example, children who have recently received high-dose cytarabine (Ara-C) are at risk for developing bacteremia with α-hemolytic streptococcus, followed by a rapidly progressive ARDS and respiratory failure. These patients are managed with appropriate antibiotic therapy along with aggressive supportive care including corticosteroids, meticulous fluid management to avoid overload, and bi-pap or endotracheal intubation with mechanical ventilation. L-asparaginase and etoposide may cause IgE-mediated bronchoconstriction and pulmonary radiation can cause inflammatory pneumonitis. Respiratory distress may also be secondary to heart failure that may occur with severe anemia (leukemia or hemorrhage), tumor thrombus in the vena cava and right atrium (Wilms tumor), or prior therapy with either anthracyclines or radiation to the myocardium.

Pulmonary complications following stem cell transplantation (SCT) occur in 30% to 50% of patients and contribute significantly to the morbidity and mortality associated with transplant. Few pulmonary complications are acute and will be discussed here, while many others (chronic graft-versus-host disease, bronchiolitis obliterans) are more indolent and therefore do not pose immediate threats. One such acute complication of SCT is engraftment syndrome, which is characterized by fever, rash, and capillary leak that often leads to respiratory distress. Pleural effusions and interstitial pulmonary infiltrates suggestive of pulmonary edema may be seen on chest radiograph. Engraftment syndrome is usually self-limited, requiring only supportive measures. Idiopathic pulmonary syndrome (IPS) defined by the acute onset of signs and symptoms consistent with pneumonia, and a diffuse interstitial pattern on imaging in the ABSENCE of infectious agents. IPS occurs 15 to 90 days following the infusion of cells, and is currently treated with solumedrol (2 mg/kg/day) and supplemental oxygen. Mortality rates of IPS as high as 70% have been reported. Studies utilizing novel agents such as etanercept (blocks TNF-α) in conjunction with corticosteroids are ongoing.

Hemoptysis in children with malignancies may be caused by several etiologies. Tumor progression causing blood vessel erosion may cause hemoptysis. Invasive pulmonary aspergillosis, *Staphylococcus aureus*, *Klebsiella*, or *Pseudomonas* represent potential infectious causes. Children undergoing radiation therapy involving the chest are also at risk of hemoptysis due to tissue damage and resultant friability. Coagulopathy

caused by the cancer or its treatment may contribute as well. Patients should be evaluated with a chest radiograph and CT scan of the chest to identify any lesions and potential sources of bleeding, and a CBC and DIC panel so that thrombocytopenia and any existing coagulopathy can be corrected. Children with massive hemoptysis must be evaluated in the intensive-care unit for respiratory management, and to facilitate bronchoscopy. Procedures including embolization and occlusion of the bleeding vessel with a balloon catheter may be performed during the bronchoscopy. Surgical resection of an area of infected lung should be considered if significant hemoptysis recurs.

Transfusion Guidelines and Emergencies

Patients with malignant diseases may require transfusion with blood products at some point in their treatment. Of course, the full clinical picture of each individual patient must be considered when making decisions to transfuse PRBC—the intensity of the current chemotherapy regimen, cardiac dysfunction, pulmonary disease, infection, and anticipated procedures. In general, PRBC transfusions should be considered in children receiving chemotherapy when their hemoglobin falls below 8 to 10 g/dL. PRBC units should be irradiated and leukoreduced to prevent transfusion-associated graft-versus-host disease and transmission of viruses such as cytomegalovirus (CMV), respectively. Washing of PRBC units is usually recommended only in children with a history of severe anaphylactic transfusion reactions.

The level at which to transfuse platelets remains somewhat controversial. Children at higher risk for bleeding include those with concurrent infections (with or without disseminated intravascular coagulation), recent surgery, central nervous system tumors, and liver disease. Frequent transfusion of platelets can result in alloimmunization and reduced efficacy. Most oncologists transfuse platelets when the platelet count falls below 10 to 20/mm^3 in the clinically stable child. When transfused, platelets should be irradiated and leukoreduced to avoid graft-versus-host disease, febrile transfusion reactions, and transmission of infectious organisms.

Transfusion reactions vary greatly in severity. Hemolytic transfusion reactions can be acute or delayed, and are likely due to IgG or IgM antibodies present in the patient's serum that can fix complement on the transfused red blood cells. Bacterial contamination of the transfused product represents another potential cause of hemolytic transfusion reactions. Patients experiencing acute hemolytic transfusion reactions may present with fever, nausea, vomiting, chills, back pain, hypotension, disseminated intravascular coagulation, and shock. Those with a delayed hemolytic reaction (may occur up to 2 weeks following the transfusion) are usually hemodynamically stable, with jaundice, hemoglobinuria, and a lower-than-expected post-transfusion hemoglobin.

Patients in whom a hemolytic transfusion reaction is suspected should be evaluated with a direct and indirect antiglobulin test, hemoglobin, DIC panel, and serum bilirubin. The transfusion should be stopped immediately, and intravenous fluids (without potassium) given. Adequate urine output must be maintained. DIC is managed with fresh frozen plasma; those who are bleeding should receive platelets (and PRBCs if necessary). Blood products should be evaluated for compatibility with the patient and for infectious organisms.

Transfusion-associated lung injury (TRALI) is a rare but potentially fatal complication following transfusion of blood products containing plasma (11). Patients experience an acute onset of respiratory distress due to pulmonary edema and hypoxemia. They may develop hypotension and fever, and may require mechanical ventilation as supportive care until symptoms improve (24 to 96 hours). Most children recover without sequelae. The mechanism of injury is thought to be through the recruitment of neutrophils and cytokines in the recipient in response to antibodies contained in the plasma of the donor. Treatment is supportive with fluid boluses and oxygen (the use of corticosteroids is controversial but may be of some value).

References

1. Gaston MH, Verter JI, Woods G, et al. Prophylaxis with oral penicillin in children with sickle cell anemia. A randomized trial. *N Engl J Med* 1986; 314:1593–1599.
2. Vichinsky EP, Neumayr LD, Earles AN, et al. Causes and outcomes of the acute chest syndrome in sickle cell disease. *N Engl J Med* 2000;342:1855–1865.
3. Vichinsky EP, Styles LA, Colangelo LH, et al. Acute chest syndrome in sickle cell disease: clinical presentation and course. *Blood* 1997;89:1787–1792.
4. Goldman SC, Holcenberg JS, Finklestein JZ, et al. A randomized comparison between rasburicase and allopurinol in children with lymphoma or leukemia at high risk for tumor lysis. *Blood* 2001;97:2998–3003.
5. Young G, Shende A. Use of pamidronate in the management of acute cancer-related hypercalcemia in children. *Med Pediatr Oncol* 1998;30:117–121.
6. Porcu P, Farag S, Marcucci G, et al. Leukocytoreduction for acute leukemia. Therapeutic apheresis 2002;6:15–23.
7. Zarkovic M, Kwaan HC. Correction of hyperviscosity by apheresis. *Semin Thromb Hemost* 2003;535–542.
8. Katzenstein HM, Kent PM, London WB, et al. Treatment and outcome of 83 children with intraspinal neuroblastoma: the pediatric oncology group experience. *J Clin Oncol* 2001;19:1047–1055.
9. Hoover M, Bowman LC, Crawford SE, et al. Long-term outcome of patients with intraspinal neuroblastoma. *Med Pediatr Oncol* 1999;32: 353–359.
10. Efrati O, Gonik U, Bielorai B, et al. Fiberoptic bronchoscopy and bronchiolar lavage for the evaluation of pulmonary disease in children with primary immunodeficiency and cancer. *Pediatric Blood and Cancer* 2007;48(3):324–29.
11. Popovsky MA. Transfusion-related acute lung injury. *Curr Opin Hematol* 2000;7:402–407.

CHAPTER 61 ■ RENAL SIGNS/SYMPTOMS AND LABORATORY ABNORMALITIES

SUE HOFFMAN

Evaluation of renal dysfunction in the pediatric patient requires the hospitalist to look at the overall condition of the patient. Signs and symptoms, laboratory, and radiologic evaluation must all be accessed to determine the child's diagnosis. Many cases do not present classically but instead require searching for clinical clues to elicit the underlying condition. A systematic approach with a functional understanding of the renal system is necessary when evaluating a patient suspected of renal dysfunction.

SIGNS AND SYMPTOMS

Some presentations of renal disease can be straightforward and the diagnosis is obvious. In the majority of the cases, the signs and symptoms are subtle and nonspecific, making the diagnosis more difficult. A high index of suspicion is important, as early diagnosis and treatment can prevent some of these disorders from progressing and becoming irreversible. Examining signs and symptoms based on the functional components of the kidney can be an efficient way to organize your approach.

The kidney is comprised of three functional components. The renal arteries first deliver blood flow to the glomeruli of the kidney. This represents the *prerenal* portion and is affected by perfusion as well as the integrity of the vessels themselves. Historical features to be considered would be those that could indicate intravascular volume loss such as vomiting, diarrhea, decreased intake, oliguria, history of hemorrhage or trauma, severe burns with excessive fluid losses, or recent surgeries. Physical findings might include signs of dehydration, (tachycardia, hypotension, prolonged capillary refill, sunken eyes, decreased skin turgor, and dry mucous membranes). Other causes of decreased perfusion affecting the kidneys are secondary to impaired cardiac performance (i.e., cardiogenic). Histories of cardiac disease, tachypnea, fatigue, or such physical signs as the presence of a murmur or peripheral or pulmonary edema suggest a cardiac etiology. Third spacing after surgery can also cause a decrease in the effective circulating volume and cause renal dysfunction.

The *intrinsic* component of the kidney is comprised of the glomeruli, which filter the blood delivered from the renal arteries producing the ultrafiltrate; and the tubules, which receive the ultrafiltrate and reabsorb and secrete solutes and/or water. History consistent with glomerular involvement would be grossly bloody urine, edema, bloody diarrhea, abdominal pain, fatigue, recent illness including pharyngitis and impetigo, rashes (especially petechial, purpuric or malar), oliguria or anuria, hearing loss, and headache as a sign of hypertension. Renal-associated hypertension is caused by hypervolemia secondary to sodium and water retention as well as an activated renin–angiotensin system. Very important signs are failure to thrive or slow growth. These can occur with any aspect of renal disorders but are more frequently seen with glomerular and tubular dysfunction. Growth charts should be obtained if possible. Changes in urinary pattern such as polyuria, oliguria, anuria, enuresis, and excessive thirst can be associated with tubular dysfunction. A history of significant hypotension can be important as well as medication/toxin history for nephrotoxic drugs such as amphotericin B, nonsteroidal anti-inflammatories, methicillin, aminglycosides, and heavy metals, as these can damage the tubular system. Family history should include a history of renal disease, deafness, or the need for dialysis or renal transplant. Physical findings that can be consistent with glomerular involvement would be rashes, pallor, jaundice, ear anomalies, hypertension, periorbital edema, and rales. Tubular dysfunction produces less specific physical findings with changes in urinary volume being most noticeable.

The *postrenal* component describes the drainage system of the kidney that relieves the body of waste. Postrenal dysfunction is primarily due to obstructive causes. History would include decreased urine output, change in urinary stream, suprapubic pain if obstructed distal to the bladder, and/or a history of stones. Physical findings can include a distended bladder and/or a palpable abdominal mass.

Meticulous intake and output must always be assessed in the hospitalized child with suspected renal disease. Normal urine output varies with age (Table 61.1). Oliguria would represent a decrease from these values and anuria would be the absence of urine. Oliguria can be a normal physiologic response to decreased renal perfusion causing decreased filtration and increased tubular reabsorption so that intravascular volume can be maintained. This is the most common cause of oliguria in children. Oliguria can also occur due to maldistribution of fluid as seen in congestive heart failure, nephrotic syndrome, and capillary leak syndromes. Intrinsic renal disease can also produce oliguria and anuria. It is imperative to keep accurate account of all intake (oral, enteral, and intravenous) and output (urine, stool, drains, ostomies, and significant skin losses). It is also mandatory to document any significant weight loss or gains.

Edema with or without associated hypertension is also an important sign of renal disease. Many times children with edema are admitted for evaluation of other diseases, such as cardiac disease, but are subsequently found to have renal involvement. Edema occurs with an increase in hydrostatic pressure in the vascular space, decreased plasma oncotic pressure, increased capillary permeability of fluid, or decreased lymphatic drainage. Increased hydrostatic pressure occurs with decreased renal excretion of sodium and water. This can be seen with intrinsic renal disease including glomerulonephritis, tubular necrosis, or interstitial nephritis. It can also occur with obstructive uropathy

TABLE 61.1

NORMAL URINE OUTPUT

Age	Normal urine output (mL/kg/hr)
First 1 to 5 days of life	0.5
Preterm post 5 days of life	2–5
Term post 5 days of life	2–4
Children	1–2
Adolescents	0.75

or chronic renal failure. Increased hydrostatic pressure can also occur from nonrenal causes as in congestive heart failure and venous obstructive states. Corticosteroids can also cause sodium and water retention leading to edema. Edema can be produced from decreased oncotic pressure as seen with excessive protein loss (hypoalbuminemia associated with nephrotic syndrome or gastrointestinal losses from protein-losing enteropathy). Additionally, decreased protein synthesis from liver disease can produce edema. Generally edema does not occur until albumin is less than 2.2 mg/dL. Additional causes of edema are increased capillary permeability (inflammation, sepsis, burns, anaphylaxis, or trauma) or decreased lymphatic drainage.

LABORATORY EVALUATION

Once the history and physical have been performed, the laboratory evaluation of the child with renal dysfunction should be initiated. When looking at renal diseases there are several screening labs that should be obtained.

The most important noninvasive test that is easily obtained and inexpensive is the urinalysis. The urinalysis should be performed on freshly voided urine, less than 30 minutes postvoid if possible. The urinalysis consists of a dipstick composed of commercially available reagents and a microscopic examination.

The dipstick portion of the urinalysis evaluates for nine abnormalities. The pH of the urine can provide a screening tool for the overall acid–base balance of the body. A low urine pH (<6.0) is suggestive of metabolic acidosis. An elevated urinary pH (>8.0) would be suspicious for renal tubular acidosis. Urine pH is also a useful tool when alkalinization of the urine is required to manage certain conditions such as tumor lysis syndrome, rhabdomyolysis, or salicylate poisoning.

The specific gravity reagent can be used to estimate hydration status, although this is not as accurate as urine osmolality. If significant proteinuria or glycosuria exists, this will affect the accuracy of the result. Leukocyte esterase tests for the presence of white blood cells. This suggests urinary tract infection, especially in conjunction with nitrites, bacteria, and white blood cells on microscopic exam. A urine culture is required for a definitive diagnosis. Leukocyte esterase can also be positive in glomerulonephritis, interstitial nephritis, acute tubular necrosis, and transplant rejection.

Protein on the dipstick is specific for albumin. Low-grade proteinuria is of concern as urine is protein free. Greater than 1+ protein is consistent with nephrotic syndrome and should be quantified with a timed specimen for protein and creatinine. Ketones are also evaluated. Elevation in ketones without associated glycosuria can be produced by dehydration, shock, starvation, ketotic hypoglycemia, strenuous exercise, and fever. Diabetic ketoacidosis results in ketonuria and glycosuria. Glycosuria without ketones is suggestive of diabetes mellitus as well but can also be seen after a large glucose load and with galactosemia. Glycosuria in the presence of normal serum glucose would suggest renal tubular dysfunction.

Elevated urinary bilirubin is found in patients with liver disease or a hemolytic process. Betadine may produce a false positive for bilirubin. Hemoglobin as a screen for red blood cells is also on the dipstick. The urine sediment should be checked for red blood cells in the presence of a hemoglobin-positive dipstick. If hemoglobin is positive but there are no red blood cells on the microscopic exam, this could indicate hemoglobin from hemolytic anemia or myoglobin from rhabdomyolysis. Further workup would be indicated in either case.

A microscopic exam is then performed to evaluate the urinary sediment. Examination for white blood cells is diagnostic of urinary tract infection, especially if bacteria are also present. If further staining is performed, urinary lymphocytes can be seen with transplant rejection and eosinophils with interstitial nephritis. When epithelial cells along with mixed cellular and granular casts are observed, the differential diagnosis includes acute tubular necrosis, hemolytic uremic syndrome, chronic glomerulonephritis, or chronic renal insufficiency. Other casts that can be seen are broad brown casts, which are classically seen in acute tubular necrosis; and red blood cell casts, which are diagnostic of acute glomerulonephritis. The presence of red blood cells (RBCs) may be caused by glomerulonephritis, especially when seen with red blood cell casts. Additional causes include infection (generally seen in conjunction with white blood cells), renal calculi, sickle-cell disease, and urinary tract obstruction. Urinary crystals are also evaluated. These can be seen with renal calculi, infection, contrast agents and certain medications such as acyclovir and sulfa-containing drugs. Nephritic syndrome exhibits urine protein >1,500 mg/d or >1,000 mg/g creatinine, RBC and RBC casts, edema, and elevated blood pressure. In nephrotic syndrome the urinary protein is >3500 mg/d or >3000 mg/g creatinine, and fatty casts and oval fat bodies can be seen with or without RBCs or RBC casts. Clinically there is significant edema, and on chemistries a decreased serum albumin and elevated serum lipids would be seen. In tubular syndromes the protein is <1,500 mg/d with normal sediment and normal imaging, but with fluid and electrolyte abnormalities and an inability to concentrate urine. For renal imaging, see Table 61.2.

The evaluation should also include complete blood count (CBC) and chemistries. The CBC will document anemia if present, and more importantly, what type of anemia. Normochromic normocytic anemia suggests chronic disease, or can indicate hemodilution. Microangiopathic hemolytic anemia with associated thrombocytopenia is indicative of hemolytic uremic syndrome. Sickle-cell disease can be diagnosed in the presence of sickle-shaped RBCs and an associated anemia.

Abnormal chemistries can lead to the diagnosis of tubular dysfunction of the kidney. A decrease in HCO_3 is a marker for renal tubular acidosis. Abnormalities in sodium or potassium, for example, should bring concern for diabetes insipidus (hypernatremia) or Bartter syndrome (hypokalemia). Blood urea nitrogen (BUN) and creatinine are the two major markers of renal disease. BUN is synthesized by the liver and is the product of protein metabolism. The BUN is increased by decreases in urea clearance (decreased intravascular volume or renal failure), excessive protein intake (such as hyperalimentation or enteral feeds), or increased protein breakdown (seen with renal failure, gastrointestinal bleeding, corticosteroid usage, and sepsis). Decreases in BUN are seen with decrease protein intake (protein malnutrition, liver disease due to a decrease in protein production) or increased urea clearance (as can be seen with volume expansion). Thus the BUN is an important but not specific marker of renal dysfunction.

The most reliable and easily obtainable serum indicator of glomerular function is the serum creatinine (Cr) level. Its interpretation also has its limitations. Creatinine is a product of skeletal muscle metabolism of creatinine and phosphocreatinine. Elevations in creatinine are seen with decreased renal clearance or muscle breakdown as seen in rhabdomyolysis, or

TABLE 61.2

RENAL IMAGING

Exam	Utility	Advantages	Disadvantages
Ultrasound	Anatomic details Size, shape, number of kidneys Evidence of obstruction	Noninvasive With added Doppler can assess renal vessels and blood flow	

VCUG
  Contrast
  Radionuclide
	Assesses presence of
	vesicoureteral reflux
	Best for grading reflux
	More sensitive for reflux
		Provides better anatomic detail
		Less expensive,
		no contrast used
			Both types require placement
			of urinary catheter
			Contrast allergy risk
			Difficult to grade reflux, more
			of a screening exam

Mag-3 renal scan (diuretic renography)	Functional study that provides a quantitative measure of renal function and drainage of the collecting system	Useful in evaluating hydronephrosis in the absence of reflux and UPJ obstruction	Requires placement of urinary catheter, IV access, and administration of furosemide
DMSA renal scintigraphy	Accurate in detecting renal scarring often associated with reflux Some urologists feel this will likely replace routine VCUGs in evaluating UTIs as if scarring is not seen then unlikely to have significant reflux	Can be used in the acute setting Several times more sensitive than IVP in detecting renal scars No contrast required Noninvasive	
CT scan Helical CT	More detailed anatomy compared to ultrasound Gold standard in the diagnosis of renal calculi	Especially good for complex cyst and tumor evaluation	Requires IV access and contrast administration Significant radiation exposure
MRI/MRA	MRA has virtually replaced renal arteriography and venography in evaluation of renal vessel and thrombotic disorders MRI useful for even greater anatomic definition, especially if ultrasound and/or CT scan is nondiagnostic	MRI good if patient has contrast allergy	MRA requires IV access and contrast Sedation is generally required in infants and young children

CT, computed tomography; DMSA, dimercaptosuccinic acid; IV, intravenous; IVP, intravenous pyclogram; UPJ, ureteropeluic junction; MRA, magnetic resonance angiogram; MRI, magnetic resonance imaging, VCUG, voiding cystorethrogram; UTI, urinary tract intection.

vigorous exercise. The normal creatinine value is age dependent. In the first 4 to 5 days of life, it is reflective of the mother's value, but with any age the trend of the serum creatinine is the most sensitive indicator of renal function. For example, if you find that the serum creatinine increases from 0.5 mg/dL to 1 mg/dL, this represents a 50% decline in glomerular filtration rate (GFR) (Table 61.3).

Determination of the GFR is important in evaluating the child with suspected renal disease or in the follow-up of a child already known to have renal insufficiency. This will require a 12- to 24-hour collection of urine. A 12-hour study requires collection during the day when urine flow is at its highest. Total daily creatinine should be 14 to 20 mg/kg. Using the equation:

$$\text{Ccr (creatinine clearance)} = (U_{cr} V)/P_{cr}$$

where U_{cr} = urinary creatinine (mg/dL), P_{cr} = plasma creatine (mg/dL), and V = urine volume (mL/min).

Or the Schwartz formula can be utilized to quickly estimate GFR using plasma creatinine:

$$\text{Estimated Ccr (mL/min/1.73m}^2) = kL/P_{cr}$$

where k = proportionality constant, as follows:

Low-birthweight infants (first year) = 0.33
Term infants (first year) = 0.45

TABLE 61.3

NORMAL CREATININE VALUES

Age	Normal creatinine values (mg/dL)
First month of life	1
Second month of life	<0.5
From 3 months to 6 years	<0.6
6 years to 15 years	<1.0

Children 2 to 2 years = 0.55
Adolescent girls = 0.55
Adolescent boys = 0.70

L = length (cm)
Pcr = plasma creatinine (mg/dL)

The value obtained correlates with a timed 24-hour specimen for creatinine clearance.

The ratio of BUN to creatinine can be useful in differentiating decreased intravascular volume from intrinsic renal disease. A normal BUN/Cr ratio is 10:1. With decreased renal perfusion (seen in volume depletion), the BUN/Cr ratio >20. With intrinsic renal disease (acute tubular necrosis, for example) the BUN/Cr < 10 due to decreased tubular function.

Another frequently utilized test is the fractional excretion of sodium (FENa). This measures the percent of filtered sodium that is excreted in the urine. It is used to differentiate prerenal from renal (intrinsic) disorders:

$$FE_{Na} = (U_{Na} \times P_{Cr})/(P_{Na} \times U_{Cr}) \times 100$$

Where Una = urine sodium, Ucr = plasma creatinine, Pna = plasma sodium, and Pcr = plasma creatinine.

- A value <1% is consistent with prerenal disease.
- A value of 1% to 2% is equivocal.
- A value >2% is consistent with renal (intrinsic) disease.

Serum proteins can be decreased and serum lipids increased with nephrotic syndrome. Complement abnormalities, especially C3, can be seen with some glomerulonephrities as well as positive streptozyme with post-streptococcal glomerulonephritis.

CLINICAL CORRELATES

A history of hypertension, periorbital edema, hematuria, proteinuria, and Coke-colored urine is indicative of acute glomerulonephritis, especially in the presence of RBC casts. When associated with a recent history (3 to 4 weeks prior) of phayngitis or impetigo, then the diagnosis of postinfectious glomerulonephritis is likely. Glomerulonephritis associated with hemoptysis is consistent with pulmonary–renal syndrome, also known as Goodpasture disease. Purpura, petechiae, abdominal pain, joint swelling, proteinuria, and hypertension suggest the diagnosis of Henoch–Schönlein purpura. A low C3, malar rash, and hypertension with symptoms consistent with glomerulonephritis suggest a diagnosis of systemic lupus erythematosis.

In the presence of severe vomiting and diarrhea, hemorrhage or sepsis, and clinical evidence of hypovolemia (tachycardia, sunken eyes, dry mucous membranes, lethargy, orthostasis, and oliguria), pre-renal failure exists. Laboratory abnormalities such as elevated specific gravity, elevated BUN, a BUN/Cr > 20, and perhaps proteinuria, are consistent with pre-renal failure or acute tubular necrosis.

Bloody diarrhea, along with oliguria or anuria, anemia, thrombocytopenia, and elevations in BUN and Cr, suggests hemolytic–uremic syndrome (see Chapter 63). Anuria, oliguria, or change in urinary stream in the newborn points to obstruction or congenital malformation with the most common cause being posterior urethral valves. Generalized edema, hypertension, significant proteinuria with associated hypertension, decreased serum albumin, and elevated serum lipids are diagnostic of nephrotic syndrome. Hypernatremia, polydipsia, and polyuria can be signs of nephrogenic diabetes insipidus, a tubular disorder. The inability to concentrate urine as is seen with polyuria, polydipsia, enuresis, decreased specific gravity, and especially dilute first morning void can be the first sign of chronic renal failure.

The indications for referral of the patient to a pediatric nephrologist include:

1. Persistent abnormalities in renal function
2. Declining renal function unresponsive to initial therapy
3. Diagnosis in question
4. Need for renal biopsy

SPECIAL TOPIC: EVALUATION OF ANTENATALLY DIAGNOSED HYDRONEPHROSIS

Fetal hydronephrosis is frequently diagnosed on antenatal ultrasounds. It can be transient or persistent. Knowing how to manage infants with this finding is very important to the hospitalist, as evaluating newborns is becoming increasingly expected.

Renal ultrasound as soon as possible after birth is indicated for newborns with the following antenatal diagnoses:

1. Severe hydronephrosis
2. Bladder distension
3. Dilated ureter
4. Presence of an ureterocele

Urology should be consulted if the postnatal ultrasound demonstrates continued abnormalities.

Those newborns diagnosed with moderate to severe hydronephrosis antenatally require institution of prophylactic antibiotics, generally amoxicillin at 15 to 25 mg/kg given daily until reflux is ruled out. Postnatal ultrasounds should be done after the infant is 48 hours old, and some pediatric urologists say it is best to wait 2 weeks, ensuring a euvolemic state. If hydronephrosis persists at the moderate to severe grade on the postnatal ultrasound, the infant should undergo a voiding cystourethrogram (VCUG) to evaluate for vesicoureteralreflux (VUR). If the VCUG is positive for VUR, prophylactic antibiotics should be continued until reflux resolves. A DMSA scan should be performed on those infants with grade III-V reflux to screen for evidence of renal scarring. These infants with high-grade reflux should be referred to a pediatric urologist for continued follow-up. If the VCUG is negative in the presence of moderate to severe hydronephrosis, a functional renal scan (mag-3 scan) should be preformed to evaluate for possible obstruction. At this point pediatric urology should also become involved.

The newborns with mild hydronephrosis antenatally do not require prophylactic antibiotics as the risk of reflux is thought to be negligible. They should have a follow-up ultrasound after 7 days of age. If at this point the hydronephrosis remains mild or not present, no antibiotic therapy is needed, but they should be reevaluated with an ultrasound at 3 months of age. If the grade of hydronephrosis progresses to the moderate to severe range on the post–7-day or 3-month ultrasound, then the workup goes to that of VCUG and prophylactic antibiotics until reflux is ruled out.

Suggested Readings

Andreoli SP. Clinical evaluation and management of Acute Renal Failure. In: Avner ED, Harmon WE, Neaudet P, eds. *Pediatric nephrology.* Philadelphia: Lippincott, Williams & Wilkins; 2004:1233.

Chan JC, Williams DM, Roth KS. Kidney failure in infants and children. *Pediatr Rev* 2002;23:47.

Greenburg A. Urinalysis. In: Greenburg A, ed. *National Kidney Foundation primer on kidney diseases.* 3rd ed. San Diego: Academic Press; 2001:28–37.

Koff SA. Postnatal management of antenatal hydronephrosis using an observational approach. *Urology* 2000;55:609.

Swan SK, Deane WF. Clinical evaluation of renal function. In: Greenburg A, ed. *National Kidney Foundation primer on kidney diseases.* 3rd ed. San Diego: Academic Press; 2002:25–28.

Woodward M, Frank D. Postnatal management of antenatal hydronephrosis. *BJU Int* 2002;89:149–156.

CHAPTER 62 ■ ACUTE RENAL FAILURE

TROY L. McGUIRE

Acute renal failure (ARF) is a frequently encountered condition in pediatric hospitalist practice, either as the primary reason for hospitalization or secondary to other systemic illness. If not already present upon admission, renal failure may develop as a consequence of progression of the underlying disease, onset of multiorgan system failure, or due to iatrogenic causes. Early recognition and treatment of ARF is vital to reverse its course and to prevent life-threatening complications. Although the simplest understanding of ARF is the sudden onset of progressive azotemia accompanied by either oliguria (urine output <1 mL/kg/hr in children; <0.5 mL/kg/hr in older adolescents) or anuria (absent urine output), any meaningful definition of ARF must also accommodate other conditions in which a decrease in glomerular filtration rate (GFR) is present even in the presence of normal or increased urine output (UOP). Moreover, even in the presence of normal glomerular filtration, renal tubular function or concentrating ability may be lost in a broadened definition of ARF. Clearly, there are situations in which azotemia and oliguria are simply homeostatic mechanisms designed to maximize water and sodium reabsorption for preservation of vital organ perfusion and blood pressure. Thus, a patient's renal function must be viewed in the context of volume status, electrolyte balance, and baseline renal function before ARF is diagnosed.

In an effort to provide clarity to the definition of ARF, the Acute Dialysis Quality Initiative group published a consensus statement in 2004. The criteria employed are: (1) serum creatinine (rise from baseline) or GFR (decrease from estimated baseline); and (2) degree and duration of oliguria/anuria. Using an acronym RIFLE (Risk, Injury, Failure, Loss, End stage) to stratify the severity of renal function compromise, acute renal failure is defined at serum creatinine >3 times baseline (or GFR <75% of predicted GFR in absence of a baseline creatinine determination) or UOP <0.3 mL/kg/hr for >24 hrs or anuria >12 hrs. Applicability to the pediatric population is uncertain at these cutoffs and, even in adults, the classification scheme is only now being validated in reported studies. However, similar schemas will surely be developed over time for pediatric patients that will help focus diagnostic certainty and permit comparisons across research populations.

When approaching the differential diagnosis of the patient presenting in ARF, a formal structure is helpful (Table 62.1). Prerenal ARF includes all of those conditions that are marked by a compromise in renal perfusion. Intrinsic ARF includes those entities in which renal parenchyma is the site of pathology. The conditions comprising intrinsic ARF may be subgrouped into acute glomerulonephritis (AGN), acute tubular necrosis (ATN), and tubulointerstitial nephritis (TIN). Finally, postrenal ARF refers to those conditions in which there is obstruction between the renal pelvis and urethral meatus. Most cases of ARF will in actuality be multifactorial, but the construct of prerenal versus intrinsic renal versus postrenal causes for ARF is extremely helpful in approaching the evaluation of the complex hospitalized patient.

PRERENAL ACUTE RENAL FAILURE

Prerenal ARF occurs in situations when there is inadequate renal perfusion to meet the body's needs for waste removal. In pediatric practice, hypovolemia is by far the most common cause of prerenal ARF. Gastrointestinal losses from vomiting and diarrhea, inadequately replaced stomal output, or inadequate dietary intake are common. Frequently encountered excess renal losses include diuretic use, diabetes mellitus, diabetes insipidus, and concentrating defects. Insensible losses through the integument and respiratory tract can be relatively large, especially in hyperpyrexia, hypermetabolic states, sepsis, respiratory distress, and extensive body surface area burns. Intravascular collapse may occur despite adequate extracellular fluid volume in states marked by third-spacing including sepsis, systemic inflammatory response syndrome (SIRS), multiple organ dysfunction syndrome (MODS), nephrotic syndrome, and hepatorenal syndrome. Redistribution of blood to capacitance vessels may cause renal hypoperfusion in septic shock and neurogenic shock, despite an otherwise previously adequate intravascular volume. In cardiogenic shock due to sepsis, congestive heart failure (CHF), congenital heart disease, myocarditis, arrhythmia, or cardiomyopathy, renal perfusion will be diminished along with other vital organ perfusion. Finally, renal artery thrombosis, pure alpha-adrenergic agents, and angiotensin-converting enzyme (ACE) inhibitors all serve to compromise renal vascular supply.

Compensatory measures are initiated in response to decreases in renal perfusion. When renal blood flow drops below the autoregulatory range at which GFR can be maintained constant, GFR falls and less sodium chloride is delivered to the distal tubule, causing renin to be released at the juxtaglomerular apparatus. Renin stimulates downstream angiotensin and aldosterone activity. Angiotensin II renally promotes generation of prostacyclin (PGI_2) and nitric oxide (NO), both vasodilatory at the glomerular afferent arteriole. The net effect of afferent arteriolar vasodilatation and efferent arteriolar vasoconstriction is a hydrostatic improvement in glomerular blood delivery and therefore glomerular filtration. In the peripheral vasculature, angiotensin II is a potent vasoconstrictor, shunting blood toward central, vital organ perfusion. Aldosterone acts on the tubules to improve sodium and water reabsorption. The subsequent increase in plasma osmolality stimulates release of vasopressin from the posterior pituitary driving a behavioral thirst response and improving water reabsorption from the distal collecting system by altering permeability.

DIFFERENTIAL DIAGNOSIS OF ACUTE RENAL FAILURE

	Prerenal	Intrinsic renal	Postrenal

Major causes	Hypovolemia
	  Inadequate intake
	  GI losses
	    Vomiting
	    Diarrhea
	    Tube drainage
	  Renal losses
	    Diuretics
	    Diabetes mellitus
	    Diabetes insipidus
	  Insensible losses
	    Burn
	    Fever
	    Respiratory distress
	Third spacing
	  Sepsis/SIRS/MODS
	  Nephrotic syndrome
	Septic shock
	Neurogenic shock
	Cardiogenic shock
	  Congestive heart failure
	  Myocarditis
	  Cardiomyopathy
	  Cardiac arrest
	Renal artery thrombosis
	Alpha-adrenergic agonist
	ACE inhibitors
		Acute Glomerulonephritis
		  PSGN
		  Postinfectious GN
		  RPGN
		  FSGS
		  MPGN
		  Diffuse mesangial sclerosis
		  Mesangial proliferative
		    GN
		  Microscopic polyangiitis
		  Lupus nephritis
		  IgA nephropathy
		  Goodpasture disease
		  Wegener granulomatosis
		Acute tubular necrosis
		  Hypoxic-ischemic insult
		    Protracted prerenal state
		    Cardiorespiratory arrest
		    ECMO/bypass
		    Near-drowning
		    Asphyxia
		  Cellular lysis
		    Rhabdomyolyis
		    Hemolysis
		    Tumor lysis syndrome
		  Renal microvascular disease
		    HUS
		    TTP
		    DIC
		    Small-vessel vasculitis
		  Drugs
		    Acyclovir
		    Aminoglycosides
		    Radiographic contrast
		    Amphotericin
		    Others
		  Tubulointerstitial Nephritis
		    Hypersensitivity
		      Penicillins
		      Cephalosporins
		      NSAIDs
		    Infectious
		  Congenital kidney disease
		  Nephrotic syndrome
		  Lab values
			UPJ obstruction
			Ureterocele
			Extrinsic ureteral compression
			Nephrolithiasis
			UVJ obstruction
			Neurogenic bladder
			Vesicoureteral reflux
			Posterior urethral valves
			Prune-belly syndrome
			Renal vein thrombosis

LAB Values			
U_{Na} (mEq/L)	<20	>40 (may be <30 in AGN)	>40
U_{osm}/P_{osm}	>1.5	1–1.5	1–1.5
FE_{Na} (%)	<1	>2 (may be <1 in AGN)	>2

U_{Na} = urine sodium, mEq/L (without forced diuresis).
U_{osm}/P_{osm} = urine to plasma osmolality ratio.
FE_{Na} = fractional excretion of sodium [$100 \times (U_{Na}/P_{Na})/(U_{Cr}/P_{Cr})$].

INTRINSIC RENAL FAILURE

Just as renal parenchyma is composed of the glomerulus, the balance of the nephron, distal collecting tubules, vascular supply, and supporting interstitial tissues, ARF can arise from disease at a glomerular, tubular, or interstitial level.

Glomerular diseases may lead to acute renal failure through either new-onset, or acute-on-chronic, changes. Poststreptococcal (PSGN) or postinfectious glomerulonephritis (GN) will be frequently encountered. Other primary glomerular diseases include rapidly progressive glomerulonephritis (RPGN), membranoproliferative glomerulonephritis (MPGN), focal segmental glomerulosclerosis (FSGS), mesangial proliferative GN, diffuse mesangial sclerosis, lupus nephritis, IgA nephropathy, Goodpasture disease, Wegener granulomatosis, microscopic polyangiitis, and other vasculitides.

Considering the extensive list of histologically distinct glomerular diseases above, most of which require nephrology and rheumatology management, it is encouraging to note that ATN is the intrinsic renal disease most often encountered in the hospitalized pediatric patient. ATN is typically secondary to protracted prerenal states. Additionally, hypoxic insult from near-drowning, asphyxia, or cardiorespiratory arrest will produce tubular injury. Myoglobin from rhabdomyolysis, hemoglobin from brisk hemolysis, and tumor lysis syndrome all have potential to precipitate and damage the tubules. Renal microvascular diseases including disseminated intravascular coagulation (DIC), hemolytic uremic syndrome (HUS), thrombotic thrombocytopenic purpura (TTP), and small-vessel vasculitis, are preferentially injurious to the tubules. ATN may complicate pharmacotherapy with acyclovir, aminoglycosides, radiographic contrast media, amphotericin, cyclosporine, tacrolimus, methotrexate, cisplatinin, and many other drugs.

Renal diseases that predominantly affect neither the glomerulus nor the tubules themselves are referred to collectively as TIN or interstitial nephritis interchangeably. Hypersensitivity reactions to penicillins, cephalosporins, nonsteroidal anti-inflammatory drugs (NSAIDs), and sulfa are the most common. Infections including bacterial pyelonephritis with vesicoureteral reflux, acid-fast bacilli, viral, and fungal infections may all be seen in interstitial nephritis.

Although they do not fit neatly into one of the three main categories of the intrinsic renal disease, polycystic kidney disease, nephrotic syndrome, hypoplastic and congenitally dysplastic kidneys, and metabolic diseases affecting the kidneys should all be mentioned in this context.

POSTRENAL FAILURE

Postrenal failure most often develops in relation to a structural or anatomic defect. Posterior urethral valves (PUV), with or without prune-belly syndrome, are not uncommon. Obstruction at the ureterovesicular junction (UVJ), an ureterocele, or the ureteropelvic junction (UPJ) may escape notice for years, as azotemia will not occur in unilateral lesions proximal to the bladder. Neurogenic bladder, vesicoureteral reflux, nephrolithiasis, and masses extrinsic to the urinary system may all cause acute renal failure. Obstruction to venous drainage from the kidney in the form of renal vein thrombosis should be included here as well.

EVALUATION

With such a broad differential diagnosis, arriving at the specific etiology for ARF requires a meticulous history, review of past medical records, thorough physical examination with particular attention to volume status and edema, and careful interpretation of laboratory results. Pertinent historical information includes onset of swelling, if present, and recent changes in weight or blood pressure. Urinary pattern should be assessed for any evidence of oliguria or polyuria. Recent fluid intake, vomiting, diarrhea, and hematochezia should be questioned. Water sources, possible contaminated food sources, toxin exposures, and medication history are important to document. Recent infections with particular attention to pharyngitis or skin/soft-tissue infection should be elicited. Fever, chills, oral lesions, photosensitivity, rash, and arthralgias should all be noted. Abdominal pain or mass, flank or suprapubic pain, and gross hematuria may suggest a specific etiology. Recent trauma,

environmental heat exposure, myalgias, or excessive exercise would raise the suspicion of rhabdomyolysis. Severe headache, altered mental status, or seizures are important to note as well.

Once hospitalized, the patient continues to be at risk for exacerbation of the presenting condition and is placed at risk for development of ARF due to medical therapy. Accurate intake and output measurements from all sources should be maintained and reviewed frequently. In an unfortunately common scenario, voluminous stool output may be recorded and misinterpreted as urinary output, delaying the identification of oliguric renal failure. Generous gastrostomy and nasogastric tube output as well as fistula or surgical drain output may also go unrecognized and under-replaced for long periods of time. Tachycardia develops in advance of oliguria such that vital signs should be regularly observed for evidence of volume depletion. Upon return from the operating room, documentation should be reviewed for net fluid balance during the procedure, intraoperative hypoxic or ischemic episodes, and medications given. Children undergoing cardiac surgery should also have their operative course reviewed for the duration of bypass pump time and duration of aortic cross-clamping. Likewise, at each interface of care, previous procedures and medications received should be evaluated for the possibility of contributing to ARF.

Past medical history should be complete, but specifically interrogated for neonatal course (umbilical vessel catheters), drug history, prior renal disease, surgical history, any previous lab studies that might be available, and prior radiographic studies. Family history of vasculitis, renal disease, hemoglobinopathies, and hypertension are helpful. Particularly in the adolescent, social history should address the possibility of laxative for diuretic abuse, dietary supplements, sexual activity, and recreational or habitual drug abuse.

Physical examination starts with vital signs carefully noting weight, general growth parameters, heart rate, and blood pressure as compared to age and height standardized charts. Orthostatic blood pressure measurements and four extremity blood pressures should be obtained when appropriate. Clinical estimate of volume status (hypovolemic, euvolemic, hypervolemic) should be made based on assessment of edema, fontanelle, tear production, mucous membranes, skin turgor, mental status, and capillary refill. As children will often display an atypical distribution of edema, it is vital to pay special attention to the periorbital area, face, sacral area, and external genitalia in addition to lower extremity–dependent edema. Auscultation of the lungs may reveal rales in pulmonary edema, diminished breath sounds or friction rubs in pleural effusions, or evidence of pneumonia. Cardiovascular examination should note activity of the precordium, perfusion, and jugular venous distention. During abdominal examination, the examiner should be alert for costovertebral angle tenderness, abdominal masses, tenderness, shifting dullness or fluid wave suggesting ascites, and auscultate for flank or abdominal bruit. The skin should be scrutinized for exanthem, petechiae or purpura, malar rash, or other stigmata of vasculitic processes.

Attention to the detail of urine output is critical, though changes in UOP do not always correlate well with changes in GFR. However, the categories of anuric, oliguric, and nonoliguric renal failure may assist in working through the differential diagnosis of ARF. Anuric ARF (UOP <0.1 mL/kg/hr) suggests postrenal obstruction, RPGN, HUS, severe renal cortical necrosis, Takayasu arteritis, or renal artery thromboembolism. Oliguric ARF (0.1–1 mL/kg/hr) suggests prerenal failure or severe AGN, while nonoliguric ARF (>1 mL/kg/hr) suggests TIN, AGN, nephrotic syndrome, loss of concentrating ability, toxins, and other intrinsic renal disease in the absence of diuretic therapy.

Laboratory evaluation for all patients with ARF should include basic blood chemistries: sodium (Na), potassium (K), bicarbonate (CO_2), blood urea nitrogen (BUN), and creatinine (P_{Cr}). Plasma osmolality (P_{osm}), and urinary osmolality (U_{osm}), sodium (U_{Na}), and creatinine (U_{Cr}) are also quite helpful. Examination of the urine must include microscopic analysis of urine sediment. Beyond this, studies ordered should be targeted.

Creatinine measurement, while imperfect, is the most specific clinically available and standard measure we have for following and trending renal function. Creatinine is synthesized from creatine and phosphocreatine in lean muscle mass. As such, a "normal" creatinine level is related to the patient's weight. In catabolic states, creatinine levels fall as less lean muscle mass is available for turnover. The typical creatinine for a healthy adolescent up to 1.2 mg/dL would be considered quite abnormal in a small infant. It must be remembered that until the 4th day of life, the newborn's creatinine level is indicative of the maternal level. Unfortunately, creatinine rise may lag well behind GFR deterioration during rapidly progressive ARF. Additionally, in acute GN, tubular secretion of creatinine, normally minimal, may be considerable leading to a lower creatinine level than would otherwise be expected for the degree of GFR decrease. These caveats notwithstanding, trending creatinine levels are quite useful in ARF. Using a single serum creatinine determination, the GFR can be reasonably estimated from the Counahan–Barratt equation:

$$\text{GFR (mL/min/1.73m}^2) = (0.43 \times \text{length}) / P_{Cr}$$

In rapidly developing and in profound renal failure, the above equation likely overestimates GFR preservation, such that it is best to assume a lower GFR for diagnostic and drug-dosing purposes. BUN is less ideal for trending renal function for a variety of reasons. BUN levels are subject to nonrenal influences including trauma, gastrointestinal bleeding, steroids, and nutritional status. Urea nitrogen, unlike creatinine, is readily reabsorbed in the tubules at a rate inversely proportional to tubular flow. In other words, in low tubular flow states, more urea nitrogen will be reabsorbed into the bloodstream from the tubular lumen such that the BUN will rise out of proportion to the serum creatinine. BUN/creatinine ratio >20 is thus indicative of prerenal azotemia in most circumstances.

Measurement of U_{Na} and osmolality of urine and serum allows several indices to be calculated that may help distinguish prerenal from intrinsic renal failure (Table 62.1). In prerenal azotemia, compensatory measures favor urinary concentration and reabsorption of filtered sodium from the tubules in order to preserve total body water. Accordingly, U_{Na} <20 mEq/L and U_{osm}/P_{osm} >1.5 are diagnostically consistent with prerenal states, whereas U_{Na} >40 mEq/L and U_{osm}/P_{osm} in range from 1.0 to 1.5 favors intrinsic or postrenal failure. A very useful measure that includes both sodium avidity and a measure of creatinine clearance, the fractional excretion of sodium (FE_{Na}):

$$FE_{Na} = 100 \times (U_{Na}/P_{Na})/(U_{Cr}/P_{Cr})$$

is <1% in prerenal failure and >2% in intrinsic renal and postrenal failure.

Important exceptions should be noted. Unique among the intrinsic renal diseases, AGN will often show U_{Na} <20, U_{osm}/P_{osm} 1 to 1.5, and FE_{Na} <1 due to intact tubular function with physiologically appropriate reabsorption of filtered sodium. Children with concentrating defects or with other causes for non-oliguric ARF will not show the physiologically expected increase in urinary sodium in response to volume depletion in prerenal ARF. If prerenal conditions persist, urinary indices will transition into those typical of ATN, where tubular necrosis will interfere with sodium absorption and U_{Na} may be quite elevated. During that transition, the indices above may be equivocal. Finally, all of the indices rely on physiologic underpinnings that are disrupted and invalidated by therapeutic maneuvers, especially forced diuresis.

Complete urinalysis is the single most important laboratory evaluation in acute renal failure. The urine color in brisk hemolysis, rhabdomyolysis, and glomerulonephritis will often be described as tea- or cola-colored. The supernatant remaining after centrifugation should allow discrimination, as hemolytic processes will generally have a pink supernatant whereas rhabdomyolysis and glomerulonephritis will continue to have a brown supernatant. Measurement of specific gravity will permit identification of urine that is inappropriately dilute or confirm suspected prerenal states. Gross hematuria will be noted in IgA nephropathy, glomerulonephritis, urinary tract infection, and traumatic injury. Proteinuria is a rather nonspecific finding, but dipstick findings of 3+ to 4+ proteinuria are consistent with glomerulonephritis and nephrotic syndrome. Leukocyte esterase is also a nonspecific finding, but may increase suspicion for pyelonephritis. Microscopic analysis of spun urinary sediment is often most revealing. Sediment will appear benign in prerenal in most instances of postrenal failure. Red blood cells (RBCs) will be seen in many types of intrinsic renal disease. When dipstick testing is positive for blood but microscopy does not reveal RBCs, either myoglobin or free hemoglobin is presumed to be present. The morphology of RBCs or presence of RBC casts is helpful: RBCs that appear as normal biconcave disks (eumorphic) have entered the urine after the glomerulus; they are consistent with infection, TIN, ATN, trauma, nephrolithiasis, and other causes of postrenal failure. On the other hand, RBC casts and mangled-appearing (dysmorphic) RBCs are pathognomonic for glomerulonephritis. Additionally, white blood cell (WBC) casts may be seen in interstitial nephritis, thromboembolism, and pyelonephritis. If stained, the WBC casts seen in pyelonephritis will be neutrophils, whereas those in interstitial nephritis or thromboembolism will most often be eosinophils. Crystals may suggest drug (acyclovir, sulfonamides, methotrexate, IV radiocontrast) nephropathy or nephrolithiasis.

Hyperkalemia, hypokalemia, hyponatremia, hypernatremia, hyperphosphatemia, hypocalcemia, and other electrolyte disturbances are all seen with acute renal failure. Of these, hyperkalemia poses greatest threat to life acutely due to cardiotoxicity. As hyperkalemia is covered elsewhere in this text (Chapter 14), only brief discussion of its management will be covered here.

Hyponatremia is often seen with nephrotic syndrome, SIADH, and dehydration with inappropriate oral fluid replacement. Hypernatremia is also seen with severe dehydration and inappropriate formula preparation in infants as well as in nephrogenic or central diabetes insipidus. Hypokalemia together with hypophosphatemia is frequently encountered in patients on diuretics, amphotericin B, and cyclosporine. The pattern of hyperkalemia, hyperphosphatemia, and hypocalcemia should raise concern for the possibility of acute-on-chronic renal failure. Complete blood count is often helpful in differentiating the causes of ARF. Leukocytosis may be appreciated in systemic infection, enterocolitis, pyelonephritis, vasculitis, and TIN. Leukopenia may be seen in association with overwhelming sepsis, viral infection, lupus, and other vasculitis. Microcytic anemia suggests anemia of chronic disease, lead poisoning, or hemoglobinopathy with chronic hemolysis. Normocytic anemia may be seen in acute hemorrhage, acute hemolysis, chronic illness, vasculitis, glomerulonephritis, IgA nephropathy, or chronic renal failure. RBC morphology should always be reviewed, as the findings of microangiopathic hemolytic forms combined with thrombocytopenia in the face of azotemia is highly suggestive of hemolytic uremic syndrome (HUS), disseminated intravascular coagulation (DIC), or thrombotic thrombocytopenic purpura (TTP). HUS, in particular, is one of the more common causes of pediatric ARF and may occur as complication of bacterial enterocolitis with *E. coli*

TABLE 62.2

ADDITIONAL SPECIFIC TESTING IN ARF

Finding	Specific testing
Recent pharyngitis or skin infection, urinary sediment consistent with glomerulonephritis	Anti-streptolysin O titer, anti-DNAse B, throat culture C3, C4
Malar rash, oral lesions, arthralgias, photosensitivity	ANA, anti-dsDNA, C3, C4, SS-A, SS-B
Sinusitis, wheezing, recurrent respiratory infection	ANCA, anti-GBM, CXR, ? high-resolution chest CT and
Gross hematuria with viral URI	IgA
Abdominal pain, arthralgias, purpura	IgA, ANCA
Crush injury, myalgias, brown urine	CK, aldolase
Thrombocytopenia	PT, PTT, fibrinogen, D-dimers, ADAMTS-13
Male, poor urinary stream	VCUG
Severe occipital headache, visual disturbance, seizure	Head CT

0157:H7, *Shigella dysenteriae*, or of pneumococcal respiratory infection. Isolated thrombocytopenia is seen most often in vasculitis, thromboembolic events, or as a drug toxicity.

Additional laboratory testing should be based on a narrowed differential diagnosis after the completion of the above evaluation (Table 62.2).

Renal ultrasound with Doppler interrogation will be negative in most cases of prerenal ARF. Increased echogenicity may be noted in ATN, AGN, and TIN. Polycystic kidney disease, dysplastic kidneys, renal agenesis, hydronephrosis, hydroureter, or other specific leads may be obtained. Doppler of the renal pedicle may reveal thromboembolic events. Voiding cystourethrogram (VCUG) should be pursued for suspicion of PUV, neurogenic bladder, or reflux nephropathy.

MANAGEMENT

Recognizing the significant morbidity and mortality burden of ARF and the fact that azotemia may not develop until >50% of baseline GFR has been lost, the goal of therapy must be preservation of the remaining viable renal units. Therapy cannot await a definitive underlying etiology and empiric supportive care must be initiated promptly while investigation continues. A rapid assessment of volume status determines need for fluid resuscitation. Especially given that prerenal failure and ATN due to prolonged prerenal states are by far the most common causes of ARF in children, it is unwise to initially restrict fluids due to theoretical concerns regarding fluid overload. Normal saline 20 mL/kg IV bolus should be followed by frequent reassessment, and additional fluids given as needed until it is clear that there is no further benefit of volume loading or contraindicated by evidence of fluid overload. Initiation of loop diuretic once intravascular volume appears replete, indwelling urinary catheterization to improve monitoring of urine output changes, and elimination of dietary and parenteral potassium sources are all appropriate steps in initial management. Any nephrotoxic drugs that the patient is currently receiving should be suspended if possible and care should be taken to assure that there is no unnecessary exposure to nephrotoxic agents going forward. Radiographic contrast media, nephrotoxic antibiotics, and NSAIDs are particularly important to avoid in this context. Any medication that must be continued should be reviewed for nephrotoxicity. Renally cleared medications should be adjusted for the esti-

mated GFR. Ongoing excessive fluid losses should be identified and replaced in addition to maintenance fluid requirements. The main treatment goal of presumed prerenal failure is prompt rehydration and reestablishment of effective urine output. Likewise, the immediate treatment goal of postrenal failure is prompt removal of obstruction if present and reestablishment of normal urine output.

In the event that oliguric or anuric ARF fails to reestablish normal urine output rapidly, appropriate fluid replacement should be limited to insensible losses (350 mL/m²/day) as D5%W in addition to urinary output, measured and replaced every 4 hours. Urine electrolytes should be measured in order to determine the correct composition of replacement fluids. For the patient who is intravascularly replete with fluid overload, avoidance of overhydration is important. Meticulous attention to fluid replacement, appropriate use of diuretics, pressors, and early renal replacement therapy for fluid removal must be considered. Fluid management in ATN merits unique attention, as a polyuric phase with persistent renal dysfunction and concentrating defect may be anticipated after 1 to 2 weeks of oliguria as tubular regeneration progresses. The massive diuresis characteristic of the recovery phase may be exacerbated by diuretics started during the oliguric phase and can lead to intravascular depletion quickly if diuretics are not stopped and fluids are not increased to match output.

Renal replacement therapy (RRT) options include peritoneal dialysis (PD), intermittent hemodialysis (HD), continuous venovenous hemofiltration (CVVH), and most recently continuous venovenous hemodialysis (CVVHD). Each modality has its own advantages and disadvantages, which are beyond the scope of this chapter. HD is more widely available and very effective at solute removal, but is associated with greater magnitude of fluid shifts. The periods of hypotension associated with these fluid shifts place the patient's injured and vulnerable renal parenchyma at risk. Less widely available but favored by many in the intensive-care unit setting, CVVH is more effective at water removal and control of uremia. Because it is continuously at work, fluid shifts are avoided and it is better tolerated in hemodynamically unstable children. CVVHD is true dialysis and therefore superior to CVVH in solute removal but maintains the advantages of continuous renal replacement therapy. Mostly of use in chronic renal failure and in infants too small for CVVH or HD, PD is technically simple, requires fewer resources, but has limited applicability in ARF because of the slower processes for solute and fluid removal. Well-accepted indications for acute RRT in ARF are hypertension with volume overload refractory to vasodilation, phlebotomy, and diuresis; severe hyperkalemia associated with electrocardiogram changes in refractory to calcium, insulin/glucose, bicarbonate, albuterol, and Kayexalate; acidosis refractory to sodium bicarbonate and phosphate binders; uremia associated with serositis, bleeding, or mental status changes; severe hyponatremia or hypernatremia; and dialyzable intoxication.

Hyperkalemia alters cardiac automaticity and provokes ECG changes in a predictable concentration-dependent fashion. Initially T-waves peak, then PR and QRS complexes widen, followed by a sinusoidal pattern, heralding asystole. The absolute potassium (K^+) level at which cardiotoxicity is inaugurated varies with pH, calcium, and magnesium levels, but in general, K^+ levels >6.0 demand cardiac monitoring and an action plan to protect the heart. In the presence of hyperkalemia and ECG changes beyond peaking of T-waves, calcium chloride (20 mg/kg up to 500 mg maximum IV) is cardioprotective (but does *not* lower the K^+ level) and rapid in onset; in the absence of ECG changes the risks of calcium infusion are not merited and other measures to reduce serum K^+ levels are more appropriate. Insulin (0.1 unit/kg) with 25% dextrose (0.5 g/kg) administered IV over 30 minutes will reduce serum K^+ by moving K^+ intracellularly though total body potassium is unchanged. Albuterol (10 mg nebulized) has been shown to reduce K^+ levels transiently in some but not all patients. Sodium bicarbonate, long a mainstay of initial treatment to lower serum potassium levels, is no longer recommended except in hyperkalemia with concomitant acidosis, as several studies have shown it to be ineffective. Regardless of the initial approach, they are temporizing measures to protect the heart from the deleterious effects of hyperkalemia and do not reduce total body potassium stores. If the patient has intact response to furosemide (1 mg/kg IV), it can be effective in inducing kaliuresis. Otherwise, the cation exchange resin, sodium polystyrene sulfonate (Kayexalate, 1 g/kg every 6 hours orally or rectally), permits excretion of potassium through dialysis across the bowel. It should be clear that neither furosemide nor exchange resins are appropriate as the initial steps in hyperkalemia from a cardioprotective standpoint, and equally clear that neither calcium, insulin/glucose, albuterol, nor sodium bicarbonate have a lasting effect or reduce total body potassium stores.

To prevent deleterious effects of hyperphosphatemia (acidosis, arrhythmia, extraosseous calcification, hypocalcemia, tetany) in ARF, intake from dietary and medication sources should be minimized and oral calcium carbonate (100 mg/kg three times per day with meals) should be given as a phosphate binder to further minimize absorption of dietary phosphates.

Metabolic acidosis in ARF can be severe and can be ameliorated by a low-protein diet. Nutritional consultation is helpful in view of the difficulty following a low-protein, low-potassium, low-phosphate diet.

COURSE

The prognosis and outcome for children with ARF are as variable as the conditions that live under its tent. Mortality rates from 10% to 50% have been reported. The vast majority of cases of prerenal azotemia and most cases of ATN will demonstrate significant to full recovery with excellent long-term prognosis. Many patients with postrenal failure will have lasting sequellae unless the duration of obstruction is brief. A nuclear diuretic renogram may help manage these patients after discharge, as it represents a functional assessment of individual kidney performance. For those patients with other intrinsic causes for ARF, outcome is more variable and close nephrology follow-up is essential.

Suggested Readings

Andreoli SP. Management of acute renal failure. In: Barratt TM, Avner ED, Harmon WE, eds. *Pediatric nephrology*. 4th ed. Philadelphia: Lippincott Williams & Wilkins; 1999:1119–1133.

Askenazi DJ, Feig DI, Graham NM, et al. 3–5 year longitudinal follow-up of pediatric patients after acute renal failure. *Kidney Int* 2006;69:184–189.

Bellomo R, Ronco C, Kellum JA. Acute renal failure—definition, outcome measures, animal models, fluid therapy and information technology needs: the second international consensus conference of the acute dialysis quality initiative (ADQI) group. *Crit Care* 2004;8:R204-R212.

Bock KR. Renal replacement therapy in pediatric critical care medicine. *Curr Opin Pediatr* 2005;17:368–371. Related articles, links.

Ellis EN, Pearson D, Belsha CW, et al. Use of pump-assisted hemofiltration in children with acute renal failure. *Pediatr Nephrol* 1997;11:196–200.

Flynn JT. Causes, management approaches, and outcome of acute renal failure in children. *Curr Opin Pediatr* 1998;10:184–189.

Goldstein SL, Somers MJ, Baum MA, et al. Pediatric patients with multi-organ dysfunction syndrome receiving continuous renal replacement therapy. *Kidney Int* 2005;67:653–658.

Kamel KS, Wei C. Controversial issues in the treatment of hyperkalaemia. *Nephrol Dial Transplant* 2003;18:2215–2218.

Klahr S, Miller SB. Acute oliguria. *N Engl J Med* 1998;338:671–675.

Korevaar JC, Jansen MA, Dekker FW. Evaluation of DOQI guidelines: early start of dialysis treatment is not associated with better health-related quality of life. National Kidney Foundation dialysis outcomes quality initiative. *Am J Kidney Dis* 2002;39:108–115.

Moghal NE, Brocklebank JT, Meadow SR. A review of acute renal failure in children: incidence, etiology and outcome. *Clin Nephrol* 1998;49:91–95.

Nash K, Hafeez A, Hou S. Hospital-acquired renal insufficiency. *Am J Kidney Dis* 2002;39:930–936.

Quan A, Quigley R. Renal replacement therapy and acute renal failure. *Curr Opin Pediatr* 2005;17:205–209.

Shilliday IR, Quinn KJ, Allison ME. Loop diuretics in the management of acute renal failure: a prospective, double-blind, placebo-controlled, randomized study. *Nephrol Dial Transplant* 1997;12:2592–2596.

Siegel NJ, Van Why SK, Devarajan P. Pathogenesis of acute renal failure. In: Barratt TM, Avner ED, Harmon WE, eds. *Pediatric nephrology*. 4th ed. Philadelphia: Lippincott Williams & Wilkins; 1999:1109–1118.

Stapleton FB, Jones DP, Green RS. Acute renal failure in neonates: incidence, etiology and outcome. *Pediatr Nephrol* 1987;1:314–320.

Star RA. Treatment of acute renal failure. *Kidney Int* 1998;54:1817–1831.

Thadhani R, Pascual M, Bonventre JV. Acute renal failure. *N Engl J Med* 1996;334:1448–1460.

CHAPTER 63 ■ HEMOLYTIC-UREMIC SYNDROME

JEFF ARMSTRONG

BACKGROUND

Hemolytic-uremic syndrome (HUS), first described in 1955, is a heterogeneous syndrome characterized by a triad of microangiopathic hemolytic anemia, acute renal failure, and thrombocytopenia. Initially thought to be a sporadic process, it is now recognized as the most common cause of acute renal failure in children. Nearly 30 years passed before the connection of the classic hemorrhagic enterocolitis caused by *Escherichia coli* O157:H7 to this triad was made in 1982 during outbreaks caused by contaminated hamburger meat. Shortly after that, in 1983, the presence of a Shiga-like toxin was elucidated. The pathophysiology remains to be fully understood.

The degree of anemia, renal insufficiency, and thrombocytopenia can be quite variable. Incomplete forms of HUS with absence of anemia, azotemia, or thrombocytopenia have been described, which may make the diagnosis more elusive. To complicate matters, the list of nonclassic forms caused by other infectious agents, drugs, and other conditions, continues to grow. Although the outcome is usually favorable, HUS does have a risk of acute mortality and chronic morbidity depending on the causative agent.

At this time, there appears to be no current therapeutic interventions available in clinical practice that can prevent the onset of HUS. Even though antibiotics effective for the organisms that cause HUS are available, their use may be associated with a potential risk of precipitating HUS. For now, the emphasis is on diagnosis, close observation, and therapeutic intervention when needed to prevent complications.

EPIDEMIOLOGY

The majority of HUS in children (90%) is related to the prototypic diarrhea-associated form (D+ HUS) predominately in previously healthy children 6 months to 4 years of age with a peak between 1 and 2 years of age. Shiga toxin-producing *E. coli* (STEC) is the major cause of diarrhea-associated HUS in the United States. Specifically, *E. coli* with the serotype O157:H7 is the bacteria most commonly associated with HUS (90%) and is the most virulent. There are a number of other non-O157:H7 strains of STEC that can cause HUS. STEC can cause a wide spectrum of disease ranging from asymptomatic carriage to hemorrhagic colitis and development of HUS. Asymptomatic infection with STEC can also lead to HUS. Of young children infected with STEC, about 5% to 10% develop HUS.

Other terms synonymous with Shiga toxin-producing *E. coli* (STEC) include enterohemorrhagic *E. coli* (EHEC) in reference to the typically bloody stools, verotoxin-producing *E. coli* (VTEC) derived from the extreme cytopathogenic effect to Vero cell culture lines grown from African green monkey kidneys, and Shiga-like toxin-producing *E. coli* given the remarkable similarity to the toxin produced by *Shigella dysenteriae*. The American Academy of Pediatrics Red Book has recently replaced the term EHEC with STEC.

E. coli O157:H7 is part of the normal bacterial flora in the intestines of healthy cattle, and contamination of beef can occur during the slaughtering process. The risk is highest in ground beef because the surface of the contaminated slabs of beef gets mixed internally throughout the meat during the process of making ground beef and accounts for the majority of food-borne infections. Up to 5% of the ground beef samples in U.S. supermarkets are positive for *E. coli* O157:H7. Thorough cooking, when done properly to achieve a sufficient internal meat temperature, kills the bacteria. However, cases of STEC-mediated HUS continue to occur despite attempts to have safer slaughterhouse, meat processing, food handling, irradiation of raw meat products, and cooking standards.

Goats, sheep, deer, pigs, chickens, and game may be other sources for STEC. Typically acquired from eating raw or undercooked ground beef, other sources include unpasteurized milk, contaminated lettuce, ice, apple cider, apple juice, uncooked vegetables, as well as contaminated swimming pools, water parks, and lakes, and person-to-person transmission within families and day-care centers. Petting zoos are another potential source of exposure. As a low-inoculum disease, it takes few organisms for spread and low level of exposure to contaminated water. The incidence is 1 to 3 cases per 100,000 each year in the United States. The rate is significantly higher in countries like Argentina, the Netherlands, and South Africa. There is a seasonal prevalence peaking in summer/early fall, which correlates with an increased rate of positive cultures in cattle stools in warmer months. Epidemics can occur. Onset is typically acute, with both genders and all races affected, and with a favorable outcome in most cases. African-Americans are rarely affected. Other pathogens for D+ HUS are listed in Table 63.1.

In contrast to D+ HUS, the atypical nondiarrheal forms of HUS (D− HUS) rarely occur in children and are more common in adults, do not have a seasonal pattern, are insidious in onset, are more likely to recur, have a higher acute mortality rate, and have a worse prognosis. A significant proportion (up to 50%) of D− HUS is idiopathic. For the remainder, the triggers include a large variety of infectious agents and other conditions (Table 63.1). *Streptococcus pneumoniae* can cause up to 40% of D− HUS. The familial forms (autosomal dominant and autosomal recessive) are associated with complement protein abnormalities often due to mutations in the gene for factor H,

TABLE 63.1

CAUSES OF HEMOLYTIC–UREMIC SYNDROME

DIARRHEA-ASSOCIATED HEMOLYTIC–UREMIC SYNDROME (D+ HUS)
  Shiga toxin-producing *Escherichia coli* (STEC), especially O157:H7
  Shigella dysenteriae
  Salmonella typhi
  Campylobacter jejuni
  Clostridium difficile
  Yersinia species
  Pseudomonas species
  Bacteroides species
  Aeromonas hydrophila
  Streptococcus pyogenes
  Entamoeba histolytica
  Microtatobiotes

NON–DIARRHEA-ASSOCIATED HEMOLYTIC–UREMIC SYNDROME (D– HUS)
  Idiopathic
  Infections
    Streptococcus pneumoniae
    Staphylococcus aureus
    Streptococcus pyogenes
    Bordetella pertussis
    Citrobacter species
    Coxiella burnetti
    Helicobacter pylori
    Mycoplasma species
    Cytomegalovirus
    Enteroviruses
    Epstein–Barr virus
    Herpes simplex virus
    Hanta virus
    Hepatitis A virus
    Human immunodeficiency virus
    Influenza virus

    Portillo virus
    Aspergillus fumigatus
  Drugs
    Mitomycin-C
    Cisplatin
    Bleomycin
    Gemcitabine
    Cyclosporine
    Tacrolimus
    OKT3
    Quinine
    Interferon
    Ticlopidine
    Clopidogrel
    Oral contraceptives
    Cocaine
  Vaccines
    Mumps
    Measles
    Smallpox
    Polio
    Diphtheria
    Pertussis
    Tetanus
    Typhoid
  Scorpion bites
  Malignancy
  Pregnancy
  Organ and bone marrow transplantation
  Malignant hypertension
  Primary glomerulopathies
  Inborn error of metabolism (e.g., cobalamin C disease)
  Immunodeficiency
  Inherited familial forms
  Collagen/vascular disease

and have a particularly poor prognosis. Fortunately, these are less common. Cases of HUS associated with urinary tract infections caused by STEC have been reported.

PATHOGENESIS

In D+ HUS, with Shiga toxin-producing *E. coli* O157:H7 infection, the toxin binds, invades, and causes destruction of colonic epithelial cells, resulting in bloody diarrhea. Presumably because of the inflamed colon allowing transmural absorption, the toxin then enters the blood circulation. There the toxin binds to a glycolipid receptor known as globotriaosylceramide (Gb3), which results in endocytosis of the toxin usually within renal glomerular endothelial cells, and at times, other target organs. The expression of Gb3 receptors appears to be higher in infants and young children, which may in part explain the age-related propensity for developing HUS. Older children and adults have lower numbers of these receptors but may develop HUS whenever the combined effect of lipopolysaccharide and cytokines upregulate the expression of these Gb3 receptors.

The presence and frequency of these Gb3 receptors in other organs may also explain the variable expression of the extrarenal manifestations of HUS (seizures, stroke, coma, pancreatitis, myocarditis, hepatitis, and diabetes mellitus).

The cellular internalization of the toxin leads to inhibition of protein synthesis. As a result, injury and/or death of the endothelial cells ensues, with release of endothelial products and detachment from the basement membrane. Adhesion and aggregation of platelets to the exposed basement membrane occurs with formation of thrombi and inhibition of fibrinolysis. The glomerular filtration rate is reduced by the swelling of the endothelial cells and fibrin deposition on the injured vessel walls. Erythrocytes and platelets are damaged as they pass through the affected narrowed glomerular capillaries. Thrombocytopenia results from consumption due to vascular injury. Microangiopathic hemolytic anemia develops as the reticuloendothelial system removes the fragmented red blood cells.

In the atypical D– *Streptococcus pneumoniae*-mediated HUS, the process is mediated by neuraminidase, which exposes the normally hidden Thomsen–Friedenreich antigen (T-antigen) on red blood cells, platelets, and glomerular endothelial cells. This allows serum anti-T antibodies present in most people to react with T-antigen causing HUS. Coombs testing during typing of blood for transfusion is typically positive in these individuals.

Given these various inciting events, the damaged renal vascular endothelium is typically the final common pathway for all types of HUS, resulting in thrombotic microangiopathy and fragmentation of RBCs involving numerous mediators (e.g., elastase, fibroblast growth factor, von Willebrand factor, platelet aggregating factor, tissue plasminogen activator inhibitor, tissue factor, thrombomodulin, thomboxane, prostacyclin, hemolysin, various interleukins, tumor necrosis factor, lipopolysaccharide, nitric oxide, and lipid peroxides). The individual variability in expression of these mediators and Gb3 receptors likely plays a role in determining which children are prone to developing severe clinical disease. The challenge with the nondiarrheal forms of HUS is the even larger variety of pathogenic pathways involved, complicating study and treatment.

CLINICAL FEATURES

With STEC infection, the incubation period is typically 3 to 4 days after exposure (range, 1 to 14 days). Initial signs of symptomatic infection are vomiting, diarrhea, and significant abdominal pain. The diarrhea is often watery like typical viral gastroenteritis for the first 1 to 3 days; then, in most cases (80%), it becomes bloody. Patients are often afebrile. Only 30% have fever and it tends to be low-grade in contrast to that seen with most bacterial enterocolitis. The hemorrhagic colitis resolves completely without any sequelae in most (90–95%) cases. Infection can also be asymptomatic. When it occurs, the triad of HUS typically follows the onset of diarrhea in 5 to 7 days (range, 1 to 14 days), often just as the colitis is resolving. This time lag may provide an opportunity for potential interventions to prevent renal failure. Lethargy, irritability, renewed vomiting, pallor, edema, hypertension, and decreased urine output are common. Hypertension occurs about 75% of the time. Renal involvement can be mild with only some microscopic hematuria and proteinuria with normal urine output, or may extend to irreversible renal failure with widespread cortical necrosis. Notably, the presence of diarrhea may mask oliguria. Oliguria occurs in many cases (about 60%) lasting typically about 1 week, with frank anuria (40%) lasting a few days.

Extrarenal manifestations, when present, can include rectal prolapse, toxic megacolon, bowel gangrene, intestinal perforation, colonic stenosis, intussusception, pancreatitis, pancreatic insufficiency (diabetes mellitus), CNS involvement (seizures, cerebral edema, hemiparesis, cranial nerve involvement, cerebral infarction), myocardial dysfunction, congestive heart failure with or without fluid overload, liver injury, and myositis. Most of the cardiovascular involvement in HUS is a result of fluid overload secondary to renal failure. Direct myocardial injury can sometimes occur. CNS involvement occurs up to 30% of the time, the most common manifestation being seizures. Often, metabolic derangements (e.g., hyponatremia, uremia) or hypertension are causative, but in some cases the seizures are the result of CNS vascular involvement. The presence of fever and CNS symptoms may make the distinction between HUS and thrombotic thrombocytopenic purpura (TTP) more difficult. TTP is mainly an adult process manifested by neurologic symptoms, fever, and mild renal dysfunction. Bloody diarrhea is uncommon. Both diseases share endothelial cell damage as the inciting event but by different mechanisms. TTP is either due to congenital absence of von Willebrand factor–cleaving protease enzyme (ADAMTS 13) activity or to an acquired antibody directed against this enzyme.

The differential diagnosis for HUS would include intussusception, inflammatory bowel disease, sepsis, meningococcemia, disseminated intravascular coagulation, vasculitis, leukemia and other malignancies, post-streptococcal glomerulonephritis, rapidly progressive glomerulonephritis, lupus nephritis, TTP, immune thrombocytopenic purpura (ITP), and immune hemolytic anemia.

LABORATORY FINDINGS

Suggested initial laboratory studies in suspected HUS would include a complete blood cell count, peripheral blood smear, electrolyte panel including blood urea nitrogen and creatinine, urinalysis, prothrombin time, partial thromboplastin time, stool occult blood, and stool culture.

Laboratory findings in HUS include anemia with fragmented red blood cells (schistocytes, burr cells, helmet cells) on a peripheral smear, thrombocytopenia, and elevated blood urea nitrogen and creatinine. The hemoglobin typically drops to 5 to 9 g/dL. Like other hemolytic processes, the reticulocyte count, total bilirubin, and lactate dehydrogenase are elevated with decreased haptoglobin levels. A direct Coombs test is usually negative except in *Streptococcus pneumoniae*-associated D– HUS. Platelets counts can initially remain above 100,000/mm^3 at the onset of disease, but then typically drop to around 40,000 to 50,000/mm^3 and can go as low as 5,000/mm^3. The degree of thrombocytopenia does not appear to correlate with the severity of the disease. Return of the platelet count to above 100,000/mm^3 may signal clinical recovery. Leukocytosis with an increased number of immature forms may be present. Prothrombin time and partial thromboplastin time are usually normal. Fibrin degradation products are elevated. Fibrinogen is increased or normal. Hyponatremia, hyperkalemia, acidosis, hyperphosphatemia, and hypocalcemia are commonly present as a result of oliguria or anuria. Hypoalbuminemia from GI losses frequently occurs. Urinalysis can reveal hematuria, proteinuria, sterile pyuria, dysmorphic red blood cells, and cellular casts.

Routine stool testing for *Shigella*, *Salmonella*, and *Campylobacter* will not detect STEC. Thus it is important to alert the microbiology lab in cases of suspected HUS so that not only the appropriate stool cultures are done, but other methods can be utilized to enhance diagnostic yield. The highest yield is from stool specimens obtained in the first week after the onset of illness and drops off significantly thereafter. It is important to recognize that stool culture alone for STEC, in general, has poor sensitivity, and especially when done at the time when HUS is being clinically suspected because by then the optimum yield from stool specimens has usually passed. Free fecal Stx from O157:H7 and non-O157:H7 STEC can be detected by other assay methods such as polymerase chain reaction (PCR) or enzyme immunoassay (EIA). Serum serologies are another method of confirming the diagnosis. Using a combination of these methods to test for the presence of STEC will give a higher diagnostic yield.

MANAGEMENT

Physicians should consider the possibility of STEC disease in children who present with diarrhea, especially with bloody stools. Goals are to quickly identify those at risk for developing HUS and to order appropriate stool studies so that potential therapeutic interventions, when made available, can help prevent HUS. Parents should be instructed for which signs and symptoms to be on the alert (e.g., lethargy, renewed vomiting, pallor, or decreased urine output). Antidiarrheal agents should be avoided (1). In terms of antibiotic treatment, the data are conflicting. A recent meta-analysis failed to both demonstrate an increased risk of HUS or significant benefit (2). Large controlled, adequately powered, prospective clinical trials to address this controversy are needed. In the absence of evidence demonstrating clear and consistent benefit, the administration of antibiotics for STEC disease is not presently recommended unless specific clinical indications are present (e.g., sepsis, peritonitis).

Monitoring stable patients with known or suspected STEC-associated gastroenteritis on an outpatient basis with serial clinical exams and labs (complete blood cell count and electrolytes) two or three times weekly for 1 to 2 weeks is recommended.

For patients developing symptoms of HUS, inpatient observation and management is indicated. Supportive care, with attention to fluid and electrolyte balance, management of renal failure with diuretics or dialysis, monitoring for and treating hypertension, nutritional support, and anticipating/managing complications is of paramount importance. Vital signs including blood pressure should be monitored every 4 hours. Intake and urine output should be continuously assessed. It is usually necessary to place a Foley catheter to get an accurate hourly urine output, especially if diarrhea is present. Electrolytes and renal function tests need to be checked every 6 hours until the patient is stable.

Renal failure protocols should be instituted (Chapter 62). Fluid overload must be avoided. If there is a colitis, pancreatitis, or other gastrointestinal process that precludes adequate enteral nutrition, total parenteral nutrition is often necessary. Furosemide drips may eliminate the need for dialysis. A dose of 1 mg/kg/hr can be initiated and then titrated downward as urine output dictates. Despite attempts at medical management of renal failure or fluid overload, dialysis may be required in 50% of patients. Both peritoneal and hemodialysis are effective as renal replacement therapy. The mode of dialysis depends on multiple factors including the age of the patient, experience and preference of consulting nephrologists, availability of various methods of dialysis, presence of GI tract complications, and hemodynamic stability.

Hypertension is commonly a result of fluid overload. If hypertension persists despite efforts to manage fluid overload with fluid restriction, a trial of diuretics is appropriate as first-line drug therapy. In persistent cases, it may be necessary to use either vasodilators (e.g., hydralazine) or calcium-channel blockers (e.g., nicardipine). Angiotensin-converting enzyme inhibitors should be avoided or used with caution in the presence of abnormal renal function during the acute phase of HUS.

Infectious complications may occur especially if indwelling catheters are in place (e.g., bladder catheters, hemodialysis catheters, peritoneal dialysis catheters, or central venous catheters). Anemia may require packed red blood cell transfusions either for symptomatic anemia or a hemoglobin concentration below 6 to 8 g/dL. In the D– *Streptococcus pneumoniae* neuraminidase-mediated disease, blood products should be washed to avoid the anti-T antibodies if screening tests are positive. Platelet transfusion should only be done when required due to continued consumption, that is, for symptomatic bleeding or prior surgical/invasive procedures. Inappropriate platelet transfusion may contribute further to the thrombotic microangiopathy.

Other therapies including fresh frozen plasma infusion, immunoglobulin infusion, fibrinolytic agents such as heparin, antiplatelet agents, and corticosteroids should not be used because of lack of demonstrable efficacy. Plasmapheresis is not usually effective for D+ HUS, and is contraindicated in *Streptococcus pneumoniae* neuraminidase-mediated disease because of the potential presence of anti-T antibodies. Plasmapheresis may be useful in certain forms of D– disease, especially in the familial types.

In severe or persistent renal disease, renal biopsy may be indicated. Angiotensin-converting enzyme inhibitors appear to be useful in patients with persistent proteinuria after the acute disease in preventing or attenuating hyperfiltration injury and development of chronic kidney disease.

NEW DIRECTIONS FOR FUTURE MANAGEMENT

Recently, a number of novel therapies to prevent HUS have been explored. The use of the enteral Shiga toxin binder SYN-SORB Pk, a synthetic molecule that binds to Stx, protects against the cytotoxic effects of the Stx and has so far shown promising results in animal models but has been disappointing in human clinical trials. The lack of efficacy could be due to the fact that the patients already had developed HUS at the time of enrollment into the study and may have had more of a beneficial effect if treatment had been initiated before the onset of HUS. There are more effective enteral toxin-binding agents available based on studies in mice. Human studies of these therapies are forthcoming. Recombinant bacteria based on a nonpathogenic strain of *E. coli* that produces a modified lipopolysaccharide that has a similar terminal sequence as the Gb3 receptor and thus functions as a receptor mimic for Shiga toxin, have even a higher binding affinity than Synsorb-Pk. The use of these probiotic recombinant bacteria will likely be limited in benefit, as they need to be given during the early course of the disease. The role of human monoclonal antibodies directed against Shiga toxin is being examined. An advantage of this approach would be potential clinical efficacy with parenteral administration even after systemic absorption of the toxin as opposed to the enteral toxin binders.

More rapid diagnostic tests to identify the presence of STEC-mediated gastroenteritis and allow earlier monitoring and treatment of patients with a potential risk of developing HUS need to be developed. This will be especially true when effective therapies to prevent the development of HUS become available.

Vaccination of either cattle, humans, or both may play a role in decreasing STEC infections and thus the incidence of D+ HUS. Ongoing research in this area is in progress.

COURSE AND PROGNOSIS

Most children with D+ HUS have a favorable outcome. The acute mortality rate during active disease is about 5%, usually due to central nervous system or cardiovascular complications. Patients presenting with oligoanuria, dehydration, leukocytosis >20,000/mm^3, and hematocrit >23% are at substantial risk for fatal HUS (3). Recurrences are rare (<1%). In up to 65% to 85% of patients, complete recovery of renal function occurs after acute HUS disease. Around 30% to 50% over the course of long term follow-up will have renal abnormalities such as proteinuria or hypertension, with about 5% eventually developing chronic kidney disease requiring dialysis. Renal sequelae can take as long as 20 years or more to develop. Therefore lifetime follow-up is appropriate for all children following an episode of HUS with regular assessment of urinalysis, blood pressure, and renal function tests. Those with persistent proteinuria, hematuria, hypertension, or renal insufficiency should be followed regularly by a pediatric nephrologist.

Children who have STEC-mediated diarrheal disease should be restricted from daycare or school attendance, until at least two stool specimens are negative. Given the significant potential for asymptomatic spread within family contacts of those with STEC, stool specimens should be checked in those contacts who go to daycare, are food handlers, or are health care workers.

Patients with D-HUS, in general, have a significantly higher acute mortality rate (around 25%), increased risk of recurrences (20–50%), and higher risk of chronic kidney disease or irreversible brain damage (30–50%). In *Streptococcus pneumonia*-associated disease the acute mortality rate is high as 50% and up to 50% develop chronic kidney disease. In the familial forms of HUS, the mortality approaches 70% to

90%, with chronic kidney disease in 50% to 60%. These patients need even closer follow-up of renal function and are more likely to require the care of a pediatric nephrologist.

PEARLS

- Precautions to prevent food-borne STEC-mediated disease and public health interventions to prevent spread during outbreaks are more effective than the currently available treatment.
- One must have a high index of suspicion for STEC-mediated diarrheal illness for diagnosis and monitoring those at risk for HUS.
- Remember to consider atypical HUS with unexpected or unusual presentations of the disease.
- Supportive care is currently the mainstay of management in HUS.
- Long-term close follow-up of patients following HUS to monitor for the potential development of renal sequelae is essential, especially in the atypical forms of HUS.

References

1. Cimolai N, Basalyga S, Mah DG, et al. A continuing assessment of risk factors for the development of *Escherichia coli* O157:H7-associated hemolytic uremic syndrome. *Clin Nephrol* 1994;42;85–89.
2. Safdar N, Said A, Gangnon RE, et al. Risk of hemolytic uremic syndrome after antibiotic treatment of *Escherichia coli* O157:H7 enteritis: a meta-analysis. *JAMA* 2002;288:996–1001.
3. Oakes RS, Siegler RL, Markham A, et al. Predictors of fatality in postdiarrheal hemolytic uremic syndrome. *Pediatrics* 2006;117:1656–1662.

Suggested Readings

Corrigan JJ, Boineau FG. Hemolytic-uremic syndrome. *Pediatr Rev* 2001;22: 365–369.
MacConnachie AA, Todd WT. Potential therapeutic agents for the prevention and treatment of haemolytic uraemic syndrome in Shiga toxin producing *Escherichia coli* infection. *Curr Opin Infect Dis* 2004;17:479–482.
Ray PE, Xue-Hui L. Pathogenesis of Shiga toxin-induced hemolytic uremic syndrome. *Pediatr Nephrol* 2001;16:823–829.
Siegler R, Oakes R. Hemolytic uremic syndrome; pathogenesis, treatment, and outcome. *Curr Opin Pediatr* 2005;17:2000–2004.

CHAPTER 64 ■ RENAL TUBULAR ACIDOSIS

KATHERINE ANDREEFF

The kidneys are an integral part of many of the body's essential functions. Disorders within the kidney may affect acid–base balance, fluid and electrolyte regulation, waste product elimination, and hormone regulation within several endocrine pathways. The tubular dysfunctions that will be discussed in this chapter are responsible mainly for acid–base disorders as well as defects in electrolyte balance.

Renal tubular acidosis (RTA) is, in general, the inability of the renal tubules to regulate the body's plasma concentration of bicarbonate as a result of impaired renal acidification. That is, the kidney is unable to secrete hydrogen ions and reabsorb bicarbonate ions appropriately, resulting in a metabolic acidosis. Due to increased losses of bicarbonate in the urine, the body retains chloride ions, resulting in more specifically a hyperchloremic metabolic acidosis, with therefore a normal anion gap. Hypokalemia may also be seen in both proximal and distal RTA. Type 4 RTA, however, is characterized by hyperkalemia as well as hyponatremia.

The pediatric hospitalist must know when to consider RTA in the differential diagnosis, how to make the diagnosis, and how to treat it once it is confirmed. These issues as well as discussion of the different types of RTA will be the focus of this chapter.

UNDERSTANDING THE PROBLEM

Renal tubular acidosis is defined by the location within the renal tubules where urinary acidification is impaired. To understand the diagnostic criteria of the different types of RTA it is important to know normal tubular physiology (Fig. 64.1). A brief overview follows.

The Proximal Tubule

In the proximal convoluted tubule, the secretion of hydrogen (H) ions results in the reabsorption of 80% to 90% of the filtered bicarbonate ion (HCO_3), thereby forming carbonic acid (H_2CO_3). Carbonic anhydrase then dissociates H_2CO_3 into water (H_2O) and carbon dioxide (CO_2). The CO_2 diffuses into the cell from the tubule lumen, where it is hydroxylated to HCO_3. Bicarbonate ion is then removed form the cell and reabsorbed into the blood by means of sodium coupling. Hydrogen ion secretion is accomplished by sodium/hydrogen (Na/H) exchange, which is maintained by sodium/potassium/ATPase (Na/K/ATPase) channels within the basolateral cell membrane, providing a Na gradient that drives the Na/H exchange. The above process is driven by H secretion; therefore anything interfering with normal H secretion affects the ability to reabsorb HCO_3. For example, if the amount of carbonic anhydrase in the tubular lumen is insufficient, H_2CO_3 accumulates, which increases the amount of H within the lumen, thereby decreasing H secretion and ultimately decreasing HCO_3 reabsorption. Any decrease in the amount of HCO_3 reabsorbed in the proximal tubule results in increased amounts of HCO_3 delivered to the distal collecting tubule. Appropriate reabsorption of HCO_3 results in a urinary pH of approximately 6.7 upon reaching the distal tubules.

The Distal Tubule

Within the collecting tubules (both cortical and medullary), the secretion of H results in the reabsorption of the remaining 10% to 15% HCO_3 as well as further titrating the major urinary buffers (ammonia, phosphates, and sulfates). Hydrogen ion secretion is stimulated both by aldosterone and potassium depletion. In normal states, acidosis stimulates while alkalosis inhibits H secretion in the distal tubules. The result is the ability of the kidney to balance the body's serum/plasma pH by means of net acid excretion in the urine under acidotic conditions and to decrease the amount of acid excreted during alkalotic conditions.

Impaired renal acidification results in the kidney failing to maintain normal bicarbonate levels in the plasma while normal amounts of acid are being produced from diet and the body's metabolism. If the problem is reduced reabsorption of filtered bicarbonate by the proximal nephron, then it is classified as proximal RTA (type 2). If the problem is reduced excretion of titratable acid and ammonium in the distal nephron, then it is distal RTA (type 1). Finally, if the reduced excretion of titratable acid is joined with hyperkalemia, then hyperkalemic RTA (type 4) is the problem.

PROXIMAL RTA (TYPE 2)

As indicated above, proximal RTA results when there is an impairment in the capacity of the proximal tubule to reabsorb HCO_3. The result is bicarbonaturia, as the distal tubule's ability to reabsorb HCO_3 is overwhelmed. Metabolic acidosis results because the increased amount of HCO_3 in the distal nephron inhibits the appropriate net acid excretion. The bicarbonaturia will continue until the plasma concentration decreases sufficiently to reduce the amount of filtered bicarbonate, and the distal tubule then is able to handle the residual bicarbonate. At this point, net acid excretion equals the body's acid production, and the urine pH decreases to less than 5.5. Hypokalemia results due to the increased amounts of bicarbonate promoting K secretion. Dysfunction of bicarbonate reabsorption may occur due to abnormal electrolyte transporters in the proximal tubule, or reduced carbonic anhydrase activity. No one mechanism has been defined.

Proximal RTA typically presents as a part of Fanconi syndrome, in which case it is accompanied by glucosuria, amino aciduria, and phosphaturia. Isolated hereditary proximal RTA is extremely rare. Other genetic causes are seen with associated

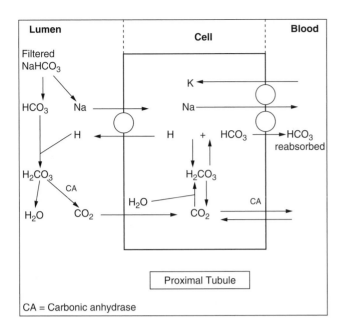

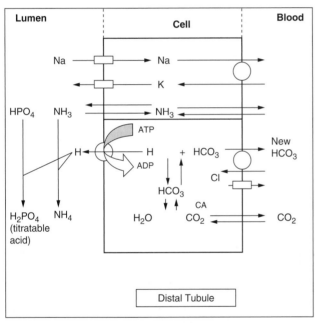

FIGURE 64.1. Diagram of renal acidification process in proximal and distal tubules.

anomalies. Mutations in the gene (SLC4A4) that codes for the Na/HCO$_3$ symporter, are associated with proximal RTA along with various ocular abnormalities such as band keratopathy, glaucoma, and cataracts. Another Proximal RTA disorder that is associated with osteopetrosis, mental retardation, and cerebral calcification is due to impaired carbonic anhydrase II activity caused by mutations in the cytoplasmic carbonic anhydrase II gene. This disorder is autosomal recessive and cases have been reported in individuals of Middle Eastern and Mediterranean descent. Proximal RTA or combined features of proximal and distal RTA are found in this situation. Additional disorders associated with proximal RTA are transient (usually occurring in young children, disappearing by age 3 years), adult onset (may be associated with multiple myeloma, congenital heart disease, or renal vascular accidents), and those due to drugs (acetazolamide, sulfanilamide, and mafenide acetate).

DISTAL RTA (TYPE 1)

In this distal RTA, dysfunctional H secretion in the distal collecting tubule results in the inability to acidify the urine. Urine pH remains inappropriately high (usually above 6.0) even in cases of severe acidosis. Persistent bicarbonaturia exists due to the inability to adequately reabsorb HCO$_3$; therefore titratable acid excretion is reduced and metabolic acidosis is the result. In infants and children the bicarbonate wasting can be severe, causing an inability to lower urinary pH below 7.0. Renal absorption of glucose, amino acids, and phosphates is not impaired as these are absorbed in the unaffected proximal tubules.

Proposed mechanisms in distal RTA include reduced H secretion from the cell to lumen due to either defects in the H secretory pump in alpha intercalated cells or to decreases in electrochemical gradients responsible for promoting H secretion. Additionally, dysfunction in cell membrane permeability may permit reverse leak of previously secreted H or HCO$_3$. Distal RTA may present alone or in association with a number of different disorders. In children it may be seen as part of an autosomal dominant disorder associated with nephrocalcinosis where metabolic acidosis is evident as early as 2 to 3 months of age. Stones are found as early as 5 years. Distal RTA associated with sensorineural hearing loss is a well-defined autosomal recessive disorder. Other genetic disorders associated with distal RTA include Ehlers–Danlos syndrome, Marfan syndrome, sickle-cell anemia, hereditary elliptocytosis, Wilson disease, Fabry disease, carbonic anhydrase II deficiency (as mentioned previously), and carnitine palmitoyltransferase type 1 deficiency. The disorder may also be seen with a variety of autoimmune disorders including hypergammaglobulinemia, Sjögren syndrome, systemic lupus erythematosus, polyarteritis nodosa, chronic active hepatitis, and thyroiditis. Drug-induced distal RTA may occur with administration of amphotericin B, rifampin, lithium, pentamidine, toluene, Cyclamate, mercury, and some analgesics.

COMBINED-TYPE RTA (TYPE 3)

For some patients the distinction between proximal and distal RTA is impossible, as they exhibit features of both. Typically there is a decrease in ability to resorb HCO$_3$ as well as an inability to acidify the urine maximally. This pattern is usually seen as a transient form of RTA in infants and children with primary distal RTA and is now no longer classified as a separate type of RTA.

HYPERKALEMIC RTA (TYPE 4)

Hyperkalemic RTA occurs as a consequence of aldosterone deficiency or impairment of its effects on renal tubules. The ability to acidify the urine is preserved during acidosis and the fractional excretion of HCO$_3$, although not normal, is not large enough to implicate the proximal tubules. Despite this, urinary excretion of ammonium and net acid is reduced. Renal potassium clearance is greatly reduced and increases in serum potassium are marked in relation to increases in dietary potassium.

The mechanism of type 4 RTA is believed to be related to aldosterone deficiency. Its function in the kidney is to directly stimulate H secretion by the alpha-intercalated cells; stimulate sodium reabsorption, thereby enhancing the secretion of H and potassium in the collecting tubules via electrical gradients; and stimulate potassium secretion directly in the collecting tubules, thereby increasing ammonium delivery to the distal tubules. Deficiency in aldosterone may be secondary to a decrease in renin occurring in older individuals with interstitial renal disease. Often diabetes mellitus, hypertension, and congestive heart failure are seen together in this disorder.

Aside from hyporeninemic hypoaldosteronism, type 4 RTA can also be seen in adrenal deficiency states such as Addison disease, secondary decreased response to aldosterone as in obstructive uropathies or with interstitial nephritities, and with potassium-sparing diuretics such as spironolactone, triamterene, and amiloride.

CLINICAL FEATURES—WHEN TO CONSIDER RTA

The clinical features of RTA are nonspecific. An untreated child with RTA may present with failure to thrive, polyuria, polydipsia, constipation, vomiting, anorexia, and/or listlessness. Additionally, rickets, osteomalacia, nephrocalcinosis, and muscle weakness may be found and are clues to specific types of RTA. Fortunately, the screening workup for most of these symptoms includes obtaining basic electrolytes, which can then lead the clinician to contemplate RTA in the differential diagnosis.

As mentioned previously, RTA is characterized by a nonanion gap hyperchloremic metabolic acidosis. Most often this abnormality is caused by gastrointestinal losses of HCO_3. Diarrhea is the most common cause in children; however, the differential diagnosis of hyperchloremic metabolic acidosis is listed in Table 64.1. It is therefore important to exclude GI losses prior to entertaining the diagnosis of RTA. The patient's history hopefully will elucidate these symptoms; however, without a significant GI history, one may utilize additional laboratory data.

TABLE 64.1

DIFFERENTIAL DIAGNOSIS OF HYPERCHLOREMIC METABOLIC ACIDOSIS

GASTROINTESTINAL LOSSES OF BICARBONATE
Diarrhea
External pancreatic or small bowel drainage
Ureterosigmoidostomy, jejunal loop
Drugs: calcium chloride, magnesium sulfate (diarrhea), cholestyramine

RENAL ACIDOSIS
Hypokalemia
    Proximal RTA
    Distal RTA
Hyperkalemia
    Hyperkalemic RTA
    Drug induced: diuretics (amiloride, triamterene, spironolactone), trimethoprim, pentamidine, ACE inhibitors, NSAIDs, cyclosporin A, tacrolimus
Normokalemia
    Early renal insufficiency

OTHER
Acid loads (hyperalimentation, ammonium chloride)
Ketosis with ketone excretion
Dilution acidosis (rapid saline administration)
Cation exchange resins
Hippurate

To rule out GI losses one must start with obtaining urine electrolytes (Na, K, Cl) to calculate the urine anion gap (Uag):

$$Uag = [Na + K] - Cl.$$

The Uag is an indirect means of measuring the urinary ammonium level. In intestinal losses of HCO_3, the urinary ammonium (NH_4) rises to provide improved buffering; therefore, the Uag will be negative (meaning that Cl $>$ Na $+$ K). With renal losses of HCO_3 there is no increase in urinary NH_4, therefore, the Uag will be positive (that is, Cl $<$ Na $+$ K). This test is only useful, however, if there is no ketonuria or large amount of anion excretion (as with medications such as penicillin). In the situation where ketonuria is present, the urinary NH_4 (UNH_4) can instead be estimated using the following equation, which requires additional urinary lab data (urine osmolarity, urea, and glucose)

$$UNH_4 = 0.5 \ (Uosm - [2(Na + K) + urea + glucose])$$

UNH_4 values of 75 mEq/L or more would indicate intact renal tubular function and therefore GI losses are more likely. Values <25 mEq/L would indicate low UNH_4, thus suggesting a renal mechanism. Once GI losses of HCO_3 as well as any other extrarenal causes of the metabolic acidosis are excluded, the diagnosis of RTA can be pursued.

MAKING THE DIAGNOSIS

Once GI losses have been eliminated as the cause of the patient's hyperchloremic metabolic acidosis, the process of confirming RTA can be initiated. The next steps involve calculating the fractional excretion of HCO_3 (FE HCO_3) as well as looking at the urine pH. The fractional excretion of HCO_3 is obtained by the following equation:

$$FE\ HCO_3 = [CO_2\ (urine) \times Creatinine\ (serum)] / [HCO_3\ (serum) \times Creatinine\ (urine)]$$

The proximal tubule is responsible for 80% to 90% of HCO_3 reabsorption; if the FE HCO_3 is $>1\%$ in an acidotic state or $>5\%$ with a normal serum HCO_3, proximal RTA is diagnosed. If, however, the serum HCO_3 is less than 16 mEq/L, the FE HCO_3 is not enough to make the diagnosis and the urine pH must be assessed.

If the urine pH is <6 (in young children) or <5.5 (older children and adolescents), proximal RTA is a possibility. Confirming the diagnosis of proximal RTA then involves supplementation with alkaline solution to bring up the serum HCO_3 so that the FE HCO_3 can be calculated. If, however, the urinary pH is >6, then distal RTA is the likely diagnosis. Additionally, if the Uag is positive, the serum K is elevated, and the urinary pH is <5.5, then type 4 RTA is likely. Table 64.2 demonstrates the diagnostic criteria for the different types of RTA.

TREATMENT STRATEGIES

In general the treatment of all types of RTA is alkali replacement. In children the ideal method is with four divided doses of sodium bicarbonate ($NaHCO_3$) or citrate salts given after feedings. In proximal RTA the amount may vary from 2 to 3 mEq/kg/day to 20 mEq/kg/day depending on the amount of urinary net base excretion. In isolated proximal RTA, bicarbonate replacement should be sufficient. Care must be taken to adjust amounts to correct acidosis to prevent short stature. Restriction of dietary sodium may be helpful in cases where the amount of replacement is excessive. Hydrochlorthiazide

TABLE 64.2

COMPARISON OF RTA TYPES

Finding	Type 1	Type 2	Type 4
Non-anion gap acidosis	Present	Present	Present
Urine pH	>5.5	<5.5	<5.5
FEHCO$_3$	<5%	>10–15%	>5–10%
Urine ammonium	Decreased	Decreased	Decreased
Serum potassium	Normal/low	Normal/low	High
Nephrocalcinosis/nephrolithiasis	Common	Rare	Absent
Osteomalacia	Rare	Frequent	Absent
Short stature	Common	Common	Possible

may also help to correct acidosis with less alkali by stimulating H secretion in the proximal tubules; however, it may increase potassium losses. In those cases where proximal RTA is associated with Fanconi syndrome, potassium replacement is a cornerstone of therapy, usually accomplished by giving 50% of the alkali replacement as potassium bicarbonate or potassium citrate. Additionally, directing treatment toward causative agents, as in Fanconi syndrome secondary to hereditary fructose intolerance, galactosemia, or Wilson disease, or RTA caused by drugs, is essential in the patient's care.

In distal RTA, the initial doses of alkali replacement should be 3 mEq/kg/day and increased every 2 to 4 days until the plasma bicarbonate is normal. As the child's growth velocity improves, the amount of alkali required to sustain correction of acidosis may range from 5 to 14 mEq/kg/day. Interestingly, after age 4 to 6 years the amount of alkali replacement required often decreases. In most cases, the correction of the bicarbonate loss alone will be sufficient to decrease renal wasting of potassium and supplementation may not be necessary. However, care should include initial replacement of potassium with careful titration, again utilizing potassium bicarbonate or potassium citrate for 20% to 50% of the correction doses. Nephrocalcinosis can be prevented with early detection and treatment of distal RTA. Rickets and osteomalacia also can be reversed with alkali therapy alone.

Hyperkalemic RTA requires smaller amounts of alkali replacement to correct acidosis, and the mainstay of therapy is dietary restriction of potassium, as well as treatment with mineralocorticoid replacement. Furosemide has also proven useful to decrease hyperkalemia in patients with renal insufficiency.

OUTCOMES AND FOLLOW-UP

As indicated above, it is important to have appropriate titration of the alkali replacement to correct acidosis and maintain normal serum bicarbonate levels as well as managing additional electrolyte abnormalities. Early consultation with a nephrologist is imperative to ensure long-term follow-up and monitoring growth velocity and for the appearance of nephrolithiasis. With appropriate treatment, growth velocity can be normal throughout puberty, and the achievement of normal adult height is likely. Treatment and management of underlying disorders may affect outcomes differently than with isolated RTA.

PEARLS

- Exclude gastrointestinal losses as possible etiology for metabolic acidosis by checking the urine anion gap.
- May need to supplement bicarbonate to be able to diagnose proximal RTA in cases where HCO$_3$ <16 mEq/L.
- Early diagnosis and treatment is essential to permit normal growth velocity and achieve normal adult height.

References

Dubose TD. Metabolic Acidosis. In: Brenner BM, Rector FC, eds. *The Kidney*. Philadelphia: Saunders; 2004:944–966.

Portale AA. Renal tubular acidosis. In: Holliday M, Barratt T, Avner E, eds. *Pediatric nephrology*. 3rd ed. Philadelphia: Williams & Wilkins; 1994:640–655.

Rodriguez-Soriano J. Renal tubular acidosis. *Pediatr Nephrol* 1990;4:286–275.

CHAPTER 65 ■ NEPHROTIC SYNDROME

TROY McGUIRE

When the normal glomerular impermeability to albumin filtration is compromised, proteinuria ensues. Although trace proteinuria is fairly common in childhood, particularly as a result of postural transitions, the normal functioning kidneys restrict protein loss into the urine to less than 100 mg/m^2/day through selective filtration and tubular reabsorption. If generalized edema occurs in association with urinary protein excretion in excess of 40 mg/m^2/hr (1 g/m^2/day), nephrotic syndrome is present. The principal findings of hypoalbuminemia, edema, and hyperlipidemia arise from direct urinary protein losses and subsequent compensatory measures. Because generalized edema is uncommon in the previously well child, whereas allergic reactions are more frequently encountered, nephrotic syndrome is often misdiagnosed as angioedema or other allergic reaction prior to arriving at the correct diagnosis. Fortunately, nephrotic syndrome has an excellent prognosis with most morbidity and mortality related to infectious or vascular complications of the condition rather than attributable to the kidney disease itself.

BACKGROUND

The incidence of nephrotic syndrome is roughly 4 in 100,000 children. The peak incidence is between 2 and 6 years of age, and it is more common in boys than in girls. Prevalence has been stable over the past several decades at 15 to 20 per 100,000 children (1–3). Negative prognostic indicators for disease severity and progression to chronic kidney disease include onset early in infancy or later in adolescence, Latin-American and African American ethnicity, and failure to respond to initial corticosteroids. As nephrotic syndrome is the final result of a variety of disturbances at the glomerular level, it does not represent a single entity in either its pathology or its response to treatment.

Idiopathic nephrotic syndrome as a group makes up 90% of pediatric nephrotic cases. Defined by pathology findings, the included types are minimal change disease (MCD), focal segmental glomerular sclerosis (FSGS), and membranous nephropathy (MN) (4). MCD accounts for the vast majority of pediatric nephrotic syndrome (80%). Most patients with MCD present before 5 years of age. MCD is marked by the absence of findings on routine light microscopy. Scant IgM deposition is occasionally encountered with immunofluorescent studies, although there is debate about whether this instead represents a separate entity, IgM nephropathy. Electron microscopy shows alteration in the foot processes of glomerular podocytes at the slit diaphragm. Response to corticosteroid therapy is predictably excellent, with >95% initial remission rate. Relapse is common during childhood, but significant adult sequellae are not.

Biopsies showing FSGS (10–15%) are marked by scattered scarring in multiple lobules. Hypertension and significant hematuria are more common in FSGS compared to MCD, though not specific for FSGS (5). Overall, the proportion of FSGS pathologic changes at biopsy appears to be increasing in reports from multiple centers (6). This may reflect a trend in reduction of early diagnostic renal biopsy such that patients undergoing biopsy are more likely to have failed steroid induction and therefore have a diminished likelihood of having MCD. Alternatively, the true incidence of FSGS may actually be increasing. The disease tends to follow a progressive course, and is much less amenable to corticosteroid treatment as less than one-fourth of FSGS lesions will be steroid responsive (5).

Finally, membranous nephropathy, though a frequent cause of nephrotic syndrome in adults, is an uncommon finding in children (5%) and carries an intermediate rate of response to corticosteroid therapy.

Secondary nephrotic syndrome, on the other hand, collectively represents approximately 10% of pediatric nephrotic cases. It is composed of various renal lesions, in isolation or in association with systemic disease. Glomerulomnephritis with distinct histopathologic findings may present with proteinuria in the nephrotic range. Lupus nephritis, other primary renal vasculitides, viral hepatitis, syphilis, drugs, toxins, allergic reactions, neoplasia, diabetes, vesicoureteral reflux, hyperfiltration states, and a variety of other systemic diseases must all be considered in the differential diagnosis of nephrotic syndrome (Table 65.1).

The best-characterized congenital nephrotic syndrome (Finnish type) merits separate discussion for a number of reasons. Whereas MCD is rare before age 1, congenital nephrotic syndrome (CNS) presents at birth or within the first 3 months of life. Protein level in the amniotic fluid is elevated, and the infant may be born hydropic. The placenta is characteristically large, generally over 25% of birth weight. The infant is often small for gestational age and may be born prematurely. Eventually, frank ascites, generalized edema, recurrent infection, and failure to thrive are universal if the condition remains undiagnosed. In contrast to the overall favorable prognosis in nephrotic syndrome, CNS predictably leads to chronic renal failure and risk of mortality is high. Recent discovery of the responsible gene NPHS1 on chromosome 19 (7) and molecular characterization of its protein product, nephrin, has implications beyond Finnish-type CNS. Together with subsequent discovery of other mutations in genes codifying glomerular structural proteins, it has provided explanation for the long-acknowledged failure of CNS to respond to immunosuppressive therapy and has additionally elucidated the structure and function of the slit diaphragm responsible for protein sieving at the glomerulus.

PATHOGENESIS

When normal permeability prevails, the glomerulus effectively prevents primary filtration of proteins larger than 65 kD,

TABLE 65.1

NEPHROTIC SYNDROME CAUSES

Type	Specific diagnoses
Congenital nephrotic syndrome	Finnish type
	Nephrin (NPHS1)
	Podocin (NPHS2)
	Alpha-actinin-4 (FSGS1)
	Syndrome-associated
	Denys–Drash syndrome (WT1)
	Lowe syndrome
	Nail-patella syndrome (LMX1B)
	Alport syndrome
	Charcot–Marie–Tooth syndrome
	Cockayne syndrome
	Frasier syndrome (WT1)
Idiopathic nephrotic syndrome	Minimal change disease[a]
	Focal segmental glomerulosclerosis[a]
	Membranous nephropathy[a]
Secondary nephrotic syndrome	Glomerulonephritis
	Post-streptococcal
	Rapidly progressive
	Membranoproliferative
	Diffuse mesangial sclerosis[a]
	Lupus nephritis
	IgA nephropathy
	Infectious
	Viral hepatitis[a]
	Toxoplasmosis[a]
	Syphilis[a]
	Rubella[a]
	Cytomegalovirus[a]
	Human immunodeficiency virus[a]
	Parvovirus[a]
	Malaria[a]
	Drug/toxin
	Heroin
	Lithium
	Penicillamine
	Mercury
	Gold
	Pamidronate
	Interferon
	Serum sickness
	Hymenoptera envenomation
	Snake envenomation
	Food allergy
	Neoplastic/paraneoplastic
	Leukemia
	Lymphoma
	Castleman disease
	Nephroblastoma
	Diabetes mellitus
	Reflux nephropathy
	Amyloidosis

[a]May present as congenital nephrotic syndrome.

changes as neighboring podocytes appear fused and flattened rather than projecting across the gap as foot-like projections. In other glomerular lesions, the changes are evident at the light microscopy level and readily explain disrupted filtration.

Much remains unknown regarding the inciting triggers for and developmental steps in the pathophysiology of nephrotic syndrome. MCD in particular, the most common pediatric variant, is less well understood than many of the less common or even rare variants. However, in the past decade, several novel discoveries have begun to improve our understanding of the normally functioning and diseased glomerular filtration barrier.

First, primary structural defects in the glomerulus are responsible for some cases of nephrotic syndrome. Genetically determined abnormality of podocyte proteins has been well described. NPHS1 mutation (recessive, 19q) coding for a defective podocyte protein called nephrin (7) produces the Finnish-type congenital nephrotic syndrome. NPHS2 mutation (recessive, 1q) results in FSGS through a dysfunctional podocyte protein, podocin (9). Mutations on 11q and 19q affecting podocyte cytoskeletal elements have been noted in dominantly inherited FSGS kindreds (9,10). These mutations and other specific anomalies in the proteins that are responsible for the integrity of the slit diaphragm or for the interaction of the podocyte with the basement membrane have emphasized the vital role of microscopic structure for intact filtration.

Second, permselectivity at the glomerulus can be altered by the action of a "factor" circulating in plasma. The rapid recurrence of markedly abnormal permeability to albumin, and subsequent progression to FSGS in the transplanted kidney, has strongly implicated a circulating humoral factor in some cases of nephrotic syndrome (11). In renal allografts for congenital nephrotic syndrome, anti-nephrin antibodies have been demonstrated post-transplantation (9). In other instances, the factor itself has not been identified, but studies have demonstrated removal of the factor by plasmapheresis and immunoadsorption. Additionally, transplacental transmission with transient neonatal nephrosis (12) supports a role for a plasma factor that might alter permeability through neutralization of the normal anionic character at the glomerulus or other means.

Third, primary dysregulation of T-lymphocytes causing overproduction of a cytokine that interferes with slit-diaphragm proteins has long been postulated. Evidence in the form of nephrotic syndrome associated with leukemia, lymphoma, Castleman disease, HIV, allergy, hymenoptera envenomation, hepatitis B, parvovirus, and other viral infection is compelling, but scrutiny of particular cytokines has been unyielding or not reproducible (13).

PATHOPHYSIOLOGY

Characteristic of all of the physiologic derangements in nephrotic syndrome is the previously described urinary loss of albumin with concomitant hypoalbuminemia. Traditionally, edema formation has been directly attributed to a decrease in oncotic pressure, resulting in third-spacing of fluid into the interstitial spaces. As intravascular depletion develops, homeostatic mechanisms are activated and exacerbate the edema: renin is stimulated by lowered renal perfusion; the angiotensin–aldosterone axis is stimulated through renin; antidiuretic hormone (ADH) is increased due to compromised intravascular volume; atrial natriuretic peptide release is downregulated early in the course as central filling pressures fall. All of these hormonal responses increase sodium and water retention. Studies in adults where renin levels have not been elevated and plasma volume is excessive rather than diminished (14) have challenged this explanation for the genesis of edema in nephrotic syndrome, but in children, it has largely been supported (15) and is a useful construct.

including immunoglobulins and albumin (69 kD). The permeability barrier is formed by a fenestrated layer of glomerular endothelial cells, the negatively charged glomerular basement membrane (collagen, heparin sulfate proteoglycans, laminin), and the slit diaphragm network comprised of interacting podocyte proteins (podocin, nephrin, and others) (8). Electron microscopy in MCD-type nephrotic syndrome shows subtle

Edema is often indolent in onset and late in recognition. Periorbital, facial, sacral, scrotal, and labial swelling may be remarkable before typical dependent edema develops. As mentioned, it is often mistaken for an allergic reaction or angioedema and treated as such. Advanced edema (anasarca) is often accompanied by significant ascites and pleural effusions, with pericardial effusions and pulmonary edema less common.

Hypercholesterolemia and hyperlipidemia occur as hepatic synthesis of lipoprotein is upregulated to compensate for other plasma proteins lost through renal filtration. This effect may persist well into remission; thus there is likely additional impetus responsible. Lipid profiles show very–low density and low-density lipoproteins elevated while high-density lipoprotein is depressed.

Humoral immunodeficiency attributable to lost immunoglobulins and complement results in functional asplenia, increasing the risk for bacterial infections. The capacity to opsonize carbohydrate antigen in particular is compromised by total and subclass IgG deficiencies and C3 loss. Propensity toward pneumonia, cellulitis, spontaneous bacterial peritonitis, and sepsis due to pneumococcal and other encapsulated bacteria requires vigilance. The risk of infection is magnified throughout treatment, owing to the immunosuppressive effects of corticosteroids. Other medical complications of nephrotic syndrome merit mention. Hypercoagulability due to renal losses of antithrombin III and plasminogen coupled with increased hepatic production of coagulation factors I, VII, VIII, X is of concern, particularly in a state of intravascular depletion, though thromboembolic events are uncommon at disease onset. Hypothyroidism is often seen, partly due to loss of thyroid-binding globulin (TBG) at the kidneys. Free thyroxine (T4) and thyroid-stimulating hormone (TSH) will allow distinction between actual hypothyroidism and euthyroid decrease in total T4 secondary to low TBG. Hypertension and microhematuria may both be present, even in MCD; if marked, glomerulonephritis should be considered.

MANAGEMENT

Diagnosis of nephrotic syndrome is clinical, resting on the constellation of proteinuria, edema, and hypoalbuminemia. Isolated elevations of spot urinary protein by dipstick are insufficient and must be quantified as nephritic-range proteinuria by analysis of spot protein/creatinine ratio >2 or a timed urinary protein excretion >1 g/m^2/24 hours. Edema is universal in nephrotic syndrome, often atypical in distribution, and may be subtle or massive. Hypoalbuminemia (serum almunin <2.5 g/dL) is also a key feature of protein-losing enteropathy, congestive heart failure, congenital defects in albumin synthesis, and disorders of systemic vascular permeability, but should not be confused as these disorders will not demonstrate the marked proteinuria of nephrotic syndrome.

Laboratory evaluation is straightforward. Urinalysis should be performed including microscopy to evaluate for significant hematuria or dysmorphic red blood cells that would suggest glomerulonephritis. Complete blood count and blood tests for urea nitrogen (BUN), creatinine, glucose, and hepatitis B are routinely obtained and may suggest a specific etiology for secondary nephrotic syndrome. Skin testing with purified protein derivative (PPD) should be placed in preparation for the eventuality of corticosteroid therapy. If azotemia, or historical or physical findings, suggest glomerulonephritis, antistreptococcal antibodies (antistreptolysin O, antiDNAse B), antinuclear antibodies, and complement assays should be obtained. Consider HIV testing and rapid plasma reagin (RPR) in the appropriate context. Finally, specific genetic testing and dysmorphology consultation should be pursued for congenital nephrotic syndrome.

Initial therapy is directed at general support, including oxygenation and cardiorespiratory support. Hypovolemia may require volume expansion despite generalized edema, whereas hypertension will generally respond to a loop diuretic alone. Antibiotic therapy including pneumococcal coverage should be undertaken if signs of bacterial disease are present. Albumin infusion (salt-poor 25% albumin 1 g/kg over 3 to 4 hours) accompanied by furosemide (1 mg/kg) as often as every 8 hours may be necessary in the presence of cardiorespiratory compromise, pleural effusions, sepsis, peritonitis with ascites, or tense scrotal/labial edema. Theoretically, albumin exerts its beneficial effects by transiently raising the oncotic potential of the intravascular space so that water may flux back into the bloodstream from the interstitium, subsequently to be delivered to the kidneys for clearance. However, albumin use is controversial, potentially harmful, and often over-employed. Neither hypoalbuminemia nor edema in isolation is an indication for albumin/dirurtic therapy, as injudicious use may cause or exacerbate hypertension and precipitate hypokalemia, requiring additional therapy, in over one-third of treatment courses (16). Albumin use may aggravate or precipitate congestive heart failure and pulmonary edema in a smaller proportion of cases. In view of sodium and water overload in the pathogenesis of nephrotic edema, additional sodium and water load may be detrimental. Albumin's expense and the fact that it is blood derived raises further concerns.

Conversely, because patients with nephrotic syndrome are hypercoagulable, excessive furosemide diuresis leading to intravascular depletion poses real potential for systemic and pulmonary clotting. Central venous catheters augment this risk and should be avoided if possible. Diuresis may further precipitate hypokalemia, hyponatremia, and hypocalcemia.

Hypertension persisting after cautious diuresis should again prompt concern for glomerulonephritis, but is seen in some uncomplicated cases of idiopathic nephrotic syndrome. Angiotensin-converting enzyme (ACE) inhibitors are an option in this situation in the absence of significant azotemia and may offer additional renoprotective benefit of ameliorating proteinuria (17,18). Additional indications for ACE inhibitors are congenital nephrotic syndrome, steroid-resistant FSGS, amyloidosis, and other nephrotic syndrome types associated with hyperfiltration. During therapy, renal function should be followed for development of azotemia.

Nutritional consultation for education of patient and family on a no-added-salt or sodium 2 g/day diet is helpful early in the course of illness. Pneumococcal immunization status should be assessed; active immunization should await stable remission and occur when the patient is off immunosuppressive therapy.

Prednisone or prednisolone is the standard for initial immunosuppressive therapy, dosed at 2 mg/kg/day or 60 mg/m^2/day for 4 weeks followed by 8 to 24 weeks of every other day (1 mg/kg/day or 40 mg/m^2/day). Shorter regimens, standard in the past, have been shown in multiple studies to be associated with higher relapse rates (19). Induction of remission within the first 4 weeks of therapy is positive prognostically and favors minimal change disease. More than half of steroid-responsive nephrotic syndrome will relapse off therapy, and further steroid courses are often effective (20).

Because the majority of patients on long-term corticosteroids for frequently relapsing disease will experience significant steroid adverse effects, steroid-sparing agents are often considered. In this context, cyclophosphamide has been used most extensively (21), but less toxic agents are being explored with promising results. Cyclosporine A (CSA) is effective in inducing remission though relapse still occurs frequently. Main adverse events of CSA include nephrotoxicity, hypertrichosis, and gingival hyperplasia (22). Mycophenolate may offer steroid-sparing benefit and preferable side-effect profile to other immunosuppressive and cytotoxic therapies (21, 23, 24). Although early results are promising, the precise role for mycophenolate awaits multicenter controlled trials. Chlorambucil, levamisole, azathioprine, and tacrolimus have all been used in trials for steroid-resistant or frequently relapsing steroid-sensitive nephrotic syndrome as well. Regardless, frequent relapses, steroid-resistance, or need for therapy beyond corticosteroids are absolute indicators for pediatric nephrology consulation and management. Renal biopsy is currently reserved for patients who either have failed (steroid-resistant nephrotic, frequently relapsing nephrotic, prolonged nephritic symptoms) or would be predicted to fail steroid therapy (congenital nephrotic syndrome, older patients). Many centers delay renal biopsy until after q trial of second-line cytotoxic therapy as well (6). Renal ultrasound is important in planning renal biopsy to assure bilateral functional kidneys and feasibility of percutaneous approach.

Congenital nephrotic syndrome requires early and highly specialized attention. By nature of its structural rather than inflammatory underpinnings, it is unresponsive to steroid or second-line immunosuppressive agents. High rates of mortality in the first 18 months of life are largely attributed to nutritional and infectious issues. Nonsteroidal anti-inflammatory agents and, increasingly, angiotensin-converting enzyme inhibitors, are used as drugs of choice to reduce glomerular filtration and thereby minimize proteinuria. Recently, unilateral rather than bilateral nephrectomy in conjunction with medical therapy has been advocated in an attempt to postpone transplantation until after 2 years of age when the likelihood of allograft survival is better. Unfortunately, even if the patient survives to transplant, there is still a 25% risk of recurrence in the allograft (9).

Nephrotic syndrome is a common pediatric illness that has favorable prognosis with appropriate management, the landscape of which has changed in recent years. Despite the good prognosis, certain etiologies have a higher risk of mortality, morbidity, and progression to chronic renal failure. Management must be tailored to the underlying cause in order to optimize outcomes.

References

1. Gulati S, Sharma AP, Sharma RK, et al. Changing trends of histopathology in childhood nephrotic syndrome. *Am J Kidney Dis* 1999;34:646–650.
2. Nephrotic syndrome in children: prediction of histopathology from clinical and laboratory characteristics at time of diagnosis—a report of the International Study of Kidney Disease in Children. *Kidney Int* 1978; 13:159–165.
3. Bonilla-Felix M, Parra C, Dajani T, et al. Changing patterns in the histopathology of idiopathic nephrotic syndrome in children. *Kidney Int* 1999;55:1885–1890.
4. Eddy AA, Symons JM. Nephrotic syndrome in childhood. *Lancet* 2003;362:629–639.
5. Abrantes MM, Cardoso LS, Lima EM, et al. Clinical course of 110 children and adolescents with primary focal segmental glomerulosclerosis. *Pediatr Nephrol* 2006;21:482–489.
6. Filler G, Young E, Geier P, et al. Is there really an increase in non-minimal change nephrotic syndrome in children? *Am J Kidney Dis* 2003;42: 1107–1113.
7. Kestila M, Lenkkeri U, Mannikko M, et al. Positionally cloned gene for a novel glomerular protein—nephrin—is mutated in congenital nephrotic syndrome. *Mol Cell* 1998;1:575–582.
8. Akhtar M, Al Mana H. Molecular basis of proteinuria. *Adv Anat Pathol* 2004;11:304–309.
9. Papez KE, Smoyer WE. Recent advances in congenital nephrotic syndrome. *Curr Opin Pediatr* 2004;16:165–170.
10. Pollak MR. Inherited podocytopathies: FSGS and nephrotic syndrome from a genetic viewpoint. *J Am Soc Nephrol* 2002;13:3016–3023.
11. Schachter AD, Harmon WE. Single-center analysis of early recurrence of nephrotic syndrome following renal transplantation in children. *Pediatr Transplant* 2001;5:406–409.
12. Kemper M, Wolf G, Muller-Wiefel D. Transmission of glomerular permeability factor from a mother to her child. *N Engl J Med* 2001;344:386–387.
13. Araya CE, Wasserfall CH, Brusko TM, et al. A case of unfulfilled expectations. Cytokines in idiopathic minimal lesion nephrotic syndrome. *Pediatr Nephrol* 2006;21:603–610. Epub
14. Schrier R, Fassett R. A critique of the overfill hypothesis of sodium and water retention in the nephrotic syndrome. *Kidney Int* 1998;53:1111–1117.
15. Vande Walle JG, Donckerwolcke RA. Pathogenesis of edema formation in the nephrotic syndrome. *Pediatr Nephrol* 2001;16:283–293.
16. Haws RM, Baum M. Efficacy of albumin and diuretic therapy in children with nephrotic syndrome. *Pediatrics* 1993;91:1142–1146.
17. Habashy D, Hodson E, Craig J. Interventions for idiopathic steroid-resistant nephrotic syndrome in children. *Cochrane Database Syst Rev* 2004;2: CD003594.
18. Bagga A, Madigoudar BD, Hari P, et al. Enalapril dosage in steroid-resistant nephrotic syndrome. *Pediatr Nephrol* 2004;19:45–50.
19. Hodson EM, Knight JF, Willis NS, et al. Corticosteroid therapy for nephrotic syndrome in children. *Cochrane Database Syst Rev* 2005;1:CD001533.
20. Ruth EM, Kemper MJ, Leumann EP, et al. Children with steroid-sensitive nephrotic syndrome come of age: long-term outcome. *J Pediatr* 2005;147: 202–207.
21. Durkan A, Hodson EM, Willis NS, et al. Non-corticosteroid treatment for nephrotic syndrome in children. *Cochrane Database Syst Rev* 2005;18(2): CD002290.
22. Frassinetti Castelo Branco Camurca Fernandes P, Bezerra Da Silva G Jr., De Sousa Barros FA, et al. Treatment of steroid-resistant nephrotic syndrome with cyclosporine: study of 17 cases and a literature review. *J Nephrol* 2005;18:711–720.
23. Moudgil A, Bagga A, Jordan SC. Mycophenolate mofetil therapy in frequently relapsing steroid-dependent and steroid-resistant nephrotic syndrome of childhood: current status and future directions. *Pediatr Nephrol* 2005;20:1376–1381.
24. Novak I, Frank R, Vento S, et al. Efficacy of mycophenolate mofetil in pediatric patients with steroid-dependent nephrotic syndrome. *Pediatr Nephrol* 2005;20:1265–1268.

CHAPTER 66A ■ HYPERTENSION

DALE A. NEWTON

Hypertension is not a common medical problem in early childhood, but occurs more frequently by adolescence. The reported prevalence varies according to the characteristics of the population surveyed and the specific definition of hypertension used. Most population studies suggest that 1% to 3% of all children have sustained hypertension, but with higher percentages in adolescents, obese children, and certain ethnic groups, especially African Americans. Recent studies have also suggested that the prevalence is increasing and can partially be explained by the increasing prevalence of overweight (1). Hypertension is also found more frequently in hospitalized children due to their underlying medical problems. Presentation may vary from the incidental finding of mild hypertension in a hospitalized child to a malignant hypertensive crisis requiring aggressive intensive care. A proper response to the former has the potential to significantly impact the related morbidities many years into that child's future. The latter example necessitates more aggressive investigation and what may be lifesaving interventions.

Temporary elevations in blood pressure measurements are sometimes found in hospitalized children related to factors such as pain, anxiety, and intravenous fluid or blood product administration. Alternatively, acute disease processes such as pneumonia, CNS infections, or acute abdominal problems such as intussusception can elevate blood pressures. Most of the discussion in this chapter is not focused on these acute and hopefully time-limited processes, but is pertinent to the appropriate response to sustained hypertension found in the hospitalized child or adolescent.

The most recent guidelines for the diagnosis, evaluation, and treatment of pediatric hypertension were published in 2004. These guidelines include data from the 1999 to 2000 National Health and Nutrition Examination Survey (NHANES), edits to create consistency with the recommendations from the Seventh Report of the Joint National Committee on the Prevention, Detection, Evaluation, and Treatment of High Blood Pressure (JNC 7), and updates in other areas.

DETERMINATION OF BLOOD PRESSURE

When possible, routine determinations of blood pressure should be based on auscultation distal to a sphygmomanometer. The below-referenced tables for normative values were determined by auscultation. Oscillometric devices are convenient, but do not give the same results. Such devices measure mean arterial pressure reasonably accurately, but are much less accurate in estimating systolic and diastolic values. Manufacturers use proprietary algorithms for the latter calculations, and these vary between manufacturers, making comparisons unreliable. In some settings and with small infants, oscillometric devices may be the only acceptable option, but comparison to the norms

must be done with care and elevated levels (>90th percentile) should be confirmed by auscultation.

Determination of blood pressure in children should start with selection of the appropriate-sized blood pressure cuff. Incorrect-sized cuffs are frequently used and can result in falsely normal or falsely elevated blood pressure determinations. The cuff should have a width that is 40% of the circumference of the midpoint of the upper arm. The air bladder should encircle 80% to 100% of the circumference of the arm. New standards for pediatric blood pressure cuffs have been established and include standardization of the ratio of width-to-length at 1 to 2. This results in seven cuff sizes ranging from newborn to adult thigh. The recommendation also includes using the fifth Korotkoff sound as the diastolic measurement. The fourth Korotkoff sound should be used only in the rare event of a failure to determine the fifth sound. The latter is best accomplished with a stethoscope bell used with gentle pressure over the cubital fossa. The technique should also include having the child seated comfortably for 5 minutes with support to the back, feet, and arm. Blood pressure values taken in the supine position compared to the standard seated position will result in slightly higher systolic and slightly lower diastolic results.

In either position, the arm should be carefully supported at the level of the right atrium. If possible, the child should not have taken stimulant drugs or foods prior to determination. Blood pressure determinations are invalid in children who are totally uncooperative. If blood pressure values are elevated (unless dangerously elevated), repeated determinations are necessary to lessen the effects of anxiety and allow for regression to the mean. Compliance with the above-recommended technique for blood pressure measurement is poor, yet it has been shown that following the recommendations significantly improves correlation of readings with other objective measures of blood pressure.

HYPERTENSION DEFINITION

Blood pressure in children and adolescents has a labile component. Many children with initially elevated levels will normalize their values when determined sequentially. Outpatient studies suggest that on initial screening, 3% to 4% of children have elevated levels. After 3 sequential determinations (not on the same day) only about 1% had sustained elevated blood pressure.

The definitions for adult hypertension are based on the levels at which interventions have been shown to improve outcomes. That is not possible in the pediatric age group because those outcomes are many years in the future. Instead, pediatric hypertension definitions are based on normative data only. Blood pressures in children have been shown to vary according to age, gender, and height; hence each of these must be considered in interpreting pediatric blood pressures. Blood pressure data tables based on these characteristics and reported by percentiles (50th, 90th, 95th, and 99th) are available in print and on the Web (www.pediatrics.org/cgi/content/full/114/2/S2/555). The 95th percentile can be *estimated* as follows (2):

- Systolic (1–17 years old) = 100 + (age years × 2)
- Diastolic
  - 1–10 years old = 60 + (age years × 2)
  - 11–17 years old = 70 + (age years)

These equations run the risk of miscategorizing children who are short or tall, and do not give adequate information about the other percentiles needed below.

To be consistent with the blood pressure recommendations for adults established in JNC 7, children with elevated blood pressure determinations are now categorized as follows:

- Pre-hypertension: average systolic or diastolic levels that are ≥90th percentile for age, gender, and height but <95th percentile, or if >120/80 and <95th percentile.
- Stage 1 hypertension: average systolic or diastolic levels are between the 95th and 99th percentiles + 5 mm Hg.
- Stage 2 hypertension: average systolic or diastolic levels are greater than the 99th percentile + 5 mm Hg.

If the category is different for the systolic and diastolic values, the higher category (whether systolic or diastolic) is used to characterize the patient and becomes the basis for subsequent evaluation and therapy.

EVALUATION

As in adults, pediatric hypertension is usually divided into primary and secondary etiologies. Primary (essential) hypertension occurs without a specific underlying disease process and has a strong familial contribution. Secondary hypertension is related to a specific underlying disease process. In the hospitalized child, the decision to proceed with evaluation of hypertension for secondary causes should be related to the age of the child, the severity of the hypertension, co-morbid diseases, and the reason for hospitalization. Pre-hypertension would rarely need an evaluation and could be followed after discharge to see if the elevated blood pressures continue. If sustained, counseling about lifestyle changes including weight control, exercise, and diet is appropriate. This may be an appropriate initial response for many children with stage 1 hypertension. If there is a known underlying problem (e.g., nephritis) that would be expected to cause hypertension, initiation of therapy while hospitalized may be appropriate. Children with sustained stage 1 hypertension who fail to respond to 6 months of lifestyle intervention should be considered for further workup and treatment.

If blood pressure elevation is sustained at or above the threshold for stage 2, evaluation for causes of hypertension is appropriate and indicates a need to initiate antihypertensive medications. Other populations to consider for further in-depth evaluation include prepubescent children (even if stage 1), or those with findings suggesting systemic diseases that could be associated with hypertension. Like adults, children can have essential hypertension related in large part to familial factors, but this more commonly occurs in adolescents. Because secondary hypertension is more commonly found in prepubescent children than in hypertensive adults, a search for secondary hypertension (Table 66.1) is appropriate.

The evaluation starts with a careful *history* focusing on eliciting information about the diseases in Table 66.1. Careful attention to a sleep history is appropriate, seeking features suggesting obstructive sleep apnea. The family history may suggest essential hypertension. Obviously careful inquiry about medications is appropriate and should include prescribed, illicit, over-the-counter, and complementary and alternative medications.

TABLE 66.1

CAUSES OF SECONDARY HYPERTENSION

Obstructive sleep apnea
Chronic or acute renal disease
  Pyelonephritis
  Acute glomerulonephritis
  Henoch–Schönlein purpura
  Congenital renal anomalies
  Hydronephrosis ± reflux
  Wilms tumor
  Polycystic kidney disease
  Renal trauma
  Nephrolithiasis
  Hypoplastic kidney
Endocrine diseases
  Primary aldosteronism
  Primary hyperparathyroidism
  Congenital adrenal hyperplasia
  Cushing syndrome
  Pheochromocytoma
  Hyperthyroidism
  Polycystic ovary disease
Cardiovascular
  Renovascular disease
  Renal vein thrombosis
  Coarctation of the aorta
  Arteriovenous fistula
  Patent ductus arteriosus
Neurologic
  Increased intracranial pressure
  Guillain–Barré syndrome
Other
  Anxiety, stress or pain
  Collagen-vascular diseases
  Neuroblastoma
  Neurofibromatosis
  Tuberous sclerosis
  Heavy metal poisoning
  Excessive fluid or blood product administration
Medications
  Nonsteroidal anti-inflammatory medications (NSAIDs)
  Sympathomimetics (ephedrine, pseudoephedrine, etc.)
  ADHD medications (methylphenidate, dexedrine, etc.)
  Illicit drugs (cocaine, amphetamines, MDMA, etc.)
  Oral contraceptives
  Steroids; corticosteroids and androgenic
  Cyclosporine or tacrolimus
  Erythropoietin
Licorice (candy, chewing tobacco)
Nicotine
Caffeine
Alcohol (in excess)
Heavy metals (lead, mercury)
Complementary and alternative medications
  Ephedra
  Ma haung
  Bitter orange

Information about the latter is often overlooked or unreported. Classic symptoms of pheochromocytoma are often lacking in children. In a child with unexplained hypertension, consideration should be given to collecting a timed urine specimen for catecholamine determination, or a random urine specimen for metanephrine/creatinine ratio.

TABLE 66.2

STUDIES TO CONSIDER IN THE EVALUATION FOR SECONDARY HYPERTENSION

Electrolytes, BUN, creatinine[a]
Urinalysis, urine culture[a]
Complete blood count with differential[a]
Fasting lipid panel[a]
Calcium, phosphorus, uric acid[a]
Renal ultrasound
Fasting glucose
Urine drug screen
Polysomnography
Plasma renin assay
Renovascular imaging
Plasma and urine steroid levels
Plasma and urine catecholamine levels

[a]Recommended screening tests for *all* hypertensive children and adolescents.

The *physical examination* should include determination of body mass index (BMI), obesity is strongly predictive of hypertension. Growth should also be ascertained (e.g., falling off on the growth curves in progressive renal disease). A blood pressure determination should be performed in all four extremities to evaluate for possible coarctation. In the normal child, blood pressure determinations in the legs will exceed the upper extremity values by 10 to 20 mm Hg. A value in the lower extremities that is more than 10 mm Hg below the values in the upper extremities should result in an evaluation for possible coarctation of the aorta. Edema may suggest fluid overload, cardiac disease, or renal disease. Certain dysmorphisms and/or skin findings may suggest associated genetic or endocrine syndromes. Careful examination of the retina is indicated to evaluate for hypertensive arterial changes and for possible papilledema. A careful cardiac exam is indicated to detect congenital heart disease. The abdomen should be carefully assessed for evidence of renal masses or bruits. Examination of the joints may reveal arthritis suggesting Henoch–Schölein purpura or systemic lupus erythematosus. Abnormal genitalia might suggest adrenal hyperplasia or endocrine problems such as precocious puberty.

Additional *laboratory tests* may be considered in the evaluation for possible secondary hypertension. The specific tests performed should be based on careful assessment of the child's history and physical findings, as noted above. Several simple screening tests (Table 66.2) are recommended in all children and adolescents with sustained hypertension. The remaining elements of evaluation (Table 66.2) should be performed only when suggested by other findings. It is usually not necessary or appropriate to perform all or even most of these tests. A determination of plasma renin activity will detect about 85% of children/adolescents with renovascular disease. If further imaging to evaluate this is necessary, consultation with your radiologist should occur to determine the best available modality, or whether referral to a center experienced in pediatric imaging is appropriate.

The final component of the initial evaluation should be an *assessment for target-organ damage*. An assessment of renal function should be performed if not already done. The retinal exam should have been completed during the initial evaluation. The most significant finding of target-organ damage is left ventricular hypertrophy (LVH). A routine CXR and ECG have poor sensitivity for detecting LVH. The guidelines suggest cardiac echocardiography to assess for LVH based on the logic that this finding could result in earlier initiation of therapy, or more aggressive efforts to control the hypertension. There are no controlled studies showing differences in outcomes based on the results of such evaluations.

THERAPY

The underlying premise for interventions to lower blood pressure in the pediatric age group is based on the adult literature. In adults there are convincing data showing decreased cardiovascular mortality and morbidity with effective therapy. Similar longitudinal data do not exist for children. Hypertensive children more commonly become hypertensive adults, but this relationship is imperfect. Elevated blood pressure will resolve over time in many children, especially children with mild hypertension. However, pediatric autopsy studies also show changes in blood vessels and end organs similar to hypertensive adults. It seems clear that hypertension can begin in childhood and can contribute to the adult cardiovascular morbidities.

Healthy habits including exercise, adequate sleep, and healthy diet are to be recommended for all children and their families. Particular emphasis is appropriate for all children when the pre-hypertension threshold (90th percentile) for blood pressure is exceeded and sustained. Effective interventions in lifestyle issues are always difficult and are more likely to be successful if family-based. Weight reduction should be sought for obese children and adolescents. Pediatric research has shown that weight reduction decreases blood pressure and decreases sensitivity to salt ingestion. Salt restriction may have some efficacy in a small percentage of patients, but the DASH (Dietary Approaches to Stop Hypertension) diet is more effective (http://www.nhlbi. nih.gov/health/public/heart/hbp/dash/). Although this diet includes salt restriction, it emphasizes fresh vegetables, fruits, and low-fat dairy. Regular vigorous physical activity (and corresponding reduction in sedentary activities) should be recommended both for the benefit in weight reduction and improved cardiovascular function including a modest decrease in blood pressure. When age appropriate, counseling should include avoidance of smoking and excessive alcohol ingestion.

Pharmacologic interventions for control of hypertension should be implemented for all sustained stage 2 hypertension and symptomatic hypertension. Medication should be considered in stage 1 hypertension that fails a 6-month trial of therapeutic lifestyle changes, has co-morbidities such as diabetes, smoking, or hyperlipidemia, or is associated with evidence of end-organ damage (usually LVH). Therapeutic options are reviewed in Table 66.3.

The JNC 7 recommendations for adults with stage 2 hypertension encourage initiation of therapy with a two-drug regimen. The pediatric guidelines have not made a similar recommendation and currently suggest initiation of therapy with a single drug from any of several classes: diuretics, angiotensin-converting enzyme (ACE) inhibitors, angiotensin-receptor blockers, calcium-channel blockers, or beta-blockers.

The clinician should consider many factors in the choice of initial therapy. Thiazides are effective but may affect hydration status in athletes, cause hyponatremia or hypokalemia, and necessitate periodic electrolyte determinations. Compliance at times is a problem with children and adolescents reluctant to take a diuretic with the accompanying need for more frequent urination. Adult studies have documented that low-dose therapy (HCTZ 12.5 to 25 mg/day) with thiazides is as efficacious as a higher dose with a marked decrease in the associated metabolic problems. Thiazides also function well when added as a second drug in therapy by potentiating the antihypertensive action of most other antihypertensive drugs. If low-dose thiazides are used, potassium-sparing diuretics should rarely be needed. The latter are specifically contraindicated in patients with renal disease or a history of hyperkalemia.

TABLE 66.3

SELECTED ANTIHYPERTENSIVE MEDICATIONS

Class	Drug[a]	Dose per day	Interval
Angiotensin-converting enzyme inhibitor	Benazepril	0.2 mg/kg/day, up to 0.6 mg/kg/day; max 40 mg/day	Daily
	Enalapril	0.08 mg/kg/day up to 0.6 mg/kg/day; max 40 mg/day	Daily or twice daily
	Lisinopril	0.07 mg/kg/day, up to 0.6 mg/kg/day; max 40 mg/day	Daily
Angiotensin-receptor blocker	Irbesartan	6–12 years: 75–150 mg/day ≥13 years: 150–300 mg/day	Daily
	Losartan	0.7 mg/kg/day, up to 1.4 mg/kg/day; max 100 mg/day	Daily
Alpha- and beta-blocker	Labetalol	1–3 mg/kg/day; up to 10–12 mg/kg/day; max 1,200 mg/day	Twice daily
Beta-blocker	Atenolol	0.5 mg/kg/day up to 2 mg/kg/day; max 100 mg/day	Daily or twice daily
	Metoprolol	1 mg/kg/day up to 6 mg/kg/day; max 200 mg/day	Twice daily
Calcium-channel blocker	Amlodipine	0.06 mg/kg/day up to 0.6 mg/kg/day; max 10 mg/day	Daily
	Isradipine	0.05 mg/kg/dose up to 0.8 mg/kg/day; max 20 mg/day	Daily (sustained release)
Central alpha-agonist	Clonidine	0.005 mg/kg/day up to 0.025 mg/kg/day; max 2.4 mg/day	Twice daily (patch available)
Diuretic	Furosemide	0.5 mg/kg/dose up to 2 mg/kg/dose; max 6 mg/kg/day	Daily or twice daily
	HCTZ	1 mg/kg/d up to 4 mg/kg/day; max 100 mg/day	Daily
Peripheral alpha-antagonist	Doxazocin	1 mg/day up to 4 mg/day	Daily (bedtime)
	Terazosin	1 mg/day up to 20 mg/day	Daily (bedtime)
Vasodilator	Hydralazine	0.75 mg/kg/day up to 7.5 mg/kg/day; max 200 mg/day	Four times daily

mg/kg/day, milligrams per kilogram (body weight) per day. The amount per dose is calculated by dividing total daily dose by the number of times given daily.
[a]Commercial liquid preparations of the diuretics are available. Compounded suspensions of the following can be prepared: enalapril, lisinopril, losartan, labetalol and amlodipine.

Beta-blockers are contraindicated in patients with asthma and heart block, and relatively contraindicated in diabetes. Propanolol in particular has a risk of CNS effects and has been largely replaced by better-tolerated medications (e.g., atenolol, metoprolol). Beta-blockers can also lead to deterioration of athletic performance. Calcium-channel blockers are usually well tolerated, but can be associated with tachycardia. The effectiveness of calcium-channel blockers appears to be modest in children when used as monotherapy.

ACE inhibitors can be used in children with normal renal function and are usually well tolerated. Children with diabetes and coexisting hypertension have a specific indication for therapy with an ACE inhibitor (or an ARB when necessary due to ACE inhibitor side effects) for the renoprotective effect. For similar reasons, this class may be indicated in children with mild renal disease, especially those with glomerular disease and proteinuria. In this setting, worsening renal function and hyperkalemia are risks and require close monitoring. Cough and angioedema are relatively uncommon with the newer drugs in this class, and are even less likely with the ARB medications. A significant problem with the ACE-I class is the risk of adverse fetal effects, especially if taken in the second and third trimesters. Hence it should not be used in pregnant adolescents or females of childbearing age who will not reliably remain on contraception. Clonidine can be used, but often causes some somnolence initially. Sudden cessation of this medication can cause a hypertensive crisis. The peripheral alpha-antagonists can cause orthostatic hypotension when first started, and hence should be started with a low dose at bedtime. Tachycardia and fluid retention can occur with hydralazine. At higher doses, drug-induced lupus can occur.

The goal for antihypertensive therapy is a reduction in blood pressure to less than the 95th percentile for both systolic and diastolic pressures. When possible, the best regimen is a single drug at the lowest effective dose and without side effects. In the presence of co-morbidities (e.g., obesity, diabetes, hyperlipidemia), the goal is a reduction in blood pressure to below the 90th percentile. Note that as a child grows, the blood pressure goals must be changed to reflect changes in the child's age and height.

Two-drug therapeutic regimens will sometimes be required. Such combinations may help minimize side effects by achieving control with lower doses of two drugs rather than a high dose of one. Certain combinations of medications seem to work best.

The adult literature notes that 85% of hypertension can be controlled by the combination of a thiazide diuretic with either an ACE inhibitor or a beta-blocker. Data about such combinations are limited in children. A decision to treat a child or adolescent for hypertension does not imply that therapy has to continue for the rest of the individual's life. Because not all hypertensive children remain hypertensive as adults, it is appropriate to consider slowly tapering therapy after 5 to 6 years of normal blood pressure. The likelihood of success in withdrawal from therapy is increased in children with stage 1 hypertension and those children with significant improvement in issues of lifestyle, weight, or perhaps even stress. If therapy is discontinued, continued monitoring of the child or adolescent for possible recurrence of hypertension is necessary.

PEARLS

- In defining hypertension in children, systolic and diastolic values are of equal importance. Severity of hypertension is based on the higher value.
- Secondary hypertension is more often found in a hypertensive child with any of the following:
  - Prepubertal age
  - Stage 2 hypertension
  - Non-obese child with negative family history for hypertension
  - An abrupt increase in blood pressure

- Obesity increases the likelihood of hypertension threefold. Note that it also increases the risk of metabolic syndrome including glucose intolerance, hyperlipidemia, and acanthosis nigricans. The increasing prevalence of pediatric obesity explains most of the increase in the prevalence of hypertension.
- Home BP monitoring should be considered a useful adjunct to improve hypertension control and compliance.
- New-onset (acute) hypertension (e.g., glomerulonephritis, acute renal failure) can cause symptoms at blood pressure levels that would otherwise be considered only mildly or moderately elevated.

Suggested Readings

Enright PL, Goodwin JL, Sherril DL, et al. Blood pressure elevation associated with sleep-related breathing disorder in a community sample of white and Hispanic children. *Arch Pediatr Adolesc Med* 2003;157:901–904.

Joint National Committee on Prevention, Detection, Evaluation, and Treatment of High Blood Pressure. Seventh report. U.S. Department of Health and Human Services; 2003: NIH pub. no. 03-5233.

National High Blood Pressure Education Program Working Group on High Blood Pressure in Children and Adolescents. The fourth report on the diagnosis, evaluation, and treatment of high blood pressure in children and adolescents. *Pediatrics* 2004;114S:555–576.

Pickering TG, Hall JE, Appel LJ, et al. Recommendations for blood pressure measurement in humans: an AHA scientific statement from the Council on High Blood Pressure Research Professional and Public Education Subcommittee. *J Clin Hypertens* 2005;7:102–109.

CHAPTER 66B ■ HYPERTENSIVE CRISIS

JASON M. KNIGHT

Hypertensive crisis, uncommon in the pediatric population, is often due to an underlying disease process (secondary hypertension). The presentation may vary from the incidental finding of markedly elevated blood pressure in a hospitalized child to an emergency requiring multidisciplinary intensive care. All hypertensive emergencies must be recognized immediately and treated in a controlled setting since there is a significant risk of end-organ damage with resultant morbidity and mortality. Once the child is stabilized, the hospitalist team should begin a thorough yet targeted investigation in an attempt to discover the etiology of the hypertension.

DEFINITION OF TERMS

Blood pressures in children vary according to age, gender, and height and are defined by age-appropriate norms (Chapter 66A). Regardless of these norms, hypertensive crisis is a clinical diagnosis that is not associated with a specific systolic or diastolic value. Hypertensive crises describe a broad spectrum of disease with or without associated end-organ pathology. *Hypertensive urgencies* are characterized by markedly increased blood pressure without evidence of end-organ damage. *Hypertensive emergencies* are defined as elevation of blood pressure in the presence of hypertension-related end-organ damage (e.g., an ophthalmologic exam with significant retinopathy denotes accelerated hypertension; retinopathy with the additional finding of papilledema is the hallmark of malignant hypertension). As such, *accelerated hypertension* implies significant potential for progressive end-organ injury, and therefore would be considered an hypertensive urgency. On the other hand, *malignant hypertension*, because of its central nervous system involvement, involves end-organ damage and thus is a hypertensive emergency. The vital organs most affected by significant hypertension are listed in Figure 66.1 and include the central nervous system, cardiovascular system, and kidneys.

ETIOLOGY

The most common causes of secondary hypertension were previously listed in Table 66.1 (Chapter 66A). Children with hypertensive crises usually have an underlying cause for their hypertension, with renal or renovascular disease being the most common. Other diagnoses to consider for children with significant hypertension include cardiovascular disease (coarctation of the aorta), neurologic disease (CVA, hemorrhage, head trauma), or drug ingestion. Eclampsia and preeclampsia must be considered in any young female patient.

Central Nervous System	Cardiovascular/Pulmonary
• Hypertensive encephalopathy	• Acute left ventricular failure and pulmonary edema
• Intracranial hemorrhage	
• Cerebral infarction	• Aortic dissection
• Seizures	Renal
• Altered mental status, coma	• Acute renal insufficiency
• Papilledema	• Hematuria, proteinuria, uremia

FIGURE 66.1. End-organ damage in hypertension.

EPIDEMIOLOGY

The syndrome of hypertensive emergency was first described by Volhard and Fahr in 1914 and was characterized by severe accelerated hypertension accompanied by evidence of renal disease with signs of vascular injury to the heart, brain, retina, and kidney, and by a rapidly fatal course ending in heart attack, renal failure, or stroke (3). The first large study of the natural history of malignant hypertension, published in 1939 before the widespread use of antihypertensive agents, found that untreated malignant hypertension had a 1-year mortality of 79% and a median survival of 10.5 months (4).

CLINICAL PRESENTATION AND EVALUATION

Pediatric patients with hypertensive crisis may present with non-specific complaints such as irritability, malaise, poor appetite, poor weight gain, or weight loss. Hypertensive crisis most commonly manifests in children with signs and symptoms of hypertensive encephalopathy that include onset of headache, nausea, and vomiting followed by severe headache, altered mental status, visual changes, seizure, focal neurologic deficits, and in severe cases, coma. Other associated symptoms include ischemic chest pain, dyspnea, renal symptoms (nocturia, hematuria, polyuria), back pain (aortic aneurysm), and gastrointestinal complaints (nausea, vomiting).

A detailed history and physical examination may reveal the cause of the hypertension in a previously normotensive child (Chapter 66A). Areas for emphasis should include the family history for cardiovascular and renal disease, as well as tumors with familial predisposition, such as pheochromocytoma. A past medical history should include perinatal course (including use of umbilical catheters in the neonatal period), failure to thrive, and the use of over-the-counter or illicit drugs.

The physical examination should include blood pressure measurements in all four extremities while the child is quiet. A comprehensive cardiovascular examination is essential, especially cardiac auscultation for murmurs or a gallop and palpation of both central and distal pulses. Particular attention should be focused on evaluation for cutaneous lesions (e.g., malar rash for SLE, café-au-lait spots for neurofibromatosis, ash leaf spots for tuberous sclerosis), any evidence of endocrine dysfunction, or abdominal masses or bruits. A careful and systematic neurologic examination is essential as it has implications relating to the diagnostic evaluation as well as the patient's morbidity and mortality. A complete and thorough retinal exam is a difficult procedure in most pediatric patients; therefore consultation with a pediatric ophthalmologist and an exam performed under conscious sedation may be warranted.

Initial diagnostic evaluation has been previously discussed (Table 66.2). In any patient with symptoms or an exam concerning for CNS involvement, computed tomography (CT) or magnetic resonance imaging (MRI) of the brain should be performed immediately. A chest radiograph, electrocardiogram, and echocardiography are indicated to determine the degree of cardiac involvement. In the older pediatric patient, a urine drug screen is necessary.

PATHOPHYSIOLOGY

Blood pressure is the product of cardiac output and systemic vascular resistance. Hypertension is generally due to an increase in systemic vascular resistance. The role of mechanical stress on the arteriolar wall appears to be critical in the pathogenesis of hypertensive crisis. Increased blood pressure above the autoregulatory zone leads to transmission of increased pressure to smaller distal vessels, causing mechanical stress and vascular wall damage. This endothelial disruption leads to vascular wall permeability, cell proliferation, and activation of the coagulation cascade and platelets, resulting in fibrinoid necrosis of arterioles and tissue ischemia. Fibrinoid necrosis of the arterioles is seen in vulnerable organs and is considered the histologic hallmark of hypertensive crisis.

Activation of the renin–angiotensin–aldosterone system contributes to the pathogenesis of hypertensive crisis. Decreased perfusion of the kidney and increased sympathetic activity stimulate the release of renin from the juxtaglomerular apparatus in the kidney. Renin converts angiotensinogen to angiotensin, which is subsequently converted to the active form, angiotensin II, by angiotensin-converting enzyme in the lung. Angiotensin II, a potent vasoconstrictor, stimulates aldosterone release, which further increases blood pressure by causing salt and water retention (5).

Activation of the renin–angiotensin–aldosterone system has been implicated in the initiation and perpetuation of the vascular injury associated with hypertensive emergencies. Angiotensin II leads to increased expression of nuclear factor-κβ (NF-κβ) (6), a transcription factor that promotes expression of proinflammatory cytokines, leukocyte adhesion, and proliferation of vascular smooth muscle cells (7). Angiotensin II promotes oxidative stress by increasing NADPH oxidase activity, which in turn generates reactive oxygen species. Reactive oxygen species injure the endothelium, leading to a decrease in nitric oxide production, which results in vasoconstriction and increased expression of NF-κβ (8). Angiotensin II further increases vasoconstriction by inhibiting the cytokine-mediated induction of inducible nitric oxide synthase (9). Adult patients with hypertensive emergencies have elevated serum markers associated with oxidative stress (lipid hydroperoxidase), endothelial damage (von Willebrand factor, soluble P-selectin, fibrinogen), and neurohumoral response (plasma adrenomedullin and natriuretic peptide). These levels declined significantly after 6 months of effective antihypertensive therapy (10).

Endothelial dysfunction, which appears to be the beginning of the final common pathway for the pathogenesis of hypertensive crisis, results not only in decreased vasodilation but also in a proinflammatory and prothrombotic state. The end result is a vicious cycle of increased vasoconstriction, oxidative stress, and inflammation leading to progressive cytotoxic effects on the vascular wall, worsening endothelial damage, and a progressive intravascular pro-coagulation state with the resultant deposition of fibrinoid material and platelet aggregation (8). These molecular events will eventually cause end-organ complications, specifically significant ischemia of the heart, brain, and kidneys.

Acute Neurologic Syndromes

Autoregulation of cerebral blood flow refers to the ability of the brain to maintain a constant cerebral blood flow as the cerebral perfusion pressure varies from 60 to 150 mm Hg (Fig. 66.2). As mean blood pressure increases in this range, cerebral vascular resistance increases in order to "protect" the brain from these elevated pressures while attempting to maintain constant blood flow. When mean arterial pressure reaches a critical level (140 to 180 mm Hg), the previously constricted vessels are unable to withstand the pressure, counter-regulation fails, and generalized vasodilation ensues. This increased cerebral blood flow leads to hyperperfusion of the brain under high pressure and results in cerebral edema and the clinical syndrome of hypertensive encephalopathy.

Patients with long-standing hypertension will have a rightward shift of the pressure–flow (cerebral, renal, and coronary) autoregulation curve (Fig. 66.2). Treatment that results in a rapid reduction in blood pressure into a range that would otherwise be considered normal will reduce blood pressure below the autoregulatory capacity of the hypertensive circulation. The resultant marked reduction in organ blood flow causes inadequate tissue perfusion, significant ischemia and infarction. In this case, a significant decrease in blood pressure may cause hypoperfusion of the brain tissue around the infarcted area, actually worsening the acute disease and eventual outcome.

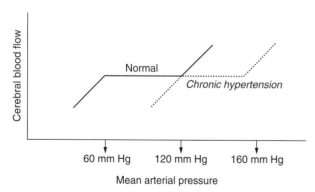

FIGURE 66.2. Cerebral autoregulation in normotensive and chronically hypertensive patients. (Adapted from Varon J, Marik PE. The management of hypertensive crises. *Crit Care* 2003;7:374–384, with permission.)

Myocardial Ischemia

When the normal heart is presented with a workload (e.g., increased systemic vascular resistance, SVR) that exceeds its capacity, the adequacy of the myocardial response is determined by the rapidity with which the hypertension evolved. The time available for compensatory ventricular hypertrophy to develop and the severity of the hypertension will dictate whether the myocardium will be able to adequately respond to an acute hypertensive emergency. The left ventricle and coronary vasculature, both exquisitely sensitive to myocardial oxygen supply and demand, are adversely affected by severe hypertension. Over time, increasing wall tension causes deposition of protein and collagen in the extracellular matrix of the ventricular wall, resulting in hypertrophy of the left ventricular myocytes and resultant increase in ventricular mass. Concurrent activation of the renin–angiotensin–aldosterone system constricts systemic vasculature, further increasing left ventricular wall tension and therefore myocardial oxygen demand and consumption. Left ventricular hypertrophy further compromises oxygen delivery by causing coronary artery compression and decreased luminal blood flow. Lastly, significant hypertension can increase the epicardial coronary wall thickness, increasing the wall-to-lumen ratio and decreasing coronary blood flow reserve (5). The end result is a hypertrophied left ventricle that is exposed to severe, ongoing afterload forces, both of which increase oxygen demand. When oxygen demand outpaces oxygen supply, coronary ischemia ensues.

Left Ventricular Failure and Acute Pulmonary Edema

The left ventricle, despite significant hypertrophy, cannot overcome the afterload forces caused by an acute rise in SVR. Neurohormonal activation of the renin–angiotensin–aldosterone system leads to increased sodium content and increased total body water. Left ventricle hypertrophy also causes focal ischemia and inadequate diastolic filling. This resultant combination, an imbalance between left ventricular contraction and relaxation and an increase in total body water, leads to pulmonary venous hypertension and acute pulmonary edema (5).

Acute Renal Insufficiency

Acute renal insufficiency may be a cause or result of rapidly progressive hypertension. Normal renal autoregulation allows the kidney to maintain a constant blood flow and glomerular filtration rate for mean arterial pressures between 80 and 160 mm Hg. With ongoing hypertension, the initially protective structural changes of the afferent arteriole become pathologic. Progressive narrowing of the preglomerular vessels results in ischemic injury, tubular atrophy, and fibrosis. The resultant impairment of the renal autoregulatory system causes systemic arterial pressure to be transmitted to the preglomerular vessels and eventually, the intraglomerular apparatus. In this situation, the kidney is exposed to elevated systemic pressures and flow, as well as any significant acute decreases associated with therapy, leading to acute renal ischemia (5).

MANAGEMENT AND THERAPY

Hypertensive crisis in the pediatric patient is life threatening and will usually require that the child be hospitalized in an intensive-care setting (Fig. 66.3). Children with a hypertensive emergency, regardless of their location (e.g., emergency department, inpatient ward), require rapid initiation of therapy and

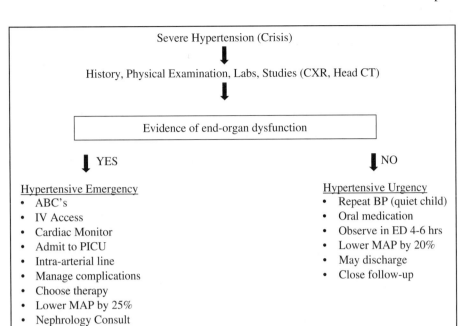

Severe Hypertension (Crisis)

History, Physical Examination, Labs, Studies (CXR, Head CT)

Evidence of end-organ dysfunction

YES   NO

Hypertensive Emergency
- ABC's
- IV Access
- Cardiac Monitor
- Admit to PICU
- Intra-arterial line
- Manage complications
- Choose therapy
- Lower MAP by 25%
- Nephrology Consult

Hypertensive Urgency
- Repeat BP (quiet child)
- Oral medication
- Observe in ED 4-6 hrs
- Lower MAP by 20%
- May discharge
- Close follow-up

FIGURE 66.3. Diagnostic approach for management of hypertensive crises. (Adapted from Suresh S, Mahajan P. Emergency management of pediatric hypertension. *Clin Pediatr* 2005;44:739–745, with permission.)

stabilization for transfer to a center with a pediatric intensive-care unit. Patients with hypertensive urgency may receive treatment and be observed for response in the emergency department (Fig. 66.3). Those hypertensive urgency patients who respond favorably to standard treatment may be stable for admission to a pediatric ward or even discharged home with close follow-up. Although noninvasive blood pressure monitoring can be considered adequate and accurate in most settings, patients with hypertensive emergency should have an indwelling arterial catheter placed. The radial artery is the preferred location, but occasionally other sites (dorsalis pedis, axillary, and femoral arteries) must be utilized. This allows the practitioner to continuously monitor the intra-arterial pressure and the patients' response to therapy. A central venous catheter may also be warranted in order to deliver continuous intravenous infusions of antihypertensive medications as well as to accurately monitor central venous pressure.

The clinician treating hypertensive crises should consider the underlying disease process when choosing initial therapy. Associated congenital or acquired heart diseases (arrhythmia or heart block), underlying renal disease (renal artery stenosis), or comorbid CNS disease (cerebral hemorrhage or infarct) are just a few of the concerns that the practitioner should attempt to address prior to initiation of therapy. *The goal for antihypertensive therapy is to safely lower the blood pressure at a rate that arrests or alleviates end-organ damage without causing ischemia of vital organs.* This usually translates to a reduction of mean arterial blood pressure by 20% to 25% over 2 to 3 hours. If the patient is clinically stable, the blood pressure may be further decreased toward normal over the next 24 to 48 hours. Nitroprusside, labetalol, or nicardipine are the typical first-line, titratable intravenous agents for treatment of a hypertensive crisis (Table 66.4).

Nitroprusside infusion causes a dose-dependent dilatation of the arterioles and venules and is easily titrated to achieve a sustained reduction in blood pressure. The initial recommended infusion rate is 0.25 µg/kg/min and may be increased by 0.25 µg/kg/min every few minutes. The drug does not have any significant direct negative inotropic or chronotropic cardiac effects. Cyanide is released nonenzymatically from nitroprusside, the amount generated being dependent on the dose

and length of administration. Effective cyanide metabolization and excretion is dependent on adequate hepatic and renal function. When high infusion rates are used for a prolonged period of time (>72 hours), treatment with thiosulfate or hydroxocobalamin (vitamin B_{12a}) infusion is safe and effective in preventing cyanide accumulation.

Beta-blockers, given as a continuous infusion, are extremely useful in managing severe hypertension. Esmolol is a $β_1$-selective adrenergic blocker with a short duration of action (about 30 minutes). The "negative" chronotropic effect may be beneficial in patients with ischemic heart disease. Labetalol produces selective antagonism at α-receptors and nonselective antagonism at β-adrenergic receptors. It has been found effective and well tolerated in myocardial infarction, neurovascular disease, eclampsia, and children with hypertensive crisis. Beta-blockers are relatively contraindicated in patients with severe asthma, heart block, and diabetes. Side effects include potential for worsening heart failure, bradycardia, orthostatic hypotension, and dizziness.

Nicardipine, a calcium-channel blocker, is an effective antihypertensive agent that decreases afterload by reducing total peripheral resistance without reducing cardiac output. Its rapid onset and short duration of action make it an ideal drug in the immediate treatment phase while invasive lines are being placed and patient stabilization is occurring. Intravenous nicardipine has been shown to reduce both cardiac and cerebral ischemia. Profound, acute hypotension can occur with even standard, recommended dosing.

Fenoldopam acts at the level of the postsynaptic dopamine (DA_1) receptors in renal, coronary, cerebral, and splanchnic vasculature resulting in arterial dilation and lowering of the mean arterial pressure. Fenoldopam is an ideal drug for hypertensive crisis because the peak effects are observed within 5 to 15 minutes, steady-state serum levels are achieved in 30 to 60 minutes, and plasma levels and clinical effects dissipate rapidly once the infusion is discontinued (11). Fenoldopam has the additional benefits of increasing renal blood flow and sodium excretion. It has been demonstrated to improve creatinine clearance, urine flow rates, and sodium excretion in severely hypertensive patients with both normal and impaired renal function (12). Although not extensively studied in children,

TABLE 66.4

SELECTED ANTIHYPERTENSIVE AGENTS IN THE ICU SETTING

Class	Drug	Dose	Duration
Alpha- and beta-blocker	Labetalol	IV: 0.2–2 mg/kg (acute); 0.2–3 mg/kg/hr continuous infusion	3–6 hr
Beta-blocker	Esmolol	IV: 500 µg/kg, then 50–500 µg/kg/min continuous infusion	10–30 min
Vasodilator	Sodium nitroprusside	IV: 0.25–10 µg/kg/min, continuous infusion	1–5 min
Arterial dilator	Hydralazine	IV/IM: 0.1–0.6 mg/kg	2–4 hr
Arterial dilator	Diazoxide	IV: 1–5 mg/kg	6–24 hr
Arterial dilator	Minoxidil	PO: 0.2–1 mg/kg/day	12–24 hr
Calcium-channel blocker	Nicardipine	IV: 1–3 µg/kg/min, continuous infusion	4–6 hr
	Nifedipine	PO/SL: 0.25–0.5 mg/kg	4–6 hr
Dopamine receptor (DA$_1$) agonist	Fenoldopam	0.2–0.8 µg/kg/min, continuous infusion	5–60 min
Central alpha-agonist	Clonidine	PO: 5–10 µg/kg/day	8–12 hr
ACE inhibitor	Enalaprilat	IV: 5–10 µg/kg q 8–24 hr	8–12 hr
	Captopril	PO: 0.1–0.5 mg/kg/dose, up to max 4 mg/kg/day	8–12 hr
Diuretic	Furosemide	IV: 1–2 mg/kg/dose	4–6 hr
	Hydrochlorthiazide	PO: 1–2 mg/kg BID	12–24 hr

there is some evidence that it can be used safely and effectively. The cost comparison for a daily infusion in a 20-kg patient shows that fenoldopam ($300) is approximately 60 times more expensive than nitroprusside (<$5) and 5 times more than nicardipine ($65) (11). This discrepancy in cost should be taken into account given the effectiveness and safety profile of the other drugs.

A majority of children with hypertensive crisis have acute or chronic renal disease and therefore diuretics may be a helpful adjunctive treatment. Characteristics and recommended dosage of other drug classes used to treat hypertensive crises are listed in Table 66.4. Grossman and associates have provided an excellent review of parenteral agents for hypertensive emergencies, including an evidence-based discussion of treatment for specific hypertensive emergencies (see Suggested Readings).

Once the child has been appropriately stabilized in the intensive-care unit, a pediatric nephrologist and pediatric cardiologist may be consulted. These specialists can help guide the diagnostic workup as well as recommend appropriate treatment for the pediatric patient with hypertensive crisis.

In summary, hypertensive crises are an uncommon but serious cause of morbidity and mortality in pediatrics. The final common cellular pathway, regardless of etiology, involves a vicious cycle of increased vasoconstriction and oxidative injury leading to worsening endothelial damage and a progressive prothrombotic and proinflammatory state with the resultant deposition of fibrinoid material. The accumulation of these molecular events will eventually manifest as significant ischemia of the heart, brain, or kidneys. It is the hospitalist's goal to recognize and safely manage the pediatric patient with hypertensive crisis.

PEARLS

- Hypertensive crisis is a clinical diagnosis that is not associated with a specific systolic or diastolic value.
- In the pediatric population, hypertensive crises are frequently due to secondary hypertension.
- The goal for antihypertensive therapy in the setting of hypertensive crisis is to safely reduce mean arterial blood pressure by:
  - "First, no harm."
  - Not hypoperfusing already ischemic organs.
  - Avoiding rapid swings in blood pressure beyond the already dysfunctional range of autoregulation of tissue perfusion.
- Initiating treatment in a monitored setting with continuously infused agents.

References

1. Muntner P, He J, Cutler JA, et al. Trends in blood pressure among children and adolescents. *JAMA* 2004;291:2107–2113.
2. Somu S, Sundaram B, Kamalanathan AN. *Arch Dis Child* 2003;88:302.
3. Volhard F, Fahr T. *Die brightsche Nierenkrankeit: Klinik, Pathologie und Atlas.* Berlin: Springer; 1914.
4. Keith NM, Wagener HP, Barker NW. Some different types of essential hypertension: their course and prognosis. *Am J Med Sci* 1939;197:332–343.
5. Aggarwal M, Khan IA. Hypertensive crisis: hypertensive emergencies and urgencies. *Cardiol Clin* 2006;24:135–146.
6. Ruiz-Ortega M, Lorenzo O, Ruperez M. Angiotensin II activates nuclear transcription factor kappa b through AT (1) and AT (2) in vascular smooth muscle cells: molecular mechanisms. *Circ Res* 2000;86:1266–1272.

7. Collidge TA, Lammie GA, Fleming S. The role of the renin-angiotensin system in malignant vascular injury affecting the systemic and cerebral circulations. *Prog Biophys Mol Biol* 2004;84:301–319.

8. Patel HP, Mitsnefes M. Advances in the pathogenesis and management of hypertensive crisis. *Curr Opin Pediatr* 2005;17:210–214.

9. Nakayama I, Kawahara Y, Tsuda T. Angiotensin II inhibits cytokine-stimulated inducible nitric oxide synthase expression in vascular smooth muscle cells. *J Biol Chem* 1994;269:11628–11633.

10. Elliott WJ. Management of hypertensive emergencies. *Curr Hypertens Rep* 2003;5:486–492.

11. Strauser LM, Pruitt, RD, Tobias JD. Initial experience with fenoldopam in children. *Am J Ther* 1999;6:283–288.

12. Shusterman NH, Elliott WJ, White WB. Fenoldopam, but not nitroprusside, improves renal function in severely hypertensive patients with impaired renal function. *Am Heart J* 1993;95:161–168.

Suggested Readings

Grossman E, Ironi AN, Messerli FH. Comparative tolerability profile of hypertensive crisis treatments. *Drug Saf* 1998;19:99–122.

Varon J, Marik PE. The management of hypertensive crises. *Crit Care* 2003;7:374–384.

CHAPTER 67 ▪ HENOCH–SCHÖNLEIN PURPURA

JEFF ARMSTRONG

BACKGROUND

Henoch–Schönlein purpura (HSP) is the most common systemic vasculitis of childhood. It was first described more than 200 years ago in 1801 by Herbeden in reference to a 5-year-old boy with abdominal pain, hematochezia, joint pain, purpuric rash, and hematuria. In 1832, Schönlein noted the presence of a purpuric rash with arthritis for which he coined the term *purpura rheumatica*. Henoch, a former student of Schönlein, reported on both the possibility for significant gastrointestinal (1874) and renal involvement (1899) with potentially serious consequences. Osler published a number of reports between 1895 and 1914 and felt that anaphylaxis played a role, eventually prompting the term *anaphylactoid purpura* as espoused by Frank in 1915. Gairdner, in 1948, noted the vasculitic nature of the disease. In 1969, Berger demonstrated that the mesangial deposits in the glomerulonephritis of HSP consist of immunoglobulin A (IgA), and prompted the eventual discovery of a similar dermal vasculitic process in the associated purpuric rash. It is still not completely clear if HSP and IgA nephropathy are separate processes with a number of similarities, or if they represent the same disease with various clinical manifestations.

HSP is a systemic leukocytoclastic small-vessel vasculitis manifested by nonthrombocytopenic purpura, arthritis, abdominal pain, and renal involvement. The definition put forth by the American College of Rheumatology is mainly clinical, requiring two or more of the following: (1) age 20 years or less, (2) palpable purpura without thrombocytopenia, (3) acute abdominal pain or GI bleeding, and (4) histologic evidence of granulocytes within the walls of arterioles or venules. Typically a self-limited process, HSP can result in life-long disease if there is significant renal involvement.

EPIDEMIOLOGY

HSP has been reported in children as young as 6 months and in adults over 80 years of age, but the vast majority of those affected are young children. The peak age is about 5 years, with 75% being between age 2 and 11 years. Overall, the incidence in U.S. children is approximately 14 cases per 100,000 children per year. HSP occurs more commonly in boys than in girls with a 1.5:1 to 2:1 ratio. All races are affected, but HSP is rarely seen in African Americans. It occurs throughout the year, but there seems to be a seasonal prevalence, with more cases from fall to spring and fewer cases during the summer months. Most large epidemiologic studies suggest that geographic or temporal clusters are uncommon. HSP is generally benign and self-limiting. The observation that respiratory infections tend to precede the onset of HSP (50–70% of the time) was first noted by Schönlein and has since been reported by many other observers.

PATHOGENESIS

Although the etiology remains far from being fully understood, it is evident that HSP is a multifactorial immune-mediated process with various potential antigenic, genetic, and environmental components. In the active disease, there are elevated levels of IgA, circulating immune complexes containing IgA, and IgA-associated deposits in renal and skin vessel walls. Specifically, one of two IgA subclasses appears to be involved, namely IgA1. Aberrant glycosylation in the hinge region of IgA1 may result in a tendency to form macromolecular complexes, thus resulting in the immunologic and histologic features of HSP. The genetic basis and mechanism for this is being explored.

As noted above, many cases of HSP are preceded by an upper respiratory illness. Group A beta-hemolytic streptococcus has been the one most extensively studied, with 30% to 45% of those with HSP having either positive throat cultures or positive serologies. However, a wide variety of other pathogens and agents have been linked potentially to the development of HSP (Table 67.1). Infections, viral and bacterial, tend to be the potential triggers in children. In adults, drugs and toxins tend to be the inciting events. Despite numerous studies, no single infectious or exposure trigger has demonstrated to be a clear and dominant cause of HSP.

As a consequence of IgA-associated immune complex deposition in the arterioles, capillaries, or venules of various target organs, a necrotizing leukocytoclastic vasculitis ensues. Numerous mediators can be involved, including prostaglandins, cytokines, elements of the complement pathway, chemotactic factors, endothelins, adhesions, polymorphonuclear cells, hematologic factors (e.g., protein C, protein S, factor XIII, thrombin–antithrombin complex, and von Willebrand factor), nitric oxide, antiphospholipid antibodies, and transforming growth factor. Various gene polymorphisms may contribute to the diversity of clinical response to inflammatory stimulation. The variety of signs and symptoms of HSP may reflect different pathophysiologic mechanisms in different patients. Ongoing research in attempt to delineate the role of all these factors is in progress.

CLINICAL FEATURES

Rash is the initial sign in more than half of patients with HSP and is almost always present (essentially 100% of the time).

TABLE 67.1

POTENTIAL TRIGGERS FOR HSP

Infections	Drugs
Streptococcus pyogenes	Penicillin
Staphylococcus aureus	Ampicillin
Salmonella	Erythromycin
Shigella	Quinidine
Campylobacter	Quinine
Yersinia	Cocaine
Legionella	Vaccines
Mycoplasma	Typhoid
Bartonella henslae	Paratyphoid
Helicobacter pylori	Measles
Kingella kingae	Yellow fever
Hepatitis virus (A, B, C)	Cholera
Human immunodefi-	Foods
ciency virus	Horse serum
Herpes simplex virus	Insect bites
Parvovirus	Cold exposure
Adenovirus	Pregnancy
Epstein–Barr virus	Malignancy
Varicella	Liver disease
Mycobacterium	Diabetes mellitus
tuberculosis	Familial Mediterranean fever
Toxocara canis	Celiac disease

Cutaneous involvement begins initially as a fixed maculopapular or urticarial rash, which often starts at the ankles and dorsal surface of the feet and then progresses to a palpable purpuric rash. Pinpoint petechiae and coalescent ecchymoses may be scattered along with these lesions. Components of the rash can resemble erythema multiforme, with typical and atypical target lesions. The rash tends to be gravity and pressure dependent and thus concentrated on the buttocks and lower extremities, but can be scattered on the upper extremities and sometimes involves the face and ears. About one-third of those affected will have nonpitting edema of the scalp, eyelids, face, and feet, more commonly in younger children. Some patients may develop hemorrhagic vesicles, bullae, or cutaneous necrosis. The diagnosis of HSP is usually straightforward when the rash is present, but up to 25% to 50% of the cases can be preceded by arthritis or gastrointestinal symptoms for as long as 1 to 2 weeks, making the diagnosis more elusive. As a result, the patient may undergo invasive diagnostic or even surgical procedures (e.g., appendectomy). It is important to keep HSP in the differential diagnosis for an acute abdomen.

Arthritis is the next most common manifestation of HSP, occurring in 65% to 80% of cases, and is the first clinical symptom 25% of the time. The knees and ankles are typically involved, with wrists, elbows, and fingers less commonly affected. Usually there is swelling and tenderness to palpation without the significant warmth, erythema, effusion, and marked decreased range of motion that would be typically present in septic arthritis. Involvement of the joints is usually transient, the pain and swelling being periarticular and without sequelae.

Gastrointestinal symptoms consisting of abdominal pain with or without hematochezia occur in 50% to 75% of cases and are the presenting symptoms 10% to 15% of the time. These have been shown to be a result of the vasculitic process occurring along the bowel wall, resulting in submucosal and subserosal edema and hemorrhages. The abdominal pain is described as sharp or colicky, sometimes mimicking an acute abdomen. Less commonly, other abdominal processes can occur

such as intussusception, frank upper gastrointestinal bleeding, appendicitis, bowel infarction, bowel perforation, pancreatitis, gall bladder hydrops, hemorrhagic ascites, hepatosplenomegaly with elevated liver transaminases, and pseudomembranous colitis. Most intussusceptions in HSP are ileoileal (70%) as opposed to ileocolic; thus abdominal ultrasound rather than barium enema may be indicated to make the diagnosis. Also the presence of inflamed and potentially necrotic segments of bowel could lead to intestinal perforation during the process of a barium enema study.

Renal involvement occurs in 20% to 50% of HSP, usually within 4 weeks of presentation, and less commonly precedes the other symptoms. The majority of renal involvement is usually transient. Notably, when present, the onset of renal abnormalities may follow the onset of other symptoms by weeks (80% within 4 weeks) or even months (97% within 3 months). The true extent of renal manifestations of HSP may be underestimated due to the fact that patients may not have their urine monitored on a regular basis. Microscopic or gross hematuria, proteinuria, nephrotic syndrome, nephritic syndrome, combined nephrotic-nephritic syndrome, hypertension, renal failure, and rapidly progressive glomerulonephritis are associated manifestations. The most frequent manifestations are microscopic hematuria and/or low-grade proteinuria. Histologic changes can range from minimal change to severe nephritis with extensive crescents. Severe nephritis, potentially leading to renal failure, occurs in 2% to 5% of patients with HSP.

Neurologic manifestations and complications can occur. The most frequent are headache, behavioral changes (e.g., apathy, irritability, and emotional lability), and seizures. Depending on the degree of the necrotizing vasculitic process, focal ischemia, diffuse encephalopathy, cerebral infarction, intracranial hemorrhage, subarachnoid hemorrhage, and subdural hemorrhage can rarely occur. Metabolic derangements and hypertension can also result in similar manifestations. Focal deficits, ataxia, altered mental status, and neuropathies can be a result.

Other less common manifestations of HSP include testicular involvement (orchitis, testicular torsion), pulmonary involvement (diffuse alveolar hemorrhage, interstitial pneumonia, interstitial fibrosis), cardiac involvement (pericarditis, myocarditis, myocardial infarction), and ocular involvement (retinal hemorrhage, anterior uveitis, optic neuritis).

A potential infantile variant of HSP, acute hemorrhagic edema of infancy (AHEI), is seen in young children typically less than 2 years old. Other terms for this syndrome are Finkelstein disease and postinfectious cockade purpura. These children often do not present with the typical palpable purpuric rash, but present with large annular ecchymotic lesions on the face and extremities with painful edema of the hands and feet. Joint and organ (gastrointestinal and renal) involvement is rare, and the process has an excellent prognosis, with a much less likelihood of recurrence. It still remains unclear if HSP and AHEI, even though they both represent small-vessel vasculitis, represent variations of the same disease process or are different diseases altogether.

Two-thirds of the time, HSP runs its course within 4 weeks of the initial symptoms without any complications. Recurrences occur 15% to 45% of the time. The symptoms are usually those of the initial presentation but milder and of shorter duration. Typically these occur early in relation to the onset of disease (e.g., within 2 to 3 months), but can occur up to years later. Recurrences are more likely to occur in patients with nephritis. Complications can occur with initial or recurrent symptoms, so careful and thorough repeated evaluations are prudent.

The differential diagnosis of HSP includes sepsis, meningococcemia, Rocky Mountain spotted fever, idiopathic thrombocytopenic purpura, disseminated intravascular coagulation and other bleeding diatheses, drug reaction, acute abdomen, leukemia and other malignancies, and other vasculitic processes. HSP is by definition a small-vessel vasculitis and therefore needs to be differentiated from other diseases involving small vessels, particularly in patients who present in an older age range than typical for HSP or who have more severe manifestations. These would include systemic lupus erythematosus, Churg–Strauss syndrome, Wegener's granulomatosis, and microscopic polyangiitis. In such cases, a rheumatology consultation would be indicated and appropriate screening labs, such as antinuclear antibodies, anticytoplasmic antibodies, antidouble–strand DNA antibodies, and antiphospholipid antibodies, would be appropriate.

LABORATORY FINDINGS

Suggested initial laboratory studies in suspected HSP would include a complete blood cell count, electrolyte panel including blood urea nitrogen and creatinine, urinalysis, stool occult blood, prothrombin time, partial thromboplastin time, and serum IgA level.

Microscopic hematuria and proteinuria may be present (35% of cases). Leukocytosis with or without a left shift is common. The platelet count is normal or increased. Inflammatory markers including erythrocyte sedimentation rate and C-reactive protein are normal or elevated. Clotting tests including prothrombin time, partial thromboplastin time, and bleeding time are usually normal. Patients with significant gastrointestinal involvement often have decreased factor XIII levels. IgA levels are elevated in 30% to 60% of patients. No association between elevated IgA and clinical symptoms has been found, thus limiting impact on clinical management. One exception would be an elevated IgA level in a patient with abdominal pain without the classic rash that might help in differentiating HSP from other causes of acute abdomen. Renal function is usually normal. Obviously, abnormalities in urinalysis or renal function need to be monitored closely and may warrant further evaluation, especially in the face of nephritis or renal insufficiency. Renal and/or skin biopsies are usually reserved for atypical or severe presentations of HSP. The renal histologic appearance of HSP is identical to that of IgA nephropathy.

MANAGEMENT

The care of children with HSP is mostly supportive with observation for complications. This includes maintenance of adequate hydration, nutrition, electrolyte balance, and pain control. Any potential triggers (e.g., drugs) should be discontinued or avoided. Urinalysis and blood pressure measurements are essential when evaluating patients with HSP. If these are abnormal, renal function tests (blood urea nitrogen, creatinine) should be checked. Even if the urinalysis is normal during the initial presentation, the urine and blood pressure should be monitored for at least 6 months.

Indications for inpatient management include significant abdominal pain, vomiting, dehydration, decreased renal function, hypertension, and the presence of complications such as gastrointestinal bleeding, neurologic manifestations, pulmonary hemorrhage, acute scrotum, intussusception and other acute abdominal processes. In such cases, careful and thorough serial examinations are an essential component of patient care. Some patients may require management in the pediatric intensive care unit. Imaging studies or subspecialty consultations, when indicated, should be obtained. The patient with significant abdominal pain requires special consideration because the abdominal pain can be due to vasculitis associated with HSP or it can be a result of a complication of HSP (e.g., intussusception or intestinal infarction/perforation).

Intussusception should be considered in the presence of colicky abdominal pain, vomiting (especially if bilious), or the presence of either bloody, mucoid, or currant jelly stools. Acetaminophen is often effective for fever, joint, or muscle pain. Nonsteroidal anti-inflammatory agents can be used for symptoms not responsive to acetaminophen, but should be avoided or used with caution in patients with significant renal or gastrointestinal disease. Histamine receptor blockers or proton-pump inhibitors may be indicated in abdominal pain with or without subclinical (occult blood positive stools) or overt gastrointestinal bleeding. Antihypertensive medications such as vasodilators (e.g., hydralazine) or calcium-channel blockers (e.g., nicardipine) may be needed to control blood pressure. In such cases, sodium and fluid restriction may be indicated. Angiotensin-converting enzyme inhibitors should either be avoided or used with caution in patients with significant renal disease during the acute phase of HSP.

The use of corticosteroids in HSP remains controversial. Many authors have reported a salutary effect of steroids on joint pain, abdominal pain, subcutaneous edema, and scrotal swelling. Prospective, randomized, placebo-controlled studies demonstrating the efficacy of steroids have not been done. It should be noted that most joint pain, abdominal pain, and painful edema resolves in 24 to 72 hours without steroids. However, steroids do appear to shorten recovery from these symptoms, usually within 24 hours. Thus steroids should be reserved for those with significant or refractory symptoms. The use of steroids does not seem to have any effect on the purpura, duration of HSP, or frequency of recurrences.

In terms of managing HSP nephritis, there has been minimal if any evidence to support the use of regular doses (1–2 mg/kg/day) of corticosteroids. Likewise, this use of steroids does not appear to prevent the onset of nephritis even if used early. However, recent studies have suggested that pulse dose intravenous steroids (30 mg/kg/day for 3 consecutive days), followed by oral steroids combined with azathioprine or cyclophosphamide, may be of benefit in patients with severe nephritis in terms of reversing the process and preventing progression of renal involvement (1). Another regimen with similar results involves the use of methylprednisolone and urokinase pulse dose therapy combined with cyclophosphamide (2). Other potential therapies with limited data include plasmapheresis, cyclosporine A, dapsone, and IV immunoglobulin. Further long-term, prospective, controlled studies are needed to support the routine use of such regimens.

Angiotensin-converting enzyme inhibitors appear to play a role in cases of persistent proteinuria after the acute phase of HSP in order to prevent or attenuate hyperfiltration injury and development of chronic kidney disease.

PROGNOSIS AND FOLLOW-UP

The majority of HSP (80%) consists of a single self-limiting episode that lasts up to several weeks requiring no treatment and is without any complications. The long-term prognosis of HSP is dictated by the degree of renal involvement. Factors associated with an increased risk of renal involvement include age greater than 4 years at onset of disease, severe abdominal symptoms, persistent purpura >1 month, and decreased factor XIII activity. Children with mild hematuria and/or proteinuria do well, with around 82% having normal long-term renal function. These abnormalities can last from a few months to a year or so. Those with a nephrotic component, nephritic component, or a combination of both have an increased risk of developing hypertension or impaired renal function (44%). Long-term studies show that in these patients, hypertension and renal failure can develop up to 20 years after the onset of HSP. Overall, 1% to 5% of children with HSP develop chronic kidney disease requiring dialysis. Even if the initial urinalysis is normal, the urine and blood pressure should be checked at least weekly during active HSP disease and then monthly for at least 6 months after the onset of symptoms. Those with an abnormal urinalysis should have renal function tests and should have more careful long-term follow-up. Regular follow-up with a pediatric nephrologist and consideration for renal biopsy, when indicated, may be appropriate. Of note, affected girls will need close monitoring of urine, blood pressure, and renal function during and after future pregnancies even if there was no evidence of HSP-associated renal involvement. They have an increased risk of pregnancy-associated complications such as proteinuria, hypertension, renal insufficiency, and fetal demise.

PEARLS

- The classic manifestations of purpuric rash, arthritis, abdominal pain, and renal involvement may either present incompletely or appear at different times, as opposed to all at once, making diagnosis more elusive.
- Careful and thorough serial examinations are an essential component of patient care.
- Most children with HSP have a benign course without any significant sequelae.

- Urinalysis, even if initially normal, should be monitored for at least 6 months. In those with persistent urinary abnormalities, renal disease and hypertension can occur many years later; such cases require careful long-term monitoring.

References

1. Singh S, Devidayal, Kumar L, et al. Severe Henoch-Schönlein nephritis: resolution with azathioprine and steroids. *Rheumatol Int* 2002;22:133–137.
2. Kawasaki Y, Suzuki J, Suzuki H. Efficacy of methylprednisolone and urokinase pulse therapy combined with or without cyclophosphamide in severe Henoch-Schoenlein nephritis: a clinical and histopathological study. *Nephrol Dial Transplant* 2004;19:858–864.

Suggested Readings

Ballinger S. Henoch-Schönlein purpura. *Curr Opin Rheumatol* 2003;15: 591–594.
Dillon MJ. Henoch-Schönlein purpura (treatment and outcome). *Cleve Clin J Med* 2002;69(suppl 2):121–123.
Narchi H. Risk of long term renal impairment and duration of follow up recommended for Henoch-Schönlein purpura with normal or minimal urinary findings: a systematic review. *Arch Dis Child* 2005;90:916–920.
Saulsbury FT. Epidemiology of Henoch-Schönlein purpura. *Cleve Clin J Med* 2002;69(suppl 2):87.

CHAPTER 68 ■ KAWASAKI DISEASE

NEQOR ASHOURI, PAUL A. CHECCHIA, AND ANTONIO ARRIETA

Kawasaki disease (KD) is a systemic vasculitis that presents as an acute self-limited febrile illness. It affects predominantly infants and young children. The constellation of symptoms that comprise KD develop over the first 1 to 2 weeks of illness and are usually self-limited. Left untreated, however, KD can lead to cardiac complications in 15% to 25% of patients, and has surpassed rheumatic fever as the leading cause of acquired heart disease in the United States.

KD was first described in 1967 by Tomisaku Kawasaki in his report of 50 Japanese children presenting with a febrile illness associated with distinct mucocutaneous changes and lymphadenopathy (LAD). Although initially thought to be a benign illness, deaths in children following the resolution of KD were soon reported, and a link between KD and subsequent cardiac complications was established. Review of autopsy records revealed that fatal KD was clinically very similar and pathologically indistinguishable from what was termed *infantile polyarteritis nodosa*, a rare vasculitis of childhood.

Prompt diagnosis and treatment within the first 10 days of illness have improved outcome. During the acute phase, treatment is aimed at decreasing inflammation in the coronary artery wall and preventing thrombosis. Long-term treatment among those patients who develop aneurysms is directed at prevention of myocardial ischemia.

EPIDEMIOLOGY AND ETIOLOGY

KD usually affects infants and children, with approximately 80% of cases occurring in children <5 year of age. It occurs less commonly in infants less than 3 months or children greater than 8 years of age; however, these groups tend to have a higher risk of coronary artery disease, likely secondary to delayed diagnosis.

KD is markedly more prevalent in Japan and in children of Japanese ancestry. In the United States, the disease is most common in children of Asian and Pacific Island descent, intermediate among African American and Hispanic children, and least among whites. A familial occurrence has been reported but primarily in Japan. An increased frequency among twins and in children of parents who had KD suggests a genetic component to the etiology of the disease. There have been numerous hypotheses as to the cause of KD but none have been proven. The most widely held belief is that KD is the result of a systemic inflammatory response to a trigger in genetically predisposed individuals. An infectious trigger is a likely candidate based on the seasonality (winter/spring) and reports of community outbreaks. The low number of cases in children >8 years and adults, suggests active immunity acquired during infancy in this group; the low frequency in infants <6 months of age suggests a role for maternal passive immunity. The importance of genetic predisposition was highlighted in a recent report of the inverse correlation of between the incidence of KD and the frequency of the CCR5-Δ32 allele in different geographic regions.

Since its description, investigators have tried to identify a definitive infectious agent as the trigger causing KD. Various bacteria including toxin-producing strains of *Streptococcus pyogenes* and *Staphylococcus aureus* and viruses have been implicated as potential etiologic agents of KD.

Despite the lack of an etiologic agent, much progress has been made in understanding the immunopathogenesis of the disease process. The result of the interaction between the trigger and the susceptible host results in activation of the inflammatory cascade, resulting in a significant increase in pro-inflammatory cytokines and chemokines including tumor necrosis factor-alpha (TNF-α), interleukin-1 (IL-1), IL-6, and IL-8. This high level of immune activation leads to vasculitis of medium and large-sized arteries, which can result in weakening of vessel walls with eventual dilatation and aneurysm formation.

CLINICAL FINDINGS AND DIAGNOSIS

In the absence of definitive diagnostic tests, clinical criteria have been established to provide objectivity to the diagnosis of KD. Laboratory findings frequently seen in KD aid in the diagnosis. These criteria are based the presence fever for 5 days or more, and 4 or more of the 5 other principal clinical features (Table 68.1).

Fever in KD is usually as high 39°C to 40°C and protracted. Without treatment, it may last for weeks; however, with therapy it usually resolves in 1 to 2 days. The rash is usually non-specific maculopapular, diffuse, and transient; occasionally the rash can be urticarial, scarlatiniform, or erythema-multiforme-like. Vesicular/bullous rashes have not been described with KD. The rash can be generalized with some accentuation of the perineal region where fine peeling may occur early in the course of the disease. The conjunctivitis is bilateral, non-exudative, affecting the bulbar conjunctiva with peri-limbic sparing. Pain and photophobia are rare. Anterior uveitis may be noted by slit-lamp exam. Mucous membrane changes include erythema, dryness and chapping/cracking of the lips, papillitis with resultant "strawberry tongue," and pharyngeal inflammation. Ulcers and exudates are not present. Extremity changes in the acute phase include swelling of the hands and feet with erythema/induration of the palms and soles, which is sometimes painful. Desquamation of finger and toes starts on the peri-ungual area usually about 2 weeks after the onset of illness in the subacute state. Approximately 1 to 2 months after the onset of illness, Beau lines (transverse grooves in the nailbed) may be seen. LAD is the least encountered of the criteria, being present in only 50% to 75% of patients. LAD is

TABLE 68.1

CLINICAL FEATURES OF KAWASAKI DISEASE

Fever persisting for ≥5 days and at least 4 of the following principal features	
Conjuctivitis	Bilateral, bulbar non-exsudative, peri-lymbal sparing.
Rash	Polymorphous, occasionally erythema multiforme-like. Not vesiculo-bullous.
Extremity changes	Acute: erythema of palm, soles; edema (sometimes painful) of hands and feet. Subacute: periungual peeling of fingers, toes during 2nd to 3rd weeks.
Mucosal involvement	Erythema and cracking of lips, strawberry tongue, diffuse injection of oral and oropharyngeal mucosa.
Lymphadenitis	Cervical, usually unilateral >1.5 cm, sometimes painful.

typically unilateral and needs to be at least ≥1.5 cm. The node is typically nonfluctuant and only mildly tender. It is important for the clinician to remember that these symptoms may be transient, and it is possible that they may not all be present at the time of diagnosis. Recent reports suggest that delay in treatment in classic KD occurs more often when the principal features are not present at the same time.

Other clinical features and common laboratory abnormalities frequently seen in KD may help with diagnosis (Table 68.2). Other cardiac features will be discussed later. Other noncardiac clinical features include intra-abdominal symptoms such as abdominal pain, vomiting, and diarrhea, which occur in up to one-third of patients; hydrops of the gall bladder, reported in about 15% of patients; arthralgias and arthritis; unusual irritability; and transient hearing loss. Laboratory findings are those consistent with an acute systemic inflammatory process. C-reactive protein (CRP) and erythrocyte sedimentation rate (ESR) are almost always elevated. White blood cell counts can be elevated, with more than 50% being over 15,000. Hypoalbuminemia is common and can be an indicator of the severity and length of disease process. In the acute phase of the disease, platelet count is usually normal. Thrombocytosis is typically seen in the second week of illness and peaks in the third week of illness. Of note, a low platelet count at onset of illness is a risk factor for the development of coronary artery aneurysms (CAA). The differential diagnosis of KD is extensive and includes infectious and noninfectious syndromes (Table 68.3).

Incomplete (Atypical) KD

Incomplete or atypical KD is diagnosed in a small percentage of cases that do not fit the classical criteria. *Incomplete* is probably the better term, as these cases did not meet all of the necessary criteria for diagnosis, yet did not have any atypical features such as thrombocytopenia or renal involvement. Incomplete KD is more common in very young infants, as clinical features are more subtle in this age group. Prolonged fever and subsequent peripheral desquamation have been reported to be the most common findings leading to the diagnosis of incomplete KD. Because CAA can occur in children with incomplete KD at the same frequency as seen in those with classical disease, appropriate diagnosis and treatment is of great importance. Laboratory findings appear to be similar in classic and incomplete KD, hence elevated acute phase reactants, such as ESR and CRP; thrombocytosis; sterile pyuria; hypoalbuminemia;or mild elevation of tranaminases; may assist in the diagnosis. Echocardiographic evaluation may also be important both in the acute phase, when ectasia and edema of the coronary arteries may be helpful to initiate preventive treatment, and in the convalescent stage, when detecting the

TABLE 68.2

OTHER CLINICAL AND LABORATORY FEATURES OF KAWASAKI DISEASE

System	Signs or symptoms
Central nervous system	Irritability, sensorineural hearing loss, cerebrospinal fluid pleocytosis
Ophthalmologic	Anterior uveitis
Cardiovascular	Tachycardia, gallop rhythm, myocarditis, pericardial effusion, mitral insufficiency, coronary artery ectasia
Gastrointestinal	Vomiting, diarrhea, pancreatitis, gallbladder hydrops, hyperbilirubinemia, elevated gamma glutamyl transpeptidase, abdominal pain
Renal/urologic	Sterile pyuria from urethritis, meatitis
Hematologic	Leucocytosis with neutrophilia and inmature forms, anemia, thrombocytosis after week one
Musculoskeletal	Arthritis, arthralgia
Other	Elevated ESR and CRP

TABLE 68.3

DIFFERENTIAL DIAGNOSIS

Infectious disease	Allergic or rheumatic disease	Toxic disease
Scarlet fever	Drug reaction	Acrodynia
Measles	Stevens–Johnson syndrome	
Epstein–Barr virus	Systemic juvenile rheumatoid arthritis	
Toxic shock syndrome	Systemic lupus erythematosus	
Scalded skin syndrome	Serum sickness	
Leptospirosis	Infantile periarteritis nodosa	
Rocky Mountain spotted fever		
Adenovirus		

presence of aneurysm may help prevent farther cardiovascular sequelae. At our institution when incomplete KD is suspected late in the disease (resolved fever, thrombocytosis, peeling of fingers), patients are started on anti-platelet doses of aspirin until an echocardiogram at 8 weeks after the onset of fever has ruled out the presence of aneurysms

Cardiac Findings

The morbidity and mortality attributed to the coronary artery abnormalities associated with KD have been studied thoroughly. Coronary artery abnormalities are recognized as the most severe complications of KD. In fact, prognosis correlates with the severity of the coronary artery involvement. Mortality is currently 0.04%, with death most common 2 to 12 weeks after the onset of illness. Scoring systems have been developed to identify children at high risk for developing CAA. Duration of fever has been identified as a strong predictor of CAA. A score developed by Harada and associates is frequently used in Japan to decide which children will receive IV gammaglobulin (IVIG). Those who meet ≥4 criteria by day 9 of illness receive IVIG. These criteria include white blood cell count >12 000; platelet count <350 000; CRP >3 g/dL; hematocrit <35%; albumin <3.5 g/dL; age <12 months; and male sex. Due to poor performance of scoring systems, IVIG is recommended in the United States for all children diagnosed with KD. Recurrence of fever after an afebrile period of at least 24 hours, or persistent fever beyond 48 hours after treatment with IVIG while on aspirin (refractory KD), has been associated with increased risk for CAA. Coronary artery abnormalities can be in the form of ectasia, fusiform or sacular aneurysms, or giant aneurysms (>8 mm internal diameter). These findings are usually first detected at day 10 of illness and the peak frequency within 4 weeks of onset.

Approximately 20% to 25% of untreated KD patients develop CAA. Serial angiographic follow-up of Kawasaki disease patients has indicated that approximately 50% of the patients with CAA showed resolution 5 to 18 months later, with giant aneurysms the least likely to regress and most likely to progress to thrombosis, rupture, and stenosis. However, Newburger and associates demonstrated that the use of IVIG reduces this incidence to <4%. It has not been demonstrated that treatment with IVIG instituted later than 10 days after onset of acute KD is effective in preventing CAA. For uncomplicated cases, echocardiography is recommended at diagnosis, 2 weeks later, and at 6 to 8 weeks from onset of illness. More frequent monitoring is needed in complicated courses.

Significant coronary artery disease still may develop in a small fraction of KD patients who are treated successfully.

These lesions include coronary aneurysmal dilatation, stenosis, and occlusion, which may lead to myocardial infarction, dysfunction, and even death. Several reports of myocardial infarction and sudden death attributable to CAA have involved patients with a history of an illness that, in retrospect, was consistent with KD or who had no known previous illness.

Serious coronary complications of KD have been treated with a variety of coronary interventions, including coronary artery bypass grafting procedures. The Japanese national experience with myocardial revascularization procedures for KD showed good long-term outcomes. More recently, a small series of KD patients underwent successful balloon angioplasty for severe coronary stenosis. However, there is a small population of patients for whom surgical or catheter revascularization procedures are not feasible because of the extent of their disease, with distal stenosis and/or extensive infarcted, nonviable myocardium. Such patients may be suitable candidates for cardiac transplantation.

In addition to the vascular findings of KD, clinical, electrocardiographic, and/or echocardiographic signs of myocarditis are recognizable in the acute phase of KD in a large number of patients. Pericardial effusion is documented by echocardiography in approximately 30% of patients. It is most often found during the acute phase of the disease, but there is no statistical correlation to development of coronary artery abnormalities. Myocarditis has been confirmed by gallium imaging, postmortem examination, and myocardial biopsy. The mechanism of myocarditis in KD is unknown. Additionally, the degree to which myocarditis is associated with the development of subsequent CAA is poorly characterized. Regardless of etiology, the diagnosis of myocarditis is based on clinical findings, echocardiographic evaluation, and endomyocardial biopsy sampling; the latter is considered the gold standard. Routine measurement of circulating troponin I appears not to be useful in acute KD.

The diagnosis of the cardiac involvement of KD is based on echocardiography. This method has a high sensitivity (near 100%) and specificity. However, the sensitivity decreases to 50% for distal lesions. In addition to its effectiveness, it is noninvasive, which makes it the standard screening test in KD. Occasionally, coronary artery angiography is required for the diagnosis.

In conclusion, the prevention of the coronary artery abnormalities associated with KD is important to a favorable long-term outcome following the disease. This can best be accomplished by the initiation of IVIG therapy early in the course of the febrile phase of the disease. However, in patients with aneurysmal findings, long-term cardiac follow up is required with a high index of suspicion for ischemic heart disease.

TREATMENT

The most important reason, as discussed above for the timely diagnosis and treatment of KD before day 10 of illness is to prevent cardiac sequelae. With high-dose IVIG, the incidence of CAA can be reduced from 20% to 25%, to 2% to 4%, of patients.

High-dose IVIG and aspirin constitute the cornerstone of therapy for KD. The possible mechanisms of actions of IVIG include modulation of cytokine production, neutralization of bacterial superantigens or other toxins, augmentation of T-cell suppressor activity, suppression of antibody synthesis, and provision of anti-idiotypic antibodies. Current recommendations are 2 g/kg of IVIG given over 10 to 12 hours accompanied by aspirin at 80 to 100 mg/kg/day divided every 6 hours. About 90% of patients will have a dramatic response to this treatment with cessation of fever and improvement of accompanying signs and symptoms including rash, irritability, and mucous membrane changes. Once the patient has defervesced and there is an improvement in clinical signs (3 to 5 days after resolution of fever), aspirin therapy can be reduced to 3 to 5 mg/kg given once a day. Aspirin therapy is continued at least 6 to 8 weeks when the follow-up echocardiogram is found to be normal or longer if there is evidence of coronary artery involvement.

Steroids were evaluated in the treatment of KD before IVIG was widely used. Initial reports suggested that steroids exerted a detrimental effect in KD patients. Several studies have since refuted those findings. A recent study showed that the addition of steroids to conventional IVIG and aspirin therapy resulted in shorter duration of fever and shorter hospital stay; however, there was no difference between groups in coronary outcomes. A larger controlled study is being conducted to evaluate the role of steroids in the treatment of KD.

Pentoxifyline, a TNF-α messenger RNA transcription inhibitor, has been evaluated as therapeutic adjunct to low-dose IVIG and aspirin, suggesting a beneficial effect on coronary outcome. The drug was well tolerated, but the role of pentoxifyline in KD at this time is uncertain.

Refractory KD

About 10% of patients will fail to respond to initial IVIG therapy or have recrudescence of fever 48 to 72 hours after completion of IVIG. A second dose of IVIG at 2 g/kg given over 10 to 12 hours is recommended. In rare cases, fevers and clinical symptoms continue beyond repeat therapy and these children are at higher risk of cardiac complications. If after careful evaluation, it is still believed that the patient has KD, there have been reports of refractory KD being treated with pulse steroids at 30 mg/kg for 1 to 3 days. A minor percentage of patients may fail to respond to repeated IVIG and steroid therapy. There is a report of a small number of patients who responded favorably to the monoclonal anti-TNF receptor antagonist, Infliximab. This option is currently being evaluated in a larger study. Abciximab, a platelet glycoprotein IIb/IIIa inhibitor, has been used to treat patients in the acute and subacute phase of

Evaluation of Suspected Incomplete Kawasaki Disease (KD)[1]

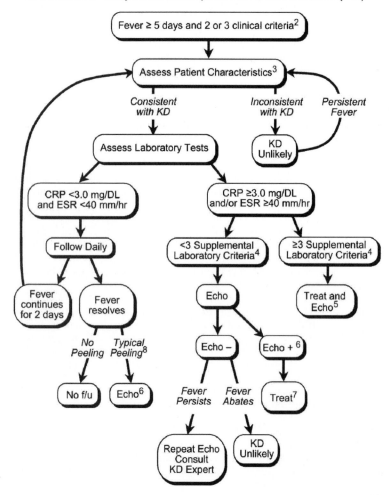

FIGURE 68.1. Evaluation of suspected incomplete Kawasaki disease. Infants ≤6 months old on day ≥7 of fever without other explanation should undergo laboratory testing and, if evidence of systemic inflammation is found, an echocardiogram, even if the infants have no clinical criteria. Supplemental laboratory criteria include albumin ≤3.0 g/dL, anemia for age, elevation of alanine aminotransferase, platelets after 7 days ≥450 000/mm³, white blood cell count ≥15 000/mm³, and urine ≥10 white blood cells/high-power field.

[5]Can treat before performing echocardiogram.
[6]Echocardiogram is considered positive for purposes of this algorithm if any of 3 conditions are met: z score of LAD or RCA ≥2.5, coronary arteries meet Japanese Ministry of Health criteria for aneurysms, or ≥3 other suggestive features exist, including perivascular brightness, lack of tapering, decreased LV function, mitral regurgitation, pericardial effusion, or z scores in LAD or RCA of 2–2.5.
[7]If the echocardiogram is positive, treatment should be given to children within 10 days of fever onset and those beyond day 10 with clinical and laboratory signs (CRP, ESR) of ongoing inflammation.
(From Newburger JW, Takahashi M, Gerber MA, et al. Diagnosis, treatment and long term management of Kawasaki disease: a statement for health profesionals from the committee on rheumatic fever, endocarditis and Kawasaki disease, council on cardiovascular disease in the young, American Heart Association. *Pediatrics* 2004;114:1708–1733.)

KD who have large aneurysms with some success in regression of aneurysm diameter, suggesting a positive effect in vascular remodeling. Other therapeutic modalities that have been evaluated in an uncontrolled manner with small numbers of patients include cyclophosphamide, plasma exchange, cyclosporin A, and unilastatin, a neutrophil-elastase inhibitor used in Japan for inflammatory conditions.

A recent consensus statement from a panel of experts developed an algorithm with criteria for the treatment of KD. It incorporates the use of clinical criteria with the timing during the acute phase of the illness. It also utilizes echocardiographic measurements of the coronaries in comparison to the population (z scores). Special emphasis is placed on the coronary arteries most likely to be affected during KD and remain normal in the population without KD (proximal right and left anterior descending coronary arteries). This algorithm should be used today for any child with prolonged fever for more than 5 days in whom KD needs to be included in the differential diagnosis (Fig. 68.1).

CARDIAC EVALUATION

Based on echocardiographic findings, patients can be stratified into risk levels according to American Heart Association (AHA) guidelines (Table 68.4). Patients should have repeat

TABLE 68.4

RISK STRATIFICATION

Risk level	Pharmacologic therapy	Physical activity	Follow-up and diagnostic testing	Invasive testing
I (no coronary artery changes at any stage of illness)	None beyond first 6–8 weeks	No restrictions beyond first 6–8 weeks	Cardiovascular risk assessment, counseling at 5-yr intervals	None recommended
II (transient coronary artery ectasia, disappears within first 6–8 weeks)	None beyond first 6–8 weeks	No restrictions beyond first 6–8 weeks	Cardiovascular risk assessment, counseling at 3- to 5-yr intervals	None recommended
III (1 small- to medium-sized coronary artery aneurysm/major coronary artery)	Low-dose aspirin (3–5 mg/kg/day), at least until aneurysm regression documented	For patients <11 yr old, no restriction beyond first 6–8 weeks; patients 11–20 yr old, physical activity guided by biennial stress test, evaluation of myocardial perfusion scan; contact or high-impact sports discouraged for patients taking antiplatelet agents	Annual cardiology follow-up with echocardiogram + ECG, combined with cardiovascular risk assessment, counseling; biennial stress test/evaluation of myocardial perfusion scan	Angiography, if noninvasive test suggests ischemia
IV (≥1 large or giant coronary artery aneurysm, or multiple or complex aneurysms in same coronary artery, without obstruction)	Long-term antiplatelet therapy and warfarin (target INR 2.0–2.5) or low-molecular-weight heparin (target: antifactor Xa level 0.5–1.0 U/mL) should be combined in giant aneurysms	Contact or high-impact sports should be avoided because of risk of bleeding; other physical activity recommendations guided by stress test/evaluation of myocardial perfusion scan outcome	Biannual follow-up with echocardiogram + ECG; annual stress test/evaluation of myocardial perfusion scan	First angiography at 6–12 mo or sooner if clinically indicated; repeated angiography if noninvasive test, or clinical or laboratory findings, suggest ischemia; elective repeat angiography under some circumstances (see text)
V (coronary artery obstruction)	Long-term low-dose aspirin; warfarin or low-molecular-weight heparin if giant aneurysm persists; consider use of β-blockers to reduce myocardial O_2 consumption	Contact or high-impact sports should be avoided because of risk of bleeding; other physical activity recommendations guided by stress test/myocardial perfusion scan outcome	Biannual follow-up with echocardiogram and ECG; annual stress test/evaluation of myocardial perfusion scan	Angiography recommended to address therapeutic options

From *Circulation* 2004:2764.

echocardiograms at 2 weeks and again at 6 to 8 weeks. Those with no coronary artery abnormalities, or transient abnormalities that resolve within the first 6 to 8 weeks, do not require further aspirin therapy, and long-term follow-up includes cardiac risk assessments every 5 years. Those with small-sized (<5 mm internal diameter) and medium-sized (5–8 mm internal diameter) aneurysms require low-dose aspirin therapy until regression of aneurysm is demonstrated as well as annual cardiology follow-up with echocardiography and ECG. Stress test and evaluation of myocardial perfusion scans are also recommended. Those with giant aneurysms (>8 mm internal diameter) require long-term anticoagulant therapy, biannual echocardiogram, ECG, and annual stress test/myocardial perfusion scans. Fusiform aneurysms less than 8 mm in internal diameter tend to have the best prognosis; the worst prognosis is associated with giant saccular aneurysms. Overall, resolution of coronary artery aneurysms is seen in approximately 50% of patients within the first 2 years following illness. Resolution with stenosis occurs in about 20% of these patients. Management of patients with CAA should be done in consultation with a cardiologist and/or hematologist.

PEARLS

- Early diagnosis and initiation of therapy are key for good long-term cardiac outcome. It is important to keep KD in the differential diagnosis of every child with prolonged fever (>5 days).
- IVIG given at the high doses for KD is thought to interfere with proper immune response to live virus vaccines. Therefore, live virus vaccines such as MMR and varicella should be deferred for 11 months following administration of IVIG.
- Children on long-term aspirin therapy are at risk for Reye syndrome; therefore it is recommended that they receive influenza vaccine yearly. If they are exposed to influenza, the patient may be switched to dypirimadole until symptoms resolve.
- Ibuprofen is thought to interfere with the antiplatelet properties of aspirin; therefore children receiving ASA should avoid concomitant administration of ibuprofen.
- Many patients with KD have discrepancies in the degree of elevation of CRP and ESR. Physicians should consider obtaining both tests when evaluating a patient for KD.

Suggested Readings

Burns JC, Shike H, Gordon JB, et al. Sequelae of Kawasaki disease in adolescents and young adults. *J Am Coll Cardiol* 1996;28:253–257.

Burns JC, Shimizu Ch, Gonzalez E, et al. Genetic variations in the receptor-ligand pair CCR5 and CCL3L1 are important determinants of susceptibility to Kawasaki disease. *JID* 2005;192:344–349.

Freeman AF, Shulman ST. Refractory Kawasaki diease. *Pediatr Infect Dis J* 2004;23:463–464.

Laupland KB, Davies HD. Epidemiology, etiology, and management of Kawasaki disease: state of the art. *Pediatr Cardiol* 1999;20:177–183.

McMaster P, Cooper S, Isaacs D. Is it Kawasaki disease? *J Paediatr Child Health* 2000;36:506–508.

McMorrow T, Tani LY, Cetta F, et al. How many echocardiograms are necessary for follow-up evaluation of patients with Kawasaki disease? *Am J Cardiol* 2001;88:328–330.

Rowley AH. Incomplete (atypical) Kawasaki disease. *J Pediatr Infect dis* 2002;21:563–565.

Stockheim JA, Innocentini N, Shulman ST. Kawasaki disease in older children and adolescents. *J Pediatr* 2000;137:250–252.

Williams RV, Wilke VM, Tani LY, et al. Does abciximab enhance regression of coronary aneurysms resulting from Kawasaki disease? *Pediatrics* 2002;109:e4.

Wright DA, Newburger JW, Baker A, et al. Treatment of immune globulin resistant Kawasaki disease with pulsed doses of corticosteroids. *J Pediatr* 1996;128:146–149.

CHAPTER 69 ■ JUVENILE IDIOPATHIC ARTHRITIS

DUNCAN M. FAGUNDUS, DALE A. NEWTON, AND MINAKSHI CHAUDHARI

In 1997, an international conference suggested a new classification scheme for juvenile rheumatoid arthritis (the Durban criteria). This included changing the name to *juvenile idiopathic arthritis* (JIA) to reflect its distinction from the rheumatoid arthritis of adults. True rheumatoid factor–positive arthritis is present in only 5% to 6% of children with chronic arthritis. JIA is by far the most common collagen vascular disease of children. Other synonyms for JIA include *juvenile chronic arthritis* and, simply, *juvenile arthritis*.

In the hospital setting, children with JIA usually present in one of three ways: the initial presentation with unexplained systemic or joint symptoms, coincidental disease in the child with chronic JIA, or complications of long-term JIA or its therapy. In the evaluation of the first scenario, often the differential is that for a child with fever without source or a child with a limp (Section III). In the latter setting, the issues may vary from antibiotic choice for the febrile child on long-term immunosuppressive therapy or with treatment-related neutropenia, to providing medical care for the child receiving corrective orthopedic surgery.

JIA is a chronic (>6 weeks) arthropathy affecting children younger than 16 years of age. The new classification divides JIA into seven categories as follows: systemic, oligoarticular, polyarticular (with subsets of positive and negative rheumatoid factor), psoriatic, enthesitis-related arthritis (spondyloarthropathy), and "other" arthritis. The latter three types are quite uncommon in the pediatric age group. Characteristics of each are discussed in following sections.

Arthritis generically is defined as joint swelling or effusion with at least two of the following: decreased range of motion, tenderness on palpation, pain with joint movement, and warmth to touch. The pattern of joint involvement and associated systemic symptoms varies between the seven types of arthritis.

Several factors including immune mechanisms and genetic and enviromental factors may be important etiologically in the development of JIA. The relative contribution of each remains unclear, in part because the role of these factors may vary between patients and types of JIA. JIA may even be a constellation of symptoms with a variety of causes. Each type should perhaps be viewed as a defined syndrome on a continuum of disease or diseases.

The development of JIA may require the combination of genetic predisposition and the appropriate "trigger." As an example of the latter, certain infectious diseases can play a role in triggering some inflammatory arthritides (e.g., arthritis following infection with *Yersinia enterocolitica* and certain other enteric pathogens). This may be related to molecular mimicry between antigens associated with the infectious organisms and host antigens. In some patients, immunologically mediated responses (T-cell and B-cell) to type II collagen or T-cell surface antigens develop. Abnormal cytokine profiles have been detected in patients with JIA. Interleukin-6 levels are increased in systemic JIA. Interleukin-1 and tumor necrosis factor alpha levels are elevated in systemic, oligoarticular, and polyarticular JIA. There is evidence that numerous other cytokines may be involved as well.

Genetic factors that may play a role in the development of JIA include human leukocyte antigen (HLA) groups. JIA subtypes have been associated with specific HLA groups or alleles: oligoarticular (HLA-A2 and -DR5, -DR6, -DR8, and -DR13, DPB1*0201), polyarticular (HLA-DR1, -DR4, -DP3) and systemic (HLA-DR4, -DR5, -DR8). JIA has a familial component with high identical twin disease concordance reported in some families. However, siblings of a child with JIA only have a mildy increased risk of developing JIA.

Even with different signs, symptoms, and genetic factors, the different types of JIA all share identical changes within the joints, resulting in synovitis. Changes within the joints include villous hypertrophy and synovial lining hyperplasia with infiltrates of lymphocytes and plasma cells. The chronic inflammatory process, if not controlled, eventually leads to destruction of articular cartilage, erosion of periarticular bone and later of pannus formation.

The age of onset of JIA can be as early as 6 months of age or as late as 16 years, but with a mean age of approximately 2 years. The incidence is approximately 1 in 10,000 children per year, resulting in a prevalence of approximately 1 in 1,000 children. There is a general trend towards a female predominance in JIA, but the actual female-to-male ratio differs according to the specific category of JIA.

CLINICAL FINDINGS

When children present with JIA, the history varies significantly according to duration of symptoms and disease type. Children usually have joint pain with associated morning stiffness and night pain. However, young children often are unable to complain about joint discomfort, so the presentation may be that of a child with a limp, refusal to walk, immobile limb, or irritability. Sometimes the presentation is as subtle as psychological regression of the child without evident reason.

Involvement of fewer than five joints is categorized as oligoarthritis, as opposed to the polyarthritis type (five or more joints). Systemic JIA has a variable number of joints involved. In addition to joint complaints (usually present), coexisting systemic symptoms sometimes are present and include fatigue, anorexia, fever, weight loss, and failure to thrive.

Uveitis usually is not clinically evident with new-onset JIA, but is most likely to develop within 5 to 7 years of onset of arthritis. This process usually is indolent and often progressive, with involvement of the iris, ciliary body, and sometimes the choroid. Uveitis usually is bilateral or becomes bilateral, and occurs most often in girls less than 6 years of age with oligoarthritis and who are often antinuclear-antibody (ANA) seropositive. Other risk factors for the development of uveitis include duration of arthritis less than 4 years and children with polyarticular JIA who are ANA seropositive. Ophthalmologic evaluation (slit lamp) and regular follow-up is necessary because of the progressive nature of uveitis and the potential for blindness (20% of affected children with uveitis). The differential diagnosis for JIA often is very extensive because of the combination of findings and usually includes trauma, infection, malignancy, and other collagen vascular diseases. (For a list of differential diagnoses for joint pain, see Chapter 20.) The considerations in the differential diagnosis often vary depending on the JIA type and associated findings (see later). Appropriate categorization of JIA type may require observation over a period of months as the pattern of a specific JIA type evolves.

Systemic

Systemic JIA (Still disease in adults) occurs in approximately 10% to 15% of all children with JIA. As the term *systemic* suggests, the non–joint-related manifestations predominate, especially at presentation. Joint symptoms may develop weeks to months after the onset of systemic symptoms. This type occurs in boys more often than the other types, resulting in an equivalent female-to-male ratio (1:1). Systemic JIA may begin during the first or second year of life, but has been reported in all age groups.

Fever usually is a prominent finding, with diagnostic criteria including daily fever for at least 2 weeks, with a documented quotidian fever pattern (sometimes with two fever spikes) for at least 3 days. Quotidian fever is notable for an afebrile baseline (without antipyretics) punctuated by temperature spikes >39°C once daily, with rapid return to baseline or below baseline. Fever spikes usually occur in the late afternoon and evening. A salmon-colored transient macular rash often accompanies the fever, and may be very evanescent. The latter characteristic makes visualization more difficult, but the rash only with fever is pathognomonic. The rash may be variable in appearance, but usually is made up of 2- to 5-mm morbilliform macules found mostly on the trunk and proximal extremities. Frequent examinations of the patient when febrile may document this rash and assist in diagnosis.

Other findings on examination may include adenopathy, hepatosplenomegaly, and findings of pericarditis (e.g., pericardial rub), pleuritis, pericardial and pleural effusions, or central nervous system involvement. Eye involvement is uncommon with systemic JIA. A variable number of joints are involved, and all joints including the cervical spine and TMJ may be affected. Laboratory abnormalities may include anemia of chronic inflammation, leukocytosis, thrombocytosis, minor elevation of liver function tests, and elevated tests for inflammation (erythrocyte sedimentation rate, C-reactive protein, and fibrinogen). An elevated serum ferritin is often found and correlates closely with systemic activity. Rheumatoid factor and ANA are rarely positive in systemic JIA.

Radiographs of appropriate joints may be helpful diagnostically and usually are necessary for long-term management. Early findings include periarticular soft-tissue swelling, juxtaarticular osteoporosis, and periosteal new bone formation. Later changes may be much more dramatic, with bony overgrowth, premature epiphyseal closure, marginal erosions, and joint space narrowing. Although a radiograph is the best initial eval-

uation in most cases, magnetic resonance imaging (MRI) is useful in detecting early articular changes secondary to arthritis.

The prognosis with systemic disease is less favorable than with other JIA types. The systemic symptoms usually are not disabling, and usually resolve over the first several years of disease. However, the joint involvement progresses in approximately 50% of affected children and can result in long-term disability. The prognosis may improve substantially with the use of newer biologic agents, including anti–tumor necrosis factor agents and autologous stem cell transplantation. Secondary amyloidosis is a long-term complication in a small number of children with systemic JIA. Secondary amyloidosis is rare in North America, but occurs in about 5% to 7% of children with chronic arthritis in certain areas of the world, including England and Europe. Death is rare with systemic JIA, but is usually associated with severe forms of the systemic type or secondary to macrophage activation syndrome or infection.

Macrophage activation syndrome (MAS) or hemophagocytic lymphohistiocytosis is a recognized complication of systemic JIA, which can be associated with significant mortality and morbidity. Typically the child becomes acutely ill with persistant fever, mental status changes, lymphadenopathy, hepatosplenomegaly, liver dysfunction, easy bruising, mucosal bleeding, and occasionally renal involvement. The laboratory findings help to distinguish between MAS and a systemic JIA flare. In MAS there is anemia, decreased leukocyte count, thrombocytopenia, low or normal ESR, elevated liver enzymes, elevated triglycerides, moderate hypoalbuminemia, prolonged PT and PTT, decreased fibrinogen levels, and presence of fibrin degradation products. In a systemic JIA flare, the leukocyte count, platelet count, and ESR are all elevated. A bone marrow aspiration will show the pathognomonic features of well-differentiated macrophages actively phagocytosing hematopoietic cells. The early administration of high-dose IV methylprednisolone dramatically improves the outcome in most patients. IV cyclosporine A is used in those cases that are refractory to IV methylprednisolone.

Oligoarthritis

This type of JIA is the most common (>50% of all children with JIA). Up to one-half of all patients have only one joint involved at presentation, most commonly the knee. Oligoarthritis is defined as involvement of one to four joints over the first 6 months of disease. This is often subdivided based on presence (~75%) or absence of ANA and the presence of uveitis (20%; more likely if ANA positive). There is a 5 to 1 female predominance. Age of onset is typically less than 5 years. Associated systemic disease is rare. Laboratory tests including complete blood count and ESR are within normal limits in the majority of patients. The associated uveitis is the major cause of morbidity, so regular eye exams screening for uveitis are recommended. There is some evidence that a moderate proportion (~40%) of children with oligoarthritis progress to polyarthritis when followed for several years.

Polyarthritis

As the term suggests, polyarthritis is defined as five or more joints involved during the first 6 months of disease. This is further subdivided into rheumatoid factor positive or negative. Polyarticular JIA occurs in about 30% of children with JIA. Age of onset is typically 1 to 3 years for children who are rheumatoid factor negative and greater than 10 years for children who are rheumatoid factor positive. Polyarticular JIA is more frequent in females. Mild to moderate systemic symptoms sometimes are present, including fever, fatigue, lymphadenopathy, and hepatosplenomegaly. Tenosynovitis and myositis sometimes complicate active polyarticular JIA.

Laboratory tests often show anemia of chronic inflammation, elevated ESR, and positive ANA (25–75%). These patients are also at a higher risk for temporomandibular joint involvement with secondary micrognathia and limited ability to open the mouth. Children with a positive rheumatoid factor are more likely to have a disease course very similar to adult-onset rheumatoid arthritis, resulting in progressive joint disease and disability in adulthood. There is a mild to moderate risk of development of uveitis, so regular eye exams screening for uveitis are recommended.

Psoriatic Arthritis

The diagnosis of psoriatic arthritis is based on the coexistence of inflammatory arthritis and evidence of psoriasis. Cutaneous findings of psoriasis need not be present at the time of diagnosis if two of the following three are present: typical nail changes consistent with psoriasis, dactylitis, or positive family history of psoriasis in a first-degree relative. Excluding factors include presence of rheumatoid factor and presence of another form of juvenile idiopathic arthritis. A positive ANA is seen in 30% to 60% of children with psoriatic arthritis. The subgroups of patients who are HLA-B27 positive or male are more likely to have sacroiliitis.

Enthesitis-Related Arthritis

This type of JIA includes children with arthritis, enthesitis, and ankylosing spondylitis. The peripheral arthritis is commonly asymmetric and predominantly affects the joint of the lower extremities. Enthesitis is caused by inflammation at the sites of attachment of ligaments, tendons, and fascia to bone. Enthesitis is most commonly noted on the knee at the insertions of the quadriceps muscles into the patella and the attachments of the patella ligament to the patella and tibial tuberosity, at the insertion of the Achilles tendon, and at sites of insertion of the plantar fascia. SEA syndrome is a term used to describe those children who are seronegative (RF and ANA negative) and have enthesitis and arthritis. These children have many of the characterisitics of juvenile ankylosing spondylitis (JAS), but lack the sacroiliac joint changes needed for a diagnosis of JAS. Some percentage of these children will go on to develop JAS. Those childen with arthritis and/or enthesitis and evidence of inflammation of the sacroiliac joints can be diagnsosed as having JAS. These children are often male and older than 8 years of age at onset. In JAS, the ANA and RF are negative and most children are HLA-B27 antigen positive. Extra-articular manifestations include uveitis, low-grade fever, and aortic insufficiency. The uveitis differs from that seen with oliquarticular and polyarticular JIA, in that it is acute and characterized by a red, painful, photophobic eye.

Other Arthritis

"Other" arthritis includes "undifferentiated" arthritis, where arthritis is present for at least 6 months but does not meet criteria for any of the aforementioned categories; and "overlap" arthritis, where criteria for more than one category are present.

MANAGEMENT

The goals of treatment are to control pain, preserve normal joint function, and promote normal growth and development. Optimal management usually is provided when care includes a multidisciplinary team. Early involvement of physical and occupational therapy for range of motion, splinting, muscle strengthening balanced with rest, and some play is necessary. The involvement of orthopedics, pediatric rehabilitation specialists, social workers, and other specialties often is needed. An important role for the hospital-based physician is to consult appropriately and coordinate the varied recommendations of this team.

If JIA findings or symptoms are limited to one or two medium to large joints such as the ankle, wrist, or knee, intra-articular injection with a corticosteroid is useful. Systemic and joint symptoms usually are significantly improved with the use of anti-inflammatory drugs. Historically, aspirin has been used, but because of the association of aspirin with Reye syndrome and the potential for gastric irritation and bleeding, aspirin therapy is now less popular and rarely used for JIA. The mainstay of therapy has now become the nonsteroidal anti-inflammatory drugs (NSAIDs) such as naproxen, meloxicam, and ibuprofen. Indomethacin is sometimes used in systemic-onset JIA and JAS. See Table 69.1 for dosing. One of these drugs often is effective as monotherapy for oligoarticular disease. Although not approved by the U.S. Food and Drug Administration for use in children, cyclooxygenase-II inhibitors (e.g., celecoxib) offer alternatives for symptomatic relief with less potential for gastrointestinal toxicity.

After the NSAIDs, the next therapeutic option usually becomes the disease-modifying antirheumatic drugs (DMARDs), including methotrexate, sulfasalazine, hydroxychloroquine, azathioprine, and pulsed cyclophosphamide. These drugs can be notably "steroid-sparing." Each of these has a spectrum of toxicities that must be carefully weighed against current disease status in a given child. Methotrexate has become the most popular second-line drug used by pediatric rheumatologists.

TABLE 69.1

NSAIDS

Use initially to control joint pain, stiffness, and swelling.

- Do not use in patients with liver or kidney dysfunction.
- Consider the concurrent use of a H_2 blocker or PPI (proton-pump inhibitor) to prevent gastric irritation.

Medication	Dosage	Maximum dosage
Naproxen (Naprosyn)	10 mg/kg/dose PO q12 hr	1000 mg PO q24 hr
Meloxicam (Mobic)	0.125 mg/kg/dose PO q24 hr	7.5 mg PO q24 hr
Ibuprofen (Advil, Motrin)	5–10 mg/kg/dose PO q6–8 hr	40 mg/kg/24 hr. Do not exceed 2,400 mg/24 hr
Indomethacin (Indocin)	1–2 mg/kg/24 hr in 2–4 divided doses	4 mg/kg/24 hr. Do not exceed 150–200 mg/24 hr

TABLE 69.2

STEROIDS

Use to control significant joint pain and swelling not controlled with NSAIDs and to control fevers and other extra-articular features (severe anemia, pericarditis, macrophage activation syndrome) associated with systemic JIA.

■ Always use concurrently with an H_2 blocker or PPI (proton-pump inhibitor) to prevent gastric irritation.

Medication	Dosage	Maximum dosage
IV methylprednisolone (Solu-medrol)	Begin with 2 mg/kg/24 hr divided q 6 hr, then slowly wean to 1 mg/kg/24 hr q 12 hr	80 mg/24 hr (may vary according to rheumatologist)
PO prednisone/ prednisolone	0.5–1 mg/kg/24 hr in 1 or 2 divided doses	60 mg/24 hr (may vary according to rheumatologist)

A new DMARD, etanercept, has been approved and has helped many previously refractory patients with polyarticular or systemic JIA. Etanercept is a genetically engineered protein that binds and inactivates tumor necrosis factor (TNF), resulting in decreased inflammation. Studies with children who have JIA have been published and show improvement in arthritis when etanercept is used alone or in combination with methotrexate. Adult studies have shown convincing evidence that etanercept retards radiographic progression of disease. Infliximab is another anti-TNF agent; although not FDA approved for children with JIA, it has been used in patients with polyarticular JIA or systemic JIA and has shown equal efficacy to etanercept for the treatment of arthritis; however, infliximab has shown increased efficacy in the treatment of uveitis. Adalimumab is a newer anti-TNF agent and studies in children are ongoing. Anakinra targets interleukin-1 and has shown benefit in patients with refractory systemic-onset JIA. Autologous stem cell transplantation has been successfully used in a limited number of children; it is usually reserved for those children with severe chronic disease refractory to all other treatments, and is associated with a 5% to 10% mortality rate.

Systemic corticosteroids should be avoided if at all possible. Children with systemic-onset JIA will usually require steroids to control symptoms, but steroids should be weaned as quickly as possible to the lowest effective dose. Short courses of oral steroids may be used intially or for acute flares in children with polyarticular JIA. Therapy usually is administered as oral prednisone. See Table 69.2 for dosing. The potential for side effects, including iatrogenic Cushing syndrome, obesity, osteoporosis, and growth delay, must be weighed carefully in the decision to use steroid therapy.

Prognosis varies according to the type of JIA and other serologic factors (see earlier). Even without systemic steroid therapy, children with severe JIA are at risk for delayed puberty, growth retardation, and severe osteopenia. Depending on the joints involved and severity, a leg length discrepancy can occur in children with asymmetric joint swelling, particularly of the knee; initially the affected leg is longer secondary to increased blood flow from inflammation to the affected leg, and later the affected leg can become shorter secondary to early fusion of epiphyses, resulting in limbs of unequal length.

All children with JIA should eventually be referred to a rheumatologist for long-term care. Hospitalized patients with significant polyarthritis or those in whom the diagnosis of systemic JIA is likely should be discussed with the local rheumatologist. Consider referral to a tertiary center where a rheumatologist is present for those cases where there is a strong suspicion of systemic JIA or polyarthritis, especially prior to starting steroids.

PEARLS

■ Early recognition of symptoms and diagnosis in combination with early aggressive therapy is key to preserving joint function and reducing morbidity from JIA.
■ Corticosteroids and some DMARDs place the patient at increased risk of infection. The lowest dose that controls the disease (and limits steroid use) is optimal.
■ Although not diagnostic, a positive ANA may be helpful in the differential diagnosis, but false-positive results frequently occur in the general population.
■ Children with polyarthritis are at risk for cervical spine involvement with atlantoaxial subluxation and apophyseal joint fusion. With cervical spine involvement, intubation for anesthesia has a high risk of cord injury.

Suggested Readings

Cassidy JT, Petty RE. *Textbook of pediatric rheumatology.* 4th ed. Philadelphia: Saunders; 2001.
Goldsmith D. Current concepts in juvenile idiopathic arthritis. *Arthritis Practioner* 2006;Jan/Feb:26–31.
Ilowite NT. Current treatment of juvenile rheumatoid arthritis. *Pediatrics* 2002;109:109–115.
Kulas DT, Schanberg L. Juvenile idiopathic arthritis. *Curr Opin Rheumatol* 2001;13:392–398.
Reiff A, et al. Long-term efficacy and safety of etanercept in children with polyarticular-course juvenile rheumatoid arthritis. *Arthritis Rheum* 2003; 48:218–226.
Dunnelly P, et al. Age-specific effects of juvenile rheumatoid arthritis-associated HLA alleles. *Arthrit Rheum* 1999;42:1843–1853.
Petty RE, Southwood TR, Baum J, et al. Revision of the proposed classification criteria for juvenile idiopathic arthritis: Durban, 1997. *J Rheumatol* 1998;25: 1991–1994.

CHAPTER 70 ■ SYSTEMIC LUPUS ERYTHEMATOSUS

SHERYL J. BOON

Systemic lupus erythematosus (SLE) is a chronic inflammatory, multiorgan disease of unknown etiology occurring in approximately 5 children per 100,000. Although less common in children than in adults, about one-fourth of all new cases present in the first 2 decades of life.

The etiology of SLE, although not fully understood, includes a complex mosaic of genetic predisposition, immune system dysregulation (including both B- and T-cell dysfunction), environmental stimuli, and hormonal factors. The genetic component is illustrated by the disease association with certain human leukocyte antigen (HLA) types, familial association (with 25% to 50% identical twin concordance), and increased prevalence in some ethnic groups (African Americans and Asians). Approximately 1 in 20 patients has a close relative with lupus. There is a marked 5:1 to 10:1 female-to-male predisposition, with the childbearing years for women showing the highest female predominance. The environmental triggers include sunlight exposure, sensitivity to certain medications (such as sulfa-containing antibiotics and ibuprofen), food sensitivity (alfalfa products), and infections.

In contrast to the causes for the disease, the pathologic mechanisms are well elucidated, SLE being the prototypic antibody-mediated autoimmune disease. Inflammation is triggered by immune complex formation and activation of the complement pathway. Most patients have many autoantibodies directed against a varied array of nuclear and cytoplasmic self-antigens. In addition, organ-specific antibodies (to skin, thyroid, blood cells, etc.) can be present. These autoantibodies are of major pathologic significance in disease activity, and provide a window for disease monitoring.

Children with SLE often receive hospital care at their initial presentation when a diagnosis is being sought, or more commonly, when the child's disease course develops severe complications (such as nephritis, pericarditis, or central nervous system involvement) or when complications of therapy occur (as in fever in a child with neutropenia from cyclophosphamide therapy). The focus of this chapter is on the myriad signs and symptoms that may be found at initial presentation or times of disease flare.

DIAGNOSTIC CRITERIA

In 1982, revised criteria for SLE were published by the American College of Rheumatology requiring that a combination of 4 of 11 clinical symptoms and laboratory criteria be met before a diagnosis of SLE is made. These criteria were modified in 1997 to include antiphospholipid antibodies within the immunoserology category (Table 70.1). Children with SLE frequently have multiple autoantibodies present, the most common being antibodies to nuclear components, including generic antinuclear antibodies (positive ANAs) and antibodies to native double-stranded (ds) DNA. The ANA test is not diagnostic because of lack of specificity, but almost all children (>98 %) with SLE have a positive test, usually in high titer and associated with a homogeneous pattern. (The immunofluorescent antibody [IFA] test is preferred over the enzyme immunoassay [EIA] test.) When evaluating the ANA test, it should be remembered that it is useful as an initial screening test but in itself does not reveal a diagnosis; it requires confirmation by other laboratory and clinical evidence of disease. Anti-dsDNA and Smith antibodies, in particular, are more specific for lupus.

Clinical diagnostic criteria include malar, discoid, or photosensitive rash; oral ulcers; arthritis; serositis; and renal, neurologic, or hematologic involvement. Because the range of clinical manifestations is varied, diagnostic criteria have been developed to assist in reaching a diagnosis based on symptom specificity and sensitivity for SLE. As the criteria suggest, multiorgan involvement with SLE is the rule, not the exception. When four (or more) criteria are positive, the sensitivity for SLE is 0.9 and specificity is 0.98. Three positive criteria are considered probable SLE. These findings can be present simultaneously or sequentially. Many clinical features of lupus are also present at times of flares of disease, but are not considered true criteria, including pathologic fatigue, fever, malaise, weight loss, arthralgia, alopecia, and Raynaud phenomenon. Although Raynaud phenomenon is commonly found in SLE, it is not a diagnostic criterion because it also has a significant presence in both the general population and in other connective tissue diseases. Low serum complement levels (C3 and C4) are seen in lupus and are useful in monitoring activity of disease, but are not specific to lupus and therefore are not useful as diagnostic criteria.

The diagnoses considered in the differential at presentation vary greatly because of the diversity of symptoms and the many organ systems that are potentially affected. SLE may cause a myriad of clinical signs, including psychosis, pericarditis, renal failure, arthritis, and cytopenias. Diseases in the differential diagnosis should include other systemic autoimmune diseases such as juvenile idiopathic arthritis; Sjögren syndrome; Henoch–Schönlein purpura; Kawasaki disease; inflammatory bowel disease; the anti-neutrophil cytoplasmic-antibody (ANCA) associated vasculitidies (Wegener granulomatosis, polyarteritis nodosa, and microscopic polyangiitis); autoimmune diseases associated with specific autoantibodies such as idiopathic thrombocytopenic purpura and Evan syndrome; postinfectious syndromes including acute poststreptococcal glomerulonephritis; acute rheumatic fever; malignancies; infections; and allergic or hypersensitivity reactions.

TABLE 70.1

CRITERIA FOR DIAGNOSIS OF SYSTEMIC LUPUS ERYTHEMATOSUS

- **Malar rash:** Erythematous fixed rash, flat or raised, over the malar area of face.
- **Discoid rash:** Erythematous raised plaques with scale and follicular plugging; may evolve into atrophic scarring with time.
- **Photosensitivity:** Skin rash secondary to sun exposure (not solar erythema); based on patient history or physician observation.
- **Oral ulcers:** Oral or nasopharyngeal mucosal ulcerations, usually painless; physician observation.
- **Arthritis:** Joint inflammation without erosions: two or more peripheral joints with tenderness, swelling, or effusion.
- **Serositis:** Including:
  Pericarditis: documented by electrocardiographic findings, rub, or pericardial effusion *or*
  Pleuritis: convincing history of pleuritic pain or documented pleural rub or pleural effusion
- **Renal disease:** Persistent proteinuria >0.5 g/day (or 4+ on dip) *or*
  Cellular casts: red blood cells, hemoglobin, granular, tubular, or mixed
- **Neurologic disease:** Seizures *or* psychosis: not secondary to drugs or metabolic derangements.
- **Hematologic disease:** Hemolytic anemia *or*
  Leukopenia (<4,000/mm^3 on at least two determinations) *or*
  Lymphopenia (<1,500/mm^3 on at least two determinations) *or*
  Thrombocytopenia (<100,000/mm^3, not secondary to medications)
- **Serologic tests:** Positive tests for any *one* of the following:
  Antiphospholipid antibody, anti-DNA antibody, anti-s antibody, or false-positive serologic test for syphilis (persisting >6 mo with negative specific test for *Treponema pallidum* (*T. pallidum* immobilization, microhemagglutination assay—*T. pallidum*, fluorescent treponemal antibody absorption assay).
- **Antinuclear antibody:** Elevated titer of antinuclear antibody by immunofluorescence or equivalent assay; absence of drug exposure known to be associated with "drug-induced lupus."

CLINICAL FINDINGS

Mucocutaneous Involvement

Cutaneous lesions are present in approximately 85% of patients with SLE. The typical malar (butterfly) rash occurs in approximately 50% of patients. It is symmetric, located over the malar eminences and the bridge of the nose, with sparing of the nasolabial folds. Rash may also occur over the forehead or the ears. The rash is vasculitic in nature, involving the epidermis, and generally is well demarcated, slightly raised, and erythematous to violaceous in color. Scarring rarely occurs (Fig. 70.1). In contrast, the discoid lupus rash (which is uncommon in children) is deeper, involving the dermis, and is not symmetrical. Discoid lupus lesions may occur on the face and the scalp, as well other areas, and may lead to atrophy and scarring with hyperpigmentation.

Vasculitic rashes (similar to those seen in HSP) can also be widely distributed over the trunk and/or extremities in patients with active SLE. Photosensitive rashes are frequently maculopapular and may occur anywhere in sun-exposed areas. Mucous membrane lesions, often on the hard palate, are associated with active disease and are usually painless, so the patient may not report any oral lesions (Fig. 70.2). Patients with coagulation disorders due to antiphospholipid antibodies may have livedo reticularis, a nonpalpable, mottled, reticular, or lacy discoloration usually seen in the extremities. Bullous or blistering lesions, erythema nodosum, or urticarial rashes can also be seen in patients with active SLE. Nailfold capillaries may become dilated and tortuous, indicating active vasculitis. Patients with severe Raynaud phenomenon may have cyanosis and digital tip ulcerations or necrosis secondary to ischemia.

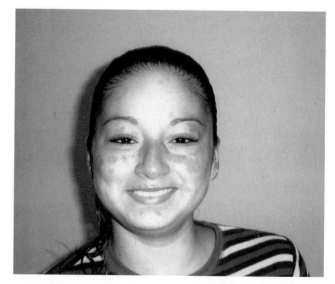

FIGURE 70.1. Classic malar rash with nasolabial sparing seen in a patient with active SLE.

Musculoskeletal Disease

Arthralgias and arthritis are frequent clinical symptoms at presentation. The arthritis in SLE is non-erosive (in contrast to that seen in juvenile rheumatoid arthritis) and often polyarticular and migratory, with pain out of proportion to the physical findings. It tends to involve the joints of the hands, wrists, and knees. The arthritis generally improves once systemic

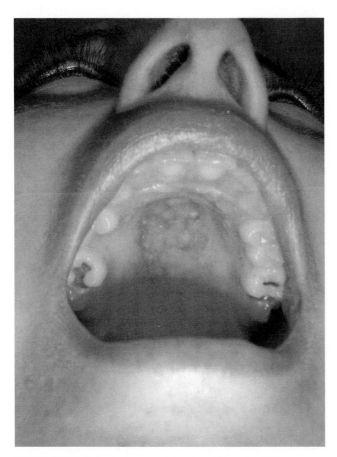

FIGURE 70.2. Palatal ulcer seen in patient with active SLE.

treatment for lupus is initiated. Myositis is also seen in active lupus and may resemble the myositis of dermatomyositis, being associated with active vasculitis and proximal muscle weakness. Serum muscle enzymes (creatine phosphokinase, aldolase, aspartate aminotransferase, and alanine aminotransferase) are elevated. Steroid myopathy can occur after prolonged therapy with steroids, and needs to be distinguished from the myositis associated with active disease. Avascular necrosis (usually of the femoral head) and osteopenia are other steroid-induced musculoskeletal manifestations that can be seen in SLE.

Serositis and Pulmonary and Cardiovascular Disease

Pleural, pericardial, and peritoneal effusions are all seen in active lupus and may be evident upon initial presentation. Other pulmonary features include pneumonitis, alveolar hemorrhage, pulmonary fibrosis with pulmonary hypertension, conduction defects (in neonatal lupus), and respiratory muscle weakness. Pulmonary function testing often demonstrates functional impairments in ventilatory capacity, and may show decreased diffusion of carbon monoxide (DLCO). Echocardiography (ECHO) is important in monitoring for elevated pulmonary pressures that may require stress testing to demonstrate. SLE may also involve the myocardium, the endocardium (Libman–Sacks endocarditis), and the coronary vessels; therefore an ECHO is indicated in patients with active lupus and any signs or symptoms of cardiovascular or pulmonary disease. Coronary artery disease may be present and due in part to lipid abnormalities and chronic corticosteroid use. Hypertension is a frequent finding in lupus and

may be secondary to cardiovascular and/or renal disease, or a result of treatment with steroids.

Renal Disease

Renal involvement is one of the most serious complications of SLE and affects up to 50% of patients at initial diagnosis to some degree. Children with SLE may have more severe and rapidly progressive renal disease than adults. In both children and adults, males have more severe disease with more complications. Acute lupus nephritis needs to be treated aggressively to prevent irreversible renal failure. Evaluation by a pediatric nephrologist is advised in any patient with renal involvement, with renal biopsy in patients who have normal bleeding studies and normal renal anatomy. The World Health Organization (WHO) classification of lupus nephritis includes an index of activity and chronicity to determine the optimal treatment. Class I denotes no detectable disease. Class II (mesangial proliferation) is present to some extent in many patients with SLE. In patients who present with renal disease and proteinuria or hematuria, the most common WHO classes are III (focal/segmental proliferative) and IV (diffuse proliferative) glomerulonephritis. In class III, focal segments of glomeruli are affected, with less than 50% of the total glomeruli involved. In class IV, the glomerular involvement is more extensive, with greater than 50% of the glomeruli affected. Class IV disease dictates aggressive treatment with steroids and immunosuppressants, usually including monthly pulsed intravenous cyclophosphamide (Cytoxan) for a minimum of 6 months, although many other regimens are being studied and may prove as effective as this one, which has established itself in the literature. Patients who present with nephrotic syndrome may have class V (membranous) glomerulonephritis, which can often be treated with steroids alone, without the use of cyclophosphamide. Class VI (sclerotic) indicates end-stage scarring and fibrosis in the kidney, and is therefore not likely to be improved with aggressive immunosuppression.

Gastrointestinal Disease

Hepatosplenomegaly develops in almost one-half of pediatric patients with SLE. Patients are also at risk for mesenteric vasculitis or thrombosis and acute pancreatitis, with potentially devastating sequelae. Abdominal pain with intestinal vasculitis can be a presenting symptom (much like HSP) or can occur with flares of disease. It is usually responsive to intravenous steroid administration. Anorexia and weight loss are frequent complaints at the time of diagnosis, but can also be associated with immunosuppressive treatment. Steroid treatment tends to have the opposite effect on appetite and frequently causes weight gain in patients who, because of their disease, may be less active.

Neurologic Disorders

Central nervous system (CNS) disease ranks second only to nephritis as a cause of morbidity and mortality in childhood SLE. It reportedly occurs in 20% to 30% of patients, although the extent is probably much greater if subtle cognitive dysfunction is included. Psychosis and seizures are the principal severe manifestations. Severe headaches occur in many children, and require a workup to differentiate migraine headaches from vasculitis or other treatable causes, such as hypertension. Patients may also manifest difficulty concentrating, poor school performance, depression, anxiety, or pain amplification. Thromboembolic disease may be seen in patients with antiphospholipid antibody-mediated hypercoagulation disorder or be secondary to treatments (steroid-induced hyperlipidemia). Peripheral neuropathy is reported in approximately

15% of patients. Eye involvement can occur and be associated with iritis, episcleritis, or retinal vascular changes (cytoid bodies). Lumbar puncture, CT, MRA, MRI, and PET scans are all useful in the evaluation of patients.

Hematologic Disorders

Many patients with lupus will initially present with anemia, thrombocytopenia, neutropenia, or pancytopenia. Thorough evaluation to rule out malignancy is necessary to avoid inappropriate treatment with steroids. Workup of anemia should include a complete blood count with manual smear, reticulocyte count, iron studies, and Coombs testing. Erythropoietin may be indicated in patients with anemia due to chronic renal failure. Autoimmune thrombocytopenia occurs in children with lupus due to antiplatelet antibodies. Steroids are usually helpful, although they may be required in high doses to correct thrombocytopenia. Intravenous immunoglobulin is also useful in treating isolated thrombocytopenia. Leukopenia (white blood cell count <4,500/mm^3) occurs both as part of SLE and as a side effect of treatment with immunosuppressants. Lymphopenia (lymphocyte count <1,500/mm^3) in particular occurs with therapy. Moderate or severe autoimmune neutropenia (absolute neutrophil count <1,000/mm^3) requires cautious treatment with immunosuppressants due to the risk of severe life-threatening infections in these patients.

Endocrine Disorders

Autoimmune thyroid disease is frequently present at some time during the disease course, and should be screened for at the time of diagnosis with thyroid hormone and thyroid-stimulating hormone (TSH) levels. Testing should include antithyroid antibody testing (including antithyroglobulin and antithyroperoxidase antibodies) if abnormal hormone levels are found. Less frequently hyperthyroidism is present, due to anti-TSH receptor antibodies. Additionally, in active lupus, there may be abnormalities in the sex hormones, and adolescent girls may report menstrual irregularities, which often persist until the lupus is well controlled. Antibodies to platelets and clotting factors can cause prolonged menstrual bleeding. Hormonal birth control may be contraindicated in some patients due to an increased coagulation risk, and should be discussed with the rheumatologist. Cortisol levels are suppressed in any patient who is on steroid therapy, so stress dosing of steroids is recommended for any patient on steroid therapy who is undergoing surgery.

MANAGEMENT

The treatment of SLE should be tailored to the individual patient. Rheumatologic consultation is almost always necessary for appropriate medical care, along with other pediatric subspecialists as indicated by the organ systems involved in a particular patient. This usually should be extended to a team approach, often including ancillary services such as physical and occupational therapy, nutrition, social work, and psychology. The therapy also has to be comprehensive and include attention not only to the medical issues, but to nutrition, exercise, and psychological well-being. Because many of these children are struggling simultaneously with adjustment to adolescence, attention to psychological support is necessary to achieve compliance and, ultimately, a good outcome.

Specific choice of medical therapy is optimally under the direction of a pediatric rheumatologist. For mild disease, nonsteroidal anti-inflammatory drugs or antimalarial drugs usually are sufficient. Hydroxychloroquine (Plaquenil) is the most commonly used antimalarial. The antimalarials have two known mechanisms to modulate immune function: they raise intracellular pH, which interferes with phagocytic function and subsequent antigen processing, and they inhibit platelet function (1). All patients receiving antimalarials require regular eye examinations by an ophthalmologist to monitor for retinal toxicity. Low-dose oral steroid therapy is commonly used for maintenance therapy between flares of disease to control symptoms. Topical steroid therapy also can help with the associated skin rashes. Steroid therapy often includes antacid therapy in some form, including calcium carbonate, histamine blockers, or proton-pump inhibitors. Because of the risk of osteopenia, regular exercise and supplements of calcium and vitamin D are recommended.

For moderate disease, steroids are used, but doses should be kept at the lowest dosage possible to minimize potential side effects, including growth retardation in children. For that reason, rheumatologists use azathioprine or methotrexate as "steroid-sparing" agents to allow tapering of the steroid dose.

For severe disease, higher dose oral and intravenous steroids and/or pulse intravenous steroids are used in combination with immunosuppressive medications, including intravenous or oral cyclophosphamide, oral mycophenolate mofetil, and oral azathioprine. The regimen of monthly intravenous infusions of cyclophosphamide (from 500 to 1000 mg/m^2) is used for class IV renal involvement and in severe CNS lupus, or other life-threatening manifestations of disease. This regimen often results in remarkable reductions in necessary steroid therapy and associated side effects, but carries its own set of risks, including significant immunosuppression and severe infections, bladder toxicity, and long-term risks of infertility and lymphoma. Newer therapies under evaluation by the NIH include use of the biologic agent Rituximab, an anti-CD-20 monoclonal antibody used in B-cell lymphoma to decrease the population of B-lymphocytes responsible for pathologic autoantibody production. All of these therapies can increase the risk of serious infection, a leading cause of morbidity and mortality in patients with lupus.

COURSE AND PROGNOSIS

The course of pediatric SLE is quite variable, with long-term remissions sometimes occurring. Most children, however, continue to have active disease requiring therapy for management of symptoms and prevention of complications. Most bad outcomes in children with SLE are related to issues of compliance, CNS involvement, infections related to the disease or the therapy (neutropenia), or progressive renal disease (especially diffuse proliferative glomerulonephritis). Less common conditions that can result in poor outcomes include pulmonary hemorrhage or hypertension, gastrointestinal bleeding, and malignant hypertension.

In the current era of therapy with immunosuppressive drugs, long-term survival of children with SLE has improved, but good data must await longer periods of follow-up because these aggressive interventions are relatively recent.

Two special situations in pediatric SLE deserve mention, neonatal lupus and drug-induced lupus. Infants born to mothers with active lupus are at risk for neonatal lupus syndrome. This risk is related to the second-trimester transplacental passage of maternal antibodies against SSA/Ro and SSB/La. Neonatal lupus syndrome may include transient development of malar rash (discoid or annular), mild hemolytic anemia, leukopenia, or thrombocytopenia (Fig. 70.3). Rarely is steroid therapy necessary, and the findings usually resolve without complication. Congenital heart block (both complete and incomplete) can occur in utero, and can be associated with severe fetal bradycardia. Surviving infants may require permanent pacemaker placement. Knowledge of Sjögren antibodies

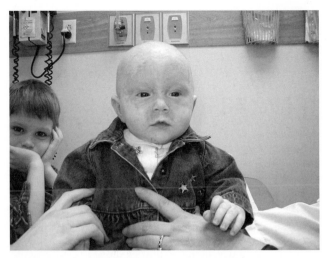

FIGURE 70.3. Young patient with cutaneous rash of neonatal lupus erythematosus.

in the mother during the pregnancy can allow fetal heart monitoring and treatment of the mother for prevention of permanent heart block in the infant.

Drug-induced lupus occurs infrequently in children on long-term drug treatment for other conditions, and symptoms tend to be milder than with SLE. A partial list of implicated drugs includes anticonvulsants, hydralazine, isoniazid, penicillins, minocycline, and sulfa-based medications. With these medications, the ANA also may be positive without clinical disease. In those with clinical findings, the features most often present include fever, rash, arthritis, pleuritis, and pericarditis. Renal and CNS involvement is quite uncommon. ANA tests may be positive with specific antihistone antibodies present. Complement levels usually remain normal. The prognosis usually is excellent, with resolution after symptomatic therapy and withdrawal from the offending medication.

PEARLS

- Children with unexplained hemolytic anemia, neutropenia, or thrombocytopenic purpura should have SLE considered in their differential diagnosis.
- Children with atypical HSP—prolonged, severe (with kidney involvement), or outside of the typical HSP age range—should have lupus and other autoimmune vasculitidies included in their differential diagnosis.
- Most lupus nephritis declares itself in the first 2 years of clinical disease. Tests of renal function may not detect mild to moderate renal involvement. Patients need to be screened for proteinuria, hematuria, and urinary casts and monitored by a rheumatologist or a nephrologist for indications for biopsy. Active nephritis is often predicted by elevated anti-dsDNA antibodies and/or hypocomplementemia.
- Thyroid function should be monitored in patients with active lupus.

Suggested Readings

Arkachaisri T. Systemic lupus erythematosus and related disorders of childhood. *Curr Opin Rheumatol* 1999;11:384–392.

Cassidy JT, Petty RE. *Textbook of pediatric rheumatology.* 5th ed. Philadelphia: Saunders; 2005.

Tan EM, Cohen AS, Fries JF, et al. The 1982 revised criteria for the classification of SLE. *Arthritis Rheum* 1982;25:1271–1277.

Wallace DJ, Hahn B. *Dupois' lupus erythematosus.* 6th ed. Philadelphia: Lippincott Williams & Wilkins; 2001.

JASJIT SINGH AND ANTONIO ARRIETA

Group A β-hemolytic *Streptococcus* (GABHS) was established as the sole etiologic agent of acute rheumatic fever (ARF) in the first half of the 20th century. The result of an autoimmune response to infection with GABHS, ARF and its chronic sequela, rheumatic heart disease (RHD), became rare in most affluent populations, but remains unabated in developing countries and in poor, mostly indigenous populations of wealthy nations. Understanding the pathogenesis of the disease; the impact of variations in virulence of diverse GABHS strains; and its interactions with susceptible hosts, which will eventually result in the acute symptoms of ARF and subsequent cardiac sequelae; will ultimately help us identify the targets for control and possible eradication of this age-old disease.

The role of vaccines in the prevention of ARF is an evolving process. In the meantime, reevaluation of traditional views is necessary, including revision of diagnostic criteria to make them applicable for populations at different risks for ARF, and developing more realistic treatment strategies focusing not only on the management of ARF but also on the development of programs for primary and secondary prophylaxis.

EPIDEMIOLOGY

Although the acute illness causes considerable morbidity and some mortality, the major clinical and public health impact arises from the long-term damage to heart valves, primarily mitral and aortic, known as RHD. Over the past century, improvement in living conditions and hygiene and, to a lesser degree, access to medical care and the introduction of antibiotics, have substantially decreased the incidence of ARF and RHD in industrialized nations. This process has not been matched in poor areas of the world. According to the WHO, as of 2004 at least 15.6 million people had RHD; 300,000 of about 0.5 million individuals who acquire ARF will develop RHD every year. In excess of 200,000 deaths are attributable to ARF or RHD. The incidence of ARF in some developing countries exceeds 50 per 100,000 children. It reaches 80 to 100 per 100,000 in Pacific Islander children in New Zealand and may reach as high as 500 per 100,000 in parts of Australia, among the Aborigine population. In contrast, the nonindigenous children of New Zealand have a rate similar to that reported in the United States in the 1960s of 10 per 100,000. Outbreaks in the intermountain region of the United States since the late 1980s have been associated with a particular mucoid strain of GABHS, M type 18.

ARF is rare in children less than 5 years old and almost unheard of in those less than 2 years of age. When it occurs, it is more likely to present as arthritis, erythema marginatum is more frequent, and carditis, when present, is moderate to severe; chorea is very rare. The first episode of ARF is most common in adolescence; incidence wanes by the end of the second decade and is rare after 35 years of age.

Recurrences are common in adolescence and early adulthood. Several studies in the United States as well as in Australian Aborigines and developing countries show a trend whereby the incidence of ARF peaks in childhood and adolescence, but the prevalence of RHD peaks in adulthood (Fig. 71.1).

PATHOGENESIS

The actual pathogenesis of ARF and RHD remains hypothetical. It was not until after the first half of the 20th century that it was established that pharyngeal infection with GABHS causes all of the manifestations of ARF, recurrent attacks, and RHD; yet not all strains of GABHS do so. Over the last few decades, it became clear that the great majority of throat infections due to GABHS do not cause ARF at all, but rather that it is caused by some unusually virulent strains. The attack rate varies with the intensity of the host response, which in turn is related to the virulence of the infecting strain.

Virulence Factors

Rebecca Lancefield and others demonstrated more than 50 years ago a marked variation in the virulence of GABHS by the content of M-protein in the cell wall, and by the degree of hyaluronate encapsulation.

M-Protein

An antiphagocytic surface constituent, M-protein protects GABHS against phagocytosis and killing by polymorphonuclear leukocytes. The M-protein is composed of two polypeptide chains, complexed in a coiled-coil configuration. The C-terminal is located within the cell membrane and is highly conserved. The N-terminal, together with the adjacent A region, constitutes the hypervariable region, which allows for the Lancefield serologic classification (Fig. 71.2). The gene (*emm*) that codes for the M-protein has been identified and allowed for organisms to be classified in one of five groups with different tissue tropisms.

Capsule

The GABHS capsule is composed of hyaluronic acid, which consists of alternating residues of N-acetyl glucosamine and glucuronic acid. Streptococcal strains vary greatly in their degree of encapsulation, and those with the most exuberant capsule production have a mucoid appearance when cultured in blood agar plates. GABHS strains rich in capsule and M-protein are extremely virulent in humans. The emergence of such strains has been thought of as a predictor of outbreaks of ARF.

Other virulent factors of GABHS are responsible for adhering, colonization, and internalization. Extracellular products

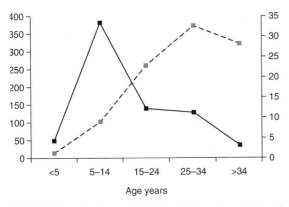

FIGURE 71.1. Incidence of ARF in 2002 and prevalence of RHD in 2003 by age in Aboriginal Australians from the top end of the Northern Territory (personal communication, Top End RHD Control Program, Department of Health and Community Services, Darwin, Australia). (From Lancet 2005; 366:156.)

such are streptolysin O and S and pyrogenic exotoxins contribute to its virulence.

Complex interactions among the different virulent factors determine the potential rheumatogenicity of particular GABHS strains. Based on the C-repeat regions of the M-protein, GABHS could fall into two different molecular classes. Class I molecules are characteristically throat strains; they do not bind fibronectin and do not produce serum opacity factor (SOF-negative). By contrast, class II binds fibronectin and is SOF-positive. They contain a much smaller M-protein and are associated with a streptococcal pyoderma and positive streptococcal glomerulonephritis. Indeed, an M-antigen, so far unidentified, has been detected in rheumatic strains, and antibodies to this antigen have been found in blood of patients with ARF.

As discussed above, the *emm* and *emm*-like genes for M-protein and other associated proteins allow for GABHS to be classified into five groups. Groups A through C are associated with throat infections and ARF, group D with skin infections, and group E with infections at either site. Although largely accepted, the notion of ARF resulting only from throat infections has been recently challenged. The low frequency of the so-called throat strains, by either classification, among children in areas of the world with a high incidence of ARF where streptococcal skin infection is present in the vast majority of children at any given time, has raised questions about the universal validity of this concept.

Host

Host factors are obviously important in the pathogenesis of ARF. Most attention has been focused in the concept of autoimmunity, or more precisely, molecular mimicry. There are several examples of antigen similarity between somatic constituents of GABHS and human tissues, including synovium, heart, and neurons of the basal ganglia of the brain. The repeated GABHS infections during childhood, with different virulent factors among and within strains and infections, may break immune tolerance in susceptible host and account for the variety of cross-reactive antibodies found in synovia, skin, basal ganglia, heart valves, and other tissues. Immune complexes may produce the nondestructive synovitis of the joints of patients with ARF and the reversible reactions on the basal ganglia observed in patients with Sydenham chorea, whereas autoimmune cell-mediated cytotoxic reactions may destroy heart valves

In the 19th century, familial clustering suggested that susceptibility to ARF and RHD was inherited. Use of molecular techniques has lead to identification of associations between

disease and HLA class II alleles; the particular alleles associated with susceptibility or protection differ by populations. Renewed interest in genetic susceptibility has been spurred by the identification of specific B-cell alloantigens, unrelated to MHC, associated with susceptibility to ARF and RHD. Murine monoclonal antibodies against B-cells elicited one (*D8/17*) that reacted with increased numbers of B-cells in all patients with ARF or RHD of different ethnic origins, but only in 10% of healthy individuals.

Clinical Manifestations

In 1944, T. Duckett Jones proposed criteria to aid in the diagnosis of ARF. These have been modified, revised, and then updated by an American Heart Association panel. These revisions increased the specificity, but decreased the sensitivity, of

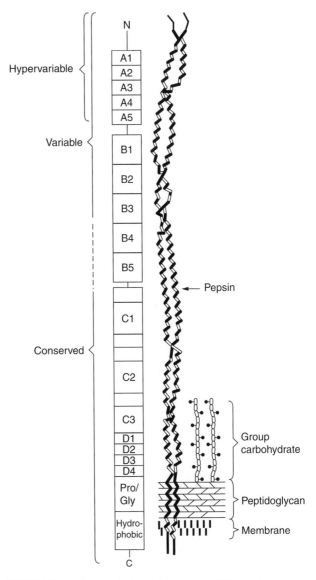

FIGURE 71.2. Characteristics of the complete M6 protein sequence. Blocks A, B, C, and D designate the location of the sequence repeat blocks. Numbers above the block indicate the number of amino acids per block. Shaded blocks indicate those to which the sequence diverges from the central consensus sequence. *Pro/Gly* denotes the protein-rich and glycine-rich region Maly located in the peptidoglycan. *Pepsin* identifies the position of the pepsin-sensitive site after aminoacid 228. The C-terminal end is located within the cell wall and membrane. (Reprinted with permission from *Lancet Infect Dis* 2003;3:192.)

TABLE 71.1

JONES CRITERIA FOR DIAGNOSIS OF FIRST ATTACK OF RHEUMATIC FEVER

REQUIREMENTS FOR DIAGNOSIS
1. Two major criteria

   Or

2. One major plus two minor criteria

   Plus

   Supporting evidence of antecedent GABHS infection
   a. Positive throat culture
   b. Positive rapid antigen test

   Or

   b. Elevated or rising streptococcal antibody titer

MAJOR CRITERIA	MINOR CRITERIA
Carditis	Previous rheumatic fever
Arthritis	Arthralgia
Chorea	Fever
Erythema marginatum	Elevated erythrocyte
Subcutaneous nodules	sedimentation rate
	Elevated leukocyte count
	Prolonged PR interval
	C-reactive protein

diagnosis, in response to the declining incidence of ARF in developed countries. These criteria (Table 71.1) are now used to aid in the diagnosis of an initial attack of ARF. The diagnosis can be established when a patient meets two major or one major and two minor manifestations, plus evidence of antecedent GABHS infection.

For the diagnosis of recurrent attacks of ARF in patients with underlying RHD, other less stringent criteria (such as the 2002–2003 WHO guidelines) might be more appropriate. ARF typically develops 2 to 4 weeks following streptococcal pharyngiitis, after the acute infection has resolved. However, one-third of patients are unable to provide a history of antecedent pharyngitis.

Migratory Polyarthritis

Approximately three-fourths of patients with ARF will present with arthritis. This will usually involve large joints, particularly the knees, ankles, wrists, and elbows. Involvement of the small joints (more typical of post-streptococcal reactive arthritis), spine, or hips, is uncommon. The affected joints are red, hot, swollen, and exquisitely tender. Arthritis can be migratory or additive. Joint fluid analysis demonstrates 10,000–100,000 white blood cells/mm³ with neutrophil predominance and normal glucose. Protein is typically about 4 g/dL, and the fluid demonstrates good mucin clot formation. The arthritis classically responds dramatically to salicylates, a feature clinically used to support the diagnosis. There are no long-term joint sequellae. There appears to be an inverse relationship between the severity of joint and cardiac involvement.

Carditis

Overall, carditis is seen in 50% to 60% of cases of ARF. Severity ranges from mild transient cardiac involvement to fulminant disease. Pancarditis is the hallmark of rheumatic carditis, with inflammation involving the pericardium, myocardium, and endocardium. Endocarditis, or valvulitis, is a universal finding, and is manifest by one or more cardiac murmurs noted on physical examination. In the vast majority of cases, mitral valve alone or mitral valve with aortic valve disease is seen. Valvular insufficiency is characteristic of acute disease, with mitral regurgitation noted as a high-pitched apical holosystolic murmur, radiating to the axilla, and aortic insufficiency characterized by a high-pitched decrescendo murmur at the upper left sternal border. Valvular stenosis develops over years to decades later. Myocarditis, pericarditis, or both, without evidence of endocarditis, is rarely due to ARF. Along with valvular disease, however, they can manifest as tachycardia, rhythm disturbances, cardiomegaly, congestive heart failure, or cardiac tamponade. The carditis of ARF, along with resulting RHD, is the most serious manifestation of illness, accounting for the majority of morbidity and mortality associated with ARF. Patients with carditis during their initial presentation are at high risk for development of carditis during subsequent attacks of ARF. Chronic progressive valvular disease, particularly stenosis, may ultimately require valve replacement. Valvular disease is also a risk factor for infective endocarditis. Electrocardiography in patients with carditis includes prolongation of the PR and QT intervals. ST segment and T-wave changes of myocarditis or pericarditis may be seen. Use of echocardiography for diagnosis of ARF is controversial, particularly if no audible murmur is present. Such subclinical carditis (valvular damage detected only by echocardiography) does not satisfy the Jones criteria for carditis. However, echocardiography may be useful to support the diagnosis in equivocal situations, assess function, establish the presence of pericardial fluid, and exclude flow murmurs and congenital heart disease.

Chorea

Sydenham chorea is a late manifestation of ARF, occurring several months after streptococcal infection. This is in contrast to the other major manifestations of ARF, which emerge 1 to 3 weeks after GABHS pharyngitis. The principal feature of chorea is involuntary movements that are irregular, rapid, flowing, nonstereotyped, and random. Motor impersistence, such as the "milkmaid's grasp," is a common feature. Mild chorea may be interpreted as restlessness or poor penmanship. Weakness and hypotonia are common, as are psychological symptoms. Emotional lability, obsessions, and compulsions may all be seen.

Sydenham chorea generally lasts 2 to 4 months with a range of 1 week to as long as 3 years. The neurologic symptoms wane in severity and completely resolve in most cases. The highest incidence is in young teenage girls.

Subcutaneous Nodules

Subcutaneous nodules occur on the extensor surface and bony prominences of the extremities, scapula, and mastoid processes. They are rarely seen, but when present, indicate severe carditis. Histopathologically, these are collections of Aschoff bodies.

Erythema Marginatum

Erythema marginatum initially appears as an area of erythema with central clearing as the margins progress. It is usually found on the trunk and proximal extremities.

Diagnosis

As mentioned above, the Jones criteria are used for diagnosis of ARF. Evidence of antecedent GABHS infection is necessary for the diagnosis of ARF. Because ARF is a post-infectious process, clinical signs of pharyngitis are often absent. Throat culture or rapid streptococcal test is positive in only 10% to 20% of cases. Supportive evidence is usually in the form of elevated or rising anti-streptococcal antibodies. These antibodies include anti-streptolysin-O (ASO), anti-deoxyribonuclease B (anti-DNAse B), anti-hyaluronidase, and anti-streptokinase. Because 80% to 85% of patients with ARF will have elevated titers if only a single antibody is measured (usually ASO), therefore some experts recommend measurement of multiple anti-streptococcal antibodies (ASO, anti-DNAse B, anti-hyaluronidase) when ARF is suspected clinically, with improved sensitivity to 95% to 100%. In most patients with ARF, symptoms correlate with peak antibody responses, the exception being patients with chorea alone.

Differential diagnosis includes other causes of fever and carditis or fever and arthritis such as autoimmune diseases (systemic lupus erythematosus, juvenile rheumatoid arthritis), infectious arthritis, serum sickness, reactive arthritis, infective endocarditis, and Kawasaki disease.

Treatment

Treatment of an ARF episode includes anti-streptococcal therapy (regardless of culture results), anti-inflammatory therapy, and if needed, cardiac medications and medications to control involuntary movements of chorea (Table 71.2). Prolonged bed rest after the acute stage of illness is not needed.

Secondary Prophylaxis

Secondary prophylaxis is aimed at preventing further episodes of streptococcal pharyngitis and hence prevention of recurrence of ARF. The risk of recurrence is highest in the first 5 years following primary ARF. For patients who are unable to tolerate either penicillin or sulfa drugs, erythromycin is recommended. Cephalosporins are felt to be likely effective as well (Table 71.2). Duration of prophylaxis is controversial. The American Heart Association (AHA) recommends lifetime prophylaxis for those with RHD. Some experts discontinue prophylaxis in those without cardiac involvement at age 21 years, or 5 years after the last attack of ARF, whichever is later. Patients with RHD require prophylaxis against IE. Complicating the assessment of newer treatments of ARF is the fact that rheumatic carditis often improves over time in the absence of recurrences. A placebo-controlled, randomized trial did not show that IV immunoglobulin (IVIG) for early ARF altered the clinical course or reduced echocardiographic evidence of acute valvular disease, or chronic cardiac damage at 1 year. A small study has suggested that IVIG might hasten recovery from chorea.

Primary Prophylaxis

Primary prevention of ARF has focused on antibiotic treatment of symptomatic GABHS pharyngitis. It has been established for some time that if antibiotics are initiated within 9 days of onset of sore throat due to GABHS, ARF can be prevented. However, up to two-thirds of patients with ARF do not have sore throat symptoms and do not seek medical attention.

TABLE 71.2

TREATMENT OF RHEUMATIC FEVER

Acute rheumatic fever

ANTISTREPTOCOCCAL THERAPY
1.2 million units of benzathine penicillin G IM (600,000 units for those <60 lb)

Or

Oral penicillin or erythromycin for 10 days

ANTI-INFLAMMATORY THERAPY
Mild or no carditis
    Aspirin 50–100 mg/kg/day in four doses for 2–4 weeks, then taper over 4 weeks
Moderate or severe carditis
    Prednisone 2 mg/kg/day in two doses for 2–4 weeks, then taper with addition of aspirin

CARDIAC MEDICATIONS (IF NEEDED)
Diuretics
Cautious use of digoxin

MEDICATIONS TO CONTROL CHOREA (IF NEEDED)
Phenobarbital

Or

Haloperidol

Secondary prophylaxis

RHEUMATIC FEVER PROPHYLAXIS (FOR ALL PATIENTS)
1.2 million units of benzathine penicillin IM monthly (0.6 million units if <60 lb)

Or

Penicillin V 250 mg PO bid

Or

Sulfadiazine 500 mg PO bid (1/2 dose if <60 lb)

Vaccines

In view of these limitations, several potential GABHS vaccines are in various stages of development. A multivalent, M-serotype specific vaccine is in phase 2 trials in North America. However, regional diversity of M-serotypes and *emm* genotypes may limit applicability of this vaccine. Alternative vaccines based on antigens common to most strains of GABHS, such as conserved regions of M-protein, or non-M protein antigens, are under development. It does not appear that a vaccine will be available for widespread use in the next few years.

CHAPTER 72A ■ UNUSUAL RHEUMATOLOGIC DISEASES: DERMATOMYOSITIS AND POLYMYOSITIS

SHERYL J. BOON

Section XI (Vasculitis/Rheumatology) of this book includes five diseases encountered by the pediatric care provider in the hospital setting: Henoch–Schönlein purpura (HSP), Kawasaki disease (KD), acute rheumatic fever (ARF), juvenile idiopathic arthritis (JIA), and systemic lupus erythematosus (SLE). In the past, ARF was the most common of these diseases, but now rarely is seen except in Utah and western Europe, due to changes in the circulating strains of group A beta-hemolytic streptococci. HSP and KD are by far the most common self-limited vasculitidies seen in the pediatric age range, with JIA and SLE being the most common chronic rheumatologic conditions in this age group. All of these diseases are addressed in separate chapters of this book.

In addition to the above diseases, children can present with a host of other autoimmune/vasculitic rheumatologic conditions that can pose a diagnostic dilemma to the pediatric hospitalist. Among these are dermatomyositis, scleroderma, mixed connective tissue disease, Sjögren syndrome, sarcoidosis, Takayasu arteritis, polyarteritis nodosa, Wegener granulomatosis, Churg–Strauss syndrome, microscopic polyangiitis, and Goodpasture syndrome. These diseases are considered here due to their autoimmune nature, along with their typically complex systemic presentation. Although each has specific findings, there is considerable overlap in the criteria for many of these inflammatory conditions. This mandates their inclusion in the differential diagnosis of most rheumatologic diseases and many infectious and oncologic diseases. Due to their low prevalence, chronicity, and specific treatments, they require management by a rheumatologist for long-term care.

DERMATOMYOSITIS

Dermatomyositis and polymyositis share clinical and laboratory findings including muscle edema with elevated muscle enzymes, weakness, and muscle tenderness. Muscular atrophy occurs with disease progression. Polymyositis, often associated with myositis-specific autoantibodies in adults, is quite rare in children. Dermatomyositis in children is primarily a vasculitic disease seen most frequently in the 2- to 12-year age range. The clinical distinction between the two is the characteristic skin involvement of dermatomyositis. The heliotrope rash is a violaceous rash over the eyelids and sometimes over the cheeks in a malar distribution, without the typical nasolabial sparing seen in systemic lupus. Gottron papules are vasculitic, dry, purpuric papules that typically occur over the extensor surfaces of the MCP and PIP joints, and the elbows, knees, and ankles

(Fig. 72.1). Nailfold capillary inflammation is another sign of active vasculitis that can be observed on examination of the hands.

Muscle involvement is proximal, with limb-girdle, truncal, and cervical weakness. Patients may initially present with complaints of difficulty going up stairs and inability to participate in sports or other activities due to weakness. They may have constitutional symptoms of fever and fatigue, along with arthralgias or frank arthritis. Gastrointestinal vasculitis is a poor prognostic sign early in the course of disease that requires aggressive treatment.

The diagnostic workup should include routine CBC, chemistries, and muscle enzyme testing (transaminases, creatine phosphokinase, lactate dehydrogenase, and aldolase levels), along with manual muscle testing. There is no specific autoantibody test that is diagnostic in dermatomyositis. ANA may be positive, but myositis-specific and myositis-associated autoantibodies are usually negative. Gower sign is often used as an indication of a child's ability to stand from a sitting position without the use of the hands for supporting the weight of the trunk. All patients should undergo physical and occupational therapy evaluations to determine the extent of weakness and tightness of the muscle groups, and the need for a PT/OT program. Respiration, speech, and swallowing

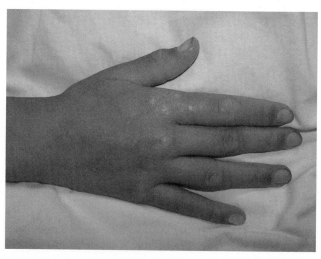

FIGURE 72.1. Cutaneous vasculitis over the extensor surfaces of the hand.

can also be affected, and therefore patients require evaluation of these muscle groups by pulmonary function testing (including inspiratory pressures), swallow studies, and speech therapy evaluations. Echocardiography is recommended to evaluate cardiac function. Magnetic resonance imaging (with contrast enhancement) using T2-weighted fat-suppressed imaging is a sensitive method used to detect muscle edema and inflammation, that is largely supplanting the need for electromyograpy (EMG) and muscle biopsy in the diagnosis of dermatomyositis.

Treatment is initially with steroids, both intravenous and oral, with steroid-sparing agents (such as methotrexate) being used as much as possible to lessen the side effects on growth and bone density associated with the long-term use of steroids in children. One of the notable long-term sequelae of dermatomyositis is dystrophic calcification or calcinosis of the subcutaneous tissues, often over the extensor surfaces of the joints in areas of skin rash. Calcinotic nodules can cause secondary joint immobility, and can erode through the skin and cause ulcerations and cellulitis.

CHAPTER 72B ■ UNUSUAL RHEUMATOLOGIC DISEASES: SCLERODERMA

SHERYL J. BOON

Scleroderma, as the name implies, is characterized by tightness of the skin. It is subdivided into systemic forms, which fortunately are extremely rare in the pediatric age range, and localized forms of morphea (patches) and linear scleroderma The localized forms of scleroderma in children are not associated with the poor prognostic outcomes of systemic sclerosis due to the lack of renal and pulmonary manifestations seen in the pediatric cutaneous forms. They often have a self-limited disease course, resulting in residual skin changes, but without continued progression. CREST syndrome (an acronym for calcinosis, Raynaud phenomenon, esophageal dysmotility, sclerodactaly, and telangiectasias—also known as limited cutaneous systemic scleroderma), is also rarely seen in children.

The pathophysiology of scleroderma is not entirely understood, but is felt to start with endothelial vascular damage, followed by platelet adhesion and recruitment of inflammatory cells. These release cytokines, which in turn stimulate fibroblast growth. This leads to collagen deposition in the vessel wall, decreased vessel lumen size, and ultimately organ, skin, and extremity ischemia, which perpetuate the inflammatory cycle.

Skin involvement occurs with initial erythema and induration followed by hardening and tightening of the skin, with hyperpigmentation and atrophy of skin and often underlying muscle. The skin changes are asymmetric with a dense texture and a shiny, scarred appearance (Fig. 72.2). The lesions of localized scleroderma may follow a dermatomal distribution. When the skin over a joint is affected, there is resulting dysmotility and contracture at that joint. The face can be progressively involved with loss of expression, and tightening of the oral aperture, with difficulty in chewing. Parry–Romberg syndrome and en coup d'sabre are facial forms of localized scleroderma that cause facial asymmetry in children.

Systemic scleroderma can involve any organ system, but skin, gastrointestinal, pulmonary, and renal are the primary systems associated with poor outcome. Gastrointestinal involvement can occur at any level of the gut but often involves the esophagus, manifesting as swallowing difficulty. Esophageal dysmotility and gastroesophageal reflux are common in systemic sclerosis. Small bowel fibrosis can be associated with malabsorption and bacterial overgrowth. Progressive renal failure and pulmonary fibrosis with pulmonary hypertension are the

major factors causing the the high morbidity and mortality associated with systemic scleroderma.

Diagnosis is based on the clinical presentation, with a diagnostic workup including evaluation of skin tightness, joint mobility, swallowing, renal function, and pulmonary function,

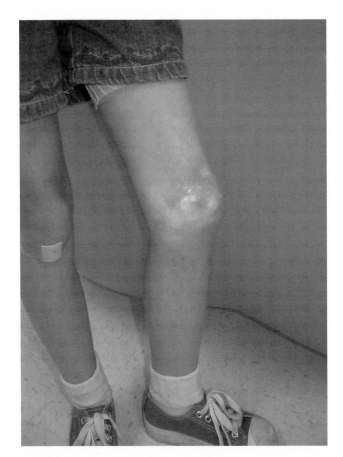

FIGURE 72.2. Linear scleroderma over a knee joint.

including echocardiography to monitor cardiac function and pulmonary artery pressures. Autoantibody testing should include testing for antinuclear antibodies (ANA), anti-Scl-70 antibodies, and anti-centromere antibodies (often positive in CREST syndrome), although specific antibodies are not usually present in the localized forms.

Therapy should be directed by a pediatric or adult rheumatologist. Antiinflammatory medications (including steroids, nonsteroidal anti-inflammatories, and immunosuppressant med-

ications such as antimalarials) are used early in the course of both systemic and localized forms. Pulse intravenous steroids, cyclophosphamide, and cyclosporine, along with other immunosuppressants, can be used in some circumstances. Specific therapy for gastroesophageal reflux (e.g., proton-pump inhibitors and prokinetic agents) and pulmonary hypertension are used when indicated. Angiotensin-converting enzyme inhibitors are useful in slowing the pace of progressive renal disease. Calcium-channel blockers and vasodilators are helpful in Raynaud phenomenon.

CHAPTER 72C ■ UNUSUAL RHEUMATOLOGIC DISEASES: MIXED CONNECTIVE TISSUE DISEASE

SHERYL J. BOON

Mixed connective tissue disease (MCTD) is an overlap syndrome associated with high-titer antibodies to uridine-rich small ribonuclear protein (U1 RNP). It can include features of systemic lupus erythematosus, dermatomyositis, rheumatoid arthritis, and scleroderma. Although it shares features of these other diseases, it is categorically unique in its HLA associations and antibody specificities, requiring high-titer anti-U1 RNP antibodies for diagnosis. Clinical manifestations include constitutional symptoms of fever, fatigue, myalgias, and arthralgias, along with myositis, arthritis, serositis, and

gastrointestinal, pulmonary, renal, endocrine, and central nervous system inflammation. Over time, sclerodermatous features can predominate, with sclerodactaly, esophageal dysmotility, pulmonary vasculitis, and pulmonary hypertension. Renal involvement tends to be less severe than in either SLE or systemic sclerosis. Autoantibodies seen in other diseases, including ANA, RF (rheumatoid factor), and anti-dsDNA antibodies, can also be seen in MCTD. Treatment is centered on immunosuppression, as in SLE, with specific organ involvement treated as indicated.

CHAPTER 72D ■ UNUSUAL RHEUMATOLOGIC DISEASES: SJÖGREN SYNDROME

SHERYL J. BOON

Sjögren syndrome in children, as in adults, can be primary or secondary to other diseases such as SLE or MCTD. It is manifested by sicca syndrome, or dry eyes (xerophthalmia) and dry mouth (xerostomia). It is associated with the presence of SS-A (anti-Ro) and/or SS-B (anti-La) autoantibodies. These are the same antibodies that cross the placenta during early pregnancy and cause the cardiac conduction defects associated with neonatal lupus. Sjögren syndrome can present with

constitutional/systemic symptoms, xerostomia and xerophthalmia, parotid gland tenderness and swelling (often mistaken for mumps), difficulty swallowing, and an increase in the number and severity of dental caries. Primary Sjögren syndrome can also involve other organ systems, including pulmonary, renal, gastrointestinal, endocrine and CNS. Treatment, again, is with immunosuppressants, along with medications for symptomatic relief of dryness (pilocarpine or cevimeline).

CHAPTER 73A ■ UNUSUAL VASCULITIC DISEASES: VASCULITIS

SHERYL J. BOON

As the term implies, *vasculitis* is an inflammatory process in the wall of blood vessels. Clinical findings secondary to vasculitis can occur in many sites throughout the body, with varied clinical presentations. Blood vessel inflammation can be secondary to numerous causes, including both antibody-mediated and cell-mediated immune mechanisms. In 1992, the Chapel Hill consensus conference on the nomenclature of systemic vasculitis revised the classification scheme for the primary systemic vasculitidies (for both adult and childhood vasculitidies), dividing them into categories based on the size of the vessels involved. These primary vasculitidies were distinguished from the secondary vasculitidies seen in other autoimmune diseases such as lupus and dermatomyositis, where vasculitis may be present but is not the predominant diagnostic feature. In 2005, a consensus conference was held in Vienna to reorder the scheme for the pediatric vasculitidies. The proposed classification includes four categories of vasculitis: large, medium, and small vessel (subdivided into granulomatous and nongranulomatous histologic types), and other or secondary vasculitis (Table 73.1).

TABLE 73.1
CLASSIFICATION OF PEDIATRIC VASCULITIS

Large vessel
  Takayasu arteritis
Medium vessel
  Kawasaki disease
  Childhood polyarteritis nodosa
  Cutaneous polyarteritis
Small vessel (granulomatous)
  Wegener granulomatosis
  Churg–Strauss syndrome
Small vessel (nongranulomatous)
  Henoch–Schönlein purpura
  Microscopic polyangiitis
  Isolated cutaneous leukocytoclastic vasculitis
  Hypocomplementemic urticarial vasculitis
Other/secondary
  Vasculitis associated with other rheumatologic conditions
  Vasculitis secondary to malignancy or infection
  Drug-induced vasculitis
  Isolated CNS vasculitis
  Cogan syndrome
  Behçet disease

CHAPTER 73B ■ UNUSUAL VASCULITIC DISEASES: TAKAYASU ARTERITIS

SHERYL J. BOON

Takayasu arteritis, or "pulseless disease," is seen in children from the ages of 1 year to young adults, with all cases occurring in patients under 40 years of age, as a diagnostic criterion. It is a vasculitis of the large vessels including the aorta and its major branches. Although rare in children, it needs to be in the differential diagnosis for unexplained hypertension. As in all of the vasculitidies, it can present with fever, irritability, and fatigue, along with hypertensive symptoms and claudication in the extremities. Physical exam reveals bruits, decreased pulses, and blood pressure differences in the extremities, localized by the affected arteries. Diagnostic evaluation includes nonspecific inflammatory labs (elevated sedimentation rate, leukocytosis, anemia, thrombocytosis, and sometimes hypergammaglobulinemia), and abnormalities on echocardiography, Doppler, and CT or MR angiography. To date, specific autoantibodies have not been identified for this condition. Cardiac catheterization is sometimes required to confirm the diagnosis, along with biopsy of the involved vessel. Treatment includes immunosuppression with steroids and other immunosuppressants, in addition to treatment of hypertension, and stinting of affected vessels as indicated. Management is optimally done by pediatric rheumatology working closely with pediatric cardiology.

CHAPTER 73C ■ UNUSUAL VASCULITIC DISEASES: POLYARTERITIS NODOSA

SHERYL J. BOON

Polyarteritis nodosa (PAN) is a medium-vessel vasculitis with multisystem involvement, that is rare in childhood. PAN presents with constitutional symptoms of fever, weight loss, arthralgias, and myalgias. Patients may have mono- or polyneuropathy, abdominal pain, testicular pain, and mottling of the skin (livedo reticularis) along with elevated blood pressure. The disease is characterized by medium-vessel fibrinoid necrosis and aneurysm formation, which can be seen on angiography. It does not have specific antibody associations, although patients may have positive anti-neutrophil cytoplasmic antibody (ANCA) titers. Treatment is with steroids and immunosuppressing agents, along with specific treatment for hypertension. A more limited form of "cutaneous" disease, often associated with poststreptococcal inflammation, is confined to the skin, muscles, joints, and peripheral nerves, without other organ involvement.

CHAPTER 73D ■ UNUSUAL VASCULITIC DISEASES: WEGENER GRANULOMATOSIS

SHERYL J. BOON

Wegener granulomatosis is a granulomatous small-vessel vasculitis associated with positive ANCA antibodies, usually cytoplasmic (c-ANCA) or anti-proteinase-3 (PR-3) antibodies. Manifestations include a purpuric rash, which can mimic the rash of HSP, SLE, or other small-vessel vasculitidies. Granulomatous lesions can be found in the nasal cavity, sinuses, and upper airway, causing obstruction of air flow. Pulmonary lesions can cavitate and bleed, causing cough and hemoptysis. Renal involvement is often progressive and severe, with pauci immune crescentic glomerulonephritis the predominant type, with few deposits of immune complexes seen on biopsy. Treatment is dependent on the extent of involvement, usually with steroids and methotrexate for disease limited to the upper airway. Antibiotics are commonly used to decrease Staphylococcal carriage in the nose, which is felt to contribute to the inflammatory cycle. In patients with pulmonary and/or renal involvement, oral cytoxan is the standard medication used, although other immunosuppressants are being evaluated for both induction of remission and for maintenance treatment.

CHAPTER 73E ■ UNUSUAL VASCULITIC DISEASES: SARCOIDOSIS

SHERYL J. BOON

Sarcoidosis in children is a multisystem inflammatory disease of unknown etiology. Like the adult form, it is associated with arthritis, uveitis (including panuveitis), and skin, pulmonary, neurologic, gastrointestinal and renal involvement. Macrophages in pulmonary lesions can convert inactive vitamin D to the active form, increasing calcium absorption in the gut, and causing hypercalciuria and renal stones. Early in the course of disease sarcoidosis can mimic polyarticular JIA, with the form of uveitis sometimes helpful in guiding differentiation. Angiotensin-converting enzyme (ACE) levels in the blood may be elevated, but can be normal.

CHAPTER 73F ■ UNUSUAL VASCULITIC DISEASES: CHURG–STRAUSS SYNDROME

SHERYL J. BOON

Churg–Strauss syndrome, or allergic granulomatosis, is another granulomatous small vessel disease with a strong association with asthma and allergic rhinitis. Eosinophilia and pulmonary infiltrates with pneumonitis are predominant features of this disease.

CHAPTER 73G ■ UNUSUAL VASCULITIC DISEASES: MICROSCOPIC POLYANGIITIS

SHERYL J. BOON

Microscopic polyangiitis (MPA) is a form of nongranulomatous small-vessel vasculitis also associated with ANCA antibodies, usually perinuclear (p-ANCA) or anti-myeloperoxidase (MPO) antibodies. It is a multisystem disease that can present with rash and constitutional symptoms, but often has renal involvement predominant at first presentation. Treatment is, as for all of these diseases, primarily immunosuppressants, with supportive and symptomatic care as indicated for hypertension and other organ involvement.

CHAPTER 73H ■ UNUSUAL VASCULITIC DISEASES: GOODPASTURE SYNDROME

SHERYL J. BOON

Goodpasture syndrome is another autoimmune, inflammatory disease, included here because it primarily presents with pulmonary and renal manifestations, and needs to be included in the differential diagnosis of any patient presenting with pulmonary/renal syndrome (along with Wegener granulomatosis, systemic lupus erythematosus, scleroderma, microscopic polyangiitis, and hemolytic uremic syndrome). It is associated with specific anti-glomerular basement membrane (GBM) autoantibodies that directly react with the collagen of basement membranes in lung and kidney. A subset of patients additionally has p-ANCA antibodies, that can be associated with CNS vasculitis. Treatment is with immunosuppressive agents and plasmaphoresis, to remove pathogenic antibodies.

Suggested Readings

Cassidy JT, Petty RE, et al. *Textbook of pediatric rheumatology.* 5th ed. Philadelphia: Saunders; 2005.
Harris ED, Budd R, et al. *Kelley's textbook of rheumatology.* 7th ed. Philadelphia: Saunders; 2006.

CHAPTER 74 ▪ ANTIMICROBIAL RESISTANCE AND JUDICIOUS USE OF ANTIMICROBIAL AGENTS

PAUL P. COOK

> Antimicrobial therapy saves thousands of lives and relieves much suffering, yet . . . untoward effects, harm, and death may occur both after logical, but especially after indiscriminate prescription. . . . The Hippocratic junction "first do no harm" or the question "Is this drug really necessary" are pertinent.
>
> —Hobert Reimann, 1961

Resistance to antimicrobial agents results from a natural process related to inherent mutation frequencies of microorganisms. Microorganisms in the environment exchange antibiotic resistance genes through plasmids and transposons. Human beings (i.e., physicians) have selected for and accelerated this process with the use of the wonder drugs of the 20th century—antibiotics. Beyond this, there are many reasons why antimicrobial resistance has increased. Factors associated with an increase in antimicrobial resistance in hospitals include (1) more severely immunocompromised patients, (2) increased use of invasive devices and procedures, (3) ineffective infection control, (4) increased use of antimicrobial prophylaxis, and (5) increased empiric polymicrobial antimicrobial therapy.

Excessive antibiotic use occurs both in the community as well as in the hospital setting. Although this chapter does not discuss the issue of excessive use of antibiotics in the ambulatory setting, it is clear that excessive use of antimicrobial agents in the community has a significant effect on the susceptibility of important hospital pathogens. Outpatient use of antimicrobials, particularly for respiratory tract infections, is a major factor in the rise in penicillin-resistant *Streptococcus pneumoniae* infections, many of which require hospitalization. Moreover, methicillin-resistant *Staphylococcus aureus* (MRSA), until recently seen only in the hospital setting, has been recognized as an increasingly common community pathogen. It is therefore imperative that appropriate use of antimicrobial agents occur both in community and hospital settings to preserve effectiveness. Judicious use of antibiotics requires that physician prescribers be aware of resistance profiles according to the pathogen as well as the hospital environment in which he or she practices. Appropriate antibiotic use will *not* prevent development of resistance, but will prolong the utility of the drugs currently available.

Antimicrobial resistance leads to increased morbidity, mortality, and health care costs. In the hospital setting, there is an indisputable association between antimicrobial usage and resistance. Areas in hospitals where antimicrobial use is high (e.g., intensive care units) have the highest rates of antimicrobial resistance. It is in these high–antibiotic-use areas where surveillance and control measures are imperative to control the spread of antimicrobial resistance.

PROBLEM PATHOGENS

Before discussing prudent use of antimicrobial agents, a brief discussion of some of the more important pathogens is needed. Each hospital has individual statistics regarding incidences and susceptibility data available in the hospital antibiogram. Problem pathogens and the risk factors for acquisition of resistant strains of organisms are listed in Table 74.1.

Since the mid-1980s, resistance rates for *Staphylococcus aureus* and coagulase-negative staphylococci have risen dramatically. MRSA were first described in 1961, but it was not until cephalosporin use became commonplace in the mid-1980s that MRSA became a problem pathogen at large tertiary-care institutions. Cephalosporins are the most commonly used class of antimicrobials at many institutions. These drugs are prescribed for a variety of conditions, including surgical prophylaxis (e.g., cefazolin) and for empiric coverage because of the broad-spectrum activity of these agents (e.g., ceftriaxone, cefotaxime, and ceftazidime). These broad-spectrum drugs facilitate overgrowth of organisms that are inherently resistant to these agents, including coagulase-negative staphylococci, MRSA, enterococci, *Clostridium difficile*, and *Candida albicans*.

A detailed discussion of the mechanisms of antimicrobial resistance is beyond the scope of this section, but the interested reader is referred to several excellent review articles at the end of the section. An understanding of the common types of resistance mechanisms is important if the physician is to make clinically important decisions regarding empiric therapy (Table 74.2). For example, if the mechanism of resistance involves a β-lactamase (e.g., *Moraxella catarrhalis*), then an acceptable empiric choice might include a β-lactam/β-lactamase inhibitor combination (e.g., ampicillin–sulbactam or amoxicillin–clavulanate). If, however, the resistance is mediated by an alteration of the target protein (e.g., MRSA), then use of an alternative class of drug (e.g., a glycopeptide like vancomycin) may be necessary.

GENERAL GUIDELINES FOR PREVENTION OF ANTIMICROBIAL RESISTANCE IN THE HOSPITAL SETTING

The Society for Healthcare Epidemiology of America and the Infectious Diseases Society of America have published guidelines for prevention of antimicrobial resistance in hospitals.

TABLE 74.1

RESISTANT ORGANISMS AND THE RISK FACTORS
FOR THEIR ACQUISITION

Resistant organism	Risk factor
Penicillin-resistant *Streptococcus pneumoniae*	Frequent otitis media Prior antibiotic use Day-care attendance
Vancomycin-resistant enterococcus (VRE)	Previous exposure to third-generation cephalosporins, vancomycin, and drugs with anaerobic actssivity Prolonged hospitalization Enteral tube feeding
Methicillin-resistant *Staphylococcus aureus* (MRSA)	Central venous catheter Prior antibiotic exposure
Extended-spectrum β-lactamase–producing *Klebsiella pneumoniae* (ESBL)	Exposure to ceftazidime and aztreonam
Azole-resistant *Candida* species	Prior fluconazole therapy Prolonged hospitalization Neutropenia

These recommendations call for an active system of antimicrobial resistance surveillance coupled with both an effective infection control program to reduce secondary spread of resistance and a program of antimicrobial use stewardship (i.e., antibiotic control). Antimicrobial stewardship includes appropriate selection, dosing, and duration of antimicrobial therapy. Ideally, an antimicrobial management program should consist of one or more hospital epidemiologists, infectious diseases clinicians, infection control practitioners, clinical pharmacists, and clinical microbiologists. To be successful, an antimicrobial management program must have the support of the hospital administration as well as the medical staff. It is incumbent on the antimicrobial

management program to prove to the medical staff that appropriate antimicrobial stewardship is not only a good idea but is a necessity to ensure the longevity of our existing antibiotic armamentarium against infectious diseases.

Methods to implement antibiotic control come in many forms. Historically, educational efforts to change physician prescribing habits have been a dismal failure. Restriction of selected antibiotics, although not popular, has been successful in certain cases. Medical record review by a clinical pharmacist is used at some institutions. Culture data usually are available at the time of the review (48 hours after the first order), resulting in implementation of appropriate focused antibiotic therapy. Guidelines for appropriate use are helpful but rarely are followed by practicing clinicians. The use of guidelines may increase with the popularity of hand-held computing devices (PDAs) that allow clinicians to obtain up-to-date guidelines that can be "hot-synced" from websites. Computerized physician order entry has been demonstrated not only to reduce antibiotic use but to reduce medical errors. Most hospitals do not yet have computerized order entry, but this is likely to change in the near future.

Specific Suggestions for Use of Antibiotics

There are a number of measures that can be taken to improve the appropriate hospital use of antibiotics. Physicians need to educate themselves regarding potential pathogens for given clinical problems. Many infections originate from the flora normally inhabiting the body site involved (Table 74.3). Neonatal infections usually are caused by maternal genital or gastrointestinal tract flora, whereas tooth abscesses contain the bacteria residing in the oral cavity and tooth plaque. Knowledge of the most likely infecting organisms for a given clinical problem simplifies decisions regarding initial antibiotic use. Pocket pharmacopoeia or "pocket drug references" and pediatric texts often list suggested antibiotics for empiric use by age and body site of infection.

Do not combine antibiotics unless indicated. Combining different agents is a common practice used by many clinicians in an effort to provide adequate coverage for the patient against all possible organisms. With the exception of serious infections caused by specific pathogens (e.g., *Pseudomonas aeruginosa*)

TABLE 74.2

MECHANISMS OF RESISTANCE FOR SELECTED ANTIMICROBIAL AGENTS

Mechanism	Antimicrobial agent/class	Representative organisms
Altered target (penicillin-binding protein)	β-Lactam	*Streptococcus pneumoniae*, methicillin-resistant *Staphylococcus aureus* (MRSA)
β-Lactamase	β-Lactam	Enterobacteriaciae, *Pseudomonas aeruginosa, Moraxella catarrhalis, Haemophilus influenzae*
β-Lactamase	β-Lactams, including carbapenems	*Stenotrophomonas maltophilia*
Enzymatic alteration	Aminoglycosides	*S. aureus*, enterococci, Enterobacteriaciae, *P. aeruginosa*
Enzymatic alteration	Macrolides, clindamycin, Quinupristin	*S. aureus, S. pneumoniae*, streptococci, Enterobacteriaciae
Efflux pump	Tetracyclines	*Escherichia coli*
Reduced permeability	Sulfonamides	*P. aeruginosa*, Enterobacteriaciae
Altered binding site	Vancomycin	*Enterococcus faecium*
Reduced permeability	Carbapenems	*P. aeruginosa*

TABLE 74.3

REPRESENTATIVE MICROORGANISMS ACCORDING TO BODY SITE

Body site	Resident and acquired organisms
Skin (other than perineum)	*Staphylococcus* sp., *Streptococcus* sp., diphtheroids
Mouth	*Staphylococcus* sp., *Streptococcus* sp., oral anaerobes (fusobacteria, *Peptostreptococcus*)
Respiratory tract	*Streptococcus pneumoniae, Streptococcus viridans, Moraxella catarrhalis, Haemophilus influenzae* (nontypeable)
Gastrointestinal tract	*Escherichia coli* and other gram-negatives Anaerobes (*Bacteriodes* sp, *Clostridium* sp.) *Salmonella, Shigella,* and other food-acquired pathogens
Genital tract	*Lactobacillus* sp. *Candida* sp. *Streptococcus* sp. (esp. group B) Sexually transmitted organisms: (gonococci, chlamydia, herpes simplex virus, genital warts)

TABLE 74.4

FACTORS THAT MAY CONTRIBUTE TO ANTIBIOTIC FAILURE

HOST RELATED
Foreign body present
Anatomic defect
Defect in host immune response to infection

DISEASE RELATED
Wrong antibiotic
Sequestered focus of infection (abscesses)
Nonbacterial infection or noninfectious cause of illness

ORGANISM RELATED
Acquired resistance (rare cause of antibiotic failure)
Superinfection with resistant organism

DRUG RELATED
Inadequate compliance
Improper dosing regimen
Inadequate diffusion into site
Drug–drug interaction

or specific clinical conditions where synergy is necessary (e.g., staphylococcal endocarditis), there is little to support this practice. Questions about appropriate antibiotics, route of administration, and duration should be referred to a pediatric infectious disease physician or clinical pharmacist for clarification.

Use fewer broad-spectrum cephalosporins (e.g., ceftriaxone, cefuroxime, ceftazidime). These agents are highly associated with gastrointestinal colonization by vancomycin-resistant enterococci. The second- and third-generation cephalosporins also are associated with acquisition of *C. difficile.* Use of broad-spectrum cephalosporins, particularly ceftazidime, is associated with outbreaks of extended-spectrum β-lactamase (ESBL)–producing organisms, such as *Klebsiella pneumoniae.* Alternatives to the broad-spectrum cephalosporins include ampicillin, ampicillin–sulbactam, piperacillin, and piperacillin–tazobactam.

Adjust antibiotics once culture results are available. Continuing broad-spectrum agents unnecessarily fosters development of antimicrobial resistance and increases the risk that the patient might contract *C. difficile* colitis or superinfections with MRSA, ESBL-producing *K. pneumoniae,* enterococci, (including vancomycin-resistant enterococci), and *C. albicans.* For example, a patient with sepsis syndrome is empirically treated with ceftriaxone and gentamicin. Blood cultures grow *Streptococcus pneumoniae* that is sensitive to penicillin (minimum inhibitory concentration = 0.03 μg/mL). The patient should be treated with penicillin unless there is a history of penicillin allergy.

Know your hospital antibiogram. If the hospital has a low rate of gram-negative resistance to aminoglycosides, these agents should be used empirically to cover for suspected gram-negative sepsis. Similarly, if the rate of MRSA at the institution is low (<20%), it may not be important to use vancomycin when infection with *S. aureus* is suspected.

Whenever possible, change intravenous antibiotics to oral antibiotics. Many oral antibiotics achieve levels in the blood that are virtually identical to levels achieved with intravenous dosing. Examples include trimethoprim–sulfamethoxazole, clindamycin, metronidazole, doxycycline, and fluconazole. There is no advantage to giving these drugs intravenously unless the patient is unable to swallow or is vomiting. In fact, there are definite disadvantages of intravenous administration, including pain, increased costs, and the potential for excessive fluid administration, phlebitis, and vascular infections with organisms such as MRSA.

Antibiotic failure: There are a number of reasons why an antibiotic regimen fails in a given patient. Failure of outpatient oral therapy may be due simply to noncompliance by the patient, but this should not be an issue in the hospitalized patient. One needs a systematic approach to the patient's failure to improve on a selected antibiotic regimen; some suggested avenues to explore are listed in Table 74.4. The patient should be thoroughly reassessed and reexamined. Substitution of one agent for another, rather than adding an agent, should be considered. Not only will it simplify the nursing responsibilities, but it will also avoid the problem of potential drug–drug interactions.

SUMMARY

In conclusion, antimicrobial resistance is a natural process that cannot be eliminated. Antibiotics do not cause mutations, nor do they create resistant bacteria. Inappropriate and excessive use of antimicrobial agents does, however, increase the selective pressure that promotes the emergence of resistant microorganisms, whether they are bacteria, viruses, or fungi. Judicious use of antimicrobial agents requires a concerted team approach involving the clinician, the pharmacy, the microbiology laboratory, and the infectious diseases consultant. In combination with effective infection control, prudent antimicrobial use will effectively treat infections and delay the development and spread of antibiotic resistance.

PEARLS

- Always focus antibiotic therapy to the narrowest-spectrum antibiotic based on culture results, when appropriate.
- Use the drug of choice for a given pathogen whenever possible.
- Use combination therapy only when indicated for a specific pathogen or a specific clinical condition.
- Know your hospital antibiogram.
- Change IV to PO medication as soon as the patient can tolerate PO.

Suggested Readings

Livermore DM. Minimising antibiotic resistance. *Lancet Infect Dis* 2005;5:450–459.

MacDougall C, Polk RE. Antimicrobial stewardship programs in health care systems. *Clin Microbiol Rev* 2005;18:638–656.

Nelson JD, Bradley JS. *Nelson's pocket book of pediatric antimicrobial therapy.* 16th ed. Buenos Aires, Argentina: Alliance for Worldwide Editing.

Paterson DL. "Collateral damage" from cephalosporin or quinolone antibiotic therapy. *Clin Infect Dis* 2004;38(suppl 4):S341–S345.

Reimann HA. The misuse of antimicrobics. *Med Clin North America* 1961;45:849–856.

Safdar N, Handelsman J, Maki DG. Does combination antimicrobial therapy reduce mortality in gram-negative bacteraemia? *Lancet Infect Dis* 2004;4:519–527.

CHAPTER 75 ■ MENINGITIS

TINA Q. TAN

Meningitis is defined as an inflammation of the leptomeninges (dura, arachnoid, and pia mater) surrounding the brain and spinal cord. It is caused by a number of etiologic agents (both infectious and noninfectious) and identified by an increased number of white blood cells (WBCs) in cerebrospinal fluid (CSF). Bacterial meningitis is caused by bacterial organisms. Aseptic meningitis lacks evidence of a bacterial organism detectable in the CSF by routine laboratory techniques (e.g., Gram stain, culture) and most commonly is attributed to a viral etiology. Encephalitis is an inflammation of the cerebral cortex. Meningoencephalitis is an inflammation of the cerebral cortex accompanied by the presence of meningitis. The most commonly found microbiologic causes of meningitis vary depending on the age of the patient (see below).

In all age groups, boys are affected more frequently than girls. Outside the neonatal age range, 90% of pediatric bacterial meningitis occurs between the ages of 1 month and 5 years, with children between 6 and 12 months of age being at the greatest risk. Data from the Centers for Disease Control and Prevention surveillance studies demonstrated that since the introduction of the conjugate *Haemophilus influenzae* type b (HIB) vaccine, the incidence of *H. influenzae* type b meningitis in children younger than 5 years of age is 2 cases/100,000. This is a 95% decline from the prevaccine era. For the other common organisms that cause bacterial meningitis in children younger than 5 years of age, the annual incidence of *Neisseria meningitidis* is 4 to 5 cases/100,000, and for *Streptococcus pneumoniae* the incidence is 2.5 cases/100,000.

Children with certain underlying conditions are predisposed to the development of bacterial meningitis. Deficiencies in the terminal components of complement lead to an increased risk for meningococcemia and meningococcal meningitis. Patients with CSF leaks, basilar skull fractures, cribriform plate fractures, cochlear implants, anatomic or functional asplenia, hemoglobinopathies, malignancy, and human immunodeficiency virus (HIV) infection have an increased risk for pneumococcal meningitis (and other invasive pneumococcal diseases). *Listeria* meningitis may be seen in children with cellular immune defects, whereas nontypeable *H. influenzae* meningitis has been associated with immunoglobulin deficiencies. Children with a dermal sinus or abnormality of the neuroenteric canal, or recent penetrating head trauma, neurosurgery, or ventriculoperitoneal shunt placement, are at increased risk for development of meningitis caused by streptococci, staphylococcal species, and gram-negative enteric bacilli, especially *Klebsiella* species, *Escherichia coli*, and *Pseudomonas aeruginosa*.

Bacterial meningitis has a peak incidence during the late fall and winter months, whereas viral meningitis tends to occur most frequently during the summer months.

The most common pediatric bacterial meningeal pathogens, group B *Streptococcus*, *E. coli* K1, *H. influenzae* type b, *N. meningitidis*, and *S. pneumoniae*, all share a similar multistep pathogenesis. The first step involves attachment of the organism to the nasopharyngeal mucosa, leading to colonization and infection of the upper respiratory tract. All of these pathogens have polysaccharide capsules that contribute to invasiveness by aiding in evading local host defenses. This allows the microorganism to invade between or through the respiratory epithelial cells into the subepithelial tissues where it can enter the bloodstream, the second step in the pathogenesis. The presence of a preceding viral upper respiratory infection seems further to aid this process. The third step involves the replication of the organism in the bloodstream, establishing a bacteremia that leads to the seeding of the meninges through the cerebral capillaries and the choroid plexus. In this protected environment, the organism can quickly multiply and spread throughout the CSF. Bacterial products (e.g., endotoxins, peptidoglycans, teichoic acid) stimulate the release of proinflammatory cytokines (e.g., tumor necrosis factor-α, interleukin-1) from endothelial cells and macrophages, leading to inflammation in the meninges and brain. Each of these cytokines in turn can stimulate the production of other inflammatory mediators (e.g., interleukin-6, platelet-activating factor, interferons, other interleukins), activate and attract leukocytes, and activate the coagulation cascade. The end result is an increased permeability of the blood–brain barrier, thrombosis of vessels with decreased cerebral blood flow, and, finally, cerebral edema with increased intracranial pressure. The administration of antibiotics can result in rapid bacterial lysis with the release of bacterial cell wall and membrane fragments, in turn further augmenting the inflammatory response and elevating intracranial pressure.

The organisms that most commonly cause bacterial meningitis vary by age as follows:

■ *0 to 3 months of age:* Almost all infectious agents, including bacteria, viruses, fungi, *Mycoplasma*, and *Ureaplasma*, can be potential causes of meningitis in this age group. Any agent isolated from CSF should be considered significant given that these young infants are considered to be immunocompromised hosts. The most common organisms that cause bacterial meningitis in this age group are group B *Streptococcus* (early and late onset), *E. coli*, *Listeria*, gram-negative enteric bacilli other than *E. coli* (e.g., *Klebsiella*, *Serratia* species, *Enterobacter*), other streptococci, fungi, nontypeable *H. influenzae*, and anaerobes. In young infants with brain abscesses, *Citrobacter diversus* should be considered as the etiologic agent. The most common CNS viral pathogens include herpes simplex virus (HSV), enteroviruses, and cytomegalovirus.

■ *3 months to 5 years of age:* Since conjugate HIB vaccine became a routine vaccination in the United States, disease caused by *H. influenzae* type b has markedly decreased. Therefore, the principal causes of bacterial meningitis in this age group are now *N. meningitidis* and *S. pneumoniae*. *H. influenzae* type b should still be considered in children younger than 2 years of age with meningitis who are unimmunized or who are incompletely immunized. Meningitis due to *Mycobacterium tuberculosis* is rare but should be considered in areas where the prevalence of tuberculosis is high and the history, clinical findings, and CSF and laboratory parameters suggest this diagnosis. The most common CNS viral pathogens in this age group include the enteroviruses, HSV, and human herpesvirus-6 (HHV-6).

■ *5 years of age to adults:* The most common bacterial organisms that cause meningitis in this age group are *N. meningitidis* and *S. pneumoniae. Mycoplasma pneumoniae* also can be a cause of severe meningitis and meningoencephalitis in this age group. Viral meningitis most commonly is caused by the enteroviruses, herpesviruses, and arboviruses. Other, less common causes of viral meningitis in this age group include Epstein–Barr virus, lymphocytic choriomeningitis virus, HHV-6, rabies virus, and influenza A and B viruses.

In the immunocompromised host with meningitis, in addition to the usual pathogens, etiologic consideration must also be given to more unusual pathogens, such as *Cryptococcus, Toxoplasma*, fungi, tuberculosis, and HIV.

CLINICAL FINDINGS

Patients with meningitis may experience a wide range of presenting signs and symptoms. Presentation may have a gradual onset of symptoms, beginning as nonspecific upper respiratory manifestations that progress over a period of several days until the disease becomes obvious. Alternatively, the course may be fulminant and result in death less than 24 hours after the onset of symptoms. Despite appropriate antibiotic therapy and intensive medical care, a significant level of morbidity and mortality continues to be associated with this disease.

Fever usually is present in children with meningitis but may be very low grade or absent in young infants. Nonspecific findings of irritability or inconsolability may evolve gradually into decreased activity or lethargy and bulging of the anterior fontanelle. Refusal to feed or anorexia increases as the disease progresses, with respiratory distress and photophobia often developing later. Children old enough to complain report headache early in the course of the disease. As the meningeal inflammation increases, back pain, stiff neck, and Kernig or Brudzinski signs may be present. As intracranial pressure begins to increase, nausea and vomiting develop. The increase in intracranial pressure ultimately may produce papilledema, confusion, or mental status changes. Seizures can occur at any time during the disease, but focal seizures or cranial nerve findings suggest central nervous system injury. In approximately 20% of children with bacterial meningitis, seizures occur before hospital admission, with another 26% having seizures within the first 48 hours after hospital admission.

Eventually, lethargy, sommolence, and shock may ensue. Petechiae, purpura, and end-organ dysfunction may develop if other areas become infected as a result of bacteremia.

Early and accurate diagnosis of bacterial meningitis is a major factor in the successful treatment of the infection. Prompt initiation of therapy with intravenous fluids and antibiotics can minimize the severity of the illness, the development of complications, and the emergence of sequelae. If there is suspicion of bacterial meningitis in a child with the appropriate signs and symptoms, lumbar puncture (LP) must be performed *immediately* to obtain CSF for analysis and culture. This is especially important in the age group most susceptible (<1 year) to meningitis. Every effort should be made to perform an LP prior to the administration of antibiotic therapy; however, if there is a delay in LP (e.g., difficult LP access, CT scan, or unstable patient), antibiotic administration should *not* be delayed until the LP is completed. The LP should be performed as soon as possible thereafter, even though the culture results may be altered.

The typical CSF parameters in infants and children are depicted in Table 75.1. The CSF in infants and children >6 months of age normally contains <6 WBC/μL and no polymorphonuclear leukocytes (PMNs). The typical CSF WBC count in bacterial meningitis is over 1,000 cells/μL (range several hundred to tens of thousands); however, WBCs may be few to none in the very early stages of infection. In bacterial meningitis, most CSF WBCs are PMNs, with the presence of immature PMNs being suggestive of a bacterial infection. In addition, the CSF glucose concentration usually is depressed (<30 mg/dL or less than two-thirds of the concurrent serum glucose), whereas the protein concentration usually is elevated (>100 mg/dL). Gram stain of the CSF specimen may be positive in 80% to 90% of patients with untreated meningitis. Detection of polysaccharide antigen in the CSF by latex agglutination may be used to aid in the determination of the etiology of meningitis (group B *Streptococcus, E. coli* K1, *H. influenzae* type b, *N. meningitidis, S. pneumoniae*), especially in patients who have abnormal CSF parameters with a negative Gram stain and culture. This is especially helpful in the setting of partially treated bacterial meningitis where the organisms are no longer viable but still can be detected by antigen methods. A positive CSF culture is the gold standard in confirming the diagnosis. For questionable cases, consultation with a pediatric infectious disease specialist may be helpful.

For patients with viral meningitis, the CSF WBC count usually is <500 cells/μL, although higher numbers of WBCs may occasionally be seen and cause confusion with bacterial meningitis. Most of the white cells are lymphocytes or mononuclear cells, but early in the illness a PMN predominance may be present. The CSF glucose concentration usually is normal and the protein concentration is normal or slightly elevated. Polymerase chain reaction is available for the detection of various viruses in the CSF, including HSV and the enteroviruses. Viral culture of the CSF (low yield) or from

TABLE 75.1

TYPICAL CEREBROSPINAL FLUID PARAMETERS IN INFANTS AND CHILDREN

Parameter	Normal newborn	Normal child	Bacterial meningitis	Viral meningitis
White cells/μL	0–30	0–6	>500	100–500
Neutrophils (%)	2–3	0	>50	<40
Glucose (mg/dL)	32–121	40–80	<30	>30
Protein (mg/dL)	19–149	20–30	>100	50–100

nasopharyngeal or rectal swabs (higher yield) may also yield the etiologic agent.

For children with possible or proven bacterial meningitis, empiric therapy is guided by the knowledge of the most likely pathogens and their current antimicrobial susceptibilities.

1. For infants 0 to 3 months of age with suspected bacterial meningitis, empiric therapy consists of ampicillin (300 to 400 mg/kg/day divided every 6 hours) and gentamicin (7.5 mg/ kg/day divided every 8 hours); *or* ampicillin and cefotaxime (200 to 300 mg/kg/day divided every 6 hours) or ceftriaxone (100 mg/kg/day divided every 12 hours). This regimen can be simplified once the organism has been identified and antimicrobial susceptibilities are known.
2. For children 3 months of age and older, empiric therapy for bacterial meningitis consists of a parenteral third-generation cephalosporin, either cefotaxime (200 to 300 mg/kg/day divided every 6 hours) or ceftriaxone (100 mg/kg/day divided every 12 hours), plus vancomycin (60 mg/kg/day divided every 6 hours). Once an organism has been identified and the antimicrobial susceptibilities are known, the antimicrobial regimen can be tailored. The initial empiric regimen provides coverage for antibiotic-resistant organisms, especially penicillin-resistant *S. pneumoniae*.

For susceptible organisms, aqueous penicillin G can be used to complete therapy for meningococcal and pneumococcal meningitis. For pneumococcal isolates that are penicillin resistant but susceptible to the extended-spectrum third-generation cephalosporins, vancomycin can be discontinued and these agents used to complete therapy. If a patient is found to have a pneumococcal isolate that is highly resistant both to penicillin and extended-spectrum third-generation cephalosporins, vancomycin and a third-generation cephalosporin are continued and rifampin should be added. However, if the patient does not clinically improve, imipenem or meropenem may be used as alternative agents.

The duration of antibiotic therapy varies by the organism isolated and the patient's clinical response. For uncomplicated cases, neonates with group B *Streptococcus* or gram-negative enteric meningitis should be treated for 14 to 21 days. Meningitis due to *S. pneumoniae* is treated for 10 to 14 days; *H. influenzae* type b, 7 to 10 days; and *N. meningitidis*, 5 to 7 days. The use of dexamethasone adjunctive therapy in the treatment of meningitis remains very controversial. Studies have shown that for patients with meningitis caused by *H. influenzae* type b, adjunctive therapy with dexamethasone significantly improved outcome, especially decreasing the risk of neurosensory hearing loss. However, with the virtual disappearance of meningitis caused by *H. influenzae* type b in the United States, the value of dexamethasone adjunctive therapy with meningitis caused by *S. pneumoniae* remains very unclear. Several studies have shown that its use in pneumococcal meningitis may negatively influence clinical outcomes. It also may reduce the penetration of vancomycin into the CSF, resulting in significantly decreased levels. There are no data to support its use in meningococcal meningitis, viral meningitis, or other infectious causes of aseptic meningitis. If dexamethasone is used, all potential benefits and possible risks need to be carefully considered. For it to have any potential benefit, it must be given *before or simultaneously with* initial antibiotic therapy.

Repeat lumbar punctures no longer are necessary for most cases of bacterial meningitis. However, there are special circumstances where repeat LP is recommended. Antibiotic-resistant *S. pneumoniae* and gram-negative infections require repeat lumbar punctures within 48 hours to ensure clearance of the organisms and guide therapy. Children without significant improvement in 24 to 36 hours, or in whom prolonged or secondary fever develops, should have a repeat LP performed as part of their ongoing evaluation. Neuroimaging likewise is recommended in any child without clinical improvement or with focal neurologic signs, seizures, or persistently abnormal CSF indices. Newborns also should have neuroimaging because many neonatal pathogens can cause abscess formation (especially *C. diversus*).

COURSE AND PROGNOSIS

The level of morbidity and mortality associated with meningitis is considerable, even with early diagnosis and appropriate therapeutic intervention. The most common complications that are seen include subdural effusions, subdural empyemas, and seizures. Subdural effusions occur in up to 30% of infants and young children with meningitis. Typically they are associated with persistent fever and may cause increased intracranial pressure due to a mass effect. Drainage usually is not necessary unless the patient has neurologic symptoms due to a mass effect. In that setting, drainage is necessary to relieve pressure. Subdural empyema occurs in approximately 1% of patients with bacterial meningitis and clinically presents with persistent fever, irritability, and other meningeal signs. This complication requires drainage and prolonged antibiotic therapy. Persistent seizures are a problem that usually requires long-term antiepileptic therapy and follow-up evaluations.

Neurologic sequelae have been detected in 25% to 56% of survivors, and death can be expected in 5% to 15% of cases. The most common neurologic sequela is neurosensory hearing loss. This is seen in approximately 30% of patients after pneumococcal meningitis and in up to 10% of patients after meningitis due to *N. meningitidis* or *H. influenzae* type b. Various degrees of impairment of motor functions and intellectual processes may occur. In more severe cases, hydrocephalus, infarction of brain or spinal cord, and/or neurologic devastation may result.

PEARLS

- Young infants with meningitis may have nonspecific findings, including paradoxic irritability, low or subnormal temperature rather than fever, and lethargy.
- The classic finding of stiff neck often is not present in children younger than 12 months of age with meningitis.
- Always administer antibiotics promptly, even if there is a delay in obtaining CSF cultures.
- There may be considerable overlap between bacterial and viral meningitis CSF parameters, especially in the first few days of illness. Always consider treatment for the "worst case" (i.e., bacterial meningitis) and administer antibiotics while awaiting culture results.
- Neurosensory hearing loss and seizure disorders are the most common sequelae of bacterial meningitis.

Suggested Readings

Feigin RD, Pearlman E. Bacterial meningitis beyond the neonatal period. In: Feigin RD, Cherry JD, eds. *Textbook of pediatric infectious diseases*. 5th ed. Philadelphia: Saunders; 2004:443–474.

Negrini B, Kelleher KJ, Wald ER. Cerebrospinal fluid findings in aseptic versus bacterial meningitis. *Pediatrics* 2000;105:316–319.

Spach D, Jackson LA. Bacterial meningitis. *Neurol Clin* 1999;17:711–735.

Wubbel L, McCracken GH Jr. Management of bacterial meningitis. *Pediatr Rev* 1998;19:78–84.

CHAPTER 76 ■ ENCEPHALITIS

DEBRA A. TRISTRAM

Encephalitis is one of the most challenging illnesses in medicine. There are a myriad of potential infectious agents and few specific tests to uncover the culprit. Compounding this diagnostic challenge is the lack of effective therapy for most forms of encephalitis. As polymerase chain reaction (PCR) technology becomes more widely available, our ability to diagnose the various causes of encephalitis will likely improve.

Encephalitis is an inflammation or infection of the parenchyma of the brain sometimes accompanied by infection of the surrounding tissues (meningoencephelitis), specifically the pia mater, the arachnoid, and the cerebrospinal fluid (CSF).

The most common agents of infectious encephalitis are listed in Table 76.1. Yearly outbreaks of encephalitis occur in the warm months in the United States and usually are associated with insect vectors, such as mosquito-born arboviruses. Eastern equine, Western equine, St. Louis encephalitis, and La Crosse are the most common arboviruses causing encephalitis. By the summer of 2005, West Nile virus had been identified in every state in the continental United States. Although several states documented only avian infections (Washington state, West Virginia, Vermont, New Hampshire, and Maine), it is only a matter of time before the human population is affected. Sporadic cases of herpes simplex encephalitis (HSV) occur year-round and always should be included in the differential of encephalitis, especially since it is one of the few treatable causes of infectious encephalitis. Rickettsial (Rocky Mountain spotted fever; RMSF) and spirochetal (Lyme disease, syphilis) agents may have encephalitis as part of the disease process.

Although the true incidence of encephalitis is unknown, it has been estimated that in the United States there are about 20,000 cases per year for all types of encephalitis. The seasonal forms of arboviral encephalitis cycle in birds and small mammals and are transmitted to humans and domestic animals by insect vectors, most commonly mosquitoes. Direct person-to-person spread does not occur. Incubation period depends on the specific virus and varies from 3 days to 14 days after exposure. Nearly all of the 100 arbovirus cases reported each year occur in children younger than 15 years of age.

Enteroviruses also are an important cause of encephalitis in children, although they more commonly cause aseptic meningitis. In temperate regions, enteroviral infections tend also to cluster in the summer months. They are spread by fecal–oral (including fomites) and respiratory routes. The incubation period for enteroviruses is 3 to 6 days.

HSV is a common cause of nonepidemic encephalitis and is identified in approximately 20% of all cases of encephalitis. Beyond the neonatal period, more than 95% of HSV encephalitis is caused by type 1 HSV. Most often, the temporal lobes are involved in nonneonatal HSV, suggesting spread by the respiratory/olfactory routes. Neonatal HSV encephalitis can involve any portion of the brain, even multiple sites, owing to spread during viremia. In neonates, HSV encephalitis tends to present between the first and sixth weeks of life. Nonneonatal HSV encephalitis may present at any age. Infection can be associated with primary (30%) or recurrent (70%) HSV infection (Chapter 84).

The differential diagnosis of encephalitis includes other infections of the central nervous system as well as noninfectious causes. Some of the other entities to consider in a patient with depressed mentation and fever are listed in Table 76.2. Central nervous system depression may occur in the context of sepsis, particularly severe sepsis in a young child. Brain abscesses, spinal abscesses, and subdural or subarachnoid infection may present with encephalopathy. Post-infectious central nervous system syndromes such as acute cerebellar ataxia, acute disseminated encephalomyelitis (ADEM) and Guillain–Barré syndrome may also mimic encephalitis, particulary if the child has a low-grade fever.

Noninfectious etiologies to consider in patients with encephalopathic presentation must include ingested toxins or drugs. Some of the more common street drugs (phencyclidine [PCP], lysergic acid diethylamide [LSD], cocaine, and amphetamines) may present with fever and altered mentation in an adolescent and be mistaken for early encephalitis. Collagen vascular disorders, particularly systemic lupus erythematosus, can present with central nervous system signs. Usually there are other associated systemic clues, such as alopecia or skin manifestations, to alert the clinician to the true diagnosis. Likewise, psychiatric conditions occasionally may be associated with altered behaviors and suggest infectious processes.

CLINICAL FINDINGS

Attention to detail when taking a history may reveal clues to the agent responsible for encephalitis (Table 76.3). The classic presentation of encephalitis is that of increasing lethargy, behavioral changes, and neurologic deficits. There is often a preceding "viral" prodrome consisting of headache, fever, and vomiting. The presence of gastrointestinal symptoms may be suggestive of enteroviral infection. Seizures are a common element at presentation.

Careful physical examination may reveal the presence of insect bites (arboviruses, Lyme disease, RMSF), rashes (RMSF, enteroviruses), scratches/bites (cat-scratch disease, possibly rabies), or vesicular lesions (enteroviruses or HSV). Nuchal rigidity is indicative of concomitant meningitis (i.e., meningoencephalitis), but is not always present. Focal neurologic deficits, if present, can suggest the area(s) of inflammation in the brain. Progression to stupor and coma often is rapid, necessitating intubation and ventilatory support.

In encephalitis, the laboratory should be used in an effort to make a specific diagnosis. However, despite careful evaluation, only a small percentage of encephalitis cases have an etiologic agent established (Table 76.4). CSF examination may reveal a modest pleocytosis with normal or elevated opening pressure

TABLE 76.1

INFECTIOUS AGENTS RESPONSIBLE FOR ENCEPHALITIS

Common	Uncommon	Rare
Herpes simplex virus	Cat scratch disease	Lymphochoriomeningitis
Arboviruses (Eastern and	Spirochetes (Lyme disease,	virus (LCM)
Western equine encephalitis,	syphilis, leptospirosis)	Jacob–Creutzfeld virus
St. Louis, La Crosse, and West	Toxoplasmosis	Mad cow disease
Nile viruses[a])	Human immunodeficiency	Variola
Enteroviruses	virus	Reoviruses
Rickettsiae: Rocky Mountain	Influenza A and B	
spotted fever, Q fever,	Adenoviruses	
Ehrlichia	Varicella-zoster virus	
Mumps[b]	Epstein–Barr virus	
Rabies	Cytomegalovirus	
	Rubella[b]	

[a]These agents are regionally distributed. Check with local health department for agents common to area of practice.
[b]These agents no longer are common owing to widespread immunizations in the United States, but may be a problem for an unimmunized person, especially from a country where preventable diseases are prevalent because of low immunization rates.

and protein, and normal or depressed glucose levels. There may be no white or red cells in the spinal fluid because the infection is present in the brain parenchyma, not the meninges. CSF should be sent for HSV PCR, and for enteroviral PCR if the season is appropriate. A specific diagnosis for either etiology allows discontinuation of antibiotics. Viral culture of CSF also should be obtained, although less than 15% of spinal fluid samples ultimately grow a viral agent. Serologies for acute and convalescent viral pathogens should be obtained and sent if

indicated by the history or season. Many state laboratories have serum immunoglobulin M (IgM) testing for arboviral infection, allowing earlier diagnosis of acute arboviral infection, as well as pathogen-specific IgM tests that can be performed on CSF. Otherwise, the diagnosis cannot be confirmed absolutely until paired sera drawn 4 weeks apart demonstrate a fourfold rise in a specific arboviral IgG. The state or local health department should have information available for test availability and requirements.

A negative computed tomography (CT) scan should not dissuade the clinician from the diagnosis of encephalitis. In the early stages of encephalitis, over half of all head CT scans are negative, only later revealing localized edema or contrast enhancement as the disease progresses. Magnetic resonance imaging (MRI) may be slightly more sensitive in early encephalitis. A rational approach to the patient with altered mentation and signs of encephalitis is an imaging procedure (CT or MRI) followed by a lumbar puncture if the scan does not demonstrate contraindications to the tap.

TABLE 76.2

DIFFERENTIAL DIAGNOSIS OF ENCEPHALITIS

INFECTIOUS
Meningitis
Brain abscess/subdural empyema/parameningeal infections
Rocky Mountain spotted fever, other tickborne infections
Embolic bacterial endocarditis
Mycoplasma pneumoniae
Spirochetes (syphilis, Lyme disease)
Cat-scratch disease

POST-INFECTIOUS
Acute cerebellar ataxia (due to varicella virus)
Acute disseminated encephalomyelitis (ADEM)

NONINFECTIOUS
Subdural hematoma
Tumor
Autoimmune/inflammatory
Toxin/drug ingestion (insecticides, cocaine, PCP, LSD, amphetamines, alcohol)
Malignant hypertension
Metabolic
  Hypoglycemia
  Hyperammonemia
  Reye syndrome
  Inborn errors of metabolism

TABLE 76.3

HISTORICAL CLUES TO THE ETIOLOGY OF VIRAL ENCEPHALITIS

TRAVEL HISTORY	IMMUNIZATION HISTORY
Arboviruses	Measles
Rickettsial disease	Mumps
	Rubella
COMMUNITY EPIDEMICS	
Arboviruses	**SEASON**
Enteroviruses	Arboviruses
Measles	Enteroviruses
Influenza	
ANIMAL EXPOSURE	**VECTOR EXPOSURE**
Rabies	Rickettsial diseases
Lymphocytic	Arboviruses
choriomeningitis	Lyme disease
Bartonella infection	

TABLE 76.4

WORKUP OF THE PATIENT WITH SUSPECTED ENCEPHALITIS

BASIC LABORATORY EVALUATION
Complete blood count/differential, blood chemistries including ammonia level, Ca, Mg
Liver function testing
Blood culture, urine culture
Lumbar puncture: cell count, chemistries, polymerase chainreaction (PCR) for herpes simplex virus/enterovirus, cerebrospinal fluid stains and cultures for bacteria, virus (fungi and mycobacteria if compromised host, tuberculosis exposure history)
Nasopharyngeal and rectal swabs for general viral isolation
Urine or blood toxicology screen, if suggested by history

BASIC IMAGING
CT or MRI
Chest radiograph
Electroencephalogram

ANCILLARY LABORATORY TESTING IF HISTORY OR PHYSICAL SUGGESTIVE
Serologies for arboviruses, enteroviruses, Rocky Mountain spotted fever, leptospirosis, Lyme disease, ehrlichiosis, *Bartonella henselae, Mycoplasma pneumoniae, Toxoplasma gondii*, Epstein–Barr virus, cytomegalovirus
Stool culture (if gastrointestinal symptoms present or history suggestive)
Malaria, thin and thick smears (travel or residence in endemic area)
Collagen vascular serologies, especially for lupus
Purified protein derivative (PPD)

Electroencephalography often reveals a focal periodicity against a diffuse, slow-wave background pattern. PLEDS (periodic lateralizing epileptiform discharges) may be present in cases of HSV encephalitis, and although suggestive, are not diagnostic of HSV infection. Additional testing to determine the etiology of encephalitis should be based on the exposure history. Travel to, or living in, endemic regions, or recent hiking or camping may be suggestive of tick- or other insect-borne diseases such as Lyme disease, RMSF, or ehrlichiosis that can have encephalitis as part of the disease process. An exposure to a kitten or its fleas may suggest the diagnosis of cat-scratch disease, especially if the patient also has old scratch marks or regional lymphadenopathy.

MANAGEMENT

Once the diagnosis of encephalitis has been suggested by the clinical features and the laboratory/radiologic evaluation, the patient should be started on acyclovir until HSV infection has been ruled out or until another specific diagnosis has been made. The dose of acyclovir is 60mg/kg/day divided every 8 hours for neonates infants and children ≤12 years of age, and 30 mg/kg/day divided every 8 hours for children >12 years of age. Often children are also begun on broad-spectrum antibiotics, such as ceftriaxone, if a lumbar puncture reveals pleocytosis. Usually empiric antibiotics can be discontinued when the CSF and blood cultures are negative. Other antibiotics or antifungals may be instituted based on the history, physical examination, and immune status of the patient.

The patient with encephalitis may require intensive care monitoring, especially if rapid clinical deterioration is present. Ancillary supportive measures for such patients include intubation and ventilation, anticonvulsants, monitoring of fluid and electrolytes (particularly early in the course to assess for inappropriate antidiuretic hormone secretion), control of cerebral edema, chest physiotherapy and suctioning, prophylaxis for stress ulcers with histamine-2 antagonists, and range-of-motion exercises to prevent contractures.

Although most cases of encephalitis are not spread person to person, any child admitted with encephalitis should be considered potentially infectious. In addition to standard precautions, contact precautions should be initiated. Although respiratory viruses are an unusual cause of encephalitis, children with respiratory symptoms also may require droplet precautions. When a specific agent is identified and isolation no longer is necessary, these measures can be discontinued.

COURSE AND PROGNOSIS

The ultimate prognosis in children with encephalitis depends on the causative agent. In general, a poorer outcome is suggested by multiple (more than three) seizures, focal neurologic findings, and more days to restoration of consciousness. Agents with better prognosis include cat-scratch disease and enteroviruses, whereas disease due to HSV and arboviruses continues to have a guarded prognosis, particularly in neonatal cases. In children with arboviral infection, prognosis depends greatly on the agent involved in the illness. All children with the diagnosis of encephalitis should have formal developmental and psychological testing when they have recovered sufficiently. Many children require long-term coordinated care, including physical therapy, occupational therapy, and intensive tutoring to regain lost milestones.

PEARLS/SPECIAL SITUATIONS

- Judicious use of the laboratory is imperative because there are numerous diagnostic tests that can be performed for encephalitis cases. Attention to detail in the history and physical examination often provides clues that direct the choice of additional tests. Not all tests should be done for all patients.
- History of swimming in stagnant fresh water may indicate *Naegleria fowleri* infection, an amoeba with a predilection for the central nervous system.
- Mollaret meningitis: Recurrent episodes of aseptic meningoencephalitis may indicate Mollaret meningitis, an entity of as yet unknown etiology. Hallmarks include recurrent changes in behavior or consciousness with CSF pleocytosis. HSV DNA has been recovered from some cases of Mollaret disease, but not all.

Suggested Readings

Whitley RJ, Kimberlin DW. Viral encephalitis. *Pediatr Rev* 1999:20:192–198.
Willoughby RE Jr. Encephalitis, meningoencephalitis, and post infectious encephalomyelitis. In: Long S, Pickering L, Prober C, eds. *Principles and practice of pediatric infectious disease*. 2nd ed. New York: Churchill Livingston; 2003:291–298.

CHAPTER 77 ■ PNEUMONIA

JOSEPH B. DOMACHOWSKE

COMMUNITY-ACQUIRED PNEUMONIA

Lower respiratory tract infections are a common cause of mortality in developing countries and represent a major source of morbidity among children worldwide. About 20% of all deaths in children under 5 years of age are due to acute lower respiratory tract infection, with 90% of these deaths due to pneumonia. Early recognition and prompt treatment and support of pneumonia is life-saving. Globally, an estimated 12 million children die from complications of pneumonia every year. Host factors, such as age, nutritional status, and underlying disease, have a major impact on mortality, morbidity, and microbial etiology associated with pneumonia. Microbial factors, especially the emergence of increasing levels of antibiotic resistance by common pathogens, are shifting epidemiologic patterns of disease. Public health factors, including ability to vaccinate against the most common etiologic agents of pneumonia, also influence these patterns.

A list of common and uncommon agents that cause community-acquired pneumonia (CAP) is given in Table 77.1. Respiratory viruses account for most lower respiratory infections in children. Bacterial causes also are prevalent, with *Streptococcus pneumoniae* remaining the most important cause of bacterial pneumonia in all age groups. *Chlamydophila pneumoniae* and *Mycoplasma pneumoniae* also have been recognized as pathogens responsible for mild to severe lower respiratory tract infections, particularly in children older than 5 years. Less common etiologic agents of bacterial pneumonia in this age group include *Streptococcus pyogenes* (group A *Streptococcus*) and *Staphylococcus aureus*. *Haemophilus influenzae*, now a rare cause of pneumonia in immunized children living in developed countries, remains a common etiologic agent of lower respiratory tract infection in underdeveloped parts of the world. *Mycobacterium tuberculosis* may cause pneumonia at any age. Patients with uncommon agents of CAP may have clues to etiology in their exposure or travel history.

Respiratory tract infections begin by the deposition and subsequent replication of viral or bacterial agents on respiratory tract mucosa. The lung also can be seeded hematogenously during bacteremia. Viral infections can impair host defenses, such as ciliary activity or alveolar macrophage activity, and predispose to secondary bacterial infection.

Uncomplicated pneumonia usually is easy to differentiate from other entities that might present with similar respiratory findings. Aspiration of a foreign body, complications of heart disease, or underlying pulmonary disease may appear as pneumonia, especially at first presentation. Toxic or occupational inhalations can result in chemical or hypersensitivity pneumonitis, and may be mistaken for a pulmonary infection if the illness is accompanied by fever. For example, ingestion and inhalation of volatile hydrocarbons can present with severe pneumonitis accompanied by fever and leukocytosis. Any underlying or preexisting lung injury is also prone to "superinfection" with bacteria.

Clinical Findings

The clinical manifestations of pneumonia are diverse and somewhat dependent on the age of the child at presentation. CAP has classically been characterized by sudden onset of fever, tachypnea, and cough. Infants may present with apnea, refusal to eat, or tachypnea. These symptoms frequently are preceded by a relatively minor upper respiratory tract infection characterized by low-grade fever and rhinorrhea. Rales and rhonchi or decreased breath sounds may be present and aid in the localization of the pneumonia. However, in young infants, assessing adventitious sounds or location may be difficult because of the small chest size. Cyanosis or pallor may be present in children with hypoxemia. Elevated respiratory rates (for age) and evidence of accessory muscle use can be helpful to assess respiratory compromise. The decision to hospitalize focuses around the child's clinical toxicity, work of breathing, and oxygen requirement (as determined by pulse oximetry). The decision to provide ventilatory support for pediatric patients in respiratory failure is based on the clinical examination and rarely relies on arterial blood gases.

Total white blood cell counts above 15,000 cells/mL suggest a bacterial infection. Elevated cold-agglutinin titers commonly are seen with *M. pneumoniae* infection. A blood chemistry panel may reveal multiple organ involvement or the presence of an underlying disease. In hospitals where the prevalence of acquired immunodeficiency syndrome is 1 per 1,000 discharges or higher, serologic testing for human immunodeficiency virus (HIV) is advocated by the Centers for Disease Control and Prevention for hospitalized patients between the ages of 15 and 54 years with CAP. Pneumonia is a common infection in HIV-infected children even when CD4 counts are normal and the HIV viral load is low.

Additional laboratory studies include a blood culture, a sputum Gram stain and culture (when possible), a pleural fluid examination (if present), and a nasopharyngeal sample for rapid diagnostic tests for viral pathogens and/or viral culture. More invasive, direct sampling by bronchoalveolar lavage is reserved for patients with severe or enigmatic forms of lower respiratory tract infections. If a child requires endotracheal intubation, a tracheal aspirate can be sent for the required microbiologic analysis, but may reflect the colonization of the upper respiratory tract and oropharynx rather than providing the true pathogen. Acute and convalescent serologic testing for *Mycoplasma* or *Legionella* should be considered. A rapid urine antigen test for *Legionella pneumophila* type 1 also is available. Because of the recent resurgence of childhood tuberculosis, a purified protein derivative (PPD) skin test is prudent in all pneumonia cases. If an unusual microbiologic cause of pneumonia is

TABLE 77.1

COMMON AND UNCOMMON ETIOLOGIES OF COMMUNITY-ACQUIRED
PNEUMONIA

Etiologic agents	Comments
COMMON VIRUSES	
Influenza A and B	Seen during epidemics; emerging concerns related to bird-to-human transmission of avian influenza strains. For current information regarding location of avian influenza outbreaks, see www.cdc.gov/flu/avian/
Adenovirus	Sporadic cases of pneumonia; associated with hepatitis, conjunctivitis occasionally
Respiratory syncytial virus	Usually presents with bronchiolitis; winter season
BACTERIA	
Streptococcus pneumoniae	Sudden onset of high fever, toxicity
Mycoplasma pneumoniae or *Chlamydophila pneumoniae*	Slow progression of clinical symptoms, "walking pneumonia," chest radiograph often worse than clinical examination
UNCOMMON VIRUSES	
Hantavirus	Contact with rodents/rodent urine or droppings
SARS Coronavirus	For current information regarding location of outbreaks, see www.cdc.gov/ncidod/sars/
BACTERIA	
Staphylococcus aureus	Recent viral infection, especially influenza
Streptococcus pyogenes (group A *Streptococcus*)	Recent viral infection; past history of strep infection
Chlamydia psittaci	Contact with psittacine birds (usually pets)
Coxiella burnetti	Contact with parturient sheep, goats, cattle, cats
Francisella tularensis	Tick bites, exposure to infected animals
Yersinia pestis	Droplet inhalation from an infected animal
DIMORPHIC FUNGI	
Histoplasma capsulatum	Eastern and central United States, Canada
Blastomyces dermatitidis	Endemic in the southeastern and midwestern United States
Coccidioides imitis	Southwestern United States, northern Mexico

suspected based on the patient's history or underlying disease, the microbiology laboratory should be consulted regarding the most appropriate specimens for submission. This type of consultation is becoming increasingly important with advances in microbiologic diagnostics such as real-time polymerase chain reaction (PCR). This and other molecular tests are increasingly available to identify microbial agents that are slow, difficult, or impossible to propagate in the laboratory.

It often is difficult clinically to distinguish children with viral pneumonia from those with bacterial disease. Chest radiographs often are used to confirm the presence and location of pulmonary infiltrates. Bacterial pneumonias are more likely to have focal infiltrates or consolidation, whereas viral pneumonias demonstrate a more diffuse, bilateral interstitial pattern on chest radiography. However, studies show that this distribution alone cannot be used to guide therapy.

Special Situations: Neonates and Young Infants

In general, a diagnosis of pneumonia without sepsis in an infant younger than 3 weeks of age is unusual; therefore, noninfectious etiologies of abnormal chest radiograph findings also should be considered. Agents known to cause sepsis neonato-

rum, such as *Streptococcus agalactiae* (group B *Streptococcus*), and gram-negative enteric organisms can cause pneumonia in this age group, but usually in combination with other signs and symptoms of sepsis. Viral etiologies such as herpes simplex virus, cytomegalovirus, adenovirus, and enteroviruses should be considered. Infants with congenital syphilis also may develop pulmonary infiltrates (pneumonia alba). Infants 3 weeks to 4 months of age more commonly contract lower respiratory tract infection in the form of viral bronchiolitis, but sometimes with concurrent pneumonitis. Pneumonia in this age group most commonly is seen as result of respiratory viruses (respiratory syncytial virus [RSV], human metapneumovirus, parainfluenza, influenza, adenovirus, and others), but bacterial etiologies, such as *S. pneumoniae* also must be considered. A maternal history of sexually transmitted diseases should increase suspicion of vertically transmitted *Chlamydia trachomatis* infection. These infants classically present with a nonproductive, staccato cough and little or no fever. Peripheral eosinophilia is seen in some of these infants. A staccato cough (often severe and paroxysmal), especially if followed by emesis, should also raise suspicion of pertussis (*Bordetella pertussis*) in this age group because pneumonia develops in 20% of infants with pertussis. Characteristically, the peripheral blood smear reveals an impressive lymphocytosis. Other causes of "pertussis syndrome" include infections caused by *Bordetella parapertussis*, RSV, and adenovirus.

Management

The management of a patient hospitalized with pneumonia should include supplemental oxygen as needed, hydration, and strict attention to pulmonary toilet. Unless the patient clearly has a viral syndrome (such as bronchiolitis), empiric antibiotic therapy usually is started after appropriate samples for microbiologic diagnosis are obtained. Findings that favor a bacterial etiology over a viral etiology include a toxic appearance, high fever, acute onset, lobar consolidation, pleural effusion, and abscess or pneumatocele formation.

Ideally, treatment of pneumonia should be focused against the specific identified pathogen, but this is often impractical. Patients hospitalized with suspected bacterial pneumonia often must be empirically treated with a parenteral second- or third-generation cephalosporin such as cefuroxime or ceftriaxone. If pertussis or a *Mycoplasma*, *Chlamydophilia*, or *Legionella* infection is being considered, a macrolide antibiotic is added to the empiric regimen until definitive diagnostic results are available. If a penicillin-susceptible *S. pneumoniae* is recovered from a blood or sputum culture, treatment should be altered to penicillin G (150,000 U/kg/day divided every 6 hours). For penicillin-resistant *S. pneumoniae*, cefuroxime or ceftriaxone should be continued. Because of the excellent levels of penicillin attained in lung tissue, there is seldom a need for vancomycin in the management of drug-resistant *S. pneumoniae* pneumonia unless the isolate has very high-level resistance (minimum inhibitory concentration ≥4 μg/mL). Questions should be directed to a pediatric infectious disease specialist for guidance regarding resistant organisms or complicated cases.

Complications of Pneumonia

In up to one-third of patients with community-acquired bacterial pneumonia, a *parapneumonic effusion* develops (Fig. 77.1). A child with pneumonia who suddenly has worsening symptoms should have a repeat chest radiograph performed because it is likely that an effusion has developed. Thoracentesis should be performed in cases of large effusions and enigmatic pneumonias, and in patients who fail to respond to standard therapy. Pleural fluid microbiologic studies should include Gram stain and routine culture, acid-fast stain and culture, and fungal stain and culture. It also is customary to measure pleural fluid pH, glucose, protein, lactate dehydrogenase, and white cell count. A low pH, low glucose, high protein, elevated lactate dehydrogenase, and a predominance of neutrophils supports a diagnosis of pyogenic pneumonia with empyema (commonly caused by *S. pneumoniae* or *S. aureus*). A pH between 7.0 and 7.3, elevated protein, and <2,000 white blood cells/mL is more characteristic of a transudative effusion. A predominance of mononuclear cells suggests tuberculous or fungal or malignant effusion.

A transudative effusion without frank pus often can be managed without placement of a chest tube, with the realization that serial thoracentesis may be required for symptomatic relief. Conversely, pus in the pleural space is an indication for aggressive drainage. In general, a chest tube is warranted if pus is present on the initial thoracentesis, especially if fluid reaccumulates rapidly or if respiratory compromise persists after the initial tap. Consultation with a pediatric surgeon is appropriate for drainage options (thoracoscopy versus serial taps versus chest tube). Even with early, aggressive drainage of pleural empyema, collections can become organized and loculated. Because of the thick, tenacious quality of the pleural fluid, regular saline irrigation through the chest tube may

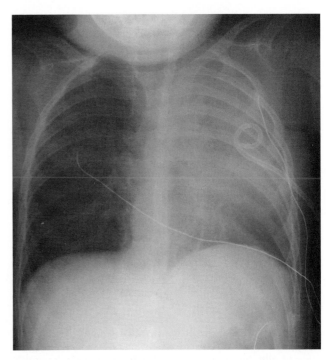

FIGURE 77.1. Chest radiograph from a 3-year-old boy with community-acquired pneumonia. A blood culture obtained on hospital admission grew *S. pneumoniae* that was resistant to penicillin, but susceptible to ceftriaxone. His pneumonia was complicated by the development of a left pleural empyema, requiring the placement of a chest tube.

facilitate drainage. Some experts recommend pleural instillation of fibrinolytics, with or without thoracoscopic exploration and debridement. Surgical pleural stripping or decortication is required only rarely for management.

Other complications of bacterial pneumonia include parenchymal abscess formation and pneumatocele formation (commonly associated with *Staphyloccocus aureus*; less commonly with organisms aspirated from the mouth, especially anaerobes). Although these entities are usually treated medically, surgical consultation may be required. Antibiotic therapy is continued for a minimum of 3 weeks. Rarely, in cases of pneumonia with empyema, a bronchopleural fistula develops. Management of this complication relies on surgical closure of the defect.

HOSPITAL-ACQUIRED PNEUMONIA

Hospital-acquired pneumonia, or nosocomial pneumonia, is considered a separate entity from CAP primarily because the etiologic agents and the respective empiric antibiotics are different. Most of these nosocomial pneumonias are ventilator associated and especially common in infants and children with chronic illnesses (particularly chronic lung disease of prematurity, neuromuscular disorders, and cerebral palsy). Among all nosocomial infections, pneumonia ranks third in overall incidence, but because these infections often are severe, mortality from nosocomial pulmonary infections exceeds mortality from infections at any other site. Currently, the most common causes of nosocomial pediatric pneumonia are enteric gram-negative bacteria (*Klebsiella*, *Enterobacter*, *Serratia*, *Escherichia coli*, and *Proteus*). Water-associated gram-negative bacteria such as *Pseudomonas*, *Acinetobacter*, *Flavobacterium*, and *Alcaligenes* also may be involved. Diagnosis of pneumonia in a ventilator-dependent child may be difficult, particularly if she has underlying lung disease. Guidelines for diagnoses of pneumonia include new or changing infiltrates on chest radiography, increased ventilatory settings or oxygen requirements, and increased pulmonary secretions with predominance of polymorphonuclear cells and organisms.

Hospital-to-hospital variations in antibiotic susceptibility patterns of nosocomial pathogens make it difficult to recommend "standard" empiric therapy for hospital-acquired pneumonia, but a broad-spectrum, antipseudomonal penicillin (e.g., piperacillin) *or* antipseudomonal penicillin plus tazobactam (Zosyn) *and* an aminoglycoside usually is acceptable while awaiting further microbiologic information. In some areas, where outbreaks of extended-spectrum β-lactamase–producing *E. coli* or *Klebsiella* have become problematic, initial coverage with a carbapenem antibiotic such as imipenem–cilastatin is prudent. Once culture and susceptibility results are available, antibiotics should be adjusted to the most narrow-spectrum effective agent.

The Child with Recurrent Pneumonia

A child admitted to the hospital with frequent or recurrent pneumonia deserves special attention, because fewer than 10% of all children hospitalized with pneumonia have this presentation. An underlying illness can be identified in up to 90% of such children and should be carefully sought. Half of the children have recurrent episodes of aspiration, 15% an underlying immune disorder (Chapter 85), 10% congenital heart disease, 8% asthma, and another 8% respiratory tract anomalies. An opportunistic infection (e.g., *Pneumocystis carinii*) or repeated bacterial infection warrants evaluation of the immune system. A partial summary of diagnostic considerations for a child with recurrent or persistent pneumonia can be found in Table 77.2.

Clinical Findings

The past medical history and physical examination are very important in the evaluation of a child with recurrent pneumonia. Specific questions should be asked about frequency, duration, and severity of all infections, respiratory or otherwise. Signs of upper airway obstruction, feeding problems and regurgitation, diarrhea, fevers, night sweats, exposures to infectious disease, allergies, immunizations, and the possibility of foreign body aspiration should be sought. Seasonal or diurnal variability of symptoms should be noted. An environmental history should emphasize contacts with home or day care infections and elucidate possible exposures to pollutants or irritants in the home, particularly second-hand cigarette smoke. Specific inquiries should be made with regard to possible exposure to tuberculosis or a personal history of a positive PPD skin test. Family history of a hereditary disorder known to be associated with recurrent lung infections warrants investigation for that particular disorder in the child. Growth parameters should be measured and plotted, including as many old values as possible.

Because the differential diagnosis of recurrent pneumonia is very broad, specific recommendations regarding diagnostic evaluations and management need to be individualized. General laboratory evaluation might include a complete blood count and chemistry panel to assess overall health. If the patient is able to produce and expectorate sputum, it should be Gram stained and cultured. All previous culture results from any source should be reviewed, remembering that certain organisms often are associated with specific

TABLE 77.2

DIFFERENTIAL DIAGNOSIS OF RECURRENT PNEUMONIA

Abnormalities resulting in pneumonia within a single lung region
Abnormalities in the airway
Foreign body
Bronchial tumor
  Adenoma
  Lipoma
  Papilloma
Abnormalities producing external compression secondary to enlarged lymph nodes
  Tuberculosis, other mycobacterial infection
  Histoplasmosis
  Coccidioidomycosis
  Blastomycosis
  Other infections
Tumors
  Direct compression
  From lymphadenopathy
Structural abnormalities that cause decreased mucus clearance
  Bronchial stenosis or atresia
  Localized bronchiectasis
  Right middle lobe syndrome
  Bronchogenic cyst
  Sequestered lobe
Abnormalities usually resulting in pneumonia of one or more contiguous lung regions
  Immunodeficiency (Chapter 85)
  Recurrent microaspiration
  Impaired swallowing
  Cranial nerve injury/central nervous system injury
    Drugs
    Seizures
    Cricopharyngeal incoordination
    Neuromuscular disorders
  Laryngeal cleft
  Submucosal cleft
  Obstructive lesions of the tongue or larynx
  Cystic fibrosis

diseases (e.g., *Pseudomonas aeruginosa* and cystic fibrosis). Sweat chloride testing should be considered for suspected cases of cystic fibrosis. For children with recurrent bacterial pneumonia, total serum immunoglobulins (IgG, IgM, IgA, and IgE) and IgG subclasses should be evaluated. HIV testing may be necessary in the initial screening if the child's or mother's history suggests risk factors for HIV acquisition (e.g., drug use, sexual activity). A tuberculin skin test also is mandatory. If radiographs and other studies have been done in the past, they should be reviewed and compared with the current studies. Recurrent pneumonia in the same anatomic location has a different list of etiologic possibilities than separate episodes of pneumonia in different segments of the lung (Table 77.2).

If an immune defect is identified or strongly suspected, consultation with a pediatric immunologist would be helpful to ascertain the latest diagnostic and therapeutic options for the child (Chapter 85). If the child does not have an identifiable immunodeficiency but has persistent problems with pneumonia, referral to a pediatric pulmonologist is appropriate.

PEARLS

- A child with bacterial pneumonia who acutely worsens should have a repeat chest radiograph to evaluate for the presence of pleural effusion.
- Pleural empyema is a closed-space bacterial infection and requires immediate drainage.
- Respiratory viral infections are very common during childhood, but more than one proven episode of bacterial pneumonia is unusual and demands further evaluation for an underlying anatomic or immune defect.

Suggested Readings

Klein JO. Bacterial pneumonias. In: Feigin R, Cherry J, eds. *Pediatric infectious diseases*. 5th ed. Philadelphia: Saunders; 2004.

McIntosh K. Community acquired pneumonia in children. *N Engl J Med* 2002;346:429–437.

Panitch HB. Evaluation of recurrent pneumonia. *Pediatr Infect Dis J* 2005; 24:265–266.

Sandora TJ, Harper MB. Pneumonia in hospitalized children. *Pediatr Clin North Am* 2005;52:1059–1081.

Septimus E. Pleural effusion and empyema. In: Mandell GL, Bennett JE, Dolin R, eds. *Principles and practice of infectious diseases*. 6th ed. New York: Churchill Livingstone; 2004.

CHAPTER 78 ■ BRONCHIOLITIS

ROBERT C. WELLIVER, SR.

Bronchiolitis is an acute obstructive respiratory illness of infancy characterized by wheezing or hyperinflation of the chest, with mononuclear cell infiltration and mucus plugging of the small airways. A similar illness occurring in older children may be referred to as *wheezy bronchitis* or *infectious asthma*.

Bronchiolitis occurs almost exclusively as the result of a viral infection. Respiratory syncytial virus (RSV) causes approximately 50% of all bronchiolitis, and virtually all of the cases resulting in respiratory failure. The parainfluenza viruses, particularly type 3 but occasionally types 1 and 2, are second to RSV in terms of frequency as etiologic agents. Other cases may be due to influenza virus infections, particularly with type A strains. Less commonly, human metapneumovirus, adenovirus, coronavirus, rhinovirus, *Mycoplasma pneumoniae*, or *Bordetella pertussis* infection may present as wheezing in infancy.

Bronchiolitis occurs infrequently during the summer months in temperate climates. The first cases of bronchiolitis are noted in the early autumn months, but marked increases in the number and severity of cases of bronchiolitis do not occur until the RSV season, which usually begins in late December in the northern hemisphere. The incidence peaks in the winter with RSV as the principal cause, and with a smaller number of influenza virus–related cases occurring during the briefer influenza virus season. RSV-related cases continue to occur through late winter and early spring, when parainfluenza activity again increases.

Because RSV represents the principal cause of moderate and severe bronchiolitis, the epidemiology of infection with this virus merits further discussion. Approximately 50% to 68% of all infants are infected with this virus before reaching 12 months of age, and virtually all children are infected before age 24 months. Most of these infections result in minor upper respiratory infections only. However, 30% of all infants with primary RSV infection acquire lower respiratory illness (LRI), mostly bronchiolitis. Recent studies from the Centers for Disease Control and Prevention estimate that 3% of all infants born in the United States are hospitalized annually with bronchiolitis, resulting in between 70,000 and 120,000 hospitalizations for RSV LRI annually.

Repeated infections with RSV occur frequently in all individuals throughout life. These infections may be associated with wheezing, but the nature of these illnesses usually is progressively milder. It is well recognized, however, that RSV infection may result in the development of LRI at any age.

Risk factors for development of LRI at the time of RSV infection in infants include crowded living conditions, day care attendance, passive smoke exposure, age 1 to 3 months at the time of infection, underlying congenital heart disease, underlying lung disease (especially chronic lung disease of prematurity, CLD), and prematurity, even without CLD. Older children with severe immune deficiency (e.g., malignancies, organ transplantation) are at high risk for the development of severe pneumonia

(but not bronchiolitis) from RSV infection. Surprisingly, human immunodeficiency virus–infected children usually tolerate RSV infection well, but may develop prolonged pneumonia.

RSV infection usually is transmitted to an infant from a school-aged child (e.g., sibling or day care center contact), probably by direct contact with the older child's respiratory secretions or by large-particle aerosols. The incubation period is probably in the range of 5 to 7 days, based on experimental challenge studies in adults and observations of the spread of infection in closed groups.

Many other conditions should be considered in the differential diagnosis of wheezing in infants. Gastroesophageal reflux frequently may manifest as wheezing, and should be considered if the infant frequently spits up, especially when this occurs hours after a feeding. Children with foreign bodies may have recurrent episodes of wheezing, but should lack signs of upper respiratory infection. The presence and location of a foreign object sometimes can be determined by comparing inspiratory and expiratory chest radiographs or bilateral decubitus films; wheezing is usually unilateral. Children with congenital heart disease as a cause of wheezing should be identifiable by heart auscultation and chest radiograph findings. Cystic fibrosis may be heralded by wheezing illnesses of unusual severity or duration, and may be distinguishable because of coexisting weight loss and edema in infancy. Infants with vascular rings may have frequent or constant wheezing, and may be identified using barium esophagrams. Bronchial malacia also presents with persistent wheezing. Children with immotile cilia syndrome may have recurrent wheezing in the context of very frequent sinus and ear infections, with or without situs inversus. Atopic asthma is rarely, if ever, diagnosed in infancy, when viral infections are the cause of most wheezing episodes. However, the eventual development of asthma may be predicted by the presence of atopy in the infant, particularly atopic dermatitis.

CLINICAL FINDINGS

The infant with viral bronchiolitis has a history of upper respiratory illness over the preceding 2 to 3 days. The onset of lower respiratory involvement is associated with frequent cough, which becomes dry and irritative. A history of premature birth (with or without CLD) should be sought because these children are more likely to have severe bronchiolitis compared to term infants. Parents who are good historians usually can describe when labored breathing began with considerable precision. Reduced oral intake may be reported, and suggests evaluation for hospitalization. In the older child, the upper respiratory illness prodrome may be shorter or absent before wheezing develops.

Episodes of apnea may be observed in infants younger than 6 months of age with RSV infection, especially those born prematurely. RSV sometimes is identified in infants dying from sudden infant death syndrome (SIDS), although the association of apnea with SIDS is uncertain. A low-grade fever (usually <39°C) may be noted in infants with bronchiolitis, although they frequently are afebrile. The presence of higher degrees of fever suggests the presence of otitis media. In bronchiolitis, other secondary bacterial infections are very uncommon (<1% of hospitalized patients). The respiratory rate is increased (60 to 80 breaths/min) in moderate or severe cases. Mild tachycardia almost always is present. Nasal flaring, use of accessory muscles of respiration, and chest wall retractions all suggest increased work of breathing. Suprasternal and xiphoid retractions suggest the presence of disease of greater severity. The chest may appear hyperinflated with an increase in the antero-posterior diameter. Cyanosis may be present in severe cases.

On chest auscultation, coarse rhonchi usually are appreciated, and diffuse or localized crackles may be heard on inspiration or expiration. Wheezing is the hallmark of bronchiolitis, but is usually harsher and of lower pitch than that heard in older children with asthma. Wheezing is audible most consistently over the upper anterior chest. Some infants may have hypoxia and respiratory distress in the absence of wheezing or any abnormal breath sounds. Therefore, particular attention must be paid to *the degree of air entry*. This is because, in severe cases, wheezing and crackles may be inaudible because of limited airflow. Finally, more severe forms of illness may be accompanied by prolongation of the expiratory phase of respiration, with reduction of the inspiratory-to-expiratory ratio.

The liver and spleen may be palpable on abdominal examination because these organs may be displaced downward by chest hyperinflation.

Although there are no specific abnormalities of routine laboratory tests in bronchiolitis, a specific diagnosis of RSV infection can be established in many ways. The most rapid method is the detection of viral antigen in respiratory tract secretions using either immunofluorescence or enzyme-linked immunosorbent assays (ELISA). Immunofluorescence tests (requires several hours to complete) may have greater reliability than the very rapid membrane ELISA (completed in minutes). Secretions are obtained by nasal washing or by aspiration directly from the nasopharynx. In infants, these tests are >95% sensitive and specific in comparison with cell culture. Identification of RSV in culture may take several days to weeks. Polymerase chain reaction (PCR) has been used to identify RSV infection, but does not add significantly to the accuracy of antigen-detection assays in infants.

Both immunofluorescence tests and ELISA are less accurate in older children, including those with immunologic deficiencies in whom RSV infection may be life-threatening. Both culture and antigen-detection techniques should be used in these patient groups. However PCR may be the preferable diagnostic method in older children, adults, and immunocompromised individuals.

On conventional chest radiographs, infants with bronchiolitis usually exhibit hyperinflation (flattening of diaphragms and blackening of air spaces), indicating expiratory obstruction of the airways. Atelectasis is commonly observed (again as a result of intraluminal airway obstruction) and often is misinterpreted as representing pulmonary infiltrates. When present, true infiltrates are patchy and diffuse. It is not essential to obtain radiographs in the management of most cases of bronchiolitis, as bacterial superinfection is decidedly uncommon.

MANAGEMENT

The optimal management of bronchiolitis remains controversial, but consensus guidelines have been developed. Most infants with bronchiolitis are treated as outpatients. Hospitalization is indicated if hypoxia or inability to maintain hydration is present. In the hospital, the administration of supplemental oxygen and adequate fluid volumes are sufficient in the considerable majority of cases. Temporary periods of deterioration after admission to the hospital probably are caused by plugging of the airway with inflammatory material, and respond to chest physical therapy or suctioning.

Continuous or intermittent pulse oximetry is effective in monitoring oxygenation. Oxygen saturations should be maintained above 92%, or high enough to prevent dyspnea, depending on the local altitude. Arterial blood gas determinations usually are unnecessary, but may be indicated if oxygen requirements are particularly great, dyspnea is marked, or the infant appears to be tiring from respiratory effort. In these cases, the pCO_2 may be unexpectedly high. Monitoring oxygenation in combination with the work of breathing is critical in identifying the small number of children who will develop respiratory failure and require mechanically assisted ventilation.

Inhaled β-adrenergic (e.g., albuterol) or α-adrenergic (e.g., racemic epinephrine) agents may provide initial reductions in respiratory effort in bronchiolitis. However, the beneficial effects are modest and usually are not observed after repeated dosing. When administered to outpatients with bronchiolitis, these agents do not reduce the eventual need for hospitalization. When administered to inpatients, these drugs reduce neither the duration of hospitalization nor the length of time supplemental oxygen is required. Infants who are unresponsive to the first dose usually do not respond to repeated or higher dosages. There is no apparent benefit from the use of bronchodilators orally, and intravenous therapy usually does not result in greater benefit than aerosol therapy.

In some of the controlled trials of β-adrenergic agents, brief periods of hypoxemia may occur shortly after treatments are administered. It is possible that β-adrenergic agents are inducing ventilation/perfusion mismatches in the lungs of some of these treated patients. Studies of α-adrenergic agents have noted the development of generalized pallor and, in one case, myocardial infarction after administration. Therefore, the use of α- and β-adrenergic agents exposes the infant to at least some risk.

Numerous studies of the efficacy of corticosteroids in bronchiolitis have appeared. In most of the studies, corticosteroid therapy has *not* been demonstrated to improve the course of the acute illness, improve lung function, or reduce the number of recurrent wheezing episodes after bronchiolitis. Infants receiving corticosteroids may excrete virus for longer periods than infants not receiving such therapy. The subset of patients with bronchiolitis that may deserve a trial of steroid therapy include those with other evidence of atopy or with repetitive episodes of wheezing.

Ribavirin is an antiviral agent with in vitro activity against RSV. Initial evaluations of this drug demonstrated only small improvements in oxygenation and minor improvements in clinical scores in treated groups. Results of a single study suggested that intubated infants receiving the drug could be removed from assisted ventilation earlier, but the control group had received inhaled water (as opposed to saline) as the placebo, therefore perhaps precipitating airway constriction. There have been no convincingly positive subsequent evaluations of ribavirin using inhaled saline as placebo. Ribavirin is also highly expensive to use. Because most infants will not derive sufficient benefit to justify the use of ribavirin, it should be considered only in life-threatening disease (respiratory failure, especially in those with preexisting lung or heart disease).

The RSV immunoglobulin preparations (RespiGam and Synagis) are effective in prevention of RSV infection (see later), but do not affect the rate of clinical recovery. Therefore, the use of these compounds as therapeutic agents cannot be defended.

Acute otitis media is a frequent finding during the course of RSV bronchiolitis. Other secondary bacterial infections are uncommon during RSV infection in developed countries, although the situation may be different in developing nations. Antibiotic therapy usually is unnecessary, but if instituted early in the course of bronchiolitis empirically, should be discontinued as soon as the diagnosis of RSV or parainfluenza virus infection has been established. The development of new infiltrates or markedly higher fevers a few days into the course of bronchiolitis may suggest that bacterial secondary infection has occurred. Therapy with an agent such as ceftriaxone or oxacillin could then be considered.

PREVENTIVE MEASURES

RSV infection appears to be spread predominantly by contact with secretions of infected individuals, and possibly by large-droplet aerosols. The possibility for spread of infection in hospitals is great. As much as possible, hospitalized infants should be placed in private rooms. Handwashing before and after patient contact is essential. Gowns should be worn by anyone whose clothing will come in contact either with the patient, his bedclothes, or other objects possibly contaminated by patient secretions. The wearing of masks is not essential in preventing nosocomial spread of infection. In the home, an infant/child at high risk for serious outcomes of RSV infection should be kept away from older siblings and adults with respiratory illnesses. Those caring for these infants should wash their hands before and after handling the infant. RSV antibody preparations (palivizumab [Synagis]) and RSV immunoglobulin (RSVIG [RespiGam]) have been used to prevent RSV infection in high-risk infants, although RSVIG is no longer available. Palivizumab is a humanized, monoclonal preparation of neutralizing antibody directed against the RSV fusion protein. The compound consists of native mouse antibody reconstructed with human amino acid sequences, so that it is more than 95% homologous with human antibodies. Protection against RSV infection can be achieved with intramuscular injections.

In infants born prematurely (both with and without CLD), injection of palivizumab at monthly intervals throughout the RSV epidemic season reduces the need for hospitalization by approximately 50%. A reduction in hospitalization rates for other respiratory viruses does not occur.

The recommended dose is 15 mg/kg of body weight intramuscularly on a monthly basis beginning just before the RSV season, and continuing until RSV activity has nearly disappeared from the community. Patient groups in whom the use of palivizumab should be considered are included in Table 78.1. Trials of the safety and efficacy of palivizumab in infants with congenital heart disease are in progress.

Attempts to develop vaccines against RSV have met with substantial issues of safety and efficacy. It is unlikely that a vaccine will be available for many years.

Families of infected infants should be educated on the importance of handwashing to prevent secondary spread of RSV infection to family contacts. Exposure to cigarette smoke may have deleterious effects on the course of bronchiolitis in infants, and avoidance of smoke exposure should be stressed. Recurrent wheezing occurs commonly after bronchiolitis. However, at least in the first few years of life, this is unrelated to exposure to agents that are known to precipitate asthma (e.g., dust, pollen, animal dander). Therefore, it may be helpful to counsel against undertaking significant asthma control measures unless another family member has asthma.

COURSE AND PROGNOSIS

Most infants hospitalized for bronchiolitis recover sufficiently (oxygen saturation >95% on room air, oral intake enough to prevent dehydration) to be discharged in 48 to 72 hours.

TABLE 78.1

PATIENT GROUPS FOR WHOM PALIVIZUMAB (SYNAGIS) PROPHYLAXIS SHOULD BE CONSIDERED

- Infants <24 months with chronic lung disease of prematurity (CLD) requiring medical intervention in the past 6 months.
- Infants born at less than 28 weeks gestation without CLD who are less than 12 months of age at the onset of the RSV season.
- Infants born at <32 weeks gestation without CLD who are less than 6 months of age at the onset of the RSV season.
- Infants born at 32–35 weeks gestation without CLD who have other risk factors (crowded living conditions including school-aged siblings in the home, exposure to pollutants in the environment, day care attendance, congenital airway abnormalities, or neuromuscular disease) making RSV LRI more likely.
- Other medical conditions in which RSV LRI may prove life-threatening.
- Children ≤24 months of age with hemodynamically significant heart disease.

Significant deterioration after hospitalization is uncommon, although transient periods in which respiratory distress increases may be encountered. As noted, these episodes usually are caused by airway plugging and respond to suctioning and chest physical therapy. Fewer than 10% of hospitalized infants require mechanically assisted ventilation. These infants almost always are recognizable at the time of hospitalization or deteriorate shortly thereafter. Therefore, once the infant appears stable, recovery can be expected.

Infants in whom respiratory failure develops, especially those with CLD, have in the past required ventilatory assistance for 1 to 2 weeks. If infants are not recovering after ventilation for 1 week, an investigation for other underlying problems (e.g., cystic fibrosis, heart disease, immune deficiency) should be initiated. It does appear that, even among those infants who require hospitalization, the use of palivizumab reduces the subsequent severity of illness. Therefore, even these more severely affected infants seem to require much shorter periods of assisted ventilation than previously required.

Although some degree of wheezing may still be present after discharge, normal health should be regained within 1 to 2 weeks. Many infants, perhaps most, have repeated episodes of wheezing through the first few years of life. The severity of these wheezing episodes (which usually are precipitated by infection with other respiratory viruses or repeat RSV infections) almost always is less than that with the primary RSV infection. Whether these repeated wheezing episodes are a result of the initial RSV infection, or whether the initial RSV-related wheezing episode is a marker of an underlying tendency to development of airway obstruction, remains unclear. Most evidence supports the latter explanation. Over time, the number of recurrent wheezing episodes continues to decline, and approaches the rate of wheezing in the general population by adolescence. Most school-aged individuals who are still experiencing recurrent wheezing after bronchiolitis in infancy are atopic. Therefore, recurrent wheezing in the older child (and many years after an episode of bronchiolitis) usually can be diagnosed as atopic asthma.

Very rarely, RSV infection in infancy can be complicated by the development of bronchiolitis obliterans. This disease is characterized by fibrous obliteration of the bronchioles. Children with this complication have, during the years after an infantile bronchiolitis episode, very frequent or continuous wheezing. Chest radiographs always reveal hyperinflation, and pulmonary function testing reveals evidence of irreversible obstructive lung disease.

PEARLS

- Acute wheezing episodes in infancy almost always are related etiologically to viral infection. Gastroesophageal reflux is another common cause in early infancy.
- Poor oral intake, reduced aeration, markedly increased work of breathing, and oxygen saturations below 92% (sea level) are the best indicators of the need for hospitalization.
- Most hospitalized infants with bronchiolitis recover with no therapeutic measures other than supplemental oxygen and fluid replacement.

- Auscultatory findings may worsen suddenly, and then improve markedly after chest physical therapy and suctioning. These phenomena probably are due to plugging of the airway with inflammatory debris.
- Repeated wheezing episodes are common in the first few years after bronchiolitis, but become less severe and less frequent during school age.

Suggested Readings

American Academy of Pediatrics. Respiratory syncytial virus. In: Pickering LK, ed. *2003 red book: report of the Committee on Infectious Diseases*. 26th ed. Elk Grove Village, IL: American Academy of Pediatrics; 2003:523–528.

Flores G, Horwitz RI. Efficacy of β_2-agonists in bronchiolitis: a reappraisal and meta-analysis. *Pediatrics* 1997;100:233–239.

Perlstein PH, et al. Evaluation of an evidence-based guideline for bronchiolitis. *Pediatrics* 1999;104:1334–1341.

Shay DK, Holman RC, Roosevelt GE, et al. Bronchiolitis-associated mortality and estimates of respiratory syncytial virus-associated deaths among US children, 1979–1997. *J Infect Dis* 2001;183:16–22.

CHAPTER 79 ■ PERIORBITAL AND ORBITAL CELLULITIS

JEAN F. KENNY

Periocular infections, which cause periorbital erythema and edema, are clinically distinguished as periorbital (preseptal) cellulitis and orbital (postseptal) cellulitis. These infections usually are unilateral. The orbital septum is a fascial extension of the periosteum that continues vertically from the orbital rim to the tarsal plates of the eyelids. This layer provides a barrier that almost totally prevents infection superficial to it from spreading to the orbit and retroorbital tissues. Infection anterior to the septum is termed *periorbital* or *preseptal cellulitis*. This presents clinically as erythema and edema of the eyelids and surrounding tissue without proptosis, ophthalmoplegia, or loss of visual acuity. With *orbital cellulitis* or infections posterior to the septum, the patient presents with periorbital erythema and edema but also with evidence of deeper infection, including proptosis or ophthalmoplegia, sometimes associated with complete or partial loss of vision. Although these two entities usually are separated based on clinical signs, occasional patients admitted with clinical preseptal disease develop signs of orbital cellulitis. Because they differ in severity and urgency of management, it is important early in a patient's course to distinguish between the two. A classification or staging system originally proposed by Chandler and associates in 1970 has been modified and continues to be used as a guide for diagnosis and treatment (Table 79.1).

Periorbital cellulitis may develop in three ways: (1) secondary to skin infections around the eye or eyelids or infections of the anterior ocular structures, (2) cellulitis resulting from bacteremic spread from the nasopharynx, and (3) sterile inflammation secondary to severe sinusitis. Trauma to facial skin with or without loss of skin integrity, infected varicella lesions or insect bites, cutaneous foreign bodies, impetigo, or other dermatitis may precede the development of periorbital cellulitis. Dacryoadenitis/cystitis, severe conjunctivitis, or hordeolum (stye) may result in periorbital inflammation. Organisms that cause these infections usually are those that infect wounds: *Staphylococcus aureus* and *Streptococcus pyogenes*. Much less often, gram-negative or anaerobic organisms are isolated.

Idiopathic or bacteremic periorbital cellulitis occurs in young children (most younger than 3 years of age) who have a viral respiratory infection. The viral infection predisposes the respiratory mucosa to invasion by pathogenic respiratory bacteria, resulting in bacteremia that seeds the periorbital area. In some patients meningitis also may develop. Before immunization against *Haemophilus influenzae* type b, most cases of periorbital cellulitis were due to this organism, with most of the remainder caused by *Streptococcus pneumoniaes*. Because of routine immunization against *H. influenzae* type b, bacteremic periorbital cellulitis is now much less common. However, these bacteria still may be the cause in an unimmunized or immunodeficient child.

Periorbital erythema and edema may occur secondary to severe sinusitis, usually ethmoiditis. Blood and periorbital tissue usually are sterile in this type of periorbital disease, which distinguishes it from the other forms. The responsible organisms most often cultured from the sinuses are those known to cause acute sinusitis: *S. pneumoniae*, nontypeable *H. influenzae*, and *Moraxella catarrhalis*. Species of *Staphylococcus* and other types of streptococci are less commonly isolated.

Most cases of *orbital cellulitis* in children are associated with severe sinusitis, usually ethmoiditis, although other sinuses may be involved, particularly in older childen. Less commonly, orbital cellulitis occurs secondary to a penetrating wound, severe infection of midfacial skin, orbital fracture, ocular surgery, dental infection, or intracranial infection. Patients may have recurrent or chronic sinusitis or a history of respiratory allergy. The ethmoid air cells are separated from the orbit by a thin connective-tissue barrier, the lamina papyracea. Infection may pass from sinus to orbit through dehiscences or vascular foramina in this membrane. Infection also may spread through valveless venous networks, which connect the sinuses, orbits, and cavernous sinus. Orbital infections may result in edema and inflammation of orbital structures only or, more often, ethmoid osteitis with subperiosteal or orbital abscess (Table 79.1). Bacteria that have been isolated from blood or pus obtained at surgery are numerous and include *S. pneumoniae*, nontypeable *H. influenzae*, *S. aureus*, *S. pyogenes*, enterococci, and respiratory tract anaerobic and microaerophilic organisms. Gram-negative bacteria, including Enterobacteriaceae and, rarely, species of *Pseudomonas*, have been isolated. Mixtures of aerobic and anaerobic flora not uncommonly are isolated from surgically obtained pus.

Because most patients with periorbital or orbital cellulitis have respiratory disease/sinusitis, these infections are more common during the respiratory virus season. The less common infections associated with trauma or skin infection may be seen throughout the year. Periorbital disease after respiratory infection usually occurs in children younger than 5 years of age, with bacteremic forms usually in children younger than 3 years of age. Orbital infections are much less common than periorbital infections and may occur from preschool to teenage years. In most series, the mean age of patients with orbital infections is older than with periorbital disease, the incidence peaking in children of elementary school age.

Other causes of unilateral periorbital edema or redness include trauma, surgical procedures, insect bites, or allergy to substances inoculated into the eye. Neoplasms (including leukemia, lymphoma, retinoblastoma, rhabdomyosarcoma, metastatic carcinoma, and neuroblastoma), ruptured dermoid cyst, histiocytosis, and others may cause periorbital fullness and proptosis. Systemic granulomatous diseases and vasculitides

TABLE 79.1

SUGGESTED STAGING AND MANAGEMENT OF ORBITAL CELLULITIS

Stage I	More likely periorbital (preseptal). Eyelid swelling with sinusitis. Occasionally febrile. CT scan normal except for periorbital swelling and sinusitis. *Management:* outpatient antibiotics (IM followed by PO), or for more ill child hospitalize with IV antibiotics followed by PO.
Stage II	Edema of orbital lining, chemosis, proptosis, limitation of extraocular movement, fever. CT scan: no subperiosteal abscess. Might see mucosal edema or swelling. *Management:* inpatient IV antibiotics.
Stage III	Occasional visual loss. Progression of changes seen in stage II. CT scan: subperiosteal abscess; globe displacement; intraconal involvement of extraocular muscles. *Management:* inpatient IV antibiotics. Surgical drainage if not improved after 24 h.
Stage IV	Ophthalmoplegia with visual loss. CT scan: proptosis; abscess formation involving the extraocular muscles and orbital fat. Periosteal rupture. *Management:* IV antibiotics and surgical drainage.

Modified from Starky CR, Steele RW. Medical management of orbital cellulitis. *Pediatr Infect Dis J* 2001;20:1002–1005, with permission.

have been associated with acute orbital inflammation. Usually, history and absence of signs of infection distinguish these entities from periorbital/orbital cellulitis.

Orbital pseudotumor, a noninfectious inflammation of orbital tissues that is responsive to steroids, may present with symptoms and signs very similar to those of orbital cellulitis. Orbital pseudotumor may be unilateral or bilateral, and usually is without associated sinusitis. A computed tomography (CT) scan may show a shaggy orbital infiltrate or a discrete mass molded to the globe or orbital nerve sheath. This is in contrast to signs of medial inflammation or abscess formation seen with orbital infection. An ophthalmologist should advise if diagnosis is uncertain.

HISTORY

Periorbital Cellulitis

In the type of periorbital cellulitis associated with superficial infection, there may be a history of penetrating or nonpenetrating trauma to the face, preceding conjunctivitis, or infection of an anterior ocular structure or surrounding facial skin. Swelling and inflammation of periorbital tissues follow over one to several days. Partial or complete closure of the involved eye may be reported. Depending on the severity of the cellulitis, fever and constitutional symptoms are variable but often minimal. In the idiopathic or bacteremic form of periorbital cellulitis, there is a history of symptoms characteristic of a viral respiratory infection followed by an acute increase in fever (usually >39°C), with

rapid swelling and inflammation of the eyelids that begins medially. Swelling and complete closure of the eye may develop overnight. The child is reported to look ill and may be irritable and anorectic. In preseptal cellulitis associated with sinusitis, the child also has a history of respiratory symptoms for several days usually followed by more gradual swelling and inflammation of the eyelids. The swelling may be intermittent at first, noted only for a few hours in the morning, but then becomes progressively worse and persistent. There may be other symptoms of sinusitis, including headache, eye pain, cough worse at night, and purulent nasal drainage. Fever may be significant but often is low grade.

Orbital Cellulitis

In most patients with orbital cellulitis there is a preceding respiratory illness with or without purulent nasal drainage followed by the development of headache and eye pain. Sudden swelling and reddening of the eye follows. The patient may report decreased or double vision, and pain with eye movement. In some patients, severe headache associated with vomiting suggests central nervous system extension of infection. Rarely, there may be a history of dental infection on the ipsilateral side or a skin infection on the malar area of the face. A rare form of posterior orbital cellulitis results in the "orbital apex" syndrome. The patient reports symptoms of sinusitis, severe visual loss, and inability to move the eye, but there may be minimal external signs of inflammation. This syndrome is associated with sphenoid and ethmoid sinusitis.

PHYSICAL FINDINGS

Periorbital Cellulitis

The physical findings of periorbital and orbital cellulitis usually differentiate the two. In periorbital disease there is swelling, warmth, and erythema of periorbital tissue. Typically, the erythema is pink to red but may be violaceous, particularly in the bacteremic form. The conjunctiva may be inflamed but usually is not edematous. Sometimes ocular secretions are purulent. The position of the eye, extraocular movements, pupillary responses, and usually vision are normal. Although tissue around the eye may be tender, pressure on the globe and movement of the eye is not painful. Sinus tenderness to percussion may be present in older children, but often is difficult to define. Meningismus may be present if the patient is one of the unfortunate few with associated meningitis.

Orbital Cellulitis

The physical findings in orbital cellulitis reflect the deep involvement of orbital structures. In addition to the findings of periorbital inflammation, the eye is proptotic and/or extraocular movements are limited. Movement and palpation of the eye are painful. The globe usually is displaced anteriorly and caudally, with limitation of upward gaze. There may be marked hyperemia and edema of the bulbar conjunctiva. Afferent pupillary reflexes and visual acuity may be impaired. Rarely there is papilledema. As the disease progresses, there may be increased orbital pressure, reduced corneal sensation, and congestion of retinal veins. An ophthalmologist should be consulted for a thorough eye examination. Patients usually have significant fever and may appear toxic and lethargic. A neurologic examination may yield evidence of complicating central nervous system disease, including meningitis, septic cavernous vein thrombosis, or cerebral abscess.

RADIOLOGIC AND LABORATORY STUDIES

The diagnosis may be made clinically, particularly in milder cases of periorbital cellulitis. However, in ill-appearing small infants, patients uncooperative with an eye examination, or patients with such severe edema that the eye cannot be visualized, radiologic scanning is necessary to differentiate preseptal from orbital disease. Because of the urgency of treating orbital infection, scanning should not be delayed. All patients with suspected orbital cellulitis must be scanned to define the extent of orbital and sinus infection and guide any surgical intervention. Both CT and magnetic resonance imaging (MRI) scans have been used, but in the young child, a thin-cut CT scan with contrast is preferable because of the briefer procedure time. MRI may be useful for complicated situations where better soft tissue characterization of the sinus or orbit is required or if there is a suspicion of intracranial extension of infection. In orbital cellulitis, findings on scan may be solely edema of orbital tissues (particularly those medially) or, more commonly, an ethmoid subperiosteal abscess or orbital abscess. Ipsilateral ethmoiditis and possibly infection of other sinuses are present. In preseptal infection, evidence of sinusitis may be present, but otherwise the CT scan is negative.

Cultures (and, where applicable, Gram stains) should be obtained from blood, purulent discharge from facial lesions or conjunctiva, purulent sinus or nasal drainage, and pus obtained at surgery. In periorbital cellulitis secondary to a skin infection or in suspected bacteremic cellulitis, a carefully obtained culture of tissue fluid may yield an organism. This is done by aspiration of the edge of the cellulitis using a tuberculin syringe containing a small amount of nonbacteriostatic saline. Extreme care must be taken not to injure the eye. The saline is not injected but serves to propel into culture medium the small amount of tissue fluid that is aspirated into the tip of the needle. Unfortunately, yield is low from many of these recommended cultures. In patients with sinusitis, the most useful pretreatment culture is that of a sinus aspirate. However, direct sinus culture requires special expertise and usually is not done before the start of therapy. Lumbar punctures were strongly recommended in the past because of the frequent occurrence of meningitis with periorbital cellulitis, usually due to *H. influenzae* type b. Recent recommendations are that this procedure no longer be routine, but be done selectively depending on the patient's clinical presentation. In the more significant periorbital and orbital infections, leukocytosis is present. White blood cell counts and erythrocyte sedimentation rates, which may be elevated initially, may be useful to monitor effectiveness of therapy.

MANAGEMENT

Periorbital Cellulitis

Children with periorbital cellulitis considered ill enough for hospital admission are treated with intravenous antibiotics after appropriate cultures. In patients with infections of skin around the eye, Gram stains of pus may be used initially to guide antibiotic choice. Because orbital cellulitis associated with a superficial skin infection is often due to *S. aureus* or *S. pyogenes*, an antistaphylococcal penicillin (e.g., nafcillin or oxacillin) or first-generation cephalosporin (e.g., cefazolin) may be used. Nafcillin (150 mg/kg/day divided every 6 hours) or cefazolin (100 mg/kg/day divided every 8 hours) should be effective. Alternatives would be clindamycin (40 mg/kg/day divided every 6 to 8 hours) or vancomycin (40 mg/kg/day divided every 6 hours as 1-hour infusions). In communities where methicillin-resistant *S. aureus* (MRSA) infections are frequent, an antibiotic other that a penicillin or cephalosporin may be preferred for initial treatment (see Chapter 93 on MRSA). If gram-negative organisms are suspected, ceftriaxone (50 mg/kg/day) or cefotaxime (150 mg/kg/day divided every 8 hours) may be substituted or added to the antistaphylococcal therapy.

For bacteremic idiopathic periorbital cellulitis or that associated with acute sinusitis, cefuroxime (150 mg/kg/day divided every 8 hours) or ampicillin/sulbactam (200 mg/kg/day divided every 6 hours) has been recommended. An alternate choice of antibiotics would be ceftriaxone with either nafcillin or vancomycin. Ceftriaxone alone has been used successfully in some patients; some experts would recommend a dose of 100 mg/kg/day divided every 12 hours to guard against meningeal inoculation. The total course of therapy usually is 7 to 14 days. Once periorbital swelling has resolved and the patient has been afebrile for 24 to 48 hours, oral therapy may be used to complete the course and the child may be followed as an outpatient.

Orbital Cellulitis

Orbital cellulitis requires urgent care. High-dose intravenous antibiotics should be started as soon as possible after cultures have been taken. Management should involve a team of physicians, including an ophthalmologist and otolaryngologist. If the CT scan shows a well-defined orbital abscess or there is severe ophthalmoplegia and loss of vision, surgical drainage of the abscess and affected sinus should be done immediately. In instances where there is only edema of orbital tissues or a small subperiosteal abscess (the most common finding), medical treatment alone suffices. However, such patients must have assessment of visual acuity, pupillary responses, and ocular motility several times a day. If they worsen or fail to improve in 24 to 48 hours, the CT scan should be repeated and surgery may be necessary.

A number of antibiotic regimens may be effective. Clindamycin (40 mg/kg/day divided every 6 hours) and cefotaxime or ceftriaxone (100 mg/kg/day divided every 12 hours) or cefepime(150 mg/kg/day divided every 8 hours) would provide coverage for the aerobic and anaerobic bacteria that might be present. Other combinations that have been used include nafcillin and ceftriaxone or cefotaxime with or without metronidazole for anaerobic coverage (30 mg/kg/day divided every 6 hours), an antistaphylococcal penicillin with ticarcillin/clavulanate (200 to 300 mg/kg/day divided every 4 to 6 hours), or chloramphenicol (50 to 75 mg/kg/day divided every 6 hours). In instances where there are geographic or patient risk factors for highly penicillin-resistant *Pneumococcus* or MRSA, or complicating central nervous system disease, vancomycin should be substituted for the clindamycin or antistaphylococcal penicillin. For central nervous system disease, the dose of vancomycin is 60 mg/kg/day divided every 6 hours. If initial cultures are positive, antibiotic therapy may be adjusted based on the results. However, if pus is obtained at surgery after the start of therapy, the subsequent cultures may not yield all flora originally present, and it is prudent to continue broad-spectrum therapy. Therapy should be continued until the patient is afebrile and the eye is normal. Total duration of intravenous therapy usually is 10 to 14 days. Longer courses may be required in some patients with especially severe disease or complications. Additional oral antibiotics may be continued for 7 to 14 days after discharge. Nasal decongestants or steroids may be used as adjunctive therapy for patients with sinusitis or allergy, but benefits are unproved.

An ophthalmologist should be consulted for all patients with orbital cellulitis and any child with periorbital disease if the eye cannot be satisfactorily examined. An otolaryngologist should be consulted shortly after admission for all patients with orbital cellulitis and selectively for patients with periorbital disease if concurrent sinusitis is severe or chronic. A neurologist or neurosurgeon should be involved with care of any central nervous system complications. An infectious disease specialist should be consulted if unusual organisms are isolated or if patients fail to respond to appropriate antibiotics.

COURSE AND PROGNOSIS

Periorbital cellulitis usually improves dramatically within a few days after initiating antibiotic therapy. With the rare exception of associated meningitis, serious complications are unusual. Orbital cellulitis resolves more slowly over a period of days, but patients appear clinically much improved soon after the start of appropriate antibiotics and any required surgery. Before the availability of antibiotics, many patients with orbital cellulitis died of central nervous system complications. These still are possible if diagnosis or treatment is delayed. Central nervous system complications include cavernous sinus thrombosis, meningitis, subdural empyema, epidural abscess, brain abscess, and osteomyelitis of the frontal bone (Pott puffy tumor). Permanent strabismus, afferent pupillary defect, and complete or partial loss of vision may occur. Pus may penetrate the orbital septum and drain through an eyelid, resulting in a chronic draining sinus. Gangrene of the eyelids and choroidal and retinal infarction due to vascular compromise have been described.

SPECIAL SITUATIONS

Neonates

Neonates rarely have ethmoiditis or dacryocystitis and more commonly have conjunctivitis, presenting with redness and swelling of the eye. A variety of bacteria have been isolated from conjunctival exudates, including *Staphylococcus* species, hemolytic *Streptococcus* (both groups A and B), enterococci, *Haemophilis* species, Enterobacteriaceae, *Pseudomonas*, and others. *Pseudomonas aeruginosa* may be particularly virulent. Marked erythema and edema of the eyelids may accompany gonococcal and chlamydial infections of the eye. Orbital cellulitis may occur in neonates. There also is a neonatal syndrome presenting like orbital cellulitis associated with maxillary osteomyelitis. Inflammation of the cheek, purulent nasal discharge, periorbital inflammation, and proptosis is characteristic of this infection.

Fungal Orbital Cellulitis

Immunocompromised patients, poorly controlled diabetic patients, and rarely immune-competent children with chronic sinusitis or allergy are at risk for fungal orbital cellulitis. *Aspergillus flavus* and *Aspergillus fumigatus* are isolated most commonly. Mucormycosis or phaeohyphomycosis of the sinuses may precede the orbital disease. In fungal orbital cellulitis, proptosis typically develops more slowly and often is painless. Diagnosis usually is made by biopsy of sinus or other infected tissue. Management includes surgical debridement and antifungal therapy but in severely immunocompromised patients, the prognosis is often poor. Consultation with infectious disease specialist is recommended.

Unusual Causes

A clinical picture of periorbital cellulitis may occur with viral infections of the eye due to adenovirus, herpes simplex virus, and herpes zoster virus. With adenovirus, there may be a history of exposure to an individual with "pink eye." The patient has conjunctival hyperemia with photophobia and abundant clear, watery discharge. On examination, preauricular adenopathy may be present. The eyelids may be swollen and a white membrane covers the palpebral conjunctiva. Punctate keratitis may be seen. In herpetic infections, vesicular or crusted skin lesions of face or eyelid and keratoconjunctivitis may be present. Cat-scratch bacillus, *Mycobacterium tuberculosis* and other mycobacteria, syphilis, *Actinomyces*, and parasites, in particular *Echinococcus granulosus*, have caused orbital cellulitis.

Cavernous Sinus Thrombosis

Patients with orbital cellulitis who have signs of contralateral paresis of ocular muscles or decreased sensation around the eye need to be assessed for cavernous sinus thrombosis. An MRI scan may be helpful.

PEARLS

- Orbital cellulitis is a medical emergency. An ophthalmologist should be consulted for all patients if the eye cannot be satisfactorily examined.
- Periorbital cellulitis usually is associated with local trauma or skin infection, bacteremic spread from the nasopharynx, or severe sinusitis.
- The physical findings of periorbital and orbital cellulitis usually differentiate the two. In periorbital disease, there is swelling, warmth, and erythema of periorbital tissue, but the eye is normal, whereas orbital cellulitis involves the globe with proptosis, impaired or painful extraocular movements, or displacement of the globe.

Suggested Readings

Chandler JR, Langenbrunner DJ, Stevens ER. The pathogenesis of orbital complications in acute sinusitis. *Laryngoscope* 1970;80:1414–1428.

Starky CR, Steele RW. Medical management of orbital cellulitis. *Pediatr Infect Dis* 2001;20:1002–1005.

Wald ER. Periorbital and orbital infections. In: Long SS, Pickering LR, Prober CG, eds. *Principles and practice of pediatric infectious diseases.* 2nd ed. Philadelphia: Churchill Livingstone; 2003:508–513.

CHAPTER 80 ■ URINARY TRACT INFECTIONS

SUE JOAN JUE

Urinary tract infection (UTI) is one of the most common bacterial infections in infants and young children and may lead to serious consequences such as renal scarring, hypertension, and end-stage renal dysfunction. Although most pediatricians are familiar with the treatment of UTI in the otherwise normal healthy child, complicated UTI (e.g., abnormal urinary system, abnormal host, frequent recurrences, and pyelonephritis) can be more of a challenge to manage. Hospitalization usually is indicated for children younger than 2 months of age, at least initially, to receive intravenous antibiotics. Other indications for hospitalization of children with suspected UTI include toxic appearance, vomiting with inability to take oral antibiotics, the presence of an abnormal urinary collecting system, immunocompromised patients (e.g., renal transplant recipients, patients on dialysis), pyelonephritis, and those who are not responding to outpatient therapy.

The prevalence of UTI varies by age and sex. In the newborn period, approximately 1% to 2% of both girls and boys have a UTI. In the first 3 months of life, UTI is more common in boys, after which it occurs more commonly in girls. The prevalence in girls 1 to 5 years of age is 1% to 3%, whereas few infections occur in boys of the same age. UTI is a common cause of fever in infants and young children, but declines as an etiology with increasing age. Although it should not be considered an indication for circumcision, during the first year of life uncircumcised infant boys have as much as a 10-fold higher incidence of UTI than circumcised boys, and more infections than girls of that age. Other risk factors for UTI include sexual activity, sexual abuse, use of bubble bath, constipation, pinworm infection, voiding dysfunction, a sibling with vesicoureteral reflux VUR, urologic abnormalities, neurogenic bladder, or the presence of an indwelling urinary catheter. Definitions used for infections of the urinary tract include the following:

> *UTI*: any microbial infection of the bladder, ureters, or collecting system of the kidneys.
> *Urethritis*: inflammation/infection of the urethra alone.
> *Cystitis*: urinary tract infection of the bladder.
> *Pyelonephritis*: UTI involving the kidney.
> *VUR*: backflow of urine from the bladder into the ureters.

Bacteria from the family Enterobacteriaceae are the most common isolates obtained from urine culture. *Escherichia coli* accounts for 70% to 90% of infections, and the other 10% are usually due to *Klebsiella*, *Enterobacter*, or *Citrobacter* species. Children with recurrent UTI or those with abnormal bladders may have less common organisms, such as *Proteus*, *Pseudomonas*, *Serratia*, or *Morganella*. The most common gram-positive organism isolated in young children with UTI is enterococcus; in adolescent girls, it is *Staphylococcus saprophyticus*, a coagulase-negative staphylococcus. Group B streptococci are unusual urinary pathogens but can be isolated from infected urine in neonates and pregnant women. Other less common causes of UTI in children include adenovirus and *Candida*.

UTI usually are caused by bacteria that normally inhabit the gastrointestinal tract, colonize the perineum, and cause infection by ascending from the urethra into the bladder. Once in the bladder, bacteria can then ascend the ureters and kidneys, particularly if VUR is present. Some strains of *E. coli* exhibit "P" pili, which facilitate mucosal attachment, enabling the bacteria to climb the ureters and avoid being washed out by the flow of urine. These virulent strains can thereby cause pyelonephritis in the absence of VUR. Bacteria without pili also can reach the kidneys in patients with VUR. The attachment of bacteria to the mucosa also may be influenced by blood group antigens expressed on the surface of the genitourinary tract mucosa. This may explain the increased frequency of the blood group P_1, Lewis blood group "nonsecretor" status, and recessive blood group phenotypes in women and children with recurrent UTI.

VESICOURETERAL REFLUX

VUR is present in 30% to 35% of children with UTI. Reflux is congenital and results from the deficiency of the longitudinal muscle of the submucosal ureter with shortening of the intramural portion of the ureter as it traverses the bladder wall. This deficiency results in the absence of the normal valvelike function of the ureter that blocks retrograde flow of urine from the bladder into the ureters and subsequently into the kidneys. VUR is graded in five stages: I, urine does not reach the kidneys; II, flow of urine extends up the renal pelvis without dilatation of the ureters; III, retrograde flow of urine extends up into the kidneys with mild dilatation of the ureter and renal pelvis; IV, moderate dilatation of the ureters with obliteration of the renal pelvises occurs; V, dilatation and tortuosity of the ureters with moderate dilatation of the renal pelvis. Grades I to III of VUR resolve spontaneously in 50% to 75% of children. Grades IV and V resolve spontaneously in only 40% of affected children and may require surgical intervention. VUR is a risk factor for recurrent pyelonephritis and renal scarring. Although controversial, some studies of pediatric pyelonephritis suggest that as many as 10% to 25% of children with renal scarring develop hypertension and 10% develop renal insufficiency.

CLINICAL FINDINGS

The signs and symptoms of UTI are variable and depend on the age of the patient. In neonates, a UTI can manifest as poor feeding, poor weight gain, vomiting, diarrhea, irritability, jaundice, or sepsis with fever. In an older infant, UTI may manifest as fever, failure to thrive, vomiting, diarrhea, colic, sepsis, jaundice, or foul-smelling urine. An older toddler may complain of abdominal or suprapubic pain, or have vomiting, diarrhea, foul- or strong-smelling urine, poor growth, constipation, or abnormal voiding patterns. By the time the child is school aged, symptoms more closely mimic that of adults and include dysuria, frequency, urgency, abdominal pain, back pain, incontinence, enuresis, and occasionally fever. It may be very difficult to distinguish between infection of the upper urinary tract and of the lower urinary tract on clinical grounds alone, especially in infants and young children. Infection in both locations can cause fever and abdominal pain, although the fever associated with pyelonephritis tends to be of higher grade. On physical examination, important findings suggesting pyelonephritis include hypertension, abdominal or flank masses, and costovertebral angle tenderness.

The symptoms of UTI in children can be mimicked by urethritis, meatal irritation, vulvovaginitis, topical irritants (e.g., bubble bath, soaps, laundry detergents, dyes/scents in clothing), medications, vaginal foreign body, pinworm infection, trauma (e.g., masturbation, sexual abuse), and emotional stress.

DIAGNOSIS

One simple laboratory test that is useful in the diagnosis of UTI is a urinalysis. Findings on a urinalysis that suggest UTI include the presence of white blood cells (WBCs) >10 to 15 per high-power field, blood RBCs, leukocyte esterase, positive nitrite test, protein, and the presence of bacteria (positive Gram stain of unspun drop of urine indicates $>10^5$ organisms/mL). Although the presence of WBCs (pyuria) alone can be very predictive of UTI in adults, their presence in children without bacteriuria is not a reliable predictor of infection.

Other than UTI, pyuria can be found in children in a number of other clinical settings, including vaginal washout with voiding, fever, viral infections, and chemical irritation from bubble baths. Less common causes of pyuria include appendicitis, glomerulonephritis, and renal tuberculosis.

Of paramount importance in the diagnosis of UTI is a properly obtained urine culture (Table 80.1). The old adage, "garbage in, garbage out" applies to the collection of urinary specimens. Urine for urinalysis and culture is obtained by one of four methods. In neonates and young infants, a suprapubic aspirate obtained from the bladder is probably the most sterile method available. Any bacterial growth from urine obtained by this method is indicative of a UTI. The next most sterile method to obtain urine for culture is by catheterization of the bladder. Usually, bacterial growth $\geq 10^4$ of a single organism is indicative of a UTI from a catheterized specimen. A clean-catch midstream urine specimen can be obtained from the older, more cooperative child, and growth of bacteria $\geq 10^5$ of a single organism is highly suspect for infection. The last method for obtaining urine, often used in young infants, is a bagged specimen, which is the least sterile method used and frequently is contaminated from the perineum. A bagged urine specimen may be helpful only if the culture is sterile (and it rarely is!).

MANAGEMENT

The choice of antibiotic to treat UTI is based on the most likely pathogen, the patient's age, and the severity of illness. Gram stain of the urine is underused and can aid in selecting appropriate empiric antibiotic therapy. Hospitalization for IV antibiotics and closer monitoring is indicated for neonates, toxic-appearing children, those with pyelonephritis, and in children at risk for complicated infections (e.g., urologic abnormalities, renal transplant recipients, immunocompromised hosts). Initial IV therapy for neonates and older children includes ampicillin (100 to 200 mg/kg/day IV divided every 6 hours) and an aminoglycoside (gentamicin 6 mg/ kg/day IV divided every 8 hours), or a third-generation cephalosporin alone (ceftriaxone 50 mg/kg/day IV divided every 12 to 24 hours, or cefotaxime 100 to 150 mg/kg/day divided IV every 8 hours). Another alternative for older infants and children with UTI is trimethoprim (TMP)–sulfamethoxazole (SMX); TMP 8 mg/kg/day, SMX 40 mg/kg/day IV divided every 12 hours. Once the urinary pathogen is identified and sensitivities are known, the antibiotic regimen can be adjusted. Duration of IV antibiotics depends on clinical response but usually is continued for at least 3 days until blood and urine cultures are negative, or for at least 24 hours after the patient has become afebrile and is able to switch to oral medications.

There are several oral antibiotics effective in treating uncomplicated UTI due to susceptible strains, such as sulfasoxazole (120 to 150 mg/kg/day PO given every 6 hours), nitrofurantoin (5 to 7 mg/kg/day PO every 6 hours), or TMP–SMX (8 mg/kg/day TMP with 40 mg/kg/day SMX, PO every 12 hours). Increasing resistance of E. coli to amoxicillin makes this drug less useful. The usual length of therapy for cystitis is 7 to 10 days, and for pyelonephritis 10 to 14 days. If the child has evidence of VUR or a history of recurrent UTI (three or more episodes per year), prophylactic antibiotics should be administered for 6 months or longer to prevent recurrences. Antibiotics used for prophylaxis include TMP–SMX (2 mg/kg of TMP up to 40 mg at bedtime), nitrofurantoin (1 to 2 mg/kg up to 50 mg at bedtime), or TMP alone (2 mg/kg up to 50 mg at bedtime). If no episodes of breakthrough infection occur, antibiotic prophylaxis can be discontinued. If infection recurs, prophylactic antibiotics should be resumed.

Based on expert opinion, imaging studies are indicated after the first documented UTI in all boys and girls younger than 5 to 6 years of age. Diagnostic imaging can be used to detect congenital or acquired abnormalities of the urinary tract, including posterior urethral valves in boys, VUR, dysplasia of the kidneys, hydronephrosis, renal scarring, and renal stones. Renal ultrasonography is a noninvasive means of accessing kidney size, shape, and position as well as detecting urinary obstruction or renal abscess. A voiding cystourethrogram (VCUG) defines the presence and grade of VUR and can be used to detect posterior urethral valves in boys. There are

TABLE 80.1

INTERPRETATION OF CULTURE RESULTS

Method of collection	Likelihood of urinary tract infection	
	Bacterial growth[a]	UTI
Suprapubic aspiration	Any growth of bacteria	Probable
Catheterization	$>10^4$	Probable
	$>10^3$	Suspect, repeat culture
	$<10^3$	Infection unlikely
Clean-catch	$\geq 10^5$	Probable
	$<10^3$	Suspect, repeat culture
	$>10^3$	Infection unlikely

[a]Single organism, colonies/mL.

two radionuclide scans available to evaluate pyelonephritis, dimercaptosuccinic acid (DMSA) and glucoheptonate, both of which are coupled to technetium-99 and injected IV. The renal tubular cells take up the isotope and defects are seen wherever there is acute inflammation of the renal parenchyma (pyelonephritis) or preexisting scars. In the past, the VCUG typically was delayed for several weeks until after the inflammation from the acute infection had resolved. Most nephrologists now advocate obtaining it at the time of the acute infection, and compliance with testing is improved.

COURSE AND PROGNOSIS

Children with uncomplicated UTI usually respond rapidly to appropriate antibiotics and defervesce within 24 to 48 hours. Any child with a documented UTI should have careful follow-up. A urine culture obtained 48 hours after starting antibiotic therapy demonstrates antibiotic effectiveness, but usually is unnecessary in the child with an uncomplicated infection responding to therapy. A repeat urine culture is deemed necessary in the child with complicated UTI, failure to respond clinically, or recurrent symptoms.

In infants younger than 6 months of age, bacteremia associated with UTI is more likely and ranges from 6% to 18%. Meningitis also can occur, particularly in infants younger than 3 months of age. Unusual complications include the development of a renal abscess or stones. Severe VUR can lead to repeated UTI with subsequent renal scarring. If renal scarring occurs, it can then lead to renal failure, growth failure, and hypertension.

Children with UTI have a risk of repeated infections, especially if they have VUR or abnormal urinary tract anatomy. From 8% to 30% of children with UTI experience one or more symptomatic reinfections, usually within the first 6 months after the initial infection. Patients with complicated UTI or with anatomic abnormalities (e.g., urinary obstruction, posterior urethral valves, hydronephrosis) should be referred to a pediatric nephrologist/urologist. For patients who are immunocompromised, or have unusual or multiresistant urinary pathogens, consultation from a pediatric infectious disease specialist should be sought. Children with VUR should be followed with yearly VCUG examinations.

PEARLS

- A properly obtained urine culture is priceless.
- Pyuria without bacteriuria is not as diagnostic of UTI in children as in adults.
- In newborns and young infants, UTI is associated more often with bacteremia. In this age group, it also is clinically difficult to distinguish between upper tract and lower tract disease.
- Renal scarring is more likely to complicate a UTI in children younger than 5 years of age.

Suggested Readings

American Academy of Pediatrics. Practice guideline: the diagnosis, treatment, and evaluation of the initial urinary tract infection in febrile infants and young children (AC9830). *Pediatrics* 1999;103:843–852.

Elder JS, Peters CA, Arant BS Jr, et al. Pediatric vesicoureteral reflux guidelines panel summary report on the management of primary vesicoureteral reflux in children. *J Urol* 1997;157:1846.

Hoberman A, Wald ER, Hickey RW, et al. Oral versus initial intravenous therapy for urinary tract infections in young febrile children. *Pediatrics* 1999;104:79. Comment.

Johnson CE. New advances in childhood urinary tract infections. *Pediatr Rev* 1999;20:335–343.

Lohr JA, Downs SM, Schlager TA. Urinary tract infections. In: Long SS, Pickering LK, Prober CG, eds. *Principles and practice of pediatric infectious diseases*. 2nd ed. New York: Churchill Livingstone; 2003:323–328.

Williams G, Lee A, Craig J. Antibiotics for the prevention of urinary tract infection in children: a systematic review of randomized controlled trials. *J Pediatr* 2001;138:868–874.

CHAPTER 81 ■ CELLULITIS AND NECROTIZING FASCIITIS

KRISTINA A. BRYANT

CELLULITIS

Cellulitis is an infection of the dermis and subcutaneous fat, with relative sparing of the epidermis. Infection may occur at any age; the median age of children with cellulitis is 5 years. Infections in boys slightly outnumber infections in girls. The lower extremity is the most common site of infection.

Group A streptococci (GAS) and *Staphylococcus aureus* account for most cases of cellulitis in immunocompetent children. Skin and soft-tissue infections with methicillin-resistant *S. aureus* (MRSA) have been increasing in many communities, even in children who lack traditional risk factors. Group B streptococci may cause cellulitis in young infants. Less common causes of cellulitis include *Streptococcus pneumoniae*, *Pseudomonas aeruginosa*, *Escherichia coli*, and *Proteus mirabilis*.

Specific exposures or mechanisms of tissue injury are associated with infection caused by unusual organisms. *Vibrio* species (especially *Vibrio vulnificus*) cause cellulitis and wound infection after contact with shellfish or seawater. *Pasturella multocida* is frequently isolated from infections caused by dog and cat bites, along with *S. aureus*, *Streptococcus intermedius*, and a host of anaerobic bacteria. Cellulitis after human bites also is polymicrobial in origin; *Eikenella corrodens* is a common pathogen, especially after "clenched fist" injuries. Anaerobic bacteria, including *Prevotella* species, *Bacteroides fragilis*, and *Peptostreptococcus* species, have been isolated from body-piercing site infections in adolescents.

Even minor disruptions of skin integrity may predispose to cellulitis. Abrasions, insect bites, and skin conditions such as eczema can lead to infection. Varicella is a common risk factor for cellulitis in children. Bacterial skin colonization usually precedes infection. Injury to the epidermis then facilitates tissue invasion. Alternatively, penetrating injuries like bite wounds may inoculate pathogenic bacteria directly into the dermis.

Cellulitis must be distinguished from other causes of red skin, including atopic or contact dermatitis, insect bites or stings with a hypersensitivity response, drug reactions, thrombophlebitis, pyoderma gangrenosa, and rarely, erythema nodosum. Osteomyelitis may present with erythema and swelling over the infected site. Swelling and redness near a joint might be confused with septic arthritis. Early necrotizing fasciitis may mimic cellulitis.

Clinical Findings

Erythema, warmth, edema, and pain are the hallmarks of cellulitis. Low-grade fever and regional lymphadenopathy may occur. The clinical findings may suggest the specific causative organism. *Erysipelas* is a distinctive form of superficial cellulitis with lymphatic involvement. It usually is caused by GAS; less commonly, group G streptococci, *S. pneumoniae*, and *S. aureus* have been isolated. An intensely red lesion with sharply demarcated, slightly raised borders is characteristic. Rapid enlargement of the lesion occurs, often several millimeters per hour. Fever, chills, malaise, and myalgias may precede or coexist with the skin findings. Bacteremia often is present. Recurrent infections may damage lymphatic channels and cause chronic lymphedema. *Ecthyma* also is caused by GAS; it can be seen as a complication of impetigo and involves invasion of the dermis as well as epidermis. A vesicle or vesicopustule appears that ruptures and crusts, leaving a central eschar surrounded by a ring of red induration. Removal of the eschar reveals a deep ulcer with a purulent base. Unlike the more superficial impetigo, ecthyma heals with scarring.

Erysipeloid is caused by *Erysipelothrix rhusiopathiae*, a gram-positive bacillus that causes disease in a variety of mammals, fish, and birds. Human infection follows contact with infected fish, animals, or animal products, and manifests as painful, purplish erythema involving the fingers and hands. Erysipeloid can be distinguished from erysipelas by a slower progression of erythema, central clearing of lesions, and minimal systemic signs.

Ecthyma gangrenosa sometimes is seen in immunocompromised children as a complication of *Pseudomonas* or *Aspergillus* infection. Hematogenous dissemination results in septic emboli that lodge in small blood vessels of the skin and subsequently establish foci of infection. Initially, these lesions appear as round, purple macules that undergo central necrosis, leaving deep, "punched-out" ulcers with a necrotic base. Scarring nearly always occurs after resolution.

Laboratory Evaluation

Aspirate cultures from the area of cellulitis yield a pathogen in up to 50% of cases. Povidone–iodine is applied to the skin and allowed to dry. A 21- to 23-gauge needle attached to a 5-mL syringe is used to aspirate from the area of maximal inflammation, often either the central zone or the leading edge. Usually, one to two drops of serosanguinous fluid are obtained. Nonbacteriostatic saline is used to flush this fluid from the needle onto culture media. If no fluid is obtained, 0.2 mL of nonbacteriostatic saline can be inoculated into the area of inflammation and withdrawn.

Only 2% of children with cellulitis have a positive blood culture. In one study, recovery of contaminants exceeded true pathogens by 2:1. Routine blood cultures in children with cellulitis are not cost-effective and should be reserved for young or toxic children.

Management

Empiric therapy for most cases of cellulitis should be directed against GAS and *S. aureus*. Knowledge of local antibiotic susceptibility patterns of *S. aureus* is crucial. In communities where MRSA accounts for 10% to 15% of community-acquired *S. aureus* isolates (CA-MRSA), clindamycin should be included in the empiric regimen. Otherwise, therapy may be initiated with an antistaphylococcal penicillin (e.g., oxacillin or nafcillin) or with a first-generation cephalosporin (e.g., cefazolin). Some communities have reported high rates of clindamycin resistance in community-acquired *S. aureus* isolates. When local clindamycin resistance rates exceed 10% to 15%, empiric therapy should also include oral trimethoprim–sulfamethoxazole for mild infections and intravenous vancomycin for severe infections. Because trimethoprim–sulfamethoxazole is not active against GAS, monotherapy with this agent is not optimal for empiric treatment of cellulitis.

Linezolid is an oxazolidinone antibiotic with activity against resistant gram-positive organisms like MRSA. It is available in intravenous and oral formulations. Although not generally recommended for empiric treatment of cellulitis, it can be used for treatment of confirmed clindamycin-resistant MRSA infections.

Because cellulitis occurring after animal bites is polymicrobial, amoxicillin–clavulanate (Augmentin) is the preferred oral empiric therapy; a parenteral formulation, ampicillin–clavulanate (Unasyn), is used if disease is severe. Treatment of penicillin-allergic patients includes clindamycin plus oral trimethoprim–sulfamethoxazole, or if intravenous therapy is needed, an extended-spectrum cephalosporin plus clindamycin. Clindamycin alone does not provide adequate coverage for *Pasteurella* species.

Course and Prognosis

Most children with cellulitis are treated as outpatients. Indications for hospital admission include inability to take oral medications or progressive disease despite oral antibiotic therapy. Intravenous antibiotics are continued until clinical improvement is noted. Cellulitis rarely is associated with sequelae. Occasionally, focal abscess formation occurs, requiring incision and drainage.

Pearls

- Cellulitis after varicella infection frequently is caused by GAS.
- Consider MRSA infection in children with cellulitis that fails to improve with intravenous oxacillin or cefazolin. Knowledge of local *S. aureus* antibiotic resistance rates should guide empiric therapy.

NECROTIZING FASCIITIS

Necrotizing fasciitis is a potentially life-threatening, rapidly progressive soft-tissue infection characterized by subcutaneous tissue necrosis. Thrombosis, vasculitis, and necrosis follow microbial and leukocytic infiltration of deep dermal tissues and superficial fascia. Necrotizing fasciitis, although uncommon, is reported with increasing frequency in children. Unlike adults, most children with necrotizing fasciitis have no chronic underlying medical conditions, although a high proportion with GAS necrotizing fasciitis have preceding varicella infection. Like cellulitis, necrotizing fasciitis often affects the extremities. Infection may arise de novo or subsequent to minor skin trauma such as a scratch or insect bite.

Some studies have suggested an association between the use of nonsteroidal anti-inflammatory drugs (NSAIDs) and the subsequent development of necrotizing fasciitis, particularly after varicella infection. Such an association is at least biologically plausible. In animal studies, NSAIDs alter granulocyte function, including chemotaxis, phagocytosis, and bactericidal activity. Alternatively, NSAIDs may mask the pain and inflammation associated with early necrotizing fasciitis and delay the diagnosis. Avoiding the use of NSAIDs when necrotizing fasciitis is suspected seems prudent. It is unknown whether limiting the use of NSAIDs with primary varicella infection decreases the incidence of necrotizing fasciitis. Type 1 necrotizing fasciitis includes polymicrobial infections with aerobic and anaerobic organisms, including *S. aureus*, *Clostridium* species, *Vibrio* species, *Aeromonas hydrophilia*, Enterobacteriaceae species, *Pseudomonas* species, and *Yersinia enterocolitica*. Type 2 necrotizing fasciitis is caused by GAS. GAS and *S. aureus* cause most cases of necrotizing fasciitis in children. Once rare as a cause of necrotizing fasciitis, community-acquired MRSA (CA-MRSA) is an emerging pathogen.

The diagnosis of necrotizing fasciitis requires a high index of suspicion. Most commonly, early necrotizing fasciitis is confused with cellulitis. When musculoskeletal pain is the prominent presenting symptom, necrotizing fasciitis may be difficult to differentiate from arthritis, tenosynovitis, bursitis, or myositis.

Clinical Findings

Like cellulitis, early necrotizing fasciitis may present with erythema, warmth, induration, and swelling. Bullae filled with clear fluid may be seen initially; these evolve into maroon or violaceous lesions. A peau d'orange appearance of the affected skin is a late finding. Crepitus due to subcutaneous air is uncommon but, when present, may suggest the diagnosis. Exquisite local tenderness, often out of proportion to the physical findings, is common and also may suggest the diagnosis of necrotizing fasciitis. The presence of coexisting fever and toxicity in combination with the local pain often points toward the diagnosis. Severe pain may give way to cutaneous anesthesia as tissue necrosis and thrombosis of blood vessels lead to destruction of superficial nerves in the subcutaneous tissues. Frank cutaneous gangrene is a relatively late finding. Because inflammation and necrosis spread rapidly along fascial planes, extensive destruction of deep tissue may occur before there is obvious cutaneous necrosis. Necrotizing fasciitis may be accompanied by severe systemic illness, including hypotension and tachycardia. Up to 50% of infections caused by GAS are associated with toxic shock syndrome. When present, generalized erythematous or scarlatiniform rash suggests necrotizing fasciitis rather than cellulitis.

Laboratory testing is nonspecific and cannot differentiate necrotizing fasciitis from less serious soft-tissue infections. Leukocytosis with increased band forms is common. An elevated creatinine kinase level is suggestive of muscle destruction, either directly by bacterial invasion or by compression from local edema (compartment syndrome). In contrast to uncomplicated cellulitis, bacteremia is common in necrotizing fasciitis, but not diagnostic.

Radiographic studies provide limited benefit in the diagnosis of necrotizing fasciitis. The presence of soft-tissue air on plain films or computed tomography may be diagnostic of infections caused by *Clostridium* species or mixed bacterial infections; it is not characteristic of necrotizing fasciitis caused by GAS (not a gas producer). A hyperintense signal on T2-weighted magnetic resonance imaging is strongly suggestive of necrotizing fasciitis. However, radiographic studies should not be undertaken if they delay surgical exploration.

Management

Necrotizing fasciitis is a surgical emergency; delayed surgical intervention is associated with mortality rates approaching

100%. Multiple debridements to remove devitalized tissue are the rule, and amputation of affected limbs may be necessary.

Empiric antibiotic therapy for suspected necrotizing fasciitis should include a penicillinase-resistant penicillin such as oxacillin or nafcillin in combination with clindamycin. A protein synthesis inhibitor, clindamycin inhibits bacterial toxin production and enhances phagocytosis of streptococci. When MRSA is suspected, empiric therapy should also include vancomycin.

Potential adjunctive therapies for necrotizing fasciitis include hyperbaric oxygen therapy and intravenous immune globulin (IVIG). Purported benefits of hyperbaric oxygen therapy include improved oxygenation of injured tissue, resulting in better wound healing, collagen deposition, angiogenesis, and epithelialization. Nonrandomized observational studies suggest that IVIG reduces morbidity and mortality associated with necrotizing fasciitis, possibly through neutralization of superantigens. Further study of both treatment modalities is warranted.

Pearls

- Exquisite pain and tenderness, out of proportion to visible physical findings, may help differentiate necrotizing fasciitis from cellulitis.
- Prompt surgical exploration confirms the diagnosis and may be life-saving.

- Clindamycin, an antibiotic that inhibits protein synthesis and downregulates toxin production by GAS, should be included in the empiric antibiotic regimens for suspected necrotizing fasciitis. MRSA is an emerging pathogen causing necrotizing fasciitis.

Suggested Readings

Danik SB, Schwartz RA, Oleske JM. Cellulitis. *Cutis* 1999;64:157–164.

Falagas ME, Vergidis PI. Narrative review: diseases that masquerade as infectious cellulitis. *Ann Intern Med* 2005;142:47–55.

File TJ, Tan JS, Ripersio JR. Diagnosing and treating the "flesh-eating bacteria syndrome." *Cleve Clin J Med* 1998;65:241–249.

Fleisher G, Ludwig S, Campos J. Cellulitis: bacterial etiology, clinical features and laboratory findings. *J Pediatr* 1980;97:591–593.

Hsieh T, Samson LM, Jabour M, et al. Necrotizing fasciitis in children in eastern Ontario: a case control study. *CMAJ* 2000;163:393–396.

Kaplan SL. Treatment of community-associated methicillin-resistant *Staphylococcus aureus* infections. *Pediatr Infect Dis J* 2005;24:457–478.

Kaul R, McGeer A, Low DE, et al. Population-based surveillance for group A streptococcal necrotizing fasciitis: clinical features, prognostic indicators, and microbiologic evaluation of 77 cases. *Am J Med* 1997;103:18–24.

Miller LG, Perdreau-Remington F, Rieg G, et al. Necrotizing fasciitis caused by community-associated methicillin-resistant Staphylococcus aureus in Los Angeles. *N Eng J Med* 2005;352:1445–1453.

Sattler CA, Mason EO Jr, Kaplan SL. Prospective comparison of of risk factors and demographic and clinical characteristics of community-acquired, methicillin-resistant versus methicillin-susceptible *Staphylococcus aureus* infections in children. *Pediatr Infect Dis J* 2002;21:910–916.

Swartz MN. Cellulitis. *N Engl J Med* 2004;350:904–912.

CHAPTER 82 ■ TUBERCULOSIS

DONALD L. JANNER

After years of decline in national rates of tuberculosis (TB) culminating in the early 1980s, public health officials and physicians were hopeful for its elimination in the United States. Unfortunately, from 1985 to 1990, there was a sharp increase in the number of reported cases, with an even more dramatic increase in children. In children aged 5 to 14 years, the number of cases during the same period increased by 39%, most likely owing to an increase in medically underserved persons, increased number of immigrants from endemic areas, and an increase in people infected with human immunodeficiency virus (HIV). Fortunately, increased infection control measures have led to a decrease in case rate of TB since 1992. However, this era of increased contagion has raised the number of people with latent disease who are at risk for the development of active infection in years to come.

Mycobacterium tuberculosis (MTB) is an aerobic, acid-fast, nonmotile organism whose only reservoir is humans. Approximately 10% of infected adults progress to active disease; infants and children have a much higher risk. Approximately 50% of infants <1 year of age develop active disease; in children <5 years, the risk is 25%. The exact reasons for this remain unclear, but it may be related to the inability of an immature immune system to respond to and/or contain mycobacterial infections.

Infection with MTB begins with inhalation of airborne bacilli that reach the pulmonary alveoli. Bacilli are then transported through pulmonary lymphatic channels to hilar lymph nodes and then to the bloodstream through the thoracic duct. MTB can also directly enter the bloodstream by way of pulmonary vasculature. Once in the bloodsteam, the organism can spread to every organ of the body. Small numbers of bacilli spreading to a variety of sites can result in clinically inapparent foci. If the immune system is compromised or the child has a large burden of bacilli spread throughout the body, the subsequent clinical presentation may be miliary or disseminated disease. Reactive tuberculin skin tests usually develop concurrently and may indicate exposure and latent infection, or possible active infection.

CLINICAL MANIFESTATIONS OF PEDIATRIC TUBERCULOSIS

Latent Infection

A patient infected with MTB but without clinical signs is classified as having latent infection. Tuberculous skin testing (TST) provides the means for diagnosing latent infection. The only reliable TST is the Mantoux test, containing 5 tuberculin units administered intradermally. Other strengths of Mantoux skin tests (i.e., 1 or 250 tuberculin units) should not be used. The TST result should be read as millimeters of induration at 48 to 72 hours by a qualified medical professional. Interpretation of an individual TST is based on epidemiologic and clinical factors, including risk factors for the acquisition of TB (Table 82.1). The use of multipronged devices (e.g., "Tine" tests) for skin testing is specifically not an acceptable technique for TB screening. The amount of antigen penetrating the skin is not reproducible, and a reactive test requires a subsequent Mantoux test for validation.

In recent years the Centers for Disease Control and Prevention (CDC) and the American Academy of Pediatrics (AAP) have turned away from universal testing of all children and recommended targeted testing of children felt to be at risk for latent tuberculosis infection (LTBI). There have been several studies that have identified risk factors for latent infection in children (Table 82.2). Examples include contact with a known case, extended foreign travel within the past year to an endemic area, or close contact with a high-risk individual. A simple series of questions can be helpful in deciding whether screening for latent tuberculosis infection is indicated. Children at risk for TB who were not skin tested in the past can and should receive skin testing while hospitalized, unless there is a contraindication to the test. Although bacille Calmette–Guèrin (BCG) vaccine is not routinely given in this country, pediatricians often have to interpret TSTs in children who have received BCG. After BCG vaccination, a positive TST may be secondary to the BCG or to latent infection. The American Academy of Pediatrics recommends that the same criteria be used for TST interpretation regardless of a past history of BCG vaccination.

Accurate diagnosis of latent tuberculosis infection is critical as it is the foundation for preventive therapy and the elimination of persons at risk for the development of active disease. The TST as described has several limitations, including adequate placement and the need for interpretation at a second reading 48 hours later. There is also the problem with cross-reactivity in persons who have received BCG vaccination. To overcome this problem, there has been active investigation into alternative methods for the diagnosis of latent TB and this had resulted in the development of a new test, QuantiFERON TB, (QFT-G). The QFT-G measures host response (by quantitation of the release of interferon-gamma from T-lymphocytes in the patient's blood) to TB antigens, ESAT-6, and CFP-10. These two antigens are unique to *M. tuberculosis* and are not found in the BCG vaccination. The assay has been studied in the diagnosis of latent infection, particularly of those patients who have previously received BCG. For diagnosis of latent tuberculous infection, a test result greater than 1.5 international units is considered positive. The test currently cannot be used to distinguish latent from active disease. In fact, some patients with active TB may have diminished T-cell responses to ESAT-6 and CFP-10, similar to the diminished PPD response seen in children with disseminated TB.

TABLE 82.1

CRITERIA FOR POSITIVE TUBERCULIN SKIN TEST

Reaction	Population
1. Greater than 5-mm induration	1. Human immunodeficiency virus positive 2. Radiographic evidence of tuberculosis 3. Contacts of contagious patients 4. Immunosuppressed individuals including organ transplant recipients or patients receiving ≥ 15 mg/day prednisone
2. Greater than 10-mm induration	1. Children younger than 4 yr of age 2. Recent immigrants (i.e., within last 5 yr) from high-prevalence countries 3. Residents of high-risk settings, including nursing homes, jails, homeless shelters
3. Greater than 15-mm induration	1. Persons with no risk factors for tuberculosis

The advantage of the new assay is that it requires only a single caretaker visit, unlike the two required for the TST administration and reading. Because the assay is a blood test, it is also less dependent on errors of placement and interpretation. Disadvantages of the assay include the need for whole blood that has to be incubated within 12-hours of collection and the current lack of validation in immunocompromised patients and children under 17 years of age. Ongoing research will likely answer questions regarding use of the QFT-G for pediatric and immunocompromised patients. The current recommendations for the use of QFT-G include all circumstances in which the TST is used, including contact investigations and serial evaluations of health care workers. A positive QFT-G need not be followed up with a TST. A positive test may be helpful particularly in those with a prior history of BCG vaccination. Patients with a positive assay should be then evaluated for active disease. Caution should be used in using QFT-G in young children and immunocompromised patients (see above).

All children with a positive TST result (see Table 82.1) require a chest radiograph. For children younger than 18 years of age with a positive TST result and negative chest radiograph, the diagnosis of latent tuberculous infection is made. Latent tuberculous infection is the only time when monotherapy is acceptable. Before or concurrently with the initiation of treatment for latent infection, an investigation for the index case should be done. In up to 50% of cases, the index case (usually an adult) can be identified and antibiotic susceptibility patterns of the specific infecting TB strain determined.

All people younger than 18 years of age who have latent infection with isoniazid-*sensitive* organisms should be treated with isoniazid for 9 months. The efficacy of isoniazid in the treatment of latent tuberculosis infection is related to duration of therapy. Treatment for less then 6 months is less effective than therapy for 9 months; therapy for 12 months offers only a slightly increased benefit. Shorter-course therapy (2 months rifampin with pyrazinimide) resulted in unacceptable side effects (high rates of liver failure and even death) and is no longer recommended. Treatment of latent TB with regimens other than isoniazid or treatment of isoniazid-*resistant* latent TB always should occur in consultation with an infectious disease specialist.

Active Disease

The most common clinical manifestation of pediatric TB is pulmonary disease, but infection in other sites such as lymph nodes, pleura, and the central nervous system (CNS) also are seen. There is an increasing proportion of extrapulmonary TB, particularly in children. As many as 30% of pediatric TB cases have extrapulmonary involvement.

Pulmonary/Endobronchial Disease

The most common presentation of active pediatric TB is pulmonary disease (Fig. 82.1). Tuberculous pneumonia is thought

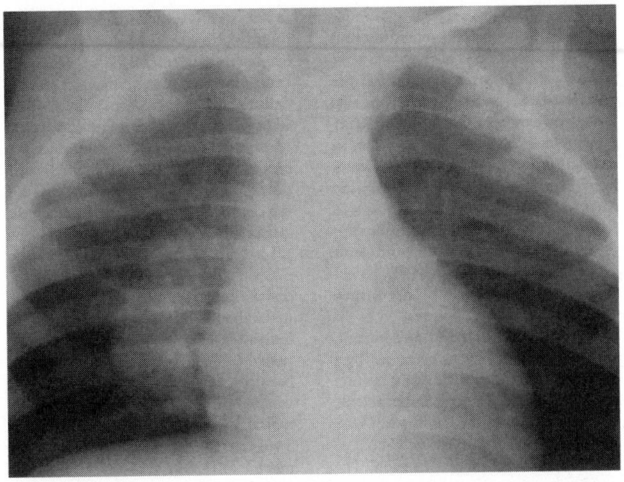

TABLE 82.2

RISK FACTORS FOR *MYCOBACTERIUM TUBERCULOSIS* INFECTION

■ Children born in or who have traveled to countries with high disease prevalence (Asia, Central and South America, Caribbean, and Pacific Islands).

■ Exposure to an adult with human immunodeficiency virus infection or tuberculosis.

■ Exposure to an adult who has lived in a correctional facility.

■ Local risk factors such as homelessness or living in certain high-prevalence neighborhoods.

FIGURE 82.1. Hilar adenopathy as the primary site in pediatric tuberculosis.

to follow reactivation of the primary infection present in hilar nodes (i.e., the Ghon complex). Endobronchial disease refers to the progression of the primary Ghon complex into the bronchus, which results in compression or atelectasis. In the younger child, pulmonary disease usually is diagnosed by chest radiography in an asymptomatic child with a positive TST result. Thus, the diagnosis of active tuberculous disease rests on the correct radiologic diagnosis of a pulmonary infiltrate and/or hilar nodes. Computed tomography (CT) has been shown to be very helpful in confirming hilar adenopathy in children and has been suggested for children with equivocal chest radiographs. Although older children with pulmonary disease or endobronchial disease often are asymptomatic, infants often present with symptomatic disease. The smaller caliber of the bronchi in infants is more easily compressed by enlarging hilar nodes, and the enlarging hilar lymphadenopathy can cause bronchial obstruction, resulting in wheezing and air trapping or complete atelectasis and even respiratory failure. Clinical assessment typically underestimates the true incidence of endobronchial compression as diagnosed by flexible or rigid bronchoscopy. Flexible bronchoscopy provides a safe and rapid means to assess the presence of endobronchial disease and determine whether adjunctive therapy (such as corticosteroids) is needed.

Miliary Disease

Miliary TB is one of the most severe manifestations of TB. Children with miliary TB may present with fever, failure to thrive, or respiratory distress. Fever and systemic symptoms can precede the development of abnormalities on chest radiography. Progressive miliary disease can produce an alveolar air block syndrome that presents with frank hypoxia and respiratory distress. The appearance of too-numerous-to-count nodules in a chest radiograph suggests a diagnosis of miliary TB (Fig. 82.2). These nodules result from unchecked hematogenous dissemination of MTB, common in the setting of a young or compromised immune system. In this setting of an ineffective immune response, TST is frequently negative.

Patients with miliary TB usually have lesions in multiple organ systems, including liver, spleen, and central nervous system. Patients can have miliary lesions in the brain without accompanying meningitis. The presence of CNS disease always should be sought in miliary disease because its presence alters medical treatment.

Rarely, a miliary pattern on chest radiography can be caused by other infectious diseases, including histoplasmosis and coccidioidomycosis, or by malignancy, especially lymphoma.

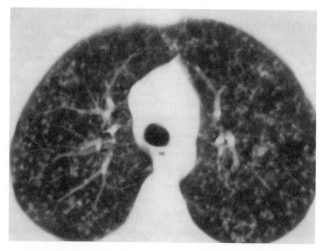

FIGURE 82.2. Computed tomography scan showing the variation in nodule size and distribution in miliary tuberculosis.

Tuberculous Pleural Effusion

A tuberculous pleural effusion typically occurs 3 to 6 months after primary infection or with reactivation of infection at any time during the life of an untreated patient. Tuberculous pleural effusion is thought to be caused by a delayed hypersensitivity reaction to mycobacteria that enter the pleural space through rupture of subpleural tubercles. Development of symptoms can be acute or insidious. Affected children present with fever, cough, and pleuritic pain. The chest radiograph shows a unilateral pleural effusion. Untreated, the natural history is complete or significant clearance of pleural fluid even without drug treatment. However, untreated patients have a high rate of development of active or extrapulmonary disease within a year. Progression to active disease is increased in young children, immunocompromised patients, and people with recently acquired disease.

This diagnosis is suggested in a patient with a unilateral pleural effusion who has exposure to TB either by travel or contact history. A one-time thoracentesis is necessary because it (1) allows examination of pleural fluid for diagnostic purposes; and (2) facilitates drainage, which can decrease the development of pleural fibrosis. Pleural fluid usually reveals several hundred white blood cells per cubic millimeter, predominantly lymphocytes. Only 30% of patients have a positive MTB culture from the pleural fluid. The yield of pleural biopsy with culture is higher and approaches 75%. After diagnosis, all patients should be treated with aggressive antituberculous therapy.

Lymphadenopathy

Enlargement of regional lymph nodes is a common extrapulmonary manifestation of TB. Tonsillar and submandibular node enlargement (historically termed *scrofula*) is a result of extension from paratracheal lymph node infection. The typical history of tuberculous adenitis is gradual enlargement of lymph nodes that become fluctuant and purplish, and often progress to fistula formation. However, most mycobacterial infections of lymph nodes in children are due to the atypical tuberculous species, most commonly *Mycobacterium aviumintracellulare*. In adenitis secondary to MTB, TST usually reveals induration greater than 15 mm, whereas in atypical tuberculous adenitis, skin testing may produce a smaller reaction. A chest radiograph should be obtained because it may reveal associated pulmonary disease. Aggressive antituberculous therapy may obviate the need for surgical resection. If the diagnosis is clear (i.e., a large cervical node with reactive TST), a course of empiric antituberculous therapy can be given. If the diagnosis is in doubt and biopsy is needed, it may be prudent to use excisional biopsy to lessen the chance for the development of a postsurgical fistula.

Central Nervous System Tuberculosis

Tuberculous meningitis arises from hematogenous dissemination of MTB, forming tubercles most commonly in the brainstem. These "Rich foci" (named after the English pathologist who initially described them) discharge acid-fast bacilli into the cerebrospinal fluid (CSF). A thick exudate develops that impedes CSF flow, resulting in hydrocephalus. A typical history is progressive lethargy and vomiting over 2 to 3 weeks as intracranial pressure increases. The chronicity of tuberculous meningitis helps the clinician distinguish this diagnosis from bacterial meningitis or self-limited illnesses such as viral meningitis. CSF examination reveals several hundred white blood cells per cubic millimeter, mostly lymphocytes. Protein usually is elevated and glucose is low. The serum CSF/serum glucose ratio is typically 20% to 25%. Brain CT shows basilar enhancement accompanied by hydrocephalus, a rare occurrence in viral or uncomplicated bacterial meningitis. Although acid-fast staining and culture of a 1-mL sample of CSF reveals organisms in only 10% of cases, obtaining larger volumes (approximately 10 to 15 mL) and cytocentrifuging this volume may yield positive results in up to 90% of cases. Surgical treatment is vital in the management of tuberculous meningitis. Patients with hydrocephalus and increased intracranial pressure are candidates for ventriculoperitoneal (VP) shunts. Because the brainstem exudate causing CSF obstruction is not likely to resolve, these patients may require VP shunting indefinitely.

Clinical outcome in tuberculous meningitis depends on the stage at the time of diagnosis. Significant permanent impairment or a fatal outcome is seen most frequently in children with advanced-stage tuberculous meningitis with significant neurologic impairment at diagnosis. Because definitive diagnosis from positive CSF culture may not be available for several weeks, initial therapy often is presumptive. Children with a clinical course of progressive neurologic compromise with a compatible CSF profile should have the diagnosis of tuberculous meningitis strongly considered.

Other forms of tuberculous CNS disease include tuberculomas and tuberculous brain abscesses. Tuberculomas are tubercles consisting of a central zone of caseating necrosis surrounded by inflammatory cells and multinucleated giant cells. They coexist with tuberculous meningitis in approximately 10% of cases. Tuberculous brain abscess is a rare but potentially devastating infection of the CNS. A tuberculous abscess may be differentiated from tuberculoma in that the former has central liquefaction and the latter is a solid, granulomatous, relatively avascular lesion. Some experts suggest that these lesions are histologic variants of the same pathologic process.

Distinguishing between the tuberculoma and abscess on neuroimaging may be difficult. Although tuberculomas may be treated without surgery, tuberculous brain abscesses may need excision (in addition to medical therapy) for resolution. The presence of focal neurologic signs should suggest the possibility of a mass effect. It has been suggested that patients with CNS opacities should be followed closely both clinically and radiographically. The development of focal neurologic findings and radiographic development of an abscess should lead to consultation with a neurosurgeon.

Skeletal Tuberculosis

TB of the bones is one of the rarest forms of infection, representing approximately 4% of total cases. Infection is the result of lymphohematogenous seeding during primary infection. Clinical manifestations of tuberculous osteomyelitis may become apparent years after initial infection. The most common site is vertebral TB (Pott disease). Symptoms of vertebral TB relate to the affected area (e.g., focal pain or inability to walk). Radiographs often reveal chronic lytic lesions. The TST usually is reactive. Definitive diagnosis is made by biopsy. TB also should be considered in the differential of a child with a chronic osteomyelitis, especially if there is a high risk history.

DIAGNOSIS OF TUBERCULOSIS

Isolation of MTB from clinical specimens remains the gold standard for diagnosis. Isolation of MTB from children with pulmonary disease is complicated because children do not produce sputum. However, the index case often can be identified by placing TSTs on all household contacts. Usually an adult with active pulmonary disease is found and sensitivities can be obtained on that isolate, rather than on the child's organism. Otherwise, an aggressive workup aimed at isolation from the child always should be attempted because this will be needed to guide subsequent therapy.

Early-morning gastric lavage from a young child with pulmonary disease contains swallowed pulmonary secretions from the previous night and yields a positive culture up to 50% of the time. Gastric lavage for the diagnosis of tuberculosis has become increasingly used as an inpatient tool for diagnosis of pulmonary TB. Use of proper technique is critical. Gastric aspirate should be performed in the early morning when the patient has been without food or fluids for at least 8 hours. Stomach contents are aspirated through an 8 French feeding tube, following which 30 mL of sterile water (not saline) is instilled and aspirated. Within 30 minutes of collection, the gastric pH should be neutralized with a 10% sodium bicarbonate solution. The specimen needs then to be refrigerated and transported to the laboratory within 4 hours of collection. Proper handling of gastric aspirates can improve the sensitivity of this test by as much as 50%. If gastric aspirate is negative, bronchoalveolar lavage is yet another alternative, yielding a pathogen in approximately 20% of infected children.

Because of the difficulties in culturing MTB, efforts have been made to develop new technology for the diagnosis of pediatric tuberculosis. A major technology being explored is nucleic acid amplification (NAA). The primary method of NAA employed in the diagnosis of pediatric pulmonary tuberculosis is the polymerase chain reaction (PCR), which amplifies specific DNA sequences for a specific pathogen. PCR has been studied in tubersulosis in adult and pediatric populations using a variety of methods and on clinical specimens including sputum, pleural fluid, and cerebrospinal fluid. In the clinical diagnosis of pediatric tuberculosis disease, the sensitivity of PCR ranges from 25% to 80% with a specificity of 80% to 100%. PCR analysis of gastric aspirates is also problematic, as studies have shown false positives in children with mycobacterium avium-intracellulare pneumonia. PCR tests on gastric aspirates should be used only when there is a strong suspicion of MTB on chest radiograph.

PCR has also been attempted for diagnosis of tuberculous meningitis. A recent meta-analysis reviewed this methodology; sensitivity was 70% with a specificity of 95%. The low sensitivity may be related to low bacilli counts (1 bacillus/mL CSF), as well as mycobacterial nucleic acid being more difficult to extract for amplification purposes.

A negative PCR never eliminates the possibility of tuberculosis; rather, it should be used in combination with a complete epidemiologic, radiographic, and microbiologic profile of the patient.

MANAGEMENT

Antituberculous Medications

Because antituberculous treatment often is initiated before MTB isolate drug sensitivity information is available, local rates of drug resistance can be helpful in determining initial treatment. In an era of increasing MTB drug resistance, and with the goal of using at least two drugs to which the infecting organism is sensitive, a four-drug initial regimen is recommended for all forms of MTB disease in children (Tables 82.3 and 82.4). Treatment of TB should be undertaken with the assistance of a pediatric infectious disease specialist or the local health department TB officer.

Adjunctive corticosteroid therapy sometimes is used in the treatment of pediatric TB disease to reduce the inflammatory response causing organ damage. The following are considered potential indications for corticosteroid treatment:

1. Tuberculous meningitis. Corticosteroids can aid patients by reducing vasculitis, inflammation, and intracranial pressure. This reduction maintains cerebral circulation and tissue perfusion, thereby facilitating medication delivery into the

TABLE 82.3

FRONT-LINE THERAPY FOR PEDIATRIC TUBERCULOSIS

Drug	Daily dose (mg/kg/day)	Twice-weekly dose (mg/kg/dose)	Adverse reactions
Isoniazid	15–25	20–30	Hepatitis Peripheral neuropathy
Rifampin	10–20	10–20	Body secretion discoloration Interference with oral contraception
Pyrazinamide	20–40	40–60	Hepatitis Hyperuricemia
Ethambutal	15	25–50	Optic neuritis; decreased red-green color discrimination
Streptomycin (intramuscular)	20–40	20–40	Nephrotoxicity Auditory and vestibular toxicity

brain. Studies have shown decreased mortality and fewer long-term sequelae in patients with tuberculous meningitis treated with steroids. The dose often used is dexamethasone 8 to 12 mg/day (or equivalent), tapered over 6 to 8 weeks.

2. Endobronchial disease. With steroid therapy, intrathoracic adenopathy involutes faster, resulting in resolution of lobar collapse and air trapping. Prednisone at doses of 2 to 5 mg/kg/day for 1 week with reduction to 1 mg/kg/day and then tapering over to 4 to 5 weeks has been reported effective.

3. Syndrome of paradoxical enlargement. This syndrome is thought to be secondary to hypersensitivity reaction (see "Special Situations," later in the chapter) and can respond to a 1- to 2-week course of prednisone 1 to 2 mg/kg/day with taper over 2 to 4 weeks.

TABLE 82.4

TREATMENT REGIMENS FOR PEDIATRIC TUBERCULOSIS

Infection/Disease	Treatment
1. Latent infection (positive tuberculous skin test, negative chest radiograph) Isoniazid susceptible Isoniazid resistant	 Isoniazid daily PO or twice weekly; 9 mo Rifampin daily PO each day or twice weekly; 6 mo
2. Pulmonary disease (usually hilar adenopathy)	a. Two months of daily isoniazid, rifampin, and pyrazinamide followed by 4 mo of daily isoniazid and rifampin *or* b. Two months of daily isoniazid, rifampin, and pyrazinamide followed by 4 mo of twice-weekly isoniazid and rifampin under directly observed therapy
3. Miliary disease, meningitis, bone/joint disease	a. Two months of daily isoniazid, rifampin, pyrazinamide, and streptomycin (ethambutal or ethionamide often substituted) followed by 10 mo of daily isoniazid and rifampin *or* b. Two months of daily isoniazid, rifampin, pyrazinamide, and streptomycin followed by 10 mo of twice-weekly isoniazid and rifampin under directly observed therapy
4. Extrapulmonary other than miliary, meningitis, or bone joint (e.g., lymphadenitis)	Same as pulmonary disease

Directly Observed Therapy

With the exception of latent infection, successful treatment of TB requires taking many drugs for a prolonged period. Most patients find taking months of daily treatment difficult and are noncompliant. This has grave implications, not only for the patient but also for the community. The noncompliant patient with active infection often develops secondary resistance, resulting in additional contacts being infected with a resistant strain. For this reason, many public health authorities advocate directly observed therapy (DOT), whereby a health care provider or other responsible person observes as the patient ingests medication (twice weekly). Successful DOT should not only include direct observation of patients taking medications, but should also provide services such as medication refills and liaison with supervising physicians.

Monitoring Pediatric Antituberculous Therapy

For patients receiving isoniazid monotherapy for latent infection, neither monthly pyridoxine supplementation nor routine laboratory monitoring is recommended. For children with active disease requiring multiple drugs, it is recommended that monthly aminotransferase levels be monitored for several months, with more extensive testing every 1 to 3 months.

The combination of rifampin and pyrazinamide should be avoided for latent infection, because there are several reports of adults with severe progressive hepatitis on this regimen. Caution is advised in patients with a history of alcohol abuse or concurrent medications associated with liver injury (e.g., anticonvulsants). Laboratory evaluation should be done at baseline and at 2, 4, and 6 weeks, with close clinical follow-up throughout the duration of therapy.

SPECIAL SITUATIONS: SYNDROME OF PARADOXICAL ENLARGEMENT

Clinicians who manage basic TB infections need to be aware of the syndrome of paradoxical enlargement of tuberculomas. During antituberculous therapy, a hypersensitivity reaction to the tuberculous antigens results in an increase in tuberculoma size. Progression of this type may be clinically important both in lungs and the brain. When faced with the clinical picture of paradoxical enlargement of lymph nodes or tuberculomas, the treating physician must determine (1) adequacy of therapy based on sensitivity patterns, (2) medication compliance, or (3) possible malabsorption of TB medications (sometimes seen in patients with acquired immunodeficiency syndrome). If paradoxical enlargement is diagnosed, a brief course of corticosteroids has been used successfully.

PEARLS

- Always read a TST based on the size of the induration (not erythema) and on the patient's risk factors.
- Use of a ballpoint pen can aid in the measurement of TST induration. Draw a short line toward the area of induration. Stop when the pen meets light resistance. Repeat this so that there are 4 lines at right angles to each other with the induration in the center, and then measure the distance across the induration to the ends of opposing lines.
- Children younger than 5 years of age have a high risk of severe TB. Always provide antituberculous medication if the child has close contact with active disease, even if the child's first TST result is negative. Medication can be discontinued if the second TST at 3 months is still negative and there are no signs of TB disease.
- Diagnosis of TB in a child indicates an active case of TB in the child's close contacts. All close contacts require TST testing.

Suggested Readings

American Academy of Pediatrics. Tuberculosis. In: Pickering LK, Baker CJ, Long SS, et al (eds). *Red book: 2006 report of the committee on infections diseases*. 27th edition. Elk Grove Village, Illinois: American Academy of Pediatrics; 2006;678–704.

Mazurek GH, Jereb J, LoBue P, et al. Guidelines for using the QuantiFERON-TB gold test for detecting *Mycobacterium tuberculosis* infection. *MMWR Morb Mortal Wkly Rep* 2005;54:49–55.

Neu N, Saiman L, San Gabriel P, et al. Diagnosis of pediatric tuberculosis in the modern era. *Pediatr Infect Dis J* 1999;18:122–126.

Small PM, Fujiwara PI. Management of tuberculosis in the United States. *N Engl J Med* 2001;345:189–200.

Starke J. Tuberculosis. In: Janson HB, Baltimore RS, eds. *Pediatric infectious disease*. Philadelphia: Saunders; 2001:396–416.

CHAPTER 83 ■ HUMAN IMMUNODEFICIENCY VIRUS

DEBRA A. TRISTRAM AND COLEEN K. CUNNINGHAM

Human immunodeficiency virus (HIV) includes two types of retroviruses: HIV-1, the primary agent responsible for the current worldwide epidemic; and HIV-2. Both HIV-1 and HIV-2 produce similar clinical disease in humans, although disease due to HIV-2 seems to progress more slowly. HIV-1 has several different subtypes, but there is little difference in the clinical disease produced. Different subtypes predominate in different regions of the world, with subtype B the most common subtype in North America and Eastern Europe. A number of other subtypes have been identified (A through H, N, and O). Subtype differences have been among the many stumbling blocks in the development of a useful worldwide vaccine.

Acquired immunodeficiency syndrome (AIDS) refers to the severe immunodeficiency disease that results from chronic infection with HIV. AIDS is defined by either clinical or laboratory evidence of immunodeficiency.

HIV is a retrovirus and is transmitted only through blood and body fluids. The virus infects predominantly CD4+ lymphocytes and macrophages, although infection can occur in other cell types. The initial steps of primary infection are not well understood; however, it is known that portions of the viral envelope (gp120) attach to CD4 receptors on the host cell surface. Subsequent conformational changes in the viral envelope lead to binding of gp120 to the cellular chemokine receptors (CCR5 and CXCR4). Further conformational changes lead to viral fusion, and the viral genome enters into the cell. After reverse transcription, viral DNA is integrated into host DNA. Infected cells can remain quiescent for years and then, on activation, produce infectious virus. When an individual becomes HIV infected, there may be an early, acute symptomatic phase (acute retroviral syndrome) followed by a clinically latent phase that may last 5 to 10 years or even longer. During the clinically latent phase, viral RNA can be detected in plasma and ongoing CD4 cell loss continues. Symptoms develop when CD4 depletion is sufficient to allow opportunistic infection and malignancy.

Worldwide, HIV is predominantly spread through heterosexual sex, with roughly equal numbers of infected men and women. It is estimated that 5.4 million new infections occur each year. In some regions (United States and Western Europe), a high proportion of those infected are men who have sex with men, and intravenous drug users (IVDU). However, the number of women infected through heterosexual contact is increasing in the United States. Women accounted for 30% of all AIDS reports in 2004, compared with <10% before 1990. Of the new HIV cases in U.S. women in 2004, over 65% identified heterosexual contact as their primary risk factor; often the male partner's possible risks for HIV infection (e.g., unprotected sex with multiple partners, bisexuality, or injection drug use) were unknown to the woman at the time of sexual contact.

Infections in youth is a persistent problem, with 25% of new infections occurring in youth 13 to 19 years of age and 50% occurring in individuals younger than 24 years.

Although infection among youth is increasing, there has been a marked decline in HIV infection among children younger than 13 years of age in developed nations because of a decrease in mother-to-child HIV transmission. Rates of perinatal transmission have decreased from >25% before 1994 to <2% in 2006 owing to the use of maternal antiretroviral treatment and infant prophylaxis. However, infection in children can still occur, and is most likely in women with highly resistant virus, children born to women who were not diagnosed as HIV infected during pregnancy, or in children born in countries where prenatal HIV testing is not consistently provided.

HIV infection and AIDS in children can present with very nonspecific findings and therefore may have a very broad differential diagnosis. In children presenting with poor growth, the differential includes all of the disorders that lead to failure to thrive. HIV may also present as chronic fever, lymphadenopathy, neurocognitive delay, immune dysfunction, malignancy, and thrombocytopenia. Laboratory testing quickly and easily establishes the diagnosis. Therefore, any child with the nonspecific symptoms possibly associated with HIV or with risk factors (either in themselves or their parents) should have HIV testing included in their laboratory evaluation. The Centers for Disease Control and Prevention (CDC) has recently recommended that routine HIV testing be incorporated into regular medical care for all patients 13 to 64 years of age.

CLINICAL FEATURES

Given current standards of HIV testing in pregnancy, most HIV-exposed infants in the United States are identified before delivery so that maternal treatment can begin during pregnancy. Children or infants known to be at risk for perinatally acquired infection should be tested for HIV before the onset of symptoms. Nevertheless, there continue to be children without recognized HIV exposure who present with nonspecific symptoms months to years after birth. Patient history may include frequent occurrence of common childhood infections, including pneumonia or *Streptococcus pneumoniae* bacteremia. Other common findings include poor growth, chronic diarrhea, and developmental delay. The identification of an opportunistic infection, in particular *Pneumocystis jiroveci* pneumonia, should suggest cellular immunodeficiency. Other symptoms that may be reported include frequent bruising (thrombocytopenia) and unexplained fevers.

Physical findings can range from normal to notable. All findings are nonspecific but should prompt diagnostic studies.

TABLE 83.1

POSSIBLE PHYSICAL FINDINGS IN CHILDREN WITH SYMPTOMATIC HIV INFECTION

- Poor weight gain
- Wasting
- Lymphadenopathy
- Hepatosplenomegaly
- Oral thrush
- Bruising
- Developmental delay or loss of milestones
- Tachypnea
- Rash

Table 83.1 includes findings that may be present in children and adolescents with symptomatic HIV infection. *Acute retroviral syndrome* is rare in infancy but may be seen when someone is first infected during childhood or adolescence. Symptoms are nonspecific, but frequently include sore throat, lymphadenopathy, fever, and rash. It often is described as "a mononucleosis-like" syndrome. In an adolescent with such findings and negative Epstein–Barr titers, the clinician should consider acute retroviral syndrome.

For adults and children older than 2 years of age, diagnosis usually is made by the identification of HIV antibody in serum with an enzyme-linked immunosorbant assay (ELISA). Screening usually is done using ELISA and confirmed by HIV Western blot testing. All currently licensed ELISAs identify both HIV-1 and HIV-2 antibody in serum. If an individual has a positive HIV ELISA and negative HIV-1 Western blot, an HIV-2 Western blot should be performed.

If an individual is suspected of having acute retroviral syndrome, antibody testing may be negative. Options for testing in that situation include testing for virus using one of the methods described below or retesting for HIV antibody in 2 to 4 weeks. Some of the methods used for testing for virus have not been well studied as a means of *diagnosing* HIV infection. Specifically, a low viral copy number in HIV RNA quantitation should not be considered diagnostic by itself. For children younger than 2 years, the presence of maternal anti-HIV antibody makes diagnosis more difficult. These children should be tested for virus using HIV DNA polymerase chain reaction. Testing should be performed in the first 2 weeks (usually done at birth), at approximately 1 month of age, and at least once more between the ages of 3 and 6 months. Some experts also confirm the loss of antibodies between 12 and 18 months. HIV RNA quantitation sometimes is used for diagnosis, but false-positive results may occur. All positive results for virus (any method) should be confirmed with a second sample obtained at a different time than the first. Other methods that can be used for diagnosis include HIV-1 culture and p24 antigen detection. Although culture is reliable, it is time consuming and expensive; P24 antigen detection has problems with sensitivity and specificity; therefore, neither assay is used often for clinical care.

TREATMENT

Treatment to Prevent Mother-to-Child Transmission

HIV-infected pregnant women who require treatment for their own HIV disease should be offered highly active antiretroviral therapy (HAART). However, such treatment should be provided by an expert in HIV care, because some antiretrovirals are con-

traindicated during pregnancy (e.g., efavirenz) and the risks and benefits of each treatment regimen must be carefully considered. In the United States, women generally receive HAART during pregnancy and IV ZDV intrapartum. This is followed by treating the infant with ZDV (2 mg/kg/dose orally given every 6 hours) for 6 weeks. Outside the United States and Western Europe, other less expensive regimens have been used.

Treatment of HIV-Infected Children

The optimal time to initiate therapy in an infected child is not known. Current guidelines in adults recommend waiting until disease is fairly advanced before starting treatment. Untreated infants are at risk for rapid disease progression and irreversible neurologic disease. Therefore, treatment with HAART is recommended for essentially all HIV-infected infants. Older children (>2 years) who have been chronically infected may have clinical or laboratory evidence that would justify holding off on HAART until disease progresses or less toxic therapy becomes available.

Available licensed antiretroviral medications can be divided into classes based on mechanism of action. For treatment of disease, medications from different classes should be given in highly active combinations with a minimum of three drugs. A summary of the currently available drugs for the treatment of HIV infection is given in Table 83.2. Knowledge of the potential side effects and drug interactions is necessary for the management of a hospitalized child with HIV infection.

When an HIV-infected child presents with fever or other evidence of an infection, evaluation and treatment depend on the immune status of the child. The most easily available measure of immune status is the CD4+ cell count. Beyond the first year of life, CD4+ cell counts for an individual do not change rapidly; therefore, a CD4+ cell result within 3 months is a good measure of immune status (Table 83.3). Children with relatively intact immune function based on CD4+ cell count are not at risk for opportunistic infection, but are much more likely than HIV-uninfected children to have pneumonia, *S. pneumoniae* bacteremia, sinusitis, and otitis. Blood cultures should be considered when the child is febrile, and treatment should be targeted to the identified source. Unless severely ill, most of these children can be managed as outpatients. Children with decreased CD4+ cells for age (Table 83.3) must be evaluated for opportunistic infection. If pulmonary symptoms are present, the clinician should consider *P. jiroveci* pneumonia. Immunodeficient HIV-infected children with fever or other evidence of significant new symptoms should be promptly evaluated and treated in consultation with a pediatric HIV specialist.

Monitoring

All HIV-infected children require frequent clinical and laboratory monitoring to evaluate for progression of disease and side effects of medications. All of the antiretroviral medications have significant toxicities and should be prescribed only by, or with the assistance, of a pediatric HIV specialist. Side effects vary with the different agents and may include pancreatitis, bone marrow suppression, peripheral neuropathy, hepatitis, hypersensitivity reactions including Stevens–Johnson syndrome, lipid abnormalities, body fat distribution abnormalities, nausea, vomiting, and diarrhea. Fusion inhibitors have the added problem of injection site reactions, including inflammation, pain, and cellulitis.

SPECIAL SITUATIONS

Every child exposed to or infected with HIV is in some respects a special situation and requires comprehensive evaluation and careful assessment of disease status, treatment options, and

TABLE 83.2

MEDICATIONS USED IN THE TREATMENT OF HIV INFECTION

Mechanism	Drug	Trade name	Pediatric form available?	Formulation[a]
Reverse transcriptase inhibitor	Zidovudine (AZT)	Retrovir	Yes	50 mg/5 mL
	Didansosine (ddI)	Videx	Yes	10 mg/mL soln
	Lamividine (3TC)	Epivir	Yes	10 mg/mL soln
	Stavuduine (d4T)	Zerit	Yes	1 mg/mL soln
	Abacavir (ABC)	Ziagen	Yes	20 mg/mL soln
	AZT/3TC	Combivir	No	N/A
	AZT/3TC/ABC	Trizivir	No	N/A
	Tenofovir	Viread	No	N/A
	Emtricitabine	Emtriva	Yes	10 mg/mL soln
	TNV/DTC	Truvada	No	N/A
Non-nucleoside reverse transcriptase inhibitor	Nevirapine (NVP)	Viramune	Yes	50 mg/5 mL
	Efavirenz	Sustiva	Yes[b]	30 mg/mL
Protease inhibitor	Saquinivir	Invirase/Fortavase	No	N/A
	Indinivir	Crixivan	No	N/A
	Ritonavir	Norvir	Yes	80 mg/mL soln
	Lopinavir/ritonavir	Kaletra	Yes	80 mg lopinavir and 20 mg ritonavir/1 mL soln
	Nelfinavir	Viracept	Yes	50 mg/scoop powder (50 mg/g powder)
	Amprenavir	Agenerase	Yes	15 mg/mL soln (contraindicated in children under 4); capsule and soln not comparable
	Atazanavir	Reyataz	No	N/A
	Tipranivir	Aptivus	No	N/A
Fusion inhibitor	Enfuvirtide (T-20)	Fuzeon	Not specifically	Pediatric dose: 2 mg/kg injected SQ twice daily to max of 90 mg twice daily

N/A, not applicable; soln, solution.

[a]Dosing varies greatly based on concurrent medications and age of patient. Dosing for an individual patient should be checked with the federal guidelines and a pediatric HIV specialist.

[b]Currently available only through expanded-access program.

treatment readiness. The importance of complete adherence to medication regimens cannot be overemphasized. All such children should be evaluated by a specialist in pediatric HIV, although in many cases such care is provided in close collaboration with a primary care provider. Furthermore, treatment options are changing rapidly and periodic reevaluation of each child is important to make sure she is benefiting from currently available testing and treatment.

TABLE 83.3

IMMUNOLOGIC CATEGORIES FOR HIV TYPE 1–INFECTED CHILDREN: NUMBER OF CD4 CELLS (PERCENTAGE OF TOTAL LYMPHOCYTES COUNTED)

Immunologic category	Age		
	<12 mo	1–5 yr	6–12 yr
No evidence of immune suppression	>1,500 CD4 cells/mm^3 (>25%)	>1,000 CD4 cells/mm^3 (>25%)	>500 CD4 cells/mm^3 (>25%)
Evidence of moderate immune suppression	750–1,499 CD4 cells/mm^3 (15–24%)	500–999 CD4 cells/mm^3 (15–24%)	200–499 CD4 cells/mm^3 (15–24%)
Severe immune suppression	<750 CD4 cells/mm^3 (<15%)	<500 CD4 cells/mm^3 (<15%)	<200 CD4 cells/mm^3 (<15%)

Adapted from Revised classification system for human immunodeficiency virus infection in children less than 13 years of age *Morb Mortal Wkly Rep* 1994;43:RR12.

PEARLS

- HIV prophylaxis of the mother and newborn is extremely effective at preventing infant infection. If the mother was not treated, the infant needs to start on oral therapy *as soon as possible* after delivery. The physician must ensure that the infant receives ZDV prophylaxis for 6 weeks *and* must confirm that the infant care provider actually has the liquid ZDV on hospital discharge followed by an early clinic visit to reinforce appropriate medication adherence.
- HIV infection should be considered in any child with failure to thrive, loss of developmental milestones, or recurrent/persistent infections.
- All sexually active adolescents should have HIV testing available as part of routine medical care. Frank discussions about HIV infection and transmission should be part of routine health maintenance.

- Any adolescent with a mononucleosis-like syndrome who does not have a documented viral pathogen deserves a test for acute HIV infection (acute retroviral syndrome).
- The field of pediatric HIV care is changing on a daily basis. Prevention, treatment, and medication side effects are becoming more and more complicated. Individuals who provide medical care to these children must work to stay current in the field.

Suggested Readings

Centers for Disease Control and Prevention. HIV/AIDS surveillance report, 2004. Washington, DC: Department of Health and Human Services, Centers for Disease Control and Prevention; 2005 Also available at http://www.cdc.gov/hiv/stats/hasrlink.htm.

Committee on Pediatric AIDS, American Academy of Pediatrics. Evaluation and treatment of the HIV-exposed infant. *Pediatrics* 1997;99:909–917.

Current pediatric guidelines and guidelines for care of adults, adolescents and for perinatal treatment can be accessed on the Web at *http://www.hivatis.org.*

CHAPTER 84 ■ HERPES SIMPLEX VIRUS INFECTIONS

SUE JOAN JUE

Herpes simplex virus (HSV) is a ubiquitous virus that has the ability to cause primary and recurrent infections. HSV infection may produce a wide spectrum of disease, ranging from trivial infections (e.g., fever blisters) to the most severe (e.g., fatal sporadic viral encephalitis, disseminated neonatal infection). The host immune status to a large extent determines the severity of the clinical manifestations.

HSV exists as two types: HSV-1 and HSV-2. HSV-1 infections typically involve the face and skin above the waist, whereas HSV-2 infections involve the genitalia and the skin below the waist in sexually active adolescents and adults. Both types, however, can infect any anatomic site and depend on the source of infection.

Immunity to HSV is not fully understood. Immunity against one strain provides some degree of protection against infection with another strain, and immunity against one type appears to provide partial protection against subsequent infection and disease from the other type. Humans are the primary hosts of HSV-1 and HSV-2, and both types are prevalent in all areas of the world. The population distribution is influenced by socioeconomic status, race, age, and virus type.

Most neonatal infections are acquired from maternal genital infection and usually are due to HSV-2. The estimated incidence of neonatal HSV infection is approximately 1 per 3,000 to 5,000 deliveries. Beyond the neonatal period, HSV-1 infections predominate and, depending on social and economic risk factors, as many as 40% to 60% of children of lower socioeconomic status are seropositive by 5 years of age. Because of sexual activity, the prevalence of HSV-2 infection increases at about the time of puberty and early adolescence.

HSV-1 and HSV-2 are transmitted from person to person through contact with infected skin lesions, mucous membranes, and secretions. Beyond the neonatal period, the incubation period ranges from 2 days to 2 weeks. Either type can be acquired in utero or perinatally, as the result of ascending infection or contact with infected cervical or vaginal secretions. The likelihood of transmission is fostered by asymptomatic viral shedding, which tends to occur more often after recently acquired HSV (primary) infection or with frequent recurrences. Transmission of HSV-2 to pregnant women is of particular concern because of the higher risk of subsequent transmission to newborns in the setting of a primary infection. Conversely, neonates most often acquire infection from asymptomatic or unrecognized maternal genital herpes (60% to 80% of infected women). The risk that an infant will acquire HSV infection when delivered vaginally is greatly influenced by whether the mother has primary or recurrent genital herpes at the time of delivery. The risk of herpetic infection is much greater (30% to 50%) if the infant is born vaginally by a mother with *primary* genital HSV (symptomatic

or asymptomatic) compared to a birth by a mother with recurrent genital HSV (3% to 5%).

HSV is a double-stranded DNA virus that enters the host through mucous membranes or abraded skin. When it infects epithelial cells, HSV gains access to and infects the regional sensory or autonomic nerves, traveling by the nerve axon to the neuron, where it establishes latent infection. During latency, the virus lies dormant and the host is asymptomatic. Subsequently, the virus may reactivate and begin replicating, usually resulting in clinical symptoms. Although not completely understood, clinical recurrences can be triggered by immunodeficiency (decreased cell-mediated immunity), physical and psychosocial stress, trauma, and exposure to sunlight.

The differential diagnosis of vesiculopustular lesions in neonates includes varicella-zoster virus, pustular melanosis, erythema toxicum neonatorum, incontinentia pigmenti, bullous staphylococcal infection, and epidermolysis bullosa. Disseminated HSV in the neonate can clinically mimic the signs and symptoms of bacterial sepsis. The differential diagnosis for skin lesions in the older child includes bullous impetigo and varicella (chickenpox); if the lesions are in a dermatomal distribution, HSV can be confused with herpes zoster (shingles).

CLINICAL FINDINGS

The site of the infection, the host's age and immune status, and any prior history of HSV infection influence the clinical manifestations of HSV infection. Primary HSV infection is diagnosed in patients without HSV antibody and with evidence of acute infection either by viral isolation or antigen positivity. Serology is not useful in diagnosing primary or recurrent HSV infection (except for research purposes) because commercial assays cannot reliably distinguish between HSV-1 and HSV-2 antibodies. HSV commonly causes six syndromes: oral/facial infections, genital infection, encephalitis, neonatal infection, skin infections other than oral/facial or genital, and eye infections (see the following sections). Other, rarer syndromes due to HSV (e.g., pneumonia, colitis, esophagitis, transverse myelitis, and Bell's palsy) are not discussed here.

Oral/Facial Infections

The most common clinical manifestation of primary HSV-1 infection in young infants and children is gingivostomatitis. Fever is common (lasting 2 to 7 days) as well as malaise, anorexia, irritability, drooling, and cervical adenopathy. Vesicular lesions are noted around and on the lips, gingiva, anterior tongue, and/or the hard palate. The vesicles break down rapidly and usually appear as 1- to 3-mm, shallow gray ulcers on an erythematous base. The gums may be mildly swollen, ulcerated, and erythematous. An exudative or ulcerative pharyngitis may be present. This illness is self-limited and of short duration. Dehydration secondary to refusal to take liquids orally (due to oral pain) is the most common complication and can result in hospitalization. Herpes labialis (i.e., fever blister, cold sore) is the most frequent form of recurrent HSV-1 infection. Usually these are short-lived and do not require specific therapy. HSV-2 also can cause pharyngitis, particularly in sexually active individuals. Herpetic pharyngitis may cause moderate to severe pain associated with systemic symptoms when it occurs as a primary infection. Although most oral/facial infections are mild and self-limited, in some patients (e.g., eczema, immunocompromised hosts) infections can be severe and should be treated with antiviral therapy.

Genital Herpes

Genital HSV infection may be asymptomatic or may be accompanied by papular, vesicular, or ulcerative lesions with symptoms of pain, itching, dysuria, and urethral or vaginal discharge. Primary infections tend to be more severe and may be associated with more extensive skin lesions, tender inguinal adenopathy, and extragenital lesions. Systemic manifestations (fever, headache, meningitis, abdominal pain) also may be more prominent in primary infections. Meningitis associated with primary genital infection occurs in 36% of women and 13% of men. This acute, self-limited form of aseptic meningitis usually is due to HSV-2 and causes headache and photophobia for 2 to 7 days. The cerebrospinal fluid (CSF) usually reveals a lymphocytic pleocytosis, sometimes with a positive HSV-2 viral culture.

Herpes Simplex Virus Encephalitis

HSV is the most common identifiable cause of sporadic acquired encephalitis and accounts for 2% to 5% of all encephalitis in the United States. Although HSV may involve any area of the brain, it has a predilection for the orbital region of the frontal and temporal lobes. HSV encephalitis, unlike the aseptic meningitis associated with genital HSV-2 infection, is a highly lethal disease with a 70% fatality rate if untreated. In 96% of cases, the encephalitis is due to HSV-1. It may be a result of primary (30%) or recurrent (70%) infection. Of 113 cases of biopsy-documented HSV encephalitis, 31% occurred in patients younger than 20 years, and 10% of patients were between 6 months and 10 years of age. Unlike other common forms of viral encephalitis (e.g., enterovirus, arbovirus), there is no seasonality to HSV encephalitis. The clinical hallmarks of acute HSV encephalitis are fever, altered mental status, and focal neurologic signs and symptoms evolving over 1 to 7 days and finally progressing to coma and often death. Signs of meningeal irritation usually are not present. There is no correlation between the isolation of HSV from sites outside of the central nervous system (e.g., oropharynx or genital tract) and encephalitis. Electroencephalographic findings may be diagnostic and demonstrate spike and slow-wave activity localized to the temporal lobes (periodic lateral epileptiform disharges, or PLEDS). A computed tomography (CT) scan or magnetic resonance imaging (MRI) study may reveal a localized lesion with edema and hemorrhage suggestive of HSV infection. The gold standard for diagnosis is histopathologic examination and culture of brain biopsy material, although the clinical use of HSV DNA polymerase chain reaction (PCR) on a CSF sample is now supplanting this procedure. In a patient with clinical symptoms suspect for HSV, empiric antiviral therapy should be instituted while diagnostic procedures are underway.

Neonatal Herpes

Neonates are particularly vulnerable to HSV infection and are more likely to develop encephalitis or dissemination with visceral involvement. In the United States, approximately 1,500 to 2,000 cases of neonatal HSV infection occur each year. Most (86%) are acquired perinatally, 10% postnatally, and rarely (4%) in utero. Approximately 75% are HSV-2 infection and 25% are HSV-1. HSV is transmitted most commonly during vaginal birth through an infected maternal genital tract, or less often from an ascending infection. Less commonly, infections result from postnatal transmission from a parent or other caregiver from a nongenital source (i.e., herpes labialis, herpetic whitlow, maternal breast lesions). Transmission postnatally from nursery personnel with fever blisters is rare.

Neonates with HSV infection present with one of three clinical patterns: disease localized to the skin, eyes, or mouth (SEM, 45%); CNS encephalitis (35%); or disseminated disease involving multiple organs (primarily liver and lungs, 20%). Infected neonates are rarely asymptomatic and often have signs and symptoms that mimic bacterial sepsis, including fever or hypothermia, lethargy, respiratory distress, poor feeding, vomiting, irritability, bulging fontanelle, focal or generalized seizures, opisthotonos, and coma. If not recognized and treated, 75% of infants presenting with SEM infection progress to CNS involvement or disseminated disease.

SEM disease typically presents in the first or second week of life and is the most easily recognized form of neonatal HSV infection. Vesicular lesions may occur singly or in clusters anywhere on the body, but typically are present on the presenting part or traumatized areas such as fetal scalp monitor sites. Vesicles due to herpes typically have an erythematous base with clear or cloudy fluid, and may even appear pustular. SEM disease is associated with little or no mortality as long as infection does not progress to involve the CNS or the viscera. These infants experience skin recurrences in 90% of cases. Even without known CNS involvement, 20% of infants who have three or more recurrences in the first 6 months of life will have developmental delay. The risk of neurologic sequelae appears to be greater with HSV-2 infections than with HSV-1 infections.

Neonatal encephalitis, with or without the presence of skin lesions, typically presents in the second to third week of life. Only 60% of these infants have skin lesions at any time during the illness. The diagnosis should be entertained in any neonate with signs and symptoms of fever, lethargy, apnea, focal or generalized seizures, and the typical CSF findings of pleocytosis and elevated protein. Untreated, neonatal HSV CNS disease has a 50% mortality rate, but with prompt institution of appropriate antiviral therapy, the mortality rate drops to 18%. Therefore, if HSV disease is suspected, appropriate therapy should be instituted promptly, even before confirmatory diagnostic testing and procedures. Despite treatment, two-thirds of survivors sustain neurologic impairment.

Disseminated HSV disease in the neonate involves multiple organs, including the brain, lungs, liver, and adrenal glands, and typically presents in the first week of life. Signs and symptoms may mimic bacterial sepsis due to group B *Streptococcus, Escherichia coli,* or *Listeria monocytogenes,* and skin lesions may not be present, or may occur late in the course. The possibility of disseminated HSV should be entertained in an infant with sepsis syndrome not responding to broad-spectrum antibiotic therapy or with the clinical picture of pneumonitis and hepatitis, with or without encephalitis. The latter findings would be unusual in sepsis due to bacteria. Without treatment, mortality due to disseminated HSV is greater than 80%. Even with appropriate antiviral therapy, mortality rates are 50% to 60%, and most survivors have neurologic sequelae.

Risk factors that increase the likelihood of neonatal HSV infection include active maternal primary infection, prematurity, absence of maternal antibody, rupture of membranes greater than 4 hours prior to delivery, procedures that interrupt skin integrity (e.g., fetal scalp monitors), and active maternal genital HSV lesions (recurrent) at delivery. Recommendations have been developed for the management of pregnant women with known genital herpes infection to decrease the risk of neonatal HSV disease. Women at risk should be thoroughly examined at delivery for the presence of active HSV lesions. If these are present, delivery should occur promptly by cesarean section, preferably before membranes have ruptured or, if already ruptured, within 4 hours. Fetal scalp monitors and other instrumentation (e.g., forceps, vacuum extractors) should be avoided. Performing genital culture for HSV as chronically infected women reach term has not been found to be a useful strategy. Treating women empirically with acyclovir in this setting has not been thoroughly studied. With the recognition that most infants with known exposure to HSV at delivery will not be infected, most experts recommend managing these infants expectantly.

While hospitalized, HSV-exposed infants should be placed in contact isolation and observed for signs and symptoms of disease. Circumcision should be delayed. If asymptomatic, these infants should have viral cultures obtained from the conjunctiva, oropharynx, and rectum at 24 to 48 hours of life. Cultures obtained before this time may reflect colonization from the maternal genital tract. Infants with positive cultures after 24 hours of life should be treated with intravenous (IV) acyclovir. If the infant is symptomatic, especially if delivered from a mother with known primary HSV infection, a lumbar puncture should be performed to assess the CSF and to obtain viral cultures and HSV PCR. These infants should be empirically placed on IV acyclovir pending final culture results.

Although rare, 4% of neonatal HSV infections are acquired in utero. Congenital infection is associated with fetal demise, preterm labor, microcephaly, hydrocephaly, hydranencephaly, microphthalmia, chorioretinitis, and vesicular skin lesions.

Skin Infections Other than Oral/Facial or Genital

In addition to the skin infection patterns discussed previously, several other skin infections are well recognized. *Herpetic whitlow* is a localized finger infection and can occur as a primary infection in health care workers or in the thumb-sucking child with herpetic gingivostomatitis. *Herpes gladiatorum* occurs in wrestlers owing to contact with infected secretions and abraded skin. Genital lesions can develop in infants and toddlers by self-inoculation. When this occurs, sexual abuse often is suspected, and viral isolation and typing may be helpful in determining the etiology of the lesion.

Eye Infections

HSV is the most common cause of corneal blindness in the United States. Keratitis may result from direct viral inoculation or from extension of facial skin lesions. Clinically, the eye infection is characterized by conjunctivitis and corneal dendritic ulcerations. HSV chorioretinitis occurs in patients with disseminated HSV infection, neonates (SEM), and patients with acquired immunodeficiency syndrome.

DIAGNOSTIC EVALUATION

Both HSV-1 and HSV-2 can be isolated by virus culture from active skin, eye, and genital lesions, usually within 48 hours of inoculation into appropriate cell lines. HSV grows rapidly (mean of 2 to 3 days, but may take as long as 5 to 7 days). When performing a culture of a vesicle, it is important that the base of the vesicle (after unroofing) or ulcer be scraped with a scalpel or plastic applicator and the resultant material placed in viral culture media. Although less sensitive and specific than viral culture, staining for viral antigens using the direct fluorescent antibody technique detects HSV more rapidly and can be used on clinical specimens from vesicular lesions, eye scrapings, and tissue such as brain. The Tzanck smear also can be performed on scrapings from skin lesions and detects multinucleated giant cells (found in both HSV and varicella-zoster virus lesions). Because available enzyme-linked immunosorbent assays cannot reliably distinguish between antibodies to HSV-1 and HSV-2, serology rarely has a role in the diagnosis of acute HSV infection.

The CSF in HSV encephalitis typically reveals a pleocytosis (up to 2,000 white blood cells/mm^3), with a predominance of lymphocytes. Early in infection, neutrophils may predominate. Although not pathognomonic, red blood cells reflecting hemorrhagic necrosis of involved areas of brain parenchyma may be seen in 75% to 85% of cases. From 5% to 25% of patients have low CSF glucose, and 80% to 88% have elevated CSF protein levels. From 2% to 3% of patients with early HSV encephalitis have normal CSF. The abnormal CSF findings are not diagnostic, and rarely is HSV isolated by CSF culture. PCR can detect HSV DNA in CSF and in serum and is highly sensitive for the diagnosis of neonatal HSV infection. In some research laboratories, PCR is 75% sensitive and 100% specific for HSV. Despite the low yield, viral culture of the CSF should still be performed.

In older infants and children, a CT or MRI of the brain characteristically shows edema and hemorrhage of the temporal lobes, while neonates may have lesions anywhere in the brain. An electroencephalogram also should be obtained in the infant suspected of having HSV and may be diagnostic, with spike and slow-wave activity localized to the temporal lobe region.

MANAGEMENT

Acyclovir is considered the drug of choice for most serious HSV infections because of its efficacy and low toxicity (Table 84.1). Parenteral acyclovir is indicated for the treatment of neonatal HSV, HSV encephalitis, and most infections in immunocompromised patients. For the neonate with HSV limited to the SEM, IV acyclovir should be administered at a dose of 60 mg/kg/day divided every 8 hours for 14 days. If the infant has chorioretinitis or keratitis, she also should be treated with trifluorothymidine 1% ophthalmic solution, 1 drop every 2 hours (up to 9 drops a day) until reepithelialization of the corneal ulcer occurs, and then 1 drop every 4 hours (5 drops a day) for 7 days. For encephalitis or disseminated disease, infants should be treated for a minimum of 21 days with IV acyclovir. For infants with frequent skin recurrences (three or more in the first 6 months of life), suppressive therapy with acyclovir 300 mg/m^2/day orally divided three times a day for 6 months has been shown to reduce the number of recurrences and therefore the risk of neurologic morbidity (see later with regard to neutropenia). For HSV encephalitis beyond the neonatal period, the dose of IV acyclovir is 30 mg/kg/day divided every 8 hours for 14 to 21 days.

Acyclovir is a safe drug whose main adverse effect is a transient rise in serum creatinine, easily reversible with drug cessation or adequate hydration. Oral acyclovir has been useful in primary genital herpes infections, but has limited impact on subsequent recurrences. For patients with 6 to 10 recurrences of genital herpes, suppressive therapy with acyclovir may be warranted. Patients on long-term suppressive therapy may develop neutropenia and should be monitored with periodic complete blood counts.

Infection-control measures also are appropriate in certain circumstances. Cesarean delivery of a woman with active HSV

TABLE 84.1

RECOMMENDED ACYCLOVIR DOSAGES FOR TREATMENT OF HERPES SIMPLEX VIRUS INFECTION

Indication	Route of therapy	Dose[a]	Doses/ Day	Therapy duration (days)
Neonatal herpes simplex virus (any form)	Intravenous	20 mg/kg	3	14 for skin, eyes, or mouth, 21 for central nervous system or disseminated disease.
Encephalitis	Intravenous	10 mg/kg	3	14–21
Primary genital	Intravenous	10 mg/kg	3	5–10
	Oral	200–400 mg	3	5–10
Recurrent genital	Oral	200 mg	5	5
Mucocutaneous in compromised host	Intravenous	5 mg/kg	3	7–10
	Oral	200–400 mg	5	7–10

[a]Adjust dose in patients with impaired renal function.
Modified from Prober CG. Herpes simplex virus. In: Long SS, Pickering LK, Prober CG, eds. *Principles and practice of pediatric infectious diseases.* New York: Churchill Livingstone; 2003:1032–1040.

genital lesions may reduce the risk of neonatal HSV if performed within 4 to 6 hours of membrane rupture. In addition to standard infection-control precautions, the following recommendations should be followed. Neonates with HSV infection should be hospitalized in a private room with contact precautions for the duration of the illness. Neonates who are exposed to HSV during delivery should be managed with contact precautions until cultures from mucous membrane sites (oropharynx, conjunctivae, rectum) obtained at 24 to 48 hours of life are negative. Continuous rooming-in with the mother in a private room is preferable. Children with mucocutaneous HSV also should be managed by contact isolation. Standard precautions are recommended for patients with infection limited to the CNS.

COURSE AND PROGNOSIS

Although neonatal HSV infections are infrequent, if untreated, death results in half the cases and neurologic sequelae in three-fourths of the survivors. Even with antiviral therapy, neonates with encephalitis or disseminated disease may succumb to disease or survive with long-term neurologic sequelae. Persistence of HSV DNA by PCR in CSF after 1 week of neurologic disease during or after completion of IV acyclovir has been associated with a poor outcome. The risk of death is increased in infants with coma, disseminated intravascular coagulopathy, or prematurity. In survivors, morbidity is most frequent in infants with encephalitis, disseminated infection, seizures, or infection with HSV-2. Although infants with SEM disease have little mortality, they often suffer from skin recurrences and subsequent neurologic impairment.

The outcome for children with HSV encephalitis is variable and ranges from normal to extensive and permanent neurologic disability or death. Untreated, the prognosis for HSV encephalitis is even worse. Even with antiviral therapy, substantial morbidity and mortality occur, and 5% to 10% of patients have a relapse. Factors associated with a poor outcome include the development of coma and clinical encephalitis for more than 4 days.

PEARLS

- Neonatal HSV infection often mimics bacterial sepsis or enterovirus infection and may occur without skin lesions.
- The clinical picture of neonatal sepsis associated with pneumonitis, hepatitis, or encephalitis would be unusual for bacterial etiologies. Viral etiologies such as HSV, enterovirus, or cytomegalovirus should be considered.
- HSV rarely presents as vesicular lesions on the first day of life; hence, other diagnoses should be sought.
- The appearance of grouped vesicles on an erythematous base is highly suspect for HSV infection.

Suggested Readings

American Academy of Pediatrics. Herpes simplex. In: Pickering LK, ed. *2000 red book: report of the Committee on Infectious Diseases.* 25th ed. Elk Grove Village, IL: American Academy of Pediatrics; 2000:309–318.

Annunziato PW, Gershon A. Herpes simplex virus infections. *Pediatr Rev* 1996; 17:415–427.

Kimberlin DW, Lakeman FD, Arvin A, et al. Application of the polymerase chain reaction to the diagnosis and management of neonatal herpes simplex. *J Infect Dis* 1996;174:162–167.

Kimura H, Futamura M, Kito H, et al. Detection of viral DNA in neonatal herpes simplex virus infections: frequent and prolonged presence in serum and cerebrospinal fluid. *J Infect Dis* 1991;164:289–293.

Overall JC. Herpes simplex virus infection of the fetus and newborn. *Pediatr Ann* 1994;23:131–136.

CHAPTER 85 ■ RECURRENT INFECTIONS AND IMMUNODEFICIENCY DISEASES

PATRICIA S. GERBER

Normal young children may have as many as nine to ten minor upper respiratory infections per year, especially if exposed to frequent viral infections in the milieu of day care. Patients with infections that are unusual, prolonged, severe, or fail to respond to appropriate therapy should raise concern about immunodeficiency.

An immunodeficiency disease may occur when part of the immune system is either absent or its function is impaired. A *primary immune deficiency* may be caused by an inborn defect resulting in abnormal functioning of one or more of the following:

■ T-lymphocytes (DiGeorge syndrome, chronic mucocutaneous candidiasis).
■ B-lymphocytes (X-linked hypogammaglobulinemia, common variable immunodeficiency, selective IgA deficiency, transient hypogammaglobulinemia of infancy, or IgG subclass deficiency).
■ Both T- and B-lymphocytes (severe combined immune deficiency, Wiskott–Aldrich syndrome, ataxia–telangiectasia syndrome).
■ Phagocytes (chronic granulomatous disease, hyper-IgE syndrome, leukocyte adhesion defects).
■ Complement (C2, C3, C5, or late complement component defects).

A primary immune disease occurs in 1 in 1,000 (e.g., IgA deficiency) to 1 in 100,000 (e.g., common variable immunodefiency, CVID) children. In general, 50% to 60% of immune defects involve B-lymphocytes, 10% to 15% T-lymphocytes, and 15% to 20% combined B- and T-lymphocytes.

A *secondary immune deficiency* may be caused by irradiation, chemotherapy, malnutrition, burns, protein loss (from the gut in malabsorption syndrome or through the kidneys in nephrotic syndrome), liver disease, and infection, such as human immunodeficiency virus. Descriptions of several more common immunodeficiencies are outlined below:

X-linked hypogammaglobulinemia is a disorder due to an arrest in B-lymphocyte differentiation, and is characterized by a defect in Bruton tyrosine kinase (Btk). Quantitative immunoglobulin levels and B-cell numbers are low, but cell-mediated immune function remains normal. Affected boys do well in the first 6 months of life and then develop chronic infections of the sinuses and lung. Serious infections, such as meningitis, sepsis, and osteomyelitis are more common than in normal children. Common pathogens include *Streptococcus pneumoniae*, *Haemophilus influenzae* type b, streptococcus, staphylococcus, mycoplasma, and enteroviral infections. Treatment includes monthly intravenous gammaglobulin infusions to prevent infection, avoidance of live virus vaccines, and prompt treatment of suspected infections.

Common variable immunodeficiency is characterized by recurrent upper respiratory and gastrointestinal infections in association with low immunoglobulin levels despite the presence of B-cells and normal cellular immune function. It is caused by one of several defects, including few or nonfunctional B-lymphocytes, inability of helper T-lymphocytes to produce certain cytokines, or excessive numbers of suppressor T-lymphocytes. Patients may have associated disorders, such as gastrointestinal problems (e.g., *Giardia lamblia* infection, inflammatory bowel disease, gluten-sensitive gastroenteropathy), nodular lymphoid hyperplasia, a variety of immune cytopenias, pernicious anemia, rheumatoid arthritis, and collagen vascular disorders. Treatment is similar to that of X-linked agammaglobulinemia.

T- and B-cell deficiency (severe combined immunodeficiency; SCID) is characterized by severe deficiency of total lymphocytes (less than 1,000), decreased T-cells (by T-cell enumeration), and low immunoglobulins. These children typically present in the first few months of life with failure to thrive, chronic respiratory and gastrointestinal infections, and/or candidal skin infections. *Pneumocystis carinii* pneumonia is often

TABLE 85.1

SIGNS OF PRIMARY IMMUNE DEFICIENCY

■ Eight or more new ear infections within 1 year
■ Two or more serious sinus infections or pneumonias (especially interstitial or with pneumatoceles) within 1 year
■ Two or more months on antibiotics for an infection without response
■ Failure to thrive or persistent diarrhea
■ Persistent, recurrent thrush
■ Need for intravenous antibiotics to clear infection
■ Recurrent deep skin or organ abscesses, periodontitis, delayed separation of umbilical cord
■ Two or more serious infections, such as meningitis, osteomyelitis, cellulitis, or sepsis
■ A family history of immune deficiency or death from infection in childhood or infancy
■ Reaction after transfusion of matched blood products
■ Clinical disease after live virus vaccination
■ Unusual rash and infection

These warning signs were developed by the Jeffrey Modell Foundation Medical Advisory Board © 2006 Jeffrey Modell Foundation.

TABLE 85.2

PHYSICAL EXAMINATION FINDINGS IN IMMUNE-DEFICIENT PATIENTS

Finding	Associated immunodeficiency diseases
Failure to thrive	Combined T- and B-cell defects
	Hypogammaglobulinemia with growth hormone deficiency
Disproportionate growth	Cartilage-hair hypoplasia
	Short-limbed dwarfism
Characteristic facies	DiGeorge syndrome
	Hyper-IgE syndrome
Purulent draining ears or nose	B-cell defects
	Combined T- and B-cell defects
Recalcitrant thrush	Combined T- and B-cell defects
Absence of lymph nodes, tonsils	X-linked hypogammaglobulinemia
	Combined T- and B-cell defects
Lymphadenopathy and splenomegaly	Common variable hypogammaglobulinemia
	Chronic granulomatous disease
	HIV or EBV infection
	Lymphoproliferative disorders
Recurrent bronchitis and pneumonia	Most immunodeficiency diseases
Pneumonia with pneumatoceles (staphylococcal)	Hyper-IgE syndrome
Interstitial pneumonia (*Pneumocystis carinii*)	T-cell defects
Cardiac anomalies	Anomalies of the great vessels; DiGeorge syndrome
Omphalitis, delayed separation of the umbilical cord (>8 wk)	Leukocyte adhesion defects
Liver abscesses	Phagocytic defects
Ataxia	Ataxia-telangiectasia syndrome
Skin manifestations	
Boils and furuncles	Phagocytic defects
Candida and herpes infection	T-cell defect
Periodontitis	Phagocytic defect
Dermatomyositis	X-linked hypogammaglobulinemia
Eczematous dermatitis	Wiskott–Aldrich syndrome
	Hyper-IgE syndrome
Seborrheic dermatitis	Omenn syndrome
	Leiner disease
Petechiae, bruising	Wiskott–Aldrich syndrome
Telangiectasia of ears and/or conjunctiva	Ataxia–telangiectasia syndrome
Hair	
Partial albinism	Chediak–Higashi syndrome
Silvery hair	Griselli syndrome
Fine hair	Cartilage hair-hypoplasia
Arthropathy	X-linked hypogammaglobulinemia
	Common variable hypogammaglobulinemia
	IgA deficiency
Hypocalcemic tetany	DiGeorge syndrome

HIV, human immunodeficiency virus; EBV, Epstein–Barr virus.

a presenting feature. There are many types of combined T- and B-cell deficiency, including common γ–chain (the most common), IL-2Rα, JAK3, RAG1 and RAG2, and ADA deficiency.

Treatment for SCID is early bone marrow transplantation and IV gammaglobulin therapy. Pneumocystis prophylaxis with trimethoprim–sulfamethoxazole is necessary. When blood products are necessary prior to transplant, they must be cytomegalovirus (CMV) negative and irradiated to prevent infection and graft-versus-host disease. Once bone marrow transplantation has been done, B-cell function remains poor and requires continued use of IV gammaglobulin for years.

Phagocytic defects are exemplified by chronic granulomatous disease (CGD) of childhood. This disorder is characterized by an inability of the polymorphonuclear leukocytes and monocytes to produce reactive oxygen products necessary to kill certain phagocytosed intracellular bacteria and fungi. Infection is common with catalase-positive organisms, such as *Staphylococcus* sp., *Escherichia coli*, *Pseudomonas* sp., *Klebsiella* sp., *Serratia* sp., *Salmonella* sp., and fungi such as *Candida* sp. and *Aspergillus* sp. There are three autosomal recessive forms and an X-linked form. These children may present at any age between infancy and late childhood. Infections commonly involve the lungs, lymph nodes, soft tissue, bone, liver, skin, and urinary tract with characteristic granuloma formation on biopsy. Treatment of CGD includes treatment of infection with appropriate antistaphylococcal antibiotics or antifungal agents, trimethoprim–sulfamethoxazole prophylaxis, and recombinant gamma interferon.

Early complement defects are characterized by sepsis, and *late complement defects* are characterized by *Neisseria* sp. infections. Prevention of infection with vaccination and prompt appropriate treatment of bacterial infections are the mainstays of therapy for complement defects.

TABLE 85.3

IMMUNE SCREENING EVALUATION

HUMORAL IMMUNITY
Absolute lymphocyte counts
Serum quantitative immunoglobulins (IgG, IgA, IgM, IgE)
IgG subclasses
Specific functional antibody titers to routine vaccination
　(diphtheria, tetanus, *Haemophilus influenzae* type b,
　pneumococcus)
B-cell enumeration (CD19, CD20)

CELL-MEDIATED IMMUNITY
Initial tests
　Absolute lymphocyte counts
　Human immunodeficiency (HIV) enzyme-linked
　　immunosorbent assay (high-risk patients)
Delayed hypersensitivity skin tests
　Candida 1:1,000, 1:100
　Tetanus 1:100
　Mumps undiluted
　Trichophyton 1:30

PHAGOCYTIC DEFECTS
White blood cell count and morphology
Nitroblue tetrazolium test (NBT; chronic granulomatous
　disease)
IgE level (hyper-IgE syndrome)
CD11/CD18 (leukocyte adhesion defects)

COMPLEMENT DEFECTS
CH50 (total pathway activity)
C3 and C4 (early classical pathways defect)

**ADVANCED IMMUNOLOGIC (IN CONSULTATION
WITH A PEDIATRIC IMMUNOLOGIST)**
T-cell enumeration
In vitro stimulation of lymphocytes
　Nonspecific mitogens: phytohemagglutinin (PHA),
　　concanavalin-A (Con A), and pokeweed mitogen
　　(PWM)
　Specific antigens: candida, tetanus
Allogeneic cells in mixed lymphocyte culture

CLINICAL FINDINGS

The history of a child with recurrent or atypical infections should be fully reviewed with attention to the type and duration of infections. For simplicity, some common signs suggesting primary immune deficiency diseases are outlined in Table 85.1.

Careful physical examination may reveal clues to the diagnosis of specific immunodeficiencies. These are outlined in Table 85.2.

Laboratory evaluation of the child with recurrent infections begins with the complete blood count with differential, platelet count, and calculation of the absolute lymphocyte count and absolute neutrophil count. A leukocytosis may suggest a phagocytic defect or bacterial infection. Large leukocyte cytoplasmic inclusions may be found in Chediak–Higashi syndrome. Howell–Jowell bodies indicate splenic dysfunction. Thrombocytopenia may be seen in Wiskott–Aldrich syndrome (very small platelets), common variable immunodeficiency, or hypogammaglobulinemia with hyper-IgM. Eosinophilia is also seen in Wiskott–Aldrich syndrome, hyper-IgE syndrome, graft-versus-host disease, graft rejection, allergic disease, and parasitic syndromes.

Routine blood chemistries may reveal a variety of suggestive abnormal findings, such as elevation of the Westergren erythrocyte sedimentation rate in infection; decreased globulin fraction of total protein (hypogammaglobulinemia, hypocomplementemia, protein loss, or malnutrition); decreased uric acid (purine pathway defects, adenosine deaminase [ADA] deficiency, and purine nucleotide phosphorylase deficiency); or hypocalcemia (frequent in DiGeorge syndrome).

Routine chest radiograph should be examined for the presence or absence of thymic shadow (T-cell defect), pneumonia (interstitial with *Pneumocystis carinii* or pneumatoceles in hyper-IgE), or lateral rib defects (ADA deficiency). Lack or presence of adenoidal tissue is useful in evaluation for X-linked (absent) or common variable (present) hypogammaglobulinemia.

The evaluation for immunodeficiency diseases is suggested in Table 85.3. Further testing of patients with suspected immune deficiency should be done in consultation with a pediatric immunologist.

MANAGEMENT

In patients with immune defects, appropriate and prompt treatment of suspected infections is fundamental, and knowledge of potential causative organisms for that disease is essential to reduce morbidity and mortality. For defects in phagocytosis or T-cell function, trimethoprim–sulfamethoxazole prophylaxis, TMP-SXT (TMP component 8 to 10 mg/kg/day, 3 days/week) is required. Patients with chronic granulomatous disease may be treated with gamma-interferon. White cell transfusions may be required during severe infections. Patients with B-cell or combined T- and B-cell defects require monthly infusions of IV gammaglobulin 200 to 600 mg/kg/dose. Routine human immune globulin IV preparations (Gamimune N, 5%; Gammar-P IV; Sandoglobulin IV: and Venoglobulin-S) are available. If a patient has a low IgA, to decrease the risk of sensitization with subsequent allergic reaction, solvent/detergent-treated human immune globulin IV preparations (Gammagard S/D or Polygam S/D) should be used. Early bone marrow transplantation with an human leukocyte antigen (HLA)-identical or a T cell–depleted haploidentical donor is indicated in some T-cell and combined T- and B-cell immune deficiencies. Bone marrow engraftment in the neonatal period prior to development of chronic infectious complications is more successful; therefore, early referral to an immunologist is important.

PEARLS

- *Immunization with live virus vaccine*, such as measles, mumps, and rubella (MMR) or varicella, or *transfusion with nonirradiated blood products*, must *never* be done when immunodeficiency is suspected.
- When treating a hypogammaglobulinemic patient with almost absent IgA, use a low-IgA preparation of IV gamma-globulin to avoid anaphylaxis.
- Early bone marrow transplantation in the neonatal period leads to better engraftment and improved survival.

Suggested Readings

Bonilla FA, Bernstein IL, Khan DA, et al. Practice parameters for the diagnosis and management of primary immunodeficiency. *Ann Allergy Asthma Immunol* 2005;94:S1–S63.

Grunebaum E, Mazzolari E, Porto F, et al. Bone marrow transplantation for severe combined immune deficiency. *JAMA* 2006;295:508–518.

Notarangelo L, Casabova JL, Fischer A, et al. Primary immunodeficieny disease an update. *J Allergy Clin Immunol* 2004;114:677–687.

Tangsinmankong N, Bahna S, Good RA. The immunologic work-up of the child suspected of immunodeficiency. *Ann Allergy Asthma Immunol* 2001;87:362–437.

CHAPTER 86 ■ OSTEOMYELITIS AND SEPTIC ARTHRITIS

TINA Q. TAN

Septic or infectious arthritis is an acute bacterial joint infection with an estimated annual incidence of 5.5 to 12 cases per 100,000 children. Infants and children less than 2 years of age represent between one-third and one-half of the reported cases. Predisposing factors for the development of this condition include trauma, joint surgery, joint injections, and surgery or instrumentation of the urinary or intestinal tracts.

Osteomyelitis is an inflammation of bone usually caused by a pyogenic organism. It is a fairly common disorder of childhood, occurring in about 1 in 5,000 children less than 13 years of age. Boys are 2.5 times more likely to develop osteomyelitis as girls, possibly related to an increased incidence of minor trauma. Overall, 50% of patients with osteomyelitis are less than 5 years of age and one-third are less than 2 years of age.

The pathogenesis of septic arthritis and osteomyelitis share many common features. Bacteria may reach either site by three routes:

1. Hematogenous spread from primary focus (primary mechanism, 90% of cases in children less than 16 years of age).
2. Contiguous spread from adjacent tissues (e.g., cellulitis).
3. Direct inoculation into the site (e.g., trauma or surgery).

Hematogenous osteomyelitis occurs as a complication of bacteremia. Blood-borne bacteria localize in the metaphyseal end of the bone shaft adjacent to the epiphyseal growth centers. The circulation of the bone in this area predisposes it to infection. The nutrient artery that supplies the bone divides into branches and then into a narrow plexus of capillaries that make sharp loops in the area of the epiphyseal plate before entering a system of large sinusoidal vessels supplying the metaphysis. Sluggish blood flow and an absence of lining reticuloendothelial cells in this area are predisposing factors for microvascular thrombosis and bacterial growth. Thrombosis of the slow-flowing vessels is caused by trauma or embolization and provides a breeding ground for blood-borne bacteria. Bacteria proliferate in this fairly avascular area, shielded from host defenses. This results in a localized cellulitis of the bone marrow. Polymorphonuclear leukocytes and bacterial products accumulate under pressure, leading to further vascular thrombosis, pressure necrosis of the bone, and death of small islands of bone. As the process continues, the infection may:

1. Spread into the metaphyseal cortex and under the periosteum, leading to the development of a subperiosteal abscess.
2. Spread along the marrow cavity and the periosteum into a joint space, resulting in a septic joint.
3. Rupture through the periosteum into adjacent muscle, resulting in a soft-tissue infection.

Staphylococcus aureus (including community-associated methicillin resistant strains, CA-MRSA) is the primary organism causing septic arthritis and acute hematogenous osteomyelitis in both children and adults. In children, it accounts for about 50% of all cases of septic arthritis and 70% to 90% of all cases of acute hematogenous osteomyelitis. Group A streptococcus is the second most common entity. Other organisms commonly associated with septic arthritis include *Streptococcus pneumoniae*, *Haemophilus influenzae* type b (<2 years old either incompletely immunized with conjugate *H. influenzae* type b vaccine or immunocompromised), *Salmonella* species (patients with hemoglobinopathies), enteric gram-negative organisms, *Kingella kingae* (children <5 years of age), and *Neisseria gonorrhoeae* (newborns and sexually active adolescents).

In addition to *S. aureus* and group A streptococci, organisms commonly associated with acute hematogenous osteomyelitis include *S. pneumoniae*, *H. influenzae* type b (children less than 2 years of age with risk factors noted above), group B streptococcus (infants <2 months old, most common serotype is III), coagulase-negative staphylococci (premature infants), *Salmonella* species (children with hemoglobinopathies), *E. coli*, *Shigella*, *Klebsiella*, *K. kingae*, *Pseudomonas aeruginosa* (associated with puncture wounds of the calcaneus and producing more of an osteochondritis), *Candida* species, and *Aspergillus* (immunocompromised host or premature infants with central venous catheters).

For contiguous focus osteomyelitis, *S. aureus* and group A streptococcus remain the most common organisms, but enteric gram-negative organisms (especially in the neonate) and polymicrobial infections may be seen.

CLINICAL FINDINGS

The clinical findings of osteomyelitis and septic arthritis vary depending on the age of the child, the duration of the process, and the location of the infection.

Neonate and Infants

In young infants, the presence of a thin cortex of bone, transepiphyseal vessels, and the extension of the joint capsule to the metaphysis allows for rapid progression of infection, rupture through the bone, and infection within a contiguous joint or muscle. The most common joints involved are the hip and knee. Clinical findings may be minimal—slight irritability, low-grade fever, and decreased feeding; or the child may appear septic with no localized findings. Physical examination may reveal diffuse edema, erythema, warmth, and swelling of a limb or joint, guarding of an affected limb with markedly decreased use (pseudoparalysis), severe discomfort with passive movement or touch, and regional adenopathy.

In neonates with osteomyelitis, up to 50% will have multifocal bone involvement. In both septic joint and osteomyelitis, a sign of hip/proximal femur involvement results in a leg that is flexed at the hip, abducted, and externally rotated—the "frog leg" position.

Osteomyelitis of the skull is most common in the neonatal population and may result from cephalohematomas, scalp monitors, intravenous (IV) lines, abscesses, and venipuncture.

Older Infant and Child

In this age group, the most common systemic symptoms for septic joint and osteomyelitis in this age group are:

- Fever up to 40°C.
- Chills.
- Malaise.
- Nausea/vomiting.
- Refusal to use the affected extremity (limp or refusal to walk), pain on passive and/or active manipulation of the involved extremity, and localized tenderness over the involved site (even prior to the appearance of swelling, erythema, and warmth).

A history of trauma (may be very minor) that occurred in the period prior to the development of septic joint or osteomyelitis may be elicited. The most common physical findings are swelling, edema, erythema, warmth, and point tenderness over the involved bone or joint; regional adenitis; or an identifiable focus of infection.

In this age group, the cortex and periosteum of the bone act as barriers to the spread of the infection so that there are fewer soft-tissue findings. After 18 months of age, joint involvement with osteomyelitis is usually not found because the physis acts as a barrier to the spread of infection. In children with septic arthritis, the most common joints involved (from most to least) are the knee, hip, ankle, elbow, shoulder, and wrist. The metaphyseal area of the long bones of the arms and legs are the most common sites of involvement in patients with osteomyelitis.

Adolescent and Adult

The findings are similar to those for a child, but the function of the affected extremity is less restricted and point tenderness may only be present at rest.

The diagnosis of a septic joint or osteomyelitis is based on a combination of factors including:

1. *Clinical evaluation*: the presence of fever, clinical symptoms, physical examination findings, and data from the patient's history.
2. *Laboratory data*: peripheral white blood cell (WBC) count (usually elevated but may be normal), erythrocyte sedimentation rate (ESR, elevated in majority of cases), C-reactive protein (CRP, elevated), blood culture (positive in 50% to 60% of cases), and joint fluid findings (Gram stain and cultures are positive in about 60% of cases; WBC count and differential, glucose level, protein level, and pH).
3. *Radiographic findings*: plain film, bone scan, magnetic resonance imaging (MRI), and/or gallium or indium scans.
4. *Surgical intervention*: open bone biopsy is the gold standard for histologic diagnosis of osteomyelitis and bacterial identification. Needle biopsy/aspiration of material from subperiosteal abscesses and associated septic joints can also provide material for cell count, culture (aerobic, anaerobic, fungal, and acid-fast bacillus), and Gram stain (positive in 70% to 80% of patients with osteomyelitis).

In the neonate, physical findings alone are sufficient to make the diagnosis of septic joint and osteomyelitis. Plain films are usually abnormal when clinical signs are present. Due to the risk of joint destruction, surgical drainage of all involved sites is considered an urgent issue, especially if the hip or shoulder joint is involved.

In the older child or adolescent, radiographic studies can be performed that confirm the diagnosis of septic joint and/or osteomyelitis:

1. *Plain film radiographs*: In septic arthritis, the findings seen on plain film are due to capsular swelling of the joint, which displaces the fat lines. For osteomyelitis, osteolytic lesions do not become evident until 40% to 50% of the bone mineral has been destroyed; therefore, at least 10 days to 3 weeks are required after the infection begins before bony changes are visible on plain radiographs. Early on in the process, soft-tissue swelling with obliteration of the tissue planes due to muscle edema is usually seen. Periosteal new bone formation does not become evident until 10 days or more from the start of the infection. However, negative plain films even at 10 to 14 days do not rule out the presence of osteomyelitis.
2. *Radionuclide imaging*: Bone scanning techniques using technetium Tc 99m phosphate or diphosphate compounds are more sensitive and can be used earlier in the infection, before bony changes are apparent on plain film. Abnormalities can be detected as early as 48 hours from the start of the infection. If septic arthritis alone is present, there will be increased uptake on either side of the involved joint during the "blood pool" phase of the scan. In osteomyelitis, increased isotope uptake is seen in areas of infection; "cold" spots (where there is no isotope uptake) are seen in areas of ischemia, necrosis, or abscess; and if there is an associated cellulitis/soft-tissue infection, uptake occurs during the early phase of the bone scan but does not persist in the later phases. The inflammation associated with cellulitis and fractures may make interpretation of the scan results more difficult. Due to the limited amount of mineralization in their bones, the sensitivity of bone scans in neonates and young infants is much lower than in older infants and children. Destruction of cortical bone and periosteal new bone formation might be seen on plain films in this age group when the bone scan result is normal.
3. *Other imaging techniques*: MRI is most useful very early in the infection, especially in osteomyelitis where bone marrow cellulitis can be seen. Gallium and indium scans use tagged WBCs to indicate the site of infection by looking for aggregation of these cells.

MANAGEMENT

For both septic arthritis and osteomyelitis, empiric therapy *must* include coverage for *S. aureus* (including CA-MRSA) and group A streptococci in all age groups. In the past, initial IV antibiotic therapy usually consisted of a penicillinase-resistant semisynthetic penicillin (oxacillin or nafcillin 200 mg/kg/day in four to six divided doses) or a first-generation cephalosporin (cefazolin sodium 75 to 100 mg/kg/day in three divided doses). However, this is changing, because of the marked increase in the amount of disease caused by CA-MRSA. Clindamycin (30 to 40 mg/kg/day IV divided every 6 hours) is suggested if the patient's isolate is susceptible; vancomycin (40 mg/kg/day IV in four divided doses) or linezolid (10 mg/kg/dose IV every 12 hours) have become recommended initial empiric therapy. This can be tailored once the organism is identified and antibiotic susceptibilities are known. In children under 2 years of age or in whom immunization status is unknown, coverage for *H. influenzae* type b should also be included. The use of cefuroxime (150 mg/kg/day IV in three divided doses) or the combination of ampicillin or a third-generation cephalosporin with oxacillin or naficillin can be considered in these cases. In patients with hemoglobinopathies, coverage for enteric gram-negative organisms should be considered. In these cases, the third-generation cephalosporins (cefotaxime sodium or ceftriaxone sodium) or ampicillin and an aminoglycoside may be used for empiric therapy. For patients who are very ill, immunocompromised, or with puncture wounds of the foot, the antibiotic chosen should also cover *P. aeruginosa*. Empiric therapy in these cases includes ceftazidime and aminoglycosides.

The duration of antibiotic therapy for septic arthritis is 3 to 4 weeks; for osteomyelitis, the duration of parenteral antibiotic therapy is a minimum of 4 weeks. Multiple studies have shown up to a 50% failure rate for *S. aureus* osteomyelitis treated less than 4 weeks. The exception to this is with puncture wound osteomyelitis due to *P. aeruginosa*. In this situation, if infection is recognized early and management is aggressive (surgical debridement), the duration of therapy can be as short as 10 to 14 days.

The treatment of acute hematogenous osteomyelitis with a combination of initial parenteral therapy followed by oral antibiotic therapy is becoming more common. Completing therapy with a course of oral antibiotics has the advantages of decreasing the cost, discomfort, and hazards of long-term parenteral therapy; however, it is not feasible for every patient. Criteria that should be met prior to changing to oral therapy include the following:

1. Afebrile for 48 to 72 hours with no other systemic symptoms.
2. Significant reduction in local signs and symptoms of infection.
3. Adequate surgical debridement.
4. Definitive identification of the organism, or response of the presumed organism to antibiotic therapy.
5. Determination of appropriate serum concentrations of the antibiotic.
6. Patient able to swallow and retain the medication.
7. A reliable caretaker.

Antibiotic therapy should be continued until the patient has a peripheral WBC count, ESR, and/or CRP that has returned to baseline, and serial radiographs indicating improvement and/or resolution of the infection. Under most circumstances, optimal therapy of these infections involves both a medical and surgical approach to completely eradicate the infection.

COURSE AND PROGNOSIS

The *complications* most commonly seen with these infections include the following:

1. Physical deformity/disability with impairment of limb growth and function.
2. Pathologic fractures at the infection site.
3. Secondary bacteremia from the infection site with seeding of secondary sites if the initial infection is not properly treated.
4. Chronic osteomyelitis, usually from inadequately treated acute osteomyelitis.

Patients with chronic osteomyelitis present with episodes of swelling, tenderness, disuse of the affected extremity, and possibly the presence of a draining sinus tract. Management usually includes surgical debridement and very long-term antibiotics (may require multiple courses).

SPECIAL SITUATIONS

1. *Vertebral* osteomyelitis is usually hematogenous and accounts for about 1% to 3% of all cases of osteomyelitis. It is more common in boys, and the presentation is usually insidious. Major symptoms may include fever, back pain and stiffness, generalized malaise, and weakness. Children may present with poorly localized chest (thoracic vertebra), abdominal, or leg pain (lumbar vertebra). The nonspecific nature of complaints associated with vertebral osteomyelitis may delay the diagnosis for several months. Vertebral osteomyelitis may mimic discitis clinically but can usually be differentiated radiographically (greater vertebral endplate involvement in osteomyelitis than in discitis) or by MRI.
2. *Pelvic* osteomyelitis often has a subacute presentation. Diagnosis may be very difficult to establish because it can mimic appendicitis and urinary tract infection. Children with pelvic osteomyelitis may present with fever, gait abnormalities, poorly localized abdominal or hip pain, and tenderness over the buttock or sciatic notch. Point tenderness and pain with hip movement can be elicited on physical examination in only 50% of patients. Like vertebral osteomyelitis, the diagnosis is often missed for a prolonged period of time.
3. *Contiguous-focus* osteomyelitis occurs through the spread of infection from adjoining infected tissue to bone. The femur and tibia are the most common sites of involvement. The microorganisms are often introduced during a traumatic injury that results in an open fracture or during open reduction and internal fixation of a fracture. Infections in the pelvis, hands (bite wounds), sinuses, and mouth may serve as the primary focus of infection.
4. *"Sneaker"* osteomyelitis is an infection of the small bones and periostia of the foot from a penetrating injury (usually stepping on a nail) while wearing sneakers. Patients tend to be older (10 to 18 years of age) than children with acute hematogenous osteomyelitis, and most commonly boys. Local debridement and antibiotics directed at *Pseudomonas* spp. (e.g., cefepime hydrochloride or ceftazidime with an antipseudomonal penicillin) are the treatment of choice. A tetanus booster is also required if not current.

PEARLS

- Fever and a limp (or refusal to use or move a limb) requires consideration of septic arthritis or osteomyelitis in the differential.
- Septic arthritis of the hip or shoulder is an infectious disease "emergency." Prompt drainage of pus is necessary to improve outcome and decrease the risk of joint damage.
- Neonates may present with multifocal disease.
- Acute osteomyelitis must be treated adequately from the onset to avoid progression to chronic osteomyelitis. When in doubt as to length of therapy, err on the side of a longer course.
- Suggestive clinical findings with absent radiographic findings do not rule out osteomyelitis.

Suggested Readings

Bradley JS, Kaplan SL, Tan TQ, et al. Pediatric pneumococcal bone and joint infections. *Pediatrics* 1998;102:1376–1382.
Burnett MW, Bass JW, Cook BA. Etiology of osteomyelitis complicating sickle cell disease. *Pediatrics* 1998;101:296–297.
Krogstad P, Smith AL. Osteomyelitis and septic arthritis. In: Feigin RD, Cherry JD, eds. *Textbook of pediatric infectious diseases.* 5th ed. Philadelphia: Saunders; 2004:713–736.
Lew DP, Waldvogel FA. Osteomyelitis. *N Engl J Med* 1997;336:999–1007.
Roy DR. Osteomyelitis. *Pediatr Rev* 1995;16:380–385.

CHAPTER 87 ■ UPPER AIRWAY INFECTIONS

SAMEER S. PATHARE

Upper airway infections in children are very common. The upper respiratory tract involves the mouth, nose, and pharynx superiorly and the glottis inferiorly. Contiguous anatomically, infections in this region result in a spectrum of disorders of the upper airway. The most common upper airway infections are rhinitis and pharyngitis, which are usually viral and self-limited. Other upper airway infections, such as epiglottitis and bacterial tracheitis, can cause respiratory distress and are potentially life-threatening emergencies. The focus of this chapter is an overview of the most common upper airway infections that result in hospitalization: croup, epiglottitis, bacterial tracheitis, and retropharyngeal abscess.

CROUP

Croup is a syndrome that encompasses many different etiologies. It is classically seen with the combination of barky "seal-like" cough, hoarseness, inspiratory stridor, and respiratory distress. Stridor is a harsh, high-pitched respiratory sound, usually inspiratory, but may be biphasic. It is a result of turbulent airflow that is caused by a partial obstruction of the airway. Croup syndrome is synonymous with laryngotracheobronchitis, and by definition involves both the upper and lower respiratory tract. The peak age for croup syndrome is in the second year of life, with a range of 3 months to 5 years. It has a prevalence of 5 per 100 children. Hospitalization is usually necessary in less than 10% of infants and children with croup.

Viral laryngotracheobronchitis is most commonly seen in the late fall and early winter, as well as in late spring and early summer. The most common viral etiology is the group of parainfluenza viruses. These account for 75% of the viral isolates. Parainfluenza type 3 is most common in the springtime, while parainfluenza 1 is most common in the winter. Other etiologies for croup syndrome include respiratory syncytial virus (RSV), influenza A & B, adenovirus, measles, rhinoviruses, and *Mycoplasma pneumoniae*.

Typically, croup begins as a viral upper respiratory tract infection (in the nasopharynx) manifested by rhinorrhea and pharyngitis. This progresses downward to the larynx, infraglottic tissues, and trachea. The cricoid cartilage encircles the airway just below the vocal cords and defines the narrowest portion of the upper airway in children younger than 10 years old. According to Poiseuille's law, airway resistance is inversely proportional to the fourth power of the radius; therefore small reductions in the airway diameter (secondary to mucosal edema) can lead to significant increases in resistance, resulting in stridor and respiratory distress.

The differential diagnosis is extensive. Some common mimickers are epiglottitis, bacterial tracheitis, retropharyngeal abscess, peritonsillar abscess, foreign body, laryngomalacia, subglottic stenosis, hemangioma, spasmodic croup, vocal cord anomalies, thermal injury, smoke inhalation, and neoplasm. Spasmodic croup is caused by noninflammatory edema in the larynx, trachea, and infraglottic tissues. Its clinical presentation is similar to viral croup with the notable exception of the absence of upper respiratory tract infection prodromal symptoms such as rhinorrhea or nasal congestion. Most people believe that spasmodic croup is an allergic reaction rather than a primary infection.

Clinical Findings

Infants and children with croup typically present with rhinorrhea, low-grade fevers, and cough that progressively worsens to the characteristic paroxysmal barking with inspiratory stridor. Low-grade fever is common, but temperatures may reach 39°C to 40°C. Fevers in this range should prompt evaluation for other possible bacterial infections. The low-grade fever is usually accompanied by respiratory distress, tachypnea, retractions, and nasal flaring. Symptoms are usually worse at night. Physical exam findings include rhinorrhea, stridor, and occasionally wheezes and crackles.

There are scoring methods for categorizing the severity of croup based on the presence of cyanosis, altered mental status, degree of stridor, quality of breath sounds, and presence of retractions. These are rarely used in clinical practice. The spectrum of disease can range from mild croup where only stridor with agitation is noted; to severe croup where the patient is cyanotic and disoriented with prominent retractions, stridor at rest, and decreased breath sounds. Cyanosis is a late sign and is consistent with impending respiratory failure.

Radiologic findings are seldom necessary or helpful in determining the diagnosis of croup. The classic radiologic finding is an AP soft-tissue view of the neck that demonstrates the "steeple sign" of the tracheal air column. This represents narrowing of the laryngeal air column below the vocal cords. Remember, the "steeple sign" may be absent in croup, may be present in patients without croup, and may be present in epiglottitis.

Management

Therapy in croup is targeted at airway management and comfort measures. Oxygen may be necessary when croup involves the lower respiratory tract, but typically when the edema is localized to the larynx, oxygen saturations do not fall until there is almost complete obstruction of the upper airway.

Analgesics, such as acetaminophen or ibuprofen, are indicated for comfort measures. Mist therapy is often used, but should be used with caution if at all. Mist tents can obscure observation of the patient and have little demonstrated benefit. Mist therapy may moisten secretions and decrease the viscosity of secretions, but may actually aggravate concurrent bronchospasm.

Nebulized epinephrine is a common therapy used in croup. Racemic epinephrine or the active L-epinephrine are both acceptable options. Epinephrine stimulates mucosal alpha-adrenergic receptors that constrict pre-capillary arterioles and lead to resorption of interstitial fluid, decreased hydrostatic pressure and decreased airway edema.

Glucocorticoids, particularly dexamethasone, in a single dose of 0.6 mg/kg (max 8 mg), either PO or IM has shown benefit. Studies have shown comparable results when dexamethasone is given parenterally or orally (1). The anti-inflammatory effect of the steroids has been shown to decrease hospitalization, decrease the need for intubation, and accelerate improvement. Inhaled steroids have also been utilized, but at much higher doses than the usual daily doses for maintenance of asthma. Studies have shown that dexamethasone is superior to inhaled steroids. In severe respiratory distress, pediatric intensive care may be necessary. Heliox ventilation has been used successfully for croup. Usually heliox is a 70/30 mixture of helium and oxygen. Heliox can increase laminar airflow, and decrease the work of respiration. As oxygen concentration increases beyond 30%, the laminar flow of heliox is lost. Therefore, the limitation of heliox ventilation is the patient's oxygen requirement. The last alternative for severe respiratory distress is endotracheal intubation. Hypercarbia, respiratory failure, worsening stridor, retractions, tachypnea, tachycardia, cyanosis, exhaustion, confusion, and failure to respond to epinephrine, are all considerations for intubation. If intubation is necessary, an endotracheal tube with a diameter one size smaller than recommended size for age should be used to allow for the airway edema.

Course and Prognosis

Croup usually resolves in 3 to 4 days. When patients have prolonged stridor or recurrent symptoms, further workup is usually necessary. The decision to consult an otorhinolaryngologist should be considered in the following situations: severe croup requiring intubation, atypical presentation such as age >3 years old, recurrent croup, minimal treatment response, or history suggesting laryngeal nerve injury. Discharge criteria include normal air entry, color, and level of consciousness along with absence of stridor at rest. The patient should have received at least one dose of steroids unless other contraindications are present. Observation for 2 to 3 hours after epinephrine nebs is usually recommended. A "rebound" of croup symptoms after inhaled epinephrine has not been substantiated, but relapse and return of symptoms can occur.

EPIGLOTTITIS

Epiglottitis is a life-threatening emergency. By definition, it is the inflammation and edema of the epiglottis and aryepiglottic folds secondary to a bacterial infection. The peak age group is 3 years of age. The range of ages is classically 2 to 8 years old, with peak seasonal incidence in the winter. The incidence of epiglottitis has fallen substantially since the advent of the H. influenzae serotype b vaccine. The incidence in 1987 was 41 per 100,000 children <5 years old. The incidence in the postvaccine era is approximately 1.3 per 100,000 in 1997 (2). Fully immunized children can have epiglottitis, but should be evaluated for possible immunodeficiency disorders. The widespread usage of vaccines has shifted the epidemiology of the pathogenic organisms. Staphylococcus aureus, Streptococcus pneumoniae, and Streptococcus pyogenes are now more common bacterial causes.

Clinical Findings

The presentation of epiglottitis is notable for sudden onset. There are associated findings and complaints of sore throat, dysphagia, drooling, and high fever. A muffled voice can also be heard, but is very nonspecific and is similar to that associated with retropharyngeal or peritonsillar abscesses.

Typically, a child with epiglottitis presents with fever and clinical toxicity. There is usually marked respiratory distress manifested by severe stridor, tachypnea, agitation, and drooling. The child will assume the most neutral position ("sniffing position") for ease of breathing. The patient will sit upright and use his arms as a tripod support for the torso, hold his airway upright, lean forward with the chin up, and hold his mouth open.

The initial examination is controversial. There have been reports of complete airway obstruction associated with oropharyngeal exam. If epiglottitis is seriously considered, this exam should be done by a skilled physician in the operating room or ICU where airway maintenance can be achieved quickly via intubation or tracheostomy. Radiologic studies are usually not needed and may actually exacerbate agitation, worsen obstruction, and potentially lead to respiratory arrest in the radiology suite. The classic "thumbprint" sign is an enlargement of the epiglottis and thickening of the aryepiglottic folds on a lateral soft-tissue radiograph of the neck.

Management

Establishing a secure airway is the priority in epiglottitis. Endotracheal intubation is indicated if the risk of obstruction is substantial. On occasion, an emergent cricothyrotomy and tracheostomy may be indicated. Postponement of phlebotomy, IV placement, and oropharyngeal inspection should be considered until after the airway is secured.

Antibiotics should be targeted to provide coverage for Staphylococcus aureus, both methicillin sensitive (MSSA) and methicillin resistent (MRSA); Streptococcus pneumoniae; and Haemophilus influenzae type b. This coverage is best provided with a second- or third-generation cephalosporin and a drug targeting MRSA (vancomycin, clindamycin, or linezolid).

BACTERIAL TRACHEITIS

Bacterial tracheitis is another potentially life-threatening emergency. It includes subglottic and tracheal edema and has the risk of upper airway obstruction at the larynx by thick, tenacious, purulent secretions. The main clinical distinction between bacterial tracheitis and viral croup is the degree of respiratory distress and toxicity. It is commonly thought to occur as a bacterial superinfection that follows viral laryngotracheobronchitis. The peak incidence is fall and winter with an age range of typically 6 months to 8 years (mean age, 5 years). The most common etiologies are S. aureus, S. pneumoniae, S. pyogenes, M. catarrhalis, and H. influenzae. Mixed bacterial infections are common and may include anaerobes. This bacterial superinfection causes bronchial mucosal edema, tissue damage, and subsequent purulent secretions. The differential diagnosis is similar to those previously mentioned— viral laryngotracheobronchitis, epiglottitis, peritonsillar abscess, retropharyngeal abscess, and foreign body aspiration.

Clinical Findings

There is usually a viral prodrome consisting of runny nose, fever, congestion, and barky cough. These progress over several days to include stridor, hoarse voice, tachypnea, dyspnea, and increasing fever. Physical exam will usually reveal a toxic infant or child with high fever in respiratory distress. However, the lung sounds are usually clear.

This diagnosis should be considered in any patient who is initially thought to have viral croup, but develops high fever with toxicity and does not respond to conventional therapies. Soft-tissue x-rays of the tracheal air column usually show a linear airway-filling defect, tracheal wall opacities, and asymmetric subglottic narrowing. However, the films may be indistinguishable from croup. Bronchoscopy usually reveals a normal epiglottis, subglottic narrowing, purulent tracheal secretions, and ulcerated tracheal mucosa. Rigid bronchoscopy can be both diagnostic and therapeutic, protecting the airway by removing the thick, tenacious secretions.

Management

Much like epiglottitis, the first priority is protecting the airway. Usually this is accomplished by rigid bronchoscopy, but occasionally tracheostomy is warranted. Blood and tracheal cultures should be obtained. Antibiotic therapy should again be targeted at *S. aureus* (MSSA and MRSA), *S. pneumoniae*, *S. pyogenes*, and *H. influenzae*. Initial antibiotics should include a second- or third-generation cephalosporin and an anti-MRSA drug such as vancomycin, clindamycin, or linezolid.

Complications of bacterial tracheitis include toxic shock syndrome, septic shock, and adult respiratory distress syndrome (ARDS).

A key distinction needs to be made between the diagnosis and treatment of bacterial tracheitis in previously normal children and children with preexisting tracheostomies. Bacterial tracheitis in a child who does not have a tracheostomy is a medical emergency. Acute infection of the trachea in a child with a pre-existing tracheostomy is somewhat less emergent. Children with tracheostomies can present with increased thickness, quantity, and change in color the of their secretions. These patients usually have increased respiratory distress, but are not toxic appearing. Easy access to the trachea allows for frequent suctioning. These children are chronically colonized with bacteria. Antibiotic choices in these children need to target *Pseudomonas aeruginosa* and *S. aureus*. It is often difficult to distinguish between tracheal colonization and infection in these children even with the guidance of cultures of tracheal aspirates. The bacterial flora present in the trachea is not necessarily different between the two clinical situations. In this setting, the Gram stain can prove useful. The presence of moderate or many white blood cells suggests substantial inflammation and supports a diagnosis of bacterial tracheitis. The presence of few white blood cells suggests minimal inflammation and is more consistent with colonization. Empiric initial treatment with piperacillin and tazobactam or Cefepime is a good choice. Once the tracheal cultures identify the bacteria present, sensitivities can guide the selection of an appropriate antibiotic. For example, the quinolones, such as ciprofloxacin, are often useful in covering pseudomonas.

RETROPHARYNGEAL ABSCESS

Retropharyngeal abscess is an infrequent infection, but is most often seen in children less than 4 years old. This type of abscess commonly originates in the lymph nodes in the prevertebral space. This chain of nodes drain the nasopharynx, paranasal sinuses, and middle ear, become infected with pyogenic bacteria, suppurate, and form an abscess. Because these lymph nodes tend to involute and atrophy by about 5 years of age, retropharyngeal abscess becomes a rare diagnosis after that age. The most common organisms include *S. pyogenes*, oral anaerobes, and *S. aureus*. In a study by Coticchia and associates (3), children younger than 1 year were more commonly infected with *S. aureus* than with group A strep. In that same study, children older than 1 year were more commonly infected with group A strep than with *S. aureus*.

Retropharyngeal abscess is also reported in children after penetrating trauma of the posterior oropharynx. Trauma is usually secondary to fish and chicken bones, but can occur after falling with an object in the mouth and sustaining an injury to the pharynx. These objects may include pen refills, pencils, and corn-on-the-cob skewers.

The presentation of this infection in children tends to be subtle because of their limited ability to verbalize their symptoms or cooperate with a physical exam. Infants may present with nonspecific findings, such as, fever, decreased enteral intake, and fussiness. Children often have a history of a recent upper respiratory tract infection. They usually progress to fever, neck pain, nuchal rigidity, torticollis, sore throat, dysphagia, odynophagia, muffled voice, and/or stridor. Studies show that children less than 4 years old frequently present with agitation, cough, drooling, lethargy, respiratory distress, retractions, rhinorrhea, and/or stridor. This age group also tends to have trismus and a positive oropharyngeal exam. Infants are more difficult to diagnose because these findings are more often absent. Lateral neck soft-tissue x-rays reveal swelling in the prevertebral space that is more than one-half the width of a vertebral body. These x-rays must be performed with the neck in slight hyperextension. A CT scan of the neck with contrast is now the imaging study of choice. It can provide the definitive diagnosis, differentiate between a true abscess and lymph node cellulitis, and guide surgical drainage. Surgical drainage usually involves intraoral incision and drainage, yet some cases are successfully treated with antibiotics alone (4). Delayed diagnosis or failure to drain a retropharyngeal abscess in a timely manner does include a risk of spontaneous rupture into the pharynx inferiorly with subsequent aspiration into the mediastinum. The severity of nuchal rigidity has resulted in some of these children receiving a lumbar puncture. In this setting, the CSF may show a mild pleiocytosis. This is due to meningeal irritation from the abscess.

Antibiotics should be targeted at *S. aureus*, *S. pyogenes*, the *S. milleri* group, and oral anaerobes (*Fusobacterium*, *Prevotella*, and *Peptostreptococcus*). Acceptable empiric antibiotic regimens include combination therapy with ceftriaxone and clindamycin. Vancomycin must be substituted for clindamycin in areas where CA-MRSA has a high prevalence of inducible clindamycin resistance (see Chapter 93). When MRSA is not prevalent in the community, ampicillin/sulbactam can be used.

Fusobacterium is a gram-negative obligate anaerobe that is normal flora in the human oral cavity. Infections with this organism alone and in combination with other oropharyngeal flora were first described by Lemierre in the pre-antibiotic era. Lemierre syndrome is an aggressive oropharyngeal infection characterized by pharyngitis, bacteremia, and suppurative thrombophlebitis of the head and neck veins, often with septic emboli (5). Thrombocytopenia secondary to a consumptive coagulopathy can also be seen. Venous Doppler studies of the jugular and subclavian veins are warranted. Some of the complications of Lemierre syndrome include dyspnea, osteomyelitis, intra-abdominal abscesses, meningitis, disseminated intravascular coagulation (DIC), and endocarditis. Therefore, recognition of this rare but potentially fatal entity is important. Treatment includes anticoagulation and an appropriate antibiotic regimen. *F. necrophorum* is susceptible to penicillin, clindamycin, and metronidazole, with variable susceptibility to the cephalosporins.

PEARLS

- The differential diagnosis for croup is extensive. Some mimickers are epiglottitis, bacterial tracheitis, retropharyngeal or peritonsillar abscess, and foreign body. These later problems are often suggested by fever, clinical toxicity, and/or pain or difficulty swallowing.
- The incidence of epiglottitis has substantially fallen after the universal adoption of Hib vaccination. The etiologic epidemiology has now shifted from *H. influenzae* type b to *S. aureus*, *S. pneumoniae*, and *S. pyogenes*.
- The diagnosis of bacterial tracheitis should be considered in any patient who was initially thought to have viral croup, but looks more toxic and does not respond to conventional therapies.

- Children with a retropharyngeal abscess have subtle presentations. Key findings are trismus, pharyngitis, and neck pain. A CT scan of the neck with contrast is the imaging study of choice.
- If *Fusobacterium necrophorum* is recovered from blood culture or from pus in a neck abscess, Doppler imaging of the jugular and subclavian veins is warranted to evaluate for Lemierre syndrome.

References

1. Rittichier K, Ledwith C. Outpatient treatment of moderate croup with dexamethasone: intramuscular versus oral dosing. *Pediatrics* 2000;106:1344–1348.
2. Rotta A, Wiryawan B. Respiratory emergencies in children. *Respir Care* 2003;48:248–260.
3. Coticchia JM, Getrick GS, Yun RO, et al. Age-, site, and time-specific differences in pediatric deep neck abscesses. *Arch Otolaryngol Head Neck Surg* 2004;130:201–207.
4. Craig F, Schunk J. Retropharyngeal abscess in children: clinical presentation, utility of imaging and current management. *Pediatrics* 2003;111: 1394–1398.
5. Ramirez S, Hill TG, Rudolph CN, et al. Increased diagnosis of Lemierre syndrome and other *Fusobacterium necrophorum* infection at a children's hospital. *Pediatrics* 2003;112:380–385.

Suggested Readings

Loftis L. Acute infectious upper airway obstructions in children. *Semin Pediatr Infect Dis.* 2006;17:5–10.

CHAPTER 88 ■ PELVIC INFLAMMATORY DISEASE

SHARON A. MANGAN

Pelvic inflammatory disease (PID) is a polymicrobial infection of the female upper genital tract that primarily affects the endometrium and fallopian tubes.

Each year, one million women are diagnosed with PID, and 20% to 30% of these cases are in sexually active adolescents. Teens are at increased risk for PID due to a variety of reasons. Biologically, the adolescent cervix is more prone to infection because the transformation zone is exposed on the ectocervix, making it more vulnerable to pathogens. In addition, teenagers have a higher prevalence of risky sexual behaviors, including engaging in uprotected intercourse, inconsistent condom use, and having multiple sex partners. Adolescents are also at increased risk for the development of sequelae due to several factors: later presentation, delay in diagnosis, and noncompliance, leading to inadequate treatment.

PID is a polymicrobial infection caused by the spread of microorganisms from the lower to the upper genital tract. *Neisseria gonorrhoeae* and *Chlamydia trachomatis* are the most commonly involved organisms. Anaerobic bacteria such as *Bacteroides fragilis*, *Peptostreptococcus*, *Prevotella bivia*, and *Prevotella disiencs*; and facultative aerobic bacteria including *Gardnerella vaginalis*, *Haemophilus influenza*, and genital tract mycoplasmas (*Ureaplasma urealyticum and Mycoplasma hominis*) are also involved.

It is often difficult to accurately diagnose PID. When an adolescent girl presents with abdominal pain, there is an extensive list of differential diagnoses that should be entertained. Gastrointestinal etiologies for abdominal pain include appendicitis, inflammatory bowel disease, and gastroenteritis. Some gynecologic entities causing lower abdominal pain are pregnancy, ovarian cysts, and dysmenorrhea. Urinary tract abnormalities, such as pyelonephritis, cystitis, and nephrolithiasis, may also present with abdominal pain. For a more complete list of differential diagnoses for acute abdominal pain, see Table 88.1.

CLINICAL FINDINGS

PID remains a clinical diagnosis. The 2006 STD guidelines (see below) from the Centers for Disease Control and Prevention (CDC) establish criteria used to aid in the diagnosis of PID. Empiric treatment of PID is advised in sexually active young women if any of the minimum criteria are present and no other cause for the illness can be identified. There are also additional criteria that may be used to support a diagnosis of PID. Use of the more definitive criteria may be warranted in selected cases where there is significant uncertainty about the diagnosis. Health care providers should have a low threshold to diagnose PID due to the potential for long-term sequelae even with mild or atypical PID.

Diagnostic Criteria

Minimum Criteria

■ Uterine tenderness
■ Adrenal tenderness
■ Cervical motion tenderness

Additional Criteria

■ Oral temperature greater than 101°F
■ Abnormal cervical or vaginal mucopurulent discharge
■ Presence of white blood cells (WBCs) on saline microscopy of vaginal secretions
■ Elevated erythrocyte sedimentation rate (ESR) or C-reactive protein (CRP)
■ Laboratory documentation of cervical infection with *N. gonorrhoeae* or *C. trachomatis*

Definitive Criteria

■ Histopathologic evidence of endometritis on endometrial biopsy
■ Transvaginal sonography or other imaging techniques showing thickened, fluid-filled tubes with or without free pelvic fluid or tubo-ovarian complex
■ Laparoscopic abnormalities consistent with PID

MANAGEMENT

In an attempt to prevent long-term sequelae (e.g., infertility), empiric treatment for PID should be started as soon as the presumptive diagnosis has been made. Treatment regimens should provide antimicrobial coverage of the likely pathogens, including *N. gonorrhoeae*, *C. trachomatis*, anaerobes, gram-negative facultative bacteria, and streptococci.

The CDC published recommendations for PID treatment in the 2006 STD guidelines. Studies of young adult women have shown no difference between inpatient and outpatient treatment of PID in terms of rates of chronic pelvic pain, ectopic pregnancy, or infertility. Most patients are initially treated as an outpatient with the following regimen: In April 2007, the CDC issued a revision to the STD treatment guidelines with regard to gonococcal infections. This change was a result of the increasing and widespread prevalence of fluoroquinolone resistance in *Neisseria gonorrhoeae*. The CDC no longer recommends using fluoroquinolones for the treatment of gonococcal infections or PID. Therefore, third-generation cephalosporins are the only

TABLE 88.1

DIFFERENTIAL DIAGNOSIS OF ACUTE LOWER ABDOMINAL PAIN

Gastrointestinal	Gynecologic	Urinary tract
Appendicitis	Pregnancy, including ectopic	Urinary tract infection
Constipation	Ovarian cyst ± torsion	Pyelonephritis
Gastroenteritis	Mittelschmerz	Nephrolithiasis
Inflammatory bowel disease	Dysmenorrhea	
Irritable bowel syndrome	Endometriosis	
Mesenteric adenitis		

class of drugs currently recommended for the treatment of *N. gonorrhoeae* and associated conditions, such as PID.

Oral Treatment (Outpatient)

■ Ceftriaxone sodium, 250 mg intramuscularly once, *or*
■ Cefoxitin sodium, 2 g intramuscularly plus probenecid, 1 g orally (given together) once, *or*
■ Another parenteral third-generation cephalosporin (e.g., ceftizoxime sodium or cefotaxime sodium in appropriate dose) *plus*
■ Doxycycline, 100 mg orally twice a day for 14 days *with or without*
■ Metronidazole, 500 mg orally twice a day for 14 days

Adolescents treated as outpatients should be reevaluated within 72 hours of the start of treatment. If they do not show clinical improvement (e.g., defervescence, decrease in abdominal tenderness, and decrease in uterine, adnexal, and/or cervical motion tenderness), then they should be admitted for further evaluation and treatment.

The 2006 CDC guidelines criteria for hospitalization include patients in whom surgical emergencies cannot be excluded, poor response to oral therapy, pregnancy, severe illness with nausea and vomiting or high fever, inability to follow or tolerate an oral regimen, and tubo-ovarian abscess. Although these guidelines do not recommend routine admission for all adolescents with PID, hospitalization should be considered whenever there is concern about noncompliance with medication or follow-up.

Recommendations from the CDC guidelines for inpatient treatment of PID are given next.

Parenteral Treatment (Inpatient)

Regimen A

■ Cefotetan disodium, 2 g intravenously every 12 hours, *or*
■ Cefoxitin sodium, 2 g intravenously every 6 hours *plus*
■ Doxycycline, 100 mg intravenously/orally every 12 hours

Regimen B

■ Clindamycin hydrochloride, 900 mg intravenously every 8 hours *plus*
■ Gentamicin sulfate, 1.5 mg/kg every 8 hours (after loading dose of 2 mg/kg; normal renal function)

The CDC recommendations include a change to oral antibiotics 24 to 48 hours after the patient shows clinical improvement. Treatment with oral therapy should be continued for a combined total of 14 days. For regimen A, continue treatment with doxycycline. If a TOA is present, consider adding clindamycin hydrochloride or metronidazole for better anaerobic coverage. For regimen B, complete the treatment course with doxycycline or clindamycin hydrochloride 600 mg PO every

8 hours. If a TOA is present, clindamycin is preferable because of more effective anaerobic coverage.

Counseling the adolescent patient about the risks associated with PID and how to avoid a future infection is extremely important. Teenagers should be advised to avoid intercourse until treatment has been completed and sexual partners (previous 60 days) have also been treated. This is also an opportunity to discuss contraception, including the use of condoms to prevent STD transmission.

COURSE AND PROGNOSIS

Tubo-ovarian abscess, peritonitis, and perihepatitis are all acute complications associated with PID.

Perihepatitis (also known as Fitz–Hugh–Curtis syndrome) is believed to occur after direct spread of microorganisms from the fallopian tubes into the peritoneal cavity, and then to the subphrenic space and hepatic surface. Therefore, the etiologic agents are similar to those found with PID. *N. gonorrhoeae* and *C. trachomatis* account for 10% and 50% of cases of perihepatitis, respectively. If not diagnosed early and treated, "violin-string" adhesions form between the hepatic capsule and the diaphragm. Patients will present with severe right-upper quadrant abdominal pain, worse on inspiration, and may have radiation of pain to the shoulder. Treatment guidelines for perihepatits are the same as those for PID.

Diagnosis of TOA, which occurs in 15% to 20% of adolescents with PID, requires a high index of suspicion, because clinical signs and symptoms are similar to those seen with uncomplicated salpingitis. However, patients are more likely to present ill-appearing and with significant pain. Of patients hospitalized for PID, approximately one-third will have a TOA. Treatment for TOA should include hospitalization for further evaluation and management. Parenteral triple antibiotic therapy with clindamycin, ampicillin, and gentamicin is the treatment of choice for TOA. More than 95% of patients will respond favorably to this regimen. Clinical response is determined by serial physical exams and pelvic ultrasonography.

The long-term sequelae of PID include chronic abdominal/pelvic pain, as well as an increased risk of ectopic pregnancy, infertility, and recurrent PID. The risk of infertility increases with the severity of the infection and the number of episodes of PID. One episode carries a 10% to 15% risk, with subsequent increases to 20% to 30% after two episodes, and 40% to 55% after three episodes.

PEARLS

■ Keep a high index of suspicion and low theshold for diagnosis of PID when evaluating adolescent girls presenting with abdominal pain and/or vaginal discharge.

- Initiate empiric treatment *early* if a diagnosis of PID is likely.
- Adolescents are at increased risk for both noncompliance with the medication regimen and complications of PID; therefore, seriously consider hospitalization.
- Routine STD screening in adolescents is extremely important to diagnose infections early and hopefully, to prevent development of PID.

Suggested Readings

Banikarim C, Chacko MR. Pelvic inflammatory disease in adolescents. *Semin Pediatr Infect Dis* 2005;16:175–180.

Centers for Disease Control and Prevention. Sexually transmitted diseases treatment guidelines, 2006. MMWR Morb Mortal Wkly Rec 2006; 55(RR-11): 56–61.

Lawson MA, Blythe MJ. Pelvic inflammatory disease in adolescents. *Pediatr Clin North Am* 1999;46:767–782.

CHAPTER 89 ■ MENINGOCOCCEMIA

BINITA R. SHAH

The prototypical meningococcal infection is characterized by fever and petechial eruption. However, the spectrum of meningococcal infections includes transient bacteremia *without* sepsis, meningococcemia (i.e., bacteremia with sepsis) *without* meningitis, meningitis *with or without* meningococcemia, meningoencephalitis, infection of specific organs (e.g., septic arthritis, osteomyelitis, pneumonia, endocarditis, purulent pericarditis) or chronic meningococcemia.

Neisseria meningitidis, the bacteria responsible for meningococcal infections, has become a leading cause of bacterial meningitis in the United States after implementation of routine vaccination resulted in dramatic reductions in the incidence of infections caused by *Streptococcus pneumoniae* and *Haemophilus influenzae* type b. An estimated 1,400 to 2,800 cases of meningococcal disease occur in the United States annually (0.5–1.1/100,000 population/year). Invasive meningococcal disease (IMD) occurs in pediatric patients with two peaks: infants <1 year and adolescents 15 to 18 years of age. Although the incidence of IMD is highest in infants, the case-fatality rate is highest in adolescents (20%).

Neisseria meningitidis is an aerobic, fastidious, gram-negative diplococcus. Among the 13 serogroups, strains belonging to groups A, B, C, Y, and W-135 account for most meningococcal disease. Serogroups B, C, and Y are the major causes of meningococcal disease in the United States (each responsible for approximately one-third of cases). The proportion of cases caused by each serogroup also varies by age group. In infants <1 year of age, more than 50% of all cases of meningococcal disease are caused by serogroup B, compared to persons >11 years of age, in whom 75% of all cases are caused by serogroups C, Y, or W-135.

Meningococcemia is usually a fulminant illness characterized by rapid multiplication of meningococci within the bloodstream leading to high concentrations of circulating endotoxin. Shock, diffuse capillary damage, disseminated intravascular coagulation, purpura, and multiorgan system failure ensue. Meningococcemia accounts for 15% to 20% of all cases of IMD. It primarily affects children younger than 5 years of age, with a peak attack rate between 3 and 5 months of age. It is more commonly seen in winter and early spring. Individuals with inherited or acquired terminal complement deficiencies (C5-9), properdin deficiency, immunoglobulin deficiency, or asplenia (anatomic or functional) are at risk for developing invasive and recurrent meningococcal infections. Asymptomatic colonization of the respiratory tract provides the focus for subsequent seeding and spread of the organisms. Transmission is from person to person through droplets of respiratory tract secretions.

Chronic meningococcemia is a rare form of meningococcal infection that is characterized by persistent bacteremia associated with fever, rash, and arthritis (acute arthritis-dermatitis syndrome). The distribution and appearance of the cutaneous lesions are identical to those seen in chronic gonococcemia.

Chronic meningococcemia should be distinguished from the recurrent episodes of meningococcal meningitis that can occur in patients with inherited deficiencies of terminal components of complement.

Differential diagnosis of meningococcemia is extensive, and it may be difficult to differentiate meningococcal infections from other forms of septicemia. Table 89.1 lists potential entities to consider in the differential diagnosis for meningococcemia-associated rash and other forms of meningococcal disease.

CLINICAL FINDINGS

Clinical findings are summarized in Table 89.2. The incubation period varies from 1 to 10 days, but the disease typically begins 3 to 4 days after exposure and establishment of nasopharyngeal carriage. The clinical findings range from fever alone to fulminant septic shock with purpura fulminans and death within hours of onset of clinical symptoms. Petechial lesions (discrete, pinpoint, nonblanching lesions) are a common harbinger of this infection, and patients need to have a careful examination of skin and mucous membranes. These lesions are commonly seen in clusters (especially at pressure points), can coalesce into larger, ecchymotic areas, and can occasionally be vesicular. A transient, nonpruritic, maculopapular rash mimicking a wide variety of viral exanthems may be a presenting sign of meningococcal infection.

Definitive diagnosis of meningococcal disease is made by isolation of the organism from a usually sterile body fluid (e.g., CSF, blood, synovial fluid). Isolation of *N. meningitidis* from the nasopharynx is not diagnostic because it can be part of normal nasopharyngeal flora. Cultures from blood, a skin lesion, and CSF should be obtained in all patients with suspected meningococcemia. In the presence of meningitis, the CSF findings usually include an elevated pressure with increased protein, decreased glucose, and pleocytosis with a predominance of polymorphonuclear leukocytes. However, CSF culture can be positive in patents with meningococcemia even in absence of clinical evidence of meningitis or CSF pleocytosis. Gram stain of a petechial skin lesion, CSF, and buffy coat smear of blood may also be positive. The latex agglutination test to detect polysaccharide bacterial antigen in the CSF is a valuable test for a rapid diagnosis and supports the clinical diagnosis while awaiting culture confirmation. However, antigen detection tests in the urine or serum are not helpful and may be unreliable for group B *N. meningitidis*. Cultures of synovial fluid, sputum, or other body fluid may be obtained as indicated. Other ancillary tests include complete blood count (leukocytosis or leukopenia, and thrombocytopenia), erythrocyte sedimentation rate (ESR), C-reactive protein (CRP), coagulation profile (elevated prothrombin time, partial thromboplastin time, D-dimer and fibrin degradation products, and decreased plasma fibrinogen), serum

TABLE 89.1

DIFFERENTIAL DIAGNOSIS OF MENINGOCOCCEMIA

DIFFERENTIAL DIAGNOSIS OF PETECHIAL/PURPURIC LESIONS
Septicemia with other gram-negative pathogens
Septicemia with gram-positive organisms
Enteroviral infections (e.g., echovirus or coxsackievirus)
Rocky Mountain spotted fever
Idiopathic thrombocytopenic purpura
Epidemic typhus
Erythema multiforme
Gonococcemia
Bacterial endocarditis
Henoch–Schönlein purpura
Measles/atypical measles
Drugs (e.g., sulfonamides)
Ehrlichia or Anaplasma infection
Erythema nodosum

OTHER CONSIDERATIONS IN DIFFERENTIAL DIAGNOSIS
Bacterial meningitis from other etiology
Viral meningitis
Leptospirosis
Collagen vascular diseases
Maculopapular rash from other etiology (e.g., rubella, streptococcal or staphylococcal toxic shock)
Acute hemorrhagic encephalitis
Encephalopathies
Hemolytic–uremic syndrome
Mycoplasma infection
Acute leukemia

DIFFERENTIAL DIAGNOSIS OF CHRONIC MENINGOCOCCEMIA
Disseminated gonococcal infection
Bacterial endocarditis
Acute rheumatic fever
Henoch–Schönlein purpura
Infectious mononucleosis
Immune-mediated vasculitis.

TABLE 89.2

CLINICAL FEATURES OF MENINGOCOCCEMIA

SYSTEMIC SIGNS/SYMPTOMS
Fever
Chills
Headache
Myalgia/weakness
Vomiting
Focal neurologic signs
Convulsion
Septic shock (tachycardia, tachypnea, cyanosis, hypotension)
Disseminated intravascular coagulation
Signs of meningitis
Nuchal rigidity
Kernig sign and/or Brudzinski sign
Changes in mental status (lethargy, stupor, coma)
Multiorgan failure

SKIN LESIONS (70% OF CASES)
Initially may present as urticaria, faint macules, papules, maculopapular, or petechiae
Petechiae may progress to ecchymosis and ischemic necrosis
Common sites
Trunk and extremities; may involve any skin area
Mucous membrane (e.g., palpebral conjunctivae)

POOR PROGNOSTIC FACTORS IN MENINGOCOCCEMIA
Hypotension
Hypothermia
Absence of meningitis
Purpura fulminans
Petechiae <12 hr before presentation
Seizures on presentation
Shock on presentation
Leukopenia
Thrombocytopenia
High levels of endotoxin
High levels of tumor necrosis factor

electrolytes (including urea nitrogen and creatinine), liver enzymes, and urinalysis (proteinuria and hematuria).

MANAGEMENT

The keys to reducing morbidity and mortality in meningococcemia are prompt recognition, stabilization, and immediate initiation of antibiotic therapy. Delays in initiating therapy while completing of diagnostic studies or awaiting admission to the intensive care unit must be avoided. Stabilization of vital signs includes the ABCs of resuscitation, cardiac and pulse oximetry monitoring, and fluid resuscitation for septic shock. Aggressive supportive therapy to maintain tissue perfusion is critical to improving survival and minimizing sequelae in patients with fulminant meningococcemia (see Chapter 34 for management of septic shock).

Intravenous antibiotic therapy options for menigococcemia include cefotaxime sodium (200 mg/kg/day) *or* ceftriaxone sodium (100 mg/kg/day). The emergence of strains with increased resistance to penicillin (i.e., with a minimal inhibitory concentration between 0.12 and 1.0 µg/mL) has been reported from Spain (highest prevalence of penicillin resistance), Africa, the United Kingdom, Argentina, the United States, and Canada. These strains are relatively resistant to penicillin but appear to be susceptible to third-generation cephalosporins, such as ceftriaxone or cefotaxime. Thus, for suspected meningococcal disease, initial therapy with these antibiotics seems prudent. Penicillin G is the *drug of choice after identification and susceptibility* testing of the cultured bacteria, and is given in high doses (300,000 to 400,000 U/kg/day divided in 6 doses). Chloramphenicol is indicated in patients with anaphylactoid-type penicillin allergy. The usual duration for therapy is 5 to 7 days. The role of corticosteroids in the treatment of meningococcemia remains controversial. Corticosteroids once were widely recommended for the treatment of adrenal insufficiency associated with fulminant meningococcemia; however, adrenal function is not impaired in all patients.

The signs and symptoms of meningococcal meningitis are indistinguishable from signs and symptoms of acute meningitis caused by *Streptococcus pneumoniae* or other meningeal pathogens.

Recommendations for empirical therapy of bacterial meningitis have been published as a practice guideline by the Infectious

Disease Society of America. For children older than 1 month of age, vancomycin plus a third-generation cephalosporin (ceftriaxone or cefotaxime) are recommended for initial therapy.

PREVENTION AND EDUCATION

Droplet precautions in addition to contact precautions are recommended for a hospitalized patient until 24 hours after the initiation of effective therapy. All confirmed, presumptive, and probable cases of invasive meningococcal disease must be reported to the local or regional department of health.

The risk of contracting meningococcal infection among close contacts is 300 to 400 times higher than the general population. Contacts need to be educated to promptly seek medical attention with any illness. Health care workers who did not have direct exposure to the patient's oral secretions (e.g., unprotected mouth-to-mouth resuscitation, intubation, or suctioning before antimicrobial therapy was initiated) do not need to panic, and they *do not* need chemoprophylaxis. Throat and nasopharyngeal cultures are of *no* value for deciding who should receive prophylaxis. Chemoprophylaxis should be inititated within 24 hours of culture-proven diagnosis of the primary case. It is given to all close contacts: household contacts, child care or nursery school contacts during the previous 7 days, any person who had contact with patient's oral secretions within 7 days prior to onset of the disease (e.g., kissing), and people who frequently sleep or eat in same dwelling as the index case. For airline flights lasting more than 8 hours, passengers who are seated directly next to an index case should be considered candidates for prophylaxis.

Regimen options include rifampin (*drug of choice* for adults: 600 mg every 12 hours for 2 days; children >1 month: 10 mg/kg to a maximum of 600 mg every 12 hours for 2 days; infants <1 month: 5mg/kg every 12 hours for 2 days), ceftriaxone sodium (single intramuscular dose: 125 mg <15 years old; 250 mg >15 years), or ciprofloxacin hydrochloride (single 500 mg dose given orally; for >18 years). Chemoprophylaxis is *required* for the index case (prior to hospital discharge) if the patient was treated with penicillin; however, it is *not* required if the patient was treated with ceftriaxone sodium or cefotaxime sodium. Patients diagnosed with a meningococcal infection should be screened for complement deficiency disorders (see above). Epidemiologic studies have shown an increased risk of IMD among college freshman living in dormitories compared to other college students and similarly aged persons in the general population. At least 75% of cases of IMD in 11- to 18-year-olds are caused by serogroups A, C, Y, and W-135; thus, IMD is pontentially preventable by immunization with quadrivalent meningococcal vaccines. A single dose of tetravalent meningococcal conjugate vaccine (A, C, Y, W-135 conjugate vaccine; MCV4; Menactra®) sure is now recommended as a routine vaccination at either 11 to 12 years (preadolescent assessment visit), or at high school entry, or at approximately 15 years of age (for those persons not vaccinated previously with MCV4). The recommendations also include administration (if not previously given) to college freshmen living in dormitories and to other populations at increased risk (i.e., patients with anatomic or functional asplenia, and patients with terminal complement deficiency, military recruits, and travelers to areas in which meningococcal disease is hyperendemic or epidemic). No vaccine is available for the prevention of N. *meningitidis* group B disease.

COURSE AND PROGNOSIS

Complications from meningococcal infection are common; 25% of patients with meningococcal disease will experience one or more complications (Table 89.3). Several scoring sys-

TABLE 89.3

COMPLICATIONS OF MENINGOCOCCEMIA

Disseminated intravascular coagulation
Purpura fulminans
   Tissue necrosis resulting in gangrene and autoamputation
    of distal extremities
Myocarditis, congestive heart failure, conduction
  abnormalities
Pneumonia, lung abscess
Neurologic sequelae from meningitis
   Deafness (sensorineural), subdural effusion or empyema,
    brain abscess
   Obstructive hydrocephalus, seizures, hemiparesis,
    or quadriparesis
Waterhouse–Friderichsen syndrome
   Adrenal hemorrhage that can result in shock, coma,
    and death
Endophthalmitis
Immune complex–mediated complications (seen 4–9 days
  after onset of illness)
   Arthritis (usually monoarticular)
   Cutaneous vasculitis

tems have been developed to aid the clinician in predicting adverse outcomes (death or severe ischemic damage resulting in loss of extremities or extensive skin gangrene). Purpura fulminans (Fig. 89.1) and shock at presentation are uniformly poor signs. Features associated with overwhelming disease, such as low WBC, low inflammatory indicators at presentation (low ESR or CRP), and absence of meningitis, also do not portend well. The overall mortality rate of meningococcemia without meningitis is 20% to 30%; for meningococcal meningitis alone, it is 2% to 13%. Morbidity in survivors includes approximately 8% with neurologic sequelae including deafness and motor

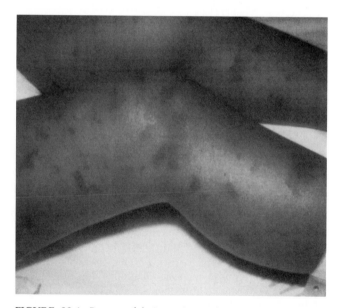

FIGURE 89.1. Purpura fulminans in meningococcemia. Purpuric lesions of less than 12 hours duration developed on the foot of a 2-year-old child who presented with septic shock, leukopenia, and thrombocytopenia with disseminated intravascular coagulation. (Reproduced with permission from Shah BR, Laude AT, eds. *Atlas of pediatric clinical diagnosis.* Philadelphia: Saunders; 2000: 105.)

dysfunction. Ischemic infarction of the skin or extremities is found in about 4% of survivors and often results in limb loss.

PEARLS

- Acute meningococcemia can mimic a virus-like infection initially presenting with fever, myalgia, headache, weakness, and pharyngitis.
- Classical signs of meningococcal infection (fever with petechiae or purpura) are seen in only 70% of cases. Patients with meningococcal meningitis (including a positive CSF culture) may lack CSF abnormalities on the initial lumbar puncture. Thus, infections caused by N. *meningitidis* (including meningitis) must be considered even in the absence of skin lesions or CSF abnormalities.

Suggested Readings

Apicella MA. *Neisseria meningitidis*. In: Mandell GL, Bennett JE, Douglas JE, eds. *Principles and practice of infectious diseases*. 6th ed. Philadelphia, PA: Churchill Livingstone Elsevier; 2005:2498–2510.

Bilukha O, Rosenstein N. Prevention and control of meningococcal disease. Division of Bacterial and Mycotic Diseases, National Center for Infectious Diseases. Recommendations of the Advisory Committee on Immunization Practices. *MMWR* 2005;54(RR07):1–21.

Gold R. *Neisseria meningitidis*. In: Long S, Pickering L, Prober C, eds. *Principles and practice of pediatric infectious diseases*. 2nd ed. Philadelphia, PA: Churchill Livingstone Elsevier; 2003:748–756.

Pickering LK, ed. *Red book 2000*: report of the Committee on Infectious Diseases. 25th ed. Elk Grove Village, IL: American Academy of Pediatrics; 2000.

Tunkel AR, Hartman BJ, Kaplan SL. Practice guidelines for the management of bacterial meningitis. *Clin Infect Dis* 2004;39:1267–1284.

Wong VK, Hitchcock W, Mason WH. Meningococcal infection in children: a review of 100 cases. *Pediatr Infect Dis J* 1989;8:224.

CHAPTER 90 ■ TICK-BORNE DISEASES

DEBRA A. TRISTRAM

Ticks and their associated diseases have become an increasingly recognized problem in many parts of the United States and continue to be a problem worldwide. Many cases of tick-borne disease are mild and self-limited, but several, such as Rocky Mountain spotted fever (RMSF), ehrlichiosis, and babesiosis, may be severe and life-threatening. Early Lyme disease is usually not an inpatient disease, but its varied late manifestations make its inclusion in the differential diagnosis of arthritis (Section X and Chapter 86), encephalitis (Chapter 76), and carditis important. This section will focus mainly on RMSF but will include babesiosis, ehrlichiosis, and Lyme disease in the discussion of tick-associated disease.

BABESIOSIS

Babesiosis is a nonspecific illness caused by an intraerythrocytic protozoa, *Babesia microti*. The protozoa is acquired by the bite of a tick vector, *Ixodes scapularis*, infected by taking a blood meal from its animal host, the white-footed mouse (*Peromycus leucopus*). Because the same tick also transmits Lyme disease, the two illnesses may occur in the same host from a single infected tick bite. Rarely the disease can be acquired by blood transfusion, or by transplacental or perinatal transmission. The disease is seen during late spring, summer, and autumn months, which are times of highest tick activity. Most cases in the United States are reported in the northeast (Connecticut, Maryland, New Jersey, New York, Rhode Island), midwest (Minnesota, Missouri, Wisconsin), and the west coast (California, Washington) and occur in persons over the age of 40. It appears that the range is continuing to expand as more cases are reported outside of the endemic regions. Although cases acquired in the United States rarely have a fatal outcome (5%, even in splenectomized patients), babesia infection acquired in Europe should be considered a medical emergency. There, the case fatality rate is close to 50%, and nearly all deaths occur in asplenic individuals.

Clinical Features

Based on serologic surveys in endemic areas, most infected individuals are asymptomatic or have mild symptoms. Among those who have symptomatic babesia infection, malaise, anorexia, and fatigue are the initial manifestations. Intermittent fever may follow, with daily spikes as high as 40°C. Other symptoms may occur, including headache, chills, sweats, myalgia/arthralgia, gastrointestinal symptoms (nausea, vomiting, weight loss), or respiratory symptoms (sore throat, cough). Occasionally, emotional lability, depression, hyperesthesia, or photophobia may be present. On physical examination, the findings are often minimal, consisting only of jaundice and mild hepatomegaly or splenomegaly, or both. Because the symptoms are not specific, the duration of illness may suggest the diagnosis. The illness may last for a few weeks to several months with a very prolonged recovery (parasites may be detected in the blood at low levels up to 18 months). Illness severe enough to come to medical attention most commonly occurs in persons greater than 40 years of age, with asplenia (including patients with sickle cell), or with immunocompromise. Fulminant illness resulting in death has been reported in such individuals, particularly in babesia infection acquired in Europe. Laboratory abnormalities seen during babesia infection may include mild to moderate anemia with reticulocytosis (depending on the degree of hemolysis) and mild elevations in liver enzymes (with elevated bilirubin and serum lactate dehydrogenase). Low or normal white counts with thrombocytopenia may be present. Hemoglobinuria and reduced serum haptoglobulin occur frequently. The diagnosis of babesiosis is made by examination of Wright or Giemsa-stained thin and thick blood smears. The organism is visible within the erythrocytes as a "ring" form (similar to malaria). The degree of parasitemia should be calculated. Individuals with normal splenic function generally have less than 20% (most patients <6%) of their erythrocytes infected with babesia, although asplenic patients have been reported with levels of parasitemia as high as 85% during severe disease. For those individuals with negative smears, serum antibody testing is available from the Centers for Disease Control and Prevention (CDC) and several commercial laboratories. Two to four weeks after acquisition, antibody titers (IgG and IgM) are generally elevated. A titer of 1:64 is considered positive, but most affected individuals have titers greater than 1:1,024.

Management

Most patients with normal immune function will not require treatment. However, those at risk of severe disease (e.g., immunocompromised or asplenic) or presenting with severe disease in the absence of risk factors should be treated. The choice of antibiotics includes oral quinine (25 mg/kg/day divided every 8 hours to a maximum of 650 mg) plus intravenous clindamycin hydrochloride (20 to 40 mg/kg/day to maximum of 1,200 mg twice daily or 600 mg orally three times a day). Those patients with high levels of parasitemia and hemolysis may benefit from exchange transfusion.

Prevention

At present, the best prevention of babesia infection is avoidance of tick-infested areas and the use of repellants if avoidance is not possible. For a more detailed discussion, see RMSF prevention.

EHRLICHIOSIS

Human ehrlichiosis is caused by at least two separate species of intracellular bacteria. Human monocytic ehrlichiosis (HME) is caused by *Ehrlichia chaffeensis*, and human granulocytic anaplasmosis (HGA) caused by *Anaplasma phagocytophilum*. Both are acquired by the bite of an infected tick; HME probably by the bite of the Lone Star tick (*Amblyomma americanum*) and HGA probably by the bite of the black-legged tick (*Ixodes scapularis*, the vector of Lyme disease) or the brown dog tick (*Dermacentor variablis*). The incubation period after a tick bite is an average of 7 to 14 days. Most cases occur between April and September (during tick activity). Coinfection with other pathogens carried by the vector is also possible, particularly RMSF and Lyme disease. The majority of cases of HME are found in the southeastern and south central United States, and HGA is reported in Connecticut, Massachusetts, Michigan, New York, California, Wisconsin, and Florida. The incidence of reported cases is increasing, possibly due to heightened physician awareness, better testing techniques, and increased exposure to the vector. Although the majority of currently reported cases have occurred in adults, children do become infected with *Ehrlichia* (and *Anaplasma*), and the features of their illness may differ somewhat from those described in adults.

Clinical Features

The clinical manifestations (Table 90.1) for both forms of human ehrlichiosis are similar in presentation to each other and RMSF, and consist of malaise, headache, myalgia, chills, anorexia, and gastrointestinal upset (nausea and/or vomiting). A few patients may present with findings suggestive of aseptic meningitis (stiff neck, confusion, and cerebrospinal fluid pleocytosis) or septic shock. In one series of HME in children, 25% required intensive care therapy. Clinically, ehrlichiosis differs from RMSF in that patients more often have leukopenia, anemia, and hepatitis, and less frequently rash. When a rash does occur, it is usually macular or papular, but occasionally may be petechial or erythematous. However, unlike RMSF, the rash occurs on the palms and soles in *less* than 10% of the cases. Physical findings in children with HME are often minimal, except in patients with rash or central nervous system involvement, but may include liver or splenic enlargement. Most children recover from HME, but there are reports of long-term neurologic sequelae (e.g., bilateral foot drop, speech impairment, impaired reading skills and fine motor skills) in children with CNS involvement. There are few reported pediatric cases of HGA documented in the literature. Adults with HGA are more likely to have a normal physical assessment; organomegaly and rash are not commonly described.

The CDC definition for a confirmed case of ehrlichiosis is a compatible clinical illness in the setting of appropriate fourfold rise in antibody titer (by indirect immunofluorescence assay [IFA]) over a 3- to 6-week period of time, identification of ehrlichial DNA by polymerase chain reaction (PCR) technology (not widely available), or identification of ehrlichial morulae (only for HGA) within white cells on a peripheral smear with a single positive IFA titer of greater than 1:64. A probable case is defined as the presence of morulae on peripheral smear or a single positive titer of greater than 1:64 by IFA.

Management

The treatment of ehrlichiosis is the same as that of RMSF. Doxycycline is the drug of choice, given at a dose of 3 to 4 mg/kg/day divided every 12 hours. Treatment should continue for 3 days past defervescence with a minimum of 5 to 7 days. Other drugs that have been alternative drugs for the treatment of RMSF, such as chloramphenicol, are not known to treat

---

TABLE 90.1

RELATIVE FREQUENCY OF VARIOUS CLINICAL AND LABORATORY FINDINGS FOR HUMAN GRANULOCYTIC ANAPLASMOSIS (HGA), HUMAN MONOCYTIC EHRLICHIOSIS (HME), AND ROCKY MOUNTAIN SPOTTED FEVER (RMSF)

Findings	HGA (adults)	HME (children)	RMSF (children)
Clinical findings			
Fever	++++	++++	++++
Malaise	++++	+++	+++
Myalgia	++++	+++	++++
Headache	++++	+++	++++
Chills	++++	++	+
Gastrointestinal (nausea, vomiting, anorexia)	++	+++	+++
Cough	+	+	+
Arthralgia	+	++	—
Rash	++	+++	++++[a]
Central nervous system signs/symptoms	++	+	++
Laboratory findings			
Serum sodium	NL	Decreased +++	Decreased +++
Peripheral white count	Leukopenia	Leukopenia +++ Lymphopenia ++++	Normal
Thrombocytopenia	++++	++++	++
Liver function testing	Mildly elevated AST and ALT	Mildly elevated AST and ALT ++++	Mild to moderately elevated AST and ALT

[a]20% may not develop rash during illness.
++++, 75–100%; +++, 50–75%; ++, 25–50%; +, <25% (but still may be seen); NL, normal; AST, aspartate aminotransferase; ALT, alanine aminotransferase.

TABLE 90.2

DIFFERENTIAL DIAGNOSIS FOR LYME DISEASE AT VARIOUS STAGES
OF PRESENTATION

Stage of Lyme disease	Finding of Lyme disease	Differential considerations
Early localized disease	Erythema migrans	Cellulitis, erythema multiforme, erythema marginatum, tinea corporis (ringworm), STARI
Early disseminated disease	Bell palsy	Epstein–Barr virus infection, central nervous system tumor
	Carditis	Myocarditis (viral), acute rheumatic fever, endocarditis
	Meningitis/encephalitis	Postinfectious meningoencephalitis, other causes of aseptic meningitis (enteroviral, arboviral infections), parameningeal infections
Late disseminated disease	Arthritis, recurrent arthritis	Pyogenic arthritis, collagen vascular disease (juvenile idiopathic arthritis, systemic lupus erythematosis), postinfectious or reactive arthritis (*Salmonella, Shigella, Yersinia*), acute rheumatic fever, serum sickness

ehrlichiosis. Furthermore, oral chloramphenicol is no longer available in the United States (since the early 1990s), and would require intravenous access. Both forms of ehrlichiosis typically last 1 to 2 weeks and recovery generally occurs without sequelae. Some reports, however, suggest neurologic complications in infected children. Fatal cases have occurred rarely (2% of cases).

Prevention

Prevention of ehrlichiosis, like that of the other tick-borne diseases (see RMSF prevention), consists of avoidance when possible. There is no current recommendation for chemoprophylaxis in the case of a tick bite nor vaccination available for preexposure prophylaxis.

LYME DISEASE (AND STARI)

Lyme disease was first recognized as a distinct disease in the mid-1970s when several children in Old Lyme, Connecticut, presented to their primary care physicians with disease complaints resembling juvenile rheumatoid arthritis. Investigation ultimately led to the identification of a new pathogen in the United States, *Borrelia burgdorferi*, a spirochete associated with the bite of an infected tick. Lyme disease primarily occurs in three distinct geographic areas in the United States. In each region, the tick vector is different: *Ixodes scapularis* in the East and Midwest, and *Ixodes pacificus* in the West. Lyme disease is also recognized in Europe, Canada, China, and Japan. Disease typically develops within 7 to 14 days after the bite of an infected tick (range, 3 to 31 days). Animal studies indicate that the feeding tick must be attached for more than 24 hours to transmit infection.

The southeastern and south central United States seem to be relatively free of classical Lyme disease but have been reported to have an illness often mistaken for early Lyme disease, STARI (southern tick-associated rash illness). STARI consists of an erythema migrans-like lesion following the bite of an *Amblyomma americanum* tick infected with *Borrelia lonestari,* but does not have the later sequelae common in Lyme disease.

The nonspecific nature of some Lyme disease features occasionally makes the diagnosis a challenge. Table 90.2 lists some of the more common entities to consider in the differential diagnosis for the various stages of Lyme disease.

Clinical Features

The clinical features and treatment of Lyme disease are outlined in Table 90.3. Early Lyme disease is usually recognized by the appearance of a characteristic skin lesion, erythema migrans (EM). The lesion consists of an initial erythematous papule at the site of the tick bite, followed by an increasing ring of erythema with partial central clearing in the days to weeks after the bite. Patients may have more than one inoculation site. In the United States, nearly two-thirds of children have EM, usually leading to the clinical diagnosis of Lyme disease. Early disseminated disease occurs approximately 3 to 10 weeks after the bite from an infected tick. This phase is characterized by multiple EM lesions (usually of smaller size than the initial inoculation lesion) and reflects "spirochetemia" similar to secondary syphilis. Other features encountered during early disseminated disease include cranial nerve palsies (especially of the facial nerve), meningitis, and conjunctivitis. Nonspecific flu-like symptoms (headache, fatigue, and low-grade fever) are also reported. Carditis, with various forms of heart block, is also possible during this stage of Lyme disease.

Late Lyme disease is most commonly characterized by recurrent pauciarticular arthritis, generally involving the large, weight-bearing joints (knees most commonly). It occurs in about half of patients not initially treated for Lyme disease. Central nervous system disease may also occur during late disease and includes subacute encephalopathy and polyradiculoneuropathy. Late complications of Lyme disease are uncommon in children previously treated for Lyme disease and mostly occur in those individuals who had unrecognized early Lyme disease (without recognized EM due to location on body or misdiagnosed as another condition). Late manifestations of Lyme disease may be included in the differential diagnosis of a variety of conditions in hospitalized patients, including encephalitis, arthritis, and acute cardiac disease.

TABLE 90.3

STAGES OF LYME DISEASE AND RECOMMENDED TREATMENT

Stage	Average timing after tick bite	Findings	Treatment
Early localized disease	7–10 days	Erythema migrans (EM)	>8 yr: doxycycline 100 mg PO b.i.d. × 14–21 days All ages: amoxicillin 50 mg/kg/day divided t.i.d. (max 500 mg/dose) × 14–21 days. For patients who cannot take doxycycline or amoxicillin, cefuroxime axetil 30–50 mg/kg/day (max 500 mg dose) divided b.i.d. or erythromycin 30–50 mg/kg/day divided q.i.d. (max 250 mg/dose)
Early disseminated disease	3–10 wk	Multiple, smaller EM-like lesions	Same as above oral regimens but for 21 days
		Cranial nerve palsies (especially CN VII)	Same as above oral regimens but for 21–28 days
		Meningitis or encephalitis	Ceftriaxone sodium 75–100 mg/kg/day (max 2 g) IV × 14–28 days or penicillin G 300,000 U/kg/day (max 20 million units) divided q4h × 14–28 days
		Carditis (especially with heart block)	Ceftriaxone sodium or penicillin as above
Late disseminated disease	2–12 mo	Arthritis	Same as above oral regimens but for 28 days
		Recurrent arthritis[a]	Ceftriaxone sodium 75–100 mg/kg/day (max 2 g) IV or IM × 14–21 days or penicillin G 300,000 U/kg/day (max 20 million units) divided q4h × 14–28 days

[a]Some experts would administer a second course of oral medication before committing to a course of IV medication.

The diagnosis of Lyme disease in the early stages can be made based on the characteristic EM lesion in the setting of tick exposure or residence in or visitation to an area where ticks are known to be infected with *B. burgdorferi*. The enzyme immunoassay (EIA) is the most widely used test for the detection of IgG and IgM antibodies to *B. burgdorferi*. All positive results are confirmed by a Western blot assay. Although patients with early localized Lyme disease are unlikely to have a positive test result, patients with early disseminated or late disease almost always have a strong antibody response to the antigens of *B. burgdorferi*. Therefore, a patient with negative serology at initial testing who is still suspected to have Lyme disease should have paired samples sent. If the paired samples fail to detect a rise in antibody response, it is highly unlikely that the patient has Lyme disease.

False-positive tests for Lyme disease are a particular problem with the EIA tests. Other spirochetes (especially syphilis and mouth spirochetes), certain viral infections (varicella), and collagen-vascular disorders (systemic lupus erythematosus) may cause false-positive tests due to the presence of cross-reacting antibodies. Physicians are advised against obtaining Lyme serology in the setting of nonspecific systemic complaints if the patient has not had travel to or residence in an endemic area. Questions regarding whom to test, the optimal timing of a test in suspect cases, or what to do with equivocal results should be directed to a pediatric infectious disease specialist.

Prevention

Prevention of Lyme disease includes avoidance of tick-infested areas (see RMSF prevention). There is no recommendation for chemoprophylaxis after a tick bite, even in endemic areas. The Lyme disease vaccine (LYMErix), consisting of recombinant outer surface protein A, was initially licensed in 1998 for individuals 15 to 70 years old at risk of contracting Lyme disease because of residence in endemic areas or working conditions that exposed them regularly to ticks. In 2002, the company discontinued the production of vaccine, citing insufficient sales to warrant further manufacture and marketing. There are no other vaccines currently available.

ROCKY MOUNTAIN SPOTTED FEVER

Rocky Mountain spotted fever (RMSF) is a rickettsial infection causing small vessel vasculitis. The infection results in myriad systemic manifestations, including fever, malaise, headache, and a diffuse rash involving the palms and soles. Although it is found in many parts of the United States and Canada, RMSF is predominately located in the southeastern, central, and Rocky Mountain states. Physicians need to be aware of the characteristic features of RMSF and of atypical or "spotless" cases.

The causative agent for RMSF is *Rickettsia rickettsii*, and it is transmitted by any of several tick vectors: *Dermacentor varibilis* (dog tick), *Dermacentor andersoni* (wood tick), or *Amblyomma americanum* (Lone Star tick). Rocky Mountain spotted fever is one of the most commonly reported tick-borne infections in the United States, second only to Lyme disease. Although cases are reported from all parts of the United States, the endemic regions in the southeastern, central, and Rocky Mountain states comprise the majority of reported cases.

The highest incidence of RMSF is noted in children in under 15 years of age. There is a seasonal predilection, with most cases occurring during the warm months of April to October when the ticks are actively feeding. Cases that occur earlier than April may not be recognized as RMSF because they are outside of the normal season. Hence, physicians in endemic areas should always maintain a high index of suspicion, even during the "off season," for tick-borne disease. For all ages, the primary risk factors include exposure to dogs, residence in wooded areas, and male gender. A history of travel to an endemic area, particularly if the child has participated in outdoor activities, should be included as a risk factor.

Rocky Mountain spotted fever is transmitted to humans by the bite of an infected tick. A feeding tick inoculates *R. rickettsii* into the dermis, where it is able to spread hematogenously. The incubation period from the time of bite to onset of disease is approximately 1 week, with a range of 3 to 12 days. Very rarely there is human-to-human transmission via blood transfusion from a patient who is incubating the disease or through an accidental needle-stick injury contaminated with infected blood.

The differential diagnosis of RMSF is broad and includes other infectious diseases with exanthema, including meningococcemia, toxic shock, measles or atypical measles, and enteroviral exanthems (particularly those in the echovirus group). Other tick-borne illnesses, such as ehrlichiosis and Lyme disease, may be in the differential (or may even cause coinfection), although the rash in Lyme disease is quite different from that in RMSF. In the southeastern United States, STARI should be included in the differential diagnosis, but usually is easy to differentiate from RMSF based on the rash. The rash is usually more EM-like, and the disease does not progress to disseminated disease as seen in Lyme disease. Secondary syphilis should always be included in the differential, particularly in the sexually active patient, because the rash of secondary syphilis also involves the palms and soles and can be maculopapular. Other noninfectious causes to include in the differential are drug eruptions (especially from sulfonamides), Henoch–Schönlein purpura, and idiopathic thrombocytopenic purpura, among others. For travelers outside of the United States, other infectious agents (e.g., dengue fever) might be included in the differential diagnosis.

Clinical Features

A history of tick bite is useful in evaluating patients with Rocky Mountain spotted fever; however, a tick bite is often painless and may be unrecognized. History of camping or hiking in an endemic area is useful. A prodrome of headache, myalgia, and abdominal pain is sometimes mistaken for a flu-like illness. After the prodrome, the abrupt onset of fever and chills in conjunction with a rash make the diagnosis more evident. The rash is usually seen 2 to 4 days into the illness and begins on the flexural areas of the ankles and wrists as an erythematous maculopapular eruption. Within hours, it can spread to the arms and legs and centrally toward the trunk. Within 1 to 3 days, the rash becomes petechial and may become confluent. Areas of skin necrosis may develop in the sites of maximal involvement. One distinguishing feature of the rash of RMSF is that palms and soles are nearly always affected (Fig. 90.1). During convalescence, the rash becomes pigmented, and desquamation may be seen over severely affected areas. It is important to keep in mind that the rash may be absent in 10% to 20% of cases. Hence, the absence of rash (or "spotless" Rocky Mountain spotted fever) should not dissuade the suspicious clinician from the diagnosis.

Although often not diagnostic early, laboratory testing can be helpful in the diagnosis of RMSF. A complete blood count should be performed, but the total white count may be normal

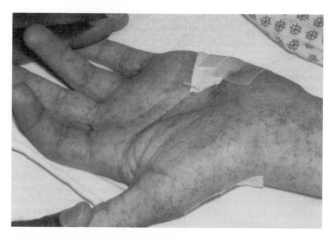

FIGURE 90.1. Child with Rocky Mountain spotted fever (RMSF) demonstrating palmar surface of left hand. A distinguishing feature of RMSF rash is the involvement of the palms and soles. (From Shah BR, Laude TA. *Atlas of pediatric diagnosis*. Philadelphia: Saunders; 2000: 82, with permission.)

or low. Elevated band count, thrombocytopenia, and anemia may be present. Serum electrolytes should be performed and may be a clue to the diagnosis if hyponatremia is present. Hypoalbuminemia may also occur due to the vasculitic nature of the illness. Liver enzymes (alanine aminotransferase [ALT or SGPT], aspartate aminotransferase [AST or SGOT]) and muscle enzymes (creatinine kinase [CK]) may be elevated. If the patient exhibits neurologic features with stiff neck or altered consciousness, a lumbar puncture should be performed. The CSF examination will usually reveal a mild pleocytosis with normal glucose and protein. Culture of *R. rickettsii* is not usually attempted due to the danger of transmission to laboratory personnel. Rather than culture, the diagnosis can be confirmed by other modalities. Many laboratories in endemic areas have RMSF tests based on either indirect immunofluorescence or indirect hemagglutination that detect the presence of IgG and IgM antirickettsial antibodies. Most of these IgG/IgM tests for RMSF are positive by 7 days after the onset of illness. Unfortunately, this is also not a universal finding, and treatment should certainly not be delayed awaiting serologic test results. Negative RMSF tests may, however, guide decisions to discontinue empiric antibiotics. Immunofluorescent staining of skin biopsy material is possible when the rash is present. There is also a PCR test for blood and biopsy specimens, but it is not widely available or currently recommended. The Weil–Felix serologic test (*Proteus vulgaris* OX-19 and OX-2 agglutinins) has been used in the past, but it is nonspecific and insensitive, and is therefore no longer recommended. The Weil–Felix test also has a high false-positive rate, particularly in the patient with a proteus or leptospiral infection.

Management

Prior to specific antibiotic treatment, the mortality from RMSF was as high as 25%. With prompt initiation of antibiotics, recovery is now the rule. The most important factor in patient survival is early diagnosis and therapy. Each year, patients who present early in the season or without rash may be misdiagnosed, and treatment is delayed with disastrous results (overall mortality in the United States is still 5% to 7%). Doxycycline is considered the drug of choice and may be given intravenously or orally. The dosage consists of a loading dose of 2.2 mg/kg given at 12-hour intervals on the first day followed by 2 to 4 mg/kg given once a day to a maximum of

300 mg/dose. This therapy is usually continued for 7 to 10 days or until the patient has been afebrile for at least 3 to 4 days. This medication may be used in all age groups and is even recommended for children under 8 years of age. Doxycycline is less likely to cause dental staining than other tetracyclines, and staining is also less likely since a prolonged course of therapy is not necessary. Alternative medications include tetracycline (30 to 40 mg/kg/day divided every 6 hours) for patients greater than 8 years of age or IV chloramphenicol (50 to 75 mg/kg/day divided every 6 hours). Because of possible concurrent infection with other rickettsial diseases in some endemic areas, doxycycline has become the drug of choice because it eradicates both RMSF and *Ehrlichia*. Chloramphenicol is less effective in RMSF and is not effective against *Ehrlichia*.

Prevention

The best way to avoid contracting RMSF is to avoid tick-infested areas. Unfortunately, this is not always possible, and families should be advised to wear protective clothing that covers arms, legs, and other exposed areas. Insect or tick repellants can be applied to clothing (permethrin spray) and exposed skin (N,N-diethylmetatoluamide [DEET] application for children older than age 2) to decrease tick attachment. During tick season, skin inspection for ticks should be completed daily for people and pets (particularly outdoor animals). If a tick is found, the recommended removal is as follows: grasp the tick with fine tweezers close to the skin and pull gently straight out without a twisting motion. If fingers are used, protect the fingers with tissue or gloves and avoid squeezing the body of the tick. Always wash hands thoroughly after tick removal to minimize any exposure to potential pathogens. Prophylactic antibiotics are not recommended after a known tick bite, even in endemic areas.

Complications

There may be numerous complications in RMSF, particularly for cases with delayed diagnosis and treatment. Most serious complications are sequelae of disseminated intravascular coagulation (DIC). Gangrene may develop in the extremities. Multiorgan dysfunction, including adult respiratory distress syndrome, hepatocelluar dysfunction, and renal failure, may also occur. Neurologic manifestations may include delirium, confusion, stupor, and seizures. Patients may also have long-term sequelae depending on the severity of the neurologic involvement, including intellectual impairment, deafness, and blindness.

Pearls

- A history of tick exposure, rash involving the palms and soles, hyponatremia, leukopenia with an elevated band count, and thrombocytopenia are important clues in the diagnosis of RMSF.
- Always include RMSF in the differential if the patient lives in or recently visited an endemic area, even if the patient does not exhibit the classical features of RMSF. Up to 20% of patients do not have the classical rash; they have "spotless" RMSF.

Suggested Readings

American Academy of Pediatrics. Babesiosis; ehrlichiosis; lyme disease; Rocky Mountain spotted fever. In: Pickering LK, ed. *2003 Red book: report of the Committee on Infectious Diseases.* 26th ed. Elk Grove Village, IL: American Academy of Pediatrics; 2003:211–212; 266–269; 407–412; 532–534.

Dumler JS, Dey C, Meyer F, et al. Human monocytic ehrlichiosis: a potentially severe disease in children. *Arch Pediatr Adolesc Med* 2000;154:847–849.

Storch GA. New developments in tick-borne infections. *Pediatr Ann* 2002;31: 200–204.

Lantos P, Krause PJ. Ehrlichiosis in children. *Semin Pediatr Infect Dis* 2002; 13:249–256.

Thorner AR, Walker DH, Petri WA Jr. Rocky Mountain spotted fever. *CID* 1998;27:1353–1360.

Shapiro E. *Borrelia burgdorferi* (Lyme disease). In: Long S, Pickering L, Prober C, eds. *Principals and practice of pediatric infectious disease.* 2nd ed. Philadelphia, PA: Churchill Livingston 2003:965–968.

Varela AS, Luttrell MP, Howerth EW, et al. First culture isolation of *Borrelia lonestari*, putative agent of southern tick-associated rash illness. *J Clin Microbiol* 2004:42:1163–1169.

CHAPTER 91 ■ STAPHYLOCOCCAL SCALDED SKIN SYNDROME

BINITA R. SHAH

Ritter von Rittershain described an exfoliative dermatitis in neonates in 1878. Appearance of large bullae and separation of extended areas of the epidermis were the characteristic features. Staphylococci were subsequently found to be the etiologic agent. This entity was referred to as Ritter disease, as well as staphylococcal scalded skin syndrome (SSSS). However, in 1956, Lyell described a toxic epidermal necrolysis (TEN) in adults that mimicked SSSS in many ways, leading to some confusion in the terminology. This entity, identified as Lyell disease, was subsequently differentiated into two subtypes: one seen most frequently in adults secondary to drug hypersensitivity (e.g., anticonvulsants) and the other occurring in infants secondary to staphylococcal infection. The latter represents what was formerly known as Ritter disease. SSSS is the most severe manifestation of infection caused by certain *Staphylococcus aureus* strains, producing an exfoliative toxin and characterized by widespread bullae and exfoliation. *S. aureus* strains belonging to phage-2 produce epidermolytic toxins called exfoliatin toxins (ETs). These toxins are capable of causing clinical diseases that include bullous impetigo (the localized form of SSSS), generalized scarlatiniform eruption without exfoliation (staphylococcal scarlatina), and exfoliative blistering skin disease (SSSS).

There are three serologic forms of staphylococcal ETs (ETA, ETB, and ETD). The ETs are antigenic and elicit an antibody response when elaborated. Only ETA and ETB have been firmly linked to human SSSS.

SSSS is most commonly seen in infants and young children. Ninety-eight percent of those infected are less than 6 years old, and 62% are less than 2 years of age. Lack of specific antitoxin antibody to exfoliative toxin and renal immaturity with poor toxin clearance are contributing factors in the younger age. Epidermolytic toxin antibody is present in about 75% of normal people over the age of 10 years, a fact that explains the rare occurrence of SSSS in adults. Infection in adults is related to a decreased renal clearance of the toxin (e.g., patients with renal insufficiency or on hemodialysis) or in association with lymphoma or immunosuppression (e.g., human immunodeficiency virus infection).

S. aureus colonizes mucous membranes of the nasopharynx, eyes, and selected areas (e.g., umbilical stump, circumcision sites), and then progresses to a localized infection. Toxin produced from that vantage point circulates widely, and then causes intra-epidermal splitting through the granular layer by specific cleavage of desmoglein-1, a desmosomal cadherin protein that mediates cell-to-cell adhesion of keratinocytes in the granular layer.

Several other skin eruptions should be included in the *differential diagnosis* of SSSS. During the initial stage of generalized erythema and scarlatiniform eruption, SSSS might be confused with staphylococcal scarlet fever, a forme fruste of SSSS that does not progress beyond the initial stage of a generalized erythematous eruption. Patients with staphylococcal scarlatina have a sandpaper rash with Pastia sign (just like streptococcal scarlet fever) but there is absence of strawberry tongue, exudative tonsillopharyngitis, and palatal petechiae (typical findings of streptococcal scarlet fever). The presence of skin tenderness and a positive Nikolsky sign in staphylococcal scarlatina, and the absence of those features in streptococcal scarlet fever, also help to differentiate the two. Diffusely erythematous skin with tenderness, Nikolsky sign around the lesions, and a negative culture from the intact bulla differentiates generalized SSSS from bullous impetigo (localized SSSS). TEN is another important consideration in the differential diagnosis of SSSS. Table 91.1 lists characteristics of SSSS and TEN that may be useful in differentiating the two entities.

CLINICAL FINDINGS

The features of SSSS are summarized in Table 91.2. SSSS begins with a localized (often inapparent) infection of the conjunctiva, nares, umbilicus, nasopharynx, urinary tract, or a superficial abrasion. This is followed by an abrupt onset of fever, skin tenderness, and a diffuse scarlatiniform rash, often accentuated in the perioral and flexural areas (Fig. 91.1). Flaccid, large, clear (sterile) bullae follow, which rupture promptly, leaving large denuded areas (Fig. 91.2). New bullae appear over a period of 2 to 3 days. In its severe form, the exfoliation can spread to cover the entire body surface area. An associated localized staphylococcal infection, such as impetigo or purulent conjunctivitis, may be present. The Nikolsky sign (Table 91.3) is positive. The diagnosis of SSSS may not be suspected early in the course, as eruption may resemble scarlet fever. Some cases of SSSS do not progress beyond the staphylococcal scarlatina stage (forme fruste of SSSS). These cases are referred as staphylococcal scarlet fever or staphylococcal scarlatina.

In SSSS, cultures from colonized sites like mucous membranes (nasopharynx or conjunctiva) or the umbilical stump may be positive for *S. aureus*. Cultures of the skin are negative for staphylococci. Cultures of the intact bullae are also negative, unlike those of bullous impetigo, in which the infecting strain is generally recovered. Blood culture is often negative in children and positive in adults.

A skin biopsy specimen (or a frozen section of an induced peel for a more rapid diagnosis) will help distinguish between SSSS and TEN. In SSSS, the splitting of the epidermis is in the stratum granulosum near the skin surface (partial split of the upper epidermis); whereas, in TEN, the bulla is subepidermal,

TABLE 91.1

FEATURES TO AID IN DIFFERENTIATION BETWEEN STAPHYLOCOCCAL
SCALDED SKIN SYNDROME (SSSS) AND TOXIC EPIDERMAL NECROLYSIS (TEN)

Feature	SSSS	TEN
Age	Infants	Older children, adults
Etiology	*Staphylococcus aureus*	Drugs
Skin tenderness	Present	Present or absent
Exfoliating skin	White	Necrotic
Skin biopsy		
Level of split	Granular layer within epidermis	Full thickness epidermis (dermal—epidermal junction)
Microscopy	Paucity of inflammatory cells	Prominent inflammatory cells
Mortality	1–10%	30%
Skin scarring	None	Frequent

TABLE 91.2

CLINICAL FEATURES OF STAPHYLOCOCCAL
SCALDED SKIN SYNDROME

Sudden onset of fever and irritability
Prominent crusting around the eyes and mouth, occurs early
May have pharyngitis, conjunctivitis, or superficial erosions on lips
Intraoral mucosal surfaces are spared
Rash
  No prodromal period at onset of rash
  Exquisite skin tenderness
  Begins as diffuse, erythematous scarlatiniform eruption with sandpaper-like texture
  Within 24–48 hr: skin wrinkles and flaccid bullae form
  Exfoliation in sheets reveals a moist, red, and shiny scalded-looking surface (Fig. 91.2)
  Borders of exfoliating skin are rolled like wet tissue paper
  Drying of exfoliated areas with flaky desquamation lasts 3–5 days
Hair and nails may also shed
Healing of rash occurs *without* scarring in 7–14 days

resulting in cleavage at the dermal—epidermal junction and full-thickness necrosis of the epidermis. Dermatology consultation may be obtained if diagnosis is unclear between SSSS and TEN.

MANAGEMENT

All patients with SSSS with widespread erosions and denuded skin require hospitalization and intravenous beta-lactamase resistant (BLR) beta-lactam antibiotic therapy (e.g., oxacillin sodium or nafcillin 150 mg/kg/day divided every 6 hours). Most *S. aureus* strains in the community or in hospitals produce beta-lactamase enzymes and are resistant to penicillin and ampicillin. Patients allergic to penicillin can be treated with a cephalosporin (if not allergic to cephalosporin [e.g., cefuroxime]), clindamycin hydrochloride, or vancomycin hydrochloride. The usual duration of therapy is 5 to 7 days, but bacteremic or immunocompromised patients require longer therapy. SSSS due to methicillin-resistant S. aureus (MRSA) has been reported. For nosocomially acquired infections due to MRSA, intravenous vancomycin remains the treatment of choice. For empiric therapy of suspected community-acquired MRSA infections, initial therapy

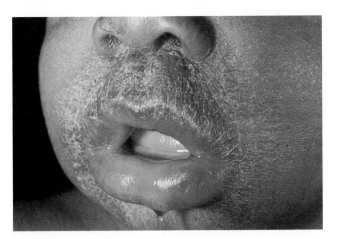

FIGURE 91.1. Staphylococcal scalded skin syndrome. Radial "sunburst" crusting and fissuring around the orifices (mouth, eyes, nose) are hallmarks of SSSS. (From Shah BR, Lucchesi M. *Atlas of pediatric emergency medicine.* New York: McGraw-Hill; 2006:101, with permission.)

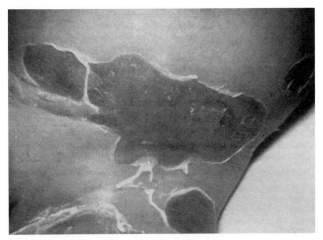

FIGURE 91.2. Staphylococcal scalded skin syndrome in a 2-week-old neonate after a wound infection from circumcision. The borders of the exfoliating skin look like rolled, wet tissue paper. (From Shah BR, Laude TA. *Atlas of pediatric diagnosis.* Philadelphia: Saunders; 2000:95, with permission.)

TABLE 91.3

NIKOLSKY SIGN: DIAGNOSIS AND ASSOCIATED
CONDITIONS

Positive sign: Slight rubbing of normal-looking skin adjacent
to lesion results in blistering
Conditions associated with a positive Nikolsky sign:
- Staphylococcal scalded skin syndrome (SSSS)
- Toxic epidermal necrolysis (TEN)
- Stevens-Johnson syndrome
- Pemphigus vulgaris

should include vancomycin and a BLR beta-lactam antimicrobial (e.g., nafcillin or oxacillin).

Subsequent therapy should be determined by antimicrobial susceptibility results. Vancomycin-intermediately susceptible *S. aureus* (VISA) strains rarely have been isolated. For seriously ill patients with a history of recurrent MRSA infections or for patients failing vancomycin therapy for whom VISA strains are a consideration, initial therapy could include vancomycin and ampicillin–sulbactam or trimethoprim–sulfamethoxazole, with or without gentamicin sulfate. For the penicillin-allergic patient, vancomycin plus gentamicin and trimethoprim–sulfamethoxazole could be considered.

Nasal swabs from the patient and immediate family members should be performed to identify asymptomatic nasal carriers of *S. aureus*. In the case of outbreaks on the ward or nursery, health care professionals should also be cultured.

Loss of the epidermal barrier requires close monitoring with fluid and electrolyte deficit replacement. Skin care includes gently moistening and cleaning the skin with isotonic saline or Burow solution and applying emollient to provide lubrication and reduce discomfort. Wet dressings may cause further drying and cracking and hence should be avoided. Application of topical antibiotics is *not* necessary. Corticosteroids (topically and systemically) are contraindicated because they interfere with host defense mechanisms. Patients with localized SSSS can be treated with oral antibiotic therapy (e.g., dicloxacillin sodium or a first- or second-generation cephalosporin, or clindamycin

or trimethoprim–sulfamethoxazole for patients with penicillin allergy).

COURSE AND PROGNOSIS

SSSS is a potentially serious but highly treatable infection with an overall mortality of 1% to 10% in children. Fluid and electrolyte losses leading to hypovolemia, faulty temperature regulation, cutaneous infection (cellulitis), pneumonia, and septicemia are some of the complications leading to morbidity or rare mortality. Long-term complications are rare because the skin lesions are superficial and heal rapidly without scarring. The mortality in adults is about 60% despite aggressive treatment, usually because of serious underlying illness.

PEARLS

- SSSS is characterized by widespread bullae and exfoliation.
- The exfoliative phase of SSSS is heralded by perioral exudation and crusting. Large radial fissures ("sunburst" crusting) around the orifices (mouth, eyes, and nose) are hallmarks of SSSS (Fig. 91.1).
- Early distinction between SSSS and TEN is extremely important, because therapy for SSSS includes antistaphylococcal antibiotics; whereas, in TEN, discontinuation of treatment with the offending drug and aggressive supportive therapy in a burn unit may be life-saving.
- Cultures from SSSS-affected skin/bullae are negative for *S. aureus*, although cultures from the colonized sites such as mucous membranes (nasopharynx or conjunctiva) or the umbilical stump may be positive.

Suggested Readings

American Academy of Pediatrics Staphylococcal Infections. In: Pickering LK, Baker CJ, Long SS, et al., eds. *Red book 2006: report of the Committee on Infectious Diseases,* 27th ed. Elk Grove Village, IL: American Academy of Pediatrics; 2006.

Swartz MN, Pasternack MS. Cellulitis and subcutaneous tissue infections. In: Mandell G, Bennett JE, Dolin R, eds. *Principles and practice of infectious diseases.* 6th ed. New York: Churchill Livingstone; 2005:1172.

CHAPTER 92 ■ TOXIC SHOCK SYNDROME

BINITA R. SHAH

Toxic shock syndrome (TSS) is a potentially fatal, systemic infection resulting from infection with toxin-producing strains of either *Staphylococcus aureus* or *Streptococcus pyogenes*. *S. aureus*–mediated TSS was first reported in 1978 in children presenting with multiorgan failure. It drew national media attention in the early 1980s because of its association with tampon use and menstruation. Super-absorbent tampons containing polyacrylate fibers were subsequently removed from the commercial market, resulting in a marked decline in menses-related TSS. *S. aureus*-mediated TSS is seen more commonly in adults than children. The highest number of cases occurs in women in the 15- to 34-year age range, with the age and sex distribution a reflection of the association with menses. Nonmenstrual cases occur in people of all ages and in both sexes. Currently, the incidence of nonmenstrual TSS exceeds that of menstrual TSS. A few examples of predisposing factors for nonmenstrual TSS include foreign body placement (e.g., nasal packing for epistaxis, tympanostomy tubes, contraceptive sponge or diaphragm, central lines), primary *S. aureus* infection (e.g., cellulitis, carbuncle, endocarditis, empyema), postoperative wound infection, skin or mucous membrane disruption (e.g., burns, insect bites, dermatitis), and vaginal or pharyngeal colonization. Menstrual TSS is related only to tampon use. *S. pyogenes*-mediated TSS is also known as toxic streptococcus or streptococcal toxic shock-like syndrome. The incidence of *S. pyogenes*-mediated TSS is highest among young children and older persons. A few examples of predisposing factors include varicella, human immunodeficiency virus infection, chronic cardiac or pulmonary diseases, diabetes mellitus, and intravenous drug use.

TSS is caused by toxins released from *S. aureus* or *S. pyogenes*. *S. aureus*-mediated TSS is usually caused by strains producing an exotoxin (toxic shock syndrome toxin 1;TSST-1). In adults, TSST-1–producing strains of *S. aureus* may be part of the normal flora of the anterior nares and the vagina. Colonization is believed to produce protective antibody, and more than 90% of adults have antibodies to TSST-1. People in whom *S. aureus*–mediated TSS develops because of TSST-1–producing strains usually do not have antibodies to TSST-1. More than 90% of menstrual TSS and about 50% of nonmenstrual TSS cases are mediated by TSST-1 production. The remainder are produced by *S. aureus* strains producing an enterotoxin B or C (SEB, SEC).

In *S. aureus*–mediated TSS, organisms colonize selected sites, where they produce exotoxins. These exotoxins are absorbed into the bloodstream through inflamed or traumatized mucous membranes, or from areas of focal infection, and transported systemically. TSST-1 acts as a superantigen, resulting in the release of cytokines (e.g., tumor necrosis factor alpha [TNF-α], interleukins 1 [IL-1] and 6 [IL-6]), which in turn are responsible for tissue injury and multiorgan failure. Host immune factors are important in the pathogenesis of TSS. Patients with TSS have low levels of antibodies to TSST-1.

A failure to generate anti-TSST-1 antibody after an episode predisposes patients to recurrent episodes. Blood cultures are often negative because the organism is usually not invasive.

S. pyogenes-mediated TSS is caused by strains producing at least one of five protein superantigenic exotoxins. These are streptococcal pyrogenic exotoxins A, B, or C (SPE-A, SPE-B, or SPE-C), streptococcal superantigen, or mitogenic factor. In streptococcal TSS, skin and soft-tissue infection by invasive *S. pyogenes* produces superantigenic exotoxins that lead to massive release of proinflammatory cytokines (TNF-α, IL-1, IL-6). These cytokines result in subsequent shock and tissue injury similar to classic *S. aureus*—mediated TSS.

The diagnosis of TSS is made from clinical presentation, laboratory data defined by the Centers for Disease Control and Prevention, and consideration/exclusion of the differential diagnoses, which include septic shock from another etiology (e.g., gram-negative sepsis), meningococcemia, scarlet fever, Kawasaki disease, measles/atypical measles, Rocky Mountain spotted fever, ehrlichiosis, and leptospirosis. Severe drug reactions including Stevens–Johnson syndrome and toxic epidermal necrolysis may occasionally present with skin findings and shock.

CLINICAL FINDINGS

The clinical findings necessary for the diagnosis of staphylococcal TSS and streptococcal TSS are reported in Tables 92.1 and 92.2. The features that make these clinically different are highlighted in Table 92.3. TSS may range in severity from a relatively mild disease, often misdiagnosed as a viral/flulike illness, to a severe, life-threatening illness. In staphylococcal TSS, onset may be abrupt or preceded by a prodromal illness lasting for a couple of days and consisting of fever, chills, and myalgia. The major manifestations are fever, rash, and hypotension (Table 92.1). The rash is almost always noted within the first 24 hours and is typically a pruritic, blanching, diffuse, macular erythroderma. The initial rash may be subtle or faint and may be mistaken for skin flushing associated with a fever. A scarlatiniform rash with flexural accentuation may also be seen. Beefy red hyperemia of mucous membranes and conjunctiva, strawberry tongue, and erythema and edema of palms and soles (findings similar to Kawasaki disease) are often seen. Desquamation of palms and soles follows in 1 to 2 weeks. The focus of staphylococcal infection may be inconspicuous in menstrual TSS because the pelvic examination is usually normal except for the presence of subtle erythema and edema of the skin of the inner thigh and perineum. Signs of inflammation in an infected skin lesion or wound may also be absent in nonmenstrual TSS. The toxins interfere locally with release of inflammatory mediators, leading to absence of inflammation. Because TSS involves virtually every organ system, a wide variety of signs and symptoms involving gastrointestinal, renal,

STAPHYLOCOCCAL TOXIC SHOCK SYNDROME CRITERIA AND
CASE DEFINITION

CRITERIA

Fever ≥38.9°C (≥102.0°F)

Rash: diffuse, macular erythroderma (scarlatiniform eruption or sunburn-like rash)

Desquamation 1–2 wk after onset (particularly palms and soles, fingers, and toes)

Hypotension:

Systolic blood pressure ≤90 mm Hg for adults

<5th percentile by age for children <16 yr of age

Orthostatic drop in diastolic blood pressure ≥15 mm Hg from lying to sitting

Orthostatic syncope or orthostatic dizziness

Multisystem involvement: (three or more of the following)

Gastrointestinal: vomiting or diarrhea at onset of illness

Muscular: severe myalgia or creatinine phosphatase kinase >2 × upper limit of normal

Mucous membrane: vaginal, oropharyngeal, or conjunctival hyperemia

Renal: blood urea nitrogen or serum creatinine level >2 × upper limit of normal or urinary sediment with ≥5 white blood cell/hpf in absence of urinary tract infection

Hepatic: total bilirubin, aspartate, or alanine aminotransferase levels >2 × upper limit of normal

Hematologic: platelet count ≤100,000/mm^3

Central nervous system: disorientation or alteration in consciousness without focal neurologic signs when fever and hypotension are absent

Negative results *if obtained*:

Blood, throat, or cerebrospinal fluid cultures (blood culture may be positive for *Staphylococcus aureus*)

Serologic tests for Rocky Mountain spotted fever, leptospirosis, or measles

CASE DEFINITION

Probable: A case with 5 of the 6 aforementioned clinical findings.

Confirmed: A case with all 6 of the clinical findings, including desquamation. If the patient dies before desquamation could have occurred, the other 5 criteria constitute a definitive case.

Modified from the American Academy of Pediatrics. Toxic shock syndrome. In: Pickering LK, ed. *Red book 2006: report of the Committee on Infectious Diseases*. 27th ed. Elk Grove Village, IL: American Academy of Pediatrics; 2006: 578. (Adapted from Wharton M, Chorba TL, Vogt RL, et al. Case definitions for public health surveillance. *MMWR Recomm Rep* 1990;39:1–43.)

hepatic, hematologic, and the central nervous system may be present (Tables 92.1 and 92.2). Menstrual and nonmenstrual TSS have similar clinical features. Menses-related cases generally develop on the third or fourth day of the menses.

Streptococcal TSS shares many features with staphylococcal TSS. The skin is often the portal of entry with underlying soft-tissue infection found in approximately 80% of patients. Patients may initially present with localized extremity pain that rapidly progresses over 48 to 72 hours to manifest both local and systemic signs. Soft-tissue involvement of this nature (e.g., necrotizing fasciitis, hemorrhagic cellulitis) is *distinctly uncommon* in staphylococcal TSS. In both forms of TSS, the complete blood count may show leukocytosis with a left shift, lymphopenia, thrombocytopenia, and anemia. Blood urea nitrogen, creatinine, and liver enzyme studies may be elevated. Other necessary studies include serum electrolytes, coagulation profile, blood culture, and cultures from the site of infection (skin/soft tissue, if appropriate). Prothrombin time and partial thromboplastin time may be prolonged with evidence of disseminated intravascular coagulation (DIC). Urinalysis may show sterile pyuria, and cerebrospinal fluid examination may show pleocytosis.

A vaginal culture will be positive for *S. aureus* in 85% of cases of menstrual TSS. Acute and convalescent streptococcal antibody titers (e.g., antistreptolysin [ASO] or antideoxyribonuclease B) may help diagnose streptococcal TSS, especially in the absence of a positive blood culture. Surgical exploration or incisional biopsy for diagnosis and culture will confirm diagnosis of necrotizing fasciitis associated with streptococcal TSS.

MANAGEMENT

Management of both forms of TSS involves stabilization followed by hospitalization in an intensive-care setting. Assessment of ABCs and simultaneous resuscitation is carried out as indicated by abnormal vital signs, including continuous cardiac and pulse oximetry monitoring. Large-volume fluid resuscitation is often required for septic shock, and pressor agents may be indicated (see Chapters 26 and 34). Multisystem organ failure needs to be anticipated and managed accordingly. Empiric IV antimicrobial therapy to cover both forms of TSS while awaiting culture results is given because it may be impossible to clinically distinguish the two forms of TSS. A beta-lactamase–resistant antistaphylococcal antibiotic (e.g., oxacillin) *and* a protein synthesis inhibitor (thereby inhibiting toxin or cytokine production; e.g., clindamycin hydrochloride) are the usual initial choices. After identification of the pathogen, therapy can be changed to

TABLE 92.2

STREPTOCOCCAL TOXIC SHOCK SYNDROME (FIG. 92.1) CRITERIA AND CASE DEFINITION

CRITERIA

    I. Isolation of *Streptococcus pyogenes*

        A. From a normally sterile site (e.g., blood, cerebrospinal fluid, peritoneal fluid, tissue biopsy).

        B. From a nonsterile site (e.g., throat, sputum, vagina, surgical wound, or superficial skin lesion).

    II. Clinical signs of severity:

        A. Hypotension: systolic blood pressure <90 mm Hg in adults *or* <5th percentile for age in children.

        and

        B. Two or more of the following signs:

        Renal: creatinine ≥ 2 mg/dL for adults or $>2 \times$ the upper limit of normal for age.

        Coagulopathy: platelets $\leq 100,000$/mm^3 or disseminated intravascular coagulation.

        Hepatic: serum alanine and aspartate aminotransferases or total bilirubin values $>2 \times$ the upper limit of normal for age.

        Adult respiratory distress syndrome (ARDS).

        Generalized, erythematous, macular rash that may desquamate.

        Soft-tissue necrosis, including necrotizing fasciitis or myositis, or gangrene.

CASE DEFINITION

  Probable: Illness fulfilling criteria IB *and* IIA and IIB, if no other etiology for the illness is identified.

  Definite: Illness fulfilling criteria IA *and* IIA and IIB.

Modified from the American Academy of Pediatrics. Toxic shock syndrome. In: Pickering LK, ed. *Red book 2006: report of the Committee on Infectious Diseases*. 27th ed. Elk Grove Village, IL: American Academy of Pediatrics; 2006: 578. (Adapted from The working group on severe streptococcal infections. Defining the group A streptococcal toxic shock syndrome: rationale and consensus definition. *JAMA* 1993;269:390–391.)

penicillin *and* clindamycin hydrochloride for streptococcal TSS, and a beta-lactam antibiotic (based on susceptibility pattern) *with* clindamycin hydrochloride for staphylococcal TSS. Therapy is continued for minimum of 10 to 14 days for staphylococcal TSS. In streptococcal TSS, therapy is continued until the patient is afebrile, hemodynamically stable, and has a negative blood culture; however, total duration depends on the underlying cause. Clindamycin hydrochloride should *not* be used alone as

TABLE 92.3

DIFFERENTIAL DIAGNOSIS: STAPHYLOCOCCAL (STAPH-TSS) VS. STREPTOCOCCAL TOXIC SHOCK SYNDROME (STREP-TSS)

Clinical feature	Staph-TSS	Strep-TSS
Age (years, usual)	15–35	20–50
Sex	Female > male	Either
Severe local pain (at site of infection)	Uncommon	Common
Hypotension	100%	100%
Blood culture (+)	<5%	>50%
Clinical features		
Erythroderma	Very common	Less common
Profuse watery diarrhea, vomiting	Frequent	Less common
Conjunctival injection	Frequent	Less common
Severe myalgia	Frequent	Less common
Local soft-tissue infection		
Cellulitis, abscess	Rare	Common
Necrotizing fasciitis, myositis	Rare	Common
Predisposing factors	Tampons, packing	Skin trauma, varicella
Mortality	<30%	30–70%
Recurrence	Seen (menses associated)	Not seen

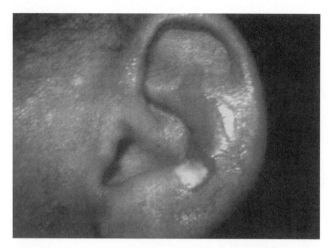

FIGURE 92.1. Streptococcal toxic shock syndrome. A 6-year-old boy admitted with fever, hypotension, an infected varicella lesion on the ear (portal of entry for GABS), and empyema. Approximately 700 mL of pus, which later grew GABS, was drained from the pleural cavity. (From Shah BR, Laude AT. *Atlas of pediatric clinical diagnosis.* Philadelphia: Saunders; 2000:90, with permission.)

initial empiric therapy because 1% to 2% of *S. pyogenes* strains are resistant to clindamycin in the United States. Vancomycin should be substituted for the beta-lactam antibiotic in areas where community acquired methicillin resistant *S. aureus* infections are common. Foreign bodies, such as tampons or nasal packs, must be removed. Intravenous immune globulin (IVIG) therapy may be considered for both forms of TSS in patients who are refractory to all therapeutic measures, have undrainable foci of infection, or have persistent oliguria with pulmonary edema. The mechanism of action of IVIG in TSS is unclear; however, antibodies to the TSST-1 and streptococcal toxins are present in IVIG and may play a role.

Surgical consultation may be indicated for debridement, exploration, and immediate resection of necrotic tissue in necrotizing fasciitis or for drainage of infected sites. Droplet and contact precautions in addition to the standard precautions are recommended for all patients with *S. pyogenes*–mediated TSS. Only standard precautions are recommended for *S. aureus*–mediated TSS (person-to-person transmission is uncommon).

COURSE AND PROGNOSIS

Renal failure and/or adult respiratory distress syndrome (ARDS) may occur in the first few days of illness and may be responsible for mortality. Other complications that may occur include overwhelming sepsis, multiorgan failure, seizures, pancreatitis, and pericarditis. Death is usually related to refractory shock, cardiac arrhythmias, and/or DIC. Streptococcal TSS carries a much higher mortality than staphylococcal TSS. Women with menses-related TSS may experience one or more recurrent episodes; therefore, tampon use should be discontinued. Internal barrier methods of birth control are also risk factors and should be discouraged (e.g., contraceptive sponge, diaphragm). Recurrences of nonmenstrual TSS are rare.

PEARLS

- TSS may be caused by toxin-producing S. *aureus* or S. *pyogenes*. Fever, rash, desquamation, hypotension, and multiorgan involvement are the hallmarks of both variants of TSS.
- TSS can be confused with many infectious and noninfectious causes of fever associated with mucocutaneous manifestations.
- An infected varicella lesion may be the portal of entry for invasive S. *pyogenes* disease.

Suggested Readings

American Academy of Pediatrics. Toxic shock syndrome. In: Pickering LK, ed. *Red book 2006: report of the Committee on Infectious Diseases.* 27th ed. Elk Grove Village, IL: American Academy of Pediatrics; 2006.

Jain A, Daum RS. Staphylococcal infections in children: Part 3. *Pediatr Rev* 1999;20:261–265.

Manders SM. Toxin-mediated streptococcal and staphylococcal disease. *J Am Acad Dermatol* 1998;39:383–398.

CHAPTER 93 ■ COMMUNITY-ACQUIRED METHICILLIN-RESISTANT *STAPHYLOCOCCUS AUREUS* INFECTIONS

WILLIAM A. B. DALZELL

Throughout the world, *Staphylococcus aureus* (SA) is part of the normal human flora. Illnesses caused by SA range from nuisance, such as recurrent boils, to life-threatening conditions associated with endocarditis and septic shock. The bacterium produces numerous extracellular products, including hemolysins, leukocidins, enzymes, and toxins, that elicit a host response when ingested or inoculated through the skin or mucosal barrier.

When penicillin was initially developed, SA was sensitive but quickly developed resistance. Subsequently, and relatively quickly, this microorganism developed resistance after exposure to many other antibiotics. SA is now divided into two major designations: methicillin-sensitive SA (MSSA) and methicillin-resistant SA (MRSA). This designation is determined by culture, and is often suggested by clinical presentation. MRSA is further divided into community-acquired MRSA (CA-MRSA) and hospital-acquired MRSA (HA-MRSA). Initial antibiotic choices are dictated by local resistance patterns to these SA groups. Final antibiotic therapy should be guided by sensitivities of the actual organism recovered from the patient. For serious infections, vancomycin remains the mainstay of therapy for MRSA, although sporadic resistance to this antibiotic has been reported.

Since the early 1990s, outbreaks of CA-MRSA have become much more common in both pediatric and adult populations, and resulted in increased awareness of its importance. The definition of CA-MRSA is not universally agreed upon, but there is often a combination of clinical features, risk factors, and laboratory data used to make this designation. Most definitions are designed for adult patients, so modifications for children are necessary. In general, HA-MRSA is more antibiotic resistant, with susceptibility only to vancomycin, trimethoprim–sulfamethasoxazole, and linezolid. CA-MRSA often retains susceptibility to gentamicin and clindamycin as well as the above antibiotics.

Both MSSA and MRSA strains can carry the Panton–Valentine leukocidin (PVL) gene. This gene is responsible for an extracellular toxin directed against polymorphonuclear leukocytes and macrophages, and leads to death of these cells in the infected host. Although it is not known if bacteria that carry this leukocidin are more virulent than others, it has been associated with necrotizing pneumonia and skin and soft-tissue infections (SSTIs), particularly in children. Beta-lactam antibiotic resistance of MRSA bacteria is mediated via the mecA gene. This gene is responsible for production of a novel penicillin binding protein (PBP-2′). This altered PBP reduces the cellular affinity for beta-lactam antimicrobials, and is not overcome by increasing doses or the use of enzyme inhibitors with standard anti-SA beta-lactam antibiotics.

CLINICAL MANIFESTATIONS

SA is commonly found as part of the normal bacterial flora in about 30%–60% of the population, mainly colonizing the skin or upper respiratory tract, and occasionally gastrointestinal or female genitourinary tract. Both MSSA and MRSA colonization are asymptomatic. If one is colonized with MRSA, there is increased risk for invasive disease if risk factors are present. The clinical conditions associated with SA infections are numerous and varied (Table 93.1). Like all SA strains, CA-MRSA may infect any organ system; however, there seems to be a predilection in children for either SSTIs with abscess formation or necrotizing pneumonia with empyema. This is particularly true if there is a predisposing condition or illness, such as eczema (for SSTIs) or concurrent influenza (for pneumonia).

SAMPLE COLLECTION AND LABORATORY PROCEDURES

When looking for simple colonization with MRSA, the samples are taken from nonsterile sites (e.g., nares, skin folds). These cultures are often obtained as part of surveillance sampling to monitor colonization rates and subsequent risk for infection. A positive culture does not confirm infection at a distant site, only that the patient carries the bacteria.

Samples from a normally sterile site (e.g., abscesses and empyemas) need collection in a sterile fashion for culture. Obtaining a needle aspiration in an aseptic manner before incision and drainage (I & D) is preferred over collecting a sample during I & D with a swab. With needle aspiration there is less chance for contamination and a clear interpretation if more than one type of bacteria is isolated (polymicrobial). The skin should be prepped and the lesion aspirated with a sterile needle and syringe. The aspirated material should be placed in a sterile transport vial; the larger the volume of sample sent to the laboratory, the better the possibility of isolating the correct pathogen. Swabs obtained from the I & D procedure are less acceptable due to the greater chance of cross-contamination with skin flora and the potential loss of viability for some organisms (other than SA) in this transport system. If anaerobic bacteria are also suspected to be part of the infection (e.g., deep neck or lung abscesses), special anaerobic transport medium is required. A discussion with the microbiology laboratory is highly recommended prior to obtaining samples in order to maximize the culture results.

TABLE 93.1

CLINICAL PRESENTATIONS AND MANIFESTATIONS OF *STAPHYLOCOCCUS AUREUS* INFECTIONS

SKIN AND SOFT-TISSUE INFECTIONS
Impetigo
Folliculitis
Carbuncle
Cellulitis
Necrotizing fascitis

TOXIN MEDIATED
Staphylococcal scaled skin syndrome
Toxic shock syndrome
Food poisoning

MUSCULOSKELETAL
Pyomyositis
Iliopsoas abscess
Obturator Internus Abscess
Septic arthritis (knee, hip, elbow most common)

RESPIRATORY TRACT
Sinusitis (acute and chronic)
Acute mastoiditis
Otitis media
Bacterial tracheitis
Pneumonia

HEAD AND NECK
Cervical adenitis
Orbital cellulitis
Ocular infections
Parotitis

CARDIOVASCULAR
Endocarditis
Pericarditis
Septic thrombophlebitis
Septicemia

VISCERAL
Liver abscesses
Renal/perinephric abscesses
Mastitis

CENTRAL NERVOUS SYSTEM
Meningitis
Epidural/subdural/cerebral abscesses
Sinus cavernous thrombosis

FOREIGN BODY/DEVICE INFECTIONS
Intravascular access device
CNS: ventricular shunt
Peritoneal dialysis catheter
Pacemaker
Prosthetic joints

The presence of staphylococcus is suggested by the finding of gram-positive cocci in clusters on the initial Gram stain of aspirated or cultured material. SA tends to grow very well on standard media in the microbiology laboratory. Identification within 24 hours is common if bacterial growth is not inhibited by prior treatment of the patient with antibiotics. Standard sensitivity testing may require as much as an additional 48 hours. These sensitivities are needed to help select antibiotics for therapy and to classify the strain as hospital or community acquired. In some labs, MRSA identification by special media or use of PCR probes for the mecA gene is used. These tests provide a shorter turnaround time, but do not give sensitivities.

Many CA-MRSA strains carry the MLS$_B$ phenotype, which has inducible resistance for clindamycin. These strains demonstrate resistance to erythromycin but sensitivity to clindamycin. Only by performing a D-test can true sensitivity to clindamycin be confirmed (see Fiebelkorn and associates in the Suggested Readings). If this test is not performed, a patient with the MLS$_B$ phenotype may fail therapy with clindamycin for CA-MRSA infection. Use of the D-test is becoming more common; it is wise to check with the laboratory to ascertain if a given MRSA isolate is truly susceptible to clindamycin before using this antibiotic.

The use of PCR probes to test for the PVL gene in SA is currently a research technique only. As noted, significance of this gene is uncertain at this time; however, it is found predominately in community strains of SA and may contribute to virulence.

MANAGEMENT GUIDELINES

Since MRSA has become a pervasive problem in many communities, the initial management of suspected infections has changed rapidly. Although rates vary, nearly 70% of SA isolates from the emergency department in our locale (eastern North Carolina) are CA-MRSA. This has prompted the development of guidelines for the initial management of these infections based upon the anatomic location of infection and the severity of illness on presentation (Fig. 93.1).

The degree of inflammation with SSTIs and/or associated co-morbidities (e.g., diabetes, dialysis, debilitation, or immunosuppression) helps to dictate management. The initial complaint of parents is often of an "infected spider bite" that fails to respond to conservative therapy. The child may have an associated cellulitis or folliculitis. If I & D is not needed, treatment of superficial skin infection with topical agents, such as mupirocin ointment, may be adequate. With simple cutaneous abscesses, I & D is often curative if the wound is adequately drained. Antibiotic therapy should be considered if the child is systemically ill. With mild systemic symptoms, I & D is performed followed by empiric antibiotic therapy directed against more common organisms (e.g., MSSA and streptococcus) with either a first-generation cephalosporin or amoxicillin–clavulanate. Close follow-up is recommended either with or without antimicrobials.

If the child is systemically ill with a deep soft-tissue infection requiring hospitalization, such as a deep abscess or necrotizing fasciitis (Chapter 81), surgery becomes an essential part of the curative therapy. Additional cultures and laboratory tests may be needed depending upon the degree of illness. Pending culture results, initial empiric therapy will then include broad-spectrum antibiotics selected based on suspected microorganisms and local sensitivity patterns. Typical initial therapy would consist of vancomycin or clindamycin plus either a third-generation cephalosporin or ampicillin–sulbactam.

For a child with a necrotizing pneumonia, hospitalization in an intensive care setting may be necessary (Chapter 77). Pertinent imaging, either ultrasound or CT, will help to guide decisions about diagnosis and management. Early surgical intervention is needed if an empyema is found. The procedure used (i.e., video-assisted thoracoscopy, open thoracotomy, closed chest tube drainage) will depend upon the surgical services available. Empiric broad-spectrum antibiotics are appropriate, such as vancomycin plus either a third-generation cephalosporin or ampicillin–sulbactam, with culture results guiding antibiotic choices when available.

Guidelines for Management of Suspected CA-MRSA and SSTIs

Case Definition

- Diagnosis of MRSA made in outpatient setting or by culture positive for MRSA within 48 hours of hospital admission and
- No history within past 12 months of: hospitalization, surgery, long term care residence, indwelling catheter or medical devices; dialysis, renal failure, diabetes, or other comorbidities and
- If <12 months of age only in regular newborn nursery after delivery

Clinical Presentation

- Looks like insect or spider bite
- Folliculitis, pustular lesions
- Furuncle, carbuncle (boil)
- Cellulitis
- Impetigo
- Infected wounds, red swollen, painful

Risk Factors Associated with CA-MRSA

- Athletes, military recruits, children, Pacific Islanders, Alaskan Natives, Native Americans, men who have sex with men, prisoners
- Close skin to skin contact (esp. abraded or non-intact skin), shared contaminated items such as towels, crowding, poor hygiene

Incision and Drainage (I & D) of abscess with culture

If I & D not performed, consider culture of draining wounds or aspirate or biopsy of central areas of inflammation

Culture & antimicrobial susceptibility testing

If erythromycin-resistant, clindamycin-susceptible, obtain "D-test" prior to clindamycin usage

Patient Education

Recommend standard contact precautions, reinforce hygiene, test knowledge of same

Mild – Moderate

Afebrile or febrile, no unstable co-morbidities

Severe – Critically Ill

Appears toxic, unstable co-morbidity, sepsis syndrome, or life or limb threatening infections (necrotizing fascitis)

Outpatient Management

- Local care, I & D – may be sufficient in mild disease
- Consider local antibiotics
- If oral antibiotics used – cephalexin or Augmentin preferred for MSSA
- If increased suspicion for MRSA (>1 risk factor), consider empiric therapy for MRSA
- Adjust antibiotics based on culture and susceptibility testing
- Monitor response to therapy

Hospital Management

- Empiric broad-spectrum IV antibiotics active against S. aureus, including MRSA (e.g. vancomycin)
- Adjust antibiotics based on culture and susceptibility testing
- Monitor response to therapy
- Consult ID specialist if no improvement and consider alternative agents
- Switch to oral therapy based on susceptibility testing if: Afebrile for 24 hours, clinically improved, able to take oral therapy, close follow-up possible

Redrawn from North Carolina Statewide Program for Infection Control and Epidemiology
www.epi.state.nc.us/epi/gcdc/ca_mrsa/ca_mrsa.html and www.unc.edu/depts/spice/CA-MRSA.html
with modification to definition according to Buckingham, et al, *Emergence of Community-Associated Methicillin-Resistant Staphylococcus aureus at a Memphis, Tennessee Children's Hospital*   PIDJ Vol 23, No.7, pg 620

FIGURE 93.1. Guidelines for management of suspected CA-MRSA and SSTIs.

There are clinical situations when combination antibiotic therapy for MRSA is recommended (e.g., persistent septicemia, endocarditis). For these, either an aminoglycoside or rifampin can be added to the vancomycin. Note that rifampin should never be used as monotherapy in MRSA infections due to the quick acquisition of resistance.

With all of these infections, oral antibiotics may be appropriate once the child has substantially improved clinically. For proven CA-MRSA, trimethoprim–sulfamethasoxazole is often effective, especially for SSTIs. Both clindamycin and linezolid have excellent bioavailability with liquid formulations, but the poor palatability of these medications may be a limiting factor for younger children. The duration of antibiotic therapy depends upon the severity of the initial clinical presentation and the child's response to treatment.

DIFFERENTIAL DIAGNOSIS

A common pitfall in the initial choice of antibiotic therapy is assuming, based on clinical presentation, that an infection is most likely caused by CA-MRSA. Although infections secondary to these bacteria have become more common, the diagnosis is ultimately based on culture results and not on clinical suspicion alone. For example, SSTIs may also be caused by MSSA, streptococci, fungi, atypical bacteria, or mycobacteria. Pneumonia with associated empyema in a child over 1 year of age is still commonly caused by *Streptococcus pneumoniae*, but may also be anaerobic if secondary to recurrent or chronic aspiration.

PREVENTION

Transmission of MRSA within the hospital setting is common. Correspondingly, prevention of transmission requires strict adherence to infection-control procedures. Contact precautions should include gown and gloves worn by all members of the hospital team providing care to these patients. For procedures where aerosolization may be a consideration (e.g., deep suctioning of an intubated patient), droplet precautions including masks may also be required to prevent transmission to the health care worker. If a patient falls into a high-risk category for MRSA (Fig. 93.1) or has suspected MRSA infection or colonization, implementation of isolation procedures pending surveillance culture results is warranted.

Eradication of MRSA nasal carriage is controversial, regarding both how and when. Most agree that the use of intranasal mupirocin for 5 to 7 days is needed for eradication of nasal MRSA carriage. In addition to the mupirocin, some experts advocate oral antibiotics (e.g., trimethoprim–sulfamethasoxazole or doxycycline) in addition to body cleansing with an antiseptic wash. There is agreement that decolonization should not occur in an uncontrolled manner, as resistance rates to mupirocin are increasing. Decolonization should be considered for specific situations such as elective surgery in a known MRSA carrier, recurrent episodes of SSTIs in an individual or within a family, and carriers with altered immune systems (e.g., immunodeficiencies, white cell dysfunction, slow healing states such as diabetes or chronic steroid use).

Although acquisition of CA-MRSA carriage or infection cannot be totally prevented, risks are decreased by adherence to hand hygiene and prompt cleansing of skin abrasions. Obviously further spread of MRSA can also be limited by rapid initiation of appropriate therapy for these infections.

PEARLS

- Even if a SA sample is sensitive to rifampin, this antibiotic should never be used as monotherapy.
- Bacterial cultures are essential to identify staphylococcal isolates as MRSA.
- Consider risk factors upon admission, as this will help facilitate infection control measures if MRSA is suspected.
- Knowledge of local antibiotic resistance patterns for both HA-MRSA and CA-MRSA is an important guide to the initial choice of antibiotics.

Suggested Readings

Daum R. A novel methicillin-resistance cassette in community-acquired methicillin-resistant *Staphylococcus aureus* isolates of diverse genetic backgrounds. *J Infect Dis* 2002;186:1344–1347.

Fiebelkorn KR, Crawford SA, McElmeel ML, et al. Practical disk diffusion method for detection of inducible clindamycin resistance in *Staphylococcus aureus* and coagulase-negative staphylocci. *J Clin Microbiol* 2003;41:4740–4744.

Jain A, Daum R. Staphylococcal infections in children. Part 1. *Pediatr Rev* 1999;20:183–191.

Jain A, Daum R. Staphylococcal infections in children. Part 3. *Pediatr Rev* 1999; 20:261–265.

Jain A, Ben-Ami T, Daum R. Staphylococcal infections in children. Part 2. *Pediatr Rev* 1999;20:219–227.

Muto C, Jernigan J, Ostrowsky B, et al. SHEA guideline for preventing nosocomial transmission of multidrug-resistant strains of *Staphylococcus aureus* and *Enterococcus*. *Infect Control Hosp Epidemiol* 2003;24:362–386.

CHAPTER 94 ■ PEDIATRIC FUNGAL INFECTIONS

DONALD L. JANNER

Fungal infections are a common part of pediatric practice but fortunately an uncommon cause of serious disease in most otherwise healthy children. Endemic and nosocomially acquired fungi continue to cause a small but significant morbidity in healthy children and substantial mortality in children with underlying conditions, particularly immunocompromise. *Candida* species are currently the third most common nosocomial bloodstream isolates, trailing only coagulase-negative staphylococci and *Staphylococcus aureus*. Other fungal pathogens, such as *Aspergillus*, are far less common, but infection with these organisms in the compromised host have significant morbidity and mortality. The last several years have seen a dramatic increase in the number of infecting fungal species and the approval of a number of new antifungal agents. Although an in-depth discussion of all of the issues relevant to pediatric fungal disease is beyond the scope of this chapter, general information on several common fungi and the clinical situations where the hospitalist pediatrician should consider them in the differential diagnosis is appropriate.

Terminology can be confusing when discussing fungal infection. Fungi can be divided into two groups based on morphology: yeast and molds. Yeasts are unicellular structures, which reproduce by budding and usually represent *Candida* species. Molds are typically multicellular and are composed of tubular structures (hyphae) that grow by branching. Typical molds include *Aspergillus* and *Zygomycetes*. Some fungi can grow as either yeasts or molds and are termed dimorphic. Dimorphic fungi can be important human pathogens, including *Histoplasma*, *Coccidioides*, *Sporothrix* and others.

Further complicating the diagnosis of true fungal infection is the issue regarding colonization versus true infection. This is particularly true for *Candida* species, especially if the isolate is obtained from a mucosal surface that is normally colonized. Invasive fungal disease often begins with the initial colonization of high-risk patients, including those undergoing immunosuppression, chemotherapy, and/or with in-dwelling catheters, followed by tissue invasion heralding true infection.

ENDEMIC FUNGI

Each region of the world has a fungus more commonly found in the soil and environment. In the United States, *Histoplasma capsulatum* is found in the Mississippi, Missouri, and Ohio River valleys, while *Blastomyces dermatitidis* and *Coccidioides immitis* are found in the southeast and southwest regions, respectively. Most of these infections do not cause symptomatic disease, but when disease does develop, each fungal infection has some characteristics that may help to differentiate the infection from other more common bacterial or viral infections. Travel to or residence in an endemic area should raise suspicion about fungal disease, especially if the patient has not been responding to antimicrobials directed at the more common cause for their clinical presentation.

Blastomyces dermatitidis

Blastomyces dermatitidis is an endemic mold found in the soil of southeastern region and midwestern states bordering the Great Lakes. Cases are usually sporadic but clusters have been documented around exposure to building and excavation sites or during prolonged dry periods, presumably due to the increased numbers of aerosolized spores. Infection occurs when the spores are inhaled and may produce asymptomatic infection, or acute, chronic, or fulminant disease. Clinical manifestations include pulmonary, dermatologic, and disseminated signs and symptoms that may be confused with a variety of other diseases. Pulmonary disease is the most common presentation. The primary care and hospitalist practitioners need to be aware of the potential for fungal pneumonia caused by this agent, because often the patient is diagnosed and treated for community-acquired pneumonia without response. Respiratory secretions (sputum, tracheal aspirates, and BAL samples) may reveal the characteristic double-walled "figure-eight" shaped, broad-based yeast forms. Serology is unhelpful. Amphotericin B is the drug of choice for serious infections, but the azoles (especially itraconazole) have been used successfully for mild illnesses and to complete oral therapy for moderate and severe illnesses initially treated with IV amphotericin.

Coccidiodes immitis

Coccidiodes immitis is the endemic mold found in the soil of the desert southwestern region of the United States and parts of Mexico, Central America, and South America. Progressive or invasive disease is present in fewer than 1% of cases. Severe disease often occurs in patients with a severe underlying T-cell deficiency (e.g., malignancy, or advanced human immunodeficiency virus infection), but may also be seen in normal children.

Progressive pulmonary disease can manifest as a diffuse miliary pneumonia, progressive pulmonary nodules, or cavitary disease. Dissemination of the disease often presents with fever, skin nodules, bone lesions, and/or lymphocytic meningitis. Large cavities or nodules can be diagnosed by biopsy where one sees the characteristic spherules. Disseminated disease is often diagnosed by complement fixation antibodies in the serum and cerebrospinal fluid. Although rare, immune-like illnesses consisting of rashes (e.g., erythema multiforme or erythema nodosum), with or without arthralgias, may also be seen.

Pulmonary disease is often treated with surgical resection and fluconazole. Nonmeningeal disseminated disease is treated with fluconazole until the complement fixation antibody titers decrease. Meningitis is an entity felt to require indefinite therapy.

Histoplasma capsulatum

Histoplasma capsulatum is the fungus endemic to the large central river valleys of the United States (Mississippi, Missouri, and Ohio), but is also found in other parts of the world, particularly Latin America. The organism thrives in moist soil, especially soil enriched by bird or bat droppings. Exposure to the aerosolized spores can occur from a variety of outdoor activities, including gardening, playing in barns, hollow trees, and caves or contact with dust from building, excavation, or cleaning of old buildings. Infection is most often asymptomatic. Clinically apparent disease, when present, may be classified by site (pulmonary, extrapulmonary, or disseminated), by duration of disease (acute or chronic), and by pattern (primary or reactivation). Acute pulmonary disease is the most common syndrome among symptomatic patients. A wide spectrum of symptoms may be seen ranging from an acute influenza-like illness with fever and mild infiltrates on chest radiographs to a severe prolonged respiratory illness with weight loss, fatigue, and diffuse nodular infiltrates on chest radiograph. Other syndromes, including progressive disseminated histoplasmosis (PDH), are less common. An unusual syndrome involving dense fibrosis of the mediastinal structures can lead to compression of the major blood vessels, esophagus, or tracheobronchial tree; this syndrome does not respond to antifungal therapy. Erythema nodosum may be seen in adolescents with acute histoplasmosis.

Diagnosis is based upon serologic tests (complement fixation), culture, and enzyme-linked immunosorbent assay (EIA) for histoplasmin antigen in the urine. The histoplasmin skin test is not useful and may cause a false-positive reaction with complement fixation antibody testing. Serology is generally positive within 4 to 6 weeks of infection and does not return to negative for 12 to 18 months. Cross-reacting antibodies may develop in both *Blastomyces* and *Coccidioides* infections, making interpretation more difficult in well-traveled children. Culture of clinical samples may take several weeks. Urinary histoplasma antigen is often positive in children with PDH syndrome and may help in immunocompromised patients who will not mount a detectable antibody response to their infection.

Treatment is rarely required in children with primary uncomplicated histoplasmosis. Progressive disseminated histoplasmosis in immunocompromised children and in otherwise healthy children should be treated with antifungal therapy. Amphotericin B is the recommended initial treatment for complicated disease, followed by oral itraconazole after clinical improvement.

FUNGAL INFECTION IN CHILDREN WITH COMPLEX MEDICAL CONDITIONS

Physicians caring for hospitalized children are increasingly confronted by children with complex chronic conditions. These patients often have underlining malignant, autoimmune, or immunodeficiency disorders requiring aggressive chemotherapy, need for long-term in-dwelling catheters, and prolonged courses of antibiotics. All of these are risk factors for invasive fungal disease (Table 94.1).

There is no consensus on when to start antifungal therapy in a patient with a positive culture from a colonization site (such as the nasopharynx or an endotracheal tube) and negative blood cultures. Various investigators have considered the following to be risk factors for the colonized patient to develop invasive disease: number of sites colonized, species of *Candida* (particularly *Candida tropicalis*), and previous gastrointestinal surgery. Often an evolving clinical context is used to decide management. The presence of negative blood cultures in the context of clinical and laboratory signs of deterioration, such as leukocytosis, increased ventilatory support, and increasing pulmonary infiltrates, should lead to consideration for empiric antifungal therapy.

The question of what antifungal agent to begin empirically while awaiting identification of the *Candida* species has not been fully resolved. In hospitals where *Candida albicans* is predominantly fluconazole sensitive, clinicians will often start this agent (Table 94.2). In cases where the patient has a history of

TABLE 94.1

RISK FACTORS AND TREATMENT OF SELECTED FUNGAL DISEASES IN PEDIATRICS

Species	Underlying conditions	Treatment
Candida species	Prolonged antibiotic use; catheter use; immunosuppression; disruption of mucosal surfaces, malnutrition	Fluconazole with the exception of *C. krusei* and *T. glabrata*
Aspergillosis	Quantitative or qualitative neutropenia	Amphotericin preparations Voriconazole Consider excision of large pulmonary masses
Fusarium species	Prolonged neutropenia, bone marrow transplantation	Complete surgical excision Voriconazole Amphotericin
Zygomycosis (*Rhizopus, Mucor, Absidia*)	Prolonged neutropenia, diabetes, malnutrition	Complete surgical excision Amphotericin Resistant to other azoles
Trichosporon asahii	Neonates	(Reported resistance to amphotericin) Fluconazole Voriconazole

TABLE 94.2

PATTERNS OF SUSCEPTIBILITY TO ANTIFUNGAL AGENTS AMONG SELECTED FUNGAL PATHOGENS

Fluconazole sensitive	Fluconazole (dose-dependent)	Fluconazole resistant	Amphotericin resistant	Voriconazole resistant
C. albicans	C. glabrata	C. kruseii	Aspergillus terreus	Zygomycetes
C. parapsilosis		Aspergillus	Fusarium spp.	
C. tropicalis		Zygomycetes	Scedosporium	
			C. lusitaniae	
			Trichosporon asahii	

prolonged fluconazole use or the hospital has a high prevalence of more resistant *Candida* species (e.g., *C. glabrata* or *C. kruseii*), fluconazole should be avoided and amphotericin, voriconazole, or caspofungin substituted.

Empiric antifungal therapy is an established part of clinical practice in the case of a *febrile neutropenic patient*. Patients with fever and neutropenia who have invasive fungal disease usually have negative blood cultures. Autopsy results from cancer patients in the 1980s found that a significant number of profoundly neutropenic patients who had persistent fever and negative blood cultures had disseminated mold infections on postmortem examination. It is for this reason that febrile, neutropenic patients with negative blood cultures often receive antifungal therapy if fever persists after 3 to 7 days on broad-spectrum antibiotics. On the other hand, choosing empiric treatment in the febrile, neutropenic patient who is growing a "mold" in culture from skin, lungs, or other tissues can be difficult. These patients can be infected with *Aspergillus*, *Fusarium*, or *Zygomycetes* and the identification of the correct fungus from culture may be delayed. Amphotericin B will treat aspergillosis but lacks activity against *Zygomycetes*. Studies have shown that predictors of *Zygomycetes* in the febrile neutropenic patient include multiple pulmonary nodules, the presence of a pleural infusion, and a history of voriconazole prophylaxis. This reemphasizes the need for biopsy and culture conformation of invasive mold species in this patient population.

NOSOCOMIAL FUNGAL DISEASE

Candidemia

Candida species is the most common cause of nosocomial fungal bloodstream infection. In the past, *C. albicans* was the most commonly isolated *Candida* species. Recently, there has been a dramatic shift: *C. albicans* currently comprises only 50% of bloodstream fungal isolates with increasing isolation of non-albicans species (e.g., *C. glabrata*, *C. parapsilosis*, and *C. tropicalis*). Duration of treatment for *Candida* bacteremia remains an area of great debate with no consensus even among infectious disease specialists. Most authorities feel a minimum of 14 days since the last positive blood culture is needed; many recommend 4 to 6 weeks of therapy to treat potential microabscesses formed during the fungemic episode. Some studies have addressed the issue of treatment duration, mostly in the neonatal population. In neonates with candidemia, 14 days of antifungal therapy was effective if (1) the blood culture was quickly sterilized, (2) there was prompt removal of an infected catheter, and (3) there was a negative workup for signs of dissemination (negative fundoscopic exam, abdominal ultrasound, and echocardiogram). Most patients in the studies had only 2 to 3 days of

fungemia and this may have been a factor in the success of shorter therapy. Patients with prolonged fungemia are candidates for longer treatment, usually in the range of 4 to 6 weeks.

Catheter infections with *Candida* pose several problems for the clinician (see Chapter 95). Fungal catheter infections do not respond well to medical management alone and require removal of the catheter. Infected catheters develop a biofilm in which the pathogens reside; fungi present in a biofilm of a catheter have an increase in their minimum inhibitory concentrations (MICs) to antifungal agents so that achievable blood levels of an antifungal cannot inhibit or kill the yeast. A patient with a positive blood culture for fungus from a catheter should also have peripheral cultures. The positive central catheter culture with a negative peripheral culture is good evidence of a catheter related infection. Persistence of positive cultures on appropriate therapy is also evidence of catheter infection and strongly suggests the need for catheter removal and investigation for more widely disseminated infection.

Candiduria

The hospitalist physician will often be confronted by a positive urine culture for *Candida*. The finding of candiduria can mean bladder colonization, cystitis, or fungal pyelonephritis. The major problem is that unlike bacterial infection (where >100,000 cfu/mL correlates with infection), no standard quantitative culture breakpoint exists for the diagnosis of fungal urinary tract infection. Attempts to achieve a quantitative cut-off have proven elusive. Studies have shown biopsy-proven renal disease with as few as 10^4 colonies/mL of urine, while greater than 10^6 colonies /mL of urine can correlate with simple colonization. Pyuria also does not correlate with fungal infections, especially in patients with indwelling catheters.

Management of candiduria should be individualized, keeping in mind the presence of catheters (which should be removed whenever possible), host factors, and the presence of symptoms. Patients with renal transplantation, anatomic abnormalities, premature infants, or patients with radiographic evidence of renal fungal disease should be treated.

Aspergillus

The classic mold infecting oncology patients is *Aspergillus*. The major risk factor remains quantitative and qualitative neutropenia. Spores are inhaled and infection usually begins in a sinus or the respiratory tract; dissemination to skin and brain often follows. Hyphae of *Aspergillus* species are typically septated and branch at acute (<90°) angles. This can aid in diagnosis when mold is seen on biopsy specimens. Blood cultures usually remain negative despite continuing fever and dissemination. This is the main reason why neutropenic patients who remain febrile after 3 to 7 days of broad-spectrum antibiotics also receive empiric antifungal therapy.

Other Molds

Zygomycetes, Fusarium, Scedosporium, and *Trichosporon* species may all be found in hospitalized children. These are often difficult to diagnose and more difficult to treat due to resistance of the organisms and poor general health of the host (e.g., neonates, oncology patients). For any unusual fungal isolate or questionable clinical situation, consultation with a pediatric infectious disease specialist may be helpful.

DIAGNOSIS OF FUNGAL DISEASE

Culture

Diagnosis of fungi and mold is traditionally made by isolation in culture media. Most species can be recovered after several days of culture on routine media (blood agar, chocolate agar). The specific fungal culture media (Sabouraud dextrose agar) may offer some advantage although the incubation time is longer. Specific "fungal culture" should be ordered when the clinical picture suggests a high likelihood of fungal disease. *Candida* spp. are the exception to this, as they readily grow on blood agar within a few days.

Radiographic Diagnosis of Invasive Fungal Disease

Because of the soil-based nature of molds, a major site for primary infection with mold is the respiratory tract in a vulnerable host. Infected patients frequently present with progressive pneumonia that can take a variety of forms. High-resolution thoracic computed tomography is the best study to characterize invasive fungal pneumonia. Radiographic findings can include cavities, nodular masses (single or multiple), and/or segmental and lobe consolidation (Fig. 94.1). A classical early sign described in invasive pulmonary aspergillosis is the "hypodense" sign, felt to be caused by vascular obstruction with secondary lung infarction and sequestration in invasive pulmonary aspergillosis. Lesions appear as a round, consolidated inflammatory reaction with the central lesion of less density. Over time it is felt that these "hypodense" lesions will progress to cavitation. In the correct clinical setting, these findings

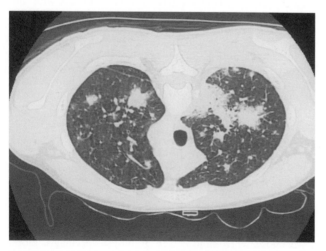

FIGURE 94.1. Computed tomography showing numerous aspergillosis nodules in a patient with chronic granulomatous disease.

should warrant consideration of empiric therapy and aggressive diagnostic measures. Studies have shown that patients with computed tomography consistent with aspergillosis pneumonia have a high yield of mold isolation on bronchoalveolar lavage (BAL). Open lung biopsy is another diagnostic option, especially if BAL is negative. Because of the heterogenous nature of molds seen in the immunocompromised host, "tissue is the issue" is a phrase repeated by infectious disease specialists to emphasize the need for definitive culture identification.

ANTIFUNGAL AGENTS USED IN INVASIVE DISEASE

Amphotericin

The "standard" antifungal agent has been amphotericin B; the traditional form has been amphotericin B deoxycholate, given at a dose of 0.6 to 1.0 mg/kg per day. Amphotericin B acts by binding to ergosterol, a cell wall membrane protein of most fungi. Binding leads to ion channel formation and cell death. There are now three lipid-associated formulations of amphotericin B: amphotericin B lipid complex (Abelcet), amphotericin colloidal dispersion (Amphotec), and liposomal amphotericin B (AmBisome). There is still no concrete proof that these newer formulations are better antifungal agents, but there is some evidence that they may decrease metabolic or renal complications. Studies have found that standard amphotericin B and the lipid formulations had equivalent efficacy, with some suggestion that the liposomal forms of amphotericin B had slightly less nephrotoxicity. Clinicians often use the lipid preparations of amphotericin B as initial therapy in children at higher risk for nephrotoxicity or electrolyte imbalance. It is important to realize that the dosing of these lipid formulations is different, at 3 to 5 mg/kg/day.

Major side effects of amphotericin B are infusion-related problems and nephrotoxicity. Reactions during parenteral administration include fever, chills, and headaches, thought to be related to release of cytokines. These reactions can often be successfully addressed by reducing the infusion rate or by premedication with acetaminophen and/or hydrocortisone.

Nephrotoxicity becomes apparent by potassium and magnesium wasting or azotemia. Azotemia can be worsened if the patient is treated with other nephrotoxic drugs. Many investigators advocate normal saline loading 10 to 15 mL mg/kg/dose to reduce risk of nephrotoxicity. Amphotericin B has activity against most *Candida* species, with *C. lusitaniae* being the major exception. It is active against aspergillosis, but lacks efficacy against *Fusarium* and *Pseudallescheria boydii*.

Azoles

The azoles, like amphotericin B, target ergosterol biosynthesis by inhibiting cytochrome P-450 dependent enzymes. Fluconazole (Diflucan) and itraconazole (Sporanox) are the azoles most frequently used.

Fluconazole

Fluconazole is available in either oral or intravenous form. The oral form of fluconazole is 90% bioavailable and achieves excellent levels even in the cerebrospinal fluid. Fluconazole clearance is more rapid in younger patients compared to adults. For children older than 3 months, the dose is 6 to 12 mg/kg/day in two divided doses. Neonates should be treated with a higher dose to compensate for their increased volume of distribution; however the interval of dosing needs to be increased because of slower elimination. For the first 2 weeks of life, fluconazole should be dosed every 72 hours; in the next 2 weeks of life, the interval is every 48 hours.

Itraconazole is fungicidal and has been in clinical use for over a decade. It is available in intravenous and oral form (suspension and capsule). The capsule form of itraconazole has erratic absorption and levels should be followed. Capsules should be taken with food while suspension needs to be given on an empty stomach. Suspension and capsules are not interchangeable and dosing needs to be specific for the oral form given.

Fluconazole and itraconazole are active against *Candida* species and coccidioidomycosis; fluconazole has less activity against *C. glabrata* and none against *C. kruseii*. Itraconazole does have activity against aspergillosis and sporotrichosis. Because of minimal data on itraconazole in candidemia, itraconazole is not considered a first-line agent for this condition. It is often used as maintenance therapy in patients with aspergillosis or coccidiomycosis. Itraconazole is frequently used as a prophylactic agent in vulnerable patients such as those with chronic granulomatous disease.

Voriconazole

Voriconazole, a recently approved second-generation triazole, is a fungicidal drug active in vitro against *Candida* species, including *C. kruseii* and *C. glabrata*. Unlike fluconazole, it has excellent activity against molds, including *Fusarium* and *Aspergillus*. The one major gap in the activity of voriconazole is resistance of the *Zygomycosis* species, the species that causes mucormycosis.

Voriconazole is available in the oral form with a bioavailability reported to be greater then 90%. Reports have cited a wide patient-to-patient absorption level, and long-term voriconazole use should be followed with blood levels. Administration with food, especially high-fat meals, reduces the absorption of oral voriconazole. Dosages of 4 mg/kg have been found to be needed in children to achieve levels consistent with adults receiving dosage of 3 mg/kg. One noted side effect of this drug is visual changes (30%), including transient blurred vision, and increased brightness. Photosensitivity, which causes erythematous and/or desquamative skin eruptions, has also been reported.

It should be noted that the intravenous and oral forms of voriconazole are excreted by different mechanisms. The oral form is excreted largely by the hepatic system, while the intravenous form is excreted renally; this should be kept in mind when dosing particular patients with various forms of voriconazole.

Caspofungin (Candicidas)

Caspofungin represents the first drug in a new class of antifungals called the echinocandins. This drug inhibits the synthesis of a separate enzyme, preventing the formation of a critical element in the fungal cell wall. This unique mechanism of action differs from two ergosterol pathways of amphotericin and azole preparations. It is available only as an intravenous medication.

Caspofungin is considered fungicidal and has good in vitro activity against all *Candida* species. It is also considered second-line therapy for refractory Aspergillosis.

Caspofungin does not have any activity against *Trichosporon* species. In addition, it has been noted the caspofungin MICs are higher for *C. parapsilosis* than other species of *Candida*, raising some concern for the use of this agent for this particular species.

FUNGAL SUSCEPTIBILITY TESTING

The role of routine fungal susceptibility testing is debated. Many clinical laboratories do not have the capability to do fungal testing and must send fungal isolates to a specialty

TABLE 94.3

ANTIFUNGAL DRUGS USED FOR TREATMENT OF INVASIVE FUNGAL DISEASE

Drug	Route	Dose
Amphotericin B deoxycholate	IV	0.6–1.0 mg/kg/day
Lipid amphotericin complex (Abelcet)	IV	3.0–5.0 mg/kg/day
Liposomal amphotericin (Ambisome)	IV	3.0–5.0 mg/kg/day
Caspofungin (Cancidas)	IV	Children: 50 mg/m^2/day Neonates: 1 mg/kg/day, × 2 days, then 2 mg/kg/day
Fluconazole	IV, PO	2 weeks: 6 mg/kg q72hr First month: 6 mg/kg q48hr Children: q 6–12 mg/kg q12hr PO: similar dosing to intravenous
Itraconazole	IV, PO	2.5–5.0 mg/kg/day divided b.i.d. PO: oral solution, 6 mo–12 yr: 5 mg/kg/day; capsules, 3–16 yr: 100 mg/day
Voriconazole	IV	Children: 6 mg/kg/day q12hr for the first 24 hr, then 4–5 mg/kg/day q12hr Infants: 8 mg/kg/day q12hr Excreted renally PO: <40 kg: 200 mg q12hr, then 200–300 mg q12hr; >40 kg: 200 mg q12hr, then 150 mg q12hr Intrahepatic metabolism

laboratory for susceptibility. Physicians should be aware of the *Candida* species present within their hospitals; sensitivity testing should be performed in the case of an unusual *Candida* species, an unusual fungal isolate, or for recurrent or persistent fungal disease despite therapy. Questions regarding treatment and susceptibility testing should be directed to a pediatric infectious disease specialist.

COMBINATION ANTIFUNGAL THERAPY

The introduction of the new classes of antifungal drugs has naturally lead to the evaluation of whether drugs used in combination offer an advantage over single-drug treatment, because some of these agents act with distinctly different mechanisms against pathogenic mold. This remains the subject of much controversy, as the azoles inhibit ergosterol formation, which could then limit the site of action against concurrently given amphotericin B. In fact, antagonism has been shown in vitro with certain azoles and amphotericin B. It is likely that in coming years further clinical studies will bring further recommendations regarding the use of combination therapy, particularly combinations using caspofungin.

SUMMARY

Serious fungal diseases are uncommon in pediatric practice, but with the increased survivorship of high-risk children, the number of fungal infections has increased in the past 2 decades. Pediatricians caring for hospitalized children need to be aware of the endemic fungi of their regions and the clinical characteristics of those diseases as well as familiarity with the patterns of more common fungal pathogens at their institutions (such as *Candida*). The ability to successfully treat fungal infections has improved with the development of new antifungal drugs (Table 94.3). Unusual isolates, persistent symptoms without clinical response, or complex issues of drug interactions and combination therapies should be referred to a pediatric infectious disease specialist.

PEARLS

- Fungal infections are of increasing importance, especially in children with risk factors.
- Deciding if a fungal culture represents true disease versus colonization may require input from a pediatric infectious disease specialist. When in doubt, first initiate treatment, and then resolve the question.
- Fungal infections are not restricted to immunocompromised children; endemic and colonizing fungi can and do cause disease in otherwise healthy children without underlying risk factors.

Suggested Readings

Bille J, Marchetti O, Calandra T. Changing face of health-care associated fungal infections. *Curr Opin Infect Dis* 2005;18:314–319.

Pappas PG, Rex JH, Sobel JD, et al. Guidelines treatment of candidiasis. *Clin Infect Dis* 2004;38:161–189.

Pfaller MA, Diekema DJ. Unusual fungal and pseuodofungal infections of humans. *J Clin Microbiol* 2005;43:1495–1504.

Spellberg BJ, Filler SG, Edwards JE. Current treatment strategies for disseminated candidiasis. *Clin Infect Dis* 2006;42:244–251.

Steinbach WJ. Antifungal agents in children. *Pediatr Clin North Am* 2005;52:895–915.

CHAPTER 95 ■ DEVICE-RELATED INFECTIONS

SAMIR S. SHAH

Medical devices such as central venous catheters (CVCs) and cerebrospinal fluid (CSF) shunts are commonly used in children. These devices increase the risk of infection by providing a portal of entry for organisms to migrate from the skin and mucous membranes to sterile body sites, and by creating a site relatively sequestered from immune system surveillance that allows bacteria to flourish unperturbed (i.e., within a foreign body). This chapter will discuss infections associated with CVCs and CSF shunts.

CENTRAL VENOUS CATHETER–ASSOCIATED INFECTIONS

CVCs are commonly used to deliver parenteral nutrition, chemotherapy, and antimicrobial agents in both the hospital and home-care settings. The presence of a CVC poses a significant risk of infection; up to 50% of children with a CVC develop a CVC-associated infection. CVC-associated infections include exit site infections, tunnel infections, pocket infections, and CVC-associated bloodstream infections (CVC-BSI). CVC-associated infections occur when bacteria gain access to the extraluminal or intraluminal surface of the device. This may occur by bacterial migration at the catheter insertion/exit site, bacterial colonization of the catheter hub, secondary seeding of the catheter following non-catheter-associated bacteremia, and bacterial contamination of fluid administered through the device. Infection rates depend on a variety of host, catheter, and environmental factors (Table 95.1). In adults, antibiotic-impregnated CVCs (e.g., minocycline, rifampin) are associated with a lower risk of CVC infection. Few data on the use of antibiotic-impregnated catheters in children are available.

Coagulase-negative staphylococci account for 40% to 50% of all isolates. Gram-negative aerobic bacilli comprise 25% of all isolates. Commonly encountered gram-negative bacilli include *Escherichia coli*, *Enterobacter* species, *Pseudomonas aeruginosa*, *Klebsiella* species, *Serratia marcescens*, and *Acinetobacter* species. Other causes include *Staphylococcus aureus*, *Enterococcus faecium*, *Enterococcus faecalis*, *Candida* species, and rapidly growing mycobacteria. Rapidly growing mycobacteria are non-tuberculous mycobacteria that produce mature growth on agar plates within 7 days rather than the weeks required for other groups of mycobacteria. The most common rapidly growing mycobacteria isolated from clinical specimens include *M. fortuitum*, *M. abscessus*, and *M. chelonae*. Isolation of less common organisms should prompt consideration of contaminated environmental water (e.g., *Burkholderia cepacia*, *Citrobacter* species, *Pseudomonas fluorescens-putida*) or conta-minated infusate (e.g., *Malassezia furfur*, mycobacteria) as the source of these pathogens.

Clinical Findings

Clinical manifestations depend on the type and location of the CVC. Fever can occur with any CVC-associated infection. *Exit site infections* are associated with erythema, induration, tenderness, or purulent discharge within 2 cm of the catheter exit site. *Tunnel infections* are associated with erythema, induration, or tenderness along the track of a tunneled catheter and more than 2 cm from the catheter exit site. *Pocket infections* manifest with purulent fluid in the subcutaneous pocket of a totally implanted venous access device. Findings in a pocket infection may include overlying tenderness, erythema, induration, visible drainage, and skin necrosis. *CVC-BSI* may manifest with fever alone or with signs and symptoms of sepsis. Catheter malfunction can be the initial presentation of CVC-BSI; thrombi and fibrin deposits on the CVC impair blood flow through the catheter and serve as a nidus for microbial colonization and subsequent infection.

Management

Blood should be obtained for culture from both the catheter and a peripheral vein in any patient with a suspected CVC-associated infection. Multiple cultures (at least two), each containing ≥ 1 mL of blood, permit detection of most clinically relevant BSIs. However, identifying the catheter as the source of a BSI can be challenging, because patients with CVCs may also develop a BSI attributable to another source (e.g., pneumonia with concurrent bacteremia). The differential time to blood culture positivity provides the most commonly used method to determine whether the catheter is the primary source of infection. Blood cultures of equal volume are drawn from the catheter and the peripheral vein within several minutes of each other. A CVC-BSI is diagnosed if the CVC culture grows 2 or more hours earlier than the peripheral blood culture.

Distinguishing between "true" BSIs and contaminated cultures can be difficult when skin flora such as coagulase-negative staphylococci (CoNS) or *Bacillus* species are isolated from culture. A study using a mathematical model of blood cultures positive for CoNS in patients with a CVC found that cultures from multiple sites facilitated interpretation of CoNS isolates. If one of two cultures was positive for CoNS, the positive predictive value (PPV) for true BSI was 20%. If both cultures were positive, the PPV was 96% if one sample was from the CVC and the other was from venipuncture. But the PPV was only 50% if both were obtained through the CVC. Other tests to consider include a complete blood count to detect anemia and

TABLE 95.1

RISK FACTORS FOR CENTRAL VENOUS CATHETER–ASSOCIATED INFECTIONS

HOST FACTORS
Immunosuppressive chemotherapy
Neutropenia
Active infection at another site
Loss of skin integrity (e.g., burns, prematurity)
Alteration of cutaneous microflora

CATHETER FACTORS
Catheter location (central > peripheral; jugular > femoral > subclavian; lower extremity > upper extremity)
Catheter type (nontunneled > tunneled > totally implanted; multiple lumens > single lumen)
Catheter care (betadine preparation > chlorhexidine preparation; frequent entries into catheter system)

ENVIRONMENTAL FACTORS
Lower nurse-to-patient ratio
Poor health care worker hand hygiene
Contaminated or multiuse topical ointments

thrombocytopenia, prothrombin and partial thromboplastin times to detect coagulopathy, and serum lactate to detect ineffective arterial circulation.

Empiric antibiotic therapy should include two agents, one with activity against gram-positive bacteria and one effective against gram-negative bacteria. Vancomycin is used empirically for gram-positive coverage at many centers given the high prevalence of methicillin-resistance among CoNS (approximately 70% are resistant) and the increasing prevalence of methicillin-resistant *S. aureus*. Options for gram-negative coverage include aminoglycosides (e.g., gentamicin, amikacin, tobramycin) and anti-pseudomonal beta-lactam agents (e.g., ceftazidime, cefepime, piperacillin-tazobactam, meropenem, imipenem). The empiric use of both an aminoglycoside and an anti-pseudomonal beta-lactam agent (with an agent for gram-positive coverage) may be appropriate in severely ill patients or when there is concern for infection with resistant gram-negative bacteria. Fluoroquinolones (e.g., ciprofloxacin, moxifloxacin) are commonly used in adults but have been approved for only limited indications in children; these agents should be considered when the use of other agents is limited by patient allergies or by antibiotic susceptibility patterns of the infecting organism.

Patients with *Candida* spp. infections should receive amphotericin B; a lipid-based preparation is preferred at some centers due to the less frequent occurrence of infusion reactions and nephrotoxicity compared with the "conventional" (deoxycholate) preparation. Fluconazole may be used for certain *Candida* species (e.g., *C. albicans*, *C. parapsilosis*). Caspofungin, an echinocandin class antifungal agent, exhibits rapid fungicidal activity against most *Candida* species. Caspofungin may be used more often if its efficacy against *Candida* species BSIs in children is proven to parallel the results in adults. Clinical trials of caspofungin involving children are currently in progress. Therapy should be modified based on the patient's clinical response and the organism's antibiotic susceptibility patterns. The therapeutic implications of commonly isolated bacteria are shown in Table 95.2.

TABLE 95.2

THERAPEUTIC IMPLICATIONS OF SPECIFIC BACTERIA CAUSING CENTRAL VENOUS CATHETER–ASSOCIATED INFECTIONS[a]

Organism	Therapeutic implications
Coagulase-negative staphylococci	Vancomycin is the drug of choice for empiric therapy; but oxacillin is appropriate for susceptible isolates. Consider addition of rifampin or linezolid for persistently positive cultures if catheter cannot be removed.
Methicillin-susceptible *Staphylococcus aureus*	Oxacillin superior to vancomycin.
Methicillin-resistant *Staphylococcus aureus*	Vancomycin is drug of choice for children. Alternate therapy: linezolid or quinupristin–dalfopristin.
Enterococcus species	Ampicillin (monotherapy) is drug of choice for susceptible isolates. Enterococcal susceptibility patterns for ampicillin are usually concordant with imipenem and piperacillin–tazobactam; therefore, these antibiotics can be substituted for ampicillin in situations where broader-spectrum coverage is required. Add gentamicin in cases of suspected endocarditis. Alternate regimens: linezolid or quinupristin-dalfopristin.
Escherichia coli or *Klebsiella* species	Monotherapy with beta-lactam agents is appropriate for susceptible isolates. Extended-spectrum beta-lactamase producing isolates may warrant carbapenem therapy.
Pseudomonas aeruginosa	Although data supporting monotherapy have emerged, combination therapy remains the standard for serious *P. aeruginosa* infections. Empiric therapy: aminoglycoside plus cefepime, piperacillin–tazobactam, imipenem, meropenem, or ceftazidime.
Candida species	*C. lusitaniae* is resistant to amphotericin B. *C. kruzei* and *C. glabrata* are often resistant to fluconazole.
Rapidly growing mycobacteria	Empiric therapy: clarithromycin plus amikacin. Other antibiotics with activity against many rapidly growing mycobacteria include imipenem, linezolid, and cefoxitin. Directed therapy depends on specific isolate.

[a]Specific therapy should account for disseminated infection, antibiotic susceptibility pattern of the organism, and host factors that may affect selection of specific antibiotics. Many uses of antibiotics discussed in this table are not included in the Food and Drug Administration product license. Consultation with an infectious disease specialist is suggested.

TABLE 95.3

APPROACH TO THE MANAGEMENT OF UNCOMPLICATED CENTRAL VENOUS CATHETER–ASSOCIATED BLOODSTREAM INFECTIONS

Organism	Duration of therapy[a]	Comments
Coagulase-negative staphylococci	10–14 days	May retain CVC unless clinical deterioration or relapsing bacteremia. If the catheter is removed, duration of therapy can be decreased to 5–7 days.
Staphylococcus aureus	14 days	Remove CVC. If echocardiogram reveals vegetations, treat for 4–6 weeks.
Enterococcus species	10–14 days	Usually treated with vancomycin, ampicillin, or penicillin. Add an aminoglycoside for persistently positive cultures.
Enteric gram-negative rods	10–14 days	Consider CVC removal/replacement for critically ill patient, persistently positive cultures, or clinical deterioration of patient during therapy.
Candida species	14 days	Remove CVC. Ophthalmologic evaluation is necessary following clearance of candidemia. Consider additional evaluation for disseminated infection.
Non-tuberculous mycobacteria	Unclear	Remove catheter. If peripheral blood cultures are positive, patient may require 6 or more weeks of therapy.

[a]Duration of therapy varies depending on presence of complications and specific underlying disease conditions. Optimal duration of therapy has not been established in children. Recommendations are extrapolated from adult data.

Table modified from Dent AR, Schreiber JR. Bloodstream infections. In: Shah SS, ed. *Blueprints pediatric infectious diseases*. Philadelphia: Lippincott Williams & Wilkins; 2005: 161, with permission.

Catheter removal is required in many but not all cases. In adult populations, non-tunneled CVCs are generally removed if the patient has erythema or purulence at the catheter exit site. In children, prompt removal of non-tunneled CVCs may not always be feasible because of limited vascular access sites and potential complications associated with reinsertion; therefore, treatment of exit site infections without removal of non-tunneled CVCs is often attempted. In patients with tunneled CVCs or implantable devices (e.g., ports), tunnel or pocket infections require immediate CVC removal. The decision to remove the catheter is more complicated for CVC-BSIs. Factors that warrant CVC removal include clinical signs of unexplained sepsis, infections caused by *S. aureus*, *Candida* spp., or mycobacteria, and infections associated with endocarditis, septic thrombophlebitis, or disseminated infection.

The duration of therapy depends in part on the pathogen, whether the catheter is removed, and whether infection is complicated by septic thrombosis, endocarditis, osteomyelitis, or other metastatic foci of bacterial infection. The duration of therapy for uncomplicated infections is summarized in Table 95.3. For complicated infections, the duration of therapy is based on the duration necessary to treat the complication. Although intravenous antibiotics are typically used for the entire duration of therapy, certain antibiotics with excellent oral bioavailability (e.g., ciprofloxacin, linezolid, fluconazole) may be considered in patients for whom compliance can be assured if the bacteremia has resolved, the patient has clinically improved, and the CVC has been removed.

Course and Prognosis

Serious complications, including endocarditis and other deep-tissue infections, have been reported in association with *S. aureus* CVC-BSI. Echocardiography should be considered in cases of *S. aureus* BSI in children with congenital heart dis-

ease, persistent bacteremia despite appropriate antimicrobial therapy, or a newly identified heart murmur.

Treatment of fungemia without removal of the catheter has been associated with poor outcomes in children and adults. Failure to promptly remove the catheter may lead to prolonged candidemia, which in turn has been associated with higher rates of disseminated infection. Disseminated infection (especially to the lung, liver, spleen, eye, brain, and heart) occurs in 10% to 20% of cases. The consensus is that catheters should be removed in patients with candidemia, whenever possible. All patients with candidemia should undergo ophthalmologic examination to evaluate for candidal endophthalmitis, preferably after resolution of the candidemia at a time when additional dissemination is unlikely. Therapy for uncomplicated candidemia should be continued for at least 2 weeks following CVC removal, as shorter treatment courses have been associated with recurrence and disseminated infection in some patients.

Pearls/Special Situations

- CVC-BSIs caused by *S. aureus*, *Candida* species, and mycobacteria require prompt catheter removal.
- CVC-BSIs caused by *Candida* species warrant ophthalmologic examination following resolution of candidemia to exclude metastatic infection.

CEREBROSPINAL FLUID SHUNT INFECTIONS

Infections associated with ventricular shunts develop in 5% to 15% of all CSF shunts, and most occur within 6 months of shunt placement. Factors associated with CSF shunt infections include premature birth, young age, neuroendoscope use during shunt insertion, and prior shunt infection. Insertion of a

TABLE 95.4

ETIOLOGY OF CEREBROSPINAL FLUID SHUNT INFECTIONS

COMMON
Coagulase-negative staphylococci
Staphylococcus aureus
Enteric gram-negative bacilli[a]

LESS COMMON
Propionibacterium acnes
Viridans group streptococci

RARE
Other streptococci[b]
Enterococcus spp.
Candida spp.
Corynebacterium spp.

[a]Usually *Escherichia coli, Klebsiella* species, *Pseudomonas aeruginosa,*
and *Proteus* species.
[b]Usually group B *Streptococcus, Streptococcus pyogenes,* or
Streptococcus pneumoniae.

TABLE 95.5

CLINICAL FEATURES ASSOCIATED WITH CEREBROSPINAL FLUID SHUNT INFECTIONS

PROXIMAL INFECTION
Fever
Headache
Malaise
Nausea
Vomiting
Irritability
Lethargy or altered mental status
Seizures
Meningismus
Paresis
Cellulitis overlying shunt reservoir or track

DISTAL INFECTION
Abdominal pain (ventriculoperitoneal shunt)
Peritonitis (ventriculoperitoneal shunt)
Intestinal obstruction (ventriculoperitoneal shunt)
Abdominal mass (pseudocyst; ventriculoperitoneal shunt)
Pleuritis/pleural effusion (ventriculopleural shunt)
Nephritis (ventriculo atrial shunt)
Hypotension/shock

ventricular–peritoneal (VP) shunt in a premature neonate (age <3 months) has been associated with a nearly five fold increase in the risk of shunt infection. Patients <1 year of age at the time of shunt placement also have a substantially higher risk of shunt infection than those older than 1 year. Insertion of a shunt after a previous shunt infection is associated with a four fold increase in the risk of shunt infection.

The etiologic agents associated with CSF shunt infections are shown in Table 95.4. Staphylococcal species account for almost two-thirds of all shunt infections. *Staphylococcus aureus* infections are associated with longer hospital stays at the time of initial shunt insertion and with prior *S. aureus* infection (replacement of a shunt). *Propionibacterium acnes* has been isolated more often in recent series of VP shunt infections, possibly due to the more frequent use of anaerobic culture media and prolonged (up to 7 days) incubation times. *Candida* species should be considered in immunocompromised patients as well as in those patients receiving parenteral nutrition, prolonged corticosteroid, or antibiotic therapy.

There are four common mechanisms of shunt infection: (1) local inoculation of bacteria at the time of surgery; (2) skin breakdown overlying the shunt with subsequent bacterial entry; (3) hematogenous inoculation of the shunt (from bacteremia); and (4) retrograde infection from the distal end of the shunt. The most common mechanism of infection, local inoculation of bacteria at the time of surgery, usually manifests within several weeks of the operation. Bacterial entry following breakdown of skin overlying the shunt may occur if the incision fails to properly heal or if the patient disrupts the healing process by scratching the open wound. Gram-positive bacteria are more likely in this scenario. Children who are relatively immobile, such as those with severe neurologic disability, may develop an overlying decubitus ulcer that permits bacteria direct access to the shunt. Rarely, accessing the shunt by needle puncture introduces colonizing skin bacteria into the shunt system. Children with VP shunts can have bacteremic seeding as a cause of shunt infections, but those with shunts in their vascular system (e.g., ventriculo-atrial shunts) are continually at risk of infection from bacteremia with retrograde spread to the ventricles. Finally, retrograde infection from the distal end of the shunt as a

consequence of viscus (e.g., bowel, gallbladder) perforation may lead to distal catheter contamination. Gram-negative bacteria are most commonly isolated in the context of bowel perforation.

Clinical Findings

The clinical features of CSF shunt infection depend on the mechanism of infection, causative pathogen, and type of shunt. The most common clinical symptoms are fever, headache, nausea, and lethargy (Table 95.5). Shunt malfunction is associated with infection in 20% of cases. Signs of meningitis such as meningismus and photophobia are less common. Children with infections caused by indolent organisms such as *P. acnes* may have an insidious course with few overt symptoms.

Signs and symptoms of distal shunt infection depend on the location of the shunt tip. Abdominal peritoneal pseudocysts can develop as a consequence of clinical or subclinical infections that cause an inflammatory reaction around the catheter tip. The pseudocysts may grow quite large because the CSF encased within the pseudocyst cannot be resorbed by the peritoneal cavity. Pseudocysts complicate VP shunt placement in 0.7% to 4.5% of cases; usually as a late complication, occurring >12 months after initial shunt placement. Small pseudocysts are more likely than large cysts to be associated with infection, presumably because pseudocysts associated with infection cause symptoms earlier than noninfected pseudocysts. Among patients with abdominal pseudocysts, the abdominal symptoms precede central nervous system complaints (e.g., lethargy, headache, and visual disturbances) by several days or weeks. Nephritis in the context of VA shunt infection can be caused by deposition of antibody–antigen complexes in the renal glomeruli. "Shunt nephritis," which can be difficult to distinguish from bacterial endocarditis, occurs in 5% to 15% of VA shunt infections. Rarely, manual compression of the reservoir or catheter track of an infected VA shunt (e.g., with shampooing of hair) can lead to intermittent bacteremia accompanied by fever and chills.

Management

Diagnosis of a CSF shunt infection requires either isolation of a pathogen from ventricular fluid, lumbar CSF, or blood (for VA shunts); or the presence of CSF pleocytosis (usually defined as >50 white blood cells/mm^3 in the context of a CSF shunt); in combination with either shunt malfunction or one or more of the signs or symptoms listed in Table 95.5. Ideally, fluid from the *reservoir* should be obtained by percutaneous aspiration under sterile conditions. Isolation of bacteria from CSF obtained by *lumbar puncture* certainly suggests CSF shunt infection in the appropriate context. However, children requiring a CSF shunt often have impaired CSF flow. As a consequence, the ventricular fluid may have little or no communication with the lumbar spinal fluid; hence, CSF obtained by lumbar puncture may not suggest infection despite the presence of ventriculitis.

The CSF should be sent for Gram stain, aerobic and anaerobic bacterial culture, cell count with differential, protein, and glucose. Although elevated CSF white blood cell counts correlate with the presence of infection, CSF pleocytosis alone is not diagnostic of infection. Pleocytosis may also be caused by postsurgical or foreign body (i.e., shunt)–associated inflammation. Furthermore, infections caused by indolent organisms may fail to induce a vigorous inflammatory response. The types of white blood cells present may also facilitate the diagnosis of infection. CSF neutrophils (>10%) are more common in shunt infections as most patients without shunt infection have very few CSF neutrophils. CSF eosinophilia (>5% of total CSF white blood cell count) has also been associated with both shunt infection and malfunction, but may also occur in response to intrathecal antibiotics or as a reaction to the shunt catheter. A negative Gram stain does not exclude the diagnosis of shunt infection.

Although most bacteria causing shunt infections grow within 48 to 72 hours, cultures should be held for 5 to 7 days because fastidious organisms such as *P. acnes* may take longer to grow. Differentiation of contamination from true infection is difficult when bacteria are identified by culture in the context of normal CSF parameters. In such cases, infection should be strongly considered and shunt aspiration should be repeated; a positive culture with the same bacteria usually indicates true infection.

Bacteremia occurs in <10% of patients with a VP shunt infection but in most patients with VA shunt infection. Therefore, blood should be routinely obtained for culture from patients evaluated for suspected shunt infection. Laboratory manifestations of shunt nephritis include anemia, azotemia, and hypocomplementemia, as well as hematuria and proteinuria. Neuroimaging studies should be performed as part of the routine evaluation of a child with a suspected CSF shunt infection. Neuroimaging studies such as computed tomography may provide evidence of shunt malfunction that accompanies some cases of infection. In rare cases, subdural empyema or brain abscess may be the first indication of shunt infection. Radiologic imaging of other areas should be considered depending on the location of the distal catheter tip. Computed tomography or ultrasound of the abdomen may identify abdominal peritoneal pseudocysts at the distal portion of a VP shunt. Some free fluid in the peritoneal cavities is normal but larger amounts should raise concern for infection. Chest radiography detects pleural effusions associated with ventriculopleural shunt infection.

The child with a ventricular shunt infection should be managed in consultation with neurosurgical and infectious disease specialists. Success rates with various treatment strategies are as follows: IV antibiotics without shunt removal, <25%; IV and intraventricular antibiotics without shunt removal, 40%; IV antibiotics with shunt removal and immediate replacement, 75%; and IV antibiotics with shunt removal and delayed replacement, >90%. Therefore, optimal management of a CSF shunt infection includes IV antibiotics and removal of the shunt with placement of a temporary external ventricular drain (EVD). The EVD facilitates resolution of the ventriculitis and permits continued monitoring of CSF parameters. Infection complicates fewer than 5% of closed external drainage systems; routine changing of the drainage catheter does not appear to reduce the infection rate.

In cases of distal shunt infection, some neurosurgeons prefer to externalize only the distal portion of the shunt. This strategy still maintains CSF flow and still offers the ability to perform frequent ventricular fluid sampling without subjecting the patient to a more extensive surgical procedure. However, early infection of the proximal portion of the shunt may be obscured by antibiotic treatment and become evident only after discontinuation of therapy and reinsertion of the distal portion of the shunt.

Empiric antibiotic therapy should include antibiotics that cover the range of potentially causative pathogens. Reasonable options include vancomycin in combination with ceftazidime, cefepime, or meropenem. In adults with severe vancomycin allergy, there are case reports of using linezolid or quinupristin-dalfopristin to successfully treat VP shunt infections due to CoNS.

Situations that may warrant additional measures include cases of delayed ventricular fluid sterilization (>3 days) and cases where the patient cannot safely undergo surgical catheter removal. First, intraventricular antibiotic administration should be considered. The Food and Drug Administration (FDA) has not approved any antibiotic for intraventricular use. However, commonly used intraventricular antibiotics include vancomycin, gentamicin, tobramycin, and amikacin. Polymixin B and colistin have also been administered directly into the ventricles to treat ventricular shunt infections caused by gram-negative bacteria resistant to many commonly used antibiotics. Penicillin and cephalosporins should *not* be instilled directly into the ventricles because intraventricular administration of these antibiotics has been associated with increased neurotoxicity, including seizures. Second, rifampin has excellent CSF penetration and should be added when the infection is caused by susceptible staphylococci. Third, neuroimaging should be performed to diagnose a concurrent intracranial abscess or empyema. Magnetic resonance imaging is preferred due to its higher sensitivity, but contrast-enhanced computed tomography is sufficient in many cases. Finally, either the trough ventricular antibiotic concentration or the ventricular fluid bactericidal titer should be measured to assess the adequacy of antibiotic therapy. No standardized values exist but many experts agree that the trough antibiotic concentration should exceed the minimum inhibitory concentration of the organism by 10-fold or more. Lower values indicate suboptimal ventricular fluid antibiotic concentrations. Bactericidal titer measurements may not be readily available because they are technically difficult and time-consuming to perform. If no broth turbidity is observed after 24 hours of growth (reflecting failure of bacteria to grow) at a dilution of 1 to 8 or higher (i.e., more dilute), then the ventricular antibiotic concentrations are probably sufficient.

The duration of therapy depends on the organism isolated. Coagulase-negative staphylococcal infections require 5 to 7 days of negative cultures prior to shunt reinsertion, while *S. aureus* and gram-negative infections require longer therapy prior to shunt replacement. If the shunt was not initially removed, therapy should be continued for an even longer period of time though the optimal duration in such cases is not known. Management strategies and duration of therapy are summarized in Table 95.6.

TABLE 95.6

SUMMARY OF MANAGEMENT OF CHILDREN WITH CEREBROSPINAL FLUID SHUNT INFECTIONS

Remove shunt

Place external ventricular drain

Administer empiric antibiotic therapy:
- Vancomycin plus ceftazidime OR
- Vancomycin plus cefepime OR
- Vancomycin plus meropenem

Obtain daily ventricular fluid samples for:
- Gram stain
- Aerobic and anaerobic culture
- Cell count and differential

Replace shunt if ventricular fluid cultures (by organism) are negative for:
- Coagulase-negative staphylococci: 5–7 days
- *Propionibacterium acnes* or streptococci: 7–10 days
- *Staphylococcus aureus*: 10 days
- Enteric gram-negative rods: 14–21 days

Delayed sterilization (positive cultures for >3 days) despite placement of an external ventricular drain, consider:
- Intraventricular antibiotics[a]
- Rifampin (orally administered) in cases of susceptible staphylococci
- Neuroimaging to detect intracranial empyema or abscess
- Ventricular "trough" antibiotic concentrations or ventricular fluid bactericidal titer

[a]Depending on the organism, consider vancomcyin, gentamicin, tobramycin, or amikacin. This is not a Food and Drug Administration–approved indication for these antibiotics.

Course and Prognosis

The mortality associated with ventricular shunt infections is low. Potential morbidity includes new or more frequent seizures and worsening neurologic impairment. Infections caused by *S. aureus* and *Candida* species have a substantially higher rate of recurrence despite adequate therapy than infections caused by other organisms.

Pearls/Special Situations

- Clinical manifestations of shunt infection are often nonspecific and prompt diagnosis requires a high level of suspicion.
- Laboratory findings of anemia, azotemia, hematuria, and proteinuria suggest shunt nephritis in a child with a ventriculoatrial shunt.
- Impaired CSF flow can result in normal CSF findings on lumbar puncture despite the presence of ventriculitis.

Suggested Readings

Anderson CM, Sorrels DL, Kerby JD. Intraabdominal pseudocysts as a complication of ventriculoperitoneal shunts. *J Am Coll Surg* 2003;196:297–300.

McGirt MG, Zaas A, Fuchs HE, et al. Risk factors for pediatric ventriculoperitoneal shunt infection and predictors of infectious pathogens. *Clin Infect Dis* 2003;36:858–862.

Mermel LA, Farr BM, Sherertz RJ, et al. Guidelines for the management of intravascular catheter-related infections. *Clin Infect Dis* 2001;32:1249–1272.

Shah SS, Smith MJ, Zaoutis TE. Device-related infections in children. *Pediatr Clin North Am* 2005;52:1189–1208.

Tokars JI. Predictive value of blood cultures positive for coagulase-negative staphylococci: implications for patient care and health quality assurance. *Clin Infect Dis* 2004;39:333–341.

CHAPTER 96 ■ INFLUENZA

KRISTINA L. SIMEONSSON

Each year in the United States, influenza causes on average 36,000 deaths and over 200,000 hospitalizations. Although the vast majority of deaths occur in the elderly, rates of hospitalization for infants and young children are similar to those for the elderly. The impact of influenza on young children has led to recent recommendations from the Advisory Committee on Immunization Practices (ACIP) that all children 6 months through 5 years of age receive the annual influenza vaccine. Monitoring for influenza-associated hospitalizations at selected sites across the United States is now part of the national influenza surveillance system. Pediatric mortality associated with influenza has recently been added to the list of nationally notifiable diseases, and many states now mandate physician reporting of pediatric deaths associated with influenza.

The two types of influenza virus that are responsible for the vast majority of human disease are type A and type B. Type A influenza viruses are further divided into subtypes based on two surface proteins, hemagglutinin (H) and neuraminidase (N). More than one strain of influenza virus can circulate during each season, but one strain often predominates. Since 1977, the three circulating strains of influenza virus have been one type B and two subtypes of A viruses (H3N2 and H1N1).

Influenza is a common midwinter respiratory illness. The majority of influenza activity peaks in the United States in January and February; however, some influenza seasons have peaked as late as May or as early as December. Because influenza circulates the globe year-round, a diagnosis of influenza can be made any time during the year, particularly in individuals who have traveled outside of the United States.

Disease is spread from person to person by respiratory droplets or by direct contact with these droplets. Children can shed influenza virus longer than adults, and are thought to be the most significant reservoir of influenza in community outbreaks.

The differential diagnosis for influenza infections includes other respiratory viruses that circulate at the same time such as respiratory syncytial virus (RSV), rhinovirus, parainfluenzavirus, and human metapneumovirus. Bacteria that can produce similar symptoms include *Chlamydia pneumoniae*, *Mycoplasma pneumoniae*, and *Streptococcus pneumoniae*.

CLINICAL FINDINGS

The classic symptoms of influenza infection include sudden onset of fever, myalgias, and respiratory symptoms (e.g., cough, rhinorrhea, and difficulty breathing). Children are more likely to manifest gastrointestinal symptoms such as vomiting and diarrhea. Infants may often present with a sepsis-like syndrome. Influenza illness typically lasts 5 days; however, the respiratory symptoms and malaise can persist for 2 to 3 weeks. If the patient develops a secondary bacterial infection such as pneumonia, there is often a brief period of improvement followed by rapid deterioration.

If a complete blood count is obtained, it may show leukocytosis with a lymphocytic predominance; platelets may also be low. Chest radiographs early in the course of illness may not provide additional information in establishing a diagnosis of influenza; however, they can be useful to rule out secondary bacterial pneumonia if the child has persistent fever or develops respiratory distress.

COMPLICATIONS

Uncomplicated influenza infection is usually not responsible for significant morbidity and mortality. The occurrence of primary viral pneumonia due to influenza virus is low compared to RSV, and viremia is not common. The morbidity and mortality associated with influenza infections is more closely related to the secondary complications that can arise. Secondary bacterial infections including pneumonia and sepsis are the leading complications of influenza that would require hospitalization. Children can also have dehydration from poor intake and/or vomiting and diarrhea associated with influenza. Individuals with certain underlying medical conditions such as chronic pulmonary or cardiac disease are at increased risk of complications due to influenza. Some common complications of influenza are listed in Table 96.1.

DIAGNOSIS

Definitive diagnosis is made by isolation of the virus from nasal or nasopharyngeal secretions. The process of confirming influenza virus by culture takes up to 7 to 10 days and is not very useful in the clinical management of patients. Fortunately there are a number of tests available to diagnose influenza infection more rapidly. Several rapid influenza diagnostic tests are commercially available in the United States that can provide results within 30 minutes. Rapid influenza testing is especially useful when deciding whether to begin treatment with antiviral medications. These rapid tests differ in the types of influenza they can detect. Some of the tests only detect type A influenza, others detect either type A or B and distinguish between the two types, and still others test for influenza generically but cannot distinguish between types A and B. These rapid tests have a lower sensitivity than viral culture; hence there is a higher likelihood of false-negative results with rapid testing alone. Providers should consider confirmation of a negative rapid test with a viral culture or another test such as an immuno-fluorescence assay. False-positive results with rapid testing can also occur, especially when influenza activity is low in the community. In these situations when the level of influenza activity is low in the community, additional testing is

TABLE 96.1

COMPLICATIONS OF INFLUENZA INFECTION

Secondary bacterial infections
    Pneumonia
    Sepsis
    Meningitis
Dehydration
Croup
Myositis
Reye syndrome
Encephalopathy
Encephalitis
Febrile seizures
Transverse myelitis
Myocarditis
Pericarditis
Disseminated intravascular coagulopathy (DIC)

recommended to confirm the diagnosis. Immunoflourescence assays are widely available in many hospitals and can provide results within 2 to 4 hours. Ideally, any testing for influenza should be performed within the first 4 days of illness.

MANAGEMENT

There are four licensed antiviral agents available in the United States for the treatment and prevention of influenza (Table 96.2). Amantadine and rimantadine are only effective against type A influenza viruses; the neuraminidase inhibitors oseltamivir and zanamivir are effective against both types A and B influenza viruses. To maximize the therapeutic benefits, antivirals should be given within 48 hours of symptom onset. Unfortunately, resistance to amantadine and rimantadine has been documented in influenza isolates from the 2005–2006 influenza season. Therefore these drugs are no longer recommended as first-line treatment or prophylaxis by the CDC or WHO. Additional measures in the management of the hospitalized patient with influenza include prompt recognition and treatment of complications such as dehydration and secondary bacterial infections.

PREVENTION

The most effective way to prevent influenza infection is to receive the yearly influenza vaccine. Influenza vaccine is indi-cated for anyone who wishes to reduce their chance of devel-oping influenza infection; however, the ACIP makes annual recommendations about certain groups of individuals who should be targeted to receive influenza vaccine. Table 96.3 lists the 2006 ACIP recommendations for the target groups to receive influenza vaccination. Most of these target groups include individuals considered high risk because of their age or an underlying medical condition. The ACIP recommenda-tions also include health care workers and household contacts of high-risk individuals because they can spread influenza virus to high-risk people if they become infected with influenza.

SPECIAL SITUATIONS

Type A influenza viruses can infect a wide range of mam-malian hosts, including migratory birds, poultry, swine, horses, and sea mammals such as seals and whales. Migratory birds are considered the natural reservoir for type A influenza viruses; there are many different subtypes of avian influenza viruses. Avian influenza viruses do not typically infect humans; however, several outbreaks of avian influenza in humans have occurred since 1997. Beginning in late 2003, an unprecedented outbreak of avian influenza A (H5N1) in poul-try and humans was identified, with human cases being reported in Asia, Eurasia, and Africa. Avian influenza viruses in humans can result in a variety of clinical manifestations. Some infections can result in conjunctivitis or an influenza-like illness with fever and myalgias, whereas more serious infections can lead to pneumonia, acute respiratory distress syndrome, and death. The index of suspicion for an avian influenza virus should be heightened if certain epidemiologic criteria are met. If patients had recent travel to a country with avian influenza (in poultry and/or humans) and/or they had direct contact with diseased poultry, testing for avian influenza viruses may be warranted.

If an avian influenza virus emerges and mutates into a form that can be easily spread from person to person, a global epidemic of influenza (pandemic) can result. Influenza pandemics occur at unpredictable intervals; there were three influenza pandemics in the 20th century. Because there would be little to no pre-existing immunity to an emerging avian influenza virus in the human population, there is potential for an increased number of hospitalizations and deaths. Pandemic influenza planning is ongoing at federal, state, and local levels of government. The United States Department of Health and Human Services released a revised Pandemic Influenza Plan in 2005 that includes clinical guide-lines for providers during an influenza pandemic. Many health care facilities are also developing plans specific to their

TABLE 96.2

ANTIVIRAL MEDICATIONS FOR INFLUENZA

	Amantadine	Rimantadine	Oseltamivir	Zanamivir
Administration route	Oral	Oral	Oral	Inhaled
Treatment indications	≥1 year Influenza A	≥13 years Influenza A	≥1 year Influenza A and B	≥7 years Influenza A and B
Prophylaxis indications	≥1 year Influenza A	≥1 year Influenza A	≥1 year Influenza A and B	≥5 years Influenza A and B
Adverse effects	Central nervous system and gastrointestinal effects	Central nervous system and gastrointestinal effects	Gastrointestinal effects	Bronchospasm

TABLE 96.3

2006 ADVISORY COMMITTEE ON IMMUNIZATION PRACTICES (ACIP) RECOMMENDATIONS FOR ANNUAL INFLUENZA VACCINATION

PERSONS AT RISK FOR COMPLICATIONS

- Persons aged ≥65 years
- Residents of nursing homes and other chronic-care facilities that house persons of any age who have chronic medical conditions
- Adults and children who have chronic disorders of the pulmonary or cardiovascular systems, including asthma
- Adults and children who have required regular medical follow-up or hospitalization during the preceding year because of chronic metabolic diseases, renal dysfunction, hemoglobinopathies, or immunosuppression
- Adults and children who have any condition that can compromise respiratory function or the handling of respiratory secretions or that can increase the risk for aspiration
- Children and adolescents (aged 6 months to 18 years) who are receiving long-term aspirin therapy
- Women who will be pregnant during the influenza season
- Children aged 6 to 59 months

PERSONS AGED 50–64 YEARS

- Recommended because this age group has an increased prevalence of persons with high-risk medical conditions

PERSONS WHO CAN TRANSMIT INFLUENZA TO THOSE AT HIGH RISK

- Physicians, nurses, and other personnel in both hospital and outpatient-care settings, including medical emergency response workers (e.g., paramedics and emergency medical technicians)
- Employees of nursing homes and chronic-care facilities who have contact with patients or residents
- Employees of assisted-living and other residences for persons in groups at high risk
- Persons who provide home care to persons in groups at high risk[a]
- Household contacts (including children) of persons in groups at high risk[a]

[a]Particularly for contacts of infants 0 to 5 months.

institutions. Providers who care for hospitalized children should take an active role in these planning efforts so that the specific needs of infants and children are addressed prior to a pandemic.

- An influenza pandemic may result in large numbers of hospitalizations and deaths; individuals from many different disciplines need to participate in pandemic influenza planning.

PEARLS

- Rates of influenza-associated hospitalizations for infants and young children are as high as they are for the elderly.
- Children are more likely to manifest gastrointestinal symptoms with influenza illness.
- The most effective way to prevent influenza infection is with the annual influenza vaccine.

Suggested Readings

Bhat N, Wright JG, Broder KR, et al. Influenza-associated deaths among children in the United States, 2003–2004. *N Engl J Med* 2005;353:2559–2567.

Peltola V. Influenza A and B virus infections in children. *Clin Infect Dis* 2003;36:299–305.

Uyeki TM. Influenza diagnosis and treatment in children: a review of studies and clinically useful tests and antiviral treatment for influenza. *Pediatr Infect Dis J* 2003;22:164–177.

Woods CR, Abramson JS. The next influenza pandemic: will we be ready to care for our children? *J Pediatr* 2005;147:147–155.

CHAPTER 97 ■ INFECTION CONTROL IN THE PEDIATRIC HOSPITAL SETTING

JENNIFER MACFARQUHAR, KRISTINA L. SIMEONSSON, WILLIAM E. CLEVE, AND JEFFREY P. ENGEL

The first hospital Infection Control and Prevention (IC) initiatives began in the 1950s due to an increase in intensive care units and in staphylococcal infections. IC programs expanded into hospitals across the United States over the next 20 years, garnered by support from agencies such as the American Hospital Association (AHA) and the Joint Commission on Accreditation of Healthcare Organizations (JCAHO). The scope of IC programs encompasses patients and health care providers, and the functions of an IC program are multifaceted. The principal functions of effective IC programs include both surveillance and practice activities, and include:

1. Management of critical data and information, including surveillance for nosocomial, or health care–associated HAIs.
2. Direct intervention to prevent infections.
3. Monitoring for risk of occupational exposure to employees.
4. Development and recommendation of policies and procedures.
5. Monitoring the use of medical devices.
6. Maintenance of the physical environment, particularly sterilization and disinfection.
7. Education of patients, families, and health care personnel (medical and nonmedical).

Several studies performed by the Centers for Disease Control and Prevention (CDC) have shown that up to one-third of HAIs can be prevented by effective IC programs (1). A comprehensive IC program in the pediatric hospital setting is essential. Children are at higher risk than adults for acquiring infectious diseases. Young children have immature immune systems. They may not have received vaccines for particular diseases such as varicella and pertussis that are highly transmissible and can cause significant morbidity and mortality. Finally, they may have congenital anomalies or immunodeficiencies that put them at increased risk for infections. Children with congenital problems frequently require invasive procedures and admissions to intensive-care units, further increasing their risk for acquiring a healthcare-associated infection (2).

SURVEILLANCE FOR HEALTH CARE–ASSOCIATED INFECTIONS

Health care–associated infections (HAIs), are those that are not present or incubating upon admission to a health care facility, and are not related to recent hospitalizations. HAIs can be related generally to the admission to the facility or specifically to a procedure performed at the facility. Nosocomial infections may be caused by microorganisms from the patient's endogenous flora; from other patients, visitors, and health care personnel; and from the hospital environment.

Active surveillance for HAIs is the foundation of any hospital infection control program. It involves the collection of data with appropriate analysis and interpretation. Active surveillance methodologies must incorporate standard definitions. The CDC provides standard definitions and also a reporting system in which hospitals may participate. The data may then be utilized for benchmarking. HAIs differ by site between pediatric and adult patient populations. According to the National Nosocomial Infections Surveillance System data summary (3), the primary site of pediatric nosocomial infections is the bloodstream. Over 90% of these bloodstream infections are associated with intravascular catheter devices.

Data obtained through active surveillance can be utilized to determine baseline rates of nosocomial infections, detect changes in these rates, and investigate any increase in rates above the baseline. In an outbreak setting, data can also be used to determine whether the recommended control measures are effective. Reporting of HAI rates to key personnel including managers and health care workers is another function of the IC program, and has been shown to be an important factor in the reduction of HAIs (4).

CHAIN OF INFECTION

The chain of infection (Fig. 97.1) describes how infectious organisms are transmitted. The primary elements of disease are considered to be the agent (infectious organism), host (person), and environment (all factors external to the host). Each component, or link, in the chain of infection is connected to another component. Prevention of infection occurs when one of the "links" in the chain of infection is broken.

The components in the chain of infection include etiologic agent, reservoir, portal of exit, mode of transmission, portal of entry, and susceptible host. *Etiologic agents*, often considered the first link in the chain, may be any microorganism that can cause infection. They consist of bacteria, viruses, fungi, protozoa, helminthes, and prions. The virulence and invasiveness of an agent affects its ability to cause disease. The *reservoir*, or second link, is the site where the microorganism resides, metabolizes, and multiplies. Reservoirs can be humans, animals, and the environment. Within the health care facility, reservoirs can include health care workers, patients, and medical equipment. Third, the *portal of exit* is the path by which the etiologic agent leaves the reservoir. The fourth link, *mode of transmission*, is how the organism reaches the susceptible host. Transmission occurs via direct or indirect contact between persons, with a contaminated object, or through ingestion of contaminated food or water; and inhalation of droplets or droplet nuclei

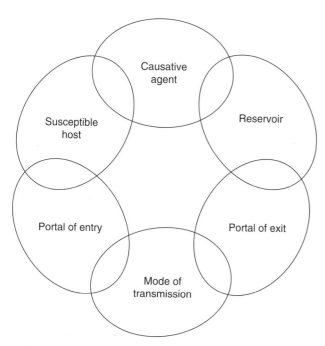

FIGURE 97.1. Chain of infection. (From Carrico R, ed. *APIC text of infection control and epidemiology.* 2nd ed. Washington, DC: APIC; 2005, with permission.)

spread by speaking, coughing, or sneezing. *Portals of entry,* the fifth link, are the paths by which an etiologic agent enters the susceptible host. Portals of entry and exit include respiratory, gastrointestinal, and genitourinary tracts, skin, mucous membranes, blood, and body fluids. The final link in the chain of infection is a *susceptible host.* Characteristics that can influence host susceptibility include age, sex, ethnicity, socioeconomic status, medical history, lifestyle, heredity, nutritional status, immunization status, occupation, medications, and therapeutic procedures.

ISOLATION PRECAUTIONS

Use of isolation precautions are an essential part of an IC program, and when implemented effectively can significantly reduce the risk of transmission of microorganisms in hospital settings. Isolation precautions prevent the transmission of microorganisms from patients to health care workers, as well as preventing transmission between patients.

The Hospital Infection Control Practices Advisory Committee (HICPAC) recommends two *isolation precaution tiers*: standard and transmission-based. Standard precautions function as the primary strategy for successful nosocomial infection control. They are designed to reduce the risk of transmission of microorganisms from both known and unknown sources. Standard precautions should be used in all patient encounters when the potential for exposure to blood and body fluid exists.

Fundamentals of Standard Precautions

Hand Hygiene

Hand-washing, also called hand hygiene, is a critical component of patient and employee safety. It is the single most important way to prevent or interrupt the transmission of infection, and reduces the incidence of HAIs. Hand hygiene technique should include either:

- Decontamination with an alcohol-based rub following the manufacturer's recommendation for adequate volume, or
- Washing with soap and warm water, rubbing vigorously for at least 15 seconds and covering all surfaces, followed by thorough rinsing and drying with a disposable towel that is then utilized to turn off water faucets (5).

Investigations of nosocomial outbreaks have often indicated an association between infections and poor adherence to hand hygiene. Outbreaks in neonatal intensive care units have been associated with poor hand hygiene and artificial fingernails. Ongoing education is important to improve compliance with hand hygiene. Noncompliance with hand hygiene has been linked to understaffing and overcrowding, so these factors should be addressed in addition to educational programs.

Patient Placement

Patient placement is another important component of isolation. State and federal codes mandate physical space requirements for patient care areas and hospital rooms in order to minimize crowding and the risk of microorganism transmission. Patients at greater risk for infection due to immunosuppression or immunodeficiency (e.g., neonates or transplant recipients) should be placed in private areas or rooms. Cohorting of patients who are colonized or infected with epidemiologically significant organisms is recommended as an outbreak control measure. Although single-room isolation for some diseases and conditions is preferred, it is not mandatory for nurseries and infant wards because these patients are confined to cribs or isolettes.

Personal Protective Equipment (PPE)

The final important component of isolation is the appropriate utilization of *personal protective equipment (PPE).* The Occupational Safety and Health Administration (OSHA) mandates that gloves be worn during all patient care activities that may involve exposure to blood or body fluids (6). Correspondingly, the CDC recommends that health care workers wear gloves in order to reduce the risk of organism transmission from personnel to patients, from patients to personnel, and to reduce the transient contamination of the hands of personnel by flora that can be transmitted from one patient to another (7). Gowns, masks, and eye protection should be utilized during procedures that may generate splashing or spraying of blood or body fluids (8).

Transmission-Based Precautions

Transmission-based precautions are designed for the care of patients with known or suspected epidemiologically significant pathogens spread by airborne, droplet, or contact routes. It is important to note that transmission-based precautions do not replace standard precautions; they should be applied in conjunction with standard precautions.

Contact precautions are designed to prevent the spread of microorganisms transmitted by direct or indirect physical contact. This includes person-to-person contact (direct), or contact with an intermediate object such as a bedrail (indirect). Droplet precautions are intended to prevent the transmission of organisms that spread via large droplets generated by coughing and sneezing that travel only short distances (generally less than 3 feet from a source to a host). Airborne precautions are designed to prevent transmission of organisms that are spread via droplet nuclei and can travel long distances on air currents.

Some infectious pathogens require a combination of these precautions. For instance, *varicella zoster* infection requires both airborne and contact precautions. Table 97.1 lists the types of isolation precautions recommended for selected infections and conditions that may be encountered in the pediatric hospital.

TABLE 97.1

TYPES OF PRECAUTIONS FOR SELECTED INFECTIONS AND CONDITIONS IN THE PEDIATRIC POPULATION

Infection/Condition	Precautions
Adenovirus pneumonia infection	Contact, droplet
Bordatella pertussis	Droplet
Enteroviral infections	Contact
Herpes simplex (neonatal; mucocutaneous, disseminated; or primary, severe)	Contact
Gastroenteritis	
Clostridium difficile	Contact
Escherichia coli, O157:H7 (diapered or incontinent)	Contact
Influenza	Droplet
Measles virus (rubeola)	Airborne
Meningitis	
Haemophilus influenzae	Droplet
Neisseria meningitidis (meningococcal)	Droplet
Meningococcal pneumonia	Droplet
Meningococcemia (meningococcal sepsis)	Droplet
Mumps (infectious parotitis)	Droplet
Mycobacterium tuberculosis	Airborne
Norovirus	Contact
Parainfluenza virus (respiratory)	Contact
Parvovirus B19	Droplet
Respiratory syncytial virus (RSV) infection	Contact
Rotavirus (diapered or incontinent)	Contact
Rubella	Droplet
Shigella (diapered or incontinent)	Contact
Varicella zoster virus (localized in immunocompromised patient, or disseminated)	Contact, airborne

Disinfection/Sterilization

Every hospital and related infection control program must have guidelines regarding the cleaning, disinfection, and sterilization of medical equipment in order to minimize the risk of infectious organism transmission to patients (9). Items in a hospital must be cleaned, disinfected, or sterilized based upon their intended use. Critical items (e.g., surgical instruments) are those that come into contact with sterile tissue; these items require sterilization. Items that come into contact with mucous membranes are semi-critical (e.g., bronchoscopes); these items require high-level disinfection. Noncritical items (e.g., blood pressure cuffs) are those that come into contact with intact skin; these items require low-level disinfection (9).

Disinfection and sterilization in the pediatric hospital setting have unique challenges. In addition to coming into contact with routine medical equipment, children are more likely to come into contact with nonmedical equipment such as toys (2). Hospitalized children may spend time in common areas such as playrooms. This increases the likelihood that toys and other equipment may be shared between patients. These items can become contaminated with infectious organisms, leading to the spread of these organisms to susceptible patients and the potential for outbreaks. No published guidelines exist for either cleaning toys or common play areas in hospitals, but a logical approach would include avoiding toys that are difficult to clean such as stuffed animals and thoroughly disinfecting toys between patients. Toys can be cleaned with a low-level disinfectant (e.g., bleach 1:100), and should be given ample time to dry. Disinfection of toys and environmental surfaces in play areas should occur at least weekly (2). Toys that are unable to be cleaned, such as stuffed animals, should not be shared or placed in common areas.

DISEASE REPORTING OF COMMUNITY-ACQUIRED INFECTIONS

Reporting of diseases of public health significance is another role that health care providers play in the control of infectious diseases. It is the duty of physicians to report certain diseases to public health authorities if they reasonably suspect or confirm one of the notifiable diseases in their patients. Physicians should report even when they *suspect* a disease because there may be public health actions that need to be taken as soon as possible to have the greatest impact. For example, contacts of a case of hepatitis A or meningococcal disease may need prophylaxis if they have been exposed, and this prophylaxis is recommended within a certain time-frame from exposure. Furthermore, the ongoing threat of bioterrorism and emerging infectious diseases necessitates early reporting when one of these diseases is suspected, giving public health officials lead time to respond to such events. Pediatric patients can be victims of bioterrorism, as witnessed during the 2001 anthrax attacks when a 7-month-old developed cutaneous anthrax after visiting an office building in New York City (Fig. 97.2).

State and local public health officials rely on health care providers, laboratories, and other public health personnel to report the occurrence of notifiable diseases to state and local health departments. Reports are used to detect unusual occurrences of diseases, monitor trends in diseases, and evaluate the effectiveness of control measures.

The list of nationally notifiable diseases is revised periodically. Diseases may be added as they emerge as public health

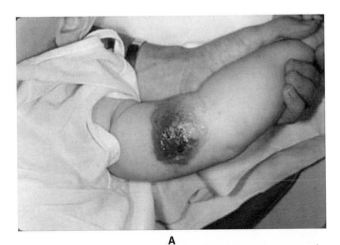

A

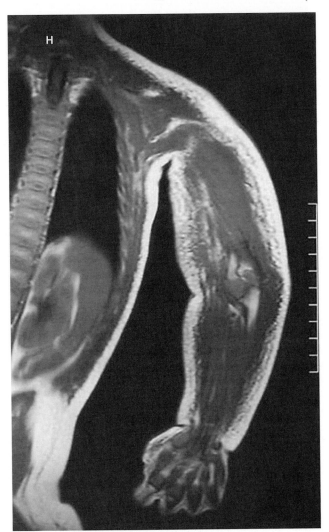

B

Copyright 2001 Massachusetts Medical Society (From Roche KJ, Chang MW and Lazarus H, Images in Clinical Medicine, The *New England Journal of Medicine*, 2001; 29; 345(22):1611, with permission)

FIGURE 97.2. Anthrax.

TABLE 97.2

NATIONALLY NOTIFIABLE INFECTIOUS DISEASES—UNITED STATES, 2006

Acquired immunodeficiency syndrome (AIDS)
Anthrax
Arboviral diseases
Botulism
Brucellosis
Chancroid
Chlamydia trachomatis, genital infections
Cholera
Coccidiomycosis
Cryptosporidiosis
Cyclosporiasis
Diphtheria
Ehrlichiosis
Giardiasis
Gonorrhea
Haemophilus influenzae, invasive disease
Hansen disease (leprosy)
Hantavirus pulmonary syndrome
Hemolytic uremic syndrome, postdiarrheal
Hepatitis, viral
HIV infection
Influenza-associated pediatric mortality
Legionellosis
Listeriosis
Lyme disease
Malaria
Measles
Meningococcal disease
Mumps
Pertussis
Plague
Poliomyelitis, paralytic
Psittacosis
Q fever
Rabies
Rocky Mountain spotted fever
Rubella
Salmonellosis
Severe acute respiratory syndrome–associated coronavirus (SARS-CoV)
Shiga toxin-producing *Escherichia coli* (STEC)
Shigellosis
Smallpox
Streptococcal disease, invasive, group A
Streptococcal toxic shock syndrome
Streptococcus pneumoniae, drug resistant, invasive disease
Streptococcus pneumoniae, invasive in children <5 years
Syphilis
Tetanus
Toxic shock syndrome
Trichinellosis
Tuberculosis
Tularemia
Typhoid fever
Vancomycin-intermediate *Staphylococcus aureus*
Vancomycin-resistant *Staphylococcus aureus*
Varicella
Yellow fever

threats; severe acute respiratory syndrome (SARS) was added to the list of Nationally Notifiable Infectious Diseases in 2003. Diseases can also be removed from the list as their incidence declines or if they no longer have public health significance. The CDC publishes standardized case definitions for these notifiable diseases. Reporting of diseases is mandated at the state level; therefore the list of reportable diseases will vary slightly in each state. Reporting of these diseases to the CDC by each state is voluntary. Table 97.2 provides a list of the nationally notifiable infectious diseases in the United States for 2006. Health care personnel should contact their local or state health department to determine the reporting requirements for their state.

ROLE OF OCCUPATIONAL HEALTH IN INFECTION CONTROL

Maintenance of appropriate immunization status is a key responsibility of health care workers. Documented immunity to vaccine-preventable diseases such as measles, mumps, rubella, varicella, and hepatitis B not only protects the health care worker from developing these illnesses, it also minimizes transmission of these illnesses from health care workers to susceptible patients. The incidence of pertussis is increasing and health care facilities are a setting in which pertussis can be transmitted from patients to health care workers and vice versa. Health care workers should receive the diphtheria-tetanus-pertussis vaccine (Tdap) in lieu of one of the tetanus boosters (Td) recommended for adults every 10 years. Finally, health care workers should receive the influenza vaccine every year. Obviously, health care workers are at risk of acquiring influenza in a hospital setting. However, of greater importance is the fact that they can also transmit influenza to hospitalized patients who are often at increased risk of influenza complications.

CONCLUSION

The scope of comprehensive IC programs includes both patients and health care workers. Whether reporting infectious diseases to public health authorities, following isolation precautions recommended for their hospitalized patients, or maintaining their immunization status to protect themselves and their patients, health care workers play an integral part in

the control of infectious diseases. Pediatric providers who work in a hospital setting should take an active role in the IC program at their facility.

PEARLS

- Hand-washing is the cornerstone of infection control; perform it frequently and scrupulously.
- Hospital infection control practitioners are excellent resources for surveillance, isolation, antibiotic utilization, patient safety, and educational activities.
- Isolation precautions are based upon the organism's mode of transmission (airborne, droplet, and contact).
- It is the duty of physicians to report either suspected or confirmed communicable diseases.

References

1. Haley RW, Culver DH, White JW, et al. The efficacy of infection surveillance and control programs in preventing nosocomial infections in US hospitals. *Am J Epidemiol* 1985;121:182–205.
2. Rosenthal A, Matlow A, Wray R, et al. Pediatrics. In: Carrico R, ed. *APIC text of infection control and epidemiology.* 2nd ed. Washington, DC: APIC; 2005.
3. Centers for Disease Control and Prevention. National Nosocomial Infections Surveillance (NNIS) System report, data summary from January 1992 to June 2003, issued August 2003. *Am J Infect Control* 2003;31:481–198.
4. Gaynes RP, Richards C, Edwards J, et al. Feeding back surveillance data to prevent hospital-acquired infections. *Emerg Infect Dis* 2001;7:295–298.
5. Guideline for hand hygiene in health-care settings. *MMWR* 51;2002:1–44.
6. Occupational Safety and Health Administration. Occupational exposure to bloodborne pathogens: final rule. *Federal Register* 1991;29 CFR Part 1910:1030.
7. Garner JS, Simmons BP. Guideline for isolation precautions in hospitals. *Infect Control* 1983;4(suppl 4):245–325.
8. Garner JS. Hospital Infection Control Practices Advisory Committee: guideline for isolation precautions in hospitals. *Am J Infect Control* 1996;24:24–52.
9. Rutala WA, Weber DJ. Modern advances in disinfection, sterilization, and medical waste management. In: Wenzel RP, ed. *Prevention and control of nosocomial infections.* 4th ed. Philadelphia: Lippincott Williams & Wilkins; 2003.

CHAPTER 98 ■ INITIAL INPATIENT STABILIZATION AND MANAGEMENT OF THE HOSPITALIZED DIABETIC PATIENT

GLENN D. HARRIS AND MARK A. SPERLING

Although diabetes mellitus has been traditionally classified as type I or type II, primary diabetes mellitus represents a spectrum of disease involving insulin deficiency or inefficacy. Causes range from autoimmune destruction of insulin-secreting beta cells (classic type 1) to relative insulin deficiency with lack of responsiveness to circulating insulin (classic type 2) particularly in the liver, skeletal muscle, and adipose tissue (Table 98.1). Diabetic ketoacidosis (DKA) is discussed in a separate chapter.

At least one of the three following criteria is necessary to make the diagnosis of diabetes mellitus:

■ A fasting blood glucose greater than or equal to 126 mg/dL (7.0 mmol/L).
■ Symptoms of diabetes mellitus (e.g. polyuria, polydipsia) plus a random plasma glucose concentration greater than or equal to 200 mg/dL (11.1 mmol/L).
■ A 2-hour oral glucose tolerance test with a 2-hour plasma glucose concentration greater than or equal to 200 mg/dL (11.1 mmol/L).

Some of the factors that can cause secondary diabetes mellitus or exacerbate insulin deficiency and/or insulin resistance include disease of the exocrine pancreas (e.g., cystic fibrosis), endocrinopathies (e.g., Cushing syndrome), certain drugs (e.g., atypical antipsychotic medications such as olanzapine; corticosteroids), genetic defects in insulin action (e.g., congenital lipoatrophy), infection (e.g., pneumonia/acute enteritis), obesity, pregnancy, puberty, and other physiologic stresses (e.g., trauma).

EVALUATION

The classic signs or symptoms of diabetes mellitus have been referred to as the "three "Ps:" polyuria, polydipsia, and polyphagia. It is important to emphasize that even with a good patient history, one or more of the "Ps" may not be present, but other clinical manifestations may be elicited, such as unexplained weight loss (or failure to gain weight appropriately), genital moniliasis, blurred vision, headache, and decreased energy. Laboratory tests to be considered include those listed in Table 98.2.

The family history should include identification of the following illnesses: diabetes mellitus, dyslipidemias, diabetic nephropathy, neuropathy, retinopathy, obesity/morbid obesity, hypertension, coronary artery disease, cerebral vascular accidents, polycystic ovary disease, and early death (and causes when known). On physical examination, adequacy of breathing, with careful differentiation between the deep sighing Kussmaul respirations of DKA from those of reactive airways disease, peripheral perfusion, and level of consciousness should be quickly assessed. If these findings are normal, the remainder of the examination should be completed and focused on identification of factors that may help delineate the cause of hyperglycemia. If a diabetic child or adolescent is admitted electively (or emergently) for surgery, special treatment considerations are recommended (Table 98.3) in addition to routine physical assessments and laboratory studies.

If mental status is compromised, unsuspected DKA may be present. Hypertension, bradycardia, irregular respirations (Cushing triad) and/or pupillary changes indicate raised intracranial pressure that requires emergency intervention (mannitol IV) and admission to a pediatric intensive care unit.

GENERAL MANAGEMENT AND MONITORING GUIDELINES

Certain principles of management apply regardless of the type of diabetes mellitus. Insulin resistance is known to be a feature of *all* forms of diabetes although its severity is variable. Diabetic patients with predominant insulin deficiency need a source of insulin at all times to prevent development of ketosis. A preferred method of insulin delivery is provision of a subcutaneous depot of a smooth long-acting insulin that will mimic normal endogenous basal insulin secretion. This is combined with mealtime doses of a short-acting insulin to mimic the normal endogenous response to carbohydrate intake ("carbohydrate exchange" doses) plus additional short-acting insulin (supplemental doses) to correct unanticipated hyperglycemia that may occur throughout the day. When such a regimen is mastered by a compliant patient, this results in the greatest likelihood of achieving excellent long-term results. We do not initiate continuous subcutaneous insulin infusion therapy ("insulin pump therapy") in the early course of diabetes mellitus.

For patients with predominant insulin resistance (classic type 2), oral antihyperglycemic agents may be instituted after adequate glycemic control is achieved (fasting blood glucose less than 200 mg/dL or 11.1 mmol/L). However, even predominantly insulin-resistant patients may require regimens similar to those who are insulin deficient until they become candidates for oral therapy. All patients with newly diagnosed diabetes should receive counseling regarding regular cardiovascular exercise and healthy eating patterns. Patients with significant dyslipidemia should be evaluated for antilipidemic

TABLE 98.1

CLASSIFICATION OF DIABETES MELLITUS

DIABETES WITH PREDOMINANT INSULIN DEFICIENCY (BETA CELL FAILURE)
- Classic type 1 diabetes mellitus
  - Autoimmune
  - Idiopathic
- Maturity-onset diabetes of youth (MODY)
- Mitochondrial diabetes
- Congenital infections

DIABETES AND OTHER SYNDROMES WITH PREDOMINANT INSULIN RESISTANCE
- Lipoatrophic diabetes
- Metabolic syndrome
- Polycystic ovary syndrome
- Type A insulin resistance
- Leprechaunism
- Rabson–Mendenhall syndrome
- Endocrinopathies (e.g., Cushing syndrome)

DIABETES RESULTING FROM COMBINED INSULIN DEFICIENCY AND INSULIN RESISTANCE
- Type 2 diabetes mellitus
  - Classic[a]
  - Classic[a] *except* susceptible to ketoacidosis (type 1.5 = double diabetes = Flatbush diabetes)
  - Type 2 diabetes mellitus with autoantibodies (type 3 = triple diabetes)
- Cystic fibrosis-related diabetes

MISCELLANEOUS CAUSES
- Medications/toxins (e.g., corticosteroids, diuretics, certain atypical antipsychotics)
- Genetic syndromes sometimes associated with diabetes (e.g., trisomy 21)
- Autoimmune polyendocrinopathy syndrome, type 1
- Diseases of the exocrine pancreas (e.g., pancreatitis)

[a]Classic: Insulin resistance associated with obesity, acanthosis nigricans, family history of type 2 diabetes mellitus, and resistance to ketoacidosis.

TABLE 98.2

LABORATORY TESTS TO BE CONSIDERED ON ADMISSION

Blood, plasma, or serum glucose
Electrolytes, serum urea nitrogen, total CO_2, creatinine
Hemoglobin A1c
C-peptide
Free and total insulin
Glutamic acid decarboxylase 65 antibody
Pancreatic islet cell antibody (ICA-512 antibody)
Insulin antibody
Fasting lipid panel (after metabolic control is achieved)
Liver enzymes
Complete blood count
Serum and/or urine ketones
Serum IgA (quantitative) and serum IgA autoantibodies to tissue transglutaminase
Urinalysis
Appropriate cultures, when clinically indicated

medications. Because hyperglycemia itself results in transient hyperlipidemia, fasting lipid values should be obtained 1 month after achieving glucose control to determine if antilipidemic medications are indicated. Hemoglobin A1c concentrations should be obtained at each hospital admission and followed every 3 to 4 months (Table 98.4).

All hospitalized patients with diabetes, regardless of type, should have bedside glucose checks at a minimum before major meals, at bedtime, and at about 2:00 AM. Additional glucose checks at midmorning and midafternoon should be considered, particularly if glycemic control is suboptimal. It is also essential to perform and teach monitoring for urine ketones, finger-stick blood glucose checks, and measurement and administration of insulin doses. Ketone meters are becoming increasingly utilized. The nursing staff should keep an intake/output record and measure the patient's weight daily, particularly if there has been significant weight loss. Consultation with a nurse diabetes educator and a nutritionist are essential. Social work intervention may be necessary if medical insurance for diabetes supplies

TABLE 98.3

MANAGEMENT OF THE PERIOPERATIVE PEDIATRIC DIABETIC PATIENT

- Discontinue all oral diabetic medications.
- NPO at the appropriate time prior to surgery.
- Insulin
  - If on an established insulin regimen with a "peakless" basal insulin such as insulin glargine, the usual evening dose may be administered.
  - If not already receiving a basal insulin, initiate continuous intravenous regular human insulin (0.025–0.05 units/kg body weight/hr), titrating to effect a blood glucose in the 90–180 mg/dL (5–10 mmol/L) range.
- Fluids for normovolemic patients
  - Preoperatively: $D_{5\%}$ 0.45% NaCl + maintenance potassium.
  - Intraoperatively: $D_{5\%}$ 0.9% NaCl (or $D_{5\%}$ Ringer lactate solution) + maintenance potassium.
  - Postoperatively: as dictated clinically.
- Blood glucose should be checked at least hourly while receiving IV insulin.
- Postoperative care includes
  - Serial vital signs, physical examination, and serial laboratory data.
  - Resume usual subcutaneous insulin regimen when alert and eating.

TABLE 98.4

PLASMA BLOOD GLUCOSE AND HEMOGLOBIN A_1c GOALS BY AGE GROUP

Children without endogenous insulin secretion (type 1 diabetes)			
	Plasma blood glucose goal range (mg/dL)		
Values by age	Before meals	Bedtime/Overnight	A_1c
Toddlers and preschoolers (<6 yr)	100–180	110–200	7.5–8.5%
School age (6–12 yr)	90–180	100–180	<8%
Adolescents and young adults (13–19 yr)	90–130	90–150	<7.5%

Pubertal children with significant endogenous insulin secretion (type 2 diabetes)		
Before meals	Bedtime/Overnight	A_1c
70–120 mg/dL	80–150 mg/dL	≤6.5%

KEY CONCEPTS IN SETTING GLYCEMIC GOALS

- Goals should be individualized and lower goals may be reasonable based on benefit–risk assessment.
- Blood glucose goals should be higher than those listed above in children with frequent hypoglycemia unawareness.
- Postprandial blood glucose values should be measured when there is a disparity between preprandial blood glucose values and A_1C levels.

[a]A lower goal (<7.0%) is reasonable if it can be achieved without excessive hypoglycemia. Modified from Silverstein J, Klingensmith G, Copeland K, et al. Care of children and adolescents with type 1 diabetes. A statement of the American Diabetes Association. *Diabetes Care* 2005;28:186–212.

is a problem, if there is no working telephone in the patient's home, or if neglect is suspected in the case of a child with poorly controlled diabetes or recurrent DKA.

In patients recovering from uncontrolled hyperglycemia, obtain serial serum potassium concentrations; potassium supplementation may be needed until serum potassium is stable within the normal range. As with all pediatric ward patients, routine vital signs and neurologic checks should be ordered.

During hospitalization, patients should walk at least twice a day for at least 20 minutes unless otherwise contraindicated. In combination with exercise, a healthy nutrition program should be planned. For children under 2 years of age, we recommend a "regular diet with no concentrated sweets." For older children, an American Diabetes Association diet is planned. If significant weight loss has occurred in a nonobese child or adolescent prior to admission, calculate caloric needs based on the ideal weight. We supply even more calories when the patient with weight loss fails to be satiated with their planned meals, particularly those who are nonobese.

How to Develop an Insulin Plan

The objective of insulin treatment is to achieve a normal, average blood glucose concentration and minimize episodes of hypoglycemia. Most newly diagnosed pubertal patients with beta-cell failure (classic type 1 diabetes) require a total daily dose of insulin of about 1 unit/kg/day; prepubertal children in that group usually require a total daily insulin dose in the range of 0.3 to 0.8 units/kg/day. We do not recommend deliberate underdosing and gradually increasing insulin, because extended hyperglycemia prolongs insulin resistance and decreases endogenous insulin secretory capacity. Patients with predomi-

nant insulin resistance will likely require insulin until good glycemic control permits institution of oral antihyperglycemic agents. Expect obese patients and patients with an underlying familial hyperlipidemia to be particularly insulin resistant; they often require insulin 1.5 to 3 units/kg/day (based on *actual*, not ideal, body weight). If moderate to large ketones are present in the urine in the absence of DKA, the daily subcutaneous insulin requirement may need to be increased by 25% or more. If the obese patient requires IV fluids, these should be calculated based on the *ideal*, not the actual, body weight.

Management of Patients with Predominant Insulin Deficiency

Highly Motivated, Capable Patients and Families

For predominantly insulin-deficient patients, provision of a minimally peaking or peakless insulin (glargine/detemir) once or twice a day along with a rapidly acting insulin (aspart/lispro or more rarely human regular) that matches ingested carbohydrate demands provides the most independence and most closely mimics endogenous insulin release.

A therapeutic substitute for endogenous basal insulin secretion can be accomplished with once or twice daily insulin detemir (Levemir) or once daily insulin glargine (Lantus) calculated as approximately 0.3 to 0.5 units/kg/day depending on age and pubertal status with the prepubertal patient receiving doses in the lower range. In conjunction with the long-acting "basal" insulin, a rapid-acting insulin (aspart or lispro) should be given based on carbohydrate to be ingested (usually 0.5 units/15 g carbohydrate in children 5 years or less, 1 unit/15 g carbohydrate for ages 6 to 11 years, and 2 units/15 g carbohydrates for those

12 years and older) at breakfast, lunch, and supper. When it is not possible to predict carbohydrate intake, as for infants and toddlers, we administer the short-acting insulin *after* the meal (within 30 minutes). Use of a portable insulin pen is the most convenient for school-age children at lunch or for those receiving insulin glargine (Lantus cannot be mixed with any other insulin).

Sliding scale or supplemental insulin doses, also termed the "insulin correction bolus," refers to the use of rapid-acting insulin to normalize elevated blood glucose values (Table 98.5). These insulin doses are administered in addition to any rapid-acting insulin administered for carbohydrate coverage. Although human insulin lispro (Humalog) is the most rapid-acting insulin, we have found it often peaks too forcefully in young children, resulting in hypoglycemia, sometimes followed by hyperglycemia. We have found rapid-acting insulin aspart (Novolog) to have a gentler initial peak and an extended "tail" activity, preventing these problems.

Highly Motivated Patients and Families Who Do Not Wish to Provide a Lunchtime Carbohydrate Injection at School

Many school-age patients prefer not to give prelunch insulin ("carbohydrate coverage") for that meal. The need for this coverage may be circumvented by use of NPH insulin prior to breakfast, because this insulin provides a peak in 5 to 7 hours, which coincides with lunch. Because most school lunches contain at least 60 grams of carbohydrate, this can be used as a guideline for the dose of NPH expected to match the anticipated meal. On this regimen, the patient will need rapid-acting insulin (Novolog, Humalog, or human regular) 0.5 to 2 units/

15 g carbohydrate at breakfast and supper, but not for lunch or daytime snacks. Insulin glargine (Lantus) 0.3 to 0.5 units/kg/day is then administered at suppertime or bedtime. Unanticipated hyperglycemia prior to main meals will still need to be treated with supplemental insulin.

Patients Who Require a Fixed Carbohydrate Meal Plan and Fixed Insulin Dosages

In patients who are unable or unwilling to match insulin with carbohydrate intake, alternate therapeutic possibilities exist. A set dose of insulin can be given before breakfast and supper, using a 0.5 to 1.5 unit/kg/day total dose of insulin, giving two-thirds of the total daily dose in the morning. Two-thirds of this morning dose (or approximately 44% of the total daily dose) is given as NPH insulin and one-third of the morning dose (or 22% of the total daily dose) is given as a rapid-acting insulin. The remaining portion of the total daily dose (one-third the total daily dose) is given in the evening, half as short-acting insulin and half as a peakless insulin (glargine or detemir). NPH insulin peaks 5 to 7 hours after injection in children, allowing for a lunchtime meal without additional carbohydrate "coverage." NPH insulin is not suited for pre-supper or pre-bedtime injection because it will peak during sleep. Thus, we recommend all children who take NPH in the morning take their supper dose as a peakless insulin, which "locks in" approximately 5 hours after injection, and does not have a classic peak, resulting in sustained overnight insulin coverage and a greatly lowered risk of hypoglycemia.

When additional short-acting supplemental insulin (for hyperglycemia) is given at night, additional blood glucose checks need to be done while the patient's individual response is being learned (1 to 2 hours after the dose if rapid-acting insulin [Novolog or Humalog] is given, or 2 to 3 hours after the dose if regular insulin is given). The presence of moderate to large ketones in the urine usually requires administration of additional insulin.

As a last-resort insulin management plan, mixed long- and short-acting insulins (e.g., Novolog Mix 70/30) twice daily may be used for glycemic control, particularly for patients who do not miss major meals. These doses also are calculated by giving two-thirds of the total daily dose prior to breakfast and one-third of the total daily dose prior to the evening meal.

For All Diabetic Patients

If multiple daily doses of supplemental short-acting insulin are required to adequately control the blood glucose, the subsequent day's AM and PM insulin doses need to be appropriately increased. Patients recently recovering from DKA may have ongoing need for supplemental potassium and rarely magnesium and/or phosphorus. If this is the case, serum levels should be monitored while adjusting supplement doses. On hospital discharge, oral electrolyte supplementation may be required for 2 to 3 days.

If activity after hospital discharge is anticipated to be greater than while hospitalized, and if blood glucose is in good control just prior to discharge, the total daily insulin dose should be reduced by 10% to 20% at the time of discharge. If blood glucose concentrations are suboptimal just prior to discharge (i.e. 200 mg/dL or 11.1 mmol/L), maintain a similar total daily insulin dose at discharge.

Management of Patients with Predominant Insulin Resistance

Patients who still possess significant endogenous insulin secretion will be ketosis resistant because only a small concentration of insulin is required to inhibit the fatty acyl–carnitine cycle in

TABLE 98.5

SUGGESTED SUPPLEMENTAL DOSES FOR SHORT-ACTING INSULIN (E.G., HUMALOG, NOVOLOG)

Blood glucose (mg/dL)	Insulin dose (units)	
	Pubertal	Prepubertal ≥5 yr
<150	0	0
150–225	2	1
226–300	4	2
301–375	6	3
376–425	8	4
>425	10	5

Blood glucose (mg/dL)	Child/Infant <5 yr
<200	0
200–300	0.5
301–400	1.0
Over 400	1.5–2.0

Another method to determine a short-acting insulin dose: the correction bolus formula:

$$\text{Insulin Supplement} = \frac{\text{Current BG} - \text{Target BG}}{\text{ISF}}$$

where BG = blood glucose

ISF = insulin sensitivity factor (the effect of 1 unit of short-acting insulin on blood glucose)

$$\text{ISF} = \frac{1500}{\text{Total daily insulin}}$$ (1700 or 1800 would be the factors more appropriate for young children and infants, respectively)

the liver. Such patients require the same laboratory evaluation obtained for the patient with predominant insulin deficiency (Table 98.2). In particular, the pretreatment total insulin, C-peptide, creatinine, and liver chemistries are important baseline values in assessing efficacy of therapy. Insulin resistance is an endogenous mechanism by which excess calories are incompletely shuttled into adipose storage, resulting in hyperglycemia with glycosuria and urinary loss of calories. Ideally, the patient will normalize C-peptide and insulin values with effective diet, oral agents, and exercise without inappropriate weight gain. Although increasing insulin sensitivity is one of the goals in the treatment of all forms of diabetes, many oral hypoglycemic agents, with the exception of metformin, are associated with rapid weight gain as insulin resistance is reversed. By increasing insulin sensitivity in the absence of exercise or decreased caloric intake, excess glucose is converted to fat. Hence, the ideal strategy for those patients would be diet and exercise without medications. Unfortunately, these measures alone are insufficient in most patients and the clinician must weigh the benefit of improving insulin sensitivity with the possible side effect of inappropriate weight gain.

Oral Therapy for Mildly Hyperglycemic (HgbA1c < 6.5%), Nonketotic, Obese Children with Predominant Insulin Resistance

In such patients with only mild hyperglycemia (HbA1c 5.9–6.5%), the goal of therapy is to achieve euglycemia by increasing insulin sensitivity without weight gain. If peripheral tissue insulin sensitivity is increased, and the available exogenous caloric load remains the same, the patient will necessarily gain weight inappropriately. Metformin hydrochloride (Glucophage) reduces the endogenously generated caloric load by inhibiting hepatic glucose release. This met-

formin hydrochloride-induced decrease in circulating glucose allows better utilization of exogenously derived calories, thus increasing insulin sensitivity often without weight gain. For the mildly hyperglycemic patient (≥10 yr) with classic type 2 diabetes, we use oral metformin hydrochloride (Glucophage) 500 mg in the morning, in addition to recommending a restricted carbohydrate intake and regular cardiovascular exercise. The dosage may be incrementally increased to 2,000 mg/day with the long-acting formulation (Glucophage XR) to control glycemia. An additional advantage to using metformin hydrochloride is that it will usually not induce hypoglycemia as a single agent and may reduce appetite in the overweight patient. Metformin hydrochloride is primarily metabolized in the kidney, and patients should be screened to ensure they do not have a serum creatinine of greater than 1.2 mg/dL. Patients should also be advised that the medication should be discontinued 24 hours prior to any intravenous contrast dye studies and for 2 days afterward. Metformin should be used with caution in patients who are prone to diabetic ketoacidosis or lactic acidosis: fatal acidosis has been reported in adults.

Oral Therapy of Moderately Hyperglycemic (HbA1c 6.5–7.5%), Nonketotic, Obese Children with Predominant Insulin Resistance

These patients often will not initially be controlled on diet and metformin hydrochloride alone, although with maintenance of a carbohydrate-restricted diet, this may be adequate therapy. During the hospital admission, there are several oral medications that may be useful in combination with diet and metformin hydrochloride to induce normoglycemia (Table 98.6). Most of these agents do not have specific pediatric indications, because their FDA approval was pending at the time of this

TABLE 98.6

ORAL MEDICATIONS USED IN DIABETES

Classification	Medication
Biguanides	Metformin hydrochloride. Major effect is in potentiating the actions of insulin in decreasing hepatic glucose productions. Its use is usually associated with decreased appetite and weight loss.
Glucosidase inhibitors	Acarbose, miglitol. These agents decrease absorption of carbohydrates from the gastrointestinal tract, and hence decrease exogenous caloric uptake. As such, they are not associated with increased weight gain as with many of the other agents. There is little or no available experience in the use of this class of oral hypoglycemic agents in children.
Thiazolidinediones	Pioglitazone hydrochloride, rosiglitazone maleate. These agents appear to directly improve peripheral insulin sensitivity, and hence dramatically improve glucose uptake in peripheral tissues. If exogenous caloric intake is not reduced, the patient will gain excessive weight, compounding obesity issues.
Meglitinides	Repaglinide, nateglinide. This is a relatively new class of insulin secretagogues that depolarizes the pancreatic beta cell, resulting in increased insulin secretion. Repaglinide has the advantage of being very short acting and should be taken with each carbohydrate-containing meal. If the patient reduces dietary intake, repaglinide may be a useful agent, because the patient is not forced to "feed" a long-acting oral hypoglycemic agent. At the time of this writing, we are unaware of studies in children.
Sulfonylureas	Glimepiride, glipizide, glyburide. This is the oldest yet effective class of oral hypoglycemic agents, and the side effects in adults are well known.

writing. However, these medications have been used in pediatric patients with diabetes who have endogenous insulin potential and are not prone to ketoacidosis. As with insulins such as lispro and glargine, the clinician needs to evaluate the potential benefit compared to the potential risk. We are most concerned with the potential hepatic toxicity of many of these agents, and liver chemistries should be monitored prior to and during therapy in all children. Given the incomplete development of certain liver detoxification enzymes, we do not use these agents in any child under 10 years of age.

Therapy in Severely Hyperglycemic (HbA1c > 8.0%), Obese Children with Predominant Insulin Resistance

In patients with severe hyperglycemia, we generally do not begin oral agent therapy upon admission to the hospital. Therapy for such patients is best initiated using an insulin regimen similar to that outlined for the primarily insulin-deficient (classic type 1) diabetic. However, the usual daily insulin dosage ordinarily will be higher than that for the classic type 1 patient because of obesity/morbid obesity and concomitant marked insulin resistance. This is the case particularly if obese patients are ketotic, an indicator of increased circulating free fatty acids. Upon discharge from the hospital, normoglycemia may be achievable with diet, an exercise program, oral antihyperglycemic therapy, and daily insulin at a dose reduced from the inpatient requirement. Within weeks after hospital discharge, patients who are involved in regular cardiovascular exercise and maintain a healthy eating pattern may be able to discontinue insulin. Administration of glucagon is an alternative strategy. In time, oral agents may also be stopped, although we have found that only a minority of these diabetic children are able to achieve good glycemic control with diet and exercise alone.

Hypoglycemia

Readily available oral glucose gel (or honey, maple syrup, cake icing) should be available in all patient care areas in case of a hypoglycemic event. If the patient is unable to ingest orally secondary to severe neuroglycopenia with or without seizures, and IV access is not available, place the patient in a lateral recumbent position, draw the glucose gel into a syringe and release it onto the buccal mucosa, then massage from the outer cheek surface; this process should be repeated on the opposite side of the mouth. If intravenous access is present or readily obtainable, 2 mL/kg of $D_{25\%}W$ IV should be given for severe reactions. In the home setting, parents should be advised to place the nozzle of regular pancake syrup into the cheek and apply the syrup after the patient is on his/her side. The parents should be warned *not* to place the syrup at the back of the mouth (because this may result in aspiration) and should be educated that the sugar is directly absorbed through the oral mucosa. The cause of the episode should be identified and appropriate adjustments made to decrease the risk of recurrence.

ERRORS IN MANAGEMENT OF PATIENTS WITH DIABETES MELLITUS

- Managing DKA outside an intermediate or pediatric intensive-care unit, where there is the potential to provide adequate treatment, monitoring, nursing, and physician support.
- Failing to recognize that leg pain and/or limp, especially in obese, sedentary patients, may be a sign or symptom of

deep vein thrombosis; underlying conditions such as deficiency of protein S, protein C, antithrombin III, antiphospholipid syndrome, and factor V Leiden mutation should be considered.
- Failing to investigate for pulmonary edema or pulmonary embolus in the event of acute respiratory distress and/or development of an oxygen requirement.
- Prolonging correction of hyperglycemia over days.
- Failing to monitor serum potassium concentrations and/or high hemoglobin A1c values.
- Inadequate replacement of electrolytes, particularly potassium and magnesium even after DKA is resolved.
- Using actual body weight instead of ideal body weight when planning fluid therapy in obese patients.
- Failing to properly monitor for hypoglycemia.
- Failing to follow-up bedside glucose when short-acting insulin is given, particularly at night.
- Failing to adjust pre-breakfast and pre-supper insulin dosing on a shift-per-shift, day-to-day basis, especially when blood sugars are consistently outside the target range (i.e. 70 to 90 mg/dL [or 3.9 to 5 mmol/L] to 160 to 180 mg/dl [or 8.8 to 10 mmol/L]).
- Using oral antihyperglycemic agents instead of insulin in type 2 diabetics who have poor glycemic control.
- Failing to educate patients regarding contraindications to use of oral antihyperglycemic agents, such as metformin hydrochloride, prior to discharge on these medications.
- Failing to tailor treatment to the individual patient.
- Failing to take seriously and show respect for a nurse's or parent's concerns about a patient.

DISCHARGE CRITERIA AND INSTRUCTIONS

The following should be accomplished prior to discharge.
    Education about diabetes care such that the main caretakers and/or the older patient can:

- Understand the basic pathophysiology of diabetes mellitus.
- Properly check blood glucose.
- Know the differences between the various insulins prescribed.
- Measure insulin doses correctly.
- Inject insulin correctly including rotation of sites.
- Know the signs and symptoms of hyperglycemia.
- Outline the necessary treatment for hyperglycemia.
- Know the signs and symptoms of hypoglycemia.
- Outline the necessary treatment for hypoglycemia (with and without significant neurologic changes).
- Know the effect of exercise on blood glucose and have a plan for decreasing insulin for extra activity.
- Understand the importance of rotating sites of insulin injection.
- Know how to contact the appropriate medical personnel for problems.

Specific discharge instructions should include the following:

- Call in for the first few days after discharge to allow a member of the diabetes team to help evaluate blood glucose control and reinforce education.
- Check blood glucose 1:00 AM to 3:00 AM for the first day or two after discharge (in addition to usual checks) to rule out overnight hypoglycemia.
- Call at any time after discharge if blood sugars are consistently high or low. It is an urgent medical situation when high blood glucose is associated with vomiting, abdominal pain, and urinary ketones; this may be DKA.
- Sick day instructions: if vomiting and/or urinary ketones occur, contact the diabetes team. Blood glucose checks will

need to be done more frequently. Short-acting, sliding-scale insulin will likely be needed throughout the day.

- Inform the school about any newly diagnosed diabetic child.
- For severe hypoglycemic reactions or seizures, one or more of the following needs to be done:
  - Glucose gel administration to inner buccal mucosal.
  - Glucagon administration.
  - Notify parent or guardian.
  - Call 911.
  - Call to diabetes team or primary care physician; after a significant hypoglycemic reaction is treated, the cause of the episode needs to be identified so as to minimize potential recurrence.
- For suspected DKA (abdominal pain, vomiting, elevated urinary ketones, and hyperglycemia) the following needs to be done:
  - Notify the diabetes team and/or primary care physician.
  - Notify the parent or guardian.
  - 911 may need to be called.
  - Immediate subcutaneous short-acting insulin administration if available (according to supplemental dosing).

- Written discharge instructions should be given to the family with a copy for the diabetes team.
- Keep the primary care physician informed.

Suggested Readings

Diabetes Prevention Program Research Group. Reduction in the incidence of type 2 diabetes with lifestyle intervention or metformin. *N Engl J Med* 2002;346:393–403.

Hathout EH, Thomas W, El-Shahawy M, et al. Diabetic autoimmune markers in children and adolescents with type 2 diabetes. *Pediatrics* 2001;107:e102.

McGarry JD. Dysregulation of fatty acid metabolism in the etiology of type 2 diabetes (Banting lecture 2001). *Diabetes* 2002;51:7–18.

Ranjana S, Fisch G, Teague B, et al. Prevalence of impaired glucose tolerance among children and adolescents with marked obesity. *N Engl J Med* 2002;346:802–855.

Silverstein J, Klingensmith G, Copeland K, et al. Care of children and adolescents with type 1 diabetes. A statement of the American Diabetes Association. *Diabetes Care* 2005;28:186–212.

Sperling M, ed. Diabetes mellitus in children. *Pediatr Clin North Am* 2005;52:1533–1804.

Steinberger J. Insulin resistance and cardiovascular risk in the pediatric patient. *Prog Pediatr Cardiol* 2001;12:169–175.

GLENN D. HARRIS AND IRMA FIORDALISI

Diabetic ketoacidosis/acidemia (DKA) is a unique metabolic derangement caused by absolute or relative insulin deficiency with varying degrees of insulin resistance, counterregulatory hormone excess, and resultant severe cellular starvation. When blood pH is relatively preserved (pH $\geq$ 7.30), we use the term *ketoacidosis*; when decompensation occurs (blood pH < 7.30), the term *ketoacidemia* applies. In the pediatric patient, DKA is also associated with varying degrees of systemic hypertonic dehydration and brain swelling.

Normally, insulin inhibits the secretion of glucagon, the release of free fatty acids (FFA) from fat cells, and ketogenesis. Insulin deficiency coupled with glucagon excess (Fig. 99.1) promotes glycogenolysis, proteolysis, and lipolysis with delivery of large amounts of FFA to the liver where they are converted to acetoacetate and B-hydroxybutyrate (ketone bodies) via the fatty acid–acyl CoA–carnitine palmitoyltransferase cycle in hepatic mitrochondria. A surge of catecholamine, cortisol, and growth hormone ensues resulting in gluconeogenesis, further lipolysis, and ketogenesis. Ketoacids cause metabolic acidosis (decreased total carbon dioxide, tCO_2) and create an increased anion gap. Initially, compensatory hyperventilation preserves a normal blood pH despite metabolic acidosis. If untreated, a decrease in blood pH (ketoacidemia) ensues.

Unless appropriate insulin replacement therapy and fluids are instituted in a timely fashion to inhibit ketoacid production, DKA progresses. Death may result from complications such as prolonged acidemia, dehydration, electrolyte disturbances, and/or brain herniation. Inciting problems, and complicating conditions or illnesses such as infection, an acute abdomen, pregnancy, or illicit drug use, should be ruled out and addressed as indicated. Noncompliance with insulin therapy and/or oral antihyperglycemic agents is the most frequent cause of DKA in children. The key to treating DKA is early provision of adequate doses of regular human insulin by continuous intravenous infusion in conjunction with appropriate monitoring and fluid and electrolyte management; infection and other precipitants that require definitive therapy should be identified and treated aggressively.

Diabetic ketoacidemia may be characterized and defined on a biochemical and clinical spectrum from very severe to minimal on the basis of both degree of depression of measured tCO_2, elevation of anion gap, elevation of serum glucose, changes in mental status, and whether shock or other complicating problems are present. Traditionally, a measured tCO_2 less than 15 mmol/L, or less than or equal to 15 mmol/L, is the defining characteristic of DKA; however, all factors need to be considered. When ketosis is present in the setting of diabetes,

whether the tCO_2 is 14 or 16 mmol/L, DKA is present, however mild its degree.

DIFFERENTIAL DIAGNOSIS

- Gastroenteritis with stress hyperglycemia and ketosis
- Starvation
- Pneumonia/primary respiratory disease
- Hypernatremic dehydration
- Hyperosmolar nonketotic coma (hyperglycemic hyperosmolar state)
- Salicylate poisoning
- Branched-chain organic acidurias
- Alcoholic ketoacidosis
- Defects in ketolysis
- Sepsis/septic shock

CLINICAL FINDINGS

Classic history includes polyuria, polydipsia, polyphagia, weight loss, vomiting, abdominal discomfort, and often a fruity odor (ketones) on the breath. As the disease progresses, hyperventilation becomes apparent, and the mental status may become altered as dehydration, acidemia, and possibly brain swelling become more severe. In the earlier stages of DKA (mild to moderate), and particularly in previously undiagnosed diabetics, the history may be nonspecific, with complaints of lethargy and weight loss; polyuria and polydipsia may escape notice or be attributed to environmental or emotional causes. Hyperventilation may be clinically imperceptible until the kP_aCO_2 is very low. A high index of suspicion is required to make the diagnosis before DKA becomes severe. A history of weight loss, vomiting, and/or dehydration, particularly without diarrhea or fever, should prompt an evaluation for DKA.

The physical examination demonstrates a spectrum from normovolemia to severe dehydration. Dry mouth is common in the presence of Kussmaul breathing (an increase in ventilation, particularly in tidal volume) and should not be used to gauge the degree of dehydration. The volume of deficit should be estimated based on the clinical and biochemical measures summarized in Table 99.1. Other findings may include altered mental status, fruity odor of the breath, mucocutaneous candidiasis, or other infections. Note that DKA is characterized by a ketoacidosis, not a lactic acidosis; serum lactate concentrations are typically normal or only mildly elevated in patients with DKA.

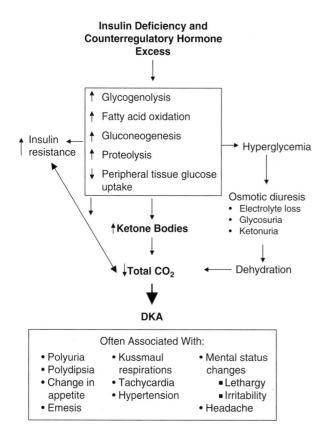

Insulin Deficiency and Counterregulatory Hormone Excess

↑ Glycogenolysis
↑ Fatty acid oxidation
↑ Gluconeogenesis
↑ Proteolysis
↓ Peripheral tissue glucose uptake

↑ Insulin resistance

→ Hyperglycemia

Osmotic diuresis
• Electrolyte loss
• Glycosuria
• Ketonuria

↑Ketone Bodies

↓Total CO_2 ← Dehydration

DKA

Often Associated With:
• Polyuria   • Kussmaul   • Mental status
• Polydipsia   respirations   changes
• Change in   • Tachycardia   ▪ Lethargy
  appetite   • Hypertension   ▪ Irritability
• Emesis   • Headache

FIGURE 99.1.

LABORATORY FINDINGS

Primary disturbances:

- Hyperglycemia
- Glycosuria
- Ketonemia
- Ketonuria
- Metabolic acidosis/acidemia
- Compensatory hypocarbia

Secondary disturbances:

- Apparent hyponatremia ("pseudohyponatremia")
- Hyponatremia or hypernatremia
- Hypokalemia or hyperkalemia
- Hypophosphatemia
- Hypomagnesemia
- Hyperamylasemia
- Increased serum urea nitrogen (SUN)
- Increased serum creatinine (may be artifactual due to cross-reactivity with ketones)

MANAGEMENT PRINCIPLES

Because DKA is a hypertonic dehydration associated with brain swelling, the objective of treatment is to progressively correct ketoacidosis/acidemia while appropriately and gradually rehydrating the patient to minimize exacerbation of brain swelling. When shock is present, it should be corrected within the first hour of therapy. The remainder of the deficit should be replaced evenly over the next 48 hours using a balanced sodium salt solution containing approximately 125 mmol/L Na⁺ plus potassium for the child and adolescent, and 100 mmol/L Na⁺ plus potassium for the infant. Although this plan suggests that rehydration will take 2 days to accomplish, patients are typically clinically rehydrated within the first 6 to 18 hours of IV therapy. By that time, DKA is resolved in the great majority of patients who are then ready for subcutaneous insulin and an appropriate diet. Any remaining intracellular fluid deficits will stimulate thirst and will be replenished by oral intake (Table 99.2).

Monitoring is essential to successful management of DKA. Pediatric patients in DKA are best monitored in an intermediate or intensive-care setting. The following factors should always be taken into consideration.

Mental Status

- If normal at presentation, mental status should remain normal. The neurologic status should be assessed at least hourly.
- If initially altered, it should improve with treatment.
- If initially normal, but deterioration occurs during treatment, urgent evaluation is indicated (see "Altered Mental Status during Treatment for DKA" later in the chapter).

Peripheral Perfusion

- If peripheral perfusion is normal at presentation, it should remain normal.
- If initially poor, peripheral pulses should improve before the end of the first hour.
- Severe ketoacidemia causes vasoconstriction; cold feet should warm with adequate emergency-phase fluids and as insulin effects improvement in ketoacidemia.

Vital Signs

- Tachycardia should improve progressively, but in severe acidemia, some degree of tachycardia will persist (even after adequate volume resuscitation) until ketoacidemia is largely corrected.
- Blood pressure should be normalized within the first minutes of treatment if low at the outset.
- Subnormal body temperature is common in moderate to severe DKA and usually normalizes with adequate insulin administration in the first few hours of treatment.
- Kussmaul respirations may take many hours to abate. This is acceptable so long as the base deficit is improving.

Laboratory Trends

Blood gases should be obtained hourly until an effective dose of insulin is established (i.e., the base deficit is improving by at least 1 mmol/L/hr). In severely ill patients, blood gases should be arterial, which are best obtained via an indwelling arterial catheter. For less severely ill patients, a freely flowing venous blood gas to monitor the correction of the base deficit should suffice. For moderate to severely ill patients, electrolytes with measured tCO_2, urea nitrogen, and creatinine should be measured at least every 2 hours. Glucose should be measured hourly when the patient is receiving IV insulin. Maintenance of a flow sheet for laboratory data is essential to assist with monitoring of biochemical and clinical data (Table 99.3).

Correct the measured concentration of serum sodium for the presence of hyperglycemia. The measured concentration of sodium in serum is decreased during hyperglycemia because glucose molecules occupy space in the serum and cause movement of water by their osmotic force.

The *predicted* serum sodium concentration may be calculated as follows. The serum sodium is decreased by 1.6 mmol/L

TABLE 99.1

GUIDELINES FOR ESTIMATING VOLUME OF DEFICIT (DEGREE OF DEHYDRATION) IN DKA

Guidelines measures	Degree of dehydration		
	Mild	Moderate	Severe
Volume of deficit (ml/kg)[a]			
≥2 yr old	30	60	90
<2 yr old	50	100	150
Clinical measures			
Peripheral perfusion			
Palpation of peripheral pulses (pulse volume)	Normal	Normal to decreased	Decreased to absent
Capillary refill time (sec)	<2	<3	≥3
Skin temperature (tactile)	Normal	Normal to cool	Cool
Heart rate	Normal to mildly increased	Moderately increased	Moderately to severely increased
Blood pressure	Normal	Normal to mildly increased	Decreased to moderately increased
Biochemical measures in serum mmol/L (mg/dl)			
Urea nitrogen	Normal to mildly increased; e.g., 7.14 (<20)	Mildly increased; e.g., 7.14–8.9 (20–25)	Moderately to severely increased; e.g., ≥9 (≥25)
Predicted Na$^+$	Usually normal	Usually normal	Normal to increased
Glucose	Mildly increased; e.g., 22.2 (400)	Moderately increased; e.g., 33.3 (600)	Severely increased; e.g., 44.4 (800)

[a]Use ideal body weight for obese patients. From Fiordalisi I, Harris GD. Diabetic ketoacidemia. In: Finberg L, Kleinman R, eds. *Saunders manual of pediatric practice*. 2nd ed. Philadelphia: Saunders; 2002;117, with permission.

for every 5.6 mmol/L (100 mg/dL) of glucose over 5.6 mmol/L (100 mg/dL).

Supplementation of Potassium, Magnesium, and Phosphorus

Generally, supplementation of these ions should be given IV until DKA is largely corrected (tCO$_2$ ≥ 15 mmol/L and/or until the anion gap normalizes). After the patient is ready for oral intake, supplementation may be given by mouth. Chronically poorly controlled patients may present with severe ion depletion and require not only IV electrolyte supplements during rehydration but often need additional oral supplementation after recovery from DKA.

Altered Mental Status during Treatment for DKA

Any deterioration in mental status, development of focal neurologic signs, or change in vital signs, such as (relative) bradycardia and/or hypertension, should suggest the possibility of raised intracranial pressure (ICP) and should be treated expectantly with hypertonic mannitol (0.5 to 1 g/kg IV over 15 minutes), assisted ventilation with hyperventilation when indicated, and a reassessment of the volume status and rate of fluid delivery. There may also be a role for the use of hypertonic saline in this setting. New complaints of headache or emesis should be assessed with the possibility of raised ICP as a cause. If raised ICP is suspected, head computed tomography (CT) scans, which may not be sufficiently sensitive to identify clinically significant swelling, should not delay definitive therapy. If tracheal intubation is required, intubation strategies for patients with raised ICP should be used. Patients with severe DKA often have profound compensatory hypocarbia in response to

extreme metabolic acidemia. If intubation is required, continued hyperventilation should be maintained to approximate the physiologic response and avoid further precipitous declines in blood and central nervous system pH.

Signs and Symptoms Suggestive of Increased Intracranial Pressure

Altered mental status (e.g. lethargy, irritability, combativeness, coma)
Diminished pupillary response to light
Anisocoria
Hypertension (with or without bradycardia)
Relative bradycardia (e.g., normal heart rate despite acidemia)
Recurrent or new-onset vomiting during treatment
Headache
Cushing's triad (hypertension, bradycardia, irregular respiration)
Seizures

Points to Remember in the Management of Pediatric DKA

- Making the diagnosis
  - Obtain adequate history; do not assume polyuria and polydipsia are always among the complaints.
  - Recognize that:
    - Nonspecific signs and symptoms, such as weight loss, vaginal or perineal candidiasis, and generalized malaise, may indicate DKA or uncontrolled diabetes.
    - Emesis, usually without diarrhea or fever, may be DKA and not gastroenteritis.

TABLE 99.2

MANAGEMENT OF DIABETIC KETOACIDEMIA

Address the following	Interventions
Airway, breathing, circulation	Provide 100% oxygen if shock is present Assist ventilation if needed Establish two peripheral IVs
If peripheral perfusion is not normal	Treat shock with 10–20 mL/kg aliquots of 0.9% NaCl or lactated Ringer solution (LR). If more than 20 mL/kg needed, consider 5% albumin in 5–10 mL/kg aliquots
If peripheral perfusion is normal	0.9% NaCl or LR 5 mL/kg/hr pending laboratory results
Measure glucose, blood gases, serum electrolytes, urea nitrogen, creatinine; complete blood count; urinalysis Weigh the patient	Estimate the degree of dehydration (Table 99.1) Emaciated patients >2 yr follow more closely; a 5%, 10%, 15% deficit for mild, moderate and severe degrees of dehydration, respectively
Insulin dosing	By end of first hour: start regular insulin 0.1 U/kg/hr by continuous infusion. Use *actual* body weight for all patients
CHOOSING A REHYDRATION SOLUTION <2 yr	NaCl 75 mmol/L (or 0.45% NaCl) plus $NaHCO_3$ 25 mmol/L plus K^+ acetate 20 mmol/L plus K^+ phosphate 20 mmol/L
>2 yr	(1) NaCl 100 mmol/L plus $NaHCO_3$ 25 mmol/L plus K^+ acetate 20 mmol/L plus K^+ phosphate 20 mmol/L *OR* (2) LR plus K^+ 40 mmol/L (as KCI or 20 mmol/L KCI + 20 mmol/L K + phosphate)
For glucose >300 For glucose ≤300	Above electrolytes in sterile water Above electrolytes in D5W
Calculate maintenance needs	Give approximately 30% more than the usual maintenance allotment for hyperventilation ($kP_aCO_2 ≤ 4$; $P_aCO_2 ≤ 30$ mm Hg) Decrease to normal maintenance once hyperventilation resolves
Calculate the volume of deficit	For obese patients use *ideal* body weight for all fluid and electrolyte calculations. Subtract any emergency resuscitation fluid given and plan to give the remainder evenly over the next 48 hr
After the first 12–18 hr of therapy	Decrease the concentration of sodium in the rehydration solution to approximately: >2 yr: 75 mmol/L; ≤2 yr: 50 mmol/L. Continue glucose and potassium as needed

INSULIN DOSING

The initial dose is 0.1 U/kg/hr. The insulin infusion may be prepared by mixing 1 unit of regular human insulin per mL 0.9% NaCl. The solution should be rinsed through any plastic connection tubing prior to infusion into the patient. If the initial glucose is ≤16.7 mmol/L (≤300 mg/dL), give glucose in the rehydration solution (e.g., D_5LR plus potassium) to permit administration of an adequate dose of insulin. The goal is improvement in the base deficit by at least 1 mmol/L/hr as calculated from blood gases. Failure to observe such a decrease in the base deficit signals insufficient insulin delivery; the insulin dose should be increased by 50 to 100% (e.g., from 0.1 U/kg/hr to 0.2 units/kg/hr, etc.) every hour until the expected improvement in the base deficit occurs. Note that the insulin dose is determined by the progress of the base deficit, *not* solely by the concentration of serum glucose. If the serum glucose concentration is <13.9 mmol/L (>250 mg/dL) and an increase in insulin is warranted by failure of the base deficit to improve, glucose delivery should be increased. For example, if the patient is already receiving D_5 LR plus potassium, change to D_{10} LR plus potassium. Occasionally, 12% or 15% dextrose-containing solutions are needed, the latter requiring central venous access.

- A patient with labored breathing, clear breath sounds, and no oxygen requirement may have Kussmaul respirations.
- Drug ingestion, pregnancy, and/or depression may be a trigger for DKA.
- Do not assume that parched oral mucosa indicates severe dehydration; Kussmaul respirations cause dry oral mucosa independent of the degree of systemic dehydration.
- Weight loss over a period of greater than 24 to 36 hours should not be attributed entirely to dehydration.
- Hourly deep intramuscular insulin injection of 0.1 units/kg is far superior to intermittent IV "pushes" of insulin when continuous IV infusion of insulin is not possible.
- A normal or nearly normal blood glucose in the continued presence of DKA requires an additional supply of dextrose in IV fluid to permit administration of adequate doses of insulin, and not simply a decrease in insulin dose.
- Recognize that the planned desired fluid rate should include all fluids administered (i.e., potassium supplementation, medications, insulin).
- For the obese patient, fluid volume is based on *ideal*, not actual body weight, but the insulin dose is based on actual weight.
- When appropriate maintenance and deficit volumes are administered, mL per mL of urine output replacement will always result in fluid overload.
- Neurotropic antiemetics, such as promethazine hydrochloride (Phenergan) to treat vomiting, may cause drowsiness and mask the mental status evaluation; vomiting caused by ketoacidosis will resolve with administration of adequate

TABLE 99.3

MONITORING OF BIOCHEMICAL DATA

Biochemical measure	Expected trend
■ Blood pH (arterial)	■ Should increase by at least 0.02–0.03 pH U/hr
■ Base deficit	■ Should improve by at least 1 mmol/L/hr
■ Measured tCO_2	■ May transiently decrease or lag behind improvement in blood pH and base deficit during the first few hours of therapy
■ Serum glucose concentration	■ Should decline by 2.8–5.6 mmol/L/hr (50–100 mg/dL/hr)
■ Serum sodium concentration	■ Should increase by 1–2 mmol/L for each 2.8–5.6 mmol/L (50–100 mg/dL) decrease in serum glucose concentration ■ Failure of the serum Na to rise appropriately requires a decrease in the rate of fluid administration (*not* an increase in salt delivery) An excessive increase in serum sodium concentration (e.g., >2 mmol/L per 5.6 mmol/L [100 mg/dL] decrease in glucose concentration) generally requires an increase in the rate of fluid delivery; if the predicted sodium is in the hypernatremic range, a decrease in the concentration of sodium in the rehydration solution may be required
■ Serum urea nitrogen (SUN)	■ Should progressively decline with therapy; if SUN fails to decrease, consider an increase in fluid delivery or rarely, renal insufficiency
■ Serum potassium	■ Should be maintained in normal range throughout treatment; potassium declines with institution of insulin and with correction of acidosis/acidemia; anticipatory supplementation should occur with these dynamics in mind
■ Serum magnesium	■ May be low either at outset or during rehydration ■ Serum magnesium should be followed at regular intervals (e.g., every 4 to 8 hours) depending on the severity of illness; provide supplementation as needed
■ Serum phosphorus	■ Usually decreases during treatment; severely ill patients commonly require phosphorus supplementation in addition to the usual K^+ phosphate 20 mmol/L in the rehydration solution

doses of IV insulin. If vomiting persists despite improvement of DKA, other causes should be considered.

Transition from IV Insulin and Fluids to SC Insulin and Oral Intake

The timing of this transition depends to some extent on practical issues (e.g., the time of day DKA is resolved) and the type of subcutaneous (SC) insulin regimen planned. For example, if DKA is resolved at 3:00 AM, we generally continue IV insulin until breakfast, giving the morning long-acting and short-acting insulin at the usual time; alternatively, regular human insulin may be given at 3:00 AM to "cover" the patient until the usual morning dose can be given. If SC regular human insulin is chosen to bridge the gap between continuous IV insulin and initiation of the long-acting insulin, the IV insulin infusion should continue for an appropriate period of time *after* the SC dose to permit enough time for the SC dose to be absorbed and effective. If insulin glargine is to be used, a

patient in DKA who presents anytime during the day may be a candidate for a late afternoon or evening dose of this long-acting insulin, which facilitates the tapering and discontinuation of IV insulin once DKA is largely corrected.

Guidelines

1. For the older child or adolescent, insulin should be given before the meal; for the infant or young child, insulin can be given just after the meal (to assure having eaten).
2. Once eating has commenced, glucose-containing IV fluids are discontinued. Hourly blood glucose should continue to be monitored as long as IV insulin is infusing.
3. Intravenous insulin should be discontinued about 1 to 2 hours after a short-acting SC dose of insulin is given. If blood glucose is relatively low at mealtime (i.e., less than 5.6 mmol/L or 100 mg/dL), the IV insulin should be discontinued by approximately one-half hour after the meal is ingested. After IV insulin is discontinued, bedside blood glucose checks are usually done every 2 to 4 hours.

4. For the patient newly recovered from DKA, our practice is to check blood glucose prior to meals, midafternoon, at bedtime, and at 2:00 AM to best assess insulin requirements.

5. If supplemental insulin is required at bedtime or later in the night, a bedside blood glucose should be checked 1.5 to 2 hours after a dose of fast-acting (Humalog or Novolog) insulin or approximately 3 hours after a dose of regular human insulin.

6. The objective of insulin therapy (along with appropriate diet and exercise) is to achieve a fasting blood glucose in the range of 3.3 to 6 mmol/L (60 to 110 mg/dL) and up to 8.3 to 9.4 mmol/L (150 to 170 mg/dL) at other times so that the eventual HbA1c value will approximate the nondiabetic range. In the young child, the goal is more often a range of 4.4 to 11 mmol/L (80–200 mg/dL).

7. Education by the diabetes team, including a nurse educator and nutritionist, should be provided throughout the hospitalization.

SUMMARY

The repair of DKA is dynamic process that requires an understanding of its pathophysiology and an appreciation for the issues surrounding fluid and electrolyte therapy in patients with hypertonic dehydration and brain swelling. Through education of patients and families and improved methods of insulin delivery, prevention of this life-threatening disorder should become increasingly achievable. When DKA does occur, appropriate monitoring, a physiologic approach to rehydration with aggressive delivery of adequate doses of insulin, and attention to associated illnesses, minimizes the risk of death from a multitude of causes including brain swelling and herniation.

Suggested Readings

Glaser NS, Wootton-Gorges SL, Buonocore MH, et al. Frequency of sub-clinical cerebral edema in children with diabetic ketoacidosis. *Pediatr Diabetes* 2006;7:75–80.

Harris GD, Fiordalisi I. Physiologic management of diabetic ketoacidemia: a 5-year prospective pediatric experience in 231 episodes. *Arch Pediatr Adolesc Med* 1994;148:1046–1052.

Harris GD, Fiordalisi I, Harris WL, et al. Minimizing the risk of brain herniation during treatment of diabetic ketoacidemia: a retrospective and prospective study. *J Pediatr* 1990;117:22–31.

Harris GD, Fiordalisi I, Yu C. Maintaining normal intracranial pressure in a rabbit model during treatment of severe diabetic ketoacidemia. *Life Sci* 1996;59:1695–1702.

Sperling M. Cerebral edema in diabetic ketoacidosis: an underestimated complication? *Pediatr Diabetes* 2006;7:73–74.

Sperling M, Dunger D, Acerini C, et al. ESPE / LWPES consensus statement on diabetic ketoacidosis in children and adolescents. *Pediatrics* 2003;113: e133–e40.

CHAPTER 100 ■ DIABETES INSIPIDUS

YING T. CHANG

Diabetes (excessive urine) insipidus (lacking flavor) (DI) is caused by the inability of the kidneys to conserve water due to an antidiuretic hormone (ADH) deficiency or resistance, leading to a large volume of diluted urine. The consequence is a reduced body fluid volume, which stimulates thirst and increases fluid intake to compensate dehydration. However, if free water intake is inadequate, hypovolemic hyperosmotic dehydration follows.

Vasopressin (VP), the ADH of most vertebrates, is synthesized in neurons located in the supraoptic and paraventricular nuclei of the anterior hypothalamus. The peptide is subsequently transported along the axons of these cells to the infundibulum and the posterior pituitary, where it is released into circulation. On the basolateral membrane of the collecting duct epithelium in the kidney, VP binds to G-protein–coupled vasopressin receptor-2 (V2-R), which generates cAMP and activates protein kinase-A, and then leads to the synthesis and assembly of aquaporin-2 (AQP2) into tetrameric water channels on the luminal membrane. Water in the collecting duct lumen passes through AQP2 into the tubular cell, and moves to the interstitial side. The higher concentration gradient in the medulla interstitium absorbs water into the interstitium via aquaporin-4 channels on the cell membrane.

REGULATION OF VASOPRESSIN RELEASE

Vasopressin is released in response to increased plasma osmolality, decreased blood pressure, or reduced blood volume. Several factors affect the secretion of VP. Among them, hypovolemia, hyperosmolality, cerebral disease, adrenal insufficiency, angiotensin II, nicotine, and upright position increase VP secretion. On the other hand, hypervolemia, hypo-osmolality, alcohol, and recumbent position decrease VP secretion.

Hypothalamic Osmoreceptor

The osmoreceptor is the most potent regulator of VP secretion. There is a strong correlation between plasma osmolality and plasma VP concentration. In a group of healthy adults, when plasma osmolality rises above 284 mOsm/kg, plasma VP level increases. This osmotic threshold for VP release lies between 275 and 290 mOsmo/kg. The plasma VP concentration in normal adults is 2.2 to 4.0 pg/mL for a serum osmolality of less than 285 mOsm/kg. The VP concentration rises approximately 1 pg/mL for every 1% increase of plasma osmolality above the set point.

Arterial Baroreceptor and Left Atrial Stretch Receptor

Plasma VP concentrations are more sensitive to changes in plasma osmolality than to changes in blood pressure or volume. The release of VP mediated by the arterial baroreceptor is sluggish when there is a minor change in blood pressure. However, plasma VP level increases exponentially when arterial blood pressure reduces by 8% (5–10%), presumably in part by decreasing tonic inhibitory impulses from the left atrial stretch receptors to the hypothalamus. VP level rises rapidly during pronounced alteration in blood volume, such as in acute hemorrhage.

Miscellaneous Regulating Factors

Nausea and vomiting raise plasma VP levels to more than 100 times those seen in ordinary circumstances. Emotional and physical stress stimulates VP secretion in regions of the forebrain. Pain, cold, hypoxia, and pharyngeal stimulation also increase VP release.

ETIOLOGIES AND CLASSIFICATION OF DIABETES INSIPIDUS

Diabetes insipidus may be divided into three categories (Table 100.1).

1. Deficiency of VP—pituitary diabetes insipidus (PDI). Other terminology includes hypothalamic DI, central DI, or vasopressin deficiency DI.
2. Renal resistance (or insensitivity) to VP—N diabetes insipidus (NDI).
3. Excessive water intake due to defects in the osmoregulation or psychiatric disorders—primary polydipsia (PP).

The most common type is pituitary DI due to a deficiency of VP-producing neurons from hypothalamic–neurohypophyseal regions, such as midline defect (or septo-optic dysplasia), holoprosencephaly, brain tumors (particularly surgical removal of a craniopharyngioma), or histiocytosis. The deficiency of VP is not necessarily absolute. Most patients have detectable plasma VP concentrations, but the levels are inappropriately low with respect to the concomitant plasma osmolalities.

When there is insufficient VP to stimulate the generation and assembly of AQP2 tetramer into water channels, water reabsorption in the renal collecting duct is decreased, resulting in large volumes of very diluted urine. Decreased body water slightly raises plasma osmolality and sodium concentration, which in turn stimulates thirst and water intake and prevents further dehydration in adults and children. However, in infants or incapacitated subjects who do not have access to water, severe hyperosmotic hypernatremic dehydration ensues.

The most common form of NDI results from defects of vasopressin receptor-2 (V2R) in collecting duct cells—either VP cannot bind to V2R appropriately, or the binding of VP and V2R

TABLE 100.1

ETIOLOGY OF DIABETES INSIPIDUS

1. Pituitary (hypothalamic)
   a. Genetic
      i. DIDMOAD (diabetes insipidus, diabetes mellitus, optic atrophy, deafness) syndrome, or Wolfram syndrome
      ii. Vasopressin-neurophysin gene (autosomal dominant and recessive)
      iii. Chromosome Xq28
   b. Congenital
      i. Midline craniofacial defects (septo-optic dysplasia)
      ii. Pituitary hypoplasia
      iii. Holoprosencephaly
   c. Acquired
      i. Trauma
      ii. Neoplasms: carniopharyngioma, pinealoma, germinoma, pituitary macroadenoma, meningioma
      iii. Granuloma: histiocytosis, sarcoidosis
      iv. Infection/inflammation: meningitis, encephalitis, toxoplasmosis, infundibuloneurohypophysitis, Guillain–Barre syndrome, vasopressin neuron antibodies
      v. Vascular: aneurysm, infaction, Sheehan syndrome, sickle-cell disease
   d. Idiopathic
2. Nephrogenic
   a. Genetic
      i. Vasopressin receptor-2 gene (X-linked recessive)
      ii. Aquaporin-2 gene (autosomal dominant and recessive)
   b. Acquired
      i. Renal: polycystic kidneys, obstructive uropathy
      ii. Metabolic: hypercalcemia, hypokalemia
      iii. Drugs: lithium, demeclocycline, cisplatin, rifampin, amphotericin B, dexamethasone, dopamine, ifosfamide, ofloxacin, orlistat
      iv. Granulomas: neurosarcoid, amyloidosis
   c. Idiopathic
3. Primary polydipsia
   a. Dipsogenic (abnormal thirst)
      i. Granulomas: neurosarcoid
      ii. Infection: tuberculosis meningitis
      iii. Trauma
      iv. Demyelination: multiple sclerosis
      v. Drug: lithium, alcohol
   b. Psychogenic (compulsive water drinking)
      i. Schizophrenia
      ii. Obsessive-compulsive disorders
   c. Idiopathic

does not initiate an appropriate signal transduction cascade. The V2R gene is located in chromosome Xq28. Because NDI is an X-linked recessive disorder, males inheriting the mutation have DI symptoms, whereas female carriers usually do not. The resultant dehydration is the same as that in PDI.

In primary polydipsia, excessive water intake slightly decreases the plasma osmolality and sodium concentration, and therefore inhibits the secretion of VP, which in turn causes diuresis and restores plasma osmolality. Subjects with dipsogenic primary polydipsia have a lower set-point of thirst; hence they feel thirsty at a lower plasma osmolality than that of normal people.

CLINICAL PRESENTATION

Infants with DI may present with constant crying, failure to thrive, vomiting, constipation, fever, hypotonic, coma, seizure, or mental retardation. Infants with PDI may also present with other neurologic manifestations including headache, nystagmus, limitation of visual field, anterior pituitary deficiency (such as growth hormone deficiency or ACTH deficiency), or craniofacial dysmorphysm. In infants, DI may not be recognized until laboratory tests for other purposes identify hypernatremia, hyperkalemia, or hyperchloremia.

Children with DI usually present with polyuria and polydipsia. A previously toilet-trained child may start bedwetting again. Almost all children with DI require water during the night, which causes sleep disturbance and tiredness during the daytime. A child may drink several liters of fluid a day. If access to water is denied, children become inconsolable and may develop dehydration rapidly. Food consumption often is decreased. Linear growth and weight gain are slow as well.

In children with DI, urine volume exceeds the normal upper limit of 150 mL/kg/day. Urine osmolality is less than 300 mOsm/kg, and often remains less than 150 mOsm/kg. Specific gravity is usually less than 1.005. Urine glucose is negative, as opposed to diabetes mellitus. Under ad libitum fluid intake, if the urine volume, osmolality, and creatinine of a 24-hour collection are normal for age, the child is unlikely to have DI unless it is masked by a concomitant adrenal insufficiency or adipsic hypernatremia. In these situations, correct the cortisol deficiency or provide water, and then repeat 24-hour urine collection.

WATER DEPRIVATION TEST

Water deprivation tests can be used to diagnose DI. The response to vasopressin at the end of the deprivation can help to differentiate PDI from NDI. The test requires careful supervision because dehydration and hypernatremia may occur. In addition, the patient must be monitored carefully to ensure that fluids are not ingested during the test (especially when the patient is using a bathroom for urine collection). In a patient having hypernatremia, the water deprivation test is not indicated.

Procedure

1. Begin the test in the morning after a 24-hour period of adequate hydration. Breakfast is withheld.
2. Collect baseline urine and blood for osmolality and electrolytes. Weigh the patient.
3. Restrict fluid intake for 4 hours for infants and 7 hours for children.
4. Measure body weight, urine specific gravity, and volume hourly.
5. Check serum osmolality and sodium and urine osmolality every 2 hours.
6. Terminate the test if weight loss approaches 5%, or if the specific gravity is greater than 1.014.
7. Obtain appropriate urine specimens for osmolality and blood for sodium, osmolality, and vasopressin when the test is complete.

Interpretation

Normal:

- Urine osmolality between 500 and 1400 mOsm/kg (some authors use >450 mOsm/kg or >400 mOsm/kg as a cutoff).
- Plasma osmolality range is between 288 and 291 mOsm/kg all the time.

- Urine specific gravity rises to at least 1.010 (or >1.015 per some authors).
- Urine osmolality: plasma osmolality ratio >2 (or >1.5 per some authors).
- Urine volume decreases significantly and there is no significant weight loss.

Diabetes insipidus (pituitary or nephrogenic):

- Urine osmolality <150 mOsm/kg.
- No significant reduction of urine volume.
- Weight loss up to 5% usually occurs.
- Serum osmolality >290 mOsm/kg.
- Serum Na >150 mEq/L.
- If plasma osmolality reaches 300 mOsmol/kg and/or plasma Na reaches 146 mEq/L, but urine is still not concentrated, then the patient has severe PDI or severe NDI, and does not have partial DI or primary polydipsia.

VASOPRESSIN TEST

The vasopressin test can be given at the end of 4-hour or 7-hour water deprivation test.

Procedure

1. Measure urine osmolality before injection of vasopressin (can use the results given at the end of water deprivation test).
2. Inject aqueous arginine vasopressin (Pitressin) 1 to 2 units, IM or SC.
3. Measure urine osmolality 1 to 2 hours later.

Interpretation

- If the urine osmolality increases by more than 50%, PDI is almost certain even though the maximum level achieved may still be subnormal due to the temporary defect in renal concentrating capacity caused by a chronic VP deficiency.
- If a rise in urine osmolality is less than 50%, this usually indicates NDI.

BRAIN MRI

In most patients with PDI, the bright spot of the posterior pituitary gland is abnormally small on a T1-weighted MRI image. In contrast, this bright spot is present in 80% to 90% of patients with primary polydipsia.

MANAGEMENT

1. Correction of dehydration
   a. Treatment for hypertonic dehydration depends on the degree of dehydration.
   b. Stabilization of circulation—severely dehydrated infants with signs of shock require volume expansion with isotonic saline.
   c. Subsequent replacement:
      i. Estimate and correct fluid deficit. Correct over 48 hours in severe hypernatremia.
      ii. Closely monitor and replace urine output, which may change dramatically after initiation of DDAVP treatment.
      iii. Replace essential water loss.
   d. In general, for every 1 mEq/L of serum Na greater than 145 mEq/L, a free-water deficit of 4 mL/kg should be replaced over 48 to 72 hours.
   e. Free water should not be given IV; it may be given by mouth. Alternatively, the amount of free water may be cal-

culated and delivered by IV infusion via an appropriate volume of 0.45% NaCl.
2. Correction of hypernatremia and hyperosmolality
   a. Caution should be taken to avoid rapid drop of serum Na concentration or plasma osmolality in severe hypernatremia to prevent brain swelling or herniation.
   b. Aim to correct Na level at <0.5 mEq/L/h and usually ≤10 mEq/L/day.
3. For PDI (the suggested dosages are for the pediatric population)
   a. Desmopressin acetate (DDAVP), a synthetic analogue of pituitary ADH. It increases cellular permeability of collecting ducts resulting in water reabsorption.
      i. Intranasal: 5 to 30 μg/day, once a day or divided twice or three times a day.
      ii. Oral: 50 to 200 μg/day, divided twice or three times a day.
      iii. IV or SC: 0.2 to 2 μg/day, divided twice a day.
   b. Vasopressin (Pitressin)—ADH activity and vasopressor effect. Use only the aqueous preparation that has a short half-life.
      i. IV: dilute in 0.9% NaCl or D5W to 0.1 to 1 U/mL, give 0.5 mU/kg/hr, continuous IV infusion initially. May increase dose, but not to exceed 10 mU/kg/hr.
      ii. IM or SC: 2.5 to 10 units, twice or four times a day, as needed.
4. For NDI
   c. In NDI, DDAVP is not effective because of the renal resistance to ADH.
   d. Hydrochlorothiazide—decreases free water delivery to distal tubule and decreases NaCl reabsorption in proximal tubule.
      i. 2 to 4 mg/kg/day, oral, once a day or divided twice a day. Maximum 37.5 mg/day for age >2 years, or 100 mg/day for age >2 years.
   e. Amiloride—potassium-sparing diuretic. In combination with hydrochlorothiazide, this exerts a synergistic antidiuretic effect.
      i. Titrate dose gradually, not to exceed 20 mg/1.73m²/day, divided twice or three times a day, oral.
   f. Chlorpropamide—a sulfonylurea promoting renal response to ADH.
      i. Limited data in pediatric patients suggests a starting dose of 50 mg/day, not to exceed 150 mg/day.
      ii. Monitor blood glucose level.
5. For primary polydipsia
   g. Mostly reassurance; identify underline causes; behavioral modification.
   h. Treatment with standard doses of DDAVP is contraindicated in primary polydipsia, because DDAVP eliminates polyuria without producing commensurate reductions in polydipsia. Therefore, it invariably produces water intoxication.

SUMMARY

PDI results from insufficiency of VP, while NDI is due to renal unresponsiveness to VP. Both result in excessive fluid intake to compensate for water loss from urine. On the other hand, in primary polydipsia, excessive water intake results in decrease of VP. If the 24-hour urine volume, osmolality, and plasma osmolality are inconclusive in making a diagnosis of DI, a water deprivation test may be helpful. A vasopressin test can differentiate PDI and NDI. DDAVP is the treatment of choice for PDI, while hydrochlorothiazide, amiloride, and chlorpropamide can be used for NDI. DDAVP is contraindicated in primary polydipsia because of the risk of water intoxication.

Acknowledgment

Thanks to Dr. Glenn Harris for his suggestions during the preparation of this chapter.

Suggested Readings

Ball SG, Baylis PH. Vasopressin, diabetes insipidus, and syndrome of inappropriate antidiuresis. In: DeGroot LJ, Jameson JL, eds. *Endocrinology.* 5th ed. Philadelphia: Elsevier Saunders; 2006:537–556.

Bode HH, Crawford JD, Danon M. Disorders of antidiuretic hormone homeostasis: diabetes insipidus and SIADH. In: Lifshitz F, ed. *Pediatric endocrinology.* 3rd ed. New York: Marcel Dekker; 1996:731–751.

Chan JCM, Roth KS. Diabetes insipidus. Emedicine from WebMD. http://www.emedicine.com/ped/topic580.htm. 2003.

Claudius I, Fluharty C, Boles R. The emergency department approach to newborn and childhood metabolic crisis. *Emerg Med Clin North Am* 2005;23: 843–883.

Ellison DH. Disorders of sodium and water. *Am J Kid Dis* 2005;46:356–361.

Garofeanu CG, Weir M, Rosas-Arellano MP, et al. Causes of reversible diabetes insipidus: a systematic review. *Am J Kid Dis* 2005;45:626–637.

Robertson GL. Clinical disorders of the posterior pituitary. In: Pescovitz OH, Eugster EA, eds. *Pediatric endocrinology: mechanisms, manifestations and management.* Philadelphia: Lippincott Williams & Wilkins; 2004:90–107.

CHAPTER 101 ■ ADRENOCORTICAL INSUFFICIENCY

CLAUDE J. MIGEON

Adrenal glands are made of two distinct parts: (1) a medulla, which secretes epinephrine; and (2) the cortex, which produces steroids: cortisol, aldosterone, and adrenal androgens.

ORGANOGENESIS OF THE ADRENAL GLANDS

At 4 to 5 weeks of fetal life, cells of mesoderm aggregate to form the primitive cortex and the primitive gonads. By 7 to 8 weeks, the cortex is invaded by ectodermal chromaffin cells, which will form the medulla.

At birth, the fetal cortex is rapidly replaced by cells that organize themselves in three distinct layers: outside, the zona glomerulosa secretes aldosterone; the zona fasciculata and zona reticularis secrete cortisol and *adrenal androgens* (androstene-dione, dehydroepiandrosterone, and its sulfate).

PHYSIOLOGY OF ADRENAL STEROID SECRETION

Cortisol Secretion

Corticol secretion is dependent upon the secretion of corti-cotropin-releasing hormone (CRH) by the hypothalamus. CRH reaches the pituitary by the short loop of the portal vessel system and activates corticotroph cells of the anterior pituitary to produce ACTH. Then ACTH is carried by blood to the adrenal gland, where it binds to specific cell-membrane receptors. This results in activation of a series of protein kinases that make stored cholesterol esters available to a set of enzymes: esterase, steroidogenic acute regulatory protein (StAR), cholesterol side-chain cleavage enzyme, 3β-hydroxysteroid dehydrogenase, 17-hydroxylase, 21-hydroxylase, and 11β-hydroxylase.

The cortisol secretion rate has been determined to be *6 to 12 mg per m² of body surface area per 24 hours*. This secretion follows a diurnal variation, with the highest plasma levels occurring at about 5 to 6 AM. In infancy, the diurnal variation is established only after the child has established a fairly regular night sleep rhythm schedule. The homeostatic regulation of cortisol is based on the negative feedback of plasma cortisol levels. When levels are high, they turn down the secretion of CRH/ACTH; and inversely, when the cortisol levels are low.

Aldosterone Secretion

The regulation of the secretion of aldosterone is quite different from that of cortisol. It binds to specific sites of the glomeru-losa cells. Angiotensin II is the trigger of secretion. The home-ostatic regulation of aldosterone results from a negative feed-back of the secretion of renin and increased blood pressure at the level of the glomerular apparatus of the kidney. However, ACTH administration has an acute, temporary effect on increasing aldosterone levels in blood. It is of interest that the secretion of aldosterone appears to be the same in infants, children, or adults (25 to 100 μg/day). Hence aldosterone replacement therapy is similar at all ages.

Adrenal Androgens

Large amounts of androgens are secreted by the fetal gland. After birth, their secretion goes down very quickly and will not resume until the establishment of the pubertal adrenarche. Levels of adrenal androgens are high in adolescence and early adulthood, and then go down to low levels by 40 to 50 years of age.

PHYSIOLOGIC EFFECTS OF ADRENAL STEROIDS

The effects of steroids require their binding to specific receptor proteins. The glucocorticoid receptor (hGR) and mineralo-corticoid receptor (hMR) have a fairly similar structure, their gene being located on chromosome 5 for the former and 4 for the latter.

Glucocorticoid effects in man are multiple. In normal metabolism, it increases gluconeogenesis and glycogenesis while inhibiting peripheral glucose utilization. It also exerts a lipolytic action. Mineralocorticoids control the excretion of electrolytes by the kidney. As to adrenal androgens, they are partially converted to testosterone.

CAUSES OF PRIMARY HYPOADRENOCORTICISM (TABLE 101.1)

Congenital Causes

The most frequent congenital form is congenital adrenal hyperplasia due to 21-hydroxylase deficiency (salt-losing, simple virilizing, attenuated or nonclassical). The salt-losing and simple virilizing forms occur in about 1 in 10,000 births. Most states in the United States screen for it at birth. Much less frequent are the 11β-hydroxylase deficiency (hypertensive form), 17-hydroxylase deficiency, and a few other rare forms.

PRIMARY HYPOADRENOCORTICISM

I. Congenital
  1. Congenital adrenal hyperplasia (CAH)
  2. Congenital adrenal aplasia
  3. X-linked adrenal hypoplasia congenita (DAX-1)
  4. Mutation of steroidogenic factor 1 (SF-1)
  5. IMAGe association
  6. Autoimmune polyglandular disorders
     a. Isolated adrenal deficiency
     b. Autoimmune polyglandular type I (AIRE gene)
     c. Autoimmune polyglandular type II
  7. Metabolic lipid disorders
     a. X-linked adrenoleukodystrophy (ALD), adreno-
        myeloneuropathy (AMN)
     b. Zellweger syndrome
     c. Volman disease (acid lipase deficiency)

II. Acquired
  1. Adrenal hemorrhage (Waterhouse–Friderichsen
     syndrome)
  2. Infections, tumors

TABLE 101.2

SECONDARY HYPOADRENOCORTICISM

I. Deficient CRH and/or ACTH
  1. Hypothalamic–pituitary insufficiency
     a. Septo-optic dysplasia (midline brain defects)
     b. Empty sella turcica
     c. Tumors (e.g., craniopharyngioma), trauma
  2. Cessation of glucocorticoid therapy
  3. Infants born to mothers treated with glucocorticoids
II. End-organ unresponsiveness
  1. Congenital adrenocortical uresponsiveness to ACTH
  2. The AAA syndrome (adrenal insufficiency, achalasia,
     alacryma)
  3. Cortisol resistance
  4. Aldosterone resistance

Autoimmune polyglandular types I and II are next in frequency. Type I includes, in order of appearance, candidiasis, hypoparathyroidism, and hypoadrenocorticism. Type II is characterized by hypoadrenocorticism in association with hypothyroidism and/or diabetes mellitus type I.

Another group of causes are related to the embryonic formation of the adrenal glands and are due to several transcription factors like DAX-1 and SF-1. X-linked adrenoleukodystrophy (ABCD-1 gene) is a catastrophic neurologic disorder of lipid metabolism that is associated with hypoadrenocorticism.

Acquired Adrenal Destruction

Acquired adrenal destruction can be due to massive, bilateral adrenal hemorrhage as sometimes seen at birth in difficult delivery or in cases of fulminating infections like meningococcemia and the Waterhouse–Friderichsen syndrome.

CAUSES OF SECONDARY HYPOADRENOCORTICISM (TABLE 101.2)

Deficient CRH/ACTH Secretion

Abnormal function of the hypothalamus and pituitary can be due to congenital brain defects such as septo-optic dysplasia or empty sella turcica. It can also be due to brain destruction as with craniopharyngioma, astrocytoma, or other brain tumors. Treatment of such tumors (surgical, radiation) can further alter brain function. Brain trauma may also result in deficient secretion of CRH/ACTH.

Glucocorticoids (cortisol, prednisone, prednisolone, and many derivatives) are used in the treatment of several conditions such as asthma and chronic arthritis. The doses used are usually many times greater than normal adrenal secretion. In such cases, the therapy will suppress CRH/ACTH secretion via the negative feedback homeostatic cortisol regulation. Recovery takes 6 weeks in half of the patients and up to 6 months in the others.

End-Organ Unresponsiveness

In congenital adrenocortical unresponsiveness to ACTH, the problem is a mutation of MC2, the gene responsible for the formation of the ACTH receptor. The triple-A syndrome is the association of adrenal insufficiency, alacryma, and achalasia. Rarely, a mutation of the cortisol receptor gene will result in cortisol resistance; whereas a mutation of the aldosterone receptor will result in aldosterone resistance.

TREATMENT OF HYPOADRENOCORTICISM

In many cases, hypoadrenocorticism is manifested by an acute adrenal crisis, as in the salt-losing form of congenital adrenal hyperplasia due to 21-hydroxylase deficiency. On occasion, it starts in an insidious fashion, because there is a progressive adrenal insufficiency as in Addison disease due to an autoimmune disorder. However hypoadrenocorticism starts, this beginning will be followed by life-long maintenance therapy with specific treatment for stress conditions.

Acute Adrenal Crisis

Acute adrenal crisis is the result of an abrupt and most complete deficiency of cortisol and aldosterone. It is characterized by marked dehydration with hyponatremic, hyperkalemic acidosis and hypoglycemia. When levels of serum electrolytes are determined, additional blood should be drawn for plasma cortisol, aldosterone, and renin activity. If CAH is suspected, blood should also be obtained for 17-OH progesterone and androstenedione.

The urgent fluid and electrolyte treatment is 20 mL per kg body weight of isotonic saline in 5% glucose given IV over the first hour of therapy. The intravenous solution should be continued to deliver about 60 mL/kg over the next 24 hours. Adjustments may need to be made in relation to fluid losses.

This therapy will correct serum electrolytes except for potassium, which often remains elevated. To correct this problem, it will be necessary to add cortisol sodium succinate (SoluCortef) to the treatment. We advise an IV bolus of 50 mg of SoluCortef per m^2 body surface area, followed by 25 mg per m^2 added to the rest of the 24-hour IV fluid. While the fluid treatment corrects the dehydration and electrolyte loss, the addition of SoluCortef will permit salt retention, as 25 mg of SoluCortef has mineralocorticoid activity of 0.1 mg 9-alfa-fluorocortisol acetate (Florinef).

Maintenance Treatment

After the acute adrenal crisis is controlled, maintenance therapy must be instituted, and will include glucocorticoid and mineralocorticoid replacement.

Glucocorticoids

Cortisol is the drug of choice, as it is the physiologic hormone. Based on a secretion rate of 6 to 12 mg/m^2/24 hours, ideal treatment would be IV infusion of the daily dose at a rate that would mimic the normal diurnal variation of cortisol. This is obviously not practical for a lifetime therapy, and cortisol (Cortef) is administered orally. Because cortisol is partially destroyed by gastric acidity, experience has shown that replacement should be about twice the secretion rate, or *12 to 24 mg/m^2/24 hr.*

Cortisol has a fairly short half-life in blood (60 to 80 minutes). In order to maintain steroid levels throughout the day, the daily dose is given as one-third of the total every 8 hours. In an attempt to mimic physiology, a little more than one-third is given in the morning and in the evening. For example, a 25-mg daily dose is distributed as 10 mg in the morning, 5 mg at noon, and 10 mg in the evening. Whether this is important and useful has never been determined by scientific data.

Problems with compliance with treatment are likely. With infants or young children in a good family, compliance can be quite good. However, this is not always the case despite medical advice. It must also be noted that small incidents that are easily taken care of by children's Tylenol can often end up in the ER with patients presenting with hypoadrenocorticism.

Experience has shown that children of school age and adolescents have even more difficulty with compliance. Fortunately, by 5 to 6 years of age, the incidents that created major problems in infancy have less severe consequences. Yet it is probably the basis for the short stature in adulthood.

The lack of compliance with older children is particularly bad in relation to the midday dose of Cortef. Two cortisol derivatives, prednisone (1-mg tablets) and prednisolone (Pediapred liquid; 1 mg/mL), are known to have a blood half-life that is about double that of cortisol. As a consequence, they can be administered at one-half of the daily dose, twice daily.

Extremely potent derivatives such as dexamethasone are rarely used for maintenance as it is difficult to adjust the dose. On the other hand, dexamethasone is used in large amounts by neurosurgeons to avoid brain edema.

Mineralocorticoids

As noted above, the secretion rate of aldosterone secretion is the same from infancy to adulthood. Hence, replacement varies little with age, ranging from 0.05 to 0.15 mg of 9α-fluoro-cortisol acetate (Florinef). It is given orally, once daily.

Because infants' salt intake is quite low (8–10 mEq Na /24 hr), it is advised to add 10 to 30 mEq of sodium per day. When infants are started on table food, the additional salt is provided by the food.

Treatment during Stress

Experience has shown that stress of various types tends to increase cortisol secretion. For this reason, we advise doubling or tripling the basic glucocorticoid dose during stress such as fever above 101°F. If the stress includes vomiting, we advise parents to administer SQ or IM Solucortef (50 mg/m^2) and then go to an ER within the next 2 to 3 hours (or repeat Solucortef IM every 6 to 8 hours).

Treatment at Surgery

We recommend giving IV Solucortef (50 mg/m^2) just before anesthesia. This is followed by a second dose (50 mg/m^2) administered as a constant infusion through the surgical procedure and a third dose (50 mg/m^2) added to IV fluids at constant rate for the remainder of the 24 hours. In both medical and surgical stress, it is important to limit the time of the increased dose to only the period of acute stress.

Cessation of Glucocorticoid Therapy

In general, glucocorticoid therapy requires amounts of steroids that are well above the normal cortisol secretion. A short course of treatment of less than 4 weeks does not require specific therapy. After more than 4 weeks of treatment, one can expect a suppression of the CRH/ACTH axis and low cortisol secretion.

To stop treatment, we advise cutting steroid administration to about one-half of the replacement amount for the patient. This is maintained for about a week. After total cessation, about 50% of patients recover the function of their pituitary–adrenal axis within 6 weeks, and all of them within 6 months. After stopping completely glucocorticoid therapy, there is no need for treatment except at times of stress, as described earlier.

Infants Born of Mothers Treated with Glucocorticoids

Mothers who require treatment usually are given prednisone, which crosses very poorly through the placenta to the fetus. Hence infants born under such circumstances are not expected to present problems. The only possible abnormality would be hypoglycemia, which can be checked for a few days.

Suggested Readings

Betterie C, Dal Pra C, Mantero F, et al. Autoimmune adrenal insufficiency and autoimmune polyendocrine syndromes: autoantibodies, autoantigens, and their applicability in diagnosis and disease prediction. *Endocr Rev* 2002;23: 327–364.

Charmandari E, Chrousos GP. Adrenal insufficiency. Chapter 13 in Endotext. com. Section on adrenal disease and function, Chrousos GP, ed.

Donohoue PA, Parker K, Migeon CJ. Congenital adrenal hyperplasia. In: Scriver CR, et al., eds. *The metabolic basis of inherited disease.* New York: McGraw-Hill; 2001:4077–4115.

Migeon CJ, Lanes RL. Adrenal cortex: hypo- and hyperfunction. In: Lifshitz F, ed. *Pediatric endocrinology.* 5th ed. New York: Marcel Dekker; 2006

Miller WL. The adrenal cortex. In: Sperling M, ed. *Pediatric endocrinology.* 2nd ed. Philadelphia: Saunders; 2002:385–438.

Moser HW, Smith KD, Watkins PA, et al. X-linked adrenoleukodystrophy. In: Scriver CR, Beaudet AL, Sly WS, et al., eds. *Metabolic and molecular bases of inherited disease.* 8th ed. New York: McGraw-Hill; 2001.

Pedreira CC, Savarirayan R, Zacharin MR. IMAGe Syndrome: a complex disorder affecting growth, adrenal and gonadal function and skeletal development. *J Pediatr* 2004;144:274–277.

CHAPTER 102 ■ DISORDERS INVOLVING THE THYROID GLAND

YING T. CHANG

THYROID ONTOGENESIS

The first thyroid structure appears when the embryo reaches 16 days as a thickening (median anlagen) between the first and second branchial arches. The thyroid reaches its final position at about 40 to 50 days of development. The fetal thyroid activity begins with the synthesis of the thyroglobulin at 8 weeks of gestation. Trapping of iodine and the iodination of tyrosine start at 10 weeks, and the pituitary gland starts to secret TSH at 12 weeks of gestation. During mid-gestation, the hypothalamic–pituitary–thyroid axis becomes functional and independent of the maternal thyroid system. Only a small quantity of maternal thyroxine passes through the placenta to the fetus, which is insufficient to prevent hypothyroidism if the fetal thyroid gland is unable to make an adequate amount of thyroid hormone. However, maternal thyroxine in the early stages of gestation is important in fetal neurologic development.

REGULATION OF THYROID SYNTHESIS

The hypothalamus secrets thyrotropin-releasing hormone (TRH), which reaches the anterior pituitary gland through the portal system. TRH binds to the TRH receptor on the thyrotroph cell membrane and stimulates the secretion of thyrotropin, or thyroid-stimulating hormone (TSH). In the thyroid gland, TSH binds to the TSH receptor, promotes thyroid follicular cells to trap and organize iodine and to synthesize thyroxine (T4). Small amounts of T4 are converted into triiodothyronine (T3), which is more potent than T4. The vast majority of circulating T4 and T3 is bound to thyroxine-binding globulin (TBG), albumin and pre-albumin. Only 0.03% of the total T4 is free T4, and 0.3% of the total T3 is free T3. Free T4 and free T3 are the active thyroid hormones. The majority of the circulating T3 comes from the deiodination of T4 in peripheral tissue such as the liver and kidney. Inside the cells of the hypothalamus and pituitary, T4 is also deiodinized into T3, which inhibits the secretion of TRH and TSH.

TSH surges to the range of 70 to 100 µU/mL in 30 minutes after birth, then declines in a day. Total T4 and T3 levels reach their peaks at 24 hours. In the newborn thyroid screening, some programs measure total T4 first, followed by TSH if the T4 level is below the 10th percentile of that assay. Some programs measure TSH, and some measure both. If a blood sample is collected too early, a high level of TSH may result in a false positive for congenital hypothyroidism.

Thyroid Function in Very-Low-Birthweight Infants

Between 20 and 40 weeks of gestation, the cord blood concentrations of T4, free T4, TBG, and TSH increase progressively with gestational age. Fetal TSH levels usually exceed maternal values during this period. Fetal T3 levels are very low throughout gestation, and only increase during the last 10 weeks. The total T4 levels are low in very-low-birthweight (VLBW) infants. The progressive maturation of the hypothalamic–pituitary–thyroid axis and the peripheral metabolism of thyroid hormones in the immature infant after birth are similar to those during intrauterine life. It is unknown if the low T4 level in VLBW infants results in adverse effects later in life. It is also not clear if routine thyroxine replacement therapy to bring the thyroxine hormone levels to a full-term level is beneficial.

A study of 104 preterm infants during the first week of life revealed free T4 levels (ng/dL) as follows: 0.6 to 2.2 for a gestational age of 25 to 27 weeks, 0.6 to 3.4 for 28 to 30 weeks, 1.0 to 3.8 for 31 to 33 weeks, and 1.2 to 4.4 for 34 to 36 weeks. The TSH levels (mU/L) were 0.2 to 30.3, 0.2 to 20.6, 0.7 to 27.0, and 1.2 to 21.6, respectively.

Another study of 128 infants of gestational age less then 30 weeks during their first 14 days of life revealed that (1) plasma total T4, free T4, and total T3 levels were much lower than in term infants; (2) the postnatal surge of thyroid hormones normally seen at 24 to 48 hours of age in term infants did not occur in these preterm infants; and (3) low free T4 and free T3 levels were associated with higher mortality rates and increased severity of lung disease.

In a study treating preterm infants with thyroxine at birth, and assessing them at an early school age, there were benefits of the treatment in the neurologic development for infants born at a gestational age less than 29 weeks, especially in infants of 25 to 26 weeks' gestation. However, in infants of 29 weeks' gestation, T4 supplementation was associated with more motor and neurologic complications. There was no convincing explanation for this difference between these two gestational age groups. Further studies are needed.

THYROID DISORDERS

In general, thyroid disorders can be grouped into four categories: hypothyroidism, hyperthyroidism/thyrotoxicosis, nodules, and other conditions associated with abnormal thyroid function tests. Table 102.1 illustrates differential diagnosis based on the results of thyroid function tests.

TABLE 102.1

THYROID FUNCTION TESTS IN THYROID DISORDERS

T T4	F T4	TSH	Conditions	Remarks
L	L	H	Primary hypothyroidism	Antibodies for autoimmune
L	L	L, N	Central hypothyroidism	Other pituitary hormone def.
L	L, N	N	Euthyroid sick syndrome	Low T3, normal or high rT3
L	N	N	TBG deficiency	Low TBG, high T3 resin uptake
H	H	L	Thyrotoxicosis	TSHR Ab; exogenous thyroxine
H	H	H	Pituitary resistance to TH	Hyperthyroid
H	H	H, N	General resistance to TH	Euthyroid or hypothyroid
H	N	N	TBG excess	OCP, pregnancy, estradiol; TBG
H, N;	H, N	L, N	Acute or subacute thyroiditis	Left lobe enlarged, pain, ESR
N	N	L	T3 thyrotoxicosis	Total and free T3
N	N	H	Compensated hypothyroidism	Treat or follow-up
N	N	N	Thyroid cancer	Nodules, ultrasound, FNA
N	N	N	Simple goiter; Hashimoto	Goiter, ultrasound, Ab; FNA?
N	N	N	Thyroglossal duct cyst	Nodule along midline of neck

H, high; L, low; N, normal; TT4, total T4; FT4, free T4; rT3, reverse T3; TH, thyroid hormone; Ab, antibody; TSHR, TSH receptor.

Hypothyroidism

Congenital Hypothyroidism

Infants with congenital hypothyroidism may show the following symptoms or signs: a patent posterior fontanelle with widely opened cranial sutures, umbilical hernias, a large size for their gestational age, prolonged jaundice, mottling skin patterns, or a hypotonic appearance; whereas many infants do not show apparent symptoms or signs. However, if untreated, typical cretinism develops in a few months: constipation, poor linear growth, doughy skin, enlarged tongue, and developmental delays.

It has been well established that delayed or inadequately treated congenital hypothyroidism results in mental development delays. One study demonstrated that the average IQ was 89, 70, and 54 if thyroxine replacement therapy started before 3 months, between 3 and 6 months, and after 6 months of age, respectively. The etiology of congenital hypothyroidism also plays a role. In thyroid agenesis, 41% of children had an IQ higher than 85. In dyshormonogenesis, it was 44% to 78%.

Primary Hypothyroidism. The incidence of congenital hypothyroidism is 1 in 3,500 to 5,000 births. The male to female ratio is 1 to 2. Congenital hypothyroidism is more common in Caucasians than in African Americans (5 to 1), and even higher among Hispanics than non-Hispanic Caucasians. The incidence is greater among Native American and Asian populations as well.

Embryogenic Defects. Embryogenic defects account for 80% of all congenital hypothyroidism. It is not hereditary in most cases, and is not associated with autoimmunity or thyroid disorders in mothers or among relatives. Diagnosis can be made by a thyroid scan using ^{123}I uptake or technetium. The defects result in thyroid agenesis, dysgenesis, or ectopia.

Dyshormonogenesis. Dyshormonogenesis is an enzymatic defect in thyroid hormone synthesis resulting from autosomal recessive mutation of several genes, or from antithyroid medications such as propylthiouracil or mathimazole. It accounts for 10% to 15% of all congenital hypothyroidism. More than 10 inborn errors have been recognized, most commonly organification defects. The disorders include defects in basolateral or apical iodide transport, defects in organification (including thyroid peroxidase, thyroid oxidase), or defects in thyroglobulin synthesis.

Pendred Syndrome. Pendrin is a protein expressed in the inner ear, thyroid, and kidney. Located at the apical membrane of thyrocytes, pendrin transports iodide from thyrocytes into follicular lumen for thyroxine synthesis. Mutations of the pendrin gene result in dyshormonogenesis hypothyroidism with goiter. However, many patients with Pendred syndrome are clinically and biochemically euthyroid unless dietary iodine intake is low. This finding, together with others, suggests that iodide may enter the lumen of thyroid follicles through another channel or other mechanisms. Patients with Pendred syndrome may also have neurosensory hearing loss.

Hyporesponsiveness to Thyrotropin. Mutations in the TSH receptor gene result in the hyporesponsiveness of thyroid to thyrotropin. The patients may present with low or near-normal T4 and T3. The defects can also be in the alpha-subunit of G-protein, as part of broader G-protein mutations found in pseudohypoparathyroidism type 1a. These patients usually have low-normal serum T4 levels and few clinical symptoms or signs of hypothyroidism.

Hypothalamic–Pituitary Hypothyroidism (Central Hypothyroidism). Hypothalamic–pituitary hypothyroidism accounts for 5% to 10% of overall congenital hypothyroidism. The prevalence is about 1 in 50,000 to 100,000. Infants may present with persistent jaundice and other pituitary deficiencies such as hypoglycemia, micropenis in males, diabetes insipidus, or other CNS abnormalities such as midline defects or ocular abnormalities. The onset is often insidious and TSH deficiency is usually partial. In this case, the T4 and free T4 levels are low while the TSH level is low or normal.

Transient Hypothyroidism. In some infants, T4 levels are low and TSH levels are high during newborn screenings. These hormones become normalized spontaneously in a few weeks or months. It may be indistinguishable from thyroid dysgenesis, which is characterized by severe hypothyroidism without goiter, and reduced or absent thyroid uptake on scan. The maternal causes include iodine deficiency or excess, antithyroid drugs, dietary goitrogen, or TSH receptor-blocking antibodies. The neonatal causes include excessive iodine, such as preparing a large skin area for surgery.

Acquired Hypothyroidism

Hypothyroidism may be acquired anytime after birth. If it occurs in infancy, children may present with symptoms and signs as those of congenital hypothyroidism. The causes of acquired hypothyroidism include autoimmune thyroiditis (Hashimoto thyroiditis), endemic iodine deficiency or environmental goitrogens, surgical excision, irradiation, drugs, hemosiderosis, and homocystinosis. Children with Down syndrome have a higher incidence of both congenital and acquired hypothyroidism, as well as hyperthyroidism.

Hashimoto Thyroiditis. Hashimoto thyroiditis is an autoimmune thyroiditis associated with antibodies against thyroglobulin and thyroid peroxidase. Lymphocytic infiltration of the thyroid gland results in thyromegaly. Patients may present with hypothyroidism, euthyroid, or transient hyperthyroidism (Hashitoxicosis). The course is often insidious in that neither the child nor the parents are aware of the symptoms, and growth retardation may be the only clue. The clinical presentations include an asymptomatic goiter, mild tenderness or a sensation of fullness in the anterior neck, sensation of obstruction in the throat when swallowing, weakness, decreased appetite, cold intolerance, constipation, dry skin, brittle hair, delayed puberty, or precocious puberty in severe cases. Children may appear chubby, but not morbidly obese. If Hashimoto thyroiditis occurs before 2 years of age, untreated children may suffer irreversible developmental delays.

Hashimoto thyroiditis may be part of an autoimmune polyendocrine syndrome (APS) which includes Addison disease, hypoparathyroidism, mucocutaneous candidiasis, hepatitis, primary hypothyroidism, Graves disease, type 1 diabetes, vitiligo, and pernicious anemia.

Compensated Hypothyroidism. In some mild asymptomatic hypothyroidism, the thyroid is able to compensate to keep normal levels of total or free T4 and T3, with an outlay of elevated TSH levels. In some cases, TSH levels may be spontaneously normalized later. In others, TSH levels remain high, and some decompensate and develop full-blown hypothyroidism. Studies have shown that the metabolic rate of children with compensated hypothyroidism is lower than normal, and thyroid hormone replacement therapy is recommended.

Nonthyroidal Illness

The changes in thyroid hormones during critical illnesses are called euthyroid sick syndrome or nonthyroidal illness. Initially, serum total T_3 (TT_3) values decline, and rT_3 values increase. When the condition deteriorates, total T_4 (TT_4) values may decline as well, but TSH levels remain normal. TBG is decreased and the free T4 levels are normal or low. Interleukin-1β (IL-1β) or tumor necrosis factor α(TNF-α) inhibits thyrotropin secretion, and induces functional changes in the rat characteristic of the "sick euthyroid" state due to cytokine-induced changes in hypothalamic and pituitary function. In children with meningococcal sepsis, both the decreased TT_3/rT_3 ratio and TT_4 levels were predictive for mortality, but were not superior to IL-6. When total T4 decreased to 4 µg/dL, the mortality rate was 50%. When total T4 was 2 µg/dL, the mortality rate was 80%. Perinatal asphyxia, recognized by low Apgar scores, is associated with a depression of TSH, T4, and T3, and the reductions are greatest in infants with hypoxic/ischemic encephalopathy. In this study, 6 of 11 infants with FT4 <2 ng/dL died. Hence, some authors argue that nonthyroidal illness syndrome is a manifestation of hypothalamic–pituitary dysfunction, and in view of current evidence should be treated with appropriate replacement therapies. However, it is still controversial.

Thyroxine-Binding Globulin Deficiency

There are three conventional carriers for the thyroid hormone: thyroxine-binding globulin (TBG), the major carrier; transthyretin (TTR); and albumin. Approximately 20,000 of 100,000 molecules of circulating TBG are occupied by T4, as compared to 300 of TTR and 3 of albumin. Deletion or mutation of the TBG gene on the X-chromosome results in TBG deficiency in boys presenting with low total T4, normal free T4, and normal TSH. Affected children are euthyroid and no treatment is needed.

Treatment of Hypothyroidism

Congenital hypothyroidism should be treated as soon as hypothyroidism is confirmed, because the thyroid hormone is crucial in the neurologic development during the first 2 years. The cognitive and motor developmental outcomes are associated with the severity of hypothyroidism, timing of the initiation of thyroxine treatment, and timing of achieving target T4 and TSH levels. The initial dose of L-thyroxine is 10 to 15 µg/kg/day. The target T4 level for congenital hypothyroidism is 10 to 15 µg/dL. If free T4 is used, the target is the upper half of the normal range for age. Initially, thyroid function tests should be followed every 2 to 4 weeks for 3 months to assure adequate treatment, and then every 3 months for the first 3 years thereafter. Children with congenital hypothyroidism need developmental evaluations to ensure normal neurologic development.

Hyperthyroidism and Thyrotoxicosis

Graves Disease

Graves disease is an autoimmune thyroid disorder resulting from stimulation of TSH receptors by TSH receptor antibodies or thyroid-stimulating immunoglobulins. Childhood Graves disease accounts for less than 5% of all Graves disease, and is rare in children less than 5 years old. The following clinical presentations are common: goiter (99%), tachycardia, nervousness, increased pulse pressure, hypertension, exophthalmos (66%), tremor, increased appetite, weight loss, thyroid bruit (53%), hyperactivity, heat intolerance, and acceleration of linear growth. Often children receive medical care because of nervousness, emotional and behavioral changes, and deteriorating school performance.

Laboratory tests reveal elevated serum total and free T4, and suppressed TSH levels. Total T3 is usually elevated if total T4 and free T4 are normal, whereas TSH levels are suppressed. More than 90% of children with Graves disease have elevated plasma TSHR-SAbs. More than 75% have a high titer of thyroid peroxidase Ab and thyroglobulin Ab. Thyroid radionuclide scans are not routinely needed. Thyroid ultrasounds may be useful to exclude nodules in the goiter.

Medical Treatment. *Thioureas.* Serving as substrates for thyroid peroxidase, thioureas block the incorporation of iodide into tyrosin residues of thyroglobulin. They also block the coupling of iodotyrosyl residues to form T4 and T3. However, they do not block the release of stored thyroid hormones. Hence, treatment requires 1 or 2 months to reach a euthyroid state. About half of all patients achieve remission in 1 to 2 years of treatment. These drugs may also exert an immunosuppressive effect and reduce serum concentrations of TSH receptor antibodies. Many people prefer PTU for initial treatment because of its ability to block the conversion of T4 to T3. However, some experts question the clinical significance of this effect and prefer methimazole because of its potency and longer half-life.

Both drugs carry side effects. More than 25% of children develop minor side effects including skin rash, arthralgia, GI symptoms, elevated liver enzymes, neutropenia, SLE, and hypoprothrombinemia. About 1% develops serious side effects such as agranulocytosis or hepatitis. Although agranulocytosis is rare and difficult to predict, a prompt evaluation is recommended if a patient develops fever and a sore throat. Cases with hepatic failure requiring a liver transplant have been encountered.

- Propylthiouracil (PTU): The initial dose is 5 to 10 mg/kg/day in 3 divided doses for young children and 300 to 450 mg/day in 3 divided doses for older children. After several weeks, the dose can be reduced by one-third or one-half of the initial dose to reach the maintenance dose. Alternatively, one may continue the initial dose until the child becomes hypothyroid, and then add L-thyroxine to maintain a euthyroid state.
- Methimazole (MMI): The potency is about 10 times stronger than PTU. The initial and maintenance doses are usually one-tenth of PTU doses.
- Carbimazole: A derivative of methimazole that has been used widely outside the United States.

Beta-Adrenergic Blockers. Blockage of adrenergic receptors provides patients with relief from symptoms of thyrotoxicosis such as anxiety, tachycardia, palpitations, tremor, and heat intolerance. The conversion of T4 to T3 is also inhibited to some degree. However, metabolic rate and oxygen consumption are not significantly altered. These drugs are used in addition to thioureas at the initial treatment, or in preparation for radioiodine ablation or surgery. Propranolol has been widely used for a long time. The dose is 2.5 to 20 mg, two to three times a day. Its use should be careful in patients with asthma because of bronchoconstriction. Newer drugs include long-acting propranolol and more cardioselective drugs such as atenolol (25–50 mg, once or twice a day) and metoprolol.

In urgent situations, iodine preparation such as Lugol solution (KI) or SSKI (saturate solution of KI) may be used.

Radioiodine Ablation. In a 26-year (107 patients) and 36-year (98 patients) follow-up study of 116 patients between 3 years 7 months and 19 years 9 months of age with Graves disease who were treated with radioiodine between 1953 and 1973, none of the patients developed cancer of the thyroid or leukemia. Over time, all but 2 patients became hypothyroid. Pregnancies did not result in an unusual number of congenital anomalies or spontaneous abortions. Treating young people with Graves disease with radioiodine appears to be safe and effective over the long term. Pretreatment with antithyroid medications is not necessary. However, if used, the drug should be discontinued 1 week prior to treatment with ^{131}I. Patients may continue beta-blockers and later resume antithyroid medications if symptoms of thyrotoxicosis are present due to the length of time the effect of radioactive iodine may take to complete.

Surgery. Near-total thyroidectomy is recommended for Graves disease patients with a large symptomatic goiter, failed medical therapy, the need for rapid reversal of hyperthyroidism such as during pregnancy, or the fear of radiation exposure. There is an increased risk for malignancy in patients with concomitant thyroid nodules. Consequently, patients with Graves disease and coexistent nodules should consider a thyroidectomy. A thyroidectomy can stabilize or improve Graves ophthalmopathy and therefore should be recommended for patients who do not get relief with medical therapy or worsen with radioiodine. Patients should be nearly euthyroid at the time of surgery to minimize surgical risks. An antithyroid drug can achieve this for several weeks. Iodide may be used for 1 to 2 weeks prior to surgery.

Neonatal Graves Disease

Neonatal Graves disease results from maternal TSH receptor-stimulating antibodies. About 2% to 3% of mothers with Graves disease deliver an affected infant. The risk factors include high maternal TSH receptor antibody titer, a need of high-dose antithyroid medication for maternal hyperthyroidism, and a history of ablation of the maternal thyroid gland. The thyrotoxicosis in infants is transient, lasting for several weeks to 6 months. In severe long-lasting thyrotoxicosis, the mortality rate may reach 20% if not treated vigorously.

A hypermetabolic state may also result in severe brain damage, premature closure of cranial fissures causing craniosynostosis, or a direct effect of excess thyroid hormones on brain maturation.

Treatment of neonatal thyrotoxicosis includes the beta-adrenergic blocker propranolol 1 to 2 mg/kg/day, in 3 divided doses, and PTU 5 to 10 mg/kg/day, in 3 divided doses. Saturated KI solution (10%), 1 drop, every 8 hours can be used in severe cases. The doses of KI and PTU may be doubled in 1 to 2 days if improvement is insufficient. Glucocorticoid may be used but is slower in achieving its effects.

Other Causes of Thyrotoxicosis

Other causes of thyrotoxicosis include TSH-induced hyperthyroidism, TSH-producing pituitary adenoma, pituitary resistance to thyroid hormone, thyroiditis, subacute thyroiditis, toxic Hashimoto thyroiditis (Hashitoxicosis), exogenous thyroid hormone, iodine-induced hyperthyroidism, tumor-produced thyroid stimulators (hydatidiform mole, choriocarcinoma).

Resistance to Thyroid Hormone

In order to express their actions, free T4 and free T3 need to bind to thyroxine receptors (TR) in the nucleus of their target cells, including the hypothalamus and the pituitary. Mutations of TR result in resistance to thyroid hormones (RTH), either generalized or selective to the pituitary.

In generalized RTH, the patients are usually eumetabolic, compensated by the high levels of thyroid hormones, and maintain a near-normal serum TSH level. Some children may present with growth retardation, delayed bone maturation, and learning disabilities suggesting hypothyroidism, particularly in the patients who are mistakenly treated with antithyroid medicines for elevated thyroid hormone levels.

On the other hand, in selective pituitary RTH, the thyroid hormone levels are equally high and TSH levels are also elevated. Patients present with restless, hyperactive behavior, and sinus tachycardia compatible with hyperthyroidism.

About half of the subjects with RTH have learning disabilities with or without attention deficit hyperactive disorder (ADHD). In contrast, the occurrence of RTH is rare in children with ADHD. No genetic linkage of these two disorders has been identified.

Goiter and Nodule

Many genes are involved in thyroid tumorigenesis. Activation of proto-oncogenes such as the *RET* gene results in papillary thyroid carcinoma, and medullary thyroid carcinoma as part of multiple endocrine neoplasia (MEN) type 2. Inactivation of tumor-suppressor genes such as *p53* and *PTEN* can cause follicular thyroid carcinoma. Other factors also play a role in tumor growth. For example, overexpression of angiongenesis stimulators (such as vascular endothelial growth factor c) is associated with papillary carcinomas. In contrast, underexpression of angiogenesis inhibitors (such as thrombostatin-1) is associated with follicular thyroid carcinomas.

Compared to other cancers, thyroid cancer is uncommon and the prognosis is favorable. However, since 1980, the incidence of thyroid carcinoma has been increasing. Women have three times the number of cases that men do. In Caucasians, 85% of thyroid cancer is papillary, 10.9% follicular, 1.7% medullary, 0.78% anaplastic, and 1.3% other carcinomas, including Hürthle cell carcinoma, lymphoma, metastatic cancer, sarcoma, teratoma, and epidermoid carcinoma. The mortality rates from 1985 to 1995 were about 7% for papillary carcinoma, 15% for follicular carcinoma, and 24% for Hürthle cell carcinoma. The three main features determining prognosis are tumor stage, age at the time of diagnosis, and treatment modality. For example, the cancer-specific mortality rate is 0.4% for a papillary carcinoma ≤1 cm (microcarcinoma), which rarely metastasizes to distant sites. In children and adolescents, overall survival rates at 20 to 30 years are over 95%. In a study of children under 16 years of age, 42% developed distant metastases, but 70% experienced complete remission. Children under 10 years of age have higher mortality and recurrent rates than adolescents.

Evaluation

The majority of thyroid cancer patients present with a thyroid mass, whereas about 14% to 29% of cancer patients present with palpable cervical lymph nodes. Thyroid function tests are normal in most cases of thyroid cancer, whereas T4 and TSH are elevated in functioning thyroid adenoma. Thyroid antibodies may help to differentiate between Hashimoto thyroiditis and Hürthle cell tumor. However, thyroid antibodies may be present in up to 25% of thyroid carcinoma. Serum calcitonin levels can be useful in identifying medullary thyroid carcinoma if there are other components of MEN 2, or a family history of thyroid cancer.

Thyroid scintiscan using ^{123}I can identify a functioning adenoma, which may have resulted from activating mutations of the TSH receptor or G-protein. A biopsy is not needed in this case.

The ultrasonographic features of benign nodules and carcinomas are similar in general. However, the following features increase the possibility of malignancy: diffuse microcalcifications, hypoechogenicity, an irregular sonolucent halo or no halo around the nodules, or an irregular margin that suggests invasion.

Fine-needle biopsy is very useful for almost all patients with thyroid nodules except thyroid adenoma, which can be identified by a thyroid scan and thyroid function tests. A biopsy is recommended if the nodule size is greater than 1 cm in its longest dimension. A length of 1 cm is used because many people have small thyroid carcinomas that never cause health problems, and the risk for missing a small carcinoma that will result in adverse health consequences is low. Patients having a thyroid carcinoma smaller than 1 cm have the same life expectancy as that of the general population. There are limitations of fine-needle biopsy: the experience of obtaining the specimen, the experience of the pathologist, inadequate specimens for interpretation, and the fact that the specimen from one nodule may not represent the pathology of the other nodules. The procedure can be more precisely done under the guidance of ultrasound. If the initial biopsy result is inconclusive, a repeated biopsy or surgery is needed for an accurate diagnosis.

Treatment

Once the diagnosis of thyroid carcinoma is confirmed, the best choice is total or near-total thyroidectomy. An experi-enced surgeon should perform the procedure, especially for children, who have a higher risk of complications than adults. Major complications include hypothyroidism, transient or permanent hypoparathyroidism, damage to the recurrent laryngeal nerve, and facial paralysis. After the thyroidectomy, patients are treated with T3, at 25 µg, every 8 to 12 hours for 4 weeks. Treatments then stop for 2 weeks to allow the thyroid gland to build up its ability to uptake radioiodine. The TSH level is expected to be higher than 30 U/mL at the end of these 2 weeks. Patients receive an rhTSH intramuscular injection every day for 2 days, followed by ^{131}I for a whole-body scan to estimate the thyroid remnant tissue or identify metastasis of the cancer. Then ^{131}I ablation treatment is given to reduce the recurrence. This is followed by thyroxine suppression therapy to keep the TSH level at or below the low normal range. The thyroglobulin level is measured every 6 months and used as an index of the recurrence of the cancer.

SUMMARY

Congenital hypothyroidism requires prompt and adequate treatment to avoid permanent neurologic damage. Normal ranges of thyroid function tests as well as thyroxine treatments in very-low-birthweight infants require further studies. Compliance, side effects, and efficacy of antithyroid medicines remain problematic in some children with Graves disease. The results of a recently published 36-year follow-up study on radioiodine treatment are encouraging. Thyroid cancers in children generally have a very favorable outcome. However, prompt diagnosis is necessary to avoid metastasis.

Suggested Readings

Adams LM, Emery JR, Clark SJ, et al. Reference ranges for newer thyroid function tests in premature infants. *J Pediatr* 1995;126:122–127.

Biswas S, Buffery J, Enoch H, et al. A longitudinal assessment of thyroid hormone concentrations in preterm infants younger than 30 weeks' gestation during the first 2 weeks of life and their relationship to outcome. *Pediatrics* 2002;109:222–227.

Briet JM, van Wassenaer AG, Dekker FW, et al. Neonatal thyroxine supplementation in very preterm children: developmental outcome evaluated at early school age. *Pediatrics* 2001;107:712–718.

De Groot LJ. Non-thyroidal illness syndrome is a manifestation of hypothalamic-pituitary dysfunction, and in view of current evidence, should be treated with appropriate replacement therapies. *Crit Care Clin* 2006;22:57–86.

Fisher DA. Hypothyroxinemia in premature infants: is thyroxine treatment necessary? *Thyroid* 1999;9:715–720.

Halac I, Zimmerman D. Thyroid nodules and cancers in children. *Endocrinol Metab Clin* 2005;34:725–744.

Kaare J, Weber KJ, Solorzano CC, et al. Thyroidectomy remains an effective treatment option for Graves' disease. *Am J Surg* 2006;191:400–405.

Kaplan MM. Clinical evaluation and management of solitary thyroid nodules. In: Braverman LE, Utiger RD, eds. *The thyroid—a fundamental and clinical text.* 9th ed. Philadelphia: Lippincott Williams & Wilkins; 2005:996–1010.

Kempers MJE, van der Sluijs Veer L, Nijhuis-van der Sanden MWG, et al. Intellectual and motor development of young adults with congenital hypothyroidism diagnosed by neonatal screening. *J Clin Endocrinol Metab* 2006;91:418–424.

Mazzaferri EL, Kloos RT. Carcinoma of follicular epithelium: radioiodine and other treatments and outcomes. In: Braverman LE, Utiger RD, eds. *The thyroid—a fundamental and clinical text.* 9th ed. Philadelphia: Lippincott Williams & Wilkins; 2005:934–966.

Rapaport R, Rose SR, Freemark M. Hypothyroxinemia in the preterm infant: the benefits and risks of thyroxine treatment. *J Pediatr* 2001;139:182–188.

Read CH, Tansey MJ, Menda Y. A 36-year retrospective analysis of the efficacy and safety of radioactive iodine in treating young Graves' patients. *J Clin Endocrinol Metab* 2004;89:4229–4233.

Selva KA, Harper A, Downs A, et al. Neurodevelopmental outcomes in congenital hypothyroidism: comparison of initial T4 dose and time to reach target T4 and TSH. *J Pediatr* 2005;147:775–780.

Van Wassenar AG, Briet JM, van Baar A, et al. Free thyroxine levels during the first weeks of life and neurodevelopmental outcome until the age of 5 years in very preterm infants. *Pediatrics* 2002;110:534–539.

CHAPTER 103 ■ DISORDERS INVOLVING THE PARATHYROID GLAND

SUDIPA BARR AND MICHAEL A. LEVINE

Control of mineral homeostasis requires the intricate interplay of parathyroid, renal, gastrointestinal, and skeletal factors. Critical in this respect is parathyroid hormone (PTH), which is synthesized and secreted from the parathyroid glands at a rate inversely proportional to the plasma concentration of ionized calcium. PTH secretion is tightly regulated through the interaction of extracellular calcium with specific calcium-sensing receptors (CaSRs) present on the surface of the parathyroid cell. In turn, PTH regulates mineral homeostasis and skeletal integrity through its actions on specialized target cells in bone and kidney that express the PTH/parathyroid hormone–related peptide (PTHrP) or type 1 PTH receptor. PTH increases bone resorption, renal calcium resorption, and decreases renal phosphate reabsorption. PTH also induces expression and activity of the renal 1α-hydroxylase enzyme that converts 25-hydroxyvitamin D to 1,25 dihydroxyvitamin D, thereby increasing intestinal absorption of calcium and phosphate as well as osteoclastic bone resorption.

The parathyroid glands are derived from the third and fourth branchial pouches and appear around the fifth week of gestation. Nearly all (84%) humans have four parathyroid glands, but the number of glands can vary from one to twelve, and it is not unusual to find three (1 to 7%) or five (3 to 13%) parathyroid glands in normal individuals. Parathyroid disorders are uncommon in children and adolescents. Deficient or absent secretion of PTH with resultant hypocalcemia is the hallmark of hypoparathyroidism, a clinical disorder that may occur in combination with other endocrine (or non-endocrine) defects or as a solitary endocrinopathy termed isolated hypoparathyroidism. By contrast, excessive and unregulated secretion of PTH from one or more enlarged parathyroid glands leads to hypercalcemia, the biochemical characteristic of primary hyperparathyroidism.

Approximately 99% of total body calcium is in the skeleton in the form of hydroxyapatite, leaving only 1% of the total body calcium within extracellular fluids and soft tissues. Calcium is distributed among three interconvertible fractions in the circulation. Approximately 45% to 50% of total serum calcium is in the ionized form at normal serum protein concentrations, and represents the biologically active component of the total serum calcium concentration. Another 8% to 10% is complexed to organic and inorganic acids (e.g., citrate, sulfate, and phosphate); together, the ionized and complexed calcium fractions represent the diffusible portion of circulating calcium. Approximately 40% of serum calcium is protein-bound, primarily to albumen (80%) but also to globulins (20%). Although conventional measurement of serum calcium implies determination of the total serum calcium concentration, more physiologically relevant information is obtained by measurement of the ionized calcium concentration. From a practical point of view, measurement of total serum calcium concentration provides a reasonable estimate of the ionized calcium concentration, but several caveats are worth noting. For example, decreased concentration of serum albumin, the major calcium-binding protein in the circulation, is the most common cause of hypocalcemia in hospitalized patients.

Plasma levels of ionized calcium can be measured in most clinical chemistry laboratories using now-standardized techniques. However, when it is not possible, or practical, to determine the ionized calcium concentration directly, a "corrected" total calcium concentration can be derived using one of several proposed algorithms that are based on albumin or total protein concentrations. None of these correction factors is absolutely accurate, but they often provide useful estimates of the true concentration of calcium in serum. One widely used algorithm estimates that total serum calcium declines by approximately 0.8 mg/dL for each 1 g/dL decrease in albumin concentration, without a change in ionized calcium.

HYPOCALCEMIA

Etiology

Sudden changes in the distribution of calcium between ionized and bound fractions may cause symptoms of hypocalcemia. Increases in the extracellular fluid concentration of anions, such as phosphate, citrate, bicarbonate, or edetic acid, will increase the proportion of bound calcium and decrease ionized calcium. Extracellular fluid pH also affects the distribution of calcium between ionized and bound fractions. Alkalosis increases the affinity of albumen for calcium, and thereby decreases the concentration of ionized calcium. By contrast, acidosis increases the ionized calcium concentration by decreasing the binding of calcium to albumen. Therefore, measurement of ionized calcium is preferred when evaluating symptoms of hypocalcemia in patients who have abnormal circulating proteins or acid–base and electrolyte disorders.

Neonatal hypocalcemia is common. Early-onset neonatal hypocalcemia is evident within the first 4 days of life and most likely represents an exaggeration of the normal physiologic calcium nadir that occurs at 24 to 48 hours of life. This is due to an inadequate release of PTH, decreased response to PTH by the kidney, or an exagerrated calcitonin release. Common associations with neonatal hypocalcemia include prematurity, low birthweight, hypoglycemia, maternal diabetes mellitus, and respiratory distress syndrome. Although hypocalcemia is self-limited, infants who are symptomatic or who have Q_o-Tc prolongation on an electrocardiogram should be treated with oral or intravenous calcium. A more severe form of transient neonatal hypoparathyroidism and tetany occurs in infants who were exposed to maternal hypercalcemia in utero. Intrauterine hypercalcemia suppresses parathyroid activity in the developing fetus and apparently leads to impaired responsiveness of the parathyroid glands to hypocalcemia after birth.

Late-onset hypocalcemia occurs on the 5th through 10th days of life and is due to relative resistance of renal tubules to PTH action. Because the kidneys do not respond to PTH, phosphate is retained and hyperphosphatemia induces hypocalcemia. This phenomenon represents an acquired form of pseudohypoparathyroidism, an unusual genetic syndrome that is associated with mutations in or near the *GNAS1* gene. These mutations lead to decreased expression or function of G_α the G protein that couples the type 1 PTH receptor to activation of adenylyl cyclase. Several observations distinguish late-onset hypocalcemia from pseudohypoparathyroidism. First, it is very unusual for the genetic form of pseudohypoparathyroidism to cause hypocalcemia during infancy. Second, neonates with late-onset hypocalcemia show normal cyclic AMP responses after administration of PTH. And third, the PTH resistance of late-onset hypocalcemia is transient.

Late-onset hypocalcemia most typically occurs in newborns who are fed humanized cow's milk-based formulas, which have much higher concentrations of phosphorous than breast milk.

Rarely, neonatal vitamin D deficiency can also manifest as hypocalcemia after the first few days of life, when intestinal absorption of calcium begins to rely on vitamin D-dependent transport. Maternal vitamin D deficiency is typically associated with this condition. Hypoparathyroidism must be considered when hypocalcemia persists beyond 4 weeks of life. Severe congenital hypoparathyroidism is most commonly due to agenesis or dysgenesis of the parathyroid glands. The velocardiofacial/conotruncal anomaly/DiGeorge sequence (DGS) is caused by an embryonic field defect that impairs the development of the third and fourth branchial pouches and the fourth pharyngeal arch. The clinical features of the DGS are highly variable between individuals; some have subtle findings, whereas others are severely affected. The most common clinical features include hypoparathyroidism, T-cell immunodeficiency, and aortic arch defects. Other features include facial dysmorphia (e.g., hypertelorism, antimongoloid slant of the eyes, low-set notched ears, short philtrum of the lip, micrognathia), palate anomalies, velopharyngeal dysfunction, renal anomalies, and speech and feeding disorders as well as neurocognitive, behavioral, and psychiatric disorders. A significant number of patients with tetralogy of Fallot, truncus arteriosus, type B interrupted aortic arch, isolated aortic arch anomalies, and perimembranous ventricular septal defects have DGS. The most common cause of DGS is hemizygosity on chromosome 22q11, which occurs in 1 out to 2,500 to 4,000 live births. A large, contiguous gene deletion can be identified by fluorescent in situ hybridization (FISH) of peripheral blood cells in 75% to 90% of patients with DGS. DGS with loss of genetic material on chromosome 22q11 is often referred to by the acronym "CATCH-22," which stands for *c*ardiac anomalies, *a*bnormal facies, *t*hymic aplasia, *c*left palate, *h*ypocalcemia, and 22q11 deletion.

The DGS critical region includes the *TBX1* gene, which encodes a transcription factor that is expressed in pharyngeal arches and pouches, and small mutations in this gene have been described in some patients with DGS who are negative for the large 22q11 deletion. DGS can also be caused by large deletions at 10p13 (DGSII), and this molecular defect can also be identified by FISH analysis. In addition to genetic defects, DGS can also occur in infants who were exposed in utero to retinoic acid, alcohol, or maternal diabetes.

Although most cases of DGS are sporadic, autosomal dominant inheritance of DGS has been documented in some families. Fewer than 10% of patients with DGS will have "complete" DGS with thymic aplasia and severe immunodeficiency due to absence of functional T-cells. These children will experience recurrent infections, often with opportunistic organisms, and failure to thrive. Complete DGS can be identified by specialized studies that analyze the number and function of peripheral blood T-cells.

Hypoparathyroidism can occur as a feature of several other complex developmental syndromes, including the autosomal recessive Kenny–Caffey syndrome (which is characterized by short stature, osteosclerosis, basal ganglion calcifications, and opthalmic defects) and the allelic Sanjad–Sakati syndrome (growth and mental retardation), both due to mutations in the *TBCE* gene. The Barakat syndrome, also termed the hypoparathyroidism, deafness, and renal dysplasia (HDR) syndrome, is due to autosomal dominant mutation of the *GATA3* gene on chromosome 10p13.

Isolated hypoparathyroidism can occur as a result of homozygous inactivation of the *GCMB* gene, which is required for development of the parathyroid glands, or due to mutations of the *PTH* gene. A milder form of hypoparathyroidism occurs in newborns who have an activating mutation in the *CASR* gene that encodes the calcium-sensing receptor. This form of hypoparathyroidism is termed autosomal dominant hypocalcemia. Affected infants have parathyroid glands, but secretion of PTH is reduced significantly due to a gain-of-function mutation that increases sensitivity of the calcium-sensing receptor to extracellular calcium. The activated calcium-sensing receptor not only reduces PTH secretion but also increases renal excretion of calcium and magnesium, and thus causes hypocalcemia with hypercalciuria. Older patients can develop essentially the same syndrome due to the presence of antibodies that bind and activate the calcium-sensing receptor.

Destruction of parathyroid gland tissue is another cause of hypoparathyroidism, and can occur secondary to an autoimmune process. Autoimmune polyglandular syndrome type 1 (APS-1) consists of the triad of hypoparathyroidism, adrenal insufficiency, and mucocutaneous candidiasis, which can be familial or occur sporadically, and is typically due to homozygous inactivating mutations of the *AIRE* gene, which is highly expressed in the thymus. Patients with APS-1 develop a variety of autoantibodies that destroy endocrine tissues, including the parathyroid glands. Hypoparathyroidism can also occur as a consequence of surgical procedures that involve the parathyroid, thyroid, or other structures in the neck, but this risk has been minimized with awareness of the parathyroid gland location prior to and during surgery. Infiltration of the parathyroid tissue with metals, such as copper (Wilson disease) or iron (secondary to genetic or acquired hemochromatosis), can also result in impaired function of parathyroid tissue.

Hypomagnesemia can cause either decresed secretion of PTH or PTH resistance.

Clinical Findings

The clinical hallmark of hypoparathyroidism is neural hyperexcitability due to hypocalcemia, which causes paresthesias and smooth and skeletal muscle contractions (i.e., tetany). The patient should be examined for the following:

- Cataracts and papilledema.
- Cardiopulmonary effects.
  - Acute hypocalcemia causes prolongation of the QT interval, which may lead to ventricular dysrhythmias. It also causes decreased myocardial contractility, leading to congestive heart failure and hypotension.
  - Smooth muscle contraction may lead to laryngeal stridor and bronchospasm, particularly in infants, as well as dysphagia.

- Peripheral nervous system findings include tetany, focal numbness, and muscle spasms.
  - A positive Chvostek sign is present when tapping over the facial nerve about 2 cm anterior to the tragus results in contracture of the associated perioral muscles. The response is graded, and typically related to the degree of hypocalcemia.
  - An even more dramatic indicator of latent tetany is the Trousseau sign, in which carpopedal spasm (manifested as flexion at the wrist and metacarpophalangeal joints, extension of the distal interphalangeal and proximal interphalangeal joints, and adduction of the thumb and fingers) is elicited by insufflation of the blood-pressure cuff on the upper arm to 10 mm Hg above systolic pressure for 3 minutes.
- Irritability, confusion, hallucinations, extrapyramidal manifestations, and seizures may occur.
  - Calcification of basal ganglia, cerebellum, and cerebrum may occur.
  - Seizures can be spontaneous or occur in individuals with preexistent epileptic foci when the excitation threshold is lowered.

Patients with APS type 1 may also manifest candidiasis, adrenal insufficiency, hypothyroidism, diabetes mellitus, pernicious anemia/atrophic gastritis, gonadal failure, and ectodermal dystrophy.

All infants with congenital hypoparathyroidism should be investigated for anomalies associated with CATCH-22 and or DGS and APS type 1.

Laboratory Evaluation

The clinician should suspect hypoparathyroidism when hypocalcemia occurs in the presence of low or normal serum concentrations of PTH. In contrast, patients with hypocalcemia and *elevated* serum levels of PTH have secondary hyperparathyroidism, and are likely to have vitamin D deficiency or (less commonly) pseudohypoparathyroidism. It is important to recognize that it is inappropriate for the serum PTH level to be "normal" in the presence of hypocalcemia, and this relationship implies abnormal parathyroid function. Decreased parathyroid "reserve" is present in many patients with DGS who "outgrow" clinical hypoparathyroidism, but who may experience transient hypocalcemia when calcium demands are high (as with rapid growth). Similarly, patients with thalassemia who have had multiple blood transfusions can develop parathyroid insufficiency due to deposition of iron in the parathyroid glands, and will be at risk of symptomatic hypocalcemia during periods of stress or illness. An important biochemical concomitant of hypoparathyroidism is hyperphosphatemia, which occurs as a consequence of deficient PTH-dependent renal excretion of phosphorus. The serum concentration of PTH provides a useful clue to distinguish hypoparathyroidism from *pseudohypoparathyroidism,* a condition characterized by target tissue resistance to PTH and high rather than low PTH concentrations.

Patients with hypoparathyroidism will have normal levels of serum alkaline phosphatase and 25-hydroxyvitamin D, but serum concentrations of 1,25-dihydroxyvitamin D will be low because of the lack of PTH-induced conversion of vitamin D to its active 1,25-dihydroxy form. Serum magnesium levels should always be checked.

These findings are in contrast to those found in patients with nutritional vitamin D deficiency rickets, where elevated serum levels of PTH activate bone resorption and depress renal tubular reabsorption of phosphate with consequent hypophosphatemia. Although serum concentrations of 25-hydroxyvitamin D are typically low, serum concentrations of 1,25-dihydroxyvitamin D may be low, normal, or even elevated. The serum level of bone-derived alkaline phosphatase is usually elevated in proportion to the mineralization defect that results from the low serum levels of phosphate and calcium.

Genetic testing is now available in many commercial laboratories, and includes FISH tests for DGS (both 22q11 and 10p13 deletions) and mutation analysis for the *AIRE* and *CASR* genes. These tests not only facilitate a proper diagnosis, but can also identify asymptomatic relatives who may be at risk and can provide important information for family planning.

Therapy

Acute neuromuscular spasm or seizures are treated emergently with intravenous administration of 10% calcium gluconate solution, 0.5 mL/kg up to a maximum 10 mL over 15 minutes. This may be repeated if spasms are not controlled after the first bolus. After controlling the hypocalcemia-induced spasms, a continuous infusion of 500 mg calcium gluconate/kg/24 hours should be started in neonates. A continuous infusion of 1 to 3 mg of elemental calcium per kg/hour should be started for infants and older children. Because too rapid an infusion of calcium can induce bradycardia, all patients should be monitored by electrocardiogram. Serum magnesium levels may indicate a need for supplemental magnesium administration, which may subsequently normalize parathyroid secretion, especially in neonates or premature infants. Infants with late-onset hypocalcemia may require no treatment beyond reducing the gastrointestinal availability of phosphorus in humanized cows-milk formula, which will normalize the infant's serum phosphorus level. This can be achieved by assuring that the infant's formula contain a calcium to phosphorus molar ratio of at least 4 to 1. For example, one can supplement a low-phosphorus formula such as Similac PM 60/40 (11.2 mg calcium/oz and 5.5 mg phosphorus/oz, calcium:phosphorus ratio of 1.6:1) with calcium (add 220 mg of calcium carbonate to 5 oz of formula) to achieve a 4 to 1 ratio.

Because PTH deficiency is associated with impaired synthesis of 1,25-dihydroxyvitamin D, long-term treatment of hypoparathyroidism requires administration of calcitriol, 50 to 90 ng/kg/day in 2 to 3 divided doses. Supplemental calcium (requirements vary with age) should be given with meals to provide a constant source of calcium and to reduce gastrointestinal absorption of phosphorous. Under some circumstances it may be reasonable to consider daily injections of recombinant human PTH instead of treatment with calcitriol. Patients with hypoparathyroidism have increased urinary calcium excretion in relation to serum calcium and are therefore prone to hypercalciuria, and this is particularly true for patients with activating mutations of the *CASR* gene. Serum and urinary calcium levels should be monitored regularly, and those patients with hypercalciuria (greater than 4 mg/kg/24 hr calcium), who are at greatest risk of nephrocalcinosis and nephrolithiasis, should have renal ultrasound examinations annually.

HYPERPARATHYROIDISM AND HYPERCALCEMIA

Etiology

Primary hyperparathyroidism is characterized by hypercalcemia, either total or ionized calcium, in the presence of an elevated concentration of PTH.

Neonates normally have high levels of calcium with an upper limit of normal of 11.3 mg/dL. The most common cause of neonatal hyperparathyroidism is neonatal severe primary hyperparathyroidism (NSPHT). This disease is related to familial hypocalciuric hypercalcemia (FHH), and although FHH is a relatively benign disorder, infants with NSPHT can present with severe, life-threatening hypercalcemia in their first few days of life. Both FHH and NSPHT result from inactivating mutations in the *CASR* gene that decrease the sensitivity of parathyroid cells to extracellular calcium levels. Patients with NSPHT have hypercalcemia with elevated PTH and alkaline phosphatase, normal to low serum levels of phosphate, normal to high serum levels of magnesium, and low fractional exretion of urinary calcium.

Neonates who have had a difficult delivery may develop subcutaneous fat necrosis. This usually is insignificant, but when present over a large area, may cause hypercalcemia within a few days or weeks of life. Skin that has endured trauma either through vacuum or forceps delivery begins to produce calcitriol by macrophages present within the granulomatous reaction that have ectopic 1α-hydroxylase activity.

Approximately 15% of children with Williams syndrome will present with hypercalcemia in infancy. The serum calcium level typically normalizes within 2 to 4 years, but hypercalciuria may persist. Features characteristic of this sporadic disorder are "elfin" facies, clinodactyly of fifth fingers, kyphoscoliosis, pectus excavatum, renal defects, and supravalvular aortic stenosis in 30% of patients. Williams syndrome can be diagnosed by FISH analysis using a probe to detect a microdeletion region on chromosome 7q11 that includes the elastin gene.

Congenital lactase deficiency can cause hypercalcemia by increasing intestinal calcium absorption due to increased gastrointestinal lactose. This presents in the first few months of life and usually resolves after dietary modifications with a lactose-free diet. Another cause of hypercalcemia in the newborn period is hypophosphatasia, an autosomal recessive disorder characterized by deficiency of alkaline phosphatase, skeletal demineralization, and premature loss of deciduous teeth. Lastly, blue diaper syndrome is due to abnormal intestinal tryptophan transport and is a rare cause of hypercalcemia in the neonate. The oxidation of indican in the urine (from metabolism of abnormal intestinal tryptophan degradation) causes the blue discoloration.

Children with Jansen metaphyseal chondrodysplasia have hypercalemia and bone lesions that are typical of primary hyperparathyroidism, but have suppressed PTH levels. This unusual disorder is due to mutations in the PTH/PTHrP receptor that lead to ligand-independent activation of the receptor. This causes increased bone resorption, metaphyseal defects, elevated serum levels of 1,25 dihydroxyvitamin D, and growth delay.

In older children and adolescents, primary hyperparathyroidism is most commonly the result of a solitary parathyroid adenoma. However, primary hyperparathyroidism with multiple gland enlargement can occur as a manifestation of several autsomal dominant syndromes. The most common of these is multiple endocrine neoplasia (MEN) type 1, due to mutation of the *MEN1* gene, and is associated with multiple enlarged parathyroid glands (90%), pancreatic islet cell (>50%) and pituitary (25–40%) adenomas, and dermal lesions (70–90%) such as angiofibromas and collagenomas. Primary hyperparathyroidism occurs with lesser frequency in patients with MEN 2a, due to *RET* gene mutations, in which medullary thyroid carcinoma and pheochromocytoma are common. Primary hyperparathyroidism is very unusual in the MEN 2b variant, in which medullary carcinoma of the thyroid and pheochromocytoma are associated with ganglioneuromas of the gastrointestinal tract and a marfanoid habitus.

Clinical Findings

The most obvious clinical features of primary hyperparathyroidism relate to hypercalcemia. General symptoms include weakness, malaise, decreased appetite, difficulty concentrating, headache, decline in school performance, behavior changes (including irritability), and diffuse muscle pain. Physical signs

of elevated calcium include abdominal pain, nausea, vomiting, constipation, flank pain (related to nephrocalcinosis or renal stones), hypertension, nonpurulent conjunctivitis, stupor, and coma. Elevated levels of PTH can induce excessive bone resorption with the consequent development of osteoporosis. Rarely, long-standing disease will lead to the development of the specific bone lesion of hyperparathyroidism termed *osteitis fibrosa cystica*. A parathyroid mass is almost never palpable or visualized on physical examination and can often be difficult to detect using imaging techniques.

Laboratory Evaluation

A diagnosis of primary hyperparathyroidism is confirmed by the demonsration of an elevated serum calcium level and an elevated, or inappropriately normal, level of serum-intact or whole-molecule PTH. Commercial laboratories provide reference ranges for circulating levels of PTH that are based on sampling large numbers of "normal" adult subjects. These normal ranges represent a nongaussian distribution, which implies that some subjects with primary hyperparathyroidism will have serum PTH levels that are "normal." Circulating levels of PTH in children have been shown to be either lower or similar to those levels in adults.

Often, but not always, the patient will also have an elevated serum level of bone-specific alkaline phosphatase and a low serum phosphorus level. Serum concentrations of 1,25-dihydroxyvitamin D are elevated due to increased PTH-induced conversion of vitamin D, and often the serum level of 25-hydroxyvitamin D is depressed. The fractional excretion of urinary calcium is less than 1% in patients with FHH or NSPHT, and increased in most patients with other causes of hypercalcemia.

Imaging studies, to identify a parathyroid adenoma, are not indicated unless minimally invasive parathyroidectomy is planned (see the "Therapy" section, below). Among imaging modalities, planar ^{99m}Tc-sestamibi (MIBI) scintigraphy (dual-phase and dual-isotope technique), often with complementary ultrasound, appears to be the method of choice for imaging an enlarged parathyroid lesion in the neck with >90% sensitivity. However, single-photon emission computed tomography (SPECT), using ^{99m}Tc-sestamibi (MIBI) scintigraphy, with co-registered CT scanning, provides superior three-dimensional anatomic information for surgery, and may be more sensitive for localization of ectopic parathyroid lesions. Other high-resolution techniques include ultrasound, computed tomography scan, and magnetic resonance imaging.

Therapy

Surgical excision is the definitive therapy for primary hyperparathyroidism, and is recommended as the principle treatment for all patients under the age of 50 years. Newborns with NSPHT may require urgent surgery, with excision of all enlarged parathyroid glands. By contrast, children with FHH are typically asymptomic, as opposed to newborns with NSPHT, and do not require any specific treatment; surgical intervention is not indicated. Emergency treatment of life-threatening or symptomatic hypercalcemia should include aggressive hydration with intravenous normal saline; loop diuretics should not be used or used with great caution as they can worsen hypercalemia by inducing a state of dehydration with reduced glomerular filtration of calcium. Other agents such as calcitonin and bisphosphonates can reduce serum calcium concentrations and may be useful prior to surgery. Calcimimetics, such as cinacalcet, increase the sensitivity of the CaSR to calcium and can lower serum calcium levels, but there is no information regarding their usefulness or safety in children and adolescents with primary hyperparathyroidism. Minimally invasive parathyroidectomy is a reasonable surgical approach in older children and adolescents with a solitary parathyroid adenoma that has been localized by an imaging study (above). However, if there is evidence of multiple-gland disease, such as MEN1, a traditional bilateral neck exploration should be performed. All enlarged parathyroid tissue should be removed, and a remnent of the most normal-appearing parathyroid gland may be left in situ or transplanted to the forearm. Function of the transplanted parathyroid tissue can be easily assessed by comparing PTH levels in opposite arms, and if the transplanted tissue becomes hyperactive, it can be easily removed or partially resected.

Careful follow-up with referral to an endocrinologist and an oncologist is required for evaluation and treatment of suspected MEN type 1 and type 2 syndromes.

Suggested Readings

Abrams SA, Griffin IJ, Hawthorne KM, et al. Relationships among vitamin D levels, parathyroid hormone, and calcium absorption in young adolescents. *J Clin Endocrinol Metab* 2005;90:5576–5581.

Carling T, Udelsman R. Parathyroid surgery in familial hyperparathyroid disorders. *J Intern Med* 2005;257:27–37. Review.

Guarnieri V, Scillitani A, Muscarella LA, et al. Diagnosis of parathyroid tumors in familial isolated hyperparathyroidism with HRPT2 mutation: implications for cancer surveillance. *J Clin Endocrinol Metab* 2006;91:2827–2832.

Kollars J, Zarroug AE, van Heerden J, et al. Primary hyperparathyroidism in pediatric patients. *Pediatrics* 2005;115:974–980.

Krebs LJ, Arnold A. Molecular basis of hyperparathyroidism and potential targets for drug development. *Curr Drug Targets Immune Endocr Metabol Disord* 2002;2:167–179. Review.

Levine MA. Hypoparathyroidism and pseudohypoparathyroidism. In: DeGroot LJ, Jameson JL, eds. *Endocrinology*. 5th ed. Philadelphia: Saunders; 2005.

Levine MA, Streeten EA. Primary hyperparathyroidism. In: Martini L, ed. *Encyclopedia of endocrine diseases*. Vol. 2. San Diego: Elsevier/Academic Press; 2004:558–566.

Levine MA, Zapalowski C, Kappy MS. Disorders of calcium, phosphate, parathyroid hormone and vitamin D. In: *Principles and Practice of Pediatric Endocrinology*. Springfield, IL: Thomas; 2005:695–814.

Mihai R, Gleeson F, Buley ID, et al. Negative imaging studies for primary hyperparathyroidism are unavoidable: correlation of sestamibi and high-resolution ultrasound scanning with histological analysis in 150 patients editors: Kappy MS, Allen DB, Geffner ME, *World J Surg* 2006;30:697–704.

Younes NA, Shafagoj Y, Khatib F, et al. Laboratory screening for hyperparathyroidism. *Clin Chim Acta* 2005;353:1–12. Review.

CHAPTER 104 ■ PANHYPOPITUITARISM

CLAUDE J. MIGEON

PHYSIOLOGY AND PATHOPHYSIOLOGY OF ANTERIOR PITUITARY HORMONES

Panhypopituitarism is, by definition, a deficiency of more than one of the hormones secreted by the anterior pituitary gland. The major pituitary hormones include growth hormone (GH), thyroid-stimulating hormone (TSH), luteinizing hormone (LH), follicle-stimulating hormone (FSH), adrenocorticotropic hormone (ACTH), and prolactin.

It is well established that the secretion of all pituitary hormones is controlled by specific "releasing hormones" from the hypothalamus. They include GH-releasing hormone (GHRH), TSH-releasing hormone (TRH), LH- and FSH-releasing hormone (GnRH), and corticotrophin-releasing hormone (CRH). The releasing hormones reach the pituitary via a short vessel loop or "portal system."

The pituitary hormones are secreted in blood and carried to their target glands. They bind to specific cell-membrane receptors, and by means of a system of "G-proteins" and of protein kinases, they will activate the secretion of IGF-1, thyroid hormones (T4 and T3), sex hormones (estrogens and androgens), and cortisol.

The hormones just mentioned are carried in blood mainly bound to proteins: IGF-1 binding proteins, thyroxine-binding globulin (TBG), sex hormone-binding globulin (SHBG), and cortisol-binding globulin (CBG). However, a small fraction of these hormones remain unbound, and can be directly transferred into the cytoplasm of the "target cells," where they recognize and bind to specific DNA-binding proteins (receptors). The union of hormone/receptor will control the expression of genes, the product of which will be the hormonal effects.

An attempt to comprehensively classify hypopituitarism is presented in Table 104.1. However, the study of panhypopituitarism usually is limited to the secretion of GH, TSH, gonadotropins, and ACTH.

SIGNS AND DIAGNOSIS OF PANHYPOPITUITARISM

In practice, the most frequent problems will be related to either congenital septo-optic dysplasia or the acquired abnormalities of the hypothalamus/pituitary. Although gene mutations of releasing hormones are not rare, they are more difficult to study at this time.

Septo-Optic Dysplasia

Septo-optic dysplasia is a mid-brain malformation that includes absence of septum pellucidum and abnormalities of hypothala-

mus and optic chiasma, resulting in an absence of secretion of some or all the "releasing hormones" and blindness. However, the degree of mid-brain malformations can be variable; the blindness may be absent, and some releasing hormones may remain.

In the newborn period an important problem can be hypoglycemia related to absence of GH and cortisol secretion. In male infants, micropenis may be present related to lack of gonadotropins and full fetal masculinization.

The work-up will include head MRI, estimation of level of vision, and determination of levels of hormones in blood.

Acquired Abnormalities

Brain tumors such as craniopharyngioma occur usually in childhood. In addition to signs of brain compression, there will often be symptoms of growth failure and/or hypothyroidism. Pituitary tumors like non-functional adenoma or Rothke cysts can result in primary panhypopituitarism.

Autoimmune hypophysitis can result in destruction of the pituitary.

Accidental head trauma, surgical trauma, and head radiation will also produce a loss of some or all pituitary function.

In all cases, head MRI with and without contrast helps to determine the extent of hypothalamus/pituitary damage, whereas hormone measurement demonstrates the extent of lack of function.

TREATMENT

Therapy will involve replacement of glandular hormones, growth hormone, thyroxine, cortisol, and at puberty, sex hormones.

Growth Hormone Replacement

Most clinics use the dose of 0.3 mg of GH, per kilogram of body weight, per week. The weekly dose is divided in 6 or 7 fractions, which are administered 6 or 7 days of each week. Usually there is some increase of dose at the time of puberty.

Thyroid Hormone Replacement

L-thyroxine is used in dosage varying in relation to age and body size. Doses of 25 to 150 μg are given once daily. Monitoring of total and unbound T_4, along with clinical signs of euthyroidism, will determine the level of replacement.

Cortisol Replacement

Cortisol replacement is described in Chapter 101. The maintenance dose of cortisol (Cortef) is equal to about twice the daily secretion rate, or 12 to 24 mg/m²/24 hours, given in 3 equal parts every 8 hours. Prednisolone at a daily dose of 1.75 to 3.5 mg/m²/24 hr, given in two equal parts every 12 hours can also be used. The stress dose is 2 to 3 times

TABLE 104.1

CLASSIFICATION OF HYPOPITUITARISM

1. Congenital malformations of hypothalamus and anterior pituitary gland
   - Anencephaly
   - Septo-optic dysplasia
   - Empty sella turcica syndrome
   - Mutation of transcription factors: SF-1, DAX-1, Pit-1, PROP-1
2. Acquired abnormalities of hypothalamus and anterior pituitary gland
   - Tumors (craniopharyngioma, astrocytoma, etc.)
   - Pituitary adenoma
   - Head trauma
   - Hypophysitis (autoimmune)
   - Therapeutic brain surgery or radiation
3. Mutation of gene for "releasing hormones": GHRH, TRH, GnRH, CRH, prolactin
4. Mutation of genes for "receptors of releasing hormones"
5. Mutation of genes for "hormones": GH, TSH, LH, FSH, ACTH
6. Mutation of genes for "receptors of hormones"
7. Mutation of genes for "glandular hormones": IGF-1, T_4 and T_3, sex hormones (estrogens and androgens), cortisol
8. Hormone insensitivity due to mutation of genes for hormone receptors

the maintenance dose. In case of stress with vomiting, Solucortef (50 to 100 mg) given SQ or IM is used.

Gonadotropin Replacement

At puberty, the absence of gonadotropins will require the administration of sex steroids. In girls, we usually start with Premarin 0.3125 mg orally, twice a week, followed by the same dose daily. After 12 to 18 months, the treatment may be changed to a contraceptive pill such as Lo-Estrin 1/20.

In boys, an IM injection of 25 mg of testosterone enanthate is given once monthly for 6 to 12 months. This is followed by progressive increases to 50, 100, and 200 mg monthly or every 3 weeks. In late puberty, a gel preparation or testosterone patches can be used.

Suggested Readings

Chung TT, Monson JP. Hypopituitarism. Chapter 12, March 28, 2003 *in* Endotext.com.

DeVille CJ, Grant DB, Hayward RD, et al. Growth and endocrine sequelae of craniopharyngioma. *Arch Dis Child* 1996;75:108–114.

Jenkins PJ. Inflammatory lesions—lymphocytic hypophysitis, sarcoid, histiocytosis, TB, Wegener's granulomatosis. In: Wass JAH, Shalet SM, eds. *Oxford textbook of endocrinology and diabetes*. Oxford: Oxford University Press; 2002:236–242.

Kovacs K, Scheithauer BW, Horvath G, et al. The World Health Organization classification of adenohypophysial neoplasms. *Cancer* 1996;78:502–510.

Radeva H, Harpal S, Schoebel J, et al. Classical pituitary apoplexy: clinical features, management and outcome. *Clin Endocrinol* 1999;51:181–188.

CHAPTER 105 ■ TERM NEWBORN EXAMINATION

PATRICIA V. LOWERY

Involvement in the examination and care of the newborn infant is usually one of the most gratifying experiences for the pediatric health care provider. With the exception of infants who have problems at birth requiring the care of a neonatologist, this provider has the first opportunity to thoroughly assess the infant.

HISTORY

The newborn assessment should include both historical elements and physical examination. The history provides information that is used to establish the infant's risk for developing problems. It is crucial that the examiner identify those infants with abnormal findings, because of the need for immediate intervention and the implications for future health. Neonatal problems are most often related to transitional physiologic changes, infection, injury, or birth defects.

Review of the maternal history by chart review and personal interview must be a key part of newborn care. The maternal history provides information regarding risk factors for the infant, such as maternal diabetes, group B streptococcal carriage, or history of sexually transmitted infection (STI). Fetal ultrasound may detect physical abnormalities warranting further evaluation in the postnatal period. Table 105.1 lists information needed about the family and the details of pregnancy, labor, and delivery needed to guide care.

The examiner should always estimate the infant's gestational age. Estimation of gestational age and plotting weight for gestational age is helpful in predicting potential problems that may occur during the transition to extrauterine life. The revised Ballard examination, based on predictable patterns of changes occurring throughout gestation, consists of neuromuscular and physical maturity ratings. When discrepancy exists between expected and actual scores, influences on gestational age assessment should be considered, such as inaccuracy of estimated date of confinement, intrauterine conditions, neonatal illness, sedation, or underlying neurologic disease. When dates are uncertain, the Ballard score remains the best method for gestational age estimation. Growth parameters are plotted on growth charts in order to classify the newborn as appropriate for gestational age (AGA), large for gestational age (LGA), or small for gestational age (SGA). By classic definition, AGA infants fall between the 10th and 90th percentiles; SGA infants below the 10th percentile, and LGA infants above the 90th percentile.

PHYSICAL EXAMINATION

When possible, the *physical examination* should occur with the parent(s) present in order to promote questions and education and strengthen the provider—parent relationship. An infant at risk of cold stress (ill infant, premature or SGA infant, or one requiring a prolonged period of being unwrapped) should be transferred to an open bed warmer. The examiner should develop procedural flexibility along with patience and gentleness necessary to complete all elements of the newborn exam, proceeding in the fashion allowed by the infant's general state.

By simple inspection and observation of the infant, overall condition and well-being can be determined. The gender, posture, color, level of alertness and activity, symmetry of movement, respiratory status, and presence of any gross dysmorphisms should be noted. Vital signs should be recorded and repeated if abnormal until transition is completed or to assess progress of required interventions. The frontooccipital circumference, length, weight, chest circumference, and abdominal circumference should be documented.

The skin of the infant should be inspected for neurocutaneous markings, benign newborn skin lesions, birthmarks, and evidence of trauma, in addition to other color variations. The plethoric infant may be polycythemic. Acrocyanosis may be physiologic and may increase with chilling. Mottling may be indicative of cold stress, hypovolemia, sepsis, or cutis marmorata. The presence of pallor should raise suspicion of anemia, or sepsis with poor perfusion. Meconium staining suggests previous fetal distress; excessively dry, cracked skin is consistent with being post-term. Nutritional status may be assessed by noting the amount of subcutaneous fat, particularly in the anterior thighs and gluteal regions, or by the amount of Wharton's jelly in the umbilical cord.

If the infant is quiet, the examiner may proceed with the cardiopulmonary exam, eye exam, and palpation of femoral pulses since these elements are more difficult in the crying infant. Increased work of breathing, manifested by use of accessory muscles, retractions, nasal flaring, grunting, tachypnea, and persistent central cyanosis, usually indicates cardiopulmonary or severe metabolic problems. Paradoxical breathing (the rib cage moves inward and the abdomen outward during inspiration) is due to increased chest wall compliance, which results from incomplete ossification of the ribs and sternum, and diaphragmatic breathing of the newborn. Auscultation of the lungs should be performed in all fields to check for symmetry of aeration and presence of adventitious breath sounds. The pattern of neonatal respiratory effort often suggests a disease process. The quality of the cry should be noted. Stridor may indicate airway obstruction (see Chapter 22).

The cardiac examination should begin with inspection of the skin color, symmetry and shape of the chest, and precordial activity. If central cyanosis, which involves the mucous membranes, fails to resolve, congenital heart disease or respiratory

TABLE 105.1

KEY ELEMENTS OF MATERNAL HISTORY

Category	Element
Prior health history	Diabetes
	Hypertension
	Seizures
	Drug use/abuse (include smoking and alcohol)
	Problems with prior pregnancies
	Medications
	Family history (immediate family, congenital disease)
	Social history (family support, work, school, preparations for baby)
Pregnancy	Pregnancy planned or unplanned
	Prenatal care (early/late)
	Estimated date of confinement (EDC)
	Plans for feeding (breast or formula)
	Sexually transmitted diseases (STDs) (and treatment if indicated): syphilis, gonorrhea, chlamydia, human immunodeficiency virus, herpes (primary or recurrent)
	Other illness during pregnancy
	Weight gain in pregnancy
	Complications: diabetes, pre-eclampsia
	Maternal laboratory data: blood type, group B streptococcal culture, screening tests for above STDs, rubella immune status
Labor	Spontaneous or induced
	Rupture of membranes: spontaneous or artificial, hrs prior to delivery
	Amniotic fluid: clear, cloudy, foul, meconium
	Complications, including findings on fetal monitoring
	Medications (especially antibiotics)
	Maternal fever
Delivery	Process: spontaneous vaginal, Cesarean section, forceps; reason for latter two
	Presentation: vertex, breech, transverse
	Apgar scores: 1 and 5 min

problems must be considered (see Chapter 13). Heart sounds should be more clearly heard and palpated in the left chest, with the point of maximal impulse (PMI) best appreciated at the left lower sternal border (LLSB), owing to right ventricular dominance. Upon palpation, one may appreciate a heave, thrill, or tap. Louder heart sounds on the right suggest dextrocardia or pneumothorax. Sinus arrhythmia or ectopic beats (PACs and PVCs) are commonly heard and are usually benign. First and second heart sounds should be distinct. Physiologic splitting of the second heart sound, which is caused by asynchronous closure of the pulmonary and aortic valves, may be appreciated after the first few hours of life. Murmurs should be carefully categorized to include location, phase of the cardiac cycle, intensity (based on a grading system of I to VI), quality, and associated findings. Palpation of pulses is fundamental to the newborn cardiac exam. Increased pulse pressure and bounding pulses with a machinery-like murmur are classic findings of patent ductus arteriosus (PDA). Features associated with innocent murmurs include intensity less than or equal to grade II heard at the left sternal border, normal pulses, absence of clicks, a normal physiologically split S2, and capillary filling time less than or equal to 2 seconds. Conversely, features generally associated with significant congenital heart disease include a murmur greater than or equal to grade III, harsh quality, pansystolic, loudest at the left upper sternal border with an single or fixed split S2, and absent or decreased femoral pulses. Murmurs associated with an active precordium are more likely to be pathologic. It is important to remember that at times no murmur is heard in infants with serious congenital heart disease.

Examination of the eyes should include inspection for intercanthal distance, width of palpebral fissures, presence of epicanthal folds, abnormal slant, pupillary size, and abnormalities of the iris such as coloboma and heterochromia. Periorbital edema from the birth process and installation of ophthalmic antibiotic ointment may hinder adequate examination, but gentle manual separation of the eyelids is usually sufficient for assessing presence of subconjunctival hemorrhages, eye movements, and the red reflex. Alternatively, by holding the infant vertically in low ambient light, the infant will often open the eyes spontaneously allowing examination. The red reflex may vary from pale pink to reddish yellow and should be symmetrical. Abnormalities of the lens, vitreous, or retina produce leukocoria, which mandates further investigation.

After examining the cardiorespiratory system and eyes, the examination can proceed cephalocaudally. Inspection and palpation of the head often reveals molding or overlapping of sutures, which occur most often with vaginal delivery. Six bony plates and six suture lines should be identified. Caput succedaneum, an area of edema over the presenting part of the head, is common and can be distinguished from the subperiosteal bleeding of a cephalohematoma, which usually develops later and does not cross suture lines. Commonly, a caput resolves as a cephalohematoma evolves, with the latter often taking weeks to months to disappear. The least frequently encountered scalp injury, the subgaleal hematoma, produces a fluctuant mass underlying large areas of the scalp. Such subaponeuronal bleeding may result in anemia and even profound shock. Both cephalohematomas and subgaleal hematomas may worsen hyperbilirubinemia and delay its resolution. Superficial bruising, abrasions, and fetal scalp monitor electrode wounds are also seen. Craniotabes may be physiologic, for example with prematurity; or pathologic, being associated with rickets or congenital syphilis. Any full and pulsating fontanelle should cause concern for increased intracranial pressure. Less frequently, encephaloceles, meningoceles, dermoid cysts, and skull fractures may be detected. Auscultation over the cranium and temporal arteries for bruits should be done, particularly in the setting of unexplained heart failure. Cranial shape and proportion should be noted. Right-sided positional plagiocephaly is most commonly noted because the more common fetal presentation is left occiput anterior. Hair whorls are single in 97.5% of infants and are most often located to the right of the parietal midline, with clockwise rotation more common. More than two whorls or a single anteriorly located whorl may be a sign of CNS abnormality.

The face may have bruising related to birth trauma or forceps-assisted delivery. Tiny pearl-like milia, resulting from retention of keratin and sebaceous material within the pilosebaceous units of the face, are frequently noted. Jaundice is usually first noted in the face and progresses in a cephalocaudal fashion. Because visual inspection of jaundice is unreliable once the total serum bilirubin exceeds 12 mg/dL, predischarge measurement of bilirubin is now advised. Asymmetry of the mouth, asynclitism, is commonly related to facial nerve palsy from in utero positioning or from application of forceps, but can also occur with syndromes such as Mobius, Poland, DiGeorge, and Goldenhar. Congenital absence of the depressor anguli oris should also be considered in the differential diagnosis of asymmetry of the mouth. Congenital muscular torticollis may result from intrauterine malpositioning or birth trauma; it presents as a sternomastoid tumor (with a mass), muscular torticollis (without a mass), or postural torticollis. The neck exam should include assessment for folds, webs, or skin redundancy, as well as for cystic lesions, tumors, or goiters.

The vertical plane of the external ear should run parallel to the long axis of the infant. A portion (10–20%) of the pinna should extend above a line defined by the medial and lateral canthus of the eye. Low-set, rotated, or malformed ears should be considered dysmorphisms. Abnormalities of the external ear are often associated with renal malformations and hearing loss. Preauricular pits and tags are common. The patency of the external auditory canal should be confirmed. Otoscopic examination of the middle ear may be limited by the presence of vernix caseosa, but should be attempted.

The nares should be inspected for patency and the presence of a midline septum. The latter is sometimes displaced from the vomerian groove and requires manipulation for correction. Upon manual depression of the tip of the nose, a dislocated septum angles within the nares. Because infants are obligate nose breathers, the ability to breathe through each naris with the mouth closed should be noted. When in question, a small nasogastric tube should be passed through each naris to rule out choanal atresia. A misshapen nose can suggest genetic abnormalities. Profuse purulent nasal discharge may be found with congenital syphilis.

Examination of the mouth should begin with assessing for cyanosis. Central cyanosis is defined by cyanosis of mucous membranes, while perioral cyanosis is more likely a result of vasomotor instability. Cleft lips may be unilateral, midline, or bilateral. The alveolar ridges, palate, tongue, and pharynx should be carefully inspected. Epstein pearls are usually in the midline at the junction of the hard and soft palate; Bohn nodules are similar in appearance, but are found on the alveolar ridges. A loose natal tooth should be removed because of the risk of aspiration; true deciduous teeth occur in fewer than one in 2,000 births and should not be extracted. Mucous retention cysts, which are sometimes found on the gums (epulis) or on the floor of the mouth (ranula), occur in about one in 3,500 live births and usually resolve. Solid tumors and large cysts require surgical consultation. Palpation of the palate may help identify a submucosal cleft, which may be suggested by a bifid uvula. Macroglossia is associated with Pompe disease, Down syndrome, and Beckwith–Wiedemann syndrome. "Tongue-tie" or ankyloglossia requires frenectomy only in the event of difficulty with feeding or speech. Micrognathia is seen with Pierre–Robin sequence.

Chest size and symmetry should be noted, along with formation and placement of the nipples. A smaller-than-normal chest is seen with pulmonary hypoplasia or neuromuscular disease. Chest asymmetry may be seen with Poland anomaly (absent pectoralis major), mass, or abscess. Clavicular fractures may be seen in settings of shoulder dystocia or breech presentation. Palpable callus formation develops in days to weeks. Treatment, if any, consists of modifying feeding position and handling to minimize pain. The sternum should be inspected for pectus excavatum or carinatum. Infants commonly have some palpable breast tissue due to maternal estrogens; breast enlargement may reach 3 to 4 cm and galactorrhea may be present. Parents should be discouraged from manual expression of this milk, due to an increased risk of mastitis. Wide-set nipples, generally defined as an internipple distance greater than 25% of chest circumference, should be considered dysmorphic. Accessory or supernumerary nipples, often noted in the nipple line and varying from a slightly pigmented dimple to a fully formed breast, occur in one in 40 newborns and are seen more often in African-American infants.

The abdomen of the newborn is normally mildly protuberant. A scaphoid abdomen may suggest diaphragmatic hernia or intestinal atresia. Mild protrusion of the abdomen between the muscles of the rectus abdominus is referred to as diastasis recti. Infraumbilical ecchymosis or fullness suggests vessel spillage or urachal leakage. Umbilical herniation or omphalocele should be considered when the cord base seems broad or fluctuant after pulsations have ceased. The umbilical cord should be examined for diameter, length, color, abdominal wall insertion, and the number of vessels it contains. The normal cord diameter at term is 1.5 cm on average; a smaller cord is seen in SGA infants. The cord should contain two arteries and one vein. Because up to 10% of infants with single umbilical artery may have underlying congenital anomalies, renal ultrasound should be considered if other dysmorphisms are found. Meconium staining of the cord should be noted. The abdomen should be auscultated for bowel sounds. Palpation of the abdomen is improved by elevating the lower extremities and pelvis with one hand, while examining the infant's relaxed abdomen with the other hand. Gentle palpation should begin in the lower quadrants and move upward to avoid missing hepatic enlargement. In the term infant, the liver edge may be up to 2 cm below the costal margin in the midclavicular line with a liver span of approximately 6 cm. The spleen is rarely palpable; one that is more than 1 cm below the left costal margin should be considered abnormal. Deep palpation is required for renal examination: by placing one hand posteriorly at the costovertebral angle and lifting anteriorly, the examiner can direct the fingertips of the other hand deeply into the flank. The left kidney is more easily palpable than the right. The kidney of a term neonate measures 4.5 to 5 cm. The bladder may be palpable 1 to 4 cm above the symphysis pubis, making suprapubic aspiration an often preferred method for obtaining a urine specimen.

Examination of the female genitalia begins with the labia majora, which are enlarged in the term infant. Gentle traction facilitates visual inspection of the clitoris, labia minora, hymen, and vagina for size, position, and patency. Maternal estrogen stimulation causes hymenal redundancy and vaginal discharge, which may be whitish or blood-tinged as the newborn's estrogen level falls. Examination of male genitalia should include inspection of the shaft and glans for abnormalities. The normal penile length should not be less than 2.5 cm when stretched to full length. The foreskin may remain variably unretractable well into childhood and should not be forcibly retracted. White sebaceous cysts at the tip of the foreskin are benign. Abnormalities such as hooded foreskin, hypospadias (urethral opening on the ventral surface), epispadias (urethral opening on the dorsal surface), or chordee (ventral curvature of the erect penis) are contraindications to circumcision. Infants with perineal or scrotal hypospadias, those with hypospadias and a nonpalpable testis, or nonpalpable testes in a phenotypic male should be evaluated for ambiguous genitalia or virilizing adrenal hyperplasia. Cryptorchidism occurs in 3% to 5% of term males and up to 33% of preterm males. Scrotal rugae are present after 37 weeks gestation. The normal testicular volume is 1 to 2 mL. Hydroceles, when present, will usually resolve over the first 6 months of life. Inguinal hernias are commonly of the indirect type and occur in 3.5% to 5% of term infants. These hernias in infants frequently incarcerate or strangulate in the first year of life; prompt surgical consultation is recommended. The infant's anus should be inspected for appropriate placement and rugation.

The musculoskeletal examination begins with general inspection of the spine and extremities for symmetry, posture, tone, and movement, both passive and active. The back should be inspected and palpated from neck to buttocks, noting curvature, neurocutaneous markers of disease such as midline hemangiomas, pigmented nevi, or hairy tufts, and obvious gross defects. Sacral dimples, pits, clefts, lipomas, or hair tufts may signal a tethered cord or spinal dysraphisms. Ultrasonographic evaluation is the study of choice for initial evaluation. Early diagnosis of congenital scoliosis associated with malformed vertebrae allows treatment to prevent progressive curvature. The upper extremities should be examined for possible brachial plexus injury, which occurs more often in the setting of macrosomia, shoulder dystocia, instrument-assisted deliveries, and malpresentations. An adducted, internally rotated arm with a flexed wrist referred to as "waiter's tip" position of the hand, suggests upper plexus injury, known as Erb palsy. Less commonly, a limp wrist and absent grasp suggests injury to the lower brachial plexus, known as Klumpke paralysis; if sympathetic fibers are also involved, the ptosis and miosis of Horner syndrome will be present as well. Injury to the phrenic nerve, which has input from the third to fifth cervical nerve roots, leads to paralysis of the ipsilateral diaphragm. Birth injury to the recurrent laryngeal nerve occurs most often on the left side; the resulting vocal cord paralysis may present with stridor, altered cry, dysphagia, or respiratory distress. Although rare, spinal cord injury may occur with traumatic deliveries and presents with the classic lower motor neuron signs of absent or decreased movement and loss of deep tendon reflexes; response to pain may be diminished as well.

Thigh fold asymmetry should lead the examiner to check for leg-length discrepancy (Galeazzi sign) due to developmental dysplasia of the hip (DDH). The Ortolani maneuver reduces the dislocated femoral head into the acetabulum by abduction of the thigh while gentle pressure is applied to the femoral head; the Barlow maneuver dislocates the femoral head posteriorly. DDH shows a 9 to 1 female predominance, occurring in one in 800 white females. Of those affected, 60% are firstborn, 30% to 50% are breech, 20% have a positive family history, 10% have associated metatarsus adductus, and torticollis may occur in up to 20%. Laxity of the hip ligaments may result in a subluxable hip after delivery but the findings should resolve by 2 weeks of age. If the hip exam remains abnormal at 2 weeks, orthopedic consultation is warranted. The shape of the tibia and feet should be noted. Intoeing commonly results from tibial torsion and metatarsus adductus, which are related to in utero positioning. The physiologic flexion contractures in the newborn's hips and knees normally resolve over the first few weeks of life. Syndactyly, most common in the 2nd and 3rd toes, is often familial. Polydactyly of the 5th toe occurs in 2 in 1,000 newborns. Clubfoot is seen in one in 1,000 births; it carries a 3% risk for subsequent siblings and a 20% to 30% risk for offspring of affected parents.

The initial neurologic assessment consists of noting the infant's state and resting posture, motor activity, integrated reflexes, and phasic postural tone. The normal newborn has increased flexor tone and maintains a moderately flexed posture. The suck, root, grasp, and Moro reflexes should be elicited. Abnormal postures include persistent extension of the neck (opisthotonus), obligate flexion of the thumb (cortical thumb), and frog-leg positioning in infants greater than 36 weeks gestation. Jitteriness is seen in up to 44% of newborns in the first few hours of life and can be distinguished from tonic-clonic seizure activity in that the rhythmic movements of jitteriness are more rapid and can be stopped with pressure or sucking.

A second detailed exam within 24 hours is desirable, and a third should ideally be performed at the time of discharge, as the dynamic physiology of the newborn demands frequent reassessment.

The pediatric health care provider's evaluation of the newborn is usually an opportunity to learn more about the infant and family. The second but equally important reason for the evaluation is to recognize, evaluate, and manage or refer those few infants with problems requiring intervention, thus improving their chance of appropriate health care and good outcomes. A renewed campaign emphasizing family-centered care has further demonstrated that the pediatric health care provider is integral to the promotion of family education and support that begins with the birth of an infant and continues throughout childhood.

Suggested Readings

Gomella TL. Prenatal testing. Newborn physical examination. In: *Neonatology: management, procedures, on-call problems, diseases and drugs*. 5th ed. New York: McGraw-Hill; 2004:1–38.

Hernandez J, Glass S. Physical assessment of the newborn. In: Thureen PJ, Deacon J, O'Neill P, et al., eds. *Assessment and care of the well newborn*. 2nd ed. Philadelphia: Elsevier Saunders; 2005:119–172.

McKee-Garrett TM. Examination of the newborn. *UpToDate*. 2006.

Narvey M, Fletcher MA. Physical assessment and classification. McDonald MG, Mullett MD, Seshia MMK. In: *Avery's neonatology: pathophysiology and management of the newborn*. 6th ed. Philadelphia: Lippincott Williams & Wilkins; 2005:327–350.

Stoll BJ, Kliegman RM. The newborn infant. Nelson WE, Behrman KE, Kliegman R. In: *Nelson textbook of pediatrics*. 17th ed. Philadelphia: Saunders; 2004:523–531.

Uhing MR. Management of birth injuries. *Clin Perinatol* 2005;32:19–38.

CHAPTER 106 ■ CYANOSIS

PAMELA G. LARSEN

Cyanosis is the visible expression of pathologically low arterial blood oxygen saturation. Arterial blood saturation depends upon:

■ Pulmonary blood flow and alveolar oxygen exchange
■ Appropriate return of oxygenated blood to the left atrium
■ The concentration of saturated hemoglobin

Acrocyanosis in the newborn (blue hands and feet with a pink body) is common and usually results from decreased peripheral perfusion due to vasomotor instability. It is frequently seen during transition or if the infant becomes cool. During transition, periodic and brief mild cyanosis ("dusky spells") may occur during crying or bathing, and may be considered normal. However, persistent central cyanosis of the trunk, mucous membranes, and tongue is always a sign of a serious condition.

Cyanosis is apparent when 4 to 5 g/dL or more of hemoglobin is deoxygenated. Profound cyanosis, usually secondary to congenital heart disease, is present if the PaO_2 is less than 50 mm Hg in room air or less than 100 mm Hg in 100% oxygen (hyperoxia test). However, it is important to remember that the actual oxygen saturation level may not correlate with the intensity of the cyanosis. This discrepancy may be exaggerated in conditions such as polycythemia (visible cyanosis more than expected based on PaO_2) or marked anemia (significant desaturation, but with less obvious cyanosis).

The cause of cyanosis may be pulmonary, cardiovascular, central nervous system (CNS), hematologic, metabolic, or anatomic (Table 106.1).

CLINICAL FINDINGS

History

Cyanosis usually requires immediate intervention, allowing little time for a complete history. A quick initial evaluation may be performed, followed by appropriate interventions; a review of the history can be obtained when the patient is stable. Key components of the history help establish a broad differential diagnosis that may be focused when integrating findings on the newborn physical examination. Most symptoms associated with newborn cyanosis are observed by providers and are discussed with the physical examination below.

Family and prenatal history should include information on maternal drug use, specifically narcotics, barbiturates, and sedative-hypnotics. Drug-induced CNS depression may cause hypoventilation, apnea, and respiratory distress, resulting in cyanosis. Prenatal ultrasound diagnosis of cardiac or CNS anomalies can facilitate the evaluation of cyanosis. Maternal morbid obesity or diabetes mellitus can cause symptomatic neonatal hypoglycemia, with clinical manifestations of apnea, cyanosis, and respiratory distress symptoms. Other maternal illnesses that may cause cyanosis in the newborn include metabolic disorders (hypothyroidism and hypoparathyroidism), hypertension (preeclampsia and eclampsia), renal disease, and systemic lupus erythematosus. Maternal systemic lupus erythematosus may cause congenital heart block, anemia, or pericardial effusion. Conditions such as oligohydramnios, post-dates gestation, or fetal malformations may also be associated with specific causes of newborn cyanosis. Finding individuals with inherited malformations of the heart in first- and second-degree relatives raises the possibility of cardiac causes of cyanosis. The inheritance pattern varies with the specific congenital heart defect. If the mother has a congenital heart defect, the recurrence risk may be significant. For example, the risk of congenital heart disease in the offspring of a mother who has a ventricular septal defect (VSD) is 9.5%, 14% if the mother has an arteriovenous canal defect, and 18% if the mother has aortic stenosis.

Events during the perinatal period may be quite relevant to the newborn's cyanosis. Fetal distress with hypoxia suggests a partial or complete lack of oxygen in the brain or blood. The resulting CNS depression or injury may cause hypoxemia to persist through transition and into the neonatal period. Intrapartum factors that may contribute to neonatal cyanosis include emergency cesarean section, abnormal fetal presentation, premature labor, prolonged rupture of membranes, precipitous delivery, prolonged labor, intrauterine infection, fetal distress, cord compression, general anesthesia resulting in respiratory depression, maternal narcotics administered less than 4 hours prior to delivery, prolapsed cord, or placenta abruptio or previa, resulting in hemorrhage and hypovolemia. A traumatic delivery (e.g., forceps or vacuum extraction) or prematurity may result in intracranial hemorrhage (ICH), CNS and respiratory depression, and concomitant cyanosis. The need for assisted ventilation after delivery, particularly with poor resolution of cyanosis, indicates a compromised infant. A low 5-minute Apgar score is helpful to evaluate resuscitative efforts, but is not considered evidence of or consequent to substantial asphyxia.

Physical Examination

The determination of whether the cyanosis is episodic or persistent should be an early priority and is usually evident on inspection. The location (peripheral or central) and severity (mild, moderate, or severe) of the cyanosis should be noted. Differential peripheral cyanosis (more evident in the lower extremities) may indicate a localized process, such as right-to-left shunting across a patent ductus arteriosus with an associated coarctation of the aorta. Central cyanosis (mucous membranes and trunk) indicates a significant illness or condition. Grading the visible cyanosis as mild, moderate, or severe will further determine the urgency of the condition.

TABLE 106.1

DIFFERENTIAL DIAGNOSIS OF CYANOSIS
IN NEWBORN

System	Disease
Pulmonary	Respiratory distress syndrome
	Sepsis
	Meconium aspiration pneumonia
	Diaphragmatic hernia
	Transient tachypnea of the newborn (TTNB)
	Pleural effusion
Cardiovascular (the 6 Ts)	Transposition of the great vessels
	Tricuspid atresia
	Tetralogy of Fallot
	Total anomalous pulmonary venous return
	Truncus arteriosus
	"Transitional circulation" (persistent fetal circulation)
Central nervous system	Maternal sedative drugs
	Asphyxia
	Intracranial hemorrhage
	Neuromuscular disease
	Seizures
Hematologic	Acute or chronic blood loss
	Polycythemia
	Methemoglobinemia
Metabolic	Hypoglycemia
	Adrenogenital syndrome
Anatomic	Choanal atresia
	Malacia of the larynx, trachea, bronchus

From Behrman RE, Kliegman RM, eds. *Nelson essentials of pediatrics*, 3rd ed. WB Saunders: Philadelphia, 1998.

If episodic, the *timin*g of the cyanosis may be key in further clarifying its cause. Cyanosis may be noted only with crying, suggesting intolerance for increased activity with concomitant increased oxygen need, or intolerance to the change in intrathoracic pressures created when crying. Cyanosis associated with feeding may point to a conducting airway abnormality (e.g., choanal atresia, subglottic hemangioma, cleft palate, or tracheoesophageal fistula), or it may be related to a lack of coordination of the infant's sucking, swallowing, and breathing.

The *duration* of a cyanotic episode may provide a clue to the source of the problem. A brief episode, occurring once or twice, lasting only a few seconds, and associated with choking, spitting, or feeding, may be benign. However, prolonged or unresolved cyanosis raises concern for serious conditions—usually cardiac, respiratory, or anatomic.

Associated symptoms, especially symptoms of respiratory distress, help narrow the differential diagnosis. Generally, cardiac lesions that result in reduction of pulmonary blood flow (e.g., pulmonary atresia, tetralogy of Fallot) will not be associated with respiratory distress until cyanosis is profound. Lesions with poor systemic output (e.g., coarctation of the aorta, hypoplastic left heart) or increased pulmonary blood flow (e.g., d-transposition, truncus arteriosus) usually result in respiratory distress symptoms. Concurrent findings of seizures,

apnea, hypotonia, or hypoventilation may be the result of CNS abnormalities or insults. Pallor or sweating may represent metabolic or hematologic abnormalities (e.g., hypoglycemia, acute or chronic blood loss, methemoglobinemia, adrenogenital syndrome).

The *time to resolution* of a cyanotic episode also assists in diagnosis. Spontaneous recovery from cyanosis, without external stimulation, oxygen, or other intervention, is reassuring. Persistent or increasing cyanosis requires immediate intervention.

Prompt placement of pulse oximetry is a priority. The overall condition of the infant should be observed, including meconium staining, size for dates, and signs of respiratory distress (e.g., nasal flaring, retractions, tachypnea). The clinician should pay careful attention to all vital signs, in particular to the core (rectal) temperature, because cold stress can be a factor in cyanosis. If physical examination will be prolonged, a thermal neutral environment should be maintained with an over-bed warmer to promote full observation of the infant. The blood pressure between extremities should vary little. Blood pressure measurements vary with gestational and neonatal age; in term infants, the average systolic blood pressure ranges from the 70s to 80s, with diastolic pressures in the 60s. A greater than a 10 mm Hg systolic difference between upper and lower extremity blood pressures suggests coarctation of the aorta.

The cardiac examination should begin with *observation* of the precordium for heaves and hyperactivity, as well as obvious abnormalities, masses, or asymmetry. The precordium is *palpated*, noting the location of the cardiac apical impulse. The amplitude of the brachial and femoral pulses is determined. Weaker and delayed femoral pulses are associated with coarctation of the aorta. Examination of the skull may identify fullness of the fontanelles; the head circumference is measured, providing possible clues for CNS problems associated with cyanosis. The liver is palpated during exam of the abdomen, because the cyanosis associated with congestive heart failure may not be evident for hours to days after birth, and is usually associated with hepatomegaly.

Auscultation of the respiratory and cardiovascular system may further narrow the differential diagnosis. The examination may reveal stridor, diminished breath sounds (e.g., in atelectasis or pneumothorax), bowel sounds audible in the chest (diaphragmatic hernia), or the presence of crackles. Diastolic and systolic murmurs may be heard. Noteworthy characteristics of a heart murmur include its timing, location of maximal intensity, radiation, intensity (grade I to VI), pitch, and quality. The quality of a murmur may change with respirations; murmurs originating in the right heart tend to vary more with respiration than left-sided murmurs. It is important to remember, however, that even severe cardiac defects may not be associated with a murmur. Other cardiac findings may include dysrhythmias, gallops, or rubs.

Laboratory Findings and Interpretation

Pulse oximetry can direct initial evaluation and interventions by offering indirect measurement of oxygenation. Confirmation of findings and better assessment of gas exchange is afforded by an arterial blood gas measurement, which may be obtained by a single arterial puncture, but in persistently cyanotic infants often requires placement of an umbilical artery line for continuous monitoring. For a normal term infant, the expected PaO_2 levels during transition are 55 to 60 mm Hg at 30 minutes of age, 75 mm Hg at 4 hours of age, and 90 mm Hg at 24 hours of age, with concurrent $PaCO_2$ of 35 to 40 and pH of 7.35 to 7.40. A complete blood count (CBC) and differential will assist in the diagnosis of sepsis, anemia, and polycythemia. A hematocrit greater than 66% to 70% indicates polycythemia, which if severe, may be associated with cyanosis. Blood, urine, and CSF cultures should be obtained to identify a possible infectious cause for the cyanosis.

Blood should also be assayed for *glucose, calcium, and magnesium*. Hypoglycemia is associated with many conditions that may lead to cyanosis, including respiratory distress, sepsis, heart disease, and hyperinsulinemia. Blood glucose should be maintained at 40 mg/dL or more. Hypocalcemia, a disturbance in homeostasis between blood and bone, is often asymptomatic, but may be associated with nonspecific symptoms, such as twitching, increased tone, convulsions, and cyanosis. Hypocalcemia may occur as a primary problem, but is more often secondary to stressors, such as respiratory distress, asphyxia, cerebral injury, sepsis, and hypoglycemia.

Radiologic Findings and Interpretation

A chest radiograph should be obtained to ascertain heart placement and size, as well as to assess the lungs. Pneumothorax, diaphragmatic hernia, and pleural effusion cause cyanosis secondary to direct respiratory compromise and/or pulmonary hypoplasia. Many congenital cardiac lesions may not affect the radiographic appearance of the heart, but in some cases cardiac shape, pulmonary vascularity, and other findings often suggest specific diagnoses. For example, the cardiac contour may show a diminutive pulmonary artery in pulmonary atresia, or a narrow upper mediastinum may indicate transposition of the great arteries. Chest films may also implicate pulmonary congestion as the cause of cyanosis: a ground glass (opaque) appearance to the lung fields suggests hyaline membrane disease, or focal infiltrates may be noted with pneumonia.

An electrocardiogram (ECG) in the first few days of life is rarely lesion-specific, because the right ventricle is dominant both in normal newborns and in those with most forms of cyanotic heart disease. An echocardiogram, on the other hand, almost always accurately defines the cardiac anatomy.

MANAGEMENT

Unless there is an immediately reversible etiology (e.g., maternal narcotics), infants who have cyanosis secondary to hypoventilation must be intubated and mechanically ventilated. A key clinical tool in distinguishing pulmonary causes of cyanosis from cyanotic heart disease is the *hyperoxia test*. An arterial blood gas is obtained while the infant is breathing 100% oxygen: if the arterial PaO_2 is greater than 150 mm Hg after 10 to 15 minutes of 100% oxygen, a cyanotic heart lesion is unlikely. Conversely, an arterial PaO_2 less than 100 mm Hg suggests cardiac disease. If immediate evaluation by a pediatric cardiologist is not possible, this determination is quite important because of the risks associated with administering supplemental O_2 to infants with cyanotic heart disease. A high concentration of inspired O_2 may cause pulmonary vasodilation and closure of the ductus arteriosus. Many infants with cyanotic heart defects are ductus-dependent (see below). When interpreting the hyperoxia test, the clinician must keep in mind that the site of blood sampling relative to the cardiac defect may also affect the oxygenation level of the results (Chapters 13 and 29).

Intravenous (IV) access should be obtained and a work-up for presumed sepsis initiated in any cyanotic infant with coexisting acidosis, respiratory distress, hypothermia, or hyperthermia. After the laboratory work (CBC with differential, blood culture, and cerebrospinal fluid [CSF] culture) is completed, antibiotic therapy should begin empirically.

Immediate pediatric cardiology consultation is imperative for cyanosis that does not resolve, especially for infants who do not have significant associated respiratory distress. Cyanosis that occurs initially with crying or feeding and then worsens over time may result from progressive closure of the ductus arteriosus and suggests ductal-dependent cyanotic heart disease. In infants with ductal-dependent cyanotic lesions, poor peripheral perfusion, profound cyanosis (PaO_2 less than 25 mm Hg), or acidosis, an infusion of prostaglandin E1 (PGE1) may be indicated. PGE1 given by continuous IV infusion helps maintain patency of the ductus arteriosus until definitive evaluation and intervention take place. If a pediatric cardiologist is not immediately available, telephone consultation prior to treatment with prostaglandin E1 is recommended. The dose is 0.05 to 1.0 μg/kg/min. *Note: Infants receiving prostaglandins should be intubated due to the potential for apnea, which occurs in approximately 20% of cases.*

If the infant is suspected to have tetralogy of Fallot, severe cyanotic episodes may be improved by placing the infant in a knee-chest position and administering intramuscular or subcutaneous morphine sulfate (0.05 mg/kg/dose). Administration of prostaglandin E1 may also be beneficial.

Once a strong likelihood of congenital heart disease has been established, subsequent care should be given in a neonatal intensive care unit. If this involves transfer to another facility, stabilization prior to transport is of utmost importance. The unstable newborn should have continuous cardiopulmonary and blood pressure monitoring, receive nothing by mouth (NPO), and have IV access. Any infant requiring oxygen supplementation should also be placed on pulse oximetry. Remember, however, that for newborns in acute distress with poor peripheral perfusion or shock, pulse oximetry may not reflect their true oxygenation status, nor does it provide information necessary to prevent hyperoxemia.

PEARLS

- Placing a cyanotic infant on oxygen may be both therapeutic (relieving hypoxia) and diagnostic (100% hyperoxia test). If cyanosis is secondary to ductal-dependent congenital heart disease, oxygen may be detrimental (accelerated PDA closure).
- Cyanosis has a wide range of causes. Remember the groups of causes by considering the path oxygen takes from the nose to the peripheral tissues: oxygen → conducting airways → diffusion (alveoli) → ventilation/perfusion match → oxygen carriage (blood flow and hemoglobin) → oxygen delivery (1).
- Infants with congenital heart disease may present with some combination of persistent cyanosis, respiratory distress (usually mild), and/or a low systemic output. The primary respiratory symptom found in infants with congenital heart disease is tachypnea without retractions or grunting.

Reference

1. Smith MBH. Cyanosis in the infant. In: Baldwin GA, ed. *Handbook of pediatric emergencies.* 3rd ed. Philadelphia: Lippincott Williams & Wilkins; 2001.

Suggested Readings

Behrman RE, Kleigman RM, Jenson HB, et al. eds. *Nelson textbook of pediatrics.* 17th ed. Philadelphia: Saunders; 2004.
Taeusch HW, Ballard RA, eds. *Avery's diseases of the newborn.* 8th ed. Philadelphia: Saunders; 2004.

CHAPTER 107 ■ HYPOGLYCEMIA

PAMELA G. LARSEN

Hypoglycemia in the newborn is a well-recognized condition, yet the definition remains elusive. Blood glucose levels vary by method and timing of feeding, type of glucose test used, condition of the infant, and prenatal, intrapartum, and neonatal experiences. The controversy about the threshold for hypoglycemia arises from physiologic fall in blood glucose levels after birth followed by spontaneous recovery in most healthy newborns.

Historically, clinical definitions of hypoglycemia for the term infant have been made based on the age of the infant. Srinivasan and associates (1986) described the normal distribution of glucose concentration levels; those more than 2 SD below the mean that were considered hypoglycemic. The infant at 1 to 3 hours old was considered hypoglycemic with a glucose level of less than 35 mg/dL; the infant 3 to 24 hours old at 40 mg/dL; and the infant 24 to 48 hours old would be hypoglycemic with a glucose level less than 45 mg/dL. Most clinicians agree that a blood sugar level less than 35 mg/dL is low in a full-term infant; others define hypoglycemia as whole blood glucose less than 40 mg/dL regardless of gestation or postnatal age. Further, many newborns with low blood glucose remain asymptomatic. Although recent studies have not found correlations between neonatal glucose levels or duration of hypoglycemia with neurologic abnormalities, untreated or prolonged hypoglycemia is associated with adverse consequences, such as mental retardation or recurrent seizure activity. This association has led to aggressive attempts to diagnose and manage this condition.

The brain is the primary site for glucose use; thus, many of the signs and symptoms of hypoglycemia represent glucose deprivation of the CNS. Hypoglycemia is categorized as transient or persistent, as well as symptomatic or asymptomatic. Transient hypoglycemia occurs after birth and is confined to the newborn period. Persistent and recurrent hypoglycemia involves extended management, usually with glucose infusions over several days, and may require other pharmacologic intervention.

At birth, with the abrupt interruption of maternal glucose support, several events occur that allow the newborn to establish glucose homeostasis. After a transient decrease in glucose levels immediately after birth, hepatic glycogen stores decrease. Lipolysis occurs with increased plasma fatty acid concentrations, and glucose levels increase. Many pathologic states can interfere with these homeostatic mechanisms, resulting in hypoglycemia in the newborn. Hypoglycemia occurs as a result of three mechanisms: limited glycogen stores, hyperinsulinemia or increased glucose use, or decreased glucose production.

Limited glycogen stores are responsible for hypoglycemia in several conditions. Stored energy in the form of glycogen rapidly accumulates near term. Glycogen is an essential source of energy the first few hours after birth. These energy stores are reduced in infants who are small for gestational age (SGA), premature, or suffer from intrauterine malnutrition. The occurrence of perinatal events such as cold stress, increased work of breathing, and hypoxia further deplete available glycogen stores. Although infrequent, glycogen storage diseases may be the cause of newborn hypoglycemia, resulting in depleted or unavailable glycogen.

Hyperinsulinemia or increased glucose use may also result in a hypoglycemic newborn. Although great advances in management of maternal diabetes have occurred in recent decades, infants may experience significant morbidity even when born to mothers with euglycemic control during pregnancy. The infant of a diabetic mother (IDM) develops significantly lower glucose concentrations, does not mobilize fatty acids from adipose tissue, and has persistent insulin action. Failure of counterregulatory hormonal results in lack of increase in circulating glucagon and catecholamine levels. Persistent neonatal hypoglycemia in the absence of maternal hyperglycemia should lead to consideration of Beckwith–Wiedemann syndrome (macrosomia, macroglossia, exophthalmos, distinctive ear lobe groove) or the rare instance of congenital hyperinsulinism (formerly nesidioblastosis).

Decreased glucose production is noted in polycythemia (mechanism undetermined), adrenal insufficiency (decreased gluconeogenesis), SGA infants (mechanism unknown but theories include placental abnormalities with starvation, polycythemia, increased breakdown of fat, and/or early depletion of glycogen stores), and inborn errors of metabolism. Glycogen storage disease, fructose intolerance, fructose 1-6 diphosphatase deficiency, galactosemia, glycogen synthase deficiency, maple syrup urine disease, and other amino and fatty acid metabolism defects are also included in the differential diagnosis for hypoglycemia, but are beyond the scope of this chapter.

Neonatal hypoglycemia can be classified as follows:

■ Transient (days). Occuring with prematurity, SGA, peripartum stress, or maternal hyperinsulinemia.
■ Transient (weeks). Due to birth asphyxia, SGA, or hyperinsulinemia.
■ Persistent. Accompanying inborn errors of metabolism, hypopituitarism, or congenital hyperinsulinemia.

The etiology of hypoglycemia is usually apparent, and affected infants are easily treated. However, for unknown reasons, some infants fail to adapt to the extrauterine environment and develop idiopathic hypoglycemia. It has been proposed that this condition is secondary to maternal obesity or mild maternal glucose intolerance. Neonatal infection is rarely associated with hypoglycemia and, in fact, is more likely to be associated with hyperglycemia. Sepsis-associated hypoglycemia may be related to depleted glycogen stores, failed gluconeogenesis, or increased peripheral glucose use. In most animal models, the response to sepsis is to increase gluconeogenesis. A decrease in this process is noted in the late stages of infection; therefore, hypoglycemia associated with sepsis should be considered an indicator of an advanced infection.

Persistent or recurrent hypoglycemia is seen much less frequently, and with significantly poorer outcomes. Hyperinsulinism is the most frequent cause of persistent hypoglycemia in the newborn and in early infancy. These infants are macrosomic at birth but do not have a history of maternal diabetes. Plasma insulin levels may be greater than 5 to 10 μg/mL, and the insulin–glucose ratio is greater than 0.4. Although this persistent hypoglycemia may present in the early days of life, it is more commonly noted between the first and fourth weeks of life. The differential diagnoses include familial and nonfamilial hyperinsulinism of infancy, β-cell hyperplasia, and β-cell adenoma (requiring genetic evaluation). Autosomal recessive forms of persistent hypoglycemia in the infant are severe and respond poorly to medical management. Autosomal dominant forms are less severe, but more likely to occur at about 1 year of age. Hypoglycemia may be associated with adrenal insufficiency, and infants with hypopituitarism may present with hypoglycemia. In boys, the notable feature may be microphallus secondary to gonadotropin deficiency.

CLINICAL FINDINGS

History

A careful history of the mother and infant is essential. Because the fetus is entirely dependent on the mother for its source of glucose, maternal conditions significantly affect the fetus and, in turn, the newborn's glucose status. Of significance in the maternal history is the presence of diabetes, eclampsia, and glucose administration during the intrapartum period. The clinician should inquire about the use of maternal medications that have known associations with newborn hypoglycemia:

- Terbutaline sulfate or ritodrine (used in management of preterm labor)
- Beta-blockers or beta-adrenergic drugs (for hypertension or cardiac arrhythmias)
- Benzothiadiazide diuretics (hypertension)
- Oral hypoglycemic agents (maternal diabetes)

Infants with associated placental abnormalities, IUGR, prematurity, or the smaller of discordant twins are particularly at risk for hypoglycemia. Further, a history of siblings with persistent hypoglycemia may reveal previous neonatal deaths, unexplained seizures, or mental retardation. The perinatal history of the neonate also contributes significantly to the assessment of transient or persistent hypoglycemia. Conditions that contribute to hypoglycemia include birth asphyxia, hypothermia, congenital cardiac malformations, polycythemia, and other iatrogenic or idiopathic conditions.

Physical Examination

Signs and symptoms of hypoglycemia in the newborn are nonspecific and can represent other pathologies that may occur independently or concurrently with hypoglycemia. These symptoms of hypoglycemia often are similar to those of sepsis or asphyxia, and the astute clinician must be alert to the myriad differential diagnoses that may be represented by such nonspecific signs. Although some hypoglycemic infants are asymptomatic, most will demonstrate one or more of the following:

- Hypothermia
- Hypotonia
- Apnea or cyanotic spells
- Grunting and tachypnea
- Irritability
- Jitteriness/tremors (most frequent symptom)
- Lethargy or stupor
- Sweating
- Tachycardia
- Feeding difficulty
- Abnormal cry
- Exaggerated Moro reflex
- Seizures

Symptoms of low blood sugar should improve or resolve when the glucose concentration is normalized.

The IDM is one of the most frequently seen hypoglycemic infants in the newborn nursery. These infants will classically present as obese, ruddy, and puffy-faced and yet may actually be premature for gestational age, as well as hypotonic and lethargic. Fetal and neonatal mortality associated with IDM has substantially declined; however, it remains more than five times that of infants of nondiabetic mothers. A three-fold incidence of certain morbidities persists:

- Congenital anomalies
- Heart failure and septal hypertrophy
- Hyperbilirubinemia
- Macrosomia
- Renal vein thrombosis
- Small left colon
- Polycythemia
- Organomegaly (liver, spleen, heart)

These infants may continue to be hypoglycemic, although only a small percentage will be symptomatic. This is usually directly proportionate to the level of glucose control sustained by the mother. In addition, 50% of IDM infants will experience hypocalcemia and hypomagnesemia, and this is usually apparent within 48 to 72 hours after birth.

Infants with persistent hypoglycemia (congenital hyperinsulinism) may have seizures, cyanosis, hypotonia, and apnea, along with the inability to maintain euglycemia. Severe forms of this condition may require pancreatectomy to avoid long-term neurologic sequelae.

Laboratory Findings

The American Academy of Pediatrics (1993) recommends testing glucose levels on all symptomatic infants and those who are at risk for hypoglycemia. The optimum method of screening is measuring plasma glucose; however, these results from the central lab are not usually available in a timely manner. Therefore, "point-of-care" devices such as a glucometer are often used in newborn and high-risk nurseries. Unfortunately, results from different types of glucometers are unreliable. These meters are designed largely for adult populations to ascertain hyperglycemia, but are less satisfactory for lower-range values. Further, agents such as fluoride, uric acid, bilirubin, acetaminophen, and isopropyl alcohol may interfere with results. Anemia falsely raises and polycythemia falsely lowers glucometer readings. At a minimum, values less than 40 mg/dL should be confirmed immediately by the laboratory. Clinicians should also be aware that results from the central laboratory may vary because ongoing glycolysis occurs during the first hour after blood sampling despite the addition of glycolysis inhibitors. Glycolysis is hematocrit and temperature dependent and the decrease in glucose concentration is unpredictable.

MANAGEMENT

The clinician should be guided by two principles as described by Williams (1997) and supported by the AAP, in the management of hypoglycemia:

- Healthy term infants do not develop symptomatic hypoglycemia merely as a result of underfeeding.
- Early, frequent, and exclusive breastfeeding meets the nutritional requirements of healthy term infants.

With these princlples in mind, there is no need to routinely monitor blood glucose in healthy term infants who are breastfeeding.

For other infants, the clinician must anticipate which infant is at risk, and then diagnose, treat, and if possible, determine the cause. Screening glucose determinations should be done on infants who are LGA or SGA, IDM, macrosomic, or acutely ill. Other clinical settings that warrant glucose screening include hypoxia, respiratory distress, cold stress, IUGR, or prematurity and infants of mothers with pregnancy-induced hypertension, or who received medications associated with neonatal hypoglycemia. Any symptomatic infant must be screened. Low findings from the heel-stick screen should be confirmed with serum glucose measurement.

Infants in the above at-risk categories whose blood sugar falls between 20 to 40 mg/dL, but who are asymptomatic and able to feed enterally, should immediately be put to breast or fed formula. Subsequent feeds should occur as often as every 1.5 to 2 hours for breastfed infants and every 2 to 3 hours for formula-fed infants. Blood glucose should be checked before feeds and monitored every 3 hours for 24 to 48 hours and/or until three consecutive values are greater than 45 mg/dL.

For infants unable to feed, who have blood glucose less than 20 mg/dL, or who are severely symptomatic, immediate peripheral venous access must be established. Peripheral access is preferred to umbilical artery access because of the possibility of catheter placement near the celiac axis. The latter can result in preferential perfusion of the pancreas, inadvertently causing an increased insulin response and further hypoglycemia. An IV bolus of 10% dextrose solution ($D_{10}W$) should be administered at the rate of 2.0 to 2.5 mL/kg over 1 minute (200 mg/kg). The bolus is followed immediately by continuous infusion of 3 to 5 mL/kg/hr (5 to 8 mg glucose/kg/min) of $D_{10}W$. In the event of seizures, a 4-mL/kg bolus infusion is indicated, followed by continuous infusion of 3 to 5 mL/kg/hr (5 to 8 mg glucose/kg/min). Serum glucose levels should be checked frequently until stable and the infant no longer requires IV glucose. If hypoglycemia recurs, the $D_{10}W$ bolus should be repeated and the continuous infusion titrated incrementally to maintain glucose levels. Oral feedings should be initiated as soon as the infant is able to drink. Hypoglycemia may recur if the IV glucose infusion infiltrates or is withdrawn before adequate feeding is established.

Persistent or recurrent hypoglycemia may require venous infusions of glucose as high as 15 to 20 mg/kg/min in addition to frequent feedings. Rarely, despite these interventions serum glucose levels remain low. In that setting, additional therapeutic modalities to consider include diazoxide and somatostatin. Diazoxide (which functions to open K_{ATP} channels) has been used in the past, but reports now suggest that it fails to control hypoglycemia. Parenteral somatostatin, which blocks calcium flux, may be somewhat more effective. Inability to normalize an infant's serum glucose levels in the newborn nursery requires transfer to a level III neonatal care unit.

PEARLS

- A hypoglycemic infant may be asymptomatic
- Hypoglycemia associated with sepsis is a sign of late infection
- The minimum desired serum glucose level is at least 40 mg/dL
- There are three categories to consider in determining the cause of neonatal hypoglycemia

  - Limited glycogen stores: IUGR, SGA, prematurity, placental malformation; perinatal stress, glycogen storage defects
  - Hyperinsulinemia or increased glucose use: IDM, glucose infusion during labor, Beckwith–Wiedemann syndrome
  - Decrease glucose production: polycythemia, adrenal insufficiency, SGA, inborn errors of metabolism

Suggested Readings

Couch RM. Hypoglycemia. In: Baldwin GA, ed. Handbook of pediatric emergencies. 3rd ed. Philadelphia: Lippincott Williams & Wilkins; 2001.

Kahlan SC, Saker F. Disorders of carbohydrate metabolism. In: Taeusch HW, Ballard RA, eds. Avery's diseases of the newborn. 7th ed. Philadelphia: Saunders; 1998: 727.

Sperling MA. Hypoglycemia. In: Nelson WE, Behrman RM, Kleigman RM, et al. eds. Nelson textbook of pediatrics. Philadelphia: Saunders; 1996.

Additional Readings

Srinivan G, Pildes RS, Cattamanchi G, et al. Plasma glucose values in normal neonates: a New look. J. Peds 109(1):114–117, 1986.

American Academy of Pediatrics Committee on Fetus and Newborn. Routine evaluation of blood pressure, hematocrit, and glucose in newborns. Pediattics 92(3):474–476, 1993.

Williams AF. Hypoglycemia of the newborn: a review. Bulletin of the World Health Organization 75(3):261–290, 1997.

CHAPTER 108 ■ JAUNDICE IN THE NEWBORN

PAMELA G. LARSEN

Jaundice is a very common newborn condition with infrequent but potentially devastating neurologic sequelae. Recognized in the early 1900s, the term "kernicterus" was used to refer to the yellow color of the basal ganglia observed at autopsy in infants who had died of extreme jaundice. Increased recognition of Rh-hemolytic disease and associated kernicterus in the United States in the 1950s through 1970s resulted in aggressive treatment of newborn jaundice. With better knowledge about kernicterus, significant improvement in control of Rh isoimmunization, and the realization that many infants were being unnecessarily treated for jaundice, the management of jaundice became less aggressive. However, controversy remains about the threshold for a response to hyperbilirubinemia in the term neonate, because the level that produces toxicity is hard to predict. It is unclear why a given level of bilirubin produces kernicterus in some infants but not in others.

Jaundice is the most common clinical condition that requires medical attention in the newborn period. In the United States, 50% to 60% of term newborns and 80% of preterm infants become clinically jaundiced. For unknown reasons, infants of Asian and American Indian descent have a higher incidence of jaundice, while African-American infants have a lower incidence of jaundice than Caucasians. Other risk factors for significant jaundice include male gender and living at high altitudes. In the vast majority of cases, jaundice is transient, mild, and requires no intervention.

Average peak serum bilirubin in a term newborn is 5 to 6 mg/dL, gradually falling to 1.5 mg/dL by the 10th day of life. Exaggerated physiologic jaundice occurs at values above these levels (7 to 17 mg/dL). Serum bilirubin above 17 mg/dL is no longer considered physiologic, and a cause of the hyperbilirubinemia should be sought in these infants. Breast-fed infants generally have a bilirubin level 1 to 2 mg/dL higher than formula-fed infants.

In the majority of infants, an elevated unconjugated serum bilirubin is the result of the normal physiologic breakdown of fetal red blood cells. Compared to older infants' and children's red blood cells, fetal red blood cells have a shorter life span (80 to 90 days), and the infant has a higher erythrocyte mass relative to body surface area than older children. Other sources of bilirubin include heme-containing compounds such as myoglobin, cytochromes, tryptophan pyrrolase, and peroxidases, as well as ineffective erythropoiesis. For poorly understood reasons, the newborn liver has a decreased capacity to handle the products of this heme breakdown. Bilirubin is also reabsorbed via the enterohepatic circulation, with bilirubin concentration in meconium as much as 50 times higher than in serum.

In the normal neonate, bilirubin is produced at the rate of 6 to 8 mg/kg body weight each 24 hours, approximately two and a half times the adult rate. The metabolic pathway for the breakdown of heme and the formation of bilirubin is complex, and sites for pathology are many. Heme is released when the hemoproteins are degraded by heme oxygenase, releasing iron and forming carbon monoxide and biliverdin. Biliverdin is further degraded to bilirubin by the enzyme biliverdin reductase. This bilirubin is taken up by the liver and conjugated with glucuronides to form bilirubin monoglucuronide (BMG) or diglucuronide (BDG). These reactions are catalyzed by uridine diphosphate and monophosphate glucuronosyltransferase. The bilirubin glucuronides (conjugated bilirubin) are excreted into the intestinal lumen, where intestinal flora catabolize bilirubin to water-soluble urobilinogen, a portion of which is reabsorbed and returned to the liver. The remaining urobilinogen is converted to stercobilin and excreted in the feces. Urobilinogen and stercobilin are responsible for most of the pigmentation of urine and stool.

CAUSES OF NEWBORN JAUNDICE

Causes of hyperbilirubinemia (Table 108.1) can be categorized by disturbances of bilirubin production, conjugation, hepatic uptake, enterohepatic circulation, or a combination of overproduction and undersecretion. *Increased bilirubin production* results in increased unconjugated bilirubin. Jaundice noted within 24 to 36 hours after birth is usually due to excessive production of bilirubin and is considered pathologic. Further, significant hyperbilirubinemia with a sudden increase in the serum bilirubin should prompt the provider to consider glucose-6-phosphate dehydrogenase (G6PD) deficiency. G6PD deficiency is an X-linked recessive disorder whose primary effect is the reduced level of the enzyme G6PD in red blood cells, causing increased destruction of the cells. Although more common in the Mediterranean area and in the Middle East, immigration and intermarriage have resulted in G6PD deficiency becoming a worldwide concern. In the United States, many more black than white people have the disorder. Approximately 10% to 14% of the black male population is affected; hence, severe hyperbilirubinemia in an African-American male infant should always raise the possibility of this condition.

Impaired conjugation of bilirubin is seen in familial nonhemolytic jaundice where there is a shortage of glucuronyl transferase, such as the lifelong conditions of Gilbert syndrome and Crigler–Najjar types I and II. Drugs and hormones also interfere with the conjugation of bilirubin and hepatic uptake by competing with binding sites in the liver cytosol. Finally, persistent jaundice in some breast-fed infants may be associated with increased amounts of the nonesterified fatty acids (NEFA) in breast milk, although the exact mechanism is

TABLE 108.1

CAUSES OF NEWBORN JAUNDICE

INCREASED BILIRUBIN PRODUCTION
  Blood group incompatability
  Rh incompatibility
  Erythrocyte enzyme deficiency
    Glucose-6-phosphate dehydrogenase deficiency
    Pyruvate kinase deficiency
    Hexokinase deficiency
    Congenital erythropoietic porphyria
  Structural defects in the red blood cells
  α-thalassemia, β-thalassemia
  Galactosemia defects
  Chronic fetal hypoxia
  Neonatal infection
  Maternal–fetal and placental transfusion (polycythemia)
  Enclosed hematoma

DEFICIENCY OF HEPATIC UPTAKE
  Persistent ductus venosus shunt
  Hyperviscosity
  Hypovolemia
  Deficient intracellular ligandin
  Saturated ligandin protein

DEFECTS OF BILIRUBIN CONJUGATION
  Crigler–Najjar types I and II
  Gilbert syndrome
  Lucy–Driscoll syndrome
  Hypothyroidism
  Galactosemia

Drugs and hormones
Breastfeeding
Dubin–Johnson syndrome
Rotor syndrome

INCREASED ENTEROHEPATIC CIRCULATION
  Biliary atresia
  Stenosis
  Hirschsprung disease
  Meconium plug syndrome
  Meconium ileus
  Fasting or poor feeding
  Pyloric stenosis

COMBINATION OVERPRODUCTION/
UNDEREXCRETION
  Perinatal infections
    Toxoplasmosis
    Cytomegalovirus
    Herpes simplex
    Syphilis
    Hepatitis
  Metabolic disorders
    Tyrosinemia (amino acids)
    Wolman, Gaucher, and Niemann–Pick diseases (lipids)
    Galactosemia, glycogen storage disease type IV
      (carbohydrates)
  Prematurity

unknown. *Deficiency of hepatic uptake* also contributes to unconjugated hyperbilirubinemia. Persistent ductus venosus shunt, hyperviscosity, or hypovolemia reduces portal blood flow through the liver sinusoids. Reduced diffusion of bilirubin into the hepatocytes may result from deficient or saturated ligandin, which binds to the bilirubin molecule. Elevated unconjugated bilirubin is also noted in infants with hypoxia, cardiorespiratory problems, and prematurity.

Increased enterohepatic circulation or mechanical obstruction results in increased resorption of bilirubin from the gut. Fasting or poor oral intake may also increase bilirubinemia by reducing peristalsis. Elevated direct bilirubin with biliary atresia is seen most frequently in full-term female infants, whereas giant-cell hepatitis with signs of fetal infection, splenomegaly, hemolysis, and small for gestational age is seen more often in male infants.

There are several circumstances that result in *a combination overproduction/undersecretion* hyperbilirubinemia. Hyperbilirubinemia seen in perinatal infections may occur with hepatosplenomegaly, hemolytic anemia, thrombocytopenia, and other evidence of hepatocellular injury. Intrahepatic bile stasis may be seen in infants who are septic, lethargic, feeding poorly, and often anemic. Jaundice associated with prematurity is multifactorial. The inadequate bile clearance mechanisms found in the term infant are even more deficient in the premature infant. There is excessive hemolysis due to ecchymosis of the skin and subcutaneous tissues in the fragile preterm infant. Bilirubin conjugation is also impaired in acidosis, hypoxemia, and hypovolemia, all of which occur more frequently in the premature infant.

CLINICAL FINDINGS

Although newborn jaundice is a very common finding, hyperbilirubinemia may be an early sign of serious neonatal disease. Important clues are found in the history. Risk factors in the maternal history include:

- Race (e.g., Asian, American Indian, Greek)
- Presence of diabetes or infection
- The use of epidural anesthesia
- The administration of oxytocin, prostaglandins, diazepam, or sulfa during labor
- Delayed cord clamping

Newborn jaundice in siblings and anemia, splenectomy, liver disease, or other genetic defects in any family member are important components in the history. The mother's and infant's blood types, Rh, and direct Coombs test provide information about Rh or ABO incompatibility diseases. When the mother is blood type O and the infant is blood type A or B with a positive Coombs antibody test, the infant has an ABO incompatibility with the maternal blood. This incompatibility occurs in 33% of O-positive mothers, and about 20% of this cohort have infants who develop severe jaundice. Rh incompatibility occurs if an Rh-negative but sensitized mother has an Rh-positive infant. This results in erythroblastosis fetalis, with predictable, usually severe jaundice and other complications, including hydrops fetalis, a life-threatening condition.

Neonatal history includes weight, gestational age, medications including vitamin K, feeding and stooling patterns, and hydration status. Difficult delivery with birth trauma, bruising, or hematoma also increases the risk for elevated bilirubin. Delayed feeding, breast-feeding, or supplementing feedings with glucose water have been associated with a higher incidence of neonatal jaundice. Delayed meconium passage results in resorption of bilirubin via enterohepatic circulation and is a major factor in physiologic jaundice regardless of the feeding method. Metabolic diseases and infection must be considered if the history includes lethargy, irritability, vomiting, or poor feeding. Acholic stool and/or bile in the urine may indicate biliary obstruction.

When performing the physical examination, specific findings should be noted, including distinctive dysmorphologies. Organomegaly, abdominal masses, and large cephalhematomas may be present. Cardiovascular examination should include assessment for murmurs, because peripheral pulmonic stenosis may be associated with arteriohepatic dysplasia. Other physical findings such as petechiae, hepatosplenomegaly, and microcephaly may be associated with hemolytic anemia, sepsis, and congenital infections; all are potential causes of jaundice.

The degree of jaundice in the skin, sclerae, and mucous membranes should be assessed no less than every 8 to 12 hours. Despite the presence of physiologic bilirubinemia of some degree in nearly all full-term infants, only about one-half will have visible jaundice in the first 3 days of life. Serum levels of bilirubin greater than 5 mg/dL usually result in visible cutaneous newborn icterus, which is first noted on the face and progresses caudally. Jaundice can be ascertained by pressing on the skin and noting where the blanching reveals the underlying yellow color. The examination should take place in a well-lit area. Historically, there have been unsuccessful efforts to correlate the progresssion of jaundice to specific serum bilirubin levels. It remains a challenge to the health care professional to correlate degree of jaundice on physical exam with a level at risk for serious outcomes. The 2004 AAP guidelines provide an algorithm for management of jaundice in the newborn nursery (Fig. 108.1).

Besides clinical jaundice, the infant with significant elevations in serum bilirubin may demonstrate lethargy, drowsiness, and poor feeding; overt neurologic signs, such as altered cry, altered muscle tone, or seizures, signal an infant at risk for kernicterus warranting immediate attention.

There is decreasing controversy about the routine laboratory investigation of physiologic jaundice, and many are advocating for routine bilirubin screening prior to discharge of the newborn. In addition to the degree of visible icterus and age, components of the history, such as race, type and frequency of feedings,

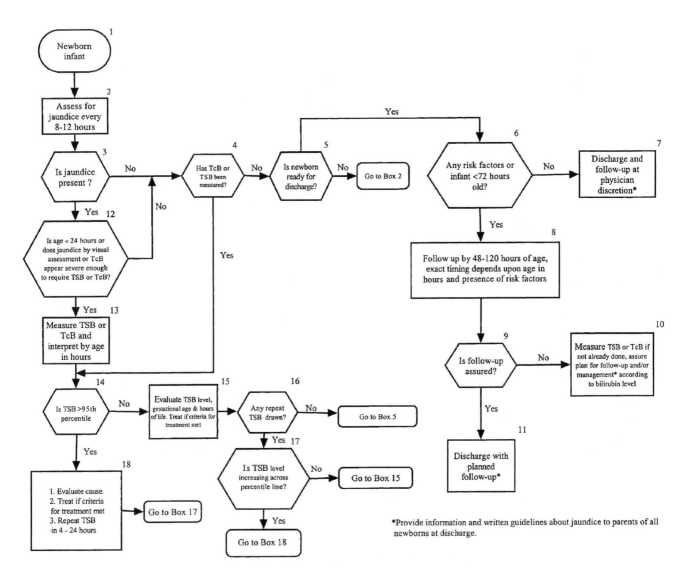

FIGURE 108.1. Algorithm for the management of jaundice in the newborn nursery. (From American Academy of Pediatrics. Practice parameter: management of hyperbilirubinemia in the newborn infant 35 or more weeks of gestation. *Pediatrics* 2004;114:297–316.)

and sex of the infant, should prompt laboratory investigation. The first, and usually only, laboratory test needed is total serum bilirubin (TSB). Other laboratory tests (e.g., direct bilirubin, liver function tests) are indicated only if the jaundice is severe, or if there is evidence of hemolysis, liver disease, or other causes of jaundice.

Acquaintance with the physiology of bilirubin metabolism facilitates the understanding of the laboratory's role in the diagnostic workup of the jaundiced infant. *Direct bilirubin* is measured if *total bilirubin* levels are markedly elevated or if there are other suggestions of nonphysiologic jaundice. In turn, this measurement can be used to estimate the *indirect bilirubin* (unconjugated and neurotoxic) by subtracting the direct bilirubin from the total serum bilirubin. This is an imprecise measurement because it is subject to interlaboratory and intralaboratory variation. The direct bilirubin level is therefore not a sensitive tool for diagnostic purposes. Generally speaking, when the direct bilirubin is over 2 mg/dL or makes up more than 20% of total bilirubin, disorders of conjugated bilirubin should be sought.

Transcutaneous bilirubin (TcB) measurement provides an estimate of the TSB and can provide a noninvasive measurement in most infants with bilirubins less than 15 mg/dL. Recent data suggest that these instruments are accurate to within 2 to 3 mg/dL of the total serum bilirubin. For infants with mild jaundice, this may be all that is required for reassurance that the infant is at low risk for future kernicterus. For

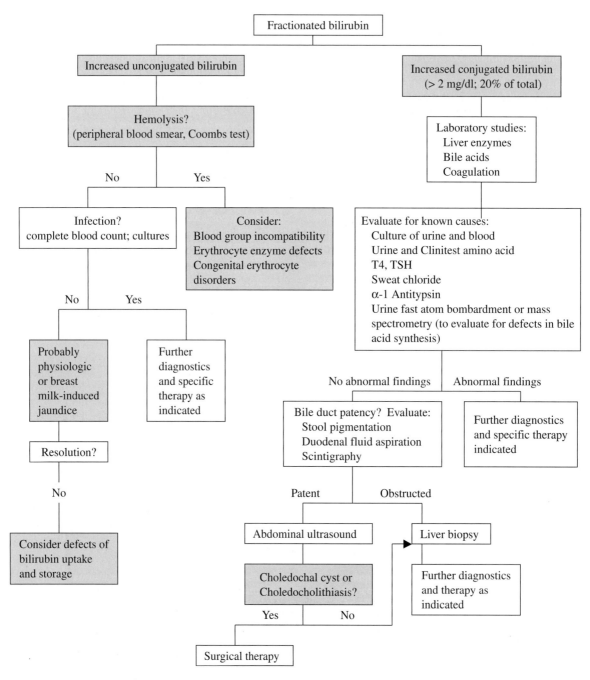

FIGURE 108.2. Algorithm presenting an approach to the evaluation of the neonate with jaundice. (TSH = thyroid-stimulating hormone.) (Used with permission from Laney DW. The gastrointestinal tract and liver. In: Rudolph AM, Kamei RK, Overby KJ, eds. *Rudolph's fundamentals of pediatrics.* 3rd ed. New York: McGraw-Hill; 2002.)

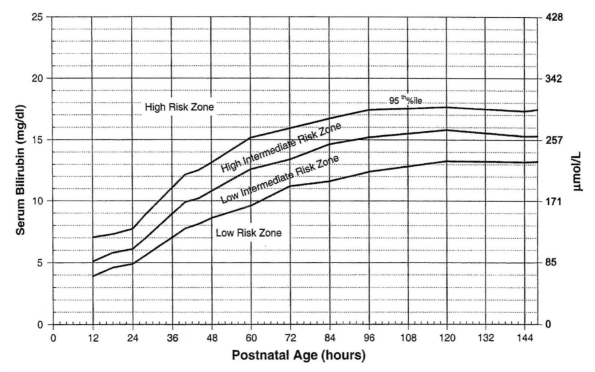

FIGURE 108.3. Nomogram for designation of risk in 2,840 well newborns at 36 or more weeks of gestational age with birthweight of 2,000 g or more, or 35 or more weeks of gestational age and birthweight of 2,500 g or more, based on the hour-specific serum bilirubin values. (From American Academy of Pediatrics. Practice parameter: management of hyperbilirubinemia in the newborn infant 35 or more weeks of gestation. *Pediatrics* 2004;114:297–316.)

infants with moderate jaundice, transcutaneous bilirubin levels are useful for determining the need for serum bilirubin measurement as well as for postdischarge monitoring. With phototherapy, however, TcB measurements are not reliable due to "bleaching" of the skin.

If the clinical picture is one of conjugated hyperbilirubinemia, the evaluation is more complicated. An algorithm for evaluation of jaundice is presented in Figure 108.2. In the investigation of nonphysiologic clinical jaundice (greater than 17 mg/dL), a key first step is the determination of unconjugated versus conjugated bilirubin. Not only is this helpful diagnostically, but recognition of direct hyperbilirubinemia and cholestasis mandates some urgency in making a diagnosis.

A peripheral blood smear and Coombs test are useful initial tests for significant hemolysis. In severe jaundice, serum albumin levels are a helpful adjunct in evaluating the risk of CNS toxicity, because bilirubin in the blood is largely bound to albumin. Although not used as frequently, end-tidal carbon monoxide levels in breath can also be determined, because carbon monoxide is a breakdown product of bilirubin converted to biliverdin. Additional laboratory studies should look for causes of neonatal cholestasis (Fig. 108.2). Blood and urine cultures for bacteria and viruses, viral titers, thyroid hormone levels, sweat chloride, and α-1 antitypsin should be ascertained. A positive urine test for reducing substances suggests galactosemia and should be confirmed by reduced levels of galactose-1-phosphate uridyl transferase activity in erythrocytes.

If the above tests are not diagnostic, the evaluation should include an assessment of bile duct patency by stool observation and biliary tract scintigraphy. Abdominal ultrasound may indicate a choledochal cyst or cholelithiasis as a cause of extrahepatic biliary obstruction. If cholestasis is ruled out,

liver biopsy should be performed to look for idiopathic neonatal hepatitis or other causes of cholestasis. Consultation with gastroenterology or pediatric surgery may be helpful.

MANAGEMENT

All infants should be evaluated for jaundice during hospitalization and prior to discharge to determine their risk for developing severe hyperbilirubinemia. The Bhutani nomogram provides a guide for predicting the rise of bilirubin by categorizing bilirubin levels into zones (Fig. 108.3). Values exceeding the 95th percentile (high-risk zone) indicate an increased risk for the infant to have a future bilirubin exceeding the 95th percentile for age, where bilirubin levels in the low or low intermediate zones provide reassurance that the infant will be less likely to have extreme hyperbilirubinemia. Hospitals are advised to develop a plan for routine assessment of jaundice at least every 8 to 12 hours. Risk is determined by using TSB or TcB, or by determining clinical risk factors as listed in Table 108.2. For most infants with unconjugated hyperbilirubinemia, no therapy is needed, and bilirubin levels gradually return to normal. The level of serum bilirubin that requires intervention depends on several factors: gestational age, etiology (e.g., hemolysis), and coexisting illnesses (e.g., sepsis). The American Academy of Pediatrics published guidelines in 2004 for management of hyperbilirubinemia in the healthy term infant.

Phototherapy is the mainstay of treatment for unconjugated hyperbilirubinemia; it rapidly reduces serum bilirubin concentrations, and apparently works by photoisomerization of bilirubin to form lumirubin, a water-soluble compound. The AAP guidelines for phototherapy should be used to plot

TABLE 108.2

RISK FACTORS FOR DEVELOPMENT OF SEVERE
HYPERBILIRUBINEMIA IN INFANTS 35 OR MORE
WEEKS GESTATION (IN APPROXIMATE ORDER OF
IMPORTANCE)

MAJOR RISK FACTORS
  Predischarge TSB or TcB level in the high-risk zone
  Jaundice observed in the first 24 hours
  Blood group incompatability with positive direct
     antiglobulin test, other known hemolytic disease
     (e.g., G6PD deficiency), elevated ETCO$_2$
  Gestational age 35–36 weeks
  Previous sibling received phototherapy
  Cephalohematoma or significant bruising
  Exclusive breast-feeding, particularly if nursing is not going
     well and weight loss is excessive
  East Asian race

MINOR RISK FACTORS
  Predischarge TSB or TcB level in the high–intermediate risk
     zone
  Gestational age 37–38 weeks
  Jaundice observed before discharge
  Previous sibling with jaundice
  Macrosomic infant of a diabetic mother
  Maternal age ≥25 years
  Male gender

**DECREASED RISK (THESE FACTORS ARE ASSOCIATED
WITH DECREASED RISK OF SIGNIFICANT JAUNDICE,
LISTED IN ORDER OF DECREASING IMPORTANCE)**
  TSB or TcB level in the low-risk zone
  Gestation age ≥41 weeks
  Exclusive bottle feeding
  Black race
  Discharge from hospital after 72 hours

bilirubin values in the high-risk zone to determine which infants require phototherapy (Fig. 108.4). Web-based tools can also assist the provider in determining the risk status for initiating phototherapy based on the AAP clinical practice guidelines (e.g., www.bilitool.org).

Phototherapy has its greatest impact in the first 24 to 48 hours, although effectiveness depends on the type and dose of light, the amount of body surface exposed, and the duration of exposure. There is a direct relationship between the irradiance used and the rate at which the serum bilirubin declines. Blue light (450 nm) is the most effective. Irradiance can be improved by bringing the lamps closer to the infant; the optimal distance is 10 to 20 cm from the infant. Halogen lamps are also available, and manufacturers' recommendations must be followed to remove the risk of burn. Fiberoptic blankets, as well as "bili-beds" effectively increase the amount of surface area exposed and the irradiance. Both of these methods allow parental contact during treatment. Phototherapy may be temporarily discontinued for breast-feeding and family visits.

The infant should be unclothed, preferably undiapered, and its eyes shielded continuously during phototherapy. The crib should be open, because an isolette's top prevents the light from being within 10 to 15 cm from the infant. If the infant's temperature is compromised from being in an open crib, improved thermoregulation is obtained with the infant in an isolette at a temperature of approximately 30°C. The isolette temperature is then adjusted based on the infant's temperature, which should be determined at least every 3 to 4 hours.

During phototherapy, the infant may experience loose stools, possibly due to the high concentration of bilirubin and bile salts excreted into the gut, so hydration status should be monitored. If the infant becomes mildly dehydrated due to increased stooling and/or poor oral intake, correction of the dehydration will be necessary. The best fluid to use in this situation is breast milk or milk-based formula, not water. Providing adequate hydration promotes good urine output and improves the effectivenss of the phototherapy. If the infant becomes dehydrated and oral rehydration is inadequate, IV fluids should be considered. Otherwise, breast milk or formula are offered every 2 or 3 hours. The skin should also be observed for rash; the diaper area may become excoriated quickly by liquid stools. Oil-based diaper rash ointments should be avoided because of the potential for burns, as they heat rapidly under phototherapy.

Phototherapy can be discontinued in the term infant after the serum bilirubin level has dropped by 4 to 5 mg/dL, or falls below 13 to 14 mg/dL. The serum bilirubin levels may decrease more slowly in a breast-fed infant because of the greater enterohepatic recirculation and the presence of NEFAs in breast milk. There is some controversy as to whether bilirubin levels rebound after phototherapy is discontinued. There is no evidence that hospital discharge need be delayed in order to monitor for rebound. Phototherapy that was initiated early and discontinued prior to 3 to 4 days of age warrants a follow-up TSB within 24 hours of discharge.

For infants with known or suspected cholestatic jaundice (conjugated hyperbilirubinemia), phototherapy is ineffective and should not be used. The infant can develop a transient gray-bronze discoloration (bronze baby syndrome), possibly due to accumulation of copper porphyrins or the retention of photooxidation bilirubin products. In the absence of hepatosplenomegaly, "bronzing" does not appear to be a serious problem, and no known lasting adverse effects are seen. Although the discoloration may last several months, it begins to clear as soon as phototherapy is stopped.

For infants with hemolytic disease or bilirubin levels that increase faster than 0.5 mg/dL/hr, exchange transfusion may be indicated to decrease the risk of neurotoxicity. Additionally, the American Academy of Pediatrics 2004 guidelines recommend exchange transfusion for a TSB level ≥5 mg/dL above the appropriate line in Figure 108.5, a TSB > 25 mg/dL, or if the infant demonstrates evidence of advanced acute bilirubin encephalopathy (e.g., hypertonia, arching, retrocollis, opisthotonos, fever, high-pitched cry). Further, if the bilirubin level at admission warrants, intensive phototherapy with triple lights and blanket should be initiated, and the bilirubin should be repeated in 2 hours while preparing for exchange transfusion. Exchange transfusion involves the removal of small aliquots of blood from the infant and replacement with the same volume of donor red blood cells (RBCs) reconstituted with plasma. The procedure is repeated until the blood volume is replaced twice. This rapidly clears both bilirubin and the circulating antibodies that cause hemolysis. Due to the risks associated with exchange transfusion, this procedure is usually reserved for the neonatologist.

For the healthy, preterm infant, the threshold for treating hyperbilirubinemia is lower than for the term infant. For the sick preterm infant (e.g., respiratory distress, infection, hypoxia, hypoproteinemia, or factors causing hemolysis), intervention levels are lowered still further, due to the immature blood–brain barrier of premature infants. Fewer guidelines are available in the literature regarding phototherapy and exchange transfusion for premature or extremely premature infants. Frequently, in determining therapy in infants weighing less than 2 kg, clinicians use the following strategy: exchange transfusion is considered in the the premature infant weighing less than 2 kg if the serum bilirubin level is 10 times the infant's weight in kilograms.

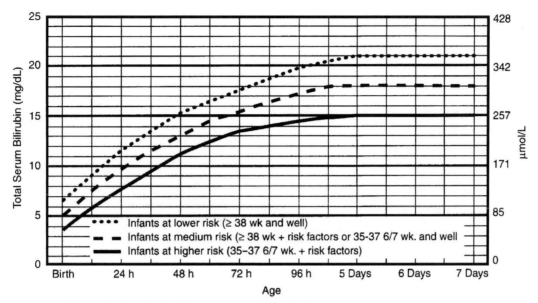

- Use total bilirubin. Do not subtract direct reacting or conjugated bilirubin.
- Risk factors = isoimmune hemolytic disease, G6PD deficiency, asphyxia, significant lethargy, temperature instability, sepsis, acidosis, or albumin < 3.0g/dL (if measured)
- For well infants 35–37 6/7 wk can adjust TSB levels for intervention around the medium risk line. It is an option to intervene at lower TSB levels for infants closer to 35 wks and at higher TSB levels for those closer to 37 6/7 wk.
- It is an option to provide conventional phototherapy in hospital or at home at TSB levels 2–3 mg/dL (35–50 mmol/L) below those shown but home phototherapy should not be used in any infant with risk factors.

FIGURE 108.4. Guidelines for phototherapy in hospitalized infants of 35 or more weeks of gestation. (From American Academy of Pediatrics. Practice parameter: management of hyperbilirubinemia in the newborn infant 35 or more weeks of gestation. *Pediatrics* 2004;114:297–316.)

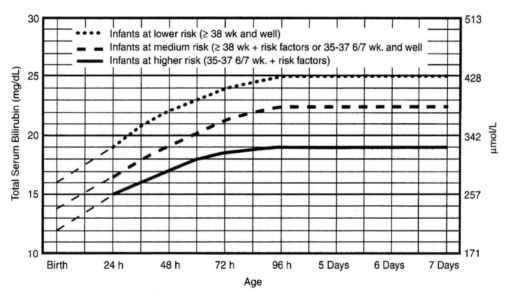

- The dashed lines for the first 24 hours indicate uncertainty due to a wide range of clinical circumstances and a range of responses to phototherapy.
- Immediate exchange transfusion is recommended if infant shows signs of acute bilirubin encephalopathy (hypertonia, arching, retrocollis, opisthotonos, fever, high pitched cry) or if TSB is ≥5 mg/dL (85 μmol/L) above these lines.
- Risk factors - isoimmune hemolytic disease, G6PD deficiency, asphyxia, significant lethargy, temperature instability, sepsis, acidosis.
- Measure serum albumin and calculate B/A ratio (See legend)
- Use total bilirubin. Do not subtract direct reacting or conjugated bilirubin
- If infant is well and 35–37 6/7 wk (median risk) can individualize TSB levels for exchange based on actual gestational age.

FIGURE 108.5. Guidelines for exchange transfusion in infants 35 or more weeks of gestation. (From American Academy of Pediatrics. Practice parameter: management of hyperbilirubinemia in the newborn infant 35 or more weeks of gestation. *Pediatrics* 2004;114:297–316.)

TABLE 108.3

MANAGEMENT OF HYPERBILIRUBINEMIA IN HEALTHY AND SICK PREMATURE INFANTS (<37 WEEKS)

Weight (g)	Healthy: Total serum bilirubin level (mg/dL)		Sick: Total serum bilirubin level (mg/dL)	
	Phototherapy	Exchange transfusion	Phototherapy	Exchange transfusion
Up to 1,000	5–7	10	4–6	8–10
1,001–1,500	7–10	10–15	6–8	10–12
1,501–2,000	10	17	8–10	15
>2,000	10–12	18	10	17

Adapted from Halamek LP, Stevenson DK. Neonatal jaundice and liver diseases. In: Fanaroff AA, Martin RJ, eds. *Neonatal perinatal medicine: diseases of the fetus and infant*. 6th ed. St. Louis: Mosby-Year Book; 1997: 1345–1389; and Gartner LM. *Pediatr Rev* 1994;15:422–432.

Phototherapy is initiated if the serum bilirubin level is 50% to 75% of the transfusion level. For example, an infant that weighs 1.8 kg will have a serum bilirubin exchange level of 18 mg/dL, and the range to initiate phototherapy would be a serum level of 9 to 14 mg/dL. Table 108.3 is used as an additional guide for phototherapy and exchange transfusion of healthy and sick infants less than 37 weeks gestation.

Some medications have also been used to treat jaundice. Phenobarbital has been favored for several decades because it increases liver glucuronyl transferase, increases hepatic uptake of bilirubin, and improves bilirubin excretion. However, phenobarbital also has other metabolic effects in addition to those on bilirubin metabolism and therefore has not been widely used except in very specific high-risk populations. A dosage of 60 mg/day is sufficient for maternal administration, to secondarily treat the fetus, and 5 mg/kg/day for neonatal treatment. The combination of phenobarbital and phototherapy has not been shown to offer any advantage over phototherapy alone.

Other pharmacologic interventions have focused on competitive heme oxygenase inhibitors (e.g., tin- and zinc-protoporphyrin and tin- and zinc-mesoporphyrin), which effectively suppress the formation of bilirubin. An untoward effect noted in these studies was transient erythema with phototherapy. Metalloporphyrins are not currently approved for use in newborn infants, and further studies are necessary before widespread use can be expected.

The healthy, term breast-fed infant may experience increased levels of serum bilirubin due to dehydration and inadequate calories from poor feeding ("breastfeeding" jaundice). Increased bilirubin levels may also be due to enterohepatic circulation. The mother should be encouraged to breast-feed the infant frequently, at least 10 to 12 times per 24-hour period. Colostrum has a laxative effect, helping to empty the gut of meconium, and colonizes the gut with beneficial bacterial flora that enhance bilirubin degradation. Supplementing with water or dextrose water does not lower serum bilirubin levels and may interfere with breast-feeding success. If the bilirubin level approaches that requiring phototherapy, a phototherapy blanket should be considered, with frequent breastfeeding sessions.

True "breast-milk jaundice" (late-onset jaundice or breast-milk jaundice syndrome) does not occur in the newborn period; it appears at 5 to 10 days of age. "Breast-feeding jaundice" may precede breast-milk jaundice. Peak serum bilirubin levels for breast-milk jaundice may be as high as 25 to 30 mg/dL. The actual cause of breast-milk jaundice is unknown. Caution must be exercised in attributing jaundice to breast-feeding; the search for other causes of jaundice must not be delayed simply because the only symptom is jaundice in a breast-fed infant. In breast-milk jaundice, indirect serum bilirubin rises; in contrast, in conditions such as biliary atresia, direct bilirubin will rise.

Home phototherapy might be considered for infants in the "optional" range for phototherapy. However, home devices do not provide adequate irradiance or surface area exposure, and should not be used for infants with higher bilirubin levels. Infants who are candidates for home phototherapy must be followed daily; this follow-up may include home health in close collaboration with the infant's health care provider. A few experts argue that if the goal is to prevent neurologic damage, the treatment should not be done outside the hospital setting; however, 24 to 48 hours of home phototherapy is usually all that is required to reduce the serum bilirubin levels.

PEARLS

- Jaundice occurs in 50% to 60% of term newborns and 80% of preterm infants.
- Normal infants produce about 6 to 8 mg/kg body weight of bilirubin each 24 hours.
- When the direct bilirubin concentration is 2 mg/dL or greater than or equal to 20% of the total bilirubin, the infant should be evaluated for disorders of conjugated hyperbilirubinemia. Caution should be exercised in interpreting direct bilirubin.
- Transcutaneous bilirubinometry is a reliable and valid estimate of serum bilirubin.
- The greatest impact of phototherapy is in the first 24 to 48 hours of therapy.
- Phototherapy can be discontinued after the serum bilirubin level has dropped by 4 to 5 mg/dL, or the level is below 14 to 15 mg/dL (term). Rebound serum levels are of little importance.
- The healthy, term breast-fed infant may have increased serum bilirubin due to increased enterohepatic recirculation, dehydration, inadequate calories, and competitive factors for conjugation. Mothers should breast-feed at least 10 to 12 times/24-hour period.

Suggested Readings

American Academy of Pediatrics. Practice parameter: management of hyperbilirubinemia in the newborn infant 35 or more weeks of gestation. *Pediatrics* 2004;114:297–316.

Dennery PA, Seidman DS, Stevenson DK. Drug therapy: neonatal hyperbilirubinemia. *N Engl J Med* 2001;344:1–17.

Hansen TWR. Neonatal jaundice. *EMed J* 2002;3:1–24.

CHAPTER 109 ■ VOMITING

GREGG M. TALENTE

The evaluation and management of vomiting in the newborn period can be challenging. Many infants will have some emesis or spitting in the first few days of life. Newborn providers must be able to separate common, benign causes from more serious ones to guide subsequent necessary interventions. Vomiting in the newborn can be caused by a wide variety of disorders; some require only simple interventions and close monitoring, while others are urgent and life-threatening. Understanding the presenting signs and the appropriate management of the various causes of emesis in the newborn period is essential for any provider working in a newborn unit.

Vomiting is defined as the forceful retrograde expulsion of the stomach's contents; it must be distinguished from *regurgitation*, which describes the passive movement of stomach contents into the esophagus. Differentiating these two processes is difficult without close examination and observation. Vomiting is a reflex controlled by the somatic nervous system. It is usually associated with nausea, which in infants manifests itself as pallor, sweating, salivation, tachycardia, and retching. These signs should not accompany regurgitation. Infants are typically undisturbed by regurgitation, although in some instances (e.g., gastroesophageal reflux disease) regurgitation can be associated with discomfort symptoms.

Vomiting is also further classified by its appearance. The most common and critical distinction is between bilious and nonbilious emesis. Bilious emesis refers to vomitus stained green or yellow by bile acids and other intestinal secretions. Although it may suggest a more serious etiology, such as intestinal obstruction distal to the ampulla of Vater, not all bilious emesis is pathologic. In some cases, nonbilious emesis can be equally serious. It is also important to note hematemesis when present.

DIFFERENTIAL DIAGNOSIS

There are many causes of vomiting in newborns (Table 109.1), some of which are not associated with a pathologic process. For example, newborn infants commonly regurgitate after a feed at some point in the first day or two of life. Regurgitation of a teaspoon or two of milk shortly after feeding without evidence of distress, called spitting, is common, benign, and does not require intervention. Newborns may also vomit from swallowed gastric irritants, including amniotic fluid, mucous, and maternal blood. In fact, swallowed maternal blood is the main cause of benign hematemesis in newborns.

Gastroesophageal reflux (GER) is a common cause of infant regurgitation. It can present in the newborn period, or the diagnosis may not be evident until later. Although it is usually benign and remits during the first year of life, reflux may be associated with esophagitis, bronchospasm, asthma, and failure to thrive.

Gastrointestinal obstruction can cause emesis in the newborn period. The various causes of gastrointestinal obstruction, listed in Table 109.2, can be differentiated by careful evaluation. Congenital abnormalities of the oropharynx, such as cleft palate and laryngopharyngeal clefts, can lead to emesis in the newborn. A cleft palate will frequently cause an infant to reflux formula or breast milk into the nasopharynx, causing choking, gagging, and possibly emesis. The emesis will consist predominantly of formula or breast milk.

Obstruction of the gastrointestinal tract at the esophageal level can be caused by esophageal atresia, vascular rings, and tracheoesophageal fistula. Prenatally, these anomalies commonly produce polyhydramnios. Infants with esophageal atresia vomit with all feedings; in addition, they often regurgitate large quantities of saliva and are described as "mucousy" babies. Infants with complete esophageal atresia will present early in the postnatal period, while infants with incomplete esophageal obstruction, such as vascular ring or tracheoesophageal fistula, will have more intermittent dysphagia and emesis. Infants with tracheoesophageal fistula may also present with respiratory symptoms, such as cough and wheezing from aspiration.

Duodenal atresia occurs in 1 in 5,000 live births. Twenty-five percent of affected infants with duodenal atresia also have Down syndrome. These infants present with emesis in the first few hours after birth and will usually vomit with every feed. The emesis is frequently bilious; however, in up to 15% of infants with duodenal atresia, the obstruction lies proximal to the ampulla of Vater, and therefore the emesis is nonbilious. Again, maternal polyhydramnios is commonly seen in this setting.

Jejunal atresia, occurring in 1 in 3,000 live births, is caused by a vascular accident during fetal life. Infants present in the first 24 hours of life with bilious emesis and abdominal distension. Incomplete obstruction, such as duodenal stenosis, will still present in the neonatal period, although vomiting may be more intermittent, the infant may feed successfully, and the diagnosis may be more difficult.

Intestinal malrotation is caused by a failure of the bowel to rotate correctly during gestation. The malrotation itself is not typically a problem; rather, it is the development of volvulus through a twisting of the malrotated bowel that leads to emesis and clinical deterioration. In malrotation with volvulus, the vascular supply to the midgut is obstructed, leading to bowel ischemia and intestinal obstruction. Volvulus will usually occur in the first week after birth, although it can happen at any time. Volvulus is an acutely life-threatening condition; without intervention, the infant's condition will deteriorate rapidly. As bowel ischemia progresses, metabolic acidosis and hemodynamic instability will develop. Occasionally, malrotation without volvulus presents in infancy, with findings of intermittent obstruction in the duodenum and proximal small bowel secondary to Ladd bands.

An annular pancreas encircles the duodenum, causing compression of the duodenal wall and secondary obstruction. The variable degree of obstruction will determine the presentation

TABLE 109.1

CAUSES OF NEWBORN EMESIS

Cause	
"Spitting"	Inborn errors of metabolism
Irritants	Maternal effects
Amniotic fluid	Drugs
Maternal blood	Illness
Mucous	Neurologic causes
GERD	Central nervous system
Gastrointestinal obstruction	hypertension
Necrotizing enterocolitis	Hydrocephalus
Infection	Kernicterus
Sepsis	
Urinary tract infection	

of infants with this abnormality. A complete or nearly complete obstruction will present in the first day of life with bilious emesis during feedings, whereas an infant with partial obstruction will have intermittent bilious emesis.

Obstructions of the gastrointestinal tract at the ileal or colonic level will present first with abdominal distension and subsequently with failed feeding and vomiting. The more distal the obstruction, the greater the degree of distension. Vomiting occurs several days later than it does in more proximal obstructions. Mechanical obstructions include atresia or stenosis of the bowel in the ileum, colon, or rectum; Imperforate anus will also result in abdominal distension and bilious emesis if not noted at birth. Hirschsprung disease, a functional obstruction presenting with a similar picture, is caused by a defect in the innervation of the rectum and distal colon. The neural ganglion cells of the submucosa of the distal intestine are absent for a variable distance, leading to impaired peristalsis and a great or lesser degree of obstruction.

Meconium ileus is a disorder in which thick meconium is retained in the distal intestine so that passage of meconium is delayed. Ninety percent of infants with meconium ileus also have cystic fibrosis. The bowel itself can be intact, or there can be an associated defect, such as volvulus, atresia, or bowel perforation (with resulting meconium peritonitis). Infants with meconium ileus develop significant abdominal distension and bilious emesis.

Meconium plugs can also lead to abdominal distension, emesis, and delayed passage of meconium, but this condition differs from meconium ileus, in that meconium plugs result from the impaction of meconium with a lower than normal water content. Meconium plugs are also associated with small left colon syndrome in infants of diabetic mothers, cystic fibrosis, rectal aganglionosis, maternal drug use, and magnesium sulfate treatment for maternal preeclampsia. Necrotizing enterocolitis (NEC) is a rapidly progressing disorder of unknown eitiology in which infants develop bowel necrosis, infection, and ultimately, bowel perforation and peritonitis. NEC is associated with prematurity and pulmonary disorders, but 10% to 35% of cases occur in full-term infants. Typically, the infant presents about 10 to 12 days after birth with abdominal distension, bilious emesis, ileus, and bloody stools. In later stages, infants develop bradycardia, hypothermia, apnea, and without intervention, rapid deterioration and death.

Emesis in newborn infants is not always related to gastrointestinal disease. Other causes of emesis in young infants include:

- Metabolic syndromes (e.g., galactosemia, phenylketonuria)
- Infection (e.g., group B streptococcal sepsis, urinary tract infection)
- Maternal drug exposure (e.g., narcotics, antibiotics, drugs of abuse)
- Neurologic disorders (e.g., hydrocephalus, kernicterus)

TABLE 109.2

CAUSES OF GASTROINTESTINAL OBSTRUCTION IN NEWBORNS

Site	Cause
Oropharynx	Cleft palate
	Laryngopharyngeal cleft
Esophagus	Esophageal atresia
	Vascular ring
	Tracheoesophageal fistula
Gastric	Antral web
Upper intestine	Duodenal atresia
	Duodenal stenosis
	Jejunal atresia
	Anular pancreas
	Choledochal cyst
	Malrotation/volvulus
Lower intestine	Ileal atresia
	Meconium ileus
	Meconium plug
	Colonic atresia
	Colonic stenosis
	Hirschsprung disease
	Imperforate anus
	Rectal stenosis

CLINICAL FINDINGS

The evaluation of an infant with emesis should aim at determining the cause of vomiting. The most useful tools for making this determination are the history and physical examination. A variety of tests can aid the investigation, but they should be used only when necessary. It is important for the newborn provider to classify newborn emesis accurately through history and examination, to separate benign causes from dangerous disorders, and to choose the correct diagnostic tests to quickly and correctly determine the cause of the vomiting.

In taking a history, the first step is to obtain a description of the emesis. When did it occur? When was the most recent feeding? How many times has the infant vomited? It is important to know what the emesis looked like; if possible, the physician should look at it directly. Is it bilious? Is it bloody? Is it mucousy? It is important to determine if the infant was distressed when vomiting. Were there signs of nausea? Was this true vomiting or regurgitation? As much information as possible regarding the specific episodes of emesis should be obtained.

A detailed maternal history is also important, because there are several causes of newborn vomiting that are related to interventions given prior to delivery or that are associated with prenatal findings, such as polyhydramnios and prematurity. The infant's risk for developing sepsis should be determined. A family history can be helpful in diagnosing inherited conditions, such as cystic fibrosis and other congenital disorders. Finally, the infant's entire postnatal history should be reviewed. Information about previous feedings, passage of meconium, presence or absence of respiratory distress, and thermoregulation can provide clues that are helpful in evaluating vomiting in a newborn.

A complete examination should be performed on any infant with vomiting. Vital signs should be reviewed for hypotension, hyperthermia or hypothermia, and tachycardia or tachypnea. Growth parameters, such as head circumference and abdominal circumference, should be remeasured to look for changes. A dramatic change in abdominal circumference would suggest either a distal intestinal obstruction or NEC. The presence of a skin rash can signal infection. Discoloration of the abdomen is associated with peritonitis. The head and neck examination may show a bulging fontanelle when there is increased intracranial pressure. The oropharynx should be examined for defects, such as cleft palate. The cardiac and respiratory examinations may indicate associated problems that are contributing to the emesis.

The abdominal examination in a newborn with emesis should be done carefully, beginning with inspection followed by auscultation. Imperforate anus, for example, can be easily diagnosed by visualizing the area. Bowel sounds may be absent or hypoactive in infants with ileus, while high-pitched, tinkling sounds accompany obstruction. The next step is palpation of all four quadrants. An infant's abdomen should remain soft and nondistended; increasing firmness or distension is suggestive of intestinal obstruction or ischemia. In distal obstruction, such as meconium ileus or colonic atresia, dilated loops of bowel may be palpable or visible. Information gathered in the course of a detailed history and physical examination will influence the next step in evaluating a newborn with emesis. Abdominal radiographs and contrast studies are the most common diagnostic tests used in evaluating infants with vomiting, but every infant that vomits does not require a radiograph. Unfortunately, determining whether the vomiting is benign or not can be challenging, because no one finding is sufficient to decide the question. Findings such as abdominal distension, persistent vomiting, bilious emesis, and delayed passage of meconium all suggest a more serious cause for a newborn's vomiting, but none of these findings is specific. Similarly, the absence of such symptoms does not exclude the possibility of intestinal obstruction or a more serious cause of the emesis. The decision to proceed with diagnostic testing should be based on the combination of findings and clinical judgment. Even when emesis appears to be benign, ongoing vigilance and periodic reevaluation are warranted.

The initial radiologic test for evaluating newborn emesis is the plain abdominal radiograph. Certain causes of newborn emesis have very distinctive radiographic findings. Duodenal atresia is known for the classic "double-bubble" sign on abdominal radiographs, caused by the dilated stomach and dilated proximal duodenum. Meconium ileus can be diagnosed by noting distended bowel loops with a ground-glass appearance (Neuhauser sign). Abdominal radiographs in infants with NEC show dilated bowel loops and pneumatosis intestinalis. Intestinal obstruction from other causes can lead to dilated bowel loops proximal to the obstruction, air–fluid levels, and a paucity or absence of bowel gas distal to the obstruction. Despite these helpful signs, however, a plain abdominal radiograph is not sensitive enough to pick up every case of intestinal obstruction or disease. Again, the provider must use clinical judgment to determine which infants should have additional tests performed and which can simply be observed closely. Usually, if further testing is required, a contrast study of the upper or lower gastrointestinal tract is ordered.

The placement of a nasogastric (NG) tube can also be a useful evaluative tool, or even diagnostic as in the case of esophageal atresia or another proximal obstruction. Inability to pass the tube into the stomach, combined with a radiograph showing the tube in the esophagus, is sufficient to diagnose esophageal obstruction. In another scenario, finding large amounts of retained material in the stomach strongly suggests a proximal intestinal obstruction; if the fluid is bile stained, the obstruction is beyond the ampulla of Vater.

When evaluating an infant with emesis, it is at times necessary to expand the evaluation to include disease outside the gastrointestinal tract. A CBC and differential can be helpful in assessing the possibility of infection, as well as assessing for anemia. Serum electrolytes and glucose should be measured whenever feeding is disrupted. These tests can also be used to identify metabolic disturbances or acid-base disturbances. Blood cultures should be drawn whenever a systemic infection, NEC, or bowel ischemia is suspected.

MANAGEMENT

The cause of a newborn's vomiting determines its treatment. When innocent causes, such as gastric irritants or GER are suspected or when the infant's spitting is felt to be benign, simple observation may be all that is indicated. However, whenever a more serious cause is suspected, immediate interventions are necessary. First, feeding should be suspended, as continued feeding of an infant with a suspected obstruction or NEC can be harmful. An NG tube should then be placed to allow decompression of the infant's stomach and prevent further emesis and discomfort. It may also provide information that is helpful in establishing the diagnosis. Finally, the infant should be given IV fluids and nutrition until the infant is hemodynamically stable; then the diagnostic workup can be completed.

The further treatment of vomiting in the newborn depends on the underlying etiology. Meconium ileus and meconium plugs can be corrected by gastrograffin enema; surgery is only necessary when this procedure fails. Stopping feeds and giving antibiotics and IV nutrition for approximately 10 days can treat NEC. If intestinal perforation, stricture, or volvulus develop, immediate surgical intervention is required. Malrotation requires surgical correction. Intestinal obstruction from stenosis or atresia is usually treated surgically, regardless of the level of obstruction.

PEARLS

■ Although bilious emesis is usually equated with intestinal obstruction, many infants with bilious emesis are in fact healthy and do not have an obstruction. In a recent study, 63 infants with green-colored emesis in the first days of life were evaluated; of these, only 24 had an obstruction due to disorders including Hirschsprung disease, jejunal atresia, malrotation, meconium ileus, and meconium plugs. Most of the other 39 infants were not diagnosed with a specific condition, and the rest were diagnosed with reflux.

Suggested Readings

Davenport M. Surgically correctable causes of vomiting in infancy. *BMJ* 1996;312:236–239.

Godbole P, Stringer MD. Bilious vomiting in the newborn: how often is it pathologic? *J Pediatr Surg* 2002;37:909–911.

Kimura K, Loening-Baucke V. Bilious vomiting in the newborn: rapid diagnosis of intestinal obstruction. *Am Fam Physician* 2000;61:2791–2798.

Murray KF, Christie DL. Vomiting in infancy: when should you worry? *Contemp Pediatr* 2000;17:81–115.

CHAPTER 110 ■ HEMORRHAGIC DISORDERS IN THE FULL-TERM NEWBORN

CHARLES W. DAESCHNER III

Assesment of hemostasis in the newborn presents a unique challenge. During the delivery process, trauma to the newborn often results in bruising, cephalhematoma, and/or petechiae. Similarly, some bleeding from the umbilical stump or from the penis after circumcision is not uncommon; therefore, the challenge to the pediatric provider is deciding when an infant has sufficient evidence of bleeding to initiate an evaluation. It is also important for the clinician to remember that the most common cause of hematochezia and hematemesis in the newborn is swallowed maternal blood, not gastrointestinal bleeding.

The evaluation of bleeding in newborns is complicated by the fact that although hemostasis is normal in most infants, some tests of coagulation function are commonly mildly abnormal in newborn infants (Table110.1). Normal infants have decreased platelet aggregation, modestly increased prothrombin time (PT), increased partial thromboplastin time (PTT), and decreased levels of the coagulation inhibitors (antithrombin 3, protein C, protein S, and heparin cofactor 2).

HEMOSTASIS IN THE FULL-TERM NEWBORN

Platelet counts and size are similar to those in the adult, with a similar half-life (3.5 to 4 days). Platelet-dense granules contain less adenosine diphosphate (ADP) and serotonin than do adult platelets, and less platelet aggregation is triggered by epinephrine, ADP, and thrombin. On the other hand, aggregation upon exposure to ristocetin is increased, possibly because of a relative excess of high molecular weight von Willebrand multimers. The bottom line is that newborns seem inclined to hypercoagulation (thrombophilia) rather than hypocoagulation, as reflected by a fairly short bleeding time, despite these platelet dysfunctions and decreased in vitro coagulation factors.

Coagulation factors with levels in the "normal" range in the newborn include fibrinogen, V, VIII, XIII, and von Willebrand factor. Fibrinogen remains in a fetal form, but this does not seem to confer on it any functional disadvantage. The four "contact factors"—XI, XII, prekallikrein, and high molecular weight kininogen—are decreased and account for the increased neonatal PTT. The vitamin K–dependent factors (II, VII, IX, and X) are present at about 50% of adult values and are reflected by the modest increase in PT. This is not reversed at birth, even with prompt administration of vitamin K. The increased PT and PTT do not translate clinically into a neonatal bleeding tendency, because they are compensated by a relative decrease in coagulation inhibitors. This is well illustrated by the short whole blood clotting time in the newborn.

As noted above, the relative decrease in coagulation inhibitors compensates for the decreased levels of some coagulation factors. The decreased physiologic coagulation inhibitor factors include antithrombin 3 (AT-3), protein C, protein S, and heparin cofactor 2. Furthermore, the inhibition of thrombin generation by AT-3 and α-2-macroglobulin is slow, and there is a low level of tissue factor protein inhibitor (TFPI), which ordinarily down-regulates the activity of VII. These procoagulant factors partly modulate the lower levels of coagulation factors described above.

Finally, fibrinolysis functions at an essentially normal level in the neonate, but again with differences compared to older children and adults. Fibrinolysis is initiated at birth, but due to low (50%) plasminogen levels, less plasmin is generated and no increased fibrinolysis develops in vivo, which ensures the persistence of a stable fibrin clot.

CLINICAL FINDINGS

Some evidence of minor bleeding is common in the newborn. The experienced clinician should have some perspective about when to initiate an evaluation for bleeding diatheses; appropriate situations might be any of the following:

- Oozing from the umbilicus (onset of oozing is delayed in XIII deficiency)
- Very large or severe scalp hemorrhages or cephalhematomas
- Bleeding from circumcision (occurs in only 30% of severe hemophilias)
- Widespread petechiae (platelet disorders)
- Massive bruises, and intracranial hemorrhage (ICH)

The initial laboratory evaluation should include PT, PTT, fibrinogen level, platelet count, and a bleeding time (if possible). If available, a PFA-100 in vitro bleeding time may be better. Platelet morphology should be examined for macroplatelets or microplatelets (e.g., Wiskott–Aldrich syndrome), in particular. If the PTT is prolonged, factor VIII and IX levels should be checked; if they are normal, factors XI and XII should be evaluated.

If emergency management for bleeding is necessary while awaiting detailed laboratory results, fresh frozen plasma (FFP), given at 10 to 20 mL/kg, will correct most coagulation abnormalities until specific replacement therapy can be used. The use of activated coagulation factor complexes should be avoided because of their ability to trigger disseminated intravascular coagulation (DIC). Platelet transfusions should be given to thrombocytopenic patients only if the etiology is not immune, or if an immune thrombocytopenia is life-threatening (see below). The "trigger value" for platelet transfusion is usually 50,000/μL or any value below 100,000/μL associated with significant

TABLE 110.1

COAGULATION TESTS IN HEALTHY FULL-TERM INFANTS

Coagulation tests	Mean (Range)			
	Day 1	Day 5	Day 30	Adult
PT (sec)	13.0 (10.10–15.9)	12.40 (10.0–15.3)	11.80 (10.0–14.3)	12.40 (10.8–13.9)
International normalized ratio	1.0 (0.53–1.62)	0.89 (0.53–1.48)	0.79 (0.53–1.26)	0.89 (0.64–1.17)
APTT (sec)	42.9 (31.3–54.5)	42.6 (25.4–59.8)	40.4 (32.0–55.2)	33.5 (26.6–40.3)
Fibrinogen (g/L)	2.83 (1.67–3.99)	3.12 (1.62–4.62)	2.70 (1.62–3.78)	27.8 (1.56–4.00)
Factor II	0.48 (0.26–0.70)	0.63 (0.33–0.93)	0.68 (0.34–1.02)	1.08 (0.70–1.46)
Factor V	0.72 (0.34–1.08)	0.95 (0.45–1.45)	0.98 (0.62–1.34)	1.06 (0.62–1.50)
Factor VII	0.66 (0.28–1.04)	0.89 (0.35–1.43)	0.90 (0.42–1.38)	1.05 (0.67–1.43)
Factor VIII	1.00 (0.50–1.78)	0.88 (0.50–1.54)	0.91 (0.50–1.57)	0.99 (0.50–1.49)
VWf	1.53 (0.50–2.87)	1.40 (0.50–2.54)	1.28 (0.50–2.46)	0.92 (0.50–1.58)
Factor IX	0.53 (0.15–0.91)	0.53 (0.15–0.91)	0.51 (0.21–0.81)	1.09 (0.55–1.63)
Factor X	0.40 (0.12–0.68)	0.49 (0.19–0.79)	0.59 (0.31–0.87)	1.06 (0.70–1.52)
Factor XI	0.68 (0.10–0.66)	0.55 (0.23–0.87)	0.53 (0.27–0.79)	0.97 (0.67–1.27)
Factor XII	0.53 (0.13–0.93)	0.47 (0.11–0.83)	0.49 (0.17–0.81)	1.08 (0.52–1.64)
PK	0.37 (0.18–0.69)	0.48 (0.20–0.76)	0.57 (0.23–0.91)	1.12 (0.62–1.62)
Factor XIII	0.79 (0.27–1.31)	0.94 (0.44–1.44)	0.93 (0.39–1.47)	1.05 (0.55–1.55)

INR, international normalized ratio; PK, pre-Kallikrein; PT, prothrombin time; APTT, activated partial thromboplastin time. All factors except fibrinogen are expressed as units per milliliter (U/mL).
From Andrew M, Paes B, Johnson M. Development of the hemostatic system in the neonate and young infant. *Am J Pediatr Hematol Oncol* 1990; 12:95–104, with permission.

hemorrhage (other than bruises and petechiae). The fibrinogen level should be above 100 mg/dL (l g/L), or coagulation factor replacement will not be effective. Cryoprecipitate or fibrinogen concentrates may be necessary if levels are low. Cryoprecipitate bags (10 to 25 mL) contain 250 mg of fibrinogen.

ABNORMALITIES OF HEMOSTASIS

Thrombocytopenia

The three most common etiologies of thrombocytopenia (low platelet count) include infection (bacterial or viral), alloimmune thrombocytopenia, and maternal immune thrombocytopenic purpura (ITP). Table 110.2 lists some of the less common causes of neonatal thrombocytopenia. The thrombocytopenia can be due to decreased production or increased destruction.

The most common cause of thrombocytopenia due to decreased production is infection, which can coincide with hypersplenism and/or antiplatelet antibodies. Other etiologies of decreased platelet production are rare and include congenital leukemia, trisomy 21, leukemoid reaction, bone marrow replacement by neuroblastoma or histiocytosis, and congenital amegakaryocytic disorders with or without radial bone abnormalities. All of these respond well to platelet transfusions; 10 to 20 mL/kg of platelet concentrate should raise the count by 25,000 to 50,000/µL.

Thrombocytopenia due to increased destruction is usually seen in one of three clinical situations: alloimmune thrombocytopenia, maternal ITP, or DIC. *Alloimmune thrombocytopenia* occurs when the neonate's platelets contain antigens different from the mother. If the mother was sensitized during the pregnancy and developed IgG antibodies, these antibodies cross the placenta and cause severe thrombocytopenia in the perinatal period. This can sometimes have devastating consequences for the infant, including in utero ICH. At birth, the baby presents with massive bruises, petechiae, and extreme thrombocytopenia (less than 10,000/µL). Even with excellent medical care, 20% of affected newborns develop severe morbidity or die. Alloimmune thrombocytopenia is mostly due to antibodies against the HPA-1 (formerly PLA-1) antigen, lacking in the mother and present in the baby and its father. Approximately 11% of mothers lack the HPA-1 antigen on their platelets, but only 1 in 2,500 pregnant women, half of whom are primagravida, present with alloimmune thrombocytopenia. If possible, the affected infant should be transfused with HPA-1 negative platelets, which are now available now from most large blood banks. Maternal washed and irradiated platelets are a practical alternative, but if the blood bank can isolate and wash platelets, it usually also has access to HPA-1 negative platelets. Because most subsequent pregnancies manifest the same alloimmune situation, serial fetal ultrasound (US) should be performed after midgestation to assess for possible ICH. If ICH is suspected on US, the fetus should be treated with intrauterine platelet infusions. A prenatal cord blood platelet count should be obtained toward the end of gestation to help determine whether vaginal or Caesarean delivery is preferable. In all cases, weekly IV immunoglobulin (IVIG) infusions should be administered to the mother starting at midgestation and to the neonate at delivery (0.5 to 1.0 g/kg/wk). Steroids (prednisone 4 mg/kg/day) are also given to the baby and sometimes to the mother at term. Thrombocytopenia may recur for several weeks or even months.

In the setting of *maternal ITP* (or a history of ITP), the mother's broad-spectrum IgG antiplatelet antibodies cross the placenta to the fetus. The newborn then presents at birth with bruises and petechiae, but is not as severely affected as in the alloimmune situation. These infants rarely develop complications, respond well to IVIG, and usually do not require elective Caesarean section. If the mother's ITP is known, then maternal IVIG treatment can be started at midgestation, as in alloimmune thrombocytopenia, even if the mother's platelet count is normal. The only fetal platelet count monitoring needed is a scalp platelet count at the time of delivery; if platelets are less than 50,000/µL, then a Caesarean section should be considered but is controversial. Thrombocytopenia usually abates in 1 to 2 weeks.

TABLE 110.2

ETIOLOGY OF NEONATAL THROMBOCYTOPENIA

Category	Disease
Increased destruction	
Immune-mediated	Maternal idiopathic thrombocytopenic purpura
	Maternal systemic lupus erythematosus
	Maternal hyperthyroidism
	Maternal drugs
	Maternal preeclampsia
	Neonatal alloimmune thrombocytopenia
Nonimmune-mediated (probably related to disseminated intravascular coagulation)	Asphyxia
	Perinatal aspiration
	Necrotizing enterocolitis
	Hemangiomas
	Neonatal thrombosis
	Respiratory distress syndrome
Unknown	Hyperbilirubinemia
	Phototherapy
	Polycythemia
	Rh hemolytic disease
	Congenital thrombotic thrombocytopenic purpura
	Total parenteral nutrition
	Inborn errors of metabolism
	Wiscott-Aldrich syndrome
	Multiple congenital anomalies
Hypersplenism	
Decreased production of platelets	
Bone marrow replacement disorders	Congenital leukemia
	Congenital leukemoid reactions
	Neuroblastoma
	Histiocytosis
	Osteopetrosis
Bone marrow aplasia	Thrombocytopenia with absence of radius
	Amegakaryocytic thrombocytopenia
	Fanconi anemia
	Other marrow hypoplastic or aplastic disorders

From Andrew M. Developmental hemostasis: relevance to newborns and infants. In: Narran DG, Orkin SH, eds. *Nathan and Oski's hematology of infancy and childhood*, 5th ed. WB Saunders, 1998:125, with permission.

DIC is a consumption coagulopathy that involves much more than thrombopenia. It accompanies other serious disorders, such as birth asphyxia, hypovolemic or septic shock, severe infections, and aspiration of meconium or amniotic fluid. The infant is terribly ill and bleeds from "everywhere." Laboratory tests show markedly prolonged PT and PTT, as well as decreased fibrinogen, factor VIII, factor V, and platelets, and evidence of microangiopathic hemolysis with fragmented red cells. D-dimers are elevated, but this very sensitive test is usually not helpful.

Treatment consists of replacing the many missing factors with FFP, platelet packs sufficient to achieve a goal of 50,000/μL, and sometimes fibrinogen components. If protein C

concentrates are available, they should be given urgent consideration, because protein C is consumed in this disorder, and replacement usually stops the consumption and thrombotic phenomena immediately; they also have important anti-inflammatory properties.

Coagulation Factor Deficiencies

The deficiencies of coagulation factors can be hereditary or acquired. The acquired deficiencies include several situations that can be due to vitamin K deficiency, liver disease, or DIC. There are several forms of *hereditary coagulation factor deficiency*; the most common are hemophilia A and B (factors VIII and IX deficiency, respectively). Both are X chromosome–linked and therefore affect only boys. Hemophilia is severe, with the level of the deficient factor less than 2% of normal in 70% of affected newborns. The less severe forms may be missed completely at birth and reveal themselves years later—after an accident, surgery, or an abnormal PTT. Clinical manifestations at birth include prolonged bleeding from puncture sites, large cephalhematomas or subgaleal hematomas, prolonged bleeding from circumcision in 30% of the patients, and ICH. Bruising also may be present.

These signs are also common to all other severe hemophilias. Factor XIII deficiency often presents with delayed umbilical bleeding on days 3 or 4. Factor XII and prekallikrein deficiencies show no abnormal bleeding at all—just a very long PTT. von Willebrand disease is extremely rarely manifested at birth or is occasionally misdiagnosed as severe hemophilia A, unless present in a girl.

Laboratory findings show a very long, often immeasurable PTT for deficiencies of factors VIII, IX, X, XI, XII, and prekallikrein, a very long PT for VII deficiency, and a somewhat prolonged PT and PTT for V, prothrombin (factor II), and fibrinogen deficiencies. Specific factor assays can be focused at these three classes of abnormalities for confirmatory diagnosis.

After obtaining appropriate coagulation studies (and citrated plasma for subsequent factor analysis if needed), treatment should always be started with FFP. The exception is a prior family history that suggests the presence of a well-defined factor deficiency (e.g., brother or maternal uncle with hemophilia A), in which case specific factor replacement would be indicated. When a sibling is known to be affected, prenatal sex determination should be attempted by fetal US and/or a search for the Y chromosome in the maternal blood. If the family history is positive for hemophilia A or B and the fetus is not clearly a girl, or if the hemophilia is not X-linked, then a factor assay should be obtained from an intrauterine umbilical sample. If factor deficiency is confirmed, plans should be made for elective caesarean section and immediate postnatal factor replacement. Nonessential circumcision should be discouraged, even in the era of recombinant coagulation products, because of the very real risk of developing antifactor inhibitors. Both Jewish and Islamic law allows dispensations from circumcision in hemophilia situations, and this should be discussed with the family and their religious counsel.

In view of the high rate of spontaneous mutation in both hemophilia A and B, mothers of newly diagnosed patients should be thoroughly investigated for possible carrier status. Several genetic markers are available for such investigations, allowing enhanced genetic counseling in many cases.

Acquired Coagulation Factor Deficiencies

DIC results in deficiencies of both coagulation factors and platelets. Further discussion occurs above under the topic of thrombocytopenia.

Vitamin K deficiency exists in three clinical forms defined by the timing of the symptoms and signs: "early," first 24 hours of life; "classical," days 2 to 7 of life in breast-fed babies (e.g., hemorrhagic disease of the newborn, HDN); and "late," 0.5 to 6 months after birth. All three manifest themselves clinically as a severe bleeding diathesis, with hemorrhages from the gastrointestinal tract and, during the first week of life, the umbilicus. ICH has been reported. Laboratory tests show a very long PT, often a prolonged PTT, and depletion of the vitamin K–dependent clotting factors.

Early vitamin K deficiency occurs during the first 24 hours of life and is secondary to maternal ingestion of drugs that affect vitamin K levels and cross the placenta. Common examples of such maternal drugs include anticonvulsants, rifampin, isoniazid, and warfarin sodium (Coumadin).

Classical HDN occurs during the first week of life (days 2 to 7) in breast-fed babies with poor intake. Such babies tend to have a sterile gut, and therefore lack the bacterial flora that manufactures vitamin K. Babies on commercial formula are relatively protected from this disorder, because all commercial formulas contain adequate amounts of vitamin K.

Late vitamin K deficiency occurs beyond the first week of life, up to 6 months of age, and develops secondary to circumstances that compromise the supply or the absorption of vitamin K, such as malabsorption syndromes, antibiotic therapy of more than 7 days, or exclusive breast-feeding.

Prevention of these disorders is best provided by IM administration of 0.5 to 1.0 mg of vitamin K1 (phytonadione) or K2 (menaquinone) at birth, which some authors advise to repeat at 1 month of age in breast-fed infants. Avoid vitamin K3 (menadione), which can cause hemolytic anemia. Pregnant women on anticonvulsants should take 5 mg vitamin K per day orally during the last trimester .

Liver disease is a rare cause of coagulation factor deficiency in the newborn. Both acute (hepatitis) and chronic (cirrhosis) liver disease can seriously deplete coagulation factors. The major issue is lack of factor production, but there is also a poorly understood element of factor consumption of all coagulation factors manufactured in the liver, as well as platelets. The diathesis that results is profound and life-threatening. In acute hepatitis (viral or toxic), short-lived coagulation factors V and VII, with a half-life of 6 hours, translate their deficiencies into an initially long PT and fairly normal PTT. On days 2 to 3 and later, the longer-lived factors (IX, half-life 20 hours)

disappear, and the PTT becomes very prolonged. Fibrinogen, with its half-life of 3 to 4 days, is the last depleted. Factor VIII, synthesized by vascular endothelial cells, remains normal or even elevated. Therefore in the bleeding neonate, low levels of factors V, VII, and VIII imply DIC with consumption of coagulation factors; normal factor V and VIII with a low factor VII implies vitamin K deficiency; and low factors V and VII with a normal to elevated factor VIII level implies hepatocellular dysfunction.

Clinically, patients range from mildly ill, with certain forms of viral hepatitis, to deathly ill, in cases of fulminant hepatitis or terminal liver failure of cirrhotic patients. Besides the usual bleeding manifestations, patients may exhibit an orange skin rash due to the combination of dermatologic hemorrhages and jaundice.

Treatment should center on clotting factor replacement, mostly with FFP, but also with specific factors (factors IX, VII, and platelets) as indicated. The use of multiple factor complexes is controversial because they may lead to sudden DIC. Extra vitamin K, although not always helpful, may be administered. Acute bleeding must be managed with factor replacement, because the effect of vitamin K will not be seen for 12 to 18 hours. DDAVP (vasopressin), at 0.3 μg/kg/dose IV, may help neonates who exhibit a prolonged bleeding time.

References

1. Bick R. Disseminated intravascular coagulation and related syndromes: clinical review. *Semin Thromb Hemost* 1988;14:299.
2. Antonarakis SE, Rossiter JP, Young M, et al. Factor VIII gene inversions in severe hemophilia A: results of an international consortium study. *Blood* 1995;86:2206–2212.
3. Aperin J. Coagulopathy caused by vitamin K deficiency in critically ill hospitalized patients. *JAMA* 1987;258:1916.

Suggested Readings

Goodnight SH, Hathaway WE. *Disorders of hemostasis and thrombosis: a clinical guide.* 2nd ed. New York: McGraw-Hill; 2001.
Nathan D, Orkin S, Look AT, et al. *Nathan and Oski's hematology of infancy and childhood.* 6th ed. Philadelphia: Saunders; 2003: chapters 36–45.

CHAPTER 111 ■ NEONATAL SEIZURES

KRISTINA L. SIMEONSSON AND KARIN M. HILLENBRAND

A seizure is defined as a paroxysmal disturbance of electrical function in the brain associated with altered neurologic function. By definition, neonatal seizures occur any time in the first month of life, though most present from 12 to 48 hours after birth. The neonatal brain is particularly susceptible to seizures; seizures are more common during the neonatal period than at any other time in life. The incidence of neonatal seizures is 0.2% to 0.5% in term infants and 15% to 20% in premature infants. Seizures in neonates present unique diagnostic and prognostic considerations. Prompt diagnosis and treatment are important to limit long-term morbidity.

Due to immaturity of the central nervous system, newborns rarely have generalized clonic seizures or the other well-defined seizure patterns seen in older children. Any paroxysmal alteration in neurologic function—whether behavioral, motor, or autonomic—may be a manifestation of seizures in the newborn. Seizure types specific to the newborn include subtle, tonic, clonic, and myoclonic seizures (Table 111.1). Subtle seizures are most common, especially in the premature infant, representing at least 75% of seizures in newborns. Persistent focal clonic seizure activity may be a clue to a focal cortical lesion, although it may also occur in association with a metabolic abnormality. Myoclonic seizures are rare in neonates, though myoclonic movements are common, especially in premature infants.

The majority of neonatal seizures are intermittent events rather than predictors of true epilepsy. Neonatal seizures are rarely idiopathic; they are a manifestation of a variety of anatomic, metabolic, or functional disorders of the neonatal brain. Most are caused by perinatal hypoxic–ischemic insult, intracranial hemorrhage, or intracranial infection. Other etiologies are listed in Tables 111.2 and 111.3.

Care must be taken to distinguish seizure activity from normal newborn behaviors. Jitteriness may be mistaken for clonic seizure activity. However, jitteriness can be provoked by tactile stimuli, and typically ceases when the limb is held in passive flexion. Jittery movements are usually symmetric, and do not involve the face or eyes, while clonic seizure activity is focal or multifocal, not necessarily symmetric, and may include facial twitching or eye deviation. Autonomic nervous system manifestations such as tachycardia and hypertension occur in association with seizures but not with jitteriness. Jittery movements occur in normal term newborns, but are seen with increased frequency in association with hypoxic encephalopathy, drug withdrawal, hypoglycemia, and hypocalcemia. The phenomenon decreases with age.

Myoclonic seizure activity should be differentiated from benign neonatal sleep myoclonus. Myoclonus occurs frequently during sleep in healthy neonates; it is typically synchronous, and may be unilateral or bilateral. Benign sleep myoclonus ceases when the infant is awakened. The electroencephalogram (EEG) should reveal a normal sleep background. The behavior resolves over several months.

Though apnea may be a manifestation of subtle seizure activity in the neonate, most neonatal apnea is not related to seizures and another etiology should be sought. Movement abnormalities that might be confused with tonic seizures include Sandifer syndrome and hyperekplexia. Sandifer syndrome is a characteristic tonic posturing seen in infants with gastroesophageal reflux. Hyperekplexia, also known as congenital stiff-man syndrome, is a rare familial disorder in which infants demonstrate an exaggerated startle reflex and sustained tonic spasms that may be associated with apnea, but are not believed to be epileptiform in nature. Treatment with clonazepam may control the episodes, which usually disappear by 2 years of age.

EVALUATION

The approach to neonatal seizures should be directed at establishing the etiology. The collection of historical data is one of the most important steps in this process. The history should begin with a description of the event, which should include noting the type of seizure activity as well as duration. The age of the newborn when seizure activity begins may provide important clues (Fig. 111.1).

A review of the prenatal and perinatal histories may provide important clues in the evaluation of neonatal seizures. Gestational age should be noted, as etiologies may differ between premature and term infants. A history of drug use during pregnancy should be investigated; seizures may occur during withdrawal from narcotic and sedative drugs or may be a clue to a cerebral infarction from cocaine use. Complications during labor and delivery may lead to a perinatal insult. Low Apgar scores and the need for resuscitation may indicate birth asphyxia. Occurrence of trauma at or after birth may result in an intracranial hemorrhage or contusion. Important elements of the family history include presence of inherited metabolic disorders, neurocutaneous disorders, or a history of seizures in the newborn period that later resolved.

Evaluation of the newborn with suspected seizures should include thorough general and neurologic examinations. Vital signs should be monitored, as alterations in heart rate, blood pressure, and respirations can occur with seizure activity. Fever or hypothermia may be a clue to systemic infection. Abnormal head circumference occurs in association with prenatal hypoxic injury, cerebral malformation, hydrocephalus, or intracranial hemorrhage. An unusual odor may be a clue to an inborn error of metabolism, and dysmorphic features may indicate a genetic syndrome. Characteristic skin lesions like café-au-lait spots, ash leaf spots, or a port wine stain may be clues to a neurocutaneous disorder. A detailed neurologic exam should be performed; tone, symmetry of neonatal reflexes, and level of alertness are particularly important.

TABLE 111.1

MANIFESTATIONS OF SEIZURES IN NEWBORNS

Type	Typical manifestations
Subtle	■ *Ocular*: eyelid fluttering, eye deviation, fixed stare, repetitive blinking ■ *Oral*: mouthing, lip smacking ■ *Motor*: pedaling, stepping, swimming ■ *Autonomic*: apnea, desaturation, tachycardia, hypertension
Tonic	■ *Focal*: sustained posturing of limbs, trunk, or neck; eye deviation ■ *Generalized*: decerebrate or decorticate posturing
Clonic	■ Repetitive, rhythmic jerking ■ Focal or multifocal; may migrate ■ Consciousness sustained
Myoclonic	■ Sudden flexor spasms ■ Focal, multifocal, or generalized

Initial laboratory analysis in the evaluation of neonatal seizures should include serum glucose, electrolytes, calcium, and magnesium. A complete blood count should be obtained; an abnormal white blood cell count may suggest infection, and anemia may be seen with intracranial hemorrhage. Analysis of cerebral spinal fluid (CSF) should be performed to rule out meningitis unless an obvious metabolic disturbance has already been identified and treated, and seizures have resolved. Blood in the CSF could indicate a traumatic tap or the presence of an intracranial hemorrhage. Additional cultures should be obtained as needed to confirm an infectious etiology. Studies for congenital viral infection should be done when there is a history of first-trimester maternal illness, and for infants with relevant physical abnormalities such as microcephaly, jaundice, rash, or hepatomegaly.

If seizure activity is persistent or recurrent, despite normal laboratory results, an inborn error of metabolism should be considered. In addition to serum glucose measurement, laboratory tests useful in the evaluation of an inborn error include serum pH, lactate, and ammonia. Further evaluation comprising measurement of serum amino acids and urine organic acids is directed by physical exam findings and abnormalities in the initial laboratory tests. A meconium toxicology screen should be considered if the history is suggestive of maternal drug use, or if another etiology has not been established. A karyotype may be helpful if congenital anomalies are present.

Neuroimaging can be performed using cranial ultrasound, computed tomography (CT), or magnetic resonance imaging (MRI). Ultrasound is useful as a first-line screening assessment because it can be performed easily at the bedside. Ultrasound can identify gross central nervous system (CNS) pathology as well as periventricular and intraventricular hemorrhages, but is of limited utility when diagnosing cerebral artery infarctions, subdural and subarachnoid hemorrhages, and cerebral malformations. If results from cranial ultrasound are normal and seizure activity continues, a head CT or MRI should be obtained. CT is especially useful in identifying acute hemorrhage and intracerebral calcifications, while MRI is superior at showing differentiation between white and gray matter. Diagnosis of CNS malformations such as schizencephaly and lissencephaly is best made with MRI.

EEG characteristics in newborns with seizures differ considerably from those seen in older infants and children. Postconceptual age and sleep state must be considered in interpretation of the EEG. Only one-third of neonates with seizures have simultaneous clinical and electrical manifestations; the EEG may be normal in infants who clearly have seizure activity, and it may show electrical seizure activity in neonates without clinical manifestations. The EEG is often normal with subtle sizures, but is more likely to be abnormal if the infant has eye manifestations during the seizure. The EEG is variable with tonic seizures, and may demonstrate characteristic high-frequency sharp waves and spikes. In infants with clonic seizures, the EEG is usually abnormal and correlates with the seizure activity. During myoclonic seizures the EEG itself is typically normal, but the background is often markedly abnormal.

The EEG in neonates with suspected seizure activity is rarely useful in identifying an etiology, but it can be useful in assessing adequacy of management and determining prognosis. The EEG can be used to monitor seizures in paralyzed infants, and may also help determine seizure treatment endpoint, though most neurologists aim for clinical control rather than electrical control. Continuous video EEG monitoring can aid in identifying ongoing seizure activity when electrographic seizures persist in the absence of clinical seizure activity. EEG findings may also be useful prognostically; while the ictal EEG pattern is not predictive of outcome, the interictal EEG may provide useful prognostic data, particularly in term infants.

MANAGEMENT

When treating neonatal seizures, the goals are rapid identification and treatment of any underlying disorder and control of ongoing seizures. For the actively seizing newborn, attention should be given to the basics of resuscitation. Prompt airway management and intravenous access are necessary because seizure activity can compromise respiratory function, alter perfusion, and may result in ongoing cerebral injury if prolonged or recurrent.

Hypoglycemia should be corrected promptly. Other specific treatments, such as calcium and magnesium, should be used as indicated to correct metabolic abnormalities. Broad-spectrum antibiotics should be administered if a bacterial infection is suspected; acyclovir is indicated if a herpes infection is suspected.

Phenobarbital is the most commonly used anticonvulsant medication in the treatment of neonatal seizures. A loading dose of 20 mg/kg should be administered intravenously; this can be followed by boluses of 5 mg/kg to a maximum total of 40 mg/kg. In the absence of intravenous access, phenobarbital can be administered intramuscularly; however, higher doses may be needed and effectiveness may be compromised by unpredictable absorption.

Fosphenytoin, the salt ester of phenytoin, is another option for treatment. Fosphenytoin is the preferred form, because it can be administered more rapidly and is soluble in glucose-containing solutions. The loading dose is 20 mg/kg, administered intravenously. Fosphenytoin can be given after the 40 mg/kg of phenobarbital if seizures are not yet controlled. It can also be used after the initial loading dose of phenobarbital if there is concern for respiratory depression, or if the infant has hypoxic–ischemic injury.

A benzodiazepine may be necessary for the acute treatment of neonatal seizures. Lorazepam is the most commonly used agent, with a recommended dose of 0.1 mg/kg, given intravenously. Diazepam is not recommended for neonates, because it may contain sodium benzoate and benzoic acid, which can displace bilirubin from protein-binding sites.

Newer anticonvulsants such as topiramate and zonisamide may be useful in the treatment of neonatal seizures if standard therapies are not effective. Decisions regarding their use should be made in consultation with a pediatric neurologist.

TABLE 111.2

ETIOLOGY OF NEONATAL SEIZURES

Etiology	Comments
HYPOXIA, ISCHEMIA	
Asphyxia	■ Seizures usually begin within 24 hours of birth.
Cerebral infarction	■ Risk is increased with cocaine use during pregnancy.
INTRACRANIAL INFECTION	
Bacterial meningitis	■ *E. coli* and group B streptococcus are the most common etiologic agents.
Viral infection	■ Herpes simplex virus is the most common viral etiology.
Congenital infection	■ Intracranial calcifications may be clues to infection with cytomegalovirus or toxoplasmosis.
INTRACRANIAL HEMORRHAGE	
Intraventricular	■ Intraventricular hemorrhage occurs most commonly in preterm infants.
Subdural	■ Risk factors include macrosomia, difficult delivery, and child abuse.
Subarachnoid	■ Subarachnoid bleeding may occur in association with vaginal delivery.
METABOLIC DISTURBANCES	
Hypoglycemia	■ Infants born to diabetic mothers and those who are small for gestation are at increased risk.
Hypocalcemia	■ Early onset is seen in low-birthweight infants and infants of diabetic mothers; later onset occurs with nutritional deficits or endocrinopathy.
Hypomagnesemia	■ This usually occurs in association with hypocalcemia.
Hypo- and hypernatremia	■ Abnormalities result most often from SIADH, dehydration, or inappropriate water intake.
Inborn error of metabolism (IEM)	■ Other symptoms include poor feeding and lethargy. Amino acid and organic acid abnormalities are the most common IEMs presenting with neonatal seizures.
Pyridoxine dependency	■ Persistent seizures refractory to anticonvulsants typically present soon after birth, but can also be present in utero.
BRAIN MALFORMATION	
Abnormal neuronal migration	■ The most frequent disorders include lissencephaly, pachygyria, and polymicrogyria.
NEUROCUTANEOUS DISORDERS	
Tuberous sclerosus	■ Characteristic skin pigment abnormalities are noted.
Neurofibromatosis	■ Seizures rarely present in the newborn period.
Sturge–Weber Syndrome	■ Affected infants have a hemifacial hemangioma and ipsilateral brain involvement. Seizures are unusual in the newborn period.
TOXINS	
Maternal drug use	■ Seizures can occur during neonatal withdrawal from narcotics and sedatives; cocaine use during pregnancy can result in cerebral infarction.
Injection of local anesthetic	■ Seizures may present in the delivery room; fixed, dilated pupils are a clue.

EPILEPSY SYNDROMES (see Table 111.3)

If seizures persist despite the administration of anticonvulsants, pyridoxine dependency may be the cause. Though rare, this autosomal recessive condition can be diagnosed by observing the cessation of seizures after pyridoxine is given and their recurrence when it is discontinued. Parenteral pyridoxine should be administered in an intensive-care setting because of the associated risk of hypotonia and apnea.

Treatment of neonatal seizures involves a difficult balance between the apparent benefit of stopping seizure activity and the known adverse effects of anticonvulsant medications. Important

TABLE 111.3

NEONATAL EPILEPSY SYNDROMES

Epilepsy type	Etiology	Description	Interictal EEG findings	Outcome
Benign familial neonatal seizures	Family history is positive; autosomal dominant inheritance	Seizures begin on the second or third day. Partial or generalized clonic seizures or myoclonic jerks may occur 15 to 20 times daily.	Normal	Seizures resolve spontaneously, usually in the first 6 months of life. Neurodevelopmental outcome is normal.
Benign idiopathic neonatal seizures ("fifth-day fits")	Unknown; acute zinc deficiency has been suggested	Multifocal clonic seizures begin on or around the fifth day in healthy term newborns. Seizures may occur 15 to 20 times in a day.	Normal	The majority have seizures less than 24 hours, and essentially all resolve within 2 weeks. Neurodevelopmental outcome is normal.
Early myoclonic encephalopathy	Multiple; most commonly inborn errors of metabolism	Onset may be in utero, or in the first weeks of life. Infants develop severe recurrent myoclonic and clonic seizures.	Characteristic burst-suppression pattern	Infants are severely neurologically impaired; many die during infancy.
Early infantile epileptic encephalopathy (Ohtahara syndrome)	Primarily associated with structural brain malformations	Onset is early in infancy. Infants develop severe recurrent tonic spasms.	Characteristic burst-suppression pattern	Progressive uncontrolled seizures with neurologic deterioration.

unanswered questions include the ideal duration of treatment, optimal drug dosing, and the benefit of eliminating all seizure activity, both electrical and clinical. Because there are potential adverse effects on brain development from anticonvulsant medications, efforts should be made to discontinue them whenever possible. Some factors that would support cessation of medication include normal physical exam, normal neuroimaging study, absence of recurrent seizures, and non-epileptiform EEG. Most neurologists recommend discontinuation of anticonvulsant drugs before discharge from the hospital, unless the infant continues to have an abnormal neurologic exam or ongoing seizures. Infants discharged on anticonvulsants should be

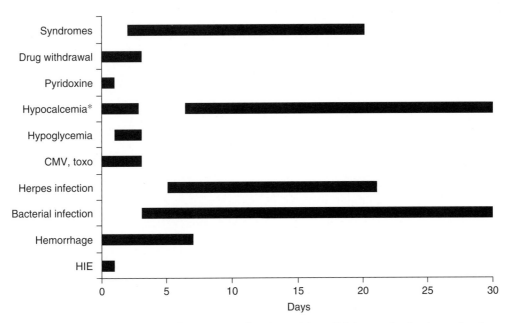

FIGURE 111.1. Typical timing of seizure onset, based on etiology. (* Seizures related to hypocalcemia may have an early or later onset, related to cause.)

reevaluated every few months to determine whether their anticonvulsant could be discontinued. Discharge planning issues include educating caregivers regarding recognition of seizure activity and basic first aid should a seizure occur. They should also be instructed on the proper dosing and administration of anticonvulsant medications. Discussion about prognosis and risk of seizure recurrence should take place before the day of discharge. Follow-up appointments with a primary care provider and a pediatric neurologist should be made; referral for early developmental intervention services may also be warranted.

COURSE AND PROGNOSIS

In many cases, neonatal seizures represent significant neurologic disease that can lead to major adverse outcomes. It is now recognized that neonatal seizures themselves can have a detrimental impact on the developing brain. Overall mortality in neonates with seizures is 15%, and adverse sequelae including mental retardation, cerebral palsy, and future seizures are noted in two-thirds of survivors. Up to 25% of neonates with seizures develop epilepsy.

Prognosis is related primarily to etiology of the seizure. Up to one-third of neonates with seizures related to hypoxic–ischemic encephalopathy die, and more than half of survivors have a handicap. Poor prognosis is also common for infants with cerebral dysgenesis and CNS infection. Other poor prognostic factors include very low birthweight and abnormal findings on neurologic exam. Prognosis is best for infants with familial neonatal seizures or transient metabolic abnormalities that are quickly recognized and treated. An abnormal interictal EEG pattern or abnormal sleep background is highly correlated with an increased risk of long-term sequelae, including epilepsy and poor neurodevelopmental outcome; conversely, a normal interictal EEG at term is associated with a normal neurodevelopmental outcome in 85%.

PEARLS

- The timing of seizure onset provides a useful clue to etiology. Seizures related to perinatal hypoxic–ischemic insult—the most common cause of neonatal seizures—usually present during the first 24 hours after birth.
- Unlike older children, neonates with persistent metabolic abnormalities like hypoglycemia or hypocalcemia tend to demonstrate intermittent seizure activity. A bedside glucose test and laboratory evaluation of electrolytes, calcium, and magnesium should be obtained in any neonate with seizures, even if the seizure has stopped.
- Anticonvulsant therapy for neonates is generally not tailored to seizure type, and begins with phenobarbital in almost every case.

Suggested Readings

Volpe JJ. Neonatal seizures. In: Volpe JJ, ed. *Neurology of the newborn.* 4th ed. Philadelphia: Saunders; 2001:178–214.
Zupanc ML. Neonatal seizures. *Pediatr Clin North Am* 2004;51:961–978.

CHAPTER 112 ■ BIRTH TRAUMA

KARIN M. HILLENBRAND

Birth trauma is defined as injury to the newborn resulting from mechanical forces during labor and delivery. Injury to the newborn is disturbing to parents, obstetricians, and pediatricians and carries the potential for long-term or permanent sequelae. The use of the term "birth trauma" should not imply that delivery has been inappropriately traumatic; in fact birth injury may occur during a difficult passage through the birth canal, may be related to obstetric manipulation of the fetus to assist delivery, or may occasionally occur in the face of an apparently normal and unassisted delivery. Many risk factors for birth trauma have been identified. Breech presentation carries the highest risk; additional risk factors are found in Table 112.1.

Improvements in prenatal care and diagnosis as well as in obstetrical management have resulted in significant reductions in birth injury. Nevertheless, traumatic injury occurs in 2% to 5% of all deliveries. Injuries can be grouped into those that involve the skin and soft tissues, injuries to the head and face, skeletal injuries, and injuries of the spine and nerves.

SKIN AND SOFT-TISSUE INJURIES

Petechiae and *ecchymoses* are common after birth and may relate to direct pressure or to increased intrathoracic pressure during passage through the birth canal. Absence of bleeding from other sites and lack of evolution of lesions over time differentiates this benign bleeding from bleeding associated with coagulation abnormalities or infection. Lesions typically resolve within 1 week. Infants with extensive bruising are at increased risk for hyperbilirubinemia.

Lacerations and abrasions may occur in association with scalp electrodes, forceps placement, contact with the maternal pelvis during passage through the birth canal, or occasionally, secondary to scalpel use during cesarean section. Most newborn lacerations and abrasions heal quickly without noticeable scarring. Full-thickness lacerations may require steri-strips or suturing. These injuries should be observed for signs of infection as they heal.

Subcutaneous fat necrosis results from ischemic injury to adipose tissue and is usually related to direct pressure. Lesions on the face are frequently associated with forceps application. Affected infants present in the first 2 weeks with irregularly shaped, firm, subcutaneous nodules that may have overlying red-purple discoloration. Common locations include cheeks, extremities, upper back, and buttocks. Lesions may become calcified and be visible on radiographs. Complete resolution is expected over 2 to 3 months.

INJURIES TO THE HEAD AND FACE

The most common head injuries related to birth trauma involve the various layers of the scalp (Fig. 112.1). Scalp injury occurs with increased frequency in association with forceps and particularly with vacuum-assisted deliveries. Other important injuries of the head and face include skull fractures, intracranial hemorrhage, eye injury, and facial fracture or dislocation.

Caput succedaneum, in which edema develops within the subcutaneous soft tissue of the newborn scalp, represents the most common scalp injury occurring at birth. On examination, a caput is usually found at the vertex; it feels soft and boggy, and the suture lines do not restrict extent. It may be associated with molding of the skull or with overlying bruising. The caput typically disappears within hours or days after delivery. In the case of a caput that seems unusually extensive or is increasing in size, subgaleal hemorrhage should be ruled out.

Subgaleal hemorrhage is an unusual but potentially life-threatening injury to the neonatal scalp. It almost always occurs as a sequela of vacuum extraction; overall occurrence in association with vacuum extraction is 0.6%. It may also occur as a complication of difficult delivery without the use of vacuum extraction; or rarely, it may be related to a coagulation disorder. In subgaleal hemorrhage, bleeding occurs beneath the galea aponeurosis and is therefore not restricted by periosteal attachment at suture lines. The hematoma may extend within the large potential space from the orbital ridges to the nape of the neck and laterally to the level of the ears. Clinically, infants present on the first day with a diffuse soft fluctuant mass over the calvarium, and this may continue to increase in size after birth. Affected infants may demonstrate signs of hypovolemia, and may develop a consumptive coagulopathy. Extent of the bleed can be characterized by CT scan, which can also be used to evaluate for suture diastasis, depressed skull fracture, and cortical hematoma.

Mortality is as high as 22%; therefore, early recognition and careful management is essential. Serial observation for fetal scalp changes and signs of hypovolemia should be done after all vacuum-assisted deliveries. Infants who develop subgaleal hemorrhage should be monitored for life-threatening complications including severe anemia, hypotension, coagulopathy, and secondary infection. Evaluation should include serial measurements of head circumference, blood pressure, hemoglobin and hematocrit, serum bilirubin, and coagulation studies. Affected infants may require intravenous volume support, treatment of coagulopathy or infection, and management of hyperbilirubinemia. The hematoma should not be aspirated or drained due to the risk of causing infection.

A *cephalhematoma* is a traumatic, subperiosteal hemorrhage of the newborn skull. It is a common injury, occurring in 1% to 3% of all deliveries, and is twice as common in boys as

RISK FACTORS ASSOCIATED WITH BIRTH TRAUMA

MATERNAL FACTORS
- Primiparity
- Small stature
- Pelvic abnormalities
- Oligohydramnios

FETAL FACTORS
- Very low birthweight
- Extreme prematurity
- Macrosomia
- Macrocephaly
- Anomalies

DELIVERY FACTORS
- Prolonged or rapid labor
- Use of forceps or vacuum
- Version with extraction

in girls. Incidence increases significantly in infants delivered by vacuum extraction or with the use of forceps. Bilateral cephalhematoma occurs in 15% of cases, and skull fracture is associated in 5% to 10%. On examination, a cephalhematoma is a firm, well-defined mass most often found in the parietal region. Because it is subperiosteal, the extent of bleeding is limited by attachment of the periosteum to the bone at suture lines. It may be difficult to distinguish a cephalhematoma from an overlying caput until the third or fourth postpartum day. Midoccipital cephalhematoma is rare and should raise the question of an encephalocele. Unlike an encephalocele, a cephalhematoma does not transilluminate, will not vary in size with crying or straining, and is not pulsatile. Diagnosis can be further clarified with ultrasound.

A cephalhematoma requires no specific treatment, although infants are at increased risk for hyperbilirubinemia. The subperiosteal blood is typically reabsorbed by 2 to 8 weeks after delivery. Abscess formation within the hematoma is rare, but may occur in relation to a fetal scalp electrode and is more common if aspiration is undertaken. Aspiration is indicated only for hematomas that are increasing in size and have associated erythema or other signs of infection.

Clinically significant *skull fractures* are quite rare. Skull fractures are most often parietal in location and linear in type. They may occur in association with an overlying cephalhematoma and probably occur more often than is recognized. Routine skull radiographs are not indicated. For infants with significant head injury, head CT is the preferred study. Linear, nondisplaced fractures are benign and heal without intervention. For depressed skull fractures, neurosurgical elevation has been the traditional approach. However, recent reports suggest that in some circumstances the newborn skull will remodel well without any intervention, and that nonsurgical approaches such as digital pressure or vacuum elevation may be successful in other cases. Leptomeningeal herniation through a dural tear is a rare late complication of neonatal skull fracture.

Intracranial hemorrhage (ICH) is uncommon and ranges from minor bleeding that may be clinically unrecognized to major, potentially fatal blood loss. Epidural and subdural hemorrhages are virtually always related to trauma; subarachnoid, intraventricular, and intraparenchymal hemorrhages may occur secondary to trauma or in relation to asphyxia, prematurity, hemorrhagic diathesis, infection, or vascular abnormalities. Infants may present with seizures, apnea, bulging fontanel, or other neurologic abnormalities resulting from irritation by subarachnoid or intraparenchymal blood, or from focal hematoma in subdural or epidural locations. Imaging with CT scan is indicated in infants with a difficult delivery associated with neurologic signs; ultrasound is inadequate for identifying ICH and parenchymal injury. Observation, with treatment of associated symptoms such as seizures, is appropriate for most infants with ICH. Surgical intervention is indicated for signs of acute brainstem compression or hydrocephalus. Most infants with subarachnoid hemorrhage recover fully; prognosis is less favorable for infants with epidural or subdural bleeds. Sequelae can include hydrocephalus, seizures, and developmental abnormalities.

Subconjunctival hemorrhages occur commonly after normal vaginal delivery and resolve spontaneously without sequelae. *Retinal hemorrhage* can occur in association with all types of delivery, although occurrence is highest with vacuum extraction and lowest with caesarean delivery. Most retinal hemorrhages are mild and resolve within days to weeks without sequelae. More significant eye injuries—including vitreous hemorrhage, corneal laceration, hyphema, and orbital fracture—are most often related to direct trauma from obstetrical instruments. An ophthalmologist should evaluate any significant eye injury.

Facial bone and cartilage injuries may present with facial asymmetry, respiratory distress, or feeding difficulty. Nasal septal dislocation is the most common facial injury and presents with asymmetry of the nares with visible septal deviation when the nasal tip is positioned centrally. Facial injuries require otorhinolaryngology evaluation and intervention in the early newborn period.

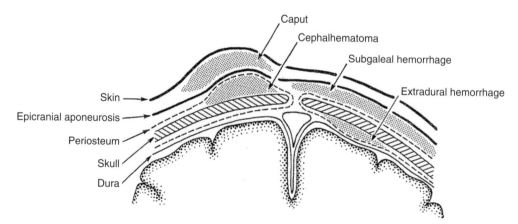

FIGURE 112.1. Sites of scalp injury and hemorrhage. (From Injuries of extracranial, cranial, intracranial, spinal cord, and peripheral nervous system structures. In: Volpe JJ, ed. *Neurology of the newborn.* 4th ed. Philadelphia: Saunders; 2001: 814, with permission.)

SKELETAL INJURIES

Clavicle fracture is the most common bone injury related to delivery, occurring in approximately 0.5% of live births. Risk is significantly increased with fetal macrosomia, with an incidence as high as 18% in vaginally delivered infants weighing more than 4,500 grams. Clavicle fracture is also more common with shoulder dystocia or breech presentation. On physical examination, there may be a visible deformity, asymmetric Moro reflex, decreased arm movement, an overlying hematoma, or pain and crepitus with palpation of the clavicle. The affected infant should be carefully assessed for a brachial plexus injury, which occurs in about 10% of infants with a clavicle fracture. If the diagnosis is uncertain after physical examination, it can be confirmed by plain radiograph or ultrasound. If the clavicle fracture is an isolated injury, it can be expected to heal without specific intervention and without long-term sequelae. Healing occurs within 7 to 10 days with formation of a visible and palpable callus that parents should be counseled to anticipate. Immobilization of the arm or shoulder is unnecessary, but parents should be instructed to handle the infant gently and limit motion of the arm and shoulder on the affected side. During healing, the infant should be positioned or bundled with the arm adducted, elbow flexed, and the forearm supinated to allow the hand to rest near the infant's face.

Humerus fracture may occur in relation to shoulder dystocia or breech presentation, or following an apparently normal delivery. Infants should be evaluated for associated brachial plexus palsy. *Fracture of the femur* is uncommon. This injury may occur with breech delivery or other difficult extraction, but may also occur during an apparently normal delivery. The infant presents with swelling or deformity of the thigh. Varying degrees of immobilization, splinting, and casting have been used for humerus and femur fractures; prognosis is excellent for uncomplicated healing within several weeks.

INJURIES OF THE SPINE AND NERVES

Spinal cord injury is a rare but devastating consequence of birth trauma. Two types of injury are described: upper cervical injury usually occurs with cephalic delivery involving extreme rotation, while lower cervical and upper thoracic injury is more likely to occur in association with breech delivery where there is hyperextension or significant traction on the head. Injury or dislocation of the vertebral bodies is unusual; the cord injury results from meningeal damage with epidural hemorrhage, laceration or avulsion of the spinal roots, or laceration or transection of the cord itself. Incidence is increased in association with intrauterine malposition (especially breech), difficult extraction, and use of forceps.

Clinically, infants may demonstrate symptoms of associated perinatal asphyxia, generalized hypotonia, absent deep-tendon reflexes, respiratory distress or apnea, and bladder distension from urinary retention. Detection of a sensory level helps to distinguish this injury from neuromuscular disorders. Ultrasound is useful as an initial imaging modality in defining the location and extent of the injury because it can be done at the bedside. Magnetic resonance imaging can be used in stable infants to further characterize the injury. Prognosis is poor, particularly if the infant lacks spontaneous respiratory function by 24 hours. Operative intervention for newborn spinal cord injury is rarely effective.

Facial nerve injury is the most common cranial nerve sequela of delivery. Forceps-assisted delivery is a risk factor, but the injury frequently occurs following an apparently uncomplicated delivery as a result of compression of the facial nerve against the maternal pelvis or fetal shoulder. Clinically, unilateral upper and lower facial weakness is noted at birth; this is most obvious when the infant cries, at which time incomplete eyelid closure is more evident, and the mouth is drawn away from the affected side. Prognosis for recovery is good, with some improvement noted within a week in most cases. During recovery, the eye should be kept lubricated. If improvement is not noticed within several weeks, referral to a neurologist is warranted.

The differential diagnosis for facial nerve injury includes the Moebius sequence, which is typically bilateral and results from congenital hypoplasia or destruction of cranial nerves six and seven. Facial nerve paralysis should also be differentiated from the asymmetric crying facies syndrome, which is the result of congenital hypoplasia or absence of the depressor anguli oris muscle, whose normal function is to draw the lower corner of the lip downward and evert it. Palpation of the thickness of the muscles lateral to the angle of the lip on either side may reveal asymmetry, suggesting this disorder. The cosmetic significance of asymmetric crying facies syndrome lessens with age; its clinical importance relates more to an associated increased likelihood of congenital heart disease, as well as other congenital anomalies.

Injury to the phrenic nerve typically occurs in association with brachial plexus injury but is occasionally an isolated finding. Phrenic nerve injury results in ipsilateral hemidiaphragmatic paralysis, with physical findings of respiratory distress and decreased movement of the hemithorax on the affected side. Although routine radiographs may reveal elevation of the affected hemidiaphragm, diaphragmatic paralysis is best evaluated using fluoroscopy or real-time ultrasound. For injuries that do not spontaneously improve, diaphragmatic plication or phrenic nerve pacing can be considered.

Brachial plexus palsy is the most common peripheral nerve injury associated with delivery, occurring in 0.1% to 0.2% of live births. Brachial plexus palsy can occur as an in utero insult, but it is most often the result of injury during delivery and is related to excessive lateral flexion or hyperextension of the neck. Associated risk factors include prolonged gestation, prolonged labor, augmented labor, fetal depression, macrosomia, shoulder dystocia, use of forceps, and breech delivery. The injury occurs in more than 5% of vaginally delivered infants with birthweight above 4,500 grams, and affects up to 10% of infants with shoulder dystocia. In most cases of brachial plexus injury, the plexus is compressed by hemorrhage and edema within the nerve sheath. Less often, an actual tear of the nerves or avulsion of the roots occurs. When related to obstetrical forces, a clavicular fracture and, less often, a humeral fracture may be associated. Causes of brachial plexus palsy unrelated to delivery include intrauterine compression, humeral osteomyelitis, hemangioma, exostosis of the first rib, neck compression, and neoplasm.

The differential diagnosis for brachial plexus injury includes fracture of the clavicle or humerus, shoulder dislocation, proximal humeral epiphyseal separation, septic arthritis, and osteomyelitis; in these situations, there is decreased motion of the upper extremity due to pain. The examiner may note the infant grimacing during attempts at passive range of motion, as well as the absence of the typical posture associated with brachial plexus palsy. In infants with bilateral upper extremity paralysis, urinary retention, or associated lower extremity weakness, a cervical spinal cord injury should be ruled out.

Injury to the brachial plexus results in varying degrees of upper-extremity paralysis. The extent of injury to the brachial plexus is best determined by careful physical examination. Clinically, an infant with brachial plexus injury may demonstrate varying degrees of abnormal tone, movement, posture, and sensation of the affected limb (Table 112.2). The injury is unilateral in 90% of cases and is twice as common on the right

TABLE 112.2

FUNCTIONS OF THE BRACHIAL PLEXUS

Nerve root	Motor	Reflex
C 5,6	Shoulder external rotation, abduction Elbow flexion Forearm supination Wrist extension	Biceps
C 7,8	Shoulder internal rotation, adduction Elbow extension Forearm pronation Wrist flexion	Triceps
C8, T1	Finger abduction, adduction	Grasp

side. Brachial plexus injuries are divided into types, depending on which portion of the plexus is involved.

- Erb–Duchenne palsy (upper plexus palsy: C5, C6, and sometimes C7) accounts for 80% to 90% of brachial plexus injuries. On examination, the arm is limp, and is internally rotated in adduction with the elbow extended, the forearm pronated, and the wrist flexed, resulting in a position described as the "Waiter's tip" posture. In a pure Erb–Duchenne palsy, the palmar grasp reflex is not affected and sensory deficit is insignificant. The Moro reflex is asymmetric, and the biceps tendon reflex is depressed or absent. In approximately 5% of cases, an associated injury of C4 fibers results in phrenic nerve palsy.
- Klumpke palsy (lower plexus palsy: C7, C8, and T1) is the least common presentation, constituting 1% or less of all brachial plexus injuries. It primarily affects the small muscles of the hand and wrist. The infant presents with flexed elbow, supinated forearm, extended wrist, and "claw" hand due to weakness of the intrinsic muscles of the hand. The triceps reflex is depressed, and palmar grip is weak or absent. There is decreased sensation over the palmar surface. An associated Horner syndrome, with ptosis and miosis on the ipsilateral side, indicates injury to the sympathetic fibers that accompany the first thoracic nerve.
- Erb–Duchenne–Klumpke palsy (complete plexus palsy: C5–T1) involves fibers from all spinal segments and results in a limb that is flaccid and motionless. Tendon reflexes, Moro reflex, and palmar grasp are absent, and sensory deficit is extensive. A Horner syndrome may be associated.

Management of an infant with a brachial plexus injury should begin with radiographic evaluation for associated injuries, which might include clavicle fracture, humerus fracture, rib fracture, or dislocation of the elbow or shoulder. Subsequent management initially focuses on preventing contractures and preserving integrity while awaiting recovery. Many authors advocate rest for the first week due to the likelihood of associated pain; the infant should be swaddled with the elbow flexed so that the hand lies near the face. This period of rest should be followed by passive range-of-motion exercises of the wrist, elbow, and shoulder to maintain joint integrity. Pediatric rehabilitation physicians, neurologists, and occupational and physical therapists are helpful in assessing the extent of injury and planning and monitoring rehabilitation. Referral to these specialists is warranted for infants with any persistent abnormality after 2 weeks.

For infants with persistent significant paralysis after an initial period of observation, microsurgical repair can be considered. The primary goal of surgical repair is to obtain reasonable hand function, improved elbow motion, and shoulder stability. Microsurgical repair is more often associated with a favorable outcome when undertaken in the first year of life. As microsurgical techniques and successes improve, earlier repair has been advocated by some. Although controlled prospective studies of outcomes are not available in the literature, evaluation for possible operative intervention is appropriate for infants who continue to have significant impairment after 3 months of age.

Most brachial plexus injuries are mild and transient. Approximately 80% to 90% of infants with Erb–Duchenne palsy recover by 3 months. Permanent sequelae are more likely for infants with lacerated rather than stretched nerve roots, complete plexus or Klumpke palsy, and paralysis related to in-utero compression or malformation rather than to traction at delivery. Return of some function within the first 2 weeks suggests a good prognosis. Full recovery is unlikely if no improvement is seen by the end of the second week. Outcome following microneurosurgical repair is variable and relates to degree of injury, timing of surgery, and whether nerves were intact or avulsed.

PEARLS

- Although risk factors for birth injury are well described, many birth injuries are both unpredictable and unavoidable. Injury at birth does not necessarily imply iatrogenic trauma; some injuries are already present in utero, while others result following apparently uncomplicated and unassisted deliveries.
- Most birth injuries are self-limited, and recovery often occurs without intervention. Serious birth injuries include subgaleal hemorrhage, spinal cord injury, and complete brachial plexus injury.

Suggested Readings

Piatt JH. Birth injuries of the brachial plexus. *Pediatr Clin North Am* 2004;51: 421–440.

Uhing MR. Management of birth injuries. *Pediatr Clin North Am* 2004;51: 1169–1186.

Volpe JJ. Injuries of extracranial, cranial, intracranial, spinal cord, and peripheral nervous system structures. In: Volpe JJ, ed. *Neurology of the newborn.* 4th ed. Philadelphia: Saunders; 2001: 813–838.

CHAPTER 113 ■ DELAYED ONSET OF VOIDING

JOHN M. OLSSON

Initiation of normal urination by the newborn is one sign of well-being and usually reflects adequate hydration and oral intake. Regardless of gestational age, approximately 92% of newborn infants have their first void by 24 hours and 99% do so by 48 hours.

Decreased urine output in the newborn should be approached in the same manner as in older children: consider prerenal, renal, and postrenal etiologies. The differential diagnosis of delayed voiding includes both fetal and maternal considerations (Table 113.1).

CLINICAL FINDINGS

Perinatal and maternal history should be reviewed for oligohydramnios, asphyxia, familial renal disorders, intrapartum medications (e.g., vasodilators, pancuronium bromide, barbiturates), and risk factors for infection.

The physical examination should determine the state of hydration, the presence of cardiovascular disease (causing renal hypoperfusion or systemic hypotension), or systemic hypertension (suggesting intrinsic renal disease). The presence of an abdominal mass or abnormalities of the spine may suggest the possibility of malformation of the urinary tract; similarly palpating a distended bladder may signal bladder outlet obstruction.

MANAGEMENT

Generally, consider obtaining relevant history and performing a thorough physical examination on any newborn who has not voided within the first 24 hours. A more extensive evaluation, including bladder catheterization and diagnostic studies, should be strongly considered in the newborn who has not voided by 48 hours.

Bladder catheterization will determine if there is bladder outlet obstruction as opposed to renal dysfunction or upper urinary tract obstruction. Anatomic abnormalities of the kidney can be assessed by use of renal ultrasound. Vascular problems of the kidneys can be evaluated with a renal scan. A voiding cystourethrogram is indicated if bladder outlet obstruction or vesicoureteral reflux is suspected. Creatinine (Cr), blood urea nitrogen (BUN), and serum and urine electrolytes and osmolality can help differentiate prerenal, renal, and postrenal causes of decreased urine output. Calculation of the fractional excretion of sodium may help differentiate prerenal from intrinsic renal failure. The fractional excretion of sodium is less than 3% in prerenal oliguria and greater than 3% in intrinsic renal failure. A BUN:Cr ratio greater than 30 may be seen in prerenal oliguria; whereas a ratio less than 20 is seen with intrinsic renal etiologies. However, BUN and Cr values early in the newborn period may reflect maternal renal function to a greater extent than newborn renal function, thus limiting the usefulness of the BUN:Cr ratio.

$$\text{FeNa (\%)} = \text{Na clearance/Cr clearance} \times 100$$
$$= \{[U_{Na} \times P_{Cr}] \div [P_{Na} \times U_{Cr}]\} \times 100$$

If prerenal oliguria is suspected (from clinical and laboratory evaluation), a fluid bolus of 20 mL/kg of normal saline given over 1 to 2 hours should produce urine output. If this is not successful, the fluid bolus should be repeated, followed by a dose of IV furosemide 1 mg/kg. After confirmation by appropriate diagnostic study, intrinsic renal disease should be managed with fluid restriction and consultation with a pediatric nephrologist.

Postrenal etiologies include obstructive uropathies and should be managed by bladder catheterization and consultation with a pediatric urologist.

COURSE AND PROGNOSIS

Based on the cause of the decreased urine output, the course and prognosis vary. In prerenal and postrenal oliguria, normal urine output is restored after normal renal perfusion has been

TABLE 113.1

DIFFERENTIAL DIAGNOSIS OF DELAYED ONSET OF VOIDING

Category	Diagnosis
Idiopathic pre-renal	Maternal medications
	Nonsteroidal anti-inflammatory drugs
	Angiotension-converting enzyme inhibitors
	Pancuronium
	Barbiturates
	Twin–twin transfusion
	Asphyxia
	Dehydration
	Sepsis
	Heart failure
	Hypotension
Renal	Renal agenesis
	Renal dysplasia/hypoplasia
	Multicystic dysplasia
	Polycystic kidneys
	Renal vein thrombosis
Post-renal	Obstructive neuropathies

established in the former and after relief of the obstruction in the latter. The course and prognosis for renal etiologies of decreased urine output depend on the diagnosis.

- Delayed voiding is more commonly missed voiding; careful review of the delivery room records and discussion with the parents often accounts for the "missing urine."

PEARLS

- Although unusual, newborn infants can present with dehydration, often as a result of cord compression, premature separation of the placenta, or maternal hypovolemia.

Suggested Readings

Clark DA. Time of first void and first stool in 500 newborns. *Pediatrics* 1977; 60:457.
Vega-Rich CR. Newborn: first stool and urine. *Pediatr Rev* 1994;15:319.

CHAPTER 114 ■ DELAYED MECONIUM STOOL

JOHN M. OLSSON

Passage of initial meconium stool within 24 hours of birth is a sign of healthy newborn transition to extrauterine life. In general, approximately 60% of healthy term newborns stool in the first 8 hours of life, 91% do so by 16 hours, almost 99% by 24 hours, and virtually all by 48 hours. Breast-fed infants tend to pass their first stool later than formula-fed infants. Gut motility is decreased in preterm newborns, and delay in passage of the first meconium stool beyond 24 hours may be seen in as many as 25% of these infants. However, like term newborns, almost all premature infants have passed their first meconium stool by 48 hours.

Conditions associated with delayed passage of the first meconium stool include the various causes of lower intestinal obstruction, as well as sepsis, hypothyroidism, and maternal drugs (Table 114.1).

CLINICAL FINDINGS

Maternal history should be reviewed for perinatal administration of medications, including magnesium sulfate and narcotics. Perinatal history should be reviewed carefully for evidence of

TABLE 114.1

DIFFERENTIAL DIAGNOSIS FOR DELAYED PASSAGE OF MECONIUM

Cause	
Idiopathic	Sepsis
Prematurity	Hypothyroidism
Lower intestinal obstruction	Maternal drugs
Meconium plug syndrome	Magnesium sulfate
Hirschsprung disease	Narcotics
Imperforate anus/anal atresia	

meconium-stained amniotic fluid or passage of meconium in the delivery room. The delivery staff sometimes overlook or fail to document these events.

Physical examination should focus on the abdomen and perineum. Evaluation of the abdomen for distension or bladder enlargement and the perineum for the presence, patency, and location of the anus are important. Forceful passage of meconium after a rectal examination should make one suspicious of Hirschsprung disease.

If intestinal obstruction is suspected, a flat plate and prone lateral radiographs of the abdomen may be obtained to look for focal distension of the bowel, air–fluid levels, and air in the rectum (which should be present by 24 hours after birth).

MANAGEMENT

An infant who has not passed meconium within the first 24 hours should be evaluated. Maternal history, physical examination, and radiologic studies should be reviewed as outlined above. Management is dictated by the diagnosis and can vary from watchful waiting to surgical intervention.

COURSE AND PROGNOSIS

The course and prognosis for specific diagnostic etiologies depend on the identity of those conditions and will not be covered here. Most of these newborns will successfully pass meconium stool by 48 hours without further intervention.

Suggested Readings

Clark DA. Time of first void and first stool in 500 newborns. *Pediatrics* 1977; 60:457.
Vega-Rich CR. Newborn: First stool and urine. *Pediatr Rev* 1994;15:319.
Verma A, Dhanireddy R. Time of first stool in extremely low birthweight (≤1,000 g) infants. *J Pediatr* 1993;122:626.

CHAPTER 115 ■ NEWBORN RESPIRATORY DISTRESS

KRISTINA L. SIMEONSSON

Respiratory distress is a common problem encountered by the practitioner who cares for newborns. It may present immediately in the delivery room or develop over several hours or days. A systematic approach to the evaluation of respiratory distress will aid the newborn provider in making an accurate diagnosis and correctly managing the problem.

Respiratory distress in the newborn is defined by the presence of one or more of the following: tachypnea, retractions, nasal flaring, grunting, and cyanosis. Although these clinical findings often occur in combination, a thorough evaluation should be undertaken if any of these signs are present. For example, the infant with congenital heart disease may manifest significant cyanosis with minimal tachypnea and no retractions, or a newborn with pneumonia may be acyanotic but display severe retractions and tachypnea.

Pulmonary disorders are the most common cause of respiratory distress; however, the differential diagnosis is lengthy and includes extrapulmonary disorders. Congenital anomalies of the airway and diaphragm can lead to respiratory distress; in addition, cardiovascular, metabolic, and neurologic disorders can have respiratory manifestations in the newborn. Table 115.1 provides a differential diagnosis of respiratory distress in term newborns. Respiratory disorders are a leading cause of morbidity and mortality in preterm infants, but review of these diseases is beyond the scope of this chapter.

CLINICAL FINDINGS

A review of the history is an important part of the assessment. The obstetrical record should be reviewed, with particular attention to the prenatal and perinatal histories. Results of prenatal ultrasounds should be reviewed for the presence of congenital anomalies (e.g., heart defects) and other problems (e.g., oligohydramnios or polyhydramnios). The type of delivery and complications associated with delivery, such as meconium-stained fluid or traumatic delivery resulting in a birth injury, may point to the diagnosis. Administration of narcotics to the mother during labor and delivery can affect the infant's ability to establish and maintain adequate respirations. Maternal factors, such as the presence of prolonged rupture of membranes, fever, or chorioamnionitis, may offer clues to an infectious etiology for the newborn's respiratory distress. Colonization of the mother's urogenital tract with group B streptococcus increases the risk of pneumonia or sepsis in the newborn.

Knowing the infant's gestational age should help to eliminate certain diagnoses: respiratory distress syndrome (RDS, also known as hyaline membrane disease) is the most common cause of respiratory distress in the preterm neonate, but occurrence in newborns over 37 weeks gestation is rare. The age at onset of symptoms also aids in the diagnosis. Respiratory symptoms that develop in the delivery room are more likely to be from congenital anomalies of the airway or lungs or from meconium aspiration. Symptoms that develop over the course of hours to days are more characteristic of infection and congenital heart disease. Congenital lobar emphysema, a very uncommon cause of respiratory distress, has a gradual onset over 2 to 3 weeks. Onset of symptoms after a feed may be secondary to aspiration, with several possible underlying etiologies.

The physical examination should include all major organ systems so as not to miss an extrapulmonary cause. Vital signs, including blood pressure, should be noted. Temperature instability, either hyperthermia or hypothermia, can indicate an infection. Tachypnea in the newborn is defined as a respiratory rate greater than 60 breaths per minute. The infant's gestational age should be assessed by physical maturity characteristics. Dysmorphic features should be identified; for example, micrognathia seen in the Pierre–Robin sequence can cause problems with upper airway obstruction. Several genetic sequences and syndromes can be associated with bilateral choanal atresia, which can be diagnosed by the inability to pass a suction catheter through the nares. Neck masses, such as a goiter, can result in compression of the airway.

The pulmonary examination should begin with observation, and respiratory rate should be counted for a full minute, given the wide fluctuations in rate depending on the infant's arousal state. Nasal flaring may be present. Subcostal, intercostal, and substernal retractions should be noted, as well as asymmetry of chest wall movement. Stridor could indicate an airway obstruction. Auscultation of the chest should focus not only on abnormal breath sounds but also on unilaterally diminished or absent breath sounds. Transillumination of the chest can be attempted if pneumothorax is suspected, although this technique may not be positive in the term newborn. If suspicion remains, a chest radiograph should be performed. Displaced or muffled heart sounds may also raise suspicion of a pneumothorax. Presence of a hyperdynamic precordium or a murmur may indicate congenital heart disease. Decreased or absent femoral pulses point to a coarctation of the aorta, which should be accompanied by a difference of at least 10 mm Hg in the systolic blood pressure of the upper versus the lower extremities. Peripheral perfusion should be noted, because poor perfusion can be a sign of congenital heart disease or sepsis. On abdominal examination, hepatomegaly could indicate heart failure or an inborn error of metabolism. A scaphoid abdomen might be a clue to a diaphragmatic hernia. The neurologic exam should focus on the infant's tone; hypotonia or hypertonia can provide additional clues to the etiology of respiratory distress. Examination of the skin

TABLE 115.1

DIFFERENTIAL DIAGNOSIS FOR NEWBORN RESPIRATORY DISTRESS

Respiratory causes		
Pulmonary/Parenchymal	**Upper airway**	**Chest abnormalities**
Hyaline membrane disease	Choanal atresia	Rib deformities
Transient tachypnea of the newborn	Pierre–Robin sequence	Rib fractures
Meconium aspiration syndrome	Laryngeal obstruction	Congenital diaphragmatic hernia
Air leak syndromes	Mass	
Pneumothorax	Web	
Pneumomediastinum	Vocal cord paralysis	
Pneumopericardium	Laryngomalacia	
Pulmonary interstitial emphysema	Tracheal obstruction	
Hypoplasia	Tracheomalacia	
Pulmonary hemorrhage	Goiter	
Chylothorax	Cystic hygroma	
Aspiration pneumonia	Vascular ring	

Nonrespiratory causes			
Cardiovascular/Hematologic	**Metabolic**	**Neurologic/Muscular**	**Infectious**
Congenital heart disease	Hypoglycemia	Intracranial hemorrhage	Sepsis
Persistent pulmonary hypertension	Acidosis	Asphyxia	Pneumonia
Hypovolemia	Hypothermia	Medications (e.g., narcotics)	Meningitis
Polycythemia	Hyperthermia	Phrenic nerve damage	
Anemia	Inborn errors of metabolism	Spinal cord injury	
		Muscular disorders	
		(e.g., neonatal myasthenia)	

should focus on the presence of cyanosis, pallor, or mottling. If cyanosis is present, it is important to distinguish between peripheral and central cyanosis. Central cyanosis affects the entire body, including the tongue and mucous membranes. Peripheral cyanosis, also known as acrocyanosis, is limited to the extremities. Peripheral cyanosis may be benign and self-limited. For example, an infant exposed to a cold environment may display peripheral cyanosis. The newborn practitioner should not dismiss peripheral cyanosis as a benign process, however, until other more serious conditions are ruled out.

A radiograph of the chest is the most useful diagnostic test in evaluating the neonate with respiratory distress. Disorders such as transient tachypnea of the newborn, pneumothorax, and meconium aspiration have distinct radiographic findings. The diagnosis of pneumonia and meconium aspiration can be supported by the presence of patchy infiltrates. The heart size and shape, as well as the pattern of pulmonary vasculature, should be noted, because abnormal findings may suggest congenital heart disease or persistent pulmonary hypertension. Reviewing the radiograph for fractures of the ribs and clavicles is important, especially if the infant had a difficult delivery.

Initial blood work should include a complete blood count to evaluate for sepsis and anemia. If an infectious etiology is the likely cause of the respiratory distress, a blood culture should be obtained. Based on other clinical findings, cultures of the urine, cerebrospinal fluid, and trachea may be warranted. Arterial blood gases are useful for assessing the degree of respiratory compromise, as well as for monitoring the disease process. A blood glucose level should be determined because hypoglycemia is an easily correctable cause of respiratory distress.

MANAGEMENT

Any infant in respiratory distress should be placed on cardiopulmonary monitors, including pulse oximetry. An infant in moderate or severe respiraory distress should be made NPO and intravenous fluids should be administered. Thermoregulatory control should be maintained in an isolette or radiant warmer. If hypoxemia is present, oxygen should be administered unless cyanotic heart disease is highly likely. Infants who do not respond to 100% oxygen most likely have a congenital anomaly of the heart or lung. These infants are best managed at a tertiary care center with neonatal intensive care and pediatric subspecialty services.

Intubation and mechanical ventilation may be necessary if the infant is in severe respiratory distress. A pH less than 7.20 or PCO_2 greater than 60 indicate the need for mechanical ventilator support for infants with acute respiratory distress. Some conditions may warrant intubation for stabilization (e.g., diaphragmatic hernia) or insertion of an oral airway (e.g., Pierre–Robin sequence).

In infants with more than minimal distress, placement of an umbilical artery catheter should be considered to allow serial monitoring of blood gas values. If hypovolemia is present, circulatory support should be maintained with the use of fluid resuscitation and pressor support. Additional management and evaluation may be necessary, depending on clinical findings and involvement of other organ systems. Antibiotics should be given for suspected bacterial infection; ampicillin plus an aminoglycoside are the broad-spectrum antibiotics of choice for newborn sepsis and pneumonia. Echocardiogram and ECG may be necessary to evaluate suspected congenital heart defects.

COURSE AND PROGNOSIS

The outcome of respiratory distress in the term newborn is highly dependent on the cause of distress. For example, transient tachypnea of the newborn is a benign, self-limited condition that resolves within 1 to 3 days. Disorders such as meconium aspiration syndrome and persistent pulmonary hypertension carry higher mortality and, often, related CNS sequelae.

A low PaO_2 while breathing high O_2, in the infant with an accompanying respiratory acidosis, usually indicates severe pulmonary disease; thus it is important to transfer the infant early if oxygen requirements are increasing or respiratory distress is not improving. Most surgical conditions, such as diaphragmatic hernia, are associated with good outcomes if the diagnosis is made early and surgical correction can take place before secondary complications occur.

Suggested Readings

Aly H. Respiratory disorders in the newborn: identification and diagnosis. *Pediatr Rev* 2004;25:201–208.

Sasidharam P. An approach to diagnosis and management of cyanosis and tachypnea in term infants. *Pediatr Clin North Am* 2004;51:999–1021.

Tyrala EE. Respiratory disorders of the newborn infant. In: Schidlow DV, Smith DS, eds. *A practical guide to pediatric respiratory diseases.* St. Louis: Mosby; 1994:127–140.

CHAPTER 116 ■ NEWBORN SEPSIS AND THE PREVENTION OF GROUP B STREPTOCOCCAL INFECTION

PAMELA G. LARSEN

Neonatal sepsis, defined as a systemic infection with positive blood or other central culture, occurs when bacteria infect the bloodstream of the "immunologically compromised" newborn host. Mortality has decreased in recent years for term, low-birthweight, and very-low-birthweight infants, possibly due to the shift in predominant organisms from gram-negative to gram-positive.

For assessment and management purposes, sepsis can be divided into early (birth to 7 days of life) or late presentation (greater than 7 days old). Approximately 50% of early-onset sepsis is clinically apparent within 6 hours of birth, and the great majority (95%) will present within 72 hours. Low birthweight is the major risk factor for early-onset neonatal sepsis, followed by prematurity, prolonged rupture of membranes, and chorioamnionitis. Early-onset newborn sepsis is usually characterized by sepsis or pneumonia, while osteomyelitis, septic arthritis, or meningitis is less frequently seen. Conversely, meningitis is more likely in late-onset disease. Group B streptococcus (GBS) remains a leading cause of newborn infections. The incidence of early-onset GBS disease has decreased by 81%, being associated with the increased use of maternal antibiotic prophylaxis in the 1990s, and now equals that of late-onset disease. Likewise, the mortality of GBS disease, which in the 1970s stood at more than 50%, has decreased, and currently is associated with a case fatality rate of 3% to 5% in term infants (somewhat higher in the premature). Black infants remain at highest risk for neonatal sepsis; boys have a higher incidence of sepsis and meningitis than girls.

Over the years, the pathogens responsible for sepsis have changed considerably. Infections in the neonate may be bacterial, viral, and fungal. The most frequently encountered bacterial pathogens are GBS, *Staphylococcus aureus*, *Escherichia coli*, *Klebsiella*, *Haemophilus influenzae*, and *Listeria monocytogenes* (Table 116.1). GBS is most common, followed by enteric pathogens; together they account for approximately 70% of early-onset sepsis in the United States. Neonatal sepsis with gram-negative organisms or fungi has a higher mortality. Pathogens reach the neonate by a variety of routes. Transplacental transmission is responsible for the earliest infections, especially for syphilis, toxoplasmosis, rubella, cytomegalovirus (CMV), herpes, and human immunodeficiency virus (HIV). Vertical transmission, however, is more common. The infection is transmitted from the mother to infant via ascending infection in utero or during descent through the birth canal. Infection may also take place after birth, accounting for most late-onset cases.

Maternal colonization with GBS is the most common source for neonatal sepsis. GBS inhabits the gastrointestinal and genitourinary tracts of up to 30% of women. The colonization rate is greatest in younger, sexually active women from lower socioeconomic strata. Women heavily colonized with GBS have the highest risk of perinatally transmitted infection, although infants have also developed heavy colonization even when the mother has a low colony count. Initial maternal colonization at 23 to 26 weeks is associated with increased risk of premature delivery, and colonization at delivery is often associated with infection of the infant. Nine serotypes of GBS exist. Types I, II, and III are commonly associated with neonatal sepsis. Type III has been associated with central nervous system (CNS) involvement in early disease, while type V is associated with non-CNS involvement in early disease.

Revised guidelines for the prevention of perinatal GBS infections were published in 2002 by the Centers for Disease Control and Prevention. After the implementation of the 1996 guidelines, the incidence of GBS infection decreased significantly with the use of anogenital GBS culture-based screening and intrapartum penicillin prophylaxis. A large, population-based study of deliveries from 1998 to 1999 demonstrated culture-based screening to be 50% more effective than the risk-based approach (Fig. 116.1). Further, there was an almost 90% decrease in early-onset disease in infants born to women without risk factors who had positive anogenital cultures and were treated with intrapartum antibiotic prophylaxis.

If cultures have not been obtained, or if the result of cultures is not known at the time of labor, antibiotic prophylaxis is recommended for the mother with any positive risk factor. For women who have ruptured membranes prior to 37 weeks gestation, but have not gone into labor, recommendations are to obtain GBS cultures if time permits, and to consider administration of antibiotics pending culture results. Planned cesarean section of the GBS-positive mother with intact membranes poses an extremely low risk of transmission, so in that situation, antibiotic prophylaxis is not recommended. The Centers for Disease Control and Prevention (CDC) guidelines include treatment of the infant based on culture results, intrapartum antibiotic prophylaxis, and symptomatology. This culture-based strategy is most likely to prevent early-onset GBS sepsis, although it seems to have little effect on late-onset infection.

CLINICAL FINDINGS

History

Recognition of *risk factors* in the history (Table 116.2) is critical for early identification and effective management of the sick

TABLE 116.1

PATHOGENS OF NEONATAL SEPSIS

Bacteroides	MRSA
Candida	Neisseria meningitidis
Clostridium	Pseudomonas
Escherichia coli[a]	Salmonella
Group B streptococcus[a]	Serratia
Groups A, C, &	Staphylococcus aureus
G streptococcus	STORCH infections
Haemophilus influenzae	Streptococcus
Klebsiella-Enterobacter	pneumoniae
Listeria[a]	Virus: adenovirus,
	enterovirus,
	coxsackievirus

[a]Most common pathogens.

neonate. For example, premature rupture of membranes may occur as a response to untreated chorioamnionitis. If signs or symptoms of chorioamnionitis (e.g., fever greater than 100°F, leukocytosis, fetal tachycardia, uterine tenderness, purulent amniotic fluid) coexist with rupture of membranes, the incidence of newborn infection quadruples.

The *clinical course* should be reviewed for early signs of sepsis, which may be nonspecific or minimal. The infant may show signs of poor feeding, hypothermia, decreased tone, decreased alertness, or ill appearance. Moreover, because early infections are usually fulminant and multisystemic, there may be evidence of fetal distress during labor, or the infant may be in distress at the time of delivery.

Physical Examination

The general appearance of the neonate should be noted. The infant may be lethargic, with pallor and distress. The septic infant is also more likely to be small for gestational age.

Temperature instability may be present, and must be assessed with reference to the chronologic age and gestational age of the infant. Within the first 6 to 12 hours after birth, the normal infant may experience difficulty in thermoregulation as part of transition. Repeated hypothermic episodes, however, should raise the index of suspicion for infection. Conversely, elevation of temperature in the term newborn is infrequent; a single brief rise is not generally associated with illness, but temperature elevation sustained for more than 1 hour often signals infection. Although temperature instability occurs commonly, poor peripheral perfusion and increased respiratory effort are better indicators of infection than hyperthermia or hypothermia.

Respiratory symptoms (tachypnea, nasal flaring, retractions, grunting, cyanosis, and apnea) are frequently seen,

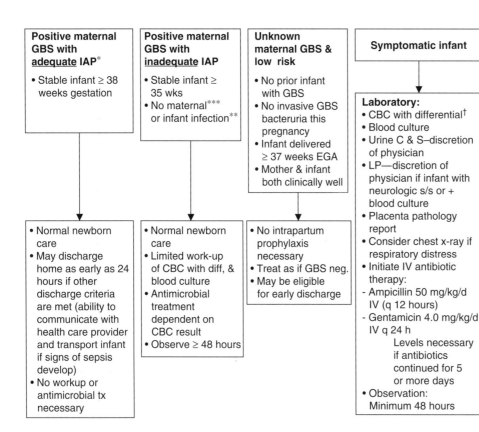

*IAP → Intrapartum Antibiotic Prophylaxis: Penicillin, 2 doses with 1 dose greater than 4 hours prior to delivery; or for penicillin allergic patients: Clindamycin, Erythromycin, Cefazolin, or Vancomycin, with 1 dose greater than 4 hours prior to delivery.

**Infant Infection → Respiratory distress, apnea, shock, poor feeding, inability to maintain temperature, lethargy, pallor

***Maternal Infection → Prolonged rupture of membranes ≥ 18 hours, intrapartum fever ≥ 38.0 , chorioamnionitis, GBS bacteriuria

FIGURE 116.1. Schematic for assessment of GBS in the newborn.

TABLE 116.2

PREDISPOSING RISK FACTORS FOR NEONATAL SEPSIS

Maternal factors	Neonatal factors
African-American race	Acidosis/asphyxia/hypoxemia
Amnionitis	Apgar score < 6 at 1 or 5 min
Antenatal steroid use	Congenital anomalies
Difficult/instrumented delivery	Fetal tachycardia
Fever >101°F/ leukocytosis	Low birthweight
	Male infant
Low socioeconomic status	Meconium staining
Poor nutrition	Prematurity
Poor prenatal care	First-born twin
Prolonged rupture of membranes (>18 hr)	
Recurrent abortion	
Substance abuse	
Urinary tract infection	
Vaginal colonization with GBS	
Young age	

because the most common manifestation of neonatal sepsis is pneumonia. Differential diagnoses include respiratory distress, metabolic disorders, congenital heart disease, and intracranial hemorrhage.

Cardiac signs are seen in overwhelming sepsis and are probably due to pulmonary hypertension, decreased cardiac output, and poor oxygenation. The infant may exhibit signs of shock, including pallor, poor perfusion, and edema.

Metabolic signs may include hyperglycemia or hypoglycemia and metabolic acidosis. The infant's reduced intake, in the face of the higher glucose requirement associated with infection, leads to hypoglycemia, often a late sign of sepsis. Paradoxically, glucose intolerance and hyperglycemia may occur due to an increased catabolism. Acidosis may result from anaerobic metabolism and the production of lactic acid. Poor thermoregulation (exacerbated by the lack of a thermal neutral environment) can both cause and worsen metabolic acidosis.

Neurologic signs are noted if the septic infant has CNS involvement. Hypotonia may be seen in sepsis, with or without meningitis. Cerebral edema may occur in meningitis, and areas of infarction and periventricular leukomalacia may evolve, but because of the neonate's open sutures, the fontanelles will rarely bulge. It is important to remember that early-onset meningitis produces nonspecific signs, such as lethargy or irritability. Late-onset disease is more likely to cause neurologic symptoms, such as stupor, coma, seizures, focal signs, and although uncommon, nuchal rigidity.

Gastrointestinal signs include abdominal distension, vomiting, diarrhea, guaiac-positive stools, and organomegaly, especially hepatomegaly. An ileus may be noted on radiologic examination.

Dermatologic signs such as petechiae or pallor may be noted in early sepsis; purpura may develop, secondary to thrombocytopenia or disseminated intravascular coagulation. Skin lesions may be present, such as vesicles, abscesses, cellulitis, or granulomas due to *Listeria* infection. Dermal erythropoiesis (blueberry muffin spots) may represent infections caused by herpes simplex virus (HSV), CMV, or rubella. Approximately one-third of septic infants have jaundice, although the incidence of jaundice is probably not significantly different than in nonseptic infants. Abrupt onset of jaundice,

however, may occur in infected neonates and is frequently associated with urosepsis.

Laboratory Findings

Laboratory studies contribute to the assessment of the septic infant, whether symptomatic or asymptomatic. Abnormal laboratory values parallel findings such as acidosis, hypoglycemia, or hyperbilirubinemia as the infection progresses. Initial laboratory studies one should consider are described in the following sections.

Cultures

A causative organism must be isolated to prove bacterial sepsis. The organism may be identified in blood, cerebral spinal fluid (CSF), urine, joint fluid, peritoneal fluid, or pleural fluid. If possible, cultures should be obtained prior to administering antibiotics. Cultures should be repeated in any symptomatic infant who does not improve.

Blood for culture should be obtained from a peripheral venous site. Reliable results may be obtained with as little as 0.2 mL of blood; it is better, however, though often not feasible, to use 1 to 2 mL or 0.5 mL from separate sites for two cultures, in order to optimize the chance of positive results. False-negative cultures are frequent, while cultures drawn from capillary sticks or umbilical catheters carry a high risk of contamination and false-positive results. Aerobic cultures are sufficient for most neonatal sepsis workups.

Urine culture is not usually helpful in early-onset sepsis, but it is appropriate for in the workup of late-onset symptoms. The culture should be obtained with sterile in-and-out catheterization or suprapubic aspiration; bagged urine specimens are not acceptable.

Lumbar puncture (LP) with CSF Gram stain should be performed in all symptomatic infants, as 25% of infants with bacterial sepsis may have meningitis. Because the LP has a low yield in asymptomatic neonates, its use in these infants is controversial. Organisms may be detected in 80% of infants with meningitis, and in 75% of these, the CSF Gram stain will aid in identifing the organism. The CSF of neonates with meningitis will usually have elevated white blood cell (WBC) counts with a polymorphonuclear predominance, elevated protein, and a low CSF/serum glucose ratio. Abnormal WBC and protein levels are more likely to be seen in late-onset and gram-negative infections. Table 116.3 lists the normal CSF values by age for WBCs, protein, and glucose. If the LP is traumatic, interpretation of the results is more difficult. Red blood cell (RBC) lysis may articificially elevate CSF protein values, and obtaining a reliable WBC is problematic. Although many formulas have been proposed to estimate the CSF leukocyte count, given a traumatic tap, a common one assumes one leukocyte for every 700 RBCs. Alternatively, the RBC to WBC ratio may be calculated from the complete blood count (CBC) and extrapolated to the CSF.

Positive *gastric aspirate*, and ear canal, rectal, skin, and amniotic fluid cultures identify potential bacterial exposure, but do not confirm sepsis; hence they have limited value.

Complete Blood Count and Differential

Normal WBC counts vary in newborns, but values less than 4,000 to 5,000 or greater than 25,000/μL are abnormal. Normal WBC counts may be seen even in culture-proven sepsis; however, the use of immature/mature WBC ratios is more sensitive in predicting sepsis. The positive predictive value of a single abnormal test in an asymptomatic infant is low. The WBC count is found to be abnormal in 94% to 100% of symptomatic, culture-positive infants and can be helpful in following the course of the illness. Neutropenia is more

TABLE 116.3

NORMAL CEREBROSPINAL FLUID (CSF) VALUES IN INFANTS

Newborn age	Values in CSF mean (range)		
	White blood cells (cells/μL)	Protein (mg/dL)	Glucose (mg/dL) *Ratio CSF:Blood
Term	8 (0–32) 60% PMN	90 (20–170)	52 (34–119) *.81 (0.44–2.48)
Preterm	9 (0–29) 0–66% PMN	115 (65–150)	50 (24–63) *.74 (0.55–1.05)
0–4 wk	10 0–15% PMN	84 (35–189)	46 (36–61)

PMN, polymorphonuclear.

predictive of infection than neutrophilia; in general, clinicians consider WBC counts of less than 5,000 worrisome, though nonspecific. Thrombocytopenia of less than 100,000/mm^3 may be seen in sepsis, especially in the late-onset variety.

The assessment of the asymptomatic infant can be a frustrating and difficult experience. For the infant without symptoms but with known risks (e.g., maternal fever or clinical course complicated by poor feeding or hypothermia), a single CBC is not very useful in screening for sepsis. The CBC may produce false-negative results, creating the misleading impression that the infant is not infected. Conversely, abnormal WBC counts are often seen in asymptomatic, noninfected infants. An elevated WBC count alone does not indicate infection, and a left shift in the differential may be associated with the stress of birth or medical procedures as often as with infection. Consequently, serial CBCs may be more useful than a single test. Rather than obtaining the CBC immediately after birth in an asymptomatic infant, delaying the CBC for 4 to 6 hours after delivery improves the probability that abnormal results are related to infection and not simply to the stresses of birth.

For every infant with proven bacteremia, 15 to 20 uninfected newborns are evaluated and treated. Because the WBC count has poor positive predictive value, other methods of improving sensitivity and specificity for sepsis have been sought. Morphologic changes in the WBCs, such as toxic granulation, Döhle bodies, and vacuolization, have been examined. Ratios (Table 116.4), such as the immature to mature (I:M), immature to total (I:T), and band to segmented neutrophils (B:S), have been only slightly more helpful in identifying the septic but asymptomatic infant. The scoring system developed by Rodwell and associates (Table 116.5) uses an array of hematologic criteria for evaluating sepsis. The combination of three or more abnormal laboratory values improves their positive predictive value.

C-reactive protein (CRP) is an acute-phase reactant that is synthesized by the liver and that increases in response to an inflammatory process. Use of the CRP in addition to the WBC count and WBC-derived ratios may help the clinician identify the newborn at high risk for sepsis. However, because of the 6- to 12-hour delay between the onset of infection and a measureable rise in CRP, it may not add useful data to the initial assessment. The CRP is more useful in monitoring potentially infected infants over time. Because it peaks in 2 to 3 days and remains elevated until the inflammation is resolved, the CRP may be a useful guide for the clinician making decisions about antibiotic discontinuation and hospital discharge in infants with suspected sepsis but who are culture-negative.

MANAGEMENT

Management of the infant at risk for sepsis varies depending on whether or not she is symptomatic. The history and physical examination findings will suggest management strategies

TABLE 116.4

RATIOS IN THE DIFFERENTIAL WHITE COUNT

Corrected WBC	$\dfrac{\text{Total WBC} \times 100}{\text{Number nucleated RBCs} + 100}$
Absolute neutrophil count (ANC)	WBC × (% Segs + % Immature cells[a])
Immature to total neutrophil (I:T) ratio	$\dfrac{\text{\% Immature cells}^a}{\text{\% Segs} + \text{\% Immature cells}}$
Immature to mature (I:M) ratio	$\dfrac{\text{Bands} + \text{Metas} + \text{Myelos}}{\text{Neutrophils}}$
Band to seg (B:S) ratio	$\dfrac{\text{Bands}}{\text{Neutrophils}}$

[a]Immature cells include bands, metamyelocytes, and myelocytes.
From Polinski C. The value of the white blood cell count and differential in the prediction of neonatal sepsis. *Neonatal Network* 1996;15:13–23.

TABLE 116.5

RODWELL SCORING SYSTEM: DERIVATION OF HEMATOLOGIC SCORES

Test	Abnormality	Score
I:T ratio[a]	↑	1
Total polymorphonuclear count[a,b]	↑ or ↓	1
I:M ratio[c]	↑	1
Immature polymorphonuclear count[d]	↑	
Total white blood cell count	↑ or ↓ (≤5000/mm³ or ≥25,000, 30,000, and 21,000, at birth, 12–24 hr, and > day 2, respectively	1
Degenerative changes in polymorphonuclear cells	≥3 for vacuolization, toxic granulation or Döhle bodies	1
Platelet count	<150,000/mm³	1

PMN, polymorphonuclear.
Abnormal values:
[a] Immature to total neutrophils >0.2.
[b] Total PMN count <3,000 or >7,000 cells/mm³; if no mature PMNs are seen on blood film, score 2 rather than 1 for abnormal total polymorphonuclear count.
[c] Immature to mature neutrophils ≥0.3.
[d] Immatures are bands, metamyelocytes, and myelocytes >1,500/mm³.
From Rodwell RL, Taylor KM, Tudehope DI, et al. Hematologic scoring system in early diagnosis of sepsis in neutropenic newborns. *Pediatr Infect Dis* 1993;12:372–376, with permission.

for the symptomatic newborn, which should also take into account the maternal intrapartum course (Fig. 116.2). The management of the infant born to a mother who has chorioamnionitis is controversial. If the mother has suspected chorioamnionitis, her infant should receive a full diagnostic workup, and empiric antibiotic therapy should be considered, depending on its condition, pending culture results. If the infant demonstrates signs of sepsis, the full diagnostic evaluation should include an LP.

The *symptomatic* infant will most commonly present with signs of respiratory distress (e.g., tachypnea, grunting, flaring, retractions, apnea) and may require transfer to a tertiary neonatal intensive-care unit (NICU). Initial antibiotic therapy (Fig. 116.2) commonly includes IV ampicillin and an aminoglycoside to cover GBS and other gram-positive organisms, as well as gram-negative bacteria, such as *E. coli*. Ampicillin 50 mg/kg/dose, given every 12 hours, and gentamicin sulfate 4.0 mg/kg/dose, given every 24 hours, are appropriate for term infants, pending further laboratory data. Antibiotic coverage can be adjusted after culture results and sensitivities are available. If the infant shows no clinical improvement, gentamicin levels should be obtained to determine whether a therapeutic level has been reached. Furthermore, if aminoglycoside coverage continues beyond 3 days, drug levels should be monitored in order to avoid ototoxic and nephrotoxic side effects. Renal function should be assessed during aminoglycoside therapy, and a hearing examination should be performed prior to discharge.

Intensive care management of the symptomatic infant, including fluid administration, packed red blood cell transfusions, and granulocyte and immune globulin therapy, are beyond the scope of this chapter. Consultation with infectious disease specialists may be useful if the infant is not responding, or if an unusual symptom (e.g., rash) develops.

Management of the asymptomatic infant at risk for sepsis is less clearly defined. Infants with risk factors who have normal laboratory studies may receive routine neonatal care (e.g., feeding, open crib, parental contact) in the normal newborn nursery. A positive blood culture, abnormal WBC count or ratio, or Rodwell score of 3 or more warrants IV ampicillin and aminoglycoside administration. Aminoglycoside drug levels may be postponed until after culture results are available. If the antibiotics are continued, levels should be drawn on day 3 to 5, and doses adjusted accordingly, with appropriate monitoring for side effects. An infant who is at significant risk but is otherwise clinically stable poses a therapeutic dilemma. Negative blood cultures after 2 days are reassuring, but a small number of infants with sepsis will have negative cultures from the initial workup, a situation that is more likely if the mother received intrapartum antibiotics. Monitoring the CRP level may assist the clinician in this decision; after it returns to normal, antibiotics may be discontinued.

Discharge of the asymptomatic at-risk infant should be deferred until at least 48 hours after birth. Obtaining a normal repeat CBC and CRP at 24 hours of age is encouraging if the initial laboratory work was inconclusive. Asymptomatic term infants delivered to mothers with *unknown* GBS status and no other identified risk factors can be considered noninfected and eligible for early discharge, if desired, with outpatient follow-up in 2 to 4 days. Given that prematurity is a risk factor for GBS infection, near-term (i.e., 35 to 37 weeks gestation) infants whose mothers have unknown GBS status require a sepsis screen and are not candidates for early discharge.

PREVENTION OF GROUP B STREPTOCOCCAL INFECTION

Following the implementation of prevention strategies initiated by the American Academy of Pediatrics (AAP), the American College of Obstetrics and Gynecology, and the Centers for Disease Control and Prevention (CDC), newborn early-onset GBS infection declined significantly. Recent data reporting further declines confirm the superiority of culture-based screening. It is also clear that the risk-based approach (mother with prior infant with GBS, GBS bacteriuria this pregnancy, infant delivered at less than 37 weeks estimated gestational age) is

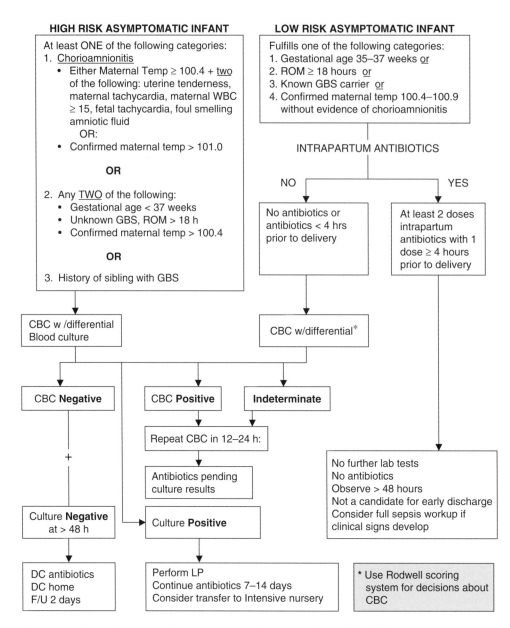

FIGURE 116.2. Management of risk assessment and treatment of the infected infant.

less effective than GBS culture screening of all women at 35 to 37 weeks gestation. Nationally, more than 2,000 cases of early-onset neonatal GBS infection occur annually, primarily because GBS-positive mothers did not receive intrapartum antibiotics. This number could be reduced with universal screening and consistent adherence to the guidelines for management of infants born to GBS-positive mothers.

Penicillin is the intrapartum drug of choice for prevention of GBS disease in the newborn. Ampicillin is an acceptable alternative if broad-spectrum antibiotic coverage is necessary. Because an increasing number of GBS strains are resistant to erythromycin and clindamycin, cefazolin sodium is the drug of choice for penicillin-allergic women at low risk for anaphylaxis. Testing of GBS isolates to determine susceptibility is recommended for penicillin-allergic women; clindamycin or erythromycin is recommended if the strain is susceptible. Vancomycin is reserved for penicillin-allergic women at high risk for anaphylaxis when erythromycin or clindamycin can-

not be used, either because of unknown susceptibility or in vitro resistance of the prenatal isolate.

Group B streptococcal bacteriuria during pregnancy is a marker for heavy colonization. Women with any GBS bacteriuria should receive chemoprophylaxis during labor, regardless of anogenital culture results. A planned cesarean delivery, without labor and without rupture of membranes, is at low risk for transmission of GBS infection. GBS prophylaxis for threatened preterm delivery is probably indicated pending culture results.

The 2002 guidelines have not affected the incidence of late-onset GBS disease. Current research is exploring the development of a vaccine that could prevent peripartum maternal disease and decrease neonatal disease by transplacental transfer of protective IgG antibodies. When administered to the mother, it would provide the newborn with protection against both early-onset and late-onset GBS. Such a vaccine offers the greatest future hope for complete prevention of GBS infection.

PEARLS

- Infants with bacterial sepsis will usually present in the first 6 hours of life.
- Infants who are septic usually present with respiratory symptoms, making recognition of the septic infant more difficult.
- A normal CBC obtained in the first few hours of life does not rule out sepsis.
- The Rodwell index improves the sensitivity of WBC count and differential in assessing an infant.

- An LP is necessary in the symptomatic infant.
- A WBC count less than 4,000/mL is ominous.
- A negative blood culture does not rule out sepsis and should be disregarded if other findings suggest sepsis.

Suggested Readings

Centers for Disease Control (CDC). Prevention of perinatal group B streptococcal disease: revised guidelines from CDC. *MMWR* 2002;51(no.RR-11):1–22.

Belling LL, Ohning BL. Neonatal sepsis. *eMedicine J* 2002;3:1–26.

CHAPTER 117 ■ THE FEEDING AND GROWING PRETERM INFANT

PAMELA G. LARSEN

The rate of preterm births continues to rise, especially for infants considered moderately premature (32 to 36 weeks gestation), but also for very preterm and very-low-birthweight infants (less than 1,500 g). The birth rate of premature infants less than 32 weeks has risen more than 16% over the last 25 years; of all births, 8.1% are low birthweight (less than 2,500 g) and 1.47% are very low birthweight (less than 1,000 g). As more infants are surviving prematurity than ever before, gestational age and birthweight are the most influential factors affecting length of hospital stay. Although these infants may require weeks to months of intensive-care hospitalization, many infants are discharged after shorter stays and at lower discharge weights than were previously thought possible. Whereas shorter stays may improve parental bonding, reduce exposure to the stress of the intensive-care environment, and lower hospital-associated morbidity and costs, discharge must come only after physiologic stability has been appropriately maximized.

Premature infants have significantly more emergency room visits, hospital readmissions, and deaths than their healthy term counterparts. Often, when premature infants no longer need intensive care but are not yet ready for hospital discharge, they are transferred to a step-down nursery. Because discharge planning for such infants involves many factors, the AAP has published discharge guidelines addressing four categories of high-risk neonates: premature infants, infants requiring technologic support, infants at high social risk, and infants with irreversible disease processes that will result in an early death. While preparing the premature infant for discharge, monitoring of feeding and growth, respiratory status, and thermoregulation must be continued. In addition, adequate time must be allowed for the family to prepare for home care and to arrange follow-up medical care. The management of the stable, growing premature infant has three components: identification of common problems of these infants, establishment of goals to be met prior to discharge, and creation of management strategies to meet these goals.

DISCHARGE GOALS AND MANAGEMENT

Continued Weight Gain

Although there is no minimum weight established for discharge, sustained weight gain must occur. The premature infant should gain 15 to 30 g daily for several days prior to discharge. Many practitioners feel comfortable discharging stable infants when their weight reaches 1,600 to 1,800 grams.

Adequate Nutrition

The infant must be able to take in sufficient calories to achieve adequate weight gain. Physiologically, the activities of suck, coordinated cheek and tongue movement, uvular closure of the nasopharynx, epiglottal closure of the larynx, normal esophageal motility, and appropriate gag reflex can be expected of the infant at 32 to 34 weeks postmenstrual age. Prior to discharge, the infant should be taking all feedings orally without associated bradycardia. Frequency of feeding is usually every 3 hours, extended to every 4 hours, and then ad lib, as tolerated. Nasogastric (NG) or orogastric (OG) tube feedings may be necessary early in the establishment of enteral feeding; infants less than 2 kg may tolerate OG better than NG tubes. A 5F feeding tube is usually of sufficient gauge. If the respiratory rate is greater than 60, or if other evidence of respiratory distress is noted, feedings should be given by tube rather than by mouth. Placement of the feeding tube in the stomach must be checked prior to infusion. If more than 10% of the previous feeding is aspirated from the stomach immediately prior to the next, the amount of the bolus should probably be reduced. The infant should be monitored closely for emesis, distension, and respiratory distress. Using both oral and tube routes may be necessary for the premature infant who becomes easily fatigued with oral feedings. Alternating oral and tube feeds promotes oral feeding with less fatigue, better weight gain, and lowered risk of aspiration. Infants may have episodes of bradycardia during oral feeding due to sucking bursts and the volume of milk generated by each suck. Because infants rarely have the ability to adjust the sucking pressure in response to the flow rate of the milk from the nipple, the oropharynx floods with milk and results in a vagal-mediated bradycardia.

The type of feeding (formula, breast milk, or combination) that will be used after discharge must be well established and well tolerated. Formula intolerance, frequent adjustments in caloric concentration, or the continued need to alternate oral and tube feeding indicates an infant not yet ready for discharge. Special premature infant formulas with increased nutrients (calcium, phosphorus, electrolytes, and vitamins) and higher caloric density (22 to 27 kcal/ounce) can provide 100 to 120 kcal/kg/day without increasing solute load. Given this caloric intake, the infant will take in 100 to 150 mL/kg/day of fluids. The infant should be observed for dehydration if caloric density is increased because of the consequent reduction in fluid intake. For infants receiving breast milk, human milk fortifier may be added to augment calories, calcium, and phosphorus.

If possible, the infant should progress to 20 kcal/ounce formula several days prior to discharge while monitoring weight gain. The infant discharged on a calorie-dense formula should be followed closely by the health care provider and changed to a standard-calorie formula (20 kcal/ounce) when stable weight gain is demonstrated. Data suggest that infants weighing less than 1,500 g at birth may benefit from continuing to take a premature formula of higher caloric density until they are 9 months old. The additional calcium and phosphorus, along with the increased calories, results in better overall growth.

In addition to calories, feedings must provide adequate protein, fat, and micronutrients. Because inability to take in sufficient calories may result in inadequate vitamin intake, a daily multivitamin (1.0 mL by mouth or tube) may be necessary. Folic acid (15 μg/kg/day, maximum dose 50 μg/day) and vitamin E (25 IU/day) may be therapeutic in treating anemia of prematurity by enhancing RBC production. Vitamin D supplementation can promote bone mineralization in premature infants. However, these supplements may be discontinued when the infant changes to regular formula.

Respiratory Stability

Respiratory criteria for discharge usually include absence of respiratory distress, a respiratory rate less than 60 breaths/min, no apnea greater than 15 to 20 seconds, no bradycardia less than 80 beats/min, and no oxygen desaturations to less than 80%. In infants of less than 28 weeks gestation, apnea persisting long after other criteria for discharge are met may represent normal postnatal maturation or may be a subtle predictor of future neurodevelopmental or sleep disturbance. Although published reports do not clearly demonstrate a relationship between reflux and apnea, a trial of antireflux treatments and medications may be attempted. An otherwise stable infant with continued apnea, especially one of less than 27 weeks gestational age or with a continued oxygen requirement, may be discharged on an apnea monitor. There is a lack of clear discharge criteria for the infant with apneic episodes, as well as considerable debate concerning the accuracy of apnea documentation in the hospital. For clinical reassurance and to decrease the probability that significant apnea will occur at home, many providers require an infant to be free of apnea for at least 5 to 7 days prior to discharge.

Infants with apnea and/or apnea-associated bradycardia may require stimulant medications. New-onset apnea must be considered pathologic and the infant assessed for hypoglycemia, infection, anemia, pneumonia, or pneumothorax. The use of xanthines (caffeine, theophylline) is widespread for idiopathic apnea (Table 117.1), although they affect bilirubin binding and should not be used in infants with hyperbilirubinemia. Xanthines are discontinued at 35 to 37 weeks postmenstrual age if apneic spells have not occurred for 1 week. When assessing the infant's stability, the practitioner must remember that the long half-life of the xanthines may delay a recurrence of apnea.

Discharge on an apnea monitor may be considered for otherwise stable infants with continued apnea. Home monitoring may also be appropriate in other circumstances, including:

- Very low birthweight
- A sibling in the family who died from sudden infant death syndrome (SIDS)
- The need for supplemental oxygen
- Previous "apparent life-threatening events" (ALTEs)

Referral to home health nursing for follow-up is necessary, and parents must be taught cardiopulmonary resuscitation (CPR).

Thermoregulation

The premature infant has imperfect thermoregulation due to CNS immaturity, lack of subcutaneous fat deposits, low heat-generating capacity, and large surface-to-volume ratio. Prior to discharge, the infant must be able to maintain a body temperature of greater than 97.8°F (36.6°C) axillary without supplementary warming. The premature infant who is unable to maintain temperature in an open crib should be provided with a thermally neutral environment in a double-walled isolette; humidity and air flow should be controlled so that heat production is minimal and core temperature is stable. The isolette temperature should initially be set at 36.5°C to 37.0°C, wtih 40% to 60% humidity, then decreased as appropriate for the infant's size and maturity. To wean the infant from the isolette, it should be dressed in clothing and a double-layered hat, wrapped in a blanket, and the isolette temperature reduced over a 24-hour period by one-half to one degree increments, checking the infant's temperature every 4 hours. The infant may be removed from the isolette when its temperature remains stable in a 27°C isolette. It has been observed that apneic episodes are reduced by maintaining the infant's temperature closer to the lower end of the thermal neutral environment and minimizing temperature fluctuations.

The Discharge Plan

The complexity of the discharge plan will vary based on the neonatal course and the degree of prematurity. Early involvement of the parents in care and decision-making facilitates the transition to home. Intensive involvement of the parents in caring for the infant prior to discharge allows for assessment of the strengths and needs of the family. Assessment tools, such as the Neonatal Discharge Assessment Tool (N-DAT), can be used to identify high-risk newborns or situations where

TABLE 117.1

XANTHINES IN THE TREATMENT OF APNEA

Medication	Oral dose	Adverse events	Monitoring
Caffeine	*Load*: 20–40 mg/kg *Maintenance*: 5–8 mg/kg/day divided q 12–24 hr	Tachycardia Cardiac dysrhythmias Reflux Sleep disturbance	*Therapeutic levels*: 8–20 μg/mL *Toxic*: >50 mg/mL
Theophylline	*Load*: 4 mg/kg/dose *Maintenance*: 4 (3–6) mg/kg/24 hr divided q 6–8 hr	GI upset Agitation Tremor	After at least 1 day of therapy: *Therapeutic*: 6–14 μg/mL *Peak*: 1 hour post-dose *Trough*: Just before dose

planning should begin well in advance of the actual discharge. Premature infants are at increased risk for abuse and neglect, especially if there is a history of parental substance abuse, a teen mother, or domestic violence. Assessment of the home situation by social services may be indicated and helpful to the discharge team. Intensive parent education and close infant follow-up are necessary to reduce the likelihood of unscheduled hospital readmissions, frequent acute care clinic visits, and early infant death. Studies on early discharge show that service coordination, home visits, transportation, sibling care, and in-home support to the family are cost-effective.

Vision Screening

Infants less than or equal to 1,500 g or 28 weeks gestational age at birth (or 1,500 to 2,000 g with an unstable neonatal course) should have vision screening for retinopathy of prematurity (ROP). The dilated fundus examination should be performed at least twice unless the first one clearly shows both retinas to be fully vascularized. The initial eye examination should take place at 4 to 6 weeks chronologic age or 31 to 33 weeks postmenstrual age, whichever is later. This ophthalmologic examination may occur prior to discharge, with a follow-up appointment, if necessary. The responsibility for examination and follow-up of the infant at risk for ROP must be carefully defined. If the infant's medical care is being transferred to a primary provider, oral and written communication about the assessment for ROP and the necessity and timing of follow-up are essential. Treatment and recommendation guidelines for follow-up examinations are well outlined. (See the American Academy of Pediatrics Committee on Fetus and Newborn. Policy statement: hospital discharge of the high-risk neonate—proposed guidelines, in the Suggested Readings list.)

Hearing Screening

Premature infants are at increased risk for hearing impairment. If any of the following conditions exist, brainstem evoked response or otoacoustic impedance audiometry is used to assess hearing:

- Abnormalities of the head, neck, nose, or throat
- Severe jaundice
- Neonatal meningitis
- Congenital infection associated with sensorineural hearing loss
- Family history of hearing loss before age 5
- Seizure activity attributed to hypoxia or neurologic abnormality
- Ototoxic medications
- Birthweight less than 1,500 g
- Apgar score of 0 to 4 at 1 minute or 0 to 6 at 5 minutes
- Mechanical ventilation for 5 or more days
- Severe acidosis

If the hearing examination is not conducted in the hospital, it should be scheduled within 2 to 4 weeks after discharge. Infants who fail the hearing examination should be retested, and intervention services should be initiated.

Laboratory Assessments

Metabolic screening of the premature infant should be obtained before the seventh day of life. A blood transfusion may interfere with the accuracy of results. Any infant receiving a transfusion should have the screening tests repeated 3 months posttransfusion. Screening for phenylketonuria (PKU) and galactosemia is most reliable when performed 48 hours or more after the infant has begun feedings (oral or enteral) totaling ≥75 cal/kg/day; a normal screen in an infant who has insufficient enteral intake does not rule out metabolic disease. Total parenteral nutrition may cause a false-positive PKU result. Soy formula may yield a false-negative galactosemia test. An abnormal screening test result should be noted in the chart, and if the premature or ill infant shows clinical signs compatible with the disorder, confirmatory testing should be done at once. If the patient shows no signs of a metabolic disorder, repeat screening should be done by 4 weeks of age or at discharge, whichever occurs first. A reminder system is recommended to assure appropriate follow-up.

Car Seat Evaluation

Proper positioning of the infant in a car seat (Table 117.2) must be ensured prior to discharge, and many hospitals have policies for conducting this evaluation. Some infants, especially small premature infants, have been shown to demonstrate apnea, bradycardia, and oxygen desaturation when placed in a semisitting position in car safety seats. Premature infants who are <37 weeks gestation or <3 kg at birth should be monitored in the specific car seat the family will use (Table 117.3). Infants with cardiorespiratory problems in the car seat should not be placed in similar equipment at home (e.g., infant swings, seats, or carriers) and may have to travel flat in a car bed that meets federal safety standards. In that case, the infant should be reassessed later before switching to a car seat.

Cardiopulmonary Resuscitation

The parents or primary caregivers should demonstrate competence in CPR, particularly if the infant has a history of apnea or is being discharged on oxygen and/or monitors. At least one alternative support person should also be trained in CPR. Sufficient planning prior to the actual discharge allows time for parents to be trained in CPR and to consolidate this complex information.

Immunizations

The immune response in very-low-birthweight infants may be reduced, but insufficient data exist to alter the recommendations. The AAP Committee on Infectious Diseases recommends starting immunizations at 2 months chronologic age with diphtheria, tetanus, acellular pertussis, H. influenzae type B conjugate, inactivated poliovirus, and pneumonccocal vaccines. Hepatitis B vaccine can be given after the infant weighs more than 2,000 g, or at discharge if less than 2,000 grams, or at 1 month of age if less than 2,000 g and stable. Some infants with a history of prematurity or related chronic lung disease should receive respiratory syncytial virus (RSV) immunoglobulin (Synagis, RespiGam) during RSV season, as well as influenza immunizations annually in the fall after they reach 6 months of age (see the criteria in the AAP Red Book).

Follow-Up Care

Coordinating post-hospitalization care requires a concerted effort on the part of the discharge team and the parents or guardians. This transition is facilitated if the physician providing the convalescent care also provides follow-up care. When this is not possible, telephone and written communication between the neonatologist or physician providing nursery care and the primary provider about the infant's course and discharge plan is essential. A follow-up appointment with the community provider should take place within 1 to 2 weeks, or

TABLE 117.2

POSITIONING OF THE PREMATURE INFANT IN CAR SAFETY SEATS

DO	DON'T
Use 3-point harness infant-only seat **OR** a 5-point convertible seat.	*Do not* use a shield, abdominal pad, or arm rest that could directly contact face or neck.
Make sure the distance from crotch strap to the seat back is <5½ inches.	*Do not* allow the infant to slump forward or the head to flop.
Place a small rolled blanket between crotch strap and infant.	*Do not* allow the harness straps to cross the infant's ears.
Make sure the distance from lower harness straps to seat bottom is <10 inches.	*Do not* allow the retainer clip to be positioned on the abdomen or in the neck area.
Place buttocks and back flat.	*Do not* place in the front passenger seat with passenger-side front air bags.
Place rolled blankets on both sides to support the head and neck.	*Do not* leave infant unattended in car safety seat.
Make sure shoulder straps are at the lowest slots, with infant's shoulders well above slots.	
Snug the harness.	
Position the seat's retainer clip at the midpoint of the infant's chest.	
Recline the seat at a 45-degree angle by using a firm roll under car seat if necessary in vehicles with high front slope.	
Position should be rear-facing, middle of back seat until 20 pounds and 1 year old.	
Arrange for adult to ride in the back seat with infant.	

sooner if the child is unknown to the provider. Providing a written discharge summary to the primary provider is vital.

Community services, such as early intervention, speech and audiology, and/or physical therapy, may be necessary. Initiation of these contacts prior to discharge decreases the likelihood that the infant will be lost to critical early intervention and assessment. Neurodevelopment of the infant may be followed in a clinic associated with the NICU or by a community agency with expertise in following at-risk infants and identifying deviations in development and growth; such referral should precede discharge. Follow-up ophthalmologic appointments should be made if the infant has ROP. If the infant failed the hearing examination, a follow-up appointment should be made within 2 to 3 months. Infants who will need follow-up care with other specialists (e.g., orthopedic, cardiologic, surgical, pulmonary) should also have appointments scheduled prior to discharge, if possible. The parents should receive very specific instructions about the importance of follow-up, including possible consequences of missed appointments.

Follow-up by experienced public health or home health nurses is recommended for complex cases or families struggling to add a medically fragile infant to an already stressful home situation. The readmission rate of infants discharged from the NICU, especially for those with respiratory infections, is much higher than that of healthy infants. Ensuring that the parents have the necessary resources to care for the infant capably increases the likelihood of good growth and development and decreases subsequent readmissions. Home health follow-up is necessary for many infants in order to assess medication administration, equipment operation, and nutrition and weight gain. The nurse can evaluate clinical status and, together with the parents, review early signs and symptoms of illness, findings specific to the infant's condition

TABLE 117.3

CAR SEAT EVALUATION PROCEDURE

- Use the specific car seat parents plan to use for transport.
- Infant should not have fed within the previous 1 hour.
- Place infant in car seat, secure all straps properly.
- Attach CP and pulse oximetry monitors.
- Monitor for 1 hour.
- *Pass*: No CP alarms; pulse oximetry maintained ≥80%.

(cardiac, respiratory, neurologic), safety issues (such as positioning during sleep), and answer questions.

PEARLS

- Premature infants have significantly more emergency room visits, hospital readmissions, and deaths than their healthy full-term counterparts.
- There is no minimum weight established for discharge. Sustained weight gain must be noted at 15 to 30 g/day.
- Coordinated sucking, swallowing, and breathing can be expected of the infant at 32 to 34 weeks EGA.
- Infants weighing less than 1,800 g at discharge may benefit from continuation of a higher caloric density premature formula for up to 8 weeks after discharge.
- An apnea-free period of at least 5 to 7 days is clinically reassuring and decreases the probability that significant apnea will occur at home.

- A written discharge summary to the primary provider is critical, as this provider is essential in the ongoing coordination of services after discharge.

Suggested Readings

American Academy of Pediatrics Committee on Fetus and Newborn. Policy statement: hospital discharge of the high-risk neonate—proposed guidelines. *Pediatrics* 1998;102:411–417.

American Academy of Pediatrics Committee on Injury and Prevention and Committee on Fetus and Newborn. Policy statement: safe transportation of premature and low birthweight infants. *Pediatrics* 1996;97:758–760.

American Academy of Pediatrics Committee on Practice and Ambulatory Medicine and Committee on Fetus and Newborn. Policy statement: the role of the primary care pediatrician in the management of high-risk newborn infants. *Pediatrics* 1996;98:786–788.

American Academy of Pediatrics Section on Ophthalmology. Ophthalmology and strabismus. Screening examination of premature infants for retinopathy of prematurity. *Pediatrics* 2006;117:572–576.

CHAPTER 118 ■ DRUG EXPOSURE IN THE NEWBORN

PAMELA G. LARSEN

Infants with intrauterine exposure to drugs of abuse may experience withdrawal symptoms within hours to weeks after birth. Estimates of the prevalence of drug use in pregnant women range from 3% to 50%, with significant variation depending on the population studied and type of drug screen. Drug use among childbearing women has reportedly decreased. The drugs used during pregnancy include cocaine, tobacco, alcohol, heroin, marijuana, inhalants, and hallucinogens. These drugs are not used in isolation but in various combinations, and the drugs of choice vary by ethnic group. African-American women are more likely to use cocaine than Caucasian women, who in turn are more likely to use alcohol and cigarettes than African-American or Hispanic women. Rates of abuse are lowest for the Asian population. It is estimated that 32% of women who use drugs during pregnancy are polydrug users.

The effect of in-utero exposure to licit and illicit drugs on the fetal brain is not clearly understood, but animal data suggest that drugs of abuse may act as behavioral teratogens. Drug-exposed infants appear to exhibit behavioral disorganization of state, alerting, and motor processes. They are also at higher risk for SIDS. Clinical studies show that prenatal drug exposure affects the fetal brain by compromising the neurotransmitter systems that control attentional and affective functions. Ongoing research is exploring the long-term outcomes of drug exposure at the level of the neurotransmitter. Data thus far, however, are inconclusive regarding the effects of fetal drug exposure on child outcomes. Although early outcome reports showed relationships between maternal drug use and certain neurobehavioral disorders (e.g., attention deficit disorder, developmental and cognitive delay), other studies have noted few differences in developmental functioning when compared with demographically similar, non-exposed, age-matched controls.

Little is known about the effects of polydrug use, but abundant data are available on the effects of individual drugs on the infant. Between 50% and 90% of infants exposed to opioids or heroin will have *withdrawal* symptoms. Clinical signs of withdrawal from methadone are more common than from heroin, although clinically significant manifestations of withdrawal are less likely if the maternal methadone dose is below 20 mg/day. Methadone withdrawal usually begins between 2 and 7 days after birth, whereas heroin withdrawal occurs within the first 24 hours. Conversely, infants exposed to cocaine appear to have abnormal behavioral symptoms secondary to *continued drug effects* rather than withdrawal symptoms. Although no current studies describe cocaine withdrawal in the newborn infant, we know that cocaine withdrawal in the adult leads to irritability, anorexia, and difficulty sleeping. These symptoms are thought to be mediated by imbalances of dopamine, serotonin, or both. Current drug therapies for cocaine withdrawal in the adult, therefore, include dopamine agonists and serotonin antagonists. Such drug therapies have not been studied in the neonate.

CLINICAL FINDINGS

The clinician caring for the newborn in the nursery often will not know the mother, and must gather objective and subjective data to determine if substance abuse has occurred. Every newborn evaluation should include a review of the medical and psychosocial history of the mother. The mother's history of drug use before delivery, the type of anesthesia and analgesia used during labor, and the infant's estimated gestational age should all be noted.

Because medical records may not be accurate, it is incumbent on the pediatric provider to ask the mother about possible drug use. The tenor of the interview will influence the information she provides: reassurance of privacy and a nonjudgmental approach are important. It is helpful to begin by asking about licit, prescribed drugs, and then tobacco and alcohol. One approach is to ask the mother about illicit drug use by those close to her, such as parents or partner; questioning can then touch on any current drug use by the mother. The amount, frequency, and time of last use must be determined. Mothers may be reluctant to answer the questions because of fear of incarceration, denial of the problem, or other psychosocial issues. Emphasizing the importance of this information may persuade the mother to respond accurately in order to provide the best care for her newborn. Data show that practitioners who routinely inquire about prenatal drug use are twice as likely to recognize drug use in their patients as those who do not. Women who abuse drugs and alcohol often have family histories of substance abuse, childhood histories of sexual victimization, domestic violence issues with past or current partners, and mental health problems. These factors concern the pediatric provider because these women are often limited in their ability to respond sensitively to their infant, further compounding the teratogenic effect of the drugs on the infant and child.

Other maternal risk factors or newborn characteristics should increase the index of suspicion for drug withdrawal as the explanation for symptoms (Table 118.1). A neonatal history of excessive weight loss, poor thermoregulation, and frequent stools may be noted. Other characteristics, such as prematurity or intrauterine growth retardation (IUGR), may indicate prenatal drug exposure including tobacco and alcohol, cocaine, amphetamines, and marijuana. If the provider does not include drug withdrawal as part of the differential

TABLE 118.1

MATERNAL OR INFANT CHARACTERISTICS THAT INCREASE THE INDEX OF SUSPICION FOR MATERNAL DRUG USE

Maternal	Infant
No prenatal care	Prematurity
Previous unexplained fetal demise	Unexplained IUGR
Precipitous labor	Neurobehavioral abnormalities
Abruptio placentae	Urogenital abnormalities
Hypertensive episodes	Atypical vascular incidents
Severe mood swings	(CVA, MI, NEC)
Myocardial infarction	Birth defects (FAS)
Cerebrovascular accident	
Repeated spontaneous abortions	

IUGR, intrauterine growth retardation; CVA, cerebrovascular accident; MI, myocardial infarction; NEC, necrotizing enterocolitis; FAS, fetal alcohol syndrome.

for certain symptoms in the neonate, other problems, such as colic, diarrhea, or infection, may be erroneously diagnosed. A history of jitteriness, lethargy, irritability, or tachypnea may be mistaken for hypoglycemia, infection, or respiratory distress.

The clinical presentation of the newborn will depend on the circumstances of in-utero exposure: the drug(s) used, timing, amount of last maternal use, and maternal and infant metabolism and excretion (Table 118.2). If more than 1 week has elapsed since the last fetal drug exposure, the incidence of withdrawal symptoms is low.

Physical examination of the newborn may reveal tachycardia, tachypnea, tremors, and hyperreflexia. Premature infants may exhibit a high-pitched cry, poor feeding, and tachypnea but are less likely to have fever or changes in stools, tone, or reflexes, perhaps because of the relative immaturity of the premature's nervous system, or to differences in drug exposure.

The infant should be examined for features of fetal alcohol syndrome (FAS), especially in the setting of polydrug use. Alcohol is the only commonly used substance clearly linked to birth defects. Microcephaly, altered palmar crease pattern, pectus excavatum, atrial septal defect, strabismus, and facial dysmorphic features (e.g., short palpebral fissure, thin upper lip, smooth philtrum, maxillary hypoplasia, and short nose) comprise the features of FAS. However, infants exposed to alcohol in utero may lack all of the foregoing features, yet display neurobehavioral and motor problems later in infancy or childhood.

In-utero exposure to cocaine, a powerful vasoconstrictor, is thought to be potentially teratogenic, causing fetal organ defects of structure and function, including necrotizing enterocolitis, renal and genitourinary malformations, and CNS infarctions and hemorrhage. Recent data, however, show that although theoretically possible, the vascular defects do not appear consistently with in utero cocaine exposure.

It is the characteristics of newborn behavior that often impel the provider to consider drug exposure. Because cocaine and methamphetamines are potent vasoconstrictors, they stimulate the release and block the reuptake of dopamine, epinephrine, norepinephrine, and serotonin. Stimulant-exposed newborns are more jittery, and have a hyperactive Moro response, excessive sucking, poor organizational response to environmental stimuli, and more stress behaviors (such as crying) than non-exposed infants.

Conversely, infants exposed to depressants (e.g., alcohol, barbiturates, diazepam, phencyclidine (PCP), and volatile inhalants) develop neonatal abstinence syndrome (NAS) (Table 118.3). NAS is a generalized disorder consisting of CNS hyperirritability, gastrointestinal symptoms (e.g., vomiting, diarrhea), respiratory distress, and autonomic symptoms (e.g., sneezing, sweating). Infants exposed in utero to heroin, prescription pain drugs containing opiates (e.g., morphine, codeine), SSRIs, or methadone may also experience NAS, although 25% to 40% of infants with known exposure are asymptomatic or display only mild symptoms. Although the majority will show symptoms from within minutes of birth to 72 hours after delivery, the onset may be delayed up to 2 weeks, especially with maternal methadone use. Infants exposed to more than 5 marijuana cigarettes per week may show marked

TABLE 118.2

CLINICAL MANIFESTATIONS OF NEONATAL ABSTINENCE SYNDROME IN THE NEWBORN

Neurologic excitability	Gastrointestinal dysfunction	Autonomic signs
Tremors	Poor feeding	Increased sweating
Irritability	Uncoordinated and constant suck	Nasal stuffiness
Increased wakefulness	Vomiting	Rhinorrhea
High-pitched crying	Diarrhea	Mottling
Increased muscle tone	Dehydration	Temperature instability
Hyperactive DTRs	Poor weight gain	Fever
Exaggerated Moro reflex		Tearing
Seizures		
Frequent yawning, sneezing		
Excoriation of knees/elbows		
Coarse/"flapping" tremors—bilateral		
Rigidity of limbs, resisting flexion or extension		
Tachypnea		

DTRs: deep tendon reflexes.

TABLE 118.3

CLINICAL SIGNS AND SYMPTOMS OF NEONATAL ABSTINENCE SYNDROME

Signs & symptoms	Heroin	Methadone	Cocaine	Amphetamines	Marijuana	Barbiturates
CENTRAL NERVOUS SYSTEM						
Irritability	√	√	Early sign		√	√
Restlessness						√
Tremors	√	√	√	√	√	√
High-pitched cry	√	√	√			
Fist sucking	√	√	√			
Yawning	√					
Abnormal sleep		√	√	√	√	√
Seizures	Less often	√				
Drowsiness			Late sign	√		
Increased sleep			√	√		
Excessive crying		√	√	√		√
Hypertonicity	√	√	√	√		
GASTROINTESTINAL						
Diarrhea	√	√				√
Vomiting	√	√				√
Poor feeding	√		√	√		
AUTONOMIC DYSFUNCTION						
Sneezing	√	√				
Stuffy nose	√	√				
Sweating	√	√				
Tachycardia			√	√		
Tachypnea	√	√				

Used with permission: Tran, JH. treatment of neonatal abstinence Syndrome. *J. Pediatric Health Care* 1999; 13:295–302.

tremors, startle, and altered visual responsiveness at 2 to 4 days of age.

In the case of prenatal depressant exposure, neurobehavioral characteristics (i.e., NAS) have been well documented, yet it is important to note that ongoing research on the neurobehavioral responses of drug-exposed infants has resulted in conflicting data. The newborn's nervous system responds similarly to a variety of stimuli: a jittery infant may be drug exposed, but he may also be hypoglycemic, hypocalcemic, septic, or have an intracranial hemorrhage. These diagnoses must also be carefully considered in the evaluation of a jittery infant. Further, because many drug-exposed infants may be asymptomatic, they are erroneously considered candidates for early discharge.

MANAGEMENT

The infant in acute distress must be assessed and its most urgent presenting symptoms(s) managed appropriately. It is important to remember that the use of naloxone hydrochloride during resuscitation of a newly delivered opiate-addicted infant is contraindicated because the opiate antagonist may precipitate abrupt withdrawal and possible seizures.

Management of the drug-exposed infant is predominantly supportive and involves swaddling, frequent small feedings, and reduction of environmental stimuli. Adding pharmacologic therapy prolongs hospitalization and exposes the infant to additional drugs that may not be indicated. Therefore, the decision to start medications to control symptoms should be based on the severity of NAS and the drugs involved. Intravenous fluids and electrolytes may occasionally be necessary to stabilize the condition of an infant in acute withdrawal.

A scoring system, such as the neonatal abstinence scoring system (NASS, Finnegan 1992), the Lipsitz tool (Lipsitz 1975), and the Neonatal Withdrawal Inventory (Zahorodny 1998) may be used for infants withdrawing from opiates. The NASS (Fig. 118.1) is the most widely used scoring system. Its applicability in cases of other drug exposures remains undefined. The NASS allows caregivers to assess signs and symptoms falling into three categories: (1) CNS disturbances; (2) metabolic, vasomotor, and respiratory disturbances; and (3) gastrointestinal disturbances. The infant is observed every 2 to 4 hours, and the score is used to grade the severity of the symptoms and to monitor the clinical course. Although widely used, the NASS carries a margin of error, due to the subjectivity of the signs and symptoms. For this reason, there are also no specific recommendations for scores that require intervention. Our experience is that scores of 8 to 12 may require intervention and that those above 12 usually need medications to control symptoms. The NASS should be seen as an approximation of the clinical course and should not be used as the sole basis for treatment decisions or changes in drug dosages, especially if only one or two scores are available. If at all possible, treatment decisions should be based on daily average scores or a trend in scores over 24 to 48 hours.

It is necessary to remember that the NASS is for withdrawal from opiates. If used in the setting of cocaine withdrawal, these scores indicate the *toxic* effects of cocaine rather than evidence of withdrawal. With intrauterine cocaine exposure, neurobehavioral abnormalities occur on days 2 and 3, which is consistent with the effects of cocaine rather than withdrawal from it. Infants exposed to stimulants (e.g., amphetamine, cocaine) appear to be less symptomatic than infants in opiate withdrawal. Infants who experience withdrawal symptoms from

Date		Weight		SCORE	AM				PM				COMMENTS
	SIGNS AND SYMPTOMS												
Central nervous system disturbances	Excessive High Pitched (or other) Cry			2									
	Continuous High Pitched (or other) Cry			3									
	Sleeps < 1 hour after feeding			3									
	Sleeps < 2 hours after feeding			2									
	Sleeps < 3 hours after feeding			1									
	Hyperactive Moro Reflex			2									
	Markedly Hyperactive Moro Reflex			3									
	Mild Tremors Disturbed			1									
	Moderate/Severe Tremors Disturbed			2									
	Mild Tremors Undisturbed			3									
	Moderate/Severe Tremors Undisturbed			4									
	Increased Muscle Tone			2									
	Excoriation (Specific area)			1									
	Myoclonic Jerks			3									
	Generalized Convulsions			5									
Metabolic/Vasomotor/ Respiratory disturbances	Sweating			1									
	Fever < 101 (99-100.8°F/37.2-38.2 °C)			1									
	Fever > 101 (38.4°C and higher)			2									
	Frequent yawning (> 3–4 times/Interval)			1									
	Mottling			1									
	Nasal Stuffiness			1									
	Sneezing (> 3–4 times/Interval)			1									
	Nasal Flaring			2									
	Respiratory Rate > 60/min			1									
	Respiratory Rate > 60/min with retractions			2									
Gastrointestinal	Excessive Sucking			1									
	Poor PO Feeding			2									
	Regurgitation			2									
	Projectile Vomiting			3									
	Loose Stools			2									
	Watery Stools			3									
	Total Score												
	Initials of Scorer												

FIGURE 118.1. Neonatal Abstinence Scoring System (NASS). (Used with permission from Finnegan LP, Kaltenbach K. The assessment and management of neonatal abstinence syndrome. In: Hoekelman RA, Nelson NM, eds. *Primary pediatric care.* 2nd ed. St. Louis: Mosby; 1992: 1367–1378.)

PCP suffer from increased wakefulness, constant sucking, and the risk of intraventricular hemorrhage. Infants exposed to marijuana and barbiturates seem to experience more neurobehavioral than physiologic withdrawal symptoms.

Infants in withdrawal need a calming environment that includes swaddling (minimizing the added stimulation of startled movements), decreased light, and decreased noise. Gentle handling and up-and-down (rather than side-to-side) rocking may soothe the irritable infant. Frequent diaper changes are necessary to reduce skin excoriation (from frequent stools). Intake, output, and weight should be checked daily to assess hydration and caloric status in the face of vomiting, diarrhea, and/or feeding problems.

Because withdrawal is a hypermetabolic state, the infant may demonstrate poor feeding and subsequent weight loss due to inadequate calorie intake. A hypercaloric formula (e.g., 22 to 27 kcal/ounce) may be necessary to meet increased caloric requirements up to 150 to 250 cal/kg/day. A pacifier should be provided for excessive sucking, and breast-feeding should be encouraged if the mother is drug abstinent (or well maintained on methadone), not abusing other substances, and HIV negative.

Because withdrawal from sedative-hypnotics or narcotics may be life-threatening, pharmacologic therapy may be necessary for the severely addicted infant (Table 118.4). Indications for starting drug therapy include seizures, poor feeding, severe diarrhea and vomiting, excess weight loss, dehydration, inability to sleep, and fever not due to an infectious etiology. Drug therapy helps decrease signs and symptoms of withdrawal, but its effects on long-term morbidity are unknown. Use of a drug in the same class as that causing withdrawal is recommended. Drugs approved by the United States Food and Drug Administration for treating drug withdrawal include benzodiazepines for alcohol withdrawal and methadone for opioid withdrawal. Other management options include tincture of opium, morphine sulfate, clonidine, phenobarbital, chlorpromazine, and diazepam. Recommended dosages are listed in Table 118.4. Tincture of opium is preferred to paregoric because of concerns about exposing infants to benzoic acid, which displaces bilirubin from binding sites and can result in kernicterus at lower bilirubin levels. Advantages and disadvantages of each of the medications must be considered. Therapy is adequate if it decreases abstinence scores, improves thermal regulation, improves sleeping between feedings and medication dosing, and decreases motor activities, such as crying, sucking, and restlessness. Stable symptoms and NASS scores for 3 to 5 days are an indication to initiate weaning from pharmacologic therapy.

LABORATORY STUDIES

With appropriate history or clinical findings, drug screening for both the mother and the infant are indicated. Urine screening may used for the mother, although the results will depend on many factors (e.g., specific drug and dosage, time of most recent use). For many drugs, remote use may not be detectable (Table 118.5). Although blood and urine drug screening have been used in the infant, screening meconium for drugs is simpler and more reliable for amphetamines, cocaine, opiates, marijuana, and PCP. Meconium starts to form in the bowels at 16 to 18 weeks gestation, and drug metabolites accumulate in it; therefore, drugs used during the last 20 weeks of gestation can usually be detected. Screening the infant's urine or blood may be reliable if maternal drug use occurred in the 24 to 72 hours prior to delivery. Meconium screening will detect drugs in smaller amounts and is easier to collect. Meconium testing is 93% sensitive and has an 82% positive predictive value.

TABLE 118.4

TABLE 118.4

PHARMACOLOGIC THERAPIES IN NEONATAL ABSTINENCE SYNDROME

Medication	Dosage	Comments
Paregoric (tincture of opium) (anhydrous morphine 0.4 mg/mL)	0.2–0.5 mL/dose q 3–4 hr PO *or* 4–6 drops q 4–6 hr; may increase by 2 drops until clinical improvement	■ Improves sucking/caloric consumption. ■ When symptoms controlled, begin to taper dose by 10–20% per day; *each* decrease only after symptoms controlled for 3–5 days.
Phenobarbital	15–20 mg/kg loading IM *then* 3–4 mg/kg/day maintenance PO divided q 12 hr	■ Maintain 4–5 days, then taper dose by 10–20% per day. ■ Mild symptoms (tremulousness) are not indications to increase dose.
Diazepam	0.3–0.5 mg/kg q 8 hr (0.9–1.5 mg/kg/day); initial dose IM, then PO	■ Allows rapid suppression of symptoms. ■ Slow excretion—up to 1 month. ■ Decreased suck. ■ Do not use in jaundice or premature infant.
Methadone	0.1–0.5 mg/kg/day divided every 4–12 hr	■ Increase by 0.05 mg/kg/dose until symptoms are well controlled. ■ Taper dose by 10–20% per day; *each* decrease only after 7 days with symptoms controlled. ■ Treatment usually longer (5 days to 4 months). ■ Long half-life (26 hours).
Chlorpromazine	0.5–0.7 mg/kg/dose loading *then* 2–2.8 mg/kg/day in divided doses q 6 hr	■ Decrease dose over 2–3 weeks.
Clonidine	0.5–1 µg/kg single dose *then* 3–5 mg/kg/day divided doses every 4–6 hr	Increase by 0.5 µg/kg over 1–2 days until maintenance dose is achieved.

Maternal screening for hepatitis B and C, as well as HIV, should be strongly considered. Tests for chlamydia, syphilis, and gonorrhea must be performed if not done prenatally. Management of the infant if any of these tests are positive is addressed in *The Red Book: Report of the Committee on Infectious Diseases* by the AAP.

DISCHARGE

The decision to discharge an infant who has been drug-exposed must be made on an individual basis. In most cases, early discharge of a known drug-exposed infant is contraindicated.

TABLE 118.5

TABLE 118.5

DETECTABILITY OF DRUGS IN URINE

Drug	Duration	Comments
Cocaine	2 days	Benzoylecgonine is the metabolite detected in urine
Marijuana	1–3 days >30 days	Occasional smoker Chronic daily smoker
Methamphetamines	1–2 days	Assays cross-react with ephedrine and phenylpropanolamine
Opiates	2–4 days	Does not distinguish between codeine and morphine Heroin is metabolized to codeine and morphine
Phencyclidine	Up to 1 week	

However, it must be reiterated that because many drug-exposed infants will be asymptomatic or mildly symptomatic, early discharge may be considered by the uninformed provider.

Social work consultation is mandatory to assess housing, baby supplies, and parenting skills of the mother; for possible child protective services referral; and to assist with referral to treatment facilities, if warranted. After discharge, outpatient follow-up should be scheduled within 1 week. Communication with the outpatient provider is essential if follow-up responsibility will be assumed by someone other than the physician caring for the infant during its hospital stay. Frequent office visits allow weight monitoring, infant behavior evaluation, and assessment of the mother's coping and parenting skills. Public health nurse referral, as well as referral to early intervention programs, is strongly encouraged.

PEARLS

■ Every newborn examination should include a review of the maternal history of drug use, and the pediatric provider should obtain a drug history directly from the mother.
■ To avoid missed diagnosis, drug withdrawal must be considered in the differential for many neonatal symptoms.
■ Newborn *behaviors* are most often the trigger for the provider to consider drug exposure.

■ Twenty-five percent to forty percent of infants with known exposure are asymptomatic or display only mild symptoms.
■ Management of the drug-exposed infant is predominantly supportive.
■ Pharmacologic therapy may unnecessarily prolong hospitalization if withdrawal symptoms are mild, but should be used with severe symptoms.
■ A tool such as the NASS should be used to determine the severity of the symptoms and to monitor the clinical course.
■ Meconium toxicology screening is accurate and reliable.

Suggested Readings

American Academy of Pediatrics Committee on Drugs. Policy statement: neonatal drug withdrawal. *Pediatrics* 1998;101:1079–1088.

Beauman, SS. Identification and management of neonatal abstinence syndrome. *J Infusion Nurs* 2005;28:159–167.

Buchi KF. The drug-exposed infant in the well-baby nursery. *Clin Perinatol* 1998;25:335–350.

Finnegan LP, Kaltenbach K. Neonatal abstinence syndrome. In: Hoekelman RA, Nelson NM (eds), *Primary Pediatric Care* 2nd ed. Mosby yearbook, Inc. St. Louis. 1992 (pp. 1367–1378).

Lipsitz PJ. A proposed narcotic withdrawal score for use with newborn infants, a pragmatic evaluation of its efficacy. *Clin. Pediator* 14:592–594, 1975.

Zahorodny W, Rom C, Whitney W, et al. The Neonatal withdrawal inventory: a simplified score of newborn withdrawal. *J Dev Behav Pediator* 19(2):89–93, 1998.

CHAPTER 119 ■ CONGENITAL INFECTION

JAMES J. CUMMINGS

Strictly speaking, the term "congenital infection" should refer to an infection present at the time of birth and, therefore, acquired in utero (i.e., transplacentally acquired), in contrast to infection that is acquired during the birth process (i.e., vertically transmitted). Although still present at delivery, the infection may have begun weeks or even months earlier. Etiologic agents are quite varied and include viruses, bacteria, and protozoa. Despite their diversity, these agents share two important characteristics:

1. The propensity to attack specific fetal organ systems.
2. The tendency to lead to a chronic carrier state that may result in complications delayed for months or even years.

Although symptomatic cases often present with a "classic" collection of clinical findings, the majority of congenital infections are asymptomatic. Nevertheless, all infants with congenital infection are at risk for long-term complications.

Although it is important to diagnose asymptomatic infants with congenital infection, it is also important not to waste time and resources evaluating infants with minimal risk of congenital infection. This chapter will help the clinician to

1. Decide which infants are at highest risk for chronic infection, whether clinically apparent or not.
2. Recognize other noninfectious conditions that may overlap clinically with congenital infection.

Finally, because many of the sequelae of congenital infection are not amenable to treatment, preventive strategies for counseling patients of childbearing potential will be reviewed.

Congenital infection is relatively common. It is estimated that intrauterine infection results in more than 30,000 infected newborns each year in the United States, and approximately half of these children will become symptomatic sometime during infancy and early childhood. Cytomegalovirus (CMV) can be isolated from the cervix or urine in approximately 3% of pregnant women, approximately half of whom have a primary CMV infection. In the United States, it is estimated that approximately 35% of the adult population have serologic evidence of previous infection with *Toxoplasma gondii*, and over 50% have evidence of CMV. Up to 40% of women of childbearing age lack immunity to parvovirus. The subsequent risk of fetal infection after active maternal parvovirus infection can be as high as 30%, depending on the stage of gestation when infection occurs. In the last 20 years, dramatic increases in tuberculosis and syphilis among women of childbearing age have been found, with attendant risks to their fetuses.

A list of microorganisms that can cause transplacental infection is given in Table 119.1. Among these, CMV, which may be isolated from urine in approximately 1% of all newborns, is by far the most common. In contrast, *T. gondii*, varicella-zoster, and herpes simple virus HSV account for less than 0.1% of all congenital infections.

In recognition of the fact that a rather heterogeneous group of infectious agents appeared to cause a somewhat homogeneous clinical pattern of disease, the acronym "TORCH" was coined in 1974. This mnemonic refers to specific organisms causing congenital infections, including toxoplasmosis, rubella, CMV, and herpes simplex virus (HSV). Unfortunately, the acronym distracts the clinician from a variety of other agents (the "O" in TORCH, a listing of that is quite long and continues to grow), and suggests a workup that may be insufficient (e.g., TORCH titers).

Despite their inclusion in Table 119.1, many viruses, including HSV, human immunodeficiency virus (HIV), and the hepatitis viruses, are rarely acquired as intrauterine infections. They are typically transmitted vertically (i.e., during the delivery process), and thus belong more appropriately in a discussion of perinatally acquired infections (e.g., group B streptococcus). Although it may cause significant disease in the developing fetus, rubella rarely occurs as a congenital infection due to efforts at worldwide vaccination. Despite its terrible morbidity, congenital rubella will probably be of only historic interest by the end of this decade. On the other hand, recent reports of dermal erythropoiesis in infants born after intrauterine parvovirus B_{19} infection makes it an important addition to the list of congenital infectious agents.

CLINICAL FEATURES

Despite the heterogeneity of organisms that can infect the fetus, the picture of subsequent developmental anomalies and clinical findings are remarkably similar. These commonly include:

■ Petechiae
■ Dermal erythropoiesis ("blueberry-muffin spots")
■ Maculopapular rash
■ Hepatosplenomegaly
■ Direct hyperbilirubinemia
■ Hemolytic anemia
■ Thrombocytopenia
■ Pneumonitis
■ Growth retardation

Numerous other findings are possible (Table 119.2), some of which may suggest specific agents, such as bone lesions with rubella or syphilis, chorioretinitis with rubella and toxoplasmosis, and intracranial calcifications in congenital CMV or toxoplasmosis.

Other findings are virtually pathognomonic for specific conditions, such as:

■ Cataracts or glaucoma with rubella
■ Myocarditis with enteroviruses
■ Cicatricial skin lesions with varicella

TABLE 119.1

ORGANISMS ASSOCIATED WITH CONGENITAL INFECTION

Group	Organism
Viruses	Cytomegalovirus
	Enteroviruses
	Hepatitis viruses (B, C, E)
	Herpes simplex
	Human immunodeficiency virus
	Lymphocytic choriomeningitis virus
	Parvovirus
	Rubeola
	Rubella
	Varicella
Bacteria	*Campylobacter fetus*
	Mycobacterium tuberculosis
	Listeria monocytogenes
	Salmonella typhosa
	Treponema pallidum
Protozoa	*Plasmodium species*
	Toxoplasma gondii
	Trypanosoma cruzi

- Koplik spots (tiny, granular, slightly raised white lesions with an erythematous halo on the buccal mucosa) with measles
- Disseminated vesicular bullous eruptions on the palms and soles with syphilis
- Microcephaly with CMV

As the list of organisms grows and additional cases are described, the overlap between clinical presentations has increased; therefore, caution must be exercised before assuming that a particular clinical finding is "diagnostic." Even so-called "classic" findings lose their diagnostic significance if other signs are missing. Thrombocytopenia, hepatosplenomegaly, growth retardation, cataracts, glaucoma, microcephaly, or even intracranial calcifications, if found in isolation, are unlikely to be the result of an intrauterine infection. Infection in utero tends to be indiscriminate and causes multiple organ injury. Thus, an isolated finding that may be part of a "classic" presentation should not automatically trigger a workup for congenital infection, particularly if another explanation for the isolated finding can be identified. For example, intrauterine growth retardation (IUGR) occurs in approximately 5% of all

TABLE 119.2

CLINICAL MANIFESTATIONS OF CONGENITAL INFECTIONS

Hepatosplenomegaly	Intracranial calcifications
Jaundice	Myocarditis
Growth retardation	Heart defects
Lymphadenopathy	Bone lesions (periostitis,
Pneumonitis	osteochondritis)
Dermal erythropoiesis	Glaucoma
Thrombocytopenia	Cataracts
Maculopapular exanthem	Chorioretinitis
Microcephaly	Optic atrophy
Hydrocephalus	Microphthalmia

pregnancies but has a noninfectious etiology in 90% to 95% of cases. Therefore, routine evaluation of IUGR infants for congenital infection is unwarranted.

PROGNOSIS

The sequelae of congenital infection can be devastating. Ninety percent of infants who are symptomatic with CMV at birth will have significant neurodevelopmental impairment. Twenty percent to forty percent of infants born to untreated HIV-infected mothers will develop acquired immunodeficiency syndrome. Most infants with congenital toxoplasmosis will be symptomatic at birth and develop serious neurodevelopmental sequelae during childhood. Virtually all infants born to women with untreated primary or secondary syphilis will become infected; even latent maternal infection results in a neonatal infection rate of up to 40%.

Most infants with congenital infection are asymptomatic but have significant risk for long-term complications. Ninety percent of congenital CMV is asymptomatic, yet 10% of these infants will develop hearing loss and/or mental retardation. Most infants with congenital toxoplasma infection are asymptomatic at birth, yet most develop sequelae during childhood or adulthood. Approximately two-thirds of infants with congenital syphilis will appear clinically normal at birth; overt clinical disease may not present until 2 years of age, followed by keratitis in 5 to 20 years, and eighth cranial nerve disease in 10 to 40 years.

APPROACH TO DIAGNOSIS

There are three key elements in the diagnosis of congenital infection: maternal history, placental pathology, and neonatal evaluation. These are covered in the following sections.

Maternal History

Certain elements of maternal history should be routinely elicited as part of every newborn evaluation. These include results of specific laboratory testing (e.g., venereal disease research laboratory (VDRL) test, rubella titer, hepatitis B surface antigen), exposures or illnesses (e.g., varicella, tuberculosis), and substance use (including tobacco, alcohol, and illicit drugs).

Even if maternal rubella status is unknown, the risk of congenital rubella is vanishingly small in the United States due to routine immunization since the 1960s. However, although rubella is on the verge of elimination in the United States, it remains a threat among women of child-bearing age from countries where routine childhood immunization is not practiced. Most U.S. cases in recent years have been among Hispanic women from Central and South America, particularly from the Dominican Republic, Peru, and Guatemala, which did not have routine rubella immunization practices until recently. Aggressive efforts in the last 5 years by the Pan American Health Organization have resulted in routine rubella immunization throughout the Americas; future cases of congenital rubella are more likely to come from Asia or Africa, which largely continue to have no routine rubella immunization practices.

When the diagnosis of congenital infection is being considered in a newborn with suggestive clinical and/or laboratory findings, additional maternal history may suggest specific infectious agents. This history might include the following:

- Mononucleosis-like syndrome and/or lymphadenopathy (CMV, syphilis, toxoplasmosis, HIV)
- Flu-like syndrome (parvovirus)
- Rash (rubella, parvovirus, enterovirus, syphilis)

- Arthralgia/arthritis (rubella, parvovirus)
- Day care exposure (CMV, parvovirus)
- Handling or ingestion of raw meat that has never been frozen (toxoplasmosis)
- Travel to malarial endemic regions
- High-risk sexual behavior (CMV, hepatitis B [HBV], HIV, syphilis, HSV)

In addition, women with HIV are often co-infected with CMV, HSV, and occasionally, *T. gondii*, and these agents tend to develop latency after a primary infection. Exposures or disease immediately prior to conception may also be important: with rubella, for example, viremia can persist for weeks. The maternal history is sometimes not helpful because some serious infections are commonly asymptomatic. For example, fewer than 10% of women who contract toxoplasmosis during pregnancy will have lymphadenopathy or other symptoms.

Congenital tuberculosis is uncommon, and affected infants are often asymptomatic; hence, the clinician must maintain a high index of suspicion. Women with known exposure to tuberculosis who then develop pleural effusion, miliary or meningeal disease, or endometritis shortly before or during pregnancy should be considered at high risk for intrauterine transmission of tuberculosis. Active pulmonary disease in the mother is much more likely to cause perinatal rather than intrauterine transmission.

Placental Pathology

Although placental pathology is not usually helpful in diagnosing a specific infection, it can often help distinguish between infection (either acute or chronic) and other, noninfectious disorders that may account for the observed findings in the neonate. Placentomegaly with evidence of inflammation is suggestive of congenital infection. A small placenta with calcifications is suggestive of noninfectious microvascular disease (i.e., placental insufficiency). This latter finding in an infant with hepatomegaly, growth retardation, and thrombocytopenia suggests conditions such as maternal hypertension or chronic placental abruption.

Neonatal Evaluation

Suspect a congenital infection in any newborn with a combination of the findings included in Table 119.2. In the absence of specific maternal indications (e.g., a positive VDRL), consider the entire spectrum of congenital infection agents. Nevertheless, be judicious in the diagnostic workup; look for patterns of organ involvement, and then search for the more common and/or treatable conditions. Clinical examination should include:

- Measurement of length, weight, and head circumference
- Careful inspection of the skin for rash or petechiae
- Eye examination
- Cardiac evaluation
- Abdominal examination, including taking care to distinguish between true (abnormal) and relative (normal organ size in small-for-dates infants) hepatosplenomegaly

Although certain clinical findings may suggest a particular etiologic agent, there is much overlap and no single clinical finding should be considered "pathognomonic."

Basic diagnostic tests that often prove useful include a CBC (with coagulation studies if the infant is thrombocytopenic or actively bleeding), liver function tests, and cardiac imaging. CMV and *T. gondii* usually result in pancytopenia, while parvovirus only infects erythroid precursors. Rubella is associated with structural heart disease, but the cardiac dysfunction seen in enteroviral (myocarditis) or parvoviral (high output failure) infection is associated with a structurally normal heart. No evidence of coagulopathy or hepatitis is found in parvovirus infection; however, enteroviral infection is usually associated with severe coagulopathy and hepatic dysfunction.

The most reliable method of diagnosis depends on the agent involved. If the agent can be detected by direct examination of infected tissue or body fluid, this is the preferred method of diagnosis. Examples of such examinations include:

- Dark-field microscopy of placental tissue or skin lesions for syphilis
- Urine culture for CMV
- Culture of nasopharyngeal secretions for enterovirus and rubella
- Culture of stool for enterovirus
- Blood culture for listeria
- Tissue culture (either placental or neonatal) for *T. gondii*

Some organisms require particular conditions for culture (e.g., parvovirus requires the S-phase of mitosis to replicate and can only be cultured in bone marrow cells), and many agents cannot be reliably cultured at all. It is also important to note that neonatal (as opposed to congenital) infection can occur as a result of contact with agents in the mother's genital tract at delivery or through ingestion of infected breast milk. Thus, only positive cultures obtained during the first 1 to 2 weeks of life should be considered an indication of congenital infection.

When direct identification is not feasible, the next step is to detect antibody or antigen. Specific IgM antibody assays for toxoplasma and rubella are available, although recent data suggest that IgA antibody may be more sensitive. With either IgM or IgA, the likelihood of a false-negative result is high if the infection occurred before the fifth month of gestation, because fetal antibody response is negligible before that stage of development. For these and other organisms for which specific serologic evaluation is problematic or unavailable (CMV, HIV, parvovirus B_{19}, HSV, *T. pallidum*, and enteroviruses), detection by polymerase chain reaction should be considered. It is important to note that treatment during pregnancy does not appear to alter the ability to detect infection in the neonate. However, with or without maternal treatment, the potential for a false-negative test is still high. For example, it is estimated that 30% of cases of congenital toxoplasmosis test negative in the neonatal period.

Measurement of nonspecific total IgM may be elevated in the newborn with a variety of noninfectious conditions. Cord blood IgM is also rather insensitive; 20% of infants with congenital toxoplasmosis and 35% of infants with congenital rubella will have normal cord IgM levels. Hence, a total IgM titer is of little diagnostic use. Likewise, so-called "TORCH titer" packages should be avoided, because the actual tests included may vary between laboratories and reliability is questionable.

Detection of specific IgG in the newborn is not helpful because of passively transmitted maternal antibodies that persist for months postnatally. Serial titers taken postnatally that show a rise at age 2 to 4 months or that persist beyond 6 to 8 months may demonstrate infection. Titers from a single time point or paired titers conducted in different laboratory runs may be highly insensitive. Except in cases of very recent infection, negative neonatal IgG serology generally excludes the possibility of intrauterine infection. However, because commercial and hospital laboratories vary widely in their ability to isolate specific agents or accurately measure serologies, interpret negative results with caution. If the clinical picture is highly suspicious, repeat testing or the use of an alternate laboratory may be warranted.

Despite a high index of suspicion, some cases of congenital infection will not be confirmed by serologies or culture during the neonatal period. Therefore, even if asymptomatic at birth, any infant felt to be at high risk needs close follow-up.

MANAGEMENT

The management of congenital infection includes preventing the disease in the mother, reducing transmission from an exposed/infected mother to her fetus, reducing severity of disease in the fetus/neonate, and reducing long-term complications. The following discussion includes each of these approaches and concludes with current recommendations for some specific conditions.

As noted earlier, most congenital infections have already resulted in significant fetal/neonatal injury by the time they are diagnosed. Thus, prevention is of primary importance. This is accomplished by immunization against rubella and varicella, education of pregnant women to avoid communicable sources (particularly raw meat, cat litter, or individuals with infectious rashes or active tuberculosis), and passive immunization after known exposure. Although helpful, preventing maternal exposure during pregnancy does not completely eliminate fetal risk, because some infections contracted prior to pregnancy can later be transmitted to the fetus when the woman becomes pregnant. Immune globulin administration after exposure to rubella, varicella, measles, or enterovirus may modify, but does not consistently prevent, clinical disease in the pregnant woman, nor does it necessarily reduce risk to the fetus.

Unfortunately, for many agents, including enteroviruses and parvovirus, there is no proven way to reduce fetal risk after the mother is infected. However, after the fetus becomes infected, treatment initiated during pregnancy may reduce the incidence of sequelae (e.g., syphilis, toxoplasmosis).

Cytomegalovirus

Recent studies have suggested that prolonged ganciclovir treatment of symptomatic newborns with congenital CMV may reduce the incidence and severity of long-term hearing loss. The rationale for systemic treatment of CMV-infected infants comes from the observation that progressive hearing impairment appears to be mediated by immune complex deposition in the inner cochlea of the ear. However, the known toxicity of ganciclovir (currently the only medication evaluated for treatment of congenital CMV) precludes its routine use and restricts it to only the most severely affected infants. Unfortunately, this will have little or no impact on CMV-induced sensorineural hearing loss, because 90% of cases occur in infants who are asymptomatic at birth. The sensorineural hearing loss (usually unilateral, high-tone deafness) associated with CMV may be a slowly progressive disorder, and longitudinal audiologic assessments are necessary.

Toxoplasmosis

Recommended treatment for symptomatic infants with suspected congenital toxoplasmosis (or asymptomatic infants with confirmed infection) includes multidrug therapy with pyrimethamine and sulfadiazine, supplemented with folinic acid, for up to 1 year. Some experts suggest adding leucovorin during the initial week of therapy, and corticosteroids if CSF protein levels are greater than 1 g/dL. Infants with suspected congenital toxoplasmosis who have chorioretinitis should be started promptly on pyrimethamine and sulfadiazine, pending serologic confirmation. Because congenital toxoplasmosis is rare in the United States and issues of diagnosis and management remain somewhat controversial, consultation with an expert is advised.

Syphilis

It is imperative that the mother's serologic status be known, or assessed if unknown. Cord blood or infant serum is inade-

quate for screening, because these sources may be nonreactive even when the mother is seropositive. False-positive nontreponemal tests (usually low titers) in the mother can result from infection with Epstein–Barr virus (EBV), IV drug use, and various autoimmune diseases. However, because of the devastating consequences of congenital syphilis, *all infants born to seropositive mothers should have a quantitative nontreponemal syphilis test.* The test should be performed on the infant's sera, because tests on cord blood have poor sensitivity and specificity; it should be of the same type as that performed on the mother so that titers may be compared. Further evaluation is indicated if the mother's titer has increased fourfold, if the infant's titer is fourfold greater than the mother's, if the infant is symptomatic, or if the mother has one or more of the following conditions:

- Syphilis untreated, treated inadequately, or treatment not documented.
- Syphilis during pregnancy treated with a non-penicillin agent, such as erythromycin.
- Syphilis during pregnancy treated appropriately, but without the expected decrease in nontreponemal antibody titer.
- Syphilis treated less than 1 month before delivery.
- Syphilis treated before pregnancy but with insufficient serologic follow-up.

Further evaluation of the infant includes a VDRL test of CSF, long-bone radiographs (unless the diagnosis has otherwise been made), and pathologic examination of the placenta or umbilical cord using specific fluorescent antitreponemal antibody staining (FTA-ABS), if available.

Infants should be treated if they have proven disease, or probable disease as demonstrated by one or more of the following:

- Physical, laboratory, or radiographic evidence of active disease.
- Positive placental or umbilical cord test results for treponemes using FTA-ABS staining or dark-field test.
- A reactive VDRL on CSF.
- A serum quantitative nontreponemal titer that is at least fourfold higher than the mother's, using the same test, and preferably the same laboratory.

The preferred treatment of congenital syphilis is IV penicillin G (50,000 U/kg/dose) every 12 hours for the first 7 days of life, and every 8 hours thereafter, for a total of 10 days. Alternatively, penicillin G procaine (50,000 U/kg/day) may be given IM in a single daily dose for 10 days; however, adequate CSF concentrations may not be achieved by this approach. In either case, if more than 1 day of therapy is missed, the entire course should be repeated.

All infants with congenital syphilis should have repeat serologic nontreponemal tests at 3, 6, and 12 months of age. Infants with congenital neurosyphilis should have a repeat VDRL test of CSF at 6 months. Note that treponemal and nontreponemal antibodies are not protective; individuals with congenital syphilis infection can later acquire syphilis from horizontal (i.e., sexual) transmission.

Tuberculosis

Women who have only pulmonary tuberculosis are not likely to infect their fetuses, but may infect their infants after delivery. Congenital tuberculosis is rare, but may occur if the mother is bacillemic during pregnancy. *If congenital tuberculosis is suspected*, a tuberculin skin test, lumbar puncture, and cultures (gastric aspirate, tracheal aspirate, urine, and blood) should be performed on the infant, and *treatment should be initiated until further evaluation is completed.* The mother should have a skin test and chest radiograph; if both are positive, the infant should be separated from the mother until her sputum is tested. Although a tuberculin skin test should be done in the infant, the chance of a false negative is high; testing of family members is much more likely to yield reliable information. Treatment of the infant should initially include isoniazid, rifampin, pyrazinamide, and streptomycin or kanamycin. If meningitis is confirmed, corticosteroids should also be given.

PEARLS

- Congenital infections are more common than most clinicians realize, because most affected infants appear normal at birth.
- Long-term consequences of congenital infection may be devastating, particularly for congenital syphilis.
- Growth retardation alone should not generate a congenital infection workup.
- A targeted approach to diagnosis is preferred. TORCH titers and total IgM levels in the infant are not helpful.
- Review of maternal history, clinical examination, and basic laboratory tests often lead to a specific diagnosis.

Suggested Readings

Barton LL, Mets MB. Congenital lymphocytic choriomeningitis virus infection: decade of rediscovery. *Clin Infect Dis* 2001;33:1445.

Duff P. Immunotherapy for congenital cytomegalovirus infection. *N Engl J Med* 2005;353:1402. Editorial.

Fischer GW, Ottolini MG, Mond JJ. Prospects for vaccines during pregnancy and in the newborn period. *Clin Perinatol* 1997;24:231.

Hageman JR. Congenital and perinatal tuberculosis: discussion of difficult issues in diagnosis and management. *J Perinatol* 1998;18:389.

Hollier LM, Cox SM. Syphilis. *Semin Perinatol* 1998;22:323.

Nelson CT, Demmler GJ. Cytomegalovirus infection in the pregnant mother, fetus, and newborn infant. *Clin Perinatol* 1997;24:151.

Noyola DE, Demmler GJ, Nelson CT, et al. Early predictors of neurodevelopmental outcome in symptomatic congenital cytomegalovirus infection. *J Pediatr* 2001; 138:325.

Pickering LK, ed. *Red book: 2003 report of the Committee on Infectious Diseases.* 26th ed. Elk Grove Village, IL: American Academy of Pediatrics; 2003.

Reef SE, Frey TK, Theall K, et al. The changing epidemiology of rubella in the 1990s. *JAMA* 2002;287:464.

Ross SA, Boppana SB. Congenital cytomegalovirus infection: outcome and diagnosis. *Semin Pediatr Infect Dis* 2005;16:44.

Sanchez PJ, Wendel GD. Syphilis in pregnancy. *Clin Perinatol* 1997;24:71.

Singh AE, Romanowski B. Syphilis: review with emphasis on clinical, epidemiologic, and some biologic features. *Clin Microbiol Rev* 1999;12:187.

Starke JR. Tuberculosis: an old disease but a new threat to the mother, fetus, and neonate. *Clin Perinatol* 1997;24:107.

Wicher V, Wicher K. Pathogenesis of maternal-fetal syphilis revisited. *Clin Infect Dis* 2001;33:354.

CHAPTER 120 ■ AMBIGUOUS GENITALIA

YING T. CHANG

Although the law clearly distinguishes between males and females, nature may not always be so precise. The term *ambiguous genitalia* refers to a birth defect in which either the external genitalia do not have the typical appearance of either sex, or normal-appearing external genitalia do not concur with the genetic sex. It may refer to ambiguity of internal sex organs as well. Many people use "intersex" or "disorders of sexual development" to cover a broader spectrum of the disorders. The finding of ambiguous genitalia is generally considered a medical and psychosocial emergency, which requires multidisciplinary evaluation.

SEXUAL DIFFERENTIATION

Sexual differentiation is a complex process that usually is divided into four phases: genetic (chromosomal) sex, gonadal sex, phenotypic sex, and gender identification. The constitutive sex in the fetus is female. A functional testis is mandatory for normal male development, whereas an ovary is not required for a female phenotype. The sex-determining region of the Y chromosome (SRY) plays a critical role in testicular differentiation. One of the earliest effects of this SRY is the somatic cell migration from the mesonephros into the XY gonad to prepare for the development of testis cords. On the other hand, no equivalent specific ovary-determining factor has been identified, although the development of the ovary requires factors such as wingless-type MMTV integration site family-4 (WNT4) and the dosage-sensitive sex-reversal adrenal hypoplasia congenital locus on the X chromosome-1 (DAX1).

In the early stages of embryogenesis, under the influence of Wilms tumor suppressor gene (WT1) and steroidogenic factor-1 (SF1), the intermediate mesoderm develops into the genital ridge, which in turn develops into a bipotential gonad. This process is influenced by a transcriptional factor, SRY-related high-mobility group box 9 (SOX9), which contains a region homologous to a sex-determining region in SRY (Fig. 120.1). At 6 weeks of gestation, if a normal SRY along with other required factors are present, the bipotential gonad differentiates into a testis. A testis contains two important cell groups, the Sertoli cells and the Leydig cells. The Sertoli cells make Müllerian-inhibiting substance (MIS) under the influence of WT1 and SF1. MIS suppresses the development of Müllerian structures into the Fallopian tubes, uterus, and upper portion of the vagina. The Leydig cells produce testosterone, which stimulates the Wolffian ducts' development into seminiferous tubules, epididymis, and vas deferens. Concurrently, testosterone is converted by 5α-reductase into dihydrotestosterone (DHT), which is the most influential hormone in the development of male external genitalia. The masculinization of external genitalia begins at 9 weeks and is completed at 11 to 12 weeks of gestation. The testes start descending at the 12th week, reach the internal inguinal ring at 22 weeks, and enter the scrotum after 28 weeks.

In the female, normal ovarian differentiation requires the presence of germ cells. Otherwise, the gonad degenerates into a fibrous streak. In a normal genetic female, the SRY gene is absent; therefore, the bipotential gonad does not develop into a testis. Although the factors directing ovarian development are not well characterized, it appears that WNT4 promotes the expression of DAX1, which antagonizes SF1 and subsequently represses SOX9, resulting in the development of granulosa cells instead of Sertoli cells. Because there are no Sertoli cells to generate MIS, Müllerian structures develop into the Fallopian tubes and uterus. On the other hand, WNT4 inhibits the transformation of bipotential interstitial cells to Leydig cells. Without Leydig cells to produce testosterone, Wolffian ducts begin to degenerate. Vaginal development starts at 11 weeks, and feminization of the external genitalia is completed at 20 weeks.

Recently, retinoic acid has been found to play an important role in ovarian development in mice. In the early embryonic stage, retinoic acid stimulates the expression of a gene called "stimulated by retinoic acid gene 8" (Stra8), which directs a bipotential gonad to develop into an ovary. However, if the gonad produces the enzyme CYP26B1, which degrades retinoic acid, the gonad develops into a testis.

During the first trimester, placental human chorionic gonadotropin (hCG) stimulates testicular testosterone production; later, gonadotropins from the pituitary gland replace placental hCG. Consequently, with a few exceptions, a deficiency of LH and FSH from the pituitary gland does not result in ambiguous genitalia, but rather causes micropenis in males and has no effect on female external genitalia.

ETIOLOGY AND CLINICAL MANIFESTATIONS OF AMBIGUOUS GENITALIA

Because of the complexity of sexual differentiation, various classifications of ambiguous genitalia have been proposed. Simplistically, ambiguous genitalia result either from overexposure to androgens, causing virilization of genetic females; or androgen deficiency or insensitivity, causing undervirilization in genetic males during the first 12 weeks of gestation. Table 120.1 gives a simplified classification for practical purposes. A revised nomenclature and classification was proposed in a consensus statement which was published in 2006 after this chapter was prepared.

Male Hermaphroditism

Classification of hermaphroditism is based on the type of gonads. In male pseudohermaphroditism, the karyotype is 46,XY and the gonads are testes. The external genitalia are

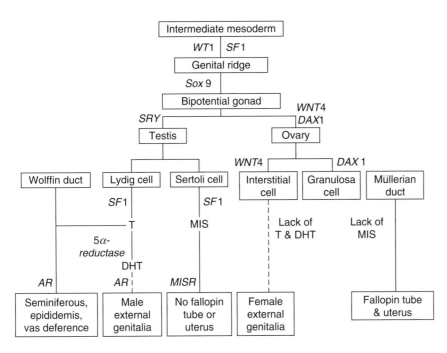

FIGURE 120.1. Sex determination and differentiation cascade. (WT1, the Wilms tumor suppressor gene; SF1, steroidogenic factor-1; SOX9, autosomal gene containing SRY-like HMG box; SRY, sex-determining region Y; WNT4, wingless-type MMTV integration site family-4; DAX1, DSS-congenital adrenal hypoplasia critical region on the X gene 1; MIS, Müllerian inhibiting substance; MISR, MIS receptor; T, testosterone; DHT, dihydrotestosterone; AR: androgen receptor.)

TABLE 120.1

DISORDERS OF SEX DETERMINATION

I. Male pseudohermaphroditism (MPH): incomplete virilization in subjects with testis. 46,XY
   A. Inadequate androgen production
      1. Testis dysgenesis or hypoplasia
         a. Dysgenetic male pseudohermaphroditism
         b. Leydig cell aplasia or hypoplasia
         c. Testicular regression syndrome
         d. Denys–Drash syndrome
         e. Frasier syndrome
         f. WAGR syndrome (Wilm's tumor, aniridia, genitourinary anomalies, and mental retardation)
         g. Klinefelter syndrome
      2. Androgen biosynthesis defects
         a. Defect in cholesterol biosynthesis
            1) 7-Dehydrocholesterol reductase deficiency (Smith–Lemli–Opitz syndrome)
         b. Defect in adrenal and/or gonadal steroid biosynthesis
            1) Congenital adrenal hyperplasia (CAH)
               a) Steroid acute regulatory (StAR) protein deficiency (congenital lipoid adrenal hyperplasia)
               b) Cholesterol side-chain cleavage (SCC) enzyme deficiency
               c) 3β-hydroxysteroid dehydrogenase (3βHSD) deficiency
               d) 17α-hydroxylase (17-OH) deficiency
               e) 17,20-desmolase (17,20-D) deficiency
               f) Cytochrome P450 oxidoreductase deficiency (Antley–Bixler syndrome)
               g) 17β-hydroxysteroid dehydrogenase (17βHSD) deficiency
         c. Defect in dihydrotestosterone (DHT) biosynthesis
            2) 5α-reductase deficiency

   B. Inadequate response to androgens
      1. Androgen insensitivity (resistance) syndrome
   C. Impaired Müllerian-inhibiting substance (MIS) effect—persistent Müllerian duct syndrome
      1. MIS deficiency
      2. MIS receptor defect
II. Female pseudohermaphroditism (FPH): virilization in subjects with ovary. 46,XX
   A. Excessive fetal androgens
      1. CAH
         a. 3βHSD deficiency
         b. 21-hydroxylase deficiency
         c. 11β-hydroxylase deficiency
         d. Cytochrome P450 oxidoreductase (POR) deficiency
      2. Aromatase deficiency
   B. Excessive maternal androgens
      1. Adrenal or ovarian tumor
      2. Luteoma of pregnancy
      3. Ingestion of androgens or progestins
III. True hermaphroditism
IV. Pure gonadal dysgenesis
V. Mixed gonadal dysgenesis
VI. Other gene mutations or chromosomal anomalies
   A. SRY: gonadal dysgenesis
   B. DAX1: gonadal dysgenesis, adrenal hypoplasia congenital
   C. SF1: gonadal and adrenal dysgenesis
   D. SOX9: campomelic dysplasia, male gonadal dysgenesis or XY sex reversal
   E. Turner syndrome

female or an undervirilized male. The Wolffian structures may not be well-formed if Leydig cells are unable to produce sufficient testosterone secondary to Leydig cell hypoplasia or impaired androgen production, or if there is androgen insensitivity. On the other hand, the Müllerian structures may be present if Sertoli cells do not secret MIS, or if there is an MIS receptor defect.

Female Hermaphroditism

In female pseudohermaphroditism, the karyotype is 46,XX and the gonads are ovaries. The external genitalia are consistent with a virilized female without palpable gonads. The Müllerian structures are present because there is no testicular tissue to produce MIS.

True Hermaphroditism

In true hermaphroditism, both testicular and ovarian tissues coexist in either the same gonad or opposite gonads. The Müllerian or Wolffian structures, as well as the external genitalia, correspond to the gonadal tissue, functions, and locations. For example, a testis on one side results in Wolffian structure and male external genitalia on that side, whereas an ovary on the other side results in Müllerian structure and undervirilized external genitalia on that side. The predominant karyotypes are 46,XX (60%); 46,XX/46,XY (13%); and 46,XY (12%); others exist in much smaller numbers.

Pure Gonadal Dysgenesis

In pure gonadal dysgenesis, a 46,XX or 46,XY subject presents with bilateral streak gonads, Müllerian structures, and normal-appearing female external genitalia. The etiology may involve mutation of the SRY or SOX9 gene.

Mixed Gonadal Dysgenesis

In mixed gonadal dysgenesis, there is a streak gonad on one side and an ovotestis containing a dysgenetic fibrotic testis on the other side. The external genitalia may be male, female, or ambiguous, depending on the functionality of the Leydig cells of the ovotestis. The Müllerian ducts are usually retained, due to a deficiency of MIS from ineffective Sertoli cells. The karyotype is usually a mosaic 45,X/46,XY, although a 46,XY karyotype is found in 40% of patients. Because of the possibility of gonadoblastoma, early removal of gonads is recommended.

Androgen Insensitivity Syndrome

Androgen effect is mediated by the binding of androgens, including testosterone, DHT, and other weaker adrenal and gonadal steroids, to androgen receptors. The binding induces a conformational change of receptors and enables receptors to bind to the DNA of the targeted genes in the cell nucleus. Androgen insensitivity syndrome (AIS) is due to an inability to express an androgen effect in a 46,XY individual who has normal androgen production. The underlying mechanism is a deletion or mutation of the androgen receptor gene, resulting in a decreased number of androgen receptors, or the inability of the receptor to bind with androgens or a target gene. Other possibilities include mutations of androgen-responsive genes. There is a wide spectrum of AIS, ranging from a complete form (CAIS) to a partial form (PAIS).

In CAIS, patients are born with normal female external genitalia with several exceptions. The vagina ends blindly, due to the suppression of the Müllerian structures by testicular MIS. The testes may be undescended, located in the inguinal region, or in the labial folds. Testicular histology is grossly normal in infants, but the seminiferous tubules tend to be small, and in adolescents there is a lack of spermatogenesis. The Wolffian structures are rudimentary or absent because of the lack of the response to local testosterone. Infants are assigned and raised as females without any doubt, unless gonads are found in the inguinal or labial area. Adolescents develop normal-appearing breasts, although the areolae and nipples are somewhat under-developed. The absence of pubic hair, axillary hair, or menstruation brings these children to medical attention. The plasma levels of testosterone and DHT are in the normal male range. LH and FSH levels are elevated. In PAIS, also called Reifenstein syndrome, the external genitalia are ambiguous. The penis is small in early childhood, although it may enlarge slightly during puberty. In adolescents, the testes are small and azoospermic due to maturation arrest. In very mild PAIS, subjects have normal male external genitalia, but are infertile.

5α-Reductase Deficiency

Testosterone must be converted by 5α-reductase to the more potent DHT to masculinize the external genitalia. In 46,XY individuals with 5α-reductase deficiency, testosterone levels are high, while DHT is low and the testosterone/DHT ratio is elevated. At birth, the phallus is quite small and appears to be a normal or slightly enlarged clitoris. Although testes can be found in the inguinal canals, the labioscrotal folds are bifid and empty. A urogenital sinus leads to a blind-ending vaginal pouch. Wolffian structures are normal and Müllerian structures are absent. At puberty, masculinization starts and the phallus grows, although remaining small. Sperm production is normal. Gynecomastia and hair-line recession do not occur.

Congenital Adrenal Hyperplasia

Congenital adrenal hyperplasia (CAH) is the most common cause of female pseudohermaphroditism. The majority of cases of CAH are due to 21-hydroxylase deficiency. There are two forms of 21-hydroxylase deficiency based on the severity of clinical presentations: the classic form and the nonclassic or late-onset form. In the classic form, three-quarters of cases are salt-wasting, with ambiguous genitalia in females or mild overvirilization in males. The remaining one-third are simple virilized. In the nonclassic or late-onset form, subjects do not have salt-wasting or ambiguity of genitalia at birth, but later develop hyperandrogenism, such as premature pubarche in childhood, or hirsutism, clitoromegaly, and polycystic ovary syndrome in adolescents. In males with 21-hydroxylase deficiency, the genitalia appear normal, enlarged, or hyperpigmented at birth. The biochemical marker of 21-hydroxylase deficiency is an elevated plasma 17-OH progesterone level (Fig. 120.2).

In 11-hydroxylase deficiency, the genitalia are similar in appearance to those seen in 21-hydroxylase deficiency, but there is no salt-wasting, because of the overproduction of deoxycorticosterone (DOC), which exerts a weak mineralocorticoid effect. In 3β-hydroxysteroid dehydrogenase deficiency, male infants present with ambiguous genitalia, while female infants' external genitalia are either normal or exhibit mild clitoromegaly.

Cytochrome P450 oxidoreductase (POR) is an enzyme that is important in electron transfer from NADPH to 17-hydroxylase and 21-hydroxylase. A mutation of the POR gene mutations results in CAH with impaired activity of 17α-hydroxylase and 21-hydroxylase, even though the genes encoding these two enzymes are normal. Individuals with POR deficiency have varying degrees of cortisol deficiency, ambiguous genitalia, primary amenorrhea, and enlarged cystic ovaries. The genital ambiguities include micropenis and undescended testes in males, and vaginal atresia, fused labia minora, hypoplastic labia majora, and a large clitoris in females. These signs of deficiency

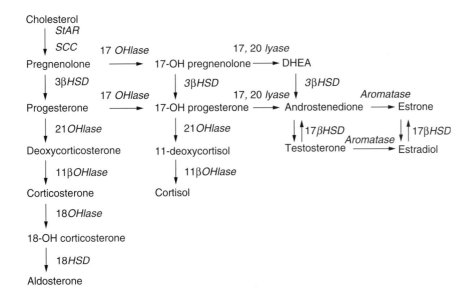

FIGURE 120.2. Pathway of steroid synthesis. (StAR, steroid acute regulatory protein; SCC, cholesterol side-chain cleavage enzyme; 3β-HSD, 3β-hydroxysteroid dehydrogenase; 21-OHlase, 21-hydroxylase; 11β-OHlase, 11β-hydroxylase; 18-OHlase, 18-hydroxylase; 18HSD, 18-hydroxysteroid dehydrogenase; 17-OHlase, 17-hydroxylase; 17β-HSD, 17β-hydroxysteroid dehydrogenase; DHEA, dehydroepiandrosterone.)

of this enzyme seem to suggest an alternative pathway in human androgen synthesis, present only in fetal life, which explains the combination of antenatal androgen excess and postnatal androgen deficiency.

SRY

Although SRY is critical in testis determination, its mechanism of action is not clearly understood. A fundamental role appears to be the regulation of SOX9 expression. In a group of 46,XX males, 80% have a SRY gene and usually present with male genitalia, whereas the other 20% do not have a detectable SRY gene. This indicates that some genes are able to induce testis differentiation without SRY. On the other hand, 15% to 20% of 46,XY females have inactivating mutations in SRY, mostly in the high-mobility-group (HMG) domain of the gene, which result in complete male-to-female sex-reversal with pure gonadal dysgenesis in the majority of cases, whereas the other 80% to 85% have a normal SRY gene. This indicates that many factors other than SRY are important in testis determination. 46,XX males with SRY, although usually short, have a normal male body habitus, normal penis, and normal testicles, and also psychologically identify themselves as male. However they are infertile because they lack other genes on the Y chromosome required for spermatogenesis.

SOX9

SRY-related high-mobility group box 9 (SOX9) encodes a transcription factor involved in chondrogenesis and testis development. SOX9 and SRY are coexpressed in the male, but not the female, urogenital ridge. SOX9 activates the transcription of MIS in the testis. Mutations or translocations of the SOX9 gene are identified in 46,XY male-to-female sex reversal, streak gonads, and skeletal malformations (e.g., campomelic dysplasia). On the other hand, duplication of the SOX9 gene results in 46,XX female-to-male reversal. These facts demonstrate the importance of SOX9 in testis determination and genital development.

DAX1

DAX1 is a nuclear-receptor protein that regulates gene expression, presumably through protein–protein interaction. Mutations of the DAX1 gene result in adrenal hypoplasia con-

genita and hypogonadotropic hypogonadism, but normal testicular development (except for small size and spermatogenetic defects) and external genitalia in 46,XY males. Infants develop signs and symptoms of adrenal crisis at birth, and in adolescence lack secondary sexual characteristics. A double-dose of the DAX1 gene in a 46,XY male results in sexual reversal from male to female. The heterozygote DAX1 mutation or deletion has no effects on females.

WT1

WT1 is important in the early steps of the differentiation of gonads and kidneys. Mutations of this gene may result in several syndromes. In Frasier syndrome, the mutation takes place at the intron-exon splicing site, resulting in decreased production of SRY and MIS. A 46,XY subject will have female external genitalia and Müllerian duct structures with focal segmental sclerosis or renal failure in infancy, and a risk of developing gonadoblastoma. In Denys–Drash syndrome, the mutations occur in exons. The testes are able to produce MIS to suppress the Müllerian ducts, but due to inadequate testosterone production, there may be varying degrees of hypospadias and undescended testes. Renal disorders include mesangial sclerosis, proteinuria, and renal failure. Wilms tumor develops before 2 years of age. In WAGR syndrome (Wilms tumor, aniridia, genitourinary anomalies, and mental retardation), a microdeletion involving several contiguous genes on chromosome 11p13, including PAX6, WT1, and other genes, is responsible for the clinical presentation.

Mayer–Rokitansky–Kuster–Hauser Syndrome

Mayer–Rokitansky–Kuster–Hauser syndrome is a failure of Müllerian development in 46,XX females, characterized by the absence of the upper four-fifths of the vagina with a rudimentary uterus; the Fallopian tubes may be developed. Renal agenesis, a pelvic kidney, or other urinary-tract anomalies may coexist. A few cases of this syndrome may be caused by inactivation of the WNT-4 gene. Secreted by the Müllerian duct epithelium, the WNT-4 protein induces the development of the Müllerian mesenchyme; the development of Müllerian ducts ceases if the WNT-4 gene is inactivated. It has been estimated that at least one in four women with primary amenorrhea have this syndrome, which should be considered as part of the VATER syndrome if the patient has associated vertebral anomalies.

Turner Syndrome

Subjects with Turner syndrome (45,X or variants) have bilateral streak gonads, Müllerian structures, but no ambiguity of external genitalia in most cases. However, the SRY gene or Y chromosome material has been identified in virilized Turner syndrome patients with the 45,X karyotype. Müllerian derivatives and intra-abdominal testes can be found, and gonadectomy is recommended to reduce the risk of future gonadoblastoma.

EVALUATION

One should raise questions of intersexuality if there are any of the following conditions:

In an apparent male:

- Bilateral nonpalpable testes in a full-term infant.
- Hypospadias with separation of the scrotal sacs.
- Undescended testis with hypospadias.

In an apparent female:

- Clitoral hypertrophy of any degree.
- Foreshortened vulva with single opening.
- Inguinal hernia containing a gonad.

The evaluation for ambiguous genitalia includes:

1. History
   - Detailed medical history of associated problems.
   - Gestational history: maternal illness, hirsutism, tumor, medications containing androgens or progestins.
   - Fetal ultrasound findings.
2. Family history
   - Sudden infant death.
   - Infants with symptoms of acute or chronic adrenal insufficiency (severe or recurrent gastrointestinal symptoms, dehydration, failure to thrive, hyperpigmentation).
   - Ambiguous genitalia, infertility.
   - Males with hypospadias, undescended testis.
   - Females with little or no pubic hair, axillary hair, menstruation.
   - Kidney diseases.

3. Physical examination
   - Careful examination of genitalia.
   - Masculinization of external genitalia.
   - Phallus: size, chordee, prepubic fat (edema, fat pad).
   - The appearance and actual length/width of phallus and the degree of descent of the testes varies by gestational age.
   - Edema or fat pad affects the appearance and size of phallus and scrotum, or labia.
   - Urogenital sinus: urethral orifice, vaginal opening.
   - Labioscrotal folds: fullness, symmetry, rugosity.
   - Gonads: if palpable, most likely testes, thus not a female with CAH.
   - Hyperpigmentation of scrotum, finger knuckles, palmar or plantar creases.
   - Any feature of a malformation syndrome or associated illness.
   - Vital sign instability, suggesting adrenal insufficiency or crisis.
4. Laboratory tests. Figure 120.3 outlines laboratory tests for the evaluation of ambiguous genitalia.

Infants with ambiguous genitalia who are suspected to have CAH should be monitored closely for the symptoms and signs of adrenal crisis. Glucose and electrolytes need to be checked within a few days after birth. In addition to obtaining plasma cortisol and testosterone levels, other steroid measurements include 17-OH progesterone for 21-hydroxylase deficiency, 17-OH pregnenolone for 3β-hydroxysteroid dehydrogenase deficiency, deoxycorticosterone and 11-deoxycortisol for 11-hydroxylase deficiency, and progesterone and 17-OH progesterone for 17-hydroxylase deficiency. An ACTH stimulation test may be needed if the results from random samples are inconclusive.

A high level of testosterone during the first few months after birth indicates a functioning testicle. In the presence of a low testosterone level, an hCG stimulation test will be needed to assess testicular function. A low DHT level or a high T/DHT ratio suggests 5α-reductase deficiency.

In an individual with a Y chromosome, ambiguous genitalia, and Müllerian duct derivatives, the differential diagnosis includes persistent Müllerian duct syndrome and testicular

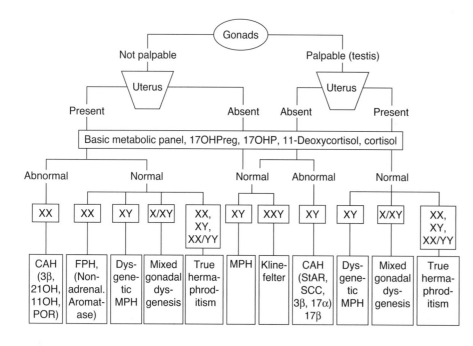

FIGURE 120.3. Initial evaluation of ambiguous genitalia. Tests also include T and DHT. (17OHPreg, 17-hydroxy pregnenolone; 17OHP, 17-hydroxy progesterone; CAH, congenital adrenal hyperplasia; 3β, 3β-hydroxysteroid dehydrogenase; 21OH, 21-hydroxylase; 11OH, 11-hydroxylase; POR, cytochrome P450 oxidoreductase; FPH, female pseudohermaphroditism; MPH, male pseudohermaphroditism; SCC, cholesterol side-chain cleavage enzyme; 17α, 17α-hydroxylase; 17β, 17β-hydroxysteroid dehydrogenase.) (Modified with permission from Forest MG. Diagnosis and treatment of disorders of sexual development. In: DeGroot LJ, Jameson JL, eds. *Endocrinology.* 5th ed. Philadelphia: Elsevier Saunders; 2006: 2779–2829.)

dysgenesis. Karyotype, specific molecular analysis, and biopsy can be used to make the diagnosis.

MANAGEMENT

Sex Assignment

Sex assignment should be a multidisciplinary decision involving the parents. The following factors need to be considered:

- Nature of the disorder.
- Fertility potential.
  - There is potential fertility in CAH females or in females exposed to maternal androgens.
  - Most other intersex individuals have reduced or no fertility.
- Capacity for sexual function.
  - Size of the phallus and its potential to develop.
  - Trial of testosterone injection.
  - Severity of hypospadias is not a deciding factor.
  - Children with very small phalluses due to PAIS are less likely to respond to a testosterone trial and may have less testosterone imprinting effect. These children are frequently raised as females.
  - For other severely undervirilized genetic males, the assignment to the female gender by surgery should only be undertaken with considerable caution.
- Testosterone imprinting.

Animal studies had shown that prenatal testosterone imprinting plays a significant role in postnatal gender identity. This phenomenon has been identified in humans and has created significant difficulty in individuals who were exposed in fetal life to high levels of androgens, but raised as females.

It appears that differing pathologies of ambiguous genitalia result in different outcomes of gender identity. There have been fewer problems with sexual identification in girls with CAH. Although they have masculine behavior patterns and may have difficulty adjusting to female gender, they usually do not overtly demonstrate problems with sexual identity. Behavioral masculinization in girls with CAH results from high levels of androgens during fetal development, but not in postnatal life. Gender identity in girls with CAH was not related to the degree of genital virilization or the age at reconstructive surgery.

Parents may desire to assign their children's gender based on their personal or cultural preference. Thorough information regarding the mechanisms of the ambiguity, the options for treatment, and the potential outcomes should be discussed with the parents and family.

Medical Treatment

In infants with salt-wasting CAH, it is essential to provide glucose-containing electrolyte solutions, hydrocortisone for cortisol deficiency, fludrocortisone (Florinef) for aldosterone deficiency, and correction of electrolyte abnormalities. Detailed medical management for CAH is discussed in Chapter 101.

Infants with small phalluses raised as males may benefit from repeated, short courses of low-dose testosterone injections from infancy throughout childhood to keep their penile size in the normal range, with increased dosage for pubertal development if needed. Females with streak gonads or ovarian insufficiency will need estrogen to support the development of secondary sexual characteristics during puberty.

Surgery

Since the early 1990s there has been a controversy about sex assignment and timing of surgery on intersex patients. Traditionally, it was proposed that "nurture" overcomes "nature" in gender identity. The gender of rearing was determined at birth or changed before 18 months of age; the external genitalia were reconstructed to be compatible with sex of rearing. However, in patients with severe ambiguity, early surgical reconstruction frequently resulted in an unsatisfactory outcome. The effect of prenatal testosterone exposure on gender identity could also be profound and troublesome. In 1993, a group of intersex people advocated that surgery for ambiguous genitalia be performed only in life-threatening situations; and otherwise that surgery should be deferred until the patient can participate in the decision-making. Some researchers have called for a moratorium on genital surgery without patient consent until comprehensive retrospective studies show positive outcomes of surgery.

On the other hand, some surgeons argued for surgery in infancy or early life using meticulous dissection that avoided a narrow introitus. The benefit of early surgery is that infant's pelvis is shorter, making the mobilization of the vagina less problematic than if the procedure is done later. Early vaginal repair using a new technique to substitute for the vaginal pull-through procedure has also been reported. However, another surgical group reported that routine neonatal assignment of genetic males to female sex because of severe phallic inadequacy can result in unpredictable sexual identification. Clinical interventions in such children should be reexamined in the light of these findings.

Some of the possible limited surgical approaches are, for girls, to perform clitoroplasty in infancy, but to postpone major genital reconstruction until the patient can participate in the decision; and for boys, to bring down an undescended testis into the scrotum at the time of gonadal biopsy. Correcting a chordee and performing repair of a hypospadias between 6 and 18 months of age is recommended. A dysgenetic, Y-chromosome-containing gonad needs to be removed to prevent gonadoblastoma.

PEARLS

- A functional testis is mandatory for normal male development, whereas an ovary is not required for a female phenotype.
- SRY is critical in testicular differentiation.
- Ambiguity of genitalia can be divided into male pseudohermaphroditism, female pseudohermaphroditism, true hermaphroditism, pure gonadal dysgenesis, mixed gonadal dysgenesis, and others.
- The key evaluation elements include karyotype, pelvic ultrasound for uterus, adrenal steroids and electrolytes for CAH, testosterone for testicular function, dihydrotestosterone for 5α-reductase activity, and possible VCUG for urogenital structure.
- The initial treatment should focus on adrenal crisis if the underlying condition is CAH. Testosterone trial may be given for evaluation and treatment purpose.
- Decisions about sex assignment should take into account the nature of the disorder, the fertility potential, the capacity of sexual function, the effect of testosterone imprinting, and the cultural background of the family.
- Perform surgery in infancy only for important functional need. Timing of major reconstruction surgery is controversial and should be evaluated carefully on a case-by-case basis. Share the informed decision-making with parents,

and later with patients, and honor their preferences for or against surgery.

Suggested Readings

American Academy of Pediatrics, Committee on Genetics. Evaluation of the newborn with developmental anomalies of the external genitalia. *Pediatrics* 2000;106:138–142.

Brown TR, Scherer PA, Chang YT, et al. Molecular genetics of human androgen insensitivity. *Eur J Pediatr* 1993;125(suppl 2):S62–S69.

Diamond DA, Burns JP, Mitchell C, et al. Sex assignment for newborns with ambiguous genitalia and exposure to fetal testosterone: attitudes and practices of pediatric urologists. *J Pediatr* 2006;148:445–449.

Forest MG. Diagnosis and treatment of disorders of sexual development. In: DeGroot LJ, Jameson JL, eds. *Endocrinology.* 5th ed. Philadelphia: Elsevier Saunders; 2006:2779–2829.

Lee PA, Houk CP, Ahmed F, et al. Consensus Statement on Management of Intersex Disorders. *Pediatrics* 2006; 118:e488–e500.

MacLaughlin DT, Donahoe PK. Mechanisms of disease: sex determination and differentiation. *N Engl J Med* 2004;350:367–378.

Meyer-Bahlburg HF, Migeon CJ, Berkovitz GD, et al. Attitudes of adult 46,XY intersex persons to clinical management policies. *J Urol* 2004;171:1615–1619.

Migeon CJ, Berkovitz GD, Brown TR. Sexual differentiation and ambiguity. In: Kappy M, Blizzard R, Migeon C, eds. *Wilkins the diagnosis and treatment of endocrine disorders in childhood and adolescence.* 4th ed. Springfield: Thomas; 1994:573–715.

CHAPTER 121 ■ COMMON GENETIC ABNORMALITIES

OPAL JEAN HOOD AND KAREN RUSSELL SCHMIDT

The diagnosis of a genetic defect or disorder in a newborn is a frequent and at times difficult problem encountered by health care providers in the nursery. Epidemiologic studies have shown that by young adulthood, genetically determined or influenced disorders will affect approximately 1 in 20 live-born children. Some will remain undetected in early childhood, but birth defects, chromosome abnormalities, dysmorphic syndromes, and hereditary diseases are major contributors to neonatal and pediatric morbidity and mortality. Progress in defining the genetic contributions to these problems has resulted in the rapid proliferation of technically sophisticated diagnostic tests that are increasingly available to practicing physicians. This section will address common presentations of genetic defects and disorders in the newborn and an approach to assessment and diagnosis that can assist the health care provider in choosing appropriate studies from among the often bewildering array of available genetic tests.

COMPONENTS OF GENETIC ASSESSMENT IN NEWBORNS

Growth Parameters

Clues that a genetic defect or disorder may be present in a newborn come to the observant health care provider from readily available sources. Genetic assessment should begin with an accurate determination of gestational age. A prenatal ultrasound done in the first trimester of pregnancy is the most accurate reference point for gestational dating, because dysmorphic features and abnormal muscle tone may affect the validity of physical assessment measures obtained after birth. If ultrasound dating is not available, information on uterine size and menstrual dating should be sought from the mother's initial prenatal care visit. The infant's standard growth parameters (birthweight, crown to heel length, head circumference, chest circumference, crown-to-rump length) should then be carefully determined. Abnormal intrauterine growth (e.g., asymmetry of birthweight, length, and head circumference) or disproportionate growth should always alert the health care provider to the possibility of a genetic defect or disorder. In the normal full-term neonate, the head circumference is greater than the chest circumference, and the chest circumference is greater than the abdominal circumference. The head circumference should measure within 1 cm of the crown-to-rump length. Although placental insufficiency from many causes and poor antepartum maternal glucose homeostasis are important nongenetic causes of abnormal intrauterine growth, they should be accepted as the etiology only with supportive pathologic or physiologic data.

Physical Examination Parameters

The identification of major congenital anomalies (birth defects) is a primary goal of the admission physical examination to the nursery. Even those major congenital anomalies that occur as isolated birth defects are likely to have a genetic component to their etiology. When a major congenital anomaly is found, the health care provider should search for others. Determination of a recognized pattern or association of birth defects is a critically important step in the diagnostic process and facilitates use of genetic reference texts and syndrome databases. The recognition of minor congenital anomalies during the physical examination can also be quite helpful in the identification of birth defects. Although minor anomalies usually do not have medical or cosmetic significance, the association between an increasing number of minor anomalies and the likelihood of birth defects is well established. Standard anthropometric measurements easily done during the physical examination may provide additional clues to the presence of a genetic defect or disorder (see Hall and associates in the Suggested Readings). For example, abnormalities in facial development, such as closely set or widely spaced eyes, may be the first clue that the baby has a structural brain anomaly. Neurologic status should be assessed (particularly resting muscle tone), as neurological abnormalities may be useful diagnostic clues.

Birth and Family History Parameters

Other useful clues in assessing the possibility of a genetic defect or disorder may be found in the prenatal history. Information on pregnancy complications, potential teratogenic exposures, abnormal amniotic fluid volume, unusual fetal position, poor fetal movement, and abnormal length of the gestation is helpful in determining the likelihood of a genetic defect or disorder. History of the delivery and ease of adaptation to extrauterine life should also be assessed. Family history is extraordinarily useful in the diagnosis of a genetic defect or disorder in the neonatal period. Points of particular importance include:

■ Information on similarly affected persons
■ Parental ages and consanguinity
■ Birth defects, epilepsy, unusual medical problems
■ Known hereditary diseases
■ Mental retardation
■ Reproductive failure such as recurrent miscarriages, stillbirths, or infertility

Information should be sought on members of the baby's nuclear family and on close relatives, including grandparents, aunts, uncles, and first cousins. The family's ethnicity should also be ascertained, because the occurrence of genetic defects varies in different ethnic groups. It is a maxim of clinical genetics that evaluation for defects or disorders in the newborn is most effectively done in the context of the infant's family and ethnic heritage.

COMMON PRESENTATIONS OF GENETIC DEFECTS AND DISORDERS IN NEWBORNS

Abnormalities of Growth

The differential diagnosis of abnormal intrauterine growth is extensive and includes many genetic and nongenetic etiologies. Success in correctly diagnosing the cause in any newborn requires a systematic approach. One of the most frequently encountered examples of abnormal intrauterine growth is *symmetric growth retardation*. For the determined gestational age, birthweight, length, and head circumference are all proportionately below the fifth percentile. The most common nongenetic etiology, placental insufficiency from many possible maternal causes, should be diagnosed only when there is confirmatory placental pathology and when genetic etiologies are not suggested by history and physical examination. The presence on physical examination of a major congenital anomaly, multiple minor anomalies, dysmorphic features, or hypotonia suggests the presence of a chromosomal abnormality, hereditary syndrome, or teratogen exposure syndrome. Chromosome analysis from a blood sample; ultrasound study of the heart, brain, and abdominal organs for major anomalies; and assessments of visual and auditory deficits are potential diagnostic tools. The prenatal history should be carefully evaluated, and specific exposures should be sought. The family history should also be reviewed for genetic risk factors including abnormal parental growth parameters.

Another commonly encountered intrauterine growth abnormality, *symmetric fetal overgrowth*, should be similarly assessed before it is assumed to be due to being an "infant of a diabetic mother," because several other overgrowth syndromes have a congenital presentation. *Asymmetric intrauterine growth abnormalities* must always be screened for genetic etiologies before a nongenetic cause is diagnosed. The genetic differential diagnosis is quite extensive, but again, the initial step in the evaluation is accurate determination of gestational age. Assignment of the primary site of the growth abnormality to the cranium (microcephaly or macrocephaly) or to the body (somatic growth retardation or somatic overgrowth) must then be made. After these steps have been taken, a reasonable diagnostic plan can be made. Genetic etiologies to be considered in the differential diagnosis include many chromosomal abnormalities, dysmorphic syndromes (e.g., Russell–Silver syndrome), and nonlethal skeletal dysplasias (e.g., achondroplasia).

Major Congenital Anomalies

Approximately 2% of all live-born children have a major congenital anomaly or *birth defect*. Congenital heart defects, genitourinary defects, orofacial cleft defects, neural tube defects, and musculoskeletal anomalies, including limb defects, are frequently encountered problems in the nursery. Most major congenital anomalies occur as isolated birth defects, have a genetic component in the etiology, and carry a multifactorial recurrence risk for the family. The needs of the child and family can be met by the primary health care provider with appropriate specialty consultation.

In other infants, nonsyndromic *association* of more than one major congenital anomaly may occur. Recognition of a tracheoesophageal fistula in an infant should prompt a search for other, often occult, anomalies, such as the hemivertebrae and renal dysgenesis that are frequently associated with this gastrointestinal defect. A major congenital anomaly may also be the presenting sign of an underlying genetic disorder. Very few pathognomonic birth defects and genetic syndrome associations are found in clinical genetic practice, although well-recognized associations, such as the frequent occurrence of atrioventricular canal defects in infants with Down syndrome, are found.

When confronted with a newborn who has a major congenital anomaly, the health care provider must consider the possibility of an underlying genetic disorder. A thorough physical examination for *minor physical anomalies, growth abnormalities, abnormal neurologic signs,* and other *birth defects* is the minimal assessment. Prenatal history, especially potential teratogenic exposures, and a thorough family history should also be sought. Diagnostic testing should be directed by the data gathered from the child, the family, and easily available genetic epidemiology data. For example, tetralogy of Fallot is one of the most frequently occurring congenital heart defects. The majority of cases represent an isolated birth defect with a multifactorial inheritance pattern and a recurrence risk of approximately 2%. However, tetralogy of Fallot occurs as a component of several genetic syndromes, including:

- Goldenhar syndrome (associated with birth defects of branchial arch–derived structures).
- CHARGE syndrome (associated with ocular colobomas, genital anomalies, choanal defects, and ear anomalies).
- Chromosome 22q11.2 deletion syndrome (associated with thymic hypoplasia, immunodeficiency, hypocalcemia, cleft palate, and dysmorphic facial features).

Recurrence risk for Goldenhar syndrome and chromosome 22q11.2 deletion syndrome depend on whether one of the parents is affected, but the recurrence risk for CHARGE syndrome is usually low. Tetralogy of Fallot is also a feature of retinoic acid embryopathy, a teratogenic syndrome associated with early first-trimester exposure to systemic retinoids used in the treatment of severe acne. Assessment of the infant with tetralogy of Fallot must include consideration of these potential associations and may require an extensive evaluation prior to hospital discharge.

A similar approach is recommended for other common major congenital anomalies such as cleft lip with or without cleft palate, hypospadias, and neural tube defects. The initial step is the search for other birth defects. An important factor to consider is the temporal relationship of the identified birth defect to fetal development. Organ systems and structures developing at the same time embryologically may be similarly affected by the causative developmental error. Another factor to consider is shared embryonic spatial orientation. Many of the common birth defects occur in organ systems that have embryonic origin in the craniocaudal midline axis of the developing fetus. Because formation of more than one midline organ system may be affected by the developmental error, associated birth defects should be sought in them. With some thought and a careful physical examination, the health care provider can identify any other birth defects present and initiate the diagnostic assessment.

Dysmorphic Features

The newborn whose appearance is described as "unusual" or "different" is a common reason for referral to a clinical geneticist. Dysmorphic features may be assumed to simply be a combination of multiple minor anomalies, especially of craniofacial development, when in fact there may also be major anomalies. For some genetic disorders, such as Down syndrome, the dysmorphic appearance of the infant is so characteristic that the presence of the underlying causative chromosome abnormality is suspected at once. More frequently, the etiology is not immediately evident from the appearance, and a systematic approach to assessment must be followed to determine the etiology, beginning with the infant's family history and ethnic heritage. Both parents and any siblings should be observed to determine whether the features are family traits or actual minor anomalies. In some situations, it may be necessary to view family photographs of close relatives whom the infant is reported to resemble or photographs of the parents as infants to clarify this point. Determination of the infant's ethnicity is also essential in the question of minor anomaly versus benign trait, because certain traits (e.g., width of the palpebral fissure) vary by ethnicity and age. The possibility that the family member whom the infant resembles may be mildly affected with the syndrome must be considered, because there is phenotypic variability in many syndromes. Examination of the family member with the most pronounced features of a suspected syndrome should help the clinician decide whether the infant deserves further evaluation. To generate a differential diagnosis, an objective description of observed features is essential for effective use of syndrome databases and genetic reference texts. Here again, accurate anthropometric measurements can provide useful information on quantifiable physical traits. The description of nonquantifiable features should be anatomic, such as "up-slanting palpebral fissures" rather than "almond-shaped eyes" to describe the typical eye orientation of an infant with Down syndrome. Although the list of possible diagnoses in dysmorphic infants is extensive, careful assessment will result in a narrowed differential to guide laboratory testing and radiographic studies toward specific diagnosis.

Genetic Causes of Severe Hypotonia in Newborns

Severe neonatal hypotonia is often a perplexing problem for health care providers. Some cases are easily explained from the perinatal history, but others require investigation. A pregnancy history of decreased fetal movement or physical findings of abnormal palmar creases, pterygia, or ankyloses are indications of long-standing hypotonia with prenatal onset. Not all infants have suggestive physical signs or clues in their prenatal and family histories. Genetic causes of severe neonatal

hypotonia are quite varied and include numerical chromosome defects, such as trisomy 21, unbalanced structural chromosome defects, Prader–Willi syndrome (an imprinted chromosomal microdeletion syndrome), and hereditary neurologic diseases (e.g., myotonic dystrophy and spinal muscular atrophy). For these disorders, specific chromosome testing or genetic tests are now readily available, allowing a definitive diagnosis to be made. However, the health care provider must first suspect the diagnosis in the hypotonic infant and request the appropriate chromosome or genetic test. There are no "molecular screening tests"; each gene must be specifically tested for mutations. Microdeletion testing is locus-specific and detects submicroscopic chromosomal deletions not visible with light microscopy by using fluorescent in situ hybridization (FISH) technology. Numerical and most structural chromosome defects can be diagnosed by readily available techniques in a cytogenetic laboratory. Several inborn errors of metabolism may present as severe hypotonia, particularly in the infant over 24 hours of age.

Suggested Readings

Amato RSS. Genetic Disorders. In: Behrman RE , Kliegman RM, eds. *Essentials of pediatrics*. 2nd ed. Philadelphia: Saunders; 1994:123–138.

Clayton-Smith J, Donnai D. Human malformations. In: Rimoin DL, Connor JM, Pyeritz RE, et al., eds. *Emery and Rimoin's principles and practice of medical genetics*. 4th ed. New York: Churchill Livingston; 2002:488–500.

DeMario FJ Jr. Genetic diseases in the etiology of the floppy infant. *Rhode Island Med J* 1989;72:357–359.

Hall JG, Froster-Iskenius UG, Allanson JE. *Handbook of normal physical measurements*. New York: Oxford University Press; 1989.

Iosub S, Fuchs M, Bingol N, et al. Palpebral fissure length in black and Hispanic children: correlation with head circumference. *Pediatrics* 1985;75:318–320.

Leck I. The contribution of epidemiologic studies to understanding human malformations. In: Stevenson RE, Hall JG, Goodman RM, eds. *Human malformations and related anomalies*. Vol. 1. New York: Oxford University Press; 1993:65–93.

Leppig KA, Werder MM, Can CI, et al. Predictive value of minor anomalies. I. Association with major malformations. *J Pediatr* 1987;110:531–537.

Rimoin DL, Connor JM, Pyeritz RE, et al. Nature and frequency of genetic disease. In: Romoin DL, Connor JM, Pyeritz RE, et al., eds. *Emery and Rimoin's principles and practice of medical genetics*. 4th ed. New York: Churchill Livingston; 2002:55–59.

Riopel DA. The heart. In: Stevenson RE, Hall JG, Goodman RM, eds. *Human malformations and related anomalies*. Vol. 2. New York: Oxford University Press; 1993:237–253.

CHAPTER 122 ■ INBORN ERRORS OF METABOLISM

PAMELA H. ARN

Individually, inborn errors of metabolism are rare. This fact makes it particularly hard for clinicians to integrate these diseases into a meaningful differential diagnosis when caring for children. As a group, however, inborn errors of metabolism are a significant source of morbidity and mortality in pediatrics. Great strides are being made in the screening of newborns for inborn errors using tandem mass spectroscopy; however the diseases screened for vary from state to state, and not all inborn errors are detected in newborn screening programs. Some children become ill before the newborn screen is reported. A clinician should never rely exclusively on a newborn screen when assessing a sick child, because these screens are designed to detect specific disorders in a well infant and are not appropriate tests for diagnosis in children suspected to have an inborn error.

In this chapter we will discuss the clinical presentation of children with inborn errors, the diagnostic workup, and the early care and stabilization in the hospital. The role of the hospital pediatrician is to suspect an inborn error, collect appropriate specimens so a diagnosis can be made, and stabilize the patient while waiting for a specific diagnosis. This can be accomplished by proper use of a good history, including a detailed family history, a few commonly available laboratory tests, and knowledge of the various groups of inborn errors. Although there are a very large number of inborn errors, most disorders fit into only a few common clinical presentations. For this purpose, the inborn errors will be divided into three groups: disorders of intoxication, disorders involving energy metabolism, and disorders involving complex molecules.

COLLECTION OF LABORATORY SPECIMENS

Initial assessment should include basic chemistries available in every hospital lab: CBC with differential, electrolytes with anion gap, liver enzymes, CK, venous pH, ammonia, and lactic acid. Urine should be examined for ketones and for reducing sugars. With these tests alone, progress can be made toward determining the likelihood of an inborn error of metabolism, deciding which category of disease the inborn error may fall into, and working toward early stabilization. If an inborn error is likely, the most helpful tests are checking plasma for amino acids, carnitine, acylcarnitine profile, lactate and pyruvate with lactate:pyruvate ratio, and urine for organic acids. Testing urine for amino acids is helpful but should be done only when plasma is tested as well, due to the difficulties in interpretation when renal function is impaired or immature. Because a spinal tap is almost always done as part of the initial sepsis workup, it is advisable to save an aliquot of frozen CSF for metabolic studies. Table 122.1 outlines the tests along with some expected findings.

DISORDERS OF INTOXICATION

Disorders of intoxication include amino acid disorders, most organic acidemias, urea cycle defects, and galactosemia.

The early signs and symptoms of these inborn errors are nonspecific in and of themselves, but the pattern of presentation among this group of inborn errors is fairly consistent. Typically, a term newborn with no risk factors for sepsis will feed well for the first 24 to 48 hours, and then will become lethargic, vomit, and will often progress to seizures and coma if no intervention is made. Because neonates have a limited variety of ways to respond to illness, this presentation could also signal sepsis or a structural congenital malformation. Because most of these diseases are amenable to treatment by removal of the toxin and maintaining a special diet, an inborn error must be considered early in the evaluation while simultaneously looking for other causes of the infant's symptoms. Although most states screen for galactosemia, babies with classical galactosemia (galactose phosphate uridyl transferase deficiency) often have jaundice, elevated liver enzymes, vomiting, and cataracts within 1 week, often prior to the newborn screen report. Urine is positive for reducing sugars but negative for glucose.

Illustrative Case 1

EF was the product of term delivery to a 25-year-old primagravida. Delivery was uncomplicated. Just prior to discharge at 2 days of age, the mother complained to the nurses of excessive spitting after breast-feeding. Family history was negative. At home, the baby continued to have vomiting; abdominal ultrasound showed no evidence of pyloric stenosis. The baby was admitted to the hospital on day 6 with severe lethargy progressing to seizures. CBC with differential was normal, as were electrolytes, liver enzymes, and CK. An ammonia test, however, was 600 µmol/L, and venous pH was 7.45.

This is a classic presentation for a disorder of urea cycle metabolism. No significant anion gap exists, and initially venous pH may be slightly alkalotic because of the effect of ammonia in stimulating the respiratory center. Hyperammonemia is a medical emergency that requires immediate consultation with an inborn errors specialist; the duration of coma is directly correlated with ultimate neurologic outcome. Hemodialysis is indicated to decrease the ammonia level while definitive diagnosis is being made.

Further metabolic tests included amino acids and organic acids. The pattern of amino acids was consistent with citrullinemia, a disorder of urea cycle metabolism. After hemodialysis,

TABLE 122.1

LABORATORY TESTS FOR INITIAL SCREENING FOR INBORN ERRORS

Laboratory tests	Clinical pearls
BLOOD	
Electrolytes, BUN, Cr	Acidosis in organic acid disorders, low BUN in urea cycle disorders
CBC with differential	Bone marrow suppression in organic acidemias, mitochondrial disorders
Liver enzymes	Raised in a variety of disorders
Bilirubin	Direct hyperbilirubinemia in galactosemia, others
Blood gas	Metabolic acidosis in organic acidemias, respiratory alkalosis in urea cycle
Ammonia	Very elevated in urea cycle disorders, moderately elevated in many other inborn errors
Lactic acid	Elevated levels should be repeated over time
URINE	
Ketones	Presence or absence is important
Reducing sugars	Positive in galactosemia and disorders of fructose metabolism
Smell	Helpful in MSUD and some organic acidurias but low sensitivity

the baby was started on IV medications to stimulate alternative pathways of waste nitrogen metabolism and was given a low-protein diet.

Genetic defects in urea cycle metabolism most often present in the first week of life. Some partial defects may present at any age, usually after a period of intercurrent illness or higher than normal protein intake. The most common of the defects is ornithine transcarbamylase deficiency, an X-linked disorder that may manifest in some females. A positive family history of male relatives on the maternal side of the family who died after short illnesses, in the neonatal period or after "Reye syndrome," should alert the clinician to the presence of this disease. All other urea cycle defects, as with most all of the other inborn errors of metabolism, are autosomal recessive.

Illustrative Case 2

BG is a 12-month-old boy who presents to the PICU with depressed mental status. By history he was well until 3 days prior when he developed URI symptoms. His mother has also weaned him from infant formula to 2% milk over the past week. He began to vomit 1 day prior to admission and became progressively more lethargic. Laboratory results on admission show a CBC with mild neutropenia, normal liver enzymes and glucose, a lactic acid level of 4 mmol/L, a HCO_3 level of 5, and a pH of 7.19. Anion gap is 26. Ammonia is 150. Urine is markedly positive for ketones and negative for sugars.

In this case, there is marked acidosis with elevated anion gap, suggesting an organic acidemia or maple syrup urine disease.

Further investigation shows normal amino acids and high levels of methylmalonic acid in the urine. On advice of the metabolic specialist, vitamin B_{12} in the form of hydroxycobalamin was given IM along with vigorous rehydration with glucose-contained fluids, and the child responded rapidly. Later testing revealed a defect in cobalamin metabolism (B_{12}), leading to the methylmalonic acidemia.

Several lessons can be learned from this case. The vitamin-responsive form of the disorder probably allowed for a later presentation of symptoms. The combination of an intercurrent illness with weaning to milk with a higher protein content led to a disruption of metabolic homeostasis and decompensation. This illustrates that, although inborn errors of intoxication most often present within the first few weeks of life, they can present later with a similar pattern of vomiting and lethargy leading to coma or seizures.

DISORDERS OF ENERGY METABOLISM

Disorders of energy metabolism are primarily due to defects in glycogenolysis, gluconeogenesis, and fatty acid oxidation. The lactic acidemias and defects in the mitochondrial respiratory chain also can be considered in this category. The pattern of presentation for this group of disorders is not as consistent as it is in disorders of intoxication. In the case of disorders of fatty acid oxidation, glycogenolysis, and gluconeogenesis, hypoglycemia is prominent, and hepatomegaly is often an accompanying feature.

Glycogen storage diseases (GSDs) present primarily with hepatomegaly and hypoglycemia. In glycogen storage disease type Ia, the hypoglycemia may be profound, but because the brain adapts to using ketones and lactic acid as fuel, the child may be asymptomatic except for hepatomegaly, poor growth, and other laboratory abnormalities including elevated uric acid, triglycerides, and lactic acid. As the child is treated, however, this adaptation is lost, and hypoglycemia will manifest symptomatically. Type III GSD includes IIIa that involves muscle and IIIb that does not. Hypoglycemia may also be marked in this disorder, although elevations in lactic acid are not seen. Other glycogen storage disorders rarely present acutely. Deficiency of fructose 1,6-diphosphatase inhibits gluconeogenesis from all precursors, but because glycogen synthesis and breakdown remain intact, hypoglycemia is seen only after glycogen stores are depleted.

Beta-oxidation of fatty acids represents an important source of energy during times of fasting and metabolic stress. Mitochondrial fatty acid oxidation metabolizes free fatty acids released into the blood by catabolism of fat stores or from dietary sources. Mitochondrial beta-oxidation involves transport of acyl-CoA moieties into the mitochondria and subsequent removal of 2-carbon acetyl-CoA units. These units are used as fuel for the tricarboxylic acid cycle or for the production of ketone bodies. There are at least 22 different defects of fatty acid oxidation described in humans. The spectra of clinical features of these defects are among the most variable within a family of metabolic disorders, although the most common clinical signs include recurrent hypoglycemia induced by fasting or stress, and hypotonia. The manifestations can range from neonatal hypotonia and acidosis to cardiomyopathy, myopathy, and rhabdomyolysis at any time in life.

Defects in carnitine palmitoyl transferase I (CPT I) are often characterized by episodic hypoketotic hypoglycemia, hyperammonemia, and multiorgan failure. Muscle and cardiac symptoms are rare. Cardiomyopathy and rhythm problems are seen in carnitine-acylcarnitine translocase deficiency, primary and secondary carnitine deficiencies, and very-long-chain acyl-CoA dehydrogenase deficiency (VLCAD).

Medium-chain acyl-CoA dehydrogenase deficiency (MCAD) is one of the most common inborn errors, with incidence estimates as high as 1 in 10,000 births in some populations. Many states now screen for MCAD deficiency, as well as some other fatty acid oxidation defects, at birth. MCAD provided much of the impetus for expanded newborn screening, because children with this defect are normal until they are stressed with an intercurrent illness. The most frequent clinical presentation, with onset between 1 and 3 years, is that of hypoketotic hypoglycemia and coma after a time of fasting with illness. Approximately 30% of undiagnosed children will die during the initial episode, and 30% more will suffer irreversible neurologic damage. Sudden death (often attributed to SIDS) has been described in numerous cases of MCAD deficiency. A single mutation, 985AG, is responsible for up to 80% of mutant alleles in the population. Presymptomatic identification of affected children through newborn screening programs can prevent death and neurologic compromise.

Illustrative Case 3

MG is a 14-month-old boy who was previously healthy and developmentally normal who presents to the Emergency Department lethargic and obtunded. The history reveals that he has had URI symptoms for 3 days, and the previous night vomited once and did not eat his dinner or a bedtime snack. Mom awoke at 4 AM to a strange cry and found him seizing. 911 was called, and a blood sugar reading was 28. At the hospital he has no ketones, mild hyperammonemia, and mild metabolic acidosis. Intravenous fluids with dextrose are given, but the child remains obtunded for the next 8 hours.

Urine organic acids show abnormal amounts of dicarboxylic acids, the plasma carnitine level is low, and an acylcarnitine profile is diagnostic for MCAD.

Diagnosis of defects in fatty acid metabolism requires knowledge of the clinical presentations and a high index of suspicion. Organic acids and carnitine levels may be normal between episodes. A fasting test should not be undertaken without the advice and supervision of a specialist in inborn errors. An acylcarnitine profile using tandem mass spectroscopy techniques, which is widely available, will detect minute quantities of abnormal intermediates even between episodes in most cases. This is the preferred initial test for diagnosis of most fatty acid oxidation defects.

Treatment depends on the specific defect. Carnitine is usually added as a daily supplement. Special care is taken during times of intercurrent illness. Intravenous glucose (8–10 mg/kg/min) can be used when oral intake is not maintained or during acute episodes.

Defects of the mitochondrial respiratory chain and related disorders include deficiencies of pyruvate carboxylase or pyruvate dehydrogenase, abnormalities of the Krebs cycle, or mitochondrial respiratory chain. Lactic acidosis is commonly seen in this group. Other common symptoms include myopathy, cardiomyopathy, arrythmias, cardiac conduction defects, hypoglycemia, mental retardation, and failure to thrive. Unlike most other inborn errors, dysmorphic features and malformations may be seen. This group of disorders is among the hardest for clinicians to diagnose and treat.

Elevated blood lactate concentrations are commonly seen in tissue hypoxia from sepsis, heart defects, and asphyxia, and these metabolic defects should always be considered when confronted with an elevated lactic acid level. Lactic acid concentrations of 4 to 6 mmol/L can be seen with seizures, tourniquet use, or simply a struggling child, so that lactic acidosis is a suggestive but nonspecific marker of mitochondrial dysfunction.

Pyruvate concentrations are useful only in cases of persistently elevated lactate. Like lactic acid, pyruvic acid concentrations are very sensitive to collection and processing variations. The clinically useful ratio of lactic acid to pyruvic acid reflects the redox state of the cell. When both lactate and pyruvate are expressed in mmol/L, the ratio is generally near 20. A decreased lactate/pyruvate ratio (<10) is suspicious for pyruvate dehydrogenase deficiency. A ratio >25 is seen in pyruvate carboxylase deficiency, mitochondrial respiratory chain abnormalities, and tissue hypoxia.

Pyruvate dehydrogenase complex deficiency is the most common of the disorders causing lactic acidosis. Its presentation may range from overwhelming lactic acidosis shortly after birth to mild to moderate lactic acidosis with psychomotor retardation and ataxia in the older child. Pyruvate carboxylase deficiency can present similarly with varying degrees of lactic acidosis combined with neurologic deficits.

Oxidative phosphorylation, the process of ATP synthesis by the respiratory chain, is the metabolic pathway that supplies most organs and tissues with energy. Consequently, defects in oxidative phosphorylation are protean in their manifestations and effects: A defect in the mitochondrial respiratory chain should be considered in children presenting with an otherwise unexplained combination of neuromuscular and other organ system defects, which may include cardiomyopathy, hepatic failure, diabetes, deafness, renal Fanconi syndrome, retinopathy, and myelodysplasia, among others.

Indirect diagnostic tests include plasma lactate with lactate/pyruvate ratio, glucose, plasma amino acids, and urinary organic acids. Alanine is often elevated with significant underlying lactic acidosis and in respiratory chain defects. Organic acid testing may show elevations in lactate, ketone bodies, and citric acid cycle intermediates. Specific diagnosis is difficult and requires specialized testing including muscle biopsy and molecular genetic studies. Treatment is generally symptomatic in these diseases; no satisfactory therapy is presently available. Many clinicians will prescribe a combination of cofactor therapies that include carnitine, coenzyme Q10, and B-complex vitamins, but these should only be started with the understanding that few patients respond to these supplements and after appropriate diagnostic studies have been undertaken.

Illustrative Case 4

MH presented to the hospital at 3 months of age with lethargy and vomiting. History revealed that she had been noted to have microcephaly at birth and has had intermittent vomiting since birth. Two days prior to admission she developed mild fever to 101°F with increased vomiting. Lab results at presentation revealed a marked metabolic acidosis with venous pH of 7.19, lactic acid level of 10 mmol/L, and glucose of 35. She was stabilized with IV dextrose and fluids and the laboratory values became normal within 24 hours. She returned to her usual state of alertness. All cultures were negative. She was sent home and returned at age 7 months with a similar episode after a prolonged respiratory infection. At that admission she was noted to be significantly developmentally delayed with hypotonia. A muscle biopsy for histology was unrevealing. Over the next year she became ataxic with episodic rhabdomyolysis requiring hospitalization. Repeat muscle biopsy with mitochondrial studies revealed a defect in complex I of the oxidative phosphorylation pathway. She has been treated with carnitine, coenzyme Q10, and B vitamins, and has remained relatively stable, though very developmentally delayed.

DEFECTS IN COMPLEX MOLECULES

Defects in complex molecules include all of the lysosomal storage disorders, peroxisomal disorders, congenital defects of glycosylation (CDG syndromes), and inborn errors of cholesterol synthesis. Each of these groups is chronic, and many are progressive. They generally do not present in an acute setting related to intercurrent illness; they are not related to diet nor are they amenable to acute treatment.

PEARLS

- The first step in diagnosis of an inborn error of metabolism is a high index of suspicion.
- Acute management generally involves providing a source of fluids and calories to reverse catabolism and to stabilize the patient.
- Even in the most experienced hands, not all children with inborn errors of metabolism survive. In cases where a child dies without a diagnosis but with a suspected inborn error, specimens should be collected including frozen serum, urine, CSF, and several dried blood spots on newborn screening cards. Urgent consultation with a metabolic specialist for further guidance is warranted.
- Because all inborn errors of metabolism are inherited in either an autosomal recessive, X-linked, or mitochondrial fashion, all carry a significant recurrence risk. Diagnosis allows a family to know the recurrence risk and to have the opportunity to prevent or treat the disease in future pregnancies.

Suggested Readings

Saudubray JM, Nassogne MC, de Lonlay P, et al. Clinical approach to inherited metabolic disorders in neonates: an overview. *Semin Neonatol* 2002;7: 3–15.

Scriver CR, Beaudet AL, Sly WS, et al., eds. *The metabolic and molecular bases of inherited disease*. 8th ed. New York: McGraw-Hill; 2001.

Vockley J, Singh RH, Whiteman DAH. Diagnosis and management of defects of mitochondrial β-oxidation. *Curr Opin Clin Nutr Metab Care* 2002;5: 601–609.

CHAPTER 123 ■ INTERPRETATION OF NEWBORN SCREENING TESTS

MARY-ALICE ABBOTT

Babies born today in the United States are tested for a variety of congenital diseases at birth. The panel of conditions tested for, and the methods of testing, vary from state to state, but the same basic principles apply nationwide. The conditions for which newborn screening has been incorporated are primarily conditions not evident at birth, but for which early intervention is believed to improve prognosis. It is generally accepted that mass screening of newborns should be applied when (1) the disease has a significant impact on the population, (2) the condition is not clinically evident at birth, (3) the disease can be detected via a reliable and affordable test, and (4) early diagnosis is beneficial. Current state screening protocols test for many types of conditions, including inborn errors of metabolism, hormonal abnormalities, common single-gene disorders, congenital infections, and hearing loss. As the panel of conditions expands, so does the pediatric practitioner's need for familiarity with his or her state's screening tests, the necessary confirmatory testing/follow-up, and the conditions' associated clinical features. Effective newborn screening requires a system that includes not only testing but also tracking (follow-up evaluation and diagnosis) and treatment (management).

History of the Newborn Screen (NBS)

In the 1930s, phenylketonuria (PKU), an autosomal recessively inherited inborn error of metabolism, was discovered to be a cause of mental retardation. Soon after, Dr. Robert Guthrie developed diagnostic testing, but treatment was not available. Decades later, treatment with a diet low in phenylalanine was attempted, and it was realized that the sooner treatment was begun, the better the outcome. The method of testing dried blood spots on filter paper made mass screening possible. Thus, newborn screening began in the 1960s, with testing for PKU. Although PKU causes severe mental retardation when untreated, initiation of a strict diet low in phenylalanine, within the first days of life, and allows an affected individual to maintain normal intelligence.

TESTING, TRACKING, AND TREATMENT

In the early neonatal period (e.g., within 48 hours of birth, or prior to discharge or transfer from the nursery) a newborn's blood is spotted on filter paper, dried, and sent to the state-designated lab for testing. Although the screening of newborns is mandated in the United States, each state has its own timing protocols, panel of conditions tested for, normal values and cutoffs for positive results, and protocols to track patients and initiate treatment. All states screen for PKU and congenital hypothyroidism; most screen for galactosemia and sickle-cell anemia and some screen for maple syrup urine disease (MSUD) and congenital adrenal hyperplasia (CAH). The American College of Medical Genetics (ACMG), in association with the Health Resources and Services Administration (HRSA), has recommended a list of 29 conditions that should be included in newborn screening programs (9 organic acidemias, 5 disorders of fatty acid oxidation, 6 amino acid disorders, 3 hemoglobinopathies, and 6 others).

Some states incorporate a second sample obtained after discharge to improve sensitivity. For some conditions, collection of a second dried blood spot is appropriate for evaluation of mildly abnormal results, whereas other conditions require referral to the appropriate specialist for even minor abnormalities.

The next component of the screening process is tracking positive results. Once a sample is shown to yield an abnormal result, the patient must be located, and the responsible physician (usually the provider of record at the time of birth), and often the state board of health, notified. There may also be a designated team of subspecialists, such as geneticists, hematologists, infectious disease specialists, and endocrinologists, who are notified of positive results and are responsible for evaluating the patient to confirm or exclude the diagnosis. Finally, in coordination with the primary care physician, the appropriate subspecialist initiates prompt treatment and management.

EXPANDED NBS

A variety of laboratory techniques are used for NBS tests, including fluorometry and fluorescent antibodies, colorimetric testing, high-performance liquid chromatography (HPLC) with isoelectric focusing, bacterial inhibition assay, and tandem mass spectroscopy (MS/MS). MS/MS has emerged as an effective means of screening for an expanding number of inherited metabolic diseases (aminoacidemias, fatty acid oxidation defects, and others) with relative ease. Increasingly, states are incorporating MS analysis of amino acids and acylcarnitines in dried blood spots into their screening protocol and thus significantly increasing the number of conditions screened for ("expanded NBS"). This is a somewhat different approach to screening, because elevation of one analyte can be due to a number of conditions, and one condition may have several metabolic markers, whereas previously each metabolic condition was identified by elevation of a single metabolite. In addition, the tests detect scores of rare diseases, not all of which have effective treatments, and in some cases the sensitivity of various markers for different metabolic diseases is unknown. Although expanded newborn screening has been in existence for a number of years, it is currently available in only a handful of states and from commercial labs. Other states have introduced pilot expanded newborn screening programs using MS/MS, and most are now investigating the prospect of offering such screening, in order to comply with the recent HRSA/ACMG recommendations.

INTERPRETATION OF NEWBORN SCREENING TESTS: GENERAL APPROACH

The majority of conditions tested for in the NBS do not result in symptoms at birth. Because the goal of testing is to identify all at-risk individuals, some number of unaffected individuals will have positive screening results. Prompt evaluation of neonates with positive screens is important for early diagnosis and treatment, as well as timely reassurance to families in cases of false positives.

A number of factors can affect the outcome of a neonate's screen. These include age at sampling, prematurity, birthweight, the infant and maternal diet, blood transfusion, ethnicity, and parental consanguinity. Age of the newborn can be important for interpreting the results, as normal ranges may vary with postnatal age or weight. An inadequately or incorrectly completed NBS card (incomplete demographic information or insufficiently dried blood spots) can delay identification of an affected infant. For some metabolic conditions, a sample collected from an affected individual in the first days of life is more likely to display a characteristic or diagnostic pattern, whereas testing the same individual at even a week of age may not reveal the same pattern, and the infant may not be identified as affected.

INTERPRETATION OF NBS TESTS: SYMPTOMATIC AND ASYMPTOMATIC CHILDREN

It is important to remember that NBS tests are just that, screening tests. In the case of a *symptomatic newborn*, a negative NBS does not exclude a condition suggested by clinical signs. Hypothyroidism, for example, has a particularly high false-negative rate. When a condition included in the NBS is suspected clinically, diagnostic testing should be pursued. Although sending a repeat sample to the NBS lab can be a useful addition to diagnostic testing, and may provide testing sensitivity information to the screening laboratory, repeating the NBS alone is inadequate.

Individuals with phenotypes characterized by a milder or atypical course or an older age of onset are often not identified by the NBS tests. The cutoffs used in the screening program are generally designed to identify individuals most likely to benefit from treatment, while minimizing the false-positive rate. In the case of an older infant or child with symptoms suggestive of a condition included in the NBS, analysis of a blood spot by the state-designated NBS lab may still be useful, although many screening labs have not established reference intervals for older infants and children. Some conditions included in current screening may not have been part of testing at the time of the child's birth. International adoptees often have limited, if any, newborn screening, and it may be appropriate after arrival in the United States to send a sample to the screening lab, even if the infant is asymptomatic.

Conversely, in an *asymptomatic neonate* with a positive screening result, the absence of clinical symptoms is not reassuring. Positive results require heightened clinical suspicion for underlying disease and further testing for confirmation or exclusion of a diagnosis. Infants who are being evaluated for a metabolic disease should be monitored closely, as they may be at risk for decompensation during periods of fasting or intercurrent illness.

- Failure to receive notification of abnormal results does not necessarily imply a normal screen. There are many possible reasons for a physician not to receive NBS results, including the test not being performed, incomplete demographics, or an error in delivery of the sample or the results.
- Evaluation of abnormal results should be done as directed by the screening lab, with repeat screening only at the request of that lab. Discussion with the appropriate subspecialist may be helpful for the workup of an infant whose results indicate the need for immediate assessment and testing, but for whom that evaluation is delayed.
- Many NBS results are not sufficiently abnormal to require confirmatory testing, and the physician will be asked to obtain a repeat blood spot for retesting by the NBS lab.

CONDITIONS INCLUDED IN NBS

Hemoglobinopathies

Early identification of sickle cell anemia (SCA) and other hemoglobinopathies allows for prompt initiation of coordinated medical care, which can decrease mortality. NBS for hemoglobinopathies measures normal and abnormal hemoglobins (Hb A, F, C, S, and others) via hemoglobin isoelectric focusing or high-performance liquid chromatography (HPLC). Not only are pathologic hemoglobin variants identified, but hemoglobin variants of limited clinical significance and carrier states are also identified.

Interpretation of the hemoglobin analysis is complex, and a number of quick reference tables for the interpretation of the hemoglobinopathy portion of the NBS are available (e.g., "Quick Reference Guide to Results from Massachusetts Newborn Screening for Hemoglobinopathies," available at www.nepscc.org/newbornscreen.html). All samples obtained in the neonatal period will show the presence of HbF (fetal), which is present at a higher concentration than HbA (normal adult hemoglobin). Reports will typically list the types of hemoglobin detected, in order of predominance (FAS is not equivalent to FSA). Thus, FA is a normal result.

The most clinically relevant hemoglobinopathies identified are sickle cell disease and beta-thalassemia. HbS is an abnormal hemoglobin found in sickle cell disease or the sickle cell carrier state. HbC is another aberrant form that in combination with other abnormal hemoglobins can be associated with sickle cell disease.

HbS is seen in various types of sickle cell disease, and when it predominates over HbA it causes clinical sickle-cell disease (FS, FSA, FSC). Sickle cell trait is identified when HbA predominates over HbS (FAS). Beta-thalassemia is diagnosed in the presence of an abnormal HbA to HbF ratio. NBS does not identify beta-thalassemia trait (carrier).

Hemoglobin Bart (HbB) is seen in individuals affected with one of a number of types of alpha-thalassemia, ranging from a silent carrier state (one of the four alpha hemoglobin alleles deleted) to hemoglobin H disease (three of the four alpha hemoglobin alleles deleted). When all four alpha hemoglobin alleles are absent, Hemoglobin Bart (HbB) is produced to the exclusion of all other hemoglobins (including HbF and HbA), a condition incompatible with extrauterine life, which presents as hydrops fetalis.

If a newborn screens positive for a hemoglobinopathy, referral to a hematologist and diagnostic testing by hemoglobin electrophoresis (except for HbB) are necessary to define the underlying condition or to identify false positives. A solubility test (sickle prep) is inadequate for follow-up of an abnormal NBS. Penicillin prophylaxis to prevent sepsis is indicated in individuals identified as having one of the types of sickle cell disease.

Genetic counseling should be provided to families of children identified as having sickle or HbC trait (carriers) or as carriers of other hemoglobin variants. Carrier status may have reproductive implications, not only for the infant upon reaching reproductive age, but also for the parents, who may be at risk for having a child with a significant hemoglobinopathy if both are carriers of a hemoglobin variant.

- The hemoglobinopathy screen may be invalid if an infant has received a blood transfusion within a certain number of weeks of the NBS. If more adult hemoglobin than expected for age is noted, a transfusion is assumed. Although a history of blood transfusion should be noted on the NBS card, it should never delay submission of a sample per usual protocol, because the majority of other NBS results can be interpreted normally. The timing of submission of a repeat sample should follow state guidelines. (See "Galactosemia" later in the chapter.)

Cystic Fibrosis

NBS for cystic fibrosis (CF), aimed at improving long-term pulmonary function and nutritional outcomes, typically involves a two-tiered approach, which can include a combination of biochemical and genetic (DNA) testing. First, the level of immunoreactive trypsinogen (IRT) in the blood spot is measured. IRT is a nonspecific marker of pancreatic function, and repeat IRT testing at a few weeks of age improves specificity. When the IRT is not elevated, the infant is presumed not to have CF. Typically, all samples with an IRT level above the 95th percentile undergo second-tier testing. In some states, samples above a cutoff IRT level are tested for the presence of the most common CF mutation(s). The number of mutations tested for is state-specific.

Sweat chloride testing remains the gold standard diagnostic test for CF. The identification of two pathogenic mutations, however, essentially confirms a diagnosis of CF. When one mutation is identified, a sweat test, usually performed 1 to 2 weeks after the positive result is reported, is used to determine the infant's CF status. When the IRT is elevated but no mutations are found, implying that the likelihood of CF is low, sweat testing is often performed nonetheless. States that perform NBS for CF have diagnostic protocols in place that also address diagnostically difficult cases, such as those in which one mutation is present with a "borderline" sweat test result; discussion of the evaluation of these variations is beyond the scope of this chapter.

- Elevated IRT is associated with pancreatic insufficiency, and may not identify the pancreatic-sufficient CF variants that may be associated with chronic sinusitis or congenital absence of the vas deferens. Often no elevation of the IRT is found in babies with meconium ileus, a common neonatal presentation of CF.
- CF is most common in the Caucasian population, but occurs in all ethnic groups. When mutation analysis is used as part of the screening protocol, it is important to realize that such testing typically includes those mutations most common in the Caucasian population. Therefore, the false-negative rate of the screening test is based on the panel of mutations used and the ethnicity of the population tested. Caution in interpreting the NBS (positive or negative) is important when the ethnic background is not Caucasian.
- One consequence of using molecular testing as part of the newborn screen is the identification of CF carriers, at about

three times the rate that affected patients are identified. As with the hemoglobinopathies, a child's carrier status has potentially important reproductive implications both for the child and for its parents; thus, accurate genetic counseling is important for the entire family.

Congenital Adrenal Hyperplasia

The goal of screening for congenital adrenal hyperplasia (CAH) due to 21-hydroxylase deficiency (21-OH) is to identify male neonates at risk for adrenal crisis due to the salt-wasting form of CAH (hyponatremia, hyperkalemia, and hypotension). CAH due to 21-OH is classified into three categories: classic salt-wasting, classic simple virilizing, and nonclassical forms. The classic forms, which are caused by severe mutations in the CYP21A2 gene, lead to increased production of adrenal androgens (17-alpha hydroxyprogesterone, DHEAS, androstenedione, and testosterone), with consequent virilization. Salt-wasting occurs if mineralocorticoid synthesis is also affected by the CYP21A2 mutation. Although infant girls with the salt-wasting form (and the non-salt-wasting form) attract medical attention soon after birth due to the associated genital virilization, infant boys (1/40,000 births) are clinically undetected until they present in adrenal crisis. Current screening methods for CAH measure the concentration of 17-alpha hydroxyprogesterone (17OHP) in the filter paper blood spot.

- The incidence of 21-OH CAH (an autosomal recessive condition) is greater in communities with higher rates of consanguinity.
- The rate of false positives is higher in premature and low-birthweight infants.
- NBS for CAH does not differentiate between classic salt-wasting CAH and the simple virilizing type. Nonclassic 21-OH CAH is not usually identified by NBS.
- NBS does not screen for non-21-OH forms of CAH (e.g., 11-OH deficiency and 3-beta HSD deficiency).

Congenital Infections

The goal of population-based screening of asymptomatic neonates for congenitally acquired infection is to allow for early diagnosis and treatment. Some states include screening for either human immunodeficiency virus (HIV) and/or the *Toxoplasma gondii* protozoan parasite as part of their NBS panel. Others attempt to identify HIV risk by testing pregnant women, testing the newborn only when there has been inadequate testing of the mother. The CDC, AAP, and ACOG support screening of all pregnant women for HIV. These screening decisions, as well as non-population-based HIV testing of at-risk newborns, are addressed in Chapter 83.

One method of screening newborns for congenital infection uses serologic immunoassay for specific antibodies. IgM-specific antibodies imply infection of the newborn. A positive screen for IgM antibodies to *Toxoplasma* in an asymptomatic neonate must be followed up with confirmatory testing. A number of different assays measuring IgA or IgM levels are available, and a combination of these is usually recommended for confirmatory testing. Treatment of asymptomatic infected newborns with pyrimethamine and sulfadiazine appears to lead to improved outcomes.

Antibody-based testing for HIV identifies the mother's HIV status and does not imply infection of the neonate. Currently, the only state using a population-based newborn screening approach for identification of HIV is New York, which employs a DNA PCR-based testing methodology. A positive DNA PCR screen in a neonate should be followed by immediate initiation of HIV antiretroviral prophylaxis. Follow-up HIV PCR-based testing is required to determine the infant's HIV status. This is typically performed at birth, repeated at 4 to 6 weeks, and again 2 to 3 months later. Testing and treatment should be coordinated through a pediatric HIV/infectious disease center.

■ Infants infected during delivery may have a negative HIV DNA PCR test during the first few days of life, and high-risk neonates require follow-up testing.

Hypothyroidism

The fact that all states screen for congenital hypothyroidism represents one of the most significant successes of NBS. Most states use a two-tiered approach, either measuring thyroxine (T4) in all blood spots, followed by measurement of thyroid stimulating hormone (TSH) in the subset of samples falling below a cutoff, or vice versa (T4 measured subsequent to an elevated TSH level). Methodologies that measure TSH only can miss cases of central hypothyroidism. Abnormalities are detected in approximately 1 in 2,500 newborns. The causes of congenital hypothyroidism are diverse, but early treatment has been shown to protect against the developmental problems seen when the disease is left untreated.

■ When TSH measurement is the primary screen, congenital hypothyroidism associated with delayed elevation of TSH will be missed if samples are obtained within the first 48 hours of life, or if they are taken from sick or premature infants.

Galactosemia

A number of inherited enzyme defects can result in the inability to metabolize galactose, causing galactosemia. The most common form of galactosemia is due to galactose-1-phosphate uridyltransferase (GALT) deficiency. Screening for galactosemia aims to prevent or reverse the early problems that can occur with severe GALT deficiency, such as increased susceptibility to bacteremia with gram-negative organisms, cataracts, and liver dysfunction. If instituted early enough, treatment with a galactose-restricted diet is effective in reversing both cataracts and liver disease.

The sugar galactose is contained in human and cow's milk—based formulas, but not in soy-based formulas. Newborn screening for galactosemia may involve measurement of galactose or use a fluorometric assay for GALT activity in RBCs. Measurement of total galactose identifies all forms of galactosemia, but only in those infants who have received galactose prior to sample collection. The GALT assay identifies GALT deficiency independent of dietary intake of galactose, but does not identify other forms of galactosemia.

Positive NBS results require follow-up with biochemical quantitative measurement of GALT activity, GALT electrophoresis/isoelectric focusing, and/or molecular testing to confirm the diagnosis and determine the presence of classic galactosemia (G) and Duarte (D) alleles. The most common classic mutation is Q188R. The presence of two classic galactosemia mutations leads to the complete absence of GALT activity. Abnormally low, but not absent, enzyme levels occur in individuals with one or two Duarte mutations (G/D or D/D). Some screening programs test samples with low GALT activity for common GALT mutations in order to distinguish classical galactosemia from milder variants such as Duarte, that do not require lifelong restriction of galactose.

■ Some states measure galactose, and false-negatives can occur in infants who have not ingested adequate galactose.
■ False negatives are rare in classic galactosemia (G/G), but Duarte variants (D/D or G/D) may not be detected. False positives can occur if blood is collected in EDTA tubes or stored at warm temperatures.

■ As with hemoglobinopathies, GALT testing may remain inaccurate for months after a blood transfusion. GALT activity can be falsely elevated into the normal range (negative) in an infant with galactosemia who has received a blood transfusion.
■ Mutation analysis cannot exclude the diagnosis, because it currently only identifies the most common mutations. If a baby is suspected to have galactosemia, but two mutations are not found, quantitative measurement of GALT in blood is required.
■ Diagnosis of the epimerase and kinase forms of galactosemia requires a specific request for these enzyme assays.

Biotinidase Deficiency

The enzyme biotinidase releases biotin from biotin-dependent carboxylases. Biotinidase deficiency results in a deficit of free biotin and a secondary deficiency of the carboxylases. Treatment with biotin can prevent the seizures, hair loss, and hearing loss caused by this form of multiple carboxylase deficiency. The NBS measures biotinidase activity directly, using a colorimetric or fluorometric assay, and identifies severe biotinidase deficiency, as well as partial deficiency (10–30% activity). Follow-up testing in positive screens is by quantitative serum biotinidase assay.

SCREENING BY TANDEM MASS SPECTROMETRY

MS/MS can be used to measure amino acids and acylcarnitines in dried blood spots. The pattern and levels of particular acylcarnitines is used to identify aminoacidopathies, organic acidemias, and disorders of fatty acid oxidation.

Phenylketonuria and Other Hyperphenylalaninemias

Classical phenylketonuria (PKU) is caused by lack of the enzyme phenylalanine hydroxylase (PAH), with consequent inability to metabolize phenylalanine, an essential amino acid, to tyrosine. Screening has been performed through the Guthrie bacterial inhibition assay, fluorimetric phenylalanine assay, or by MS/MS measurement of phenylalanine and tyrosine. A high phenylalanine level identifies hyperphenylalaninemia (HPA), but additional testing is required to confirm a diagnosis of PKU. An elevated phenylalanine/tyrosine ratio can help distinguish between true abnormalities of phenylalanine metabolism and transient elevations in phenylalanine in postprandial samples. HPA can be seen in the first days of life in infants born to mothers with PKU, but phenylalanine levels rapidly normalize, unless the infant also has PKU. Abnormalities in the metabolism of tetrahydrobiopterin (BH4), a cofactor for PAH, can also cause persistent HPA.

Treatment of PKU should be initiated as soon as further testing confirms the diagnosis, but testing for BH4 defects (by urine pterins and blood dihydropteridine reductase assay) should precede treatment with a phenylalanine-restricted diet, because BH4 replacement is indicated for BH4-responsive HPA. Mutation analysis has limited usefulness in PKU because of the great number of mutations and lack of common mutations.

■ Feeding is not necessary to detect PKU on NBS. In an infant with PKU, the concentration of phenylalanine in the blood begins to rise after separation from the placenta. The most accurate results are obtained from samples collected after 24 hours of age.
■ Infants of mothers with PKU will have an abnormal NBS. If the infant is unaffected the phenylalanine level will fall within a few days, but if affected (1 in 200 chance), the level will remain abnormal.

■ A phenylalanine-restricted diet will retard growth in an infant who is able to metabolize phenylalanine. Initiation of a phenylalanine-free formula prior to obtaining adequate confirmatory testing samples is not recommended, as it may lead to inaccurate diagnostic testing results and poor growth.

■ Hyperalimentation or postprandial samples can result in elevation of blood phenylalanine. If initial testing reveals elevated phenylalanine, repeat testing should be obtained preprandially or after stopping parenteral nutrition for 30 to 60 minutes.

■ Antibiotic contamination of the sample can affect results when the bacterial inhibition assay is used, even in the presence of elevated blood phenylalanine. Antibiotic use does not interfere with diagnosis of PKU by other methods, however.

■ The urine ferric chloride screening test is unreliable for the detection of PKU.

■ Persistent mild elevations of phenylalanine may not be detected by newborn screening, which may miss some individuals with abnormalities of biopterin metabolism ("non-PKU HPA"). Rarely, mild hyperphenylalaninemia in an infant has significance later in life, including potential fetal exposure to a mother's elevated phenylalanine during pregnancy, with possible teratogenic effects.

Tyrosinemia

The goal of screening is to identify neonates at risk for hepatorenal tyrosinemia (tyrosinemia type 1, a condition particularly common in Quebec), which untreated results in liver failure, coagulopathy, proximal tubulopathy, and eventually hepatocellular carcinoma. Treatment with both a tyrosine-restricted diet and Orphadin, if started in the first month, greatly reduces the risk of hepatocellular carcinoma.

MS/MS screening for tyrosinemia includes measurement of tyrosine concentration. The measurement of tyrosine alone will identify infants with tyrosinemia types 2 and 3 and benign transient tyrosinemia, seen in premature and some term infants; but is unlikely to identify tyrosinemia type 1, because plasma tyrosine is only mildly elevated prior to the development of liver disease. To improve identification of tyrosinemia type 1, some screening programs test samples with mildly elevated tyrosine for succinylacetone, a compound pathognomonic for tyrosinemia type 1 that rises before hepatic dysfunction develops.

■ A normal tyrosine level at the time of screening does not rule out tyrosinemia type 1.

■ Elevated tyrosine levels can also result from liver disease.

Homocystinuria

Homocystinuria can result from a number of defects in the metabolism of methionine. The most treatable form of homocystinuria is due to deficiency of cystathionine beta synthase (CBS) and is detected through the identification of elevated methionine.

■ Hypermethioninemia may not be present during the first few days of life when the blood spot is typically obtained. The B6-responsive type of CBS deficiency the most readily treatable form, is not often missed by current NBS protocols.

■ Elevated methionine is also seen in liver disease, transient hypermethioninemia of the newborn, and methionine adenosyltransferase deficiency.

■ Homocystinuria due to abnormalities of folate or vitamin B_{12} metabolism is not identified by newborn screening, as methionine levels tend to be low in these conditions.

Maple Syrup Urine Disease

Screening for maple syrup urine disease (MSUD) is aimed at preventing the life-threatening effects of untreated MSUD, which can present as irritability advancing to encephalopathy and coma within the first 2 weeks of life. The branched-chain amino acids leucine, isoleucine, and alloisoleucine are all elevated in this disorder, due to defects in branched-chain alpha-ketoacid dehydrogenase complex (BCKD). NBS for this condition traditionally has been performed by the Guthrie bacterial inhibition assay for leucine, the amino acid most significantly elevated in infants with MSUD. MS/MS cannot distinguish among leucine, isoleucine, and alloisoleucine, so the reported results include the concentrations of all three of these amino acids, as well as hydroxyproline. Classic MSUD, the intermediate form of MSUD, and deficiency of E3 (one of the components of BCKD), can be detected by NBS. The intermittent form and the thiamine-responsive types may be missed by NBS.

Infants with MSUD often become ill during the first 2 weeks of life, and prompt evaluation is required following a positive NBS or if an individual presents with symptoms, including the distinctive odor of maple syrup or burnt sugar detected on wet diaper or in ear wax. Diagnostic testing is through plasma amino acid and urine organic acid analyses. The branched-chain amino acids are greatly elevated in blood, CSF, and urine; the presence of alloisoleucine in particular is pathognomonic for MSUD. High levels are always present in classic MSUD, and in milder forms will persist in the plasma for several days following an episode of decompensation.

■ The urine DNPH (2,4-dinitrophenylhydrazine) test identifies alpha-keto acids including acetoacetate, which is not a good screening test for MSUD.

■ Parenteral amino acid solutions are especially high in branched-chain amino acids and often result in false-positive results. Calculation of a leucine/phenylalanine ratio can help distinguish true MSUD from a false positive due to parenteral nutrition.

■ The urine from breast-fed newborns can have a sweet odor from spices or curry in the mother's diet. A similar odor can be noted when the umbilical stump is cleaned with Betadine. Some disposable diapers have even been noted to emit this odor in older infants.

Urea Cycle Disorders

MS/MS measurement of citrulline and arginine levels can identify some urea cycle disorders. In their most severe forms, most urea cycle disorders present in the neonatal period with coma that may be mistaken for sepsis if the associated hyperammonemia goes unnoticed. Elevated citrulline is seen with citrullinemia (argininosuccinate synthetase deficiency) and argininosuccinic acidemia (argininosuccinyl-CoA lyase deficiency), while low citrulline levels can identify infants with ornithine transcarbamylase deficiency. Elevation of plasma arginine may indicate argininemia (arginase deficiency), a rare disorder of the urea cycle. Infants with positive NBSs for urea cycle disorders should be referred to a metabolic center for plasma ammonia levels, plasma amino acid analysis, and urine organic acid analysis. Morbidity and mortality in these conditions can be high, and it remains unclear whether early identification by NBS will improve outcomes. Treatment with a protein-restricted diet and ammonia conjugating agents improves survival of individuals with urea cycle disorders.

Organic Acid Disorders

Organic acid disorders result from abnormalities in the metabolism of various amino acids. Often, neonates affected with an organic acidemia are well for the first few days of life, and

TABLE 123.1

TABLE 123.1

ORGANIC ACID DISORDERS RECOMMENDED FOR NBS BY ACMG/HRSA

Condition	Abnormal acylcarnitines	Comments
Isovaleric acidemia	C5	Presentation can range in severity, but is characterized by metabolic acidosis and the characteristic "sweaty feet odor." The condition may progress to coma and death.
Glutaric acidemia, type I	C5-DC	The incidence of this condition is high in Old Order Amish. False negatives can occur. Results can normalize on repeat acylcarnitine screening. One clinical presentation is rapid head growth and later macrocephaly.
3-Hydroxy-3-methylglutaryl-CoA lyase deficiency (HMG)	C5-OH	May present from the neonatal period to childhood with symptoms resembling Reye syndrome.
Multiple carboxylase deficiency (MCD)	C5-OH	These enzymes are dependent on biotin, so most children respond to treatment with oral biotin supplementation.
Methylmalonic acidemias (MMA), (mutase deficiency, Cb1 A,B)	C3	There are a variety of types of MMA, ranging from a milder, vitamin B_{12}-responsive type with good outcomes to severe, B_{12}-unresponsive types.
3-Methylcronyl-CoA carboxylase deficiency (3MMC)	C5:1, C5-OH	The clinical course is quite variable. Abnormal test results may be from an affected, asymptomatic mother.
Propionic acidemia	C3	Neurologic damage can occur during metabolic crises. May not respond consistently to treatment.
Beta (3)-ketothiolase deficiency	C5:1, C5-OH	Clinical course is variable, ranging from asymptomatic to severe ketoacidosis, coma, and cardiomyopathy.

then become ill; some present later, with failure to thrive or neurologic problems. Early initiation of treatment may improve outcomes, so infants with an abnormal NBS profile suggestive of an organic acid disorder should be evaluated immediately. In rare cases, follow-up testing may simply involve sending plasma acylcarnitines or a repeat sample to the NBS lab if the child is well. However, most abnormalities suggesting an organic acidemia require prompt, definitive testing through urine organic acid analysis, urine ketones, and plasma amino acid analysis. The pattern of organic acids in the urine will point to the diagnosis, which is then confirmed with enzyme assays. Diets low in protein with diagnosis-specific amino acid restrictions and avoidance of catabolism, including early treatment of illnesses, are the mainstay of treatment. Although severely affected individuals will often be symptomatic before the results of newborn screening are available, this testing also identifies individuals with milder enzyme deficiencies so that they can begin treatment before they suffer permanent neurologic injury (Table 123.1).

Fatty Acid Disorders (β-Oxidation Defects)

Fatty acid oxidation disorders (FAOD) result from abnormalities in the mitochondrial breakdown of fatty acids, used for energy during fasting. Acylcarnitines are metabolites of this process; the pattern and levels of particular acylcarnitines detected by MS/MS are used to identify disorders of fatty acid oxidation.

Newborns who are suspected to have a fatty acid oxidation defect are at high risk for metabolic decompensation (often accompanied by hypoketotic hypoglycemia) during fasts or illness, so they should be fed regularly. FAODs can be fatal in the neonatal period in infants who are poor feeders and in breastfed infants when the mother's milk has not come in. Diagnostic testing may include plasma acylcarnitines, plasma free and total carnitines, plasma fatty acid (free and total) profile, and

urine acylglycine and organic acid analyses. Diagnosis is confirmed with enzyme assays and molecular mutation analysis. Treatment typically involves avoidance of fasts, disease-specific recommendations for low fat intake, and early evaluation and treatment of acute illnesses, including IV glucose support during periods of decreased oral intake. Long-chain FAODs may require treatment with medium-chain triglycerides to prevent or reverse the cardiac symptoms commonly seen in these disorders (Table 123.2).

■ Because acylcarnitines can normalize in some infants with FAODs after the first few days of life, normal plasma acylcarnitines should not be used as the sole criteria to exclude an FAOD in an infant with an abnormal newborn screen.

CONCLUSIONS

■ NBS can identify newborns at risk for treatable diseases prior to the onset of symptoms.

■ With new testing strategies, carrier states and conditions with limited information about natural history and utility of treatment are reported.

■ Interpretation of "normal newborn screening" can be difficult, due to the state-to-state variability of the diseases tested for and different methods for identifying at-risk newborns. Each state has designated subspecialists to assist in the diagnosis and treatment of conditions identified through newborn screening, and many states have developed guidelines, often Web-based, for clinicians.

■ The lack of symptoms in a neonate with an NBS suggesting metabolic disease does not exclude the diagnosis.

■ Symptomatic newborns require prompt diagnostic testing and management. In some cases, the results of their NBS may aid in diagnosis.

TABLE 123.2

FATTY ACID OXIDATION DISORDERS (FAOD) RECOMMENDED
FOR NBS BY ACMG/HRSA

Condition	Acylcarnitines	Comments
Medium-chain acyl-CoA dehydrogenase (MCAD) deficiency	C0, C6, C8, C10	Most common FAOD. At high risk for hypoglycemia with fasting.
Very-long-chain acyl-CoA dehydrogenase (VLCAD) deficiency	C14:1, C16, C18:1	Hypertrophic cardiomyopathy common.
Long-chain 3-hydroxy acyl-CoA dehydrogenase (LCHAD) deficiency or trifunctional protein deficiency (TFP)	C14:1, C16-OH C18:1-OH	A pregnant mother carrying a fetus with LCHADD is at risk for HELLP syndrome. Hypoglycemia may not be seen in acute crisis. Pericardial effusion and pigmentary retinopathy are common later findings.
Carnitine uptake defect (CUD)	C0, C16	A low level of free carnitine (C0) may indicate CUD, causing hypoketotic hypoglycemia and cardiomyopathy, or may be due to a diluted sample.

Recommended Readings

American College of Medical Genetics/American Society of Human Genetics Test and Technology Transfer Committee Working Group. Tandem mass spectrometry in newborn screening. *Genet Med* 2000;2:267–269.

National Newborn Screening and Genetics Resource Center website: GeNeS-R-US (Genetic and Newborn Screening Resource Center of the United States), http://www.genes-r-us.uthscsa.edu/index.htm. Accessed Feb. 2, 2006.

Newborn screening fact sheets. American Academy of Pediatrics. Committee on Genetics. *Pediatrics* 1996;98:473–501.

Newborn screening: toward a uniform screening panel and system. *Genet Med* 8(suppl 1);2006,15–115.

Rose SR, Brown RS, Foley T, et al. Update of newborn screening and therapy for congenital hypothyroidism. *Pediatrics* 2006;117:2290–2303.

Seashore MR, Seashore CJ. Newborn screening and the pediatric practitioner. *Semin Perinatol* 2005;29:182–188.

CHAPTER 124 ■ STABILIZATION OF THE NEWBORN FOR TRANSPORT

SCOTT S. MACGILVRAY

Of the nearly 4 million infants born in the United States each year, the majority are delivered in community hospitals. As a result of the regionalization of perinatal care, many of the infants who require tertiary care are identified prenatally and delivered in a tertiary care medical center. However, there will always be infants born in community hospitals who will require transfer to a tertiary care medical center. One reason is that mothers may arrive at the community hospital in advanced premature labor with insufficient time to transfer them to the tertiary care medical center where specialized neonatal services are available. In other cases, the conditions requiring specialized neonatal services have escaped prenatal detection, may not develop until late in pregnancy, or do not develop until after birth. Under these circumstances arrangements to transfer infants to a facility where they can receive the services they need is made once they have been identified as requiring a higher level of care than can be provided at the birth hospital. One of the most important phases in the successful transfer of a newborn infant is the stabilization of the patient prior to transport.

The process of stabilizing a neonate for transport begins with the identification of the problem in the infant, and continues until the transport team departs the referring hospital with the patient. Neonatal outcomes are enhanced by the timely provision of appropriate interventions to the patient. Given that it may take several hours for the transport team to arrive and assume care of the patient, the physicians and staff at the referring hospital play a vital role in the stabilization of the newborn for transport. As such, it is critical that physicians and staff in the community hospitals work to enhance their procedural skills and knowledge to optimize the care of these patients.

The importance of the resuscitation and stabilization team has been highlighted by several reports in the literature. In 1996 Kronick and colleagues reported the observations of the Children's Hospital of Western Ontario transport team (1). They noted that there was a significant inverse correlation between the number of procedures and interventions performed by the transport team and the length of time the referring physician had been in practice. They also noted that there was a greater need for procedures and therapeutic interventions when the referring physician was someone other than a pediatrician. This complemented a report in 1993 by Whitfield and Buser detailing the experience of the Children's Emergency Transport Service in Denver (2). They reported that the time the transport team spent stabilizing the infant in the referring hospital varied based on the severity of the infant's condition; it was an average of 70 minutes for nonventilated patients and an average of 136 minutes for patients requiring mechanical ventilation and inotropic support. Although not addressed in their report, it

follows that the more stable the patient is when the transport team arrives, the more rapidly the patient can be transferred to the tertiary care medical center.

McNamara and colleagues reported in 2005 on the experience of the Acute Care Transport System of the Hospital for Sick Children, University of Toronto (3). They compared the outcomes of premature infants resuscitated by the community hospital team with those resuscitated by the transport team who had been called to attend the delivery in the community hospital. They found that 40% of the infants resuscitated by the community hospital providers were hypothermic, and that the transport team was able to intubate and secure vascular access significantly more rapidly than the community hospital providers. Taken together, these reports support the need for continuing education and training in neonatal resuscitation and stabilization, including technical skills such as intubation and vascular access, for physicians and staff in community hospitals.

There are several programs available that can help meet these educational needs, including the Neonatal Resuscitation Program (NRP), the Perinatal Continuing Education Program (PCEP), and the S.T.A.B.L.E. transport education program (STABLE). All of these programs offer practical approaches to neonatal stabilization in the context of the community hospital setting. Many neonatal centers also offer outreach educational programs in addition to the above programs, including workshops that teach the various procedures that may be needed to successfully resuscitate and stabilize a neonate. Participation in these programs has the added benefit of establishing a relationship between the physicians at the referring and accepting institutions, enhancing communication that is imperative when caring for a critically ill neonate.

RECOGNITION OF THE NEED FOR TRANSPORT

The most important step in the stabilization of a neonate is the recognition that she needs a level of care that cannot be provided in the current hospital, and therefore requires transfer to another facility where that care is available. In some instances this need is immediately apparent, as in the case of small premature infants or infants with major congenital anomalies. In other instances the need for transport, while not initially present, may evolve over a period of time as the patient's condition changes. The decision on whether a particular infant needs to be transferred will depend on the capabilities of the community hospital and should be individualized. Although it may be appropriate to care for a child on continuous positive airway pressure (CPAP) in one hospital, another may be

637

unable to provide needed intravenous (IV) fluids to an infant, and it would therefore be inappropriate to care for the patient in that facility. When management questions arise and the need for transfer is considered, early telephone consultation with a physician at a receiving tertiary care hospital can be very helpful. Even if the collaborative decision is that the patient does not require transfer at that moment, the discussion often leads to improved patient care and facilitation of the patient's transfer should it become necessary.

Antenatal Screening and Monitoring

The optimal time for transferring a newborn to a tertiary care facility is prenatally. This will allow specialized neonatal services to be present from the moment of birth and provides for optimal outcomes. In order to identify as many high-risk pregnancies as possible, all pregnancies should be screened for risk factors, such as those listed in *Guidelines for Perinatal Care*, 4th edition (see the Suggested Readings); and when appropriate, referral made to the tertiary center before delivery. An accurate determination of gestational age should be documented as early as possible to aid in this process. Maternal and fetal status must also be monitored during labor, as approximately 25% of pregnancy complications are first identified at that time. In keeping with the NRP guidelines, if risk factors or complications that increase the probability of difficulties with the delivery and transition to newborn life are identified, at least two individuals skilled in neonatal resuscitation should attend the delivery.

Evaluation of the Newborn

The evaluation of a newborn infant begins at the time of delivery and continues through the transition period. This period may last for several hours, but for most infants will be completed in 15 to 30 minutes. Although most infants who require transfer will develop symptoms within the first several minutes to hours of life, depending on the underlying disorder, some may not do so for several days. In general, infants who require significant or ongoing resuscitation are of very low birthweight, or have major congenital anomalies should undergo resuscitation and stabilization while preparations for transport to a tertiary center are made (see below). Infants who are apparently healthy and successfully complete the transition to newborn life should have a comprehensive evaluation by the nursery staff within the first 2 hours of life. This should include a review of maternal risk factors, physical examination with measurement of weight, length, and head circumference, vital signs, and gestational age assessment. This information can then be used to classify the infant as well, at risk, or sick, as described in the PCEP:

Well

- Term
- Weight appropriate for gestational age
- No maternal risk factors
- Normal physical examination and vital signs
- Normal feeding and activity

At Risk

Normal physical examination, vital signs, feeding, and activity, but also one or more of the following:

- Preterm or postterm
- Small or large for gestational age
- Presence of maternal risk factors
- Abnormal labor and delivery or need for resuscitation (e.g., low Apgar score)
- Previous abnormal examination or vital signs, which are now normal

Sick

- Abnormal physical examination, vital signs, feeding, or activity

Subsequent management is guided by this classification. Infants categorized as "well" are provided with standard newborn care with periodic observation, feeding, and routine treatments and diagnostic evaluations (e.g., vitamin K administration, eye prophylaxis, newborn metabolic screening). Infants categorized as "at risk" may undergo more frequent assessments and specific diagnostic testing, depending on what risk has been identified: for example, the monitoring of serum glucose levels in an infant born to a diabetic mother. Many of these infants will be stable with no immediate problems, and as such require no special care beyond the more frequent evaluations. However, in certain instances where complex or unusual diagnostic procedures are needed, these infants may require transfer to a referral center to complete their evaluation. Infants categorized as "sick" require immediate diagnostic and therapeutic intervention to provide basic support and to identify and treat the underlying pathology. Many of these infants will require transfer to a tertiary care medical center. A key point is that the provision of diagnostic and therapeutic interventions should begin immediately, and not wait for the arrival of a transport team. Specifics of the required interventions can be discussed with the tertiary center to begin the stabilization process.

GENERAL SUPPORT AND EVALUATION

Thermal Support

All newborn infants, but especially those who are ill and premature, have impaired thermoregulation and may experience excessive heat loss during resuscitation or procedures. This leaves them at an increased risk of hypothermia and its consequences, which include a significant increase in morbidity and mortality in the very premature newborn. These risks can be reduced by providing a warm environment, avoiding drafts, and monitoring the infant's temperature. Covering the infant's head with a stocking cap will significantly decrease heat loss, as will promptly drying infants with warm towels or blankets. To minimize heat loss during the initial resuscitation and observation, and during procedures, infants should be placed on radiant warmers with servo-regulated temperature control. After stabilization they may be moved into prewarmed incubators. In order to maintain normal body temperature, the incubator temperature can either be set manually according to the infant's estimated "neutral thermal environment," or automatically, using the servo-control mechanism in the incubator with a surface electrode placed on the patient.

Observation and Monitoring

When an infant is ill with rapidly changing status, it requires nearly continuous monitoring and observation. In order to monitor color, perfusion, respiratory status, and other important parameters, the infant should not be clothed or swaddled in blankets. For this reason sick infants are best observed in an open servo-controlled radiant warmer. This allows them to be easily observed, with ready access for any needed procedures, while maintaining their body temperature. Cardiorespiratory monitors and a pulse oximeter should be applied for continuous monitoring of heart rate, respirations, and oxygen saturation. Serial assessments should be done at least hourly until the patient is stable. These include recording vital signs with blood pressure, as well as assessments of respiratory effort, oxygen saturation, perfusion, neurologic status, and abdominal girth. Any infant with respiratory difficulty or possible abdominal pathology should have a gastric decompression tube placed, and the amount and appearance of any drainage from the tube should be documented. If oxygen is administered, the concentration or fraction of inspired oxygen (FiO_2) should be documented with each assessment, as should auscultation of the lungs with attention to the equality and character of air entry in all lung fields. Transillumination of the chest should be considered in patients experiencing acute cardiorespiratory deterioration (see "Pneumothorax" later in the chapter).

Diagnostic Studies

Most sick infants (those with an abnormal physical examination, vital signs, feeding, or activity) will require some diagnostic laboratory tests to help determine the nature of their condition. The initial evaluation of a sick neonate often includes a complete blood count with differential and platelet count, serum glucose determination, and if respiratory distress is present, either an arterial or capillary blood gas. If there is a concern that sepsis may be present, a blood culture with at least a 1-mL blood sample should be obtained before any antibiotics are started. However, if there is a high index of suspicion, antibiotic therapy should not be unduly delayed because of difficulty in obtaining a blood culture. Depending on an individual patient's particular condition and the expected length of time before the transport team arrives, repeated blood glucose determinations and/or blood gases may be required to monitor the patient's course. Chest radiographs should be obtained in any infant who exhibits respiratory distress or cyanosis, and abdominal radiographs in those exhibiting abdominal distention or feeding intolerance.

Antibiotics

Early-onset neonatal sepsis is a potentially life-threatening condition that may initially present with very subtle and nonspecific signs and symptoms. Accordingly, it is a part of the differential diagnosis for most neonatal illnesses, and consequently many infants are begun on antibiotic therapy pending the results of blood cultures and other screening tests for sepsis. Empiric antibiotic therapy directed against the most common bacterial pathogens responsible for neonatal sepsis should be chosen based on the prevailing antibiotic resistance patterns in the community. One possible combination that is widely used consists of initial doses of ampicillin (50 mg/kg) and gentamicin sulfate (4 mg/kg).

RESPIRATORY SUPPORT

In sick neonates, the organ system most likely to exhibit derangements in function is the respiratory system. As a result of this, respiratory distress, manifested by tachypnea, grunting, nasal flaring, and retractions, with or without hypoxemia, is one of the most common reasons for neonatal transports. Infants with respiratory distress require gastric decompression and may require additional supportive measures, including supplemental oxygen, CPAP, or endotracheal intubation and positive pressure ventilation. Respiratory distress and hypoxemia may be exacerbated by handling; therefore, bathing and repeated examinations should be minimized. For some patients requiring respiratory support, judicious sedation may reduce agitation, thus improving ventilation and oxygenation.

Oxygen

Oxygen without distending airway pressure is best administered via a head hood, although it may also be given via nasal cannula. A head hood allows for a more precise determination of the FiO_2 delivered and better humidification of the respiratory gases than a nasal cannula. The need for supplemental oxygen is indicated by the presence of central cyanosis, and it may be confirmed by the measurement of an oxygen saturation less than 90% by pulse oximetry or by arterial blood gas with a partial pressure of arterial oxygen (PaO_2) less than 50 mm Hg in room air. The delivered FiO_2 should be adjusted to the lowest concentration of oxygen that eliminates cyanosis or produces oxygen saturations of 90% to 94% by pulse oximetry or a PaO_2 of 50 to 80 mm Hg on an arterial blood gas.

Continuous Positive Airway Pressure

Nasal continuous positive airway pressure (CPAP) provides distending airway pressure without the need for endotracheal intubation, thereby helping to maintain airway stability and prevent alveolar collapse. Indications for CPAP include rising oxygen requirements (a fixed FiO_2 greater than 0.60 to 0.80, or rapidly increasing FiO_2), worsening respiratory distress (respiratory rate greater than 60 to 80, moderate to severe retractions), progressive hypercapnia (PCO_2 greater than 60), and periodic apnea. Nasal CPAP is contraindicated in patients with suspected diaphragmatic hernia, abdominal wall defects, or other conditions in which intestinal distention should be minimized. CPAP is also unlikely to be effective for patients with apnea or hypoventilation due to severe neurologic depression.

Mechanical Ventilation

Endotracheal intubation with mechanical ventilation is indicated for patients with acute respiratory failure, who have not responded to a trial of CPAP, or in whom CPAP is contraindicated. Because of the limited ability for physical assessment of patients and the difficulty intubating a patient during transport, an infant may be intubated prior to transport in order to provide a secure airway for the trip. Decisions about the most appropriate type of respiratory support in such cases should be based on the patient's condition, the skill and experience of the community hospital staff, and the expected delay before the arrival of the transport team. It should be emphasized that most infants can be effectively ventilated using a bag-valve-mask system for extended periods of time without the need for intubation, as long as there is no contraindication to CPAP, and a large-caliber orogastric tube is in place to prevent gaseous distension of the abdomen. After intubation, the patient should be placed on a mechanical ventilator with settings that minimize respiratory distress and improve oxygenation. An initial ventilator rate of between 30 and 40 breaths per minute and positive end-expiratory pressure (PEEP) of 4 or 5 cm H_2O will usually be sufficient to accomplish this when coupled with an appropriate peak inspiratory pressure (PIP). The PIP should initially be set somewhere between 18 and 22 cm H_2O; this initial pressure is then quickly adjusted to provide a comfortable chest rise, approximating that seen with a normal breath in healthy infants. After the initial ventilator settings have been selected, the chest wall movement, breath sounds, work of breathing, oxygen requirement, blood gases, and chest radiograph will guide any needed adjustments. After intubation, proper endotracheal tube position is indicated clinically by the presence of bilaterally equal breath sounds and radiographically by locating the tip of the endotracheal tube midway between the clavicles and the carina.

Artificial Surfactant Treatment

Although commonplace in tertiary centers, surfactant replacement therapy is not currently available in most community hospitals. Safe use of this therapy requires experience in identification of patients most likely to benefit from it, proper administration of the drug, adjustment of ventilatory support after dosing, and observation for complications. It should therefore only be undertaken by trained respiratory therapists, nurses, and physicians who use it regularly.

Pneumothorax

A pneumothorax may occur spontaneously, as a complication of an underlying disease process such as meconium aspiration, or as a complication of positive airway pressure ventilatory support. It should be suspected in any infant with respiratory distress, especially if there is a sudden change in respiratory or hemodynamic status. Transillumination of the chest with a high-intensity fiber-optic light should be performed with the room darkened to increase the likelihood of detecting a pneumothorax. If transillumination of the chest is consistent with the presence of a pneumothorax, and the patient is hemodynamically stable, an emergency chest radiograph should be obtained for confirmation. However, intervention to evacuate the pneumothorax should not be delayed for the confirmatory radiograph in patients with severe oxygen desaturation and hemodynamic instability, as these patients usually have a tension pneumothorax causing their hemodynamic compromise. Needle thoracentesis with aspiration of the affected hemithorax will often temporarily alleviate the cardiorespiratory embarrassment while preparations are made for placement of a chest tube. Following evacuation of the pneumothorax by needle aspiration and/or chest tube insertion, the patient's oxygen saturation and blood pressure should improve immediately. Repeated transillumination of the chest can help determine the effectiveness of the intervention and monitor for the return of the pneumothorax.

Patients with a pneumothorax that is not under tension often experience less severe deterioration of respiratory status and frequently have no hemodynamic instability. In these patients, the decision to intervene may be delayed while chest radiographs are obtained to confirm the presence of the pneumothorax and consultation sought from the accepting tertiary center staff. These non-tension pneumothoraces may resolve spontaneously, especially in patients with mild respiratory distress not requiring mechanical ventilation. However, if the patient is to be transported by air with significant changes in altitude, an initially asymptomatic pneumothorax may become significant as the intrapleural air expands with increasing altitude. In this instance, evacuation of the pneumothorax may need to be performed prior to the air transport.

CIRCULATORY SUPPORT

Hypotension/Shock

Patients who are unable to maintain an adequate circulatory volume are at risk for developing metabolic acidosis and hypoperfusion injury to various organs. Hypovolemia may be suspected based on the presence of certain risk factors such as abruptio placenta. In other cases, it may present unexpectedly due to late or unseen complications, such as fetal–maternal transfusion. Signs include pallor, tachycardia, hypotension, weak pulses, and delayed capillary refill. Hypovolemia should also be suspected in patients requiring delivery room resuscitation who fail to respond quickly to positive pressure ventilation and chest compressions.

Infants with signs of hypovolemic shock should initially be treated with attempts at volume expansion. This can be accomplished by the provision of 20 mL/kg of a crystalloid volume expander such as 0.9% saline. Although colloid solutions such as 5% albumin may also be used, they have not been shown to be any more effective than 0.9% saline solutions. In cases where the hypovolemia is the result of an acute blood loss, transfusion with emergency-released un-cross-matched O-negative packed red blood cells may be lifesaving. Further fluid resuscitation may be indicated depending on clinical response and laboratory studies.

For term infants whose mean blood pressure is less than 40 to 50 mm Hg, or preterm infants whose mean blood pressure is less than 25 to 30 mm Hg, consideration should be given to the possibility that they might be relatively hypovolemic. If so, they may benefit from the administration of a 10 mL/kg dose of a volume expander as noted above. Infants who remain hypotensive after initial volume expansion and are felt to have a normal intravascular volume may benefit from the infusion of an inotropic vasoconstricing medication such as dopamine. Initial infusion rates of dopamine at 10 µg/kg/min are often adequate to raise the mean blood pressure into the desired range. Detailed instructions for concentration, infusion rates, and routes of infusion are available in STABLE; alternatively, assistance should be sought from the referral center providing transport.

Fluids and Glucose

Most infants requiring transport should not be fed. Fluids with glucose should therefore be administered via either the peripheral intravenous (PIV) route or umbilical catheters. Insertion of an umbilical venous catheter (UVC) is usually the quickest way to achieve dependable venous access. When placed in a central location in the inferior vena cava, UVCs can be used as a route for administering several types of fluids and medications beyond standard glucose and electrolyte-containing fluids. They can be used to infuse glucose concentrations greater than 12.5%, volume expanders, blood products, sodium bicarbonate, antibiotics, vasopressors, or prostaglandin E1 infusions. Umbilical arterial catheters (UACs) are more difficult to insert, but they allow sampling of arterial blood gases and continuous blood pressure monitoring. They are particularly useful in patients with respiratory problems and hemodynamic instability, in whom frequent monitoring of blood gases and blood pressure is imperative.

Term infants who require IV fluids can often be successfully started on a 10% dextrose in water solution (D10W) at 60 to 70 mL/kg/day. Preterm infants have higher insensible water losses and are less tolerant of glucose loading. Extremely small infants weighing less than 1,000 g should therefore be started on higher maintenance fluid rates of between 100 and 120 mL/kg/day of 5% dextrose in water solution.

Serum glucose levels can be readily monitored using one of several available bedside screening methods, but it is important to remember that these are only screening tools, and their accuracy can vary considerably, especially at low serum glucose levels. The goal of glucose therapy is to prevent hypoglycemia by maintaining the serum glucose level above 50 mg/dL. This can be accomplished by adjusting either the rate of the infusion or the glucose concentration of the fluid being infused. In infants whose glucose levels are less than 40 mg/dL, a 2-mL/kg bolus of D10W should be given, and the glucose infusion rate increased to correct the hypoglycemia. The serum glucose level should then be rechecked in 15 to 30 minutes and further adjustments made when necessary until the serum glucose has stabilized above 50 mg/dL. If needed, glucose concentrations greater than 12.5% should only be infused via a UVC or UAC because of the significant risk of phlebitis and tissue necrosis from infiltration of PIV infusions of these hyperosmolar solutions.

INFANTS WITH SPECIAL PRETRANSPORT STABILIZATION NEEDS

Although all sick neonates need thermal, respiratory, and circulatory support, some have special problems that should be addressed prior to the arrival of the transport team. Guidance should be sought from the staff at the accepting tertiary care unit for patients with unusual or difficult complications.

Congenital Heart Disease

Neonates with congenital heart disease usually present with either cyanosis or signs of circulatory failure. They often appear normal at birth but develop problems on the second or third day of life after closure of the ductus arteriosus. Cyanotic infants with minimal respiratory distress, who fail to show significant improvement in oxygen saturation when placed in high concentrations of oxygen, are likely to have cyanotic heart lesions (Chapter 106). Infants with obstruction to left ventricular output may deteriorate on the second or third day of life, manifesting decreased perfusion and blood pressure, oliguria, and metabolic acidosis. Prostaglandin E1 (PGE1) may be helpful in both types of congenital heart lesions by maintaining or increasing ductal patency. The use of PGE1 should only be undertaken with guidance from the receiving tertiary care center or a pediatric cardiologist. Starting infusion rates are usually 0.05 to 0.1 µg/kg/min, but the consulting tertiary care medical center or pediatric cardiologist may suggest specific instructions regarding the dosage, concentration, and route of administration. Apnea and hypotension are common side effects of PGE1. Therefore, patients receiving a PGE1 infusion should be closely monitored and ventilatory and/or blood pressure support provided if necessary.

Birth Asphyxia

Infants with birth asphyxia should be evaluated for signs of hypoxic-ischemic organ injury. Feedings should initially be withheld while the infant is observed for seizures, neurologic abnormality, respiratory distress, apnea, and hypotension or heart murmur; additionally, urine output should be monitored. Reduced fluid volumes should be given to patients with a history of asphyxia, especially if they are oliguric. In these infants, initial IV fluid rates of 40 to 60 mL/kg/day may be appropriate. Infants with perinatal asphyxia are at increased risk for developing seizures. Should seizures develop, the initial therapy consists of phenobarbital with an initial intravenous loading dose of 20 mg/kg. Subsequent doses of phenobarbital, 10 mg/kg each, may be given intravenously up to a total dose of 50 mg/kg for persistent seizures, but ventilatory support may then be necessary as a result of the central respiratory depressant effect of the phenobarbital.

Abdominal Wall Defects

Infants with open abdominal-wall defects (gastroschisis or ruptured omphalocele) are at increased risk for infection, hypothermia, and dehydration. The abdominal contents should be carefully covered with sterile plastic wrap in such a way that there is no kinking of the mesenteric blood vessels as they traverse the abdominal wall. It may also be helpful to position these infants on their right sides after covering the intestines, thereby lessening pressure on the mesenteric vessels.

These infants will also require a higher than usual IV fluid infusion rate to compensate for increased fluid losses from the exposed intestines and prevent dehydration.

Nasogastric suction should be started immediately, with a large-bore gastric decompression tube to prevent gaseous distension of the intestines. If positive pressure ventilatory support is needed, the patient should be intubated, rather than being placed on nasal CPAP or given bag/mask ventilation. Broad-spectrum antibiotic therapy should be started, and the infant's temperature must be closely monitored.

Gastrointestinal Obstruction

Infants with known or suspected intestinal obstruction should be placed on gastric decompression, usually with a large-bore nasogastric tube connected to low intermittent suction. Appropriate fluid and glucose support should be provided via either PIV or UVC.

Neural Tube Defects

Infection and fluid loss are also concerns in infants with neural tube defects, such as myelomeningocele. Open neural tube defects should be immediately covered with a saline-moistened sponge to avoid rupture of the sac and drying of the exposed neural placode. The infant should be maintained in the prone or side-lying position to avoid placing pressure on the defect. Intravenous fluids should be started, and the infant should not be fed until he has been evaluated at the tertiary care medical center. Finally, broad-spectrum antibiotic therapy should be started. One commonly used regimen consists of initial doses of ampicillin 100 mg/kg and gentamicin 4 mg/kg. The higher dosage of ampicillin is recommended to maximize penetration into the central nervous system and minimize the risk of meningitis or ventriculitis.

Hyperbilirubinemia

Otherwise healthy infants with hyperbilirubinemia are sometimes transferred to tertiary centers for possible exchange transfusion. These infants may not need special care or monitoring before or during transport. Intravenous fluids are not necessary unless the patient is dehydrated, and enteral feedings may prove beneficial by stimulating gastrointestinal motility and bile excretion. Indications for transfer vary, depending on the etiology and timing of the hyperbilirubinemia, the patient's size and gestational age, and any associated clinical conditions.

DOCUMENTATION AND COMMUNICATION

Good communication between referring and accepting caretakers is essential to assure the best possible care for the sick neonate. Accurate, complete, and legible records for both infant and mother are important to the tertiary center staff that will be receiving the infant. These records should include physician and nursing notes and records of orders, medications, laboratory results, procedures, and any other pertinent information. Copies of all radiographs, rather than reports of interpretations, should also be sent.

FAMILY SUPPORT

The parents of sick neonates should be kept informed of their child's condition, treatment plans, and prognosis. The reasons for transport should be explained, emphasizing the differences in the roles of the referring and accepting institutions. The parents should be provided with telephone numbers of the tertiary center neonatal intensive care unit (NICU), and given any available information about visitation policies, family support services, and affordable lodging (e.g., Ronald McDonald houses). Every effort should be made to ensure that the parents have seen and touched their infant prior to transport. This is especially important for mothers who have had cesarean sections or whose hospital discharge may be delayed because of complications.

References

1. Kronick JK, Frewen TC, Kisson N, et al. Influence of referring physicians on interventions by a pediatric and neonatal critical care team. *Pediatr Emerg Care* 1996;12:73–77.

2. Whitfield JM, Buser MK. Transport stabilization times for neonatal and pediatric patients prior to interfacility transfer. *Pediatr Emerg Care* 1993;9:69–71.

3. McNamara PJ, Mak W, White HE. Dedicated neonatal retrieval teams improve delivery room resuscitation of outborn premature infants. *J Perinatol* 2005;25:309–314.

Suggested Readings

Hauth JC, Merenstein GB, eds. *Guidelines for perinatal care*. 4th ed. American Academy of Pediatrics and American College of Obstetricians and Gynecologists; American Academy of Pediatrics Elk Grove Village, Illinois 1997.

Karlsen KA. The S.T.A.B.L.E. program: transporting newborns the S.T.A.B.L.E. way. Park City, Utah; Publisher: Kristine A. Karlsen 2001.

Kattwinkel J, Cook LJ, Hurt H, et al. Perinatal continuing education program. Vol. 1: *Maternal and fetal evaluation and immediate newborn care*. Vol. 2: *Maternal and fetal care*. Vol. II: *Neonatal care*. Vol. III: *Complex perinatal care*. Vol. IV: *Specialized newborn care*. Charlottesville: University of Virginia Health System; 2002.

CHAPTER 125 ■ PREOPERATIVE AND POSTOPERATIVE CARE OF PEDIATRIC SURGICAL PATIENTS

RONALD M. PERKIN, KARIN M. HILLENBRAND, AND KRISTINA L. SIMEONSSON

Despite the increase in outpatient surgery, 10% or more of children admitted to a hospital have problems requiring surgery. Patient care is optimized by communication and cooperation between anesthesiologists, surgeons, and providers of primary care. The primary care provider has a role both in providing preoperative assessment and stabilization and in aiding in postoperative recovery. Surgical care of neonates and of children with congenital heart defects and cancers is typically done in tertiary care and children's hospitals, with consultation by appropriate subspecialists and support by intensive-care units for children.

PREOPERATIVE EVALUATION

The pre-anesthesia assessment is directed toward minimizing the risk of anesthesia and surgery by maximizing health and identifying risk factors. Although the anesthesiologist and surgeon have specific expertise in the management of surgical patients, the provider of primary care for the child often is best suited to review those aspects of the history and physical examination that can affect the course of anesthetic and perioperative management. In this role, the primary provider should assess the child's medical and family history, perform a physical examination, ensure appropriate nothing-by-mouth (NPO) guidelines, and obtain laboratory studies if indicated. For chronically ill children and those with complicated underlying disabilities, the primary care provider may be best suited to determine whether a child is at baseline, maximize health before surgery, and facilitate continuity and coordination of care. This individual also can serve as a resource to the family for explanations and support.

The preoperative evaluation begins with the medical history. The American Society of Anesthesiologists has defined physical status categories that help characterize underlying health before the current illness or condition necessitating surgery (Table 125.1). Higher physical status categories are associated with an increased risk of complications from anesthesia and surgery. Any child with a physical status of 3 or higher requires a preoperative anesthetic evaluation, ideally 1 week or more before surgery to allow time to arrange appropriate workup if needed. Risk also is increased for children undergoing emergency surgery and for those with multiple coexistent medical problems.

Past medical history and underlying medical conditions can have a significant impact on a patient's care during the surgery, as well as the preoperative evaluation and the postoperative recovery period. Knowledge of the patient's past medical history and underlying medical conditions enables the primary care physician to keep the surgeon and anesthesiologist well informed of potential intraoperative and postoperative complications that could arise. Many conditions require preoperative adjustments in medications and specific evaluations before surgery (Table 125.2).

All prescription or over-the-counter medications that the patient is currently taking or has taken recently should be noted; alternative and complementary therapies should not be overlooked. Anesthesiology should be informed of all pharmacologic therapies. Most medications can be continued until the morning of surgery, up to 2 hours before anesthesia. Exceptions include tricyclic antidepressants, which should be discontinued 2 or 3 weeks before elective surgery because of an increased risk of arrhythmias; and chronic aspirin therapy, which increases the risk of postoperative bleeding. Children who have received chemotherapeutic agents should be managed in consultation with an oncologist. Allergies to drugs, foods, latex, or other substances should be documented in the chart. If the patient has had surgery before, any past complications with anesthesia such as postoperative nausea and vomiting, prolonged recovery, or body temperature instability should be investigated. Family history should focus on reactions to anesthesia and presence of bleeding disorders.

The preoperative physical examination is intended to identify abnormalities that increase anesthesia risk, and should focus particularly on the airway, cardiorespiratory risk, and neurologic status. In addition, the system relevant to the surgical procedure should be carefully examined. Evaluation of hydration status is necessary so that fluid imbalance can be corrected. Morbid obesity is associated with increased risk of cardiovascular difficulties, obstructive and postanesthesia apnea, restricted pulmonary function, delayed gastric emptying, aspiration during anesthesia, and difficulty in positioning and maintenance of the airway. Obstructive sleep apnea (OSA) is a common problem in children characterized by frequent episodes of upper airway obstruction during sleep. Snoring is an extremely common finding and may be a sign of OSA. OSA is often associated with episodes of desaturation and hypoventilation of varying degrees and importance. Long-standing hypoxemia and hypercarbia in patients with chronic OSA can lead to pulmonary hypertension and eventually right ventricular failure. Patients suspected of having severe obstructive symptoms with possible cardiac effects should be evaluated with preoperative polysomnography, ECG, and echocardiography. Polysomnography can delineate the severity of OSA in terms of number of significant episodes associated with hypoxemia (described as the apnea index). Residual

AMERICAN SOCIETY OF ANESTHESIOLOGISTS
PHYSICAL STATUS CATEGORIES

ASA PS 1	Normally healthy
ASA PS 2	Mild illness
ASA PS 3	Serious illness
ASA PS 4	Life-threatening illness
ASA PS 5	Moribund; not expected to live

anesthetic gases and sedating pain medications, especially the narcotics, can reduce tone in upper airway muscle, thus increasing the potential for significant upper airway obstruction in the postoperative period. Signs may not appear until some time after the anesthesia and surgery, especially after the patient falls asleep. All patients with symptoms of OSA should be monitered until free of the effects of pain medications and residual anesthetic, whereas those patients with severe OSA should be monitored in the intensive-care unit.

Other physical examination findings that affect airway management include jaw mobility and size, glossoptosis, marked scoliosis, dwarfism, and musculoskeletal abnormalities. The integrity of the dentition should be noted before intubation. Heart murmurs should be evaluated for etiology before anesthesia unless the murmur is known to be functional. A baseline neurologic examination should be done so that postoperative abnormalities can be detected. The child's current medical condition should be reviewed. Any acute illness, especially upper respiratory infection (URI), increases the risk of anesthesia, and surgery may need to be rescheduled. This is particularly true when URI is associated with fever, purulent nasal discharge, or lower respiratory abnormalities like cough, wheeze, or crackles. If surgery will be undertaken without intubation (e.g., myringotomy), a URI may not preclude the procedure. The condition for which the child is undergoing surgery may have resulted in vomiting, dehydration, or electrolyte abnormalities; these problems should be identified and treated before surgery.

Various guidelines for fasting before surgery have been proposed, but no uniform recommendations exist. It is generally accepted that infants and children may take clear liquids and breast milk until 3 or 4 hours before surgery. An unnecessarily prolonged fast should be avoided. Table 125.3 provides a sample NPO guideline.

Preoperative laboratory evaluation is not always required, but should be undertaken in specific circumstances. A baseline hemoglobin should be recorded if significant blood loss or large fluid shifts are anticipated or the patient has an underlying condition such as prematurity or chronic disease that increases the risk of anemia. Coagulation studies should be obtained for patients who have recently or chronically taken nonsteroidal anti-inflammatory drugs or aspirin, and for those with a personal or family history of unusual bleeding. They should also be obtained if the surgical procedure involves anticoagulation, such as cardiac bypass, or if a serious complication could arise from even a small amount of postoperative bleeding, such as with neurosurgical or ophthalmologic procedures.

Laboratory assessment of serum electrolytes, blood urea nitrogen, and creatinine should be considered for patients with significant systemic illness; those receiving intravenous fluids, diuretics, digoxin, or antihypertensive agents; and for those with vomiting or diarrhea. Glucose should be checked for all infants as well as for children with diabetes or malnutrition. A urine pregnancy test should be obtained on menarchal girls who may be sexually active. If recent levels of anticonvulsants,

antiarrhythmics, and theophylline are not available, they should be obtained before surgery. The possibility of blood transfusion and the hospital policies concerning autologous or donor-directed transfusion should be discussed.

The primary care provider plays an essential role in preparing the family for the surgical experience. Anxiety affects all children and families about to undergo anesthesia and surgery. Common parent stressors include loss of control, fear of failure of the surgery, fear for the child's safety or survival, a lack of information or understanding, and financial concerns. A child's level of anxiety is a function of developmental stage. Children may be aware of and distressed by parental anxiety, suffer from separation anxiety (especially from 6 months to 5 years), fear being "put to sleep," and dread needles, mutilation, or disfigurement. Adolescents often suffer a disturbance of body image. In addition, surgery results in disruption of routine and places the child in unfamiliar surroundings. A primary care provider who is familiar to the child and family may be best suited to assist in their psychological preparation before surgery. The primary provider should explain what the child and family can expect before and after surgery. As much as possible, the child should be given explanations that are completely truthful and age appropriate, but that avoid graphic terms as well as technical ones. An advance tour may be helpful to increase child and family comfort in the hospital environment; in addition, child life therapists may be very helpful in orienting the family and child and preparing them for the surgical experience. The most distressing moment for the child and family usually occurs when the child is taken from the parent. Whenever possible, a parent should be included during anesthesia induction and should be present when the child wakes up.

POSTOPERATIVE MANAGEMENT

The surgeon and anesthesiologist retain a central role in the child's postoperative recovery from anesthesia and surgery. The primary care provider is also an essential part of the team, with integral roles in the provision of appropriate fluids, nutrition, and pain relief, in the detection and management of common postoperative problems, and in discharge planning.

Fluid needs in the postoperative period are comprised of maintenance fluids, replacement of ongoing losses, and compensation for third-space losses. Maintenance requirements include the replacement of water and electrolyte losses through evaporative losses and urine output; fluid losses are decreased with use of humidified air and increased with hyperthermia or tachypnea. Excessive losses from the gastrointestinal tract, the urinary tract, or from drains should be assessed for volume and electrolyte content, with replacement of both. Third-space losses in the interstitium and gut may require additional fluid replacement of approximately 3 to 5 mL/kg/hr with minor procedures, and up to 10 or 15 mL/kg/hr with major abdominal surgery. Children who have undergone intracranial surgery have an increased postoperative risk for both syndrome of inappropriate antidiuretic hormone secretion and diabetes insipidus; fluid intake and output should be monitored especially closely for these children.

Provision of appropriate nutrition in the postoperative period aids in recovery, and enhances return to health. The commencement and frequency of postoperative feeds probably does not influence the rate of vomiting after nonintraluminal abdominal surgery. Initial feeding with electrolyte solutions or 5% dextrose in water instead of milk is a common practice, but has not clearly been shown to decrease acid aspiration. After pyloric stenosis repair, accelerated or ad libitum feeding slightly increases the incidence and frequency of vomiting but usually shortens hospital stay; patients who tolerate two consecutive full feedings may be safely discharged. Volvulus repair and other major abdominal surgeries may significantly delay resumption

TABLE 125.2

PERIOPERATIVE MANAGEMENT CONSIDERATIONS FOR SPECIFIC MEDICAL CONDITIONS

Problem	Considerations
PULMONARY	
Prematurity	■ Increased risk of postanesthesia apnea, inversely related to age. ■ Defer elective surgery until 60 wk postconceptual age (4–5 mo corrected age). ■ If earlier surgery is necessary, use apnea monitoring for 24 hr after surgery. ■ Chronic lung disease/bronchopulmonary dysplasia: maximize therapy with bronchodilators, diuretics, or corticosteroids. ■ Consider a chest radiograph and hematocrit.
Asthma	■ Continue usual medication regimen. ■ Begin use of bronchodilator medication 24 hr before surgery. ■ If recent exacerbation, consider corticosteroid therapy 2–3 days before surgery (e.g., prednisone 1–2 mg/kg/day). ■ Cancel elective surgery if upper respiratory infection or wheezing is present.
Cervical spine abnormalities	■ More common in children with Down syndrome, achondroplasia, rheumatoid arthritis, mucopolysaccharidoses. ■ Increases airway complications. ■ Screen by history for long tract signs. ■ Consider flexion/extension films before intubation. ■ Caution the operating and recovery room personnel about danger of extreme neck flexion.
ENDOCRINE	
Diabetes	■ Document usual insulin regimen, compliance, and blood sugar control. ■ Early morning surgery typically better for glycemic control. ■ Insulin should be taken the morning of surgery: half the usual dose may be appropriate. ■ Monitor glucose during surgery and during recovery; anesthetics may mask signs of hypoglycemia. ■ Provide dextrose infusion, insulin based on monitoring.
HEMATOLOGIC	
Sickle-cell disease	■ Hypoxia, hypovolemia, stress, and acidosis increase the risk of sickling, and may lead to stroke, myocardial infarction, or acute chest syndrome. ■ Perioperative transfusion may be required. ■ Consult patient's hematologist to help coordinate care.
Hemophilia	■ Factor replacement before surgery to attain 25%–50% of normal levels.
NEUROLOGIC	
Seizures	■ Document seizure type, frequency, medications, and compliance. ■ Continue anticonvulsant medications. ■ Obtain recent anticonvulsant levels. ■ Seizure threshold is decreased during anesthesia: develop plan for management of perioperative seizures.
Increased ICP	■ Anesthesia may further increase ICP.
Central nervous system stimulant use (e.g., methylphenidate)	■ May increase anesthetic requirements.
Myelodysplasia (spina bifida)	■ Increases the risk of latex sensitization and anaphylaxis. ■ Use latex-free products.
Neuromuscular disorders	■ Associated with increased anesthesia side effects. ■ Muscle degeneration increases risk of malignant hyperthermia.
CARDIAC	
Murmur; congenital heart defect	■ Document cause, innocent vs. pathologic. ■ Innocent murmurs pose no risk. ■ Assess pathologic murmurs for hemodynamic compromise. ■ Intracardiac shunt increases risk of paradoxical embolus. ■ Provide subacute bacterial endocarditis prophylaxis based on American Heart Association guidelines.
Arrhythmia	■ Risk increased with an underlying rhythm abnormality, underlying heart defect, or if patient is on arrhythmogenic drugs (e.g., epinephrine, theophylline).

ICP, intracranial pressure.

TABLE 125.3

PREOPERATIVE NPO GUIDELINE

	Length of fast		
	Clear liquids	Breast milk	Formula, milk, and solids
Neonates	2 hr	3–4 hr	4 hr
Infants	2 hr	3–4 hr	6 hr
Children	2 hr	NA	6 hr

NA, not applicable.

of bowel function; parenteral nutrition should be provided for postoperative patients unable to resume enteral feeds.

Postoperative pain relief should be given at regular intervals or continuously; it is inappropriate to give medications "as needed" because this makes it inevitable that the child will have pain. The most commonly used options for pain relief include regional techniques, opioid medications, and nonsteroidal anti-inflammatory and nonopioid analgesics. The pediatrician should work with the anesthesiologist or surgeon to develop and implement a plan for pain management (see also Chapter 112 for guidelines and dosing).

Self-administration of intravenous medication for analgesia is known as patient-controlled analgesia (PCA). Built in safety benefits include a programmed dose with built-in lock-out time between PCS doses and a maximum number of doses per unit time, which decreases the potential for dosing errors.

The effective use of PCA is limited by the patient's level of understanding and coordination rather than simply patient age. The patient must be capable of understanding that a seemingly unassociated action—pushing a button—triggers a pump to administer medication when the patient percieves pain of significant magnitude to warrant a response. Most patients need to be at least 10 years old, but there are children who can effectively operate PCAs at 4 years of age, especially those who might be very experienced with pain and its treatment (e.g., sickle-cell patients).

Problems that are commonly encountered in the postoperative period include vomiting, bleeding, fever, and complications of intubation. Nausea and vomiting is the most common complication of anesthesia. It is especially common after eye surgery, tonsillectomy, middle ear procedures, scrotal or testicular surgery, and abdominal procedures, and it is increased when perioperative narcotics are used. Adequate perioperative hydration decreases the risk of postoperative emesis. Most emesis that occurs after surgery can be handled as gastroenteritis would be, with a 2- to 4-hour NPO period followed by small sips of clear liquids. Antiemetic medications may be indicated; a common side effect is increased drowsiness. For patients undergoing same-day surgery, mandatory oral intake before discharge increases the chance of emesis, and does not decrease the possibility of vomiting once the child goes home.

Fever occurring in the first 24 hours after surgery is usually associated with atelectasis; early ambulation, deep breathing, and coughing help to prevent its occurrence. A careful history and physical examination should lead to identification of other causes, which include wound infection, urinary tract infection, dehydration, and infected intravascular access.

Patients should be observed closely for bleeding after surgery. Serosanguinous drainage in small amounts is expected. Bleeding that persists longer than 8 hours after surgery, or which results in two or more blood-soaked dressings in the first 8 hours, should prompt reevaluation by the surgeon.

A sore throat is common for children who have been intubated during surgery; it can be managed with popsicles or lozenges. Stridor may occur as the result of subglottic edema, and is treated similarly to croup with humidification, nebulized epinephrine, and corticosteroids. Careful discharge planning is essential to ensure that parents and children will be able to provide self-care at home and are aware of necessary follow-up. Caregivers must be able to provide wound care; in most cases they should be advised to keep the wound dry and dressed for 48 hours; it can be washed with soap and water by postoperative day 4. Sun exposure can lead to permanent hyperpigmentation of a surgical scar for up to a year after surgery, so sun protection strategies should be recommended. Parents or patients must be taught the care of catheters, tubes, and ostomies and must have appropriate equipment. Rehabilitation and home health services may assist in the transition home for children with complicated postsurgical care or equipment. Parents should be counseled about potential postoperative complications and must know what to do if they occur. Appropriate activity and the length of restriction should be clarified. Finally, surgical and primary care follow-up should be arranged before discharge.

Suggested Readings

American Academy of Pediatrics, Section on Anesthesiology. Evaluation and preparation of pediatric patients undergoing anesthesia. *Pediatrics* 1996;98: 502–508.

Anshuman S, Jones MB, Hirshberg GE. Pediatric anesthesia, pain management, and procedural sedation. In: Olham KT, Columbani PM, Foglia RP, et al., eds. *Principles and practice of pediatric surgery*. Philadelphia: Lippincott Williams & Wilkins; 2005:313–333.

Doyle L, Colletti JE. Pediatric procedural sedation and analegesia. *Pediatr Clin North Am* 2006;53:279–292.

Feldman D, Reich N, Foster JMT. Pediatric anesthesia and postoperative analgesia. *Pediatr Clin North Am* 1998;45:1525–1537.

Ferrari LR. Cleared for anesthesia: what it means, how to do it. *Contemp Pediatr* 1997;14:81–89.

Kain ZN. Psychological aspects of pediatric anesthesia. In: Motoyama EK, Davis PJ, eds. *Smith's anesthesia for infants and children*. Philadelphia: Mosby; 2006:241–254.

Krane EJ, Davis PJ. Preoperative preparation for infants and children. In: Motoyama EK, Davis PJ, eds. *Smith's anesthesia for infants and children*. Philadelphia: Mosby; 2006:255–271.

CHAPTER 126A ■ SURGICAL EMERGENCIES: MALROTATION AND VOLVULUS

TIMOTHY M. WEINER

Malrotation and midgut volvulus is an absolute pediatric surgical emergency. It is imperative that the clinician rapidly diagnose and initiate treatment when this condition is suspected.

Malrotation of the intestines, as the name suggests, is an abnormal twisting of the small and large intestine. It is a congenital abnormality and occurs in utero, but it is not known what precipitates it. Four weeks after conception, the primordial gut of the fetus begins to lengthen. Initially there is not enough room for this to occur, and the gut pushes out into the umbilical cord, where it further elongates. Between the eighth and tenth week of gestation, the bowel begins a specific 270-degree pattern of twisting and folding so that it can return to the abdomen and fix in place. (Imagine putting 25 feet of garden hose into a small box for winter storage.) This extrasomatic rotation and subsequent fixation occurs in a very particular way in order for the gut to end up in the correct position with the *start* of the small intestine (the duodenaljejunal junction or so-called ligament of Treitz) in the left, upper part of the abdomen and the *end* of the small intestine (the ileocecum and appendix) moving into the lower, right part of the abdomen. The axis around which this rotation occurs is the main blood supply to the small intestines, the superior mesenteric artery (SMA). If this rather complicated event does not happen properly, the child will be born with some form of malrotation of the intestine. The general term "malrotation" therefore includes everything from no twisting of the gut (nonrotation) to various degrees of incomplete (<270-degree) rotation.

More significantly, the normally widely spaced mesentery of the midgut is much narrower when malrotation has occurred (Fig. 126.1). As bowel loops fill with fluid and air, this narrow mesenteric pedicle is more likely to volvulize and compromise the vascular supply for the entire small bowel within spiraled and kinked SMA. (Think of the mesentery as a window curtain with the small bowel as the ruffle at the bottom of that curtain. The more narrow the curtain, the higher the likelihood that the ruffle will twist and flip.) A midgut volvulus can therefore cause the entire small intestine to infarct and/or perforate.

It is important to appreciate that *once the volvulus has occurred, the bowel is immediately at risk* for losing its blood supply. Furthermore, there is no way to predict if and when a volvulus will occur in a patient with malrotated bowel (though 80% of volvuluses occur in children under 1 year old). The only thing that can be said with any certainty is that bowel that is malrotated is capable of twisting at some point in a person's life; normally rotated bowel cannot undergo a midgut volvulus. Though the bowel may untwist itself in some cases and survive, this possibility should not be expected or relied on. The view that must be taken is that the "clock is ticking" for the twisted, volvulized bowel and a delay of even a few hours can result in a catastrophic and tragic outcome. A timely diagnosis and surgical therapy is imperative. More simply put: *a midgut volvulus is a surgical emergency*.

PATHOPHYSIOLOGY OF VOLVULUS

Intestines that are malrotated do not necessarily mean that a child will suffer a midgut volvulus. In fact, such children may grow to be adults without ever coming to medical attention for this abnormality. To understand why malrotation is of great concern and why many surgeons would recommend an operation for this condition, it is important to appreciate the potentially catastrophic sequence and results that occur with a midgut volvulus.

Recall that in the more common form of malrotation, the counterclockwise twist of the intestines around the SMA fell short of the necessary 270 degrees, resulting in the duodenum and cecum in close proximity. Often the cecum will establish tissue bands to the retroperitoneum in an attempt to anchor itself, and these may cause extrinsic compression and duodenal obstruction as they cross the duodenum (Ladd's bands).

CLINICAL PRESENTATION

The unfortunate thing is that because volvulus is not a common problem and because it can present itself in atypical or confusing ways, it may not be immediately recognized. In fact, a child with this condition can present in a relatively unremarkable way with symptoms that are be mistaken for more usual childhood illnesses such as stomach flu, feeding intolerance, reflux, or constipation. *However, serious consideration to malrotation and volvulus must be given to any child, and particularly any infant, who throws up bile-stained fluid*. Although most such children will ultimately be found not to have this condition, ignoring this possibility can clearly have devastating consequences. Pediatric surgeons and pediatricians must therefore have an aggressive and proactive approach to diagnosing a suspected volvulus. Particular attention should be given to children with conditions that occasionally are associated with malrotation such as midline atresias (duodenal, esophageal), situs inversus, and dextrocardia. Children

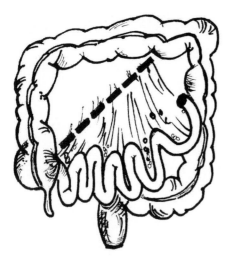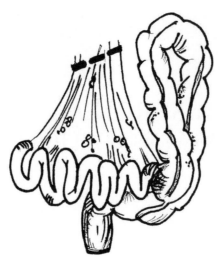

FIGURE 126.1. Normally rotated bowel (*right*) with widely spaced midgut mesentery. Malrotated bowel (*left*) with narrowed mesenteric pedicle more prone to volvulus.

with omphaolcoele, gastroschisis, and diaphragmatic hernias by definition have nonrotation or malrotation of the gut; however this rarely seems to cause volvulus.

The mainstay of diagnosis is an upper GI study to determine if the duodenaljejunal junction is properly positioned in the left, upper abdomen (crosses the spine and reaches the level of the pylorus) (Fig. 126.2). Although a contrast enema may demonstrate a normally positioned cecum and can exclude an acute volvulus, no study other than an UGI or exploratory abdominal surgery can definitively rule out malrotation and volvulus. Ultrasound and CT scan may document a flip of the superior mesenteric artery and vein or a spiraling of the mesentery suggestive of malrotation and/or volvulus, but these are not the preferred first test of choice. Occasionally, in a very ill child in whom the surgeon has a high index of suspicion that the illness may be due to a midgut volvulus, surgery may be undertaken directly (bypassing any time in the radiologic suite) to avoid any further delay and jeopardy of the midgut.

In brief, any infant or child with bilious emesis, particularly in the first year of life and especially in the first week of life, must be considered to have malrotation and volvulus until proven otherwise by UGI or surgical exploration.

MANAGEMENT

The treatment of malrotation with a suspected acute midgut volvulus is rapid and emergent surgical exploration. The patient is typically explored by a right upper quadrant transverse incision. If the bowel is volvulized, it is detorsed in a counterclockwise direction until the mesentery is flat. The compromised bowel is then observed. If its viability remains in question, the detorsed intestine is returned to the abdomen, the incision closely temporarily, and plans made for a second-look operation in 12 to 24 hours. The patient is taken to an ICU where he is aggressively resuscitated, including broad antibiotic coverage for the next 8 to 24 hours. At reexploration, nonviable bowel will be removed and anastomoses or ostomies created based on the extent and pattern of the damage and the clinical judgment of the surgeon.

If the bowel recovers during intaoperative observation or if the child had malrotation without volvulus, a classic Ladd's procedure is done. It is important to recognize that this does not reestablish normal rotation, but rather positions the bowel on a more widely spaced mesentery in order to minimize the future risk of volvulus. This is accomplished by straightening the duodenum (Kocher maneuver), incising and widening the mesenteric tissues, positioning the small intestine in the right abdomen and the large intestine in the left abdomen, and removing the appendix.

Many pediatric surgeons believe that the several forms of malrotation always carry a significant degree of risk for a future midgut volvulus. Therefore in patients in whom malrotation is found but who have not suffered a volvulus and who are often asymptomatic, surgery to minimize the risk should be very seriously considered. Some pediatric surgeons feel that any form of malrotation seen or suspected during an upper GI study should be operated upon and a Ladd procedure performed.

Laparoscopy may emerge as a useful tool for several scenarios of this condition:

- In a sick child in whom volvulus is suspected but not certain, and in whom a delay for an upper GI study may be detrimental.
- To further evaluate the child with a "slightly abnormally placed duodenum" in whom a form of malrotation cannot be excluded.
- In malrotated patients for whom a prophylactic Ladd procedure is appropriate but who wish to avoid the morbidity of a full open operation.

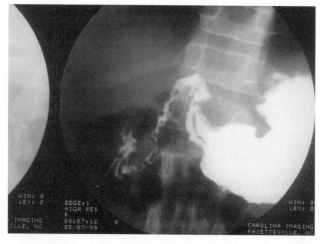

FIGURE 126.2. Upper GI study demonstrating abnormally positioned duodenal–jejunal junction (duodenal "sweep" does not cross the spine).

As pediatric surgeons gain experience with this technique and smaller instruments are developed, this minimally invasive therapy may be more frequently applied to this condition.

COMPLICATIONS AND OUTCOMES

Generally, children recover uneventfully from the Ladd procedure, especially if bowel resection was not necessary. Although the intent of the Ladd's procedure is to in fact create some postoperative adhesions in order to fix the widened mesentery in place, occasionally these adhesions can create mechanical small bowel obstructions later in life.

Children who require extensive bowel resection, sometimes including the entire midgut, face a more uncertain outcome. Early death from sepsis is not uncommon, and if they survive this insult, there is a later and significant possibility of "short gut syndrome." Children who lose more than 60% of their small bowel have a high likelihood of needing TPN long-term often for life. The only hope for survival in some of these patients is small-bowel/liver transplants.

SUMMARY

Malrotation and volvulus, though uncommon, remains a feared medical and surgical problem. Although bilious emesis is the hallmark symptom, it is also a condition that may be hard to recognize in up to 20% of patients. Its potential for catastrophic consequences leaves very little room for a delay in its diagnosis and treatment, however. Clinicians who take care of children must be aware of it and its ability to present in atypical ways, and must be willing to accept a high percentage of negative tests (especially upper GIs) in order to rapidly identify the occasional child with this problem. The management of asymptomatic malrotation without acute volvulus is debated, with many pediatric surgeons recommending surgical correction.

CHAPTER 126B ■ SURGICAL EMERGENCIES: APPENDICITIS

J. DUNCAN PHILLIPS

Acute appendicitis is the most common pediatric abdominal surgical emergency, affecting approximately 85,000 American children every year. Roughly 1 in 13, or 7%, of persons in the United States will undergo appendectomy during their lifetimes. The peak incidence of appendicitis occurs in children between the ages of 8 and 18 years. Although potentially life-threatening, with prompt medical and surgical intervention, most of these patients recover relatively quickly, with a low risk of long-term morbidity.

PATHOPHYSIOLOGY

Most cases of acute appendicitis are presumed secondary to luminal obstruction of the vermiform appendix by a fecalith (also called an appendecolith by some). The obstructing entity (Table 126.1), which is typically a piece of incompletely digested foodstuff and/or vegetable matter, blocks the usual egress of mucous, produced by the Goblet cells of the appendiceal mucosa, into the cecum. It is felt that pressure eventually builds within the appendiceal lumen, progressively blocking normal venous and lymphatic drainage and causing eventual impairment of arterial inflow from the tiny branches of the appendiceal artery. With impaired circulation within the appendiceal wall, bacteria within the appendix begin to infiltrate the mucosa, triggering an inflammatory reaction and then ulceration and actual infection of the appendiceal tissue. Progression of this process may lead to gangrene and eventual perforation.

Pearls

- Obstruction of the appendiceal lumen by *Enterobius vermicularis* (pinworm) is a not-unusual cause of acute appendicitis in young children. Treatment still requires appendectomy (see below), but affected children and their families also require postoperative treatment with antihelminthics.
- Occasional children will present with clinical evidence of acute appendicitis following a recent presumed viral illness (that is, a brief illness characterized by fever, myalgias, headache, possibly vomiting and diarrhea). Presumedly, lymphatic tissue within the wall of the appendix and/or cecum becomes hypertrophied, obstructing the lumen of the appendix and triggering the above-described sequence of events.

SIGNS AND SYMPTOMS

Most children who develop acute appendicitis are previously healthy and not chronically ill. The first symptom is typically that of abdominal pain (Table 126.2), which usually begins as a rather diffuse, poorly localized sensation throughout the abdomen and then gradually localizes, over a period of 6 to

TABLE 126.1

PATHOPHYSIOLOGY OF ACUTE APPENDICITIS

- Lumen obstruction
- Continued secretion of mucous
- Venous/lymphatic/arteriole obstruction
- Mucosal ulceration
- Bacterial invasion
- Infection
- Necrosis/gangrene
- Perforation

TABLE 126.2

CHARACTERISTICS OF ABDOMINAL PAIN OF
PEDIATRIC APPENDICITIS

The pain . . .

1. Usually precedes other symptoms.
2. Usually begins periumbilical and gradually goes to the
   right lower quadrant.
3. Usually is constant in character.
4. Usually progressively worsens with time.
5. Usually worsens with walking/jumping/coughing.
6. Usually causes the child more distress than all other
   symptoms.

10 hours, to the right lower quadrant. Occasional children deny the usual "diffuse" nature of the initial pain, despite repeated questioning by multiple physicians, and insist that the pain began in the right lower quadrant. Typically, the pain is constant and does not fluctuate in severity, but gradually increases in intensity. The pain is typically exacerbated by movement and by coughing/sneezing.

Children suffering from acute appendicitis have been said to have the "appendicitis walk." That is, because movement is painful, they shuffle across the floor and slowly crawl onto the examining table (and may require assistance to do so). Children who smile, laugh, run around the room, and jump up onto the examining table are unlikely to have appendicitis.

Associated with the pain is usually a sensation of anorexia, although occasional children with acute appendicitis deny this and insist that they are very hungry. Most children experience at least some nausea and even mild vomiting. Children with acute appendicitis will typically vomit just a few times. Prolific vomiting is uncommon. Low-grade fever is common, although high fever should prompt the physician to consider either perforated appendicitis (see below) or other diagnoses.

Occasional children will present with typical signs and symptoms of acute appendicitis and parents will relate a history of similar previous episodes. These episodes are described as having been less severe and may or may not have prompted visits to emergency rooms and/or physician offices.

Diarrhea is uncommon in early appendicitis, but may become manifest later in the course of the disease if the appendix perforates and/or becomes adherent to the side of the superior rectum or sigmoid colon (see below).

Pearls

- Be suspicious of the diagnosis if the abdominal pain is something elicited by the examining physician after listening to a list of patient symptoms. That is, if a child complains of nonspecific symptoms such as headache, fever, and fatigue or even gastrointestinal symptoms such as nausea and vomiting, and only later admits to abdominal pain, following careful questioning by the physician, it is unlikely that the patient is suffering from acute appendicitis.
- Be suspicious of the diagnosis if the patient appears to have developed appendicitis during a hospitalization for treatment of another acute illness. For example, if a patient has been hospitalized for treatment of bacterial pneumonia and only later develops abdominal pain, it is unlikely that the pain is due to onset of appendicitis during the hospitalization but, more likely, that the pain is somehow secondary to the underlying disease entity responsible for the initial hospital stay.

The typical time course of acute appendicitis, from onset of symptoms to perforation of the appendix, is roughly 24 to 36

hours. Occasional children will develop acute appendicitis that will progress more slowly, and not perforate for up to 72 to 96 hours.

DIFFERENTIAL DIAGNOSIS

The list of "appendicitis mimics" is extremely lengthy (see Table 126.3 for a partial listing). A detailed history and physical examination, as well as a few simple laboratory tests, will often help the physician to distinguish between these other illnesses and achieve the correct preoperative diagnosis of acute appendicitis.

It should be noted, however, that because the lists of mimics is so extensive, and because there remains no perfect test for the evaluation of appendicitis (with 100% sensitivity, specificity, and accuracy), children still undergo appendectomy from time to time for removal of a normal appendix. A reasonable "negative appendectomy" rate in adult patients has been felt to be roughly 15%. In children, most experienced pediatric surgeons report a "negative appendectomy" rate of between 5% and 10%.

Common mimics of acute appendicitis include:

1. *Acute gastroenteritis.* The etiology of this illness may be viral or bacterial. It is one of the most common reasons for children to seek medical attention. Typically the vomiting and/or diarrhea are more pronounced (and more bothersome to the patient) than the abdominal pain and frequently precede the pain by minutes or hours. There may be a history of eating something "suspicious" at a restaurant, family picnic, or other outing. Other family members may be ill with similar symptoms. The associated abdominal pain is typically more diffuse and usually fails to localize to the right lower quadrant as it does with acute appendicitis.
2. *Mesenteric lymphadenitis.* This is perhaps the most difficult illness to distinguish from acute appendicitis in children, because signs and symptoms are so similar. Indeed, in the experience of most pediatric surgeons, this entity is probably the most common cause for negative appendectomy (surgical removal of a normal appendix in a child with the preoperative diagnosis of acute appendicitis). Although found throughout the abdominal cavity, mesenteric lymph nodes are especially prominent along a branch of the superior mesenteric artery known as the ileocolic artery, the branches of which supply blood to the distal ileum, cecum, and ascending colon. Because of proximity of the ileocolic artery to the appendix, nodal hypertrophy and inflammation

TABLE 126.3

PEDIATRIC ACUTE APPENDICITIS: DIFFERENTIAL
DIAGNOSIS

(partial list, not comprehensive)

1. Acute gastroenteritis
2. Mesenteric adenitis
3. Ruptured ovarian cyst
4. Urinary tract infection/pyelonephritis
5. Salpingitis/pelvic inflammatory disease
6. Meckel's diverticulitis
7. Acute small bowel obstruction
8. Severe dysmenorrhea
9. Unsuspected blunt abdominal trauma (including child
   maltreatment)

may cause pain and tenderness indistinguishable from that of appendicitis.

3. *Ruptured ovarian cyst.* This is probably the second most common cause for negative appendectomy in children. Girls with symptomatic ovarian cysts typically relate a history of fairly sudden onset of pain (that is, over a period of 10 to 15 minutes), which begins in the lower abdomen. This may be associated with other gastrointestinal symptoms, such as vomiting, but is often just associated with anorexia and/or nausea. Although previously felt to only occur in girls who have undergone menarche, it is now known to affect even much younger girls.

4. *Urinary tract infection*, including pyelonephritis. Although often accompanied by dysuria and high fever, occasional children will present with abdominal pain as the primary manifestation. A paucity of "intestinal symptoms" (nausea, vomiting, anorexia) may help point the clinician toward this disease, as well as a history of documented urinary tract infections in the past.

5. *Salpingitis* (pelvic inflammatory disease, or PID). This is typically a disease of sexually active females, and is usually caused by sexually transmitted organisms such as gonorrhea. Girls with PID usually present with the gradual onset of lower abdominal or pelvic pain, which can be accompanied by anorexia, nausea, and vomiting. Fevers are often quite high. Bimanual pelvic examination may reveal cervical motion tenderness and a speculum examination may show cervical discharge.

WORKUP

Because most children with acute appendicitis will be treated with urgent appendectomy (see below), consultation with a pediatric surgeon (or, in some medical communities, a general surgeon with extensive pediatric experience) early in the evaluation of a child with possible appendicitis is prudent. Input from an experienced surgeon can be invaluable in guiding the workup, minimizing unnecessary laboratory and/or radiographic tests, and in addition, preparing the child for surgical treatment. *Note*: If the clinical suspicion of acute appendicitis is high, and if a surgeon competent in the treatment of children is not available at your institution, transfer to another facility with the appropriate personnel should be arranged as quickly as possible, preferably after telephone consultation with the accepting surgeon.

Evaluation should not preclude resuscitation. The surgical dictum of REO (resuscitate, evaluate, operate) *in that order* should usually be followed. Children are rarely in respiratory distress. However, severe acute appendicitis, especially if associated with perforation and peritonitis, may cause bacteremia, hypotension, septic shock, multisystem organ failure, and even death. Optimal evaluation of these "sick" patients should typically begin with the establishment of intravenous access and fluid resuscitation. Insertion of a Foley catheter may be needed to guide fluid management. Placement of a nasogastric tube to suction may be required in patients with excessive nausea. Rare patients may even need preoperative stabilization in a pediatric intensive-care unit.

Empiric treatment with broad-spectrum intravenous antibiotics is usually discouraged until the presumed diagnosis of appendicitis has been made, because the antibiotics can mask the symptoms of appendicitis and make the physical examination by the consulting surgeon unreliable. Giving small doses of intravenous narcotics was formerly discouraged by most surgeons for similar reasons. However, several recent studies in children have suggested that small doses do not significantly interfere with the physical examination, increase

---

TABLE 126.4

TYPICAL WORKUP FOR SUSPECTED PEDIATRIC APPENDICITIS

1. History and physical examination (If appendicitis strongly suspected at this point, surgical consultation)
2. Complete blood count, urinalysis (If appendicitis strongly suspected at this point, surgical consultation)
3. Advanced radiographic imaging (ultrasound or computed tomography) (If appendicitis strongly suspected at this point, surgical consultation)

TESTS RARELY INDICATED (PRIMARILY USED TO EXCLUDE OTHER DISEASE PROCESSES)
1. Liver function tests
2. Tests of pancreatic function (amylase, lipase)
3. Urine culture
4. Various other radiographic tests, including MRI, angiography, nuclear medicine

---

the risk of misdiagnosis, or increase the risk of progression to perforation.

Many children with acute appendicitis require no further workup, other than a thorough history and physical examination. Indeed, previously healthy boys with classic signs and symptoms of appendicitis may need no laboratory testing and no radiographic studies (Table 126.4).

Laboratory Tests

Most children being evaluated for possible appendicitis undergo urinalysis (to exclude an obvious urinary tract infection) and a complete blood count, to assess for leukocytosis. Most children with appendicitis have an elevated white blood count, with values between 10,000 and 20,000 and a "left shift" (increased percentage of neutrophils and possibly a bandemia). It should be noted, however, that a normal white blood count does *not* exclude the diagnosis of appendicitis and the severity of the leukocytosis has *not* been shown to correlate with the severity of the appendicitis. Laboratory tests such as liver function tests (bilirubin, ALT, AST, alkaline phosphatase) and pancreatic enzymes (amylase and lipase) are typically not helpful in diagnosing acute appendicitis and are typically ordered only if the physician is suspicious for biliary tract disease or pancreatitis.

Pearls

■ An inflamed vermiform appendix, stuck to the right ureter from inflammatory adhesions, can cause leukocytes to appear in the urine and thus a "positive urinalysis." This is also true for a perforated, inflamed appendix adherent to the urinary bladder.

■ A dramatically elevated white blood count (that is, greater than 25,000 or 30,000) is unusual with acute appendicitis, unless there is perforation and peritonitis, which typically takes several days to occur following onset of symptoms. Thus, if a child presents with a brief history of abdominal pain (just a few hours) and a white blood count of greater than 30,000, she is unlikely to have acute appendicitis.

■ A urine pregnancy test should probably be obtained on any postmenarchal girl presenting with acute lower abdominal pain, for several reasons. First, it may help exclude intrauterine pregnancy as a cause of the pain. Second, a positive test (in a girl who also happens to have acute appendicitis) alerts the treating surgeon and anesthesiologist, so that they can discuss the risks of the surgical procedure to the fetus and possibly alter the choice of anesthetic agents, antibiotics, postoperative analgesia, and even surgical technique.

■ Although perioperative blood transfusions are rarely indicated during the treatment of acute appendicitis, many hospital operating room protocols require that patients undergoing invasive surgical procedures have blood typing performed, just in case emergency transfusion is required. Therefore, when a child with suspected acute appendicitis undergoes venipuncture for complete blood count sampling, it is reasonable to obtain an extra tube of blood for possible "type and screen," if necessary.

Radiographic Tests

Plain Radiographs

The KUB (kidneys, ureters, and bladder) radiograph is often obtained in children with abdominal pain to assess for the possible existence of a fecalith obstructing the appendix. Unfortunately, only 20% of patients with documented histologically proven appendicitis will have calcified fecaliths visible on KUB x-rays, thus limiting the sensitivity of the test. However, if a child presents with classic appendicitis by history and physical examination, has a somewhat elevated white blood count and a normal urinalysis, and has a calcified right lower quadrant fecalith identified on KUB, the chance that the child has appendicitis is quite high.

The value of the KUB in evaluation of a patient with possible acute appendicitis is probably its ability to assess for other illnesses such as small bowel obstruction, fecal impaction, and the rare patient with pneumoperitoneum ("free air") after perforation of an abdominal viscus. In addition, calcifications from other diseases, such as those seen in ovarian teratomas, can be identified.

Ultrasound

Since the early 1980s, many authors have advocated the routine use of ultrasound to diagnose acute appendicitis in children. Successful diagnosis has varied, depending on the skill and experience of the examining radiologist. Ultrasound is felt to be the most "user-dependent" radiographic test and is highly dependent upon the experience of the radiologist.

Computed Tomography (CT)

Perhaps no diagnostic tool has stirred more interest (and controversy) than abdominal and pelvic CT (Fig. 126.3), advocated by many since 1998 for routine use in the diagnosis of appendicitis, following the landmark study by Rao and associates. In that study of 100 patients with suspected acute appendicitis, CT was 98% accurate in diagnosing the disease, resulted in treatment changes in 59% of patients, and resulted in significant cost savings by reducing unnecessary surgical procedures and hospitalizations for observation. Many have criticized that study for various reasons, including (1) the high negative appendectomy rate of the treating surgeons (a full 28%); (2) the fact that "triple contrast" (venous, oral, and rectal) was used in all patients, with a special protocol of very fine cuts through the right lower quadrant; and (3) the fact that specially trained radiologists were available throughout the day and night, in the hospital, to interpret the images immediately after they were obtained. Despite these criticisms, numerous studies since then have reached similar conclusions.

Garcia Pena and colleagues, from the Boston Children's Hospital, published a series of five reports between 1999 and 2004 describing the routine use of preoperative CT to diagnose suspected acute appendicitis in children. These reports

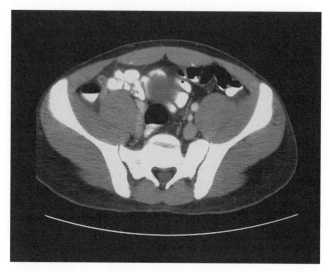

FIGURE 126.3. CT scan of pediatric patient with acute appendicitis.

all concluded that CT was very accurate in the diagnosis of suspected appendicitis in children and advocated its routine use in suspected cases. It should be noted, however, that these authors were careful to note that children with the "clinical diagnosis" of acute appendicitis do not need *any* sort of imaging study, and that surgical consultation should be obtained *before* imaging studies are ordered.

As a result of the reports by Rao, Garcia Pena, and others, the routine use of preoperative CT scanning in children with suspected appendicitis has skyrocketed, from near zero in 1997 to well over 50% in 2005. At some centers, almost 90% of children with suspected acute appendicitis are now evaluated with CT. Unfortunately, radiation exposure to the child can be significant, raising fears of long-term harm such as increased risk of cancer. In addition, undergoing CT increases hospital charges dramatically, adding an average of 26% to the child's hospital bill; and may delay definitive surgical treatment, by an average of 7 hours in one study.

The above concerns, and others, have generated the beginning of an "anti-CT" backlash, with several authors advocating a return to the clinical diagnosis. Koslaske and associates, in 2004, reported a 97% accuracy rate for the diagnosis of appendicitis in children based on classic clinical history and physical, reserving CT only for unsure cases.

The most vocal critics of CT scanning for the diagnosis of appendicitis in children have noted that its diagnostic accuracy depends, to some extent, on the ability to detect inflammatory changes in the fat and other soft tissue around the appendix itself. Several recent reports have indicated that children under age 10 years and those with decreased amounts of body fat (low BMIs) have been shown to have high false-negative rates when being evaluated by CT.

The general consensus, among practicing pediatric surgeons and general surgeons experienced in the care of children, is that CT is probably the test of choice for equivocal cases (that is, children who are felt to possibly have acute appendicitis but with atypical histories and/or equivocal physical examinations), but should not be used routinely to evaluate *all* children who present with possible appendicitis. The radiologist evaluating the CT should be given as much clinical information about the patient as possible, in order to make a more informed interpretation. Rather than ordering a test, the clinician should consider himself obtaining a *radiologic consultation*. In addition, the clinician who orders the CT should personally review the radiographs and challenge the radiologist over controversial and/or unclear interpretations.

TREATMENT

Once the diagnosis of presumed acute appendicitis has been made, treatment should be instituted immediately. Patients should be made NPO (nothing by mouth), if this has not already been done. Resuscitation with intravenous fluids (see above) should be continued and infusion of broad-spectrum intravenous antibiotics should be started.

Numerous trials have been performed to compare various antibiotic regimens. Most drugs have been shown to be clinically equivalent, as long as the agent (or combination of medications) has broad coverage against a variety of enteric flora. Bacteria within the appendiceal lumen are the same as those found within the cecum and remainder of the large intestine. That is, a large number of enteric gram-negative rods, anaerobes, and gram-positive aerobic cocci. Perhaps the most common "cocktail" in use is that of gentamicin (an aminoglycoside, for treatment of the gram-negative aerobes), ampicillin (for use against the enterococci), and metronidazole or clindamycin (for treatment of the anaerobes). Similar success has been achieved with combinations of second- and third-generation cephalosporins and even single-agent therapy.

Most children with acute appendicitis undergo urgent appendectomy following resuscitation, usually within several hours of diagnosis. The traditional right lower quadrant incision (that is, open appendectomy) has been utilized for many decades with an acceptable, low risk of perioperative morbidity (Fig. 126.4). This procedure, performed under general

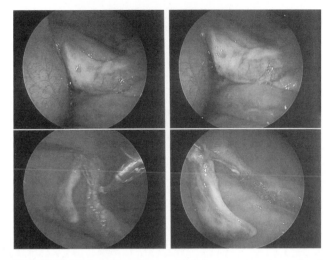

FIGURE 126.5. Laparoscopic appendectomy (grasper on appendiceal artery, adjacent to appendix).

anesthesia, typically takes 30 to 90 minutes. Drains are sometimes placed if the appendix has perforated and/or the infection has caused abscess formation.

The open procedure has recently been challenged by the newer laparoscopic approach (Fig. 126.5), initially reported in the late 1980s and early 1990s. Initially, most series in the surgical literature failed to demonstrate a statistical advantage with the laparoscopic technique, when assessing postoperative hospital stay, length of utilization of postoperative narcotic analgesia, and time to resumption of full diet and activity. However, these surgical reports have been criticized for including the surgical learning curve, in which surgeons with little laparoscopic experience unfairly compared results with their open procedures, with their lengthy track records. More recent series have excluded this learning curve and have often documented shorter lengths of stay and faster returns to full diet. Despite this, most surveys indicate that only about one-third of children in the United States with acute appendicitis currently undergo their surgical procedures laparoscopically.

Several recent reports have challenged the generally accepted dogma that appendicitis is a surgical emergency requiring immediate surgical intervention, even if that involves operating in the middle of the night. Studies from both the University of Michigan and the University of California at Irvine have advocating delaying appendectomy in children "until the daylight hours" and performing the procedure within 24 hours of hospitalization, at a time convenient to the surgeon and personnel of the operating room. The studies have shown no increase in perforation rates, readmission rates, length of stay, and complications.

Occasional children will present with "missed appendicitis" without diffuse peritonitis. In this situation, children may have developed appendicitis that becomes progressively inflamed and gangrenous and/or perforated, but is walled off by omentum, loops of small intestine, and/or cecum. This process, which typically takes 3 to 7 days, usually results in a right lower quadrant or pelvic abscess. In such cases, a number of authors have documented successful treatment with a protocol involving (1) hospitalization for treatment with intravenous antibiotics, typically for 7 to 10 days; (2) CT or ultrasound-guided abscess aspiration and drainage, with placement of a drainage catheter into the abscess cavity; (3) discharge home on a longer course of oral (or intravenous) antibiotics; and (4) interval appendectomy (either "open" or laparoscopic) roughly 6 weeks later. Candidates for such a treatment strategy

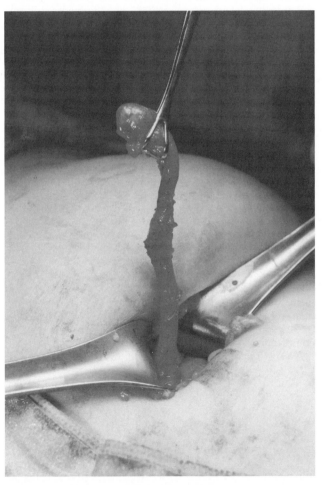

FIGURE 126.4. Open appendectomy (via right lower quadrant transverse incision) for acute appendicitis in a child.

should not have evidence of diffuse perforation nor other complications, such as adhesive intestinal obstruction.

Suggested Readings

El Ghoneimi A, Valla JS, Limonne B, et al. Laparoscopic appendectomy in children: report of 1,379 cases. *J Pediatr Surg* 1994;29:786–789.

Fishman SJ, Pelosi L, Klavon SL, et al. Perforated appendicitis: prospective outcome analysis for 150 children. *J Pediatr Surg* 2000;35:923–926.

Garcia Pena BM, Taylor GA, Lund DP, et al. Effect of computed tomography on patient management and costs in children with suspected appendicitis. *Pediatrics* 1999;104:440–446.

Gilchrist BF, Lobe TE, Schropp KP, et al. Is there a role for laparoscopic appendectomy in pediatric surgery? *J Pediatr Surg* 1992;27:209–214.

Kokoska ER, Minkes RK, Silen ML, et al. Effect of pediatric surgical practice on the treatment of children with appendicitis. *Pediatrics* 2001;107:1298–1301.

Kosloske AM, Love CL, Rohrer JE, et al. The diagnosis of appendicitis in children: outcomes of a strategy based on pediatric surgical evaluation. *Pediatrics* 2004;113:29–34.

Muehlstedt SG, Pham TQ, Schmeling DJ. The management of pediatric appendicitis: a survey of North American pediatric surgeons. *J Pediatr Surg* 2004;39:875–879.

Pearl RH, Hale DA, Molloy M, et al. Pediatric appendectomy. *J Pediatr Surg* 1995;30:173–181.

Rao PM, Rea JT, Novelline RA, et al. Effect of computed tomography of the appendix on treatment of patients and use of hospital resources. *N Engl J Med* 1998;338:141–146.

Yardeni D, Hirschl RB, Drongowski RA, et al. Delayed versus immediate surgery in acute appendicitis: do we need to operate during the night? *J Pediatr Surg* 2004;39:464–469.

CHAPTER 126C ■ SURGICAL EMERGENCIES: INTUSSUSCEPTION

J. DUNCAN PHILLIPS

Intussusception is a not-uncommon condition in which a thickened segment of intestine invaginates or "telescopes" into the next "downstream" (distal) segment of intestine. Waves of peristaltic intestinal muscular contractions propel the "upstream" segment of intestine (the intussusceptum) into the next segment of intestine (the intussuscipiens). As the intussusceptum travels into the intussuscipiens, it becomes entrapped there and may gradually become swollen, edematous, and thickened. It may swell to the point that it eventually blocks the passage of digested foodstuffs through the intestine and thus causes partial or complete intestinal obstruction.

Although patients of any age can develop intussusception, it occurs only rarely in adults. It typically affects children between the ages of 5 and 12 months. The incidence is approximately 2 to 4 cases per 1,000 children.

PATHOPHYSIOLOGY

"Idiopathic intussusception" accounts for about 95% of all cases (Table 126.5). In this condition, scattered microscopic areas of lymphoid tissue within the wall of the intestine may swell as part of the body's response to infection. A recent viral illness often precedes the intussusception episode. Lymphoid tissue called Peyer's patches is especially abundant in the terminal ileum. Thickening of the terminal ileum, caused by enlarged Peyer's patches, is the usual reason that intussusception develops. The intestine is essentially "fooled" into believing that the thickened intestine is a piece of undigested food—the intestine attempts to propel this "undigested food" downstream, hence causing the intussusception. The most common location for idiopathic intussusception is the ileocecal junction, with thickened ileum intussuscepting into the cecum as an "ileo-colic" intussusception. Less common types of idiopathic intussusception include ileo-ileal and colo-colic.

Approximately 5% of intussusception patients have an actual "lead point." That is, they have an abnormality of the intestine other than thickened Peyer's patches causing the intussusception. The most common cause is a Meckel's diverticulum, a small congenital outpouching of the terminal ileum which looks like an extra appendix. The Meckel's diverticulum is often referred to as "the organ of 2's" because it is found in approximately 2% of the overall population, is typically about 2 inches long, and is typically located on the ileum, about 2 feet from the large intestine.

Other unusual lead points for intussusception include intestinal polyps, hematomas within the wall of the intestine, other congenital intestinal lesions, ingested foreign bodies, and intestinal tumors.

If intussusception develops and is not promptly treated, obstruction of the intestine can progress from partial to complete, causing partially digested food to back up into the proximal intestine. As the intussusceptum is pushed more tightly into the intussuscipiens, the mucosal blood supply may be compromised. If the mucosa loses its blood supply, it will begin to slough off of the inner wall of the intestine and be carried distally. If the sloughed mucosa is passed through the anus, it can appear frankly bloody or can appear almost like currant jelly in color and consistency.

The intussusceptum can be squeezed so tightly by the surrounding intestine that it can actually be deprived of its blood supply and *die* (Fig. 126.6). Bacteria and bacterial toxins from the ischemic intestine can enter the bloodstream and travel, by way of the circulation, throughout the child's body. Bacteria and their toxins can cause sepsis, which is a severe systemic illness that can affect all of the organ systems of the body. If

TABLE 126.5

PATHOPHYSIOLOGY OF INTUSSUSCEPTION

- Lymphoid tissue thickening (Peyer's patches)
- Propelled distally by peristalsis
- Impaction within distal intestine
- Intestinal obstruction
- Mucosal ischemia, necrosis, gangrene
- Bacterial translocation
- Septicemia

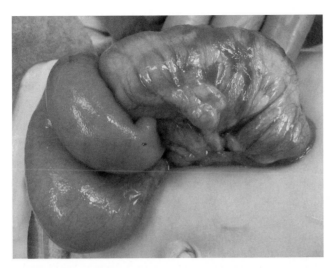

FIGURE 126.6. Infarcted ileum, intussuscepted, and "trapped" within ascending colon, as seen at time of laparotomy.

TABLE 126.6

DIFFERENTIAL DIAGNOSIS OF INTUSSUSCEPTION

(partial list)
- Acute gastroenteritis
- Acute appendicitis
- Acute intestinal obstruction for other reasons (tumor, hematoma, etc.)
- Meckel's diverticulitis
- Incarcerated hernia

---

in 40% to 70% of patients as a large sausage-shaped mass of tissue.

Patients with intussusception that has progressed to infarction may present with somnolence, lethargy, and even shock.

DIFFERENTIAL DIAGNOSIS

Many conditions that affect the gastrointestinal tract, such as acute viral gastroenteritis and acute food poisoning mimic intussusception (Table 126.6). Therefore, in most instances, the diagnosis is confirmed with an x-ray study (see below). Common mimics of intussusception include the following:

1. Acute gastroenteritis. Vomiting is one of the most frequent presenting complaints of infants and toddlers seeking medical attention in emergency departments, walk-in clinics, and physician offices. Distinguishing the common "GI bug" from a case of intussusception can be extremely difficult. Obtaining a history of similar symptoms in other affected family members (or other children in the same day care environment) may be helpful. In addition, children with acute gastroenteritis are often somewhat older (for example, 2 to 4 years of age). In addition, a history of profuse diarrhea is unusual with intussusception.
2. Acute appendicitis. This disease most commonly affects children between the ages of 8 and 18 years and is quite rare in children below the age of 2 years. Children with appendicitis typically present with abdominal pain that is more constant in quality, with gradual progressive worsening and localization to the right lower quadrant. Vomiting is typically mild, and usually occurs three or fewer times.

---

untreated, this can cause hypotension, respiratory failure, heart failure, kidney failure, and even death.

In addition to bacteremia, the child is at risk for developing hypotension and hypoperfusion for other reasons. This can occur when, as a result of intestinal blockage, a patient is unable to eat or even keep down oral fluids. Dehydration can quickly develop and, if untreated, cause hypovolemic shock.

SIGNS AND SYMPTOMS

Because intestinal contractions typically occur in "waves" of peristaltic activity, the intestine usually contracts quite forcefully for several minutes and then relaxes for 15 to 30 minutes. When intussusception occurs, the intestine continues to contract above the obstruction and often gradually forces more intestine into the intussuscipiens. With each series of intestinal contractions, there is stretching of the intestinal wall, which causes severe, crampy pain. The typical patient with intussusception develops the sudden onset of crying and screaming and pulls the knees up toward the abdomen. When the attack ends, after several minutes, the baby may initially appear quite normal, with the resumption of normal activity. These attacks, which can occur every 10 to 30 minutes, can be quite dramatic and frightening to parents and others. Occasionally, however, the attacks may be mild and just "crampy" in nature, and thus unsuspecting parents may be rather shocked when told that their child may have a serious illness.

As the intussusception continues, the obstructed intestine eventually "backs up" with undigested food and bile, causing the child to vomit. The vomited material initially appears to be undigested food, but gradually becomes yellowish in color and bitter tasting. Eventually, the child may vomit dark green bile.

Most children with intussusception are somewhat distended and tender. However, the abdominal examination may be remarkably "benign" with many examiners reporting a soft, nontender abdomen. The intussusceptum may be palpable in the right upper quadrant or right mid-abdomen

---

TABLE 126.7

WORKUP FOR SUSPECTED INTUSSUSCEPTION

- Surgical consultation
- Intravenous access
- Fluid resuscitation and nasogastric decompression
- Consider broad-spectrum intravenous antibiotics
- Plain abdominal radiograph to exclude pneumoperitoneum ("free air")
- Possible screening ultrasound
- Contrast enema (air or barium) for diagnosis and/or attempted reduction

WORKUP

Intussusception, if present, is a true emergency, requiring urgent diagnosis and treatment because the disease can quickly progress to intestinal infarction, bacteremia, perforation, peritonitis, and even death (Table 126.7). Standard evaluation (and possible treatment) is typically undertaken with the assistance of a radiologist capable of performing a diagnostic (and potentially therapeutic) contrast enema (see below). A child suspected of having intussusception should be managed at a facility with the capability of both proper evaluation and treatment of this problem. If such capability is not available at your facility, urgent consultation with the appropriate specialist in order to arrange transfer to another facility should be undertaken immediately.

If intussusception is suspected, the surgical dictum of "REO" (Resuscitate, Evaluate, and *then* Operate) should be followed. The child should usually have intravenous access obtained expeditiously and begin receiving intravenous fluids to treat probable dehydration. In addition, a nasogastric or orogastric tube should probably be placed in order to assist with gastric decompression. Although somewhat controversial, most children should also receive intravenous antibiotics to treat possible bacteremia.

Pearl

■ When placing the intravenous catheter, if possible utilize the same venipuncture to obtain blood for a complete blood count and to obtain a "clot" for type and screen procedure. Most children with intussusception will have evidence of leukocytosis. Occasional children will be anemic from blood loss (sloughed intestinal mucosa—see above) and require perioperative blood transfusions.

Surgical consultation should be obtained before a diagnostic contrast enema is obtained. Some pediatric surgeons prefer to be physically present and participate in this process with the radiologist.

A plain abdominal x-ray (kidneys, ureters, and bladder; KUB) may suggest intestinal obstruction by documenting the presence of air-filled, dilated small bowel segments. Occasionally, a soft-tissue mass is seen (or, at least a paucity of air is seen) in the right upper quadrant to suggest the presence of the intussusception. An upright x-ray (or lateral view) may show small intestine air–fluid levels. Many radiologists insist on this study before performing a contrast enema as a screen for free air (pneumoperitoneum) so that there is no radiographic evidence of intestinal perforation.

Some radiologists advocate abdominal ultrasound as a diagnostic screening tool for atypical cases. A target sign is looked for, and if present, a contrast enema is then performed.

Definitive diagnosis of intussusception is typically made by either barium or air-contrast enema. Using fluoroscopy, the radiologist can watch the barium pass backwards, up the large intestine, to the area of the intussusception (if present). If one raises the barium bag about 3 feet above the level of the patient, one can often use the column of barium as if it were a long flexible snake to "push" the intussusceptum backwards and into its normal location. This is called hydrostatic reduction and is successful, depending on the duration of the patient's symptoms, about 50% to 80% of the time.

Pearl

■ To be considered negative for intussusception, barium from the enema *must* pass proximal to the ileocecal valve and fill the most distal loops of terminal ileum. Unfortunately, many children with idiopathic intussusception develop edema and swelling of the tissue at the ileocecal junction, making it quite difficult for the radiologist to reflux barium into the ileum following successful reduction. It is not unusual to have an experienced, competent radiologist report that an intussusception was present and that it was "probably completely reduced." Depending upon the clinical situation, this may prompt the responsible physician to admit the patient to the hospital for observation (see below) or even consider laparoscopic evaluation (see below).

Hydrostatic reduction, although transiently painful to the child, avoids the need for surgical reduction (see below). Complications of attempted hydrostatic reduction are rare. However, because hydrostatic reduction can result in intestinal perforation, it should only be performed at an institution where either a pediatric surgeon or a surgeon with special expertise in the care of children is immediately available should surgery be necessary (see below).

Air can be used instead of barium. Using a similar tube, attached to a pressure gauge, an experienced radiologist can pump air under pressure retrograde up the large intestine and demonstrate the intussusception. Again, the intussusception can be relieved by the radiologist using air instead of barium. This is called pneumatic reduction and has been reported to be somewhat faster than hydrostatic reduction and may have a higher success rate (80–90%). However, specialized equipment and training is required to learn this technique—it is not currently available in many hospitals but is recently gaining increasing acceptance.

Following either hydrostatic or pneumatic reduction, children with intussusception are typically admitted to the hospital and observed for 24 to 48 hours. This is done for several reasons. First, intestine that has been transiently obstructed will often be dilated and have a somewhat diminished capacity to contract and function normally. Children will therefore typically require at least some amount of intravenous fluid supplementation as they begin a liquid diet and progress gradually to their usual diets. Second, about 3% of children will develop another intussusception (see below) and need further in-hospital treatment. Third, if a child suffers an intestinal perforation during a nonoperative reduction and if that perforation is missed by the radiologist doing the procedure, the child could develop peritonitis and become hemodynamically unstable.

Pediatric surgeons in the recent past recommended that children who had undergone successful hydrostatic or pneumatic reduction be given nonabsorbable charcoal by mouth upon admission to the hospital. In this way, when charcoal appeared in the child's stool, the child's nurse or family members could joyfully announce that there was objective evidence of relief of the child's intestinal obstruction and thus the child could safely be discharged home. Few surgeons currently continue this practice.

Rarely, children with intussusception progress so quickly to the development of severe intestinal ischemia that the segment of intestine dies before the child is seen by a physician. If that has occurred, the affected intestine can rupture, spilling intestinal contents throughout the abdominal cavity, causing diffuse inflammation of the abdomen and peritonitis. If peritonitis is present, x-ray studies can be dangerous because of the risk of barium or air leaking from the intestine into the abdominal cavity. In this case, urgent surgical treatment is usually performed immediately (discussed next).

TREATMENT

If intussusception is confirmed by x-ray study and if hydrostatic or pneumatic reduction is unsuccessful, or if diffuse peritonitis is present (see above), the child requires urgent surgical treatment. This is performed in the operating room by either a pediatric surgeon or a general surgeon experienced in the surgical care of children. The operation requires general anesthesia, induced either by a pediatric anesthesiologist or an anesthesiologist with expertise in the care of pediatric patients.

Typically, a transverse incision is made in the right lower quadrant of the abdomen and the intussusception is reduced by the surgeon by gently squeezing the intestine just past the intussusception and thereby pushing the intussusceptum backwards, out of the intussuscipiens and into its normal location (Fig. 126.7).

The incision is quite similar to that used to perform an appendectomy. Thus, if a patient who has undergone surgical reduction of an intussusception ever develops abdominal pain many years (or decades) later and is examined by a physician who does not have access to the medical history, a physician might assume that the patient had already undergone appendectomy. To avoid this potential confusion, most surgeons also remove the appendix when reducing an intussusception surgically.

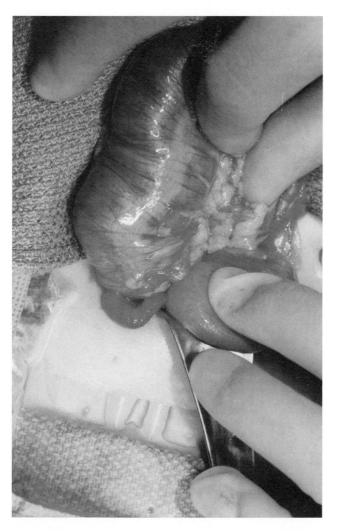

FIGURE 126.7. Laparotomy for intussusception.

Occasionally, the intussuscepted intestine will have become so swollen that, despite attempts by the surgeon, it cannot be safely reduced. This usually means that the involved intestine has been squeezed so tightly for so long that it has died. In that case, the involved segment of intestine is resected. Intestine proximal and distal to the intussusception can usually be connected together during the same operation, using either sutures or a surgical stapling device.

Rarely, dead intestine involved in an intussusception can rupture, or perforate, either before surgery or during gentle manipulation of dead intestine during surgery. This can cause diffuse inflammation of the abdominal cavity, or peritonitis. In this case, connecting the intestine together could be very risky—the connection, or anastomosis, would be at an increased risk of not healing and possibly leaking intestinal contents into the abdomen. Therefore, if peritonitis is detected at the time of surgery, most surgeons advocate removal of the involved intestine and creation of diverting stoma, or ileostomy, proximally. A plastic bag called an appliance is fitted over the ileostomy after surgery. Intestinal contents flow into the appliance, which can be emptied into the toilet several times each day. After the peritonitis subsides, which typically takes 5 to 10 days, most children with ileostomies can be discharged home and then rehospitalized 6 to 8 weeks later for a second operation. At the second operation, also performed under general anesthesia, the abdominal cavity can be reopened, the ileostomy can be taken down, and the intestine can be reconnected.

In about 3% of patients, following either hydrostatic or pneumatic reduction, symptoms of crampy abdominal pain will recur. This usually happens within 1 to 2 days following the initial reduction. If this occurs, most patients can be returned to the radiology suite for a second reduction. The recurrence rate following surgical reduction is similar and can be treated by hydrostatic or pneumatic reduction if intestinal resection (with the creation of a "fresh" intestinal anastomosis) was not performed at the time of surgery. Occasionally, recurrent intussusceptions require surgical reduction.

Most children with intussusception, who are promptly diagnosed and treated, respond well with no long-term sequellae. Survival is over 95%.

Several new treatments have emerged for intussusception during the past several years. First, it has long been known that the adequacy of hydrostatic or pneumatic reduction (see above) can be difficult to assess. Some patients will have their intussusceptions completely reduced by the radiologist, but the x-ray studies will appear as if the reductions were incomplete. Indeed, at the time of surgery, about one-fourth of those children felt to have incomplete hydrostatic reductions will actually have been reduced. For that reason, some surgeons have recently advocated a less invasive surgical approach that involves laparoscopy (Fig. 126.8). With this technique, a small incision is made in the umbilicus and a laparoscope is inserted. A small video camera is then attached to the laparoscope and the image is transmitted to a television monitor in the operating room. If the intestine is visualized and the intussusception has been completely reduced, the laparoscope can then be removed and the operation concluded. Second, during the past several years specialized instruments have been developed to allow laparoscopically-assisted manipulation of the intestine in small children. These instruments can be inserted into the child's abdomen through small incisions and, using the laparoscope to visualize the inside of the abdomen, these small instruments can sometimes be used to reduce the intussusception and remove the appendix.

Laparoscopy and laparoscopic surgery still require general anesthesia, with all of its risks and potential complications, and are done in an operating room. Specialized training in

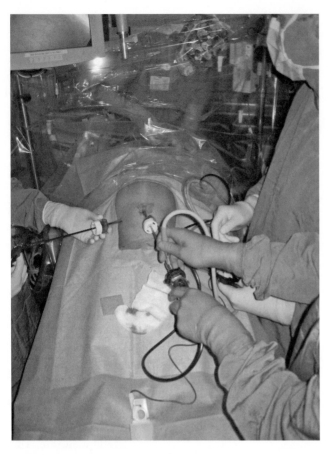

FIGURE 126.8. Laparoscopy for intussusception.

pediatric laparoscopic surgery is required to master these techniques.

On August 31, 1998 the Wyeth-Lederle pharmaceutical company began marketing a vaccine for rotavirus, a virus that can cause a diarrhea-type illness in small children. The vaccine, called RotaShield, was supposed to be given to children at ages 2, 4, and 6 months and was recommended by the American Academy of Pediatrics, the Advisory Committee on Immunization Practices of the Centers for Disease Control and Prevention (CDC), and the American Academy of Family Physicians. As of September 1999, after an estimated 1.5 million doses of the vaccine were administered, 23 cases of intussusception were reported in these children. Children affected tended to be somewhat younger than typical intussusception patients, and have a higher likelihood of requiring surgical reduction. The CDC investigated these cases and, because of the possible increased risk of intussusception, recommended that physicians temporarily suspend administration of this vaccine. The manufacturer voluntarily removed its product from the market. As of January 2006, several new rotavirus vaccines were reported, having undergone extensive human testing, with no increased risk of intussusception compared to placebo. Future rotavirus vaccines will likely be scrutinized closely by pediatricians and other responsible physicians.

Suggested Readings

Ein SH, Palder SB, Alton DJ, et al. Intussusception: toward less surgery? *J Pediatr Surg* 1994;29:433–435.

Grosfeld JL. Intussusception then and now: a historical vignette. *J Am Coll Surg* 2005;201:830–833.

Guo JZ, Ma XY, Zhou QH. Results of air pressure enema reduction of intussusception: 6,396 cases in 13 years. *J Pediatr Surg* 1986;21:1201–1203.

Kia KF, Mony VK, Drongowski RA, et al. Laparoscopic vs. open surgical approach for intussusception requiring operative intervention. *J Pediatr Surg* 2005;40:281–284.

Schier F. Experience with laparoscopy in the treatment of intussusception. *J Pediatr Surg* 1997;32:1713–1714.

Verschelden P, Filiatraut D, Garel L, et al. Intussusception in children: reliability of ultrasound in diagnosis—a prospective study. *Radiology* 1992;184:741–744.

CHAPTER 126D ■ SURGICAL EMERGENCIES: PYLORIC STENOSIS

DANIEL VONALLMEN

Pyloric stenosis was described as early as the 17th century, and was specifically characterized by Harald Hirschsprung in 1888. It has subsequently been recognized as one of the most common surgical conditions in young children. It develops in roughly 2 to 7 cases 1,000 children. More common in whites than nonwhites, it is far more common in males, with a male to female ratio of 4 to 1, and most commonly presents between the 3rd and 5th week of life. It has been reported in patients up to several months of age and as early as in fetuses on prenatal ultrasound.

PATHOPHYSIOLOGY

Hypertrophy of the pyloric muscle causes progressive narrowing of the pyloric channel and subsequent progressive blockage of forward flow of liquid from the stomach to the duodenum. Although the cause of this idiopathic pyloric hypertrophy remains unknown, there is clearly a genetic component, although the exact genetic mutations have not been fully characterized and are probably polygenic. The risk of developing hypertrophic pyloric stenosis (HPS) in the children of an affected mother is 20% for a daughter and 7% for a son. The risk to the offspring of an affected father is 5% for a daughter and 2.5% for a son.

SIGNS AND SYMPTOMS

The overwhelming majority of patients with HPS present with progressive nonbilious emesis. Although the vomiting is often described as "projectile," this cannot be used as a reliable indicator of the presence or absence of HPS. The most important characteristic is the absence of bile in the emesis.

DIFFERENTIAL DIAGNOSIS

Bilious emesis implies a possible obstruction distal to the ampulla of Vater and necessitates emergent evaluation for malrotation with volvulus, and in turn, requiring immediate surgical intervention. In the neonate and infant, the differential diagnosis of nonbilious emesis is much less urgent than bilious emesis, allowing careful fluid resuscitation and further evaluation before considering surgery. The differential for nonbilious emesis includes infectious etiologies (e.g., sepsis, urinary tract infection) as well as other mechanical issues. With HPS, the infants typically appear well and are often vigorous with feedings. Gastroesophageal reflux disease (GERD) and simple overfeeding are more common than HPS, and notable for absence of progressive severity and associated dehydration, electrolyte abnormalities, and even malnutrition. Overfed children maintain or exceed their growth curves, and most infants with GERD continue to thrive. Without early recognition and intervention, all infants with HPS ultimately develop issues with hydration, nutrition, and electrolytes. Gastric webs and preampullary duodenal atresia remain in the differential but are decidedly less common.

WORKUP

The diagnosis of HPS in many centers has shifted from one based on physical exam to one relying on radiologic workup. This in part is due to increasing availability of more sophisticated radiologic tools (e.g., ultrasound), and also likely reflects earlier recognition related to a more aggressive diagnostic approach by primary care physicians. Historically, infants with pyloric stenosis presented late with severe metabolic abnormalities and malnutrition. This contributed to a high complication rate with surgery and a substantial mortality rate. Fortunately with earlier diagnosis and more sophisticated perioperative care, the mortality rate is now less than 0.1%.

The diagnosis of pyloric stenosis can usually be made with the physical exam. Doing so requires patience and experience. On simple observation one may note peristaltic waves in the epigastrium, and with careful palpation the characteristic pyloric mass can be palpated to the right of midline below the liver edge. When the stomach is full the pylorus rotates posteriorly, making palpation more difficult. Placement of a nasogastric tube to decompress the stomach increases the likelihood of palpating the "olive." Physical exam alone carries a sensitivity of 72% and specificity of 97%. The positive predictive value of a positive exam is 98%. Thus, in an appropriate clinical presentation with a characteristic epigastric

mass noted on physical exam, no additional diagnostic testing is needed. When palpation is negative, additional testing is indicated.

The two most common radiologic tests used to confirm the presence of HPS are the ultrasound and the upper gastrointestinal (UGI) study. Ultrasound has become the test of choice in most institutions, although there are some studies suggesting that in the evaluation of all infants presenting to a primary care physician with nonbilious vomiting, the UGI is a more cost-effective initial test. In a study involving 246 infants evaluated for possible HPS, UGI had a positive predictive value of 1.0 compared to 0.98 for ultrasound. The UGI offers the advantage of providing alternative diagnoses. In comparison, ultrasound is less traumatic, avoids the radiation exposure, and decreases risk of aspiration (i.e., secondary to filling the stomach with contrast material before a general anesthetic). The quality and interpretation of both ultrasound and UGI are somewhat dependent on the experience of the radiologist performing the exam.

LABORATORY EVALUATION

Electrolyte abnormalities are not uncommon with HPS. Persistent vomiting results in a hypokalemic, hyponatremic metabolic alkalosis, and this must be corrected prior to surgery. The metabolic alkalosis especially raises concerns for postoperative apnea following a general anesthetic; hence most anesthesiologists require that the chloride level be greater than 100 mmol/L and the bicarbonate level less than 30 mmol/L prior to going to the operating room. In severe cases, the infants are dehydrated, with chloride levels in the 50s and bicarbonate levels near 40 mmol/L. Although hypokalemia is expected with HPS, as many as one-third of patients will have normal or elevated potassium levels at diagnosis. Initial resuscitation is usually done with intravenous normal saline followed by half-normal saline with potassium once the patient demonstrates adequate renal function. Electrolytes are typically rechecked every 8 to 12 hours to document resolution of the metabolic alkalosis prior to induction of general anesthesia.

TREATMENT

There are two main treatment options for patients diagnosed with HPS. The vast majority of patients in the United States undergo surgical treatment with a pyloromyotomy. However, medical therapy does exist. Atropine given either orally or intravenously can stop the vomiting and eventually allow the child to return to normal oral intake. Therapy may be required for days to weeks, and usually requires inpatient hospital stays significantly longer than infants treated with surgery.

Although there are several different approaches to the operative treatment of HPS, the basic techniques are similar. A longitudinal seromuscular incision is made extending from the antrum of the stomach across the pylorus to the duodenal junction. The thickened muscle fibers are then split longitudinally, allowing the intact mucosa to bulge out between the muscle layers. When properly completed, the two halves of the pylorus can be moved independently, confirming adequate separation of the muscle fibers.

Although the actual pyloromyotomy technique is common to all surgical treatment, the manner in which the pylorus is accessed through the abdominal wall is variable. There are three primary approaches to the operation. Classically, the pylorus is approached through a right upper quadrant muscle-splitting incision. The advantage of this approach is excellent visualization, rapid exposure of the pylorus, and direct manipulation of the pylorus. The drawbacks include a highly visible scar that grows with the patient, and potentially increased postoperative pain.

In the early 1990s the technique was modified to approach the pylorus through a periumbilical incision similar to that used for umbilical hernia repair. The advantage of this approach is mostly cosmetic in that the right upper quadrant scar is avoided. Critics of this approach note more difficult access to the pylorus resulting in more trauma to the antrum, theoretically resulting in delayed return of postoperative gastric function. Several studies have also documented higher rates of wound complications with this approach.

Most recently, minimally invasive techniques have been applied to the treatment of HPS and many pediatric surgeons now perform the operation laparoscopically. With this approach, a 3- or 4-mm laparoscope is inserted through a small incision at the umbilicus. The pylorus is visualized, and two laparoscopic instruments are inserted through 2- to 3-mm incisions in the upper abdomen. The pyloromyotomy is completed with the pylorus in situ, thus theoretically reducing the trauma from the traction needed to bring it out of the abdomen for the open approaches. Compared to the open approach, studies have shown a more rapid return to full diet after laparoscopic surgery, but a randomized controlled trial has not yet been done. Although the cosmetic result is excellent, there is a learning curve involved and a higher rate of duodenal perforation has been reported using the laparoscopic approach. Ultimately the complication rate should be similar for both techniques.

POSTOPERATIVE CARE

The postoperative management of patients after pyloromyotomy primarily focuses on the feeding regimen. Regardless of the surgical approach, infants usually leave the operating room without a nasogastric tube, and postoperative pain is usually easily controlled with moderate doses of intravenous narcotics (morphine 0.05–0.1 mg/kg) and oral acetaminophen. Discharge from the hospital requires resumption of full enteral feedings, and a wide variety of feeding regimens are employed by pediatric surgeons. Classically infants are started on small amounts of oral glucose/electrolyte solutions and then slowly advanced to formula feedings based on a predetermined feeding schedule. Advances are held if the patient vomits. Discharge from the hospital occurs when full feedings have been achieved.

Others have employed a more aggressive feeding regimen in which ad lib formula feedings are started within 2 hours after completion of surgery. Studies have shown that although there is an increase in the number of episodes of vomiting, these infants reach full feedings faster thus allowing earlier hospital discharge. The latter can usually be achieved within 24 to 48 hours of the surgery. In a few infants, resumption of full feedings is delayed during several days of slowly advancing feedings.

COMPLICATIONS

The complication rate for routine surgery for HPS is quite low. Reliance on ultrasound for the diagnosis introduces the possibility of false-positive or false-negative results. These misinterpretations are more common with inexperienced radiologists. False-positive results may lead to unnecessary surgery and false-negative results may delay treatment. Studies may need to be repeated when the results of the initial workup are equivocal or unreliable.

Operative complications include the standard operative risks of bleeding and wound infection as well as more serious complications related directly to the pyloromyotomy. Wound infections occur in 2% to 6% and are treated with local care. Perforation of the mucosa of the pyloric channel or duodenum occurs in approximately 4% of cases. The incidence is higher when the operation is performed by inexperienced or non-pediatric surgeons and higher with the laparoscopic approach. When the perforation is noted at the time of surgery, it can be repaired primarily followed by nasogastric tube drainage for 24 hours postoperatively. Delayed diagnosis may result in more serious intra-abdominal infections and a more prolonged hospital course.

Although mucosal perforation is the result of a pyloromyotomy that is too aggressive, an inadequate myotomy is also possible. This typically occurs at the antral end of the myotomy and may prevent the patient from being able to advance on a diet postoperatively. Repeat myotomy is warranted in these cases. Recurrent pyloric stenosis has been reported but is extremely rare.

PEARLS

- In infants with *progressive nonbilious emesis*, hypertrophic pyloric stenosis should be strongly considered in the differential diagnosis.
- Surgical repair is not an urgency and should be delayed until fluid and electrolyte abnormalities are corrected.
- The diagnosis of HPS can often be made based on an appropriate history and a good physical examination with palpation of the enlarged pylorus. When uncertainty remains, upper gastrointestinal imaging with barium (string sign) or ultrasound (muscle thickness ≥3 mm or pyloric length ≥13 mm) can be diagnostic.

Suggested Readings

Brain AJ, Roberts DS. Who should treat pyloric stenosis: the general or specialist pediatric surgeon? *J Pediatr Surg* 1996;31:1535–1537.

Godbole P, Sprigg A, Dickson JA, et al. Ultrasound compared with clinical examination in infantile hypertrophic pyloric stenosis. *Arch Dis Child* 1996;75:335–337.

Hall NJ, Van Der Zee J, Tan HL, et al. Meta-analysis of laparoscopic versus open pyloromyotomy. *Ann Surg* 2004;240:774–778.

Hulka F, Campbell JR, Harrison MW, et al. Cost-effectiveness in diagnosing infantile hypertrophic pyloric stenosis. *J Pediatr Surg* 1997;32:1604–1608.

Kawahara H, Takama Y, Yoshida H, et al. Medical treatment of infantile hypertrophic pyloric stenosis: should we always slice the "olive"? *J Pediatr Surg* 2005;40:1848–1851.

Kim SS, Lau ST, Lee SL, et al. The learning curve associated with laparoscopic pyloromyotomy. *J Laparoendosc Adv Surg Tech A* 2005;15:474–477.

Ladd AP, Nemeth SA, Kirincich AN, et al. Supraumbilical pyloromyotomy: a unique indication for antimicrobial prophylaxis. *J Pediatr Surg* 2005;40:974–977; discussion, 977.

Olson AD, Hernandez R, Hirschl RB. The role of ultrasonography in the diagnosis of pyloric stenosis: a decision analysis. *J Pediatr Surg* 1998;33:676–681.

Poon TS, Zhang AL, Cartmill T, et al. Changing patterns of diagnosis and treatment of infantile hypertrophic pyloric stenosis: a clinical audit of 303 patients. *J Pediatr Surg* 1996;31:1611–1615.

Safford SD, Pietrobon R, Safford KM, et al. A study of 11,003 patients with hypertrophic pyloric stenosis and the association between surgeon and hospital volume and outcomes. *J Pediatr Surg* 2005;40:967–972; discussion, 972–973.

CHAPTER 126E ■ SURGICAL EMERGENCIES: INCARCERATED AND STRANGULATED INGUINAL HERNIA

TIMOTHY M. WEINER

Hernias are a common pediatric surgical condition, with a four to one male preponderance and an increased incidence in premature infants. In the pediatric population, hernias typically result from a persistent patency of the *processus vaginalis*, a so-called "indirect" hernia. This occurs as the testes pass through the internal ring of the abdominal wall in the 7th gestational month and the inguinal tissues fail to close behind the descending testicle. A patent processus has been reported in up to 80% of newborns, with persistence of up to 20% of these into adulthood. If the processus obliterates after birth, fluid may be trapped in the distal scrotum, resulting in a *noncommunicating hydrocoele*. A small opening in the processus that allows fluid to ebb and flow across it is deemed a *communicating hydrocoele*. If this opening enlarges to allow the entry of abdominal viscera into the inguinal canal and scrotum, a hernia has developed, and the individual is at risk for this viscera to incarcerate, strangulate, and infarct (Fig. 126.9).

In infants and children, the majority of incarcerations occur in the first year of life. It has been reported in several series that up to 30% of hernias will incarcerate by age 2 months. Over 90% of these incarcerated inguinal hernias in children can be reduced nonoperatively.

The dilemma for the clinician is the differentiation of an incarcerated hernia from other similar scrotal conditions, such as acute inguinal lymphadenopathy, testicular torsion, or acute swelling of a hydrocoele. The clinician must also be able to recognize whether an incarcerated hernia has been effectively reduced as well as the features and urgency of ischemic or infarcting viscera.

ing towards the labia or scrotum. Crying or straining often demonstrates the bulge, which may reduce spontaneously as the child relaxes. Restraining an infant across the torso and knees can often induce sufficient straining to cause protrusion of an occult hernia.

A hernia is of immediate concern if it contains viscera that is entrapped and cannot be easily reduced with gentle steady manual manipulation. Such an incarcerated hernia usually contains small bowel but can also entrap the appendix, omentum, a Meckel diverticulum, ovary and/or tube, colon, or even a projection from the bladder. A child with an incarcerated hernia presents with symptoms that can include general irritability and inguinal tenderness, erythema, and firmness. Incarceration of bowel will cause obstructive symptoms such as abdominal distension and vomiting. Compromise of this bowel can lead to fever, peritonitis, and toxemia.

A good clinical exam is usually sufficient to achieve a diagnosis and determine the level of concern and urgency. Transillumination may help differentiate an incarcerated hernia from an acute hydrocoele. Abdominal films may demonstrate bowel loops projecting into the scrotum and air–fluid levels suggestive of a mechanical small bowel obstruction. Physical findings that appear exclusive to the hemiscrotum and do not seem to refer into the inguinal canal should raise a suspicion for testicular torsion. In females, a palpable irreducible mass in the inguinal canal is discovered to be a (viable) ovary in 15% of cases. However, it may not be possible to distinguish a torsed and strangulated ovary from incarcerated bowel without operative inspection.

CLINICAL PRESENTATION

An indirect inguinal hernia is typically noted by a parent or health care provider as a bulge in the lower abdomen extend-

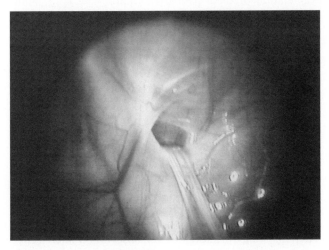

FIGURE 126.9. Right hernial orifice at the internal ring as seen from within the peritoneal cavity by laparoscopy.

MANAGEMENT

Nonoperative

A patient and diligent attempt should be made to reduce an incarcerated hernia provided the child is stable, nontoxic, and without signs of peritonitis. Most surgeons believe that an attempt is warranted even if there is evidence of obstruction as long as there is no peritoneal irritation.

Sedation, elevation of the lower torso and legs and gentle, steady manipulation are the mainstays of a nonoperative reduction. The clinician should appreciate the oblique trajectory of the inguinal canal and apply pressure in that vector (Fig. 126.10). Much like guiding a balloon into the neck of a bottle, the bowel should be maneuvered with three fingers of the practitioner's nondominant hand into the neck of the hernia at the overlap of the internal and external inguinal rings. Slow, consistent pressure—rather than a rapid, "cramming" approach—will allow bowel gas and edema to decompress and promote the reduction. Patience and the recognition that persistence over 10 to 20 minutes may be necessary should yield a successful reduction in 9 of 10 cases.

Sedation using small doses of short-acting analgesics and anxiolytics is a useful adjunct but commits the patient to a period of inpatient observation even if the reduction is successful.

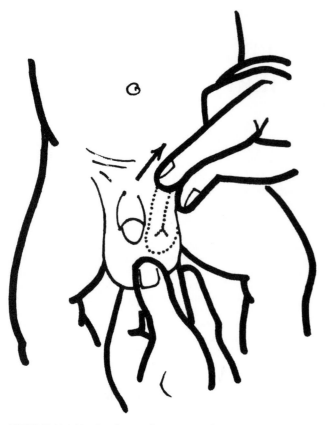

FIGURE 126.10. Gentle, steady pressure of incarcerated bowel in direction of the inguinal canal (*arrow*) to achieve reduction.

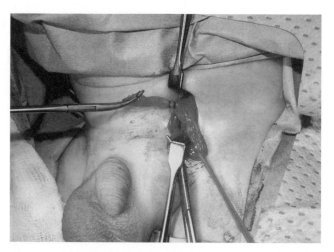

FIGURE 126.11. Surgical ligation of the hernia sac with preservation of the spermatic cord structures in the vessel loop (on the right).

In cases in which the reduction and repair are straightforward, many surgeons will attempt to assess the contralateral inguinal ring via a small laparoscope placed through the hernia sac prior to its ligation.

Many surgeons prefer to admit the child after nonoperative reduction of an incarcerated hernia and repair the hernia within 24 hours when the edema of the inguinal canal has subsided. Clearly, if the reduction was not successful or if there is uncertainty about whether a complete reduction was achieved, the child is prepared for urgent operative exploration.

Operative

If attempts at reduction were unsuccessful or uncertain, or if the patient presented with signs of physiologic instability and/or peritonitis from the incarcerated hernia, they are taken directly to the operating room. In some cases, the hernia will reduce spontaneously with the induction of anesthesia.

Typically, a small inguinal incision in the lowest abdominal crease is made, the hernia and adjacent cord structures are isolated, and the herniated viscera are reduced under direct visualization. The hernia sac is then skeletonized away from the testicular vessels and vas deferens, divided, and a "high" suture ligation is done at the internal inguinal ring (Fig 126.11). Repair or reinforcement of the tissues of the inguinal canal is usually not necessary in pediatric patients. If the entrapped bowel appears to be of questionable viability; or cloudy, bloody, or foul-smelling fluid is noted within the hernia sac; an attempt to fully examine the bowel should be made. This may require extending the hernial incision and orifice to recapture the viscera in question or even making a second transperitoneal incision higher on the abdomen. Infarcted, necrotic tissue is resected and anastomoses done as needed.

OUTCOMES AND COMPLICATIONS

Uncomplicated repairs are typically discharged to home within 24 hours of surgery with premature infants being closely observed for postanesthetic apnea and bradycardia. Patients who suffer a bowel obstruction or resection as a result of the incarcerated hernia may require longer hospitalization while the postoperative ileus resolves. Fewer than 1% of all incarcerated hernias and between 4% and 7% of irreducible hernias require intestinal resection. The majority of these patients recover uneventfully and without prolonged gastrointestinal problems.

Depending upon the study, there is between a 2% and 14% incidence of ipsilateral testicular infarction and atrophy after incarceration of a hernia. A plan for regular follow-up and examination of these patients is appropriate and should include thorough examination of testicular size and location.

The chance of a recurrence of the hernia is less than 1% after an uncomplicated repair. This incidence rises to about 3% if the hernia was incarcerated, and is further exacerbated if the child was a premature infant.

SUMMARY

Indirect inguinal hernias in males are a common condition, with incarceration tending to occur in the first year of life. An irreducible inguinal bulge is the typical presentation but must be distinguished from lymphadenopathy, testicular torsion, and acute hydrocoele. The majority of incarcerated hernias can be reduced nonoperatively with steady manipulation and sedation, but children who receive sedation for a reduction should be admitted for observation and elective repair

Any child with an incarcerated hernia and signs of instability and/or peritonitis should go urgently to surgery.

CHAPTER 126F ■ SURGICAL EMERGENCIES: MECKEL'S DIVERTICULUM

DANIEL VONALLMEN

Meckel's diverticulum (MD), named for the 19th century physician Johann Friedrich Meckel, arises as a remnant of the omphalomesenteric duct. Although most MDs are asymptomatic, those that become symptomatic can present with obstruction, infection, or bleeding. The initial diagnosis is sometimes delayed as other etiologies are considered more likely.

PATHOPHYSIOLOGY

Meckel's diverticulum is one of a number of congenital abnormalities with an origin in the embryonal connection between the distal small bowel and the umbilicus. This duct usually disappears via complete resorption by the end of the 7th week of gestation. A failure of this involution can result in a patent duct or solid cord of tissue connecting the terminal ileum to the umbilicus. Alternatively, when the bowel end resorbs completely but the distal end persists, an umbilical cyst or sinus tract may result. However, when the distal end resorbs leaving a portion of the duct attached to the distal small bowel, the result is an MD. This is a true diverticulum composed of all three layers of the bowel wall (mucosa, submucosa, and muscle), and arises from the antimesenteric surface of the small bowel. In adults, the MD is typically located 80 to 120 cm proximal to the ileocecal valve, but in infants and small children it will be much closer.

MDs are present in 1% to 3% of the population and, although equal in frequency in males and females, are more likely to become symptomatic in males. Complications occur in 4% to 8% of patients with an MD and present in one of three ways: infection, obstruction, or bleeding. The majority of complications occur before the age of 10 years. Bleeding is the most common complication followed by obstruction and infection. An unusual presentation of MD is when it is found in an inguinal hernia sack (Littre hernia).

INFECTION

Signs and Symptoms

As a bowel diverticulum similar to the appendix, an MD can present as an infected diverticulitis. The presenting symptoms may be identical to those seen with acute appendicitis, although the localizing pain may be in a somewhat atypical location. Fever, anorexia, and abdominal pain that becomes localized are typical. In severe Meckel's diverticulitis, perforation and peritonitis may develop.

Workup

Ultrasound may be useful, but the findings of a tubular structure with features of acute inflammation may be difficult to distinguish from acute appendicitis. Many are only identified at the time of surgery for presumed acute appendicitis. Conversely, a surgeon should inspect the terminal ileum if the history and physical exam suggests appendicitis but the appendix appears normal at the time of laparotomy (or laparoscopy).

Treatment

Treatment for an infected MD is resection, often accomplished by simple transection at the base of the diverticulum using a surgical stapling device. Laparoscopic staplers allow a minimally invasive approach for patients with infection localized to the tip of the diverticulum leaving a suitable base for excision. If inflammation or perforation near the base of the diverticulum prevents safe diverticulectomy, a segmental bowel resection with primary anastomosis is the preferred treatment. Recovery is similar to complicated appendicitis.

OBSTRUCTION

An MD can also present with intestinal obstruction. A persistent omphalomesenteric cord extending from the bowel wall to the umbilicus can provide a pivot point for a segmental small-bowel volvulus. More commonly, the diverticulum serves as a pathologic lead point for an ileoileal intussusception, often becoming ileocolic (see Chapter 126C).

Signs and Symptoms

Patients typically present with cramping abdominal pain, and may have dark bloody stools if the intussusception has been long-standing. A pathologic lead-point such as an MD should be suspected in any child presenting with intussusception outside the typical 3-month to 3-year age range for idiopathic intussusception, or in any patient with recurrent intussusception.

Workup

A contrast enema may make the diagnosis but is not likely to be therapeutic. The diagnosis may also be missed if the intussusception is limited to the small bowel. In many centers, ultrasound has become the diagnostic test of choice. It is painless, noninvasive, and can accurately identify an intussusception regardless of which segment of bowel is involved. As with any other ultrasound examination, the test is somewhat dependent on the experience of the radiologist performing the study.

Treatment

The treatment is based on the condition of the bowel at the time of surgery. If the intussusception cannot be reduced or the viability of the bowel is questioned, a segmental bowel resection with primary anastomosis is appropriate. A simple diverticulectomy is less likely to be technically feasible but can be considered if the anatomy is amenable to this approach.

BLEEDING

The most common complication of a Meckel's diverticulum is bleeding. It accounts for approximately two-thirds of the cases of small bowel bleeding in men under the age of 30, and is one of the most common causes of significant gastrointestinal bleeding from any site in children.

Signs and Symptoms

Classically patients present with significant painless rectal bleeding. The bleeding episodes are usually self-limited but recurrent, often resulting in a transfusion requirement. The bleeding caused by an MD is a manifestation of the presence of ectopic gastric mucosa within the diverticulum. The gastric mucosa secretes acid that causes peptic ulceration either within the MD or in the adjacent small bowel. In severe cases, perforation of the ileum may occur. Ectopic pancreatic tissue is also frequently found within an MD but is not associated with bleeding complications.

Workup

Diagnosing an MD as the source of gastrointestinal bleeding can be quite difficult. It is not uncommon for patients to undergo extensive workups with multiple endoscopic procedures, bleeding scans, and even arteriograms in an effort to identify the source of blood loss. However, in young patients with a history of significant painless rectal bleeding, MD should be high on the differential diagnosis and the workup should be directed toward confirming that diagnosis.

The most specific study for making the diagnosis is the "Meckel's scan," a nuclear medicine study employing radiolabeled 99-technetium pertechnetate. The label is preferentially taken up in the ectopic gastric mucosa, and the accumulation of radioisotope is visible on the gamma camera image. The sensitivity has been reported to range from 50% to 92%. Pretreating patients with histamine type-2 receptor antagonists increases the sensitivity of the study by mechanisms that are not clearly defined. One study has suggested that a false-negative rate of almost 40% could be decreased to about 12% after pretreatment with ranitidine for 24 hours prior to study. It is also important to obtain lateral scan views of the abdomen in order not to miss a Meckel's diverticulum in the pelvis, sometimes obscured by the accumulation of isotope in the bladder. However, even with these modifications, the test still has a significant false-negative rate. Hence a negative Meckel's scan should be followed by a more complete workup to rule out alternative causes.

Colonoscopy and upper endoscopy are most helpful in identifying or ruling out other causes for the bleeding. Capsule endoscopy has also been used to identify small-bowel bleeding sites and may demonstrate an MD. However, the patient must be large enough and old enough to swallow the capsule, limiting its usefulness. In patients with painless gastrointestinal bleeding, a negative evaluation, and history, laboratory studies, and physical exam consistent with the diagnosis of MD, a diagnostic laparoscopy may be indicated.

Treatment

As with the intussuscepted and infected MDs, the treatment is resection. This is usually accomplished laparoscopically with an endoscopic stapling device if possible. If not, once the MD is identified with the laparoscope, it can be brought out through a small laparotomy incision and the diverticulum resected using open techniques. It is also important to consider that if a bleeding ulcer is present, it typically occurs adjacent to the ectopic gastric tissue and thus may be in the small bowel rather than the diverticulum itself. A segmental ileal resection including the diverticulum is a more definitive method of treating both the inciting ectopic tissue and the actual bleeding site. Regardless of which technique is used, the patients typically recover quickly and can be discharged from the hospital as soon as they are tolerating a diet.

ASYMPTOMATIC MECKEL'S DIVERTICULUM

A surgeon confronted with an asymptomatic MD during a laparotomy for another indication must decide whether or not to resect the diverticulum. The decision hinges on the risk of that patient developing a complication from the MD versus the risk of resection. The answer to that question is not clear-cut, hence a range of different approaches have been described including universal resection, universal observation, and resection of only those lesions with palpable ectopic mucosa. The complication rate for resection of an MD is estimated to be as high as 5% to 10%, underscoring the fact that there is a small but real risk to resecting an asymptomatic lesion. Conversely, the complications from an MD left in place are potentially life threatening. Several authors have proposed criteria to assist in the decision at the time of surgery based on the size of the MD or the age of the patient. Patients with longer MDs are more likely to develop complications, as are patients less than 8 years of age, but these criteria are rarely applied.

PEARLS

- An asymptomatic Meckel's diverticulum is much more common than a symptomatic one. Appropriate intervention for the incidental (asymptomatic) Meckel's diverticulum is poorly defined
- Symptomatic presentation of a Meckel's diverticulum is usually one of three clinical scenarios
  - Painless gastrointestinal bleeding (most common)
  - Inflammation and infection
  - Obstruction (volvulus or intussusception)
- Massive painless bleeding in a small child, requiring blood transfusion, is often due to a Meckel's diverticulum
- Atypical appendicitis (often localized tenderness at some site other than the right lower quadrant) may be the initial presentation of a Meckel's diverticulum

Suggested Readings

Baldisserotto M, Maffazzoni DR, Dora MD. Sonographic findings of Meckel's diverticulitis in children. *AJR Am J Roentgenol* 2003;180:425–428.

Onen A, Cigdem MK, Ozturk H, et al. When to resect and when not to resect an asymptomatic Meckel's diverticulum: an ongoing challenge. *Pediatr Surg Int* 2003;19:57–61.

Rerksuppaphol S, Hutson JM, Oliver MR. Ranitidine-enhanced 99m-technetium pertechnetate imaging in children improves the sensitivity of identifying heterotopic gastric mucosa in Meckel's diverticulum. *Pediatr Surg Int* 2004; 20:323–325.

Schmittenbecher P. Ranitidine-enhanced 99m-technetium pertechnetate imaging in children improves the sensitivity of identifying heterotopic gastric mucosa in Meckel's diverticulum. *J Pediatr Surg* 2005;40:892.

Shalaby RY, Soliman SM, Fawy M, et al. Laparoscopic management of Meckel's diverticulum in children. *J Pediatr Surg* 2005;40:562–567.

Yau KK, Siu WT, Law BK, et al. Laparoscopy-assisted surgical management of obscure gastrointestinal bleeding secondary to Meckel's diverticulum in a pediatric patient: case report and review of literature. *Surg Laparosc Endosc Percutan Tech* 2005;15:374–377.

CHAPTER 126G ■ SURGICAL EMERGENCIES: TESTICULAR TORSION

WILLIAM T. ADAMSON

A boy who complains of sudden pain in the scrotum demands urgent attention. Testicular torsion must be considered. Scrotal pain is particularly worrisome if it is accompanied by swelling, tenderness, or erythema. The consequences of testicular torsion, including loss of the testicle and risk of infertility, can be devastating. Rapid diagnosis of testicular torsion can usually be made by clinical evaluation by a urologist or surgeon. Diagnostic ultrasound can be a fast, reliable means of diagnosis in many cases. Urgent surgery to restore blood flow to the testicle within 3 hours is usually successful, while delay in surgery more than 6 hours is associated with a dramatic decrease in testicular salvage(1). Although there are other more common diagnoses presenting as an acute scrotum, ruling out testicular torsion remains the burden of the primary or emergency pediatric caregiver. Testicular torsion and its complications is one of the four most common reasons for lawsuits involving the children's emergency room (2).

PRESENTATION

Testicular torsion is relatively uncommon, occurring in 4 to 8 per 100,000 males (3). Testicular torsion usually presents prior to age 3 years or around the time of onset of puberty. It is rare after age 25 years. Not infrequently, a child will present with a history of previous pain attacks or trauma (4). Intermittent torsion should be suspected in recurrent sudden attacks of scrotal pain that resolve quickly. As many as 50% of boys with acute testicular torsion have had a prior episode of testicular pain (5). Even if the pain has resolved at the time of evaluation, the caregiver should suspect intermittent torsion and consider ultrasonographic evaluation.

Clinical diagnosis of testicular torsion can be made based on the sudden onset of scrotal or lower abdominal pain. Nausea or vomiting frequently accompanies the pain. Pain can occur during activity or can wake the boy from sleep. Boys report a sickening feeling similar to being hit in the testis. These symptoms can be vague and difficult to localize in a toddler. As a result, younger boys with testicular torsion frequently present with a testicle that is beyond salvage.

DIAGNOSIS

On exam, the torsed testicle is retracted or elevated in the scrotum. It frequently lies transversely or horizontally in the upper scrotum with a lack of the cremasteric reflex on that side. Tenderness is usually diffuse throughout that side of the scrotum. The scrotum can be erythematous and swollen. If the testicle is compromised, the mass may appear dark or purplish through the scrotal skin. When the exam strongly suggests testicular torsion, the patient should be referred for surgical evaluation without delay.

If the clinical diagnosis is unclear, urgent radiologic evaluation with ultrasound can be helpful. Diagnostic ultrasound can evaluate perfusion of the testis and can also identify swelling of the tunica and thickening of the scrotum. Abnormal findings may suggest a diagnosis of testicular torsion and a need for surgical exploration. In many cases of testicular torsion, twisting of the spermatic cord can be identified. An untwisted spermatic cord effectively rules out torsion (6). Sensitivity of ultrasound for testicular torsion is 60% to 70%, while specificity approaches 100% (7). Ultrasound is adequate to evaluate the testis in most cases (8). Magnetic resonance imaging may have a higher sensitivity for testicular torsion than ultrasound (9), but the time necessary to obtain an MRI may compromise its clinical usefulness to rule out testicular torsion expeditiously. Many authors caution that ultrasound should not be solely relied on to exclude the diagnosis of testicular torsion. If torsion is suspected, surgical evaluation should not be delayed.

PATHOPHYSIOLOGY

The pathophysiology of testicular torsion has been suggested for many years to result from abnormal attachments of the testicle to the wall of the scrotum (10). The testicle is formed by the 6th week of gestation, but does not generally descend from an abdominal position to the opening of the inguinal canal until the 28th week. The processus vaginalis, the outpouching of the peritoneum at the internal inguinal ring, is formed by the 8th week of pregnancy and extends into the scrotum, creating the inguinal canal. The testicle and most but not all of the epididymis are invested within a sac of the outpouching peritoneum, the tunica vaginalis. As the testicle and epididymis drop through the inguinal canal within this peritoneum, the tail of the epididymis and trailing spermatic cord, which are not invested in the peritoneal sac around the testicle, become attached to the scrotal wall. These attachments are secure enough to fix the testicle in position and keep it from twisting.

If the entire epididymis and spermatic cord are free within the peritoneal sac that surrounds the testicle, there are no attachments to keep the testicle from twisting on itself. This arrangement is called the "bell-clapper" deformity and is present in 12% of men (10). This bell-clapper deformity is thought to predispose the testicle to torsion. No data suggest that the attachments of the epididymis to the scrotum mature as the child grows older; thus the risk of torsion of the bell-clapper testicle does not improve with time.

MANAGEMENT: SURGICAL EXPLORATION

Once a diagnosis of testicular torsion is suspected and cannot be ruled out, immediate surgical exploration is necessary to attempt salvage of the testicle. Physical manipulations of the testicle cannot reliably untwist the testicle; surgery is necessary to reestablish blood flow to the testicle. Even if presentation is late, surgery is indicated to remove the nonviable testicle and to perform orchiopexy on the contralateral side.

Open exploration through a scrotal incision is the most common surgical approach. The testicle is assessed for viability. Orchiectomy is performed for a nonviable testis. If the testis appears viable, it is untwisted and an orchiopexy is performed.

Many different variations on orchiopexy have been reported, most of which involve fixation of the testicle to the scrotal wall. Sutures are used to secure the tunica albuginea to the lateral wall of the scrotum, the medial septum, or to the dartos muscle in a subcutaneous pouch. Orchiopexy prevents recurrence in most boys. Yet even with direct suture of the tunica albuginea to the scrotal wall, recurrent torsion may occur with any of these techniques (11).

Testicular salvage rates as high as 80% after exploration are reported. Unfortunately, despite apparent early salvage, the reperfused testis may atrophy over time. Development of late atrophy likely depends upon the duration of ischemia during torsion. Even if the duration of torsion appears to be well beyond the limits of viability for the testicle, urgent exploration is indicated. Testicular salvage of a small percentage of patients who present many hours after the onset of pain is often explained as partial or intermittent torsion.

If the testicle is not viable, removal of the testicle is advocated. The presence of a dead testicle results in an increased risk of infertility, presumably through an inflammatory reaction to the nonviable testis that activates an immune response against the remaining testicle. Stimulation of apoptosis of the seminiferous epithelium of the contralateral testicle has also been suggested to result from stimulation of pro-apoptotic enzymes called caspases (12). Even with prompt removal of the torsed testis, fertility is decreased in patients with testicular torsion. Release of damaging reactive oxygen radicals increases with ischemia time and may play a role in ischemia--reperfusion injury and the consequent oxidative insult to the contralateral testis (13).

Urologists and pediatric surgeons advocate exploration and orchiopexy of the normal testis on the unaffected side to prevent torsion of the remaining testicle. Exploration of both sides at the time of the initial operation can be performed through a midline scrotal raphe incision or through bilateral, symmetric scrotal incisions. If the contralateral testis is undescended, laparoscopy to identify the other testis and subsequent orchiopexy may be appropriate.

DIFFERENTIAL DIAGNOSIS

A boy with pain, swelling, and redness of the scrotum has testicular torsion until proven otherwise. Imaging studies such as ultrasound for a patient with an acute scrotum can be very helpful in identifying other diagnoses in the differential of testicular torsion such as torsion of the appendix testis, epididymitis, and testicular tumors. The duration of symptoms and age of the patient are important historical data that may suggest a diagnosis other than testicular torsion.

Torsion of the Appendix Testis

The appendix testis is a relatively small structure that is frequently found at the top of the normal testis adjacent to the epididymis. It is a vestige of the Müllerian duct and is normally only a few millimeters in size. The appendix testis may enlarge in response to estrogen and testosterone. Thus stimulated, the swollen appendix testis may have an increased tendency to twist on its narrow pedicle. A peak incidence of torsion of the appendix testis is seen in 7- to 10-year-old boys, perhaps in response to rising prepubertal hormone levels (14).

Torsion of the appendix testis presents as a tender, painful "blue dot" seen through the scrotal skin. Pain is often localized to this area in the upper scrotum, in contrast to the pain of testicular torsion, which involves the entire testicle. Ultrasound is effective in confirming a clinical diagnosis of torsion of the appendix testis (4). When the diagnosis of torsion of the appendix testis is clear, most urologists will treat this condition with nonsteroidal analgesics. A few authors recommend exploration for torsion of the appendix testis, but most agree that exploration is usually not necessary for torsion of the appendix testis, as long as *testicular* torsion can be ruled out.

Epididymitis

Ten to fifteen percent of patients who present with acute pain, swelling, and erythema of the scrotum will have epididymitis. Inflammation of the epididymis is frequently found at exploration for a presumed diagnosis of testicular torsion. Onset of epididymitis is often more gradual than testicular torsion and is more likely associated with urinary symptoms. It can be associated with urinary anomalies; therefore, urinalysis and urinary culture should be obtained if epididymitis is suspected.

Scrotal ultrasound is very accurate in confirming a diagnosis of epididymitis. Ultrasound or other imaging modalities may also be helpful in evaluating for other anatomic anomalies of the urogenital system that may be associated with epididymitis (15). Treatment is supportive and nonsurgical.

Testicular Tumors

Testicular tumors are often discovered during evaluation of the acute scrotum. Although tumors are usually painless, any mass in the scrotum demands further workup. Ultrasound is the initial imaging modality. Approximately 15% of tumors are identified during an ultrasound obtained for suspected testicular torsion (16). With an incidence of a little more than 1 per 100,000, tumors of the testicle are less common than testicular torsion (3). Intraoperative handling of the testicle is markedly different during resection of a testicular tumor than in exploration for testicular torsion. Suspected tumors are approached through a groin incision, so that control of the blood supply to the mass can be secured prior to manipulation of the tumor. Suspicion of a tumor, therefore, is an important element in formulating the operative plan for exploration of the acute scrotum.

OTHER TYPES OF TESTICULAR TORSION

Perinatal Testicular Torsion

Occasionally, newborn boys will present with a large, firm, painless mass in the scrotum. This finding should prompt an emergent ultrasound to evaluate the testicles for the possibility of perinatal torsion. Ultrasound findings of unequal testicular volume, tunica swelling, and scrotal thickening suggest a diagnosis of perinatal torsion and prompt emergent scrotal exploration.

Usually, the testicle has undergone complete torsion in utero and is not viable. As there is an increased risk of tumor in the case of a painless mass, exploration is frequently performed through a groin incision. Perinatal torsion of the testicle is thought to be a twist of the spermatic cord outside of the tunica vaginalis, which is a more proximal level than that of torsion of the testicle in an older boy. The entire cord can be exposed and evaluated through a scrotal incision.

Some authors advocate contralateral exploration and orchiopexy in perinatal torsion as well. One study has documented a 22% incidence of contralateral torsion of the supposedly normal testis in cases of perinatal torsion (17). Evidence of testicular atrophy of the asymptomatic side is also a common finding in perinatal torsion.

Torsion of the Undescended Testis

Torsion of an undescended, cryptorchid testis is rarely reported. Clinical signs and symptoms of torsion are difficult to identify in a testicle that remains within the peritoneal cavity. Scrotal findings are absent. Torsion of the left undescended testicle is more common than of the right. When intra-abdominal testes are found to be torsed, approximately 60% are associated with testicular tumors (18). Orchiopexy for salvage of a potentially viable cryptorchid testis has a poor outcome. These poor results support prophylactic laparoscopic or open exploration of an undescended contralateral testis during exploration of a torsed testicle.

CONCLUSIONS

The primary or emergency room caregiver must have a high index of suspicion for the diagnosis of testicular torsion. The boy presenting suddenly with pain in the scrotum should be referred early for surgical evaluation. Ultrasound of the scrotum can confirm suspicion of testicular torsion and rule out other causes of the acute scrotum. Results of testicular salvage at the time of surgical exploration are quite good overall. Parents should be counseled that salvage rates, while relatively high, depend upon the duration of time from onset of symptoms to surgical correction. Even with appropriate early surgical management, recurrence of torsion and impact on fertility cannot be completely mitigated.

References

1. King PA, Sripathi V. The acute scrotum. In: Ashcraft KW, Holcomb GW, III, Murphy JP, eds. *Pediatric surgery* 4th ed. Philadelphia: Saunders; 2005: 717–721.

2. Selbst SM, Friedman MJ, Singh SB. Epidemiology and etiology of malpractice lawsuits involving children in U.S. emergency departments and urgent care centers. *Pediatr Emerg Care* 2005;21:165–169.

3. Mansbach JM, Forbes P, Peters C. Testicular torsion and risk factors for orchiectomy. *Arch Pediatr Adolesc Med* 2005;159:1167–1171.

4. Ciftci AO, Senocak ME, Tanyel FC, et al. Clinical predictors for differential diagnosis of acute scrotum. *Eur J Pediatr Surg* 2004;14:333–338.

5. Eaton SH, Cendron MA, Estrada CR, et al. Intermittent testicular torsion: diagnostic features and management outcomes. *J Urol* 2005;174:1532–1535; discussion 1535.

6. Kalfa N, Veyrac C, Baud C, et al. Ultrasonography of the spermatic cord in children with testicular torsion: impact on the surgical strategy. *J Urol* 2004;172:1692–1695; discussion 1695.

7. Karmazyn B, Steinberg R, Kornreich L, et al. Clinical and sonographic criteria of acute scrotum in children: a retrospective study of 172 boys. *Pediatr Radiol* 2005;35:302–310.

8. Dogra V, Bhatt S. Acute painful scrotum. *Radiol Clin North Am* 2004;42: 349–363.

9. Terai A, Yoshimura K, Ichioka K, et al. Dynamic contrast-enhanced subtraction magnetic resonance imaging in diagnostics of testicular torsion. *Urology* 2006;67:1278–1282.

10. Caesar RE, Kaplan GW. Incidence of the bell-clapper deformity in an autopsy series. *Urology* 1994;44:114–116.

11. Mor Y, Pinthus JH, Nadu A, et al. Testicular fixation following torsion of the spermatic cord—does it guarantee prevention of recurrent torsion events? *J Urol* 2006;175:171–173; discussion 173–174.

12. Said TM, Paasch U, Glander HJ, et al. Role of caspases in male infertility. *Hum Reprod Update* 2004;10:39–51.

13 Filho DW, Torres MA, Bordin AL, et al. Spermatic cord torsion, reactive oxygen and nitrogen species and ischemia-reperfusion injury. *Mol Aspects Med* 2004;25:199–210.

14. Samnakay N, Cohen RJ, Orford J, et al. Androgen and oestrogen receptor status of the human appendix testis. *Pediatr Surg Int* 2003;19:520–524.

15 Haecker FM, Hauri-Hohl A, von Schweinitz D. Acute epididymitis in children: a 4-year retrospective study. *Eur J Pediatr Surg* 2005;15:180–186.

16. Wittenberg AF, Tobias T, Rzeszotarski M, et al. Sonography of the acute scrotum: the four T's of testicular imaging. *Curr Probl Diagn Radiol* 2006;35:12–21.

17. Yerkes EB, Robertson FM, Gitlin J, et al. Management of perinatal torsion: today, tomorrow or never? *J Urol* 2005;174:1579–1582; discussion 1582–1583.

18. Zilberman D, Inbar Y, Heyman Z, et al. Torsion of the cryptorchid testis—can it be salvaged? *J Urol* 2006;175:2287–2289; discussion 2289.

CHAPTER 127A ■ TRAUMATIC INJURIES: MINOR CLOSED HEAD INJURY

PATRICIA A. LANGE

Nearly 500,000 children sustain traumatic brain injury per year in the United States, with 95,000 hospital admissions, 7,000 deaths and 29,000 children with permanent disabilities. Most children have minor closed head injuries (CHIs), but even these can be associated with intracranial injuries. The goal of the treating physician should be recognizing deterioration, preventing secondary injuries, and avoiding unnecessary imaging studies.

Motor vehicle collisions and falls make up the majority of head injuries in children. Other mechanisms include nonaccidental trauma, violence, and penetrating wounds in older children and adolescents. Compared to adults, children are more prone to injuries to the head because of the disproportionately large head compared to the remainder of the body. Child abuse may account for up to 25% of closed head injuries in children less than 2 years of age. The severity of the mechanism does not always correlate with the severity of the injury, thus necessitating a high index of suspicion in all children with trauma to the head. The definition of minor traumatic brain injury is generally considered an injury caused by blunt acceleration/deceleration forces that may cause brief loss of consciousness (less than 20 minutes), Glasgow Coma Scale score of 13 to 15, no focal neurologic deficit, and normal computed tomography (CT) scan findings. Definitions of other types of intracranial injuries are listed below.

GLOSSARY OF SPECIFIC TYPES OF INJURIES

A *scalp hematoma* is a collection of blood under the skin. The scalp is highly vascularized, and a large volume of blood can be lost from lacerations or hematomas to the scalp due to trauma. Often urgent stapling of a laceration in the emergency room is required to achieve hemostasis.

Concussions result from the brain shifting within the confined space of the skull cavity. A concussion may cause a brief depressed level of responsiveness or actual loss of consciousness. Often patients have headaches, nausea, vomiting, and/or dizziness following a significant blow to the head. Most concussions do not lead to any long-term deficits but on some occasions, memory and cognitive deficits can persist.

A *skull fracture* (Fig. 127.1) may be isolated or associated with underlying parenchymal injury. Temporal and parietal regions have thinner bones and are more prone to fractures. Similarly, the skull base is prone to injury due to the many foramina. Fractures are classified as open or closed. Open fractures are associated with lacerations or breaks in the skin. Depressed skull fractures are those in which a fragment of bone protrudes into the cranium. Most fractures do not require any surgical intervention but significantly depressed fragments may need elevation by the neurosurgical team.

A *subdural hematoma (SDH)* is a collection of blood underneath the lining of the brain but external to the brain parenchyma. Subdural hematomas typically form when bridging veins are torn. Patients often lose consciousness when there is a significant-enough trauma to the head to cause a SDH. The mortality for SDH ranges from 20% to 50%. Interhemispheric SDHs are sometimes associated with child abuse.

An *epidural hematoma (EDH)* occurs when there is an accumulation of blood between the dura and the skull. Epidural hematomas are usually seen in the temporoparietal region, where a traumatic blow causes injury to the middle meningeal artery. Most EDHs are associated with a skull fracture. Patients who are found to have an EDH often present with loss of consciousness and impaired Glasgow Coma Scale. Some patients may have a lucid interval from the time of the traumatic event until they begin to have neurologic deterioration. Mortality ranges from 3% to 43% and may be higher in children less than 5 years of age.

Subarachnoid hemorrhage (SAH) (Fig. 127.2) is bleeding beneath the innermost lining of the brain in the space that typically contains the cerebrospinal fluid. Patients with SAH may have loss of consciousness, seizures, associated fractures, and signs of increased intracranial pressure.

Diffuse axonal injury (DAI) results from shearing forces transmitted to the brain during a deceleration injury. Injury to the nerves leads to edema (Fig 127.3) and leakage of fluid from the axons. Mortality for patients with DAI is relatively low, but morbidity is very high, often leaving patients in a persistent vegetative state. Noncontrasted head CT scans may appear normal in patients with DAI. The recommended study to further evaluate for this type of injury is a brain MRI.

Seizures may be seen in approximately 10% of patients sustaining trauma to the head, the majority of which are self-limited. Seizures can increase the intracranial pressure therefore prompt and effective medical management is needed.

INITIAL MANAGEMENT OF CLOSED HEAD INJURIES

As in any trauma, the initial assessment begins with the ABCs (airway, breathing and circulation). These constitute the primary survey. The spine should be stabilized in the field with use of a backboard and cervical collar, and should be maintained until cleared by clinical examination and/or radiographic studies. The fit of the cervical collar should be carefully inspected and adjusted as needed, as these are often not sized

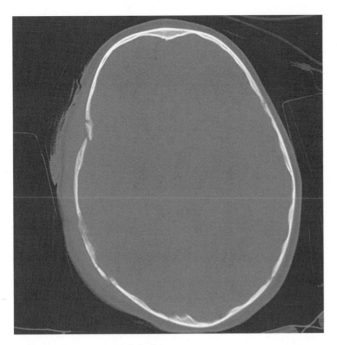

FIGURE 127.1. Temporal skull fracture.

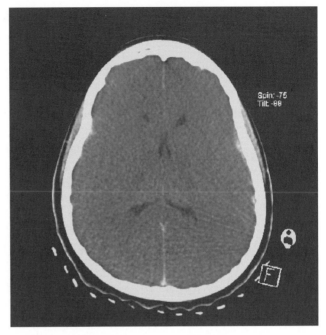

FIGURE 127.3. Edema from diffuse axonal injury (DAI).

correctly in young children. Maintaining oxygenation is the first priority, and thus assessing and assuring an adequate airway takes precedence over all other parts of the exam. The need for intubation and mechanical ventilation due to depressed mental status may indicate a more serious head injury.

Next, the lungs should be ausculted to assess for equality of breath sounds and signs of pulmonary contusion. Nasal flaring or use of accessory muscles in children indicates respiratory distress, and etiology should be determined. One of the best ways to assess for adequacy of circulation is to check for capillary refill on the toes or fingers. A refill time greater than

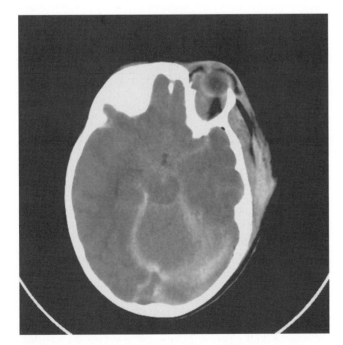

FIGURE 127.2. Subarachnoid hemorrhage (SAH).

2 seconds is generally thought of as delayed and indicates diminished perfusion.

The secondary survey consists of a head-to-toe examination for associated injuries. The head exam includes careful inspection of the scalp, especially in areas hard to visualize like the occiput and the area under the cervical collar. Scalp lacerations can bleed profusely and need prompt attention. Direct pressure on the wound is the first step in controlling the bleeding. Sutures or staples can then be used to repair the wound and obtain hemostasis. The skull should be palpated for fractured edges or depressed fractures. The pupils should be carefully inspected for reactivity to light and should have equal responsiveness. Pupil asymmetry is often an early sign of increased intracranial pressure. Battle's sign or periorbital ecchymosis should alert the examiner to possible basilar skull fracture. The midface and jaw should also be carefully palpated for signs of fracture or instability. The remainder of the secondary survey is completed after the head exam—please see Chapter 127B for specifics about the secondary survey.

The exam should now focus on determining the Glasgow Coma Scale (GCS) score. This score allows for some prognostic information and gives practitioners a reliable way to relay information. The values have been modified for children (Table 127.1). A score of less than 8 is considered a coma and usually necessitates airway protection with endotracheal intubation. The goal of initial management should be to stabilize the patient as quickly as possible and proceed to head CT scan within the first 30 to 45 minutes.

IMAGING FOR MINOR CLOSED HEAD INJURIES

Skull Radiographs

In the era of CT scanning, plain x-rays of the skull are now rarely used. Skull x-rays may show fractures but they cannot give any information about intracranial injuries. Intracranial injuries may be more common in the presence of skull fractures,

TABLE 127.1

GLASGOW COMA SCALE FOR CHILDREN

EYE OPENING

Spontaneous	4
To voice	3
To pain	2
None	1

VERBAL RESPONSE

Verbal Patient		**Nonverbal**
Oriented	5	Appropriate words, smiles, coos
Confused	4	Inappropriate words, cries, consolable
Inappropriate words	3	Persistent cries and screams
Incomprehensible sounds	2	Grunts, agitated, restless
None	1	None

MOTOR RESPONSE

Obeys commands	6
Localizes pain	5
Withdraws (pain)	4
Flexion (pain)	3
Extension (pain)	2
None	1

but not all fractures indicate an underlying intracranial lesion. The specificity for showing intracranial injuries with the use of skull radiographs has been reported to be about 53% to 97%. Given these numbers, the majority of patients with minor head trauma would have x-rays read as abnormal when in fact they have no intracranial injury. The sensitivity of skull x-rays is also low, meaning that some patients would have x-rays read as normal even though they do have an intracranial injury. The Pediatrics Subcommittee American Academy of Pediatrics Committee on quality improvement consensus is that skull radiographs have only a limited role in management of a child with brief loss of consciousness. CT scanning is the study of choice if available and the practitioner believes that imaging is indicated. CT scans have a much greater sensitivity and specificity as compared to plain skull radiographs.

CT

The use of CT scans in children with minor head injuries and no loss of consciousness is not typically indicated; however, there are children who later develop signs of intracranial injury necessitating imaging. Children with intracranial injuries after minor head injury are not easily clinically distinguishable from those children without intracranial injuries. Some children may present with headaches, vomiting, or lethargy, and these may be signs of intracranial injury, although the majority of children with these symptoms do not have any intracranial anomalies. No data exist that demonstrates improved outcome in children who undergo early CT scan after minor head trauma with brief loss of consciousness compared to children who are closely observed. CT scanning is generally safe with low risks; however, in small children sedation is often required, and this may add to complications. Additionally, routine CT scanning may demonstrate incidental anomalies that lead to unnecessary surgery or treatment. Cost of medical care must also be evaluated with any treatment regimen. Added costs that provide no additional diagnostic or therapeutic benefit will be poorly tolerated.

MRI

MRI imaging provides additional information regarding cerebral injuries but is more time consuming, less sensitive for detecting intracranial hemorrhage, and usually more costly compared to CT scan. The committee consensus is that CT offers more advantages over MRI in evaluating acute intracranial injuries in children.

The American Academy of Pediatrics has developed practice parameters for the management of children with minor closed head injuries. This management guideline is for children from age 2 years to 20 years and defines minor closed head injury as "normal mental status at the initial evaluation, no abnormal or focal findings on neurologic examination and no physical evidence of skull fracture (such as hemotympanum, Battle's sign or palpable bone depression)." (See reference for American Academy of Pediatrics.)

MANAGEMENT BY CATEGORY

1. *Evaluation and management of child with minor closed head injury and NO loss of consciousness*
   a. Observation in clinic, office, ER or at home under competent caregiver.
   b. Observation implies regular monitoring by adult who would be able to recognize neurologic abnormalities and seek appropriate assistance.
   c. Use of CT and MRI not recommended for initial evaluation.
   d. Fewer than 1 in 5,000 patients with minor CHIs and no LOC have intracranial injuries that require medical or neurosurgical intervention.
   e. In two smaller studies of children with minor CHI and no LOC, amnesia, vomiting, headache, or mental status abnormalities, no children had abnormal CT scan findings.

2. *Evaluation and management of child with minor closed head injury and BRIEF loss of consciousness*
   a. Loss of consciousness <1 minute, the child may be carefully observed in the office, clinic, ER, hospital, or home under care of a competent caregiver.
   b. Head CT may be used in addition to observation.
   c. Use of skull x-rays or MRI in the initial management of children with minor closed head injuries and brief loss of

consciousness is not recommended. There are limited situations in which these are options.
   d. No known evidence suggests that immediate neuroimaging study improves outcomes in children with minor closed head injuries compared to children managed primarily by examination and observation.

3. *Management of ASYMPTOMATIC patients with intracranial hemorrhage*
   a. Surgery is not always indicated for intracranial hemorrhage, and usually close observation is the management of choice.
   b. Factors to consider include size of bleed, shift of parenchymal structures, and patient clinical status.

Generally, neurology and/or neuosurgery teams are consulted to help in the management decision.

DISPOSITION

The majority of children with minor closed head injuries and normal neurologic exam are at very low risk for having subsequent deterioration in their condition, and therefore observation in an appropriate setting is recommended. Most life-threatening complications occur in the first 24 hours after injury, so some advocate observation during this period in a hospital setting. The setting for the observation period must take several factors into consideration. The time it would take the family to bring the patient to a medical facility, the ability of the caretaker to appropriately observe the child and recognize deterioration in clinical status, or other caretaker and/or patient concerns may dictate where the child resides during the observation period. The caretakers should be adequately assessed as to their ability to understand instructions, provide transportation if needed, and recognize worrisome symptoms before releasing the child. The health care providers must provide the caretakers with written and verbal instructions of how to carefully observe the child and which symptoms necessitate prompt medical attention.

If the child underwent CT scan evaluation after minor head trauma and the CT scan and neurologic exam remain normal, the likelihood of subsequent problems is extremely low. The child should still be observed carefully for 24 to 48 hours, as there are rare reports in children who do not undergo CT imaging of delayed intracranial bleeding after an initial stable period.

OUTCOMES

The majority of children who sustain minor head injuries recover completely within 1 month and have no long-term neurologic sequelae. However, approximately 10% to 20% of children with minor to moderate head injuries have memory problems. In addition, almost half of patients with minor head trauma experience postconcussive symptoms (headache, dizziness, and memory problems). Those patients who continue to have any of these symptoms beyond 3 months should undergo neuropsychological testing. This would allow for identification of potential deficits that may be improved with the assistance of rehabilitation specialists.

Suggested Readings

Adams J, Frumiento C, Shutney-Leach L, et al. Mandatory admission after isolated mild closed head injury in children: is it necessary? *J Ped Surg* 2001;36:119–121.
Cacey RG Jr, Alves WM, Rimel RW, et al. Neurosurgical complications after apparently minor head injury. Assessment of risk in a series of 610 patients. *J Neurosurg* 1986;65:203–210.
Committee on Quality Improvement, American Academy of Pediatrics. The management of minor closed head injury in children. *Pediatrics* 1999;104:1407–1415.
Cushman JG, Agarwal N, Fabian TC, et al. Minor closed head injuries. *East Guidelines on Trauma.*www.east.org
Mattei P, ed. *Surgical directives: pediatric surgery*. Philadelphia: Lippincott Williams & Wilkins; 2003.
O'Neil JA, Rowe MI, Grosfeld JL, et al. *Pediatric surgery*. 5th ed. St. Louis: Mosby; 1998 321–330.
Schutzman SA, Greenes DS. Pediatric minor head trauma. *Ann Emerg Med* 2001;37:65–74.
Spencer MT, Baron BJ, Sinert R, et al. Necessity of hospital admission for pediatric minor head injury. *Am J Emerg Med* 2003;21:111–114.

CHAPTER 127B ■ TRAUMATIC INJURIES: BLUNT ABDOMINAL TRAUMA

PATRICIA A. LANGE

Trauma is the leading cause of death and morbidity in children and accounts for approximately 20,000 deaths per year in the United States. The abdomen is a common site for injury, which is most often due to blunt forces from motor vehicle collisions, falls, sports-related injuries, and nonaccidental trauma. Abdominal injuries are the third most common site of injury due to blunt trauma. The majority (~95%) of abdominal injuries can be treated without surgery; however, signs and symptoms of intra-abdominal injuries may be subtle and therefore require an astute clinician to recognize them. The abdomen is the most common site of unrecognized fatal injury in children involved in trauma. Radiographic imaging has markedly improved over the last few decades and greatly aides in evaluation of intra-abdominal trauma.

The abdominal cavity in children differs from the adult abdomen in several ways, making it more susceptible to blunt forces. The shape of the child's abdomen is more square and the organs are relatively larger than in the older child or adult. The musculature of the abdominal wall is thinner, and there is less fat surrounding the solid organs. Ribs are more flexible in children, which means that a significant force exerted on them may be transmitted to the underlying organs, especially the upper abdominal organs such as the liver and spleen. At birth, the bladder extends to the level of the umbilicus and gradually descends lower in the pelvis with age. In the adolescent child, the rapid growth rate of the spine makes it vulnerable to flexion and/or extension injury.

INITIAL EVALUATION AND MANAGEMENT

Every child with confirmed or suspected abdominal trauma should be evaluated in a systematic manner according to the Advanced Trauma Life Support system. As with any significantly injured patient, the exam begins with the ABCs (airway, breathing, and circulation). The child's spine should be stabilized in the field and the airway should be assessed immediately. Following the immediate ABC assessment, a thorough head to toe examination is performed. The head exam includes careful inspection of the scalp, especially in areas hard to visualize like the occiput and the area under the cervical collar. The skull should be palpated for fractured edges or depressed fractures. The pupils should be carefully inspected for reactivity to light and should have equal responsiveness. The midface and jaw should also be carefully palpated for signs of fracture or instability. The exam continues to the neck, checking that the trachea is midline and assessing for cervical spine tenderness. In addition to listening for breath sounds in the primary survey, the chest is examined for sternal and rib stability and/or tenderness. The abdominal exam involves palpating the entire abdomen looking for tenderness, distension, or bruising from seat-belt force. A careful inspection of the genitourinary and perineal regions should be done next. Digital rectal exams should be reserved for older children in whom abdominal or rectal injury is suspected by exam. All four extremities should then be inspected for any bony or joint abnormalities and for perfusion status. The child should then be carefully rolled onto her side while a trained clinician keeps the cervical spine in a stable alignment. The spine should then be palpated from the base of the skull to the coccyx looking, for any step-offs or point tenderness in the spinous processes.

Specific to the abdominal exam, any external signs of injury such as bruising, discoloration, lacerations, or masses should be noted. Abdominal distension, guarding, or tenderness may signal an intra-abdominal injury. Spine, pelvic, or rib fractures in children generally indicate significant forces have been applied and intra-abdominal injuries are more likely.

Resuscitation in children is very important, and intravenous or intraosseus access should be obtained as soon as possible. Hypotension in children is a late finding in shock. A bolus of appropriate fluid, usually normal saline at 20 mL/kg, should be given as soon as intravenous access is obtained. Vital signs should be carefully monitored throughout the evaluation and resuscitation phases of management.

SPECIFIC ORGAN INJURIES

Diaphragm

A sudden increase in intra-abdominal pressure may lead to rupture or laceration of the diaphragm, more commonly on the left side (Fig 127.4). Diaphragmatic injuries can be difficult to diagnose and often have other associated abdominal injuries. Respiratory symptoms related to injury of the diaphragm often do not manifest right away. A chest x-ray may suggest asymmetry of the diaphragm, or air lucencies in the chest cavity may be noticed. Additionally, a nasogastric tube coiled within the stomach above the diaphragm confirms the diagnosis. An ultrasound or CT scan of the chest may also be used to confirm the diagnosis. Surgical repair of the diaphragmatic injury should be performed as soon as the diagnosis is made in order to prevent possible incarceration of intra-abdominal organs.

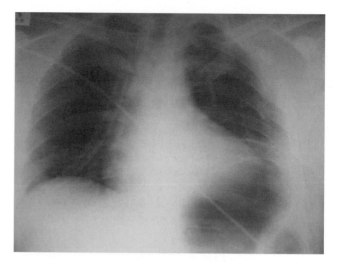

FIGURE 127.4. Chest x-ray showing air lucencies in the left chest, indicating diaphragmatic rupture.

Spleen

The spleen is the most commonly injured organ in the setting of blunt abdominal trauma. Currently, the standard of care for a hemodynamically stable child with an isolated splenic injury documented by computed tomography scan is nonoperative treatment with close monitoring by an experienced surgical team. Experience with nonoperative treatment began approximately 30 years ago when clinicians realized the increased morbidity and mortality associated with postsplenectomy sepsis. Imaging for intra-abdominal injuries has improved greatly over the last two decades, allowing for more standardized grading of injuries (Fig 127.5). Review of the National Pediatric Trauma Registry shows that only 11% of children from 1995 to 1999 with spleen injuries required operative intervention. The American Pediatric Surgical Association has proposed management guidelines for isolated splenic injuries (Table 127.2). These recommendations are

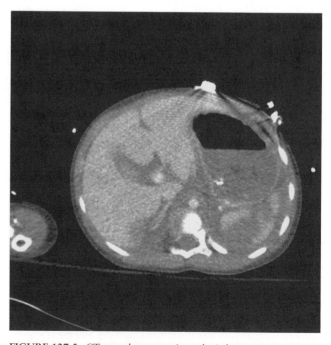

FIGURE 127.5. CT scan demonstrating splenic laceration.

TABLE 127.2

APSA GUIDELINES FOR ISOLATED SPLENIC OR LIVER INJURIES

	CT Grade			
	I	II	III	IV
ICU stay (days)	None	None	None	1
Hospital stay (days)	2	3	4	5
Activity restriction (weeks)[a]	3	4	5	6

[a]Return to full-contact, competitive sports (football, wrestling, hockey, lacrosse, mountain climbing) should be at the discretion of the individual pediatric trauma surgeon. The proposed guidelines for return to unrestricted activity include "normal" age-appropriate activities.
Modified from Stylianos S. Outcome studies and practice guidelines in trauma. *J Pediatr Surg* 2000; 35:164–169.

based on the grading of the splenic injury by CT scan imaging and based on the patient's clinical status (i.e., patients must be hemodynamically stable). A child with an isolated splenic injury who is hemodynamically stable can be closely monitored in the ICU or on the ward based on the grade of injury. Typically, serial hemoglobin is obtained every 8 to 12 hours until stabilized. The patient is kept NPO and on bed rest until the blood counts are stable and the pain is well controlled. The patient should be continued to be monitored for pain and hemodynamic status during initiation of feeding and increased activity.

Children who may require operative management include those who cannot be stabilized with crystalloid or blood product administration, those with associated injuries that may make determination of bleeding from the spleen difficult, those with coagulopathies, and those who may require exploration for other abdominal injuries. Surgical options for splenic injuries include placing surgical gauze packs around the spleen to tamponade any bleeding, partial splenectomy, splenorrhaphy using mesh to encircle and compress the spleen, and total splenectomy.

There are currently no studies that have shown a benefit in outcomes or management in children who have follow-up imaging for splenic injuries. Clinical evaluation should guide whether or not additional imaging is required. Rarely, delayed splenic rupture or hemorrhage can occur after previous blunt trauma. Typically, restriction of activities that may lead to repeat trauma of the left upper quadrant for several weeks to months after injury is adequate to allow complete healing of the splenic parenchyma.

Liver

The liver is also commonly injured in children who are subjected to blunt trauma (Fig 127.6). The frequency of hepatic injury is less than that of the spleen, but hepatic injuries are more likely to lead to significant hemorrhage. Injuries to the liver carry a higher mortality rate than injuries to other intraabdominal organs. As with the spleen, most liver injuries can be managed nonoperatively. The APSA guidelines for isolated liver injuries are also listed in Table 127.2. Immediate and adequate fluid resuscitation is paramount in the management of children with intra-abdominal injuries. Children should be closely monitored in the ICU or on the ward dependent on their clinical condition and CT grade of injury according to the APSA guidelines.

Surgical management of hepatic injuries includes direct ligation of bleeding vessels, cauterization of vessels and/or parenchyma, topical hemostatants (Surgicel, Thrombin spray,

etc.), and in cases where the child is hemodynamically unstable and/or has other associated intraabdominal injuries, packing the liver to provide a tamponade effect with reexploration a day or two later, after adequate stabilization, is sometimes required.

Kidney

The retroperitoneal organs in children are not as fixed as they are in adults, making them more prone to injury during blunt abdominal force. Renal injuries are often diagnosed by the presence of macroscopic or microscopic hematuria or by CT scan evidence. Hematuria is nonspecific but is typically present in patients with significant renal trauma. However, approximately 2% to 20% of renal injuries do not present with hematuria. Any child with gross hematuria or with greater than 50 red blood cells per high-power field should undergo abdominal CT scan with contrast to evaluate for kidney injury. Most renal injuries can be managed nonoperatively. Indications for surgery include renal vessel transection/dissection as evidenced by nonenhancement of unilateral kidney; contrast extravasation, persistent hypertension, or large urinoma. Rarely is nephrectomy

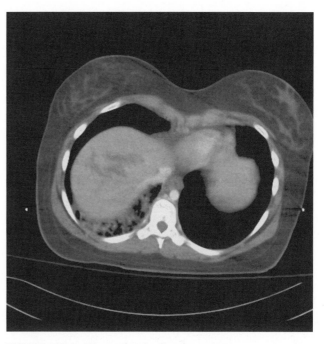

FIGURE 127.6. CT scan showing liver laceration.

required immediately after blunt trauma, but it may be required later for pain or abscess formation due to renal ischemia.

Bladder/Ureter/Urethra

As previously mentioned, the bladder in an infant reaches higher in the abdomen than in the older child or adult. Therefore, any signs of abdominal injury should lead to evaluation of the bladder and urethra. In boys sustaining blunt forces to the abdomen or pelvis, a rectal exam should be performed before placing a Foley catheter to evaluate for a high-riding prostate that may indicate urethral injury. If this is suspected, a cystourethrogram should be obtained as well as a post-evacuation x-ray. Treatment of urethral tears often includes suprapubic tube drainage with follow-up urethrogram prior to catheter removal.

Bladder rupture commonly occurs when significant blunt forces compress a full bladder. These injuries can be divided into intraperitoneal and extraperitoneal injuries, and can be evaluated by a CT cystogram or by cystourethrogram. Intraperitoneal ruptures are treated surgically with a two or three-layer closure and bladder decompression via Foley catheter for 1 to 2 weeks. Extraperitoneal rupture is managed by Foley catheter decompression alone for 7 to 10 days.

Ureters are retroperitoneal structures and are rarely injured during blunt abdominal trauma. Pelvic fractures, however, may cause injury to the ureteropelvic junction or the ureterovesical junction. When a ureteral injury is discovered, primary surgical repair is usually undertaken.

Pancreas

Pancreatitis and pancreatic injury in children are most often caused by blunt abdominal trauma. The force may compress the pancreas against the spine causing contusion or transection of the pancreas. Signs of pancreatic injury include abdominal wall bruising from seat belts or handlebars and ecchymosis of the flanks. Pancreatic injuries are often difficult to diagnose, but contrasted CT scans are the studies of choice and may show peripancreatic fluid, edema, or pancreatic disruption (Fig 127.7). Laboratory values such as amylase and

lipase do not correlate well with the degree of injury or the need for surgical intervention. Most pancreatic injuries are treated non-operatively with nasogastric decompression, total parenteral nutrition (TPN), and IV fluid resuscitation. Resolution of pain and return of bowel function are often indicators of pancreatic healing.

Early surgical intervention is often recommended for distal pancreatic transection or evidence of ductal disruption and typically includes spleen-sparing distal pancreatectomy. This may help to avoid late complications of pancreatic injury such as pseudocyst formation or ductal scarring leading to chronic pancreatitis. Proximal ductal injuries or trauma to the head of the pancreas are more difficult to manage due to their relationship to the duodenum and superior mesenteric vessels. Often percutaneous drainage of fluid collections and prolonged TPN are used as treatment options.

Duodenum

Injuries to the duodenum are often difficult to diagnose, and delayed presentation of duodenal perforation is often noted. CT scans may demonstrate a duodenal hematoma (Fig 127.8), retroperitoneal air, or free fluid in the abdomen. Duodenal hematomas are best managed by nasogastric decompression and TPN initially, followed by nutrition administered via transpyloric feeding tube for several weeks while the hematoma resolves. For simple duodenal lacerations, primary repair with an omental patch can be performed. Complex duodenal injuries require more extensive surgical intervention that may include duodenal exclusion, placement of drains, and gastrojejunostomy.

Small Bowel/Colon

Hollow viscus injuries carry a high mortality rate if they go unrecognized. The overall incidence of bowel injury from trauma in children is about 1% but increases to 15% to 25% in those with seat belt bruising. CT scans with oral and IV contrast are the most sensitive for identifying hollow viscus injuries, but oral contrast is difficult to administer in the acute setting due to nausea/vomiting and delays the imaging while awaiting contrast

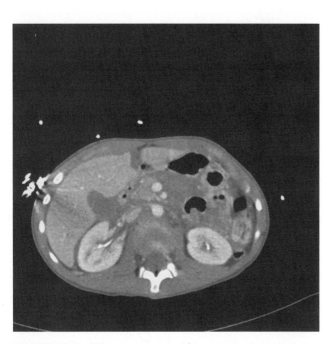

FIGURE 127.7. CT scan consistent with pancreatic transection.

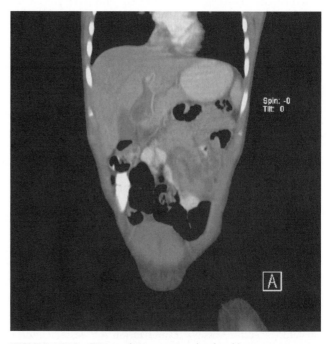

FIGURE 127.8. CT scan demonstrating duodenal hematoma.

to pass through the bowel. CT scans with IV-only contrast may demonstrate free intraperitoneal fluid, and patients with abdominal wall signs of trauma and free fluid in the abdomen have a higher likelihood of hollow viscus injuries. However, when free fluid is noted on CT scan of a child with no external signs of trauma, only 15% to 20% actually have an intestinal injury. A high degree of suspicion is always needed in children with either external or radiographic signs of trauma. Repeat CT scans with oral and IV contrast 12 to 24 hours after injury is sometimes helpful in evaluating for hollow viscus injury.

Surgical intervention is indicated in any child with hemodynamic instability in whom no other signs of blood loss are found; in patients with evidence of peritonitis; in patients with free intraperitoneal fluid and no solid organ injury who have fevers, vomiting, or abdominal distention; and in patients who have obvious intestinal injury on radiographic imaging. Diagnostic peritoneal lavage (DPL) is used less frequently now with the advent of advanced ultrasonography and CT scanning. In patients unable to go immediately to the CT scan who are suspected of having an intra-abdominal injury, DPL is an appropriate diagnostic tool. DPL is a surgical procedure that can be performed at the bedside and includes insertion of a drainage catheter into the peritoneal cavity followed by 20 mL/kg of saline or lactated Ringer solution. The bag is then placed on the floor for gravity drainage. Indications for laparotomy include gross blood or succus; more than 100,000 red blood cells per mL; more than 500 white blood cells per mL, and presence of bacteria or elevated amylase.

Exploration of the abdomen in the setting of trauma is typically done through a midline incision to allow exposure of all four quadrants. Some pediatric surgeons are beginning to use minimally invasive techniques to evaluate and even treat some hollow viscus injuries. Simple small bowel and even colon injuries can be repaired primarily. More complex injuries may necessitate intestinal resection and temporary diversion with an ostomy.

A high degree of suspicion, frequent abdominal exams, and repeat radiographic imaging, if indicated, are necessary in diagnosing hollow viscus injuries. Delayed diagnosis carries high morbidity and mortality rates.

Suggested Readings

Alonso M, Brathwaite C, Garcia V, et al. EAST guidelines on trauma, 2003. www.east.org.

Mattei P, ed. *Surgical directives: pediatric surgery*. Philadelphia: Lippincott Williams & Wilkins; 2002: 113–118.

Nance M, Stafford PW. Pediatric trauma is a surgical disease. *Ann Emerg Med* 2003;41:423–424.

O'Neill JA, Rowe MI, Grosfeld JL, et al. *Pediatric Surgery*. 5th ed. St. Louis: Mosby; 1998: 261–280.

Potoka DA, Schall LC, Ford HR. Risk factors for splenectomy in children with blunt splenic trauma. *J Pediatr Surg* 2002 37; 294–299.

Stylianos S. Outcome studies and practice guidelines in trauma. *J Pediatr Surg* 2000;35:164–169.

Ziegler MM, Azizkhan RG, Weber TR. *Operative pediatric surgery*. New York: McGraw-Hill; 2003: 1125–1142.

CHAPTER 127C ■ TRAUMATIC INJURIES: RECOGNITION OF CHILD ABUSE IN THE PEDIATRIC TRAUMA PATIENT

ELAINE S. CABINUM-FOELLER

Trauma remains the most common cause of pediatric deaths and results in more deaths than all other etiologies combined. Furthermore, for each infant or child death, approximately 10 more children are permanently disabled. Considering all presentations and mechanisms, 1 of every 6 hospitalized children is hospitalized secondary to trauma. In turn, and varying according to community and hospital characteristics, most estimates indicate that of all children hospitalized with traumatic injuries, approximately 10% received those injuries from a nonaccidental mechanism (i.e., child abuse). When hospitalized, these infants and children may be in a number of clinical settings (e.g., ward, pediatric intensive care unit, burn unit) or on any of several services (e.g., orthopedics, neurosurgery, trauma surgery, pediatric surgery, general surgery, pediatric service) with the pediatric hospital care provider as a consultant or as the primary responsible physician.

When children or infants present with traumatic injuries, often the history and injuries leave no doubt as to the manner and mechanism of injury. A witnessed high-velocity motor vehicle collision that causes fractures, contusions, lacerations, or other injuries usually results in a straightforward approach to management and causes little or no concern about possible nonaccidental trauma. However, there are many other children whose injuries, either due to their nature (e.g., closed head injury to an infant) or to characteristics of the history (e.g., absence of a history of appropriate trauma, inconsistent history over time), should result in consideration of child abuse as the mechanism of injury. It is very important that child abuse be appropriately considered and evaluated. Failure to appropriately diagnose child abuse may result in a failure to protect the child or his siblings. In turn, this failure to protect can result in future additional injuries to the child (and/or siblings) and an increased risk of death at the hands of the perpetrator. Compared to children with accidental injuries, children with injuries from child abuse have higher severity of injury scores, more severe injuries of the head and skin, longer hospital stays, higher risk of mortality, and greater risk of permanent disability.

The diagnosis of inflicted injury should be approached like diagnosing any other medical problem. The health care provider should thoughtfully obtain and consider the history, physical examination, laboratory results, and radiography. In some cases, additional information can be and should be obtained from outside sources such as child protective services investigators (CPS) or law enforcement personnel (LE). Information about the in-hospital evaluation of the possibly abused child is reviewed in detail in Chapter 136. Elements of the evaluation are briefly highlighted below.

HISTORY

When any child presents with traumatic injuries, the evaluation starts with the history. Children are active, and accidental injury is common. However, when a child presents with significant injury, historical clues that suggest inflicted trauma include the following:

- No history of trauma
- Changing versions of the history
- A history of activities that the child is not yet developmentally able to perform
- A history that does not include the biomechanical forces needed to sustain the injury

To correctly identify accidental and inflicted injuries, the physician must have some knowledge of the forces needed to sustain various injuries. In most children presenting with an injury, physical child abuse can often be removed from the differential diagnosis quickly with a thorough history and complete physical exam. It is important to obtain and record a complete history of the events surrounding the injury, including who was present, what exactly happened, when it occurred, where it occurred, and the circumstances surrounding the injury (e.g., playing around the house, motor vehicle crash, rolling off a couch). Historical detail should always be obtained from the parent or caretaker who initially presents with the child. However, sometimes the person who brings the child for medical care was not present when the injury occurred and is unable to directly report the mechanism of injury. The history obtained at a later time from the parent/caretaker must also be documented thoroughly.

With possible inflicted injury, detailed historical information should be recorded. Reporting specific important details verbatim in "quotes" is often useful to CPS and LE and for later recall if the case does go to court. History should also include a good past medical history, family history, social history, and review of systems. Additional characteristics that are associated with an increased risk of child abuse are reported in Table 127.3.

PHYSICAL EXAMINATION

When examining possible victims of inflicted trauma, every inch of skin should be examined for possible marks, bruises, and scars. Any such lesions should be documented completely with words, diagrams, and/or photographs including measurements, color, and any other features (e.g., swelling, abrasions, lacerations). Although photographs can be helpful in documentation, technology isn't perfect. Photographs may be improperly exposed or later misplaced. A good description and injury diagram is advised with every child.

LABORATORY

Laboratory evaluations are often necessary and can help to differentiate accidental and inflicted trauma. Occasionally children who present with trauma have an underlying medical condition that is important to the mechanism or nature of the injury. Medical conditions that can mimic inflicted trauma findings (e.g., bleeding disorders, glutaric acidemia type I) have to be considered. Additional tests and indications for consideration are listed below:

TABLE 127.3

RISK FACTORS ASSOCIATED WITH CHILD ABUSE IN PEDIATRIC TRAUMA

HISTORY
  No history of injury provided
  Changing history of injury
  History provided is developmentally inappropriate
  History of prior abuse in the family
  Delay in presenting for care
  Parent
    Single
    Family stress (e.g., marital issues)
    Socially isolated (e.g., military)
    Poverty
    Young maternal age
  Child
    Age <2 years
    History of previous injuries
    Disability
    Prematurity
    Hyperactivity

FINDINGS (WITHOUT A HISTORY OF HIGH-VELOCITY ACCIDENT)
  Fracture of base of skull
  Contusion of eye
  Rib fracture (especially posterior or lateral)
  Intracranial bleeding
  Multiple burns
  Patterned skin injuries
  Femur fracture < age 3
  Retinal hemorrhages
  Metaphyseal fractures (tibia/fibula, radius/ulnar)
  Hollow viscus injury (bowel and bladder)

- A complete blood count and screening coagulation studies (PT, PTT) are indicated if bruises or bleeding is present. More specialized coagulation studies may be indicated for some head trauma injuries or based on family history. Refer to Chapter 137 for further details on abusive head trauma.
- Liver function tests, amylase, and lipase should be obtained if the history or findings suggest blunt abdominal trauma. Abnormal results should trigger additional imaging of the abdomen for possible liver, pancreatic, or duodenal injuries.
- Urinalysis for blood or myoglobin can be useful for muscular or flank injuries.
- Urine for toxicologic analysis is sometimes indicated, especially for children presenting with coma or other altered mental states. The specific assays in the "tox screen" vary between institutions and do not test for all drugs. The provider needs to know the specifics of the testing at her hospital, and order more directed testing based on the clinical syndrome.

RADIOLOGY

Radiographic studies are useful to help differentiate between inflicted trauma and accidental trauma or underlying medical problems. Such studies should be ordered on a case-by-case basis and depend on the age of the child, the history, the type of injury, and even the specific technology (e.g., MRI) available at the hospital. There are a variety of radiologic studies available for assessing injuries or possible injuries. Considerations include skeletal survey, radionuclide bone scan, CT scan, and MRI.

The skeletal survey includes radiographic images of all bones in a child's body. These surveys are often obtained in children under the age of 2 years who have injuries suspicious for inflicted trauma. The survey can detect unexpected fractures or fractures of varying ages that are suggestive or diagnostic for inflicted injury. Rarely are skeletal surveys necessary in children after age 2 years because the child is capable of reporting pain associated with bony injuries. The older child may also report the mechanism and manner of injury. Accordingly, only selected radiographs based on the history of specific areas that might be injured are usually appropriate in older, verbal children, thereby avoiding unnecessary radiation exposure. Very rarely are skeletal surveys indicated in children over the age of 5 years. Radionuclide bone scans can be an adjunct to skeletal surveys in certain situations with possible inflicted trauma. "Hot" spots are present at the epiphyseal plates of long bones on normal growing children and may not help define injuries at those sites. The scan can sometimes detect unexpected injuries at other sites and those findings may be suspicious or even definitive (e.g., posterior rib fractures, vertebral body fractures). Consultation with a pediatric radiologist is often helpful.

Computed tomography (CT) scans often provide additional information and usually are the first choice for imaging head, chest, or abdominal injuries. CT is available at most hospitals and scans are quickly performed. The obtained information may not only help with diagnosis, but may determine a need for additional medical interventions. Occasionally the CT will reveal an old injury (e.g., callused rib fracture) that was not previously known. However, plain bone radiographs are the best modality for determining the approximate age(s) of bone fractures. Magnetic resonance imaging (MRI) is helpful in detecting subtle or small intracranial injuries not seen on CT. Sometimes with subdural hematomas, the MRI will also detect evidence of bleeding of more than one age. The MRI can also better diagnose axonal shear injury or brain contusions than CT. MRI usually has the best yield when performed 3 to 4 days after a brain injury. Extra sequences such as fluid-attenuated inversion recovery (FLAIR) can be added at the discretion of the radiologist to look for other subtle findings.

PATTERNS OF INFLICTED INJURY

Any injury to a child can be from abuse. Without becoming cynical, the health care provider should continue to consider abuse in the differential diagnosis. Injury patterns will be considered under the following headings: soft-tissue injury, fractures, abdominal organ injury, thoracic injury, urinary tract injury, brain injury, and other injuries.

Soft-Tissue Injury

Bruises are the most common type of soft-tissue injury seen in victims of abuse. Bruises and related marks may be in areas of the body or have a pattern that suggests a mechanism of injury in general or abuse specifically. Any bruise or mark on a child not yet cruising (walking while holding to a stationary object) is unusual (<2% of normal pre-ambulatory infants) and should be concerning. Once children are mobile and able to cruise and walk, they often sustain bruises from normal activity. Approximately 50% of all toddlers presenting for health care have one or more bruises. "Normal" bruises usually occur over bony prominences such as elbows, shins, and forehead. Other locations are more often associated with inflicted injury, such as contusions on the pinna, cheeks, inner thighs, genitalia, or central buttocks. Specific patterns of injury

sometimes suggest abuse; examples include loop marks (from electric cords), slap marks, linear bruises along the gluteal cleft, ligature marks on wrists or ankles, gag marks at the corners of the mouth, and belt marks.

A specific bruise that should cause concern is the presence of one or more bite marks. Children often bite, especially in day-care settings. However, it is usually easy to distinguish bites from older children and adults from pediatric bites. The distance between the canine teeth (usually easily identified on the arc-shaped bruise) should be measured. Three centimeters or more indicates that a person with permanent dentition made the bite. The injury sometimes becomes more evident 2 to 3 days after the injury. Careful photographic documentation may help identify a perpetrator with the assistance of a forensic dentist. Note also that human teeth are dull and result in bruising and abrasions. Animal bites involve sharper teeth that are more likely to result in puncture wounds or lacerations.

Bruises are sometimes confused with Mongolian spots (congenital birthmarks). These can occur anywhere on the body, but are often found on the lower back and buttocks and are more common in children of African-American or Asian ancestry. With bruising, other medical conditions to consider include idiopathic thrombocytopenic purpura, hemophilia, vitamin K deficiency, or other less common bleeding diatheses. A longer list of skin conditions to consider in the differential diagnosis is provided in Table 127.4. Laboratory testing should include a complete blood count and screening coagulation studies such as prothrombin time (PT) and partial thromboplastin time (PTT). Further coagulation studies such as von Willebrand factor or proteins induced by vitamin K antagonism (PIVKA II) should be considered based on the patient's personal history of bleeding and/or the family history. The PIVKA II test is more specific for vitamin K deficiency. It is a modification of PT and detects deficiencies in factors II, VII, and X.

Previous reports suggesting that bruises can be accurately aged based on appearance have been refuted by more recent research. In general, a yellow tint is not seen until 18 to 24 hours after the injury. Otherwise in children, dating an injury based solely on the appearance of a bruise is relatively unreliable.

TABLE 127.4
DIFFERENTIAL DIAGNOSIS OF SKIN LESIONS AS ALTERNATIVES TO CHILD ABUSE

BRUISES
Mongolian spots
Stains from clothing
Phytophotodermatitis (may show shape of hand)
Ethnic therapies (cupping, coining, spoon scraping)
Henoch–Schönlein purpura
Erythema multiforme
Erythema nodosum
Ehlers–Danlos syndrome
Hemangiomas

BURNS
Bullous impetigo
SSSS (staphylococcal scalded skin syndrome)
Phytophotodermatitis
Ethnic therapies (cupping, moxabustion)
Epidermolysis bullosa
Fixed drug eruption
Diaper dermatitis (severe)

Burns are often accidental, but can be inflicted (see Table 127.4 for differential diagnosis). Some burn patterns such as the stocking, glove, and donut are highly suspicious for inflicted injury seen in immersion burns. The stocking pattern is a circumferential burn of the foot and/or leg in the distribution of a sock or stocking. The glove pattern is a circumferential burn of the hand/arm in the distribution of a glove or mitten. The donut pattern is on the buttocks and shows an area of central sparing with surrounding burned tissue. These are often seen when a child is forcibly immersed in hot water. In burns, it is important to accurately and completely document the areas of skin that are injured and not injured.

By analyzing the pattern of the injury, investigators can often deduce some information about the mechanism of the burn and assess the validity of the history. Burns can also be inflicted with objects such as irons or cigarettes. The former usually shows a pattern consistent with some part of the hot flat ironing surface. The latter shows a punched out discrete (average diameter 8 mm) burn that heals with scarring. Occasionally bullous impetigo, a common skin infection, is confused with a cigarette burn. However, it is usually easy to differentiate by an experienced clinician, and ultimately by culture or by the presence or absence of scarring. Rarely seen but other reported burn injuries include microwave oven burns (infants) and stun gun burns. Children with burns secondary to abuse also require careful evaluation for other inflicted injuries.

Abrasions and lacerations can also be present as a result of child abuse. Abrasions are also seen with many of the injuries associated with bruising. Lacerations are much less common. Again, specific patterns may suggest a mechanism leading to the diagnosis of inflicted injuries (see above). Linear parallel abrasions may suggest deliberate scratching with fingernails. Small parallel abrasions (and contusions) across the tip of a digit can be secondary to applying force with a tool such as pliers.

Fractures

In abused children, fractures are often present. The challenge to pediatric providers is that while most fractures are accidental, any fracture can be the result of abuse. As noted above, a careful evaluation with history, physical examination, and pertinent other tests are indicated when the suspicion is present. Certain fractures are more suggestive of abuse as a cause (see Table 127.3). Assessing fractures necessitates an understanding of the forces needed to cause bones to break. Spiral fractures occur when a bone is under torsion or twisting forces as it breaks leading to the spiral or oblique picture when viewed on x-ray; hence such fractures should often be cause for concern, especially in young nonmobile children. The exception to this concern is a *toddler's fracture*. This is an accidental fracture seen in young ambulatory children and sometimes confused with an abusive fracture. The injury is a nondisplaced spiral fracture of the distal third of the tibia. It often presents with a history of a child who will not bear weight on the affected leg and no other history or findings suggesting nonaccidental injury.

Fractures of different ages or multiple fractures (in the absence of a history of motor vehicle collision) are highly suspicious for abuse. In children with fractures, diseases that must be considered in the differential include osteogenesis imperfecta, rickets, congenital syphilis, scurvy, Menkes kinky hair syndrome, and others. In addition to the thorough history and physical examination, characteristic radiographic findings usually assist the clinician in eliminating most of these diseases from consideration. Children under the age of 2 years should have a full pediatric skeletal survey to look for other old or subtle bony injuries. Particular attention should be paid to the metaphysis of the long bones in the extremities looking for the

characteristic chips (corner fractures or bucket handle fractures) that are highly suspicious for inflicted injury. The lack of other fractures on a skeletal survey does not rule out abuse. In the setting of a negative survey, and depending on the specifics of the presentation, repetition of the skeletal survey 2 weeks later sometimes yields useful information with callus formation now identifying fractures not evident on the initial examination.

Abdominal Organ Injury

After closed head injuries, abdominal injuries are the second leading cause of death from child abuse. Of all children admitted to the hospital with blunt abdominal trauma, child abuse is the second most common etiology behind motor vehicle collisions and ahead of falls. Compared to adults, children have less protection for the abdominal organs because of their relatively small rib cage and pelvis combined with less well-developed abdominal wall musculature. The prototypical child abuse abdominal injury is a *duodenal hematoma* as a result of blunt trauma to the abdomen. The child may present with peritonitis, shock, and no history of trauma. Alternatively, the child may develop progressive problems with vomiting and anorexia that initially is thought to be a viral gastroenteritis. Only with further evolution of symptoms is the diagnosis discovered, most often with additional imaging (usually CT).

Blunt trauma to the abdomen may also cause injury to the liver, stomach, small intestine, mesentery, kidneys, bladder, or pancreas. The *liver* is the intra-abdominal organ most commonly injured in child abuse, usually from blunt trauma. Injuries can include contusion, laceration, rupture, subcapsular hematoma, or disruption of the biliary duct system. Presentation may be obvious with shock and abdominal pain, or subtle with vague abdominal symptoms, perhaps presenting days after the injury. Especially in the latter setting, obtaining liver function tests, hemoglobin levels, amylase, and lipase provide clinical clues to these underlying important and yet sometimes subtle injuries. The *spleen* is less often injured, but has a similar presentation and need for rapid recognition and response.

In addition to the possibility of duodenal hematoma as above, *intestinal perforation* can occur secondary to blunt direct trauma. Again, in the absence of a suitable history, this injury has to be considered highly suspicious for child abuse. Caretakers often report that the child fell down stairs. However, published case series suggest that such falls are very unlikely to cause intestinal perforation.

As soon as intra-abdominal injury is suspected, an abdominal CT should be obtained. This imaging is very useful in the evaluation for blunt abdominal injury and can demonstrate suggestive or diagnostic findings (e.g., fractured liver or spleen, pancreatic edema). Contusions of the overlying abdominal wall are usually not present.

Thoracic Injury

Injuries to the chest can result in chest wall contusions and fractured ribs, but less commonly may cause direct injury to lungs, heart, esophagus, and thoracic duct. The *lungs* can be contused by blunt trauma or lacerated by blunt trauma, penetrating trauma, or displaced rib fractures. Children with severe injuries are at risk of developing acute respiratory distress syndrome (ARDS).

The *heart* can be injured in a similar variety of ways. Cardiac contusion can result from direct blunt trauma to the precordium or from being thrown against an object. This injury can result in abnormal electrocardiography findings and elevated troponin levels. Echocardiography of the heart can be diagnostic, with findings of an area of poorly contractile injured myocardium, pericardial effusions, and even valvular or septal disruption. If direct blunt trauma to the precordium occurs at just the right point in the cardiac cycle, the child can develop a potentially fatal arrhythmia (ventricular fibrillation or asystole) from commotio cordis.

The *esophagus* is less commonly involved, but can be injured by blunt or penetrating trauma from nonaccidental causes. Other mechanisms of esophageal injury to consider include forced ingestion of caustics or foreign bodies. The *thoracic duct* can also be severed by blunt trauma or shaken baby syndrome. If a child presents with a chylothorax without an appropriate history of accidental trauma, child abuse should be considered suspicious.

Urinary Tract Injuries

The kidney, bladder, and ureters in children are uncommonly injured by child abuse. Compared to adults, the pediatric *kidney* is more vulnerable to trauma because of its relatively larger size, lower position in the abdomen, and less perirenal fat. Injuries can vary from renal contusion to subcapsular hemorrhage, fractured kidney, or disruption of the vascular supply (directly or by thrombosis). The *bladder* can also be ruptured when direct impact is delivered to the suprapubic area in the presence of a full bladder. The dome of the bladder can rupture, with urine displaced into the peritoneal cavity. In addition to developing peritonitis and ileus, these children may also have pseudorenal failure secondary to the resorption of the urine. When this injury is suspected, abdominal CT is often insufficient and retrograde cystography is required. The *ureter* is rarely disrupted, but can be injured by direct penetrating trauma or severe truncal hyperextension. The adrenal glands are rarely injured, but lacerations and hematomas have been reported secondary to inflicted injury.

Injuries to these organs are often suspected based on associated injuries (e.g., contusions over the costovertebral angles), anuria, or findings on laboratory evaluations. The latter may include hematuria, elevated blood urea nitrogen, and/or elevated creatinine. In the setting of abuse with muscular injury, the clinician should also consider the possibility of rhabdomyolysis as a cause of renal dysfunction, especially if myoglobinuria is present with pigmented granular casts in the urine.

Brain Injury

Inflicted head injury is the leading cause of death from child abuse. It has been estimated that as many as 80% of deaths due to head trauma in the first 2 years of life are because of child abuse. In children less than 3 years of age presenting with a subdural hematoma, more than one-half are found to be from abuse, and this increases to approximately 75% if those with obvious accidental etiologies are excluded. Signs of head injury in children can be subtle, ranging from mild (vomiting and lethargy) to severe (seizures, coma, and death). Unfortunately, because some of the milder symptoms are also often seen in children with common viral illnesses, at the time of first assessment by a physician, the diagnosis of child abuse is missed almost one-third of the time.

The intracranial injuries may include subdural hematomas, intracerebral hemorrhage, ischemic stroke, epidural hematoma, subarachnoid hemorrhage, and acute cerebral edema. The mechanism of such injuries (shaking versus impact) remains controversial, but does not change the fact that adults all too often cause abusive brain injuries in children. The most common victims are the youngest and most dependent. (See Chapter 137 for more details on abusive head injury)

Other

Other forms of injuries from trauma can also be related to child abuse. These include asphyxia, drowning, traumatic alopecia, hypo- or hyperthermia, and deliberate poisoning (including excessive water or salt). In any child felt to have been physically abused, sexual abuse should also be evaluated, even though it is uncommonly concurrently present (see Chapter 138). Finally, the physician treating a child for traumatic injuries should always consider the possibility of *child neglect*. Did the injuries occur because the child was not properly supervised? Did the care provider place the child (or allow the child to be) in a dangerous situation that resulted in injury? Has the parent or caretaker failed to present the child for appropriate and timely care for traumatic injuries? Conversely, has there been a failure to comply with necessary and very important care subsequent to accidental injuries? Is such neglect due to a misunderstanding or willful? Diagnosing child abuse is difficult, but ascertaining neglect to the satisfaction of social services and/or law enforcement is even more difficult. However, reporting and providing information during the subsequent investigation is necessary in the hope that ultimately the child will be protected and receive all appropriate and necessary care.

PEARLS

- Obtain and document a careful and thorough history of any suspicious injury including who, what, where, and when.
- Document the child's developmental level as reported, and as observed.
- Document injuries both with word and diagrams. Photographs are optional.
- Keep child abuse in the initial differential diagnosis of all pediatric injuries.
- The "tin ear syndrome" is the combination of bruises on the pinna, retinal hemorrhage, and closed head traumatic injury.
- Report suspicious injuries to child protective services. They have the responsibility for investigating and, when appropriate, protecting the child.

CHAPTER 128 ■ INTRODUCTION, DEFINITIONS, PREVALENCE, AND SERVICE NEEDS

CHARLES F. WILLSON, RONALD M. PERKIN, AMY J. JONES, AND JUDY W. WOOD

As outpatient methods and therapies have become more effective, the need for hospitalization of children has diminished. As a result, a quick tally of diagnoses on a pediatric ward in a community or tertiary care hospital shows a high percentage of children with a chronic or disabling condition. The general pediatric ward also is serving as a step-down unit for children coming from a pediatric or neonatal intensive care unit before discharge. These children have many of the same needs as the child with a chronic medical or surgical condition.

Therefore, although many children need to use hospital services at some time, a growing percentage of children have illnesses or disabilities that require care over many years and involve recurring hospital admissions and consultation with a wide range of pediatric specialists (1,2). In these long-term relationships, factors important to total quality management and consumer satisfaction relate to continuity, communication, and partnership. However, there is evidence that the health care and welfare systems for those with chronic conditions and disabilities are instead frequently experienced as fragmented and characterized by poor coordination and communication. Health care in the United States has been characterized as provider-centric, where the preferences and needs of the providers and staff take priority over the needs of the patients whom we serve (3). Hospitals are organized into fairly independent specialist areas, a situation that has both positive and negative effects on service provision to the population of children with chronic disability. Although it increases the level of specialist expertise available to children with complex health care needs, the presence of multiple service providers reduces the likelihood of coordination between providers occurring easily and comprehensively. By default, families often must take major responsibility for ensuring that specialist areas are aware of each other's treatment plans. Professionalism dictates that physicians caring for a mutual patient communicate with each other in a timely and effective manner.

Indeed, families are the daily caregivers between hospitalizations and should be recognized as the ultimate experts on their child's health and care. This is the central tenet family-centered care. On admission, a simple acknowledgement of the family's central role in the care of the child both at home and during the hospitalization will empower the family to stay involved. Hospitalization should be considered a (hopefully) brief interruption in a child's life to provide a service or intervention not possible to receive in the home setting. At all times, the preferences and desires of the child and the family should be solicited and respected. The results of tests and procedures and any change in the child's condition should be

immediately shared with the family in order to formulate the next steps in the care plan. A care plan developed jointly by the caregivers and the family has a much better chance of compliance and success.

Any relationship between a family with a sick child and a health care provider is complex, with issues of anxiety, gratitude, control, anger, and hopelessness in evidence. If the child has a chronic condition, these issues are likely to be accentuated and may lead to considerable conflict between staff and parents. Often parents feel upset and angry with the difficulties in dealing with "the system" and attitudes toward disability, as well as the prognosis itself. For this population, it is necessary to view conflict as an intrinsic part of a complex working relationship, rather than an unfortunate and unpleasant burden. When conflict is seen as part of the continuum of a developing relationship, movement toward partnership becomes possible through ongoing dialogue between patient (if able), parents, and health professionals.

A model of care that addresses the complex needs of the acutely and chronically ill child must have several elements. Although technical expertise is vital, empathy, continuity, and coordination of care, with partnership between parents and health professionals, must also be present. The model must recognize the contribution to care of a disease orientation while ensuring that the patients' and families' broader needs are not sacrificed (Table 128.1). This approach, therefore, is not just organ or treatment specific, but is child and family centered: actively acknowledging and using parents' knowledge of their own child and his condition. Such a model, which presents challenges to the ever-increasing specialization of pediatric hospital practice, is unlikely to arise spontaneously, but instead requires organizational vision and determined commitment (4). Financial considerations and limitations of resources often impede the model from reaching ideal. Fortunately, family-centered care is as much attitudinal as it is structural, so that an energized staff of health professionals can make great strides in a short period of time. Changes in bricks and mortar can be part of a longer planning process.

Because of the complexity and uniqueness of each child with a chronic illness, a team approach with a system of care should be developed. The system relies on evidence-based practices where available. The team may include family, primary care physician, hospitalist physicians, case-appropriate specialty physicians, case manager, nurses, therapists, mental health specialists, social workers, child life specialists, educators, and other child advocates. The admission should be viewed as a brief intensification of care along the continuum of a child's life.

TABLE 128.1

FACTORS IMPORTANT TO PARENTS IN A
LONG-TERM RELATIONSHIP WITH HEALTH
CARE PROVIDERS

- Technical expertise.
- Easy access to the hospital.
- Clear information about the child's illness, the hospital system, and other relevant resources.
- Acknowledgment of the parents' expertise with their own child and her condition.
- Partnership between professionals and parents.
- An advocate to coordinate the various parts of the "system."
- Flexible negotiation of roles, especially when the child is an inpatient.
- Professional willingness to see the child as a person, not as a disability.
- Recognition that the child's illness affects all members of the family.
- Time, empathy, and attentive listening.
- Staff willingness to learn of the child's condition.
- Continuity of care with known, trusted, and respected professionals.

The admitting physician's traditional role continues to be the correction of the derangement of clinical status necessitating the admission. Ideally, the admitting physician is the physician who cares for the child at the primary care medical home. If not, communication with the primary care physician should be established immediately and repeated often. Also, under ideal circumstances, the parents are able to provide the admitting physician with a copy of the child's comprehensive care plan, listing ongoing diagnoses, current medications, outpatient therapies, specialty consultations, school regimens, family strengths, community resources, and so forth. The inpatient admission should be viewed as an opportunity to reevaluate and update the care plan and remedy any lapses that have occurred. In the all too common situation where a comprehensive plan does not exist, such a plan should be developed in concert with the patient, family, primary care medical home, and local resources. Discharge planning should commence at the moment of admission. An initial discussion of any ongoing hassles and barriers to care for the family is often helpful in improving care for the future.

In an effective management model, continuity and coordination need to be promoted in several areas: between the hospital and community agencies; between specialist areas within the hospital; and between inpatient and outpatient departments. It is crucial that continuity and coordination be viewed as intrinsic elements of each hospital stay at the ward level, with a negotiated and consistent plan for each inpatient period.

The inpatient physician's or hospitalist's role is critical and involves developing or renewing links between parent, hospital administration, all hospital health care providers, and community-based professionals and organizations. "Seamless" care will be possible when there are effective mechanisms for communication between hospitals, community-based health care providers, schools and families; this is as relevant to the provision of acute care as it is for the care of those who have longer-term needs. This requires the compilation of different kinds of documentation, such as care manuals (general and disease-specific for each child), staff training, and the facilitation of planning sessions between health care professionals and parents. A wise hospitalist will become familiar with the primary care medical homes, ancillary service agencies, and other community resources in her referral areas. Where deficiencies are perceived, the hospitalist will advocate for the development of high-quality resources for children with chronic and complex conditions.

The task outlined is clearly an evolutionary process and requires changes in attitudes and "culture" as well as new procedures and systems, some of which will employ emerging information technologies. Ultimately, the success of the hospitalist care management system depends on the ability of health professionals to work within models of care that may differ considerably from those in which they were originally trained. Future training program need to incorporate these emerging holistic models of care that require professionals to cross traditional service and role boundaries. There is a great deal of thinking and planning to be done to establish the structural, training, and cultural changes needed for a comprehensive care management system.

Although case-mix funding requires administrative emphasis on length of stay and discharge planning, increasing attention also is being paid to consumer satisfaction and to the balance between cost and quality. Recent experience indicates that a hospitalist management approach is consistent with efficiency and fiscal accountability. There can be a strong argument made for funding an inpatient physician or hospitalist program as long as it promotes continuity of care between hospital, community, and family. There is an ever-present risk that the primary care physician no longer caring for the hospitalized care may feel overwhelmed by the complex patient, or the parents may interpret the physician as inadequately trained to handle the complexity of the chronically ill child. The result is a default model of care that bypasses the primary care medical home and uses the emergency department as an entry back to the hospitalist. The hospital physician must be an ardent advocate for the primary care medical home, and work to build capacity there if lacking.

Clinical pathways, critical paths, and care map systems all provide a database for continuous quality improvement and research, case management through collaborative care, and a degree of patient centeredness. These databases serve as springboards for quality improvement. Often an item not measured is not done. Although these systems are used currently for relatively straightforward conditions and procedures, they may well provide a useful model for achieving better outcomes in more complex illnesses, especially if patients and their families take part in the development. In addition, the evaluation of the introduction of these systems increasingly includes consumer satisfaction measures.

Clear goals for the admission must be established and agreed upon by the child (if able) and the family. Every attempt must be made to develop self-management skills with the ultimate goal of the child achieving a productive, satisfying, and hopeful life. Once the immediate clinical derangement is overcome, issues relating to physical strength and stamina, proper nutrition, and adequate rest should be addressed. An assessment should be made of the impact of any new physical impairment or required therapy on the patient's previous roles in the family, at school, and in the community.

As the discharge from the hospital approaches, the outpatient system of care should be assessed. Barriers to continuity of care and success of the care plan include:

- Lack of a care plan
- Lack of understanding of the care plan by the parent
- Lack of transportation to primary care or specialist visits
- Proposed appointment times when transportation or child care is not available

Appendix A

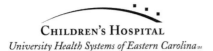

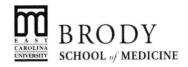

Center for Children with Complex and Chronic Conditions (C5)

My Care Plan

Please call me: _____

My family and I speak: ☐ English   ☐ Spanish   ☐ Other:_____

Full Name:_____   DOB:_____

Parent/Caregiver:_____   Relationship: _____

Address:_____

_____

Phone: (home): _____   (work):_____

(cell): _____   Best time to reach:_____

Emergency Contact: _____   Phone:_____

Insurance: _____

Primary Care Provider/Medical Home:_____ (PCP)Address:_____	Phone:_____ Fax: _____

Diagnosis (es):   _____   _____

  _____   _____

Baseline vital signs: _____HR _____RR _____Temp _____ O2 sats _____BP

  Other:_____

Baseline physical findings: _____

_____

Baseline neurological status:_____

_____

☐ Deaf   ☐ Blind   ☐ Non-verbal

☐ Hearing Impaired   ☐ Visually Impaired   ☐ Ambulatory   ☐ Nonambulatory

FIGURE 128.1. Care plan example, from the Center for Children with Complex and Chronic Conditions at the Brody School of Medicine.

- Inability of school systems to comply with medical care regimens
- Lack of comprehensive health care insurance or inability to pay for items not covered

Is the primary care medical home set up to handle patients with chronic illness of the severity and complexity involved? Telephone contacts made with the primary care physician during the child's hospital stay will give many valuable clues regarding the capability of that medical home. To be effective, acute care offices may need to make adjustments in physical plant, scheduling, appointment timing, and protocol for the disabled patient. Physicians need to stay educated regarding best practices and evidence-based care for these complex patients. In larger practices, a physician champion for children with special health care needs may be designated within the practice to facilitate care and communication across the care continuum. A care plan should be developed that includes regularly scheduled follow-up, systematic assessments, and

documentation of achievement of self-management goals. Ideally, physician extenders and case managers are used to relieve physicians of some of the time-intensive visits required to address these predictable needs (5). These case managers may be practice- or hospital-based. In some communities, public health or school nurses may fill or supplement this role. When appropriate, a plan for school reentry should be established.

Successful outcomes require ownership of the treatment plan by the patient/family, primary care physician, specialty physician, and other therapists. In one study, over 50% of admissions to a pediatric intensive care unit for a chronically disabled child were due to either poor decisions by the caregiver or a breakdown in the system of care for the child (6). For most children with chronic illness or disabling conditions, hospitalizations should be viewed as preventable events. For each hospitalization, breakdowns in outpatient care should be identified and remedied.

A well-designed Care Plan is the complex child's passport to a seamless continuum of care. The Care Plan can be generated

Specialists				
Name	Specialty	Clinic/Hospital	Phone	Fax

Medications		
Medicine	Dose	How often

Allergies: Medications and Foods to be avoided and why	
Medication/Food	Why

Procedures and Activities to be avoided and why	
Procedure/Activity	Why

Pharmacy: _____   Phone:_____

Home Care Provider:_____   Phone:_____

Durable Medical Equipment Company: _____Phone:_____
Telehomecare   ☐ Yes   ☐ No

Therapies			
Type	Therapist	Phone	Private (P) or School (S)

FIGURE 128.1. *Continued*

in the primary care physician's office, at the end of a necessary hospitalization, or as an outcome of an evaluation at a clinic designed for comprehensive evaluation and planning for the child with special health care needs, such as the Center for Children with Complex and Chronic Conditions at the Brody School of Medicine (C5). The Care Plan is generated with direct input of the family, patient (when possible), physician, care coordinator, and community service agencies. Our C5 care plan template (Fig. 128.1) will be available at the BSOM website so that area physicians can download the tool for use in their offices in either paper or electronic format. The Care Plan is entered as part of the permanent record, but will be a living document that will change as the child grows or new problems arise.

A Care Plan serves many purposes:

1. It avoids duplication of services and tests, allowing seamless care coordination by all individuals involved in the child's care to be aware of the scope of diagnoses, therapies, and services. Medication errors due to duplication or incorrect dosing can also be avoided.
2. It alerts medical staff unfamiliar with the child's unique aspects of care such as family wishes, traditions, and nicknames that may personalize a potentially traumatic experience

in the ED, Urgent Care Center, or hospital, making it less stressful for the child and family.
3. It relieves the parent/caretaker or older patient from having to repeat past medical history multiple times in medical centers where learners are involved in the care of the patient.
4. It provides valuable and up-to-date information about the special child's medical home, home health providers, therapies and equipment, school teachers, medical subspecialists, and care coordinators.
5. It allows the majority of the complex child's care to be provided within the medical home by linking all aspects of care back to the primary care physician.

As informatics technology advances, we would envision a day when the care plan is placed on an electronic disk, an identification card, or even an embedded computer chip.

Abundant research opportunities are available, including the assessment of the impact of the hospitalist on health care services, involvement in the development and evaluation of inpatient care paths, prospective intervention trials among hospitalized patients, and retrospective reviews of clinical experiences. Research opportunities also exist within the realm of educational interventions.

Education-Evaluation Information				
	Contact Name	Phone	Fax	Effective Dates
Early Intervention				
CDSA				
Childcare				
Preschool				
School				
School Nurse				

Current equipment and assistive technology (please check all that apply and use lines below to explain)

☐ gastrostomy
size:_____

☐ adaptive seating

☐ wheelchair

☐ tracheostomy
size:_____

☐ communication device

☐ orthotics

☐ suction

☐ monitors: _____ apnea _____ O_2

☐ crutches

☐ nebulizer

_____ cardiac _____ glucose

☐ walker

☐ ventilator

☐ urinary catheter   ☐ other: _____
size:_____

_____

_____

☐ See additional information sheet(s) on equipment/assistive technology

Unique Immunization Needs (for full immunization record, see chart)				
Date:				
Influenza				
Pneumococcal				
RSV				
Other				

Prior Surgeries/Procedures		
Surgery/Procedure	Date	Where this was performed

Most recent labs/diagnostic studies		
	Date	Where this was performed
Labs:		
Drug Levels:		
EKG:		
EEG:		
MRI/CT:		

FIGURE 128.1. *Continued*

DEFINITION

Who are the children with disabilities and chronic conditions? More than 200 disabilities and chronic conditions can affect children and adolescents, including asthma, diabetes, cerebral palsy, and spina bifida. A variety of approaches have been used to describe this population, including the diagnosis of a chronic condition and the presence of functional limitations and increased service needs. In general, they are categorized in one of four groups:

1. Children with disabilities (e.g., cerebral palsy).
2. Children with chronic physical illnesses (e.g., diabetes).
3. Children with congenital defects (e.g., cleft lip and palate, congenital heart defect).
4. Children with health-related educational and behavioral problems (e.g., learning disability, attention deficit/hyperactivity disorder).

State and federal Maternal and Child Health Bureau (MCH) programs adopted the phrase *children with special health care needs* to refer to this population (5). A group convened by the MCH developed the following definition of this term:

Children with special health care needs are those who have or are at risk for a physical, developmental, behavioral, or emotional condition and who require health and related services of a type or amount beyond that required by children generally.

In 1987, the U.S. Office of Technology Assistance defined the technology-dependent child as "one who needs both a medical device to compensate for the loss of a vital body function and substantial and ongoing nursing care to avert death or further disability" (6). In an effort to clarify the population considered technology dependent, the U.S. Office of Technology Assistance defined four groups:

1. Ventilator-dependent children.
2. Children requiring prolonged intravenous medications and parenteral nutrition.
3. Children dependent on other device-based respiratory or nutritional support.
4. Children dependent on other medical devices and daily or near daily nursing.

PREVALENCE

Of the children younger than 18 years of age whose families participated in the 1994 National Interview Survey on disability, 18% had a chronic physical, developmental, behavioral, or emotional condition and required more than the usual level

X-Rays:		
Other:		
Other:		

Formula and feeding instructions:

Current needs and Plan of Care:

Review Date No later than:_____Will be reviewed by:_____

Care plan developed by the following members of the health care team:

Patient signature: _____ Date: _____

Parent signature: _____ Date: _____

Staff signature: _____ Date: _____

PCP signature: _____ Date: _____

I give my permission to share the information on the care plan with all of my child's

providers except:_____

Parent/Caregiver signature:_____ Date:_____

FIGURE 128.1. *Continued*

---

of health and related services (7). Approximately 11% of these children were uninsured, and 13% had one or more unmet health care needs in the year before the survey.

SERVICE NEEDS

In general, the service needs of children with disabilities and chronic conditions are complex, costly, and enduring. Services may be provided in all settings of the child's life including home, school, community, region, and nation. Children with disabilities and chronic conditions require 1.5 times more visits to the primary care office, twice the time per visit, 5 to 10 times more hospitalizations, and 2 to 3 times more physician time overall (8). These children manifest twice the number of behavioral problems and miss at least twice the number of school days compared to children without disabilities and chronic conditions.

The care provided to children with disabilities and chronic conditions and their families should be community-based, family-centered, culturally competent, comprehensive, coordinated, and compassionate. Each child is unique, and family members are the experts in managing the care of their child. Families are partners with service provider; they are essential contributors to and participants in all treatment decisions. The family is defined as who the caregiver and patient say they are. Each family has specific strengths that may be called upon to improve the child's care and weaknesses that must be addressed that, without attention, will foil the best treatment

plan. Services are provided in or near these children's home communities when possible, and the system of care honors and respects each family's cultural beliefs, values, and experiences. Curriculum guidelines have been developed for culturally sensitive and competent health care for use in family practice and pediatric residency programs. Table 128.2 presents the likely elements of family-centered care.

Health services for children with disabilities and chronic conditions can be categorized as primary care, secondary care, and tertiary care. A child with a disability or chronic condition is first and foremost a child and has all the acute illnesses and preventive care needs of other children. Children with disabilities and chronic conditions must have access to primary health care through a medical home. The American Academy of Pediatrics' Ad Hoc Task Force of the Medical Home (9) listed the following characteristics of a medical home:

- Provision of preventive care.
- Assurance of ambulatory and inpatient care.
- Provision of care over an extended period of time.
- Identification of the need for subspecialty consultation and referrals.
- Interaction with school and community agencies.
- Maintenance of a central record and database containing all pertinent medical information.

Secondary-level health care refers to the comprehensive management of children with disabilities and chronic conditions by the primary care physician in a medical home, in collaboration with parents and other community service providers and

TABLE 128.2

KEY ELEMENTS OF FAMILY-CENTERED CARE

- Incorporating into policy and practice the recognition that the family is the constant in a child's life, while the service systems and support personnel within those systems fluctuate.
- Facilitating family—professional collaboration at all levels of hospital, home–and community care.
- Exchanging complete and unbiased information between families and professionals in a supportive manner at all times.
- Incorporating into policy and practice the recognition and honoring of cultural diversity, strengths, and individuality within and across all families, including ethnic, racial, spiritual, socioeconomic, educational, and geographic diversity.
- Recognizing and respecting different methods of coping and implementing comprehensive policies and programs that provide developmental, educational, emotional, environmental, and financial supports to meet the diverse needs of families.
- Encouraging and facilitating family-to-family support and networking.
- Ensuring that hospital, home, and community service and support systems for children needing specialized health and developmental care and their families are flexible, accessible, and comprehensive in responding to diverse family-identified needs.
- Appreciating families as families and children as children, recognizing that they possess a wide range of strengths, concerns, emotions, and aspirations beyond their need for specialized health and developmental services and support.

Modified from Nickel RE. Children with disabilities and chronic conditions and their service needs. In: Nickel RE, Desh LW, eds. *The physician's guide to caring for children with disabilities and chronic conditions.* Baltimore: Paul H. Brookes; 2000: 1–14.

medical subspecialists as needed. It requires a commitment by the physician champion and nurse case-manager to serve this population; an expanded knowledge of disabilities and chronic conditions; and changes in office procedures, including the provision of comprehensive care coordination. It can and should be provided by all interested primary care providers. Regrettably, reimbursement by commercial insurers and governmental payers is often woefully inadequate to compensate these individuals for the extraordinary amount of time and skill required to meet the complex needs of these patients and their families. The following set of competencies is needed to provide secondary-level health services:

- Developmental screening and surveillance.
- Diagnosis of the disability or chronic condition (often in conjunction with specialists).
- Development and periodic updates of a management plan.
- Knowledge of education programs and other community services.
- Child and family education, support, and counseling, which should include the provision of written information regarding the condition and community services.
- Care coordination.
- Preparation of the patient and family for transition at an appropriate age to adult care providers.

Tertiary care is provided by pediatric subspecialists. It requires a specific level of knowledge and technology that may only be found at regional medical centers or in children's hospitals.

Children with disabilities and chronic conditions require a wide array of medical and related services:

- Adequate primary and specialty medical and surgical care (inpatient and outpatient).
- Specialized nursing and support services.
- Mental health services.
- Assistive technologies.
- Nutritional counseling and services.
- Specialized dietary products.
- Home health care.
- Palliative care (including hospice care).
- Care coordination.
- Long-term physical and occupational therapy (habilitative and rehabilitative services).
- Long-term speech-language and hearing services.
- Adaptive equipment and supplies.
- Medications.
- Specialized evaluations.
- Enabling services (e.g., transportation to appointments with specialists, respite care).

Pediatricians should advocate for managed care contracts that provide a broad, comprehensive array of services for children with disabilities and chronic conditions. Medical expenses will often require a family to qualify for governmental assistance through Medicaid or Medicare.

Both primary care and specialty care providers require specialized knowledge and experience to serve well children with disabilities and chronic conditions. Specialists must have training and ongoing, regular experience specific to the diagnosis of, treatment of, and procedures for caring for disabled children of specific age groups. Referral to an adult specialist who is untrained or inexperienced in treating children with a particular disability or chronic condition is not recommended. In addition, there is a growing research base for clinical decision-making in all disciplines with regard to providing care to children with disabilities and chronic conditions. Primary care physicians and specialists must participate in relevant continuing education activities to stay current with this information.

In general, it is inappropriate for hospitalists and specialists to provide primary care to children with disabilities and chronic conditions. In a few rare instances, the medical home may be provided by a medical subspecialist who offers specialty and all necessary primary care to the child and family. These subspecialists can enhance the effectiveness of the primary care physician by emphasizing the importance of their role in the care plan continuum.

References

1. Neville B. Tertiary pediatrics needs a disability model. *Arch Dis Child* 2000; 83:35–38.
2. O'Neill C, Cuntole J, Bryan D, et al. Partnership in chronic health care: care management as an integral part of the pediatric hospital system. *J Paediatr Child Health* 1997;33:4–6.
3. Johnson BH, Eichner J. Family-centered care and the pediatrician's role. *Pediatrics* 2003;691–696.
4. Dosa NP, Boeing NM, Kanter RK. Excess risk of severe acute illness in children with chronic health conditions. *Pediatrics* 2001;107:499–504.
5. Farmer JE, Clark MJ, Sherman A, et al. Comprehensive primary care for children with special health care needs in rural areas. *Pediatrics* 2005;116: 649–656.
6. Newacheck PW, Strickland B, Shonkolt JP, et al. An epidemiologic profile of children with special health care needs. *Pediatrics* 1998;102:117–123.
7. U.S. Congress, Office of Technology Assessment. *Technology-dependent children: hospital v. home care—a technical memorandum.* OTA-TM-H-38. Washington, DC: U.S. Government Printing Office; May 1987.
8. Nickel RE. Children with disabilities and chronic conditions and their service needs. In: Nickel RE, Desh LW, eds. *The physician's guide to caring for children with disabilities and chronic conditions.* Baltimore: Paul H. Brookes; 2000:1–14.
9. American Academy of Pediatrics. The medical home. *Pediatrics* 1992;90:774.

CHAPTER 129A ■ SPECIFIC DISORDERS: OBESITY

DAVID N. COLLIER, CARRIE E. WALLER, AND RONALD M. PERKIN

The proportion of children and adolescents who are overweight has tripled in the past three decades. With 1 of every 2 or 3 children in the United States now exceeding a healthy weight, overweight has become the most common chronic medical condition of childhood in the United States and many other countries. As a predisposing factor for the development of type 2 diabetes mellitus, cardiovascular disease, cancer, and other chronic diseases, obesity has been estimated to account for about 117,000 preventable deaths annually and more than $100 billion per year in treatment costs. At current rates of childhood obesity, about 1 of every 3 children born in the United States in 2000 are expected to develop diabetes during their lifetime, foreshadowing an impending public health crisis (1,2).

Obesity is not only an important early risk factor for much of adult morbidity and mortality, but medical problems are common in obese children and adolescents (Table 129.1). These problems can affect cardiovascular health, the endocrine system, and mental health. The pulmonary, musculoskeletal, gastrointestinal, and central nervous systems can also be negatively impacted by excess adiposity. Such problems may directly result in hospitalization, or may complicate the management of the obese child hospitalized for other reasons (3,4). See Table 129.2 for an evaluation of the obese pediatric patient.

Weight Assessment

Body mass index (BMI), defined as weight (kg) divided by height (m)^2, is a convenient means for assessing weight status. Although BMI is not a direct measure of adiposity, it correlates well with more direct measures of adiposity, is correlated with weight-related health risks, tracks into adulthood, and uses measures that are routinely obtained clinically. BMI charts and the rationale for using BMI are readily available at www.cdc.gov.

In adults, overweight is defined as a BMI $\geq$ 25 but < 30, and obesity as a BMI $\geq$ 30. In contrast, the thresholds for defining obesity vary by gender and age in children and adolescents, with a BMI > 85th but < 95th percentile for gender and age considered "at-risk for overweight," while a BMI $\geq$ 95th percentile for gender and age is considered "overweight." *At-risk for overweight* and *overweight* are the preferred terms for discussing weight status with a patient (3). Here the term *obesity* refers to the condition in which BMI > 85th percentile.

Determining a BMI$_{score}$, or the ratio of the actual BMI to a target BMI, is a means of normalizing the raw BMI value so that it can be interpreted without plotting it on a gender-specific chart. This facilitates the comparison of weight status of boys and girls of varying ages as well as tracking an individual's weight status over time. For example, a 5-year-old girl with a BMI of 24 has a BMI$_{score85}$ of 143% (normalized to 16.8 kg/m^2, the value corresponding to the 85th percentile for age and gender, ×100); while a 15-year-old girl with a BMI of 24 kg/m^2 has a BMI$_{score85}$ of 100% (normalized to 24 kg/m^2, the value corresponding to the 85th percentile for a 15 year old girl, ×100).

ENDOCRINE CONSEQUENCES OF OBESITY

Type 2 Diabetes

Type 2 diabetes is being increasingly diagnosed within the pediatric population. Although the exact prevalence is not known, one study has documented a tenfold increase, paralleling the increased prevalence of pediatric obesity. Type 2 diabetes now accounts for as much as one-half of newly diagnosed cases of diabetes in children age 10 to 21 years (5). The mechanism(s) by which excess adiposity, particularly visceral or central adiposity, promotes the development of diabetes is the subject of intensive research. It is now clear that adipose tissue synthesizes and secretes numerous factors, often referred to as adipokines, which can have both direct and indirect effects on peripheral and central tissues. Adiponectin is an example of a circulating adipokine produced exclusively in adipose tissue, but at levels inversely proportional to the degree of adiposity. A major activity of adiponectin is the stimulation of insulin action, as evidenced by improved insulin sensitivity associated with either direct adiponectin administration or the up-regulation of its synthesis by thiazolidinediones (6). Hence an important mechanism for obesity-associated insulin resistance is the decline in adiponectin levels associated with increased adiposity. Other factors, such as decreases in insulin action associated with increased free fatty acid levels that accompany visceral adiposity, also contribute to obesity-related insulin resistance. Diabetes develops once the insulin resistance exceeds the ability of the pancreas to compensate by hypersecretion of insulin (see Chapter 98).

Early signs of insulin resistance such as acanthosis nigricans, a thickened hyperpigmented skin condition found on the neck, axillae, fingers, or groin; or acrochordons (skin tags); warrant further screening including fasting insulin and glucose levels. According to the 2005 standards of the American Diabetes Association, a fasting plasma glucose (FPG) of 100 mg/dL to 125 mg/dL (5.6 mmol/L–6.9 mmol/L) is considered an impaired fasting glucose, while an FPG $\geq$ 126 mg/dL (7.0 mmol/L) is diagnostic of diabetes. The homeostasis model assessment (HOMA) of insulin resistance is a simple and reliable index utilizing fasting insulin and glucose levels ([glucose

TABLE 129.1

HEALTH IMPLICATIONS OF CHILDHOOD OBESITY

System affected	Potential consequences
Metabolic	Insulin resistance, dyslipidemia
Endocrine	Type 2 diabetes mellitus, advanced physical maturation
Reproductive	Polycystic ovary syndrome
Cardiovascular	Hypertension, obesity cardiomyopathy (adipositas cordis), coronary artery disease
Renal	Microalbuminuria, obesity-focal segmental glomerulosclerosis, IgA nephropathy, increased GFR, altered pharmacokinetics
Respiratory	Sleep apnea, obesity hypoventilation syndrome, asthma
Immune	Chronic inflammation
Musculoskeletal	Slipped femoral capital epiphyses, Blount disease, fractures
Gastrointestinal	Cholelithiasis, hepatic disease, gastroesophageal reflux
Psychosocial	Depression, low self-esteem, low quality of life
Neurologic	Idiopathic intracranial hypertension

(mg/dL) $\times$ insulin (μ units/mL)] $\div$ 405) to quantitate insulin resistance and has been validated in obese children and adolescents. Although values greater than 2.5 are indicative of insulin resistance in adults, 3.16 has been proposed as an appropriate cutoff point to define insulin resistance in children and adolescents (7).

Advanced Maturation

Primary obesity is associated with accelerated linear growth rates, advanced bone age, higher bone density, and in girls early menarche. In overweight girls, the onset of puberty is most commonly marked by thelarche, whereas in lean girls, pubarche normally occurs first. In contrast, puberty tends to occur later in obese boys than in lean boys. These pubertal effects are due in large part to the increased production of estrogens that results from the peripheral conversion of androgens to estrogens by aromatase, an enzyme that is located within the adipocyte. Postmenopausal production of estrogens by adipose tissue also predisposes obese women to develop estrogen-dependent breast cancers (8,9).

Polycystic Ovary Syndrome

Polycystic ovary syndrome is a complex disorder characterized by hyperandrogenemia, infertility, hirsutism, and menstrual disturbances that is primarily associated with excess abdominal fat. Adipose tissue produces sex hormones; hence excess adiposity can result in the overproduction of testosterone. Insulin resistance associated with central adiposity also up-regulates production of estrogen by the ovaries and androgens by the adrenal glands. This effect is amplified by an obesity-associated down-regulation of sex hormone–binding globulin that results in excessive concentrations of the free, biologically active fractions of sex hormones.

Weight loss may normalize ovulation in some women and should be an important component of therapy. Metformin has also been shown to restore normal menses in the majority of patients, presumably through restoration of insulin sensitivity. In the hirsute patient who does not desire pregnancy, excess androgen production can be suppressed with oral contraceptives, luteinizing hormone-releasing hormone analogues, or antiandrogens (spironolactone). If the patient is non-hirsute,

TABLE 129.2

EVALUATION OF THE OBESE PEDIATRIC PATIENT

SYMPTOMS TO EVALUATE

Depression or suicidality	Orthopnea
Snoring, apnea, restless sleep	Headaches
Daytime somnolence, inattentiveness	Hirsutism, acne
New-onset/worsening nocturia or enuresis	Cold intolerance
Exercise intolerance	Constipation
Polydipsia, polyuria	Reflux
Abdominal pain	Menstrual irregularities
Joint pains	Skin rashes/lesions
Dyspnea	Developmental delay

IMPORTANT EVALUATION IN PHYSICAL EXAMINATION OF THE OBESE CHILD

Degree of obesity (BMI, BMI$_{score}$) and its distribution (truncal, peripheral, generalized)
Developmental status of the patient
Size of the tonsils in relation to the nasopharynx
Oral exam looking for generalized gingivitis, caries, pus pockets in gums
Thyroid size and consistency
Presence of acanthosis nigricans (hyperpigmented velvety skin in area of neck or axilla)
Presence of any right upper quadrant tenderness
Liver size
Sexual maturity rating (Tanner stage) of genitalia and appropriateness for age
Skin examination for hirsutism, acne, striae, "buffalo hump"
General mood and affect of patient
Gait and musculoskeletal exam

then monthly withdrawal bleeding should be induced to reduce the risk for endometrial neoplasia (4,10).

CARDIOVASCULAR CONSEQUENCES OF OBESITY

Hypertension

Obesity is the most common cause of hypertension in children. The prevalence of elevated blood pressure is approximately 20% to 30% in obese children; and compared to controls, obese children have a 2.4-fold risk for elevated blood pressure. Central (abdominal) adipose distribution is a particularly strong risk factor for elevated blood pressure in children. The risk for obesity-related hypertension tracks into adulthood, with obese adolescents at 8.5-fold to 10.0-fold risk for adulthood hypertension (11,12).

Sleep apnea, a common co-morbidity of obesity (see Chapter 42 and below), is frequently associated with pulmonary hypertension as well as systemic hypertension. These hemodynamic changes can lead to the development of cardiomyopathy with the attendant risk for congestive heart failure, cor pulmonale, and arrhythmias (4,13,14).

Blood pressure should be properly measured and interpreted using age-, gender-, and height-specific standards. If stage 2 hypertension is diagnosed in the hospitalized patient, then an appropriate diagnostic workup and medical intervention should be considered (see Chapter 66). Unless contraindicated, weight loss through physical activity and dietary changes should be recommended for prevention and treatment of hypertension in all obese patients.

Atherosclerosis

Results of the Bogalusa heart study have shown that the formation and extent of atherosclerotic lesions in children are correlated with BMI, blood pressure, smoke exposure, and dyslipidemia (11). As the most common cause of elevated cholesterol and triglycerides in children, obesity contributes to the development of atherosclerotic lesions in childhood, both as an independent risk factor as well as through elevations in blood pressure and lipid derangements. These risk factors have a strong tendency to track from childhood into adulthood (4,15).

Though unlikely to cause overt disease in the child, obesity-related dyslipidemia should be aggressively addressed through dietary intervention, particularly targeting reductions in saturated fat intake (<7% of calories) and cholesterol, as well as increases in dietary fiber and physical activity. If total or LDL cholesterol remain above acceptable levels (Table 129.3), then pharmacologic treatment with niacin or a statin should be considered.

TABLE 129.3

AHA CONSENSUS GUIDELINES FOR DIAGNOSIS OF DYSLIPIDEMIA IN CHILDREN

Component	Borderline (mg/dL)	Abnormal (mg/dL)
Total cholesterol	170–199	≥200
LDL cholesterol	100–129	≥130
HDL cholesterol		<40
Triglycerides		≥200

Adipositas Cordis

In addition to the structural changes induced by the altered hemodynamics associated with obesity, obesity is associated with the formation of fatty infiltrates that accumulate as cords of fat cells between the cardiac myocytes. These cords result in myocyte degeneration and defects in cardiac conduction. Like atherosclerosis, this process may not cause overt disease in the pediatric patient, but is likely initiated during childhood.

RESPIRATORY CONSEQUENCES OF OBESITY

Sleep-Disordered Breathing

The association between obesity and disturbed breathing during sleep in children has been recognized since Charles Dickens described in *Pickwick Papers* the messenger boy Joe, who was overweight , snored loudly, had excessive daytime sleepiness, and heart failure. In 1956, Burwell and associates coined the term *Pickwickian syndrome* for patients with extreme obesity and alveolar hypoventilation. The syndrome of obstructive sleep apnea (OSA), characterized by periods of repeated partial or complete airway collapse and increased airway resistance during sleep, is also included in the spectrum of sleep-disordered breathing (SDB).

In cross-sectional studies of adults, obesity has been shown to be a significant risk factor for OSA. Prospective studies have shown that a 10% weight gain over a 4-year period is associated with a six-fold increase in the odds of developing SDB. The relationship between weight gain and SDB risk is essentially a linear dose–response curve, with a 3% increase in the apnea–hypopnea index (AHI; defined as number of apnea and hypopnea events per hour) associated with every 1% increase in weight. This graded risk indicates that SDB is not a complication found exclusively in the morbidly obese patient (16,17).

Obese adult subjects with SDB have an increase in the size of the tongue, soft palate, and lateral pharyngeal walls. The degree of severity of SDB expressed as the AHI is positively correlated with the volume of adipose tissue adjacent to the pharyngeal airway. Specifically, obese subjects with SDB have large deposits of fat in the posterior and lateral aspects of the oropharyngeal airspace at the level of the soft palate. A result of these abnormalities is that obese subjects are more likely to have obstruction of their airway at the level of the velopharynx rather than at the level of the velopharynx and oropharynx, as is the case of subjects with OSA due to craniofacial abnormalities (18).

The risk of SDB is four to five times higher in obese children than in non-obese children. Although assessment of airway structures and dynamics in obese children with SDB has not been fully investigated, it is likely that obesity in children is associated with the same types of structural changes as those observed in obese adults. Such structural effects may pose an even greater risk for SDB in children, because their lymphoid tissues are proportionally larger and their airway structures relatively smaller than adults and hence more prone to obstruction (19).

Current knowledge suggests that there is a closed, feed-forward loop between SDB and obesity whereby the initial development of obesity might contribute to SDB by physical factors promoting airway obstruction during sleep, with poor sleep in turn promoting the development of obesity through hormonal effects. The observation that short sleep duration is associated with elevated ghrelin (an orexigenic incretin produced in the stomach), reduced leptin (anorexigenic adipokine), and increased BMI provides a plausible mechanism (20), as does the observation that SDB in obese patients is associated with higher levels of insulin and insulin resistance (21). Obstructive sleep apnea, with carbon dioxide retention and hypoxia, may lead to (1) pulmonary hypertension with associated right-ventricular (RV) hypertrophy, RV failure, and possibly pulmonary embolism; (2) systemic hypertension and associated left-ventricular hypertrophy and its consequences; (3) polycythemia and sludging syndromes; (4) nocturnal enuresis; and (5) behavioral problems including daytime somnolence, irritability, inattentiveness, hyperactivity, poor school performance, and neurocognitive defects (22). Hence the consequences of SDB may require hospitalization to manage, or may complicate the overall management of the hospitalized patient.

When compared to evaluation by overnight polysomnography (PSG or sleep study), elements of the clinical evaluation are of low specificity and only moderately high sensitivity for diagnosing OSA (Table 129.4) (23). However, parents or other caregivers should be asked if the patient snores habitually, is a mouth breather or a noisy breather, if the caregiver has witnessed apnea, or if the patient experiences severe daytime somnolence, inattentiveness, or behavioral problems. Assessment of nasal passage patentcy, and inspection of the oropharynx for tonsil size, the presence of redundant soft palate tissue, enlarged uvula, micrognatha, macroglossia, retroglossia, or other structural features that may obstruct air flow, should be performed. Because OSA is associated with systemic hypertension in children, a high index of suspicion should be maintained for OSA in the obese hypertensive child (14). Although not sufficient for making a diagnosis, repeated nocturnal blood oxygen desaturations detected by pulse oximetry in the hospitalized patient is also evidence of OSA.

A sleep study should be obtained for all children and adolescents with a history suspicious for SDB. In most circumstances this can be obtained on an outpatient basis. However, urgent inpatient consultation with a sleep specialist (neurologist, pulmonologist, intensivist) or an otolaryngologist to determine if immediate initiation of continous positive airway pressure/bilevel positive airway pressure (CPAP/BiPAP) is warranted or if urgent surgical therapy is required to relieve airway restriction. Although not a substitute for definitive treatment, short courses (6–24 weeks) of topical glucocorticoid nasal sprays such as fluticasone proprionate and beclomethasone can significantly reduce the severity of apnea, particularly in the obese patient with adenotonsillar hypertrophy and/or allergic rhinitis (24). In case studies nasal budesonide was

shown to not only improve snoring and polysomnography findings, but also to completely resolve nocturnal enuresis associated with mild obstructive SDB (25). In contrast, oral corticosteroids have not proven to be useful for treating sleep apnea associated with adenotonsillar hypertrophy. Treatment of OSA in obese children with enlarged lymphoid tissues by tonsillectomy and/or adenoidectomy will improve the OSA but may not help with weight reduction and may even exacerbate the obesity. When OSA complicates obesity, attention must be paid to reducing weight by such measures as exercise, diet, and behavior therapy, in addition to treatment of the OSA.

Asthma

The increasing prevalence of asthma has coincided with an increase in the number of both children and adults who are overweight. Furthermore, high BMI is associated with an increased risk of asthma, with relative risk of asthma in the highest BMI quartiles ranging from 1.6 to 3.0 times that in the normal weight category (26).

The association between high BMI and asthmatic symptoms could be due to a variety of factors, such as low physical activity, dietary factors such as increased trans-fat, hormonal influence, immune modification, and/or mechanical factors. Bronchoscopy reveals that fat deposition in the chest wall frequently results in narrowing of the airways, a widening of the bifurcation at the carina, and a loss of cartilage ring definition in obese patients. Low physical activity is clearly associated with being overweight and the reduction in deep breathing associated with a sedentary lifestyle may lead to a "latching state" of airway smooth muscle, and in turn to airway obstruction and hyperreactivity. Whether being overweight causes asthma symptoms through low physical activity, or whether asthma symptoms result in avoidance of exercise, which then leads to weight gain, cannot be determined from cross-sectional studies. However, several prospective studies indicate that high BMI appears to be a risk factor for the future development of asthma. Consistent with the contention that there is a causal relationship between obesity and asthma, airway obstruction and peak expiratory flow variability in obese asthmatics were improved after moderate weight loss (26,27).

Airway Management

Obesity is associated with physiologic and anatomic derangements that place the obese patient at greater risk for requiring endotracheal intubation to manage his airway, as well as render placement of the endotracheal tube more difficult. First, there can be a decrease in chest wall and diaphragmatic excursion secondary to fat deposits over the chest and abdomen that leads to decreased pulmonary compliance and increased work of breathing and oxygen requirement. This is reflected in the tendency of morbidly obese patients to desaturate more quickly than non-obese patients. Second, decreased lung volume, increased airway resistance, and reduced total respiratory volume frequently results in decreased tidal volume, alveolar hypoventilation, hypoxia, and hypercapnia. This process is exacerbated by the tendency of obese patients to experience some ventilation–perfusion (VP) mismatch (perfuse lower pulmonary segments while preferentially ventilating upper segments). Obesity-related VP mismatch is exacerbated in the supine position. Third, the larger volume of gastric fluid, increased intra-abdominal pressure, and higher incidence of gastroesophageal reflux associated with obesity increases the risk of aspiration in this patient population. Finally, reduced pulmonary compliance, increased chest wall and airway resistance, and abnormal diaphragmatic position makes bag-valve-mask ventilation of the obese patient more difficult. Sedation,

TABLE 129.4

SENSITIVITY AND SPECIFICITY[a] OF COMPONENTS OF CLINICAL EVALUATION FOR DIAGNOSING OBSTRUCTIVE SLEEP APNEA

Characteristic	Sensitivity (%)	Specificity (%)
Snores nightly	44–97	4–58
Witnessed apnea	47–88	17–90
Mouth-breathing	29–78	27–56
Severe daytime somnolence	20–61	0–92
Tonsil size greater than 3+	12–93	35–89

[a]Compared to OSA diagnosed by polysomnography.
Adapted from Brietzke SE, Katz ES, Roberson DW. Can history and physical exam reliably diagnose pediatric obstructive sleep apnea/hypopnea syndrome? A systematic review of the literature. *Otolarngol Head Neck Surg* 2004;131:827–832.

paralysis, or placement in the supine position can markedly exacerbate these pulmonary function changes (28–30).

Fatty infiltration of muscles and subcutaneous fat deposits may exert anteroposterior and lateral forces on regional structures in the neck that can narrow the upper aerodigestive tract and increase the risk of a difficult intubation by blocking the view of the glottis and other laryngeal structures (29). In an awake spontaneously breathing patient, the Mallampati scale, an objective measure of the pharyngeal structures visible with the patient's mouth wide open, can be helpful in predicting the likelihood of a difficult oral intubation. Limited neck mobility, limited mouth opening, and micrognathia are other potential predictors of a difficult intubation.

Prior to intubation, preoxygenation should be maximized by allowing the patient to sit upright or semirecumbent for as long as possible (minimizes VP mismatch). Monitoring blood oxygen saturation with the pulse oximeter probe on the finger may be unreliable due to excessive tissue thickness on the fingers. Placement on the ear, which has less tissue and is well perfused, may prove more reliable (28). Many obese patients have marked thoraco-cervical lipodystrophy ("buffalo hump") that can cause hyperextension of the neck and compression of the upper airway when in a supine or even a semirecumbent position. Hence positioning the patient in the appropriate sniffing position in preparation for intubation may require the placement of towels under the head, rather than under the back as is often required with smaller children in whom the occiput is relatively large.

Children with Down syndrome are frequently obese and represent a special subset of obese patients who are at increased risk for obstruction secondary to associated problems of micrognathia, macroglossia, midfacial hypoplasia, and hypotonia. Because 10% of patients with Down syndrome have atlantoaxial instability, assessment with flexion-extension neck radiography prior to elective intubation is indicated.

Once intubated and on positive pressure ventilation, ideal body weight should be used to calculate initial tidal volume, because use of the patient's actual weight may result in excessive peak airway pressure and overdistention of the alveoli. Changes in tidal volume, peak airway pressures, and ventilator rate should be guided by arterial blood gases. Arterial oxygenation and respiratory compliance may be improved by placing the patient in the prone position, or by the addition of positive end-expiratory pressure (PEEP) (28,29).

MEDICATIONS

Obesity can influence the pharmacokinetics of drug metabolism in complex and often unpredictable ways. For example, the increased glomerular filtration rate in obese patients with normal kidneys is associated with increased clearance of compounds eliminated by the kidney. In contrast, the increasingly prevalent forms of obesity-mediated renal failure (see below) decrease clearance. Changes in hepatic metabolism associated with obesity also have variable effects on different drugs (28,31,32).

A common problem is deciding if total body weight (TBW), ideal body weight (IBW), or a hybrid of these two values is appropriate for calculating drug dosages. Ideally, such decisions would be based on clinical research data for the drug of interest in obese subjects. Such data are scarce for obese adults and virtually nonexistent for obese pediatric patients. In lieu of such data, a generally useful approach is to determine the loading dose of lipophilic drugs based on TBW, and the loading dose of hydrophilic drugs based on IBW or dosing weight (DW). The formula for DW can vary for different drugs, but is calculated empirically as IBW + X(TBW − IBW), where X is usually between 0.3 and 0.4, reflecting the fact that about 30% of adipose tissue is water. Suggested dosing strategies for selected drugs are shown in Table 129.5. These dosing strategies do not supplant the need for frequent evaluation of clinical response, determination of drug levels where necessary, and monitoring for signs of toxicity (28,32).

CHRONIC INFLAMMATORY STATE

It is well known that obesity has an impact on the traditional risk factors for the development of cardiovascular disease (CVD)—hypertension, lipid abnormalities, and diabetes. However, it appears to promote CVD independent of these effects, and the American Heart Association has declared that obesity is a major independent risk factor for CVD. Although the mechanism(s) by which obesity promotes CVD independent of traditional risk factors is not yet elucidated, the production of cytokines by adipocytes, particularly by centrally located (visceral) adipocytes, promotes a chronic inflammatory

---

TABLE 129.5

DOSING GUIDELINES FOR OBESE PATIENTS

Medication	Loading dose	Maintenance dose
Succinylcholine	TBW	N/A
Vecuromium	IBW	IBW
Benzodiazepine	TBW	IBW
Phenobarbital	TBW	IBW
Propofol	IBW + (0.4 × TBW)	6 mg/kg/hr
Ketamine	IBW	IBW
Morphine	IBW	IBW
Fentanyl	TBW	0.8 × IBW
Methylprednisolone	IBW	IBW
Phenytoin	IBW + (1.33 × TBW − IBW)	IBW
Propranolol	IBW	IBW
Lidocaine	TBW	IBW

IBW, ideal body weight ($2.396e^{0.01863}$ × height in cm); TBW, total body weight.
Adapted from Brunette DO. Resuscitation of the morbidly obese patient. *Am J Emerg Med* 2004;22:40–47.

state characterized by overproduction of tumor necrosis factor-α (TNF-α). TNF-α promotes the release of interleukin-6, which in turn stimulates the production of acute-phase reactants such as C-reactive protein (CRP) by the liver. Elevated CRP is now recognized as an independent risk factor for CVD. Hence inflammation associated with obesity contributes to the link between obesity and CVD (33,34).

PERIODONTAL DISEASE

In adults, obesity has been shown to be a predictor of periodontal disease and it appears that this relationship is mediated through obesity-related insulin resistance (35). In turn, the inflammation associated with periodontal disease can exacerbate insulin resistance associated with obesity-mediated inflammation, resulting in significant insulin resistance. This contention is bolstered by a series of elegant studies demonstrating that when the levels of inflammatory cytokines in type 2 diabetics with periodontal disease are reduced via aggressive treatment of their periodontal disease, insulin resistance declines, as reflected by significant improvements in HgA1c levels (without changing the medical management) (36). Hence the highly inflammatory nature of periodontal disease appears to contribute to insulin resistance by augmenting the levels of cytokines that are already elevated by excess adiposity. Periodontal disease likely plays an important role in the development of frank type 2 diabetes in many obese individuals. Although it is not yet know what role periodontal disease plays in the pathophysiology of obesity-related co-morbidities in children and adolescents, poor oral health is common in children in many areas, and a complete physical exam of the hospitalized obese child should include an evaluation of the teeth and gums looking for caries, gingivitis, abscesses, and pus pockets. This is particularly important in an obese patient presenting with diabetic ketoacidosis, where a cryptic infection can further reduce insulin sensitivity sufficiently to precipitate hyperglycemia.

ORTHOPEDIC CONSEQUENCES OF OBESITY

Overweight children and adolescents are four times as likely to have musculoskeletal (MSK) pain and to experience significant restrictions in mobility than are children with BMI values between the 5th and 95th percentiles. Overweight is also associated with about a four-fold increase in the prevalence of malalignment of the lower-extremity joints. These observations suggest a mutually reinforcing relationship between pre-existing joint malalignment or MSK pain and weight gain, where MSK deficits result in decreased physical activity and hence weight gain, and excessive weight gain exacerbates or creates MSK problems that in turn promote sedentary behaviors and further weight gain. An exercise program involving swimming or biking to minimize lower extremity joint loading, or an exercise prescription obtained from a physical therapist or other trained specialist, should be considered for obese children with MSK complaints and/or children who are extremely obese (37).

Although obese children have higher bone mineral density than lean children (8), the greater forces generated by falls in obese children, even from low heights, result in a significantly higher rate of fractures in obese children (odds ratio 4.5) (37). Idiopathic tibia vara or Blount disease and slipped capital femoral epiphysis (SCFE) are also serious orthopedic complications that are overrepresented in obese children (37,38). The varus deformity of Blount disease is the result of decreased growth of the posteromedial aspect of the proximal tibial physis

and the concomitant medial angulation and internal rotation of the proximal tibia. The infantile form, presenting between 2 and 4 years of age, is the most common form and accounts for about 1% of all bowed legs. This form is more common in girls, is usually associated with a history of early walking and early childhood overweight, and is characterized by significant lower extremity bowing, little pain, and is usually bilateral. The adolescent form, generally presenting between ages 6 and 18, is much less common, is more prevalent in boys, and is characterized by significant knee pain, scant bowing, and may be unilateral. The differential diagnosis includes hypophosphatemic rickets, normal physiologic bowing, trauma, osteochondroma, and cartilaginous dysplasias. Evaluation should include laboratory studies to rule out rickets and standing anteroposterior radiographs of the legs to evaluate the mechanical axis of the leg and the tibiofemoral angle. A tibial metaphyseal–diaphyseal angle in excess of 15 degrees is significant for Blount disease. The presence of a medial physis bar indicating fusion of the metaphysis and epiphysis is associated with more advanced disease. An orthopedic consultation should be obtained to determine if bracing, osteotomy, and/or complete closure of the proximal tibial physis is warranted.

Slipped capital femoral epiphysis (SCFE) occurs when "slippage" across the femoral physis allows the femoral head to be displaced relative to the femoral metaphysis. SCFE is the most common hip disorder of adolescence, and if undetected and untreated can have severe long-term consequences resulting from osteonecrosis of the femoral head and severe degenerative joint disease. SCFE can be classified as either atypical or idiopathic. Atypical SCFE is associated with endocrinopathies such as hypothyroidism, metabolic disorders such as renal osteodystrophy, or a history of radiation or chemotherapy. Idiopathic SCFE is the more common form, and typically presents in pubertal youth (girls 10–14, boys 10–16) during the growth spurt when growth hormone levels are relatively high. Growth hormone reduces the strength of the physis; hence this is a period when adolescents are particularly susceptible to growth plate injuries. Though not limited to overweight children, more than 80% of children diagnosed with idiopathic SCFE have a BMI greater than the 85th percentile (38).

Symptoms of SCFE include pain in the groin, thigh or knee. Decreased internal rotation of the affected hip, maintaining the affected hip in an externally rotated position, and limp or other gait abnormality are typical signs. The differential diagnosis includes Perthes disease, femur fracture, and septic joint. Anteroposterior and lateral radiographs of the hips should be obtained and evaluated for an apparent varus angulation of the epiphysis on the femoral neck, widening of the physis or other radiographic abnormalities. Immediate management of the patient with diagnosed or suspected SCFE should include complete avoidance of weight-bearing and urgent orthopedic consultation to confirm the diagnosis and stabilize the femoral head if necessary.

GASTROINTESTINAL CONSEQUENCES OF OBESITY

Nonalcoholic Fatty Liver Disease

Nonalcoholic fatty liver disease (NAFLD) is thought to be the most common liver disease of childhood. It is characterized histologically by the accumulation of large droplets of fat within hepatocytes, the proliferation of inflammatory cells within the liver parenchyma, and in some cases hepatic fibrosis and cirrhosis. The high lipid levels result in the production of lipid peroxides and oxygen free radicals that induce the production of proinflammatory cytokines with resulting inflammation and fibrosis. Obesity, and in particular obesity-associated insulin resistance, are strong risk factors for NAFLD in children, with 10% to 16% of obese children having elevated aminotransaminases, 35% having histologic evidence of steatosis or steatohepatitis, and 50% with sonographic evidence of steatosis. Gender and race both influence the prevalence of NAFLD (boys > girls, Hispanic > Caucasian > African American) (39). NAFLD will eventually progress to cirrhosis in about 15% of cases with the attendant risk of portal hypertension and necessity of liver transplant (40).

NAFLD usually presents silently and is therefore underdiagnosed. About 50% of children with NAFLD have hepatomegaly, but the habitus of the obese child renders detection challenging (40). Transaminases may be elevated two- to five-fold, usually with ALT levels exceeding AST levels. Alkaline phosphatase, albumin, bilirubin, and prothrombin time remain normal in NAFLD, and when normal help rule out other causes of steatohepatitis. Normal transaminase levels do not rule out NAFLD, as many children with normal ALT and AST levels have sonographic evidence of NAFLD (39). However, compared to liver biopsy, even ultrasonography has only 67% sensitivity and 77% specificity (41).

The treatment of choice for NAFLD is weight loss through diet and physical activity. Small clinical trials also support the use of the insulin sensitizer metformin (500 mg twice daily) and the antioxidant vitamin E (400 to 1,200 IU/day). Treatment with metformin improves both steatosis and liver enzyme levels without significant weight loss, while vitamin E reduces liver enzyme levels without reducing liver echogenicity. The efficacy of ursodeoxycholic acid is uncertain (39,42).

Cholelithiasis

Cholelithiasis occurs with increased frequency among obese adults and paradoxically may occur even more frequently with weight reduction. Increased cholesterol synthesis and cholesterol saturation of bile occurs in obesity. Although gallstones are a less frequent occurrence among obese children and adolescents than adults, almost 50% of cases of cholecystitis in adolescents may be associated with obesity. Furthermore, as in adults, cholelithiasis in adolescents may be associated with weight reduction. Cholelithiasis should be high on the differential diagnosis of the obese pediatric patient presenting with right upper quadrant pain, particularly if pain is recurrent, colicky, or radiates to the right scapula or there is associated intolerance of fatty foods. Ultrasonography is the best imaging modality for diagnosis of cholelithiasis.

RENAL CONSEQUENCES OF OBESITY

Obesity is an independent risk factor for developing renal disease, including IgA nephropathy as well as an obesity-related form of focal segmental glomerulosclerosis (O-FSGS) that is distinct from idiopathic FSGS. With the rise in the prevalence of obesity, the prevalence of O-FSGS has increased ten-fold (43). Obesity also induces functional abnormalities including increased renal blood flow, increased glomerulofiltration rate, and microalbuminuria. These effects are due in part to both direct effects of adipokines such as leptin on the kidney, as well as indirect effects mediated by adipokine stimulation of the sympathetic nervous system (31).

Renal function should be carefully evaluated in the obese hospital patient, particularly if medications excreted by the kidneys are to be used (see Chapter 61). Angiotensin-converting enzyme (ACE) inhibitors may reduce the risk of progression to renal failure associated with obesity-hypertension and should be considered a first-line therapy for the obese hypertensive patient requiring treatment with antihypertensive medications (31). Because ACE inhibitors are contraindicated in pregnancy, any female of child-bearing age using an ACE inhibitor should be using reliable contraception. Fortunately modest weight loss results in a significant reduction in proteinuria caused by various chronic renal diseases.

PSYCHOSOCIAL CONSEQUENCES OF OBESITY

Obese children are at significantly higher risk than normal weight children for experiencing poor psychological well-being, including low self-esteem, depression, and low health-related quality-of-life (QOL) scores (44–46). In fact, obese children have QOL scores similar to those of children diagnosed with cancer and receiving chemotherapy. The extent of obesity, as determined by BMI Z score (Z score indicates the number of standard deviations from the mean), and QOL scores are inversely correlated, and obese children with symptomatic co-morbidities such as obstructive sleep apnea or orthopedic complications have significantly lower QOL scores than obese children without complications (47).

Studies demonstrating a correlation between obesity and psychological complications are generally cross-sectional in nature, and therefore cannot determine if depression is a consequence of obesity, of if depression predisposes to obesity, although there is strong evidence that schizophrenia and bipolar disorder are independent risk factors for obesity. Regardless of the causal relationship, restoring the obese child to good health requires that psychological co-morbidities are identified and addressed. Hence a psychological evaluation utilizing age-appropriate screening instruments, such as the PedsQL, Beck Depression Inventory, or Child Behavior Checklist, or consultation with a clinical psychologist or other mental health professional, should be considered for the hospitalized obese patient. Finally, certain psychotrophic medications, such as the second-generation antipsychotics, promote excessive weight gain, hyperglycemia, and dyslipidemia (clozapine, olanzapine, quetiapine > risperidone > amisulpride), while others such as fluoxetine and buproprion are associated with small but statistically significant weight loss. Hence when possible, the bariatric side effects should be considered when choosing medications for treatment of depression, bipolar disorder, mania, or schizophrenia (48).

IDIOPATHIC INTRACRANIAL HYPERTENSION

Idiopathic intracranial hypertension (IIH), also known as pseudotumor cerebri, is a disorder associated with increased intracranial pressure (ICP). The most common symptoms are headaches, transient visual obscuration, vomiting, and diplopia. Less common symptoms include pulsatile tinnitus, somnolence, or other vague complaints such as shoulder pain. Headaches, which are the most common presenting complaint, can be attributed to IIH if they develop in close temporal proximity to increased ICP and have at least one of the following features: occur daily, are diffuse and/or constant nonpulsating, or are worsened by straining or coughing. These headaches are typically unresponsive to standard therapy (49,50)

Obesity and female gender are strong risk factors for IIH in adults (49). In young children, IIH is rare, and displays neither a marked gender preference nor a close association with obesity. However, in pubertal adolescents the majority of cases are associated with obesity (50). It is currently unclear how obesity promotes IIH.

The diagnosis of IIH is a diagnosis of exclusion and requires that appropriate clinical, laboratory, and radiographic studies have ruled out intracranial or systemic pathology including cerebral venous sinus thrombosis, AV malformations, neoplasms, infections, coagulation disorders, sleep apnea, and other hypoventilation syndromes. A thorough fundoscopic exam, including fundus photography and perimetry to detect papilloedema and differentiate it from pseudopapilloedema, should be performed. MRI with magnetic resonance venography should be obtained, and if normal, then opening lumbar CSF pressures determined and CSF sent for appropriate studies. Opening pressures of ≥ 200 mm H_2O in a nonobese patient, or ≥ 250 mm H_2O in an obese patient, are consistent with this diagnosis (49). Tonsillar herniation during LP may complicate the evaluation (50).

Treatment of IIH is centered on reducing ICP through serial LP and/or inhibition of CSF production with the carbonic anhydrase inhibitor acetazolamide. Weight loss is also effective at lowering ICP, and therefore aggressive lifestyle interventions based on medical nutrition therapy and physical activity should be implemented with the assistance of professional nutritionists and exercise counselors (49). Oral corticosteroids may be indicated for the short-term treatment of severe cases, but the potential for side effects, including exuberant weight gain, preclude their long-term use. With a timely diagnosis, most children respond favorably to treatment with complete resolution of symptoms and no long-term sequelae (50). However, close ophthalmic follow-up following resolution of symptoms is prudent.

SUMMARY

Over the past two to three decades obesity has emerged as the most common chronic medical condition of childhood. Changes in lifestyle have led to significant reductions in the energy expenditure of children and have encouraged overconsumption of calorie-dense but nutrient-poor foods. The resultant positive energy balance, coupled with an individual's genetic and/or epigenetic predisposition (influence of intrauterine exposures on the lifelong propensity to develop obesity, insulin resistance, and hypertension), are thought to be major factors driving this epidemic.

Like exposure to tobacco smoke, obesity should be recognized as an important risk factor contributing to the morbidity and mortality of the hospitalized pediatric patient. Obesity and its co-morbidities should be screened for, and when identified, included on the problem list. And just as initiation of smoking cessation is now considered an integral component of care for the hospitalized patient who smokes, efforts to address a patient's obesity problem should be initiated in the hospital. Finally, extreme care should be exercised to prevent the development of iatrogenic obesity in chronically ill, technologically dependent children who may be unable to naturally regulate their energy balance because they are nonambulatory, are tube fed, or are receiving total parenteral nutrition.

PEARLS

- Obese children with normal or accelerated linear growth trajectory most likely have primary obesity, not obesity due to a rare genetic or metabolic cause.
- Striae and buffalo hump are common physical findings in obese adolescents and are rarely associated with Cushing disease or syndrome (especially if linear growth is normal)
- Acanthosis nigricans is frequently associated with hyperinsulinemia/insulin resistance.
- Obese patients with hypertension are much more likely to have sleep-disordered breathing (apnea) than normotensive obese patients.

CHAPTER 129B ■ SPECIFIC DISORDERS: CEREBRAL PALSY

DANIEL P. MOORE AND LAURA E. PETER

DEFINITION

Cerebral palsy (CP) is a descriptive term that identifies children with static encephalopathy. It involves insult to the immature brain, and results in alterations in muscle tone, deep tendon reflexes, primitive reflexes, and postural reactions (51). Although gross motor abnormalities are considered prerequisite, there are other impairments (e.g., gastroesophageal reflux, mental retardation, recurrent otitis media, seizures, strabismus) associated with this central nervous system (CNS) disorder (52,53). It is a diagnosis that is made primarily by clinical assessment. Despite all the technology available, the history and physical examination are mandatory to make the diagnosis. Technology is more helpful to exclude other disorders. Survival of most of these children into adulthood requires an understanding and willingness of health care providers to treat and provide education about and to this patient population.

Classification of CP has been difficult because of the wide variations in the clinical presentation. Historically, a neurologic system was used, but more recently a functional system has grown in popularity. Children with CP can be placed initially into two groups, spastic (pyramidal) or nonspastic (extrapyramidal; Table 129.6). Although this appears to be an easy system to use, in the clinical setting there often is crossover between the groups, and classification is based on the distribution and abnormal tone of the extremities. A child with greater spasticity in the lower than the upper extremities and relatively intact cognition may be classified as having spastic diplegic CP. Children with involvement of the ipsilateral arm and leg would be classified as having hemiplegic CP, and those with four-extremity involvement as having spastic quadriplegic CP. Classifications

TABLE 129.6

TOPOGRAPHIC CLASSIFICATION OF CEREBRAL PALSY

	Clinical	Associated findings
PYRAMIDAL/SPASTIC		
Spastic monoplegia	Single extremity	Rare, usually hemiplegia misdiagnosed
Spastic hemiplegia	Arm and leg, one side	Congenital, unilateral lesion, seizures, shortened limb(s), sensory impairment
Spastic diplegia	Legs > arms	Common in prematurity, intraventricular hemorrhage, periventricular leukomalacia
Spastic triplegia	Three extremities	More involved child
Spastic quadriplegia	Four extremities	Most severely involved child, seizures, cognitive impairment
EXTRAPYRAMIDAL/DYSKINETIC		
Ataxia	Uncoordinated	Hyperbilirubinemia, sensorineural loss
Athetoid	Slow, writhing	Increases with emotion or activity
Choreiform	Abrupt, irregular	
Choreoathetoid	Combination	Visual and auditory disturbances
Dystonic	Slow, rhythmic	

in children with extrapyramidal or nonspastic CP include choreiform, athetoid, and ataxic CP. There can be a mixture of spastic and nonspastic, or crossover, within a group. Also, although CP is a static encephalopathy, the results of clinical examination may vary considerably during the course of the day based on factors including environment and condition of the child at the time of the exam, thus making classification more difficult.

EPIDEMIOLOGY

Epidemiologic information varies and is influenced by the population and survey team. Variation in definitions, severity of findings, and exclusion criteria complicate the data. Studies in a number of developed countries have a prevalence of 1.2 to 2.5 per 1,000 children of early school age (54,55). Cerebral palsy has been noted to be more common in boys, African Americans, and in infants born to women older than 40 years of age or teenage mothers (56,57). Because the diagnosis is arrived at by physical examination, interpractitioner variability must be considered. Also, with improved neonatal care, the incidence of CP may change. Improving the survival rate of premature infants may result in a greater number of children with CP (58–60).

ETIOLOGY

The injury to the brain is often classified by the period in which the injury likely occurred, including the prenatal, perinatal, or postnatal periods (Table 129.7) (61). Most CP is thought to be prenatal in origin, although a percentage of CP cases have an unknown origin (53). In the past, many children with CP were thought to have a brain insult in the immediate perinatal period. However, when investigated thoroughly, risk factors often were found to be present before birth. This is especially true in children born with CP at term (55). The major known risk factor for CP is low birthweight. A significant number of children with CP have birthweights under 2,500 g (62). Although survival of preterm infants has improved, the prevention of preterm birth has not changed as significantly. There are multiple other risk factors associated with CP, some of which are listed in Table 129.8 (53).

PATHOPHYSIOLOGY

The pathophysiology of CP is as variable as its etiologies. Patients with similar brain lesions by modern imaging techniques still may have different clinical presentations. Cerebral palsy is most commonly associated with prematurity. Intraventricular hemorrhages (IVH) are common in the premature newborn and are thought to be related to the fragility of the vasculature in the premature neonate, especially in the region of the germinal matrix. A classification of IVH has been developed to assist in grading its severity (63). Bleeding into the germinal matrix is considered a grade I hemorrhage; bleeding into the ventricle, grade II; subsequent enlargement of the ventricles, grade III; and bleeding into the parenchyma, grade IV. This classification has some prognostic value (64). Brain lesions associated with CP can be divided into three main groups: (1) cerebral malformation, which occurs early in fetal development; (2) periventricular lesion, which occurs in the most vulnerable part of the brain between 24 and 32 weeks gestational age; and (3) cortical/subcortical lesions, which occur in areas of the brain that are most vulnerable at term (65).

DIFFERENTIAL DIAGNOSIS

The differential diagnosis of CP is extensive. Other CNS, peripheral nervous system, metabolic, and genetic disorders are included in the differential diagnosis. The history and physical examination are important, along with early ultrasonography, if IVH is suspected, to confirm the diagnosis. Often the diagnosis cannot be made at birth, even if there is evidence of a CNS abnormality, because the physical examination must show evidence of a gross motor delay that is not progressive. The gross motor skills available to evaluate the newborn child with suspected CP are limited; therefore serial examinations are performed over ensuing months to determine if a persistent motor delay is present. Neuromotor deficits manifest themselves as the child grows because additional gross motor skills are not met as the child develops. In some cases, the diagnosis can be made as early as 6 months via observation of primitive reflexes. Most cases should be diagnosed by 18 months of age.

TABLE 129.7

MRI ABNORMALITIES IN CHILDREN WITH CEREBRAL PALSY BASED ON PRETERM, TERM, AND POSTNATAL ONSET OF INSULT

Abnormalities	Preterm (n = 335)	Term (n = 272)	Postnatal (n = 29)
ACQUIRED LESIONS	261	178	22
PVL with other areas of injury	227	45	—
Diffuse encephalopathy (cortical/subcortical atrophy/ ventriculomegaly)	14	71	—
Focal ischemic/hemorrhagic (e.g., infarct porencephaly)	14	52	10
Multicystic encephalomalacia	3	10	—
Trauma (at birth or later)	0	0	4
Infection	3	0	8
MALFORMATIONS[a]	48	55	0
Cortical dysplasia/polymicrogyria	8	18	—
Schizencephaly	6	11	—
Pachygyria/lissencephaly	5	9	—
Complex brain malformation	22	6	0
Agenesis/hypoplasia of the corpus callosum	3	3	—
Arachnoid cyst	1	0	—
Vermian/cerebellar hypoplasia	1	2	—
Hydrocephalus/holoprosencephaly/ hydraencephaly	2	2	—
MISCELLANEOUS/UNKNOWN	23	18	1
Miscellaneous etiologies	22	9	1
Delayed/abnormal myelination	1	9	0
NORMAL	3	21	6

[a]The data in the malformations section of this table are separated into preterm, term, and postnatal as that is how they were presented in the original reports. It is believed, however, that these malformations occur prenatally.
PVL, periventricular leukomalacia.
Reproduced with permission from Ashwal S, Russman BS, Blasco PA, et al. Practice parameter: diagnostic assessment of the child with cerebral palsy. Neurology 2004;62:851–863. Copyright 2004 Lippincott, Williams & Wilkins.

HISTORY

The history is a key component in diagnosing a child with CP. Refer to Table 129.8 to help plan history-taking, with the following additional information. Questions should be focused on the prenatal, perinatal, and postnatal risk factors. Fetal movements, prenatal care, and family history should be reviewed. Information obtained about the perinatal period should include Apgar scores, birthing complications, delivery, IVH, intubation, feeding, and tone. The postnatal history should include questions about developmental milestones, educational needs, equipment, and medical/surgical history.

PHYSICAL EXAMINATION

The entire well-child examination should be performed because these children often require treatment of other medical problems. The neurologic examination should include an evaluation of tone (movement of the joint through passive range of motion) and should be performed with the head initially in neutral position because variations in the examination can occur.

Examination with the head rotated to the right and left, flexed and extended, with documentation of the postural changes associated with these movements, is necessary. The hypotonia present at birth often becomes hypertonia in children with CP, but many infants with hypertonia suspect for CP later have normalization of their tone. Deep tendon reflexes usually are increased in the spastic or mixed spastic–athetoid type of CP, but may not be in the other types. Hyperreflexia, the presence of ankle clonus, Babinski reflex, variable tone with change in posture, and contractures also support the diagnosis of CP.

The traditional neurologic examination should be supplemented by the neurodevelopmental evaluation because the diagnosis is based on a delay in gross motor function. Primitive reflexes are the first group of infant automated responses that appear during late gestation and are present at birth, but most are suppressed by 6 months age (i.e., Moro, asymmetric tonic neck reflex, symmetric tonic neck reflex, positive support reaction, tonic labyrinthine response). They

TABLE 129.8

RISK FACTORS ASSOCIATED WITH CEREBRAL PALSY

PRENATAL
Abdominal trauma to mother
Congenital malformations
Intrauterine infections
Maternal factors (mental retardation, hyperthyroidism,
 seizures)
Multiple births
Placental complications
Reproductive inefficiency
Socioeconomic factors
Teratogenic agents

PERINATAL
Abnormal presentations
Birth weight <2,500 g
Bradycardia and hypoxia
Growth retardation
Hyperbilirubinemia
Intracranial hemorrhage
Infection
Prematurity <32 weeks' gestation
Seizures
Trauma

POSTNATAL
Coagulopathies
Infection
Intracranial hemorrhage
Trauma

Modified with permission from Matthews DJ, Wilson P. Cerebral palsy. In: Molnar GE, Alexander MA, eds. *Pediatric rehabilitation*, 3rd ed. Philadelphia: Hanley & Belfus, 1999:194.

are important to help detect motor abnormalities, either by presence beyond normal age of suppression (6 months) or by their presence in an obligatory pattern even if at the normal age of appearance. Care should be taken with the early diagnosis of CP, with emphasis on gross motor abilities. An 8-month-old child with hypertonia and hyperreflexia would not be in the high-risk category for CP if gross motor skills of sitting and crawling were normal.

LABORATORY FINDINGS

There are no laboratory findings diagnostic of CP, but findings related to factors that may have caused CP can be identified. Metabolic and some genetic diseases can be diagnosed with serum, urine samples, and chromosomal testing. Some tests to consider should include serum amino acids; lactic, organic, and pyruvic acids; blood pH; and chromosomal analysis. Elevated white blood cell counts in the cerebrospinal fluid may reflect an infectious state.

RADIOLOGIC FINDINGS

Radiologic testing has advanced over the years, and there are multiple options available to support the diagnosis. The use of cranial ultrasonography in the neonatal unit is standard practice. It allows visualization of the ventricles and surrounding parenchyma and can confirm the presence of brain hemor-

rhage. It is a noninvasive test and can be performed in the unit without transport of the child. Computed tomography can more clearly define structural features, including masses and congenital abnormalities of the brain. Transport to the radiology department must be feasible. Magnetic resonance imaging (MRI) provides the best resolution of the brain parenchyma, especially of white matter disease, but sedation and a metal-free environment are limitations. Magnetic resonance spectroscopy is becoming more widely available and can be performed after MRI. A section of the brain is analyzed using a spectroscopic pattern that allows identification of relative quantities of metabolites such as *N*-acetylaspartate (NAA), choline, creatine, and lactate. NAA is located almost exclusively in neurons and axons. It has been shown in animal models to be reduced in some neurodegenerative processes, and an absolute or relative (to creatine) decrease of this peak is usually considered to be an indicator of neuronal or axonal damage (66,67). It also may be an indicator of normal oligodendroglial development. Some facilities may have access to positron emission tomography, which is used to define blood flow and glucose metabolism, or single-photon emission computed tomography, which is used to measure cerebral perfusion using radioactive tracers.

MEDICAL MANAGEMENT

Medical treatments, specifically pharmacologic options, often are directed to the management of spasticity. Any upper motor neuron lesion can produce spasticity. In an extremity with spasticity, the joint has resistance to passive range of motion that increases as the joint is ranged more quickly. Associated findings may include hyperreflexia, excessive spread of a reflex response, and clonus. These abnormal patterns can interfere with functional activities and also may lead to contractures and discomfort. Treatment therefore may be warranted. Baclofen, diazepam, dantrolene, and more recently, tizanidine are commonly used off label in children as options for the reduction of spasticity. Phenol nerve blocks are also used to reduce spasticity in specific muscle groups. These blocks are used less frequently due to the requirement for nerve stimulation to localize nerves before injection, poor patient tolerance of the procedure, and the potential for significant side effects, including intravascular injection and painful dysesthesias. Although expensive, the availability of botulinum toxins A and B allow the more convenient and comfortable intramuscular route of injection to be used to block the neuromuscular junction and decrease spasticity.

Intrathecal Baclofen

Normal inhibitory signals are lost with upper motor neuron lesions; this may result in spasticity (hypertonicity, hyperreflexia, spread of reflexes, velocity-dependent range of motion). Baclofen, a GABA analogue, is one of the medications utilized orally to decrease hypertonicity with the goal of improved function. Baclofen's use is limited due to side effects such as sedation and hepatotoxicity. Intrathecal infusion of baclofen via an internalized pump allows for excellent compliance and dosing adjustment by programming the pump electronically. Microgram doses can be utilized, which minimizes systemic side effects. Prime candidates for intrathecal baclofen include those who have the potential for ambulation but who exhibit lower extremity hypertonicity. Lower limb contractures and/or orthopaedic surgical history are relative contraindications. Clinical evaluation, intrathecal test dose administration, and pump adjustments can be performed by rehabilitation physicians and other MDs.

Sialorrhea

Sialorrhea is a common social and medical problem, especially for patients with cerebral palsy. Skin breakdown can occur, dental hygiene is more problematic, and social stigma is of real concern if interactions with peers and vocational opportunities are to be pursued. Initial treatment for sialorrhea should include referral for proper dental hygiene, as this commonly contributes to excessive salivation. A stepwise approach should ensure that adequate swallowing function is present and that positioning of seating devices is utilized to assist posterior displacement of secretions. Some medications can be used in an attempt to decrease saliva production (e.g., Scopolamine and Robinul—off-label uses). Scopolamine can be compounded into a gel and applied topically (e.g., posterior to the ear). More aggressive treatment options include sectioning of the salivary ducts or removal of the glands.

THERAPY

Involvement of an experienced interdisciplinary pediatric therapy team is important for enhancing the functional progress of children with CP. The "neurodevelopmental" treatment approach is the most common form of physical therapy in the United States in use today for children with CP, although some therapists use a blend of styles (52). The neurodevelopmental approach is based on the concept that normal postural control against gravity is significantly compromised by cerebral damage. The child is positioned to inhibit the primitive reflexes and reduce the hypertonicity. Normal postural reactions are facilitated simultaneously to give the child the experience of normal movements.

Other methods include the Rood, Doman–Delacato, sensory integration, and conductive education (Peto) systems. Conductive education has not been shown to be an effective treatment option in controlled studies, and the other methods have not shown an advantage over each other in the limited research available (68).

Other treatments include the use of early interventionists who work with the infant and family as early as possible to prevent or minimize adverse developmental outcomes. Orthotics are used in conjunction with therapy to prevent progressive contractures and scoliosis. They also facilitate function by augmenting or substituting for weak muscle groups and by reducing the effect of spasticity. Depending on the severity and distribution of involvement, occupational and speech therapists, child life specialists, psychologists, social workers, nutritionists, and nurses are potential team members. Regardless of the team members and treatment approach, transition to a home program with the parents becoming active participants in the daily therapy needs of the child is paramount.

Constraint-induced (CI) movement therapy has recently been advocated to improve functional use of the affected upper limb in hemiplegic CP. Children with hemiplegic CP typically experience difficulties with grasping, releasing, and manipulating objects when utilizing the involved hand. These difficulties are associated with characteristics of the hemiplegic hand, which include slow, weak, and uncoordinated movement; spasticity; and impaired tactile sensation. Perhaps more importantly, impairment of the upper limb translates to difficulties performing self-care and academic, vocational, play, and leisure activities.

Elements of CI therapy are (1) constraint of the normal hand to encourage use of the affected hand, (2) massed practice of the affected hand, and (3) use of intensive techniques to train the affected hand. Studies that have examined the effects of CI therapy in children and adolescents with hemiplegic CP have indicated positive outcome with improved hand function (69).

Hyperbaric Oxygen Therapy

Hyperbaric oxygen therapy (HBOT) has been used by several centers in the United States, Canada, Germany, and the United Kingdom in an attempt to improve functional outcomes in patients with CP. This application of HBOT therapy is based upon the theory that "the hypoxic–ischaemic penumbra zone surrounding" the static encephalopathy "may be reactivated metabolically or electrically by increasing the oxygen level mainly in plasma" (70). The Undersea and Hyperbaric Medical Society (UHMS) monitors and regularly reviews published medical literature for reports on the use of HBOT. Based on this review, they attempt to provide guidance to the medical community as to those medical conditions likely to benefit from HBOT. An objective review of the available published literature funded by the U.S. Agency for Healthcare Research and Quality states that (1) there is insufficient evidence to determine whether the use of HBOT improves functional outcomes in children with CP; (2) the results of the only truly randomized trial were difficult to interpret because of the use of pressurized room air in the control group; and (3) because both the HBOT group and the pressurized air group improved, further studies on both interventions should be carried out (71).

SURGICAL TREATMENTS

One neurosurgical option includes selective dorsal rhizotomies for treatment of spasticity. The CP patient with the greatest potential to benefit from this procedure is 3 to 8 years of age and has good family support, spastic diplegic involvement with severe, pure spasticity involving predominantly the lower limbs, no fixed contractures, voluntary motor control, good trunk control, the ability to walk with good underlying strength and balance, and reasonable intelligence and motivation to carry through a rehabilitation program. Again, central control of balance is usually unchanged, but decreased lower motor neuron activity results in a reduction in spasticity.

After selective dorsal rhizotomy, in the early postoperative period, the patient is weaker than before surgery and requires intensive physical therapy (PT). As a result, availability of and cooperation with postoperative PT are prerequisites for a successful outcome. The multidisciplinary approach provided in an acute inpatient rehabilitation facility is ideally suited to address the needs of these patients.

ORTHOPAEDIC CONSIDERATIONS

Two considerations are of paramount importance when evaluating/treating a patient with spastic quadriplegia who has global involvement. These are (1) the priorities of the patient and (2) realistic goals for orthopaedic care. Priorities for the patient, in order of importance are communication with others, the ability to take care of activities of daily living (especially personal hygiene), mobility in the environment, and walking (72). Given that the majority of patients with global involvement will be nonambulatory, realistic goals for their orthopaedic care are related to maintaining balanced, comfortable sitting.

A comprehensive discussion of orthopaedic treatment for the numerous musculoskeletal abnormalities associated with CP is beyond the scope and intended purpose of this text. The following is an overview of important considerations for some of the more common and problematic orthopaedic diagnoses, including scoliosis, hip problems, and spasticity of the upper limb.

General Postoperative Concerns Related to Orthopaedic Surgical Procedures

Immediately postoperatively, the major concerns are pain management, relief of superimposed muscle spasm, and minimization of anxiety. Overall postoperative management goals include restoration of joint motion and muscle strength as well as improving gait.

Scoliosis

Scoliosis occurs more frequently in all types of CP (about 25%) than in the general population. Scoliosis in patients with CP is different from idiopathic scoliosis. It develops earlier, tends to be more progressive and to progress beyond skeletal maturity (especially when the curve is >40 degrees), and is significantly less responsive to treatment with orthoses. All of these factors combine to make scoliosis in patients with CP more likely to require surgical intervention. Important considerations for providers caring for postoperative scoliosis patients include maintaining adequate nutrition for healing, being cognizant of the extent of blood loss associated with the procedure, the potential for postoperative hyponatremia, and the potential for postoperative pulmonary problems. The potential for problems associated with traction on neurovascular structures resulting from straightening (and thereby functionally lengthening) the spine (e.g., nutcracker syndrome) should also be considered.

Patients with gastroesophageal reflux and/or malnutrition should have these problems addressed preoperatively to minimize risk of wound infection and delayed healing. Intraoperative blood loss should be carefully calculated and appropriately replaced to avoid hypovolemia and potentially dangerous coagulopathies. In patients with previously normal renal function, postoperative hyponatremia due to SIADH is felt to be related to administration of hypotonic saline during and after the corrective procedure (73). Postoperative pulmonary complications include hypoventilation, atelectasis, aspiration pneumonia, and adult respiratory distress syndrome. Nutcracker syndrome is associated with entrapment of the left renal vein between the aorta and the superior mesenteric artery (SMA). This may occur as a result of change in the relative positions of these structures when the spine is straightened. SMA syndrome (entrapment of the 3rd part of the duodenum between the aorta and the SMA) and acute mesenteric ischemia can also occur by similar mechanisms.

Hip Problems

Hip problems are frequently seen in CP patients with spastic quadriplegia. These include limitation of motion, contractures, and the hip at risk with potential sequellae of subluxation and dislocation. Surgical intervention is indicated to prevent hip dislocation or to treat dislocated hips that are painful or are interfering with seating/positioning. Abduction splinting, applied at night and limited to the patient's range of comfortable abduction, is frequently utilized postoperatively to avoid recurrent contractures.

Upper Limb Spasticity

In patients with upper extremity involvement, surgical intervention is indicated for specific functional goals. These include improving the ability to position a functional hand in space, improving hygiene, preventing skin breakdown, and improving cosmetic appearance. Characteristics of CP patients most likely to benefit from upper extremity surgery include good intelligence, good hand placement capability with voluntary control, adequate passive range of motion of all upper limb joints, good hand sensation (including proprioception and stereognosis), and a stable trunk and body position.

COURSE AND PROGNOSIS

The expected course of CP is variable because of the wide spectrum of clinical presentations. In addition, secondary problems can arise over time, such as contractures, increasing tone, pulmonary disease, scoliosis, and malnutrition, that can further reduce the function of the child. Productive years can be enjoyed by less-involved children, and vocational opportunities should be considered for such children, with referral to the local vocational counselor when they are ready to enter college or pursue a career. Counselors are available to train adults and career-age teenagers to enter the workforce and provide support to promote more independent living. Predictors for successful employment include independent ambulation, hand use close to normal, IQ greater then 80, and speech patterns that are no worse than "hard to understand" to normal (74).

COMPLICATIONS

Problems associated with CP seen later in life include neck pain, back pain, pain in weight-bearing joints, contractures, carpal tunnel syndrome and other repetitive use syndromes, scoliosis, fractures, constipation, gastroesophageal reflux, and sialorrhea. All of the usual medical problems seen in the nondisabled population also should be considered. Limited research has been conducted on the life span of the child with CP, but it appears to be lower than in the general population (75,76). They do have increased mortality rates secondary to breast cancer, brain cancer, respiratory diseases, circulatory and digestive diseases, drowning, and "being hit by motor vehicles" (77). Some of these problems could be improved with better detection, prevention, and treatment.

PEARLS

- Independent sitting by 2 years of age is a good predictor of eventual ambulation (with or without assistive devices) in spastic diplegic/quadriplegic and athetoid patients with CP (78).
- If a loss of milestones, as opposed to a delay only, is documented, the diagnosis of CP should be questioned because by definition it is a static lesion.
- If a child is suspected of having diplegic CP, but has *no* upper extremity involvement, a spinal cord injury should be considered in the differential diagnosis. All children with diplegic CP have some involvement of the upper extremities, even though the most prominent motor abnormalities are in the lower extremities.
- Sialorrhea is a common, treatable symptom in CP.

Suggested Readings

Kuban KCK, Leviton A. Cerebral palsy. *N Engl J Med* 1994;330:188–195.

Matthews DJ, Wilson P. Cerebral palsy. In: Molnar GE, Alexander MA, eds. *Pediatric rehabilitation.* 3rd ed. Philadelphia: Hanley & Belfus; 1999: 193–217.

Moore DP. Helping your patients with spasticity reach maximal function. *Postgrad Med* 1998;104:123–135.

Renshaw TS. Cerebral palsy. In: Morrisey RT, Weinstein SL, eds. *Lovell & Winter's pediatric orthopaedics.* 4th ed. Philadelphia: Lippincott-Raven; 1996:469–502.

CHAPTER 129C ■ SPECIFIC DISORDERS: HYDROCEPHALUS, CEREBROSPINAL FLUID SHUNTS, AND THEIR COMPLICATIONS

HERBERT EDGAR FUCHS

Hydrocephalus is the pathologic accumulation of cerebrospinal fluid (CSF) in the cerebral ventricles, with an associated increase in intracranial pressure (ICP). Hydrocephalus has been recognized for centuries, but the understanding and treatment of hydrocephalus have significantly improved over the last 70 years. This chapter will review the normal CSF physiology and the pathologic entities leading to hydrocephalus. In addition, the treatment of hydrocephalus, and the complications resulting from different treatment modalities, will be reviewed.

Normal CSF Physiology

Normal CSF physiology involves production, circulation, and absorption. Abnormalities in each of these phases can result in hydrocephalus. CSF is produced in the cerebral ventricles, circulates throughout the ventricular system and then into the subarachnoid space, and is finally reabsorbed primarily through the arachnoid villi into the superior sagittal sinus.

Production

Cerebrospinal fluid is produced by the choroid plexus in the cerebral ventricles, and as a by-product from cerebral metabolism for a total of approximately 0.3 to 0.35 mL/min (79). This rate is relatively constant except at extreme ICP elevations. The choroid plexus accounts for approximately 50% to 80% of CSF production, in a process that is energy dependent and utilizes the enzyme carbonic anhydrase (80). This portion of CSF production can be almost completely blocked with acetazolamide. The remaining 20% to 50% of CSF production is the passive byproduct of cerebral metabolism. This extracellular fluid flows centrally through the ependymal lining into the ventricles to mix with choroidal CSF.

Circulation

Cerebrospinal fluid produced in the lateral ventricles flows through the two foramina of Monro into the midline third ventricle, and then through the aqueduct of Sylvius into the fourth ventricle. Flow continues through the midline foramen of Magendie and the two lateral foramina of Luschka, into the subarachnoid space. Flow continues throughout the subarachnoid space, and eventually over the cerebral convexities to be reabsorbed through the arachnoid villi into the superior sagittal sinus.

Absorption

The absorption of CSF through the arachnoid villi into the superior sagittal sinus is a passive process via bulk flow. The rate of CSF absorption is dependent on ICP. At ICP less than 5 mm Hg, there is no absorption. The rate of absorption increases linearly above this point, which is the opening pressure for the arachnoid villi. The curves for rate of CSF production and absorption cross at approximately 10 mm Hg, the normal physiologic state.

Abnormal CSF Physiology

Hydrocephalus may result from abnormalities in each phase of CSF physiology. The cause of hydrocephalus has implications in possible therapies that may be utilized.

Production

Overproduction of CSF occurs very rarely in cases of the tumor, choroid plexus papilloma, or in villous hypertrophy of the choroid plexus. Cerebrospinal fluid production rates up to several times normal have been reported with these tumors. In addition, these tumors may block CSF circulation, resulting in obstructive hydrocephalus.

Circulation

The flow of CSF may be obstructed at many levels. Obstruction of the foramen of Monro may occur either unilaterally or bilaterally, resulting in dilatation of one lateral ventricle, or both, respectively. Lesions commonly associated with occlusion of the foramen of Monro include colloid cyst, subependymal giant cell astrocytoma in tuberous sclerosis, hypothalamic astrocytoma, and craniopharyngioma. The classic form of obstructive hydrocephalus is occlusion of the aqueduct of Sylvius, resulting in dilatation of the lateral ventricles in addition to the third ventricle. Common causes of aqueductal occlusion include tectal plate gliomas and aqueductal atresia. Occlusion of the outlets of the fourth ventricle results in dilatation of all four cerebral ventricles and is commonly caused by fourth ventricular or cerebellar tumors, such as medulloblastoma, ependymoma, or astrocytoma.

Absorption

Impaired absorption of CSF is commonly found in post-hemorrhagic or post-meningitic hydrocephalus. The arachnoid villi become occluded with debris from hemorrhage or infection, and CSF absorption is inadequate. Increased pressure in the superior sagittal sinus or in the transverse sinus, such as occurs with either occlusion or stenosis, will also lead to increased ICP secondary to decreased absorption.

DIAGNOSIS OF HYDROCEPHALUS

Children with hydrocephalus commonly present with lethargy, nausea, vomiting, and may also manifest "sunsetting" or paresis of upward gaze, or isolated sixth cranial nerve palsies. In infants, increased head circumference and full fontanelles are common findings.

The diagnosis of hydrocephalus requires cranial imaging with ultrasound, computed tomography (CT), or magnetic resonance imaging (MRI). CT and MRI scanning provide better anatomic detail and when combined with intravenous contrast, may delineate tumors or other lesions associated with hydrocephalus.

TREATMENT OF HYDROCEPHALUS

The treatment of hydrocephalus would ideally recreate the natural physiologic state with an ICP of approximately 10 mm Hg, with CSF production and absorption matched. Unfortunately, none of the current treatments completely meets these criteria, and each introduces new potential complications.

MEDICAL THERAPY

The medical therapy of hydrocephalus is directed at decreasing CSF production by the choroid plexus. Acetazolamide decreases CSF production by interfering with the function of carbonic anhydrase, and may significantly decrease CSF production both acutely and chronically. Furosemide appears to decrease CSF production by interfering with chloride transport rather than any direct effect on carbonic anhydrase. Neither of these drugs has any effect on the 20% to 50% of CSF production from cerebral metabolism. Glucocorticoids may or may not decrease CSF production, as various studies have shown conflicting results (81).

SURGICAL THERAPY

Surgical procedures to treat hydrocephalus are primarily designed to drain CSF, and may be classified as either short term or long term. In communicating hydrocephalus, lumbar puncture or lumbar drain insertion will provide temporary treatment of hydrocephalus. These techniques are particularly useful for short-term management of hydrocephalus that is expected to resolve. External ventricular drain (EVD) insertion provides short-term management for either communicating or obstructive hydrocephalus, and is particularly useful for treatment of hydrocephalus secondary to tumors, where resection is expected to potentially cure the hydrocephalus. Ventricular reservoirs, which are placed subcutaneously, are commonly used in the treatment of post-hemorrhagic hydrocephalus in premature infants, with serial tapping until the infant is of adequate size and medically stable for shunting.

SHUNTS AND COMPLICATIONS

The classic treatment for both communicating and obstructive hydrocephalus, and the only long-term treatment option, is shunting. Cerebrospinal fluid is either returned directly to the bloodstream in the case of ventriculoatrial shunting, or diverted to a site where reabsorption into the bloodstream can occur, as in ventriculo-peritoneal or ventriculo-pleural shunting. Unfortunately, current shunts do not restore normalcy to the CSF physiology. Because the cerebral ventricles and the distal drainage sites are at different heights in the erect position, there is an overdrainage or "siphoning" effect in virtually all shunted patients. Despite this, the development of valve-regulated CSF shunts in the 1950s transformed the treatment of hydrocephalus, and is the cornerstone for our modern treatment of hydrocephalus.

There are a number of different shunt systems on the market today, with a number of creative engineering solutions to the problem of regulation of CSF drainage. Most of these valves work as strict differential pressure valves. A few are flow regulated, with higher resistance at higher flow rates to limit overdrainage and overshunting. A randomized trial of cerebrospinal fluid shunt valves in pediatric hydrocephalus was published in 1998, with a conclusion that there was no one ideal valve system, and that further work was needed to improve shunt failure rates (82). The typical shunt system consists of a ventricular catheter, valve, and distal catheter, typically peritoneal. It is imperative that the system contain a tapping chamber, in order to sample CSF for workup of shunt infection, and to check flow rates for evaluation of shunt malfunction.

The ventriculo-peritoneal shunt is the most commonly used shunt in use today. The peritoneal cavity has excellent absorptive capacity, and allows the placement of excess tubing to allow for growth of the pediatric patient. The pleural cavity is used on occasion, when other sites are not available. The ventriculo-atrial shunt diverts CSF from the ventricle directly back to the bloodstream, and could potentially be an ideal shunt if a valve with an opening pressure of 5 to 10 mm Hg were used, and the patient remained in a horizontal position. It is the assumption of the upright position that leads to many potential shunt complications.

In normal patients, the superior sagittal sinus pressure is 3 to 8 mm Hg when recumbent. On standing, the pressure falls to −10 mm Hg. This would result in an increase in CSF absorption, but the jugular veins collapse, with venous drainage diverted to collaterals to try to maintain superior sinus pressure. In shunted patients, there are similar pressure changes on standing. For patients with ventriculo-atrial shunts, with the distal catheter tip in the right atrium of the heart, there is a large fluid column pressure gradient, as much as 10 to 20 mm Hg negative. In patients with peritoneal shunts, the fluid column pressure gradient is even greater, easily exceeding −20 mm Hg. The result of these pressure gradients is overshunting, resulting in either subdural hematomas or slit ventricle syndrome.

In infants with massive hydrocephalus, rapid CSF drainage may result in collapse of the cerebral hemispheres and subdural hematomas (Fig 129.1). Treatment consists of drainage of the subdurals and valve upgrade. Long-term overdrainage in these infants may result in inadequate head growth, and eventually, brain growth results in obliteration of the ventricles and subarachnoid spaces, resulting in the slit ventricle syndrome (Fig 129.2).

The slit ventricle syndrome is defined as headaches in a shunted patient with very small, unchanged ventricles on CT or MRI scan. Headache may be due to intermittent or chronic shunt obstruction, overdrainage of CSF causing low-pressure headaches, or headache unrelated to ICP. Workup for these patients includes nuclear medicine shunt flow study and possible ICP monitoring. Surgery involves increasing the resistance of the valve and incorporating an antisiphon device into the shunt system, both measures aimed at preventing overdrainage. If these measures fail, cranial expansion or addition of a lumbar shunt to drain CSF from the subarachnoid space may be considered.

Complications of shunting include injury to brain parenchyma from catheter positioning, loculation of CSF spaces, most commonly associated with foramen of Monro occlusion, and catheter occlusion, usually due to choroids plexus. Additional complications vary with the distal site chosen. Peritoneal shunts may erode through an abdominal viscus, resulting in infection, or may become walled off, resulting in a pseudocyst. Complications of atrial shunts include pulmonary emboli, autoimmune glomerulonephritis, and cardiac arrhythmias. Pleural shunts may result in significant pleural effusions, which compromise respiration. For a more detailed discussion of various shunts, the reader is directed to an excellent text, *The Shunt Book* (83).

Shunt Malfunction

Shunt malfunction is one of the banes of treatment of patients with hydrocephalus, with up to 40% shunt failure rate in the first year after implantation. Symptoms of shunt malfunction include headache, lethargy, irritability, lack of developmental progress, poor school performance, nausea, vomiting, and forced downgaze (sunsetting sign). Patients with increased ICP may present with hypertension, bradycardia, and irregular respirations

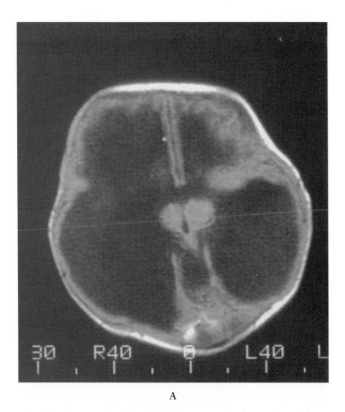

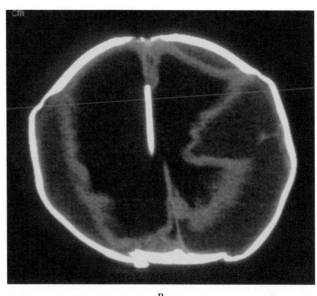

A   B

FIGURE 129.1. T1-weighted axial MRI scans of an infant with massive hydrocephalus. **A.** Pre-shunting. Note thin cortical mantle. **B.** Post-shunting. Cortical mantle has collapsed, leading to bilateral chronic subdural hematomas.

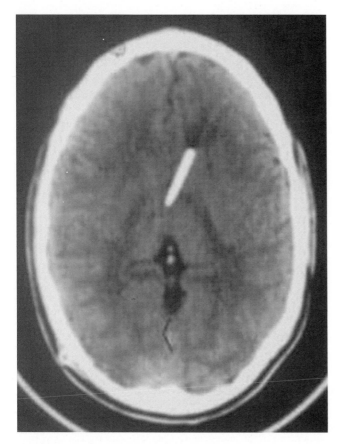

FIGURE 129.2. CT scan of patient with slit ventricle syndrome. There is virtually no CSF space surrounding the ventricular catheter.

(Cushing triad). This is a neurosurgical emergency. Workup of shunt malfunction includes CT or MRI scanning to assess ventricular size, shunt series x-rays to rule out disconnection or dislocation of shunt tubing, and, potentially, shunt tap or nuclear medicine shunt flow study. It is critical to obtain a history of prior shunt malfunctions, and to inquire whether the clinical presentation was the same as present, and if the ventricles previously dilated with a malfunction. An unchanged CT scan in a patient who does not dilate his ventricles with shunt failure does not rule out a shunt malfunction. The most common cause of shunt malfunction is ventricular catheter obstruction. Valve and distal catheter obstruction are somewhat less common. It is rare for an atrial catheter to become occluded with clot in the absence of proximal catheter malfunction. Failure of absorption in pleural shunts may lead to massive pleural effusion. The treatment of shunt malfunction is shunt revision, with replacement of the occluded component, and perhaps revision of the valve, to decrease further malfunctions.

Shunt Infection

Infection rates in shunts for hydrocephalus vary from 1% to 40% in published series, with most in the range of approximately 5% to 10% (84). Greater than two-thirds of all shunt infections are due to staphylococcal species, with *Staphylococcus epidermidis* most common (47–64%), and *S. aureus* at 12% to 29% (84,85). Gram-negative organisms, especially *Escherichia coli* and *Klebsiella* species, are responsible for 6% to 12% of shunt infections. These infections almost always present within 6 months of shunt surgery, with the gram-negative and *S. aureus* infections seen earliest, followed by *S. epidermidis* most commonly by 1 to 3 months. After 6 months since shunt manipulation by either surgery or tapping, the incidence of shunt infection decreases markedly. In atrial shunts, however, the risk of shunt infection continues, due to the presence of hardware within the bloodstream, and the potential for contamination with bacteremia.

Patients with shunt infection may present with or without fever, and may only manifest shunt malfunction symptoms. Shunt tap should be performed in any patient within 6 months of shunt manipulation, and CSF sent for Gram stain, culture, glucose, protein, and cell count. The treatment of shunt infection involves removal of infected hardware, placement of a temporary external ventricular drain to handle CSF drainage, and intravenous antibiotic therapy. Occasionally, intrathecal antibiotic therapy is required as well. The duration of antibiotic therapy for shunt infection is a matter of debate, but usually with sterilization of the CSF, the shunt can be replaced within 7 to 14 days of removal. Prolonged antibiotic therapy after shunt reinsertion is not required.

OBSTRUCTIVE HYDROCEPHALUS

For patients with obstructive hydrocephalus, several additional therapies are available, in addition to shunting. If the normal flow of CSF can be restored, and CSF absorption is adequate, then no shunt may be required, and the patient may be shunt independent. With modern microsurgical and ventriculoscopic surgical techniques, removal of obstructive lesions, or ventricular fenestrations are becoming commonplace. The prototypical condition associated with obstructive hydrocephalus is aqueductal stenosis. With ventriculoscopic third ventriculostomy, involving perforation of the floor of the third ventricle, and communication of the third ventricle with the prepontine subarachnoid space, there is an 80% chance of achieving shunt independence (86). Figure 129.3 illustrates a

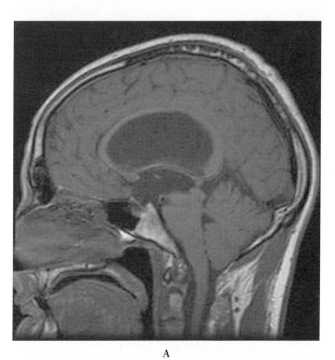

A

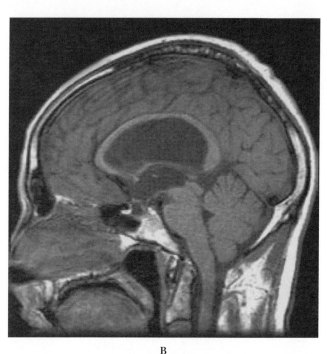

B

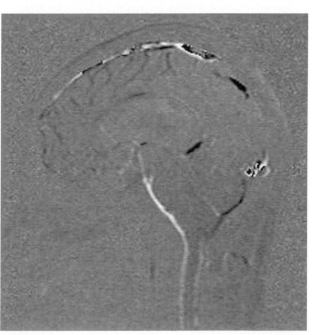

C

FIGURE 129.3. Sagittal MRI scans of patient with aqueductal stenosis. **A.** T1-weighted image showing occlusion of the aqueduct and bulging floor of the third ventricle. **B.** T1-weighted image status post-ventriculoscopic third ventriculostomy. Note defect in third ventricle floor anterior to the brainstem. **C.** Cine-MRI showing CSF flow from the third ventricle through the third ventriculostomy to the prepontine CSF space.

patient with aqueductal stenosis who underwent third ventriculostomy, with resolution of hydrocephalus. Infants under 6 to 12 months of age are not good candidates for third ventriculostomy, most likely due either to poorly developed CSF absorption pathways, or improved healing, resulting in closure of the stoma in these young infants (87). Third ventriculostomy may also be effective in patients with shunted obstructive hydrocephalus, and may result in shunt independence in these patients as well. In patients with history of extensive infection or hemorrhage, the procedure is less successful, most likely due to impairment of CSF absorption pathways. In patients with colloid cysts obstructing the foramen of Monro, resection via craniotomy or ventriculoscope will likely lead to shunt independence. Resection of pineal tumors or posterior fossa tumors causing obstructive hydrocephalus may also result in normalization of CSF physiology.

SUMMARY

The treatment of hydrocephalus in children is complex, and is an ongoing process. There are many issues related to hydrocephalus that we do not fully understand (80). The ideal treatment would simply restore normal CSF physiology. Unfortunately, this ideal treatment does not exist, with the exception of some cases of obstructive hydrocephalus, where removal or bypass of the obstructing lesion may be successful. The majority of patients with hydrocephalus will require shunt placement, and continued neurosurgical care for a lifetime. Although shunts may enable patients to lead fairly normal lives, there is always the potential for shunt malfunction or other complications, and vigilance on the part of physicians of many specialties is required.

CHAPTER 129D ■ SPECIFIC DISORDERS: MUSCULAR DYSTROPHIES

RONALD M. PERKIN AND DANIEL P. MOORE

Muscular dystrophy is a collective group of inherited, noninflammatory, progressive muscle-wasting diseases. The initial pathologic feature is an abnormality in the genetic code for dystrophin or one of its associated glycoproteins, which leads to the various clinical syndromes. Despite minor variations between the different types, all muscular dystrophies have in common progressive muscle weakness, which is best typified by Duchenne muscular dystrophy (DMD). A classic Gower sign may be present due to the proximal muscle weakness, but more subtle findings like weakness of neck flexion or macroglossia may be present earlier.

The weakness occurs in a proximal-to-distal direction and can compromise ambulatory status as well as cardiopulmonary function. An exception is myotonic muscular dystrophy, which has distal muscle weakness. In addition, structural soft tissue contractures and spinal deformities may develop from poor posturing secondary to the progressive muscle weakness and imbalance. The rapidly developing scoliosis and its associated pelvic obliquity can even compromise sitting. Recent advances in molecular biology and gene therapy research raise the hope for a cure for muscular dystrophy in the near future. Until that time, a multidisciplinary team must work to preserve or prolong the functional status of the patient with muscular dystrophy for as long as possible.

DMD is an X-linked recessive disorder characterized by diffuse skeletal and cardiac muscle involvement beginning in childhood. It is the second most common lethal genetic disorder, affecting approximately 1 in 3,300 live male births. The genetic abnormality in DMD is associated with an abnormality of the Xp21 chromosome, which controls synthesis of dystrophin, a muscle protein absent in patients with DMD.

Workup should include creatine kinase and aldolase, which are very sensitive for DMD. Enzyme evaluations of myopathies are not always abnormal; for example, congenital myopathies (e.g., myotubular myopathy) do not typically display elevated muscle enzyme levels.

Electromyoegraphy (EMG) is a useful physiologic test that can help diagnose the presence of a myopathy when characteristic low-amplitude polyphasic motor unit potentials, early recruitment pattern, and spontaneous potentials are present. This should be performed by a physician who has had adequate training in their application and interpretation. Mild transient elevation of muscle enzymes may occur after an EMG. If a muscle biopsy is to be performed after needle EMG, it should occur on the contralateral extremity, as microtrauma to the muscle occurs as part of the normal insertion process during needle EMG.

RESPIRATORY FAILURE

Respiratory failure is the major cause of death in patients with DMD. Respiratory impairment is manifest in the advanced stages of the disease, usually in late adolescence. Death occurs secondary to pneumonia, retained secretions, atelectasis, or simply respiratory muscle fatigue and eventual failure. Deterioration in respiratory function parallels the deterioration in muscle strength and overall functional capabilities of the patient. The patient and family should be educated about benefits and alternatives to trach and ventilator placement prior to the time they are needed.

Ventilatory abnormalities during sleep resulting in nocturnal hypoventilation also may be associated with the development of respiratory insufficiency and cor pulmonale. In patients with weak bulbar musculature, aspiration of secretions aggravates and accelerates respiratory problems. The presence of an underlying cardiomyopathy contributes to the development of hypoventilation and orthopnea.

The development of respiratory failure during wakefulness usually is preceded by hypoventilation during sleep, which appears to be a consequence of the combined effects of sleep-induced decreased ventilatory drive and respiratory muscle weakness. Although often nonobstructive in origin because of weakness of the respiratory pump muscles, the sleep-related hypoventilation may have an obstructive component because of upper airway muscle weakness, particularly when other predisposing factors, such as obesity, are present. Sleep-related hypoventilation/hypoxemia due to neuromuscular disorders may be accentuated in the presence of obstructive sleep apnea.

Potential consequences of sleep-related hypoventilation include sleep disruption with diurnal lethargy, hypoxemia, and hypercarbia. Untreated, sleep-related hypoxemia and hypercarbia may have a causal role in the development of respiratory failure because of disordered ventilatory control resulting from adaptation and down-regulation of the ventilatory responses to these stimuli. Uncontrolled studies suggest that treatment of sleep hypoventilation with noninvasive ventilation can improve daytime gas exchange and prolong survival of patients with established respiratory failure.

The speed and severity of respiratory and cardiac decompensation with hypoventilation make early diagnosis important; however, patients and their physicians may not be aware of the significance of such symptoms. Many have symptoms for weeks or months before seeking help or before the severity of the problem is recognized. Cyanosis, abnormal respiratory muscle activity, and right heart strain are important diagnostic clues. In patients with neuromuscular disorders, vital capacity is an important measurement of respiratory function, and can be conveniently monitored with simple portable equipment.

Sleep-related hypoventilation can be predicted by daytime respiratory function in patients with DMD and appears to be implicated in the pathogenesis of respiratory failure. It is recommended that arterial blood gases be performed in patients with DMD when the forced expiratory volume in 1 second (FEV_1) is <40% of the predicted normal value. Polysomnography should be considered when the $PaCO_2$ is ≥45 mm Hg, particularly if the base excess is ≥4 mmol/L, because significant sleep hypoventilation is likely to be present, requiring consideration of noninvasive ventilation.

Any dysfunction of the diaphragm—whether neurogenic as in motor neuron disease or phrenic nerve paralysis, neuromuscular as in myasthenia gravis or the muscular dystrophies, or extrinsic as in morbid abdominal obesity—will interfere with breathing during rapid eye-movement (REM) sleep. In consequence, REM sleep will be aborted, causing REM sleep deprivation, or in less severe cases will be fragmented by multiple arousals and awakenings. In general, diaphragmatic insufficiency is more noticeable when the individual sleeps supine, because in this position the contents of the abdomen displace the flaccid, weak, or dysfunctional diaphragm cranially, compressing the lungs and placing an additional burden on ventilation. Aborted REM sleep and fragmentation of sleep are not the only consequences of diaphragmatic insufficiency. Hemoglobin desaturations of oxygen are profound, translating weak respirations and hypoventilation. Desaturations are so conspicuous that REM sleep can be identified in the polysomnogram and more readily in the hypnogram by the evolutions of the oxygen saturation graph. In addition to hypoventilation, the interplay between weak intrathoracic negative pressures and oropharyngeal muscle collapsibility determines the presence of apneas.

The identification of REM sleep hypoventilation requires polysomnography. This test should be considered for patients with a known neurogenic or neuromuscular disorder who complain of excessive daytime sleepiness with multiple awakenings at night. In severe cases, patients will develop orthopnea, nocturnal and early morning headaches, vomiting, and cyanosis, particularly when sleeping supine, all in the context of signs of progressive cardiopulmonary morbidity.

Because all respiratory complications of DMD are mechanical in nature (i.e., weak cough, dysphagia, hypoventilation), mechanical techniques for clearing the airway and improving ventilation are indicated. The concept of respiratory therapy should be introduced at diagnosis. Therapists can instruct parents in chest percussion and assisted cough. Bronchodilators may improve drainage, as will chest percussion. Intermittent positive-pressure breathing may reverse atelectasis.

Ventilatory support can reverse or prevent may of the physiologic difficulties associated with respiratory muscle weakness in patients with DMD.

The application of bilevel positive airway pressure is the accepted mode of treatment in individuals with REM sleep-related diaphragmatic insufficiency because continuous positive airway pressure (CPAP) is less well tolerated by patients with neuromuscular disease. The suggestion has been made that autoCPAP, capable of changing pressures from breath to breath, may be more amenable for treatment of patients whose respiratory pressure requirements change significantly from non-REM to REM sleep. All of these considerations require confirmation with appropriate clinical trials.

Among patients with a neuromuscular disorder and nocturnal ventilatory compromise, positive airway pressure applications during sleep vastly improve the quality of sleep, and in consequence the overall quality of life.

CARDIAC FAILURE

Although cardiac muscle is histologically abnormal in most patients with DMD, symptoms from cardiomyopathy develop in only approximately 10%. Those patients who become symptomatic do so in early to middle adolescence and usually die of congestive heart failure within 2 to 3 years from the onset of symptoms. Thus, this subgroup has a markedly shortened life span relative to most patients with DMD, and therefore it is imperative to discuss with the patient and family both the respiratory and cardiac complications of muscular dystrophy once the diagnosis is established.

Assessment of prognosis, both pulmonary and cardiac, is essential in planning long-term therapy. Although numerous means of evaluating pulmonary function are available and easy to use, no similar noninvasive, readily available indicator for the onset of cardiac failure is apparent. As opposed to respiratory problems, cardiac abnormalities do not correlate with the severity of skeletal muscle disease. Thus, a need exists to assess independently cardiac function in patients with DMD, especially if any form of long-term treatment with mechanical ventilation is under consideration. The patient with DMD and severe cardiomyopathy does not benefit from long-term assisted ventilation.

Detailed electrocardiographic findings in the dystrophic myocardium have been reported, but their ability to predict morbidity and mortality have not been well defined in patients with DMD. Echocardiography can provide adequate evaluation of cardiac function and is a relatively simple method for follow-up. Proper performance of echocardiography in patients with DMD may not be easy owing to limitations imposed by thoracic skeletal deformities.

SPINAL DEFORMITY

Scoliosis, another common problem in muscular dystrophy, develops early and tends to be rapidly progressive, especially when patients become nonambulatory. The curve usually is thoracolumbar or lumbar, with associated pelvic obliquity, thoracic kyphosis, and lumbar hyperlordosis. The abnormal sagittal alignment may cause problems with seating systems, even modified systems, and the rapid progression requires frequent wheelchair adjustments. Braces are not effective in progressive paralytic or neuromuscular curves. Rigid braces cause pressure areas on the skin and result in poor patient tolerance, and the softer braces are ineffective. Early spinal stabilization often is indicated in patients with muscular dystrophy when the curve reaches 30 degrees, before the onset of severe cardiopulmonary muscle weakness, which can make surgery more risky.

The technique of choice is an isolated posterior spinal fusion to L-5 or the sacrum, using the Harrington technique or, more commonly, the Luque–Galveston technique. Fusions stopping short of the sacrum usually occur because of the diffuse osteopenia in the sacrum and concern about pull-outs of the instrumentation. Failure of fusion to the sacrum, however, leads to recurrence of pelvic obliquity and necessitates further revision surgery.

Recent reviews of the Luque technique for instrumentation and fusion to the sacrum in patients with severe dystrophic curves found a high incidence of minor or temporary complications. Early severe complications occurred in 27% of patients, consisting of cardiac arrest, pseudoarthroses, ventilation problems, colonic perforation, bladder dysfunction, superior mesenteric artery syndrome, and distal weakness. Isolated cases of major cardiopulmonary complications such as ventricular fibrillation and fatal fat embolism also have been reported. Minor complications such as wound infection, urinary tract infection, and limb and trunk hypoesthesia occurred in 16% of patients, but all resolved within a few weeks to 2 months. Overall, however, the results were very satisfactory for all patients in obtaining spinal correction, achieving fusion, and restoration of sitting balance in their wheelchairs.

Before surgery, all patients with muscular dystrophy should have a detailed cardiac assessment, a pulmonary evaluation with pulmonary function tests (including arterial blood gases), and hematologic studies. Because of potential cardiomyopathy, intraoperative monitoring is an essential component of the anesthetic. Intraoperative blood loss usually is substantial in patients with muscular dystrophy because the muscle abnormalities cause ineffective constriction of the vessels. Another anesthetic complication is malignant hyperthermia, which is found in patients with muscle diseases. This risk is minimized with the use of nitrous oxide, intravenous narcotic sedatives, and nondepolarizing muscle relaxants.

NEUROMUSCULAR COMPLICATIONS

Because of the progressive muscle weakness and atrophy that occurs during adolescence, all patients with DMD at this stage of the disease have very limited forearm and intrinsic hand muscle use. Paraspinal muscle weakness results in kyphoscoliosis as well as poor head control, problems that can be helped with the use of several of the newer orthotic devices that improve seating and allow better head control. Ultimately, by their late teens or early twenties, the rate of progression in most patients appears to decrease, so that many patients reach a stable plateau with further deterioration occurring at a slow rate; however, by this stage almost all patients are completely dependent on their caregivers.

Orthotic treatment is helpful, but not as simple as evaluating a weak extremity and placing it with an antigravity position. One must have an understanding of gait analysis. DMD patients with quadriceps weakness use excessive knee extension to maintain ambulation. Plantar flexion of the ankle during foot strike causes an extension moment at the knee. Therefore, the clinical team must be very careful when attempting to correct plantar flexion positioning at the ankle. A patient who is placed into a solid ankle–foot orthosis (AFO) to improve clearance during swing phase of the gait cycle will actually cause a knee flexion moment. With limited quadriceps strength, the knee flexion moment cannot be opposed, and the child will become nonambulatory *after* initiating the brace.

Exercise has been shown to improve endurance in patients with DMD. It is important to remember that exercise prescriptions should not be written without directions or precautions. Persons with neuromuscular disease should not undergo exercise to exhaustion, as this could exacerbate symptoms. They should perform submaximal exercise only.

GASTROINTESTINAL INVOLVEMENT

Involvement of the gastrointestinal tract because of smooth muscle degeneration can be associated with severe symptoms in patients with DMD. Forms of intestinal pseudo-obstruction presenting with vomiting, abdominal pain, tenderness, and distention may be extremely serious. Many patients with DMD have a variety of gastrointestinal symptoms, such as dysphagia, reflux, choking, and heartburn due to upper gastrointestinal dysmotility. In some of these patients, such symptoms cause poor weight gain and eventually may lead to some degree of emaciation. More commonly, moderate to marked obesity is present, which adversely affects respiratory function.

PSYCHOLOGICAL INVOLVEMENT

Patients with DMD suffer a variety of emotional disturbances, most commonly depression and anxiety, particularly during adolescence. The erosion of the hope of normality and its effects on family dynamics have a wide-ranging impact on all involved. Over time, the patient with DMD lives in a "smaller world" as physical limitations preclude participating in many family, educational, and social activities both outside and in the home. The development of increasing dependence on others, realization of the limitations that the disease imposes, as well as its ultimate outcome, frequently require individual or family counseling or participation in local support groups.

FUTURE DEVELOPMENTS

DMD was thought of for a long time as a disease that could not be cured. Palliative treatments with steroids, physical therapy and orthotics were the main treatment options. Now, the possibility of treating DMD has transitioned from basic science research to the clinical realm. In the early 1990s, gene therapy was initiated using adenoviral vectors that contained genes encoding dystrophin. Patients received multiple muscle injections with the hope of repairing the gene or replenishing the dystrophin. Over a decade progress was made, but the clinical trials were stopped due to the development of adenovirus vector-induced shock syndrome and leukemia in some of the patients. The development of a nonpathogenic, adeno-associated vector, and the use of limited local injections, should eliminate future problems, with hope renewed to offer these patients a cure in the future.

Suggested Readings

Carroll JL, Marcus CL, eds. *Sleep and breathing in children.* New York: Dekker; 2000: 691–736.

Culebras A. Diaphragmatic insufficiency in REM sleep. *Sleep Med* 2004;5: 337–338.

Do T. Orthopedic management of the muscular dystrophies. *Curr Opin Pediatr* 2002;14:50–53.

Givan DC. Sleep and breathing in children with neuromuscular disease. In: Loughlin GM, Hilton T, Orr RD, et al., eds. End of life care in Duchenne muscular dystrophy. *Pediatr Neurol* 1993;9:165–177.

Hukins CA, Hillman DR. Daytime predictors of sleep hypoventilation in Duchenne muscular dystrophy. *Am J Respir Crit Care Med* 2000;161: 166–170.

Kelly BJ, Luce JM. The diagnosis and management of neuromuscular diseases causing respiratory failure. *Chest* 1991;99:1485–1493.

Russman BS. Rehabilitation of the child with a neuromuscular disorder. In: Jones HR, DeVivo DC, Darras BT, eds. *Neuromuscular disorders of infancy, childhood, and adolescence, a clinician's approach.* Philadelphia: Elsevier; 2003: 1275–1278.

CHAPTER 129E ■ SPECIFIC DISORDERS: MENINGOMYELOCELE

GEORGE W. CROWL AND DANIEL P. MOORE

Meningomyelocele is one of the most common congenital anomalies in the United States. Its incidence declined from 1.3 in 1,000 births in 1970, to 0.6 in 1,000 births in 1989, due in part to efforts to increase perinatal intake of folic acid and increased availability of prenatal screening (89). It is estimated that 70% of all neural tube defects can be prevented by daily intake of folic acid by all females of child-bearing age (90). Meningomyelocele is a chronic condition with multiple problems that requires a team of medical specialists to manage appropriately. The decline of multidisciplinary clinics has had a negative effect on the health care of this population (91). The challenge for the inpatient physician involved in the acute care of a patient with spina bifida is to understand his acute illness within the context of his chronic condition, and to coordinate the patient's continuing chronic care needs during his hospital admission.

Meningomyelocele is one of the most severe of the neural tube defects collectively known as spinal dysraphisms. Neural tube defects also include anencephaly and spina bifida occulta. Neural tube defects result from a failure of neurulation between the third and fourth week after conception. It is not certain whether the failure is due to a lack of closure or to a reopening of the canal, but it may be both or either. Several theories exist, including Padget's neuroschisis theory, Gardner's hydrodynamic theory, and Daniel and Strich's arrested development theory, but there is no current human research to prove the theories (92). These lesions are seen at all levels of the spine affecting motor function below the level of the lesion as well as sensation and bowel and bladder function. It is not entirely a spinal disease and has other significant effects on the central nervous system including the brain. Ninety percent of persons with meningomyelocele also have an Arnold–Chiari malformation requiring further intervention, usually surgery to place an indwelling shunt to relieve hydrocephalus (93). Though the disease is nonprogressive, the lifetime course can have ongoing complications that require the careful and thoughtful management of a large team of health care professionals including but not limited to neurosurgeons, urologists, orthopedists, rehabilitation physicians, ophthalmologists, nurse specialists, nutritionists, as well as school and vocational counselors.

The inpatient physician admitting the child with meningomyelocele needs to be aware of the variant physiology and anatomy that challenge the child and make the patient's presentation unique. Spina bifida is characterized by a vertebral defect with an open lesion or covered epithelial sac containing meninges, nerves, and cerebral spinal fluid (CSF). This lesion is usually closed surgically within a few days after birth. The closure is meant to prevent central nervous system (CNS) infection and does not change the functional course of the spinal cord lesion. In utero surgery is now being attempted at some institutions to alter the course of the disease, reduce the need for shunting, and decrease morbidity due to early infection. One hundred percent of children with meningomyelocele have an associated Arnold–Chiari malformation, which may cause an obstruction of the flow of CSF from the fourth ventricle or posterior fossa, resulting in dilatation of the ventricles and hydrocephalus (93).

The neurosurgeon may choose to place a cerebrospinal fluid shunt at the time of the closure of the spinal defect due to the presence of hydrocephalus. Alternatively, the patient may have little evidence of hydrocephalus at birth, due to the presence of an open lesion that decompresses the CNS. When the lesion is closed, the patient may develop progressive ventriculomegaly and require shunting. For most infants, a ventriculoperitoneal shunt is placed within the first 2 to 3 weeks of life.

SHUNT OBSTRUCTIONS AND INFECTIONS

A common reason for hospital admission beyond the newborn period and a major cause of morbidity and mortality is shunt infection or obstruction. The neurosurgeon caring for the patient is usually contacted for assessment upon admission, and if there is an infection present the shunt is externalized and the infection treated until the CSF is sterilized prior to reinsertion. If there is an obstruction or other mechanical problem related to the shunt, it may be replaced. In a recent study, 120 out of 189 (64%) children with meningomyelocele experienced a first shunt failure with a median time of 303 days; 24% were due to shunt infection. Sixty-one experienced a second shunt failure, 38 a third, and 36 had four or more. Shunt complications continue to be an important cause of morbidity and mortality in patients with meningomyelocele (94). For a more complete discussion of shunt problems, see Chapter 129C.

SLEEP-DISORDERED BREATHING

The patient with meningomyelocele may present with central sleep apnea and lower cranial nerve dysfunction due to a symptomatic Arnold–Chiari malformation that may require shunting or decompression. Separately, other types of sleep-disordered breathing (SDB) have been described in these patients, including obstructive apnea, central hypoventilation, and sleep-exacerbated restrictive lung disease characterized by hypoxia without apnea or central hypoventilation. The prevalence of moderate to severe SDB in patients with meningomyelocele may be as high as 20% (95). Polysomnography is used to determine the type and severity of the disease, and treatment may include supplemental oxygen, noninvasive positive pressure ventilation, and occasionally, tracheostomy and positive-pressure ventilation. The patient with sleep-disordered breathing is discussed in some detail in Chapter 42. An experienced multidisciplinary team can best treat the patient with meningomyelocele and sleep-disordered breathing.

SPINAL DEFORMITIES

The patient with meningomyelocele may have other spinal complications due to the congenital lesion and the defect of the vertebral anatomy. Scoliosis may be due to either neuromuscular weakness and/or asymmetric spasticity of the back musculature. A tethered spinal cord may present with scoliosis in addition to asymmetric weakness. It may also be caused by vertebral abnormalities including wedge vertebrae, hemi-vertebrae, congenital bars, or block vertebrae. Severe kyphosis may require surgical kyphectomy and fusion to prevent respiratory and abdominal compromise.

Diastematomyelia is a splitting of the spinal cord by a bony ridge or fibrous septum. The bony spicule may act as a fulcrum for tethering. Another more common cause of the tethered cord syndrome is the scarring down and adhering of the spinal cord to the closed spinal lesion. Tethered cord will be discussed separately later in this chapter.

ARNOLD–CHIARI MALFORMATION

Arnold–Chiari malformation (ACM) has, as its principal features, a caudal displacement of the medulla, lower pons, and cerebellar vermis and elongation of the fourth ventricle through the foramen magnum. In addition, the posterior fossa is small and the cisterna magna is obliterated. The cervical spinal cord is also displaced and the medulla kinked in spina bifida patients (96). It is type two of four types of hindbrain herniations called Chiari malformation described in the 1890s. Type I causes only caudal displacement of the cerebellar tonsils and type IV is a hypoplasia of the cerebellum. Chiari type III is a caudal displacement of the inferior cerebellum and brainstem into a cervico-occipital meningomyelocele (96). ACMs may become symptomatic after the newborn period during the first 2 to 3 months of life. Table 129.9 reviews symptoms of ACM during infancy.

TETHERED CORD SYNDROME

Tethered cord syndrome is a late presentation in patients with spina bifida. It is the result of skeletal growth and traction on the spinal cord. MRI of the spinal cord in a patient with meningomyelocele is likely to discover a tethering, but not all tethered cords are symptomatic and require intervention. The

most common signs and symptoms of a tethered cord are increased weakness (55%), worsening gait (54%), scoliosis (51%), pain (32%), orthopedic deformity (11%), and urologic dysfunction (6%) (97). Intervention consists of surgical release of the cord. After release, symptoms usually stabilize and back pain improves; however, some symptoms may persist, including any loss of bladder function or muscle weakness.

SYRINGOMYELIA AND HYDROMYELIA

Syringomyelia and hydromyelia are possible late complications of meningomyelocele and hydrocephalus. Syringomyelia is a central tubular cavitation within the spinal cord that is accompanied by an obstruction of the outlet of the fourth ventricle. This differs from hydromyelia, which communicates with the fourth ventricle. Syringomyelia is often present in the asymptomatic child and its presence often confuses the diagnosis of a shunted patient with spina bifida (who may also have a tethered cord) when he presents with a change in mental status or function. When the syringomyelia becomes symptomatic it requires surgical intervention. See Table 129.10 for selected signs of a symptomatic syringomyelia.

GROSS- AND FINE-MOTOR FUNCTION

Problems with upper-extremity coordination, fine graphomotor dexterity, and speeded fine-motor performance have been well documented in children with spina bifida.

Upper-extremity dysfunction is attributable to hydrocephalus, Chiari-related cerebellar and pyramidal tract abnormalities, or progressive cervical myelopathy (98,99). Gross motor function is only partially dependent on the physical level of the spinal lesion as the actual motor and sensory levels assessed by thorough manual muscle testing may vary somewhat from an absolute spinal level. Upper motor neuron spasticity is often mixed with lower motor neuron paralysis, causing muscle imbalance that affects both bone growth and joint anatomy (e.g., hip dislocation). The most important variable affecting ambulation is the level of paralysis. In the child with a L3 or

---

TABLE 129.9

SYMPTOMS OF CHIARI TYPE II MALFORMATION IN INFANTS

Feeding problems
  Choking
  Nasal regurgitation
  Poor suck
  Prolonged feeding time
  Aspiration
  Failure to thrive
  Depressed gag
Apnea (central, obstructive)
Weak cry
Bradycardia
Laryngeal stridor due to abductor paralysis of vocal cords
Cyanotic breath holding spells
Upper extremity weakness or hypotonia
Stiff hands (will not open to hold bottle)
Arching of the neck (opisthotonus)
Hypoventilation

Modified from Nickel RE. Meningomyelocele and related neural tube defects. In: Nickel RE, Desch LW, eds. *The physician's guide to caring for children with disabilities and chronic conditions*. Baltimore: Paul H. Brookes; 2000: 425–476.

TABLE 129.10

SELECTED SIGNS OF SYRINGOMYELIA AND HYDROMYELIA IN CHILDREN WITH MENINGOMYELOCELE

- Neck and occipital pain
- Weakness of the upper extremities
- Sensory loss in the arms
- Atrophy of hand muscles
- Headache
- Hyperextension of head and neck (retrocollis)
- Loss of deep tendon reflexes in the arms
- Onset or worsening of spasticity of legs
- Onset or worsening of hip and knee flexion contractures
- Onset or worsening of scoliosis
- Cranial nerve and brainstem dysfunction (onset can be rapid)

Modified from Nickel RE. Meningomyelocele and related neural tube defects. In: Nickel RE, Desch LW, eds. *The physician's guide to caring for children with disabilities and chronic conditions*. Baltimore: Paul H. Brookes; 2000: 425–476.

L4 neurosegmental function it is important that the quadriceps be sufficiently strong and the hips have full extension. Dislocation of the hips affects both quality of gait and, when asymmetric, causes pelvic obliquity. Pelvic obliquity contributes to scoliosis. Bilateral hip dislocations will affect the quality of gait but do not alone eliminate the possibility of functional ambulation. The child with spina bifida will often have foot and ankle deformities: equinovarus, cavus, calcaneus, and calcaneovalgus deformities. These deformities are managed with early serial casting when appropriate; orthotics are prescribed to position the foot and prevent further deformity; and surgery, when necessary, is performed to improve positioning, balance the musculature, and reshape and fuse the foot for weight-bearing and ambulation when appropriate. Usually these are ongoing orthopedic issues in the lives of children with meningomyelocele and are not addressed during admissions for acute medical issues. On the other hand, the child with spina bifida who is in school and is already receiving ongoing therapy services is often overlooked as he progresses when he might benefit from reevaluation and receive a new prescription for acute rehabilitation. His disease is often seen as chronic and nonprogressive. A short course of intensive therapy, at times, might return significant benefit. The benefits of therapy and physical training may be observed in a relatively short period of time. A 10-week structured exercise program in children aged 8 to 13 with spina bifida resulted in gains versus controls on measures of self-concept, cardiovascular endurance, and isometric strength (100). Neuromuscular electrical stimulation applied to *functioning* muscles (quads) by surface stimulation for 30 minutes a day over an 8-week period resulted in peak torque production and improvements in functional tasks (timed walking, timed step ascent and descent) (101).

BLADDER MANAGEMENT

Not all of the complications caused by the congenital lesion are confined to the central nervous system. Most notable are the effects on the sensory and motor nerves that innervate the bladder and the muscles of the perineum, including the pelvic muscles and sphincters of bladder and bowel. The effect is varied; some children have balanced bladders that empty with the usual signals of stretch of the detrusor and relaxation of the external sphincter; others experience detrusor-sphincter dys-synergy, or more generally, a hypertonic or hypotonic bladder with a spastic or incompetent external sphincter.

Although there is some controversy with regard to the sensitivity and specificity of the voiding cystourethrogram versus urodynamics for determining the proper management of the child during the early years of development, most urologists agree that clean intermittent catheterization is the proper treatment for children over 4 years of age who have a tight external sphincter, in preparation for school attendance. By age 6 most children can perform self-catheterizations with proper teaching and support (102). Normal bladder volumes for children can be estimated by the simple formula (103):

$$\text{Bladder volume} = (2 + \text{age}) \times 30\text{mL}.$$

Pharmacologic management includes anticholinergics (oxybutinin and propantheline) to aid in relaxation of smooth muscle in the bladder detrusor to decrease intravesical pressure and increase bladder capacity. Imipramine, a tricyclic antidepressant, may also be used for this purpose, with the added advantage of increasing the outlet resistance by an effect on the bladder neck. Alpha-sympathomimetics (ephedrine, pseudophedrine) also can increase outlet resistance by a tightening effect on the bladder neck.

Surgical interventions may be necessary to provide an appropriate reservoir (augmentation) due to a hyperspastic bladder, or for urinary diversion to allow the patient to self-catheterize if the patient has a high spinal lesion (cervical or thoracic) or other anatomic challenge. The Mitrofanoff procedure uses the appendix as a competent valve for self-catheterization. Another popular diversion, the Indiana pouch, is made by bringing the distal ileum to the skin, and uses the ileocecal valve for urinary continence.

A new implantable neuroprosthesis can replace the incompetent external sphincter function by inflating a valve to prevent leakage. It must be switched off to allow passage of urine.

BOWEL MANAGEMENT

Bowel management usually consists of a high-fiber diet and adequate fluid intake, and some physical manipulations as necessary. Sometimes stool softeners, cathartics, and suppositories are necessary. Constipation is often an accepted part of the patient's disabilities by family, but their acceptance is a result of resignation and lack of assistance more than satisfaction. It is often a social obstacle for the child when he reaches school age, and may result in rectal prolapse or megacolon with poor toileting and chronic constipation. Biofeedback training has been used with some success when there is some preservation of sensorimotor function in the perianal region. An enema continence catheter has been used to empty the rectosigmoid every 48 hours, allowing some children social continence. Electrical stimuation of the pudendal nerves using a neuroprosthetic device has been used in some patients (104). The pudendal nerve is stimulated continuously to achieve continence. The stimulation is discontinued only for stooling.

SKIN INTEGRITY

Absent or diminished sensation, particularly in the lower extremities and back, along with spinal deformities including pelvic obliquity from scoliosis or asymmetric dislocation of the hips, combine to increase the risk of decubiti, or pressure sores, due to compromised vascular perfusion in the tissue over a bony prominence. The loss of perfusion for as little as 20 minutes can cause necrosis of skin and muscle, which is often underestimated when first discovered due to depth of the most compromised tissues. Decubiti are the most common and the most costly cause of inpatient hospital admissions in these children. Over 70% of total hospital time and overall cost expenditures are associated with problems of skin integrity (105). Wheelchair seating, protection of the feet at home where some of these children crawl on the floor with erosion of the subcutaneous tissues, and protection from extremes of heat and cold are important primary care and health maintenance issues that need to be reemphasized when a patient with meningomyelocele is admitted to the hospital. Physical and occupational therapy consults are important for evaluation of equipment, range of motion, and transfers. Wheelchair seating evaluations are important when a patient is admitted for pressure sores. Allied health professionals may be able to assist in preventing future admissions for the same issues.

LATEX ALLERGIES

Children with meningomyelocele should be assumed to have a latex allergy, because the incidence is very common (47%) even compared to other children with latex exposure and similar surgical histories (106). Anaphylaxis is a rare, but very real, complication of exposure. Due to cross-allergen reactivity, diet restrictions should include bananas, avocados, chestnuts, kiwis, and tomatoes. ELISA studies can be used to document antibody production if necessary, but given its prevalence among the spina bifida population all patients with such lesions should be treated as if they are allergic.

OBESITY

Obesity is common among children with meningomyelocele. Because their lower extremities are often paralyzed, the long bones of the lower extremities are often shorter due to a lack of normal weight-bearing forces. Precocious puberty is also common and promotes early closure of the growth plates. Measurement of the skin folds at the scapula is a more accurate measurement of adiposity than linear height in these children.

Nutritional consultation should be sought early to assist families in adjusting diets for the relatively reduced physical activity and metabolism. In a Japanese study, 58% of patients above 6 years had an increased percentage of body fat compared to controls (107).

PRECOCIOUS PUBERTY

Precocious puberty is common and, on the average, female children experience the beginning of menstruation 1 to 2 years before their normal counterparts. This is possibly due to abnormalities in the hypothalamic–pituitary axis. Counseling for sexual activity and birth control should take into consideration the earlier menstrual onset.

AUTONOMIC DYSREFLEXIA

Autonomic dysreflexia is not commonly seen in children with meningomyelocele. Most meningomyelocele lesions are in the lumbosacral or sacral region. Autonomic dysreflexia should be considered in any children with a cervical and thoracic spinal level above T6.

Autonomic dysreflexia presents with diaphoresis, headache, blurred vision, stuffy nose, hypertension, and either tachycardia or bradycardia. Autonomic dysreflexia is a neurologic emergency when present, and should be treated by first searching for noxious stimulants such as an overfull bladder, urinary tract infection, constipation, or decubiti.

Elevation of the head of the bed on a patient at bed rest and bladder catheterization may quickly relieve symptoms. Severe hypertension (hypertensive crisis) should be quickly controlled to prevent serious sequelae such as stroke. Nitroglycerine paste is a useful treatment that can quickly control blood pressure and can be quickly removed when blood pressure normalizes.

SCHOOL AND EDUCATIONAL SERVICES

Most children with spina bifida are receiving special services in the school system. Each child has an Individualized Education Program (IEP) because of learning disabilities as well as fine-motor and gross-motor disability. They often receive physical, occupational, and speech therapies as part of their IEP. Children from 0 to 3 years of age receive Early Intervention services in the home. Children from 3 to 5 years of age should receive preschool services including therapy and medical equipment.

VISION AND HEARING

Vision and hearing should be evaluated. Most of the problems are related to hydrocephalus. When the hydrocephalus is treated and comprehensive eye care is available, 94% of the patients will have 6/12 visual acuity or better (108). Strabismus is common in this population. Changes in vision can be a sign of shunt obstruction or symptomatic AC malformation. Hearing abnormalities are found in up to 13% of children with spina bifida (109).

LANGUAGE DEVELOPMENT AND INTELLIGENCE

Developmental delay and mental retardation are fairly common findings in meningomyelocele. Delays in acquisition of gross- and fine-motor milestones by children with meningomyelocele have been documented across all lesion levels including those with minimal or no paralysis. Wide variations occur within lesion level groups. Delays are seen in those children with axial hypotonia, delayed integration of primitive reflexes, and delayed acquisition of protective reflexes, suggesting a CNS etiology (110).

Language development in the child with spina bifida is adequate in the areas of form and content, so much so that a superficial examination of their speech may seem age-appropriate. The social personality of the child with spina bifida who has a normal speech pattern but often reduced relevant content is sometimes described as "cocktail chatter."

Most children with spina bifida have problems using language appropriately for meaning construction and semantic-pragmatic communication and would benefit from therapy specifically focused on these areas (111). There are significant learning disabilities in the area of arithmetic. Despite this, the majority of children with spina bifida are felt to be in the low normal range of intelligence, testing (75%) above 80 on IQ testing. Only 9% are found to have scores below 70 on IQ testing (112).

VOCATIONAL PLACEMENT AND INDEPENDENT LIVING

In the United States, one-third of adults with spina bifida live with their families. Most children with spina bifida complete high school and 50% go on to further education. Employment rates range from 25% to 50%. Failure of both society and families to prepare their adolescent children for independent living is cited more than inability as a cause for this current situation.

Adolescents with meningomyelocele, in general, are felt to be happy and optimistic, but counseling in psychosocial areas, such as sexuality, vocational counseling, and decision–making, are noted to be underserved (113,114).

SUMMARY

The inpatient physician may be called upon to manage the patient with meningomyelocele who is admitted for a diagnosis-related problem, that is, neurologic emergencies, such as symptomatic Arnold–Chiari malformation, tethered cord, or shunt infection or obstruction. She may be called upon to manage a child with a severe decubitus or with urosepsis or in renal failure. She may be faced with an obstructed bowel or megacolon, or be consulted to manage his primary care needs when admitted for an elective orthopedic surgery to improve his musculoskeletal alignment for motor functioning. In each case, she must assess the complex interplay of a generally healthy static chronic condition and his daily care needs against the disturbance of acute illness or challenging surgery. The child and his family often have socioeconomic as well as psychosocial challenges. The inpatient physician has the potential for positively affecting their lives during their hospital stay.

PEARLS

- It has been estimated that two-thirds of all neural tube defects can be prevented by prescribing folic acid 0.4 mg orally on a daily basis to all women of child-bearing age.
- Spina bifida is not only a spinal cord lesion but also a brain and brainstem anatomic abnormality.
- Urologic problems are the most common cause of morbidity and mortality.
- Decubiti are the most common reason for admission and the most costly single complication in spina bifida. More attention should be paid to maintaining skin integrity through anticipatory guidance.
- Tethered cord syndrome can happen in the "innocent" spina bifida occulta lesion. Not all tethered cords are symptomatic. Not all syringomyelias are acute.
- Almost all children with meningomyelocele, who eventually ambulate in the community, achieve unsupported sitting by 15 months, crawl on all fours before 18 months, pull to stand by 24 months, and ambulate outside by age 4 (115,116).
- Children with lesions at L4 and more caudally are possible candidates for community ambulation.
- Arnold–Chiari malformation complications are the number one leading cause of death under the age of 2 in meningomyelocele.

References

1. Ogden CL, Carroll MD, Curtin LR, et al. Prevalence of overweight and obesity in the United States, 1999–2004. *JAMA* 2006;295:1549–1555.
2. Mokdad AH, Marks JS, Stroup DF, et al. Actual causes of death in the United States, 2000. *JAMA* 2004;291:1238–1245.
3. Barlow SE, Dietz WH. Obesity evaluation and treatment: Expert committee recommendations. *Pediatrics* 1998;102:e29.
4. Speiser PW, Rudolf MCJ, Anhalt H, et al. Consensus statement: childhood obesity. *J Clin Endocrinol Metab* 2005;1871–1887.
5. American Diabetes Association. Consensus statement: type 2 diabetes in children. *Diabetes Care* 2000;23:381–389.
6. Ahima RS. Central actions of adipocyte hormones. *Trends Endocrinol Metabol* 2005;16:307–313.
7. Keskin M, Kurtoglu S, Kendirci M, et al. Homeostasis model assessment is more reliable than the fasting glucose/insulin ratio and quantitative insulin sensitivity check index for assessing insulin resistance among obese children and adolescents. *Pediatrics* 2005;115:e500–e5003.
8. De Simone M, Farello G, Palumbo M, et al. Growth charts, growth velocity and bone development in childhood obesity. *Int J Obes Relat Metab Disord* 1995;19:851–857.
9. Biro FM, Khoury P, Morrison JA. Influence of obesity on timing of puberty. *Int J Andrology* 2006;29:272–277.
10. Ibanez L, Valls C, Ferrer A, et al. Sensitization in insulin induces ovulation in nonobese adolescents with anovulatory hyperandrogenism. *J Clin Endocrinol Metab* 2001;86:3595–3598.
11. Freedman DS, Dietz WH, Srinivasan SR, et al. The relation of overweight to cardiovascular risk factors among children and adolescents: the Bogalusa heart study. *Pediatrics* 1999;103:1175–1182.
12. Styne DM. Childhood and adolescent obesity: prevalence and significance. *Pediatr Clin North Am* 2001;48:823–854.
13. Hanerold C, Waller J, Daniels S, et al. The effects of obesity, gender, and ethnic group on left ventricular hypertrophy and geometry in hypertensive children: a collaborative study of the International Pediatric Hypertension Association. *Pediatrics* 2004;113:328–333.
14. Perkin RM, Lin JJ. Obstructive sleep apnea and hypopnea in hypertensive obese pediatric patients. *Chest* 2003;124:73S.
15. Li S, Chen W, Scrinivasan SR, et al. Childhood cardiovascular risks factors and carotid vascular changes in adulthood: the Bogalusa heart study. *JAMA* 2003;290:2271–2276.
16. Peppard PE, Young T, Palta M, et al. Longitudinal study of moderate weight change and sleep-disordered breathing. *JAMA* 2000;284:3015–3021.
17. Young T, Peppard PE, Taheri S. Physiology and pathophysiology of sleep apnea: excess weight and sleep-disordered breathing. *J Appl Physiol* 2005;99:1592–1599.
18. Watanabe T, Isono S, Tanaka A, et al. Contribution of body habitus and craniofacial characteristics to segmental closing pressures of the passive pharynx in patients with sleep disordered breathing. *Am J Respir Crit Care Med* 2002;165:260–265.
19. Redline S, Tishler PV, Schluchter M, et al. Risk factors for sleep-disordered breathing in children. Associations with obesity, race, and respiratory problems. *Am J Respir Crit Care Med* 1999;159:1527–1532.
20. Taheri S, Lin L, Austin D, et al. Short sleep duration is associated with reduced leptin, elevated ghrelin, and increased body mass index. *PLoS Med* 2004;1:e62.
21. Amin R. Relationship between obesity and sleep-disordered breathing in children: is it a closed loop? *J Pediatr* 2002;140:641–643.
22. Rhodes SK, Shimoda KC, Wald LR, et al. Neurocognitive deficits in morbidly obese children with obstructive apnea. *J Pediatr* 1995;127:741–744.
23. Brietzke SE, Katz ES, Roberson DW. Can history and physical exam reliably diagnose pediatric obstructive sleep apnea/hypopnea syndrome? A systematic review of the literature. *Otolarngol Head Neck Surg* 2004;131:827–832.
24. Brouillette RT, Manoukian JJ, Ducharme FM, et al. Efficacy of fluticasone nasal spray for pediatric obstructive sleep apnea. *J Pediatr* 2001;138:838–844.
25. Alexopoulos EI, Kaditis AG, Kostadima E, et al. Resolution of nocturnal enuresis in snoring children after treatment with nasal budesonide. *Urology* 2005;194e.14–194e.16.
26. Ford ES. The epidemiology of obesity and asthma. *J Allergy Clin Immunol* 2005;115:897–909.
27. Hakala K, Stenius-Aarniala B, Sovijärvi A. Effects of weight loss on peak flow variability, airways obstruction, and lung volumes in obese patients with asthma. *Chest* 2000;118:1315–1321.
28. Brunette DO. Resuscitation of the morbidly obese patient. *Am J Emerg Med* 2004;22:40–47.
29. Ray RM, Senders CW. Airway management in the obese child. *Pediatr Clin North Am* 2004;48:1055–1063.
30. Pelosi P, Croci M, Ravagnan I, et al. The effects of body mass on lung volumes, respiratory mechanics, and gas exchange during general anesthesia. *Anesth Analg* 1998;87:654–660.
31. Wolf G. After all those fat years: renal consequences of obesity. *Nephrol Dial Transplant* 2003;18:2471–2474.
32. Erstad BL. Dosing of medications in morbidly obese patients in the intensive care unit setting. *Intensive Care Med* 2004;30:18–32.
33. Ford ES, Galusta DA, Gillespie C, et al. C-reactive protein and body mass index in children: findings from the third National Health and Nutrition Examination Survey, 1988–1994. *J Pediatr* 2001;138:486–492.
34. Yudkin JS, Stehouwer CD, Emeis JJ, et al. C-reactive protein in healthy subjects: associations with obesity, insulin resistance, and endothelial dysfunction: a potential role for cytokines originating from adipose tissue? *Arterioscler Thromb Vasc Biol* 1999;19:972–978.
35. Jenco RJ, Grossi SG, Ho A, et al. A proposed model linking inflammation to obesity, diabetes, and periodontal infections. *J Periodontol* 2005;76(suppl):2075–2084.
36. Grossi, SG, Skrepcinski FB, DeCaro T, et al. Treatment of periodontal disease in diabetics reduces glycated hemoglobin. *J Periodontol* 1997;68:713–719.
37. Taylor ED, Theim KR, Mirch MC, et al. Orthopedic complications of overweight in children and adolescents. *Pediatrics* 2006;117:2167–2174.
38. Manoff EM, Banffy MB, Winell JJ. Relationship between body mass index and slipped capital femoral epiphysis. *J Pediatr Orthop* 2005;25:744–746.
39. Alfire ME, Treem WR. Nonalcoholic fatty liver disease. *Pediatr Ann* 2006;35:290–299.
40. Flack-Ytter Y, Younossi ZM, Marchesini G, et al. Clinical features and natural history of nonalcoholic steatosis syndromes. *Semin Liver Dis* 2001;21:17–26.
41. Graif M, Yanuka M, Baraz M, et al. Quantitative estimation of attenuation in ultrasound video images: correlation with histology in diffuse liver disease. *Invest Radiol* 2000;35:319–324.
42. Marchesini G, Brizi M, Bianchi G, et al. Metformin in non-alcoholic steatohepatitis. *Lancet* 2001;358:893–894.
43. Kambham N, Markowitz GS, Valeri AM, et al. Obesity-related glomerulopathy: an emerging epidemic. *Kidney Int* 2001;59:1498–1506.
44. Goodman E, Whitaker RL. A prospective study of the role of depression in the development and persistence of adolescent obesity. *Pediatrics* 2002;109:497–504.
45. Friedlander SL, Larkin EK, Rosen CL, et al. Decreased quality of life associated with obesity in school-aged children. *Arch Pediatr Adolesc Med* 2003;157:1206–1211.
46. Zeller MH, Helmut RR, Modi AC, et al. Health-related quality of life and depressive symptoms in adolescents with extreme obesity presenting for bariatric surgery. *Pediatrics* 2006;117:1155–1161.
47. Schwimmer JB, Burwinkle TM, Varni JW. Health-related quality of life of severely obese children and adolescents. *JAMA* 2003;289:1813–1819.
48. Citrome L, Blonde L, Damatarca C. Metabolic issues in patients with severe mental illness. *South Med J* 2005;98:714–720.
49. Skau M, Brennum J, Gjerris F, et al. What is new about idiopathic intracranial hypertension? An updated review of mechanism and treatment. *Cephalagia* 2005;26:384–399.

50. Kesler A, Fattal-Valevski A. Idiopathic intracranial hypertension in the pediatric population. *J Child Neurol* 2002;17:745–748.

51. Blasco PA. Primitive reflexes: their contribution to the early detection of cerebral palsy. *Clin Pediatr* 1994;33:388–397.

52. Capute AJ, Accardo PJ. Cerebral palsy. In: Capute AJ, Accardo PJ, eds. *Developmental disabilities in infancy and childhood*. 2nd ed. Baltimore: Paul H. Brookes; 1996:81–94.

53. Matthews DJ, Wilson P. Cerebral palsy. In: Molnar GE, Alexander MA, eds. *Pediatric rehabilitation*. 3rd ed. Philadelphia: Hanley & Belfus; 1999:193–217.

54. Pharoah POD, Cooke RWI. A hypothesis for the aetiology of spastic cerebral palsy: the vanishing twin. *Dev Med Child Neurol* 1997;39:292.

55. Kuban KCK, Leviton A. Cerebral palsy. *N Engl J Med* 1994;330:188–195.

56. Cummins SK, Nelson KB, Grether JK, et al. Cerebral palsy in four northern California counties, births 1983 through 1985. *J Pediatr* 1993;123:230–237.

57. Murphy CC, Yeargin-Allsopp M, Decoufle P, et al. Prevalence of cerebral palsy among ten-year-old children in metropolitan Atlanta, 1985 through 1987. *J Pediatr* 1993;123:S13–S19.

58. Hagberg B, Hagberg G, Olow I. The changing panorama of cerebral palsy in Sweden: VI. Prevalence and origin during the birth year period 1983–1986. *Acta Paediatr Scand* 1993;82:287–293.

59. Nicholson A, Alberman E. Cerebral palsy: an increasing contributor to severe mental retardation? *Arch Dis Child* 1992;67:1050–1055.

60. Stanley FJ. Cerebral palsy trends: implications for perinatal care. *Acta Obstet Gynecol Scand* 1994;73:5–9.

61. Ashwal S, Russman BS, Blasco PA, et al. Practice parameter: diagnostic assessment of the child with cerebral palsy. *Neurology* 2004;62:851–863.

62. Nelson KB. Epidemiology and etiology of cerebral palsy. In: Capute AJ, Accardo PJ, eds. *Developmental disabilities in infancy and childhood*. 2nd ed. Baltimore: Paul H. Brookes; 1996:73–79.

63. Papile L, Munsick-Bruno G, Schaefer A. Relationship of cerebral intraventricular hemorrhage and early childhood neurologic handicaps. *J Pediatr* 1983;103:273.

64. Volpe JJ. *Neurology of the newborn*. Philadelphia: Saunders; 1995.

65. Wiklund LM, Uvebran P. Hemiplegic cerebral palsy: correlation between CT morphology and clinical findings. *Dev Med Child Neurol* 1991;33:512–523.

66. Higuchi T, Graham SH, Fernandez E, et al. Effects of severe global ischemia in *N*-acetylaspartate and other metabolites in the rat brain. *Magn Reson Med* 1997;37:851–857.

67. van der Knaap MS, Valk J. *Magnetic resonance of myelin, myelination, and myelin disorders*. 2nd ed. Berlin: Springer; 1995.

68. Bairstow P, Cochrane R, Hur J. *Evaluation of conductive education for children with cerebral palsy: final reports* [parts I and II]. London: Her Majesty's Stationery Office; 1993.

69. Taub E, Ramey SL, DeLuca S, et al. Efficacy of constraint-induced movement therapy for children with cerebral palsy with asymmetric motor impairment. *Pediatrics* 2004:113;305–312.

70. Jain KK. The use of hyperberic oxygen in treating neurological disorders. In: Jain KK, ed. Textbook of hyperbaric medicine. Seattle: Hogrete and Huber Publishers, Inc. 1996:236–251.

71. Oregon Health & Science University Evidence-Based Practice Center. Agency for Healthcare Research and Quality Evidence Report/Technology Assessment no. 85 *Hyperbaric oxygen therapy for brain injury, cerebral palsy, and stroke*. September 2003. Full report and summary may be accessed on line at www.ahrq.gov.

72. Renshaw TS. Cerebral palsy. In: Morrisey RT, Weinstein SL, eds. *Lovell & Winter's pediatric orthopaedics*. 4th ed. Philadelphia: Lippincott-Raven; 1996:469–502.

73. Brazel PW, McPhee IB. Inappropriate secretion of antidiuretic hormone in postoperative scoliosis patients: The role of fluid management. *Spine* 1996; 21:724–727.

74. Robinson R. The frequency of other handicaps in children with cerebral palsy. *Dev Med Child Neurol* 1973;15:305.

75. Crichton JU, MacKinnon M, White CP. The life expectancy of persons with cerebral palsy. *Dev Med Child Neurol* 1995;37:567.

76. Blair E, Watson L, Badawi N, et al. Life expectancy among people with cerebral palsy in Western Australia. *Dev Med Child Neurol* 2001;43:508–515.

77. Strauss D, Cable W, Shavelle R. Causes of excess mortality in cerebral palsy. *Dev Med Child Neurol* 1999;41:580–585.

78. Molnar GE, Gordon SU. Cerebral palsy: predictive values of selected clinical signs of early prognostication of motor function. *Arch Phys Med Rehabil* 1976;57:153.

79. Cutler R, Page L, Galicich J. Formation and absoption of cerebrospinal fluid in man. *Brain* 1968;91:707–720.

80. Milhorat T, Hammock M, Fenstermacher J, et al. Cerebrospinal fluid production by the choroids plexus and brain. *Science* 1971;173:248–252.

81. Rekate H. Hydrocephalus classification and pathophysiology. Editor: McLone DG. In: *Pediatric neurosurgery. Surgery of the developing nervous system*. 4th ed. Philadelphia: Saunders; 2001.

82. Drake JM, Kestle JRW, Milner R, et al. Randomized trial of cerebrospinal fluid shunt valve design in pediatric hydrocephalus. *Neurosurgery* 1998;43:294–303.

83. Drake JM, Sainte-Rose C. *The shunt book*. Cambridge: Blackwell Science; 1995.

84. Ersahin Y, McLone DG, Storrs BB, et al. Review of 3017 procedures for the management of hydrocephalus in children. *Concepts Pediatr Neurosurg* 1989;9:21–28.

85. Choux M, Genitori L, Lang D, et al. Shunt implantation: reducing the incidence of shunt infection. *J Neurosurg* 1992;77:875–880.

86. Pollock I, Pang D, Albright A. The long term outcome in children with late onset aqueductal stenosis resulting from benign intrinsic tectal tumors. *J Neurosurg* 1994;80:681–688.

87. Buxton N, MacArthur D, Mallucci C, et al. Neuroendoscopic third ventriculostomy in patients less than 1 year old. *Pediatr Neurosurg* 1998;29:73–76.

88. Bergsneider M, Egnor MR, Johnston M, et al. What we don't (but should) know about hydrocephalus. *J Neurosurg* (suppl pediatrics) 2006;104:157–159.

89. Yeh IH, Khoury MJ, Erickson JD, et al. Study of genetics, epidemiology and vitamin usage in familial spina bifida in the United States in the 1990s. *Neurology* 1994;44:65.

90. Spina Bifida Association website. www.sbaa.org

91. Kaufman BA, Terbrock A, Winters N, et al. Disbanding a multidisciplinary clinic: effects on the health care of myelomeningocele patients. *Pediatr Neurosurg* 1994;21:36–44.

92. Tarby TA. Clinical view of the embryology of myelomeningocele. In: Rekate HL, ed. *Comprehensive management of spina bifida*. Boca Raton: CRC Press; 1991:29–48.

93. Menkes JH, Till K. Malformations of the central nervous system. In: Menkes J, ed. *Textbook of child neurology*. 5th ed. Baltimore: Williams & Wilkins; 1995:240–324.

94. Tuli S, Drake J, Lamberti-Pasculli M, et al. Long-term outcome of hydrocephalus management in myelomeningoceles. *Childs Nerv Syst* 2003;19:286–291.

95. Kirk VG, Morielli A, Gozal D, et al. Treatment of sleep disordered breathing in children with myelomeningocele. *Pediatr Pulmonol* 2000;30:445–452.

96. Griebel , ML, Oakes WJ, Worley G, et al. The Chiari malformation associated with myelodysplasia. In: Rekate HL, ed. *Comprehensive management of spina bifida*. Boca Raton: CRC Press; 1991.

97. Hudgins RJ, Gilreath CL. Tethered spinal cord following repair of myelomeningocele. *Neurosurg Focus* 2004;16:E7.

98. Grimm, RA. Hand function and tactile perception in a sample of children with myelomeningocele. *Am J Occup Ther* 1976;30:234–240.

99. Jansen J, Taudorf K, et al. Upper extremity function in spina bifida. *Childs Nerv Sys* 1991;7:67–71.

100. Andrade CK, Garben M. Changes in self concept, cardiovascular endurance and muscular strength of children with spina bifida aged 8 to 13 years in response to a 10-week physical activity programme: a pilot study. *Child Care Health Dev* 1991;17:183–196.

101. Karmel-Ross K, Cooperman DR, et al.The effect of electrical stimulation on quadriceps femoris muscle torque in children with spina bifida. *Phys Ther* 1992;72:723–730.

102. Bailey RR. Urologic management of spina bifida. In: Rekate HL, ed. *Comprehensive management of spina bifida*. Boca Raton: CRC Press; 1999:185–214.

103. Berger RM, Maizels M, Moren OC, et al. Bladder capacity (ounces) equals age (yr) plus 2 predicts normal bladder capacity and aids in diagnosis of abnormal voiding patterns. *J Urol* 1983;129:347–349.

104. Younoszai MK. Stooling problems in patients with myelomeningocele. *South Med J* 1992l;85:718–724.

105. Harris MB, Banta JV. Cost of skin care in the myelomeningocele population. *J Pediatr Orthop* 1990;10:355–361.

106. Pittman T, Kiburz J, Gabriel K, et al. Latex allergy in children with spina bifida. *Pediatr Neurosurg* 1995;22:96–100.

107. Mita K, Akataki K, Itoh K, et al. Assessment of obesity of children with spina bifida. *Dev Med Child Neurol* 1993;35:305–311.

108. Biglan AW. Ophthalmologic complications of meningomyelocele: a longitudinal study. *Trans Am Ophthalmol Soc* 1990;88:389–462.

109. Radke J, Gosky GA. Hearing and speech screening in hydrocephalus myelodysplasia population. *Spina Bifida Ther* 1981;3:25.

110. McDonald, CM. Rehabilitation of children with spinal dysraphism. *Neurosurg Clin North Am* 1995;6:393–412.

111. Fletcher JM, Barnes M, Dennis M, et al. Language development in children with spina bifida. *Semin Pediatr Neurol* 2002;9:201–208.

112. McLone DG. Continuing concepts in the management of spina bifida. *Pediatr Neurosurg* 1992;18:254–256.

113. Alexander MA, Steg NL. Myelomeningocele: comprehensive treatment. *Arch Phys Med Rehabil* 1989;70:637–641.

114. Rinck C, Berg J, Hafeman C. The adolescent with myelomeningocele: a review of parent experiences and expectations. *Adolescence* 1989;24: 699–710.

115. Findley TW, Agre JC, et al. Ambulation in the adolescent with myelomeningocele I: early childhood predictors. *Arch Phys Med Rehabil* 1987;68:518–522.

116. Souza JC, Telzrow RW, Holm RA, et al. Developmental guidelines for children with myelodysplasia. *J Am Ther Assoc* 1983;63:21–29.

Suggested Readings

Alexander MA, Steg NL. Myelomeningocele: comprehensive treatment. *Arch Phys Med Rehabil* 1989;70:637–641.

McDonald CM. Rehabilitation of children with spinal dysraphism. *Neurosurg Clin North Am* 1995;6:393–412.

Molnar GE, Murphy KP. Spina bifida. In: Molnar GE, Alexander MA, eds. *Pediatric rehabilitation*. 3rd ed. Philadelphia: Hanley & Belfus; 1999: 219–244.

Rekate HL, ed. *Comprehensive management of spina bifida*. Boca Raton: CRC Press; 1991.

CHAPTER 130 ■ ASPIRATION PNEUMONITIS AND ASPIRATION PNEUMONIA

RONALD M. PERKIN

Aspiration is defined as the inhalation of oropharyngeal or gastric contents into the larynx and lower respiratory tract. Several pulmonary syndromes may occur after aspiration, depending on the amount and nature of the aspirated material, the frequency of aspiration, and the host's response to the aspirated material. Aspiration pneumonitis is a chemical injury caused by the inhalation of sterile gastric contents, whereas aspiration pneumonia is an infectious process caused by the inhalation of oropharyngeal secretions that are colonized by pathogenic bacteria. Although there is some overlap between these syndromes, they are distinct clinical entities.

DEFINITIONS

Aspiration pneumonitis is defined as acute lung injury after inhalation of gastric contents. Aspiration of gastric contents results in a chemical burn of the tracheobronchial tree and pulmonary parenchyma, causing an intense parenchymal inflammatory reaction. There is a biphasic pattern of lung injury after acid aspiration.

The first phase peaks at 1 to 2 hours after aspiration and presumably results from the direct, caustic effect of the low pH of the aspirate on the cells lining the alveolar–capillary interface. The second phase, which peaks at 4 to 6 hours, is associated with infiltration of neutrophils into the alveoli and lung interstitium, with histologic findings characteristic of acute inflammation. The mechanisms of the lung injury after gastric aspiration involve a spectrum of inflammatory mediators, inflammatory cells, adhesion molecules, and enzymes. However, neutrophils and complement appear to have a key role in the development of lung injury.

Because gastric acid prevents the growth of bacteria, the contents of the stomach are sterile under normal conditions. Bacterial infection therefore does not have an important role in the early stages of acute lung injury after the aspiration of gastric contents. Bacterial infection may occur at a later stage of lung injury, but the incidence of this complication is unknown. Colonization of the gastric contents by potentially pathogenic organisms may occur when the pH in the stomach is increased by the use of antacids, histamine-2 receptor antagonists, or proton-pump inhibitors. In addition, there may be gastric colonization by gram-negative bacteria in patients who receive enteral feedings as well as in patients with gastroparesis or small bowel obstruction. In these circumstances, the inflammatory response in the lungs probably results both from bacterial infection and from the inflammatory response to the particulate gastric matter. Patients who have aspirated gastric material may present with dramatic signs and symptoms. There may be gastric material in the oropharynx as well as wheezing, coughing, shortness of breath, cyanosis, pulmonary edema, hypotension, and hypoxemia, with rapid progression to severe acute respiratory distress syndrome and death. However, many patients have only a cough or a wheeze, and some patients have what is commonly referred to as *silent aspiration*, which manifests only as arterial desaturation with radiologic evidence of aspiration.

Aspiration pneumonia develops after the inhalation of colonized oropharyngeal material. Aspiration of colonized secretions from the oropharynx is the primary mechanism by which bacteria gain entrance to the lungs. The term *aspiration pneumonia*, however, refers specifically to the development of a radiographically evident infiltrate in patients who are at increased risk for oropharyngeal aspiration.

In patients with aspiration pneumonia, unlike those with aspiration pneumonitis, the episode of aspiration usually is not witnessed. The diagnosis therefore is inferred when a patient at risk for aspiration has radiographic evidence of an infiltrate in a characteristic bronchopulmonary segment. Swallowing difficulties occur frequently in patients with cerebral palsy and neurologic impairment, and in the chronically ill.

Assessment of the cough and gag reflexes is an unreliable means of identifying patients at risk for aspiration. A comprehensive swallowing evaluation, supplemented by either a video fluoroscopic swallowing study or a fiberoptic endoscopic evaluation, is required. A speech–language pathologist can perform this evaluation at the bedside. In patients found to be at risk for aspiration, further behavioral, dietary, and medical management to reduce this risk can be initiated. Tube feeding usually is recommended in patients who continue to aspirate pureed food despite these strategies.

Feeding tubes offer no protection from colonized oral secretions, which are a serious threat to patients with dysphagia. Furthermore, scintigraphic studies have revealed evidence of aspiration of gastric contents in patients fed by gastrostomy tube. Over the long term, aspiration pneumonia is the most common cause of death in patients fed by gastrostomy tube.

MANAGEMENT

Aspiration Pneumonitis

The upper airway should be suctioned after a witnessed aspiration of gastric contents. Endotracheal intubation should be considered for patients who are unable to protect their airway (e.g., those with a decreased level of consciousness). Although it is common practice, the prophylactic use of antibiotics in patients in whom aspiration is suspected or witnessed is not recommended. Similarly, the use of antibiotics shortly after aspiration in patients in whom a fever, leukocytosis, or a pulmonary infiltrate develops is discouraged because the antibiotic may select for more resistant organisms in patients with an uncomplicated chemical pneumonitis. However, empiric antibiotic therapy is appropriate for patients who aspirate gastric contents and who have small bowel obstruction or other conditions associated with colonization of the gastric contents. Antibiotic therapy should be considered for patients with aspiration pneumonitis that fails to resolve within 48 hours after aspiration. Empiric therapy with broad-spectrum agents is recommended; antibiotics with anaerobic activity are not routinely required. Sampling of the lower respiratory tract (with a protected specimen brush or by bronchoalveolar lavage) and quantitative culture in intubated patients may allow targeted antibiotic therapy and, in patients with negative cultures, the discontinuation of antibiotics.

Although corticosteroids have been used in the management of aspiration pneumonitis, the existing data do not support their use, and therefore use of corticosteroids is not recommended.

Aspiration Pneumonia

Antibiotic therapy is unequivocally indicated in patients with aspiration pneumonia. The choice of antibiotics should depend on the setting in which the aspiration occurs as well as the patient's general health. However, antibiotic agents with activity against gram-negative organisms, such as third-generation cephalosporins, fluoroquinolones, and piperacillin, usually are required. Penicillin and clindamycin, which often are identified as the standard antibiotic agents for aspiration pneumonia, are inadequate for most patients with aspiration pneumonia. Antibiotic agents with specific anaerobic activity are not routinely warranted and may be indicated only in patients with severe periodontal disease, putrid sputum, or evidence of necrotizing pneumonia or lung abscess on radiographs of the chest.

Suggested Readings

Brambaugh DE, Accurso FJ. Persistent silent aspiration in a child with trisomy 21. *Curr Opin Pediatr* 2002;14:231–233.

Lundy DS, Smith C, Colangelo L, et al. Aspiration: cause and implications. *Otolaryngol Head Neck Surg* 1999;120:474–478.

Marik PE. Aspiration pneumonitis and aspiration pneumonia. *N Engl J Med* 2001;344:665–671.

Mercado-Deane M, Burton EM, Harlow SA, et al. Swallowing dysfunction in infants less than 1 year of age. *Pediatr Radiol* 2001;31:423–428.

CHAPTER 131A ■ LONG-TERM CENTRAL VENOUS CATHETERS

RONALD M. PERKIN

The long-term use of indwelling central venous catheters has become a mainstay in the management of infants and children with critical and chronic illnesses. Central venous lines (CVLs) have been developed to infuse fluids and drugs, to provide total parenteral nutrition, and to obtain samples of blood for study. Implantation of catheters for periods of months and years has been a significant advance in the management of patients with cancer and other diseases that require prolonged and intensive intravenous chemotherapy. Management of these indwelling lines demands meticulous attention to rote guidelines and procedures to ensure a functioning system free of complications.

TYPES OF CATHETERS

Three general types of catheters for long-term placement are:

1. External partially implanted (Broviac, Hickman, Groshong)
2. Totally implanted with a subcutaneous port (Portacath, Mediport, Infusaport)
3. Percutaneously inserted (PICC line)

Whereas the first two CVLs are inserted for long-term access, with reported durations of 12 to 32 months, PICC lines are used for briefer periods, with reported average durations varying from 16 to 72 days.

Broviac–Hickman Catheter

In 1973, Broviac and colleagues described a silicone rubber (Silastic) catheter for use in long-term intravenous alimentation. The original Broviac catheter was 90 cm long with a thin and flexible intravascular portion allowing it to float in the superior vena cava. This part of the catheter is attached to a thicker extravascular portion with a Dacron cuff in its midportion. The extravascular portion is placed in a subcutaneous tunnel and exits about 35 cm from the venous entry. After placement, the Dacron cuff becomes fixed by fibrous tissue, which in turn serves as a barrier to the migration of microbes from the skin along the catheter tract. A Broviac catheter was modified by Hickman to provide a larger bore. The Hickman catheter is available in one size only and may be used in older children and adults. The Broviac catheter is made in different sizes for infants, children, and adults.

Once it is in place, meticulous care and attention must be given to the catheter. Because of the long-term use, spanning months or years, involvement of the patient, parents, or other family members is often required. The most successful approaches to management come through specific, ritualistic, and even obsessive attention to details of dressing changes, drug and fluid administration, and maintenance of catheter

patency. Manufacturers of the catheters provide guidelines for care, and medical centers where these catheters are in frequent use establish a team and guidelines to meet their specific needs.

Implantable Ports

Implantable ports ("ports of entry") may be preferred for some older children and adolescents. The implantable device consists of a self-sealing injection port with a preconnected or attachable silicone catheter that is inserted into a large vein. These units are placed entirely under the skin. The Portacath has two major parts: (1) the subcutaneous port, used for entry into the system, is a silicone-covered metallic chamber with a self-sealing silicone septum; and (2) the plastic catheter. The installment of the Portacath is similar to that of the Broviac–Hickman catheters. The catheter is inserted into the large central vein, such as the superior vena cava, and the port is placed under the skin and sutured to the chest wall. The target surface of the port is easy to locate and access. The skin covering the port must be in a healthy condition. The self-sealing septum can withstand at least 2,000 punctures with a 22-gauge noncoring needle or 1,000 punctures with a 10-gauge noncoring needle.

Only special noncoring needles are used for accessing the port. The needles are available in several shapes and sizes. The 90-degree noncoring needle is angulated and may be secured into the port with a dressing for infusions. The maximum time that the needle can be left in place is approximately 7 days.

The unit should always be filled with heparinized saline after each use. The heparin lock helps prevent thrombotic occlusion of the catheter.

The system is flushed the first 3 days after surgery once per day with 5 mL heparinized saline (100 U/mL heparin), or by continuous infusion of fluids. When there are extended periods between injections, infusions, or blood sampling, the system must be flushed with heparinized saline once every 2 weeks.

COMPLICATIONS

Infection

One of the main risks of a central line is that of line infection. This risk is increased if sterile technique is not maintained during procedures. Although accessing a line or withdrawing blood can introduce organisms into the line, infection from the line also may be the presenting problem. Precipitating organisms cultured from infected lines include *Staphylococcus aureus*, *Staphylococcus epidermidis*, *Streptococcus viridans*,

Pseudomonas aeruginosa, Klebsiella pneumoniae, Escherichia coli, and *Enterobacter cloacae* as well as fungi. The risk of introducing line infection remains in patients even when sterile technique is done well.

Catheter infections include line sepsis (at least bacteremia) and skin infections at the skin exit site, subcutaneous tunnel, or the skin overlying the implanted devices. Common organisms implicated in skin infections include *S. aureus* and *S. epidermidis*. Skin infections involving gram-negative bacilli such as *P. aeruginosa* appear to be more likely in neutropenic patients. Management should involve obtaining a blood culture from both the line and a peripheral site. Appropriate intravenous antibiotic therapy is initiated, and a decision about exploring for distal sites of infection is required.

Air Embolism

Because these catheter systems end in blood vessels near the heart, the risk of air embolism is present. It is vital to keep the system clamped whenever installation of fluid or withdrawal of blood is not taking place to minimize this risk. Signs and symptoms of air embolism include the sudden onset of tachypnea, hypotension, and loss of consciousness. Treatment includes clamping the system immediately, placement of the patient on the left side in a Trendelenburg position, administration of oxygen, and providing intravenous access.

Catheter Occlusion and Embolization of a Catheter Thrombus

A risk of thrombus formation at the tip of the catheter exists. Studies have shown fibrin sheaths around occluded catheters, and one study measured thrombi that were aspirated from occluded catheters after the instillation of urokinase. These thrombi can occlude the catheter or increase the risk of embolization. Although these thrombi are small fragments, a large one can result in pulmonary embolism if dislodged during flushing. Signs and symptoms include tachycardia, tachypnea, hypoxemia, and chest pain. Diagnosis can be confirmed by a ventilation–perfusion scan, and therapy initiated.

Resistance to saline instillation or a failure to see a blood return can be due to catheter malposition (against a vein wall), catheter malfunction, or a fibrous clot at the distal tip. Noninvasive methods to evaluate for this include altering the patient's position, raising the patient's hands above head, having the patient cough or performing a Valsalva maneuver, or placing the bed in reverse Trendelenburg. All of these interventions may change the venous pressure gradient along the catheter and improve patency.

Importantly, the clinician should not try to flush the catheter by forcefully pushing saline into it or by overzealous withdrawal, but rather instill saline or aspirate for blood after trying one or more of the previously mentioned maneuvers.

If fluid cannot be instilled or no blood returns, either a clot in the catheter or a fibrin clot at the tip may be present. In such cases, attempts to declot the catheter should be made, unless the patient is actively bleeding or has cerebrovascular disease. (It is the practice in some hospitals to require a physician directly to perform this procedure.) One method is to use a fibrinolytic such as urokinase to restore catheter patency. However, the U.S. Food and Drug Administration issued an "Important Drug Warning" about urokinase; hence it is unavailable for use to restore CVL patency. Both alteplase and streptokinase have been used to restore CVL patency. However, the producers of streptokinase released a letter in December of 1999 warning of the risk of allergic reactions to streptokinase and that streptokinase is not indicated for restoration of CVL patency.

There is limited clinical experience with alteplase for restoration of CVL patency. One study using alteplase in children (0.5 mg for children <10 kg; 1–2 mg for children >10 kg) showed that it appears to be a safe and effective thrombolytic agent for CVL patency restoration in children.

Tissue plasminogen activator (TPA) 0.5 to 1 mL, left to rest in the catheter for 2 hours before attempting aspiration, can restore function. A study that evaluated the efficacy of TPA in clearing CVLs showed 86% success with the first dose and 95% with two attempts.

CVLs must be flushed regularly with heparinized saline to reduce incidence of thrombotic occlusion.

Catheter Breakage

Catheter breakage can result inadvertently from cutting the catheter with scissors while trying to remove the dressing, from a needle piercing the catheter, from a child pulling away during access, from children who play with the implantable port site (twiddler syndrome), or from injury to it from contact sports. The catheter can separate from the port of the implanted device. For partially implantable devices, it is important to clamp the catheter proximal to the break and cover the torn region with a sterile gauze if available. If no external catheter is present, pressure should be applied at the catheter entrance site into the vein (not at the exit site). Repair kits are available for partially implantable catheters. For totally implanted devices, a radiograph should be obtained to determine the integrity of the system. Both the primary physician and the surgeon needed to be contacted.

Other catheter-related complications result from catheter migration. These include arrhythmias, cardiac tamponade, pneumothorax, and superior vena cava syndrome.

PICC Line Complications

Complications with PICC lines are reported to be as high as 40%, with occlusion and infection being the most frequently reported. Complications more common with PICC lines include external breaks, shoulder pain, phlebitis without infection, exit site irritation, dislodgement, and occlusion. A study that compared PICC line function with non-central tip location versus central tip location showed comparable results and complication rates, with the exception that non-central PICC lines failed sooner, and fewer patients completed their course of therapy.

Suggested Readings

Choi M, Massicottee P, Marzinotto V, et al. The use of alteplase to restore patency of central venous lines in pediatric patients. *J Pediatr* 2001;135: 152–156.

Marino C, Aslam M, Kamath V, et al. Life threatening complications of peripherally inserted central catheter (PICC) in a newborn. *Neonatal Intensive Care* 2006;19:63–65.

Ryder MA. Peripherally inserted central venous catheters. *Nurs Clin North Am* 1993;28:937–971.

Shah SS, Smith MJ, Zaoutis TE. Device-related infections in children. *Pediatr Clin North Am* 2005;52:1189–1208.

Srivastava R, Stone BL, Murphy NA. Hospitalist care of the medically complex child. *Pediatr Clin North Am* 2005;52:1165–1187.

Thiagarajan RR, Bratton SL, Gettmann T, et al. Efficacy of peripherally inserted central venous catheters placed in noncentral veins. *Pediatrics* 1998;152: 436–439.

Yeung CY, Lee HC, Huang FY, et al. Sepsis during total parenteral nutrition: exploration of risk factors and determination of the effectiveness of peripherally inserted central venous catheters. *Pediatr Infect Dis J* 1998;17: 135–142.

CHAPTER 131B ■ TECHNOLOGY-DEPENDENT CHILD:TRACHEOSTOMY

SANA AL-JUNDI AND PAUL LUBINSKY

CHILDREN WITH SPECIAL HEALTH CARE NEEDS

In the United States, the number of children with special health care needs (CSHCN) has been increasing, and is currently estimated to be over 12 million or between 13% and 18% of all children (1).

CSHCN are defined as "those who have or are at increased risk for a chronic physical, developmental, behavioral, or emotional condition and who also require health and related services of a type or amount beyond that required by children generally" (1). Technology-dependent children are a subgroup of CSHCN and are dependent on certain devices for survival. Recent advances in medical technology have enabled more children to survive the complications of premature birth, congenital abnormalities, and chronic illnesses. The trend is for these children, who otherwise would have required a prolonged hospital stay, to be cared for at home. This means more frequent visits to the emergency department and more hospitalizations for recurrent complications.

Patients with chronic lung disease, severe neurologic disorders, or muscle diseases often require mechanical ventilatory assistance via a tracheostomy, while others require a tracheostomy to maintain a patent airway. These patients are cared for either at home or in a chronic care facility. A significant proportion of all pediatric hospitalizations come from admission of technology-dependent children as they experience acute exacerbation of their underlying diseases. Up to one-fourth of all pediatric emergency department (ED) visits are related to chronic illnesses (2). Many of these technology-dependent children have a tracheostomy in place and some require home mechanical ventilation. Hospitalists need to be familiar with the equipment involved and the specific complications these patients encounter. Hospitalists are often involved in the initial decision to place the tracheostomy and need to be familiar with the indications and timing of placement, available sizes and types of tracheostomy, the insertion techniques, appropriate care for the tracheostomy tube and site, complications of tracheostomy, and the use of a Passey–Muir valve.

TRACHEOSTOMY TECHNIQUES

Tracheostomy is the procedure in which an artificial airway is surgically created to bypass upper airway obstruction, or to provide a long-term access to the trachea for mechanical ventilation and suctioning. It is an ancient procedure that has been cited in documents dating back to 400 BC (3). It became a standard surgical procedure after 1909 when Chevalier Jackson published his article in *Laryngoscope*, where he described this procedure with specific indications, techniques, and complications (4).

Tracheostomy can be inserted by open surgical technique or percutaneously. Percutaneous dilational tracheostomy (PDT) is done using Seldinger technique with bronchscopic guidance . It is often done at the bedside by the critical care physician, hospitalist, or pulmonologist. This technique is becoming more common in adults compared to open surgical technique (5),

and seems to be safe when performed by an experienced practitioner (6). This technique still has some limitations and is contraindicated in patients with coagulopathy. PDT is less common in pediatric patients and considered contraindicated in patients less than 12 years old (7). A few case reports suggest the applicability of PDT in pediatric patients (8,9). PDT can be a good choice for older children and teenagers.

More common in the pediatric population is the open surgical technique performed in the operating room by a general surgeon, or a head and neck surgeon. A midline vertical incision is created from the inferior border of the thyroid cartilage to the sternal notch. The trachea is then exposed by midline dissection to minimize injury to lateral structures such as the carotid artery, jugular vein, and their tributaries. The isthmus of the thyroid is either clamped and divided or retracted inferiorly. The trachea is entered normally between the second and the third tracheal rings; one ring in small children is commonly divided (10). The lateral tracheal walls are secured to the skin and an appropriate-size tracheostomy tube is inserted and secured by ties (usually cloth or Velcro) around the neck. Many surgeons leave the traction sutures they place in the operating room in each side of the tracheal incision; they are labeled for right and left and taped to the patient's skin, so they can be pulled up to facilitate tube replacement in the event of accidental decannulation. Others (7) do not advocate this technique, because use of traction sutures to blindly replace a fresh tracheostomy tube can easily lead to misplacement of the tube into the mediastinum.

There have been no standards and little published research in the field of tracheostomy care in children. Tracheostomy tube type, composition, and size are usually selected based on preference of the surgeon. In January 2000, the Pediatric Assembly of the American Thoracic Society published a consensus statement to serve as standard of pediatric tracheostomy care that provides detailed guidelines on tube selection and the evidence supporting it (11).

TRACHEOSTOMY INDICATIONS AND TIMING

Tracheostomy is indicated in patients who are unable to breathe normally due to disorders that may involve the function of the central nervous system and brainstem, diaphragm and intercostal muscles, upper and lower airways, and those with cardiopulmonary dysfunction requiring positive-pressure ventilation.

A list of common indications for tracheostomy in children is given in Table 131.1.

In addition to the categories listed in the table, an emergency tracheostomy is indicated in respiratory failure patients in whom direct laryngoscopy fails to provide successful intubation. When a patient is predicted to need long-term mechanical ventilation, an early tracheostomy is beneficial in improving patient comfort, decreasing amount of sedation used, improving patient's ability to communicate with staff, and allowing for earlier use of oral nutrition (4). Controversy exists regarding the timing of this procedure in

TABLE 131.1

COMMON INDICATIONS FOR TRACHEOSTOMY IN PEDIATRIC PATIENTS

Upper airway obstruction	Congenital and acquired subglottic stenosis
	Acute upper airway edema: burns, infections, anaphylaxis
	Airway compression: tumors, abscess, or trauma
	Vocal cords paralysis
	Congenital airway abnormalities
	Congenital vascular abnormality
	Severe facial deformity: micrognathia
Neuromuscular diseases	Muscular dystrophy
	Spinal cord injuries
Chronic lung diseases	Prematurity
	Prolonged mechanical ventilation
	Pulmonary hypertension
Central nervous system disorders	Chiari malformation
	Central hypoventilation syndrome
	Brain tumors
	Lack of airway protection reflexes: chronic aspiration
	Hypoxic ischemic brain injury
	Traumatic brain injury

adults (12). Published guidelines by the American College of Chest Physicians (13), in which a review was made of all published studies regarding the impact of tracheostomy timing on the duration of mechanical ventilation, have failed to confirm the need to perform a tracheostomy after a specific period of mechanical ventilation. A recent prospective randomized study (14) compared the benefits and risks of percutaneous tracheotomy within 48 hours versus 14 to 16 days in 120 critically ill adult patients who were projected to require ventilation for ≥ 14 to 16 days. This study found that early tracheostomy group showed statistically significant less mortality, pneumonia, accidental extubations, shorter duration of mechanical ventilation, and reduced length of stay in the intensive-care unit compared to the late tracheostomy group.

The timing and indications for tracheostomy in children are less well defined. Recent advances in neonatal and pediatric critical care along with the increasing use of chronic mechanical ventilatory support via tracheostomy, and the growing use of noninvasive ventilatory techniques, will change the characteristics of this group of pediatric patients. The decision to place a tracheostomy remains based on individual case presentations and should be tailored to accommodate the specific needs of each patient.

TRACHEOSTOMY EQUIPMENT

Tracheostomy equipment includes the tube itself, which is connected to a swivel device that connects to a heat and moisture exchanger. Patients with tracheostomies can breathe either humidified room air, oxygen by a "trach collar," or they can be on mechanical ventilation (Fig. 131.1).

There are many different commercial brands in the market each with certain advantages and disadvantages. *Tracheostomy tubes* are made of polyvinyl chloride or silicone, which is more flexible. Metal tubes are rarely used. All tubes consist of the main shaft and neck flanges with holes for the tracheostomy ties. All tracheostomies have a 15-mm universal adapter that connects to the ventilator tubing or to an ambu-bag or anesthesia bag.

Tracheostomy tubes are sized based on three dimensions: the inner diameter, outer diameter, and length. The inner diameter is usually printed on the outer flange and ranges from 2.5 to 10.0 mm. Some tracheostomy tubes have removable inner cannula, which can be removed for cleaning while the outer cannula remains in place to maintain the airway. Cuffed tracheostomies are occasionally used in pediatric patients if high pressure is needed during mechanical ventilation, or in case of chronic translaryngeal aspiration. Uncuffed tubes are generally preferred (11), and facilitate the use of a Passey–Muir valve, optimizing the patients ability to speak.

The *Passey–Muir* valve is a unidirectional flanged valve that opens on inhalation and occludes on exhalation, reestablishing laryngeal and vocal cord airflow as the power source for vibratory sound production. Some patients benefit from the extra airflow with minimum resistance provided by a fenestrated tracheostomy tube. This is a tracheostomy with perforations allowing egress of respiratory gasses to the trachea above the tracheostomy tube and out through the vocal cords.

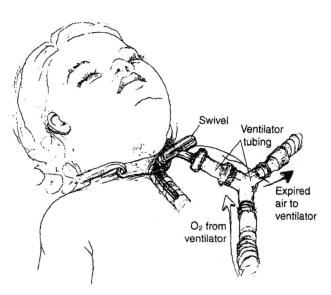

FIGURE 131.1. Tracheostomy parts. (From Fleisher GR, Luwing S, eds. *Textbook of pediatric emergency medicine.* 4th ed. Philadelphia: Lippincott Williams & Wilkins; 2000.)

Fenestrated tracheostomy tubes also have an inner cannula that occludes the fenestration and must be removed for the fenestration to become patent. A fenestrated tube may facilitate weaning from the tracheostomy tube as it reduces airflow resistance. The Passey–Muir valve is contraindicated in the presence of upper airway obstruction, patients who require inflated cuffs, and tubes with snug fits if there is no ability for air to egress. A Passey–Muir valve or similar device is not required for all patients. Optimizing speech is a complex process that should involve an experienced speech and language pathologist and may require adjustments of PEEP, inspiratory time, and tidal volume in ventilated patients.

Swivel devices are used when the tracheostomy tube is connected to a mechanical ventilator to avoid disconnection when traction is applied to the tracheostomy; they also provide an additional few centimeters of extension from the neck, which helps prevent tube occlusion when the neck is flexed.

The *heat and moisture exchanger* is a small plastic device that connects to the swivel device. It has a hygroscopically active membrane that captures the heat and humidity of the patient's exhaled gasses, moisturizing and warming the inspired gasses. These are practical and convenient in outpatient settings, allowing for a greater degree of mobility, but are usually replaced with heated humidifiers when the patient is hospitalized.

POSTOPERATIVE CARE FOR PATIENTS WITH A NEW TRACHEOSTOMY

Patients who undergo tracheostomy tube placement are observed in the pediatric intensive-care unit (PICU) until their stoma wound is epithelialized and the open edges of the tracheal wall secured to the subcutaneous tissues. This is referred to as a "mature stoma." Once the stoma is "mature," the tracheostomy tube can be safely changed with less concern for the development of a false passage. The time required for this maturation and duration of PICU observation is variable and ranges from 4 to 8 days. Immediate postsurgical care consists of continuous monitoring of vital signs and oxygen saturation, frequent physical examination, frequent assessment of breath sounds, and providing adequate sedation to avoid excessive movements. Table 131.2 gives a checklist for the physician caring for patients immediately after tracheostomy surgery.

Secretion management is important in tracheostomy patients. Underlying lung disease is often responsible for much of the secretions, but the tracheostomy tube may induce mucus production. The tracheostomy tube impairs mucociliary clear-

ance, reducing the ability of the patient to clear secretions and pathogens. The tracheostomy tube also compromises the patient's ability to cough, and they often require suctioning to help clear secretions. Frequent routine suctioning is not recommended, and it has been suggested that this may introduce some of the bacteria colonizing the tracheostomy into the patient's tracheobronchial tree. The depth of suctioning must be measured, and it is usually not necessary for the tip of the catheter to be passed beyond the end of the tracheostomy tube, where it will induce mucosal damage. Glycopyrolate is initiated in many instances to reduce secretions. It is important to ensure that secretions are not excessively thickened and to monitor for anti-cholinergic side effects.

EARLY COMPLICATIONS

Early complications and their management are listed in Table 131.3. They include bleeding, tube displacement, pneumomediastinum, pneumothorax, and rarely esophageal perforation and nerve damage. Transient tracheitis and stomal cellulitis may occur, and can be minimized with strict local hygiene. Severe infections such as mediastinitis, osteomyelitis, and necrotizing fasciitis are rare, but have been reported and must be treated aggressively.

A small amount of bleeding from the stoma can be controlled by changing the dressing as needed and suctioning blood from the airways to avoid airway obstruction. Accidental removal of the tracheostomy tube before the stoma is healed can be problematic; the tracheostomy tube should be replaced by reinserting it gently through the stoma. As discussed earlier, if traction sutures are left in place, they can be used by pulling them up and to the sides when reinserting the tracheostomy tube. In a "fresh" tracheostomy, if severe respiratory distress or cyanosis develops after tube reinsertion, if unable to confirm equal breath sounds with adequate chest expansion with bagging, or if the ETCO$_2$ detector does not confirm correct placement (measured exhaled CO$_2$, or colorimetric detector changes color from purple to yellow), then orolaryngeal intubation should be performed emergently. Caution should be taken when intubating patients in whom tracheostomy was indicated for airway abnormalities and obstruction. The otolaryngologist should be called immediately to reestablish the airways.

A spare tracheostomy tube and a tube that is one size smaller should always be available at the bedside in case of complete obstruction that requires emergency tracheostomy tube change. In addition, there should be scissors to facilitate removal of the tracheostomy ties. In the event of acute tracheostomy obstruction, suctioning and clearing the tracheostomy tube should be attempted first. If this does not resolve the obstruction, the tracheostomy should be replaced. If it is a cuffed tracheostomy tube, the cuff should be deflated first. If tracheostomy tube displacement causes respiratory compromise and deterioration of vital signs, standard endotracheal intubation using direct laryngoscopy can be lifesaving. The tracheostomy stoma can close in a short period of time ranging from hours to a few days if the tracheostomy tube remains out. In the event oral intubation is necessary, the surgeon should be called to reestablish the tracheostomy as soon as possible.

LATE COMPLICATIONS

Pediatric patients with tracheostomy will develop complications in 25% to 50% of cases. Complications are more common in younger children, premature infants, and patients with prolonged cannulation time (11).

Late complications include bleeding, which is usually a small amount from the stoma. Rarely, catastrophic bleeding occurs due to tracheal wall erosion or tracheal erosion into the

TABLE 131.2

POSTOPERATIVE CARE OF PATIENT WITH A NEW TRACHEOSTOMY TUBE

- Physical exam (identify tracheal stoma surgical threads when present).
- Check for equal breath sounds.
- Check for subcutaneous air.
- Check for bleeding.
- Control pain and agitation.
- Check chest x-rays for pneumothorax or pneumomediastinum.
- Institute continuous-pulse oximetry.
- Maintain a "spare" tracheostomy tube, scissors, and light source at the bedside.
- Rule out esophageal perforation if acute hemodynamic deterioration.

TABLE 131.3

COMMON EARLY COMPLICATIONS FOLLOWING INSERTION OF TRACHEOSTOMY

Complication	Symptoms	Management
Bleeding	Excessive bleeding from the stoma	Change dressing and suction blood from airways
	If severe, compromised hemodynamics	If severe, call the surgeon immediately to investigate, check measures of coagulation, including platelets, and start volume replacement
Subcutaneous air	Crepitus and swelling	No specific management but minimize respiratory effort and/or ventilator pressures
Tube displacement	Respiratory distress, unequal breath sounds, cyanosis	Replace through stoma or perform oral intubation
Tube occlusion	Respiratory distress, cyanosis, sudden vocalization	Suctioning, ambu-bagging, and trach tube change if needed
Pneumomediastinum	Facial and neck swelling and cepitus	None, if hemodynamically stable; confirm with chest x-rays
Pneumothorax	None, if small unequal breath sounds, respiratory distress, cyanosis if large	Confirm with chest x-rays, check tube position, thoracotomy tube if large
Stoma infection and trachetis	Erythema and in duration at the site, fever, leukocytosis	Obtain cultures, appropriate antibiotic therapy

Innominate artery. This rare complication can be fatal and requires immediate surgical intervention.

Granulomas are common and their management is controversial unless they are found distal to the tracheostomy tube, or if they cause obstruction and excessive bleeding. Symptomatic granulomas are generally treated with laser removal. Suprastomal granulomas are often not removed because they are asymptomatic and tend to reoccur.

A life-threatening complication that can occur at home or in the hospital is tracheostomy tube obstruction and/or dislodgement; this can be fatal if not managed properly. Any patient with a tracheostomy whose respiratory distress does not abate after suctioning must have the tracheostomy tube changed immediately, even if this has been done recently.

When patients are admitted for any respiratory tract infection or pneumonia, they are at risk for tracheostomy tube obstruction with thick secretions. Figure 131.2 illustrates the steps for replacing the tube. If a tube of the same size is difficult to pass through the stoma, a tube that is half a size or a full size smaller should be tried. If not immediately available, an endotracheal tube through the stoma is an acceptable temporizing measure that will maintain the patency of the stoma and allow ventilation. A useful technique to facilitate replacement of a tracheostomy when difficulty occurs is to pass a suction

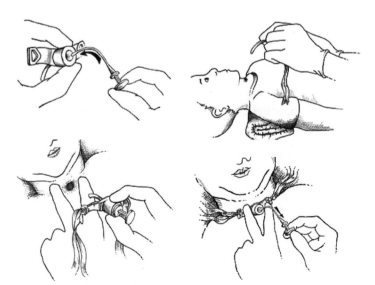

FIGURE 131.2. Tracheostomy tube change steps. 1. Insert obturator into new tracheostomy tube. Attach ties and lubricate end with water-based lubricant. 2. Remove old tube after placing a towel under child's shoulders. 3. Gently insert it pushing back then down in an arching motion. 4. Remove the obturator as you hold the tube in place. (Modified from Shiley® *Parent's guide to pediatric tracheostomy home care*. 2005 Nellcor Puritan Bennett Inc.)

TABLE 131.4

LATE COMPLICATIONS OF TRACHEOSTOMY

Complication	Cause	Management
Bleeding	Dryness of the mucosa Granulomas	Use humidification daily
Granuloma	Reaction to foreign instrumentation Aggressive suctioning	(Controversial): Removal if obstructive None if suprastomal and small
Tracheostomy tube dislodgement	Tension from ventilator tubing and suctioning Loose tracheostomy ties	Replacement See Figure 131.2
Tracheostomy tube obstruction	Tracheal secretions	Suctioning, humidification
Tracheitis and pneumonia	Colonization with bacteria Reduced cough Aspiration Poor hygiene at home care	Obtain tracheal aspirate cultures Antibiotic therapy
Impaired swallowing and airway protection	Reduced laryngeal function and gag reflex Reduced cough Esophageal compression from over inflated cuff	Speech and langauge pathologist assessment and treatment, including swallow studies

catheter through the tracheostomy to then insert the tip of the suction catheter through the stoma into the trachea, and to then feed the tracheostomy in over the catheter guide. In a spontaneously breathing patient it may be possible to hear air passage through the suction catheter, confirming placement in the tracheal lumen.

Pneumonia and re-recurrent tracheitis may occur more frequently in the presence of a tracheostomy tube. Patients with a tracheostomy are frequently colonized with pathogens such as *Staphylococcus aureus*, *Pseudomonas aeruginosa*, and *Candida albicans*. Many develop resistant strains. Because tracheal aspirate culture will reveal positive results, the physician should treat based on associated clinical signs and symptoms such as fever, leukocytosis, change in the quality and quantities of tracheal secretions, and chest x-rays changes. Culture results can be useful to guide the choice of antimicrobial agents.

Some complications may present only after decannulation such as tracheomalacia and tracheal stenosis, and should be investigated before considering removal of the tracheostomy tube permanently.

Other rare complications are tracheoesophageal fistula and tracheocutaneous fistula. Table 131.4 summarizes the common late complications, their causes, and their management.

TRACHEOSTOMY PATIENTS WITH CHRONIC LUNG DISEASE

Chronic care includes routine changing and cleaning of the tracheostomy tube weekly. If an inner cannula is present, it is cleaned daily. Cleaning solutions are half-strength peroxide or a dilute solution of saline and detergent. A tracheostomy brush to remove encrustations is often required.

When tracheostomy patients are admitted to the hospital for respiratory distress, the etiology can be related to either proximal or lower airways disease. In addition to performing a thorough physical exam, the admitting physician needs to obtain a detailed history regarding triggering event, associated symptoms, whether the patient has recently had airway instrumentation, change in tracheal secretions, an increased oxygen requirement, or a change in air leak around the tube.

Review of the patient's past medical history is important. See Table 131.5.

Patients with chronic lung disease on home ventilation may experience a worsening of their pulmonary condition and may develop respiratory distress, increased oxygen requirement, and a change in their tracheal secretions. As pulmonary compliance decreases there may be an increased loss of delivered tidal

TABLE 131.5

RESPIRATORY DISTRESS IN TRACHEOSTOMY PATIENTS

History	Possible clinical diagnosis
Recent tracheostomy tube change	Possible false passage Pneumomediastinum, pneumothorax
Associated symptoms: fever, lethargy, cough, increased secretions	Tracheitis, pneumonia
Previous history of recurrent granulomas	Possible obstruction from granulomas
Last bronchscopic exam by otolaryngologist?	
Increase air leak from stoma	Acute lower airway disease, increased pulmonary resistance
Bleeding from tracheostomy stoma	Granulomas or infections

volume around the tracheostomy stoma. If the air leak is significant and cyanosis is present, assisted ventilation with a larger tidal volume is necessary. It may be necessary to replace the uncuffed tracheostomy tube with a either a larger tracheostomy tube or a cuffed tracheostomy tube, or with a cuffed endotracheal tube inserted through the stoma. In an emergency situation, if sufficient ventilation cannot be accomplished by means of the tracheostomy stoma, orotracheal intubation utilizing direct laryngoscopy is the next step.

DECANNULATION

When the tracheostomy tube is no longer required, the patient should be evaluated for possible decannulation. If the patient is able to maintain an adequate airway and has no need for mechanical ventilation, the tracheostomy tube may be removed. Traditionally, the tracheostomy tube is downsized sequentially and often occluded for a few days before it is removed, to ensure the patient's ability to breathe without it.

The one-stage method is generally preferred. It involves endoscopic examination of the airways during spontaneous breathing; if anatomic and functional patency is found to be adequate, the patient is decannulated. Observation and monitoring in the hospital is appropriate for some patients for 24 to 48 hours after decannulation (11).

ETHICAL ISSUES

Hospitalists are often the primary physician for patients with chronic illnesses because of the significant period of time these patients are hospitalized. Discussions regarding need for tracheostomy, home mechanical ventilation, and end-of-life decisions should involve all medical care team members including the hospitalist. The hospitalist and pulmonologist or intensivist will have the most experience determining the need and benefits of tracheostomy, and addressing issues of futility. The home setting must be carefully evaluated to ensure adequate resources. In some instances, the establishment of chronic tracheostomy or ventilatory support may preclude the patient's return to his prior residence.

Families of children with severe chronic illnesses need guidance in making these decisions. It is difficult to address the do-not-resuscitate (DNR) orders during emergencies, but these issues should be addressed before patient discharge in a multi-disciplinary team approach.

CHAPTER 131C ■ TECHNOLOGY-DEPENDENT CHILDREN: GASTROSTOMY TUBE

PAMELA G. LARSEN

A gastrostomy is the creation of a gastrocutaneous fistula into which a tube is placed for the purpose of administrating nutrition or medications, or for decompression (venting). Gastrostomy tubes (GTs) are placed in children with a variety of conditions when oral feeding is not possible, or when nutrition cannot be adequately consumed orally. Children may require partial or total enteral feeding through the GT to provide adequate nutrition for growth and development.

INCIDENCE

For over a century, the gastrostomy has been used as enteral access for nutritional support to the child or adult with chronic conditions affecting the ability to feed orally (e.g., tracheoesophageal fistula, cerebral palsy, and other neurologic or disabling conditions). Over 200,000 gastrostomy tubes are placed yearly. Since the early 1990s, significant increases have been seen in the number of children for whom long-term enteral access is required. Reports show that as many as 15% to 75% of children with neurologic impairment, oral-motor impairment, gastroesophageal reflux (GER), delayed gastric emptying, or constipation may require long-term enteral access. Central nervous system (CNS) dysfunction may increase or decrease gastrointestinal motility, result in persistent activation of the emetic reflex, or be associated with dysfunction of the lower esophageal sphincter.

Lower esophageal sphincter dysfunction and GER are seen more often in children with hiatal hernia, prolonged supine positioning, or increased intraabdominal pressure as a result of spasticity, scoliosis, or seizures. GER may cause esophagitis, aspiration pneumonia, and failure to thrive from malnutrition and vomiting.

Feeding GTs are increasingly used to improve nutritional status of disabled children. Because these children also frequently experience reflux, it often has been assumed that this is a complication of GT feeding. Because conventional antireflux measures, including modifications of feeding time and position and medical management, often are unsuccessful, many of these children also undergo surgical antireflux procedures such as fundoplication. Data show, however, that postoperative complications of fundoplication are higher in disabled patients, and the procedure may not be efficacious, especially in the very young child. Initial placement of a GT without a protective antireflux procedure currently is the favored approach for neurologically impaired children without preoperative evidence of GER. Newer procedures, such as percutaneous endoscopic gastrostomy (PEG; PEG placement does not require laparoscopy), have made the issue of an antireflux surgical procedure a decision separate from the decision to place a GT. The PEG procedure for placement of the GT is an important innovation in the care of this high-risk group of pediatric patients and allows the avoidance of celiotomy with its related morbidity and mortality.

TABLE 131.6

INDICATIONS FOR GASTROSTOMY

Alimentary anomalies
Bowel obstruction
Chronic diseases (cystic fibrosis, cerebral palsy, head trauma, tumors, degenerative diseases)
Central nervous system disorders
Developmental delay
Esophageal atresia
Injuries to mouth/esophagus
Intestinal strictures
Malrotation
Necrotizing enterocolitis
Severe gastroesophageal reflux disease
Short bowel syndrome
Supplemental feedings for failure to thrive
Tracheoesophageal fistula
Underlying pulmonary cardiac diseases

INDICATIONS FOR GASTROSTOMY TUBE PLACEMENT

Some of the indications for GT placement are listed in Table 131.6. Cerebral palsy (CP) is a common neurologic disability in children. Despite gains in perinatal care, the incidence of CP does not appear to be declining, and actually is increasing secondary to survival of very-low-birthweight premature infants. Feeding problems among these children are frequent, and total or near-total inability to swallow (inanition) is the main reason for gastrostomy placement. Further, there are significant associated stresses for both child and parent surrounding feeding. In as many as one-third of children with special needs, feeding problems such as anorexia, oral aversion, dysphagia, aspiration, or vomiting develop. Children with gastrointestinal tract anomalies or with chronic diseases (e.g., cystic fibrosis or degenerative disorders) also may require gastrostomy for correction of malnutrition. Children with complications of prematurity, CNS injury, cancer, or gut disorders (e.g., necrotizing enterocolitis, malrotation, malabsorption syndromes, tracheoesophageal fistula, or bowel obstruction) also may be candidates for gastrostomy. Further, data show that parents of children with special needs reported improved weight gain, less stress surrounding feeding, and easier medication administration after a gastrostomy was placed, and many caregivers had more time to devote to themselves and other children.

TYPES OF GASTROSTOMY TUBES

The GT itself may be a tube such as a simple Foley (urinary) catheter, or a Malecot or Robinson rubber catheter. Many children (and their parents) prefer GTs that are shorter with less protrusion from the abdomen, usually at the level of the skin. These GTs include the MIC-KEY "button" (similar to those made by Bard, Ross, Corpak, and others), are easier to clean and more aesthetically appealing, and were designed specifically for gastrostomy feedings. Further, in a study assessing silicone versus polyurethane PEG tubes, the polyurethane button lasted significantly longer.

The primary health care provider may be one of the first to recognize the physical, developmental, or emotional need for GT placement. In turn, this same provider often must trou-

bleshoot and treat subsequent complications with the GT. The GT can be placed by (1) a percutaneous procedure using endoscopic pull-through (*pull* PEG); (2) a radiologic percutaneous procedure (*push* PEG); (3) laparoscopy; or (4) an open procedure (Stamm gastrostomy or Janeway gastrostomy).

COMPLICATIONS AND MANAGEMENT OF GASTROSTOMY TUBES

Complications of GTs can be divided into complications arising early (within the first 1 to 2 weeks after placement), and late (>2 weeks). Many of these complications overlap the time period distinction. An early complication is injury or perforation of the gastric wall. This is unintended and may occur immediately after surgery, or with replacement of the GT before healing (maturation) of the stomal tract. Leakage of gastric contents into the peritoneum may cause peritonitis if the gastric wall separates from the abdominal wall. If the child is poorly nourished or has difficulty healing (e.g., steroid therapy or immunosuppression), wound separation or dehiscence may occur. Waiting for 3 to 4 weeks or longer after initial placement before changing the GT allows the stoma tract to mature. Securing the GT snugly at the abdominal wall reduces complications of leakage, separation, and wound trauma. Excessive pressure, however, may result in tissue ischemia and pressure necrosis of the gastric or stomach wall.

Postoperative infection occurs in approximately 10% of the children, and prophylactic antibiotics frequently are prescribed to reduce wound infection. Pathogens include bacteria (staphylococci), viruses, and fungi. Infection presents as spreading erythema, edema, and peristomal wound drainage. Consultation with the pediatric surgeon should be pursued immediately.

Hemorrhage may result from inadequate hemostasis. This may occur within 48 hours or as late as 6 or 7 days after surgery. Superficial gastric mucosal erosion with secondary bleeding also may occur if there is excessive tension on the GT.

Accidental dislodgement is the most common complication. If the dislodgement occurs in the first 2 or 3 weeks after surgical placement, replacement may require surgery or radiologic guidance. After 2 to 4 weeks, the stoma tract is healed and the outer gastric wall has adhered to the inner peritoneum. Tube replacement can then take place safely and easily. Mature stomas may close quickly, within minutes to hours, and therefore replacement with the same or a new tube should be attempted as soon after the dislodgement as feasible. For children with a skin-level "button," a back-up Foley catheter may be used until the correct button can be inserted. Prolonged dislodgement may require dilatation with a smaller tube, or reoperation may be necessary. Difficulty in replacing a tube may warrant a radiopaque contrast dye injection to confirm that the GT is in the stomach and the tract has not been disrupted.

Local infection around the GT is common, and scrupulous skin care is important. Daily cleansing with soap and water usually is adequate. For crusting or drainage at the GT site, half-strength hydrogen peroxide solution cleansing followed by clear water rinse may help dissolve the debris. The clinician should be alert for a contact dermatitis from a silicone tube or related devices such as tape, foam, or bumpers used to secure the tube. Frequently, there is a clear to slightly purulent discharge from the stoma, an inflammatory foreign body response to the GT. Frequent cleansing is necessary to prevent excoriation of the local skin area. If the surrounding skin develops a cellulitis, a 7- to 10-day course of oral antibiotics is indicated. Likely pathogens include *Staphylococcus aureus* and group A *Streptococcus*. A first-generation cephalosporin (i.e., cephalexin) should be prescribed.

Skin breakdown may result from gastric contents leaking around the GT. Excess movement or a GT that is too long may cause the stoma to enlarge, with subsequent leakage of gastric contents or formula resulting in skin irritation. In addition to keeping the site clean, prophylactic skin barriers can be applied, or a topical agent can be applied around the tube to neutralize the stomach acid. Erythema or swelling of the stoma site can be treated with a topical antibiotic such as or neomycin or bacitracin (e.g., Neosporin). Monilial infections (maculopapular rash with a weepy appearance) should be treated with an antifungal such as nystatin (Mycostatin). The powdered form of nystatin may help keep the area drier. Blister-like lesions surrounding the stoma may be treated with a hydrocolloid barrier powder such as Stomahesive. Placement of a wafer (flat disk that adheres to and seals the skin) may reduce contact of acid liquids with the skin. Frequent dressing changes are necessary to promote healing and reduce further breakdown.

Migration of the distal end of the GT occurs from inadequate stabilization of the GT, or excessive length, especially if a Foley catheter is used. Migration may be into the esophagus or the pylorus. In the esophagus, the GT may cause vomiting and increase the possibility of aspiration. Migration into the pylorus results in gastric outlet obstruction with abdominal distention and pain. Although infrequent, distal migration of the GT may result in a "dumping-like" syndrome with nausea, diarrhea, bloating diaphoresis, and pallor. Further, if the balloon on the migrating GT is inflated, mucosal erosion of the esophagus, duodenum, or bowel may result. Proximal stabilization of the GT is essential both to prevent migration and to reduce stomal site irritation, which may cause granulation tissue to form. Stabilization may be accomplished using a foam or plastic bumper, hypoallergenic tape, or a "T" stabilizer (Figs. 131.3 to 131.5).

Granulation tissue usually is the result of the body's reaction to a foreign body—the GT. The leakage of gastric contents is an additional factor in granulation tissue formation. Granulation tissue develops in nearly 50% of GTs. The inflamed epithelial tissue extrudes out of the GT stoma and is friable. Movement of the GT against the stoma worsens the problem. Chemical cautery with silver nitrate shrinks the granulation tissue. Application once or twice daily for several days may be required, and causes the tissue to turn gray and slough. Caution must be used to avoid direct contact with intact skin. Skin that is excoriated around the stoma may need application of a protective barrier cream, wafer, or other adhesive dressing (DuoDerm). Application of a steroid cream such as triamcinolone 0.5% TID has been recommended for hypergranulation tissue.

Bleeding at the GT site usually arises from the aforementioned friable granulation tissue. However, bleeding from

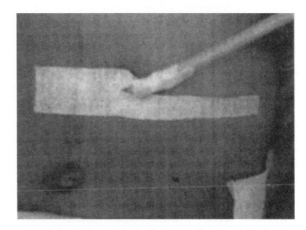

FIGURE 131.4. Securing gastrostomy tube with hypoallergenic tape.

along the stoma tract or gastric mucosa must be considered. Excessive mobility or tension may lead to gastric irritation, mucosal bleeding, and hematemesis. Upper endoscopy may be required for bleeding not resolved by stabilization of the tube. Treatment of the granulation tissue is reviewed earlier.

GT blockage may occur if the tubing becomes clogged with formula, medications, or other debris. Failing adequately to flush the GT usually is the cause of the blockage, and is easily prevented. Gently "milking" the tube usually loosens the matter in the tubing. After GT medications and formula, the tubing should be flushed with 5 to 10 mL of water for an infant, or 15 to 20 mL for a child. An air flush can be used for children on fluid restrictions. Many children are more comfortable if the GT is vented for 10 to 15 minutes after feeding. If the GT cannot be cleared with water, a small amount of carbonated beverage allowed to sit in the tube for 5 to 10 minutes may free the tubing of the obstruction. This may be repeated as necessary to clear the GT. Clamping the GT proximally reduces clogging of the tube with larger formula or medication particles. Medications administered through the gastrostomy tube must be liquid (i.e., pills must be crushed or otherwise dissolved in liquid, and capsules must be opened and diluted).

Peristomal leakage of gastric contents usually is noted if the stoma site has enlarged around the GT. Enlargement of the stoma occurs if the GT, particularly a long G-tube such as a Foley catheter, is allowed excessive movement. The temptation is to place a larger tube to stop the leakage; however, this does not solve the problem, and in fact often worsens the enlarging stoma. Gradually downsizing the GT allows the stoma to shrink and corrects the dilatation. Placing a hydrocolloid dressing or barrier powders helps reduce the likelihood of the leakage resulting in excoriation of the stoma site.

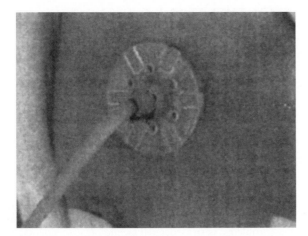

FIGURE 131.3. Securing gastrostomy tube with plastic bumper.

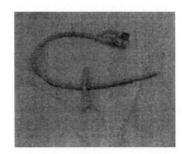

FIGURE 131.5. Securing gastrostomy tube (GT) with "T" slit. Cut 1½ to 2 inches off second Foley, and make a slit into the rubber. Before inserting Foley into stoma, slide GT Foley through the slit to form a "T." After insertion into the stoma, slide the "T" close to the abdomen to secure GT in place.

Leakage also can be reduced by increasing the size of the intragastric balloon. After ensuring that the balloon is fully inflated with 5 mL of water, the water in the balloon is gradually increased by 2-mL increments, to a total of 10 mL. Leakage also may be noted if there is overfeeding, delayed gastric emptying, or gastric outlet obstruction. The provider may consider providing antacids, histamine-2 blockers, or proton-pump inhibitors to reduce skin irritation and promote gastric emptying. Topical application of a barrier cream may reduce skin irritation. A radiologic study for gastric outlet obstruction should be considered for copious leakage of gastric contents.

Beyond the immediate postoperative period, complications associated with GTs include bowel obstruction, bowel perforation, exacerbation of GER, and gastrocutaneous fistula. Parents should be informed that the need for gastrostomy revision is seen in about 6% of children, and is usually related to concurrent fundoplication at the time of gastrostomy, percutaneous placement of the GT, or infants younger than 18 months. Bowel obstruction may result from migration of the GT if a longer tube such as the Foley or Robinson catheter is used. Surgical placement of a button GT in the distal stomach also may occlude the bowel by obstruction of the gastric outlet or the duodenum. Bowel perforation occurs typically during surgical placement and may cause postoperative peritonitis. If the gastrostomy is placed incorrectly into the bowel, a milky diarrhea may occur; alternatively, feculent peristomal discharge may be noted. Because the GT alters the angle of the gastroesophageal junction, new or recurrent GER may be seen.

For GTs that have been removed, the stoma is expected to close spontaneously. GTs that have been in place for an extended period of time (>9 months) may have a gastrocutaneous fistula that requires surgical closure. Temporarily, a drainage bag such as a colostomy bag may be placed over the site to collect gastric secretions and reduce skin excoriation from gastric secretions. Cauterization with silver nitrate may promote closure; however, if closure is not complete within 4 weeks, surgical consultation should be considered.

GASTROJEJUNAL FEEDING TUBES

A transgastric jejunal feeding tube is an alternative in children with feeding difficulties who also have GER or gastroparesis.

There is a paucity of information describing the use of gastrojejunal feeding tubes in children.

Several techniques have been described for the nonsurgical insertion of gastrojejunal tubes in children. The gastrojejunal tube may be placed by an endoscopist (a percutaneous endoscopic gastrojejunal tube) or a radiologist using a percutaneous technique. Alternatively, the gastrojejunal tube can be inserted through an existing gastrostomy track. In all cases, the tube is manipulated into position using fluoroscopy or endoscopy. Difficulty intubating the jejunum frequently is encountered.

Although gastrojejunal tube feedings have been shown to have nutritional benefits, they are associated with a high incidence of complications. Some children have evidence of duodenogastric reflux of bile and GER despite correct positioning of the tube beyond the ligament of Treitz. Other complications are primarily mechanical and include tube migration, fracture, dislodgement, and blockage. Continuous feedings and frequent flushing of gastrojejunal tubes reduces the likelihood of blockage.

PEARLS

- Although less expensive to use, Foley catheter GTs are more likely to cause granulation tissue, be associated with leaking, and result in enlarging stomas.
- Placing a larger GT into a leaking stoma worsens the problem with leaking in the long run.
- Meticulous care of the GT avoids many of the more minor but irritating complications of GTs.

Suggested Readings

Borkowski S. Pediatric stomas, tubes, and appliances. *Pediatr Clin North Am* 1998;45:1419–1435.
Burd RS, Price MR, Whalen TV. The role of protective antireflux procedures in neurologically impaired children: a decision analysis. *J Pediatr Surg* 2002;37:500–506.
Crawley-Coha, T. A practical guide for the mangagement of pediatric gastrostomy tubes based on 14 years of experience. *J Wound Ostomy Continence Nurs* 2004;31:193–200.
Godbole P, Margabanthu G, Crabbe DC, et al. Limitations and use of gastrojejunal feeding tubes. *Arch Dis Child* 2002;86:134–137.

CHAPTER 131D ■ TECHNOLOGY-DEPENDENT CHILDREN: MECHANICAL SUPPORT OF VENTILATION (MECHANICAL VENTILATION IN CHRONIC RESPIRATORY FAILURE)

JAMES P. CAPPON AND NICK G. ANAS

Advances in bystander cardiopulmonary resuscitation (CPR), pre-hospital emergency medical systems, (EMS), emergency medicine, and intensive and subspecialty pediatric care have led to a growing population of children who previously would

not have survived their acute illness, injury, or condition. Many of these children do not survive unscathed; chronic medical problems, with associated technology dependency, are increasingly the norm. Recurrent illnesses, deteriorations in baseline function, and scheduled visits and procedures result in frequent returns to the acute hospital setting from the chronic care environment. It is therefore prudent for the pediatric hospitalist to be prepared to manage these "chronic" children when they return to the acute care setting.

With increasing survival of preterm infants, infants with congenital malformations, and infants and children with a wide variety of severe chronic diseases, a small but growing cohort of patients with chronic respiratory insufficiency has developed. Such infants and children suffer from impaired oxygen delivery or carbon dioxide retention while breathing unassisted in room air, and they require support to prevent or correct these deficiencies. Chronic respiratory insufficiency includes infants and children with disorders of (1) airway, (2) control of breathing, (3) neuromuscular system with subsequent abnormalities of breathing, (4) chest wall and spine, (5) lungs, and (6) heart.

Therapy for respiratory failure is successful if a positive energy balance between supply and demand regarding the respiratory muscles can be reestablished. Treatment is designed to decrease energy demands as much as possible by reducing the work of breathing and enhancing muscle strength and efficiency, while optimizing nutrition, hemoglobin, oxygenation, and cardiac output. Chronic respiratory failure is present if the balance cannot be permanently restored, and respiratory muscle fatigue supervenes unless mechanical ventilatory support is continued.

The technologies available to support these children in environments outside of the acute care setting have dramatically improved. Both function and mobility of chronic care equipment, particularly ventilators and monitoring equipment, have progressed to the point that technology that was commonly considered the domain of the intensive-care unit (ICU) has become commonplace in the non-ICU chronic care setting.

BACKGROUND

Healthy People 2010 calls for all children with special health care needs to receive coordinated, ongoing, comprehensive care within a medical home. The Institute of Medicine in 2001 (*Crossing the Quality Chasm*) identified overly complex and uncoordinated care as a major reason for "a chasm . . . that exists between the health care that we now have and the health care that we could have." Data support the fact that children with special health care needs account for a substantial amount of health services utilization. Special-needs children are estimated to account for 13% of all children, yet they represent 70% of health care expenditures.

Data are unavailable on the number of adults and children in the United States who are managed on chronic mechanical ventilation, but estimates range from 10,000 to 20,000. A national survey in France of all children managed at home for chronic respiratory failure revealed that this age group compromised 3.2% of the total number of pediatric and adult patients during that period. In that study, 39% required long-term oxygen therapy, 59% required mechanical ventilation, and 2% received continuous positive airway pressure (CPAP). Six percent of such children were managed with tracheostomy without oxygen or need for mechanical ventilation.

TRACHEOSTOMY

Tracheostomy has been known and described for 2,000 years. Approximately 1.5 million tracheostomies are performed in the United States each year. Earlier studies of pediatric tracheostomies show two to three times more morbidity and mortality than in adults. There is an increasing trend of tracheostomies at younger ages, related to more neonates surviving with chronic respiratory failure related to complications of prematurity. Although tracheostomy is more thoroughly presented elsewhere (see Chapter 131B), any discussion of chronic respiratory failure would be remiss without its inclusion.

Perhaps two decades ago, there were simply, in most countries, no options for long-term ventilatory support of children. When offered, chronic mechanical ventilation has traditionally involved the placement of a tracheostomy tube. Newer practice includes the use of noninvasive ventilatory support on occasion, thereby avoiding the complications associated with tracheostomy care, and to some degree, complex positive-pressure ventilators.

The overall mortality rate for tracheostomized children with respiratory failure in one series was 53%, but is more often reported as 7% to 36%. Mortality rates vary by as much as 40% depending on the population studied, and tracheostomy-related mortality is 0% to 6%. Among patients in the first year of life, mortality rates range from 12% to 75%. In one pediatric intensive care unit (PICU), despite accounting for only 2.5% of admissions, and 7.3% of patients requiring mechanical ventilation, these patients accounted for 62% of patient mechanical ventilation days and 33% of all PICU days.

Mean duration of tracheostomy in all children is 18 to 24 months. Planned tracheostomy decannulation rates in the first 5 years of life have been reported to be as high as 61%. Tracheal granulations are so common as to be routine findings rather than complications (20% to 80%). After tracheostomy decannulation, 41% of children require primary or secondary stomal closure. This need should not be seen as a complication but rather a consequence of the duration of the tracheostomy.

Tracheostomy tube obstruction continues to be the most common cause of tracheostomy-related death. Tracheostomy tube displacement is usually more apparent than obstruction, but is functionally equivalent, and essential to identify early and correct. The importance of regular suction, the use of humidification, and interval tube changes cannot be overemphasized to nursing and respiratory staff and parents. Rule Number One remains: *In respiratory distress, the tracheostomy tube is considered obstructed until proven otherwise.*

Fortunately, the procedure of surgical laryngotracheal separation, after which the trachea cannot be intubated via the oronasal cavity, has been abandoned. This procedure, which prevented aspiration by eliminating the pharyngeal–glottic pathway, thus "sealing off" the glottis superiorly, mandated such patients to be completely tracheostomy dependent for airway. It is thus essential for families, emergent responders, and health care providers to be aware of this particular anatomic state.

NONINVASIVE VENTILATION

Noninvasive ventilation refers to techniques of augmenting alveolar ventilation without an artificial airway. The traditional use of tracheal intubation and mechanical ventilation for acute respiratory failure continues, but has recently been reevaluated in both adult and pediatric medicine. Complications may occur with intubations and with artificial airways; therefore, noninvasive ventilatory support is becoming an increasingly popular first choice, particularly in chronic diseases. Using noninvasive forms of ventilatory support in patients in stable condition with chronic respiratory failure may be expected to improve physiologic function and quality of life.

Children with chronic, often progressive, respiratory insufficiency are characterized by at least intermittent central and obstructive apnea, hypoxemia, and hypercarbia. Treatment with noninvasive ventilation may improve quality of life, and reduce early morbidity and mortality of the underlying condition. Nasal intermittent positive-pressure ventilation and bilevel positive pressure have been used successfully in the treatment of hypoventilation in patients with apnea, central hypoventilation, and chronic neuromuscular and pulmonary parenchymal respiratory failure of many etiologies.

The two types of noninvasive ventilation are positive pressure and negative pressure (NNPV). Negative-pressure ventilators are increasingly of more historical than clinical importance, but their use still continues in limited settings. Varieties include tank (e.g., iron lung), shell, and vest or cuirass ventilators. All varieties are designed for children who require only partial chronic support—for example, nighttime ventilation. Substantial disadvantages to this technique exist. Foremost is lack of airway control and secretion clearance. During lower respiratory tract infections, lack of access to an artificial airway prevents optimal diagnosis and management. Furthermore, obstructive sleep apnea may result with this ventilatory mode. Common and necessary activities such as patient mobility, positional change, and bathing are challenging. All of these devices suffer from variable air leak at the sealing sites, leading to a wide variation in effective ventilation, often from hour to hour. Finally, as patient growth (a primary aim) occurs, cuirass shells need to be modified or replaced. Although the importance of NNPV in the history of respiratory medicine cannot be overstated, the above concerns as well as the development of noninvasive positive-pressure ventilation techniques has led to a recent widespread shift to the latter.

Noninvasive positive-pressure ventilation (NPPV) is defined as the use of a mask or nasal devices to provide ventilatory support through a patient's nose and/or mouth. By definition, this technique is distinguished from those ventilatory methods that bypass the patient's upper airway with an artificial airway (endotracheal tube, tracheostomy tube, or rarely, laryngeal mask airway). Since its introduction in the late 1980s for nocturnal hypoventilation, NPPV has seen increasing popularity for pediatric patients with both chronic and acute respiratory failure of many etiologies.

The primary advantage of NPPV is the avoidance of endotracheal intubation or tracheostomy. Secondary advantages of avoiding an invasive airway include decreased risk of nosocomial pneumonia, potential ability to manage such patients in the non-ICU setting (with associated cost reduction), decreased or absent sedation requirement, improved ability to tolerate enteral feeds, and in selected cases, increased ease of ambulation. Regardless of setting, NPPV patients require close monitoring, skilled observation by trained caregivers, and established parameters for further assessment and intervention.

The noninvasive delivery of positive-pressure ventilation requires a positive-pressure ventilator connected to an interface (nasal device or mask) that directs air through the upper airway into the lungs. Among the available interfaces for NPPV are nasal masks, nasal pillows, mouthpieces, and face masks (oronasal masks). Continuous positive airway pressure (CPAP) is the most traditional form of NPPV. In this mode, a single level of positive airway pressure is provided, which is maintained above atmospheric pressure throughout the respiratory cycle. Benefits include alveolar recruitment and maintenance of lung inflation. Typical CPAP pressures range from 5 to 8 cm H_2O.

Bilevel positive airway pressure (BiPAP) provides an inspiratory positive airway pressure for ventilatory assistance as well as an expiratory pressure. Breaths are typically initiated by patient inspiration. Initial settings to normalize ventilation and oxygen saturations are typically adjusted in the sleep laboratory or monitored bedside, with adjustments made during serial evaluations as the patient's requirements change with time. The assist control mode is most often used. The machine

(backup) rate is set to approximate the spontaneous breathing rate. Setting the rate slightly lower than the spontaneous rate may encourage patient triggering of the ventilator, thus improving patient–ventilator synchrony. Conversely, increasing the machine rate during sleep periods may suppress spontaneous breathing, and allow respiratory muscle rest. Inspiratory pressure in children is typically begun at approximately 12 cm H_2O, and adjusted incrementally upward to achieve desired ventilation. Patient tolerance, and/or mask leak, are typically the limiting factors, and pressures rarely exceed 24 cm H_2O. PEEP is typically set at physiologic levels, and maintained ≤8 cm H_2O.

Improvements utilizing noninvasive positive-pressure ventilation include increased survival, increased quality of sleep, reduced daytime sleepiness, improved well-being and independence, improved gas exchange, and a slower rate of pulmonary decline. An intriguing trend of NPPV use in children with impending acute respiratory failure has been recently described in small studies, with NPPV success rates of approximately 80% in selected patients. NPPV in chronic respiratory failure in is general quite successful in older children who tolerate daily periods of time without ventilation. Failure in this setting is usually due to acute cardiopulmonary illness, or patient intolerance of the modality.

Complications of NPPV include eye irritation, conjunctivitis, skin ulceration, gastric distention, and emesis into a full face mask. Facial complications can be reduced by barrier devices, and regular assessment of mask fit. In patients with fragile pulmonary status, mask displacement is poorly tolerated, with rapid onset of hypoxemia and hypercarbia. Some bilevel and CPAP machines do not have alarms; thus additional monitoring, such as pulse oximetry, is a useful adjunct.

INVASIVE POSITIVE-PRESSURE VENTILATION

Despite the recent inroads of NPPV, invasive positive-pressure mechanical ventilation (IPPV), delivered via endotracheal tube or tracheostomy tube, continues to support the vast majority of patients with respiratory failure characterized by inadequate ventilation of acute or chronic nature. A recent survey estimated that >100,000 positive-pressure ventilators are used annually, with half being applied in North America. Approximately 1.5 million patients in the United States receive mechanical ventilation outside of operating and recovery rooms each year.

There is no question that the improved survival of infants and children with chronic illnesses and injuries, primarily of pulmonary or neuromuscular nature, has resulted in thousands of children receiving long-term IPPV. All current evidence suggests that the number is growing. A portable positive-pressure ventilator, via a tracheostomy patient interface, remains the most common means of providing chronic ventilatory support in children and adults.

An important tenet of long-term ventilatory care is that, once the decision has been made to provide chronic ventilation, medical care should utilize the ventilator in similar fashion to any other chronic therapy, such as medications. With the possible exception of severe static or progressive conditions, most long-term illnesses will logically benefit from patient growth and development. Mechanical ventilation greatly helps to create a stable "platform" of cardiopulmonary function that allows the more usual aspects of a child's life to be addressed and prioritized.

Continuous invasive ventilation can be provided using a tracheostomy when other devices and interfaces are poorly tolerated, or endogenous airway control cannot be assured. Advantages of a tracheostomy include a more secure ventilator–patient interface, the ability to deliver more effective ventilation in patients with advanced stages of acute or chronic lung disease, and as access to allow direct tracheal suctioning during events of increased secretion production (e.g., infections). However, tracheostomies have many potential complications, including generating more secretions, impairing swallowing, increasing the risk of aspiration, and bypassing airway defenses, thus increasing the risk of infection. Moreover, the risk of airway obstruction by mucus plug is increased. In addition, vocalization is typically challenged, although this may be overcome with the aid of expiratory occlusion valve speaking assist devices. Many patients and families are concerned with the potential communication and cosmetic implications of tracheostomy. Conversely, once a stable tracheostomy is established, patient mobility, participation in daily activities, and opportunities for ventilator liberation are often markedly enhanced.

A more thorough description of mechanical ventilation for acute respiratory failure is provided elsewhere in this text (Chapter 41). Chronic IPPV generally utilizes smaller, less sophisticated, and more portable ventilators than used in the acute setting. Chronic ventilators usually use volume control mode, with pressure limits. Tidal volumes are typically set at 8 to 10 mL/kg, and adequacy of ventilation is subsequently confirmed by blood gas analysis and/or end-tidal CO_2 monitoring. Ventilation goals may vary considerably, depending on the underlying condition(s). Children with chronic lung disease often have $PaCO_2$ values in the 50- to 65-mm Hg range, while patients with encephalopathy are more often managed at normal $PaCO_2$ levels. Interestingly, conscious, communicative patients with chronic neuromuscular disease often prefer hyperventilation to a $PaCO_2$ range of 30 to 35 mm Hg; the reason for this is unknown. Favorably, this degree of ventilation does allow margin for growth and intercurrent illness.

Most children with IPPV are managed with uncuffed tracheostomy tubes to facilitate speech and minimize mucosal injury. The tracheostomy tube lies distal to the subglottis, which is the narrowest portion of the pediatric airway. Thus, a certain degree of air leak around the tube is expected in ventilated patients, usually during mid- to late-inspiration, when peak airway pressures result in airway dilation. Consequently, a portion of the delivered ventilator tidal volume leaks around the tracheostomy tube, and does not ventilate the lungs. At times, particularly in younger, active, or labile children, this leak is variable in size and compensation by tidal volume adjustment can be difficult. Episodic hypoventilation can ensue. If a larger tracheostomy tube is not possible, a pressure control ventilator control mode can be considered in this situation. As in acute ventilatory care, a peak inspiratory pressure (PIP) >30 cm H_2O is undesirable, and >35 cm H_2O unacceptable, with rare exceptions.

Some commercially available portable ventilators have a high-pressure limit adjustment that can be reduced to the desired PIP. An appropriate tidal volume is then set, and the ventilator functions as a time-cycled, pressure-limited device. If and when the PIP is reached, the remainder of the set tidal volume is "vented" to the room, thereby avoiding potentially injurious high PIPs and the cascade of ill effects leading to ventilator-induced lung injury (see Chapter 41).

Oxygen is typically delivered in portable IPPV via cylinder tanks, which can reliably deliver up to 30% concentrations. An oxygen generator is used for home settings. If a higher oxygen concentration is required, liquid nitrogen is most often used. In general, patients requiring >40% inspired oxygen are not candidates for chronic outpatient or subacute care. The delivery of positive end-expiratory pressure (PEEP) has become increasingly common in long-term IPPV. Traditionally, patients were managed without PEEP, due to mechanical limitations of the ventilator circuits. In the situation of continuous flow ventilators, a "PEEP valve" is used to partially occlude the expiratory circuit and allow the well-established benefits of PEEP. Modern portable IPPV ventilators typically contain a PEEP setting within the primary ventilator control settings. Physiologic PEEP of 5 cm H_2O is a reasonable default setting for IPPV patients, and it is the rare child who requires more than 8 cm H_2O. Notable exceptions include patients with severe tracheal and/or bronchial malacia, who often require relatively high PEEP for airway stenting.

Pressure support ventilation (PSV) is another newer adjunct to the treatment of chronic ventilatory failure, and many newer IPPV ventilators offer the modality. PSV "rewards" the patient's self-initiated breath with an inspiratory positive-pressure support. The duration of the support is typically time or flow limited. Typical pressure support values in endotracheally intubated children with acute respiratory failure are 5 to 15 cm H_2O. Similar to acute respiratory failure, the exact indications for PSV in chronic IPPV remain unproven. It can be expected to aid as a weaning mode in patients without static respiratory failure, particularly in neuromuscular disease states or chronic lung disease. In the presence of a tracheostomy tube, artificial airway resistance is generally much less than with an ETT, lessening the benefit of PSV for this indication. Patients with static respiratory failure, particularly those with abnormal respiratory drive and consciousness, will usually not benefit from PSV. If a patient-triggered mode is desired in these children, assist control is more often indicated.

The humidification of inspired gas in all forms of IPPV, and often in NPV as well, is a routine aspect of care of patients with tracheostomy tubes. As the nasal mucosal surfaces are bypassed, lack of humidification predisposes the patient to mucociliary dysfunction, mucus plugging, and atelectasis. Three common humidification systems are used in chronic respiratory failure. The most efficient technique of humidification is the heated "pass-over" or "bubble-through" humidifier, in which a gas flow source is directed through a heated water bath. Gas temperatures can be controlled at or above body temperature at 100% relative humidity. This method is commonly associated with chronic ventilator usage. A second technique more often used with spontaneously breathing patients uses compressed gas to nebulize water, which is sometimes also heated to physiologic temperatures and delivered into the gas flow circuit. Lastly, available for use in the tracheostomized patient during periods of ventilator liberation are small, simple humidification devices (i.e., artificial nose) that attach to the outside of the tracheostomy tube. While in place, these disposable devices passively trap water vapor in exhaled air, allowing partial humidification of room air during subsequent inspiration. Although less efficient than the above active devices, patient mobility is greatly enhanced when this method is tolerated and used. Modern devices also have bacteriostatic qualities.

NON-ICU CARE OF CHRONICALLY VENTILATED PATIENTS

Step-Down Units/Ventilator Units

Specialized units, which have fewer resources and are generally designed for stable patients who still require close attention, are appropriate sites for weaning ventilated patients, as well as supporting patients with chronic respiratory failure readmitted for acute medical or surgical conditions. Recent experience suggests that the ICU environment is not needed for long-term ventilator care and may even interfere with optimization of functional potential. A non-ICU setting that avoids intensive medical care and provides for a multidisciplinary rehabilitative approach (when appropriate) may not only reduce the cost of care but also improve the functional status and quality of life of the ventilator-dependent child.

Prior to admission, patients should have stabilization of nonrespiratory organ function, and a treatment plan that emphasizes simplified medical regimens. Ideally, such individuals are enterally fed, and are managed without parenteral medications. Respiratory stability also is essential. Patients require a secure airway (e.g., tracheostomy) or are stable with noninvasive ventilatory support. Airway secretions should be manageable, ventilatory changes infrequent, and there should not be episodes of apnea, oxygen desaturations, or dyspnea.

It has been demonstrated that stable chronic ventilator-dependent children can be hospitalized successfully and safely in a non-ICU setting. Hospitalization of medically stable ventilator-dependent children in a specific area designed for this purpose does not increase the risk of unexpected ICU transfers and does not increase the risk of death, provided proper monitoring and care are instituted. Key features to success include the availability of trained personnel who are skilled in the care of such children and the availability of physical resources that would provide close monitoring of these patients and assist the staff in giving emergency care if required.

Home Care

The role of continuous home monitoring for children with chronic ventilator support remains controversial, and there are no controlled studies to appropriately guide the decision-making process. It is unclear that the goal of decreased morbidity and mortality in this population has been achieved, and clinical practice patterns vary. Chronic ventilatory support in the home is a safe and relatively inexpensive alternative for many patients that optimizes overall health, rehabilitative potential, psychosocial development, and family well-being.

Core guidelines for discharge to home have been outlined, and an example is given in the following paragraphs.

Oxygen requirement should be ≤40%. $PaCO_2$ levels should be proven to be stable and maintained on the home equipment, without frequent adjustments, prior to discharge. The patient should demonstrate appropriate growth, and all other medical conditions should be stable. The family home must be evaluated for appropriate utilities and equipment space. Home nursing and durable medical equipment (DME) supplies must be arranged and confirmed before discharge. Rehabilitation services and transportation arrangements must be established. Most importantly, *caregivers must demonstrate proficiency in the use of home equipment and complete patient care before discharge.*

Once at home, patient goals vary. Children with chronic, stable disease, such as a spinal cord injury, may not require a significant change in their home ventilation. Others with progressive disease may require regular reassessment of ventilatory and other support. Alternatively, many children with bronchopulmonary dysplasia or other types of congenital and acquired lung disease of infancy may improve and need less support over time, even to the point of liberation from mechanical ventilation. Regular assessment and adjustments in chronic ventilation needs are the responsibility of the physician prepared to manage long-term respiratory failure, typically a subspecialist in pulmonary, critical care, or neonatal medicine.

Chronic Subacute Care Units

Chronic subacute care units, which may be located within acute care hospitals or be freestanding, typically admit patients who are medically complex and/or who require physiologic monitoring. Patients in such facilities are in stable condition no longer needing acute care, but require treatment too complex for conventional skilled nursing facilities. Goals may include interval support of the patient transitioning to the home setting, or long-term care of the complicated or fragile patient.

The spectrum of disease processes in subacute care units may be wide, and supports the concept of multidisciplinary team care. Currently in California, the hallmark of pediatric subacute units is the long-term support of encephalopathic, tracheostomized children with one or more components of respiratory failure. Although most patients in pediatric subacute facilities require some degree of chronic respiratory support, in many cases neurologic, nutritional, or rehabilitative concerns are of equal or higher priority. In general, such patients are chronically ventilated via tracheostomy for insurance of airway patency, secretion management, and reliable ventilation. On occasion, subacute care permits the use of "acute-care" ventilators, more commonly considered "ICU ventilators," thus permitting care of patients of a higher level of respiratory insufficiency. These devices are traditionally nonportable, technologically sophisticated, and significantly more expensive than ventilators designed for chronic use. Recent advances in ventilator technology and design, however, continue to blur this distinction.

There is an increasing number of such units in many parts of the country. It is noteworthy that states with active and successful organized home care programs typically have much lower usage of subacute facilities. The impact of prolonged hospitalization or institutionalization on the life of the child and family must be carefully considered as decisions regarding location and duration of long-term care are made.

Acute Hospitalization

The growing number of chronically ventilated children inevitably leads to hospital readmission for acute illness or disease progression. A "therapeutic cycle" of sorts is created with these children: they move forward from illness or injury stabilization through acute care to the chronic care setting, ideally making overall progress, only to return periodically to the acute setting as their natural history dictates. At least 75% of chronically ventilated children are rehospitalized in the first 5 years of support. In many pediatric centers, particularly PICUs and ventilator units, the number of inpatient days for chronically ill children is steadily increasing. Certainly not all readmissions require ICU care, and it is the responsibility of each facility and physician managing such children to have advanced preparations in place for the care of acutely ill, technologically dependent children.

Similarly, the presence of "high-tech kids" in the community requires additional training and resource utilization by pre-hospital personnel. Training and familiarity with tracheostomy and home mechanical ventilation vary widely; some jurisdictions do not allow pediatric tracheostomy changes in the field by EMS personnel. The complex, chronic child in extremis is among the most daunting of challenges facing prehospital providers of care.

In the accidentally decannulated tracheostomy patient in whom the tracheostomy tube cannot be replaced, ventilation can be immediately supported with mouth-to-tracheostomy, and mouth-to-mouth (with the tracheostomy stoma externally occluded) breaths. More definitively, ventilation should proceed with traditional bag-valve-mask techniques, and/or endotracheal intubation (again, with tracheostomy stomal occlusion). It is important to note that an appropriate-size endotracheal tube can easily be used as a substitute tracheostomy tube should the need arise.

Tracheostomy obstruction or occlusion must be ruled out as a possibility in every such patient who presents in acute respiratory distress, or with other signs of respiratory deterioration (i.e., hypoxemia, hypercapnia, decreased respiratory system compliance.) Although ease of suctioning through the tracheostomy tube rules out complete intraluminal obstruction, obstructive plugs are often attached to the distal end of the tube, where they may act in a ball-valve manner to occlude the tracheostomy tube during exhalation. *The replacement of the tracheostomy tube in such children developing respiratory distress eliminates this simple problem as an etiology, and is often life-saving.*

Once the airway is proven clear, attention is directed toward the respiratory pump and lung parenchymal function. Ventilators used in the chronic setting (i.e., "home vents") may not be available in the inpatient setting. Furthermore, portable ventilators may not be sufficient in situations of poor lung compliance or elevated airway resistance. Conversion to an acute care ventilator is often required, and when baseline ventilator settings are used, typically *but not always* improves ventilation of the chronically supported patient due to increased sophistication of the device. It is thus prudent to document satisfactory gas exchange by pulse oximetry and blood gases whenever the ventilator type is changed, regardless of the indication. Oxygen is delivered as needed to maintain safe arterial oxygen saturation, typically >90%. If the necessary inspired oxygen concentration exceeds 50%, PEEP should be incrementally increased as well.

The most common reason for acute hospitalization of children with chronic respiratory failure is lower respiratory tract infection (LRTI). All children with tracheostomy tubes become colonized with bacteria; as nasal pharyngeal immune system structures are bypassed, humidification of air may be suboptimal, cough is usually poor, and musculoskeletal deformities and/or patient immobility predispose to inadequate lung inflation. Among the most common colonizers of the respiratory tract are *Staphylococcus* and *Pseudomonas* species. Depending on the setting, *Haemophilus* spp. and additional aerobic gram-negative organisms, traditionally considered as nosocomial, may be commonly identified.

Given the above, it can be difficult to accurately identify the cause of acute clinical infection. Close attention should be given to caregiver description of secretion quality and quantity, as well as fever, oxygen requirement, and overall appearance of the patient. Viral infections generally increase the amount of secretions more than any qualitative change. Bacterial infections are more likely to be associated with fevers and significant changes in qualitative secretion characteristics. A tracheal aspirate is recommended; ideally, via a clean, replaced tracheostomy tube. As opposed to colonization, both viral and bacterial infections can be relied upon to increase to a large number the amount of white blood cells detected on Gram stain of tracheal secretions. Colonization may cloud the diagnostic accuracy of the tracheal culture; however, results may well lead to new microbial diagnosis, document the presence of concerning resistant microorganisms (see below), and establish sensitivity and resistance status of selected antibiotics. In select cases of focal pulmonary consolidation, a directed bronchoalveolar lavage specimen via flexible bronchoscopy may be of use.

The distinction between tracheitis and pneumonia is usually of more descriptive than clinical use. Clinical history and examination is often the same. A chest radiograph is required to reliably document the presence of alveolar infiltrates associated with the latter, as the auscultatory exam, particularly in small children, is challenging in this category of patients due to an overall high incidence of adventitial airway sounds. There is no established evidence that antibacterial therapy should differ in intensity, method of delivery, or duration

between any type of LRTI. Viral detection tests, even in the properly immunized child, may establish diagnosis or co-diagnosis early, and prevent unnecessary or undesirable further therapies. Enteral or parenteral antibiotic choices should cover the spectrum of likely organisms including the above, with narrowing of coverage as culture results dictate.

Airway clearance management is always of high priority in the management of chronically ventilated children. This is particularly true of the acutely ill patient, due to the higher incidence of pathologically produced tracheobronchial secretions. Ineffective airway clearance can hasten the onset of respiratory failure and death, whereas early intervention to improve airway clearance can prevent hospitalization and reduce the incidence of pneumonia. Traditional initial methods of airway clearance and reduction of lung collapse are increased chest physical therapy and frequency of suctioning. Mechanical techniques include insufflator-inexsufflators, which simulate a cough by providing a positive-pressure breath followed by a negative-pressure exsufflation. Peak cough expiratory flow rates and airway clearance have been proven superior to manual techniques alone. This device has been shown to be well tolerated and effective in pediatric patients with neuromuscular disease and ineffective cough. Tracheotomized patients managed in this way benefit from improved secretion clearance from peripheral airways, avoidance of mucosal trauma from direct tracheal suctioning, and improved patient comfort. Reported complications include transient nausea, abdominal distention, bradycardia, and tachycardia.

Intrapulmonary percussive ventilation delivers brief durations of high-frequency, low-amplitude oscillations superimposed on CPAP. Additionally, high-frequency chest wall oscillation has been used in patients with neuromuscular respiratory failure. Neither technique has established success, but may be considered for supplemental use. Bronchoscopy is generally used for cases of persistent atelectasis and suspected mucus plugging but has not been of proven benefit, and should be reserved for patients who have failed noninvasive therapy.

Hospitals and other health care institutions are increasingly identified as reservoirs of resistant strains of bacteria, notably methicillin-resistant *Staphylococcus aureus* (MRSA), vancomycin-resistant *Enterococcus* (VRE), and extended-spectrum beta-lactamase (ESBL) producing organisms. Both individual patients and larger populations are detrimentally affected by such colonization, which on occasion becomes acute infection. Although there currently are antibiotic options to adequately treat almost all acute infections with the above organisms, appropriate concerns about our future ability to do so have been raised. Screening for resistant organisms is recommended, as the resistant organism burden in terms of absolute numbers of infected patients is correlated with the difficulty in achieving institutional eradication of the microorganism. It has long been the policy of our children's hospital, and many others, to screen all admissions of chronically ill patients from long-term care facilities and the home setting, as well as all patients with a previous history of one of the above resistant organisms. As a sign of the times, and in an effort to identify community-acquired MRSA, our hospital has extended this screening to all ICU admissions. The role of prevention and treatment of colonization by these resistant organisms is unclear. Regimens of enteral antibiotics, nebulized antibiotics, and tracheostomy site and intratracheal anti-infective agents have all demonstrated mixed success, with concerns over long-term efficacy and development of resistance.

During acute illness and rehospitalization of the chronically ill child, it is imperative for the clinician to be attentive as well to the nonmedical needs and wishes of the patient and family. In many cases, rehospitalizations are a return to the setting, if not the same site, as the initial scenario that set in motion the cascade of events leading to the child's current status. Emotions can run high; a calm and realistic approach to care can restore appropriate order and decision-making priorities to the situation.

These occurrences are also the appropriate time to confirm, or in some cases seek for the first time, limitations of care, including decisions not to intervene (DNI) or resuscitate (DNR). Input from the primary care clinicians and multidisciplinary team is invaluable in this regard. In most cases, patients and/or families have had adequate time to consider such options prior to interval rehospitalization. It is of the highest importance that "transportable" DNR/DNI orders should be actively sought out at the initiation of care, in order to avoid treatment and interventions that are not desired by the patient and/or family. Respecting the end-of-life wishes of a chronically ill child is perhaps the finest example of supportive care that the acute care clinician can provide.

References

1. Newache PW, Strickland B, Shonkoff JP, et al. An epidemilologic profile of children with special health care needs. *Pediatrics* 1998;102:117–121.
2. Fein JA, Kronan K, Posner JC. Approach to the care of the technology-dependent child. In: Fleisher G, Ludwig S, eds. *Textbook of pediatric emergency medicine.* 4th ed. Philadelphia: Lippincott Williams & Wilkins; 2000.
3. Morgan CE, Dixon S, Tracheostomy. *eMedicine* article. June 2002.
4. Heffner John E. Tracheostomy application and timing. *Clin Chest Med* 2003;24:389–398.
5. Ernst A, Critchlow J. Percutaneous tracheostomy—special considerations. *Clin Chest Med* 2004;24:409–412.
6. Wright SE, vanDahm K. Long-term care of the tracheostomy patient. *Clin Chest Med* 2003;24: 473–487.
7. David G, Bhatti N. Management of the impaired airways in the adult. In: Cummings CW, ed. *Otolaryngology: head and neck surgery.* 4th ed. St. Louis: Mosby; 2005.
8. Zawadzka-Glos L. Percutaneous tracheotomy in children. *Int J Pediatr Otorhinolaryngol* 2004;68:1387–1390.
9. Toursarkissian B, Fowler CL, Zweng TN, et al. Percutaneous dilational tracheostomy in children and teenagers. *J Pediatr Surg* 1994;29: 1421–1424.
10. Wood R. Diagnostic and therapeutic procedures in pediatric pulmonary patients. In: Taussig, ed. *Pediatric respiratory medicine.* St. Louis: Mosby; 1999.
11. Johnston J, Davis J, Sherman JM, et al. Care of the child with a chronic tracheostomy. This official statement of the American Thoracic Society was adopted by the ATS Board of Directors, July 1999. *Am J Respir Crit Care Med* 2000;161: 297–308.
12. Freeman BD, Borecki IB, Coopersmith CM, et al. Relationship between tracheostomy timing and duration of mechanical ventilation in critically ill patients. *Crit Care Med* 2005;33:2513–2520.
13. MacIntyre NR, Cook D, Ely E, et al. Evidence-based guidelines for weaning and discontinuing ventilatory support: a collective task force facilitated by the American College of Chest Physicians; the American Association for Respiratory Care; and the American College of Critical Care Medicine. *Chest* 2001;120(suppl): 375S–395S.
14. Rumbak MJ. A prospective, randomized, study comparing early percutaneous dilational tracheotomy to prolonged translaryngeal intubation (delayed tracheotomy) in critically ill medical patients. *Crit Care Med* 2004;32:1689–1694.

Suggested Readings

American Academy of Pediatrics Council on Children with Disabilities. Policy Statement. Care coordination in the medial home: integrating health and related systems of care for children with special health care needs. *Pediatr* 2005; 116:1238–44.

American Thoracic Society. Care of the child with a chronic tracheostomy. *Am J Respir Crit Care Med* 2000; 161:297–308.

Cheifetz IM. Invasive and noninvasive pediatric mechanical ventilation. *Respir Care* 2003;48:442–453.

Fauroux B. Home treatment for chronic respiratory failure in children: a prospective study. *Eur Respir J* 1995;8:2062–2066.

Make BJ, Lipton P, Alexander J, et al. Mechanical ventilation beyond the intensive care unit. Report of a consensus conference of the American College of Chest Physicians. *Chest* 1998;113:289–344.

Mallory GB, Stillwell PC. The ventilator-dependent child: issues in diagnosis and management. *Arch Phys Med Rehabil* 1991;72:43–55.

Perkin RM. Invasive positive-pressure ventilation. In: Perkin RM, Swift JD, Newton DA, eds. *Pediatric hospital medicine.* Philadelphia: Lippincott Williams & Wilkins; 2003:733–736.

Tantinikorn W, Alper C, Bluestone C, et al. Outcome in pediatric tracheotomy. *Am J Otolaryngol* 2003;24:31–37.

CHAPTER 132 ■ TRANSITIONAL CARE OF CHILDREN WITH CHRONIC DISEASES

NATHAN ANDREW BRINN AND GREGG M. TALENTE

In the past there were many diseases that could be thought of almost exclusively as pediatric because most of the patients affected by them rarely survived into adulthood. The examples are many, and would include diseases such as cystic fibrosis and congenital heart problems. Advances in the care of those patients, however, have dramatically and rapidly changed that paradigm. Now over 90% of children with chronic illnesses survive into adulthood. This development, although obviously welcome, is presenting new challenges to the health care system; challenges both for primary care providers in the outpatient setting and to hospital providers caring for complex and often chronically ill children as they progress toward adulthood.

These issues are being addressed in the emerging field of transitional care. Transitional care can be most simply and accurately described as "the purposeful, planned movement of adolescents and young adults with chronic physical and medical conditions from the child-centered to adult-oriented health care systems" (1).

Although transitional care has obvious importance to the outpatient world, it is equally important and often problematic in the inpatient setting. As any experienced practitioner knows, chronically ill children can at any given time consume the majority of a pediatric ward's time and resources. One of the unintended consequences of numerous admissions for a pediatric patient can be the development of deep-rooted expectations and even dependency upon familiar and beloved providers. These expectations may then go unmet with an abrupt change to adult providers and staff, leading to problems in the therapeutic alliance between health care provider and patient.

A common and illustrative example of a formerly "pediatric" disease now presenting to adult providers would be cystic fibrosis CF. In the early 1970s, the mean childhood survival for CF was 7 years. Now, with the improvements in antibiotics, technology, and team-oriented care, the mean survival for patients is more than 30 years and continues to increase. To adult providers and hospital administrators this means inheriting an adult patient population not only unique in its health care needs (e.g., specialized respiratory care, specific epidemiologic precautions), but also in the long-term personal relationships built up over many years with pediatric physicians and staff. How that transition is managed on the inpatient setting may have a dramatic influence on the health and quality of life experienced by the patient.

The *Healthy People 2010* initiative has stated as one of its goals that "young people with special health care needs will receive the services needed to make necessary transitions to all aspects of adult life . . . ." So why do they feel that transitional care is important? Moving young adults with chronic health care needs from a pediatric to an adult system is warranted for

several reasons. First, many insurance providers will limit payment for pediatric services after a certain age. Second, many institutions, needing to fulfill their primary duty to children, feel the need to close their units to patients now in their upper teens or twenties. Third, many pediatric-trained providers may feel uncomfortable dealing with adult disease processes not related to the patient's primary diagnosis. Fourth, young adults desire access to services appropriate to their age. Finally, and perhaps most importantly, is the need for adolescents and young adults to achieve their own autonomy and independence, which may sometimes be a difficult task in the pediatric environment.

Much has been written about the subject of transitional care and several excellent reviews are available. Most of the literature has to do with transitioning patients as outpatients. The American Academy of Pediatrics published a consensus statement in 2002 on the subject that was subsequently approved by the American College of Physicians and the American Academy of Family Practitioners (2). Their recommendations are summarized in Table 132.1. The focus of these recommendations is on the overall management of these patients and a primary care approach to transitions. The pediatric hospital care provider should be familiar with these recommendations and, when appropriate, incorporate the underlying principles including preparation, good communication between providers, age-appropriate service, and promotion of patient autonomy into his patient care.

BARRIERS TO TRANSITION

In implementing successful strategies for transitioning patients, it is vitally important to understand the barriers that can hinder successful transitions. Common barriers include factors related to the patient and her family, factors related to the pediatric provider community, factors related to the adult health care provider community, and systemic factors (i.e., health care coverage). These factors are summarized in Table 132.2.

Examples of patient-related factors include familiarity that may evolve into dependence, immaturity, poor self-image resulting in unwillingness to enter new environments, and lack of trust. Family factors include a pervasive need for control that is almost universally unavailable in the adult world, overprotective attitudes, codependence with a child who is chronically ill, and issues of trust. Barriers related to the pediatric staff and physicians may include strong emotional bonds with the patient and family. Pediatricians may also become comfortable with the status quo, not feel a compelling need to move a transition along, and may overestimate their ability to manage adult health problems. Internists are often reluctant to take on

TABLE 132.1

2002 AAP CONSENSUS STATEMENT

STEPS TO ENSURE SUCCESSFUL TRANSITION

1. Ensure that all young people with special health care needs have an identified health care professional who attends to the unique challenges of transition and assumes responsibility for current health care, care coordination, and future health care planning.
2. Prepare and maintain an up-to-date medical summary that is portable and accessible.
3. Create a written health care transition plan by age 14 together with the young person and family.
4. Apply the same guidelines for primary and preventive care for all adolescents and young adults including those with special health care needs.
5. Ensure affordable, continuous health insurance coverage for all young people with special health care needs throughout adolescence and adulthood.

new and complicated patients due to a perceived lack of financial reimbursement and unfamiliarity with the underlying diseases (often more pediatric). Financial concerns are also paramount as a chronically ill and perhaps disabled child approaches adulthood. As many as one-fourth or more of all young adults with a history of a chronic childhood illness lack health care insurance coverage.

Another transitional barrier that must be acknowledged is the inherent cultural difference between adult and pediatric health care settings. Internists tend to solve problems, focus on disease, expect and demand autonomy, and expect patient participation. Pediatricians are more focused on general health and development. They are family centered and frequently focus on a relationship with the parent. Pediatricians are also more nurturing and understanding, responding to patient noncompliance by looking for ways to provide more assistance and help to the patient. Without orientation to the differences between the comfortable setting the patient is leaving and the frightening new health care setting they are entering, it is not surprising that patient satisfaction is frequently low, resulting in disruption of the physician–patient relationship and less adequate health care.

RECOMMENDATIONS

Knowing more about transitional care and the barriers that can prevent successful transitions, what should a pediatric hospital care provider do? What steps should this physician take in order to accomplish the goals of transition to adult-oriented care? Regardless of where they work, all pediatric hospital care providers should evaluate their practices and determine ways in which the principles of good transitional care can be implemented for their patients. Relationships with local adult and pediatric primary care providers and adult hospitalists should be developed. Finally, partnership with providers in other disciplines such as nursing and social work should be sought, as these health care professionals can also improve transitions for chronically ill children.

In many settings and at many institutions transitional care programs have been developed. Transitional care programs can be disease specific or focused on the general care of all adolescents with special health care needs. Medical providers for children working in institutions where these programs exist should make contact with these programs and collaborate to assist with transition issues specific to the inpatient setting. The managers of these programs can provide significant assistance in developing protocols for adolescents during their hospitalization that can support their transitional care plan.

If there is no local transitional care program, pediatric inpatient providers should try to partner with the local primary care physicians and adult hospitalists to formalize a plan for assisting patients with this difficult step in the lifetime management of their illness. Some specific recommendations for steps that can be taken with every adolescent admitted to a pediatric unit are described in Table 132.3.

In summary, transitioning the care of chronically ill pediatric patients is an essential part of good health care. As such, it is imperative that hospital providers be able and willing to assist and promote such transitions.

PEARLS

- All pediatric providers, both inpatient and outpatient, have a responsibility to facilitate transitional care for appropriate chronically ill adolescent patients.
- Pediatric hospital care providers should encourage increased autonomy in their adolescent patients.

TABLE 132.2

BARRIERS TO TRANSITIONING CARE

Factors related to patient	Factors related to parents	Factors related to pediatricians	Factors related to adult medicine	Factors related to financial concerns
Dependence on current providers	Need for control	Strong emotional bonds with patient	Concerns about reimbursement	Lack of insurance coverage
Low self-esteem	Codependence between family and child	Comfort with the status quo	Lack of familiarity with disease processes	Confusing insurance laws for adults with chronic illness
Fear of new environments	Overprotection on the part of the family	Overconfidence in managing adult health problems	Failure to orient patients to the adult setting	Differing adult community services
Lack of trust in adult providers	Lack of trust in adult providers	Lack of relationships with adult providers	Lack of relationships with pediatric providers	

TABLE 132.3

SPECIFIC RECOMMENDATIONS FOR TRANSITION

STEPS TO TAKE WHEN ATTEMPTING TRANSITION IN AN INPATIENT SETTING

1. Ask all patients age 14 and older with chronic health care issues if they have a transition plan in place.
2. If not the patient's primary care provider, the physician should maintain an ongoing relationship with the patient's primary care provider and adult providers in the community, and should partner with them in facilitating transitions for patients.
3. All patients age 14 and older with chronic health care issues should be offered a tour and orientation to adult floors and units where they would likely be admitted or have contact with in the future, including the opportunity to meet staff.
4. Ask the families of all patients 14 and older with chronic health care issues if they want/need a social work consult to discuss future financial issues.
5. Keep in mind the goal of developing autonomy in adolescent patients with chronic health care issues, and make an effort to provide opportunities for decision-making and self-efficacy.

- Pediatric hospital care providers should develop relationships with pediatric and adult primary care providers and adult hospitalists to develop systems to make transitions easier and more successful for their patients.
- Pediatric hospital care providers should work with the social worker(s) at their institution to provide adolescents with special health care needs counseling about medical insurance coverage as they approach adulthood.

References

1. Blum RW, Garell D, Hodgman CH, et al. Transition from child-centered to adult health-care systems for adolescents with chronic conditions. *J Adolesc Health* 1993;14:570–576.
2. AAP, AAFP, ACP-ASIM. A consensus statement on health care transitions for young adults with special health care needs. *Pediatrics* 2002;110:1304–1306.

Suggested Readings

Callahan ST, Fienstein-Winitzer R, Keenan P. Transition from pediatric to adult-oriented health care: a challenge for patients with chronic disease. *Curr Opin Pediatr* 2001;13:310–316.

Coleman EA, Berenson RA. Lost in transition: challenges and opportunities for improving the quality of transitional care. *Ann Intern Med* 2004;141:533–536.

Rosen D. Between two worlds: bridging the cultures of child health and adult medicine. *J Adolesc Health* 1995;17:10–16.

CHAPTER 133 ■ PEDIATRIC HOME CARE

MARK S. McCONNELL AND RUSSELL C. LIBBY

WHAT IS HOME CARE?

In its simplest terms, home care is the delivery of necessary medical care in the patient's home or another comfortable surrounding outside of the hospital. The concept of home care includes home visitations by physicians, nursing home visits to assist with medical care after hospital discharge, interventions by therapists to assist patients in meeting their rehabilitation goals, social work visits to provide psychosocial support for families affected by their child's disease process, infusion of medications to continue therapies initiated in the hospital, or the delivery of medical equipment to a patient at home for physiologic monitoring or continued medical therapy.

HOME CARE DELIVERY MODELS

Typically, as pediatric home care is delivered today, physicians order home care services for a patient on discharge from the hospital, and then hospital discharge planners make arrangements for private or public home care agencies to complete the ordered services in the home. The type of home care services a patient needs dictates which type of home care agency the discharge planner contacts to provide the necessary medical services.

Home care services usually are described according to the types of services provided. Home nursing agencies provide skilled and nonskilled nursing services to patients in the home. Nursing agencies may provide or arrange for specific therapies (e.g., occupational, speech, or physical therapies) or social work services themselves or by contract with specialty providers. Home infusion companies focus on delivering pharmaceuticals to the home that are administered by a nurse, the patient, or the family. Home infusion agencies frequently have their own nurses, but sometimes they contract with home nursing companies to provide the nursing functions required for home infusion services. Durable medical equipment (DME) suppliers deliver medical equipment to the home. Typically, the set-up of equipment and instruction on the use of the equipment is accomplished by respiratory therapists or nurses; however, other licensed personnel sometimes fill this role. Integrated home care providers provide all of these services—nursing, home infusion, and medical equipment—under the umbrella of one agency. This kind of integrated home care provider usually is more convenient for the family and the hospital discharge planners. In delivering home care to children, working with an integrated home care provider who focuses on delivering care to children may be important for improving satisfaction for the patient's family.

HOME CARE IN THE CONTINUUM OF CARE

The pediatric hospitalist should view home care as one option in the spectrum of medical care environments. Home care can be used to prevent a hospitalization for some patients who require medical therapies but do not need close nursing monitoring. As an example, a pediatrician faced with a child in the emergency department with acute gastroenteritis and mild dehydration has several choices available; he can (1) try oral rehydration, (2) give IV hydration and watch the patient in the emergency department or discharge the patient home, or (3) admit the patient to the hospital for bowel rest and IV hydration. Another possibility would include IV hydration at home if the family is willing and skilled nursing services are conveniently available to care for the child.

Pediatric home care also can be used to shorten a hospital stay when a patient achieves physiologic stability and requires only ongoing medical therapies to complete a prescribed treatment course. Examples of this type of home care include home IV antibiotics for infections or home oxygen therapy for infants with chronic lung disease. In some cases, home care can substitute for long-term hospital or institutional care. An example of avoiding long-term institutionalization would include patients who receive mechanical ventilation or total parenteral nutrition in the home.

Because some studies have shown that patients and families tend to do better at home (1), the pediatric hospitalist should make every attempt to keep or return the patient to the more comfortable surroundings of the home environment whenever possible. The home environment promotes healing, provides a more nurturing environment, and reduces the degree of "hospitalitis."

THE PEDIATRICIAN'S ROLE

The pediatrician plays a crucial role as the director of home care services for the patient. Many primary care pediatricians have competing priorities and practical impediments that prevent their participation in the care of hospitalized patients, particularly when it has been provided in the PICU or NICU. It is extremely important for the hospitalist to bridge the transition of patient care from the hospital to the primary pediatrician so that he or she can effectively assume management of the continuing course of treatment. In addition to keeping the primary pediatrician informed of the patient's condition during a hospitalization, the pediatrician needs to understand the nature of the patient's problems and the approach to treatment. The primary pediatrician needs to be involved in the discharge-planning process. This involvement may be a simple process requiring a short phone call, or for more complex patients, a formal discharge-planning conference. The discharge-planning conference should include all medical disciplines as well as the patient and her caregivers, if appropriate. The discharge planning conference helps to establish realistic goals and expectations for home care, reviews the roles of all members of the home care team, and allows the patient and caregivers opportunity to ask questions.

Whether or not your patient is provided a discharge planning conference prior to discharge, it is very important that the hospitalist contact the primary care physician directly to transition care of the patient who needs home care services. Information that should be communicated during this transition conversation, in addition to the patient's condition and treatment in the hospital, should include the discharge plan, type of home care services ordered, goals for home care, frequency and expected number of home visits, and any clinical issues that require follow-up.

Home care services must be ordered by a licensed physician and the orders should clearly indicate the type of services that will be necessary, duration of services, and frequency of visits. Prescribing medical equipment in the home usually requires a certificate of medical necessity (CMN). The CMN is a statement by the ordering physician, required by federal law, that a patient requires a specific piece of equipment to meet his medical needs. The CMN usually is time-limited and requires the physician to indicate the duration of time that the patient will need the equipment. Orders for home medical equipment should be specific (e.g., "oxygen concentrator for nasal cannula oxygen at 2 liters per minute," not "oxygen titrate to effectiveness"). For certain pieces of medical equipment, like cardiorespiratory monitors and ventilators, the physician should indicate high and low alarm settings in addition to other settings.

Orders for nursing or therapy visits should include the date visits are to begin, the frequency and duration of visits, whether additional or "as-needed" visits are allowed, the skill level of the visiting professional (licensed practical nurse or registered nurse, or home health aide), and the type of specific orders or interventions required (e.g., teaching, dressing changes, infusing medications, patient assessment). Even though the pediatrician may never visit the patient in the home, the pediatrician remains responsible for all aspects of care for that patient in the home. Therefore, it is important that the physician and home nurse or therapist establish clear communication so that important changes in the patient's condition can be quickly and effectively communicated.

Pediatricians also may play a role in home care by visiting patients in the home to render care. The hectic pace of a busy office or hospital practice may seem to preclude home visitation, but many physicians have designed their practice to incorporate home calls, much to the satisfaction of their patients and themselves. An effective home care practice requires good staff support, creative schedule organization, a flexible medical records system, and transportable medical supplies. Such organizational requirements, however, should not discourage the hospitalist from occasional home visits to meet with families in their native environment, especially patients with chronic medical conditions who frequently require hospital admissions. Observing the home environment may give the hospitalist more insights into the patient's care needs and prevent future hospitalizations. *CPT* codes are available for physicians to bill for home care visits and oversight of the patient's plan of care.

WHAT CAN YOU DO AT HOME?

A host of medical services have been developed for home care. Partly as a response to rising health care costs, partly in response to bed capacity problems in some communities, and partly from the desire of patients to receive their care at home, an increasing number of therapies and diagnostic tests now can be performed in the home. Home care services span the medical spectrum from simple parent education to home dobutamine infusions and mechanical ventilation. In the past, pediatricians were reluctant to embrace home care services for a variety of reasons, including unfamiliarity with home care in general, lack of competent pediatric home care providers, a perceived increased risk of morbidity in children who have a smaller margin for error, lack of published research on home care outcomes in children, and a fear of losing control of the patient. Most of these fears are unfounded, and many pediatricians have successfully integrated home care services into their daily practice.

Although initially home care services were driven by payers seeking to reduce the financial burdens of continued care in the hospital, improved patient satisfaction and outcomes are now the driving force for physicians utilizing pediatric home care. Recent research in specific clinical situations has demonstrated better outcomes in pediatric patients who receive ongoing medical care in the home. A recent study of pediatric bone marrow transplant recipients demonstrated that patients discharged home earlier to a specialized home care program had less graft-versus-host disease, lower transplantation-associated mortality rates (RR = 0.22), and lower costs compared with controls who remained in the hospital (2). A novel "Hospital-at-Home" Program in England randomized 399 pediatric patients suffering with breathing problems, vomiting, diarrhea, or fever to hospital care or hospital-at-home care with 24-hour nursing availability. Although patients in the hospital-at-home program spent one extra day in care, there were no differences in hospital readmission rates. Patient and parent satisfaction were much higher in the hospital-at-home group compared with the hospitalized group (3).

Almost any medical therapy, apart from invasive procedures that must be done in the hospital, usually can be performed safely in the home. For example, rehabilitation services including physical therapy, occupational therapy, and speech therapy can be provided in the home and may shorten a patient's hospital stay and improve her functional outcome. Table 133.1 lists the types of home care services for children that can be performed in the home. Although the medical literature does not contain many well-designed outcome studies about pediatric home care, numerous observational studies have shown that various types of home care services for children can be provided safely and effectively in the home. The main factor limiting pediatricians from using many of the services listed in Table 133.1 is the lack of qualified pediatric home care agencies or personnel in their service area.

SPECIAL PEDIATRIC HOME CARE PROGRAMS

Certain home care services for children have become so well established in the medical literature and pediatric practice that they deserve special mention. These services include phototherapy, apnea monitoring, care of low-birthweight (LBW) infants, home infusion therapy, and mechanical ventilation. These home care programs are used routinely in pediatric practice, and competent home care agencies should have policies and procedures that allow for the care of children requiring such services in the home.

Phototherapy

Children with hyperbilirubinemia frequently are cared for in the home. Advances in phototherapy technology have allowed

TABLE 133.1

RANGE OF HOME CARE SERVICES

HOME INFUSION
Antibiotics
Antivirals
Antifungals
Antirejection medications
Chemotherapy
Intravenous hydration
Erythropoietin
Pain medications
Intrathecal baclofen
Total parenteral nutrition
Blood transfusions
Clotting factors
Hormones
Prostacyclin
Vasoactive agents

DURABLE MEDICAL EQUIPMENT
Phototherapy
Cardiorespiratory (apnea) monitors
Pulse oximetry
End-tidal capnography
Oxygen therapy
Mechanical ventilation
Bilevel positive airway pressure
Assistive technology

THERAPIES
Speech therapy
Occupational therapy
Physical therapy
Social work services

DIAGNOSTIC TESTING
Apnea testing
Multichannel sleep studies
Radiography
Electrocardiograms
pH probes
Phlebotomy/blood analysis

children with hyperbilirubinemia to be safely and effectively cared for in the home by their parents. Phototherapy lights are now lighter and more compact to allow for more mobility at home, increasing the time that the infant remains in contact with the light source. A home care phototherapy program typically includes a visit by a home care nurse for parent education and patient assessment, and delivery of a phototherapy blanket or light source. The patient and family either receive daily home visits by a nurse who checks serum bilirubin levels and completes a patient assessment, which is then communicated to the pediatrician, or the patient is seen by the pediatrician in her office on a regular basis.

The hospitalist should determine whether the patient and family are appropriate for home care services. The physician should establish that no significant pathologic causes for hyperbilirubinemia exist (e.g., sepsis or hemolysis) that may require exchange transfusions or closer physiologic monitoring (Section XIV). In addition, premature infants <35 weeks EGA, infants younger than 96 hours of age, infants with total serum bilirubin greater than 20 mg/dL, those with an increase in serum bilirubin greater than 0.25 mg/dL/hr, or those at risk

for neurologic complications should be treated and monitored in the hospital setting. Likewise, if the parents are unwilling or incapable of providing the care, or the home situation is unsafe or inappropriate (e.g., no electricity) for home phototherapy, then the patient should be treated in the hospital.

The ordering pediatrician should ensure that the phototherapy equipment sent to the home is appropriate and meets the minimum standards for light intensity and irradiance (wavelength 430 to 490 nm and >30 μW/cm^2/nm). Typically, overhead spotlights, used in hospitals in the past, are inappropriate for home use. Phototherapy blankets or newer-generation banked fluorescent lights are safer and more effective for home phototherapy. The most recent AAP guidelines (2004) on the management of hyperbilirubinemia suggest that home phototherapy can be instituted at total serum bilirubin levels that are 2 to 3 mg/dL below the suggested treatment levels (4). The treatment time for phototherapy varies depending on the intensity and irradiance of the light source, the surface area of the patient exposed to the light, and the time of exposure to the light. In patients with uncomplicated hyperbilirubinemia, phototherapy can be discontinued when the total serum bilirubin is <13 mg/dL. In most cases of uncomplicated hyperbilirubinemia, patients require 2 to 4 days of therapy.

Apnea Monitoring

Cardiorespiratory monitors are one of the most common medical devices prescribed for the home. The causes of infant apnea are diverse, and therefore the indications for apnea monitoring at home remain uncertain. Although there is a lack of medical research data regarding the efficacy of home apnea monitoring in preventing morbidity and mortality in infants believed to be at risk for apnea or sudden infant death syndrome (SIDS), many pediatricians still prescribe apnea monitors to alleviate parental anxiety or reduce the perceived threat of medical malpractice claims.

The purpose of the home cardiorespiratory monitor is to alert a caregiver, by an auditory alarm, to the presence of apnea or heart rate variations that deviate from preset values. Most home apnea monitors attach to an infant by electrodes or a Velcro monitor belt. These electrodes determine both heart rate and respiratory rate when placed appropriately. The DME supplier can then set an audible alarm to sound when the heart rate is above or below settings determined by the ordering physicians (typically <80 or >200 beats per minute in infants). An apnea delay alarm also can be set to alarm when the monitor does not sense any respiratory activity for a certain time (typically 15 to 20 seconds in infants). This type of monitor is not used in patients with obstructive apnea because the monitor will continue to sense respiratory effort even though the patient's airway is obstructed. False alarms are frequent with the current generation of monitors and often lead to parental noncompliance with monitoring. In addition, lead failure or misplacement can cause false alarms or inaccurate sensing, which may cause the monitor to miss an important cardiorespiratory event. Most monitors have the ability to record data that then can be downloaded and reviewed by a clinician to determine the incidence and severity of any cardiorespiratory events. Some monitors can even communicate with data centers over telephone lines to alert clinicians of events as they occur. It is usually best to ask for a monitor that has memory capability when ordering one for the home.

Appropriate children for home apnea monitoring include infants with apnea of prematurity or apnea of infancy with significant episodes of braycardia, infants who have experienced an acute life-threatening event, infants with chronic lung disease, siblings of children who died of SIDS, infants with seizures, infants of substance-abusing mothers, children on mechanical ventilation, children with tracheostomies or anatomic airway abnormalities, children with cardiac dysrhythmias, and children with certain neuromuscular disorders. Patients who are the best candidates for home cardiorespiratory monitoring are those infants with a disease process that causes infrequent episodes of central apnea, who require monitoring for a relatively short period (<3 months), who respond to interventions available in the home, and who have motivated caregivers. The routine use of home monitoring of children determined to be at a higher risk of SIDS remains controversial. No data have shown an improvement in outcome of children who have been placed on monitors, and home monitoring places emotional and financial burdens on the family. Recent AAP guidelines (2003) do not recommend apnea monitoring for children at risk for SIDS. The decision to use home cardiorespiratory monitoring in this setting should be a decision made with the family after carefully weighing the risks and benefits of this technology.

The home cardiorespiratory monitor is not a substitute for a careful diagnostic evaluation of an infant after an acute life-threatening event. Treatable causes for apnea, such as gastroesophageal reflux or seizures, should be evaluated before discharging a patient home on a cardiorespiratory monitor. A brief course of home monitoring may be indicated for certain infants with treatable causes of apnea to document the success of treatment or to alleviate parental anxiety. Apnea associated with respiratory syncytial virus infections is short-lived, and usually does not recur; therefore these children should not require home apnea monitoring. In general, the length of time a patient requires home monitoring is determined by the natural history of the disease that caused the acute life-threatening event. Patients with treatable causes of apnea should require only a short period of monitoring to document the success of treatment. An apnea-free period of 6 weeks has been used as a general rule of thumb in determining when to terminate apnea monitoring. Patients who continue to experience acute life-threatening events should have further diagnostic evaluation done to determine the causes of the events, or if these are known, monitoring should continue until the events have ceased. Infants with apnea of prematurity or infancy usually require monitoring until they reach 43 weeks postconceptional age, at which time their apnea usually resolves (5).

Orders for home cardiorespiratory monitoring should include an initial nursing visit so that the nurse can complete a home evaluation, including a home safety review; review apnea monitoring goals; and review interventions with the family in response to monitor alarms. The parents or patient caregivers should receive CPR training prior to discharge. The need for additional home nursing visits should be determined by the patient's clinical status and family situation.

Low-Birthweight Infants

The care of premature and LBW infants in the home is a well-established practice that has garnered some medical research interest. Most studies find that infants discharged early from the neonatal intensive care unit (NICU) have clinical outcomes similar to those of infants who are held in the NICU for longer periods until they achieve predetermined weight or growth guidelines. In addition, earlier care in the home decreases the total cost of care for these infants and improves parental bonding and satisfaction, as well as maternal psychosocial functioning (6,7).

Before discharge, the infant should achieve some level of physiologic stability, including resolution of apnea/bradycardia spells, adequate growth, maintenance of normal body temperature, and stabilization of organ dysfunction. Infants do not necessarily need to achieve predetermined weight goals before

discharge, but should demonstrate an adequate growth rate on the home nutritional program. Likewise, infants do not need to be nippling all feedings because nurses and parents usually can safely administer gavage or nasogastric feedings in the home. Infants who require continuous nasogastric feedings by pump should be placed on a home apnea monitor to alert caregivers in case the feeding tube becomes dislodged. Ongoing oxygen requirements should not be a barrier to earlier discharge home, because oxygen can be easily and safely delivered in the home setting.

Premature or LBW infants may be discharged home once they become physiologically stable. The discharge process should begin soon after birth so that parents can be psychologically prepared to care for their newborn once he achieves stability. Care for premature infants in the home should be entrusted only to nursing agencies with experience caring for these infants, and the home setting should be assessed for appropriateness prior to discharge.

Once the infant appears stable for discharge and the parents have been adequately trained in their infant's care, then arrangements should be made for medical follow-up, including identification of the primary care physician and any subspecialty physicians. In addition, the discharge planners should identify appropriate community resources, including parent support groups, social workers, early intervention programs, and any available financial resources. The first home nursing visit should occur on the day of discharge or soon thereafter. The frequency and duration of nursing visits vary depending on the infant's age, chronic medical conditions, and parental anxiety and competence. Normally, parents quickly become skilled at caring for their child, and nursing visits can be decreased accordingly. The importance of nursing resources available 24 hours per day cannot be overemphasized in providing new parents with comfort and support after discharge from the NICU. A good nursing agency can provide a safe and effective transition to home for the family and significantly reduce the number of nuisance calls to the pediatrician.

Home Infusion Therapy

Home infusion of total parenteral nutrition, antibiotics, and other antimicrobial agents is one of the most common reasons for using home care services. The delivery of IV medications and nutrition in the home has been one of the main driving forces in the development of the home care industry. Children who are physiologically stable and who require ongoing hospitalization only to complete a prescribed course of IV antibiotics or other medications are now commonly cared for in the home.

The pediatric hospitalist caring for children requiring prolonged courses of infused medications should be familiar with home infusion services in his area. Most medications delivered IV in the hospital can be safely delivered in the home. Medications ranging from simple IV solutions to dobutamine infusions have been safely administered to patients in the home. Other IV therapies that can be delivered in the home include analgesic infusions, IV immune globulin (IVIG) preparations, antiviral/antibacterial medications, anti-transplant rejection medications, clotting factors and other blood products, chemotherapy, and antifungal medications. A competent home infusion company partnering with a motivated and educated family should allow the hospitalist to consider any patient a potential candidate for home infusion therapy.

One of the greatest risks to the patient receiving medications in the home is allergic reactions. The risk of allergic reactions can be mitigated by delivering the first or second dose of a new medication to the patient in a more controlled setting, like the hospital or clinic. In addition, when delivering medications that have a high incidence of allergic reactions, such as IVIG, home nurses should be authorized to carry and deliver emergency medications like subcutaneous epinephrine, diphenhydramine, methylprednisolone, and normal saline, in the event of an unexpected reaction. Other common problems associated with home infusion therapies include programming errors with infusion pumps, mixing or calculation errors by the pharmacist or family, and breaks in line antisepsis techniques leading to catheter-associated infections. These errors can be mitigated by using a home infusion company or pharmacy that is familiar with dispensing parenteral nutrition and medications for children, and through careful education of the family caregivers.

The greatest barrier to accessing home infusion services is obtaining reliable IV access, especially in children. There are a variety of IV access devices that are appropriate in the home. Simple IV catheters may be appropriate for older children who do not require prolonged therapy or in younger children who require only short courses of therapy (e.g., less than 3 days). Typically, a midlength or longer peripherally inserted catheter is placed before discharge home, which allows for more stable IV access and greater patient mobility. Sometimes a central venous catheter needs to be placed when peripheral IV access is limited, if the infused medications are vesicants or have a significant potential for morbidity if they extravasate, or if the patient requires prolonged or repeated IV access. Usually a surgeon places a tunneled catheter (e.g., Hickman or Broviac) into a larger central vein such as the jugular or subclavian vein. Temporary central venous catheters like those used in the pediatric intensive care unit usually are inappropriate for the home because they typically are stiffer and pose a risk for erosion through the vessel, and can be more easily dislodged accidentally than tunneled catheters.

Planning a discharge of a patient requiring home infusion services requires a coordinated effort among the family, hospitalist, primary care pediatrician, discharge planner, and home infusion company. Once a patient has been identified as a good home infusion candidate, the discharge planners should locate a home infusion company that has pediatric nurses who are experienced with home infusion therapy in children. The home care nurse should ensure that the home is appropriate for home infusion therapy, including the presence of a refrigerator, running water, electricity, and a working telephone. The nurse should determine a medication schedule that is convenient for the family. In some cases, this may mean the hospitalist will have to substitute medications that require less frequent dosing (e.g., substituting ceftriaxone every 24 hours for cefotaxime every 6 hours). The primary care physician should be involved with the development of the home care plan and be aware of any drug or laboratory monitoring that is needed.

Home Mechanical Ventilation

The preparation for discharge of a child dependent on mechanical ventilation is a complex task requiring careful coordination between the primary care physician, family, social worker, discharge planner, repiratory therapists, home nurses, and the medical equipment supplier. The psychosocial, financial, and technologic barriers that must be overcome to transition successfully a child dependent on technology into the home are great, but not insurmountable. Discharge planning should begin the moment a child is anticipated to need home mechanical ventilation because the process of transitioning a patient to the home may take many months. The following factors need to be addressed before discharge: patient, home environment, financial, technological, and psychosocial.

TABLE 133.2
COMMON REASONS FOR CHRONIC VENTILATORY SUPPORT
NEUROMUSCULAR DISORDERS Muscular dystrophy
CHRONIC AIRWAY OBSTRUCTION Bronchomalacia Tracheomalacia Subglottic stenosis
CENTRAL APNEA/HYPOVENTILATION Central hypoventilation syndrome
BRONCHOPULMONARY DYSPLASIA
METABOLIC DISORDERS
PERIPHERAL OR CENTRAL NERVOUS SYSTEM DYSFUNCTION Spinal cord trauma Phrenic nerve injury
CHEST WALL ABNORMALITIES Kyphoscoliosis
PARENCHYMAL LUNG DISEASE Cystic fibrosis

The Patient

Patients require home mechanical ventilation because they are unable to maintain adequate ventilation or oxygenation on their own. Common reasons for chronic ventilatory support are given in Table 133.2. The underlying medical condition sometimes determines the type of long-term mechanical ventilatory support that will be used at home. Patients with central or obstructive apnea or progressive neuromuscular disorders may be able to tolerate noninvasive ventilation with continuous positive-airway pressure delivered by mask, although this mode of ventilation is most effective when used only during sleep. Less commonly used today, some patients may achieve adequate ventilation using a negative-pressure generator like a cuirass or negative-pressure tank (i.e., "iron lung") that allows adequate tidal ventilation usually without the need for a tracheostomy tube. However, most children requiring long-term mechanical ventilatory support require the placement of a tracheostomy tube. The placement of an artificial airway exposes the child to additional risks such as infection, tracheal obstruction, or vascular erosion, but these risks are outweighed by the benefit of a stable airway that allows for long-term ventilation.

A patient should be considered stable for discharge only after an initial tracheostomy change in the hospital by the surgeon, and once the parents or caregivers have demonstrated competency in all aspects of tracheostomy care. In addition, the patient should have been maintained on stable ventilator settings for 1 to 2 weeks before discharge. It is advisable to place the patient on the same mechanical ventilator she will be using in the home for a period of time before hospital discharge.

Patients preparing for home mechanical ventilation should have achieved some level of medical stability before discharge. Their other medical problems must be addressed and they should have demonstrated adequate growth and nutrition on the proposed home nutritional regimen. The child should have a primary care physician who will coordinate specialty care and provide routine pediatric care including immunizations. Children should have their hearing tested before discharge, and a plan for communication and speech development should be made before discharge.

Home Environment

The home needs to be prepared for the patient who requires mechanical ventilation. A predischarge evaluation of the home should be done by the home nursing agency and the respiratory therapist or medical equipment supplier. Rooms may need to be modified to accommodate the equipment necessary for home mechanical ventilation. The home evaluation should consider electrical needs, oxygen storage, and accessibility needs. Older children who can be mobile with a wheelchair may need to have ramps or lifts installed in their homes. Local emergency medical services agencies and utility companies should be alerted to the presence of a child who is dependent on technology.

Technological Issues

The main technological factor to be considered before discharge is the type of mechanical ventilation and ventilator to use at home. The simplest mode of ventilation is noninvasive ventilation using a continuous positive-airway pressure generator. These generators can deliver both inspiratory and expiratory pressure as well as oxygen. For these devices to be used noninvasively, the patient must wear a tight-fitting mask over his nose or face that is secured with straps around the head. Children often have difficulty maintaining a good seal with the masks and therefore fail this type of ventilation. Noninvasive ventilation is not appropriate for many disease processes like central apnea.

The other type of noninvasive ventilation is provided by negative-pressure ventilators. These ventilators work by isolating the chest in an airtight cavity and then applying negative pressure in that cavity that allows for inspiration through the patient's airway. Various types of negative-pressure ventilators have been developed, including flexible jackets made of cloth, hard shells or cuirasses that clamp around the thoracic cavity, and tanks that envelope the whole body except for the head. Negative-pressure ventilators are less invasive but tend to isolate the child from his environment and limit mobility.

More commonly, children are sent home with positive-pressure ventilators that require invasive airway access by tracheostomy. A new generation of small, lightweight, portable mechanical ventilators have come into the marketplace. These new ventilators work similarly to the latest generation of hospital ventilators and are easy to operate, with multiple modes of ventilation available. Portablility of the ventilator allows for the most reasonable lifestyle for the patient; they can attend school, play outdoors, and spend the night with friends, for example. The ventilator settings for discharge will be determined by the patient's disease process and are best established with the help of a pediatric pulmonologist or intensivist. The ventilators should come with internal or external battery backup power supply that can be used for travel or in the event

of power utility interruption. In addition, a second backup ventilator usually should be available in the home.

Psychosocial Issues

Fortunately, the amount of time required to prepare a child dependent on technology for discharge to home allows the family and the patient to adjust to their new living situation. Often, parents demonstrate the stages of grief when faced with the prospect that their child will require long-term mechanical ventilatory support. They should be allowed ample opportunity to cope with the reality of the situation and deal with their feelings of grief.

Caring for a child on mechanical ventilation requires a significant adjustment to normal life routines. Nurses are required to live in the home up to 24 hours per day with the rest of the family. Running errands requires a coordinated effort between caregivers so that someone is always available to the child. Family outings require extra planning time to ensure safe transportation of the affected child and her equipment. Families may need to purchase a different vehicle that can accommodate the patient and equipment. These are only a few of the practical psychosocial issues that families must address as they prepare to care for their child at home.

Financial Issues

The cost of caring for a child who requires home mechanical ventilation can be burdensome to the family. Not uncommonly, families have exhausted much of their insurance resources before discharge home because of prolonged or frequent hospitalizations. Government programs like Medicaid provide a safety net for most families; however, the approval process for home mechanical ventilation can take months. The patient's family should have a good financial plan in place before hospital discharge.

References

1. Wilson A, Wynn A, Parker H. Patient and carer satisfaction with "hospital at home": quantitative and qualitative results from a randomized controlled trial. *Br J Gen Pract* 2002;52:413.
2. Svahn BM, Remberger M, Myrback KE, et al. Home care during the pancytopenic phase after allogenic hematopoietic stem cell transplantation is advantageous compared with hospital care. *Blood* 100:2002;4317–4324.
3. Sartain SA, Maxwell MJ, Todd PJ, et al. Randomised controlled trial comparing an acute pediatric hospital at home scheme with conventional hospital care. *Arch Dis Child* 2002;87:371–375.
4. American Academy of Pediatrics. Clinical practice guideline. Management of hyperbilirubinemia in the newborn infant 35 or more weeks of gestation. *Pediatrics* 2004;114:297–316.
5. American Academy of Pediatrics. Policy statement. Apnea, sudden infant death syndrome, and home monitoring. *Pediatrics* 2003;111:914–917.
6. Merritt TA, Pillers D, Prows SL. Early NICU discharge of very low birth weight infants: a critical review and analysis. *Semin Neonatol* 2003;8:95–115.
7. Casiro OG, McKenzie ME, McFaden L, et al. Earlier discharge with community-based intervention for low birth weight infants: a randomized trial. *Pediatrics* 1993;92:128–134.

Suggested Reading

American Academy of Pediatrics, Section on Home Health Care. *Guidelines for pediatric home health care.* Elk Grove Village, IL: American Academy of Pediatrics; 2002.

CHAPTER 134 ■ ACUTE PAIN MANAGEMENT IN INFANTS AND CHILDREN

DAVID M. POLANER

In the past decade, the recognition and understanding that acute pain in infants and children is a common problem that deserves both treatment and study has finally reached the mainstream (1). Numerous studies and anecdotal reports have documented the undertreatment of pain in our smallest and most vulnerable patients, a situation that is thankfully becoming less common. Indeed, the pendulum has swung, in some cases, so far to the opposite pole that we may lose sight of the fact that a measure of discomfort is sometimes unavoidable, and that we must balance the provision of analgesia with the risks that such treatment can at times entail. Nevertheless, the treatment of pain in pediatric inpatients has evolved to allow effective analgesia with minimal risk and side effects for the majority of patients. An understanding of the pharmacology of analgesics, neurophysiology of pain, developmental pediatrics, and anatomy are all necessary to formulate a plan of analgesia for a given patient.

ASSESSMENT OF PAIN

Assessment of pain in infants and children is often more challenging than in adults due to the limitations of cognitive development and of communication in the preverbal or developmentally delayed child. Even children who are able to verbalize their pain are often unable to cooperate with assessments that are designed for more mature children or adults, and may be unable to utilize some modalities that are appropriate for older children. They may have different and disturbing reactions to some of the side effects of our therapies, such as numbness from local anesthetics or dysphoria from opioids, which make meaningful measurements of the adequacy of analgesia difficult.

Infants

It is axiomatic that pain is a subjective experience, and follows logically that the ideal means of measuring it would rely on self-assessment. This is, of course, impossible in preverbal children and infants, where we must rely on validated observational instruments to measure the adequacy of analgesia. Several scales have been developed and validated in this age group that can be used to score pain so that analgesic need and effectiveness can be assessed. Of necessity, these scoring systems rely on observation of behavior and facial expression, which may not always prove accurate (2). These scales are often used clinically in combination with signs of autonomic activation, such as blood pressure and heart rate, to facilitate decision-making about analgesic management. The two most commonly used scales in infants are the FLACC and CHEOPS scales. The FLACC scale, which is an acronym for *Facial expression, Legs, Activity state, Crying,* and *Consolability,* was developed in postoperative patients and has been used, but not validated, in other settings (3). It assigns a 0 to 2 score for each of the parameters, which are added to give a total score. The scale descriptors are shown in Table 134.1. This scale has been validated from ages 2 months to 7 years, although like all of the observational scales, it is often employed for older nonverbal developmentally delayed children. Its principle virtue is ease of use—scoring is relatively easy to learn and apply in the clinical setting.

The CHEOPS (Children's Hospital of Eastern Ontario Pain Scale) was developed to provide an observational pain scale for nonverbal children from 1 to 7 years old (4). It too was developed for measuring postoperative pain, but has also been validated for procedural pain. It employs a somewhat more complex scoring scheme and may require more training to use properly, but it has been used extensively in research on pediatric pain as well as in the clinical arena. The scale descriptors are shown in Table 134.2.

School-Aged Children

The CHEOPS scale has been validated in children up to 7 years of age, and can be used in younger children. In addition to this observational scale, there are several self-reporting scales that are easily employed in children, and can be used effectively by even some preschoolers. When a self-reporting scale can be used effectively, it is preferable to an observational scale, although in situations where there is doubt about the accuracy or comprehension of self-reporting scores, an observational scale can be used to confirm the self-reported score. Several variations of the faces scale are available, but we prefer the modified Bieri scale (Fig. 134.1), because it has been best validated to correspond to the 10-point verbal numeric and visual analog scales (5). The child is asked to point to the face that best reflects how they feel. It is important to note that the scale is not intended to be used as an observational scale; that is, the faces are not designed to reflect the child's own facial expression. We use this scale in preschool and school-aged children, especially those who have trouble giving accurate or consistent verbal numerical scores. It has been reported by some clinicians that some younger school-aged children may use the verbal numerical score better in reverse (i.e., 10 = no pain, 0 = worst pain imaginable) because they

TABLE 134.1

FLACC PAIN SCALE

Category	Score		
	0	1	2
Face	No particular expression or smile	Occasional grimace or frown; withdrawn, disinterested	Frequent to constant quivering chin, clenched jaw
Legs	Normal position or relaxed	Uneasy, restless, tense	Kicking or legs drawn up
Activity	Lying quietly, normal position, moves easily	Squirming, shifting back and forth, tense	Arched, rigid, or jerking
Cry	No cry (awake or asleep)	Moans or whimpers, occasional complaint	Crying steadily, screams or sobs, frequent complaints
Consolability	Content, relaxed	Reassured by occasional touching, hugging, or being talked to, distractible	Difficult to console or comfort

From Merkel SI, Voepel-Lewis T, et al. The FLACC: A behavioral scale for scoring postoperative pain in young children. *Pediatr Nurs* 1997;23: 293–297.

TABLE 134.2

CHILDREN'S HOSPITAL OF EASTERN ONTARIO PAIN SCALE (CHEOPS)

Item	Behavior	Score	Definition
Cry	No cry	1	Child is not crying.
	Moaning	2	Child is moaning or quietly vocalizing, silent cry.
	Crying	2	Child is crying but the cry is gentle or whimpering.
	Scream	3	Child is in a full-lunged cry; sobbing: may be scored with complaint or without complaint.
Facial	Composed	1	Neutral facial expression.
	Grimace	2	Score only if definite negative facial expression.
	Smiling	0	Score only if definite positive facial expression.
Verbal	None	1	Child is not talking.
	Other complaints	1	Child complains but not about pain, e.g., "I want to see my mommy" or "I am thirsty."
	Pain complaints	2	Child complains about pain.
	Both complaints	2	Child complains about pain and about other things, e.g., "It hurts; I want my mommy."
Torso	Positive	0	Child makes any positive statement or talks about other things without complaint.
	Neutral	1	Body (not limbs) is at rest; torso is inactive.
	Shifting	2	Body is in motion in a shifting or serpentine fashion.
	Tense	2	Body is arched or rigid.
	Shivering	2	Body is shuddering or shaking involuntarily.
	Upright	2	Child is vertical or in upright position.
	Restrained	2	Body is restrained.
Touch	Not touching	1	Child is not touching or grabbing at wound.
	Reach	2	Child is reaching for but not touching wound.
	Touch	2	Child is gently touching wound or wound area.
	Grab	2	Child is grabbing vigorously at wound.
	Restrained	2	Child's arms are restrained.
Legs	Neutral	1	Legs may be in any position but are relaxed; includes gentle swimming or serpentine-like movements.
	Squirming/kicking	2	Definitive uneasy or restless movements in the legs and/or striking out with foot or feet.
	Drawn up/tensed	2	Legs tensed and/or pulled up tightly to body and kept there.
	Standing	2	Standing, crouching, or kneeling.
	Restrained	2	Child's legs are being held down.

From McGrath P, Johnson G, et al. CHEOPS: A behavioral scale for rating postoperative pain in children. In: Fields H, ed. *Advances in pain research and therapy*. New York: Raven Press; 1985: 395–402.

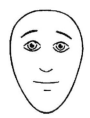 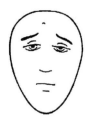 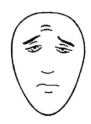 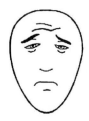 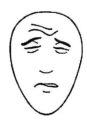 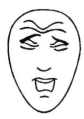

FIGURE 134.1. The Bieri Faces Pain Scale. The faces are intended to measure how the child feels, not how her face looks. The child is told "These faces show how much something can hurt. This face (point to the face on the left) shows no pain. The faces show more and more pain up to this one (the face on the far right)—it shows very much pain. Point to the face that shows how much you hurt." The child's choice is scored 0, 2, 4, 6, 8, 10 from left to right. Intermediate scores, based on the spaces between the faces (odd numbers), may be given. This revision of the original Bieri scale has been validated to correspond with verbal digital and visual analog 0–10 pain scales.

associate better scores with better performance on tests in school, and therefore a better score is associated with feeling better. This strategy is worth trying if a child seems to have trouble reporting accurate scores with the verbal numeric scale, although no data on this have yet been published.

Teenagers

Teenagers can use any of the scales devised for adults. We most commonly employ either a verbal numeric scale (0 = no pain, 10 = worst pain imaginable) or a visual analog scale (a 100-mm line marked "no pain" at one end and "worst possible pain" at the other, on which a mark is made by the patient corresponding to her level of pain).

Developmentally Delayed Older Children

There are no scales that have been devised specifically for older developmentally delayed children. Most clinicians, therefore, use the CHEOPS or a modification of the FLACC scale for nonverbal developmentally delayed children, although in this setting they are used outside the parameters for which they were validated. The FLACC in particular includes criteria that may be inappropriate for older children (the "legs" parameter), and one should be hesitant to use it in this age group.

NONOPIOID ANALGESICS

Nonopioid analgesics are the mainstay for the management of mild to moderate pain. Palatable pediatric oral formulations of most agents are available, and the lack of alterations in sensorium and of respiratory depression makes them the first line of therapy in many children. They are also highly effective when combined with opioids for more severe pain, and may significantly reduce opioid requirements in those patients. Suggested doses for nonopioid analgesics are shown in Table 134.3.

Acetaminophen is the most commonly used nonopioid agent for pediatric analgesia. It potency and effectiveness is often underestimated, but its use as a sole agent is limited to mild pain. It is also a very effective adjunctive agent, particularly when used in conjunction with opioids (6). It has a wide margin of safety when used in appropriate doses, and has been found to be safe even in newborns, where the immaturity of hepatic glucuronidation pathways may actually confer a decreased risk of toxicity. The current recommendation for oral dosing is 10 to 15 mg/kg every 4 hours, with a total daily dose not to exceed 4 g/day regardless of patient weight, or 100 mg/kg/day in children or 60 mg/kg/day in infants (7). Oral absorption is rapid, with effective blood levels being reached within 20 minutes of administration. Rectal dosing is quite different, as acetaminophen's absorption via this route is less effective than when orally administered. Several studies have demonstrated that 40 mg/kg will result in therapeutic blood levels after an initial loading dose, with maintenance of those levels being best achieved by administering subsequent doses of 20 mg/kg every 6 hours (8,9). Absorption of rectally administered acetaminophen is more erratic and slower than via the oral route, with peak blood levels appearing between 60 and 180 minutes. There is also significant variability in the absorption between different brands of suppositories, and it is important to note that the drug may not be evenly distributed in the suppository. This means that cutting suppositories to achieve fractional doses may result in the delivery of either higher or lower doses of drug, and should be considered an unreliable practice (10). In Europe, a parenteral formulation of acetaminophen is available; it has not yet been released in the United States.

Ibuprofen is the prototypic oral nonsteroidal anti-inflammatory agent. Like all drugs of this class, it inhibits peripheral cyclooxygenase (COX) and thereby reduces the production of prostaglandins. It is absorbed readily from the gastrointestinal tract. Because COX is ubiquitous in many tissues, its inhibition can lead to numerous undesirable side effects or toxicities, such as decreased platelet function, gastritis, and diminished renal blood flow (11,12). Although the newer COX-2 inhibitors, which have specificity for the inducible rather than the constitutive isoform of the enzyme, cause much less gastric irritation and platelet dysfunction than the nonspecific COX inhibitors, renal toxicity is still a concern. Other nonsteroidal agents, such as ketoprofen, are also highly effective analgesics for mild to moderate pain and have been successfully used in children (13).

Ketorolac is the only intravenous COX inhibitor available in the United States (14). Although it has been reported to be as effective as morphine in equipotent doses, we have found that the claim of equipotency is difficult to assure in all clinical situations because its mechanism of analgesic action is different than the opioids (15). Ketorolac, like the oral COX drugs, can have numerous undesirable side effects. Most prominent among these is its effect on renal blood flow and the risk of nephrotoxicity. Therefore, great caution is mandated for the use of this drug in patients with renal impairment, and our institution recommends that a course of therapy should not exceed 48 hours without monitoring renal function. A second caveat is that ketorolac, like other COX agents, inhibits platelet function (16,17). In patients who had undergone tonsillectomy there was an increased incidence of bleeding complications, and its use is not recommended in that setting (18). In a study of 70 children who had undergone open heart surgery

TABLE 134.3

SUGGESTED DOSES FOR NONOPIOID ANALGESICS

	Route	Dosage guidelines	Onset	Peak effect	Half-life	Duration
Acetaminophen	PO	10–15 mg/kg/dose every 4–6 hr, maximum dose 4,000 mg/day	30 min	30–60 min	Neonates: 2–5 hr Adults: 2–3 hr	4 hr
	PR	40 mg/kg loading dose, followed by 10–20 mg/kg/dose every 6 hr				
Ibuprofen	PO	4–10 mg/kg/dose every 6–8 hr, maximum dose 40 mg/kg/day, no greater than 2,400 mg/day	45–90 min	2–4 hr, peak serum level 1–2 hr	Children 1–7 yr: 1–2 hr Adults: 2–4 hr	6–8 hr
Ketoprofen	PO	0.5 mg/kg/dose every 8 hr	15 min	30 min, peak plasma level	2 hr (6 mo– adults)	6–8 hr
Ketoralac	IV	0.5 mg/kg/dose every 6 hr, maximum of 30 mg/dose, maximum course of 2–3 days	10 min	1–2 hr	Children: ~6 hr Adults: ~5 hr	4–6 hr

there was no increase in postoperative bleeding complications (19). A study of pharmacokinetics of ketorolac in children ages 1 to 16 found similar blood levels to those achieved in adults following a single intravenous dose of 0.5 mg/kg (20).

OPIOID ANALGESICS

Opioid analgesics are used for moderate to severe pain, and are the mainstay of most analgesic programs in the acute hospital setting. Aside from the obvious advantage of potency, opioids also have the advantage of numerous routes and strategies of administration, which bring with them great flexibility for almost every clinical situation. Suggested starting doses for opioid analgesics are shown in Tables 134.4 and 134.5.

Regardless of how an opioid is administered, there are two primary dosing goals. The first is to keep the blood level of the drug within the therapeutic window, and the second is to tailor the dose to the patient's analgesic need. The therapeutic window is a blood level range of the drug that exceeds the threshold of analgesia (the level below which there is inadequate analgesia) but remains below the threshold of respiratory depression, above which potentially serious complications may develop. This concept is depicted in Figure 134.2. All opioids at any clinically effective dose may produce some degree of respiratory depression, and the addition of other central nervous system depressants may have additive or synergistic effects on central respiratory drive.

Tolerance must always be born in mind when administering opioids (21,22). Tolerance develops more rapidly with more potent opioids, and may develop more rapidly with infusions compared to intermittent doses. Tolerance is a particular problem when very high doses are required for long periods of time. In these cases, it is important to wean the dose gradually, not more than 10% to 15% per day, to avoid precipitating abstinence symptoms (23). The use of adjunctive drugs such as clonidine can be very helpful in this situation (24).

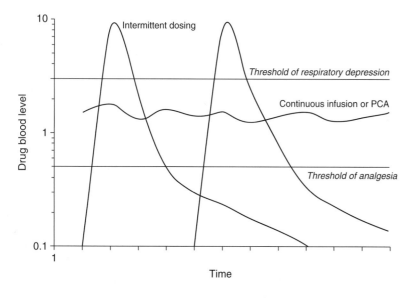

FIGURE 134.2. An idealized representation of continuous infusion versus intermittent dosing of opioids. Note that with infrequent intermittent doses the blood level (represented on the vertical axis) peaks above the threshold for respiratory depression soon after the administration of the drug, and falls below the threshold of analgesia before the next dose is given. With continuous infusions (or PCA) the blood level stays in the target window.

TABLE 134.4

SUGGESTED STARTING DOSES OF INTRAVENOUS OPIOIDS IN INFANTS AND CHILDREN[a]

Opioid drug	Route	Dosage guidelines	Onset	Peak effect	Half-life	Duration
Hydromorphone	IV	Children: 0.015 mg/kg/dose every 3–6 hr Adolescents: 1–4 mg every 3–6 hr	15 min	15–30 min	2.5 hr	4–5 hr
Fentanyl	IV intermittent	0.5–1 µg/kg/dose (best for intermittent short-duration analgesia; titrate to effect)	1–3 min	5–10 min 2.4 hr	5 mo–4.5 yr: Adults: 2–4 hr	30–60 min
	IV continuous	1 µg/kg/hr	1–3 min (following loading dose)			
Methadone	IV	0.1 mg/kg/dose every 4 hr for 2–3 doses, then every 6–12 hr	10–20 min	1–2 hr	~23 hr	6–8 hrs (22–48 hr after repeated doses)
Morphine	IV intermittent	0.05– 0.1 mg/kg/ dose every 2–4 hr	5–10 min	20 min	Neonates: 7–8 hr 1–3 mo	2–4 hr
	IV continuous	0.01–0.03 mg/kg/hr	5–10 min		old: 6 hr 6 mo–2.5 yr: 3 hr	
			15–60 min		3–19 yr: 1–2 hr Adults: 2–4 hr	

[a]These doses assume an opioid-naïve patient, and must be modified up or down based on the individual clinical situation of each individual patient and on the concurrent administration of other drugs. See the text for more complete information. Note that due to its short duration of action, intermittent doses of fentanyl are best used for episodic, rather than ongoing, pain, and that small frequent doses should be administered and titrated to effect. For intermittent administration in ongoing pain situations, consider the use of an intermediate or longer-acting agent.

Rational Use of Intermittent Dosing

Intermittent doses of intravenous opioids have been used commonly to good effect in infants and children for years, but better understanding of these agents can lead to more effective dosing schemes. Intermittent doses are best used when analgesic needs are not continuous. For continuous pain, such as postoperative pain, an infusion technique or a long-acting drug may be better (25). One should choose a drug for intermittent administration based on the duration of action of both the drug and the pain, the desired speed of onset, and the potential for side effects. For example, if episodic pain is spasmodic in nature, comes on rapidly, but lasts less than an hour, fentanyl may be a good choice. It has a rapid onset (within 2 minutes), a relatively short duration of action (under an hour), and does not release histamine. Morphine or hydromorphone can be chosen if an intermediate duration of action is desired. Because of the rapid peak in the plasma level that occurs after the administration of a short or intermediate-acting intermittent opioid, the risk of respiratory depression may be greater than with continuous infusions, and monitoring and observation of the patient during the period of peak effect is necessary to detect and reduce the risk of respiratory depression. It is critically important to assess both the effects of the administered dose and the total drug used during each 24 hour period to optimize the dose and interval. Patients receiving concomitant sedating agents, patients with drug metabolic organ dysfunction, or patients with altered potential for drug binding or elimination must have dose and interval carefully titrated to take these factors into account (26).

When the kinetics of an infusion is desired but an infusion cannot be used, a long-acting opioid such as methadone, sometimes used with a technique referred to as "reverse PRN," can be employed. Methadone has a long half-life with a slow peak, making it ideal for intermittent dosing when a steady level of analgesia is needed (27). For reverse PRN dosing, a patient's pain is scored on a regular (e.g., every 4 hour) basis, and a variable dose administered based on a sliding scale linked to the pain score. In this manner, the dose, and therefore the blood level, of drug is titrated to the patient's analgesic needs. The same strategy can be employed for the intermediate-acting opioids; however, the smoothness of drug level is harder to achieve due to the rapid peak after injection. Methadone accumulates slowly, and takes several days to reach a steady state. This must be born in mind when escalating the dose.

Continuous Infusions

Continuous infusions are the most efficacious way to achieve steady-state drug concentrations. Clinicians unfamiliar with using infusions outside of the intensive-care unit have concerns about drug accumulation and oversedation that can be

TABLE 134.5

SUGGESTED STARTING DOSES OF ORAL OPIOIDS IN INFANTS AND CHILDREN[a]

	Route	Dosage guidelines	Onset	Peak effect	Half-life	Duration
Codeine	PO	0.5–1 mg/kg/dose every 4–6 hr, maximum of 60 mg/dose	30–60 min	60–90 min	2.5–3.5 hr	4–6 hr
Hydrocodone (in Vicodin, Lortab elixir)	PO	Children: 0.15–0.2 mg/kg/dose every 4–6 hr				
		Adolescents: 1–2 tabs q 4–6 hr (limited due to acetaminophen content; see acetaminophen recommendations in text)	10–20 min	2 hr	3.8–4.5 hr	3–6 hr
Methadone	PO	0.1 mg/kg/dose every 4–6 hr for 2–3 doses, then every 6–12 hr	30–60 min	2–4 hr	~ 23 hr	6–8 hr (22–48 hr after repeated doses)
Hydromorphone	PO	Children: 0.03–0.1 mg/kg/dose every 4–6 hr	15–30 min	30–90 min	1–3 hr	4–5 hr
		Adolescents: 1–4 mg every 3–4 hr				
Morphine	PO-IR	0.2–0.5 mg/kg/dose every 4–6 hr	15–60 min	1 hr	Neonates: 7–8 hr	3–5 hr
	PO-ER	0.3–0.6 mg/kg/dose every 12 hr	1–2 hr	3–4 hr	1–3 mo old: 6 hr 6 mo–2.5 yrs: 3 hr 3–19 yr: 1–2 hr Adults: 2–4 hr	8–12 hr
Oxycodone	PO-IR	0.05–0.15 mg/kg/dose every 4–6 hr	15–60 min	1 hr	IR: 2–10 yr old: 1.8 hr	4–5 hr
	PO-ER	Adolescents: Initial 10 mg every 12 hr with IR for breakthrough pain; adjust ER dose based on IR usage after 24–48 hr	1–2 hr	3–4 hr	Adults: 3.7 hr Adults: 4.5–8 hr	12 hr

[a]These doses assume an otherwise healthy opioid-naïve patient, and must be modified up or down based on the individual clinical situation of each individual patient and on the concurrent administration of other drugs. See the text for more complete information. Note that codeine, hydrocodone, and oxycodone are available in fixed-combination preparations with acetaminophen, which may restrict the amount of opioid that can be administered due to the dose limitations of the acetaminophen component. IR = immediate release, ER = extended release.

best addressed by understanding the kinetics of the drugs (25). The goal in choosing an infusion rate is to maintain an even drug level by replacing the drug cleared from the bloodstream with an equal rate of infusion. Pharmacokinetic studies of morphine and fentanyl have demonstrated the infusion rates that will maintain a therapeutic blood level while avoiding respiratory depression. For morphine, a rate of 0.02 to 0.025 mg/kg/hr will achieve this goal with pCO_2 levels close to the normal range in most term infants older than 6 months. Lower infusion rates (0.01–0.015 mg/kg/hr) are recommended for younger infants. Neonates, particularly those under 1 week of age, may have significantly prolonged elimination of morphine; their elimination of fentanyl is highly variable (28). In contrast, fentanyl clearance in older infants and children appears to be high, and there is no increase in respiratory depression in term infants older than 3 months (29,30).

When using a continuous infusion, it should be remembered that it takes three half-lives of the drug to achieve steady state, so if a higher blood level is desired, a small bolus should precede the increase in infusion rate to reach that new level faster. Similarly, a loading dose should precede the start of the infusion.

Patient-Controlled Analgesia

Patient-controlled analgesia (PCA) uses a microprocessor-controlled programmable pump that permits a patient to deliver his own intravenous analgesia in small incremental boluses. The opioid can thus be self-titrated to a patient's analgesic needs. Analgesic needs, best judged by the patient himself, vary for each individual and at different times during the day. The patient is best able to respond to the changing intensity of pain by choosing when to deliver a dose, resulting in rapid onset and a blood level of opioid that is kept within the therapeutic range. In anticipation of physiotherapy, for example, the patient may chose to administer an extra dose, while less analgesic may be needed during sleep or when resting in bed. When the pump settings are optimized for the patient's size and underlying medical conditions there is inherent safety in PCA, because the patient will fall asleep when over-sedation occurs and is thus unlikely to self-administer too much drug. Most patients will administer their PCA demand doses in a manner that balances sedation or other side effects with comfort, and there are wide interpatient variations in the amount of opioid use, which probably reflects individual variations in the tolerable pain levels and individual "style" of usage by each patient (31). PCA avoids the "overshoot" that can occur when a large intermittent bolus is administered by the nurse by using small but frequent incremental doses, and is reported to result in both better analgesia and lower opioid consumption (32). The larger doses can result in a high peak drug level, which may actually increase the risk of side effects as compared to a properly set up PCA regimen.

Preoperative teaching is an integral and essential component of this therapy because both the child and the parents must understand the concept of PCA in order to use it safely and properly (33). The child is taught to deliver a dose whenever he feels pain, and that the pump is programmed to prevent the delivery of either too high a dose or too many doses. The child should be instructed not to wait for the pain to become severe before actuating a PCA demand dose. The child can also deliver a dose in anticipation of a painful event such as ambulation or chest physiotherapy. The child and family must be instructed that control of "the button" rests solely with the child and not the parent. Only the child should decide when to deliver a demand dose. Most developmentally normal children over 6 or 7 years of age can be taught to use PCA properly (32,34). Older children, however, may be more effective in their use of PCA. A study comparing PCA with continuous infusions found that although all children over the age of 5 years were able to use PCA, the age 5- to 8–year-old cohort had no greater analgesia with PCA as compared to continuous infusions. The older children, however, did have better analgesia with PCA, suggesting that their understanding of how to optimally utilize PCA was better (35). The sense of command over analgesic management that a child has with PCA is one of the most attractive features of this modality and makes it an especially useful mode of therapy for older children and adolescents, for whom loss of control during hospitalization can be very discouraging.

There are five parameters to set on the PCA pump (Table 134.6). All recommended doses below refer to morphine.

1. A *loading dose* of opioid must be administered if the child is in pain so that the child begins with a therapeutic blood level. Because the PCA demand (patient actuated) doses are small, optimal effectiveness of the technique is predicated on the patient having a reasonable level of analgesia when therapy is turned over to her. For the opioid-naïve patient who is not receiving other sedating agents, this loading dose is usually in the range of 0.05 to 0.1 mg/kg, delivered in incremental doses until comfort is achieved. Further increments of 0.02 mg/kg can be added at 5- to 10-minute intervals if needed. Titration to effect, the governing principle of any intravenous opioid technique, is necessary to provide a sufficient interval between incremental doses to allow the morphine to reach peak effect and thereby avoid overdose.

2. A *patient demand dose*, that is, the dose that will be administered with each patient activation of the pump, must be set. These small boluses are usually in the range of 0.01 to 0.025 mg/kg.

3. A *lockout interval* must be set. This prevents a patient from activating the pump before the previous bolus takes effect, and is a critical safeguard against overdosing. The demand button can be pressed, but the pump will not deliver a dose until the lockout period has passed. For morphine (and hydromorphone) we chose 10 minutes.

4. A *basal infusion rate* can be used to deliver a continuous background dose of opioid. This may assist in maintaining the drug level within the therapeutic range, especially during the night so that the patient is not awakened in pain, and can moderate the number of times a patient needs to deliver a demand dose. Although some studies have suggested that this is not needed, many have shown that a judiciously chosen basal infusion rate improves analgesia and sleep patterns, and results in less respiratory depression than intermittent dosing (32). In one controlled study, however, more opioid was used by the PCA plus basal group, and some side effects were increased; but this was likely due to the higher infusion rate of 0.02 mg/kg/hr in this protocol (36). At our institution we recommend a starting rate of 0.01 to 0.015 mg/kg/hr for morphine. In pain states that are characterized by intermittent, rather than continuous, analgesic needs, the basal rate may be eliminated. During weaning from PCA to oral analgesics, the basal rate should be discontinued, leaving only demand doses as a rescue modality for breakthrough pain.

5. A *maximum hourly (or 4-hour) dose* may be chosen. Some physicians chose not to use this limit, relying on modest ranges of the other settings to limit the total drug used. The physician can set a limit on the cumulative amount of drug a patient may administer, often ranging from 0.05 to 0.2 mg/kg/hr (on some pumps, a 4-hour limit, rather than an hourly limit, is set). This amount may be chosen based on the average hourly use of morphine during the past 24 hours or, in patients started on PCA as the primary analgesic intervention, at the lower range of the dosage scale. Once this limit is reached, the patient is unable to activate the pump until the hour has passed.

Recently the use of PCA pumps has been extended to allow the activation of the demand dose by either the patient's nurse (where the activation criteria are based on observational pain scoring) or the patient's parent (where the criteria are less

---

TABLE 134.6

DOSING GUIDELINES FOR PATIENT-CONTROLLED ANALGESIA

	Morphine	Hydromorphone	Fentanyl
Concentration	1 mg/mL	100 µg/mL	10 µg/mL
Basal rate	0.01–0.02 mg/kg/hr	1.5–3 µg/kg/hr	0.1–0.2 µg/kg/hr
PCA dose	0.01–0.02 mg/kg	1.5–3 µg/kg	0.1–0.2 µg/kg
Booster or	0.05–0.1 mg/kg	15 µg/kg	0.5–1 µg/kg
loading dose	q 2–3 hr prn	q 2–3 hr prn	q 1 hr prn
Lock-out	10 min	10 min	6–10 min

objective) (37). In one situation, a patient who is unable to activate the demand dose by himself has a parent push the button on his behalf and at his request. This is still well within the rubric of PCA—the decision to activate a demand dose is made by the patient, who is simply not able to push the button. In other situations, the benefits of small, frequent titrated doses of opioid are applied to titrate analgesia for younger children or children with cognitive and developmental delays. Although there have been reports of significant success with this technique, there have also been some anecdotal reports of critical incidents where inadvertent overdosing has occurred (38,39). It is probably best applied to palliative care settings and in oncology, where the patients are opioid-tolerant. Careful selection of parent and patient, and extensive education, are essential for safety with this technique. One should recognize that the primary inherent safety feature of PCA—that the patient will fall asleep before administering a significant overdose—is eliminated with this technique.

Oral Opioids

For the child able to take oral medications with moderate pain, an oral opioid analgesic is often the treatment of choice. Numerous drugs are available in both pill and liquid form so that dosing is easy. Codeine is probably the best known and most commonly used of the oral opioids; however, it may be the least efficacious. Approximately 10% of the Caucasian population lacks the enzyme to demethylate codeine to its active form (40). Better choices for an oral opioid include hydrocodone and oxycodone. Both of these drugs have greater potency than codeine and may produce less nausea as well. Oral morphine and hydromorphone preparations are available in liquid form that can be easily dosed for children, and methadone is available as an elixir as well. None of these drugs has as fast an onset as its intravenous counterpart, so one should take this into account when converting from intravenous to oral therapy. These drugs are often administered concurrently with acetaminophen, as discussed above. Tramadol is a synthetic codeine analog with both mu receptor activity as well as inhibition of serotonin and norepinephrine uptake, a unique combination that offers multimodal analgesic properties in a single agent. It is well absorbed orally and has been studied in children for up to a month of administration (41).

Transmucosal and Transdermal Opioids

There has been increasing interest in the delivery of opioids by novel routes. The potential application for the application of these delivery technologies in children, where vascular access is often difficult, is obvious; however, most of these delivery systems still have limited use or data in pediatrics.

Transmucosal fentanyl has been available for several years in a lollypop-like matrix delivery vehicle. It has rapid uptake and good bioavailability, especially as compared with the oral transmucosal administration of the intravenous fentanyl preparation (42). Some studies have reported a higher incidence of nausea and vomiting when it was used as a premedicant before surgery or painful procedures (43). It has been specifically studied in adults as a therapy for cancer breakthrough pain; pediatric studies for this indication are not yet available. It is dosed at 10 to 15 µg/kg, and should not be used in the opioid-naive patient or in younger children. Transdermal delivery of fentanyl has also been studied in children. Fentanyl patches are available in relatively limited doses, which limits the flexibility and ability to provide size-appropriate dosing in children. Despite the thinner skin of children, the pharmacokinetics were found in one study to be similar to adults (44). Transdermal fentanyl has been used in children mostly in the setting of cancer or palliative care (45).

REGIONAL ANALGESIA

Although the placement of regional blocks is generally the purview of the anesthesiologist, analgesic care after the block is established may be shared with the hospitalist in some institutions. It is therefore prudent for the pediatric hospitalist to understand the anatomy and physiology of regional blockade and the techniques of management of continuous blockade for analgesia. There are numerous clinical scenarios beyond postoperative analgesia where regional blockade can be effectively employed to manage pain in pediatric patients with a minimum of undesirable side effects (46,47).

Epidural and Caudal Analgesia

Epidural and caudal analgesia are the most commonly used methods of regional analgesia in pediatric patients (48,49). With both techniques, a catheter is threaded into the epidural space, either via the caudal canal through the sacral hiatus, or via a midline or paramedian approach through spaces between bones of the lumbar or thoracic spine (50). Because the caudal canal is contiguous with the epidural space, a caudal block can be considered a "low" approach to the epidural space, and behaves identically in virtually all respects to an epidural block. Caudal blockade is the most commonly performed regional anesthetic in children, in large part due to its ease of performance and its high success rate. Both of these blocks may be contraindicated in patients with neural tube defects, although an epidural can be placed above the level of the defect in these patients with CT or MRI confirmation of the anatomy.

The epidural space is bounded externally by the ligamentum flavum and internally by the dura mater, and is filled with fat and a vascular plexus. Long, thin epidural catheters (usually 20 g) are threaded into the epidural space through a needle and held in place with an adherent dressing such as Tegaderm or OpSite. When a catheter is threaded into the space it may inadvertently enter a vessel in the vascular plexus, leading to intravascular injection of local anesthetic and possible toxicity, or pierce the dura, entering the subarachnoid space and causing a high level subarachnoid block (spinal anesthetic) or, in the case of an opioid, respiratory depression (the effective intrathecal dose of both local anesthetic and opioid is much less than the epidural dose). Therefore, a test dose (a small dose of local anesthetic containing epinephrine) is injected prior to the therapeutic dose to detect an intravascular catheter placement and reduce the risk of intravascular injection of the larger therapeutic dose. Intrathecal injection is usually apparent due to the rapid onset of a very dense motor and sensory block, although this may be difficult or impossible to detect if the block is placed and test dosed during general anesthesia, as is most commonly done (51).

Drugs infused into an epidural catheter fall into three categories: local anesthetics, opioids, and adjunctive agents. *Local anesthetics* block both sensory and motor function of a nerve (52). For postoperative or other analgesic use, any motor effects and dense sensory blockade are undesirable—the goal is to attain analgesia with the lowest concentration of local anesthetic possible. For this reason, the addition of other drugs to the epidural infusion, which may act in a synergistic manner, can be used to reduce the amount of local anesthetic required to achieve adequate pain control. It is important to recognize that the analgesic effect of local anesthetic is dependent on two factors: the *density* of blockade (i.e., how insensate the patient is) is dependent on local anesthetic concentration, but the *spread* of blockade (i.e., how many dermatome segments are affected) is dependent on *volume* of drug infused. In order to achieve analgesia of a particular region of the body, the spinal dermatomes that innervate that region must be blocked. A certain volume of local anesthetic must be injected into the epidural space to remain in contact with the spinal nerves of those dermatomes. The lack of understanding of this principle leads to the erroneous concept that an epidural can be "weaned" by turning down the infusion rate. In reality, such a strategy will lead to a fall in the dermatome level of the block and the return of pain once the nerves supplying the dermatomes of the area in pain are no longer bathed by local anesthetic. The concept of volume as the primary determinant of choosing local anesthetic dose also means that if high volume is required to achieve adequate analgesia (i.e., an effective dermatome spread of blockade), the concentration of local anesthetic may need to be decreased to avoid toxicity with that volume, particularly in smaller children.

The goal of catheter placement is to have the catheter tip, where drug delivery occurs, in the middle region of the dermatomes that need to be blocked. This will permit the lowest volume of local anesthetic to achieve blockade of the desired dermatomes. When a block is too "low" (i.e., the level of blockade is caudad to the highest dermatome needed to achieve analgesia), it may be driven higher by the addition of more volume. This is usually done by administering a bolus, followed by an increase in the infusion rate. However, if the catheter is placed much lower than the dermatomes that need to be blocked (e.g., a caudal catheter is placed for a thoracic operation or for acute chest syndrome in a sickle-cell disease patient), it may prove to be nearly impossible to maintain the block high enough, and local anesthetic toxicity concerns alone may prevent adequate volumes of drug from being infused.

Local anesthetic toxicity is a significant concern with continuous blocks in children. These concerns begin with the initial dose of drug when the block is established, and the bolus must be calculated to take into account not only patient weight and age but also issues such as other local anesthetics administered at the same time to other sites. The usual starting doses and hourly limits for local anesthetics are listed in Table 134.7. Note that infants under age 6 months should have the maximal doses reduced by about 25%. This is due to their lower blood levels of ?-1 acid-glycoprotein. This plasma protein is the primary binding protein for local anesthetics, and a decreased level can result in higher free fractions of drug, resulting in the potential for greater toxicity (53). Data on toxic levels of bupivacaine and ropivacaine are lacking in infants and children, and most clinicians believe that greater caution is indicated in these patients.

There are several choices of local anesthetic for postoperative analgesia (52). *Bupivacaine* is perhaps the most commonly used agent. It is an amide with a long duration of action and produces less motor blockade than sensory blockade. Its toxicities at high doses include cardiac dysrhythmias (usually ventricular bradydysrhythmias, because of its effect on fast sodium channels) and seizures, so infusion rates should not exceed 0.5 mg/kg/hr (0.3 mg/kg/hr in infants

under 6 months of age) (54). There is a risk of accumulation in infants when higher infusion rates are used, particularly after 48 hours. For continuous epidural blockade, a concentration of 0.1% is used; this may be reduced further if motor block is present. *Levobupivacaine* is the levo-enantiamer of bupivacaine. Its major benefit is that the toxicity risk is markedly reduced; however, it has recently become difficult to obtain in the United States. Dosing is identical to bupivacaine, although the toxic thresholds are probably about 20% higher. *Ropivacaine* is a new amide that has two advantages over bupivacaine—it has a greater toxic threshold (probably 20% to 30% higher than bupivacaine) and is reported by some investigators (but not all) to produce less motor blockade (55,56). It is usually used in concentrations of 0.1% to 0.2%. *2,3 chloroprocaine* is an ester local anesthetic that is sometimes used in infants for infusions because there is little to no risk of drug accumulation; its termination of action is via hydrolysis of the ester bond by nonspecific plasma esterases. A concentration of 1% is usually adequate to provide analgesia with minimal motor blockade.

Other continuous regional blocks can be performed for analgesia. Catheters can be placed in the fascia iliaca space for analgesia of femur injuries, in the axillary sheath or infraclavicular space to block the brachial plexus, and numerous other sites. Infusions into these sites are generally limited to local anesthetics, for which the same dosage limitations described above apply (57,58). The interested reader is referred to one of the standard textbooks of pediatric anesthesia for more information.

ADJUNCTIVE AGENTS

Clonidine is an alpha adrenergic agonist that was originally developed as an antihypertensive agent. It has been found to be a highly useful adjunctive drug for potentiating the effect of opioid analgesics, retarding the development of opioid tolerance, and treating opioid withdrawal (59,60). It appears to have only very limited analgesic properties of its own, although it can cause sedation, particularly at higher doses. Clonidine can be administered by several different routes— orally, intravenously, transcutaneously, and in the epidural space. Caution should be used in ambulatory patients, who may experience orthostatic hypotension or near-syncope if they change from a recumbent to an upright position too quickly. Usual starting doses are 1 to 1.5 μg/kg q 8 hours.

NMDA receptor antagonists, such as low-dose ketamine, have recently been used more frequently for pain (61,62). Although it is by no means a first-line therapy, there are case reports in which continuous infusions in combination with an opioid have been useful in patients with difficult-to-control pain. The dysphoric side effects can be problematic, and its use should be limited to monitored settings until more experience is published.

TABLE 134.7

USUAL DOSES OF LOCAL ANESTHETICS AND ADDITIVES FOR REGIONAL ANESTHESIA

	Bupivacaine or ropivacaine	Fentanyl	Hydromorphone	Clonidine
Concentration	0.05–0.1% (0.5–1 mg/mL)	1–3 μg/mL	3-5 μg/mL	0.5–1 μg/mL
Suggested dose	Less than 6 mo of age: 0.2–0.3 mg/kg/hr Older than 6 mo of age: 0.2–0.4 mg/kg/hr	0.2–1 μg/kg/hr	1 μg/kg/hr up to 2.5 μg/kg/hr	0.1–0.5 μg/kg/hr
Maximum dose	Less than 6 mo of age: 0.3 mg/kg/hr Older than 6 mo of age: 0.5 kg/kg/hr			

NONPHARMACOLOGIC ADJUNCTS

The mention of hypnosis may bring to mind entertainment rather than therapy, but medical hypnosis is a well-established and effective therapeutic modality for many indications (63). This highly underutilized intervention has virtually no side effects and is particularly effective in children, who commonly make excellent hypnotic subjects. It can be used with great success in both acute painful interventions, such as injections and intravenous line placements, and for chronic painful conditions including cancer pain; however, it is not a substitute for pharmacologic therapies in all cases (64–69). Hypnosis and other cognitive therapies require a skilled practitioner and can form a very useful adjunct in pain treatment.

MONITORING AND SAFETY

The most worrisome complication of opioid therapy is *respiratory depression*, so respiratory monitoring is an important consideration. It is worth noting that respiratory depression from central neuraxis opioids is often characterized by a fall in respiratory depth prior to respiratory rate. Two types of monitoring are in common use on inpatient wards, both of which have significant limitations in the early detection of respiratory depression. Pulse oximetry, which detects hypoxemia, will warn of hypoventilation relatively late, and will be even more delayed if supplemental oxygen is being administered. Impedance respirometry is what is commonly used to compute respiratory rate on an electrocardiographic (ECG) monitor. It measures the impedance change between ECG leads as the chest expands with each inspiration. Thus, it measures chest wall motion, not gas exchange, and cannot detect airway obstruction. The best monitor remains observation of the patient by a trained clinician, and nursing vigilance is the key to validating and supplementing the continuous electronic monitors that we have come to rely on with perhaps excess faith.

Sedation scales have been devised to quantify the degree of sedation of a patient receiving opioids and other sedating drugs. These should be recorded along with pain scores at regular intervals by the nursing staff, and excessive sedation should be promptly dealt with by decreasing the dose of sedating agents.

Motor blockade from local anesthetics in continuous regional analgesia can cause both pressure sores and peripheral nerve injuries when patients are not properly positioned and moved. The Bromage score, a scale devised to measure motor function, should be employed at regular intervals to detect motor block (Table 134.8).

Infections of regional anesthetic catheters are rare but can occur (70). Most of these infections begin at the insertion site

and can track along the catheter to deeper tissues if undetected. Daily or twice-daily inspection of the catheter site for signs of inflammation is imperative, and a catheter should be removed at the first sign of skin infection.

TREATMENT OF UNTOWARD EFFECTS

Pruritus is common in infants and children receiving opioids by any route, and may occur for two reasons. Some opioids, particularly morphine, release histamine. For this situation, an antihistamine such as diphenhydramine may be very effective, although many antihistamines are sedating and should be used with some degree of caution in infants and children receiving higher doses of opioids, and the author usually recommends starting these drugs at the lower end of the dose range. In some pediatric patients excitement, rather than sedation, may be seen with antihistamines. Even those opioids that do not release histamine, like fentanyl, can cause pruritus from central nervous system effects. This is particularly common (about 20%) in patients receiving central neuraxis opioids, and is more effectively treated with opioid antagonists. Two approaches have been used: a partial antagonist, like nalbuphine (0.05 mg/kg q 4 hr) can be administered as needed, or a low-dose infusion of an antagonist like naloxone (1 µg/kg/hr) can be continuously infused (71). Both of these approaches are effective at relieving any of the opioid-induced side effects, but when used at these doses do not adversely alter the analgesic effects of the drug.

Nausea is another common untoward effect of opioids, and can be quite problematic. Although stimulation of the central chemotactic trigger zone is a potential effect of any opioid via any route of administration, it appears that clinically some opioids may be worse in this regard than others. Unfortunately, which drug is more "emetogenic" than another varies from patient to patient and cannot be predicted in any individual based on population data. There are several treatment options for this most unpleasant reaction. As mentioned above, the use of low-dose antagonists is effective. Several classes of antiemetics are available for administration via different routes. We usually favor the first-line therapy with a 5-HT blocking agent such as ondansetron, dolesatron, or granesitron. Although these drugs are more expensive, they are highly effective and have fewer side effects (especially less sedation or dysphoria) than older agents of other classes. Prokinetic agents like metoclopramide can be used as a second-line therapy. We usually reserve the use of older drugs of the phenothiazine-derivative class such as prochlorperazine as a last-line treatment. The route of administration of antiemetics is important, since oral agents are obviously less desirable when a patient is nauseated. We tend to favor either the intravenous route or the use of oral dissolving tablets, which do not need to be swallowed. *Urinary retention* is another side effect of opioids, and can be particularly problematic with central neuraxis (epidural and intrathecal) opioids. This can be effectively treated with low-dose antagonists or agonist–antagonists as described above, or bladder catheterization can be performed.

Ileus and constipation are common side effects of opioids, and should be anticipated, especially in patients who are in bed much of the time. The preemptive administration of a stool softener may help in preventing the problem, as may adequate hydration and early ambulation. The addition of nonopioid analgesics when possible can reduce the dose requirement of opioid. *Sedation* is not always an undesirable side effect of systemic and central neuraxis opioid therapy, but excessive sedation certainly can be. Sedation is also commonly seen with other drugs given concurrently with opioids—some

TABLE 134.8

MODIFIED BROMAGE SCORE FOR MOTOR BLOCKADE

Score	Motor response
0	No evidence of motor block, able to lift extremity to gravity
1	Able to move extremity, but cannot sustain lift against gravity
2	Unable to move extremity

antiemetics, antihistamines, and alpha-adrenergic agonists such as clonidine. Most of the time dose reduction is the treatment of choice, along with the addition of a nonopioid analgesic such as acetaminophen or a nonsteroidal agent when possible.

Respiratory depression, when detected early, can usually be dealt with by reducing the dose of opioid and increasing the vigilance of monitoring until it resolves. Severe respiratory depression requires immediate intervention: the administration of oxygen and (if necessary) assisted ventilation, and the administration of an opioid antagonist (naloxone). It is rarely necessary to give a large dose of naloxone, especially if the airway is properly managed. Incremental doses of 1 μg/kg IV given every few minutes will reverse respiratory depression without adversely affecting analgesia. One must remember that the duration of naloxone is commonly shorter than that of the opioid, and a continuous infusion and transfer to a higher acuity ward may be necessary.

Dysphoria can occur with opioids, and may be difficult to treat. Often the best strategy is to switch to another opioid. It may be difficult to pinpoint whether the opioid is to blame for the problem, because many of these children are on other drugs, such as antiemetics, that can cause the same symptoms.

Motor blockade should be treated by reducing the concentration of local anesthetic. Until the block is resolved, exceptionally careful attention must be paid to the positioning of the child's extremity so that there are no pressure points that could lead to skin breakdown or peripheral nerve compression injury. Sometimes the infusion needs to be stopped for an hour to allow the motor block to recede. If this is necessary, supplemental analgesia may need to be provided until the block is reestablished with a lower concentration solution.

Local anesthetic toxicity can occur due to accumulation of drug or acute overdosage after a bolus of local anesthetic. Because of the severity of the consequences of overdosage, it is best to be extremely compulsive about calculating the maximum allowable dose of local anesthetic and ensure that it is not exceeded. Early signs of local anesthetic toxicity may include irritability, restlessness, and somnolence. If a catheter has migrated into a blood vessel there may be loss of analgesia. Verbal children may complain of a metallic taste and of tinnitus. Higher blood levels can precipitate seizures and ventricular dysrhythmias, and cardiac arrest may ensue. Cardiac arrest from bupivacaine is especially difficult to treat; the drug interacts with fast sodium channels and is refractory to most of the usual treatments. The best results have been reported with an infusion of 20% intralipid, which appears to act as a "lipid sink" to remove bupivacaine from myocardium (72,73). Phenytoin has also been shown to be effective (74).

References

1. Berde CB, Sethna NF. Analgesics for the treatment of pain in children. *N Engl J Med* 2002;347:1094–103.
2. Beyer JE, McGrath PJ, Berde CB. Discordance between self-report and behavioral pain measures in children aged 3–7 years after surgery. *J Pain Symptom Manage* 1990;5:350–356.
3. Merkel S, Voepel-Lewis T, Malviya S. Pain assessment in infants and young children: the FLACC scale. *Am J Nurs* 2002;102:55–58.
4. McGrath P, Johnson G. CHEOPS: A behavioral scale for rating postoperative pain in children. In: Fields H, ed. *Advances in pain research and therapy*. New York: Raven Press; 1985:395–402.
5. Hicks CL, von Baeyer CL, Spafford PA, et al. The Faces Pain Scale-Revised: toward a common metric in pediatric pain measurement. *Pain* 2001;93:173–183.
6. Korpela R, Korvenoja P, Meretoja OA. Morphine-sparing effect of acetaminophen in pediatric day-case surgery. *Anesthesiology* 1999;91:442–447.
7. Hahn TW, Henneberg SW, Holm-Knudsen RJ, et al. Pharmacokinetics of rectal paracetamol after repeated dosing in children. *Br J Anaesth* 2000;85:512–519.

8. Birmingham PK, Tobin MJ, Fisher DM, et al. Initial and subsequent dosing of rectal acetaminophen in children: a 24-hour pharmacokinetic study of new dose recommendations. *Anesthesiology* 2001;94:385–359.
9. van der Marel CD, van Lingen RA, Pluim MA, et al. Analgesic efficacy of rectal versus oral acetaminophen in children after major craniofacial surgery. *Clin Pharmacol Ther* 2001;70:82–90.
10. Birmingham PK, Tobin MJ, Henthorn TK, et al. Twenty-four-hour pharmacokinetics of rectal acetaminophen in children: an old drug with new recommendations. *Anesthesiology* 1997;87:244–252.
11. Lesko SM, Mitchell AA. Renal function after short-term ibuprofen use in infants and children. *Pediatrics* 1997;100:954–957.
12. Litalien C, Jacqz-Aigrain E. Risks and benefits of nonsteroidal anti-inflammatory drugs in children: a comparison with paracetamol. *Paediatr Drugs* 2001;3:817–858.
13. Kokki H, Karvinen M, Jekunen A. Pharmacokinetics of a 24-hour intravenous ketoprofen infusion in children. *Acta Anaesthesiol Scand* 2002;46:194–198.
14. Forrest JB, Heitlinger EL, Revell S. Ketorolac for postoperative pain management in children. *Drug Saf* 1997;16:309–329.
15. Lieh-Lai MW, Kauffman RE, Uy HG, et al. A randomized comparison of ketorolac tromethamine and morphine for postoperative analgesia in critically ill children. *Crit Care Med* 1999;27:2786–2791.
16. Bean-Lijewski JD, Hunt RD. Effect of ketorolac on bleeding time and postoperative pain in children: a double-blind, placebo-controlled comparison with meperidine. *J Clin Anesth* 1996;8:25–30.
17. Splinter WM, Rhine EJ, Roberts DW, et al. Preoperative ketorolac increases bleeding after tonsillectomy in children. *Can J Anaesth* 1996;43:560–563.
18. Gallagher JE, Blauth J, Fornadley JA. Perioperative ketorolac tromethamine and postoperative hemorrhage in cases of tonsillectomy and adenoidectomy. *Laryngoscope* 1995;105:606–609.
19. Gupta A, Daggett C, Drant S, et al. Prospective randomized trial of ketorolac after congenital heart surgery. *J Cardiothorac Vasc Anesth* 2004;18:454–457.
20. Dsida RM, Wheeler M, Birmingham PK, et al. Age-stratified pharmacokinetics of ketorolac tromethamine in pediatric surgical patients. *Anesth Analg* 2002;94:266–270.
21. Suresh S, Anand KJ. Opioid tolerance in neonates: mechanisms, diagnosis, assessment, and management. *Semin Perinatol* 1998;22:425–433.
22. Puntillo K, Casella V, Reid M. Opioid and benzodiazepine tolerance and dependence: application of theory to critical care practice. *Heart Lung* 1997;26:317–324.
23. Yaster M, Kost-Byerly S, Berde C, et al. The management of opioid and benzodiazepine dependence in infants, children, and adolescents. *Pediatrics* 1996;98:135–140.
24. Deutsch ES, Nadkarni VM. Clonidine prophylaxis for narcotic and sedative withdrawal syndrome following laryngotracheal reconstruction. *Arch Otolaryngol Head Neck Surg* 1996;122:1234–1238.
25. Pounder DR, Steward DJ. Postoperative analgesia: opioid infusions in infants and children. *Can J Anaesth* 1992;39:969–974.
26. Richtsmeier AJ Jr., Barnes SD, Barkin RL. Ventilatory arrest with morphine patient-controlled analgesia in a child with renal failure. *Am J Ther* 1997;4:255–257.
27. Berde CB, Beyer JE, Bournaki MC, et al. Comparison of morphine and methadone for prevention of postoperative pain in 3- to 7-year-old children. *J Pediatr* 1991;119:136–141.
28. Koehntop DE, Rodman JH, Brundage DM, et al. Pharmacokinetics of fentanyl in neonates. *Anesth Analg* 1986;65:227–232.
29. Singleton MA, Rosen JI, Fisher DM. Plasma concentrations of fentanyl in infants, children and adults. *Can J Anaesth* 1987;34:152–155.
30. Hertzka RE, Gauntlett IS, Fisher DM, et al. Fentanyl-induced ventilatory depression: effects of age. *Anesthesiology* 1989;70:213–218.
31. Tyler DC, Pomietto M, Womack W. Variation in opioid use during PCA in adolescents. *Paediatr Anaesth* 1996;6:33–38.
32. Berde CB, Lehn BM, Yee JD, et al. Patient-controlled analgesia in children and adolescents: a randomized, prospective comparison with intramuscular administration of morphine for postoperative analgesia. *J Pediatr* 1991;118:460–466.
33. Kotzer AM, Coy J, LeClaire AD. The effectiveness of a standardized educational program for children using patient-controlled analgesia. *J Soc Pediatr Nurs* 1998;3:117–126.
34. Birmingham PK, Wheeler M, Suresh S, et al. Patient-controlled epidural analgesia in children: can they do it? *Anesth Analg* 2003;96:686–691.
35. Bray RJ, Woodhams AM, Vallis CJ, et al. A double-blind comparison of morphine infusion and patient controlled analgesia in children. *Paediatr Anaesth* 1996;6:121–127.
36. Doyle E, Robinson D, Morton NS. Comparison of patient-controlled analgesia with and without a background infusion after lower abdominal surgery in children. *Br J Anaesth* 1993;71:670–673.
37. Monitto CL, Greenberg RS, Kost-Byerly S, et al. The safety and efficacy of parent-/nurse-controlled analgesia in patients less than six years of age. *Anesth Analg* 2000;91:573–579.
38. Anghelescu DL, Burgoyne LL, Oakes LL, et al. The safety of patient-controlled analgesia by proxy in pediatric oncology patients. *Anesth Analg* 2005;101:1623–1627.
39. Patient controlled analgesia by proxy. *Sentinel Event Alert* 2004:1–2.
40. Fagerlund TH, Braaten O. No pain relief from codeine? An introduction to pharmacogenomics. *Acta Anaesthesiol Scand* 2001;45:140–149.

41. Rose JB, Finkel JC, Arquedas-Mohs A, et al. Oral tramadol for the treatment of pain of 7–30 days' duration in children. *Anesth Analg* 2003; 96:78–81.
42. Wheeler M, Birmingham PK, Dsida RM, et al. Uptake pharmacokinetics of the Fentanyl Oralet in children scheduled for central venous access removal: implications for the timing of initiating painful procedures. *Paediatr Anaesth* 2002;12:594–599.
43. Schutzman SA, Burg J, Liebelt E, et al. Oral transmucosal fentanyl citrate for premedication of children undergoing laceration repair. *Ann Emerg Med* 1994;24:1059–1064.
44. Paut O, Camboulives J, Viard L, et al. Pharmacokinetics of transdermal fentanyl in the peri-operative period in young children. *Anaesthesia* 2000;55: 1202–1207.
45. Noyes M, Irving H. The use of transdermal fentanyl in pediatric oncology palliative care. *Am J Hosp Palliat Care* 2001;18:411–416.
46. Collins JJ, Grier HE, Kinney HC, et al. Control of severe pain in children with terminal malignancy. *J Pediatr* 1995;126:653–657.
47. Yaster M, Tobin JR, Billett C, et al. Epidural analgesia in the management of severe vaso-occlusive sickle cell crisis. *Pediatrics* 1994;93:310–315.
48. Pullerits J, Holzman RS. Pediatric neuraxial blockade. *J Clin Anesth* 1993;5:342–354.
49. Wood CE, Goresky GV, Klassen KA, et al. Complications of continuous epidural infusions for postoperative analgesia in children. *Can J Anaesth* 1994;41:613–620.
50. McBride WJ, Dicker R, Abajian JC, et al. Continuous thoracic epidural infusions for postoperative analgesia after pectus deformity repair. *J Pediatr Surg* 1996;31:105–107. Discussion 7–8.
51. Desparmet J, Mateo J, Ecoffey C, et al. Efficacy of an epidural test dose in children anesthetized with halothane. *Anesthesiology* 1990;72:249–251.
52. Berde C. Local anesthetics in infants and children: an update. *Paediatr Anaesth* 2004;14:387–393.
53. Luz G, Wieser C, Innerhofer P, et al. Free and total bupivacaine plasma concentrations after continuous epidural anaesthesia in infants and children. *Paediatr Anaesth* 1998;8:473–478.
54. Luz G, Innerhofer P, Bachmann B, et al. Bupivacaine plasma concentrations during continuous epidural anesthesia in infants and children. *Anesth Analg* 1996;82:231–234.
55. Ivani G, DeNegri P, Conio A, et al. Comparison of racemic bupivacaine, ropivacaine, and levo-bupivacaine for pediatric caudal anesthesia: effects on postoperative analgesia and motor block. *Reg Anesth Pain Med* 2002;27:157–161.
56. Ivani G, De Negri P, Lonnqvist PA, et al. Caudal anesthesia for minor pediatric surgery: a prospective randomized comparison of ropivacaine 0.2% vs levobupivacaine 0.2%. *Paediatr Anaesth* 2005;15:491–494.
57. Paut O, Sallabery M, Schreiber-Deturmeny E, et al. Continuous fascia iliaca compartment block in children: a prospective evaluation of plasma bupivacaine concentrations, pain scores, and side effects. *Anesth Analg* 2001;92: 1159–1163.
58. Malawer MM, Buch R, Khurana JS, et al. Postoperative infusional continuous regional analgesia. A technique for relief of postoperative pain following major extremity surgery. *Clin Orthop* 1991:227–237.
59. Murkin JM. Central analgesic mechanisms: a review of opioid receptor physiopharmacology and related antinociceptive systems. *J Cardiothorac Vasc Anesth* 1991;5:268–277.
60. Meert TF, De Kock M. Potentiation of the analgesic properties of fentanyl-like opioids with alpha 2-adrenoceptor agonists in rats. *Anesthesiology* 1994;81:677–688.
61. Subramaniam K, Subramaniam B, Steinbrook RA. Ketamine as adjuvant analgesic to opioids: a quantitative and qualitative systematic review. *Anesth Analg* 2004;99:482–495.
62. Tsui BC, Davies D, Desai S, et al. Intravenous ketamine infusion as an adjuvant to morphine in a 2-year-old with severe cancer pain from metastatic neuroblastoma. *J Pediatr Hematol Oncol* 2004;26:678–680.
63. Stewart JH. Hypnosis in contemporary medicine. *Mayo Clin Proc* 2005; 80:511–524.
64. Chen E, Joseph MH, Zeltzer LK. Behavioral and cognitive interventions in the treatment of pain in children. *Pediatr Clin North Am* 2000;47:513–525.
65. DuHamel KN, Redd WH, Vickberg SM. Behavioral interventions in the diagnosis, treatment and rehabilitation of children with cancer. *Acta Oncol* 1999;38:719–734.
66. Foertsch CE, O'Hara MW, Stoddard FJ, et al. Treatment-resistant pain and distress during pediatric burn-dressing changes. *J Burn Care Rehabil* 1998; 19:219–224.
67. Harper GW. A developmentally sensitive approach to clinical hypnosis for chronically and terminally ill adolescents. *Am J Clin Hypn* 1999;42:50–60.
68. Huth MM, Broome ME, Good M. Imagery reduces children's post-operative pain. *Pain* 2004;110:439–448.
69. Patterson DR. Non-opioid-based approaches to burn pain. *J Burn Care Rehabil* 1995;16:372–376.
70. Strafford MA, Wilder RT, Berde CB. The risk of infection from epidural analgesia in children: a review of 1620 cases. *Anesth Analg* 1995;80: 234–238.
71. Maxwell LG, Kaufmann SC, Bitzer S, et al. The effects of a small-dose naloxone infusion on opioid-induced side effects and analgesia in children and adolescents treated with intravenous patient-controlled analgesia: a double-blind, prospective, randomized, controlled study. *Anesth Analg* 2005;100:953–958.
72. Weinberg GL, Ripper R, Murphy P, et al. Lipid infusion accelerates removal of bupivacaine and recovery from bupivacaine toxicity in the isolated rat heart. *Reg Anesth Pain Med* 2006;31:296–303.
73. Rosenblatt M, Able M, Fischer G, et al. Successful use of a 20% lipid emulsion to resuscitate a patient after a presumed bupivacaine-induced cardiac arrest. *Anesthesiology* 2006;105:217–218.
74. Maxwell LG, Martin LD, Yaster M. Bupivacaine-induced cardiac toxicity in neonates: successful treatment with intravenous phenytoin. *Anesthesiology* 1994;80:682–686.

CHAPTER 135 ■ SEDATION

JOSEPH P. CRAVERO

Each year millions of children require sedation for diagnostic and therapeutic procedures that are performed in the hospital. The manner in which these procedures are accomplished (drugs used and providers involved) varies widely from one institution to another. In all cases the goals remain constant— the provision of safe, effective sedation that provides optimal conditions for the procedure that needs to be accomplished.

In recent years, no field of pediatric care provision has seen more change in practice patterns than sedation. This field, which was previously the domain of sedation nurses and (occasionally) anesthesiologists, has blossomed into a dynamic practice that includes emergency medicine providers, intensivists, hospital-based pediatricians, and others. In addition, the medications used by providers other than anesthesiologists changed from long-acting oral agents to potent short-acting sedative hypnotic and analgesic agents that allow truly excellent sedation care for a wide variety of patients and procedures. With these changes in care, the level of expectations and potential risk for sedation care have been raised significantly.

Perhaps now more than ever it is imperative that professionals who provide sedation clearly understand the concepts that are the key of sedation practice including the nature of sedation depth, monitoring during sedation, pharmacology/pharmacokinetics of the sedative agents currently available, core competencies for sedation management, and issues involving recovery of patients after sedation. It is only with a clear understanding of these concepts along with the risks involved in sedation that the goal of eliminating pain and anxiety from the experience of hospitalization can be realized for children.

LEVELS OF SEDATION

Professional organizations have defined sedation in different ways. Across the board, all these organizations have defined different "levels" of sedation ranging from minimally impaired consciousness to complete unconsciousness or general anesthesia. Any provider who delivers sedation should recognize that different levels of sedation are possible and they are *not specific to a given drug*. Any sedative (given a large enough dose) will produce obtundation. Likewise, even the most powerful intravenous sedative hypnotic can produce minimal sedation when given in a very small dose.

Sedation providers should recognize that these definitions are arbitrary and there is no clear demarcation between the different levels, and children can easily "slip" between one level and another. In recognition of these facts, the current recommendations from the JCAHO state that a provider of sedation should be able to manage or "rescue" a patient from one level of sedation "deeper" than that which is intended. Clearly, the expertise required to manage patients varies with the level of sedation, as outlined below (1):

- *Minimal sedation* (previously referred to as conscious sedation). A medically controlled state of depressed consciousness that (1) allows protective reflexes to be maintained, (2) retains the patient's ability to maintain a patent airway independently and continuously, and (3) permits appropriate response by the patient to physical stimulation or verbal command such as "open your eyes." Although cognitive function and coordination may be impaired, ventilatory and cardiovascular functions are unaffected.
- *Moderate sedation/analgesia.* A drug-induced depression of consciousness during which patients respond purposefully to verbal commands, either alone or accompanied by light tactile stimulation. No interventions are required to maintain a patent airway, and spontaneous ventilation is adequate. Cardiovascular function is usually maintained.
- *Deep sedation.* A medically controlled state of depressed consciousness or unconsciousness from which the patient is not easily aroused. It may be accompanied by a partial or complete loss of protective reflexes, and includes the inability to maintain a patent airway independently and respond purposefully to physical stimulation or verbal command. Patients may require assistance in maintaining a patent airway and spontaneous ventilation may be inadequate. Cardiovascular function is usually maintained.
- *Anesthesia.* Consists of general anesthesia and spinal or major regional anesthesia. It does *not* include local anesthesia. General anesthesia is a drug-induced loss of consciousness during which patients are not arousable, even by painful stimulation. The ability to independently maintain ventilatory function is often impaired. Patients often require assistance in maintaining a patent airway, and positive-pressure ventilation may be required because of depressed spontaneous ventilation or drug-induced depression of neuromuscular function. Cardiovascular function may be impaired.

PLANNING FOR SEDATION

Multiple factors impact the nature of the sedation that should be provided for a given patient. These factors can be divided into those related to the individual patient, the procedure, and the person providing the sedation.

Factors Relating to the Patient

Past Experience

When planning to sedate a child, the previous experiences of the patient to be sedated should be elicited. Both good and bad experiences should be reviewed along with the drugs that were previously administered. Obviously, patients who became combative with a given dose of oral midazolam would *not* be well served by repeating that drug and dose for another procedure. Similarly, the provider should elicit some indication of the anxiety that the patient and family have regarding the upcoming procedure and sedation. The severely anxious patient will often need significant sedation, where a relaxed patient may only need support or distraction. Although these facts may seem self-evident, a sedation history is often completely neglected by many providers.

Allergies

It is imperative that a good drug allergy and adverse reaction history be elicited prior to providing sedation. If a patient states an "allergy" is present to a given medication, a history of what type of reaction occurred should be obtained. Drugs that were associated with urticaria or shortness of breath should obviously be avoided.

Adverse Reactions

As mentioned above, many patients will have paradoxical reactions to sedative medications such as chloral hydrate where crying and combative behavior is elicited rather than sedation.

Aspiration Risk

A history of last oral intake is required before providing sedation. Although the data on aspiration injury associated with pediatric sedation cases is not definitive, most experts advise fasting guidelines (NPO) for elective procedures that mimic those required for anesthesia. The reasoning behind these recommendations follows the thought that it is often very difficult to predict the exact depth of sedation that will result from a dose of a sedative in a small child—therefore it should be assumed that airway reflexes may be lost and steps to minimize risk should be taken.

Generally accepted guidelines differentiate between clear liquid intake and heavy meals in a graded fashion, as outlined in Table 135.1.

In addition to the history of intake, prior to sedation the provider should elicit a history of gastroesophageal reflux disease. Patients who have a history of severe reflux disease (with associated growth failure or daily vomiting) may not be completed safely under significant sedation unless their airway is protected. At the very least, these patients should have an assured fasting interval, and some experts will insist on securing their airway with an endotracheal tube prior to sedation rather than sedating with an unprotected airway.

With the recommendations outlined above in mind, each provider will need to weigh the urgency of the procedure against the relative risk of the "full stomach." Emergency departments routinely do not abide by these fasting guidelines, and there is little indication that aspiration is a significant problem in this setting (2). In spite of this, it seems prudent to strive for a reasonable fasting interval when sedating pediatric patients—in particular those having elective procedures.

General Health

The general health status of each patient undergoing sedation should be considered. The child should undergo a general physical examination with focus on the airway, cardiovascular system, and respiratory system. Most institutions require the physical examination be completed by a licensed practitioner prior to sedation.

The AAP guidelines for sedation (3) recommend that the presedation physical include the following:

1. Age and weight.
2. Health history, including (a) allergies and previous allergic or adverse drug reactions; (b) drug use including dosage, time, route, and site of administration for prescription, over-the-counter, or illicit drugs; (c) relevant diseases, physical abnormalities, and pregnancy status; (d) a summary of previous relevant hospitalizations, (e) history of sedation or general anesthesia, and any complications; and (f) relevant family history.
3. Review of systems—including sleep apnea and current upper respiratory symptoms.
4. Vital signs, including heart rate, blood pressure, respiratory rate, and temperature.
5. Physical examination.
6. Physical status evaluation.
7. Name, address, and telephone number of the child's or family's physician.

For hospitalized patients, the current hospital record may suffice for adequate documentation of pre-sedation health; however, a brief note should be written documenting that the chart was reviewed, positive findings were noted, and a management plan was formulated.

To aid in assessment of anesthesia risk, the American Society of Anesthesiologists has a classification system for patients that categorizes individuals on a general health basis. It is one of the most important factors used to assess the overall perioperative risk (Table 135.2).

This physical evaluation should be reviewed by the sedation provider and particular attention should be paid to issues described in the following sections.

Airway Issues

Specific abnormalities of the airway should be noted. A small or malformed mandible or a large tongue are often associated with difficult spontaneous as well as assisted ventilation. Teeth that are protruding or particularly loose should be noted, as they may hinder airway visualization or be knocked free during manipulation. Any syndrome that results in an "unusual facies" should be carefully noted as they may also be associated with an airway that is difficult to manage. It may be helpful to give each child a Mallampati classification as part of the pre-sedation workup. This examination (which classifies the relative size of the tongue in the mouth) may be used as a trigger for referring a patient for "expert" sedation (Fig. 135.1). In general, a high (III to IV) Mallampati classification associated with any other abnormality of the head and neck is indicative of an airway that may well be difficult to manage.

Developmental Issues

The neurodevelopmental status of the child should be noted. Requirements for sedation will change greatly for any child who is severely delayed. Some of these patients will require

TABLE 135.1

FASTING GUIDELINES FOR SEDATION OR ANESTHESIA

Food	Hours of fasting required
Clear liquids	2
Breast milk	3 or 4 depending on mother's diet
Formula or light meal (no fat)	6
Full meal	8

TABLE 135.2

ASA CLASSIFICATION

ASA class	Description	Examples
1	A normal, healthy patient, without organic, physiologic, or psychiatric disturbance	Healthy with good exercise tolerance
2	A patient with controlled medical conditions without significant systemic effects	Controlled hypertension, controlled diabetes mellitus without system effects, cigarette smoking without evidence of COPD, anemia, mild obesity, age less than 1 or greater than 70 years, pregnancy
3	A patient having medical conditions with significant systemic effects intermittently associated with significant functional compromise	Controlled CHF, stable angina, old MI, poorly controlled hypertension, morbid obesity, bronchospastic disease with intermittent symptoms, chronic renal failure
4	A patient with a medical condition that is poorly controlled, associated with significant dysfunction and is a potential threat to life	Unstable angina, symptomatic COPD, symptomatic CHF, hepatorenal failure
5	A patient with a critical medical condition that is associated with little chance of survival with or without the surgical procedure	Multiorgan failure, sepsis syndrome with hemodynamic instability, hypothermia, poorly controlled coagulopathy
6	A patient who is brain dead and undergoing anesthesia care for the purposes of organ donation	
E	This modifier is added to any of the above classes to signify a procedure that is being performed as an emergency and may be associated with a suboptimal opportunity for risk modification	

more sedation than a similar patient their age, while others may actually not require sedation at all. Input from the primary care givers of these patients is critical in determining the amount of intervention that will be required for a given procedure—they can often predict the response a patient will have to a situation.

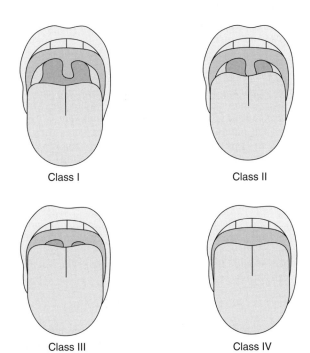

Class I   Class II

Class III   Class IV

FIGURE 135.1. Mallampati classification.

Cardiac and Respiratory Systems

As mentioned above, the cardiac and pulmonary systems must be assessed prior to beginning the sedation. Patients with a history of significant congenital heart disease deserve to have sedation provided by a true expert. In particular, patients with pulmonary hypertension may have significantly adverse reactions to hypoventilation and increased CO_2—or hypoxia. The presence of a corrected valve or shunt will require prophylactic antibiotics for minor procedures that otherwise would be the case for a well child. Finally, the amount of left-to-right shunting may be changed by pulmonary or systemic vasodilation that can be the result of medication administration.

Asthma

Respiratory issues usually involve the presence of asthma or upper respiratory tract infections (see below). Although few data exist concerning the risk of sedation for patients with asthma, experts agree that any time there is the chance of manipulating the airway (as is the case with any significant sedation), an asthmatic should be in his best possible condition prior to beginning the procedure. Generally this includes taking all usual inhalers prior to the sedation and assuring that the child is not actively wheezing.

Upper Respiratory Tract Infections

Children with upper respiratory tract infections should also be considered separately from those who are well when assessing sedation risk. Unfortunately, during the winter months as many as 20% of the pediatric population may have some symptoms of a respiratory infection. There are few clear data to help us categorize the exact increase in risk associated with a current respiratory infection, but several studies have found an increase in airway and respiratory complications after anesthesia is given to patients who have significant cough and mucous production. Prudent practice would dictate that children who have a fever, or those with a significant cough with or without sputum production, are best off postponing an elective sedation. Likewise, children with wheezing or croup-like symptoms should not be given routine sedation.

Factors Relating to the Procedure

Duration of the Procedure

When choosing a sedation medication or technique, the provider should consider the amount of time that the procedure will require to be accomplished. It would seem ill-advised to give a sedative medication that lasts for several hours to a child who is having a procedure that only takes several minutes.

Pain as a Side Effect of a Procedure

Another important aspect of sedation that must be considered is the presence or absence of pain with a given procedure. Many of the sedatives that are commonly used for sedation, such as chloral hydrate and the benzodiazepines, have no analgesic component. Adequate movement control is difficult to attain when these medications are employed for painful procedures. Other medications such as fentanyl will provide powerful pain control for procedures while not offering the same sedative potency. In general, analgesic medications should be included if the procedure is going to be painful while they may be omitted for nonpainful procedures.

Position Required for the Procedure

In planning the depth of sedation, each provider must consider the position that the patient will be in during the procedure. The average child will maintain an open airway in the supine position even when deeply sedated as long as the neck can be slightly extended and jaw lifted slightly forward. If the head must be flexed during a procedure or a scan, obstruction of the airway will be much more likely and care should be taken to avoid deep sedation unless the provider is ready to provide positive-pressure ventilation. In general, when children are placed on their side or in a prone position, the airway is at least as easy to maintain—or easier—than when in the supine position.

Anxiety/Stress/Inability to Cooperate as a Side Effect of the Procedure

Sedation may be required for procedures that are not particularly painful and do not require a great deal of movement control. There are several procedures that are particularly emotionally stressful (such as bladder catheterization required for a voiding cystourethrogram) where a brief period of unconsciousness will allow the patient to avoid an emotionally harmful experience. Often these procedures involve invasion or examination of the genitalia (sexual abuse evaluations); the same amount of discomfort involving an extremity would be trivial.

Factors Related to Person(s) Delivering Sedation

Dedicated Sedation Monitor

The use of moderate or deep sedation shall include provision of a person, in addition to the provider, whose responsibility is to monitor appropriate physiologic parameters and to assist in any supportive or resuscitation measures, as required. It is strongly encouraged that this individual be trained in pediatric basic life support. The support person should have specific assignments in the event of an emergency, and thus current knowledge of the emergency cart inventory (1).

Skills Related to Depth of Sedation

Prior to sedating a child or to writing sedation protocols, an honest appraisal of the expertise of the sedation provider must be made. As stated above, the JCAHO has recommended that the provider must have the skills necessary to "rescue" a patient from the consequences of sedation one level "deeper" than that which is intended. Following this logic, if a sedation provider desires moderate sedation for a pediatric patient, she should be readily able to perform bag-mask ventilation and ultimately to perform endotracheal intubation. She should understand how to quickly and effectively suction the airway and provide intravenous access in an expeditious manner.

BACKUP SYSTEMS AND ABILITY TO RESCUE

As important as any provider-related issue is the availability of a highly trained and reliable backup system. Studies of sedation-related critical events have shown that sedation accidents are clearly most common in venues where a good backup or rescue system is not available (4,5). The depth of sedation that is sought for any procedure should take this factor into account. A protocol for accessing the backup help for sedation critical events (most often the "code" team) should be clearly laid out and tested on a regular basis.

EQUIPMENT NEEDS FOR SEDATION

Before undertaking sedation of a pediatric patient there are some key pieces of equipment that must be in place, regardless of the desired depth of sedation that is intended. A mnemonic that is useful to remember the equipment needs is **SOBA MDI** (suction oxygen bag-mask airways monitors drugs IV-access). We prefer to have the sedation providers think in terms of categories of equipment that are crucial.

Suction

Suction apparatus must be available during any pediatric sedation. Suctioning comes in handy as a way to clear the airway of secretions that can inhibit spontaneous ventilation and cause coughing and desaturation. The best general-purpose option is an appropriately sized Yankhaur suction device that will readily suction food material and secretions from the upper airway.

Oxygen

In cases where deep sedation or anesthesia is to be induced (and oxygen delivery is critical), a second "backup" source of oxygen is helpful in case the institutional supply fails. Most often this would take the form of an "E"-sized cylinder of oxygen with an oxygen flow meter attached.

Bag and Mask

A bag and mask for positive-pressure ventilation must be present for any pediatric sedation. This may take the form of an "anesthesia" bag or self-inflating bag. If the anesthesia bag is to be used, the provider must understand how to adjust the flow rates and valves to allow good positive-pressure ventilation (PPV). Likewise, the provider should be familiar with the self-inflating bags that are often supplied with pop-off valves that may need to be closed for positive-pressure ventilation. The exact arrangement of the "tail" on this bag that allows for high inspired fraction of oxygen should also be reviewed. A variety of different-sized masks should be available. Bag-mask ventilation should be practiced (and proficiency should be documented) with the type of bag and mask that is available at the site of the sedation.

Airways

Because PPV is made much easier in infants and children when an appropriate oral airway is in place, a variety of sizes of oral airways should be present to assist with ventilation.

Monitoring Devices

The current AAP guidelines do not specifically require a particular set of monitors. They do state, however, that "vital signs, including oxygen saturation and heart rate, must be documented at least every 5 minutes in a time-based record." The most commonly used array of monitors for sedation includes pulse oximetry, electrocardiogram, and noninvasive blood pressure monitoring. Recently, the use of ventilation monitoring in sedation has become generally accepted and is highly recommended in the latest version of the AAP Sedation Guidelines.

Pulse Oximetry

Pulse oximetry monitors work by comparing the relative amounts of oxygenated versus deoxygenated hemoglobin in the pulsing blood of an extremity or digit. This is accomplished by analyzing the amount of light absorbed of different wavelengths that correspond with these different forms of hemoglobin. The readout of the pulse oximeter includes the percent saturation of hemoglobin with oxygen and the pulse rate.

Anything that obstructs arterial blood flow may disrupt sensing by the pulse oximeter. This technology will also not work when compounds such as dyes or unusual forms of hemoglobin confuse the calculation mentioned above.

Ventilation Monitors

Although the pulse oximeter yields information on oxygen saturation, it does not give the status the patient's ventilation, or exchange of CO_2. Although these two physiologic variables often go together (if your oxygen saturation is low you are probably not ventilating well), this is not always the case. In fact, a child may be apneic for 30 to 90 seconds (depending on size) before the oxygen saturation changes. The AAP guidelines on sedation are clear on this point. "The use of a precordial stethoscope or capnograph to aid in monitoring adequacy of ventilation is encouraged."

Precordial stethoscopes are placed over the chest or trachea so that the provider can listen to air movement and detect partial obstruction or complete apnea. They are accurate and inexpensive, although (depending on the procedure to be performed) they may not be particularly convenient to use.

Capnography refers to measuring the CO_2 level expired by a patient and processing that data graphically. These units are available from a variety of manufacturers and most use a "side stream" detection technique in which a small amount of gas is continuously sampled from the nasal cannula or inside of the mask that the patient is breathing. The monitor then measures the level of CO_2 in the gas and graphically displays the CO_2 content.

The capnograph can be used to confirm air exchange with each breath. Apnea can be detected as soon as it occurs. The absolute accuracy of the CO_2 level detected will vary with the monitor used, type of oxygen delivery device, and oxygen flow rates used; therefore it cannot be considered completely reliable (Fig. 135.2).

Plethysmography, or the measure of chest wall movement, has also been used as a respiratory monitor. Unfortunately this monitor will not detect the situation where the airway is obstructed and no air exchange is taking place but the chest wall is moving. Because airway obstruction is a major risk during sedation, this monitor is considered somewhat insensitive during sedation.

ECG and Blood Pressure

The standard monitors for sedation include an ECG, pulse oximeter, and noninvasive blood pressure monitors. The ECG gives information on the heart rhythm and rate, and can be used to confirm the accuracy of the pulse oximeter in that it

A normal capnogram

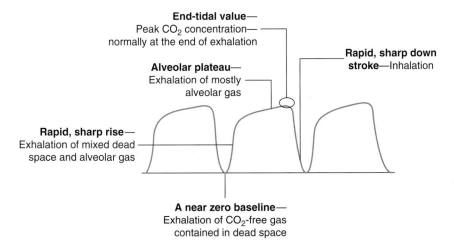

End-tidal value—
Peak CO_2 concentration—
normally at the end of exhalation

Rapid, sharp down
stroke—Inhalation

Alveolar plateau—
Exhalation of mostly
alveolar gas

Rapid, sharp rise—
Exhalation of mixed dead
space and alveolar gas

A near zero baseline—
Exhalation of CO_2-free gas
contained in dead space

FIGURE 135.2. Key aspects of the capnogram.

can confirm the accuracy of the pulse rate. Blood pressure monitoring is most helpful for deep sedation.

OVERVIEW OF DRUGS USED FOR SEDATION

Hypnotic Medications (Sedatives)

Oral Chloral Hydrate

Chloral hydrate is a halogenated hydrocarbon that has been used for sedation of pediatric patients during painless procedures for many years. The usual dose is 20 to 75 mg/kg orally. The drug has a bitter taste that may not be tolerated by all children (rectal administration is also effective). Most practitioners limit the dose to 100 mg/kg or a total dose of 2 g (6). The peak effect may take as long as 60 minutes and the plasma half-life is 4 to 9 hours. The drug can result in prolonged sedation, particularly in infants, with peak effect occurring well after the intended time of desired sedation(7,8). One of the main advantages of chloral hydrate is its lack of associated respiratory depression (9). Although rare, the potential for respiratory depression does exist, however, and is most marked when the drug is combined with opioids or other sedatives. Deaths have been reported with doses of chloral hydrate in the recommended range; thus adherence to the sedation guidelines mentioned above, as well as monitoring during the procedure and recovery period, is imperative (7).

The use of chloral hydrate for procedural pain is limited by the fact that it lacks analgesic properties, and the behavioral effects with stimulation can be highly variable at moderate doses (hyperactivity and agitation is not unusual).

Recommended Use. Chloral hydrate is well established as an agent for sedation in painless procedures such as diagnostic radiology; its usefulness in painful procedures is limited by patient movement and agitation even when sedated, especially in the young (less than 1 year old) child. The long half-life indicates a need for prolonged supervision prior to discharge.

Rectal Chloral Hydrate

Because of its somewhat bitter taste, oral chloral hydrate is not tolerated by all patients. In these cases, the drug may be administered by the rectal route. Although data on this route of administration is not abundant, the recommended dosage and effectiveness of the drug is apparently not changed (50–100 mg/kg).

Recommended Use. Sedation for minimally painful procedures in toddlers who will not tolerate the oral medication.

Oral Midazolam

Midazolam is a short-acting, water-soluble benzodiazepine devoid of analgesic properties. The drug has become particularly popular because of its short duration, predictable onset, and lack of active metabolites. It is effective in eliminating the stress response largely by binding with gamma-aminobutyric acid (GABA) receptors to inhibit spinal afferent pathways. This results in skeletal muscle relaxation, amnesia, and anxiolysis (10). Although originally formulated for intravenous use, the same medication used orally has proven very successful in producing light sedation and amnesia (11,12). The recommended oral dose is 0.5 to 0.75 mg/kg, with onset of sedation in approximately 15 minutes, with a rapid offset approximately 30 minutes after the peak effect is noted. Midazolam is highly lipid soluble and redistributes rapidly. It is highly metabolized in the liver, undergoing a large first-pass effect, and has a beta elimination half-life of 106 ± 29 minutes. Allowing self-administration through a prefilled syringe in a

comforting environment (parent's arms) has met with the most success in these authors' experience. Respiratory depression is rare with oral administration of midazolam. As a general rule, this medication and mode of administration come the closest of any of the current sedatives available to providing true conscious sedation—providing a sedated yet arousable and cooperative patient at the indicated doses. One of the most desirable side effects is the anterograde and (less frequent) retrograde amnesia that is produced, although the extent of this effect will vary with the age of the patient and the dose employed. Slurred speech has been shown to coincide with the onset of anterograde amnesia (10).

Recommended Use. Oral midazolam is most useful as a sole agent for children who will drink liquid medication. Anxiolysis and cooperation are excellent for minor invasive procedures such as intravenous catheter placement.

Rectal Midazolam

Midazolam may be administered rectally at doses of 0.3 to 0.7 mg/kg. A dose of 0.3 mg/kg has been shown to give reliable levels of sedation with a mean time of 16 minutes to maximal blood level (13). After 30 minutes, blood levels were generally low but sedation and anxiolysis effects remained. Cautions and monitoring advised for other modes of midazolam delivery apply to this route of administration as well.

Nasal Midazolam

Midazolam may be given by the intranasal route at doses of 0.2 to 0.4 mg/kg (14). Onset time is intermediate between the oral and IV routes of administration (10–15 minutes). The effectiveness of this route of administration is well established as a premedicant for anesthesia, but its use is limited by burning on application to the nasal mucosa, which most children find very objectionable, as well as the bitter taste of midazolam reaching the oropharynx.

Recommended Use. For sedation and anxiolysis in young children who either refuse or cannot take an oral dose of midazolam.

Intramuscular Midazolam

Midazolam may be given as an intramuscular bolus of 0.08 mg/kg. Good sedation and cooperation scores were recorded at 15 minutes after this dose in one study (15). Persistent sedation was minimal 60 minutes after the dose.

Intravenous Midazolam

Intravenous midazolam is titrated to effect with fractionated doses of 0.05 to 0.10 mg/kg that may be repeated at intervals of 3 to 4 minutes to a total dose of 0.7 mg/kg. As opposed to the oral route of administration, intravenous midazolam reaches peak effect in 2 to 3 minutes and is redistributed more rapidly. Slow IV administration is recommended, with close observation for respiratory depression. When combined with intravenous opioids for painful procedures, midazolam has potent sedative effects and the use of cardiorespiratory monitoring is imperative. A maximum IV dose of 0.05 mg/kg has been recommended when combining the drug with narcotics. A constant infusion of the drug (0.05–0.20 mg/kg/hr) may be used particularly for ICU patients requiring prolonged sedation or anxiolysis (16).

Certain underlying conditions or medications may prolong the effects of midazolam. Heparin decreases protein binding and increases the free fraction. Hepatic metabolism is inhibited by cimetidine, which prolongs the elimination half-life. Patients in renal failure may have three times the free fraction of the drug secondary to decreased protein binding.

Recommended Use. IV midazolam is an excellent agent for sedation and anxiolysis in patients for minor procedures when an intravenous line is in place. It provides complementary sedation for patients receiving opioids for very painful procedures but extreme caution is warranted when combining the drugs.

Intravenous Pentobarbital

Pentobarbital is a barbiturate with a long history of successful use in the radiology venue to induce sleep for nonpainful procedures. As a barbiturate, pentobarbital has potent sedative hypnotic properties, but it has no analgesic properties. Onset of action is rapid—generally within 3 to 5 minutes. The effective dose ranges from 3 to 6 mg/kg for over 98% of patients (17). Highest success rates are reported when the drug is used for patients under 12 years old and 50 kg. The incidence of respiratory depression is less than 1% when pentobarbital is used as a sole agent at the recommended dosages (9). Failure to achieve sedation rates have been reported in 1.2% of patients when confined to this population. Paradoxical reactions occur in approximately 1% of patients. Prolonged sedation can occur, but is most common when the recommended dosage is exceeded.

Recommended Use. Pentobarbital is a good choice for young school-aged patients undergoing radiologic procedures not associated with pain.

Intravenous Propofol

Propofol is a 2,6-diisopropylphenol compound that has potent sedative and hypnotic properties. Because it is only slightly soluble in water, the drug is dissolved in a solution of soybean oil. The nature of this solution requires that the drug be handled in a sterile manner and used quickly once it is opened. Onset of action is extremely rapid, and induction of anesthesia may be achieved with 2 to 3 mg/kg in 95% of patients within 60 to 90 seconds. Sleep may be induced by as little as 1.5 mg/kg, and maintenance of sedation is usually accomplished through the use of an intravenous infusion at 50 to 150 µg/kg/min. Recovery from the drug is faster than with any other intravenous sedative (2- to 3-minute redistribution time), and the incidence of prolonged sedation or vomiting is extremely low. A dose-related decrease in blood pressure is noted that is similar to that found with other anesthetics (18). Propofol causes pain on injection; this may be prevented by administering a small dose of lidocaine (1 mg/kg) through the IV catheter prior to administration of the drug, or administering the drug through a fast-flowing intravenous line into a large vein such as an antecubital vein.

Because anesthesia, with its complete loss of airway reflexes, respiratory depression, and cardiovascular depression, can be induced rapidly with propofol (19), some hospitals limit its use to anesthesia personnel. The role of this drug in the ICU and emergency department remains to be defined—clearly only individuals skilled in airway management should be administering the drug (20–22). Unexplained metabolic acidosis and cardiac failure have occurred in some patients on long-term propofol infusions in the ICU (23).

Recommended Use. Propofol is an ideal agent for brief periods of deep sedation. Minimal nausea/vomiting and rapid awakening are unique among currently available agents. Extreme caution is advised in using this drug as general anesthesia is induced rapidly.

Intravenous Dexmedetomidine

Dexmedetomidine has been used for several years by adult anesthesiologists and intensivists for sedation and anesthesia. The characteristics of this drug are remarkable for its production of a smooth sedated state with good analgesia and little decrease in respiratory drive. This drug is an α2-agonist with a short half-life that is generally given in a bolus (0.5 to 1 µg/kg over 10 minutes) followed by constant infusion (0.5 to 1 µg/kg/hr) (24,25). In the last year, reports of its use in pediatric sedation by non-anesthesiologists are starting to emerge, and the growth of its use appears to be exponential. Effective use of dexmedetomidine has been reported for sedation of children on ventilators in the pediatric intensive-care unit and as a sedative for invasive procedures (25). Reports of the effectiveness of this drug in noninvasive procedures have also appeared (26). Caution is warranted, as there is a possibility of decreased blood pressure and bradycardia with this drug; but the incidence of these side effects seems to be relatively infrequent in children.

Recommended Use. Although the total reports of the use of dexmedetomidine are still relatively few in number for any specific recommendations, the possibilities for its use are exciting. Just as enticing is the possibility of its use for procedural sedation either alone or in combination with some the agents we now employ.

Analgesic Medications

Sucrose Pacifier

Before the advent of modern pediatric anesthesia, sugar-dipped pacifiers or "whiskey nipples" were used in conjunction with restraints for surgical operation such as pyloromyotomy in neonates. A recent study evaluated sterile water and three different concentrations of sucrose in infants 1 to 6 days of age prior to undergoing heel prick sampling (27). There was a significant reduction in crying time with the use of this maneuver, with a greater reduction in those infants who received the highest concentration of sucrose.

Oral Transmucosal Fentanyl Citrate (OTFC)

Fentanyl is a powerful synthetic opioid, which is 100 times more potent than morphine. It has a very high degree of fat solubility that allows for very rapid penetration of the blood–brain barrier (7). The sedation effects are relatively brief, as the offset of the drug is dependent on redistribution rather than elimination. Oral transmucosal fentanyl (OTFC) is available as a sweetened lozenge on a plastic stick of various strengths (200 µg and 400 µg). The recommended dosage is 15 to 20 µg/kg orally (28). Generally there is excellent and rapid uptake of the drug from the oral mucosa, although the effectiveness of a given dose varies with how much of the drug is swallowed by the patient rather than allowed to absorb transmucosally. Sedation reliably occurs within 15 to 30 minutes (29). Pruritus occurs in 44%. Nausea and vomiting occurs in approximately 15% to 50% of patients and is not prevented by the administration of antiemetics (30). Respiratory depression with oxygen desaturation to less than 90% has been reported in 5% of children but usually resolves with verbal prompting (31).

Recommended Use. OTFC offers a painless method of delivering opioid, which may be of particular use in patients without an intravenous line undergoing painful procedures. Associated nausea and vomiting, and the need for more intensive monitoring and observation than with other oral sedatives, have limited its popularity to date. The use of pulse oximetry is mandatory in these patients even when they appear awake and alert.

Intravenous Fentanyl

As mentioned above, fentanyl is a very potent synthetic opioid. The IV dose recommendation is 0.5 to 1 µg/kg/dose, titrated to a total dose of 4 to 5 µg/kg. Fentanyl as a sole agent offers excellent pain relief with mild sedation at these doses.

Maximal effect occurs within 5 minutes when administered intravenously. Opioid effects last for 30 to 40 minutes.

Strict adherence to monitoring standards is mandatory. Chest wall rigidity may occur with intravenous fentanyl dosing and is particularly problematic when the drug is rapidly administered (32). Respiratory depression is *markedly* increased when the drug is combined with midazolam or other sedative, and increased vigilance for possible airway management requirements should be made when the drugs are administered together (33).

Bradycardia may occur from stimulation of the central vagal nucleus and prolongs both the atrioventricular node conduction and refractory period. In spite of this, fentanyl has the fewest hemodynamic effects of any opioid. The adverse effects of the drug are reversed by naloxone, which should be readily available when this drug is administered. Metabolism may be prolonged in neonates and patients with hepatic dysfunction, but children older than 6 months are actually less likely than adults to suffer respiratory depression at equivalent doses (34).

Recommended Use. Intravenous fentanyl offers excellent analgesia and mild sedation with a short duration of action, ideal for very painful procedures in children with an IV in place. Careful respiratory and cardiac monitoring is mandatory, especially when the drug is combined with other sedatives.

Oral Ketamine

Ketamine is a unique medication of the phencyclidine class that binds to opioid receptors and possesses intense analgesic, sedative, and amnestic qualities. It has a long track record of safety as a sedative for painful procedures in children, particularly those undergoing burn debridement or tubbing (35,36). The oral dose recommendation is 5 to 6 mg/kg. Onset of sedation occurs in 15 to 30 minutes and effects may be prolonged with this route, lasting 3 to 4 hours. A functional dissociation is created between the cortical and limbic systems of the brain. Spontaneous respirations and airway reflexes are maintained. The eyes remain open, with a slow nystagmic gaze and intact corneal and light reflexes. Patients may exhibit random tonic movements of the extremities that make this drug inappropriate for procedures where the patient must lie perfectly still (e.g., CT and MRI scans). Ketamine generally causes an increase in heart rate, blood pressure, cardiac output, and intracranial pressure. The drug should be used with caution (or not at all) in patients with suspected increased intracranial pressure or open globe injuries. Oral secretions are mildly increased with oral ketamine, although administration of an antisialagogue is rarely required. This drug also has bronchodilator qualities. Ketamine causes hyperactive airway reflexes, with a risk of laryngospasm. Prolonged emergence may occur, but postsedation emesis and dysphoria are rare with oral ketamine (37).

Recommended Use. Oral ketamine provides excellent analgesia, amnesia, and sedation for painful procedures. Oral dosing is much less reliable and has less favorable kinetics when compared to other routes of administration. Nausea and vomiting are bothersome but infrequent.

Intramuscular Ketamine

Intramuscular ketamine reaches peak blood levels and clinical effect in 5 minutes after a 3- to 10-mg/kg IM injection. Recovery from dissociation occurs within 15 to 30 minutes, with coherence and purposeful neuromuscular activity returning in 30 to 120 minutes. The elimination half-life is 1 to 2 hours in children. Elimination may be prolonged when the drug is administered with other medications that undergo hepatic metabolism. The 100-mg/mL formulation of ketamine is preferred for IM administration in older children to minimize volume-related injection site discomfort. Because of associated salivary and tracheobronchial secretions, most authors recommend administering a concurrent anticholinergic if the larger doses of ketamine are administered. The anticholinergic may best be added directly to the syringe with ketamine. Antisialagogues are not necessary if ketamine 3 mg/kg is employed intramuscularly.

Experience with intramuscular ketamine is extensive. Sedation is accompanied by the same excellent analgesia as mentioned above for IV and oral administration. Cautions concerning increased intracranial pressure, airway protection, dysphoria, and vomiting apply with IM administration, as mentioned above (38).

Recommended Use. IM administration of ketamine is an excellent means of sedating the "out-of-control" patient for IV placement or moderately painful procedure. A dose of 3 mg/kg is usually all that is required if the procedure is brief.

Intravenous Ketamine

Ketamine may be given in small IV doses of 0.05 to 1 mg/kg. Peak concentrations occur within 1 minute, and rapid absorption by the highly perfused cerebral tissue allows almost immediate induction of clinical effects. Ketamine then slowly redistributes into the peripheral tissues; this decrease in CNS levels correlates with return of coherence, generally averaging 15 minutes if no additional doses are given (39). Deep levels of sedation are achieved and maintained—"conscious sedation" is not possible with ketamine. Remarkably, painful procedures are tolerated well following administration of ketamine because of its profound analgesic properties as well as the sedation it affords.

Intravenous ketamine has been shown to be effective in accomplishing a multitude of minor procedures (36,40–43). The relatively short action of the IV form of the drug allows this drug to be used in small doses (0.05–0.1 mg/kg) in the ambulatory pediatric patient without delaying discharge. Because of higher blood levels with intravenous use, ketamine administered by this route may have more problems than oral or intramuscular administration. Oral secretions may be avoided by the administration of an antisialagogue (atropine 0.01 mg/kg or glycopyrrolate 0.005 mg/kg IV). Increases in intracranial pressure, heart rate, and blood pressure may be concerning. Although patients will continue to breathe and maintain airway tone, silent pulmonary aspiration of oral contents has been reported with deep levels of sedation. Patients may continue to move during sedation and eyes remain open.

Recommended Use. Ideal for painful procedures such as burn debridement, foreign body removal, abscess incision, and orthopedic procedures. More often administered intravenously to hospitalized patients rather than ambulatory patients.

Nitrous Oxide

Nitrous oxide (N_2O) is a colorless, odorless gas that has both analgesic and anxiolytic effects. The drug must be delivered with oxygen to avoid a hypoxic gas mixture. This may be accomplished though the use of flow meters from separate sources or through the delivery of a fixed 50% mixture of N_2O/oxygen (Entonox). The drug may be delivered alone at concentrations of 30% to 50% for moderately painful procedures or in combination with a mild sedative at lower concentrations for similar effect (44). Onset of sedation and analgesia occurs in minutes, and is terminated rapidly when the gas is discontinued. Nitrous oxide has minimal cardiovascular and respiratory effects when not combined with a potent sedative or opioid. Studies in large groups of patients (some with mild IV sedation) have failed to show any significant risk of

TABLE 135.3

SEDATION REGIMENS

Propofol	50–200 µg/kg/min IV	Ideal agent for nonpainful diagnostic procedures. Only for use by expert airway managers with good backup systems.
Pentobarbital	3–6 mg/kg IV or PO	Long history of effective use in radiology imaging. Emergence can be prolonged.
Midazolam	0.5–0.75 mg/kg PO 0.025–0.5 mg/kg IV 0.2 mg/kg intranasal	Track record of safe use both PO and IV. Paradoxical reactions are not infrequent. Intranasal route is so irritating we do not recommend it.
Chloral hydrate	50–100mg/kg PO	Still the most popular agent for radiologic sedation in community hospitals. Prolonged sedation and paradoxical reactions are reported. Monitoring required (45–47).
Dexmedetomidine	0.5–1.0 µg/kg bolus (over 10 min) followed by 1 µg/kg/hr infusion	There are only emerging data at this point on usage of this agent for procedural sedation. Respirations are maintained but hypotension and bradycardia have been reported.
Propofol with fentanyl	Fentanyl 1–2 µg/kg IV with propofol 50–150 µg/kg IV	Best for deep sedation/anesthesia–risk of requiring advanced airway management is high (48).
Midazolam with fentanyl	Midazolam 0.020 mg/kg IV with fentanyl 1–2 µg/kg IV	Most common combination for painful procedures in the emergency department—risk of apnea and hypoxia is significant (49,50).
Ketamine	3–4 mg/kg IM 1–2 mg/kg IV	Effective sedation and analgesia for painful procedures. Relatively common nausea and vomiting postprocedure. Laryngospasm reported (36,51,52). Best if combined with an anticholinergic for control of secretions. Combination with midazolam is common although effectiveness in treating emergence dysphoria is debated.

cardiopulmonary depression when nitrous oxide is used at the concentrations cited here.

Recommended Use. Nitrous oxide is useful for brief painful procedures and may be combined with a mild sedative. Expensive equipment and ventilation apparatus required for delivery will limit its widespread use.

Reversal Agents

Specific reversal agents exist for benzodiazepines and opioids. Sedation providers must understand their use in order to responsibly utilize either of these classes of agents.

Flumazenil

Flumazenil can be used to reverse the effects of benzodiazepines and should be immediately available when using benzodiazepines for sedation. A dose of 0.01 mg/kg may be repeated 4 times as needed. Although rare, resedation may occur, and additional doses of flumazenil may be required. Careful observation for this resedation should be maintained for at least an hour following the administration of flumazenil.

Naloxone

Naloxone (Narcan) is an opioid antagonist and can be given intravenously, intramuscularly, or subcutaneously; but the preferred route of administration is intravenous. The drug should be given in a slowly titrated manner when possible.

The standard preparation contains 0.4 mg/mL of naloxone. The neonatal preparation, which contains 0.02 mg/kg, is not recommended. The dose for children is 0.1 mg/kg for children under 20 kg. The dose for children over 20 kg is 2 mg. See Table 135.3.

DISCHARGE

Appropriate discharge guidelines are a key element of safe sedation practice.

Recovery Area and Equipment

Recovery should take place in a well-lit area that is not too removed from the sedation site itself. The recovery area should be equipped with suction, oxygen, and equipment for positive-pressure ventilation. Monitoring equipment including pulse oximetry, ECG, blood pressure, and ventilation monitoring should be available as well. A record of vital signs should be kept at regular intervals until the child is awake and interactive.

Discharge Criteria

Patients should be discharged only when they have met specific criteria; this should be consistent regardless of the procedure that was performed or the drugs that were used for sedation. The criteria for discharge should include (1) stable vital signs, (2) pain under control, (3) a return to the level of consciousness that is similar to the baseline for that patient, (4) adequate head control and muscle strength to maintain a patent airway, (5) control of nausea and/or vomiting, and (6) adequate hydration. It should be noted that even when these criteria are used, children have been found to be discharged with residual sedation effects (53). It is imperative that providers in charge of discharge are extremely cautious and use some objective criteria to indicate readiness to leave the hospital.

Of particular note are those children who have received large doses of long-acting sedative medications. When significant effort must be made to wake these children up post-sedation (shouting or shaking), it should be noted that they will often become resedated if left alone for a period of time (riding in the car). These children are not safe for discharge. Obstruction of the airway while in a car seat has been described in children who have experienced exactly this scenario.

Similarly, children who have had their sedation reversed with flumazenil or naloxone should be observed for an extended period of time due to the fact that resedation can occur as the reversal agent wears off and the sedative agent still has a therapeutic blood level.

Discharge Documentation

At the time of discharge the status of the child should be documented and the time of discharge should be recorded. Specific instructions should be given to the family of the child instructing them what to do if the child should appear sedated or have any other medical problems in the time immediately following discharge.

FINAL COMMENTS

Painful procedures cause not only pain, but fear in pediatric patients. This occurs prior to the anticipated procedure as well as during the procedure. It is always important to maximize the intervention for the first procedure, so that anticipatory anxiety does not increase with each procedure. Whether to add pharmacologic intervention to the psychologic and behavioral tools employed for every patient should be determined by the level of anxiety and context of the procedure. Parental education is always valuable, and parental presence is frequently an aide to the child's coping and ability to cooperate.

Psychologic intervention and local anesthesia may be sufficient for pain control and enhancing the child's mastery and feelings of self-esteem. However, if the procedure is expected to be very painful, prolonged, or repeated, pharmacologic adjuncts should be considered. The goals of procedure-related pain management are to make the procedure as nonthreatening and comfortable as safely possible.

References

1. Joint Commission on Accreditation of Healthcare Organizations. Sedation and anesthesia care standards. Oakbrook Terrace, IL: JCAHO; 2003.
2. Roback MG, Bajaj L, Wathen JE, et al. Preprocedural fasting and adverse events in procedural sedation and analgesia in a pediatric emergency department: are they related? *Ann Emerg Med* 2004;44:454–459.
3. American Academy of Pediatrics Committee on Drugs. Guidelines for monitoring and management of pediatric patients during and after sedation for diagnostic and therapeutic procedures. *Pediatrics* 1992;89:1110–1115.
4. Cote C, Notterman D, Karl H, et al. Adverse sedation events in pediatrics: a critical incident analysis of contributing factors. *Pediatrics* 2000;105:805–814.
5. Cote CJ, Karl HW, Notterman DA, et al. Adverse sedation events in pediatrics: analysis of medications used for sedation. *Pediatrics* 2000;106:633–644.
6. Greenberg S, Faerber E, Aspinall C. High dose chloral hydrate sedation for children undergoing CT. *J Comput Assist Tomogr* 1991;15:467–469.
7. Cote CJ. Sedation for the pediatric patient. A review. *Pediatr Clin North Am* 1994;41:31–58.
8. Malviya S, Voepel-Lewis T, Prochaska G, et al. Prolonged recovery and delayed side effects of sedation for diagnostic imaging studies in children. *Pediatrics* 2000;105:E42.
9. Sanborn P, Michna E, Zurakowski D, et al. Adverse cardiovascular and respiratory events during sedation of pediatric patients for imaging examinations. *Radiology* 2005;237:288–294.
10. Kain Z, Hofstadter M, Mayes L, et al. Midazolam: effects on amnesia and anxiety in children. *Anesthesiology* 2000;93:676–684.
11. McMillan C, Spahr-Schopfer I, Sikech N. Premedication of children with oral midazolam. *Can J Anaesth* 1992;39:545.
12. Malinovsky J-M, Populaire C, Cozian A. Premedication with midazolam in children. Effect of intranasal, rectal, and oral routes on plasma midazolam concentrations. *Anaesthesia* 1995;50:351.
13. Saint-Maurice C, Meistelman C, Rey E, et al. The pharmacokinetics of rectal midazolam for premedication in children. *Anesthesiology* 1986;65:536.
14. Harcke H, Grissom L, Meister M. Sedation in pediatric imaging using intranasal midazolam. *Pediatr Radiol* 1995;25:341–343.
15. Rita L, Frank L, Mazurek A, et al. Intramuscular midazolam for pediatric preanesthetic sedation: a double blind controlled study with morphine. *Anesthesiology* 1985;63:528.
16. Alexander E, Carnevale FA, Razack S. Evaluation of a sedation protocol for intubated critically ill children. *Intens Crit Care Nurs* 2002;18:292–301.
17. Greenberg S, Adams R, Aspinall C. Initial experience with intravenous pentobarbital sedation for children undergoing MRI at a tertiary care pediatric hospital: the learning curve. *Pediatr Radiol* 2000;30:689–691.
18. Hertzog JH, Campbell JK, Dalton HJ, et al. Propofol anesthesia for invasive procedures in ambulatory and hospitalized children: experience in the pediatric intensive care unit. *Pediatrics* 1999;103:E30.
19. Gottschling S, Meyer S, Krenn T, et al. Propofol versus midazolam/ketamine for procedural sedation in pediatric oncology. *J Pediatr Hematol Oncol* 2005;27:471–476.
20. Guenther E, Pribble CG, Junkins EP Jr., et al. Propofol sedation by emergency physicians for elective pediatric outpatient procedures. *Ann Emerg Med* 2003;42:783–791.
21. Bassett KE, Anderson JL, Pribble CG, et al. Propofol for procedural sedation in children in the emergency department. *Ann Emerg Med* 2003;42:773–782.
22. Barbi E GT, Marchetti F, Neri E, et al. Deep sedation with propofol by nonanesthesiologists: a prospective pediatric experience. *Arch Pediatr Adolesc Med* 2003;157:1097–1103.
23. Cray SH, Robinson BH, Cox PN. Lactic acidemia and bradyarhythmia in a child sedated with propofol. *Crit Care Med* 1998;26:2087–2092.
24. Tobias JD, Berkenbosch JW, Russo P. Additional experience with dexmedetomidine in pediatric patients. *South Med J* 2003;96:871–875.
25. Tobias J, Berkenbosch J. Initial experience with dexmedetomidine in paediatric-aged patients. *Paediatr Anaesth* 2002;12:171–175.
26. Berkenbosch J, Wankum P, Tobias J. Prospective evaluation of dexmedetomidine for noninvasive procedural sedation in children. *Pediatr Crit Care Med* 2005;6:435–439. Quiz 440. See comment.
27. Haouari N, Wood C, Griffiths G, et al. The analgesic effect of sucrose in full term infants: a randomized, controlled trial. *BMJ* 1995;310:1498.
28. Schechter N, Weisman S, Rosenblum M, et al. The use of oral transmucosal fentanyl citrate for painful procedures in children. *Pediatrics* 1995;95:335–339.
29. Nelson P, Streisand J, Mulder S, et al. Comparison of oral transmucosal fentanyl citrate and an oral solution of meperidine, diazepam and atropine for premedication in children. *Anesthesiology* 1989;70:616.
30. Epstein RH, Mendel HG, Witkowski TA, et al. The safety and efficacy of oral transmucosal fentanyl citrate for preoperative sedation in young children. *Anesth Analg* 1996;83:1200–1205.
31. Ashburn M, Streisand J. Oral transmucosal fentanyl: help or hindrance? *Druf Saf* 1994;11:295.
32. Scamman F. Fentanyl-O_2-N_2O rigidity and pulmonary compliance. *Anesth Analg* 1983;62:332–334.
33. Kennedy RM, Porter FL, Miller JP, et al. Comparison of fentanyl/midazolam with ketamine/midazolam for pediatric orthopedic emergencies. *Pediatrics* 1998;102:956–963.
34. Koehntop D, Rodman J, Brundage D, et al. Pharmacokinetics of fentanyl in neonates. *Anesth Analg* 1986;65:227–229.
35. Green SM, Nakamura R, Johnson NE. Ketamine sedation for pediatric procedures: part 1, a prospective series. *Ann Emerg Med* 1990;19:1024–1032.
36. Green SM, Denmark TK, Cline J, et al. Ketamine sedation for pediatric critical care procedures. *Pediatr Emerg Care* 2001;17:244–248.
37. Gutstein J, Johnson K, Heard M, et al. Oral ketamine preanesthetic medication in children. *Anesthesiology* 1992;76:28.
38. Green S, Rothrock S, Lynch E, et al. Intramuscular ketamine for pediatric sedation in the emergency department: safety profile in 1,022 cases. *Ann Emerg Med* 1998;31:688–697.
39. Clements J, Nimmo W. Pharmacokinetics and analgesic effect of ketamine in man. *Fr J Anaesth* 1981;53:27.

40. Slonim AD, Ognibene FP. Sedation for pediatric procedures, using ketamine and midazolam, in a primarily adult intensive care unit: a retrospective evaluation. *Crit Care Med* 1998;26:1900–1904.

41. Luhmann JD, Kennedy RM, McAllister JD, et al. Sedation for peritonsillar abscess drainage in the pediatric emergency department. *Pediatr Emerg Care* 2002;18:1–3.

42. Ng KC, Ang SY. Sedation with ketamine for paediatric procedures in the emergency department—a review of 500 cases. *Singapore Med J* 2002;43: 300–304.

43. Mason KP, Michna E, DiNardo JA, et al. Evolution of a protocol for ketamine-induced sedation as an alternative to general anesthesia for interventional radiologic procedures in pediatric patients. *Radiology* 2002;225:457–465.

44. Litman R, Kottra J, Verga K, et al. Chloral hydrate sedation: the additive sedative and respiratory depressant effects of nitrous oxide. *Anesth Analg* 1998;86:724–728. Comment.

45. Greenberg SB, Faerber EN, Aspinall CL, et al. High-dose chloral hydrate sedation for children undergoing MR imaging: safety and efficacy in relation to age. *AJR Am J Roentgenol* 1993;161:639–641.

46. Merola C, Albarracin C, Lebowitz P, et al. An audit of adverse events in children sedated with chloral hydrate or propofol during imaging studies. *Paediatr Anaesth* 1995;5:375–378.

47. Rooks VJ, Chung T, Connor L, et al. Comparison of oral pentobarbital sodium (Nembutal) and oral chloral hydrate for sedation of infants during radiologic imaging: preliminary results. *AJR Am J Roentgenol* 2003;180):1125–1128.

48. Bauman LA, Cannon ML, McCloskey J, et al. Unconscious sedation in children: a prospective multi-arm clinical trial. *Paediatr Anaesth* 2002;12: 674–679.

49. Kennedy R, Porter F, Miller J, et al. Comparison of fentanyl/midazolam with ketamine/midazolam for pediatric orthopedic emergencies. *Pediatrics* 1998;102:956–963.

50. Pitetti RD, Singh S, Pierce MC. Safe and efficacious use of procedural sedation and analgesia by nonanesthesiologists in a pediatric emergency department. *Arch Pediatr Adolesc Med* 2003;157:1090–1096.

51. Dachs RJ, Innes GM. Intravenous ketamine sedation of pediatric patients in the emergency department. *Ann Emerg Med* 1997;29:146–150.

52. Kim G, Green SM, Denmark TK, et al. Ventilatory response during dissociative sedation in children-a pilot study. *Acad Emerg Med* 2003;10: 140–145.

53. Malviya S, Voepel-Lewis T, Ludomirsky A, et al. Can we improve the assessment of discharge readiness? A comparative study of observational and objective measures of depth of sedation in children. *Anesthesiology* 2004;100:218–224.

CHAPTER 136 ■ IN-HOSPITAL EVALUATION

ELAINE S. CABINUM-FOELLER

Child abuse and neglect are not uncommon, and most medical providers who see children encounter anywhere from several to many cases during a career. Child abuse is defined by federal legislation that provides minimum guidelines for states to incorporate into their criminal and civil statues. Subsequently, each state in the United States has a working legal definition of child abuse and neglect. The medical practitioner who deals with children should be aware of the specifics of those definitions for his or her state.

The true incidence of child abuse is not known because the history often is lacking and many cases are never diagnosed. This is one of the few clinical situations in medicine where history often is falsified or not known. The latest statistics from the National Child Abuse and Neglect Data System (calendar year 2004) show that 872,000 U.S. children were substantiated as victims of child abuse and neglect in cases investigated by Child Protective Services (CPS). CPS is the branch of public social services that investigates reports of child abuse and neglect where caretakers are involved as possible perpetrators. Law enforcement is involved in many of these cases, but also has primary responsibility for investigating cases where strangers and noncaretakers are the alleged perpetrators.

There are four basic types of child maltreatment—physical abuse, sexual abuse, emotional abuse, and child neglect. Child neglect is the main form of child maltreatment investigated by CPS and is failure to provide for a child's basic needs. This can include physical, emotional, medical, supervisional, and educational neglect. Each state has different definitions that help CPS to determine if a given situation meets the standard for neglect. CPS has to investigate any reported child maltreatment and then provide support services to the family if indicated.

Physical abuse and sexual abuse probably are the most common types of child maltreatment seen in hospitalized children, although neglect can be seen with some children with failure to thrive. The medical provider in the hospital setting has the responsibility of recognizing clues to abuse or neglect and reporting to appropriate agencies. Depending on services available in the hospital or community, the provider may be the physician performing the medical portion of the child abuse assessment, or referral to a specialized child abuse team may be appropriate. Medical providers must be very familiar with their state's reporting laws covering child maltreatment. All states list health care workers as mandated reporters of child maltreatment. To report a case to CPS, the provider need only have a suspicion that maltreatment or neglect has occurred, not proof. CPS is given the job of investigating any report when the agency believes the report meets a minimal standard of likelihood. All states mandate reporting without risk of liability if the report is made without malicious intent. A medical provider can *incur liability for failing to report* a case of suspected child maltreatment. It is important to emphasize to parents (or other caretakers) that reporting is not an accusation, but is a legal requirement based on the assessment to that point.

In calendar year 2004, the National Child Abuse and Neglect Data System estimated that almost 3 million reports of child abuse and neglect were made to social service agencies. Of these, CPS substantiated for 872,000 child victims. In that same year, approximately 1,490 children died from child abuse and neglect. Forty-five percent of the fatalities were children younger than 1 year of age, and 80% were children younger than 4 years of age. This underlines the importance of pediatric medical providers in recognizing child abuse/neglect and reporting appropriately when necessary.

The important factors to assess in possible abuse or neglect are the history, the child's developmental abilities, the complete physical examination findings, and the presence or absence of other risk factors. These risk factors include, but are not limited to, young age (<5 years), prior social service investigations, prior law enforcement involvement, substance abuse in the family, and domestic violence. It also is important to remember that *lack of risk factors does not rule out abuse*, and is not a reason to fail to report if suspect findings are present.

The most common injuries to present in the hospital are burns, bruises, and fractures. Although these injuries may be seen in the office, they at times require inpatient hospitalization, or are incidental findings in children hospitalized for other reasons.

BURNS

Burns occur when tissue is damaged by heat, chemicals, sunlight, electricity, or nuclear radiation. The history related to how burns occurred and how that correlates with the burn pattern is more important than the depth of burns. But in investigating burns, records must include specific details about pattern, location, and degree. Burns can be classified into first, second, third, and fourth degree based on the depth and severity of the burn.

First-degree burns are the most common and rarely require hospitalization. There is superficial tissue damage often characterized by painful erythema without blisters. These usually heal without scarring. An example would be common sunburn. Other than raising issues of possible neglect, this severity of burn usually is not related to abuse.

Second-degree burns are considered partial-thickness burns. They are characterized by clear fluid-filled blisters that are very painful and sensitive to temperature and air. The lesions often blanch with pressure. They usually heal within 1 to 2 weeks and sometimes scar.

Third-degree burns involve the full thickness of the skin. The injury is characterized by the finding of charring or translucent white tissue with mottling. Over time, the overlying tissues may develop a leathery, dry appearance. Underlying muscle and bone may be involved or destroyed. There is minimal pain in the charred tissue because the nerve endings have been damaged. There often is marked edema, and the color can vary from white to gray to red to black or charred. These burns always scar and often require excision and grafting.

Fourth-degree burns involve not only the skin, but also the underlying tissues and muscle. In child abuse, these can occur when a body (a child) is placed in an operating microwave oven. There are only a handful of case reports describing this in the literature, all involving infants. In such cases, the tissue injury often is worse than it appears because microwaves cook from the inside out. A child with this particular injury must be closely monitored for complications, preferably in a specialized burn unit.

Burns also can be classified as thermal, electrical, chemical, or radiation. The form most commonly seen in abuse are thermal burns. Electrical burns can be seen in children when electrical cords are chewed (corners of the mouth) or outlets explored (fingertips). Chemical burns are sometimes seen, and radiation burns are virtually never seen. Depending on the severity and location of burns, some children do need to be transferred to the nearest burn facility.

In evaluating burns in children, there are several factors to consider. These include the history, physical examination, the child's developmental level, and the presentation of the injury to medical care.

When obtaining a history, the clinician first investigates the reported mechanism for the burn. Did the child pick up a curling iron, spill hot water, or step into a campfire? This is vital to the evaluation of whether the injury is abusive. It is important to note in the medical record the reported history and who reported it. In abuse cases, the history of the injury sometimes changes over time or with different witnesses. This can sometimes occur with accidental injuries, but such inconsistencies should raise a red flag for possible abuse.

The examiner also should look at the child's developmental level—both reported and observed. The caretaker is asked what the child can do: sit? roll over? walk? run? pick up objects? The clinician should remember to observe whether details provided by the caretaker are similar to those observed in interactions with the child. In evaluating burns, the examiner must ask himself or herself such questions as: "Could that child have reached up and grabbed that cup of hot tea?" Is the history compatible with the child's developmental level? In some situations, scene visits can provide additional valuable information in investigating an injury. CPS or law enforcement agencies usually can provide this evaluation when necessary.

With possible child abuse, the physical examination is more than gathering information to assess the patient's injuries and provide care; it is a source of very valuable information about mechanisms of injury and possible abuse. What is the pattern of the burn injury—immersion, flow, or contact? Does this pattern match with the reported history? As an example, the stocking-and-glove distribution seen in immersion burns is fairly specific for nonaccidental injury. These have a clear line of demarcation between the burned and unburned skin that looks like a sock line. There often are no splash marks. This is indicative of the limb being held forcefully in hot water. A donut distribution on the buttock area also can be seen with immersion burns. This is seen when the child is held in hot water in a tub (or sink). The donut appearance of central sparing and peripheral burns is related to the surface (usually of the tub) protecting the central skin, and the fluid in contact with the periphery resulting in second-degree burns. Skin in contact with other skin (e.g., between buttocks, behind knees) also is spared. By noting the burn pattern, the position the child was in at the time of the burn often can be reproduced. As a protected area of the body, genital burns are

uncommon accidental injuries. They often are seen in abusive situations, especially those involving toileting accidents.

How the child presented to medical care is also important. Did the child receive what appears to be a second-degree burn 4 days ago and is just now coming for treatment? Who is bringing the child for treatment? In abuse situations, there often is a delay in seeking appropriate medical care.

In completing the physical examination, the provider should be alert to other signs of trauma or neglect, such as failure to thrive or other injuries and scars. The physical examination should be fully documented with diagrams and pictures, if possible. This can help with longitudinally following healing of the burn and can assist greatly with recall in court if needed.

Pearls

- The key question is whether the burn is *consistent* with the history provided by the caretaker or child.
- Impetigo sometimes is confused with cigarette burns. Impetigo is uniform in width and depth and does not scar.
- Remember that lack of social risk factors does not rule out abuse.
- The severity of the burn is a combination of temperature and contact time. For example, it take approximately 10 minutes to sustain a full-thickness burn when the water if 120°F. This decreases to 5 minutes at 122°F, 30 seconds at 130°F, 5 seconds at 140°F, and 2 seconds at 150°F.

BRUISES

A bruise is an area of skin discoloration caused by the escape of blood from ruptured underlying blood vessels after an injury. They are a common injury in children and often are accidental. However, bruises may be a sign of physical abuse. To evaluate whether a bruise is abusive or accidental, it is important again to look at the history, the child's developmental level, the pattern of the bruising, and other findings on physical examination.

In general, bruises are very difficult to age by appearance alone, especially in children. A yellow color to the bruise indicates that it is probably over 18 to 24 hours old. However, red, blue, purple, and brown can be seen at any time. The healing of bruises is affected by the area of skin involved, the depth of the bruise, the amount of blood in the bruise, and other factors. The history of the bruise is important—both from the caretaker and the child, if obtainable. When was the first time the bruise was noted? What is the reported mechanism—fall, play, sports? Does the mechanism of injury match the bruise seen? Could the child do what is reported?

In the physical examination, it is important to look at all areas of skin and document any injuries. The area of the body affected is important because some areas are more suspect for abuse than others. Soft areas of the body such as the back, buttocks, neck, cheek, ear, thighs, genitalia, and hands are atypical areas for accidental bruises. Grab marks sometimes are seen on the upper arms. Some bruises may appear patterned. Patterns of concern for abusive injury are looped cord marks, handprints, and other patterns that could be matched to an object such as a shoe, belt, or other implement. Bite marks often are seen on children. If the intercanine distance is greater than 3 cm, the bite was inflicted by a person with permanent teeth. In some cases, consultation with a forensic odontologist may be necessary and sometimes can confirm the inflictee.

The differential diagnosis for bruises is long. Mongolian spots often are confused with bruises. Mongolian spots do not fade or change over days to weeks. A repeat examination can make the diagnosis if there are questions. Minimal accidental

TABLE 136.1

FRACTURE PATTERNS AND CHILD ABUSE

Highly suspicious for inflicted injury	Somewhat suspicious for inflicted injury
Classic metaphyseal fractures— "corner/bucket handle"	Fractures of different ages
Sternal fracture	Multiple fractures
Posterior rib fractures	Digital fractures
Scapular fractures	Complex skull fractures
Spinous process fractures	Vertebral body fractures

trauma may result in dramatic bruises suggesting nonaccidental trauma in some medical problems such as idiopathic thrombocytopenic purpura, hemophilia, and vitamin K deficiency. In settings of inappropriate bruising, it sometimes is appropriate to obtain a complete blood count and coagulation studies such as prothrombin time (PT) or partial thromboplastin time (PTT). In some cases with a suspect family history, studies including von Willebrand factor, proteins induced by vitamin K antagonism (PIVKA-II), platelet function, platelet function activator (PFA-100), or others may be needed. In some instances, a hematologist may be able to help guide the workup. In some cultures, there are practices that can be confused with abusive bruising. Some of these are cupping and coining. These cultural practices are done with the intent of helping the child, and some report that it feels good.

As with burns, the key question remains, "Is this injury consistent with the history provided by the caretaker and is it consistent with the child's developmental abilities?" Several studies have looked at bruises in relation to development. Based on their research, Sugar and associates reported, "Those who cannot cruise don't bruise"(1). They found that those children who are not yet cruising (walking while holding onto furniture) do not have significant bruises on their bodies. There may be one or two isolated bruises over bony prominences (e.g., forehead, knee), but most of these children do not have bruises when examined. Bruises on the face and head necessitate a good history owing to the concern for physical abuse.

Pearls

- The key question is whether the bruise is *consistent* with the history and the child's developmental level.
- Bruises cannot be precisely aged by coloration alone.
- Lack of social risk factors does not rule out physical abuse.

FRACTURES

Fractures often are seen in physical abuse cases. They also are a common accidental childhood injury. As in the preceding cases, the clinician must ask, "Is the injury consistent with the history and developmental stage?"

Abusive fractures are more common in younger children (<4 years), often present without a history of trauma, and often are characterized by delay in seeking medical care. Any fracture can be the result of abuse. It is the history, physical examination, and additional evaluation that are crucial in differentiating accidental from inflicted trauma. In children younger than 2 and selectively in children younger than 5 years of age, a skeletal survey is in order to look for other injuries, some of which may be occult. The American College of Radiology has established and published standards for performing skeletal surveys.

Radiographically, some fractures are more suspect for abusive injury than others. Fractures that are highly specific for abusive injury in infants include the following: posterior rib fractures, scapular fractures, spinous process fractures, sternal fractures, and classic metaphyseal lesions. The classic metaphyseal lesions often are called *bucket handle* or *corner* fractures, and occur at the end of the long bones at the growth plate. Fractures with moderate specificity for abuse are complex skull fractures, digital fractures, vertebral body fractures, epiphyseal separations, fractures of different ages, and multiple fractures. Fractures common in childhood with low specificity for abuse are linear skull fractures, long bone fractures, and clavicular fractures. The appearance of subperiosteal new bone formation in infants also is common, but can be a normal variant. A pediatric radiologist may help with this evaluation when appropriate (Table 136.1).

When a fracture (or other injury) raises the suspicion of physical abuse, depending on the child's age, the workup usually should include a full skeletal survey. In some cases, a bone scan may be helpful in delineating questionable areas seen on the skeletal survey, or the skeletal survey can be repeated in 10 to 14 days. The American Academy of Pediatrics has published a policy statement on "Diagnostic Imaging of Child Abuse" with guidelines for radiologic workup of possible abuse cases (2).

Pearls

- Any fracture can be the result of abuse.
- The key question is whether the history provided contains the biomechanical forces necessary to cause the fracture in question.
- Skeletal surveys are widely available and quite helpful in evaluating young children with concerning fractures.
- The lack of social risk factors does not rule out physical abuse.

References

1. Sugar NF, Taylor JA, Feldman KW. Bruises in infants and toddlers: those who don't cruise rarely bruise. *Arch Pediatr Adolesc Med* 1999;153:399–403.
2. American Academy of Pediatrics, Section on Radiology. Diagnostic imaging of child abuse. *Pediatrics* 2000;105:1345–1348.

Suggested Readings

Carpenter RF. The prevalence and distribution of bruising in babies. *Arch Dis Child* 1999;80:363–366. Available at *http://www.aap.org*.
Kleinman PK. *Diagnostic imaging of child abuse.* 2nd ed. St. Louis: Mosby; 1998.
National Clearinghouse on Child Abuse and Neglect Information. Available at: *http://nccanch.acf.hhs.gov/.* Accessed 2006.
Reece RM, Ludwig S, eds. *Child abuse: medical diagnosis and management.* 2nd ed. Philadelphia: Lippincott Williams & Wilkins; 2001.

CHAPTER 137 ■ ABUSIVE HEAD TRAUMA

STEPHEN E. BOOS

Abusive head trauma is a tragedy that affects nearly 30 of every 100,000 infants each year. The majority of these patients are under 2 years of age. Death is a common outcome, and most who do not die suffer permanent neurodevelopmental disabilities. Abused, head-injured children are complicated patients who are hospitalized longer and generate higher hospital bills than children with head injuries from other causes. The resuscitation, support, monitoring, and neurosurgical management of these children resembles that of other head-injured children, and will not be discussed in this chapter. Rather, we will discuss medical challenges and tasks that make these children distinctive. When appropriate, abuse must be included in the initial differential diagnosis, additional signs of child abuse identified (if present), conditions that may alter this analysis diagnosed or excluded, and the medical provider must report to and work with a variety of agencies.

DEVELOPING DIAGNOSTIC SUSPICION

See Table 137.1. Unlike most other cases of head injury, abusive head trauma nearly always presents without a truthful history. Most commonly, the child is brought for care of symptoms without a trauma history. Somewhat less commonly, a history of minor trauma, such as a short household fall, is given. Such false histories may lead the clinician to not consider traumatic head injury in the differential.

Jenny and associates found that one-third of children ultimately diagnosed with abusive head trauma had been evaluated and given another diagnosis by a medical provider (see suggested Readings). Other studies have found that 20% to 40% of neurologically asymptomatic infants evaluated for abuse had evidence of trauma on head CT (computed tomography) or MRI (magnetic resonance imaging). Multiple studies have found that approximately one-third of children with recognized abusive head trauma had evidence of prior intracranial injuries. Head injury, without obvious signs, is both common and likely to be overlooked.

The child who presents with acute loss of consciousness, seizure respiratory arrest, or external evidence of serious trauma is likely to raise suspicion of traumatic injury, or to receive imaging that identifies the expected effects of trauma. In children who present with irritability, unusual somnolence, or persistent emesis, particularly in the absence of diarrhea, the possibility of trauma may be overlooked in favor of a more common diagnosis such as acute viral illness, otitis media, or another atraumatic diagnosis. The occurrence of mild external head injury (e.g., contusion) is sometimes a clue to diagnosis. Bruises are uncommon in children who do not

pull to a stand and walk holding onto objects or "cruise." Finding a bruise on the calvarium of a nonmobile infant, accompanied by systemic symptoms, should prompt head imaging. A spinal tap, done to rule out meningitis, may reveal blood. If the cell count from early and late tubes is the same, the red cells are crenated, or the supernate is xanthochromic, subarachnoid hemorrhage should be suspected and imaging ordered. This conservative approach will lessen the likelihood of missing the effects of occult head trauma.

Once head trauma is recognized, the next step is to consider whether it is well explained. Subdural hemorrhages in infancy are abusive in etiology a majority to a significant minority of the time. Barring significant, publicly confirmed traumatic cause (e.g., motor vehicle collision), abuse must enter into consideration. Although exceptions may exist, short indoor falls rarely result in symptomatic subdural bleeding. Whether a trauma history is absent, forthcoming but minor, or delayed and speculative, subdural hemorrhage should put abusive head trauma on the differential diagnosis.

Skull fracture, epidural hematoma, and contusions have been described as a consequence of household falls. Each of these findings may also occur as the result of inflicted trauma. In the absence of a trauma history, the medical provider must strongly consider the possibility of inflicted trauma. In the presence of a forthcoming trauma history, the physician has the difficult task of deciding whether the given history is consistent with the objective findings and is otherwise credible. When the credibility of the history or suggested mechanism is in question, it is appropriate to proceed with the full medical evaluation for possible abusive head trauma.

Before proceeding, it should be noted that as questions of trauma and abuse are addressed, the mechanism of trauma usually has not been proposed yet. "Abusive head trauma" is not a synonymous term for the "shaken baby syndrome." Both genuine and manufactured controversies surround the concept of injury by shaking. Early use of the term "shaken baby syndrome" is likely to unduly constrain both medical assessment and investigation by law enforcement and child protective agencies. This issue will be revisited after discussing a thorough medical assessment.

INITIAL MEDICAL EVALUATION

At this point the medical provider will likely be assessing a child whose CT scan shows an acute subdural hematoma. The available history often includes no trauma, or a short fall from a raised household surface. Other findings may include chronic subdural hematoma, skull fracture, subarachnoid hemorrhage, and focal or diffuse brain swelling. The differential diagnosis will include inflicted trauma, but also medical conditions that

TABLE 137.1

SITUATIONS THAT SHOULD PROVOKE SUSPICION FOR POSSIBLE INFLICTED HEAD TRAUMA

- Infant with irritability, somnolence, or vomiting AND bruising of the head or face
- Respiratory arrest (ALTE), seizure, or loss of consciousness without apparent cause
- Infantile subdural hematoma without severe trauma (e.g., motor vehicle crash)
- Other head injuries, epidural hematoma, or skull fracture, without trauma history

make the child more susceptible to trauma or may simulate trauma. An assessment must be crafted to differentiate these possibilities. The medical provider will require the family's assistance in completing this assessment, assistance that may be lost once the concept of child abuse has been broached and protective agencies notified. For this reason, a broad and thorough history should be obtained early in the medical assessment.

History

The history of present illness should begin with information about when the child was last awake, healthy, and performing her best (Table 137.2). It should be complete for at least 72 hours before presentation for medical care. From that time to the present, any perceived illness, any trauma event, and the care and activities of the child should be documented in detail. The child's condition at transfers of care (e.g., parent to day care) may become particularly important, and should be confirmed with both parties if possible. Ultimately some change in the child led an adult to seek medical care for the child. The nature of this change, its timing, and pace of evolution should be scrupulously documented. The response of the adult should also be documented, including attempts at home treatment, calls for advice, and alerting emergency services.

The significance of the past medical history may not be apparent until additional studies are performed, so it should not be truncated. Birth history should include birthweight, route of delivery, the use of forceps or vacuum extractors, and administration of vitamin K. Apparent birth trauma, and the subsequent neonatal course, complete the birth history. Following this, every perceived trauma and illness should be explored. History of minor irritability and emesis take on new importance when evaluating subacute or chronic intracranial injury. Essentially no observation can be assumed to be insignificant. Past treatment in the home, medical evaluations, and folk medical practices complete this review of the child's health.

TABLE 137.2

HISTORICAL ELEMENTS

- Detailed history of reported trauma event
- Detailed history of reported deterioration event
- Child's care provider, symptoms, behaviors for 72 hours AND until awake and well
- Birth history
- Nutritional history
- Past health and trauma events
- Developmental history
- Family medical history

The family medical history may yield evidence of inherited diseases that can simulate trauma, or make the child more vulnerable to trauma. Coagulopathy and osteogenesis imperfecta are the most commonly discussed disorders. A family history of hemophilia, excessive bleeding following surgical or dental procedures, or easy bruising should be sought. Heavy menstrual flow and anemia in female relatives may be the only hint of von Willebrand disease. Osteogenesis imperfecta has been reported in association with intracranial and retinal hemorrhages as well as fractures. Along with fractures, blue sclerae, early hearing loss, short stature, and odontogenesis imperfecta may be found in the family history. Glutaric aciduria type 1, a metabolic disorder, may present with a subdural hematoma, frontotemporal atrophy of the brain, and limited retinal hemorrhages. Other signs of this rare disorder include macrocephaly and neurodevelopmental handicaps. The family history may also yield risk factors for child abuse. Young single parents, drug involvement, mental illness, and child caretaking by mother's paramours are significant risk factors. The occurrence of domestic violence and past involvement with children's protective services provide direct evidence of violence and dysfunction in the family.

A few additional historical points may prove important in evaluating a case. Exclusive breastfeeding without vitamin supplementation increases the chance of rickets, particularly for dark-skinned children in northern climes, and of vitamin K deficiency, particularly among mothers treated with antiepileptic drugs. A developmental history will help in judging the reported behaviors of the child, but should be interpreted with caution. It is occasionally asserted that a child who cannot yet roll over cannot fall off of a bed or sofa surface. Although this may reflect a true relative likelihood, such an absolute judgment would be overreaching.

Physical Examination

Vital signs and anthropometric data play an important part in questions of child abuse. A large head circumference may be a family trait, a sign of underlying metabolic disease, or a consequence of growing intracranial fluid collection, such as a chronic subdural hematoma. A dramatically underweight child may suffer from a chronic medical condition, or may simply be malnourished as a consequence of neglect. Body temperature at presentation should be noted. Fever will certainly trigger a search for an underlying infection. Hypothermia is often noted in abused children. This is neither specific nor well understood, but may be a reflection of delay in care seeking, or attempts to revive an injured child.

A patient hospitalized with a serious condition is likely to receive a very complete physical examination. When that child has serious but ill-explained head injuries, certain findings deserve extra scrutiny. A thorough search of the calvarium for evidence of trauma may reveal findings crucial to understanding the mechanism of injury. Bruises may be difficult to find under thick hair, and scalp swelling may not be apparent without careful palpation. Identifying easily overlooked signs of impact, or signs of multiple impacts, will affect the final diagnosis. The converse is not absolutely true. Impact that results in a skull fracture or findings on autopsy is sometimes inapparent on external exam. The presence of skull fracture without associated scalp swelling is one hint that the trauma may not have been acute.

Although there are only a few published descriptions, there is much anecdotal evidence of an association between ear bruising and child abuse. Small petechial bruises in the recesses of the ear, and marks at the apex or behind the pinna, are very concerning for inflicted trauma. Fingernail impressions and lacerations may also be found. These findings are easily overlooked, and should be actively sought. The oral exam should focus on the frenulae of the lips and tongue, the palate, and posterior pharynx. Each site is at risk of injury by a harried care provider forcing a bottle or spoon into the mouth of a crying or recalcitrant baby. The conjunctivae should be examined for petechiae. These may attest to forceful vomiting, coughing, or screaming, but may also occur during strangulation. A direct ophthalmoscopic exam by the provider is necessary to search for retinal hemorrhage(s), but this exam has limited sensitivity and specificity and does not substitute for an ophthalmologist's exam. Bruises on the neck may attest to strangulation injury. If a cervical collar is in place it should be removed briefly to allow a careful examination of the neck.

A similarly detailed examination should cover all areas of the body. In the youngest children (those not yet pulling up and walking along objects), any bruise can be significant. Certain areas, however, have special significance. Abdominal bruising is notable both because it is rare, and because it attests to abdominal trauma that must be further evaluated. Bruising of the buttocks is notable because this area is usually padded with a diaper, but is a frequent target for inflicted trauma. When a bruise has a shape, that shape may be significant. Some shapes have obvious significance, such as bites, hand imprints, belt marks, looped cord marks, or other identifiable objects. Others, such as grip marks and pinches, are less intuitively obvious, but no less significant. Some shapes may only make sense when further details of the case are known, and so should be noted. The genitals should be included in this complete survey. Any irregularity of the genital exam should prompt examination by a professional experienced in the examination of sexually abused children. This may include a child abuse physician, a sexual assault nurse or forensic nurse examiner, or a pediatric gynecologist.

So far, this section has focused on the search for additional trauma. The search for additional evidence of nontraumatic diagnoses is equally important. Facial dysmorphology may be a clue to an underlying genetic condition. A blue or muddy gray cast to the sclerae or dark translucent fragile teeth may suggest osteogenesis imperfecta. Oozing from needlesticks, extensive or palpable purpura, or hemarthroses speak strongly to the possibility of a serious bleeding disorder. Excess bruising that lacks the patterns associated with child abuse may be a clue to a milder underlying bleeding disorder.

In addition to thorough written documentation of all physical findings, graphic documentation is highly recommended. Drawing cutaneous findings on a body diagram is a good start, and will back up photodocumentation if a technical problem destroys those images. Photographs of findings should be well focused and well exposed with a close-up as well as a regional view. The plane of the film should parallel the dominant plane of the lesion. A size standard should be included in the picture at the same distance and parallel with the dominant plane of the mark. If color is to become an issue, a color standard should be included as well. Users of conventional film should shoot multiple images and bracket the exposure. Users of digital equipment should not trust the small image on the camera screen as an indication of picture quality and should view images at full resolution before accepting them as adequate.

Initial Imaging and Laboratory Studies

CT scanning is the most common initial imaging modality for head-injured children (Table 137.3.) Occasionally a child will have an MRI as their initial head-imaging study. For the child who is seriously impaired, CT scanning of the chest and abdomen should be considered to look for occult visceral injuries. External evidence of orthopedic injury will prompt clinical radiography of the affected area. Otherwise, further imaging can await the secondary assessment. Initial laboratory testing may include blood counts, basic chemistries, transaminases,

TABLE 137.3

ACUTE ASSESSMENT COMPONENTS

- CT and/or MRI scan
- Visceral CT if unconscious, multiply traumatized, or symptomatic
- Blood count with platelets
- Basic metabolic profile
- PT, PTT, factor XIII, fibrinogen, von Willebrand panel
- Liver function tests
- Amylase lipase
- Follow-up of positives

amylase/lipase, urinalysis, and a coagulation panel. Anemia is commonly identified in abusive head trauma patients, and seems disproportionate to the amount of blood identified in the head. A consumptive phenomenon or preexisting anemia may explain this finding. Hyponatremia may develop in some brain-injured patients, and can worsen brain swelling. Though no reliable temporal relationship has been established, this finding typically occurs a day or two following the traumatic event. The presence of hyponatremia at presentation may suggest a delay in seeking care, and may explain delayed onset of severe symptoms. Mildly prolonged PT and PTT values may be the result, rather than the cause, of the apparent head injury. Evidence of intravascular coagulation documents a consumptive etiology. Secondary coagulopathy may complicate severe primary head injury and serves as a marker of poor outcome. Elevated transaminases, elevated amylase or lipase, or hematuria on urinalysis may be the initial, or indeed the only sign of visceral injury. Transaminases are usually elevated very early following an injury. Amylase, on the other hand, may rise in a delayed fashion. If initial laboratory tests are performed less than 4 hours following the suspected time of injury, the amylase should be repeated at a later time.

Blood counts may also provide the first hint that a child suffers from leukemia or another cause of severe thrombocytopenia, resulting in internal bleeding that can be confused with inflicted head injury. Basic chemistries can identify renal failure (may become important if fractures are identified) or hypernatremia (a possible cause of intracranial bleeding and brain swelling). Severe coagulopathy has significant implications for patients with intra-cranial or intra-retinal bleeding. Any coagulopathy will need urgent treatment; hence it is very important to obtain baseline values before initiating treatment that can alter the results. Coagulation studies such as factor levels, proteins induced by vitamin K absence (PIVKA-II) levels for vitamin K deficiency, von Willebrand testing, fibrinogen, D-dimer, and fibrin split products may be beneficial. In the absence of prolonged clotting times, many centers order additional clotting studies including factor XIII, fibrinogen, and a von Willebrand panel. Liver disease may contribute to coagulopathy. Alagile syndrome has resulted in the mistaken diagnosis of child abuse, so elevated transaminases require follow-up, with additional evaluation for persistent elevation.

THE SECONDARY ASSESSMENT (TABLE 137.4)

Imaging

Magnetic resonance imaging can be a very helpful tool in evaluating these patients. MRI images are more sensitive to small blood collections, better at differentiating the location of

TABLE 137.4

SECONDARY ASSESSMENT

MRI if not obtained
Skeletal x-ray survey
Dilated indirect ophthalmoscopy by a qualified
   ophthalmologist
Early evaluation and treatment of coagulopathy, fibrin split
   products, D-dimers, PIVKA-II, specific clotting factor levels
Subspecialty consultation for differential diagnoses
   Coagulopathy
   Osteogenesis imperfecta
   Metabolic bone disease
   Glutaric aciduria type I and other metabolic disorders
Consider repeat skeletal x-ray survey in 2 weeks
Consult early with a child abuse pediatrician if one is available

extra-axial collections, provide additional clues to the timing of injuries, are more sensitive to parenchymal brain injury, and more likely to pick up vascular abnormalities. The American Academy of Pediatrics Section on Radiology has recommended MRI imaging in cases of suspected abusive head trauma 5 to 7 days following the acute injury (1). Magnetic resonance arteriography or venography may be recommended when there is other evidence of vascular disease, vascular area infarct, intra-parenchymal bleeding, or when intra-cranial bleeding is the only evidence of trauma.

A skeletal x-ray survey should be ordered in all children with suspected inflicted head injury. A skeletal x-ray survey is not a "babygram." Dedicated views of the axial and appendicular skeleton, including the hands and feet, will require many films. A nuclear bone scan may supplement but not replace the conventional x-ray survey, as it is insensitive to changes in the skull, pelvis, and metaphyses of the long bones. Repeating the skeletal x-ray survey in 2 weeks often adds greater information and certainty to the evaluation.

Laboratory Testing

Abnormalities in initial testing require both further investigation and longitudinal follow-up until resolution. Where an abnormality suggests a possible differential diagnosis, definitive testing should be ordered. Coagulopathy has already been mentioned in greater detail, because this dynamic issue is best assessed acutely. Other concerns, such as osteogenesis imperfecta, other metabolic bone disease, and metabolic diseases such as glutaric aciduria type I, are best assessed with the input of the appropriate consultant.

Consultation

When the case assessment has suggested a possible alternative diagnosis rather than abusive head trauma, consultation with the appropriate specialist is warranted. However, every child with possible inflicted head injury should be assessed by an ophthalmologist. Dilated, indirect ophthalmoscopy is necessary to definitively diagnose or exclude retinal hemorrhages. With this tool, the ophthalmologist can identify details in retinal hemorrhaging that are more specific for abuse or suggestive of other diagnoses. Ophthalmologists will routinely document the findings with drawings, but retinal photographs can significantly augment this practice. Photographs also allow consultation with a pediatric ophthalmologist where one is not available. Consultation with a child abuse pediatrician is available at some locations. Early involvement of these specialists

can significantly impact the in-hospital assessment and subsequent legal challenges unique to abusive head trauma.

DISCHARGE PLANNING AND PUBLIC HEALTH

As noted above, the care of the anatomic and physiologic problems of head-injured children are discussed elsewhere. The special management problems of abusively injured children revolve around discharge planning and public health. Returning a child to the environment in which they sustained an abusive injury risks repeat abuse and further injury (or death). Discharge planning must assure that a child is being released to a safe environment. Other children living in an abusive environment, or who may come into that environment in the future, are also at risk. This is a problem of public health that the treating physician is obligated to help address. As with any community and environmental problem, the treating physician cannot address these problems alone.

The law mandates that all medical providers report any reasonable suspicion of child abuse to child protective authorities. Apart from this legal mandate, these agencies, both children's protective services (CPS) and law enforcement (LE), can be allies in resolving remaining diagnostic uncertainty, and addressing the discharge planning and public health problems, which are the proper province of medical care. The medical provider will receive the best help from these agencies if reporting is thorough, and the provider remains available to help the agency understand and resolve difficult medical questions. Ultimately the treating provider, or a consultant, will need to address the issues listed in Table 137.5.

Diagnosing Abuse

Following the inpatient evaluation, any consideration of conditions that can be confused with abusive head trauma should be resolved. The presence of multiple old and new injuries accompanying classic abusive head injuries and retinal hemorrhages can safely be attributed to child abuse. These children are as correctly diagnosed with "the battered child syndrome" as with abusive head trauma. Serious acute traumatic head injury, with evidence of impact and no history of trauma, presents little problem. There is little doubt that a traumatic event occurred in these children, and that the trauma was a severe one. Given the very young age of these children, it is largely inconceivable that the trauma would be unrecognized. When an infant or young child with subdural hematoma

TABLE 137.5

CHILDREN'S PROTECTIVE SERVICES
REPORTING ISSUES

- Express level of certainty of abuse, not just suspicion, and basis for that impression
- Provide mechanism of injury where known and basis for that impression
- Indicate likely timing of trauma, level of certainty, and basis for that impression
- Identify remaining uncertainty or outstanding elements of the evaluation
- Identify needed follow-up care and evaluation
- Give a short-term prognosis
- Prescribe long-term developmental and behavioral monitoring

(or similar closed head injury) and a history of mild non-inflicted trauma presents without old and new injury or other suspicious injury, carefully considered diagnostic reasoning is required. At times, uncertainty as to whether a given injury is the result of accidental or nonaccidental trauma will remain.

Epidemiologic comparisons of abusive and nonabusive head injuries have defined the following associations. During infancy, between 40% and 80% of subdural hematomas result from inflicted injuries. Retinal hemorrhages can occur in a small minority of patients with noninflicted head injury and are not diagnostic for abuse. In studies that examined the eyes of all injured children, between 55% and 100% of the retinal hemorrhages noted were the result of abuse. Furthermore, retinal hemorrhages found after noninflicted head injury are usually limited in number and extent, and confined to the intraretinal layer and to the posterior pole.

The identification of additional and/or healing traumatic injuries is associated with abuse. These discriminating injuries include skeletal injuries, particularly the classic metaphyseal lesions, rib fractures, and old intracranial injuries. Although the presence of bruises is equally likely in children with abusive and nonabusive head injuries, patterned bruises will help to identify child abuse. Absent explanatory history, changing history, or history of a short household fall, favors abuse, whereas major traumatic events (e.g., automobile accidents) are reported in most cases that clearly are nonabusive. In cases where subdural hematoma is the only traumatic finding, but severe trauma is not reported, careful investigation is highly likely to identify serious environmental risk factors that create concern for inflicted injury.

It is clear that falls are a common etiology of noninflicted head injury. These injuries are typically minor. Simple isolated skull fracture is fairly common with short falls. Epidural hematoma uncommonly accompanies skull fracture or occurs in isolation. Complex fractures, depressed fractures, and brain contusions result from more significant household falls, often involving bunk beds or stairs. Subdural hematoma or severe and fatal brain injury are rare consequences of household falls. Studies of over 350 children with documented falls from hospital beds identified no cases of symptomatic head injury. Even a study published to show that fatal head injury could occur following short falls only found 18 fatal head injuries out of more than 75,000 falls, a rate of 0.024% (2). These were playground falls reported to the U.S. Consumer Product Safety Commission, and probably reflect a much greater number of actual falls (and a correspondingly even lower risk). Playground falls are likely to be higher and more complicated that an infant rolling off a bed or sofa.

The science of biomechanics was initially greeted as a possible way to distinguish consistent from inconsistent histories. Instead, it has fostered disagreement over the adequacy of shaking to cause the injuries referred to as "shaken baby syndrome." Although biomechanics still holds its initial promise, any current argument needs to be carefully analyzed for the adequacy of its modeling and assumptions, particularly regarding injury thresholds. Such analysis will usually show that strongly stated arguments should be rejected as overreaching.

Abuse Mechanism

Two-thirds of children with abusive head injuries have objective evidence of impact. When obvious signs of impact are found, diagnosis should reflect impact to the head. Diagnosing a child exclusively with "shaken baby syndrome" when there are skull fractures, scalp hematomas, and contusions is incomplete and misleading to investigators.

The questions that remain include the following: What causes injuries in the absence of evident impact? What injuries

are specific for violent shaking? It is clear that head impact can occur without outwardly apparent signs. The presence of subdural hematoma without external injuries is not enough to diagnose "shaken baby syndrome." These children may have been shaken or impacted, and reports should acknowledge both possibilities.

Extensive, multilayer retinal hemorrhages, with or without retinoschisis or retinal folds, are rarely found outside of abusive head injury. Crush injury of the head may lead to similar findings, but impact injury following motor vehicle crash does not. Based on clinical experience, these classic retinal findings are believed to call for a shaking event. Thus classic, but not more limited, retinal hemorrhages call for a diagnosis of shaking injury. Abuser or witness reports of violent shaking that lead to neurologic collapse also support this diagnosis. Rib fractures, grip marks on the chest, and classic metaphyseal lesions provide supportive evidence, but are also consistent with slamming injuries. At times both the possibility of impact and shaking must be acknowledged.

Abuse Timing

Medical clues to timing of the injury may help investigators identify the abuser. Rarely, a history will include an abusive act that identifies the assailant. Radiologic or pathologic findings may provide clues to timing, but usually the time scale is too wide to identify a single assailant. The best clue to the timing of injury is the timing of symptom onset. In the most seriously injured children, those who die or become comatose, unconsciousness is usually immediate and sustained. Exceptions to this presentation occur, but infrequently. The most classic cause of delayed deterioration is accumulating intracranial mass. Delayed onset seizure, particularly with status epilepticus, can result in severe deterioration following lucidity. Natriuresis or antidiuresis can provoke hyponatremia and brain swelling, with severe delayed deterioration. If these conditions are not present, the time of symptom onset becomes by far the most likely time of injury.

Complicating Conditions

In a child who is abused or possibly abused, the presence of other medical conditions that have been diagnosed or are pending further evaluation must be included in the reports to CPS and LE. An awareness of these conditions must be factored into the legal handling of the child's case, as they may affect certainty in the occurrence, nature, and timing of abuse. Additionally, if the child is taken into protective custody, CPS will have to supervise the child's medical care and the completion of any pending evaluation. At discharge, special laboratory tests may be pending, and others may need repetition. Additional tests for possible inflicted injuries, such as a repeat skeletal x-ray survey in 2 weeks, may also be necessary. These should be part of the CPS report.

EXPECTED OUTCOME

Overall, the outcome of inflicted head injury is bad, and worse than in accidental head injury. Approximately one-fourth to one-third of the victims of inflicted head trauma die. A minority of survivors demonstrate good short-term recovery, with the remainder demonstrating neurodevelopmental deficits early after discharge. The presence of intraparenchymal lesions predicts poor outcome. Neuromotor, cognitive, and visual deficits are particularly common. The long-term outcome for victims of abusive head injury is guarded. Disabilities that are evident early are likely to persist. Even children who go home from the hospital apparently symptom free are at risk for difficulties.

This has particular importance when discussing discharge plans and the child's future living arrangement. In addition to recognized residua, families and agencies receiving children discharged following inflicted head trauma must be prompted to initiate long-term developmental follow-up.

CONCLUSIONS

All forms of head injury are management challenges. In addition to the management of the significant injuries, abusive head trauma presents special legal and clinical problems. This chapter has attempted to develop a clinical pathway to assist the pediatric hospital provider in efficiently negotiating these special problems. Some portion of the additional expense for taking care of these children comes from added days in the hospital awaiting a discharge plan. Reporting to the CPS early, and being available to answer salient questions, may result in an earlier discharge and more satisfactory placement.

PEARLS

- Think about head trauma in infants with irritability, somnolence, or vomiting.
- Never accept a bloody spinal tap as "traumatic;" look for crenated cells, xanthochromic supernate, and a stable cell count from first to last tube.
- Get a thorough history from the family before announcing your suspicion of abuse.
- Try to meet with the family to obtain a history even if they are excluded from the hospital.
- Examine all skin surfaces carefully.
- A skeletal survey has a minimum of 19 films and sometimes more.
- Consider repeating the skeletal survey in 2 weeks.
- Get a radiologist's guidance with reading head CTs and MRIs.
- Short indoor falls rarely cause SDH or retinal hemorrhage.
- "Shaken baby syndrome" and abusive head trauma are not synonymous. Assign your diagnosis carefully and be able to defend it.
- Report to authorities early and communicate frequently.
- Even children who "do well" clinically remain at risk for developmental, behavioral, and educational sequelae from their trauma.

References

1. Sane SM, Kleinman PK, Cohen RA, et al. Diagnostic imaging of child abuse. *Pediatrics* 2000;105:1345–1348.
2. Plunkett J. Fatal pediatric head injuries caused by short-distance fall. *Am J Forens Med Pathol* 2001;22:1–12.

Suggested Readings

Duhaime AC, Alaria AJ, Lewander WJ, et al. Head injury in very young children: mechanisms, injury types, and ophthalmologic findings in 100 hospitalized patients younger than 2 years of age. *Pedatrics* 1992;90:179–185.

Duhaime AC, Christian CW, Rorke LB, et al. Nonaccidental head injury in infants—the "shaken baby syndrome." *N Engl J Med* 1998;338:1822–1829.

Feldman KW, Bethel R, Shugerman RP, et al. The cause of infant and toddler subdural hemorrhage: a prospective study. *Pediatrics* 2001;108:636–646.

Jenny C, Hymel KP, Ritzen A, et al. Analysis of missed cases of abusive head trauma. *JAMA* 1999;281:621–626.

Ophthalmology child abuse working party. Child abuse and the eye. *Eye* 1999;13:3–10.

Ophthalmology child abuse working party. Update from the ophthalmology child abuse working party: Royal College ophthalmologists. *Eye* 2004;18:795–798.

CHAPTER 138 ■ SEXUAL ABUSE IN CHILDREN AND ADOLESCENTS

LORI D. FRASIER

Child sexual abuse is an unfortunately common problem. Retrospective studies indicate that as many as 1 in 4 girls and 1 in 8 boys are sexually abused prior to age 18 (1). Definitions of sexual abuse are very broad and can range from unwanted touching and intercourse to a perpetrator "exposing" himself for the sexual gratification of the perpetrator.

Concerns about possible sexual abuse may be found in a hospitalized child or adolescent during the course of treatment for unrelated medical problems, or she or he may be admitted to the hospital primarily for medical issues related directly to sexual abuse. In either setting, concern might be caused by anal or genital injuries, bleeding, certain infections, suspected sexually transmitted diseases, behavioral problems, or spontaneous disclosures. A concern may be raised by parents or family members. Children can be hospitalized for somatic complaints such as chronic abdominal pain where a thorough medical workup does not reveal an organic etiology. A careful psychosocial assessment may uncover physical and/or sexual abuse. Behavioral and psychiatric problems that lead to inpatient hospitalization can have roots in child sexual abuse.

Behaviors can also be specific or nonspecific. Specific behaviors include sexual activities or sexual knowledge beyond what is expected for the child's developmental level. This child is at risk for having been exposed to sexual matters, whether directly through abuse or indirectly through exposure to adult sexual acts via pornography or poor boundaries with adults. Alternatively, many childhood stressors can cause nonspecific symptoms such as nightmares, developmental regression, undue fear of strangers, or other symptoms of posttraumatic stress disorder. A psychological assessment by a skilled mental health professional may serve to uncover the basis of a child's behavioral symptoms.

ADOLESCENT ISSUES

Adolescents often have sexual knowledge obtained from peers or popular media. They also have relationships outside the direct supervision of parents that may involve consensual sex. Adolescents are also vulnerable to sexual advances from older teens and adults who seek to exploit their desire for independence. As a result of risk-taking behaviors and this desire for independence, they may place themselves in dangerous situations. This is confirmed by a study that indicated most adolescent sexual assaults occur between 10 PM and 4 AM, involve alcohol or drugs, and involve social interactions with strangers (1). However, a great deal of sexual abuse occurs within the family, extended family, or with close acquaintances. A teen may deny sexual activity for a variety of reasons. There may be fear of parental reaction for being sexually active, or fear of retaliation if incest is revealed. Adolescents

presenting with symptoms such as vomiting or abdominal pain should be assessed for pregnancy. Pregnancy in a very young adolescent may be the first sign of intrafamilial sexual abuse. A teen's denial of sexual activity should never preclude a pregnancy test if symptoms suggest it, or if radiologic procedures are being considered for gastrointestinal complaints. Pelvic inflammatory disease may signal a sexually transmitted infection in a child who does not want her parents to know she is sexually active. Drug or alcohol intoxication may result from a pattern of adolescent behaviors that often also includes underage sex. Or a sexual assault may occur when the teen is physically compromised by substance abuse or alcohol.

Adolescent males can also be victimized or engage in high-risk behaviors with peers or adults. Males may be reticent to disclose sexual abuse by another male, fearing they will perceived by others as homosexual. Homosexual teens may seek same-sex relationships where they are or can be exploited sexually. Signs and symptoms of penile discharge, rectal pain, injury, or bleeding must be explored with these teens in a compassionate and nonjudgmental manner.

TALKING WITH CHILDREN AND ADOLESCENTS ABOUT SEXUAL ABUSE

Many physicians are reticent to talk to a child or adolescent about issues of sexual abuse. When abuse is suspected, physicians fear being accused of "tainting" a subsequent forensic interview with a child. There are highly specialized forensic interviewers who work with law enforcement or child protective services. However, in certain medical settings it may be necessary (and appropriate) to talk to a child for immediate protective or health care reasons. All physicians should have a basic knowledge of the "rules" of speaking with children and adolescents.

The following are general guidelines for talking with parents and children in situations where sexual abuse may be suspected.

■ Speak to the parent alone first. Parents will share more of their concerns openly if the child is not present. Do not forget a complete medical, social, and family history, as well as a review of physical and behavioral symptoms. Determine from the parent what terms the child uses for his genital or anal anatomy.
■ If possible speak to the child alone. A careful explanation to the parent may facilitate this.
■ Younger children may need some time to "warm up" to the physician who is questioning them. Begin with neutral topics

such as school, a recent holiday, or a birthday. This also allows the physician to assess language development and emotional state of the child.

- Begin with open ended, nondirected questions such as "Can you tell me what happened to you?" or "Do you know why you are here?"
- Younger children may need some direction, such as "Has anyone ever touched you in a place they were not supposed to?" Follow-up questions may be necessary so the child understands what this means.
- Avoid leading questions: "Did your daddy touch your pee pee?"
- The physician's language should be developmentally appropriate.
- Do not make promises that cannot be kept in order to obtain information from a child or adolescent, such as a promise that the information obtained will not be revealed to anyone.
- Be honest with teenagers about the information that will be shared with other professionals or their parents.
- Do not force a child to tell what happened.

DOCUMENTATION

Document what the child said in the child's own words. If the child says, "Big Joe put his weiner in my privacy," use those exact words. Too often the physician states, "The child alleged penile vaginal penetration." It is important to state the facts as they are related to the physician, without judgment on whether the facts could be true or not (2).

THE MEDICAL ASSESSMENT

Most pediatric hospitals will have access to specialists who can perform sexual abuse assessments of children. Those professionals may be part of developed hospital or community-based programs (such as Children's Advocacy Centers). Familiarity with referral resources is helpful. However, even for the nonspecialist, knowledge of how to examine a child or adolescent may be necessary in certain cases. Prior to an exam being attempted, the clinician should be acquainted with basic normal anatomy and what constitutes a concerning or suspicious examination finding. If the physician providing inpatient care is uncomfortable with such an evaluation, a child maltreatment specialist should be consulted to assist in coordinating and/or performing the examination. If at all possible, the child or adolescent should be examined only once and by the most skilled available professional.

Children

Prepubertal and early pubertal children rarely need invasive genital examinations such as a speculum examination. The vast majority of examinations can be performed easily with good preparatory explanation to the child and parent, and a careful, gentle and unhurried approach. A child life specialist is often priceless as an assistant to prepare the child and provide distraction during the exam. With good support and preparation, sedation for an exam is rarely needed. Specific indications for an exam under sedation may include acute injuries with bleeding, possible vaginal foreign body, a severe genital discharge, or a child with developmental delays or severe behavioral disorders.

The examination for possible sexual abuse may occur on the inpatient unit or in the clinic setting. If on the inpatient unit, the patient's room and bed should be avoided. The child should be able to consider their room a "safe" area. The

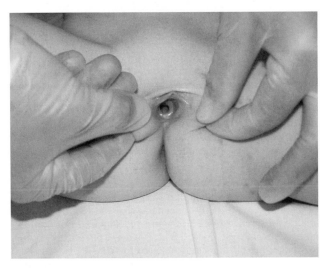

FIGURE 138.1. An example of an external examination of a prepubertal child using labial traction.

exception would be if the child is sedated or comatose in the PICU, or cannot be moved for any reason. If sedation is planned for another procedure, a sedated genital examination may be done concurrently if medically indicated. Under no circumstances should the patient be forced or held for a genital examination. Also, the clinician should explain to both the parent and child (if she is able to understand) that examination should be neither traumatic nor painful.

In general, the child may be examined on a typical examination table and in a "frog leg" position. An assistant or the physician may carefully and gently grasp the labia majora and gently pull outwards and downwards to expose the vestibular contents (traction technique; Fig. 138.1). Careful assessment of the anatomy in a sequential manner will ensure that all structures are evaluated (Fig. 138.2). The perineum and anus can be easily examined in the supine knee chest position by having the child grasp his or her legs and pull them to the chest.

If a colposcope is not available for magnification, a gooseneck lamp, magnifying glass, or otoscope light may be used. Also, as an alternative to a colopscope, a hand-held digital camera with zoom capabilities can be an adequate substitute. Knowledge of the camera's controls and functions will enable

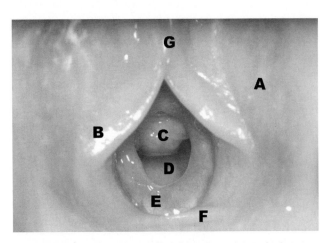

FIGURE 138.2. Typical prepubertal anatomy. **A.** Labial majora (retracted). **B.** Labia minora. **C.** Anterior vaginal wall. **D.** Vagina. **E.** Hymen. **F.** Posterior fourchette. **G.** Clitoris. (The urethra is not visualized in this picture.)

the examiner to take quality, interpretable digital images for documentation of either normal or abnormal findings. Digital images are ideal for obtaining second opinions because they can be emailed to a consultant for review. It is better to take multiple digital images at the time of the initial examination rather than attempt to describe or recreate the findings in drawings and diagrams. A brief written report is necessary, because technical problems can and do arise with cameras and colposcopes resulting in loss of pictures. Drawings and diagrams should be considered a backup, and at times a substitute if some type of imaging is not available.

Findings

It is important for any clinician examining a patient for concerns of sexual abuse to understand that the vast majority of children examined nonacutely (greater than 72 hours following last sexual contact) will have normal exams. Also, a normal examination does not preclude the possibility of sexual abuse, even anal or genital penetration. Children presenting acutely, especially those with symptoms of pain and/or bleeding, may have much higher rates of specific findings such as bruising, abrasions, or tears of the hymen, perineum, or anus.

Very few nonacute anogenital findings are *diagnostic* of penetrating vaginal or rectal injury. These include:

- Absence of the hymen (confirmed with at least two different techniques to define the hymen).
- Complete transection of the hymen below the 3 to 9-o'clock position. (A transection is an area of the hymen that is absent completely to the base without any tissue remaining.)
- Anal scarring. (Some examiners suggest that because anal scars are rare and difficult to diagnose, one should only call a finding a scar if the acute injury has been documented initially.)
- The size of the vaginal opening is not significant due to the fact that it is a dynamic parameter, neither age nor weight standards have been adequately established, and it varies significantly with the position of the child and the degree of relaxation.

Adolescents

Because the hymen is estrogenized and much less sensitive to touch, menstruating adolescents may undergo a speculum examination. However, when there are external genital injuries, this may be difficult or painful. Standard gynecologic examinations traditionally do not carefully include an assessment of the hymenal anatomy. A careful examination of the vestibular contents is necessary *prior* to the insertion of a vaginal speculum. If there are no hymenal or vestibular injuries and there is no ongoing bleeding, it is unlikely that a speculum examination will reveal additional internal injuries. However, a speculum is helpful in evidentiary collections when obtaining specimens from the vaginal pool or endocervical canal. Also, cultures from the endocervix may be necessary. In the nonacute setting, sampling for cervical cytologic analysis can usually be done with a speculum examination. In early pubertal children who are not yet sexually active but with evidence of sexual assault, it remains rarely necessary to perform cervical cytology.

Especially in adolescents, the absence of findings of hymenal injury does not preclude the possibility that penetration occurred. The estrogenized hymen and vagina are very resilient and full intercourse can occur without tearing or injuring the hymen. A recent study by Kellogg and associates demonstrated that 34 of 36 pregnant adolescents were found to have "normal" hymens without signs of acute or chronic injury (3).

Anal anatomy is also resilient and anal scars are rare. Acute anal penetrative injuries can result in bruising, abrasions, and tears that heal quickly and completely without scarring. Caution should be exercised in interpreting a small fissure as a sign of abuse unless the clinical history supports it.

EMERGENCIES, SURGICAL/ ACUTE INJURIES

When a child presents with a possible acute penetrating anal or vaginal injury, there is a risk of vaginal or bowel perforation. This situation constitutes a surgical emergency. A complete trauma assessment should not be overlooked in a child who may have been acutely anally or vaginally penetrated. Other injuries such as blunt force injuries to the head and abdomen may accompany particularly violent sexual assaults.

Acute Sexual Assault

A child with vaginal bleeding or apparent significant injury from an acute sexual assault with vaginal or anal penetration may require examination emergently in the operating room. A pediatric or gynecologic surgeon should be in attendance. The physician may assist in obtaining forensic specimens and cultures as well as taking photographs before and after surgical repair. In both children and adolescents, the more proximate the examination to the time of the sexual assault the greater the likelihood of visualizing and photographing injuries. Healing can occur very quickly. Forensic evidence can also be obtained with higher yield when done within hours of the assault. Protocols for acute forensic collection in both children and adolescents should be established. This may include the availability of "rape kits," and maintaining the "chain of evidence" for forensic specimens to protect their admissibility in court.

Careful interviewing in a child who is neither bleeding nor requiring emergent medical care may help direct the forensic collection and reduce the need for unnecessary collections. Even under optimal circumstances, forensic materials such as perpetrator's semen or saliva is rarely found in or on the child's body beyond 24 hours post-assault (4). In fact, the child's clothing and bed linens are more likely to yield such evidence.

Antibiotic prophylaxis for sexually transmitted diseases (STDs) in children is usually unnecessary. Infections are rare, excellent follow-up is usually facilitated through Child Protective Services (CPS), and prepubertal children are unlikely to have ascending infections or ongoing sexual activity. The forensic value of a diagnosed STD in a child outweighs the potential risk of the child developing an infection. However, HIV prophylaxis should be considered in cases of stranger assault, multiple assailants, a high-risk perpetrator, or anogenital injuries with bleeding.

Adolescent rape and sexual assault are much more likely to be typical penetrative sexual intercourse (as in adult rape). Protocols for collection of forensic specimens are available and should be followed. Semen is often recovered from the vagina, cervix, anus, or mouth if there is history or evidence of assault in those areas. Swabs of bite marks and "hickies" can yield DNA evidence of a perpetrator. All injuries should be photographed (genital, anal, and extra-genital). Postexposure prophylaxis for STDs including HIV is important. Teenagers may be lost to follow-up, have additional sexual contacts, and are at risk for ascending infections. Emergency contraception and HIV prophylaxis should also be offered. The Centers for Disease Control and Prevention (CDC) current recommendations for STD treatment, including prophylaxis in cases of sexual assault, can be found on the CDC website:

http://www.cdc.gov/mmwr/preview/mmwrhtml/rr5106a1.htm

SEXUALLY TRANSMITTED DISEASES

For a list of sexually transmitted infections and their significance, see Table 138.1. The CDC still considers STD cultures the gold standard in forensic cases because of their high specificity. Properly obtained cultures in children require that examiner place a swab intravaginally and leave in place for a few seconds. This may be difficult for the examiner to achieve and painful for the child. Adolescents tolerate this procedure much better, but for best results endocervical cultures are preferable to blind vaginal cultures.

Chlamydia trachomatis and *Neisseria gonorrhea* are fastidious organisms, requiring proper media and temperature. For example, *Chlamydia* transport media should be kept cold, while gonorrhea cultures should be plated immediately on selective media and kept at room temperature. Calcium alginate, cotton, and wood may be toxic to *Chlamydia*, and so only swabs made of rayon or Dacron with metal or plastic shafts can be used. All of these factors can reduce the sensitivity of cultures.

The American Academy of Pediatrics has developed recommendations regarding the evaluation of children for STDs when they present for allegations of sexual abuse (see Kellogg in the Suggested Readings). Fewer than 5% of children evaluated for allegations of sexual abuse have STDs resulting from sexual abuse. Factors to consider in the decision to culture/test should include the age of the child, type of sexual contact alleged, signs or symptoms suggestive of an STD, an abuser with risk factors for an STD, a family concern or request that STD testing be performed, and the prevalence of STDs in the community. Fortunately sexually transmitted diseases are rare in sexually abused children. Most vaginal redness and discharges are the result of poor hygiene or common bacterial or viral agents that are not sexually acquired.

New technologies of DNA amplification, specifically nucleic acid amplification tests (NAATs), are now available. Because they detect very small numbers of organisms, they have superior sensitivity to cultures in detecting STDs such as gonorrhea and *Chlamydia*. They have not been approved for forensic use, but there is some evidence that using urine- or swab-based amplification tests in children may be helpful as screening tests. However, because of the low population prevalence of STDs in children, these tests have a low positive predictive value, and any positive NAAT should not be acted on without confirmation with additional testing (5). Cultures should be obtained prior to treatment. NAATs appear to be preferable in adolescents who have higher rates of STDs, and studies have established their superiority to the sensitivity of cultures. If the teen is already sexually active, the forensic value of a positive STD is limited and NAATs can be used exclusively.

REPORTING

Most states only require a "reasonable" suspicion that abuse has occurred for a report to be made. Every physician providing care to hospitalized children should be well acquainted with his state reporting laws and the appropriate phone numbers for reporting. Physicians are granted immunity from liability if they report in good faith, and can be subject to criminal and civil liability if they do not report a suspected case of child abuse. Some experts would suggest that an allegation or concern by a parent is enough to constitute a report. Because the vast majority of children have normal exams, a report should not hinge on physical findings of sexual abuse. Physicians also need to be aware of statutory rape laws in their states. Families sometimes pressure physicians not to report, on a promise they will "handle it themselves." This approach protects no one, places others at risk from an unrecognized sex offender, and leaves the physician at risk of liability.

The physician should also be aware of her own hospital's policy for reporting suspected abuse or neglect. If the physician is the recipient of first-hand information from the parent or the child, or has specific medical information to provide, it is helpful to personally make the report to CPS or law enforcement. Too often, a nurse or social worker is instructed to make the report with sketchy or secondary information. Physicians are partners with child protection authorities in their communities and should be available to take phone calls and explain medical issues.

TESTIMONY

Physicians should be willing to provide care to a child or adolescent who may be a victim of sexual abuse. Whether or not a

TABLE 138.1

SEXUALLY TRANSMITTED INFECTIONS AND SIGNIFICANCE

Organism confirmed	Relationship to sexual abuse	Report to child protective services
Neisseria gonorrhea	Diagnostic	Yes (if neonatal infection ruled out)
Human immunodeficiency virus (HIV)	Diagnostic	Yes (if neonatal infection ruled out and no other HIV risk factors)
Chlamydia trachomatis	Diagnostic	Yes (if neonatal infection ruled out)
Trichomonas vaginalis	Highly suspicious	Yes (if neonatal infection ruled out)
Condyloma acuminatum	Suspicious	Yes (unless vertical transmission ruled out)
Genital herpes simplex (1 or 2)	Suspicious	Yes
Bacterial vaginosis (includes *Gardnerella vaginalis*)	Inconclusive	Medical follow-up

From Kellogg N. The evaluation of sexual abuse in children. *Pediatrics* 2005;116:506–512.

TABLE 138.2

DIFFERENTIAL DIAGNOSIS OF GENITAL FINDINGS

Sign or symptom suggesting sexual abuse	Differential diagnosis
Vaginal discharge	Common pathogens
	Group A beta-hemolytic strep
	Haemophilus influenzae
	Common respiratory pathogens
	Gram-negative enterics/bowel contamination
	Respiratory viruses
	Gastrointestinal viruses
	Vaginal foreign body
	Sexually transmitted diseases
	Pinworms
	Poor hygiene
	Physiologic leukorrhea
Vesicles or ulcers	Herpes simplex virus 1 or 2
	Varicella-zoster (chickenpox, shingles)
	Epstein–Barr virus
	Nonspecific viral infections
	Behçet disease
	Contact dermatitis; allergic/irritant (e.g., nickel, perfumes, latex)
	Impetigo
Bruising	Trauma
	Accidental
	Sexual
	Lichen sclerosis et atrophicus
	Hemangiomas
	Coagulopathy
	Thrombocytopenia
	Prominent or superficial blood vessels
	Dye from clothing
	Nevi/Mongolian spots
Genital/vaginal bleeding	Tumor: ovarian, vaginal
	Infection
	Shigella enterocolitica
	Group A beta-hemolytic *Streptococcus*
	Foreign body (vaginal)
	Precocious puberty
	Trauma
	Accidental
	Sexual
	Menstruation
	Genitourinary
	GI bleeding
Papules/nodules	Human papilloma virus
	Perianal pseudoverrucous papules and nodules
	Crohn disease
	Condyloma lata
	Molluscum contagiousum
	Skin tags
	Linear epidermal nevus
	Syringoma
	Darier disease
	Langerhans cell histiocytosis
Redness	Poor hygiene
	Use of irritating products
	Masturbation
	Minor trauma
	Psoriasis
	Other dermatologic conditions

physician considers herself an expert in child maltreatment, she may provide a tremendous service to the court (see Chapter 140). The physician should go to court well prepared after thoroughly reviewing the records. She is there to provide information and to educate the judge and/or jury as to the facts of the case. Testifying clearly and honestly to those facts is the physician's responsibility *regardless of whether one is called by the prosecutor or the defense*. If the physician does not consider herself a child maltreatment expert or is unsure of the significance of a certain clinical finding, it is appropriate to defer the expert opinion testimony to the child maltreatment specialist.

MIMICS OF SEXUAL ABUSE

Many so called "mimics" of sexual abuse have been reported in the literature. These conditions may lead to an inaccurate impression that a child has been sexually abused, and may result in false accusations. Table 138.2 provides a list of common mimics and how they may present. For example, lichen sclerosis et atrophicus is an autoimmune genital skin condition that is the most widely reported mimic of acute trauma. The superficial layers of the epidermis become atrophic resulting in pale skin, bruising, hemorrhagic bullae, and fissures similar to acute trauma. Accidental anal and genital injuries also must be differentiated from acute sexual assault. Straddle injuries often have a clear and detailed history, external and sometimes internal trauma, and bruising. Most experienced clinicians can differentiate accidental genital injuries from those caused by sexual assault.

Vaginal and perianal infections caused by group A beta-hemolytic *Streptococcus* are another commonly misinterpreted mimic. These infections can result in genital bleeding and discharge, giving the appearance of trauma (erythema) or raising the suspicion of a sexually transmitted disease. Perianal strep dermatitis is often confused with trauma.

SUMMARY

Hospital-based physicians or any physician providing care to hospitalized children should be aware that sexually abused children and adolescents may require inpatient care either for acute anogenital injures, physical/psychological sequelae of past or chronic abuse, and occasionally temporary protection. It may be necessary to provide care to such children either prior to, or in conjunction with, a child maltreatment specialist. Adolescents may have distinctly different medical (and perhaps psychological) needs than younger children. This is especially true in cases where pregnancy or sexually transmitted

infections are found. Physicians may need to talk to children prior to formal forensic interviewing, in order to meet urgent medical and protective needs. Protocols should be in place for obtaining forensic evidence and assessing injuries in the setting of acute sexual assault. Excellent documentation using photography and diagrams is essential. Physicians must also be prepared to provide medical testimony in the legal setting as an ongoing obligation for child protection and criminal prosecution.

PEARLS

- Child sexual abuse is common.
- Talk with the parent and the child separately if possible.
- Use developmentally appropriate, nonleading questions if possible.
- Never force a genital exam on a child or adolescent.
- A normal exam does not preclude sexual abuse even when penetration is alleged.
- Follow protocols for testing and treating STIs.
- Be familiar with state child abuse reporting laws or have resources that provide that information.
- Excellent writing and photographic documentation of injuries is preferred.
- Communication with Child Protective Services and law enforcement is essential to proper care of sexually abused children and adolescents.
- Physicians are a resource to the courts in child abuse cases.

References

1. Jenny C. Adolescent risk-taking behavior and the occurrence of sexual assault. *Am J Dis Child* 1988;142:770–772.
2. Frasier LD. The pediatrician's role in child abuse interviewing. *Pediatr Ann* 1997;26:306–311.
3. Kellogg ND, Menard SW, Santos A. Genital anatomy in pregnant adolescents: "normal" does not mean "nothing happened." *Pediatrics* 2004;113: e67–e69.
4. Christian CW, Lavelle JM, De Jong AR, et al. Forensic evidence findings in prepubertal victims of sexual assault. *Pediatrics* 2000;106:100–104.
5. Hammerschlag MR. Appropriate use of nonculture tests for the detection of sexually transmitted diseases in children and adolescents. *Semin Pediatr Infect Dis* 2003;14:54–59.

Suggested Readings

Frasier LD. The pediatrician's role in child abuse interviewing. *Pediatr Ann* 1997;26:306–311.
Kellogg N. The evaluation of sexual abuse in children. *Pediatrics* 2005;116: 506–512.

CHAPTER 139 ■ MÜNCHAUSEN SYNDROME BY PROXY (PEDIATRIC CONDITION FALSIFICATION/FACTITIOUS DISORDER BY PROXY)

SARA H. SINAL

Münchausen syndrome by proxy (MSBP) is an unusual form of child abuse. In 1977, Roy Meadow, a British pediatrician, described several children whose mothers fabricated their illnesses, causing them to undergo unnecessary hospitalization and medical procedures. In his seminal article, entitled "Münchausen Syndrome by Proxy: The Hinterland of Child Abuse," Dr. Meadow clearly recognized this clinical phenomenon as a form of child abuse (1). In 1987, Donna Rosenberg (2) reviewed all the published cases of the syndrome and defined MSBP as

> (1) Illness in a child which is simulated (faked) and/or produced by a parent or someone who is *in loco parentis*; and (2) Presentation of the child for medical assessment and care, usually persistently, often resulting in multiple medical procedures; and (3) Denial of knowledge by the perpetrator as to the etiology of the child's illness; and (4) Acute signs and symptoms of the child abate when the child is separated from the perpetrator.

A provocative article by Donald and Jureidini published in 1996 suggests that MSBP differs primarily from other forms of child abuse "by the active engagement of the medical profession in the production of morbidity." In addition, they suggest that our medical system is highly specialized and has many tests and procedures available to investigate unusual diseases in light of suspicion regarding the reported medical history, making it likely that MSBP will go undetected (3).

The *Diagnostic and Statistical Manual for Mental Disorders*, fourth edition (DSM-IV) has given the syndrome the title of "Factitious Disorder by Proxy," and points out that the symptoms can be physical or emotional and that the victim does not have to be a child. The perpetrator is given the diagnosis of Factitious Disorder by Proxy and the victim, if a child, Physical Abuse of a Child (995.5), or if an adult, Physical Abuse of an Adult (995.81). The diagnostic term MSBP has been criticized by experts in the field and other diagnostic terms suggested as substitutes for MSBP include Pediatric Condition Falsification and Fabricated or Induced Illness. It is felt that these terms more accurately describe the pattern of behavior instead of a psychiatric syndrome.

This chapter's focus is on the hospitalized victim of MSBP. Ninety-five percent of MSBP victims admitted to the hospital continue to be victimized in the hospital (2).

EPIDEMIOLOGY

MSBP is still a relatively uncommon form of child abuse; however, with heightened awareness and better diagnostic techniques, it is estimated that a minimum of 600 cases per year may be seen in the United States. A study in the United Kingdom and the Republic of Ireland in 1992 reported an annual incidence of MSBP, nonaccidental poisoning, and nonaccidental suffocation of 0.5 per 100,000 children younger than 16 years of age (4). The median age of victims at diagnosis is 20 months (4). Boys and girls are equally victimized (2,4). Diagnosis is difficult. Rosenberg's review article gave 14.9 months as a time to diagnosis in recognized cases, but there are cases that take years to recognize and many probably never are recognized (2). However, in institutions with child abuse specialists and multidisciplinary MSBP teams, rapid recognition has become more common. There also is increasing awareness of serial perpetrators of MSBP, with frequent reports of prior sibling abuse and death (5).

Most of the perpetrators are biologic mothers, but adoptive mothers, stepmothers, fathers, nurses, and babysitters have been recognized as perpetrators.

In Rosenberg's review, 25% of the cases involved simulation (faking of symptoms) only, 25% involved production (doing something to the child to cause symptoms), and 50% involved both simulation and production (2).

By definition, 100% of MSBP victims undergo unnecessary medical care and procedures and suffer short-term morbidity (2). Psychological morbidity has been recognized as well, but is harder to quantify. Mortality rates vary depending on the type of abuse, and deaths may not be recognized as due to MSBP. MSBP should be taken seriously, because mortality rates have been said to vary from 10% to 30%.

CLINICAL FINDINGS

The Perpetrator

The characteristics of the perpetrator offer diagnostic clues to the clinician. The perpetrator, usually the mother, frequently is someone with a medical background, or one who reports falsely that she is a nurse, or elevates her level of training. The perpetrator is the primary caregiver, and is always present or has been recently present when the child's symptoms develop. The perpetrator does not exhibit overt psychopathology and often initially gives the appearance of being a dedicated, caring parent of an ill child. Family members frequently report a lack of honesty in other areas of the perpetrator's life (e.g., the perpetrator has passed bad checks, misrepresented his or her own illness, or lied about relationships). Speaking about her daughter, the perpetrator, one woman observed, "I don't think she knows what is the truth. She is so convincing when she tells me something, that if I didn't know it was a lie, I would believe it—it's as if she believes it herself." The perpetrator seems to be too trusting and supportive of the physician in the face of an ill child and inability of the physician to establish a diagnosis.

Another common characteristic is that the perpetrator becomes overly friendly with the medical staff. The perpetrator relates more as a colleague than as a parent, and may represent themselves as a close friend of the physician. However, the perpetrator can become demanding and controlling if the evaluation and treatment are not what the perpetrator wants.

Although the DSM-IV suggests that there should be no secondary gain with MSBP, child abuse specialists have noted the contrary. The father often is distant, detached, or even planning to separate from the family. The mother may use the child's illness to draw the father closer or to substitute a more satisfactory relationship for the poor relationship with the father. In some cases at our institution, the secondary gain seems to have been that the mother did not have to return to work, friends were attentive, or funds were raised to help with the child's illness. Nationally, families have at times received significant media exposure because of their child's illness. The psychological motivation of the MSBP mother has been described in detail by Schreier and Libow (see the Suggested Readings). The mother does not have serious psychopathology. She tends to be diagnosed (if at all) as having a personality disorder. Schreier and Libow describe it as "impostor disorder"—these mothers are masquerading as excellent, attentive, even perfect mothers, but if observed without their awareness, they often are cold, detached, and even physically abusive to their children. The mother often has suffered abuse or disappointment in her childhood, often in some way related to her own father, and seems to need to establish a positive relationship with someone she sees as powerful. In the medical setting, this usually is the physician. The victim serves as a dehumanized object that the mother uses to satisfy her own needs and to control her relationship with the physician. At times, particularly if the relationship is threatened, the mother becomes almost compulsive in her risk-taking with the child (e.g., multiple suffocation episodes) to control the relationship with the power figure. If the child dies, the event usually is unintended. In one case, when the mother admitted to suffocating her child, instead of grief she expressed annoyance: "I've done it a lot of times, I don't know why she had to die this time."

Medical History

The history in the MSBP victim may initially appear similar to that of other patients. Over time, however, several factors make the history of MSBP stand apart. These factors are summarized in Table 139.1. The MSBP victim's course is unusual and unresponsive to standard treatment. The past medical history or family history may seem unusual or even unbelievable. For example, in one case, the mother claimed that every other one of the father's seven siblings had died of leukemia. The perpetrator exaggerates symptoms and previous medical treatment—for example, "The doctors at University Hospital said she was the worst case of _____ that they had ever seen." The perpetrator seems unconcerned about the lack of a diagnosis as long as testing is being done. Invasive tests are accepted with eagerness and almost with excitement in some cases. If test results prove normal and reassurance is provided, the symptoms often change or worsen.

Presenting Symptoms

In Rosenberg's original review, the most common presenting symptoms were bleeding, seizures, central nervous system

TABLE 139.1

CLINICAL FINDINGS IN PATIENTS WITH MÜNCHAUSEN SYNDROME BY PROXY

- Very frequent medical visits
- Failure to respond to usual treatments
- Symptoms gradually become worse or more complex
- Inability to tolerate multiple foods and medications
- Erratic drug levels, especially with anticonvulsants, including frequent intoxication
- Unusual or unbelievable family history or past medical history
- History of apnea, failure to thrive, or death of sibling
- Unusual parental response: seems to be excited by/or enjoy child's illness, particularly if tests are being done
- Relapse if hospital discharge imminent
- Feeling on part of physician: "never seen a case like it"

depression, apnea, vomiting, fever, and rash (2). With improved recognition of MSBP, apnea, seizures, and other "spells" of altered consciousness seem to be the most common complaints. Documented apnea often is due to manual suffocation that places the child at significant risk for death. By the mother's report, seizures may be unresponsive to multiple medications and victims often present with symptoms of medication overdose, but when hospitalized in an epilepsy monitoring unit, drugs can be withdrawn without the appearance of seizures. The perpetrator may give an over-the-counter emetic (usually syrup of ipecac) or a laxative to induce vomiting or diarrhea, respectively. Altered consciousness often is related to poisoning with a sedative. Other presenting symptoms include (1) fever, either factitial or due to injection of contaminated material into the child; (2) bleeding caused by trauma to the child or contamination of the specimen with maternal or animal blood or a fluid simulating blood; and (3) rash that is produced by trauma and usually easily recognized as factitial. Many bizarre types of MSBP have been reported and reviews are available.

DIFFERENTIAL DIAGNOSIS

The major barrier to the detection of MSBP is the failure of the physician to include it in the differential diagnosis. Siegel and Fischer point out that there is a strong resistance in society to the recognition of child abuse, and subsequently, for a doctor to accept that a parent is causing their child's illness is "unthinkable" to the physician (see Suggested Readings). The physician's chief concern with the diagnosis of MSBP is that an unusual illness is being missed. Subspecialty consultation is recommended in this situation. Overanxious and difficult parents are in the differential diagnosis. Meadow wrote an excellent article on distinguishing these conditions from MSBP (see Suggested Readings). A good rule of thumb is to involve a child abuse specialist if MSBP is in the differential diagnosis.

DIAGNOSIS AND MANAGEMENT IN THE HOSPITAL

If MSBP is suspected as the reason for symptoms in an outpatient, hospitalization often is necessary to confirm the diagnosis. This can be a dangerous time for the child because the perpetrator may feel the need to produce symptoms, as illustrated by the following case. A 2-year-old child with a 4-month history of severe, blood-streaked diarrhea, but good growth, was admitted to the hospital for evaluation. He then developed intermittent explosive diarrhea, resulting in weight loss. The timing of the recurrent diarrheal episodes just before planned discharge led to the suspicion of MSBP, and it was discovered that the mother had administered a laxative to the child in the hospital.

TEAM APPROACH

When MSBP is suspected, a safety plan must be implemented promptly. Failure to do so can be fatal to the child. For example, a child was admitted for recurrent apnea. MSBP was listed in the differential diagnosis, along with seizure disorder, gastroesophageal reflux with aspiration, and other disorders. On a weekend, while waiting for placement in an epilepsy monitoring unit, the child was suffocated by the mother.

Development of a multidisciplinary team and MSBP protocol is recommended for the management of MSBP in the hospital. The composition of our team and hospital protocol is given in Fig. 139.1. The child abuse consultant/team serves an integral role in suspecting and identifying MSBP, but the multidisciplinary MSBP team is needed because of the complexity and special needs of these cases. At our institution, if the child abuse consultant suspects MSBP or a life-threatening form of MSBP before or after hospital admission, the team is convened. This may take several hours, and in the interim, if the child is already in the hospital, she is transferred to a unit with a nurse in the room at all times, to assure the safety of the child. The team's primary job is to devise a management strategy. Each team member has specific tasks. The attending physician and the child abuse specialist as well as the nursing staff provide the medical history and outline the case for MSBP. The nursing staff limits the perpetrator's access to the medical record, food, and medications and helps carry out the management plan. The hospital intensivist is involved if the child is admitted to the pediatric intensive-care unit. The hospital social worker provides a social and family history and communicates with the county social worker. The county social worker hears the evidence and determines if the department of social services has enough information to intervene and protect the child without further evaluation. The police obtain the suspected perpetrator's criminal records and, if a crime is committed, become directly involved in the investigation. Police may also be able to obtain search warrants in some cases. The hospital administrator, risk management, and legal staff help weigh the responsibilities of and risks to the hospital and the patient. Hospital security staff are responsible for any monitoring techniques that may be undertaken. The psychiatrist on the team evaluates the child and the family. The timing of that assessment varies. The hospital's public relations representative assists with the news media if a crime is committed and the perpetrator is charged. The team reconvenes as necessary during the remainder of the hospitalization. Team support is valuable in dealing with these complex cases and the feelings they generate.

A major value of the multidisciplinary team is that professionals from different desciplines see MSBP in different ways. For example, the pediatrician sees it as suspected child abuse, the psychiatrist sees it as a mental health disorder, and law enforcement sees it as a crime. This enables the team to brainstorm regarding diagnoses and management much more effectively than an individual could alone. In addition, more investigative tools are available with a multidisciplinary team. As an example, a 12-year-old girl was hospitalized with severe secretory diarrhea and vomiting that continued even while on intravenous hyperalimentation. She was getting cholestyramine by mouth and it was suspected that the mother might be giving

her daughter an emetic. Nursing staff was aware that the mother occasionally visited a local pharmacy. When the team became aware of this, the police visited the pharmacy and inquired about anyone buying syrup of ipecac. They were told that a woman fitting the mother's description had made such a purchase. They obtained the pharmacy security tape and were able to confirm the mother making the purchase. When confronted with that evidence, the mother confessed to poisoning her daughter daily with syrup of ipecac.

An important responsibility of the MSBP team is to encourage rapid recognition of MSBP through education of hospital staff. In our hospital, education has been directed at those most likely to be responsible for diagnosing cases: pediatric nurses, gastroenterologists, apnea specialists, neurologists, and surgeons. Educational efforts also have been directed at those managing the suspected cases in the hospital, such as security personnel. Other hospital protocols have been published.

REVIEW OF MEDICAL RECORDS

An important part of the MSBP evaluation is to secure and examine as many old medical records of the child, the perpetrator, and other family members, particularly siblings, as possible. If record review confirms falsification of the medical history on any family member, this casts doubts on the perpetrator as a reliable historian. Attention should be paid to the records of any sibling deaths, particularly from sudden infant death syndrome or apnea. A history of a sibling on an apnea monitor also is suspect. It also is helpful for the treating physician to communicate in person or by telephone with other physicians. The physician accumulating the information should disclose that MSBP is being considered and ask if that seems possible or likely to the other physician. Often, concerns are shared that are not in the medical record. In one case, when the author mentioned MSBP to the primary care physician, she said, "That's what's wrong with this mother! My partners have refused to see her because she has lied about advice they have given her. I knew something was strange, but somehow I never thought of MSBP."

INTERVIEW OF FAMILY MEMBERS OR EYEWITNESSES

The child abuse specialist or social worker arranges interviews with close family members without the suspected perpetrator's knowledge. The interviewer attempts to get information about the social situation and understand what the perpetrator has told others about the child's illness. In one case, an estranged father related that he had come to the hospital to consider a liver donation because the mother had reported that the child was dying of cancer and needed a liver. The child was in fact hospitalized for evaluation of nosebleeds. It also is important to ask any eyewitnesses to apnea, spells, or seizures what they have seen. Often the perpetrator states that others have seen the apnea or seizures, but this cannot be confirmed.

DIAGNOSTIC TECHNIQUES

Presentation of MSBP and appropriate techniques and diagnostic clues for the most common forms of MSBP are listed in Table 139.2. There are two diagnostic techniques that require further discussion.

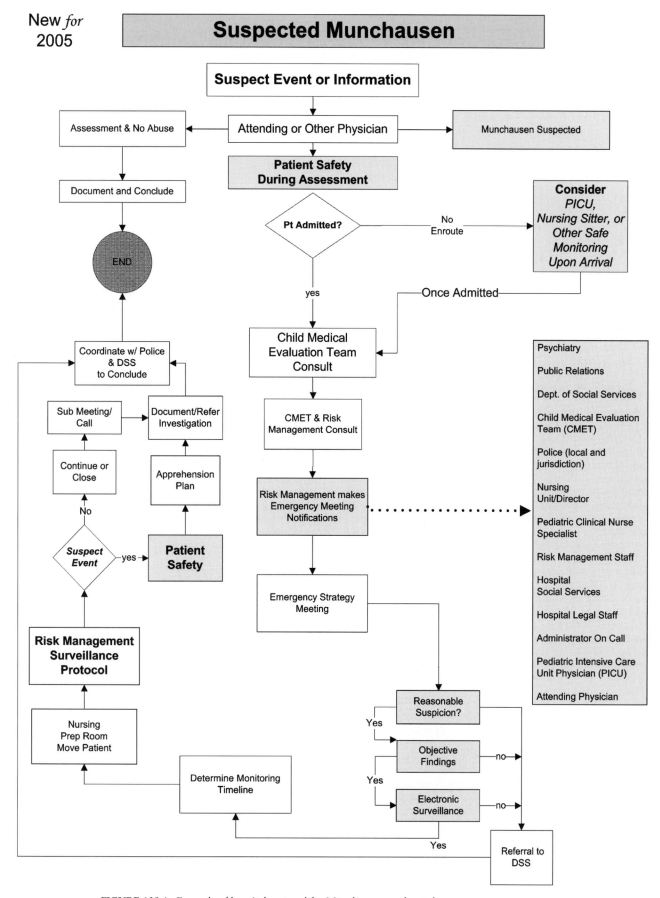

FIGURE 139.1. Example of hospital protocol for Münchausen syndrome by proxy.

TABLE 139.2

COMMON MÜNCHAUSEN SYNDROME BY PROXY PRESENTATIONS, DIAGNOSTIC CLUES, AND TECHNIQUES

Presenting symptoms	Diagnostic clues	Diagnostic technique
Apnea or unresponsive spell	Frequent and repetitive Outside of usual age >6 mo of age Blood from mouth or nose, petechiae or bruising of the face or neck	Video monitoring Interview eyewitnesses
Vomiting	Episodic, recurrent—resolves rapidly	Toxicology studies, CK, aldolase, echocardiogram
Diarrhea	Episodic, recurrent—resolves rapidly	Toxicology studies
Seizures	Unresponsive to multiple anticonvulsants Frequent toxicity on medications	Video monitoring and epilepsy monitoring Interview eyewitnesses
Central nervous system depression	Child appears drugged, resolves in 12–24 hr	Toxicology studies

Video Monitoring

Video monitoring without the patient's and parents' permission is being used increasingly. Although the ethical and legal issues surrounding privacy are complex, many hospitals believe the benefits to the child outweigh the violation of privacy. When abuse is documented, the videotaped evidence is very powerful in protecting the child. In our institution, the MSBP team has felt that there should be objective findings establishing "reasonable suspicion" of life-threatening abuse before videotaping is used. Approximately one-third of these videotapes have revealed abuse within 24 hours. In cases where the videotape was not positive for abuse, the child's safety in the hospital was ensured while further assessment and investigation was being completed. Protocols for videotaping should insist on continuous monitoring so that abuse can be interrupted in 20 seconds or less. An alternative to videotaping is separation of the child and perpetrator for a trial period, either by appealing to the family for voluntary separation by placing the child in a one-on-one nursing situation, or convincing the department of social services and a juvenile court judge to place the child outside the home. Although these techniques can confirm the suspicion of MSBP, in our experience, courts are less accepting of this evidence, and long-term protection of the child is difficult. Without firm evidence, there often seems to be a concern on the part of the courts that the child may have had an undiagnosed illness that happened to resolve spontaneously at the same time the child was removed from the family.

Toxicology/Laboratory Studies

When poisoning is suspected, it is helpful to know what is the likely agent. Medications prescribed for the child or family members, and over-the-counter medicines, should be considered. A list of agents and their presenting clinical features in MSBP cases has been published (6). All available body fluids—blood, vomitus, stools, and urine—should be collected and stored for analysis. The clinician can then consult with a toxicologist about the symptoms and likely agents, and send the specimens for appropriate testing. Searching the child's hospital room and family belongings is controversial, but often

rewarding, and the MSBP team should establish a policy regarding searches. Law enforcement personnel on the MSBP team can attempt to obtain a search warrant for the hospital room. When there is blood in stool or vomitus, it can be typed and compared with the patient's and suspected perpetrator's blood types. Other laboratory test results such as hypernatremia may suggest salt poisoning or water restriction or, in the case of hyponatremia, forced water drinking. In the previously mentioned syrup of ipecac case, the muscle enzymes (creatinine kinase and aldolase) were elevated and an echocardiogram was abnormal. This type of supportive information can be helpful, as a toxicology study to detect syrup of ipecac takes several weeks to process.

CONFRONTATION

Attention needs to be given to how to confront the perpetrator. At the time of the confrontation, in most cases the attending physician and social worker should meet with the suspected perpetrator alone. Other family members can be involved later. If in the opinion of the police a crime has been committed, the perpetrator is taken to police headquarters for questioning. A safety plan needs to be addressed for the perpetrator because suicide has been reported after confrontation.

DISCHARGE PLANNING

The child abuse specialist and MSBP team need to work with the department of social services to develop a discharge plan for the child and family. Long-term follow-up by the provider and social service worker is essential. There needs to be close coordination with a mental health provider skilled in MSBP cases. Prognosis is guarded. Suggestions for long-term management and criteria for reunification are available (7).

SUMMARY

MSBP requires a complete paradigm shift for the medical staff. The perpetrator, usually the mother, is no longer the child's greatest advocate, no longer has the child's best interest at heart, and no longer is an important part of the health care team, but in fact has become the child's biggest enemy and the physician's worse nightmare. Recognizing the characteristics of the typical perpetrator, thoroughly investigating a suspect history, and use of the MSBP team can lead to the correct diagnosis and rapid protection of the child.

Acknowledgment

The author wishes to acknowledge the role of J. T. Moser, Associate Director of the Department of Risk Management of Wake Forest University Baptist Medical Center, for developing the Hospital Protocol for Management of Suspected Münchausen Syndrome by Proxy.

References

1. Meadow R. Münchausen syndrome by proxy: the hinterland of child abuse. *Lancet* 1997;2:343–345.
2. Rosenberg DA. Web of deceit: a literature review of Münchausen syndrome by proxy. *Child Abuse Negl* 1987;11:547–563.
3. Donald T, Jureidini J, Munchausen Syndrome by Proxy. *Arch Pediatr Adolise* 1996;150:753–758.
4. McClure RJ, Davis PM, Meadow SR, et al. Epidemiology of Munchausen syndrome by proxy, non-accidental poisoning and non-accidental suffocation. *Arch Dis Child* 1996;75:57–61.
5. Bools CN, Neale BA, Meadows SR. Co-morbidity associated with fabricated illness (Münchausen syndrome by proxy). *Arch Dis Child* 1992;67: 77–79.
6. Henretig F. The deliberately p0oisoned child. In: Levin AV, Sheridan MS, eds. *Münchausen Syndrome by proxy.* New York: Lexington Books; 1995: 143–160.
7. Schreier HA, Libow JA. Management of MSBP. In: *Hurting for love: Münchausen syndrome by proxy.* New York: Guilford Press; 1993:201–220.

Suggested Readings

Levin AV, Sheridan MS. *Münchausen syndrome by proxy.* New York: Lexington Books; 1995

Meadow R. What is and is not, Münchausen syndrome by proxy? *Arch Dis Child* 1995;70:534–537.

Schreier HA, Libow JA. The perversion of mothering: the damages of being ignored. In: *Hurting for love: Münchausen syndrome by proxy.* New York: Guilford Press; 1993:83–102.

Siegel PT, Fischer H. Münchausen by proxy syndrome: barriers to detection, confirmation, and intervention. *Children' Services: Social Policy Research and Practice* 2001;4:31–50.

Whelan-Williams S, Baker TD. A multidisciplinary hospital response protocol. In: Parnell TF, Day DO, eds. *Münchausen by proxy syndrome.* Thousand Oaks, California: Sage; 1998:253–264.

CHAPTER 140 ■ THE PEDIATRICIAN IN COURT: TESTIMONY IN CHILD ABUSE CASES

BETTY S. SPIVACK

Many physicians fear and dread the prospect of court testimony. They feel, and rightly so, that neither medical school nor residency training has prepared them for the courtroom experience. Although fear of the unfamiliar is understandable, physicians may enhance their presentation in court by following some simple rules (see Table 140.1).

RULE 1: UNDERSTAND THE LEGAL SETTING

All testimony is not the same. Child abuse cases frequently involve both civil and criminal courts. Standards of proof generally differ in these types of proceedings.

Civil courts decide issues of child custody, adjudication of abuse or neglect, requirements for possible reunification, and termination of parental rights. The name given such courts differs from state to state and may be called family court, dependency court, juvenile court, district court, or something else. Generally the prosecutor in such cases is either an attorney employed by the child protection agency, or a state or county attorney. The parents or legal guardians will have attorneys, and often one will be appointed to represent the interests of the child as well. The standard of proof in civil courts is generally *a preponderance of the evidence*. This means that abuse or neglect is more likely to have occurred than not. In most cases, it is not necessary to prove that the parents or guardians inflicted the abuse themselves, merely that it occurred and they failed to protect the child. If the court determines that abuse or neglect occurred, it will decide on remedies to ensure the protection of the child. There may be several hearings in the same case; hearings on temporary custody, adjudication of abuse or neglect charges, and termination of parental rights, if no progress has been made toward reunification in a reasonable period of time. A physician's testimony may be preserved from one hearing type to another within civil court; this would permit testifying once rather than twice or three times. Nevertheless, on occasion, physicians may find themselves testifying in more than one of these hearings. If this situation arises, the physician should make an opportunity to review prior testimony.

Criminal court decides issues relating to punishment for crime. Once again, the name of the trial court will differ from state to state and may be circuit court, superior court, or something else. The prosecutor may be called a district attorney, state's attorney, attorney general, or something else. The criminal defendant will have an attorney, but generally no other attorneys will be present. The general standard of proof in criminal cases is *proof beyond a reasonable doubt*. This does not mean beyond all doubt, but that there is no reasonable basis to doubt that a crime has occurred, and that the defendant has committed the crime. In this case, the identity of the perpetrator is important, rather than merely proving that abuse has occurred.

In some states, criminal indictments are made by *grand juries*. In testimony before a grand jury, there is no cross-examination. Nevertheless, the physician is testifying under oath and should be just as careful about the accuracy of testimony as in any other legal setting.

On rare occasions, a civil or criminal trial may have a *Daubert hearing* where a judge decides whether one or more types of scientific evidence can be presented in court. In such a hearing, questions are asked about the scientific rigor and reliability of the underlying data. Important information includes publication in peer-reviewed journals, adherence to general principles of scientific research, and ability to estimate degree of error or reliability. Sometimes epidemiologic data is characterized as anecdotal rather than scientific. It is important to state that populations, cohorts, and case-control studies can generate standard deviations, 95% probability limits, and correlation coefficients that adequately indicate the degree of reliability and susceptibility to error. Physicians called to testify in a Daubert hearing should bring as much of the relevant scientific literature as is feasible.

RULE 2: UNDERSTAND THE PHYSICIAN'S ROLE

All witnesses are not the same. Some are *fact witnesses*, and testify only to what they observed or did. Other witnesses may be *expert witnesses*; expert witnesses may express their opinions within the area of their expertise. What makes someone an expert, for the purposes of court testimony? In general, an expert has, by virtue of training or experience, knowledge that may assist the court or jury in understanding the issues of the case. In many states, any licensed physician can be accepted as an expert without the publication of articles or status as faculty of a medical school. However, any additional expertise may cause the judge or jury to give more credence to an expert's opinions. Expert witnesses should provide the court with a copy of complete, up-to-date, and accurate curriculum vitae.

Upon receiving a subpoena, the physician needs clarification as to whether testimony will be as a fact witness or as an expert. If testifying as a fact witness, comments will be restricted to only what was seen or done. Opinions about

TABLE 140.1

TWELVE RULES FOR COURTROOM PRESENTATION

1. Understand the legal setting.
2. Understand the physician's role.
3. Know the case.
4. Review the relevant literature.
5. Prepare the attorney.
6. Bring relevant materials.
7. Be prepared to wait.
8. Listen carefully to the questions.
9. Be prepared to teach.
10. Be aware of cross-examination techniques.
11. Wait for rulings by the judge.
12. Be polite but firm.

diagnoses or other elements of the case will not be sought or allowed. This occurs only rarely. More typically, treating physicians are called as expert witnesses. They are asked whether they have an opinion as to the cause of the child's condition, and what that opinion is. In most states, the standard for forming such an opinion is a *reasonable degree of medical certainty*. This means the physician has considered possible alternatives and thinks them unlikely given the circumstances of this case.

Physicians who are fact witnesses must have had direct contact with the case. However, expert witnesses need not have been treating physicians. They may be retained by prosecution or defense to review the case materials and offer their opinions. The standards for testimony in either case should be the same. Expert witnesses are supposed to lend their professional expertise toward enhancing the ability of judge or jury to decide the issues at hand. They should not be advocates for either prosecution or defense; that is the role of the attorneys in the case.

RULE 3: KNOW THE CASE

A physician called to testify in a case with direct professional involvement should review all relevant records. In the setting of testimony in a case as a consultant, the same rule applies–all relevant records should be reviewed. This should also include review of x-rays, photographs, or other material relevant to the case. The physician who knows dates, names, and other details of the case will be much more credible than one who has to search through endless reams of paper to answer each question.

RULE 4: REVIEW THE RELEVANT LITERATURE

It is important to review the literature relevant to the case before testifying. The testifying physician must be aware of papers that support or contradict any stated conclusions. Disagreement with published papers may be appropriate, but as an expert, testimony should include reasons for that disagreement.

RULE 5: PREPARE THE ATTORNEY

The attorney must understand the case as well as the testifying physician does. This should include a discussion between the physician and the attorney prior to going to court, ascertaining that the attorney understands the conclusions about abuse/neglect and the underlying reasons. The attorney should be provided copies of the important articles supporting

any position. This is also an opportunity to share with the attorney any opinions about shortcomings of the opposing points of view.

RULE 6: BRING RELEVANT MATERIALS

The physician should take to court all appropriate reports and notes along with any other materials provided by the attorney or subpoenaed by the court. This should include an updated curriculum vitae and copies of any articles provided to the attorney. Tab markers placed in important places may help find information rapidly. Because the opposing attorney may ask to see anything brought to the witness stand, any confidential information that has not been subject to subpoena or provided by the attorney should be left in the office.

RULE 7: BE PREPARED TO WAIT

For many physicians, the most frustrating part of courtroom testimony is waiting to testify. Most physicians have busy schedules with little flexibility. Attorneys are generally cognizant of this and sympathetic. A discussion with the attorney about a specific time for testimony may result in the least conflict with schedules. The subpoena will generally state the time the trial begins, but the attorney may not even want testimony until later in the trial or hearing. Often, they will arrange for a physician to be "on call" for court. In this way, waiting time in the courtroom may be minimized. Nevertheless, the physician should be prepared to wait, and also be prepared for testimony to take longer than the attorney predicted.

RULE 8: LISTEN CAREFULLY TO THE QUESTIONS

When placed on the stand, the first rule for the testifying physician should be to slow down. Let the attorney finish the question before beginning a response. Words should be chosen carefully. Do not shade the truth. If the answer to a question isn't known, the physician should simply say so. If the question isn't clear, the physician should request that it be repeated or restated. If a question cannot be answered in the manner requested, this should be clearly communicated to the court. Alternatively, if asked for an explanation, it can be as full and complete as necessary. In general, the testifying physician should remember that the audience (jurors and court officials) have little scientific training. Things should be explained at the level that is used to explain a medical condition to a parent. Try to avoid medical jargon, or explain it in simpler words immediately after. For example, "He had a fractured femur—a broken thigh bone." In this manner, medical vocabulary used by other witnesses or in the medical records can be restated, but in terms that still make sense to a jury or judge with little medical expertise.

RULE 9: BE PREPARED TO TEACH

When called as an expert witness, because of training and/or experience, the physician has an understanding of issues in a case exceeding that of the general population. The physician needs to impart this information in a manner that enables the judge or jury to come to a reasonable conclusion about the evidence. In other words, the physician needs to be a teacher. Testimony should consist of simple, understandable language, which relates to everyday experience. For example, analogy to a boxing match can explain how the lack of a bruise does not mean that no impact occurred. Comparison of the folded structure of the anus to an accordion file can help a jury understand why anal intercourse might leave few or no permanent findings. It is very important for the physician on the stand to not be perceived as arrogant or patronizing. Responses should be addressed to the jurors, and their reactions watched to ascertain boredom or puzzlement as a guide in further testimony.

RULE 10: BE AWARE OF CROSS-EXAMINATION TECHNIQUES

Direct examination should be a well-choreographed dance. The physician and the attorney who subpoenaed the physician should both be aware of what points need to be made. The attorney will ask questions in a manner that allows the presentation and explanation of this information. Cross-examination, on the other hand, is used to attack credibility in general or specific points of testimony. In order to do this, the opposing attorney will use several types of tactics.

First, this attorney will attempt to minimize the expertise of the testifying physician. If the case involves abusive fractures, and the testimony is from a pediatrician, the expert may be asked whether he or she is a radiologist or an orthopedist. The appropriate response is for the witness to readily and politely acknowledge that he or she is not. The opposing attorney would do the same thing to any such witness; he would ask a radiologist whether she was an orthopedist or a pediatrician. Such questioning implies a lack of training in recognizing or classifying broken bones. If the attorney is unwise enough to state this explicitly, for example, "So doctor, you have no training in identifying rib fractures," a response about training in medical school and during residency in recognition of pediatric fractures is appropriate. Physicians with additional training, such as attendance at conferences, literature study, and work experiences related to these issues should say so. If the question is not asked explicitly with the concomitant opportunity for the expert to explain her training in interpreting fracture patterns, the attorney who called the witness will usually provide that opportunity during *redirect examination*.

The cross-examining attorney will often attack the physician witness's motives for being present at court. Generally, this will start with a question about payment for testimony. The implication, of course, is that the witness is saying what she was paid to say. If the witness is receiving an expert witness fee, it should be acknowledged in the context of reimbursing for time and expertise, but explicitly not for specific testimony. Sometimes an attorney will ask whether pediatricians have a vested interest in diagnosing child abuse. Although laughable, the expert should note the many pressures to not to make such a diagnosis, including allowing the witness to not have to be present in court.

Expert witnesses in child abuse cases are often asked whether a textbook, journal, or scientific paper is *authoritative*. The answer to this is always "No," even if it is the best book, journal, or paper on a subject. Calling something "authoritative" in the courtroom means that every word, phrase, sentence, and conclusion is inarguably correct. Science doesn't work that way, and this should be stated. The witness may, however, state *reliance upon* the data in the paper in reaching conclusions.

Another courtroom gambit is to ask the expert to read a highlighted section from a textbook or paper, often taken out of context. If the witness doesn't know the work, this should be stated. If the cited report is known to the witness and the highlighted section is not representative of the conclusions of the author, the witness should indicate that it is taken out of context. The judge will rule on whether the witness is to be allowed to complete a paragraph to highlight the intended meaning. Even if the bench rules against this, the attorney who called the witness should generally provide an opportunity to clarify the point during redirect examination. Opposing attorneys often ask questions about a hypothetical situation. For example: "Doctor, are there any other reasons a child might have a fractured femur?" The witness should feel free to agree, and then list the many situations where this might occur. At some point, the attorney will jump from the hypothetical to the actual case. At this point, the witness will need to identify why the answer to the hypothetical situation does not apply to the case at hand.

The attorney will attempt to ask questions that allow only "yes" or "no" responses. If it is not possible, the expert should say so. The judge may allow answers to be framed in a different format or even to a restated question. If the judge does not allow that leeway, the attorney who called the witness should provide that opportunity during redirect examination.

RULE 11: WAIT FOR RULINGS BY THE JUDGE

Whenever there is an objection from any attorney, the witness should wait for the judge to rule. The question may not need to be answered. If the judge overrules the objection, the witness may ask for the question to be repeated.

RULE 12: BE POLITE BUT FIRM

It is important for the witness to remain polite and professional on the stand, even when the witness's knowledge and integrity have been questioned. It is important to maintain the respect of the judge and jurors by responding with an appropriate measured professional demeanor and carefully chosen words to sometimes deliberately provocative questions or statements. Finally it is important to avoid jokes about people or situations related to the case.

Sometimes it is difficult for a witness in such a situation to maintain his composure. It may be helpful to have a glass of water available. Often one is present at the witness stand. If not, the witness should ask for one before testimony begins. Alternatively, if the witness has been on the stand for a period of time, a request for a brief recess to go to the lavatory may be appropriate. Either of these strategies may give the witness an opportunity to regain control of emotions and prepare for the remainder of the testimony.

SUMMARY

Although court testimony can be an unnerving experience, a physician witness—whether fact or expert—should try to approach the court proceedings with some degree of calm. Whatever the role, the witness should remember that he or she is there on behalf of the child, not for the prosecution or the defense. Accordingly, all testimony should be honest and impartial. And it is important for the witness, especially in criminal proceeding, to remember that it is not the witness's duty to obtain a conviction, only to provide the best possible evidence and opinions. Providing needed information to the court or jury that can assist it in reaching decisions extends the role of the physician.

CHAPTER 141 ■ GENERAL PRINCIPLES OF NUTRITIONAL ASSESSMENT

KRISTIN J. BROWN AND JOHN M. OLSSON

Nutritional assessment of the pediatric patient involves interpretation of data divided into five major categories: anthropometric, physical, laboratory data, as well as social and dietary history. There is no single marker for assessment of nutritional status at this time, and health care professionals must evaluate information from each of these categories to determine nutritional status and develop a plan of care. This chapter's intent is briefly to review these categories and discuss ongoing controversies in interpretation. Children with special health care needs often require intensive nutrition therapy, and therefore some of this population's unique nutritional needs are discussed in summary.

ANTHROPOMETRIC DATA

Accurate gathering of anthropometric data is essential. The standard data collected on admission should include weight, length/height, abdominal girth, and head circumference. Children older than 3 years of age do not require abdominal girth and head circumference measurements unless clinically indicated. Standard growth charts are available from the National Center for Health Statistics and the National Center for Chronic Disease Prevention and Health Promotion (www.cdc.gov/growthcharts). These tools allow the health care professional to compare each patient measurement with those of the general population of this country and to track growth patterns over time. Each measurement is best used when it is evaluated in relation to the other anthropometric measurements. For example, weight for age is useful, but when the weight-to-length ratio is reviewed concurrently, the two together give a greater understanding of the growth characteristics of the child. Length (supine) is recorded for children up to age 2 years, whereas height (standing) is recorded for older children and adolescents. The weight-to-length ratio is recorded for infants and toddlers, whereas the body mass index (BMI) and weight-to-height ratio are used for children older than 2 years of age:

$$BMI = Weight\ (kg)/Height\ (m)^2$$

It is of particular importance to assess serial growth measurements whenever possible; growth history is a key factor in nutritional assessment. Many infants move into different age-specific growth percentiles over time, changes that may be determined by genetic potential and nutritional support. Assessing patterns of all anthropometric measurements is useful. For example, in undernourished children the weight percentiles will slow first, then length, and last of all the rate of growth of head circumference. Additional nutrition support via enteral or parenteral routes may enable a child to grow along a given percentile; this growth pattern may be different from genetic potential, and therefore care must be taken when weaning nutrition support to set appropriate and individualized nutritional goals. Consideration must also be given to patients whose anthropometrics indicate obesity. Selecting an adjusted body weight on which to base pharmacologic and nutritional decisions is of great importance in the acute-care setting. There are several methods available; however, a widely utilized calculation for adolescents is:

$$[(ABW - IBW) \times 0.25] + IBW = Adjusted\ Body\ Weight$$

where ABW is the actual body weight and IBW is the ideal body weight. Ideal body weight is the 50th percentile weight for the child's height as noted on the standard pediatric weight-for-height chart.

Some infants and children have medical conditions with special health care needs that affect their growth pattern and warrant the use of specific growth charts. Such growth charts include, but are not limited to, those for children with prematurity, low or very low birthweight, cerebral palsy, Down syndrome, and Prader–Willi syndrome (http://depts.washington.edu/growth/cshcn/text/page6a.htm). There also are growth charts specific for race and ethnic background. An extensive medical evaluation for failure to thrive may be avoided by plotting anthropometric data on appropriate growth charts and by accounting for prematurity. Additional measurements, such as midarm circumference, midarm muscle circumference, and triceps skinfold, may be useful to assess muscle and adipose tissue stores in children with special health care needs. Because using the triceps skinfold is controversial, caution should be taken in interpreting results from a single measurement. Although there are standard techniques for obtaining measurements such as triceps skinfold, application of these techniques may vary slightly between clinicians, which in turn may lead to a wide range of results. These types of measurements can only be helpful in monitoring body composition if the same experienced individual is able to obtain serial measurements for a given child.

PHYSICAL EXAMINATION DATA

The physical assessment should focus on identifying potential anomalies related to energy, protein, vitamin, and mineral deficiencies. Particular findings on examination may suggest nutrient deficiencies or toxicities (Table 141.1). Some children may present with abnormal growth patterns resulting from a change in nutritional intake, energy expenditure,

TABLE 141.1

PHYSICAL EXAMINATION FINDINGS ASSOCIATED WITH DEFICIENCY AND TOXICITY OF ESSENTIAL NUTRIENTS[a]

Nutrient	Deficiency (inadequate nutrient)	Toxicity (excessive nutrient)
Carbohydrate	Ketosis	Obesity, diarrhea, dental caries
Protein	Edema, easy hair pluckability, skin degradation, poor wound healing, lymphopenia, impaired immune function, fatty liver, growth retardation	Acidosis, azotemia, hyperammonemia
Fat	Poor growth, poor wound healing, eczema, hair loss	Obesity, coronary artery disease, cancer, abnormal lipid panel
Vitamin A	Growth retardation, retinal degeneration, hyperkeratosis, Bitot spots, follicular hyperkeratosis, night blindness	Hair loss, dry itchy skin, jaundice, fatigue, bone pain, abdominal pain, headache, hepatomegaly, vomiting, hypercalcemia
Vitamin D	Osteomalacia, rickets	Impaired renal function, hypercalcemia, anorexia, impaired growth, emesis
Vitamin E	Retinopathy, neuropathy, increased hemolysis, myopathy, peripheral neuropathy	Impairs normal physiologic response of iron; may interfere with vitamin K activity
Vitamin K	Hemorrhages, cirrhosis, prolonged clotting, ecchymoses, petechiae	Hemolytic anemia, kernicterus
Ascorbic acid (C)	Scurvy, inadequate wound healing, joint tenderness, capillary hemorrhaging, gingivitis, petechiae	Increased uric acid excretion, gastrointestinal distress
Thiamin (B_1)	Beriberi, cardiac failure, edema, anorexia, increased intracranial pressure, confusion, neuropathy, muscle tenderness	None known
Riboflavin (B_2)	Photophobia, itchy eyes, cheilosis, glossitis, scrotal skin changes, seborrheic dermatitis	None known
Niacin (B_3)	Pellagra, apathy, cheilosis, angular stomatitis, anorexia, peripheral neuropathy, encephalopathy, diarrhea, dermatitis	Dilation of the capillaries (flushing), tingling, dizziness, nausea, diarrhea
Pyridoxine (B_6)	Microcytic hypochromic anemia with high serum iron, weakness, convulsions, depression, oxalate stone formation, nervousness, insomnia, glossitis, stomatitis, cheilosis	Sensory neuropathy, progressive ataxia
Cyanocobalamin (B_{12})	Megaloblastic anemia, leukopenia, thrombocytopenia, neurologic deterioration, stomatitis, glossitis	None known
Folic acid	Megaloblastic anemia, leukopenia, thrombocytopenia, poor growth, glossitis, stomatitis, diarrhea, malabsorption	None known
Biotin	Anorexia, nausea, vomiting, glossitis, depression, hypercholesterolemia, insomnia, dermatitis, thin hair	None known
Pantothenic acid	Infertility, abortion, slow growth, depression, vomiting, fatigue, abdominal distress, insomnia, muscle cramps, burning/tingling feet	Diarrhea, water retention, hemochromatosis, hemosiderosis
Iron	Hypochromic microcytic anemia, malabsorption, irritability, tachycardia, anorexia, pallor, lethargy, koilonychia	Vomiting, sweating, dizziness, copper deficiency
Zinc	Decreased wound healing, decreased growth, diarrhea, hypogonadism, mild anemia, decreased taste acuity, decreased cellular immunity, rash	Nausea, vomiting, headache, diarrhea, cramping, Wilson disease, anemia
Copper	Hemolytic microcytic anemia, neutropenia, Menkes syndrome	Neuropsychiatric disorders in very high doses
Manganese	Impaired growth, skeletal anomalies, neonatal ataxia, poor reproductive function, defects in fat and carbohydrate metabolism	Hair loss, brittle nails, fatigue, irritability, tooth decay, peripheral neuropathy
Selenium	Cardiomyopathy, nail changes, myalgia, muscle tenderness	Thyroid enlargement
Iodine	Endemic goiter, hypothyroidism, cretinism	
Chromium	Hyperglycemia, negative nitrogen balance, impaired growth, peripheral neuropathy, increased low-density lipoprotein cholesterol	None known
Fluoride	Dental caries	Mottling of teeth
Molybdenum	None known	Gout-like symptoms, antagonist to copper

[a]Arsenic, boron, nickel, silicon, and vanadium are ultratrace elements. There are inadequate reports to define deficiencies and toxicities for inclusion in this table.

TABLE 141.2

GENERAL GASTROINTESTINAL SECRETION AND
ABSORPTION SITES

Site	Secretion	Absorption
Mouth/ esophagus	Salivary amylase	Carbohydrate
Stomach	Gastric lipase Pepsin Hydrochloric acid Intrinsic factor	Alcohol
Duodenum	Pancreatic enzymes Bicarbonate Bile	Iron Chloride Sulfate Calcium Magnesium
Jejunum	Intestinal brush border enzymes	Glucose, galactose, fructose Vitamin C Thiamin Riboflavin Pyridoxine Folic acid
Ileum	None	Protein Vitamins A, D, E, K Vitamin B_{12} Fat Cholesterol Bile salts Sodium Potassium
Colon	None	Vitamin K (formed by bacterial action) Water
Rectum/anus	None	

DIAGNOSTIC/BIOCHEMICAL DATA

There is no single laboratory test for malnutrition, and therefore the clinician must rely on several biochemical indicators to help determine nutritional status. The analysis of serum protein levels such as albumin, prealbumin, retinol-binding protein, and transferrin, along with bone minerals, is a reasonable screening process for malnutrition. Each of these laboratory values is affected by the function of certain organ systems, and normal values may vary by laboratory. Renal or liver disease, infection, dialysis, altered nutrient intake, and catabolism all affect serum protein values. Albumin is a serum protein that functions as a transport protein and as a determinant of oncotic pressure. Its half-life of 14 to 20 days makes it useful as a screening tool for chronic undernutrition, but not as useful in acute malnutrition. Transthyretin, or prealbumin, with a half-life of 2 to 3 days, is suited to assess trends in response to acute changes in therapy. Transferrin (half-life of 8 to 10 days) is a sensitive indicator of iron balance as well as visceral protein status. Because it is affected by inflammation, infection, catabolism, hepatic or renal disease, state of hydration, iron deficiency, and pregnancy, it is not a good single indicator of protein status.

Retinol-binding protein is more sensitive than albumin and transferrin to changes in protein intake or to metabolic stress, although care should be taken in interpreting its value in patients with renal failure or possible vitamin A and zinc deficiencies. C-reactive protein is indicative of inflammatory response and may help in distinguishing acute inflammation from nutritional deficiency in the evaluation of serum protein values.

Urine studies also are useful in determining the appropriateness of the nutrition care plan. Creatinine-height index is used to estimate lean body mass and to screen for malnutrition. The creatinine level from a 24-hour urine collection is compared with those of reference children of similar age, height, and sex. Difficulties encountered with this diagnostic tool are the accuracy of urine collection and skewing of normal values by data from patients with compromised renal status, patients in catabolic states, patients with abnormal thyroid function, unusual activity levels, or abnormal dietary intake of protein. Assessment of urine electrolytes and osmolarity can also help identify the source of growth anomalies.

Nitrogen balance studies are a useful diagnostic tool to monitor adequate protein supply in hypercatabolic patients. In the acute state, it may be difficult to determine the actual amount of protein needed to maintain a zero or positive nitrogen balance. Zero nitrogen balance occurs when the amount of nitrogen (e.g., protein) consumed equals the amount that the body is currently excreting. A positive nitrogen balance indicates that protein provision is ample for growth and tissue repair. Complicating nitrogen balance studies is the need to account for the nitrogen excreted in other systems (wounds, ostomy output, feces), and for altered excretion in patients with renal insufficiency. Most facilities have the ability to run a standard nitrogen balance and possibly a total urinary nitrogen study.

Indirect calorimetry (sometimes referred to as a *metabolic cart study*) uses measures of heat and oxygen consumption in comparison with carbon dioxide output to determine the basal metabolic rate (BMR) or resting energy expenditure (REE). This may be useful for children with complicated problems that have not responded to administration of previously calculated caloric estimates. The BMR is a measure only of the energy expended in a resting state, and does not include energy used in storage or growth, or lost in excretion. The limitation of this diagnostic tool is that it is a snapshot of the energy expenditure during the 30-minute study, whereas

metabolism, or absorption of nutrients. This may occur because of individual or cultural preferences, or as a result of acquired physical disabilities. Physical limitations may be as obvious as those associated with surgical interventions, or they may be as subtle as enzyme deficiencies. During the physical exam, presence of ascites; enlarged organ size; abnormal hair, nail, or skin quality; reflexes; tone; dentition and mucosa; and bone age or density can all help in interpretation of nutritional status.

Vitamin deficiencies often are associated with malfunction of specific absorption sites in the gastrointestinal tract, either as a result of physical manipulation or faulty enzymatic processes. Table 141.2 outlines the general secretion and absorption sites in each section of the gastrointestinal tract. The boundaries of secretion and absorption are not discrete, and labeled areas may overlap.

Children with special health care needs are particularly at risk for nutritional toxicities or deficiencies; aggressive identification and treatment of these is essential for achievement of full growth potential. Children with chronic medications including, but not limited to, anticonvulsants, anticoagulants, steroids, diuretics, or narcotics should be regularly evaluated for anomalies due to medication interactions. Children with intestinal resections, liver disease, chronic inflammatory states, allergies, renal diagnoses, or lymphatic involvement are at higher risk for vitamin and mineral deficiencies and toxicities.

TABLE 141.3

ESTIMATED ENERGY REQUIREMENTS, INFANTS TO YOUNG ADULTS

Category	Age (yr)	Reference weight (kg)	REE[a] (kcal/kg)	RDA[b] (kcal/kg)	Energy (kcal/day)
Infants	0.0–0.5	6	55	108	650
	0.5–1.0	9	55	98	850
Children	1–3	13	55	102	1,300
	4–6	20	45	90	1,800
	7–10	28	40	70	2,000
Males	11–14	45	30	55	2,500
	15–18	66	25	45	3,000
	19–24	72	25	40	2,900
Females	11–14	46	30	47	2,200
	15–18	55	25	40	2,200
	19–24	58	25	38	2,200

[a]REE, resting energy expenditure computed from WHO equations.
[b]From *Recommended Dietary Allowances*. 10th ed. Washington, DC: National Academy Press; 1989.

temperature, activity, stress, neuromuscular blockade, respiratory status, dialysis, and even feeding routes can alter the child's moment-to-moment energy expenditure. Careful documentation of the patient's clinical status and treatments at the time of the test can help to provide the clinician with a better analysis. General estimates of a patient's caloric requirement, if a measurement of REE is not available, are found in pediatric nutrition references. See Table 141.3 for estimates of caloric requirements for children, birth through young adulthood.

DIET AND SOCIAL HISTORY

The dietary history helps identify eating habits, composition of meals, food intolerances, allergies, cravings, cultural influences, and medication or nutrient supplementation of a child. A food recall history often is useful for identifying grossly abnormal intakes. This method usually is a good indicator of quality of food eaten, but the quantity of portions usually is subjective. It is important to ask not only what the child is eating, but how it is prepared. For example, the cause of undernutrition may be as simple as the dilution of formula with extra water, or the addition of large volumes of rice cereal, which displace the nutrient-rich formula. In an older child, evaluation of the beverages the child drinks may reveal the source of excess weight gain. Food jags (e.g., eating macaroni and cheese for every meal) or picky eating may trigger an investigation into possible vitamin and mineral deficiencies. Food may be a comfort for a depressed or emotionally abused child.

With the wide use of herbal supplements and super-dosing of vitamins and minerals in the adult population, it seems prudent to inquire about these items when taking a pediatric diet history. These products may provide a desirable effect, although there is little medical literature on proper dosing, and product purity often is questionable. Herbal supplements also may interfere with prescribed medications. Dosing mishaps may occur when a patient is prescribed a larger dose of a specific vitamin while in the hospi-

tal, and the family does not realize that it is intended for short-term use only, so that the child presents with physical signs of toxicity at a follow-up visit.

A careful developmental assessment should be part of the dietary history. An infant or child's developmental level determines both the types of foods she can eat, as well as her feeding skills. Nutritional supplements may be required if the child is not able to consume an age-appropriate diet (Table 141.4).

The social history, also a very important part of the nutritional assessment, should identify potential neglect, evaluate the parenting skills of the primary caregivers, and determine any financial strains on the family. Medical plans will fail if the family is not able to provide the recommended nutritional intervention. It should be kept in mind that many children today are effectively their own caregivers owing to parents' work schedules. Special consideration may need to be given to identifying high-quality nutritional resources, safe cooking facilities, governmental assistance (e.g., WIC or AFDC), and community resources for safe food and exercise opportunities. Social work and discharge planning professionals are essential in assisting children and their families in meeting these needs.

CHILDREN WITH SPECIAL HEALTH CARE NEEDS

Children with various diagnoses fall under the umbrella of "special health care needs." These children may have special needs because of congenital anomalies or acquired disorders, and may require more than the general pediatric plan of care. A good nutritional assessment can help identify these patients for intervention. Special health care needs children often present with atypical growth patterns or delay in mastering developmental milestones. For example, unexplained weight loss or growth failure and delayed gross motor skills may be seen in children with cystic fibrosis, celiac disease, bronchopulmonary dysplasia, and seizure disorders. Conversely,

TABLE 141.4

DEVELOPMENTAL STAGES OF FEEDING FROM BIRTH TO 3 YEARS

Gestational age	Foods	Skills
Birth to 4 mo	Breast milk or infant formula	Appropriate latch-on to breast with good suck and swallow mechanism Hand to mouth while holding object
4–6 mo	Breast milk or formula Iron-fortified baby cereal (optional)	Head and neck control Sitting with support Can hold bottle independently
6–8 mo	Breast milk or formula Iron-fortified baby cereal: 4–8 tbsp[a] Bread: offer Crackers: 2[a] Fruit: 4–6 tbsp[a] Fruit juice: 3 oz from cup[a] Vegetables: 4–6 tbsp[a]	Finger feeding initiated Hold handled cup
8–12 mo	Add: Cheese, yogurt, cottage cheese Chicken, beef, pork Cooked, dried beans or egg yolks	Finger feeding independently Early spoon to mouth Holds cup with some spilling Mechanically altered textures
12–24 mo	Add: Whole milk Cereal, pasta, rice, muffins Whole fruits and vegetables Fish, turkey Egg	Independent scooping of food to mouth with spoon Drinks entirely from cup Increased textures Food jags Preferences Booster chair
24–36 mo	Full diet	Feeds independently with utensil, palm up Pours liquids from small container Early use of fork to stab food

[a]Per-day limit.

examples of lower energy needs populations, with the risk of becoming overweight, include children with Down syndrome, Prader–Willi syndrome, or spina bifida, or children confined to bed or wheelchair. Table 141.5 lists the basal metabolic needs of infants and children. A child's physical activity, muscle tone, stress, and thermal factors must be taken into account when determining total energy needs. Bed rest adds 10% to caloric requirements, whereas light, moderate, and heavy activity call for 30%, 50%, and 75% increases, respectively. Fever requires a 12% increase in calories per degree centigrade elevation. The thermal effect of the digestion of food is thought to account for a 10% increase in caloric expenditure. Bone fractures and traumas can cause a 20% to 40% increase in total caloric expenditure, whereas burns can increase caloric needs by 50% to 100%. These are general guidelines to initiate care; monitoring weight and biochemical data allow fine-tuning of each patient's energy needs.

There are a number of issues that enter into planning for these children's nutritional care:

- The patient's *growth pattern*. The clinician should start with the growth history and the child's individual pattern, comparing it with disease-specific norms if available. Conditions like Down syndrome, Prader–Willi syndrome, cerebral palsy, and spina bifida may not present with standard linear growth, so the weight-to-height ratio becomes more important than weight for age.

- The patient's *skeletal muscle activity*. High muscle tone, seizures, tics, and hyperactivity increase energy expenditure dramatically.

- The patient's *method of feeding*. Patients with a swallowing dysfunction who are fed by mouth may not necessarily have higher energy needs, but may simply be unable to consume enough calories to meet their needs. Feeding tubes or parenteral nutrition may also be used in conjunction with oral feeding for extended lengths of time. Selection of product and route of nutritional support may vary based on the family dynamic to ensure continued compliance.

- *Metabolic anomalies* and *drug/nutrient interactions* may be present in the patient. Once the dysfunctional metabolic process is corrected, children usually regain weight much more efficiently. For example, children with cystic fibrosis need pancreatic enzymes to use dietary fat, children with celiac disease need restriction of gluten to prevent destruction of the intestinal villi, and children on some anticonvulsants need supplemental vitamin D and B-complex vitamins.

- *Environmental factors* may affect the patient, as described in the social history section. Implementation of and compliance

TABLE 141.5

BASAL METABOLIC RATES FOR INFANTS AND CHILDREN

Age 1–10 mo		Age 11–36 mo			Age 3–16 yr		
Weight (kg)	M/F kcal/hr	Weight (kg)	Male kcal/hr	Female kcal/hr	Weight (kg)	Male kcal/hr	Female kcal/hr
3.5	8.4	9.0	22.0	21.2	15	35.8	33.3
4.0	9.5	9.5	22.8	22.0	20	39.7	37.4
4.5	10.5	10.0	23.6	22.8	25	43.6	41.5
5.0	11.6	10.5	24.4	23.6	30	47.5	45.5
5.5	12.7	11.0	25.2	24.4	35	51.3	49.6
6.0	13.8	11.5	26.0	25.2	40	55.2	53.7
6.5	14.9	12.0	26.8	26.0	45	59.1	57.8
7.0	16.0	12.5	27.6	26.9	50	63.0	61.9
7.5	17.1	13.0	28.4	27.7	55	66.9	66.0
8.0	18.2	13.5	29.2	28.5	60	70.8	70.0
8.5	19.3	14.0	30.0	29.3	65	74.7	74.0
9.0	20.4	14.5	30.8	30.1	70	78.6	78.1
9.5	21.4	15.0	31.6	30.9	75	82.5	82.2
10.0	22.5	15.5	32.4	31.7			
10.5	23.6	16.0	33.3	32.6			
11.0	24.7	16.5	34.0	33.4			

From Johnson HL. Energy metabolism at various weights: man. In: Altman PL, Dittmer DS, eds. *Metabolism*. Bethesda: Federation of the American Societies for Experimental Biology; 1998: 344. With permission.

with the care plan can be confirmed by normalizing growth patterns, increased muscle and adipose tissue on subsequent triceps skinfold measurements, improved stool quality, improved biochemical markers, or improved developmental skills.

Suggested Readings

American Academy of Pediatrics. *Pediatric nutrition handbook*. Elk Grove Village, IL: American Academy of Pediatrics; 1993.

American Society of Parenteral and Enteral Nutrition. *Nutritional considerations in the intensive care unit: science, rationale, and practice*. Dubuque, IA: Kendall Hunt; 2002.

American Society of Parenteral and Enteral Nutrition. *The science and practice of nutrition support: a case-based core curriculum*. Dubuque, IA: Kendall Hunt; 2001.

Mahan KL, Escott-Stump S, eds. *Krause's food, nutrition, and diet therapy*. 9th ed. Philadelphia: Saunders; 1996.

Wessel J. Standards for specialized nutrition support: hospitalized pediatric patients. *Nutr Clin Pract* 2005;20:103–116.

Wilmore D. *The metabolic management of the critically ill*. New York: Plenum; 1977.

Zitelli BJ, Davis HW. *Atlas of pediatric physical diagnosis*. 3rd ed. St. Louis: Mosby-Wolfe; 1997.

CHAPTER 142 ■ ENTERAL NUTRITION

SEEMA SINGLA AND JOHN M. OLSSON

Enteral nutrition is defined as the delivery of nutrients by tube to the gastrointestinal (GI) tract. Infants and children who are unwilling or unable to ingest, digest, or absorb an adequate amount of nutrition orally are candidates for enteral nutrition.

Pediatric patients with a variety of diseases are at nutritional risk, and have been shown to benefit from enteral nutritional support (Table 142.1). There are a few contraindications to enteral nutrition, and these include:

■ Necrotizing enterocolitis
■ GI obstruction
■ Intestinal atresia
■ Severe inflammatory bowel disease
■ Severe effects from GI radiation therapy
■ Severe acute pancreatitis

The many commercial infant and pediatric formulas available often make it difficult to decide which formula to use for feeding. Ideally, breast milk is the first choice for feeding both premature and term infants. When breast milk is not available, commercial formulas can be used. Product selection depends on a variety of factors, including the age of the child, the medical condition, GI function, nutrient requirements, feeding route, fluid needs, activity level, any specific allergies, feeding intolerance, formula osmolality or renal solute load, calorie concentration, and formula cost.

SELECTION OF ENTERAL FORMULAS AND INDICATIONS FOR USE

Human Milk

Human milk (Table 142.2) is the preferred source of nutrition for all infants, although the decision to provide breast milk ultimately lies with the mother. Pediatricians and other health care professionals should offer education and encouragement to help a mother decide if breast-feeding is a good choice for her and her infant. Human milk is the gold standard on which all other formulas are modeled and compared. Unlike formula, the composition of human milk varies within a single feeding and throughout the course of lactation. The milk from mothers of preterm infants, especially during the first 2 weeks after delivery, contains higher levels of energy, fat, protein, and sodium, and slightly lower concentrations of lactose, calcium, and phosphorus, compared with milk from mothers of term infants. Use of hind milk, which is higher in fat and calories, may improve weight gain in low birthweight infants fed human milk. When human milk is provided as a tube feeding, it is necessary to follow optimal delivery methods to ensure maximum nutrient delivery. Continuous drip feedings of human milk have been associated with considerable fat losses, as the fat in human milk is not homogenized, which results in calorie deficits. The delivery of essential fatty acids, phospholipids, cholesterol, and fat-soluble vitamins may also be diminished. Ingestion of a large fat bolus when residual milk is flushed causes a problem in tolerance when gastrointestinal function is impaired.

If continous feeding of expressed breast milk is necessary, combining the expressed milk with human milk fortifier (HMF), or other liquid formulas, can promote more efficient delivery of breast milk. In the absence of contraindications, however, intermittent bolus feeding of human milk, in contrast, does not result in significant loss of fat in the tubing, and is therefore the preferred method of delivery for human milk.

Human Milk Fortifiers

Human milk can be fortified by adding commercially available liquid or powdered fortifiers, to provide additional protein, minerals, and vitamins for premature infants (Table 142.3). Details of the clinical condition of the infant, such as prematurity, low birthweight (<1,500 g), low intake of calcium or phosphorus, risk of osteopenia from long-term total parenteral nutrition, or the use of diuretics and steroids, should be considered when HMF is used. The premature infant should continue with fortfied breast milk, if available, until she reaches a weight of 2,000 to 2,500 g. The intake of fortified milk should be monitored after discharge to avoid excessive consumption of nutrients, especially fat-soluble vitamins, as volume increases beyond 360 to 400 mL/day.

Premature Formulas

Premature formulas are specially designed for premature infants to provide the higher calories, protein, electrolytes, and minerals needed to support rapid growth of the preterm infant (Table 142.4). Although these formulas are available with iron-fortified and low-iron options, the American Academy of Pediatrics (AAP) recommends that all infant formulas be fortified with iron (>6.7 mg/100 kcal; 4–12 mg/L). Premature formulas should be continued until the infant reaches a weight of 2,000 to 2,500 g, after which it can be transitioned to discharge formula. The fatty acids docosahexaenoic acid (DHA) and arachidonic acid (ARA) are added to both premature and discharge formulas.

Nutrient-Enriched Discharge Formulas

After hospital discharge, premature infants may have low body stores of nutrients, deficient bone mineralization, and a deficit of accumulated energy (Table 142.5). The use of discharge formula to a postnatal age of 9 months results in greater linear growth, weight gain, and bone mineral content than the use of term formula. No additional supplements are needed, as these formulas are fortified.

TABLE 142.1

INDICATIONS FOR USE OF ENTERAL NUTRITION

DECREASED ABILITY TO INGEST FOOD
Prematurity
Neurologic disorders
  Coma
  Head injury
  Cerebral palsy affecting oral motor skills
Congenital anomalies
  Tracheoesophageal fistula
  Pierre–Robin syndrome
  Severe cleft palate
Craniofacial trauma
  Wired jaw
Head and neck obstructive lesions
  Rhabdomyosarcoma of the nasopharynx
Postoperative surgical patient

DECREASED ABILITY TO MEET CALORIC NEEDS
Increased caloric requirements
  Burns
  Sepsis
  Trauma
  Congenital heart disease
  Chronic lung disease
Anorexia due to chronic disease
  Acquired immunodeficiency syndrome
  Cancer
  Chronic renal disease
  Chronic liver disease
Eating disorders

vitamins, and trace elements are comparable with other iron-fortified, milk-based formulas (Table 142.7). These formulas can be fed to infants with lactose intolerance, because they contain only minute amounts of lactose. Although the amount of lactose is small, it is of sufficient quantity to make these formulas inappropriate choices for infants with galactosemia.

Soy-Based Formulas

Soy formulas differ from standard cow's milk–based formulas in carbohydrate and protein content (Table 142.8). The total protein in soy formulas is slightly higher than that in the milk-based formulas, to compensate for the lower biologic value of soy protein. Soy formulas contain soy protein isolate with L-methionine added to make its quality more comparable to that of casein in cow's milk. Soy formulas are lactose-free and are appropriate for use in infants with galactosemia and hereditary lactase deficiency. The AAP does not recommend using soy formulas for preterm infants who weigh less than 1,800 grams, or for prevention of colic or allergy.

Elemental and Semielemental Formulas

Elemental and semielemental formulas are recommended as the preferred formula for infants who are intolerant of cow's milk and soy protein, or those with significant malabsorption (Table 142.9). The variable fat, protein, and carbohydrate composition of the semielemental and elemental formulas may affect their use. Fat in these formulas contains differing amounts of medium-chain triglycerides (MCT) to facilitate absorption. Most of these formulas are lactose free, and are considered to be hypoallergenic.

Special Milk-Based Formulas

Some milk-based formulas have special compositional features and are used in specific clinical situations (e.g., Portagen is used in infants with biliary atresia; Table 142.10).

Formulas beyond the First Year of Life

Formulas designed for children beyond the first year of life are nutrient-dense formulas (30 cal/oz) for children 1 year of age or older (Table 142.11). They are used primarily for tube feeding or to supplement oral feedings. Only children who weigh 10 kg or more are candidates for these feedings, because the formulas' protein and renal solute loads are too high for a child of lower weight.

Standard Term Formulas

Standard term formulas are the feeding of choice when breast-feeding is not possible, or to supplement breast-feeding (Table 142.6). Milk-based formulas contain lactose as the carbohydrate source. The AAP recommends using milk-based formulas unless there is proven lactose intolerance. Standard infant formulas are available in low-iron and iron-fortified options; the AAP recommends using iron-fortified formulas.

Milk Protein–Based, Lactose-Free Formulas

Milk-based, lactose-free formulas contain glucose polymers as the source of carbohydrates; levels of protein, fat, minerals,

TABLE 142.2

HUMAN MILK PRODUCTS

Product name	Cal/fluid oz	Indications for use	Osmolality (mOsm/kg water)	Specifications of milk
Preterm human milk	20	Ideal for premature infants	290	Premature infants may need human milk fortifier. Milk from mothers who deliver prematurely may differ from mothers who deliver at term.
Mature human milk	20	Ideal for growing term and preterm infants	286	Premature infants may need human milk fortifier.

TABLE 142.3

HUMAN MILK FORTIFIERS

Product name	Cal/fluid oz	Indications for use	Osmolality (mOsm/kg water)	Specifications of formula
Enfamil Human Milk Fortifier powder (Mead Johnson)	14 cal/4 pk[a]	Designed to be added to human milk low-birthweight infants.	4 packets mixed with preterm human milk (410–440)	Mixing instructions: ■ 1 pk/50 mL = 22 cal/fl oz ■ 1 pk/25 mL = 24 cal/fl oz ■ Not to exceed 1 pk/25 mL ■ Iron 1.44 mg/4 pk
Similac Human Milk Fortifier powder (Ross)	14 cal/4 pk[a]	Designed to be added to human milk for low-birthweight infants.	4 packets mixed with preterm human milk (374–384)	Mixing instructions: ■ 1 pk/50 mL = 22 cal/fl oz ■ 1 pk/25 mL = 24 cal/fl oz ■ Not to exceed 1 pk/25 mL ■ May need additional iron ■ Iron 0.4 mg/4 pk
Similac Natural Care Advance Low Iron Liquid Human Milk Fortifier (Ross)	24 cal/fl oz	Designed to supplement human milk for premature infants of mothers whose milk supply is limited.	280	Mixing instructions: ■ Liquid fortifier may be mixed 1:1 dilution with human milk = 22 cal/fl oz. It is not intended to be used as the sole source of nutrients. ■ Iron 0.4 mg/100 cal

[a]Calories contained (total) in four packets.

Elemental and Semielemental Formulas Beyond the First Year of Life

Some elemental and semielemental formulas are designed for children 1 year of age or older with GI disorders, malabsorption, or severe food allergies (Table 142.12). The standard dilution for Vivonex Pediatric is 0.8 cal/mL, whereas for the other formulas it is 1 cal/mL.

Increasing the Calorie Concentration of Formulas

Some infants may require increased calorie concentration beyond 20 cal/oz for multiple reasons:

■ Fluid restriction that does not allow adequate calorie intake from standard formula

TABLE 142.4

PREMATURE FORMULAS

Product name	Cal/fluid oz	Indications for use	Osmolality (mOsm/kg water)	Specifications of formula
Enfamil Premature Lipil ready-to-feed (Mead Johnson)	20	Designed for growing premature and low birthweight infants. Available with iron or with low iron.	240	Includes DHA and ARA. Milk based formula. Nucleotide levels patterned after breast milk.
Enfamil Premature Lipil 24 ready-to-feed (Mead Johnson)	24	Designed for low birthweight infants. Concentrated to 24 cal/oz. Available with iron or with low iron.	300	Includes DHA and ARA. Milk-based formula. Nucleotide levels patterned after breast milk.
Similac Special Care Advance with Iron 20 ready-to-feed (Ross)	20	Designed for growing low birthweight infants. Available with iron or with low iron.	235	Contains DHA and ARA.
Similac Special Care Advance with Iron 24 ready-to-feed (Ross)	24	Designed for growing low birthweight infants. Concentrated to 24 cal/oz. Available with iron or with low iron.	280	Contains DHA and ARA.

TABLE 142.5

NUTRIENT-ENRICHED PREMATURE DISCHARGE FORMULAS

Product name	Cal/fluid oz	Indications for use	Osmolality (mOsm/kg water)	Specifications of formula
Similac Neosure Advance ready-to-feed or powder (Ross)	22	Designed to meet the nutritional needs of premature infants after discharge from the hospital. Higher levels of protein, vitamins, and minerals per 100 calories than the standard-term formula.	250	Contains DHA and ARA. Can be concentrated to provide more calories, depending on the infant's energy requirements and fluid restrictions.
Enfamil Enfacare Lipil ready-to-feed or powder (Mead-Johnson)	22	Designed to meet the nutritional needs of premature infants after discharge from the hospital. Higher levels of protein, vitamins, and minerals per 100 calories than the standard-term formula.	260 powder 250 liquid	Contains DHA and ARA. Can be concentrated to provide more calories, depending upon the infant's energy requirements and fluid restrictions.

TABLE 142.6

STANDARD-TERM FORMULAS

Product name	Cal/fluid oz	Indications for use	Osmolality (mOsm/kg H$_2$O)	Spefications of formula
Similac Advance with Iron 20, ready-to-feed, powder, or concentrated liquid (Ross)	20	Designed for feeding term infants for the first 12 months of life.	300	Milk-based iron-fortified formula with free nucleotides added (72 mg/L). Contains DHA and ARA.
Enfamil Lipil with Iron 20 ready-to-feed, powder, concentrated liquid (Mead-Johnson)	20	Designed for feeding term infants for the first 12 months of life.	300	Milk-based iron-fortified with free nucleotides added (28 mg/L). Includes Lipil blend of DHA and ARA modeled after human milk. Gluten free.
Good Start Supreme DHA and ARA ready-to-feed, powder, concentrated liquid (Nestle)	20	Designed for feeding term infants for the first 12 months of life.	250	100% whey protein, partially hydrolyzed formula. Enriched with DHA and ARA.
Store brand milk formulas ready-to-feed, powder, or concentrated liquid (Wyeth Nutritionals)	20	Designed for feeding term infants for the first 12 months of life.	296	Store brand formulas from Albertsons (Baby Basics), Target (Healthy Baby), Walmart (Parent's Choice) are made by Wyeth. Nutritional content is based on the former SMA formula.

TABLE 142.7

MILK PROTEIN–BASED, LACTOSE-FREE FORMULAS

Product name	Cal/fluid oz	Indications for use	Osmolality (mOsm/kg water)	Specifications of formula
Similac Lactose Free Advance, ready-to-feed, powder, or concentrated liquid (Ross)	20	Designed for infants when lactose is a concern and a milk protein–based formula is preferred to a soy-based formula.	230	Not for infants with galactosemia. Contains DHA and ARA. Lactose free.
Enfamil Lactofree Lipil, ready-to-feed, powder, or concentrated liquid (Mead Johnson)	20	Designed for infants when lactose is a concern and a milk protein–based formula is preferred instead of a soy-based formula. Milk-protein base, iron fortified formula	200	Not for infants with galactosemia. Lactose-free, sucrose-free; contains Lipil blend of DHA and ARA.

TABLE 142.8

INFANT SOY FORMULAS

Product name	Cal/fluid oz	Indications for use	Osmolality (mOsm/kg water)	Specifications of formula
Similac Isomil powder or concentrated liquid (Ross)	20	Designed for infants with galactosemia, hereditary lactase deficiency, lactose intolerance, parents seeking vegetarian diets, documented IgE-mediated allergy, or sensitivity to cow's-milk protein.	200	Lactose-free formula. Soy formulas are not recommended for preterm infants with birthweight <1800 g.
Similac Isomil DF ready-to-feed (Ross)	20	Designed for the nutritional management of diarrhea in infants older than 6 months and toddlers.	240	Lactose-free with added soy fiber. Contains 0.9 g of added fiber per 100 cal. Low osmolality.
Similac Isomil Advance ready-to-feed, powder, or concentrated liquid (Ross)	20	Formula for infants with feeding problems such as fussiness, gas, spit-up, lactose intolerance, and for infants with IgE-mediated allergy or sensitivity to cow's-milk protein.	200	Contains DHA and ARA. Low osmolality. Soy formulas are not recommended for preterm infants with birthweight <1800 g.
Enfamil Prosobee Lipil ready-to-feed, powder, or concentrated liquid (Mead Johnson)	20	Soy-based formula for the first 12 months, milk free. Designed for infants with lactose intolerance, galactosemia, and most infants with IgE-mediated allergy or sensitivity to cow's-milk protein.	200 liquid 170 powder	Contains Lipil blend of DHA and ARA. Lactose-free and sucrose-free. Soy formulas are not recommended for preterm infants with birthweight <1800 g.
Good Start Supreme Soy DHA and ARA ready-to-feed, powder, or concentrated liquid (Nestle)	20	Ideal for birth to 12 months of age if a soy supplement is required.	180	Iron fortified, lactose free, milk free, containing easy-to-digest supreme soy proteins.
Store brand formulas, ready-to-feed, powder or concentrated liquid, (Wyeth Nutritionals)	20	Designed for infants with IgE-mediated allergy or sensitivity to milk protein, lactose intolerance, and for vegetarian families.	296	Lactose-free.
RCF carbohydrate free concentrated liquid 1:1 dilution with water (Ross)	Standard dilution is 20 cal/fl oz	For patients who are unable to tolerate the type or amount of carbohydrate in milk or infant formulas or for patients with seizures requiring a ketogenic diet.	Osmolality depends upon type and amount of carbohydrate added.	Carbohydrate-free, soy-based, iron-fortified formula, provides 12 cal/fl oz (40.6 cal/100 mL).

- Increased calorie expenditure
- Inadequate volume of intake

Term formula powder or concentrate provides an easy method of concentrating breast milk to provide nutrient-dense feeds for term infants. The protein and mineral content of breast milk mixed with term powder formula is inadequate for preterm infants. It is more appropriate to use premature discharge powder formula when concentrating breast milk for preterm infants. Cow's milk–based or hydrolysate formulas may be used, depending on the medical diagnosis. If insensible water losses are high, the formula can be concentrated to 24 cal/oz; if desired, the concentration can be increased further by adding modulars. The use of carbohydrate (e.g., Polycose) or fat (e.g., MCT or vegetable oil) does not increase the renal solute load, but additional carbohydrate does increase the osmolality; additional fat may prolong gastric emptying time. The clinician should not increase the carbohydrate content to greater than 0.5 to 1.0 g CHO/ounce, or the fat content to greater than 0.5 to 0.75 g of fat/ounce, when concentrating formula from modulars. Adding modulars to increase calories will change the percentage of calories from carbohydrates and fat, as well as the amount of protein per 100 calories. Patients on concentrated formulas, either from added modulars or increased concentration of the formula itself, should be monitored for appropriate distribution of macronutrients.

TABLE 142.9

ELEMENTAL AND SEMIELEMENTAL INFANT FORMULAS

Product name	Cal/fluid oz	Indications for use	Osmolality (mOsm/kg water)	Specifications of formula
Enfamil Pregestimil Lipil ready-to-feed, powder (Mead Johnson)	20	Designed for infants with fat malabsorption, intractable diarrhea, and for infants sensitive to intact proteins.	330 powder 280 liquid 330 (24 cal/fl oz)	Hypoallergenic protein hydrolysate formula with MCT oil as 55% of its fat blend. Lactose- and sucrose-free. Can be concentrated to increase caloric density. Pregestimil Lipil is available with DHA and ARA. Iron-fortified.
Similac Alimentum, Advance ready-to-feed or powder	20	Designed for infants with severe food allergies, sensitivity to intact proteins, and malabsorption.	370	Hypoallergenic protein hydrolysate, 33% of fat as MCT. Lactose-free and corn-free. Contains DHA and ARA. Iron-fortified.
Nutramingen Lipil, ready-to-feed, powder or concentrated liquid (Mead Johnson)	20	Designed for infants sensitive to intact protein in milk-based and soy-based formulas. Appropriate for infants with galactosemia.	320 powder 300 liquid	Hypoallergenic protein hydrolysates. Lactose-free and sucrose-free. Iron-fortified. Contains Lipil blend of DHA and ARA.
Neocate Infant Formula Powder (SHS North America)	20	Designed for infants with multiple food protein intolerances, cow's-milk allergy, and allergy to hydrolyzed formula.	375	100% free amino acids, hypoallergenic formula, lactose-free, and sucrose-free.

TABLE 142.10

SPECIAL MILK-BASED FORMULAS

Product name	Cal/fluid oz	Indications for use	Osmolality (mOsm/kg water)	Specifications of formula
Portagen powder (Mead Johnson)	20	Designed for infants with difficulty digesting long-chain fatty acids, impaired fat absorption, bile deficiency, and chylothorax. Supplementation with essential fatty acids and ultra trace minerals should be considered when used for extended time.	350	Milk-based protein powder with MCT. 87% of calories as medium-chain triglycerides.
Enfamil AR Lipil ready-to-feed or powder (Mead Johnson)	20	Designed for full-term infants who spit up frequently or for whom physician recommends thickened formula. Enfamil AR is thickened with added rice starch and has increased viscosity.	240 liquid 230 powder	Not recommended for premature infants because of increased viscosity. The manufacturer does not recommend concentrating greater than 24 cal/oz.
Similac PM 60/40 powder (Ross)	20	Designed for infants with renal problems or those requiring low mineral content. Calcium:phosphorus ratio = 2:1	280	Low-mineral, low-solute formula. Mineral level closely approximating the mineral content of human milk. Low-iron formula; additional iron should be supplied from other sources.

TABLE 142.11

FORMULAS USED BEYOND THE FIRST YEAR OF LIFE

Product name	Cal/fluid oz	Indications for use	Osmolality (mOsm/kg water)	Specifications of formula
Pediasure, ready-to-feed (Ross)	30	Designed for oral feedings for children 1–10 years of age. NOT for children with galactosemia.	430	Milk-based, lactose-free, gluten-free. Pediasure meets or exceeds the 100% of the NAS-NRC RDA for protein, vitamins, and minerals for children 1–6 years of age in 1,000 mL, and children 7–10 years of age in 1,300 mL. Available with fiber. 1.2 g total dietary fiber from soy fiber per 8 fl oz. Available in vanilla, banana cream, strawberry, chocolate, and orange cream.
Pediasure Enteral Formula, ready-to-feed (Ross)	30	For tube feeding children 1–13 years of age. NOT for children with galactosemia.	335	Meets or exceeds 100% of DRI for children 1–8 years of age in 1,000 mL and for children 9–13 years of age in 1,500 mL. Milk-based, gluten-free, lactose-free.
Pediasure with Fiber Enteral Formula ready-to-feed (Ross)	30	For tube feeding children 1–13 years of age.	345	Same as Pediasure Enteral Formula, except provides 1.9 g of total dietary fiber per 8 fl oz.
Enfamil Kindercal Beverage ready-to-feed (Mead Johnson)	30	Tube or oral formula for children 1–10 years of age.	440 vanilla 520 chocolate	Available with or without fiber. Isotonic, lactose-free, gluten-free. Fiber content 6.3 g/1,000 mL. Meets 100% of NAS-NRC RDA for ages 1–10 years in 946 mL.
Enfamil Kindercal TF ready-to-feed (Mead Johnson)	30	Tube formula for children 1–10 years of age.	345	Isotonic, lactose-free, available with or without fiber. Meets at least 100% of NAS-NRC RDA for ages 1–10 years in 946 mL.
Nutren Junior ready-to-feed available with or without fiber (Nestle Nutrition)	30	Tube or oral formula for children 1–10 years of age.	350	Isotonic, lactose-free, gluten-free formula. Protein blend: 50% whey and 50% casein. Nestle flavor packets provide multiple flavoring options for oral use. Meets NAS-NRC RDA for ages 1–10 years in 1,000 mL. Nutren Junior with fiber has 5.1 g fiber per 1,000 mL.
Resource Just for Kids ready-to-feed (Novartis)	30	Tube or oral formula for children 1–10 years of age.	390	Lactose-free, low-residue, may be suitable for gluten-free diet, available with or without fiber. Meets NAS-NRC RDA in 1,000 mL for ages 1–10 years. Resource Just for Kids with fiber has 6 g fiber per 1,000 mL.
Compleat Pediatric ready-to-feed (Novartis)	30	Tube formula for children 1–10 years of age.	380	Isotonic, lactose-free. May be suitable for gluten-free diet. Meets NAS-NRC RDA for 1–10 year olds in 900 mL. 6 g fiber per 900 mL. Made from traditional foods including meat, vegetables, and fruit.

Although increasing the caloric density of the formula also increases its osmolality, most infants are able to tolerate a gradual increase in the concentration of the formula. The AAP recommends concentrations no greater than 450 mOsm/kg water for infant formulas. Most infants have no difficulty tolerating formulas up to 30 cal/oz if the concentration is increased gradually by increments of 2 to 4 cal/oz/day. Increasing the concentration of formula, rather than the use of modulars, is the preferred method of increasing caloric density, because the addition of modulars may dilute nutrients in the formula. The clinician should remember that medications, vitamins, and electrolyte supplements in the formula can also

TABLE 142.12

ELEMENTAL AND SEMIELEMENTAL FORMULAS BEYOND THE FIRST YEAR OF LIFE

Product name	Cal/fluid oz	Indications for use	Osmolality (mOsm/kg water)	Specifications of formula
Neocate One + powder (Nutricia North America)	30	Elemental formula for children with cow's-milk protein intolerance and multiple food protein intolerances.	610	Hypoallergenic, 100% free amino acids.
Neocate Junior powder (Nutricia North America)	30	Malabsorption, multiple food protein intolerances, cow's-milk protein intolerance.	607 unflavored 690 tropical fruit	Hypoallergenic, 100% free amino acids, high protein and extra vitamins and minerals.
Peptide one + powder (Nutricia North America)	30	Malabsorption, whole-protein intolerance. For oral or tube feeding.	430 unflavored 440 banana	44% free amino acids, 56% low-molecular-weight peptides. Extra vitamins and minerals for malabsorptive conditions.
Pediatric E028 ready- to-feed, 8-oz tetra pack, comes in flavors (Nutricia North America)	30	Malabsorption, GI tract impairment, or protein allergy.	820	100% free amino acids.
Vivonex Pediatric powder (Novartis)	24	Gastrointestinal disorders, malabsorption syndrome, cow's-milk protein enteropathy/sensitivity. Designed specifically for children 1–10 years.	360	Lactose-free, low-residue, may be suitable for gluten-free diet. 100% free amino acids. 100% NAS/NRC RDA 1–6 years in 1,000 mL, 7–10 years in 1,170 mL.
Elecare powder (Ross)	30	Malabsorption, severe food allergies, protein maldigestion, and GI tract impairment.	360	Meets 100% of the NAS-NRC RDA for children 1–6 years in 1,000 mL; 7–10 years in 1,170 mL; elemental formula for children >1 year. Milk protein-free, lactose-free, gluten-free, soy protein-free, galactose-free, fructose-free. Flavor packets are available for oral use. Amino acid-based formula with iron. Standard dilution (30 cal/fl oz) is 4 unpacked, level scoops of powder for each 5 fl oz of water. Do not heat.
Peptamen Junior ready-to-feed (Nestle)	30	Peptide-based elemental formula for impaired GI function.	260 unflavored 360 vanilla flavor	100% whey-based peptides and an antioxidant and optimal lipid blend. Isotonic, lactose-free and gluten-free.

increase the osmolality of the formula and may affect the infant's tolerance of it.

Although a reference may be used (Table 142.13), simple equations can be applied to mix formulas of different concentrations from powdered formulas and liquid concentrates.

Concentrating formula by mixing from liquid concentrate:

$$\frac{a \times b}{c} - a = y$$

where a = amount of formula to be diluted (constant: 13 oz/can), b = caloric density of formula (constant: 40 cal/fl oz),

c = desired caloric density (cal/fl oz), and y = amount of added water needed (fl oz).

For example, to calculate a 24-cal/oz formula: $(13 \times 40) \div 24 - 13 = 9$ fluid ounces of water that needs to be added to the can of concentrate.

Concentrating formula by mixing from powder:

$$\frac{a}{b} - c = x$$

where a = calories per scoop (44 calories per scoop, except 48.5 calories for Enfacare), b = desired concentration of formula

TABLE 142.13

PREPARATION OF FORMULAS FROM POWDER AND LIQUID CONCENTRATES

Cal/fluid oz from powder	Cal/mL	Volume of water mL (fluid oz) to add to 1 scoop powder[a]	Formula yield (fluid oz)
20	0.68	59 (2.0)	65 (2.2)
22	0.74	53 (1.8)	59 (2.0)
24	0.81	48 (1.6)	54 (1.8)
26[a]	0.88	44 (1.5)	50 (1.7)
27[a]	0.91	42 (1.4)	48 (1.6)
28[a]	0.95	40 (1.4)	46 (1.6)
30[a]	1.01	37 (1.3)	43 (1.5)

[a]When accuracy is essential, mL measurements should be used. Fluid ounce measures are provided for convenience when larger variance in prepared dilution is acceptable. Fluid ounce measures in above table are rounded to nearest 0.10 fluid ounce. One fluid ounce = 29.57 mL.

Volume of water (fl oz) to add to 13 fluid oz (384 mL) can of formula

Cal/fluid oz[a]	Cal/mL	Concentrate[b]	Yield (fluid oz)
From liquid concentrate			
20	0.68	13	26
22	0.74	10.5	23.5
24	0.81	9	22
27	0.91	6	19
30	1.01	4.5	17.5

[a]Enfamil AR should not be concentrated higher than 24 cal/oz because of viscosity.
[b]Each can of concentrated liquid provides 520 calories (40 cal/fl oz).

mixture (cal/oz), c = water displacement per scoop (constant 0.2 fl oz), and x = amount of water to use per scoop (fl oz).

For example, for calculating a 24-cal/oz formula: (44 ÷ 24) − 0.2 = 1.6 fluid ounces of water to be added to each scoop of powder.

The nutrient-enriched discharge formulas Similac Advance Neosure and Enfamil Enfacare Lipil are prepared differently than the standard formulas; see Tables 142.14 and 142.15.

Modular Supplements

Formulas can be concentrated by adding modular supplements, such as fats or glucose polymers, although these supplements alter the nutrient ratio of the formula composition by providing nonprotein calories. Modular supplements can be added when other nutrient needs have been met and only additional calories are needed, or to increase the concentration of a particular nutrient. When adding modulars to formula, special attention should be paid to the percentage of calorie distribution. Providing more than 60% of calories from fat may induce ketosis. Protein intake making up less than 6% of total calories ingested may result in protein deficiency; in contrast, protein calorie intake greater than 16% of the total may lead to azotemia.

Table 142.16 gives a list of modular supplements. These additives do not contribute vitamins or minerals.

ROUTE OF FEEDING

Once the the choice of formula has been made, the next step is to decide on the route and method of administering feedings.

Common routes for administration include nasogastric, nasoduodenal, nasojejunal, gastrostomy, and jejunostomy. Enteral nutrition is preferred because of its immunologic benefits, lower cost, stimulation of the GI tract, and fewer infectious complications. Parenteral nutrition should be considered when enteral nutrition fails or is contraindicated.

Two key factors must be taken into account when choosing the route for providing enteral nutrition. Table 142.17 compares the features of gastric and transpyloric feedings.

TABLE 142.14

MIXING OF SIMILAC NEOSURE ADVANCE POWDER

The following table shows the quantity of water to mix with the quantity of unpacked level scoop(s) (9.6 g) of Neosure Advance Powder to arrive at the caloric densities shown. Use only the scoop (9.6 g) provided in the can.

Cal/fl oz desired	Water (fl oz)	Unpacked level scoopful	Approximate yield (fl oz)
20	4.5	2	5
21	10.5	5	12
22[a]	2	1	2
23	9.5	5	11
24	5.5	3	6.5
25	3.5	2	4
26	5	3	6
27	8	5	9

[a]22 cal/fl/oz is the standard mixture.

TABLE 142.15

MIXING OF ENFAMIL ENFACARE LIPIL POWDER

Cal/fluid oz desired	Water (fluid oz)	Unpacked level scoopful	Approximate yield (fluid oz)
20	2.2	1	2.4
22	2.0	1	2.2
24	1.8	1	2.0
27	1.6	1	1.8

One unpacked level scoop of Enfacare lipil powder (9.8 g) provides 48 calories.
One unpacked level scoop of Enfacare lipil powder displaces 6 mL or 0.2 fl oz of water.

- If tube feeding is going to last longer than 4 to 6 weeks, a feeding enterostomy should be considered. Use of a nasoenteric tube is appropriate if tube feeding will be used for a shorter time.
- If the patient is at risk for pulmonary aspiration, transpyloric placement of the tube is recommended. A nasogastric tube is acceptable for the patient who is not at risk for pulmonary aspiration.

Preferred Features of a Pediatric Nasoenteric Tube

The following features are important in choosing a pediatric nasoenteric tube. It should be:

- Made of Silastic or polyurethane.
- Available in small diameters.
- Available in a variety of lengths, with markings to aid in determining the depth of tube insertion.
- Radiopaque, to verify placement location.
- Compatible with the administration set and with a variety of sizes of feeding containers, to accommodate use in neonates and older children.

In addition:

- The tube may have a weighted tip to help with secure placement secure.
- The tube should have a smooth point to facilitate easy insertion and removal.

Administration of Tube Feeding

The specific method used for delivery of enteral nutrition depends on the clinical condition of the patient and the distal location of the feeding tube (gastric or transpyloric). The methods most often used are continuous-drip feedings and

TABLE 142.16

MODULAR SUPPLEMENTS

Name of product	Type	Source	Kcal/Unit	Comments
Polycose powder (Ross)	Carbohydrate	Glucose polymer	8 kcal/tsp 23 kcal/tbsp	Increases osmolality.
Polycose liquid (Ross)	Carbohydrate	Glucose polymer	2.0 kcal/mL	Increases osmolality.
Corn syrup (Store brands)	Carbohydrate	Corn syrup	3.8 kcal/ml	Increases osmolality.
Karo syrup (Store brands are available)	Carbohydrate	Polysaccharides, glucose, maltose, fructose	3.9 kcal/mL 1 tbsp 58 kcal	Increases osmolality.
Moducal powder (Mead Johnson)	Carbohydrate	Glucose polymer	30 kcal/tbsp	Increases osmolality.
Promod powder (Ross)	Protein	Whey protein	28 kcal/scoop 5 g protein/ scoop 17 kcal/tbsp 3.0 g protein/tbsp	Increases renal solute load.
Casec powder (Mead Johnson)	Protein	Calcium caseinates	17 kcal/tbsp 4.1 g protein/tbsp	Provides additional protein. Increases renal solute load.
MCT oil (Mead Johnson)	Fat	Lipid fraction of coconut oil	7.7 kcal/mL	Absorbed directly into portal system. Bile salts and lipase not necessary for digestion and absorption. Does not contain essential fatty acids. Nonemulsified.
Corn Oil/ Safflower oil (Regular store brands)	Fat	Corn, safflower	8.4 kcal/mL	Nonemulsified, consists mainly of oleic and linoleic unsaturated fatty acids.
Microlipid (Mead Johnson)	Fat	Safflower	4.5 kcal/mL	High in linoleic acid, mixes well into solution.

TABLE 142.17

GASTRIC FEEDINGS VERSUS TRANSPYLORIC FEEDINGS

Site of feeding	Route of feeding	Indications	Advantages	Disadvantages
GASTRIC FEEDINGS Preferable because of normal digestive process. The stomach serves as a natural reservoir, regulates delivery of nutrients to the small intestine, and allows the digestive process to begin in the stomach.	Orogastric Nasogastric	Short-term use Prematurity Supplement diet Inability to suck and swallow Intact gag reflux No esophageal reflux Normal emptying of gastric and duodenal contents.	Easy to insert. Large reservoir capacity in stomach.	Increased risk of aspiration. Patient self-conscious because of appearance. Choking if gag reflux is present.
	Gastrostomy	Long-term use (>6 wk) Swallowing problems due to neurologic disorders Esophageal injury or obstruction	Low risk of medication occlusion. Large reservoir capacity. Home tube feedings. Allows greater mobility. No obstruction of airways.	Surgical procedure (percutaneous). May increase gastroesophageal reflux.
TRANSPYLORIC FEEDINGS Transpyloric enteral nutrition is a suitable method of nutritional support for critically ill pediatric patients. In these feedings, the tube is passed through the pylorus into the small intestine. No bolus feedings are recommended and feedings are given continuously.	Nasoduodenal Oroduodenal Nasojejunal Jejunostomy Gastrojejunal	Patients with increased risk of aspiration, diminished gag reflux, severe gastrointestinal reflux, frequent vomiting, delayed gastric emptying, and inadequate gastric motility	Reduced risk of aspiration. Feedings can be initiated sooner after injury.	Tube displacement. Limited choice of feeding schedule.

intermittent/bolus feedings. Table 142.18 compares the two methods of feeding and makes specific recommendations concerning their use.

Complications of Tube Feeding

Complications of tube feeding fall into the following categories: mechanical, GI, respiratory, metabolic, and psychological/behavioral (Table 142.19). In general, these complications can be prevented or easily solved. Securing feeding tubes can prevent mechanical problems, and particular care should be taken to anchor feeding tubes in children with copious nasal and oral secretions.

Dissolving crushed tablets in warm water or using liquid medications helps keep tubes from becoming clogged. Flushing the tube with saline or water appropriate for the type of feeding being administered also helps maintain patency of the tube. The feeding tube should be replaced if it becomes clogged or is improperly placed.

Each step in providing tube feeding should be carefully considered to prevent (or treat) GI complications of tube feeding. Formula is administered at room temperature and is kept free of bacterial contamination. The osmolality of the formula and its rate of infusion affect tolerance. Air should be eliminated from the feeding system to reduce gas, bloating, and cramps. Lactose or fat intolerance may cause vomiting or diarrhea. Continuous-drip feeding and transpyloric feeding may be helpful if vomiting is a major problem, though the clinician must always be mindful of the possibility that intestinal obstruction is causing the vomiting. Transpyloric feedings are a preferred option for the infant or child at risk for aspiration pneumonia. Metabolic complications can be avoided by providing appropriate free water, monitoring electrolytes, and providing caloric intake appropriate for the patient's clinical needs.

Using nighttime tube feeds and gastrostomy devices that are less visible may help with psychological issues. Oral feeding should be initiated at the earliest opportunity, and for those infants in whom oral feeding may need to be delayed, oral stimulation provided.

The following are sources of information about nutritional content of formulas and other nutritional products:

Mead Johnson Nutritionals, Evansville, IN
Ross Products Division, Abbott Laboratories, Columbus, OH
Nutricia North America, Gaithersburg, MD

TABLE 142.18

CONTINUOUS FEEDING VERSUS INTERMITTENT/BOLUS FEEDING

Method of administration	Advantages	Disadvantages	Suggested guidelines
CONTINUOUS FEEDINGS The feedings are administered over a period of several hours or entire by pump. Continuous feedings always are used with transpyloric feeding.	Infusion of nutrients at a constant rate. Patients with altered gastrointestinal function tolerate better. Suitable for transpyloric and nocturnal feedings. Critically ill patients tolerate better than bolus feedings. Volume of formula can be increased rapidly. Minimize risk of high gastric residuals and pulmonary aspiration. If poor tolerance to intermittent/bolus. May facilitate respiratory stability in small premature infants recovering from respiratory distress syndrome. Well tolerated.	Expensive because pump is required. Restricts ambulation. Associated with nutrient loss when providing human milk.	Initiation of feedings, rate of advancement, and final goal vary child to child. The following suggested guidelines may be individualized according to the child's clinical condition. Premature infants: ■ Begin 0.5–1.0 mL/kg/hr advancing every 12–24 hr by 1–2 mL/kg/hr as tolerated. Full-term infants/children: ■ Begin 1–2 mL/kg/hr advancing by 0.5–1.0 mL/kg/hr every 8–24 hr as tolerated until final goal is achieved, or begin. ■ Full-term infants and toddlers 10–20 mL/hr. ■ Children 20–40 mL/hr. ■ Adolescents 25–50 mL/hr. Advancement every 8–12 hr: ■ Full-term infants 5–10 mL/hr. ■ Children 10–20 mL/hr. ■ Adolescents 25 mL/hr.
INTERMITTENT/ BOLUS FEEDINGS	Freedom from infusion pump. More physiologic; less expensive due to less equipment. More flexibility of feeding regimen.	Longer time to reach goal. Risk of complications such as aspiration, nausea, abdominal pain, and distention. Not appropriate for transpyloric feedings.	Premature infants: ■ <1,000 g, initiate 10 mL/kg/day every 2 hr, advancing by 10–15 mL/kg/day. ■ 1,000–1,500 g initiate 10–20 mL/kg/day every 2–3 hr, advancing by 10–15 mL/kg/day. ■ >1,500 g initiate 20–30 mL/kg/day every 3 hr, advancing by 20–30 mL/kg/day as tolerated to a goal volume. Full-term infants/children/adolescents: ■ Calculate the amount of total formula needed. ■ Begin delivery at 25–50% volume initially and dividing that volume into 6 or 7 feedings in a day. ■ Drip slowly over 15–20 min. ■ Advance every 12–24 hr depending on the tolerance by 25% of volume. ■ Monitor for abdominal distention, diarrhea, and emesis.

TABLE 142.19

COMPLICATIONS OF TUBE FEEDING

Mechanical	Metabolic
Clogged tube	Dehydration
Tube displacement	Electrolyte disturbance
Gastrointestinal	Too little/too much weight gain
Vomiting	Psychological/behavioral
Diarrhea	Altered body image
Bloating/gas	Loss of normal ability
Dumping syndrome	to engage in oral feeding
Respiratory	
Aspiration pneumonia	

Novartis Nutrition, St. Louis Park, MN
Nestle USA, Nutrition Division, Glendale, CA
Wyeth Nutritionals, Philadelphia, PA

Suggested Readings

American Academy of Pediatrics, Committee on Nutrition. *Pediatric nutrition handbook*. 5th ed. Elk Grove Village, IL: American Academy of Pediatrics; 2004.

Baker BS, Baker DR, et al. *Pediatric enteral nutrition*. New York: Chapman & Hall; 1994.

Cox JH. *Nutritional manual for at-risk infants and toddlers*. Chicago: Percept Press; 1997.

Samour PQ, King K. *Handbook of pediatric nutrition*. 3rd ed. Sudbury, MA: Jones &Bartlett; 2005.

Wargo SG, Thompson M, Cox JH, et al. *Nutritional care for high-risk newborns*. Chicago: Percept Press; 2000.

CHAPTER 143 ■ PARENTERAL NUTRITION

CASSIE A. BILLINGS

Parenteral nutrition is the intravenous provision of nutrients, including carbohydrates, protein, fats, electrolytes, vitamins, minerals, and trace elements.

The first report of successful use of parenteral nutrition (PN) in an infant appeared in the medical literature in 1944. Since then, PN has become an important adjunctive therapy in a variety of disease states in adults and children. This support is especially necessary in children, in whom nutritional deficiencies occur much more quickly than in adults and for whom deficiencies can have many more negative consequences.

INDICATIONS

PN is indicated when an infant, child, or adolescent is unable to meet ongoing nutritional needs via the gastrointestinal tract, whether by oral intake or tube feedings. Specific indications for PN are listed in Table 143.1.

PN is considered invasive therapy with inherent risks. There are few data that show decreased mortality from the use of PN aside from its use in extremely premature, low-birthweight neonates; therefore, nutrition should be provided enterally whenever possible in any patient with a functioning gastrointestinal tract. Advantages of enteral nutrition include reduced cost, better maintenance of gut integrity, reduced infection, and decreased length of hospital stay. The complications associated with PN will be discussed later in this chapter.

VENOUS ACCESS

PN may be provided via peripheral or central venous access. Peripheral access is used when the patient needs short-term PN support or supplemental, not total, nutritional support. Patients with peripheral venous access must be able to tolerate large fluid loads to receive adequate calories. All PN solutions, even at low dextrose concentrations, are relatively hypertonic solutions. If it is anticipated that a patient may need total PN support or supplemental PN support for longer than 7 days, establishing central venous access is recommended.

Central venous access allows the delivery of hypertonic solutions for long-term nutritional support (>7 days). It is especially helpful for those patients who are fluid-restricted, have limited peripheral access, or are being considered for home PN therapy.

ENERGY REQUIREMENTS

Energy requirements vary from child to child with age, gender, body size, disease process, stress, trauma, and the use of drugs that cause changes in muscle activity. The caloric estimates are generally related to the patient's age and weight (Table 143.2).

These estimates are general guidelines, and individual patients should have their caloric intake modified as indicated by monitoring weight and appropriate laboratory markers (see Chapter 141). Both excessive and inadequate caloric intake can contribute to a variety of health problems, including delayed wound healing, prolonged ventilator dependence, and glucose intolerance.

COMPONENTS OF PARENTERAL NUTRITION

Fluid

Maintenance fluid requirements are listed in Table 143.3. In addition to weight, fluid requirements depend on hydration status, environmental factors (e.g., radiant warmers, ultraviolet light therapy), and disease (e.g., fever). Maintaining adequate fluid status is essential because complications of under- or overhydration can be serious. Due to their large body surface areas for body weight and greater insensible losses, neonates and infants require proportionally more fluids to maintain appropriate hydration. Although most infants can tolerate up to 120 to 150 mL/kg/day, caution must be exercised in premature infants, in whom complications of bronchopulmonary dysplasia (chronic lung disease), patent ductus arteriosus, intraventricular hemorrhage, and necrotizing enterocolitis have been associated with administration of excessive fluids. Other patients may require fluid restriction, including patients with cardiac defects, renal disease, or head trauma. Patients with high ostomy output, high urinary output, diarrhea, or vomiting may require supplemental replacement fluids in addition to maintenance requirements. Fever and the use of radiant warmers or ultraviolet lights have been estimated to increase fluid losses by 20% to 25%.

Carbohydrate

Dextrose is the usual source of carbohydrates in PN solutions. Peripheral administration of dextrose solutions over 12.5% is associated with an increase in infiltration and phlebitis. If older patients can tolerate large fluid loads and maximal fat doses (see below), then maintenance caloric needs may be able to be met peripherally for short periods of time.

Neonates are usually started at 5 g/kg/day (3–4 mg/kg/min) of dextrose; increases of 3 g/kg/day (2 mg/kg/min) are made until caloric goals are met. Older infants and children may be started on 10 g/kg/day (4–7 mg/kg/min) with increments of 5 g/kg/day (3–4 mg/kg/min). Stated otherwise, in an older infant or child who is receiving maintenance fluids of dextrose 5%, PN may be started at dextrose 10% and advanced by 5% each day (if central access is obtained) until the nutritional

TABLE 143.1

INDICATIONS FOR PARENTERAL NUTRITION IN PEDIATRIC PATIENTS

- Prematurity
- Severe protein–calorie malnutrition
- Congenital gastrointestinal anomalies requiring surgery
- Necrotizing enterocolitis (NEC)
- Intractable diarrhea
- Intestinal obstruction
- Paralytic ileus
- Short gut syndrome
- Radiation enteritis
- Anorexia nervosa
- Chylothorax
- Severe Stevens–Johnson syndrome
- Burns
- Severe acute pancreatitis
- Severe trauma
- Severe sepsis

goals are met. Glucose tolerance may be assessed by checking fingerstick glucose measurements and/or by dipstick urine measurements.

Calculating the glucose infusion rate (GIR, mg/kg/min) is a helpful way to measure glucose delivery, because using percentages may be misleading in a fluid-restricted patient. To calculate GIR:

$$GIR = [\text{Fluid Rate (mL/hr)} \times \% \text{ Dextrose} \times 0.167]/\text{Weight (kg)}$$

The ability of the liver to oxidize glucose is limited, and exceeding its capacity can contribute to the development of hepatic steatosis. Neonates and infants should not receive more than 14 mg/kg/min of dextrose delivery.

Carbohydrates (CHO) in the diet deliver 4 kcal/g; however, dextrose monohydrate delivers 3.4 kcal/g. To calculate calories (kcal) from dextrose:

$$CHO \text{ kcal} = [\text{Total Volume (mL)} \times \% \text{ Dextrose (g/100 mL)} \times 3.4 \text{ kcal/g}]/100$$

Protein

Crystalline amino acids are the only form of PN protein currently marketed for patient use. Early amino acid solutions consisted of protein hydrolysates, which often produced hyperammonemia and resulted in poor nitrogen retention.

TABLE 143.2

GENERAL ENERGY REQUIREMENTS FOR THE PEDIATRIC PATIENT

Age	Energy requirements (kcal/kg)
Preterm neonate	90–120
<6 mo	85–105
6–12 mo	80–100
1–7 yr	75–90
7–12 yr	50–75
>12–18 yr	30–50

TABLE 143.3

MAINTENANCE FLUID REQUIREMENTS FOR PEDIATRIC PATIENTS

Body weight (kg)	Total fluid/day
<1.5	130–150 mL/kg
1.5–2	110–130 mL/kg
2–10	100 mL/kg
>10–20	1,000 mL + 50 mL/kg for each kg >10 kg
>20	1,500 mL + 20 mL/kg for each kg >20 kg

Early amino acid formulations also consisted of hydrochloride salt forms, which often resulted in metabolic acidosis. Current amino acid formulations contain the acetate salt whenever possible.

Each patient's protein needs are based on age, development, and disease state. Amino acid doses in neonates and infants should aim at achieving appropriate percentile growth rates but are often modified by catabolic disease states and ongoing losses. Achieving an optimal positive nitrogen balance is necessary to sustain growth. Parenteral protein requirements are listed in Table 143.4.

Standard amino acid solutions are composed of essential and nonessential amino acids and are based on adult requirements. Because particular enzyme systems are immature in neonates, certain amino acids have been considered essential in this population. These amino acids include cysteine, taurine, tyrosine, and histidine. One pediatric-specific parenteral amino acid solution (TrophAmine, B. Braun Medical Inc., Irvine, CA) contains less methionine, phenylalanine, and glycine, which can accumulate in neonates, but increased concentrations of histidine, taurine, and tyrosine. This specialized solution produces plasma amino acid concentrations more similar to those of healthy breast-fed and formula-fed infants (as compared with adult amino acid formulations). L-cysteine hydrochloride must be added as an admixture just prior to parenteral nutrition administration because it is unstable in solution for prolonged periods of time. The most commonly recommended dose is 40 mg of L-cysteine hydrochloride per gram of amino acids, but the optimal dose has not been established. Addition of L-cysteine hydrochloride to PN solutions increases the solubility of calcium and phosphorus, thereby allowing for increased delivery of these minerals to preterm neonates (who require high doses), or to patients who are fluid-restricted.

TABLE 143.4

DAILY PROTEIN REQUIREMENTS FOR PEDIATRIC PATIENTS

Age	Amino acids (g/kg/day)
Premature neonate	3–4
Infant (1 mo to 1 yr)	2–3
Child (1–10 yr)	1–2
Adolescent (11–18 yr)	0.8–1.5

Caution must be exercised in patients with end-organ dysfunction such as renal or hepatic insufficiency, for whom excessive amino acids are potentially toxic.

Fat

Intravenous fat emulsions (IVFE), composed of soy or soy/safflower emulsions, are administered to prevent essential fatty acid deficiency (EFAD) and to provide a concentrated source of calories. Premature neonates have limited fat stores and may develop biochemical evidence of EFAD in less than 7 days, resulting in poor growth, dry skin and hair, impaired wound healing, and thrombocytopenia. Providing 2% to 4% of total daily calories as fat will prevent the clinical signs of EFAD.

In addition to the prevention of EFAD, the infusion of lipids with PN solutions can be helpful for patients who cannot tolerate large glucose loads and for patients who are limited to peripheral venous access (because these formulations are isotonic). The coadministration of fat emulsion and peripheral PN may prolong the viability of peripheral veins. For use in neonatal and infant populations, the 20% IVFE is preferred over the 10% formulation. The 20% emulsion contains a lower amount of surface-active agents (phospholipids from eggs) per gram of fat, resulting in more normal concentrations of circulating lipoprotein components, especially low-density lipoproteins. In addition, the 20% emulsion has a greater caloric density per unit volume. Because egg phospholipids are used to emulsify fat, patients beginning IVFE should be monitored for hypersensitivity reactions including fever, chills, dyspnea, cyanosis, nausea, headache, dizziness, chest pain, and back pain.

It is recommended that fat infusions begin at low doses and advance based on serum triglyceride measurements (see "Monitoring Parameters" later in the chapter). Most patients will tolerate starting with 1 g/kg/day and advancing by 1 g/kg/day (as directed by serum triglyceride assessment) until the caloric goal is reached. For small-for-gestational-age (SGA) neonates and preterm neonates less than 32 weeks gestation, 3 g/kg/day is the accepted maximum. For older infants and children, the American Academy of Pediatrics recommends no more than 4 g/kg/day delivered over a minimum of 20 to 24 hours; however, few patients require more than 3 g/kg/day. To calculate calories from IVFE (kcals):

$$\text{Fat kcal (20\% Fat Emulsion)} = \text{Total Volume (mL)} \times 2 \text{ kcal/mL}$$

Fat emulsions may often be administered as 3-in-1 solutions (total nutrient admixtures, TNA), in which all nutrients (protein, dextrose, lipids) are included in a single container. Limitations to the use of TNA include the particular protein solution, the total concentration of divalent cations, and IV access. Solutions containing TrophAmine cannot be mixed as TNA because the low pH of the amino acid solution destabilizes the emulsion if mixed together for long periods. These solutions may, however, be administered through a Y-site as separate infusions. The higher content of calcium and phosphate in neonatal and infant PN increases the risk of precipitation, which can go undetected because of the opacity of TNA. High concentrations of divalent cations (Ca^{++}, Mg^{++}) can reduce the particle zeta potential (negative surface charge), resulting in coalescence of lipid particles, which is dangerous to patients. In addition, most pediatric patients have only single-lumen IV access and must receive additional medications such as antibiotics, many of which are compatible with PN solutions but may not be compatible with IVFE. Separate administration allows the IVFE to be turned off for the duration of the medication administration while allowing the PN solution to continue.

Electrolytes and Minerals

Daily electrolyte and mineral requirements are shown in Table 143.5. In addition to daily maintenance requirements, electrolyte losses resulting from excessive body fluid losses (e.g., nasogastric suction, ostomy outputs, diarrheal stools) should be replaced separately with a comparable electrolyte solution. The standard electrolyte concentrations of body fluids are readily available.

Calcium and phosphorus requirements are substantially higher in neonates and infants than in older children, and are dramatically higher than in adults. Providing sufficient quantities to the premature neonate is difficult because of calcium and phosphorus solubility limitations in PN solutions. Precipitation can occur with increasing temperature, pH, or increasing concentrations of calcium and phosphorus. As the dextrose and amino acid concentrations increase, the pH of the solution falls, thereby increasing the solubility of calcium and phosphorus. Because calcium can produce severe tissue necrosis if concentrated solutions infiltrate peripherally, limitation of calcium concentration to 10 mEq/L of fluid is recommended for peripheral PN solutions.

In monitoring adequate calcium and phosphorus delivery in neonates and infants, serum calcium levels may appear normal due to the activity of parathyroid hormone, which stimulates mobilization of calcium from bone; therefore, serum calcium concentrations may not reflect actual calcium needs for growth.

TABLE 143.5

DAILY ELECTROLYTE AND MINERAL REQUIREMENTS[a]

Electrolyte	Preterm neonates	Infants/Children	Adolescents
Sodium	2–5 mEq/kg	2–5 mEq/kg	1–2 mEq/kg
Potassium	2–4 mEq/kg	2–4 mEq/kg	1–2 mEq/kg
Calcium	2–4 mEq/kg	0.5–4 mEq/kg	10–20 mEq
Phosphorus	1–2 mmol/kg	0.5–2 mmol/kg	10–40 mmol
Magnesium	0.3–0.5 mEq/kg	0.3–0.5 mEq/kg	10–30 mEq
Acetate	As needed to maintain acid–base balance	As needed to maintain acid–base balance	As needed to maintain acid–base balance
Chloride	As needed to maintain acid–base balance	As needed to maintain acid–base balance	As needed to maintain acid–base balance

[a]Assumes normal end-organ function.

TABLE 143.6

PARENTERAL MULTIVITAMIN PREPARATION

Vitamin	Pediatric dose (5 mL)	Adult dose (10 mL)
Vitamin A	2,300 IU	3,300 IU
Vitamin C (ascorbic acid)	80 mg	100 mg
Vitamin D	400 IU	200 IU
Vitamin E	7 IU	10 IU
Vitamin K	200 μg	150 μg
Folic Acid	140 μg	400 μg
Thiamin (B_1)	1.2 mg	3 mg
Riboflavin (B_2)	1.4 mg	3.6 mg
Niacin (B_3)	17 mg	40 mg
Pyridoxine (B_6)	1 mg	4 mg
Cyanocobalamin (B_{12})	1 μg	5 μg
Pantothenic acid	5 mg	15 mg
Biotin	20 μg	60 μg

In patients who are severely malnourished, the refeeding syndrome may occur. With aggressive refeeding, as the body mobilizes phosphorus, potassium, and magnesium to produce energy, serum levels may plummet, resulting in cardiac arrhythmias and sudden death. For patients at risk for refeeding syndrome, it is recommended to start nutrient repletion slowly and titrate carefully over several days while maintaining adequate serum levels of phosphorus, potassium, and magnesium.

When determining adequate electrolyte and mineral requirements for patients, risk factors for depletion should be taken into account. Medications (e.g., diuretics, amphotericin B, prior chemotherapy regimens), end-organ function (e.g., renal insufficiency), and baseline nutritional status should influence dosing. In general, children weighing over 50 kg should be dosed according to adolescent/adult guidelines for electrolytes and minerals.

Vitamins and Trace Elements

Vitamins play a key role in the metabolic processes in the body (for requirements, see Table 143.6). Many parenteral vitamins have greater bioavailability than oral forms; therefore, a lower dose than the Recommended Daily Allowance (RDA) is required to meet the body's metabolic needs. PN orders need not specify each vitamin individually (as with electrolytes and minerals); rather, age and weight are the main determinants for the dosage of parenteral supplementation. General dosing recommendations are as follows:

- Neonates weighing less than 2.5 kg require 2 mL/kg up to a maximum dose of 5 mL pediatric preparation.
- Neonates weighing more than 2.5 kg, term infants, and children 1 to 11 years of age require 5 mL pediatric preparation.
- Children older than 11 years of age require 10 mL of the adult preparation.

Vitamin D supplementation should be used with caution in patients with hypercalcemia or renal/cardiac anomalies. Hemodialysis patients and patients receiving hypertonic dextrose are at greater risk for thiamine deficiency. Vitamin C supplementation may be useful in wound healing and burn victims. Folate deficiency may be a side effect of methotrexate therapy. See Chapter 141 for further discussion of nutrient deficiencies and toxicities.

Trace element supplementation (for requirements, see Table 143.7) may need to be modified for neonates, surgery patients, and patients with kidney, intestinal, or liver dysfunction. Zinc supplementation may be needed in children with intractable diarrhea or high ostomy output. Supplementation ranges from 12 to 17 mg/L of ostomy losses. In septic children, the liver may sequester zinc, resulting in decreased serum levels. Zinc supplementation may benefit wound healing and treatment of burns in patients with zinc deficiency. However, prolonged high-dose zinc supplementation may interfere with copper uptake; therefore, assessment of zinc needs may need to be addressed after 2 weeks of supplementation beyond the RDA. In children with cholestasis, copper and manganese supplementation may need to be held or given less frequently (see the discussion of PN-associated cholestasis under "Complications of Parenteral Nutrition" later in the chapter). In cases of renal failure, chromium and selenium may need to be held or given less frequently. It is important to be familiar with the product that individual facilities utilize, as selenium and molybdenum may not be added to all parenteral pediatric preparations, especially neonatal ones. See Chapter 141 for further discussion of nutrient deficiencies and toxicities.

Monitoring Parameters

Several parameters should be monitored, both to ensure efficacy of parenteral nutrition and to screen for complications (Table 143.8).

TABLE 143.7

DAILY REQUIREMENT OF TRACE ELEMENTS[a]

Trace element	Preterm neonates <3 kg (μg/kg/day)	Term neonates 3–10 kg (μg/kg/day)	Children 10–40 kg (μg/kg/day)	Adolescents >40 kg (per day)
Zinc	400	50–250	150–125	2–5 mg
Copper	20	20	5–20	200–500 g
Manganese	1	1	1	40–100 μg
Chromium	0.05–0.2	0.2	0.14–0.2	5–15 μg
Selenium	1.5–2	2	1–2	40–60 μg

[a]Assumes normal age-related organ function and normal losses. Recommended doses cannot be achieved with the use of a single pediatric multiple trace element product. Only by using individualized trace element products can recommended doses be delivered.

TABLE 143.8

TABLE 143.8

SUGGESTED MONITORING PARAMETERS FOR PATIENTS RECEIVING PARENTERAL NUTRITION

Parameter	Frequency
Weight	Daily
Length and head circumference	Weekly
Input and output	Daily
Electrolytes	Baseline, daily × 2–3 days, then twice weekly
Calcium, magnesium, phosphorus	Baseline, phosphorus × 2–3 days if at risk for refeeding syndrome; weekly thereafter
Liver function tests	Baseline, then weekly
Albumin	Baseline, then weekly
Prealbumin	Baseline, then 1–2 times a week as needed
Triglycerides	Daily with changes in lipid dosing, then weekly
CBC with differential	As needed
Iron studies	As needed

COMPLICATIONS OF PARENTERAL NUTRITION

Metabolic

Patients receiving PN support should be monitored for development of hyperglycemia, hypoglycemia, metabolic acid-base imbalance, azotemia, hypo and hyperkalemia, volume overload, hypocalcemia, hypophosphatemia, hypomagnesemia, and hypertriglyceridemia (see Table 143.9).

Azotemia may develop in patients who are receiving inadequate amounts of nonprotein calories. Electrolyte imbalances can result from certain medications, disease states, excessive losses due to high output states, or inadequate supply. As

TABLE 143.9

COMPLICATIONS OF PARENTERAL NUTRITION

Metabolic
- Glucose abnormalities (hyperglycemia, hypoglycemia)
- Acid-base imbalance
- Azotemia
- Potassium abnormalities (hyperkalemia, hypokalemia)
- Hypocalcemia
- Hypophosphatemia
- Hypomagnesemia
- Hypertriglyceridemia

Cholestasis

Mechanical
- Catheter occlusion
- Pneumothorax, hemothorax, hydrothorax
- Vascular injury/perforation
- Cardiac injury/arrhythmias
- Embolic events (air, thrombus)
- Misdirection of catheter

mentioned previously, serum calcium levels are not always an accurate reflection of calcium requirements and may appear normal, even in a deficiency state, due to the action of parathyroid hormone.

As previously discussed (see electrolyte requirements), cardiac arrhythmias and sudden death from metabolic complications associated with refeeding syndrome may occur if PN is initiated too aggressively in a severely malnourished patient.

Hypertriglyceridemia may occur in SGA neonates due to their limited ability to metabolize fat. Carnitine facilitates transportation of long-chain fats across the mitochondrial membrane to the site of fat oxidation. SGA neonates often have limited stores of carnitine and may require addition of exogenous carnitine to PN solutions. Carnitine doses of 10 to 20 mg/kg/day added daily to PN solutions may improve fat utilization in this population. Carnitine supplementation has also been suggested for any pediatric patient receiving long-term PN supplementation (greater than 2 weeks).

In neonates with hyperbilirubinemia, administration of IVFE is controversial. Because bilirubin and fatty acids compete for binding sites on serum albumin, bilirubin may be displaced by free fatty acids, thereby increasing the concentration of unconjugated bilirubin and the likelihood of kernicterus. For patients with a bilirubin level greater than 15 mg/dL, limitation of IVFE to 1 g/kg/day to prevent EFAD is recommended, although the optimal dose has not been established.

Cholestasis can be a serious complication of PN, occurring most often in younger patients, particularly in neonates. After catheter infections, it is the second-most common reason for premature PN discontinuation. The development of cholestasis is multifactorial but is typically associated with prolonged use of PN. Possible factors include toxicities and deficiencies of the PN solution, absence of enteral feedings, overfeeding, prematurity, and sepsis. Clinically, cholestasis associated with PN presents as a gradual increase in total bilirubin, aspartate aminotransferase, and alkaline phosphatase. The most clinically important biochemical change is an increase in the conjugated bilirubin to 40% of the total bilirubin in association with PN therapy of more than 2 weeks. Because many patients in whom PN-associated cholestasis (PNAC) is suspected have other underlying risk factors for the development of hepatic dysfunction, it is considered a diagnosis of exclusion. In most cases, signs of hepatocellular damage will resolve upon discontinuation of PN, but later development of gallstones does occur. Transplantation is the only therapeutic option for patients in whom cholestasis progresses to cirrhosis and liver failure.

Prevention of PNAC includes avoidance of overfeeding, cycling off PN for part of the day, provision of some enteral nutrition, and removal of potentially hepatotoxic trace elements from PN for patients at risk. Overfeeding of all substrates, particularly carbohydrates and protein, has been associated with the development of cholestasis. The use of TrophAmine and carnitine in PN has been reported to minimize the development of PNAC, but these findings remain controversial. Cycling the patient off PN for part of the day is thought to prevent or delay the development of PNAC by decreasing the metabolic load on the liver. Results have been mixed, and any benefit has been suggested to be due to initiation of enteral feeds during the PN rest period. Failure to feed enterally has been linked to bacterial overgrowth in the gastrointestinal tract and a decrease in hormonal and neural stimulation of hepatic bile secretions, resulting in intrahepatic accumulation. Enteral feeds stimulate hormonal secretions, which enhance intestinal development and growth. Provision of as little as 10% to 20% of total calories enterally improves and/or reverses PNAC. Copper and manganese are trace elements that are excreted in the bile and may become hepatotoxic in patients with compromised hepatic function. Some institutions limit the administration of copper and manganese to once or twice a week in the PN solutions of patients who may be at risk of developing PNAC.

Numerous pharmacologic therapies for PNAC have been tried with limited success. Choleretics (phenobarbital), ursodeoxycholic acid (ursodiol, Actigall by Novartis, East Hanover, NJ), hormonal stimulants of bile flow (cholecystokinin analogues and glucagon), bile acid binders (cholestyramine and colestipol), and antibiotics (metronidazole) have all been reported to be somewhat helpful but are considered adjunctive. Prevention is the best management of this complication of PN therapy.

Mechanical

Mechanical complications of parenteral nutrition most commonly occur with placement or maintenance of a central venous catheter (Table 143.9). Occlusion of the catheter is the most common complication, and may necessitate removal of the catheter. Treatment of mechanical complications is specific to the mechanical problem encountered.

Infectious

Sepsis in a patient receiving parenteral nutrition may present with new onset of fever, recent glucose or lipid intolerance, and/or glycosuria. Other signs and symptoms of sepsis may also be present. The patient should be carefully examined for a focus of infection, including the catheter site. A blood culture should be obtained from the catheter and from an additional peripheral site. Pending the results of the cultures, appropriate antibiotics should be considered based on local epidemiology. True sepsis is demonstrated by positive blood cultures from the peripheral site in addition to a positive blood culture from the catheter; a positive blood culture from the line alone suggests a line infection. In either case, definitive antibiotic therapy is determined by the culture results and the sensitivities of the organisms. Many bacterial infections can be eradicated by administering antibiotics through the infected catheter without removal of the catheter. If the patient continues to be symptomatic, or if blood cultures continue to be positive in spite of 24 to 48 hours of appropriate antibiotics, the catheter should be removed. However fungal infections (e.g., *Candida* spp.) and some bacterial infections require immediate removal of the catheter to clear the infection. Removal of the catheter is also necessary in those patients who are seriously compromised by the septic event.

TRANSITIONING FROM PARENTERAL TO ENTERAL FEEDING

Transitioning from parenteral to enteral nutrition is patient-dependent and often relates to the diagnosis and length of time without enteral feeding. Generally feeding is initiated at 1 mL/kg/hr. Enteral product selection is discussed further in Chapter 142. Advances of 10 to 20 mL/kg/day in preterm infants, 1 to 2 mL/kg every 2 to 8 hours for term infants, 1 mL/kg every 2 to 8 hours for children 1 to 6 years, and 25 mL every 2 to 8 hours for children over 7 years, is a conservative practice. While advancing enteral feedings, the parenteral support must be decreased accordingly to maintain total fluid and calorie goals. This transitional period can last from 2 days to several weeks, depending on the child's tolerance of dietary advancements. Close monitoring of gastric residuals, stool consistency, reducing substances, stool pH, and nausea or emesis should provide any evidence of feeding intolerance.

Suggested Readings

American Society for Parenteral and Enteral Nutrition (ASPEN). Safe practices for parenteral nutrition formulations. *JPEN* 2004;28:S55–S57.

American Society for Parenteral and Enteral Nutrition (ASPEN) Board of Directors and The Clinical Guidelines Task Force. Guidelines for the use of parenteral and enteral nutrition in adult and pediatric patients. *JPEN* 2002;26:13SA–21SA, 25SA–50SA, 97SA–138SA.

Baker RD, ed. *Pediatric parenteral nutrition.* Silver Spring, MD, ASPEN; 1997.

Baumgartner TG, ed. *Clinical guide to parenteral micronutrition.* Fujisawa, LTD Deerfield, IL (Now called Astellas Pharma Ltd.), 2nd ed. 1991.

Cochrane EB, Phelps SA, Helms RA. Parenteral nutrition in pediatric patients. *Clin Pharm* 1988;7:351–366.

Kerner KA, ed. *Manual of pediatric parenteral nutrition.* New York: Wiley; 1983.

Shulman RJ, Phillips S. Parenteral nutrition in infants and children. *J Pediatr Gastroenterol Nutr* 2003;36:587–607.

CHAPTER 144 ■ ANAPHYLAXIS

EMILY FONTANE

Case reports of rapidly progressive and often fatal reactions in humans to a variety of substances have been published since the 17th century. However, it was in 1902 that Drs. Paul J. Portier and Charles R. Richet named and described the potentially life-threatening condition known as *anaphylaxis* (Greek for "without protection"). During an experiment expected to provide prophylaxis to dogs by injecting the dogs with anemone venom immunotherapy, they instead observed anaphylaxis after re-exposing the sensitized dogs to subsequent doses of venom.

EPIDEMIOLOGY

Anaphylaxis is estimated to occur in 1% to 15% of the U.S. population. The true incidence of anaphylaxis in children is unknown, but is estimated to be approximately 68.4 per 100,000 person-years.

DEFINITION

Recently, representative members of allergy and immunology organizations convened to develop a universal definition of anaphylaxis and to create a universal set of clinical guidelines for the diagnosis of anaphylaxis. Experts purposely chose a broad definition to encompass as many cases as possible. They agreed that anaphylaxis is a serious allergic reaction that is rapid in onset and may cause death. Specifically, *anaphylaxis* is described as a severe, potentially fatal, systemic allergic reaction that occurs suddenly after a patient comes into contact with an allergy-causing substance.

ETIOLOGY/PATHOGENESIS

A patient may be exposed to allergens by a variety of routes including oral, inhalational, parenteral, and transdermal. The most common known allergy-causing substances are food, medications, and insect venom. The clinical manifestations of anaphylaxis are caused by the action of histamine and other potent inflammatory mediators on epithelial and vascular tissue. Typically cross-linking of cell surface IgE on tissue mast cells and peripheral blood basophils will cause cell degranulation and subsequent release of histamine and other mediators when sensitized cells are re-exposed to antigen. Another way mast cells and basophils release mediators is through the direct effect of circulating antigen on these cells. IgE antibody-mediated reactions, also known as *type 1 hypersensitivity reactions*, are called *anaphylactic reactions*. Reactions that are not IgE-mediated are called *anaphylactoid reactions*. Mucocutaneous edema and inflammation, bronchospasm, smooth-muscle spasm, and increased capillary permeability usually occur rapidly (minutes to hours) after antigen exposure regardless of the mechanism of histamine and other mediator release. Clinically, the term anaphylaxis is used to identify patient cases due to both anaphylactic (or IgE mediated) and anaphylactoid (or non-IgE mediated) reactions because the symptoms, exam findings, and treatment are essentially the same.

The terms uniphasic, biphasic, and protracted are used to describe the variable courses of anaphylaxis. A *uniphasic reaction* may last as long as 1 to 2 hours, will completely resolve with appropriate treatment, and not recur. A *biphasic reaction* has a symptom-free period in between an early phase similar to a uniphasic reaction and a late phase that may occur hours to days after the resolution of the early phase. Biphasic reactions are reported to occur in 1% to 20% of all anaphylaxis cases. Although it is difficult to predict which patients will experience biphasic reactions, patients who have oral allergen exposures, patients with severe presentations requiring multiple doses of epinephrine, and patients in whom administration of epinephrine is delayed are reported to be at increased risk of having biphasic reactions. A *protracted reaction* may last for days without resolution of symptoms despite aggressive therapy. Protracted reactions are reported to occur more commonly after intravenous allergen exposures. Although the majority of cases of anaphylaxis are caused by food, medications, insect venom, latex, and exercise, up to a third of anaphylaxis cases have no known trigger and no identified agent. These cases are called idiopathic anaphylaxis, which can be determined only after a rigorous historical, physical, and laboratory search for the inciting agent in consultation with an allergist-immunologist.

CAUSES

Anaphylaxis to Food

Food-induced anaphylaxis is responsible for approximately 200 deaths per year in the United States. In children, most cases of anaphylaxis are caused by food. The most commonly implicated foods are peanuts and other tree nuts (most common), fish, shellfish, milk, and eggs. These reactions almost always occur minutes after ingestion. Allergen exposure via the oral route increases the risk of biphasic reactions. Children may be sensitized to food items in utero and during breast-feeding.

Anaphylaxis to Drugs

Antibiotics and nonsteroidal anti-inflammatory drugs are the most common causes of drug-induced anaphylaxis in children. Although penicillin is credited with causing the most cases of drug-induced allergy, most patients with a reported penicillin allergy have a negative skin test for penicillin. Furthermore, the extent of allergic cross-reactivity between penicillin and cephalosporins appears to be low. Only 4% of skin-test-positive penicillin allergic patients reacted to cephalosporin challenges. Atopy is considered a risk factor for contrast material-induced anaphylaxis.

Anaphylaxis to Insect Venom

Insect venom from *Hymenoptera* (bees, wasps, fire ants) causes about 50 deaths per year in the United States. Insect venom allergy has been noted to be amenable to immunotherapy.

Anaphylaxis to Latex

Children with spina bifida are at increased risk for latex-induced anaphylaxis (thought due to a unique predisposition in these patients). Children who have undergone multiple urologic surgeries, probably due to early (during infancy) exposure to latex in the hospital setting, also have an increased risk for latex allergy. Children known to have spina bifida, congenital urologic abnormalities requiring multiple surgeries, and those with a known history of latex allergy should have all medical procedures performed in a latex-free environment that has no latex gloves or latex medical equipment (catheters, adhesives, tourniquets, and sedation equipment). Atopy is considered a risk factor for latex-induced anaphylaxis. Medications and latex are likely to be the cause of anaphylaxis in the hospital setting.

Food-Associated Exercise-Induced Anaphylaxis

Food-associated exercise-induced anaphylaxis only occurs when food that is commonly associated with anaphylaxis is ingested within 2 hours prior to exercising. The food or exercise alone will not induce symptoms.

DIAGNOSIS

Anaphylaxis is a true medical emergency because it is a serious allergic reaction and may cause death. Preparedness, prompt recognition, and appropriate and aggressive treatment are essential to good outcome. A targeted history should elicit known allergies, history of atopy or anaphylaxis, offending agent and route of exposure if known, symptoms and time of onset, self-administered or ambulance treatment prior to hospital arrival, and comorbidities and routine medications. Treatment may be warranted in a patient with a history of previous severe reactions and known recent exposure despite mild symptoms.

The most frequently noted symptoms and exam findings in anaphylaxis, from the most common to the least common, include the following:

- Mucocutaneous (seen in the majority of cases): urticaria and angioedema, flushing, pruritis without rash.
- Respiratory (seen in the majority of cases): upper airway angioedema, dyspnea, wheeze, rhinitis.
- Cardiovascular: dizziness, syncope, hypotension.
- Gastrointestinal: nausea, vomiting, diarrhea, cramping pain.
- CNS: headache, seizure.

Cutaneous symptoms are reported in approximately 95% of patient case series in children. Although the majority of cases of anaphylaxis report cutaneous manifestations, the absence of cutaneous manifestations does not rule out an anaphylac-

TABLE 144.1

ANAPHYLAXIS SYMPTOMS BY SYSTEM

System	Symptoms
Oral	Labial, lingual, palatal pruritis; angioedema; metallic taste
Cutaneous	Flushing, pruritus, urticaria, morbilliform rash, pilo erection
GI	Nausea, vomiting, colic, diarrhea
Upper respiratory	Aural, nasal and pharyngeal pruritis, rhinorrhea, cough, sneezing, stridor, dysphagia, tightness in throat, hoarse voice
Lower respiratory	Shortness of breath, wheezing, chest tightness, retractions
Cardiovascular	Light-headedness, syncope, chest pain, hypotension, bradycardia/tachycardia
CNS	Anxiety, sense of impending doom, headache, decreased level of consciousness, seizures
Other	Conjunctival injection and tearing, uterine contractions, low back pain

tic event. Cutaneous signs or symptoms may be delayed or absent in rapidly progressive anaphylaxis. For a more complete list of symptoms and exam findings by systems, see Table 144.1.

Risk factors for anaphylaxis include a history of anaphylaxis, asthma, and atopy. The diagnostic criteria developed and accepted by worldwide experts in the field are predicted to identify greater than 95% of all cases of anaphylaxis. It is the hope of the international expert community that a universal definition and widely accepted clinical criteria will not only help the medical community at large to better identify patients with anaphylaxis, but also facilitate research in the epidemiology, pathophysiology, diagnosis, and treatment of anaphylaxis.

Diagnostic Criteria

Expert panelists agree that anaphylaxis is highly likely when any *one* of the following three criteria is fulfilled:

1. Acute onset mucocutaneous symptoms and one of the following:
   - Respiratory symptoms
   - Cardiovascular symptoms
2. Rapid development of two or more of the following symptoms after exposure to a likely allergen for that patient:
   - Mucocutaneous symptoms
   - Respiratory symptoms
   - Cardiovascular symptoms
   - Gastrointestinal symptoms
3. Acute-onset hypotension after exposure to known allergen for that patient.

MANAGEMENT AND TREATMENT

The standard of care for the treatment of patients suspected of having anaphylaxis comes from a practice parameter developed by specialty task force members and reviewed by experts on anaphylaxis. In the hospital setting, all patients should have ready access to emergency medications and equipment as well as readily available care from a team of health care professionals prepared to act in an emergency situation. Standard approach to and documentation of management and treatment of all emergencies is valuable to both the patient and the health care team. Regular practice drills for anaphylaxis as for other emergencies (cardiopulmonary arrest, multisystem trauma) may improve team response and success.

As in all emergency situations, the patient's airway, breathing, circulation, and disability (level of consciousness) are evaluated while interventions to protect and optimize neuro-cardio-pulmonary systems are simultaneously implemented. Epinephrine directly blocks the inflammatory effects of histamine, dilates bronchioles, constricts vessels, increases both heart rate and blood pressure, and improves contractility of the heart. It prevents ongoing capillary leakage and inhibits continued cell-mediator release. As soon as the diagnosis of anaphylaxis is suspected, or any of the three above criteria is fulfilled, epinephrine (0.01 mg/kg of 1:1000 up to 0.3 mg; see Table 144.2) should be administered as an intramuscular injection into the anterolateral thigh musculature every 5 minutes as needed. IM epinephrine injected into the lateral thigh provides more rapid absorption and higher plasma levels of epinephrine than subcutaneous dosing in children. The data supporting this practice comes from studies of healthy individuals not experiencing anaphylaxis, but it is the best evidence to date. Administration of epinephrine via alternate routes (subcutaneous, inhaled, sublingual, and endotracheal) for the initial treatment of anaphylaxis is not recommended despite case reports of anecdotal success. Delay in the administration of IM epinephrine should be avoided, because delay in first-line treatment has been associated with an increase risk of biphasic reactions and poor outcome.

TABLE 144.2

MEDICATIONS FOR ANAPHYLAXIS

PRIMARY MEDICATION

Drug	Dose	Route
Epinephrine 1:1000	0.01 mg/kg, max 0.3 mg, repeat every 5 minutes if no response	IM route of choice

SECONDARY TREATMENTS

Drug	Dose	Route
Methylprednisolone	2 mg/kg, max 125 mg	IV, IM, IO
Dexamethasone	0.2 mg/kg, max 10 mg	IV, IM, IO
IVF: normal saline	20-mL/kg bolus	IV, IO
Diphenhydramine	1–2 mg/kg, max 50 mg/dose	IV, IM, IO
Ranitidine	1 mg/kg, max 50 mg	IV, IO
Albuterol	0.5–1.0 mL, 0.5% solution nebulized in 2–3 mL NS	Inhaled
Epinephrine 1:1000	0.5 mL/kg diluted in 3 mL NS nebulized, max <4yr: 2.5 mL/dose, >4 yr: 5 mL/dose	Inhaled

REFRACTORY HYPOTENSION

Drug	Dose	Route
Epinephrine 1:10,000	0.1 μg/kg/min continuous infusion	IV titrated to effect

ALTERNATE HISTAMINE-BLOCKING AGENTS

Drug	Dose	Route
Hydroxyzine	0.5–1 mg/kg, max 2 mg/kg/day	IV, IM
Famotidine	0.25 mg/kg, max 20mg	IV

FOR PATIENTS ON BETA-BLOCKER THERAPY

Drug	Dose	Route
Glucagon	0.02–0.03 mg/kg, max 1mg over 5 minutes followed by a continuous 5–15 μg/min infusion titrated to clinical effect	IV, IM, IO

PRESCRIPTION FOR ALL PATIENTS WHO HAVE BEEN DIAGNOSED WITH ANAPHYLAXIS

Drug	Dose	Route
EpiPen	0.3 mg for children >30 kg 0.15 mg for children <30 kg	IM

Subsequent treatment is determined on the basis of the response to epinephrine. If identified, the allergy-causing substance should be removed or discontinued. Physicians caring for patients with suspected anaphylaxis should individualize care when needed while ensuring that the standard of care is upheld. As in multisystem trauma and cardiopulmonary arrest, the goal of a standard approach is improvement of the quality of care for all patients.

Airway

The upper airway is assessed for abnormal sounds (stridor, hoarseness) and angioedema (lip-tongue-uvula-pharyngeal-laryngeal swelling). Intramuscular (IM) epinephrine, given in the anterolateral thigh every 5 minutes, is the treatment of choice in anaphylaxis and should be given as soon as the diagnosis is suspected. The patient's airway should be cleared and supplemental oxygen should be provided via endotracheal tube for patients in respiratory failure or arrest or with airway edema unresponsive to epinephrine. Oxygen by nonrebreather mask should be provided for all patients with any respiratory symptoms, any cardiovascular symptoms, a history of pulmonary problems such as asthma, a history of anaphylaxis, and in any patient suspected of having a moderate or severe course. Oxygen therapy is guided by continuous pulse oximetry and/or arterial blood gas analysis. Inhaled epinephrine in doses used for croup may be administered to patients with stridor and upper airway edema. Patients with severe, unresponsive upper-airway edema who have failed an endotracheal intubation attempt should have an alternative advanced-airway maneuver performed such as needle cricothyrotomy or surgical airway by a health care professional skilled in the procedure.

Breathing

After the airway is secure, the quality and quantity of breaths is assessed. Tachypnea, bradypnea, nasal flaring, grunting, retractions and seesaw respirations are signs of respiratory distress. In addition to IM epinephrine, albuterol should be administered to patients with lower airway bronchospasm or wheezing unresponsive to epinephrine. Although corticosteroids are not proven to improve outcome in anaphylaxis and are not effective for up to 4 to 6 hours after administration, they may help decrease the risk of late-phase reactions. Steroids should be administered early to prevent late-phase reactions. Methylprednisolone (2 mg/kg, maximum 125 mg) is given IM or IV.

Circulation

A patient's appearance, color, heart rate, and blood pressure should be rapidly evaluated. A decrease in systolic blood pressure (SBP) of greater than 30% of normal for a particular patient, or an SBP lower than the lowest acceptable SBP for age (see below), should be treated immediately and aggressively with IM epinephrine given in the anterolateral thigh every 5 minutes as needed.

- <60 mm Hg in term neonates (0 to 28 days)
- <70 mm Hg in infants (1 month to 12 months)
- <70 mm Hg + (2 × age in years) in children 1 to 10 years
- <90 mm Hg in children ≥10 years of age

All patients should have cardiopulmonary monitoring and an IV line started. Patients with anaphylaxis may require multiple boluses of crystalloid fluids to counter the effects of proinflammatory mediators on the cardiovascular system. Normal saline bolus therapy may improve the course in patients with cardiovascular insufficiency initially unresponsive to epinephrine. A 20-mL/kg bolus of normal saline is given over 5 to 10 minutes. Up to 100 mL/kg of normal saline may be needed.

Less aggressive fluid replacement is required in cases with purely respiratory symptoms and in patients with only mild or immediately responsive circulatory symptoms. An intravenous or intraosseous epinephrine infusion may be started in patients who remain profoundly hypotensive or progress to cardiac arrest despite several doses of IM epinephrine and aggressive intravenous volume replacement. Although there is no established dose or regimen for intravenous epinephrine in the treatment of anaphylaxis, the experts recommend a continuous low-dose epinephrine infusion titrated to desired effect to avoid inducing lethal arrhythmias. Vasopressin therapy may be needed for intractable distributive shock. Transcutaneous pacing may be attempted in cases of pulseless electrical activity and/or asystole.

Disability

A decrease in level of consciousness in a patient in anaphylactic shock suggests impaired CNS perfusion. The patient should be placed in the recumbent position with lower extremities elevated as tolerated to help shunt effective circulation from the periphery to the central circulation. Patients who are short of breath or vomiting may not tolerate this positioning. Upright position should be avoided in those with circulatory compromise due to anaphylaxis because upright posture has been associated with poor outcome in some cases.

It is important to stress that epinephrine is considered first-line therapy for anaphylaxis and that all other medications recommended for the treatment of anaphylaxis are considered second-line therapies. These other medications will not work as quickly as epinephrine and therefore should never be used alone as treatment for anaphylaxis.

LABORATORY FINDINGS

Serum tryptase and urinary histamine levels may help diagnose unclear cases of anaphylaxis. The best time to measure serum tryptase levels is approximately 1 hour after symptom onset but no later than 6 hours after the event. Urinary histamine metabolites may be measured up to 24 hours after the onset of symptoms. Treatment should not be delayed while awaiting laboratory confirmation. Anaphylaxis is a clinical diagnosis, and delay in treatment is associated with biphasic reactions and generally poor outcome. It is more important to obtain a thorough history of the event. The history is considered by allergist-immunologists to be the most important tool one can use to help establish the diagnosis and cause of anaphylaxis.

DIFFERENTIAL DIAGNOSIS

The differential diagnosis of anaphylaxis includes other causes of distributive shock such as sepsis, moderate to severe asthma, seizure disorder, hypoglycemia, acute poisoning, foreign-body aspiration, spasmodic croup, vasodepressor (also known as vasovagal) syncope, panic attacks, hereditary angioedema, systemic mastocytosis, metastatic carcinoid syndromes, and scombroid poisoning.

COURSE

Respiratory failure and cardiovascular collapse are the most frequent causes of fatalities. Rapid progression of symptoms is associated with a more severe and potentially life-threatening course. The allergy-immunology literature states that anaphylaxis often produces signs and symptoms within 30 minutes of exposure to an offending agent, but some reactions develop after 30 minutes. The distributive shock seen in anaphylaxis due to increased vascular permeability may evolve over minutes and require aggressive crystalloid replacement. Beta-blocker use may complicate anaphylaxis by reducing the effectiveness of epinephrine. Patients should be admitted to a monitored or intensive-care unit bed depending on severity of initial course and patient condition prior to disposition.

Patients requiring higher doses of epinephrine to treat their symptoms, patients who did not receive timely epinephrine treatment, and patients who experienced severe symptoms should be admitted because they are more likely to have a biphasic reaction. Patients with a history of atopy or asthma should be considered for admission regardless of course because fatalities occur more commonly in these patients. Only those patients with mild mucocutaneous and gastrointestinal symptoms and complete resolution of symptoms within 2 to 4 hours should be considered for discharge. The recommended observation period for patients with complete resolution of symptoms is 4 to 6 hours before discharge.

PATIENT EDUCATION AND PREVENTION

Patient and patient family education is a very important preventative strategy. Recurrence is not uncommon. Prior to discharge, patients treated for anaphylaxis should be instructed to avoid any known triggers and should be encouraged to wear medical-alert jewelry indicating any known allergens. Patients should receive instructions on the indications and use of an epinephrine auto-injector along with a prescription for an auto-injector. Bright clothes and perfume attract insects and should be avoided. Follow-up with an allergist-immunologist should be arranged for all patients treated for anaphylaxis. Patients should be instructed to read food labels for ingredients and to avoid eating any food for which preparation is uncertain.

Suggested Readings

Nougat AI, Ghana AT, Miller RL. Anaphylaxis in the United States: an investigation into its epidemiology. *Arch Med* 2001;161:15–21.

Sampson HA, Muñoz-Furlong A, Campbell RL et al. Second symposium on the definition and management of anaphylaxis: summary report—second National Institute of Allergy and Infection Disease/Food Allergy and Anaphylaxis Network symposium. *J Allergy Clin Immanual* 2006: 311–117.

Zibners L, Laddis D, Berger K. Pediatric anaphylaxis: critical aspects of ED management. *Pediatr Emerg Med Rep* 2006;11:53–64.

CHAPTER 145 ■ ERYTHEMA MULTIFORME, STEVENS–JOHNSON SYNDROME, AND TOXIC EPIDERMAL NECROLYSIS

JAMES D. KORB

The evaluation and treatment of erythema multiforme (EM), Stevens–Johnson syndrome (SJS), and toxic epidermal necrolysis (TEN) have been fraught with misdiagnosis and confusion. The precise diagnostic criteria for each of these diseases, and the relationships of the diseases to one another, have been areas of controversy and uncertainty for many years.

For many years, all three of these were felt to be manifestations of the same disease process. Recently, however, EM has been shown to be a separate and distinct disease from SJS and TEN. In the vast majority of cases, EM represents a hypersensitivity reaction to herpes simplex virus (HSV). The skin rash is characterized by fixed erythematous papules, and the appearance of true target lesions that demonstrate epithelial destruction centrally. Mucosal involvement is mild, and usually confined to the oropharynx. EM is a self-limited illness with minimal morbidity (1,2).

SJS and TEN are felt by most experts to be different parts of the spectrum of the same disease. They are caused by similar precipitating factors, most commonly drugs or infection. Both are characterized by significant blistering, widespread erythematous or purpuric macules, and severe mucous membrane (especially eye and mouth) involvement. True target lesions are not seen. Current definitions apply the term SJS when the extent of blistering is <10% of the skin surface, and TEN when it is >30%. Blistering involving 10% to 30% of the skin surface is termed an "overlap SJS-TEN" (3,4). A prolonged course with significant mortality is typical of severe forms of SJS and of TEN.

The above definitions are more closely in line with the original descriptions of the diseases by von Hebra, Lyell, Stevens, and Johnson. Using these definitions, significant clinical differences can be shown between EM and SJS/TEN with respect to the distribution and extent of the skin lesions, the presence of target lesions or purpura or blisters, the extent of mucosal involvement, the precipitating factors, and outcomes. In addition, the histologic appearance and cytokine profile are also different in the two groups. All of this strongly suggests that EM is a different disease from SJS/TEN (5,6). In addition, patients with an initial diagnosis of SJS may evolve into typical TEN; patients with EM do not progress to either SJS or TEN. The use of older terms, such as EM major (for SJS and TEN) and EM minor (for EM), should be avoided (Table 145.1).

ERYTHEMA MULTIFORME

EM is a very uncommon disease in children, despite the frequent use of the term for any impressive, polymorphous skin rash. It is most commonly seen in young adults, with only 20% of cases occurring in children. There does not appear to be any racial or genetic predisposition. It occurs slightly more frequently in boys than girls, and the mean age, in one series, was 8.1 years old.

The most common precipitating factor is herpes simplex virus (HSV) type 1. A preceding herpes infection (usually oral or labial) can be demonstrated in over 50% of cases. The herpes infection usually precedes the onset of the rash by 3 to 14 days, although the two can be present concurrently. In those patients without a history of an antecedent herpes infection, HSV DNA can be detected by PCR in papules or target lesions 80% of the time (7). Hence, most cases of EM are secondary to a clinical or subclinical infection with HSV. In adolescents, HSV type 2 has also been reported as a precipitating factor.

Other infectious agents that have been infrequently associated with EM include histoplasmosis, orf, Epstein–Barr virus, and varicella-zoster. Whether or not *Mycoplasma pneumoniae* is associated with EM continues to be hotly debated in the literature, but it probably should be considered a less frequent, but possible, cause (8,9). The difficulty in making a rapid and accurate diagnosis of *Mycoplasma* has been one of the reasons for the controversy. Of note, pneumonia does not have to be present in patients with EM associated with *Mycoplasma*. The role of medications as a cause is also debated. Studies suggest an association with a preceding drug in up to 5% to 10% of cases.

Clinical Presentation

The rash begins abruptly with the development of erythematous papules that are fixed in location. The lesions are symmetrically distributed, and usually begin distally on the arms and hands. They can spread to the palms, neck, face, and trunk, but the rash still retains a predominantly acral distribution. There may be some mild itching or burning. Importantly, all of the lesions develop over the first 72 hours of the illness. Blistering, when present, will cover <10% of the skin surface area, and widespread blistering or sheet-like epidermal separation is not seen.

Some of the papules will develop into target lesions. Classic target lesions are raised and circular, with a dusky or purpuric center. They are surrounded by either a single erythematous ring, or by a middle pale edematous ring with an outer erythematous ring. The number of rings present is not clinically significant. Epidermal destruction, in the form of blisters, crusts, or erosions, is seen within a few days in the

TABLE 145.1

KEY QUESTIONS TO ASK

- Was there a recent illness consistent with HSV or *Mycoplasma pneumoniae*? Have there been prodromal symptoms?
- Were medications, especially those associated with SJS/TEN, started within the last 1 to 8 weeks?
- Are macular or papular lesions fixed in location, or do they migrate over time? Does the child have edema of the hands or feet?
- Are true target lesions present?
- Is the rash centrally or acrally distributed?
- Is the rash continuing to progress after 3 to 4 days?
- Is blistering or sheetlike separation of the epidermis present, and how much of the skin surface area is involved?
- What is the extent and nature of the oral mucous membrane involvement? Are other mucous membranes involved?
- Is the child toxic-appearing?
- Is there evidence of multiorgan system failure?

center of some of the target lesions, and is an important feature in making the correct diagnosis.

Lesions on the elbows and knees are often grouped. Lesions can also occur at the site of recent skin trauma (Koebner phenomenon).

In about half of the cases, there are oral lesions. These shallow ulcerations are few in number, and involve the lips, buccal mucosa, and tongue. The gingiva is spared. There is usually little pain associated with the lesions. Rarely, large target lesions involving the lips can resemble the crusted, hemorrhagic changes seen in SJS (10). Involvement of other mucous membranes has been reported but is uncommon.

With the exception of a preceding herpetic infection, there is usually no prodrome, and little or no fever. The children are generally well-appearing (Table 145.2).

Differential Diagnosis

The most common condition confused with EM is urticaria. Large urticarial wheals are commonly misdiagnosed as target lesions, and can frequently develop a purplish to brownish discoloration in the center as they fade. Urticaria will not show, however, the characteristic signs of epidermal damage centrally (ulcers, crusts, or bullae) seen in a true target lesion. Additional features of urticaria that help make the correct diagnosis include the transient nature of the urticaria (individual lesions last <24 hours), the frequent presence of extremity edema, and the development of new lesions beyond 72 hours. Urticaria may also improve with oral antihistamines (1,3).

TABLE 145.2

KEY FEATURES OF ERYTHEMA MULTIFORME

Usually secondary to an HSV infection
Fixed popular lesions, predominantly acral in distribution
True target lesions with central crusting, blisters, or ulcers
Mucosal involvement is mild, if present

Both SLE and urticarial vasculitis may present with lesions that resemble the target lesions of EM. Other clinical features, as well as an elevated ESR and low serum complement, will usually suggest these diagnoses. A polymorphous light eruption (PMLE) can also be confused with recurrent EM, as both can present with a papular rash on sun-exposed areas. Further changes over time will usually make the proper diagnosis clear.

Laboratory Studies

There are no routine studies needed for EM. In cases without a clear preceding HSV infection, specific testing for *Mycoplasma pneumoniae* could be considered. A skin biopsy is not routinely needed to make the diagnosis of EM, but can be done when vasculitis is clinically suspected.

Treatment and Course

EM is a self-limited condition, with most cases resolving within 2 weeks. The lesions heal without sequelae. Recurrences are often seen, and generally occur once or twice a year for several years. Patients on immunosuppressive drugs, including oral corticosteroids, may have more frequent and longer-lasting recurrences. As mentioned previously, EM does not progress to SJS or TEN.

Treatment is primarily symptomatic. Oral antihistamines are recommended for any itching or burning. The oral lesions usually do not interfere with the child's ability to drink or eat. Topical and oral acyclovir is not effective, even when started at the onset of the rash. In patients with frequent recurrences of EM associated with HSV, daily oral acyclovir (10 mg/kg/day) given over 6 to 12 months has been shown to decrease the number of recurrences or lead to remission (11).

There is no evidence that oral corticosteroids hasten the resolution of the disease, and they should not be used. Unfortunately, many children are inappropriately treated with corticosteroids in the erroneous belief that this will prevent the disease from progressing to SJS. There are no studies evaluating antibiotic treatment for possible *Mycoplasma*.

STEVENS–JOHNSON SYNDROME AND TOXIC EPIDERMAL NECROLYSIS

SJS and TEN are currently felt to represent different parts of the spectrum of the same disease. It is very uncommon, with reported incidences of 1 in 30,000 for SJS and 1 in 100,000 for TEN (1,12). The majority of cases occur in children, usually in adolescence.

The cause in most cases is either a drug or infection. Many different drugs have been associated with SJS/TEN, with nonsteroidal anti-inflammatory drugs (NSAIDs), anticonvulsants, antibiotics, and allopurinol most commonly implicated. Among the antibiotics, sulfonamides confer the greatest relative risk; aminopenicillins, tetracyclines, quinolones, cephalosporins, and macrolides have all been associated with SJS/TEN. Among anticonvulsants, carbamazepine, phenytoin, phenobarbital, lamotrigine, and valproic acid are frequently cited. Importantly, those drugs that have been started recently, from 1 to 8 weeks before the onset of the rash, are most likely to be causative. SJS/TEN is not commonly seen in the first week after starting a new drug, or after a drug has been given for more than 2 months (1,13,14).

The best-documented infectious trigger for SJS (and to a lesser extent TEN) is *Mycoplasma pneumoniae*. Other infectious agents have been sporadically reported in association

TABLE 145.3

KEY FEATURES OF STEVENS–JOHNSON SYNDROME
AND TOXIC EPIDERMAL NECROLYIS

Usually secondary to drugs or infections (*Mycoplasma*)
Severe oropharyngeal/conjunctival involvement with crusted,
hemorrhagic lips
Macules and papules without true target lesions, in a central
distribution
Bullae and areas of epidermal separation (<10% of skin surface area in SJS, >30% in TEN)
Respiratory, gastrointestinal, and urogenital tract involvement often present and severe

with the disease. Unlike EM, HSV is not commonly associated
with SJS/TEN. TEN is associated with drugs in 80% to 95%
of cases; both infection and drugs are important in SJS (1,12).

A genetically determined inability to detoxify aromatic
drug metabolites has been suggested as a possible mechanism
of disease with NSAIDs, some anticonvulsants, and sulfonamides. Other studies have suggested a role for autoantibodies
to desmoplakin I and II in the skin. Both SJS/TEN are much
more common in patients with acquired immunodeficiency
syndrome (1/1,000 versus 1.2/1,000,000). SJS seems to be
more common in patients with systemic lupus erythematosus.

Clinical Presentation

The clinical features are similar, but with some differences as
noted above (Table 145.3).

Stevens–Johnson Syndrome

Most cases of SJS begin with a prodrome that can include any of
the following: fever, cough, rhinorrhea, sore throat, headache,
vomiting, diarrhea, arthralgias, and myalgias. Many of these
symptoms probably reflect the preceding infectious precipitant.
At the time of presentation, most patients are febrile and ill-
appearing.

Mucous membrane involvement develops 1 to 14 days
later. By definition, at least two mucosal surfaces are affected.
The mucous membrane involvement is significant and clinically impressive. A severe stomatitis is seen with edema and
painful erosions throughout the oropharynx. The lips develop
hemorrhagic crusts with areas of necrosis and denudation.
Oral intake is severely limited secondary to the stomatitis.
Most patients (85% to 90%) have conjunctival involvement
as well, with conjunctival injection, erosions, purulent discharge, and photophobia. Other mucosal surfaces can be
involved, including the anogenital area. This can lead to additional problems such as vaginal or rectal bleeding from
painful erosions, dysuria, and urinary retention. Less commonly, the esophageal and respiratory tracts can be affected;
GI bleeding and pneumonia have been described.

The rash develops at the same time or after the onset of
mucous membrane involvement. Red macules develop rapidly
into a widespread morbilliform or papular eruption. Bullae
may develop in these areas, and widespread areas of epidermal necrosis can develop. By definition, the bullae in SJS
involve <10% of the skin surface area. The bullous lesions are
often large and flaccid, and tend to coalesce. The skin is tender, and lateral pressure on the skin will lead to further separation of the epidermis (positive Nikolsky sign). The skin
lesions tend to be more centrally distributed, as opposed to the
acral distribution of EM. Skin lesions increase in number over
3 to 5 days, and then slowly heal over 1 to 2 weeks. Some

patients with an initial diagnosis of SJS will subsequently be
diagnosed as having TEN because of continuing progression
of epithelial separation. Reports of SJS with only mouth
involvement also exist.

Target-like lesions are sometimes seen, consisting of an erythematous macule with a dusky center. They are flat, tend to
be centrally located, do not show the classic concentric ring
pattern of EM, and the borders are less well defined than in
EM. If a blister develops, it is usually oval or elongated in
shape, as opposed to the round blisters seen in EM. The classic target lesions of EM are rarely, if ever, seen (1).

Patients usually have generalized lymphadenopathy at presentation, and may also have hepatosplenomegaly. Arthralgias
are also common; arthritis can occasionally be seen.

Toxic Epidermal Necrolysis

TEN begins 1 to 8 weeks after exposure to the precipitating
drug, with drugs introduced 1 to 21 days before the onset of
the rash being most suspect (15). There is a brief prodrome of
high fever and tender skin that lasts 1 to 3 days. Patients
quickly become toxic in appearance, and the fever can continue for a week or more. Skin lesions begin as painful erythematous or dusky macules. Oval or elongated bullae can
develop within the macules. Over time, extensive necrosis and
widespread peeling of sheets of epidermis develops, leaving a
moist, erythematous base. Areas of normal appearing skin can
appear within the rash. TEN is defined by blistering or epidermal loss over 30% of the skin surface area. A positive Nikolsky
sign is present. True target lesions are not seen. In some
patients, the child can present with a diffuse erythroderma that
mimics staphylococcal scalded skin (SSS); this will progress,
however, to widespread epidermal loss. As noted above, some
patients will initially be diagnosed as SJS, but will evolve into
TEN. Healing in TEN is much more prolonged than in SJS, and
re-epithelialization usually takes 3 to 8 weeks. Involvement of
the oral mucosa and conjunctiva is similar to SJS. In TEN,
severe involvement of the respiratory and gastrointestinal
mucosa often occurs, as well as multiorgan failure.

Differential Diagnosis of SJS and TEN

In most cases, the diagnosis of SJS and TEN are easily made.

Kawasaki disease can present with oropharygeal changes,
conjunctivitis, and a rash. Unlike SJS/TEN, the conjunctivitis is
not purulent, and the oropharyngeal changes are limited to
erythema, a strawberry tongue, and red, cracked lips. The
hemorrhagic and ulcerative oropharyngeal changes of SJS are
not seen. Bullae and large sheets of epithelial separation are not
seen in Kawasaki disease.

Staphylococcal scalded skin is often included in the differential diagnosis, but is usually easily differentiated. SSS usually
occurs in children <5 years of age (or in older children with
renal failure), does not show oropharyngeal involvement, has
a characteristic perioral peeling, and presents with an irritable,
but nontoxic, child. Biopsy of SSS will show intraepidermal
separation as opposed to the complete loss of the epidermis
seen in SJS/TEN.

Other diseases that can present with some of the features of
SJS/TEN include bullous lupus erythematosus, graft-versus-
host disease, paraneoplastic pemphigus, and linear IgA disease.

Laboratory Evaluation

Confirmation of the diagnosis by biopsy is recommended by
many experts, but often is not done in typical cases. Further
laboratory studies are done to rule out other diseases, as discussed above, or to manage the complications and multiorgan
failure that occur.

Treatment and Course

The key to the treatment of both SJS and TEN is good supportive care of the complications of the disease. Patients with TEN require admission to a burn unit, often for many weeks. Milder cases of SJS can be managed in a PICU setting, but more severe cases should also be referred to a burn unit. The skin disease is treated in the same manner as a major burn, with topical antibiotics, surveillance for and treatment of secondary skin infection, nonadherent moist dressings, and the use of biologic or synthetic membranes. Other significant problems include dehydration and electrolyte abnormalities, hypothermia, poor nutrition, and sepsis. Many patients with TEN will develop multiorgan failure, as a consequence of epithelial damage internally to the respiratory tract, esophagus, intestines, biliary and pancreatic ducts, urethra, vagina, and rectal mucosa. Pulmonary complications include obstruction from mucosal sloughing, interstitial edema, hemorrhage, pneumonia, pulmonary edema, and ARDS. Ileus, pancreatitis, and GI bleeding reflect the gastrointestinal failure. Pancytopenia or isolated anemia, thrombocytopenia, or neutropenia are also seen. Mortality ranges from 5% in SJS to 30% in TEN; most deaths are caused by secondary infections.

If the disease is secondary to a medication, the drug should be withdrawn as quickly as possible. Prompt withdrawal of the causative medication has been shown to markedly decrease the risk of death in TEN [16]. In patients on multiple drugs, it may be difficult to ascertain which drug is causing the syndrome. In these cases, the length of time the drug was given before the symptoms began, and the strength of the association of the drug with SJS/TEN, will be most helpful. In general, any suspect drug should be stopped if at all possible. Do not forget to consider over-the-counter medications, such as NSAIDs, as causative factors. Drugs with longer half-lives are associated with a higher risk of death.

Ophthalmalogic complications deserve special comment. The cornea and conjunctiva will slough, leaving behind painful ulcerations that are often exacerbated by dessication, the formation of adhesions to the lids, and secondary infection. Consultation with an ophthalmologist is crucial. Pain control, eye lubrication, manual separation of the lids and eye to prevent adhesions, along with topical CS and topical antibiotics as indicated are the mainstays of treatment [12].

The use of corticosteroids is controversial, and confounded by the lack, until recently, of strict definitions for EM, SJS, and TEN. In addition, most reports are limited by small numbers of patients, the lack of good controls, the retrospective nature of the studies, and the small number of studies involving children. Authors supporting the use of corticosteroids recommend a short course of IV methylprednisolone (4–20 mg/kg/day for 3–4 days), given early in the disease [17,18]. Most experts do not feel that there are good data to support the contention that early steroid administration will abort the development of widespread skin involvement, and most do not recommend use of steroids [1,12]. Indeed, the long-term administration of corticosteroids has been shown to increase the risk of secondary infection and prolong the hospital stay in children with TEN. Corticosteroids may also impede epithelial healing. Finally, SJS has been reported to develop in children who are already on high-dose corticosteroids for treatment of other underlying diseases, indicating no preventive effect [1,12].

IVIG has also been used extensively, again with much controversy. Analysis of these studies is confounded by the same issues as noted above with corticosteroid treatment. Early case series of small numbers of patients suggested that IVIG could halt the progression of the disease. An open trial of 34 patients treated with IVIG 2 g/kg over 2 days did not show any measurable effect on the course of the disease [19].

Another retrospective review of 48 cases of TEN suggested improvement in those patients given 1 g/kg/day for 3 days, but only if given within the first week after the onset of symptoms [20]. Another retrospective study demonstrated a decrease in the expected mortality rate in patients given 1 g/kg/day for 4 days [21]. A more recent retrospective study of IVIG compared with historical controls did not show any significant differences between the two groups in any significant clinical outcomes [22]. Given these results, recommendations on the use of IVIG vary widely. Because of the significant morbidity and mortality associated with SJS/TEN, some experts recommend the use of IVIG early in the course of the disease [23].

Plasma exchange has not been shown to be of value. There are small retrospective studies or case reports showing some efficacy with the use of plasmaphoresis, cyclophosphamide, and anti-TNF alpha [24].

As noted above, mild forms of SJS can heal over 2 weeks, with TEN taking several months. The most common serious sequelae in survivors involve ophthalmologic complications (in about 30%). This includes corneal scarring with decreased visual acuity, eyelash abnormalities, lacrimal duct scarring with subsequent increased tearing, dry eye syndrome, and photophobia. Nail deformities and pigment changes are also common; scarring and contractures are less common.

Patients should avoid any drugs suspected of causing SJS/TEN in the future, including potentially cross-reacting drugs. Because of the potential that SJS/TEN can occur in genetically susceptible individuals, first-degree relatives of the patient should also avoid the same medications.

SUMMARY

- Erythema multiforme is an acute, self-limited disease that is largely secondary to HSV. Fixed papular lesions and true target lesions (showing central epidermal destruction) are seen. EM does not progress to SJS/TEN.
- Urticaria can be differentiated from EM by the lack of true target lesions, the transient nature of the lesions, and presence of extremity edema.
- SJS and TEN represent different parts of the spectrum of the same disease, and are usually secondary to infections or drugs. New drugs started 1 to 8 weeks before the onset of the rash are likely to be causative, and should be stopped.
- Treatment for SJS/TEN is the same as for an extensive burn, with similar complications and morbidities. Corticosteroids have not been shown to be beneficial, and IVIG use remains controversial.

References

1. Burch J, Weston W. Serious drug rashes in children. In: Kappy MS, ed. *Advances in pediatrics.* Vol. 52. St. Louis: Mosby; 2005:207–222.
2. Shin HT, Chang MW. Drug eruptions in children. *Curr Probl Pediatr* 2001;31:207–234.
3. Bastuji-Garin S, Rzany B, Stern RS, et al. Clinical classification of cases of toxic epidermal necrolysis, Stevens–Johnson syndrome, and erythema multiforme. *Arch Dermatol* 1993;129:92–96.
4. Leaute-Labreze C, Lamireau T, Chawki D, et al. Diagnosis, classification and management of erythema multiforme and Stevens–Johnson syndrome. *Arch Dis Child* 2000;83:347–352.
5. Auquier-Dunant A, Mochenhaupt M, Naldi L, et al. Correlations between clinical patterns and causes of erythema multiforme majus, Stevens–Johnson syndrome and toxic epidermal necrolysis: results of an international prospective study. *Arch Dermatol* 2002;138:1019–1024.
6. Assier H, Bastuji-Garin S, Revuz J, et al. Erythema multiforme with mucous membrane involvement and Stevens–Johnson syndrome are clinically different disorders with distinct causes. *Arch Dermatol* 1995;131:539–543.
7. Weston WL, Brice SL, Lester JD, et al. Herpes simplex virus in childhood erythema multiforme. *Pediatrics* 1992;89:32–34.

8. Tay YK, Huff JC, Weston WL. *Mycoplasma pneumoniae* infection is associated with Stevens–Johnson syndrome, not erythema multiforme (von Hebra). *J Am Acad Dermatol* 1996;35:757–760.
9. Schalock PC, Brennick JB, Dinulos JGH, et al. *Mycoplasma pneumoniae* infection associated with bullous erythema multiforme. *J Am Acad Dermatol* 2005;52:705–706.
10. Weston WL, Morelli JG, Rogers M. Target lesions on the lips: childhood herpes simplex associated with erythema multiforme mimics Stevens–Johnson syndrome. *J Am Acad Dermatol* 1997;37:848–850.
11. Weston WL, Morelli JG. Herpes-simplex virus-associated erythema multiforme in prepubertal children. *Arch Pediatr Adolesc Med* 1997;151:1014–1016.
12. Sheridan RL, Liu V, Anupindi S. Case 34-2005: a 10-year old girl with a bullous skin eruption and acute respiratory failure. *N Engl J Med* 2005;353: 2057–2066.
13. Roujeau JC, Kelly JP, Naldi L, et al. Medication use and the risk of Stevens–Johnson syndrome or toxic epidermal necrolysis. *N Engl J Med* 1995;333:1600–1608.
14. Mockenhaupt M, Messenheimer J, Tennis P, et al. Risk of Stevens–Johnson syndrome and toxic epidermal necrolysis in new users of antiepileptics. *Neurology* 2005;64:1134–1138.
15. Rasmussen JE. Erythema multiforme: a practical approach to recent advances. *Pediatr Dermatol* 2002;19:82–84.
16. Garcia-Doval I, LeCleach L, Bocquet H, et al. Toxic epidermal necrolysis and Stevens–Johnson syndrome: does early withdrawal of causative drugs decrease the risk of death? *Arch Dermatol* 2000;136:323–327.
17. Martinez AE, Atherton DJ. High-dose systemic corticosteroids can arrest recurrences of severe mucocutaneous erythema multiforme. *Pediatr Dermatol* 2000;17:87–90.
18. Kakourou T, Klontza D, Soteropoulau F, et al. Corticosteroid treatment of erythema multiforme major (Stevens–Johnson syndrome) in children. *Eur J Pediatr* 1997;156:90–93.
19. Bachot N, Revuz J, Roujeau JC. Intravenous immunoglobulin treatment for Stevens–Johnson syndrome and toxic epidermal necrolysis. *Arch Dermatol* 2003;139:33–36.
20. Prins C, Kerdel FA, Padilla RS. Treatment of toxic epidermal necrolysis with high-dose intravenous immunoglobulins. *Arch Dermatol* 2003; 139:26–32.
21. Trent JT, Kirsner RS, Romanelli P, et al. Analysis of intravenous immunoglobulin for the treatment of toxic epidermal necrolyis using SCORTEN. *Arch Dermatol* 2003;139:39–43.
22. Shortt R, Gomez M, Mittman N, et al. Intravenous immunoglobulin does not improve outcome in toxic epidermal necrolysis. *J Burn Care Rehabil* 2004;25:246–255.
23. Metry DW, Jung P, Levy ML. Use of intravenous immunoglobulin in children with Stevens–Johnson syndrome and toxic epidermal necrolysis: seven cases and review of the literature. *Pediatrics* 2003;112:1430–1436.
24. Hunger R, Hunziker T, Buettiker U, et al. Rapid resolution of toxic epidermal necrolysis with anti-TNF-α treatment. *J Allergy Clin Immunol* 2005;116; 923–924.

CHAPTER 146 ■ DRUG OVERDOSES AND TOXIC INGESTIONS

DAVID L. ELDRIDGE AND ADAM K. ROWDEN

There are many misconceptions about the evaluation and management of the poisoned pediatric patient. Movies and television suggest that managing poisoned patients is based on interpreting "tox screens" and treating with antidotes.

In reality, the evaluation and management of a poisoned pediatric patient is much the same as any with sick child. Key to this investigative process is a detailed history and a careful, focused physical exam searching for telltale signs that certain drugs provide. Only after this indispensable information is gathered should selective laboratory information be obtained. Fortunately, the management of these patients often begins and ends with good supportive care. Some ingestions and exposures do require specific interventions and antidotes, but most patients will do very well with careful attention to their airway, breathing, and circulation and awareness and anticipation of common complications that occur with poisonings.

This chapter will discuss the basic evaluation and management strategies of the poisoned pediatric patient. Although some specific poisonings will bear extra discussion, a thorough discussion of such specifics is beyond the scope of this chapter. For more explicit advice, pediatric hospitalists are encouraged to either consult their inpatient medical toxicology service or call their regional poison control center.

PEDIATRIC POISONINGS

When managing poisonings, the pediatric hospitalist will encounter two different populations. The first is young children (generally under the age of 5 to 6 years old) in whom such exposures will be either dosing errors or accidental ingestions occurring when inquisitive children are left unobserved. Luckily, most of these children suffer very little harm as a consequence. The second group is adolescents. Children in this age group are more likely to suffer a fatality. Like their adult counterparts, they will often be displaying effects of recreational drug abuse and suicidal ingestions.

HISTORY

Obtaining an acceptable history in the poisoned patient can be difficult. The first priority is to identify the exposure. The patient may arrive for evaluation unconscious and unaccompanied. Young children may be unable, and adolescents may be unwilling, to communicate this information. There is also the concern that suicidal patients may purposely provide erroneous information. However, every attempt should be made to identify the nature of the ingestion or exposure. Other sources of information (family, friends, emergency responders, law enforcement) should be utilized if the patient is incapacitated or for confirmation if the patient's cooperation is questionable. If an exact drug cannot be identified, an inventory of medications in the household is extremely valuable. Besides prescription medications, inquiry should be made into available over-the-counter medications, herbal medications, household cleaning products, and cosmetics. Having at least a list of suspects can help guide the hospitalist as to how closely the patient needs to be observed. If this list includes a particularly concerning medication, interventions like activated charcoal may be more strongly considered.

Other historical elements should be obtained if possible. Determining the number of pills or quantity of a substance ingested can be very helpful, as there are some medications (e.g., acetaminophen) for which there are minimal toxic quantities. Unfortunately this information is frequently unavailable. In these cases, it is better to assume a "worst-case scenario" and direct observation and management in that fashion. The time of ingestion is helpful if it can be trusted. This can be based on when the ingestion was witnessed, but often is estimated on a point of reference such as when a toddler was left unattended or when an adolescent was last seen without altered mental status. Knowing a timeline may help the physician judge the usefulness of gastrointestinal decontamination and the timing of laboratory levels (as in the case of acetaminophen). The circumstances of the ingestion also must be investigated. In the case of toddlers, ingestions are usually unintentional. If the child is very young (<1 year old), poisoning by a family member should be investigated. In the case of adolescents, it must be determined if suicidal ideation was a factor. Social work and psychiatric consultations may be necessary. The presence of certain drugs should trigger more concern then others (Table 146.1). These particular drug classes and medications can be extremely poisonous even in small doses (e.g., 1 or 2 tablets or a swallow) taken accidentally by a toddler. With these substances, close clinical observation may be required even in cases where a patient initially appears asymptomatic.

PHYSICAL EXAM

For poisoned patients, a focused physical exam can be used to identify clusters of physical findings that indicate a specific toxic syndrome (Table 146.2). This approach can often be more helpful then extensive laboratory testing to aid in diagnosis and guide management.

The patient's overall mental status must be addressed. The general level of consciousness, which can range from alert and

TABLE 146.1

TABLE 146.1

MEDICATIONS AND SUBSTANCES TOXIC TO
TODDLERS EVEN IN SMALL AMOUNTS

Alcohols
  Ethylene glycol
  Methanol
Antiarrhythmics
  Disopyramide
  Flecainide
  Procainamide
  Quinidine
Antidepressants
  Monoamine oxidase inhibitors (MAOIs)
    Selegiline
    Tranylcypromine
  Tricyclic antidepressants
    Amitriptyline
    Desipramine
    Imipramine
Antihypertensives
  β-blockers
  Calcium-channel blockers
  Clonidine
Antimalarials
  Chloroquine
  Hydroxychloroquine
  Quinine
Opioids/opiates
  Lomotil (diphenoxylate/atropine)
  Codeine
  Hydrocodone
  Methadone
  Morphine
Sulfonylureas
  Chlorpropamide
  Glibenclamide
  Glipizide
  Glyburide
Others
  Benzocaine
  Camphor
  Lindane
  Theophylline

wildly agitated to comatose, should be assessed. The clinician should also take note of slurred or mumbling speech, confusion, hallucinations, and paranoia. An ocular exam should include assessing pupil size and reactivity and checking for presence of nystagmus and dysconjugate gaze. The skin and mucous membranes should be examined to see if they are wet or dry. The presence of transdermal medicinal patches or pressure sores from prolonged immobility may also be discovered. The presence of rhonchi or rales on pulmonary exam may heighten suspicion for aspiration, which is a frequent complication of comatose patients. The abdomen should be assessed for presence or absence of bowel sounds and for the presence of a full bladder on palpation. Placement of a urinary catheter may help confirm urinary retention. Certain findings on the neurologic exam are also helpful. Sympathomimetic drugs may impart such findings as increased motor tone, tremors, clonus, and hyperreflexia in a child. Medications that cause ataxia may lead to any of the following presentations: difficulty sitting unsupported; refusal to attempt to walk or stand; presence of a wide-based gait; inability to grasp a favorite toy

or transfer it from one hand to another. Focal neurologic findings are unusual with poisonings and should prompt the clinician to search for an alternative diagnosis.

LABORATORY TESTING

When evaluating the poisoned patient, laboratory testing should be focused and logical. The "shotgun" approach is rarely productive and may in fact confuse the investigation. If the patient is a toddler, with a known ingestion that is likely accidental, few if any laboratory tests may need to be done. On the other hand, if the patient is an adolescent and a suicidal ingestion is suspected or the veracity of the history is suspected, broader testing may be necessary. Even in the latter case, usually only a few tests need to be ordered initially to help aid in the initial diagnostic approach and to help assess clinical stability. After this preliminary assessment, the need for further testing can be determined. Suggested diagnostic studies in the evaluation of the poisoned patient are listed in Table 146.3.

Specific Drug Levels

Obtaining drug levels for every possible drug exposure is not practical in the initial management of the poisoned pediatric patient. Relatively few drug levels are performed by a typical hospital laboratory. If a sample must be sent to another specialty laboratory, the result may take days if not weeks to obtain. When finally obtained, the results will be unlikely to change the acute management. If a drug level is pertinent, but the results will not immediately be available (as is often the case with both methanol and ethylene glycol), appropriate treatment must not be delayed. Even when a concentration is obtained, relatively few drugs have defined clinical correlation with a given serum concentration. In these cases, values can only be interpreted qualitatively (i.e., "the drug is present"). On the other hand, if the drug in question is one in which drug levels are routinely drawn, and the level may correlate with clinical symptoms, it may be useful. For example, ordering a phenobarbital level in a comatose patient who has access to this drug may simplify the clinical investigation. Finally, if the patient has access to certain prescription medications, it may be advantageous to know if they are present from the outset—even if the patient is asymptomatic at presentation. Some medications, such as digoxin, theophylline, and lithium, are extremely toxic in overdose. If their presence is detected early, the physician will be that much more vigilant and prepared for clinical decline.

Acetaminophen and *salicylate* (i.e., aspirin) levels are recommended in all potentially suicidal patients. This is particularly true if the nature of an ingestion is unknown, the patient or their family is unable to give a satisfactory history, mental status is altered, or either medication is even remotely suspected. These two drugs are ubiquitous and are available as an active ingredient in a cornucopia of over-the-counter products. They both remain in the top rankings of overdose fatalities.

Acetaminophen is a special challenge. In addition to its wide availability, an acetaminophen overdose may present with no, or very nonspecific, symptoms early after the ingestion. More severe symptoms and hepatoxicity may only become clear after the first 24 hours. By obtaining an acetaminophen level early, one may identify this toxin at a point when its antidote, N-acetylcysteine, will provide the best chance for preventing hepatoxicity. Acute salicylate poisoning should be more obvious clinically then acetaminophen poisoning and has some telltale symptoms (e.g., tinnitus and hyperventilation). However,

TABLE 146.2

COMMON TOXIC SYNDROME (TOXIDROMES)

	Sympathomimetic	Anticholinergic	Cholinergic	Sedative/Hypnotic	Opioid
Vital signs	Tachycardia Hypertension	Tachycardia	Bradycardia Hypoxia	Nonspecific	Respiratory Depression
Mental status	Agitated, euphoric Paranoid	Agitated Hallucinations	Anxious	Depressed	Depressed Euphoric
Eyes	Dilated pupils	Dilated pupils	Pinpoint Tearing	Nystagmus Pupils nonspecific	Pinpoint
Skin	Warm Diaphoretic	Warm and dry	Diaphoretic	Nonspecific	Nonspecific
Bowel sounds	Normal to increased	Decreased	Increased	Normal	Normal
Neurologic exam	Increased tone Hyperreflexia Myoclonus	Ataxia	Possible paralysis and fasciculations	Ataxia Decreased tone	Decreased tone
Other	Hyperthermia and rigidity possible	Urinary retention	Bronchospasm Bronchorrhea Drooling Diarrhea Vomiting		

it also may not be easily recognized on presentation initially and early identification will direct management.

Basic Metabolic Panel

Checking a standard set of serum electrolytes can be very helpful in assessing the poisoned patient in a number of ways. With any patient presenting with altered mental status, it is important to assess serum electrolytes and glucose. Electrolyte abnormalities may suggest a particular overdose. For example in the agitated patient, a finding of hyperglycemia, hypokalemia, and metabolic acidosis (low bicarbonate) may indicate a sympathomimetic poisoning (e.g., amphetamines or cocaine). Toxicity from these stimulants can cause a large adrenergic reaction in the central nervous system, which leads to this pattern on the basic metabolic pattern. On the other hand, profound hypoglycemia may indicate a sulfonylurea overdose.

Discovery of a metabolic acidosis with a wide anion gap can also be of particular assistance to the pediatric hospitalist. The anion gap is calculated by subtracting the concentration of chloride and bicarbonate from the concentration of sodium, as shown below:

$$[Na^+] - ([Cl^-] + [HCO_3^-])$$

The normal value of this gap varies between laboratories, but the upper limit of normal is generally reported as 12 to 16. This concentration gap represents anions that, unlike chloride and bicarbonate, are not measured directly by the laboratory. In the case of an elevated, or wide, anion gap, these "unmeasured anions" are either substances normally found in the body (e.g., lactic acid) that are present in larger quantities than normally expected or foreign substances newly introduced into the bloodstream. Some of the common causes of this type of metabolic acidosis are often described by the MUDPILES mnemonic (Table 146.4). Though it does not name every possible cause of a wide anion gap metabolic acidosis, it is a useful starting point in the differential diagnosis. Some of the members of this list (such as diabetic ketoacidosis, uremia, and lactic acidosis) are easily confirmed or eliminated by laboratory testing. Many of the components of the MUDPILES mnemonic are medications or other toxins that

TABLE 146.3

COMMON SUGGESTED LABORATORY TESTS IN EVALUATING THE POISONED PATIENT

Dextrostick
Basic metabolic panel (Chem 7)
Serum acetaminophen level
Serum salicylate level
Electrocardiogram
Creatinine phosphokinase (CPK)
Arterial blood gas with co-oximetry panel
Other drug levels (e.g., anticonvulsants, lithium, digoxin, toxic alcohols)
Osmol gap
Urine drug screen

TABLE 146.4

CAUSES OF INCREASED ANION GAP METABOLIC ACIDOSIS (MUDPILES)

Methanol, Metformin
Uremia
Diabetic ketoacidosis
Paraldehyde, Phenformin
Iron, Inborn errors of metabolism, Ibuprofen, Inhalants (e.g., carbon monoxide and cyanide gas), and Isoniazid
Lactic acidosis
Ethylene glycol
Salicylates, Starvation ketoacidosis, Solvents (e.g., toluene), and Stimulants (e.g., amphetamines)

are potentially fatal. Therefore, the discovery of a wide anion gap metabolic acidosis should provide a sense of urgency and lead the pediatrician to return to the history and physical, obtain more details when available, and dig deeper to search for clues to its origin. Without a clear explanation, its presence may necessitate further, more extensive laboratory testing (e.g., serum iron level). In the case of methanol, ethylene glycol, aspirin, and iron, specific interventions and antidotes are available. Confirming their presence early can prevent morbidity and mortality by starting these therapies promptly.

Osmol Gap

An osmol gap is also frequently mentioned in the laboratory assessment of poisoned patients. The osmol gap is the difference between the measured osmotic concentration of serum (Osm_m) and calculated serum osmolarity (Osm_c). Osm_m is usually obtained by a freezing point depression method, while Osm_c is based on the serum concentrations of sodium, glucose, and blood urea nitrogen (BUN) and calculated by the following equation:

$$Osm_c = 2[Na^+] + [BUN]/2.8 + [glucose]/18$$

A substantial difference between Osm_m and Osm_c could signify the presence of foreign chemicals in the blood. Toxic alcohols are an example of chemicals that can raise the overall osmotic concentration of serum. There are many problems with using the osmol gap in clinical decision making, but perhaps the greatest is the lack of a truly defined normal range. Traditionally, the upper numerical limit was set at 10. However, multiple studies in normal patients have shown that gaps of 20 can occur in healthy patients. Negative numbers in this range have also been reported in healthy patients. Furthermore, elevated osmol gaps are nonspecific and can occur with medications (e.g., mannitol), drug additives (e.g., propylene glycol), or disease states (e.g., chronic renal failure). At best, if an osmol gap is markedly elevated, it may provide supporting evidence that a poison such as methanol or ethylene glycol is involved. However, treatment should never be withheld, particularly in the case of toxic alcohols, based on a normal osmol gap. Definitive laboratory testing (e.g., a methanol or ethylene glycol level) should be obtained and treatment started (e.g., fomepizole/ethanol drip or hemodialysis) if clinical suspicion is high.

Electrocardiogram

Some of the most concerning overdose scenarios involve drugs or substances that are toxic to the cardiovascular system. Many of these drugs or substances (Table 146.5) will cause characteristic interval changes or cardiac arrhythmias that can be seen on an electrocardiogram (ECG). If prompt intervention is not initiated in these patients, cardiovascular collapse may ensue. Early recognition of these cardiac rhythm disturbances may be lifesaving. An ECG is a useful tool in the evaluation of the overdose patient. If the exact identity of a toxin is unknown, recognition of characteristic patterns on an ECG will help narrow the differential. Furthermore, even when the exact identity of the causative substance is unknown, recognition of certain interval changes (e.g., prolonged QSR interval) or cardiac arrhythmias (e.g., torsades de pointes) will help guide therapy in the overdose patient.

Toxicology Screens

When presented with an overdose patient, most physicians seem to reflexively ask for a blood or urine toxicology screen. These tests are ordered with the hope of identifying the intoxicant and allowing the physician to more effectively care

TABLE 146.5

ECG FINDINGS WITH EXAMPLE TOXINS

Finding	Example toxin
Bradycardia	β-blockers Calcium-channel blockers Clonidine Digoxin
Tachycardia	Amphetamines Anticholinergic poisons Cocaine Theophylline
Prolonged QRS interval (Na^+-channel blockers)	Cocaine Diphenhydramine Propoxyphene Tricyclic antidepressants
Prolonged QTc interval and torsades de pointes (K^+-channel blockers)	Antipsychotics Arsenic Citalopram Tricyclic antidepressants

for the patient. In reality, however, these screening tests have many limitations and often provide little, if any, assistance in acute patient management.

There is wide variability in the number of substances included in a given toxicology screen. Most screens look for a relatively small number of commonly abused classes of drugs including barbiturates, benzodiazepines, cocaine, amphetamines, marijuana, opioids, and phencyclidine (PCP). Before ordering this test, the hospitalist should inquire as to what is included in the toxicology screen provided by his institution's laboratory. More "comprehensive" drug screens are available that can detect the presence of hundreds of drugs of abuse and prescription medications, but it is impossible for even these tests to be all-inclusive. It must be remembered that a negative "tox screen" does not mean that a toxin has been definitively ruled out of the differential diagnosis.

Care should be taken in interpreting a positive result. The results of toxicology screens are qualitative only and not quantitative. A positive toxicology screen only indicates that a substance is present above a certain concentration of detection, but it does not indicate that it is present in a sufficient amount to cause symptoms. For example, if a patient is found in a coma and, in the course of evaluation, the urine toxicology screen is positive for benzodiazepines, this does indicate the presence of a benzodiazepine but does not signify that this is the cause of the coma. The patient may have only been taking the medicine as directed. Other possible causes of altered mentation should be investigated. Toxicology screens are also fraught with false positives. For example, false-positive results for PCP have been caused by dextromethorphan. Negative toxicology screen results should also be regarded warily. A negative result indicates that, at the time of screen, the drugs included in the screen are not present in sufficient quantities to be detected by the assay. It does not mean the patient has never been exposed to substances in the screen. False-negatives are also a common problem. Not all members of a given drug class will not be detected by all toxicology screens. In the case of benzodiazepines, lorazepam and alprazolam are not detected in many toxicology screens. Most screens for opioids do not detect the presence of commonly abused synthetic opioids, such as methadone and oxycodone.

Many clinical studies have examined the role of toxicology screens in the management of poisoned patients. The vast majority of these studies have come to the same conclusion—that toxicology screens (even when "comprehensive") typically do not change the clinical management of these patients. Results of comprehensive toxicology screens may not return until after a patient is discharged. A patient's overall clinical picture and other laboratory data collected (e.g., wide anion gap metabolic acidosis or prolonged QRS interval on ECG) should guide acute management. Clinical correlation must be sought with any positive result before clinical interventions are undertaken. Negative results should be viewed skeptically in the presence of symptoms consistent with a suspected overdose.

Although the routine use of toxicology screens is discouraged, there is a subset of pediatric patients for whom they may be useful. In cases of suspected abuse or neglect where a child may present with altered mentation, toxicology screens may have a role. In these cases, the presence of a drug of abuse in a young child may affect the disposition of the child. Even in these cases, the pediatric hospitalist will likely find it more productive to decide first if the child's symptoms could be explained by a particular drug or drug class before ordering a toxicology screen.

Other Tests

Any patient who presents with altered mental status of unknown origin ("found down") should have a *dextrostick* done immediately to assess for hypoglycemia. Another laboratory test that may be useful in the agitated patient or the patient who has been found unconscious for an unknown amount of time is a serum *creatinine phosphokinase level* (CPK) to look for the presence of rhabdomyolysis (see the discussion of rhabdomyolysis below).

An *arterial blood gas* not only will reveal acid–base disturbances; the accompanying co-oximetry panel will reveal the presence of carbon monoxide or methemoglobinemia.

Plain radiography of the abdomen, looking for the presence of pills in the abdomen, is a test that is often brought up in discussion. This study has a very limited role in this capacity. Most tablets are not radiopaque in the abdomen. Even if a pill is radiopaque in air, this does not indicate that plain film will reveal its presence in the abdomen. Some tablets, like prenatal vitamins, that contain large amounts of certain forms of iron (e.g., ferrous sulfate and ferrous fumarate) may be detectable on radiography. This finding of large quantities of radiopaque pills on x-ray may lead to whole-bowel irrigation (discussed in the next section) in an attempt to evacuate the iron pills before absorption. Even iron, however, is inconsistently visualized by radiography and such films should be interpreted cautiously.

TREATMENT

The multitude of different drug overdoses and the precise management of each is beyond the scope of this chapter. Luckily, most cases may be managed with close attention to the tenets of the ABCs (airway, breathing, circulation) and appropriate supportive care. There are certain complications common to many overdoses that can be anticipated and guarded against. Other initial management strategies will be discussed here, as will some basic guidelines for the initial management of acetaminophen and salicylate overdoses. When confronted with a specific toxin or ingestion, the pediatric hospitalist is encouraged to contact the regional poison control center in her area or discuss the case with an available medical toxicologist. Detailed recommendations such as time required for observation after the ingestion, expected clinical symptoms, need for intensive cardiopulmonary monitoring, and specific recommended interventions can be obtained from these sources.

Common Complications of Poisonings

Though direct toxic effects from poisonings can and do occur, the complications that result secondary to drug effects (e.g., altered mental status) are often a more grave and immediate threat to many poisoned patients. Decreased level of consciousness and loss of protective airway reflexes are common consequences of many types of intoxications. In this vulnerable state, the patient is vulnerable to *aspiration*. Aspiration pneumonitis of stomach contents carries a high mortality rate, estimated by some to be as high as 60%. This risk should also be considered before attempts at gastrointestinal decontamination (e.g., administration of activated charcoal) are made. Though not a fail-safe measure against aspiration, intubation should be considered in an obtunded patient in order to maximize airway protection.

Rhabdomyolysis is another feared complication of many poisonings. This may occur from a variety of mechanisms, including sustained muscle activity, as with seizures or severe agitation from amphetamines; direct toxicity to muscle tissue, as from carbon monoxide; or prolonged inactivity leading to an immobility-related pressure necrosis, as with phenobarbital. Any of these clinical settings should prompt the ordering of a CPK level. An elevated serum CPK and discoloration of a patient's urine (classically "tea-colored") are both indications of muscle breakdown. Appropriate intravenous fluid management in this setting may help to preserve renal function.

Besides generalized rhabdomyolysis, prolonged immobility secondary to a loss of consciousness may lead to more localized muscle breakdown. This pressure-related phenomenon may be limited to a single extremity or fascial compartment. Severe damage of this type can lead to *compartment syndrome* and compromise blood flow to the involved region. If this is suspected clinically by virtue of erythema, swelling and tightness of the local area, severe pain (once patient is arousable), poor perfusion, or other evidence of neurovascular compromise, surgical consultation should be expeditious.

Basic Management Guidelines

Though antidotes frequently come to mind when an overdose patient is mentioned, their use is generally the exception. Most cases truly may be managed with close attention to the tenets of the ABCs (airway, breathing, circulation). With this careful supervision most drug effects will resolve with time, and the best outcome possible will occur. The complications resulting from compromise of any component of the ABCs (discussed above) are generally a much greater threat to the patient then the drug itself. Often the history may be unclear or unavailable. The patient's evolving clinical status will in many cases provide clues to the nature of an ingestion and guide specific therapy. In the initial stages of such an evaluation, continuous cardiopulmonary monitoring with frequent vital checks is recommended. Reliable intravenous access should be obtained.

Some poisonings, such as by cocaine and amphetamines, produce patients who are extremely agitated and combative. These patients can be dangerous to themselves and medical staff. Administration of benzodiazepines to the agitated patient is usually an appropriate therapy in these cases. Titrating these medications to desired effect can produce a more calm and manageable patient. One caveat is to use care not to compromise respiratory effort. Salicylate overdoses, for example, cause a metabolic acidosis that is often compensated by hyperventilation. Removing this respiratory compensation can be fatal.

The patient who presents with depressed mental status presents another scenario. In this case, one cannot go wrong with a careful survey of ABCs and appropriate supportive care (including endotracheal intubation when necessary). Many advocate the automatic use of the "coma cocktail"—a series of antidotes used to revive a comatose patient. Caution should be used with some of these interventions, however. If the patient has signs of opioid intoxication (e.g., miosis), administration of *naloxone* may be considered. In small children, who are more likely to be naïve to opioids, there are probably few drawbacks to this intervention. However, in the older child who may abuse these drugs, the induction of withdrawal is a possibility. Also, removal of the sedating effects of opioids may unmask an agitated patient. The goal of dosing naloxone should be slow titration of the total dose, looking for improvement in respiratory effort (not complete awakening). Finally, it must be remembered that the half-life of naloxone is shorter then many oral opioids (like methadone). Therefore, even if the patient responds well to naloxone, he may have to be observed overnight for resedation. *Flumazenil*, the reversal agent for benzodiazepines, should *never* be used in this setting. The withdrawal syndrome it may precipitate (including intractable seizures) is potentially fatal.

Seizures are another common presentation in the poisoned patient. If hypoglycemia has been ruled out as a cause, benzodiazepines are the first choice in an unknown poisoning. Loading with phenobarbital is usually the next step if necessary. There are concerns with using phenytoin in the setting of some poisonings, so it is generally not utilized in poisoned patients.

After the hospitalist's initial evaluation and stabilization, it is recommended that a regional poison control center be contacted, and the case discussed with a medical toxicologist. This consultation often provides invaluable, individualized assistance with managing specific poisonings and guidance regarding duration of observation and disposition (general pediatric ward versus pediatric intensive care unit).

Gastrointestinal Decontamination

For many years, it has been a commonly held treatment principle to treat overdoses by expediting the evacuation of the toxin from the body before absorption of drugs could occur. Though this principle seems logical, this concept has received increased critical scrutiny. Conclusive evidence that any of the methods of gastrointestinal (GI) decontamination change clinical outcomes is lacking. However, to be fair, studies to conclusively evaluate these techniques are difficult to design and perform, as the number of children who die or even suffer significant morbidity from poisonings is small. Therefore, there may be a small subset of patients that might benefit from these techniques, but will not be discovered in clinical studies. For this reason, many continue to use these techniques—especially if the poisoning is particularly threatening and there is little else to offer. Some of these techniques have largely fallen out of favor, and those that remain in common use should probably be used selectively.

Oral administration of s*yrup of ipecac*, once the standard-bearer for treating poisoned children, is generally agreed now to be contraindicated. Concerns over safety, efficacy, and abuse have lead for some (such as the American Academy of Pediatrics) to advise against its use. It is not recommended by the authors.

Gastric lavage is another decontamination method that has been used empirically for decades. It involves placement of a large orogastric tube with subsequent insertion of aliquots of normal saline, which are then withdrawn in hopes of removing

pill fragments. This is an invasive, labor-intensive technique that requires intubation in order to minimize one its greatest risks—aspiration. GI tract perforation is another reported complication. Any potential benefit from gastric lavage has been shown to decrease rapidly with time, and it is generally agreed that it is probably useful only within the first hour after ingestion. In the case of ingested corrosives or hydrocarbons, it should not be used. There is no evidence that gastric lavage improves clinical outcome. Gastric lavage should only be considered if the patient presents within the first hour, medical personnel are familiar with the technique, and the overdose is considered particularly life-threatening.

Activated charcoal (AC) is the most commonly used method of gastrointestinal decontamination at this time. AC is a substrate with a large relative surface area and high absorptive capacity. It is taken (or given) enterally with the hope that it will come in contact with a drug and bind it before it is absorbed. Like gastric lavage, it seems to be most successful when given within 1 hour of ingestion. It is dosed at 1 g/kg (maximum 25–50 g) orally. Making this substance palatable is a challenge. For this reason it may be given via a nasogastric (NG) tube. Depending on the toxin, repeat doses may be given. AC is not without risk. A patient's airway needs to be protected before administration as aspiration is a serious concern. If the decision is made to give it via NG tube, great care should be taken to assure that the tube is properly placed. Repeated dosing has also been reported to lead to constipation and obstruction (especially if bowel peristalsis is decreased as in anticholinergic poisoning). AC has been shown to lower drug absorption but, like other methods of GI decontamination, there is no evidence that AC changes clinical outcomes. Therefore, it is not a mandatory intervention in all poisonings. Particular instances where the use of activated charcoal is contraindicated are listed in Table 146.6. If the poisoning is particularly concerning or life-threatening, there are no risks to administration, and it is not otherwise contraindicated, AC administration can be considered.

Whole-bowel irrigation (WBI) involves the enteral administration of polyethylene glycol electrolyte solutions (PEG ES) in an attempt to evacuate the bowels of toxins before they can be absorbed. Generally large amounts of PEG ES are given (1.0–2.0 L/hr in adults; 1.0 L/hr in children 6–12 years old; and 500 mL/hr in children 9 months to 6 years old). As with the other methods that have been discussed, no evidence of improved clinical outcome exists. Still WBI has a hypothetical benefit in some circumstances. In some life-threatening overdoses where AC has no role (as with lithium and iron), WBI has been extensively reported in the literature. It has also been utilized to speed the evacuation of packets of narcotics from the GI tracts of patients smuggling these drugs ("body packers"). As with any method of GI decontamination, potential benefits must be balanced with potential risks. A patient's airway must be secure, the integrity of the GI tract must be assured (no perforation, hemorrhage, ileus, or obstruction), and the patient must not be suffering nausea or vomiting for WBI to be safely attempted.

TABLE 146.6

INGESTIONS WHERE ACTIVATED CHARCOAL IS INEFFECTUAL OR CONTRAINDICATED

Alcohols (e.g., ethanol, ethylene glycol, isopropanol, methanol)
Corrosives (alkali and acid)
Hydrocarbons
Metals and minerals (e.g., iron and lithium)

TABLE 146.7

ANTIDOTES AND CORRESPONDING
POISON EXAMPLES

Poison	Antidote/method of increased elimination
Acetaminophen	N-acetylcysteine
β-blockers	Glucagon
Calcium-channel Blockers	Calcium chloride/gluconate
Digoxin/digitoxin	Digoxin-specific antibody fragments
Ethylene glycol and Methanol	Ethanol drip Fomepizole Hemodialysis
Iron	Deferoxamine
Na$^+$-channel blocking cardiotoxins (e.g., cocaine)	IV sodium bicarbonate
K$^+$-channel blocking cardiotoxins (e.g., tricyclic antidepressants)	IV magnesium sulfate
Opioids	Naloxone
Organophosphate pesticides	Atropine Pralidoxime
Salicylates	Urine alkalinization
Sulfonylureas	Octreotide

Antidotes

The treatment of some specific drug overdoses is best served with antidotes. Commonly held antidotes and methods of increased elimination of some toxins are given in Table 146.7. It is advised that use of any of these antidotes or methods be done in consultation with a hospital's medical toxicologist or by phone with a regional poison control center.

Treatment of Specific Toxins

Acetaminophen Overdose

Clinical Presentation. Acetaminophen (APAP) toxicity should be suspected in all intentional overdoses because of the ubiquitous nature of APAP and the inaccurate histories often provided by the suicidal patient. The early symptoms of APAP ingestion are often vague or absent, leading to concern that potentially toxic ingestions can be missed. The first 24 hours is considered the first phase of APAP poisoning, and is characterized by nonspecific findings such as nausea, vomiting, anorexia, pallor, and lethargy. In this phase, however, the patient may appear normal. In the second phase, usually 24 to 48 hours after ingestion, the patient begins to develop clinical and laboratory evidence of hepatotoxicity (e.g., elevated aspartate and alanine transaminases). In the third phase, from 48 hours to 72 hours, the patient may progress to fulminant hepatic failure (FHF) with all of its associated complications. Phase four, usually 72 to 96 hours after ingestion, sees the resolution of liver function and complete recovery if the patient does not progress to FHF or survives its complications.

Diagnosis. Potentially lethal APAP ingestions frequently do not manifest clinical signs of toxicity for 24 hours. Unfortunately, antidotal therapy with N-acetylcysteine (NAC)

is most effective at preventing mortality when started within 8 hours of ingestion. To minimize the potential for adverse outcomes, most authors recommend universal screening for APAP in all overdoses. The Rumack–Matthew treatment nomogram is the primary tool used to guide treatment after acute ingestion of APAP. Its axes are serum APAP levels versus time passed since acute ingestion. It is a well-validated and useful tool to guide treatment for acute APAP ingestions. Acute poisoning is generally defined as a single ingestion of APAP over less than a 4-hour time period. In those who present within 24 hours after an acute ingestion, a single serum APAP level may be obtained. If the time of ingestion is known (and is reliable), this single APAP level may be plotted on the nomogram. Those with levels that fall above the probable toxicity line are treated with a course of NAC and those with levels that fall below do not need treatment.

Other than in an acute ingestion, as defined above, the nomogram does not offer any guidance in the management of these patients. This includes cases where children have received repeated supratherapeutic doses of APAP over time (i.e., chronic APAP toxicity) and those who have taken a single large ingestion but do not present within 24 hours. The management of chronic APAP toxicity is complex, with little in the medical literature to guide therapy. Consultation with a regional poison control center's medical toxicologist can aid in the management of these difficult cases.

Treatment. The treatment for APAP ingestion is NAC. Once the decision to treat is made for acute ingestions, there are two treatment protocols for NAC approved by the Food and Drug Administration (FDA). The oldest is an oral, 72-hour regimen starting with a loading dose of 140 mg/kg followed by 70 mg/kg every 4 hours for 17 additional doses. The second protocol, recently approved, is a 20-hour intravenous (IV) protocol. In this 20-hour protocol, NAC is administered as a loading dose of 150 mg/kg over 15 minutes followed by 50 mg/kg of NAC infused over 4 hours. Over the remaining 16 hours an additional 100 mg/kg is administered as a constant infusion. Both protocols are effective in acute ingestions. Although oral NAC is effective, its taste and smell make it unpalatable, and if the patient is vomiting, delivery may be especially difficult. IV dosing is attractive because nausea and vomiting do not affect drug delivery; however, there is a slightly increased incidence of adverse drug reactions (ADRs) with IV administration versus oral.

Most adverse drug reactions appear to be anaphylactoid in nature and are dose and rate related. ADRs tend to occur during the initial loading dose. The overall rate of ADRs from either oral or IV NAC ranges from 3% to 25%. Nausea and vomiting are the most frequently reported ADRs of NAC therapy. The most commonly reported ADR after nausea and vomiting is cutaneous skin reactions, but more serious ADRs such as bronchospasm, angioedema, and hypotension have been rarely reported.

Prognosis. Patients who are started with NAC within 8 hours of ingestion have an excellent prognosis. Those who present later are at increased risk of FHF and death. Although not discussed here in detail, NAC therapy offers some benefit no matter how late the patient presents and should never be withheld. Elevated liver enzymes are markers of liver injury but provide no prognostic information. The King's College Criteria (Table 146.8) are useful in determining who is at risk of death without liver transplantation and needs referral to a facility capable of transplantation.

Salicylate Overdose

Although the use of salicylate (ASA) products therapeutically in the pediatric and adolescent population is uncommon, there is potential for serious toxicity from both accidental and

TABLE 146.8

KING'S COLLEGE CRITERIA

pH less than 7.3 after fluid resuscitation
PT greater than 100
Creatinine greater than 3.3 mg/dL
Hepatic encephalopathy grade III of IV

TABLE 146.9

CLINICAL SCENARIOS REQUIRING HEMODIALYSIS FOR SALICYLATE POISONING

Salicylate level ≥100 mg/dL
Signs/findings of severe CNS toxicity (e.g., seizures, altered mental status, cerebral edema)
Renal failure
Pulmonary edema
No response or contraindications to other therapies (e.g., urine alkalinization)

intentional exposures. Many over-the-counter products contain ASA, including pain relievers and cough and cold preparations. Products that contain oil of wintergreen, such as liniments and aromatherapy agents, also represent a source of exposure.

Clinical Presentation. The clinical effects of ASA poisoning can be subtle. Initially, gastrointestinal symptoms predominate. ASA has a direct irritant effect on the stomach mucosa and can cause spasm of the pylorus, both of which can cause nausea and vomiting. Tachypnea is common secondary to ASA's direct simulation of the respiratory center of the brain. Salicylates are themselves acids and will produce a metabolic acidosis with a large anion gap. CNS effects include the classic finding of tinnitus, although this disturbance in hearing may not be described as ringing by patients and may present as a deficit that is hard for them to describe. Other CNS effects include confusion, agitation, and seizures. In severe cases, clinical findings may include pulmonary edema, cerebral edema, coma, hyperthermia, and muscle rigidity. These findings are dire and should prompt aggressive intervention (i.e., hemodialysis).

Diagnosis. ASA poisoning should be suspected in all suicidal ingestions, and in all cases of unexplained anion gap metabolic acidosis. Due to direct stimulation of the brain's respiratory center, the classic finding on an arterial blood gas is a mixed state with respiratory alkalosis and metabolic acidosis. However, in small children with relatively small respiratory reserves, this finding may not exist, and the metabolic acidosis will predominate. Because the early clinical findings may be subtle and due to the ubiquitous nature of ASA, the authors recommend routine ASA screening of all intentional overdoses unless close observation for clinical change followed by appropriate laboratory testing can be assured. ASA levels greater than 30 mg/dL are toxic. However, an initial level below this may reveal initial absorption only and a higher peak may be apparent later. If any salicylate is detected, repeat levels are warranted until a consistent decrease in concentration is shown. In the case of chronic ASA poisoning, ASA levels may be normal even in the face of overt clinical symptoms. In these cases, diagnosis should be based on supporting clinical data (e.g., altered mental status and a metabolic acidosis with large anion gap).

Treatment. Once the patient is initially stabilized, treatment focuses on prevention of absorption, enhancement of elimination, and managing the anticipated complications. Because of ASA's ability to cause pyloric spasm, large concretions (bezoars) of drug may form in the stomach and lead to delayed absorption. For this reason, administration of activated charcoal (if it can be given safely) is recommended even if it has been more than 1 hour since ingestion. If ASA levels continue to rise despite aggressive therapy, repeat doses of activated charcoal (usually every 4 hours) and whole-bowel irrigation can be considered. ASA levels should be repeated often until levels are trending down significantly.

Enhanced elimination is accomplished by alkalinization of the urine. Bolusing the patient with 1 to 2 mEq/kg of sodium bicarbonate followed by continued alkalinization with an IV infusion of sodium bicarbonate is recommended to achieve this goal. One IV preparation for continuous infusion recommended by the authors is made by combining 150 mEq of sodium bicarbonate with a liter of 5% dextrose in water (D5W) along with 40 mEq of potassium. This mixture results in an isotonic solution and is infused at 1.5 to 2 times a calculated maintenance rate. The addition of potassium is key, and its concentration should be monitored serially. Hypokalemia is common with ASA poisoning. In the setting of hypokalemia, urine alkalinization loses its effectiveness. In situations where this method of elimination is contraindicated (e.g., renal failure) or where urgent removal of ASA is needed due to signs of rapid deterioration, hemodialysis is needed (Table 146.9).

There is no standard treatment guideline tool for the initiation of specific therapy based on a given ASA level (like the Rumack–Matthews treatment nomogram and NAC). Even "normal" levels (<30 mg/dL) may be unreliable. In the setting of chronic toxicity or if the patient is far removed from her ingestion, the ASA may have redistributed from the blood compartment to the CNS, and the level may not accurately reflect toxicity. Clinical symptoms and the presence of metabolic acidosis should guide therapy in these situations. Sodium bicarbonate infusions are typically started for levels above 40 mg/dL. Hemodialysis is needed for ASA levels 100 mg/dL or above.

Suggested Readings

American Academy of Pediatrics Committee on Injury, Violence, and Poison Prevention. Poison treatment in the home. *Pediatrics* 2003;112:1182–1185.

Bar-Oz B, Levichek Z, Koren G. Medications that can be fatal for a toddler with one tablet or teaspoonful: a 2004 update. *Paediatr Drugs* 2004;6:123–126.

Barry JD. Diagnosis and management of the poisoned child. *Pediatr Ann* 2005;34:937–946.

Bryant S, Singer J. Management of toxic exposure in children. *Emerg Med Clin North Am* 2003;21:101–119.

Eldridge DL, Dobson T, Brady W, et al. Utilizing diagnostic investigations in the poisoned patient. *Med Clin North Am* 2005;89:1079–1105.

Greene SL, Dargan PI, Jones AL. Acute poisoning: understanding 90% of cases in a nutshell. *Postgrad Med J* 2005;81:204–216.

Hoffman RJ, Nelson L. Rational use of toxicology testing in children. *Curr Opin Pediatr* 2001;13:183–188.

Holstege CP, Eldridge DL, Rowden AK. ECG manifestations: the poisoned patient. *Emerg Med Clin North Am* 2006;24:159–177.

Kirk M, Pace S. Pearls, pitfalls, and updates in toxicology. *Emerg Med Clin North Am* 1997;15:427–449.

Michael JB, Sztajnkrycer MD. Deadly pediatric poisons: nine common agents that kill at low doses. *Emerg Med Clin North Am* 2004;22:1019–1050.

Rowden AK, Norvell J, Eldridge DL, et al. Updates on acetaminophen toxicity. *Med Clin North Am* 2005;89:1145–1159.

Yip L, Dart RC, Gabow PA. Concepts and controversies in salicylate toxicity. *Emerg Med Clin North Am* 1994;12:351–364.

CHAPTER 147 ■ TOXIC EXPOSURES: CHEMICAL AND ENVIRONMENTAL

DAVID L. ELDRIDGE AND ADAM K. ROWDEN

As children develop, they naturally become inquisitive and investigate their environment. Although this exploration is part of sound intellectual growth, it places them in contact with a variety of chemical exposures both in and around the home. In the outdoors they may accidentally encounter environmental dangers in the form of some plants and animals. Adolescents are at risk for exposure to these same dangers, although their exposure may be intentional, either through recreation or suicidal intention. The focus of this chapter will be to discuss a general approach to manage these exposures and also discuss some of these exposures in more detail. It is beyond the scope of this chapter to discuss all possible scenarios in great detail. It is encouraged in these types of exposures to contact a regional poison control center to discuss specific management issues for individual exposures.

CHEMICAL EXPOSURES

Chemical exposures causing illness can occur in a variety of situations. Although adults can have chemical exposures in the workplace or at home, most chemical exposures in small children will be from contact with household products (e.g., cleaning products). There are many routes of exposure including ingestion, inhalation, and dermal contact. Often the route of exposure will determine symptoms. In general, these household exposures should be safer than contact with industrial-strength chemicals that occur in many adult settings. However, morbidity and mortality can still occur.

Young children have certain vulnerabilities to consider with chemical exposures. From a respiratory standpoint, it should be remembered that small children have higher metabolic rates that drive more gas exchange during inhalation. This leads to them receiving proportionately higher dosage exposure to inhaled toxins (e.g., carbon monoxide). If the chemical gas is heavier than air, small children, being closer to the ground, will also have a greater exposure then their adult counterparts. Exposure to skin can carry greater perils for children as well. They have a relatively increased body surface area compared to their weight, effectively increasing their contact area. Chemical absorption is further facilitated by the fact that their dermal layer has a greater lipid component.

Management of chemical exposures hinges on ending the contact with the chemical. Although this seems relatively straightforward, there can be several steps to achieve this depending on the route of exposure. For example, if the exposure is from inhaling a dangerous gas such as carbon monoxide, the patient needs to be taken to an area of fresh air or taken upwind from the source. Also, when a patient has received a dangerous topical exposure, contaminated clothing needs to be promptly removed and disposed of safely, and the patient should carefully and completely shower with copious amounts of soap and water. Eyes should generally be rinsed with copious amounts of water if exposed. This approach to decontamination can be used in most chemical exposure scenarios. As always, assessing and supporting airway, breathing, and circulation (ABCs) will be of vital importance in each case. Depending on the nature and identity of the exposure, the child may need to be admitted for continued close observation, support, and at times, specific medical therapies.

Chemical Toxic Syndromes

There are an infinite number of chemicals to which children may come into contact. Fortunately, many of these chemicals produce stereotypical symptom patterns. These chemical toxic syndromes (Table 147.1), also known as "toxidromes," allow rapid recognition of certain chemical families (e.g., acetylcholinesterase inhibitors). The purpose of this classification system is to guide initial management while more information is obtained. If the identity of the chemical is subsequently discovered, there may be separate specific interventions and medical therapies that apply. Contacting a regional poison control center at this point is very useful to obtain this sort of specific information on individual chemicals.

Chemical Burns

The first of these toxic syndromes is chemical burns. There are many chemicals that can damage skin and mucosa on direct contact including acids and bases that cause corrosive damage and certain hydrocarbon chemicals that cause damage by defatting tissue. Clinically, skin or mucosa will likely be erythematous or ulcerated depending on the severity of the burn. The affected tissue will likely be painful as well.

If burns occur in direct contact with a chemical, prompt decontamination of the involved area is the initial management. Contaminated clothing should be promptly removed so that continued contact with skin is ended, and the affected area should be thoroughly flushed with abundant amounts of water. Some substances that produce chemical burns (e.g., hydrofluoric acid) have other specific interventions that may aid in their management. The identity of the chemical should be ascertained as quickly as possible to help direct management appropriately. Once decontaminated, most chemical burns can then be treated similarly to thermal burns. Fluid losses based on the existing burns should be anticipated and addressed appropriately with intravenous fluids. Vigilance for subsequent infection should be exercised and treated as appropriate.

TABLE 147.1

CHEMICAL TOXIC SYNDROMES (TOXIDROMES)

Toxidrome and examples	Symptoms and findings

Chemical burns
    Acids
    Alkaline corrosives
    Phenol
    Degreasers
	Mucosa and skin with erythema, ulceration, pain, and irritation
	Specific systemic effects may exist depending on the chemical

Acute solvent syndrome
    Aliphatic hydrocarbons
    Toluene
    Benzene
    Trichlorofluoromethane
	Burning and irritation of mucous membranes
	Confusion, headaches, nausea, dizziness, faintness
	Shortness of breath, chest pain/tightness
	Some chemicals carry risk of arrhythmia

Acetylcholinesterase inhibitors
    Organophosphates
    Carbamates
    VX
    Sarin
	Miosis, bronchorrhea, bronchospasm, sialorrhea urinary incontinence, diarrhea, tearing, rhinorrhea,
	Muscle fasciculations, weakness, paralysis
	Confusion, hypotonia, coma, and seizures
	Tachycardia or bradycardia

Asphyxiants
    Simple
      –Methane
      –Propane
      –Carbon dioxide
    Chemical
      –Carbon monoxide
      –Cyanide
      –Hydrogen sulfide
      –Phosphine
	Mild exposure: headache, nausea, dizziness, fatigue
	Severe: syncope, coma, seizures, cardiac ischemia
	↓Oxygen saturation on pulse oximetry
	↓Arterial oxygen pressure
	
	Similar symptoms to simple asphyxia
	May cause swift deterioration ("knock-down")
	Lactic acidosis
	Arterial oxygen pressure and pulse oximetry may be normal

Irritant gas syndrome
    Chlorine
    Ammonia
    Hydrochloric acid
    Phosgene
	Tearing and burning eyes
	Coughing, wheezing, shortness of breath, stridor, pulmonary edema

Acute Solvent Syndrome

There are many volatile solvents and substances (e.g., benzene, toluene, and chloroform) that can cause illness if intense or continued inhalational exposure occurs. This may occur accidentally or through intentional abuse ("huffing"). Although there are symptoms that are specific to each solvent, a cluster of symptoms (termed *acute solvent syndrome*) may be seen in most solvent exposures. Many will cause irritation and a burning sensation on contact with mucous membranes. The key organ system affected by these volatile substances is the central nervous system (CNS). Effects are generally depressive, but will depend on the severity of the exposure. Some patients may suffer only confusion, headaches, nausea, and dizziness or faintness. This lightheadedness can be desirable to some and may produce a euphoric sensation. Others may suffer profound CNS depression and coma. Seizures are possible. Some may suffer chest pain and tightness and shortness of breath. Cardiac arrhythmias are also possible, particularly with some of these volatiles. Trichlorofluoromethane (Freon) has been known to induce fatal ventricular arrhythmias. Toluene may produce a renal tubular acidosis.

Initial management of acute solvent syndrome starts with management of ABCs and appropriate supportive care. All of the patient's clothes should be removed and safely sealed in a bag or disposed of. If volatile chemicals remain on the clothes, the continued release could affect health care providers.

Because fatal cardiac toxicity is possible, an electrocardiogram (ECG) should be obtained, especially if the patient has obvious CNS symptoms. While assessing the patient, cardiopulmonary monitoring should be continued. Other testing may be needed depending on the specific identity of the chemical (e.g., toluene). Specific therapies may also be warranted depending on the chemical's identity.

Acetylcholinesterase Inhibitors

Acetylcholinesterase inhibitors include the organophosphate and carbamate pesticides as well as the nerve agents (e.g., VX and sarin gas) designed as chemical weapons. The symptoms caused by these chemicals result from inhibiting the enzyme acetylcholinesterase, leading to persistent high levels of acetylcholine and resulting cholinergic excess throughout the body. A primary finding of this extreme cholinergic stimulation is increased secretions of every sort, involving multiple organ systems. Clinically, patients may present with sialorrhea, diarrhea, profuse tearing, rhinorrhea, nausea and vomiting, sweating, and urinary incontinence. Increased fluid production in the lungs is an especially concerning finding, as this bronchorrhea, with accompanying bronchospasm, is often fatal. Also prominent on initial exam is the finding of miosis, which is a very helpful clue as relatively few chemicals or drugs cause this finding. These pinpoint pupils may be accompanied by eye pain. Muscle effects are also prominent with fasciculations, weakness, and in the extreme, paralysis. Cardiovascular symptoms usually include tachycardia and hypertension, but bradycardia may also be seen. CNS effects are also prominent and may include confusion, hypotonia, coma, or seizures. In children, one case series of these poisonings has suggested that CNS symptoms (particularly hypotonia and coma) may predominate in this population and "classic symptoms" (e.g., miosis and increased secretions) may be absent (1). Therefore a high index of suspicion may be needed to identify these poisonings in the pediatric population

There are three medical therapies available for the treatment of acetylcholinesterase poisonings. *Atropine* is the first choice for an acutely ill patient in respiratory distress. Repeated doses of atropine should be given every 5 to 10 minutes until respiratory symptoms (including bronchorrhea and bronchospasm) are controlled in order to prevent respiratory failure. Very large cumulative doses of atropine may be needed to accomplish this goal. *Pralidoxime* can also be of use, particularly with organophosphate and nerve agent poisonings. If given promptly, in the right situation, it can remove the toxin from acetylcholinesterase enzyme and reactivate it. If seizures occur, *benzodiazepines* are the anticonvulsant of choice.

Asphyxiants

Any chemical or substance that deprives tissue of oxygen can be termed an asphyxiant. The mechanism by which this occurs varies, however. *Simple asphyxiants* are chemicals, typically gases that physically displace oxygen from ambient air. Good examples are methane, carbon dioxide, and nitrogen. Hypoxemia should be evident on pulse oximetry and arterial blood gas (ABG) and may be seen clinically with loss of consciousness and cyanosis. *Chemical asphyxiants* produce hypoxemia through hindering oxygen delivery or consumption at a cellular level. Cyanide, carbon monoxide, and hydrogen sulfide are classic examples of this class of chemical toxin. With chemical asphyxiants, inspired air may still contain adequate amounts of oxygen and be delivered to the blood. Therefore, normal pulse oximetry values and normal partial pressure of oxygen on ABG may be found. However, because the body cannot use oxygen appropriately, lactic acidosis may be found. Low-grade, brief exposures may cause relatively mild symptoms: nausea, vomiting, lightheadedness, and headache. However, these chemicals have more catastrophic "knockdown" capabilities, where they can cause rapid loss of consciousness and clinical deterioration (coma, seizures, cardiac arrhythmias, hypotension, and death).

If rescued promptly, those exposed to simple asphyxiants should respond well to removal from the source of exposure and administration of 100% oxygen. In the case of chemical asphyxiants, supplemental oxygen should also be applied, but other toxin-specific therapies are also indicated. For example, sodium thiosulfate and sodium nitrite are components of a cyanide antidote kit that may be used. Hyperbaric oxygen has been studied extensively for carbon monoxide and has been proposed for hydrogen sulfide and cyanide poisoning as well.

Irritant Gas Syndrome

Profound irritation to the respiratory tract can occur with the inhalation of some chemical gases, producing an irritant gas syndrome. This phenomenon can occur with certain industrial substances and household products alike. The level of the respiratory tract affected depends largely on the water solubility of the chemical in question. Chemicals such as ammonia and hydrochloric acid are highly water-soluble, and tend to be absorbed upon contact with the upper respiratory tract, quickly producing cough and mucous membrane irritation (e.g., tearing and burning of the eyes) that alerts the patient to the presence of noxious stimuli. These warning symptoms often allow the patient to avoid further exposure and escape further lower respiratory tract involvement. Upper airway swelling with stridor and airway compromise is possible.

Chlorine has a more intermediate water-solubility, and in significant exposures is prone to produce lower respiratory tract irritation (e.g., bronchospasm) and acute lung injury (e.g., pulmonary edema). Some chemicals, like phosgene, are poorly water-soluble. Phosgene's aroma may not be pungent enough and its upper airway irritation not noticeable enough to provide sufficient forewarning that the chemical is present. Some hours later, dyspnea and pulmonary edema may result from delayed acute lung injury. Large or continued exposures to any of these chemicals can cause both upper and lower airway irritation regardless of solubility.

Treatment starts with removal from the irritant gas. Close attention to airway, breathing, and circulation follows next. Any signs of potential airway compromise or acute lung injury (e.g., stridor, hoarseness, wheezing, or fatigue) should cause concern and raise the possibility of endotracheal intubation. Supplemental oxygen should be provided as needed. Bronchospasm may respond to inhaled β-agonist bronchodilators. Any eye or skin irritation should be addressed by flushing affected areas generously with water. Corticosteroids in this setting are controversial in most cases. Prophylactic antibiotics are not generally recommended.

Specific Chemical Exposures

Hydrocarbon Ingestion

Hydrocarbons are a broad category of chemicals and household products that have carbon and hydrogen as the chief components of their molecular backbone. This group of substances includes kerosene, solvents, furniture polish, gasoline, and cleaners. Accidental ingestion and subsequent aspiration of hydrocarbons is a potentially fatal childhood poisoning.

These compounds possess certain varying chemical properties that help determine their toxicity: *viscosity, surface tension,* and *volatility*. These first two contribute to the likelihood and severity of aspiration and subsequent lung injury. Hydrocarbons with low viscosity, such as furniture polish, flow easily and can lead to deeper, distal penetration of the fluid into the respiratory tract. With low-viscosity hydrocarbons, this aspiration can occur during swallowing. If it possesses a low surface tension (e.g., gasoline), a hydrocarbon will spread quickly upon contact with the respiratory tract. Those with high volatility (tendency to swiftly evaporate) likely create damage in two ways. First, by replacing alveolar gas with its gaseous form, the hydrocarbon can cause hypoxemia. Second, these hydrocarbons are more likely to enter the central nervous system and cause neurologic symptoms.

Clinical Effects. There is variability in clinical symptoms. Direct mucosal irritation to the gastrointestinal (GI) tract leads to abdominal pain, nausea, vomiting, and diarrhea. Neurologic symptoms also occur and may be relatively benign, such as headache, dizziness, and euphoria; or as severe as seizures and coma. The most feared symptoms of hydrocarbon ingestion are those of the respiratory system. Irritation of the proximal airway, clinically reflected as choking and coughing, will indicate the need for further observation. A chemical pnuemonitis may ensue. If the lower airways are involved, tachypnea, crackles, wheezing (bronchospasm), decreased breath sounds, and symptoms of respiratory distress (e.g., retractions, grunting, and nasal flaring) can develop. Fever is commonly seen in these situations as well. Lower respiratory symptoms and fever may develop as quickly as 30 minutes after the exposure or may be delayed for several hours.

Diagnostic Testing. Chest x-rays can be very helpful in the evaluation of these patients and should be performed if any respiratory symptoms exist. Radiographic abnormalities may be seen within 30 minutes and almost always within 12 hours of ingestion if lung involvement exists. Findings can include alveolar infiltrates extending from perihilar regions to involve any segment but predominantly the lower lobes. Other results include pulmonary edema, atelectasis, pleural effusions, and consolidation. Bilateral abnormalities are common. Chest x-ray findings tend to peak by day 3 and clear within 7 to 10 days.

Complete blood count (CBC) may reveal leukocytosis. An arterial blood gas may reflect elements of respiratory distress. Hepatic and renal toxicity is a possibility with hydrocarbon exposure, and this may be reflected in liver function tests, basic metabolic panel, and urinalysis. This kind of damage is unusual with a single acute exposure.

Treatment. Some children will be asymptomatic after a suspected hydrocarbon ingestion. If no respiratory symptoms or vomiting develop 6 to 8 hours after ingestion, discharge of the patient is appropriate. If symptoms exist initially but are minor and improve over 6 to 8 hours, discharge is also appropriate.

If symptoms are persistent or worsen, a chest x-ray should be obtained and the patient admitted. Appropriate supportive care (proper attention to airway, breathing, and circulation) is the main goal. Oxygen should be provided as necessary. If bronchospasm appears present, bronchodilators may be beneficial. If admitted, cardiopulmonary monitoring is appropriate. In cases of severe pneumonitis, intubation and transfer to an intensive-care unit may be necessary. Due to the risk of aspiration and lack of efficacy, all attempts at gastrointestinal decontamination (including activated charcoal, gastric lavage, and syrup of ipecac) are contraindicated. There is no evidence to suggest any benefit from prophylactic steroids or antibiotics.

Symptoms usually peak in the first 24 hours and then decrease in severity over the next 1 to 4 days. Length of stay will usually mirror this pattern.

Caustic Ingestion

Caustic chemicals, both acidic and alkaline, are a possible source of morbidity and mortality in the pediatric population. Even accidental ingestion of these corrosive compounds in small children can cause extensive GI damage. Examples of common acidic products include chlorine bleach, silver nitrate, and toilet bowl cleaners. Alkalis include drain cleaners, ammonia, and denture cleaners. The severity of tissue damage is based on several factors, including pH, concentration, quantity, and duration of contact with the mucosa.

Tissue damage occurs in areas of direct contact with the caustic agent. The mechanism of injury depends on the type of corrosive ingested. If the substance is acidic, the tissue damage occurs by coagulation necrosis, and the depth of penetration is limited. On the other hand, alkaline chemicals cause liquefaction necrosis. Alkaline ingestions lead to deeper infiltration and cause greater damage to tissues.

Clinical Effects. Caustic substances generally cause burns in areas of direct contact with the GI tract. Initial exam will often reveal pain, swelling, erythema, or ulceration of the lips, oral mucosa, tongue, and pharynx. A white exudate over affected mucosa is also seen. Burns of the esophagus and stomach are also common. Clinical signs include sialorrhea, dysphagia, abdominal pain, vomiting, and refusal to eat or drink. Although most cases of esophageal burns will also have oropharyngeal burns, it is important to remember that absence of visible burns does not exclude esophageal burns. In the worst ingestions, the patient with esophageal or gastric perforation may present with symptoms of peritonitis or shock. Mediastinitis is also possible. Besides damage to the gastrointestinal tract, aspiration is also possible. The presence of

cough, tachypnea, wheezing, stridor, or hypoxia may indicate that the caustic substance has come in contact with the respiratory tract. These symptoms indicate the need for close observation and vigilance for possible worsening respiratory status.

Exam of the skin may also reveal topical burns. The severity of these injuries may mirror the severity of internal damage.

Diagnostic Testing. Consultation with a specialist (pediatric gastroenterologist or pediatric surgeon) skilled in endoscopy is recommended. Endoscopy is vital in determining extent of injury to the gastrointestinal tract. Erythema, exudates, ulceration, and edema of the GI tract may be seen. Those with more severe burns are more likely to have complications (e.g., strictures) in the future. The ideal timing of endoscopy in theses injuries is debated and should be promptly discussed with the consultant. Some advocate waiting 24 hours before endoscopy as the full scope of injury may be more evident at this point (2). It is cautioned not to wait much beyond this point to perform endoscopy. There is concern that the natural progression of injury will lead to weakening of esophageal tissue and increase the risk of perforation during the procedure. Some advocate not waiting longer than 4 days to perform endoscopy if it is to be done (2). Direct visualization of the respiratory tract by laryngoscopy or bronchoscopy can also be considered if damage to this mucosa is clinically suspected.

Other studies may be considered. If perforation of the gastrointestinal tract is suspected, radiographs of the abdomen and chest are appropriate. Some caustic ingestions have other serious systemic effects as well. Hydrofluoric acid is known to produce profound, life-threatening hypocalcemia, hyperkalemia, and hypomagnesemia. If this chemical is involved, serum electrolytes, and an electrocardiogram should be ordered. A regional poison control center should be consulted to discuss if other diagnostic testing specific to the substance involved are recommended.

Treatment. Most important to the management of patients who have ingested caustic substances is appropriate supportive care in regard to the ABCs. A symptomatic patient should be carefully observed in an inpatient setting, kept from eating or drinking, and placed on cardiopulmonary monitoring. If airway damage is suspected by symptoms (e.g., stridor), respiratory compromise may occur and transfer to an intensive-care setting should be discussed. It is strongly recommended that the patient be discussed immediately with a regional poison control center. Some caustics, such as hydrofluoric acid, have specific concerns and pitfalls beside the expected burns, and specific advice regarding individual chemicals may be obtained from this resource.

All attempts at inducing emesis (e.g., syrup of ipecac) are strongly contraindicated. Activated charcoal is also contraindicated. Oral administration of fluids or other attempts at neutralization are not beneficial and are more likely to induce damage through the generation of heat. There has also been no definitive benefit shown in the use of corticosteroids in these cases, although adverse effects are reported. Their use is not recommended. Prophylactic antibiotic use, especially in those with evidence of gastrointestinal injury on endoscopy, is advocated by some but is debated. Use of H_2 antagonists or similar medicines has also been advocated to help minimize further damage from continued gastroesophageal reflux or gastritis.

Close consultation with a pediatric gastroenterologist or surgeon is strongly recommended in these cases. Many complications involving the GI tract, including stricture and perforation, are possible with these injuries. Surgical interventions may be necessary for these complications. Patients with few symptoms and evidence of injury on endoscopy may require only short periods of observation. Severe injuries may have prolonged hospital stays with the patient unable to take anything by mouth for some time. Close outpatient follow-up for these patients may be needed after discharge, especially if strictures occur, as repeated intervention is sometimes needed.

Lead

Lead has been a well-recognized toxin for hundreds of years. It has been used extensively in a variety of ways during this time. Perhaps its widest environmental dissemination occurred in the last hundred years or so with the extensive use of lead-based paint and the use of a tetraethyl lead fuel additive to gasoline. Since the abandonment of these practices, blood lead levels (BLLs) in children overall have been found to be in decline in the United States. However, even though active release of lead into the environment has decreased dramatically over the last few decades, preexisting lead remains perpetually in the environment.

Though cases of severe lead toxicity have decreased with these and other public health interventions, the problem of lead toxicity persists. It remains a chronic public health issue. Lead may exist in the body at levels that can cause serious neurologic and cognitive impairment without overt clinical symptoms. In the United States these subclinical cases make up the bulk of lead toxicity cases in children today. Most of these cases are treated with environmental investigation and removal of the source of contamination. These children rarely require admission. A thorough discussion of all the issues involved in the management of these cases is beyond the scope of this chapter. Some severe cases of lead toxicity still occur and require admission. Managing lead toxicity of this variety will make up the bulk of this chapter's discussion.

Clinical Symptoms. Children discovered to have elevated BLLs most typically do not have any specific physical exam findings or complaints indicative of lead poisoning even though neurologic and developmental impairments may be possible. This is one of reasons the strategy of BLL screening is employed.

As levels steadily exceed 60 µg/dL, symptoms are more likely to become evident. Irritability, headaches, abdominal colic, constipation, anorexia, and lethargy may be seen. Symptoms of anemia, such as pallor, may be seen as well. The onset of persistent vomiting, coma, or seizures is concerning for lead encephalopathy. Papilledema on ophthalmologic exam may also be evident.

Diagnostic Testing. Obtaining BLLs remains the standard for the diagnosis of lead toxicity. It is with this testing that lead poisoning is often first discovered. Lead toxicity is currently defined as a child possessing a BLL of 10 µg/dL or above. Levels are usually considerably higher then this before clinical symptoms may be evident, but there is still concern for developing neurologic and cognitive impairment at lower levels. For this reason, lead screening of children at about 1 year of age (when BLLs generally begin to increase) and about 2 years old (when BLLs tend to peak) is performed during regular well-child visits. This screening is primarily focused on those with risk factors making them epidemiologically at highest risk for lead poisoning (e.g., children eligible for Medicaid, those who have a sibling with lead poisoning, and those living in older dwellings with lead-based paint). This blood screening may be done initially with a capillary finger stick. However, any elevated BLL obtained in this manner must be confirmed with a venous sample, as capillary samples are prone to error from a variety of sources, including external contamination of skin with lead particles or dust. Any clinical or public health action should be based on a venous confirmation sample.

Other tests may be considered, especially at higher BLLs (>20 µg/dL). If there is concern based on a history of pica or the ingestion of a foreign body, a plain abdominal radiograph may reveal the presence of radiopaque material. It is strongly suggested to perform an abdominal radiograph for any sudden, unanticipated rise in lead levels to assure that there is no lead in the gastrointestinal tract, which will lead to continued absorption. A complete blood count (CBC) may reveal the presence of anemia that is typically microcytic and hypochromic. Basophilic stippling may be seen on a peripheral blood smear. Lead's interference with heme synthesis also causes the buildup of certain protoporphyrins. Measuring the free erythrocyte protoporphyrin (FEP) and zinc protoporphyrin (ZPP) in red blood cells are the typical techniques used to identify elevated protoporphyrin levels. The measurements of FEP and ZPP are not typically done unless BLLs are significantly above 25 µg/dL. With the treatment of lead poisoning (end of lead exposure or chelation therapy), some chose to follow their decline as an indicator of clinical improvement.

Treatment. Treatment of any patient begins with cessation of exposure. A thorough history of possible exposure and environmental investigation of the patient's home and any other locations where exposures could occur (e.g., a babysitter's house) must be done. The local health department should be informed and their help enlisted in this investigation. This lead exposure can be from a traditional source, such as lead-based paint, and may be easily ascertained, but the source may not be immediately apparent. Some sources that deserve inquiry are certain imported products that include ceramics, folk remedies, foods, and cosmetics. Some vinyl miniblinds (especially bought before 1997) may also be a cause of lead poisoning. Parental occupation and hobbies (e.g., making stained glass or fishing and hunting) may provide clues. Once a source is found, interventions to end it must occur. This may be as straightforward as removing a foreign body from the gastrointestinal tract. However, it may be as dramatic as removing that child and their family from an older house that is contaminated with lead dust and paint.

Management is guided by BLLs as well as symptoms. At the time of this writing, a BLL <10 µg/dL is considered nontoxic. Management of toxic BLLs <45 µg/dL require outpatient management that involves thorough history from the family, environmental investigation, appropriate removal of the source, and serial BLLs over time to assure cessation of exposure and gradual elimination of lead from the body. Chelation therapy for patient with BLLs <45 µg/dL has not been shown to change neurodevelopmental outcomes and is not indicated. Precise guidelines for the management of these outpatient cases are outlined by the Center, for Disease Control and Prevention (CDC) and the American Academy of Pediatrics (see the Suggested Readings).

Chelation therapy is indicated for BLLs >45 µg/dL. Before starting chelation, a physician (either a pediatrician or medical toxicologist at a regional poison control center) versed in the use of these agents should be consulted. Identifying such a physician can usually be facilitated by contacting a state or local health department. It is also vital that the lead exposure be identified and ended before initiating chelation therapy. If this level is <70 µg/dL and the patient has no symptoms of encephalopathy, this can generally be performed on an outpatient basis. However, admission may be necessary to end the exposure if the patient would otherwise continue to be exposed to lead (e.g., the family cannot leave their house). Outpatient therapy is generally performed with *succimer* (meso-2,3-dimercaptosuccinic acid or DMSA), an orally administered chelating agent. Side effects of succimer include abdominal pain and liver enzyme elevation. It also has a strong odor and may be difficult to give orally. Close outpatient follow-up is required with these patients.

If the patient's BLL is >70 µg/dL, or if the patient has any symptoms concerning for lead encephalopathy, the patient must be admitted emergently. Appropriate supportive care should be given as needed to maintain ABCs. An intensive-care setting is indicated if encephalopathy is present. If lead foreign bodies are evident on abdominal radiograph, whole-bowel irrigation with polyethylene glycol electrolyte solutions (PEG ES) or even endoscopy may be used to remove them. Chelation therapy is given emergently in these cases, but it is stressed again to consult a physician familiar with these medications before utilizing them. Depending on the individual patient's clinical symptoms, one chelating agent may be preferable to another, and each carries with it potential risks and toxicities that are beyond the scope of this chapter. Lead encephalopathy is a particularly concerning scenario that generally requires the use of two agents in particular. The first is *British anti-Lewisite (BAL)*, a painful intramuscular (IM) medication that should be first line in the management of lead encephalopathy (or BLLs >70 µg/dL) and given before other chelators. Peanut allergy is a contraindication for the use of BAL, as it is diluted in peanut oil. Typically IV *calcium disodium ethylenediaminetetraacetic acid (EDTA)* is then started 4 hours after BAL therapy is initiated. EDTA carries with it the risk of nephrotoxicity. Serial BLLs should be checked during hospitalization to assess response to therapy.

Carbon Monoxide

Carbon monoxide (CO) is the leading cause of poisoning deaths in the United States. Sadly, only 30% of these deaths are estimated to be unintentional. Motor vehicle exhaust contributes the bulk of exposures, but any combustion of fossil fuels has the potential to produce CO and many sources have been reported. Carbon monoxide binds to hemoglobin, causing a shift of the oxygen–hemoglobin saturation curve to the left. This causes a relative anemia and disrupts oxygen delivery to tissues. The full mechanism of toxicity appears more complicated, however, with evidence to suggest that CO has direct cellular toxicity.

Clinical Presentation. It is useful to divide carbon monoxide poisoning into two phases. The acute phase occurs soon after exposure. A second, delayed phase is also possible. In delayed poisoning, the time frame is ill defined but usually follows 2 to 40 days after an exposure. Interestingly, delayed toxicity may follow complete recovery from acute poisoning.

Acute CO poisoning manifests itself primarily with neurologic symptoms. Early symptoms are often vague and include headache, fatigue, and dizziness. In more severe exposures, symptoms may progress to include syncope, confusion, and altered mental status. Seizures are common and can be an isolated finding in children. Focal neural deficits are possible.

Cardiovascular effects are also common in acute CO exposures. Effects are likely from a combination of hypoxia and direct myocardial toxicity. Dysrhythmias, hypotension, and cardiac arrest are possible. Ischemia and infarction are possible but seem to be more common in those with underlying cardiovascular disease.

Delayed CO toxicity is an entity of neurocognitive deterioration after recovery from an acute exposure. The constellation of symptoms ranges from minor concentration difficulties and ataxia to debilitating dementia, parkinsonism, and psychosis. The incidence has been reported to be around 10% of all those hospitalized for CO poisoning and seems to occur more commonly in those with loss of consciousness. Delayed toxicity appears uncommon in those less than 30 years old.

Fetal exposure to CO is particularly concerning. Carbon monoxide readily crosses the placenta and is tightly bound to fetal hemoglobin. Fetal demise, anatomic malformations, and delayed neurologic development have been reported after apparent minor maternal exposure. Due to the vague, flu-like symptoms of accidental exposure, they are frequently missed on initial presentation. Hopefully, as home CO detectors become more popular, fewer exposures will go undiagnosed. Many poisoned patients are victims of structure fires or victims of intentional automobile exposure where the history should prompt a carboxyhemoglobin level. Patients with unexplained syncope and acidosis could also represent CO exposures. Percutaneous pulse oximetry plays no role in the diagnosis of CO poisoning, as it cannot reliably discriminate between carboxyhemoglobin and oxyhemoglobin.

Although many texts suggest that blood levels correlate with symptoms, this cannot be relied upon. Frequently, long periods of time have passed, usually with oxygen therapy, between exposure and hospital presentation, making levels difficult to interpret. High levels are clearly concerning; however, low levels in the setting of loss of consciousness are also concerning. When possible, the environment should be sampled to confirm exposure.

Treatment. After stabilization and supportive care, the treatment for CO poisoning is oxygen. The half-life or carboxyhemoglobin at room air is over 300 minutes. When 100% oxygen is administered to the patient at normal atmospheric pressure, the half-life drops to 90 minutes. Administration of 100% oxygen should be initiated with anyone suspected of CO poisoning while awaiting confirmation.

The role of hyperbaric oxygen (HBO) therapy in CO poisoning is controversial. The half-life of carboxyhemoglobin drops to 20 minutes under HBO conditions (3 atm of pressure with 100% oxygen), but the role in acute management is unclear. Many patients are improving clinically with the administration of normobaric oxygen therapy by the time HBO therapy is considered. There is, however, some evidence that HBO therapy may decrease the risk of delayed neurologic symptoms of CO poisoning after an apparent recovery. That is to say, patients with trivial levels and no persistent symptoms may still benefit from HBO therapy if there was evidence of a significant exposure. Although still a matter of debate, HBO therapy should be considered in those with a significant exposure as evidenced by syncope, altered mental status, focal neurologic deficits, or seizures. It should also be considered for pregnant women with carboxyhemoglobin levels greater than 15% despite symptoms due to the risk of fetal exposure.

ENVIRONMENTAL EXPOSURES

Snake Envenomations

There are two families of indigenous venomous snakes in the United States. The family responsible for the majority of envenomations is the Crotalid (*Crotalidae*) family or the pit vipers. These include the rattlesnakes, copperheads, and cottonmouths. These snakes all share common traits, which are sometimes helpful in distinguishing venomous snakes from nonvenomous ones. Obviously, the presence of a rattle is indicative of a pit viper, but copperheads and cottonmouths (which lack rattles) are also in the same family, with similar but less potent venom. All the pit vipers are so named because the have heat sensing pits lateral and posterior to their nostrils. These organs are used to locate and strike prey. The crotalids also have arrow-shaped heads and vertical pupils. Although handling snakes, even dead ones, is dangerous and to be discouraged, these features are sometimes helpful in determining the type of snake involved in an envenomation should a specimen be available for cautious examination.

The elapids (*Elapidae*) make up the other family of venomous snakes in the United States, and include coral snakes. These snakes do not share the characteristics noted above for pit vipers. The eastern coral snake is one of the most dangerous of these snakes in the United States, and is found in southeastern states. Coral snakes have a red, black, and yellow color pattern. Many harmless snakes have a similar color pattern, but unless the snake can be identified with absolute certainty, it should be assumed that anyone bitten by a red, black, and yellow snake has been envenomated by a coral snake.

Although not a taxonomic class, exotic snakes make up the third group of venomous snakes found in the United States and bring their own particular management challenges. Exotic venomous snake collections are common in the United States both in zoos and private settings. Identification of exotic snakes can be challenging because collectors are sometimes hesitant to divulge information for fear of legal repercussions.

The unsuspecting clinician may assume an envenomation from a local snake and make suboptimal treatment decisions. Even when bites by exotics are identified, treatment is hampered by lack of clinical expertise for the bites of these unusual animals. Although further discussion of exotic snake envenomation is beyond the scope of this text, antivenin for exotic snakes is sometimes available. Regional poison control centers can help locate antivenin and aid in treatment recommendations.

The epidemiology of snake envenomation is quite interesting. In most studies, victims of envenomation are overwhelmingly male, with alcohol playing a role in a majority of bites. Those aged 20 to 40 years are disproportionately represented as snakebite victims. The majority of bites occur on the upper extremities, which may imply attempts at handling the snake. Luckily, children make up a minority of snakebite victims and appear to have a more even distribution of lower versus upper extremity bites.

Clinical Effects

Crotalids. Venom from pit vipers contains a host of enzymes and inflammatory modulators that can result in local tissue swelling and necrosis and, in the case of rattlesnakes, life-threatening systemic effects. The swelling at the bite is often quite rapid, with the affected extremity increasing in circumference by several centimeters within minutes. Serous and hemorrhagic blister and bullae formation are possible, which may progress to necrosis and ulceration. Ecchymosis is common and can be profound. Pain is also commonly reported. These local effects usually progress distally and proximally from the bite as venom spreads via the lymphatic system. Due to the pain and swelling, the diagnosis of compartment syndrome is likely to be entertained; however, truly elevated compartment pressures are rarely encountered, and fasciotomy is rarely needed. Approximately 25% of pit viper bites are "dry" bites without envenomation. If no local effects are seen within 6 to 8 hours, it is likely a dry bite.

Systemic symptoms are common after rattlesnake envenomation but rarely occur after copperhead or cottonmouth envenomation. These systemic symptoms are at first vague and nonspecific and may include nausea, vomiting, chest tightness, palpitations, abdominal pain, and dizziness. Due to the anxiety invoked by a snakebite, these symptoms should be interpreted with caution. Patients may frequently complain of a metallic taste, which may be due to the metalloproteinases that comprise a portion of crotalid venom. This symptom should be taken seriously and is indicative of more severe, impending systemic effects. Serious systemic symptoms include coagulopathy, thrombocytopenia, disseminated intravascular coagulation (DIC), shock, and cardiovascular collapse.

The Mojave rattlesnake's venom is capable of neuromuscular paralysis, which may manifest first as muscle fasciculation, diplopia, or ptosis and may progress to respiratory collapse.

Elapids. Coral snake venom lacks significant proteolytic enzymes, so there is little local tissue damage. Furthermore, coral snakes lack true fangs for the delivery of venom, relying instead on their grooved back teeth for envenomation. Therefore, the bite site is likely to be unimpressive and may even appear to lack obvious fang marks. The systemic effects of coral snakebites are of primary concern and can be delayed for up to 12 hours. Coral snake venom is neurotoxic, blocking neural transmission mediated by acetylcholine, leading to muscle paralysis. The first signs may be subtle and include fasciculations, diplopia, and ptosis. Eventually frank muscle paralysis, including the diaphragm, is possible, and death results from respiratory failure.

Treatment

Crotalids. The effective field management of crotalid envenomations can be easily summarized. The patient should try to remain calm, immobilize and splint the affected extremity for comfort below heart level, and seek medical care as quickly as possible. Unfortunately, most attempts at more aggressive first aid provide no benefit and in most cases actually worsen local injury. The time-honored "cut and suck" technique risks introducing bacteria through an extended wound while removing nominal amounts of venom. Commercially available suction devices have been shown to worsen wound outcome with minimal venom extraction. Ice packs intuitively seem helpful, but have been shown to worsen local wound effects. Tourniquets should be avoided.

Once at the hospital, and after the patient's ABCs have been addressed, the wound should be observed for progressive swelling. Circumferential measurements every 15 to 30 minutes at the site and at distal and proximal sites provide objective points to gauge progression of swelling. The wound should be thoroughly cleaned, and tetanus status should be confirmed. Currently, prophylactic antibiotics are not recommended. Immobilizing the wound and elevating it may aid in pain control but opioid analgesics are frequently required. Laboratory testing should include a complete blood count (CBC) with platelet count, coagulation studies (prothrombin time and partial thromboplastin time), and fibrinogen to check for the presence of a coagulopathy. If these laboratory studies are normal and the patient has no symptoms (swelling or pain) after 6 to 8 hours, it is safe to assume a dry bite. The patient may be discharged with instruction to seek medical attention immediately if any symptoms develop.

The indications for antivenin therapy are progressive local tissue swelling or signs of systemic toxicity. Initial antivenin should be given slowly, and the patient should be monitored for any signs of an allergic reaction. Equipment and medical therapies should be readily available to manage an acute allergic reaction. If swelling continues to progress, more antivenin should be administered until control is achieved. It should be noted the antivenin does not reverse systemic or local effects of venom but only prevents further progression. Purified ovine polyvalent Fab immunoglobulin (CroFab) is the antivenin of choice due to its improved safety profile (much lower risk of anaphylaxis and serum sickness) over the older equine-derived antivenin, which should only be used as a last resort for serious systemic toxicity.

After stabilization and antivenin administration, the critically ill envenomated patient should receive standard supportive care. Blood products, especially those for treating coagulopathy, unless emergently needed, should be withheld until antivenin has been administered, because unbound venom will likely make their benefit temporary. Respiratory support should be provided should the patient show any signs of neuromuscular toxicity.

There is some controversy regarding the use of antivenin for copperhead and cottonmouth bites because systemic effects are so rare with envenomations from these snakes. Likewise, rigorous studies showing benefit from CroFab use are lacking. It has been used in children and adults and appears to be safe. Cottonmouth venom is used in the making of antivenin, and in-vitro studies demonstrate that antivenin is capable of binding copperhead venom. Specific recommendation regarding antivenin use can be obtained from a physician versed in its use or from a medical toxicologist by contacting a regional poison control center.

Elapids. Field treatment of elapids mirrors that for crotalids. Aggressive first-aid measures, other than immobilization and transport to the hospital, should be avoided.

Once at the hospital, the ABCs should be addressed and local wound care should proceed as described above. The initial appearance of an eastern coral snake bite is misleadingly subtle. There are no local tissue effects from the venom as impressive as the swelling and blister formation associated with crotalid envenomation. In this setting, the clinician may be tempted to suspect a dry bite. Although dry bites are possible with coral snakes, the systemic effects can be delayed up to 12 or more hours. Therefore, all suspected coral snake bites should be treated with antivenin. Because coral snake antivenin is equine derived and only partially purified, the risk of severe allergic reactions is high, so epinephrine and airway equipment should be readily available. Antivenin does not reverse symptoms; it only arrests their progression.

Spiders

Black Widow Envenomation

Black widow spiders (*Latrodectus* spp.) are found in many parts of the United States and other parts of the world. They commonly have a red hour-glass shape on the abdomen and have a shiny black appearance. Males are smaller than females and lack jaws large enough to effectively deliver venom; hence females account for the majority of clinically important envenomations.

Clinical Effects. The initial bite of the black widow is may be described a pinprick and may show a local area of erythema. Subsequent clinical effects (latrodectism) are caused primarily by a neurotoxin, α-latrotoxin, which is a component of black widow venom. Systemic symptoms are common after black widow envenomation and include muscle pain, cramping, and spasm. Usually this profound discomfort starts at the bite site and migrates proximally. Abdominal pain and muscle spasm along with nausea and vomiting can mimic an acute abdomen. Palpitations, anxiety, chest tightness, tachycardia, hypertension, and diaphoresis are typical as well. Symptoms can sometimes last for days.

Treatment. The bite should be cleaned and tetanus status confirmed. The pain of latrodectism can be severe, so liberal use of analgesics is appropriate. Anti-inflammatory agents are sometimes effective but intravenous opioids are frequently required. Due to the muscle spasm, diazepam or other muscle relaxants may provide some benefit. An equine-derived antivenin is available and is a highly effective treatment. Due to the risks of anaphylaxis and serum sickness, it is reserved for those who do not respond to conservative management.

Brown Recluse Envenomation

The venom of the brown recluse spider contains many enzymes, but the component thought to be most toxic is sphingomyelinase D2. There is no pain immediately after the bite, but pain, redness, and pruritus may develop inside 6 hours. The wound may then blister and ulcerate, forming a necrotic lesion. Very rarely, systemic symptoms (e.g., hemolysis) have been attributed to the bite.

The ability of the brown recluse spider's bite to cause large, necrotic, slow-healing wounds has elevated this spider's reputation to a near mythic level. Many large or poorly healing wounds with other plausible explanations (e.g., diabetic wounds or ulcers) are frequently blamed on the brown recluse spider. This perception perpetuates even in locations that are hundreds of miles from the spider's natural geographic range (generally the south central United States including Arkansas, Kansas, Missouri, and Oklahoma). Although this bite can cause clinically impressive wounds, it must be remembered to consider other possible causes for such lesions. In reality, the prevalence and clinical relevance of brown recluse bites may be exaggerated. Although this spider's venom can cause large wounds, causality is impossible to prove unless the spider responsible is captured and can be identified by a reliable entomologist. The bite itself is frequently painless, making capture and identification difficult.

Though many medical therapies have been suggested (e.g., dapsone), none have sufficient clinical evidence to routinely support their use. The wound of a suspected brown recluse bite should be cared for as any other wound. Likewise, alternative explanations for slow healing (e.g., diabetes) should be explored.

Plants

The overwhelming majority of accidental plant ingestions in young children result in no symptoms. Minor gastrointestinal symptoms may follow any ingestion, but few plants are truly toxic. Serious morbidity or mortality is exceed-

TABLE 147.2

COMMON TOXIC PLANTS

Classes	Clinical effects	Treatment	Comments
Cardiac glycosides: foxglove, white oleander, red qquill, lilly of the valley	Bradycardia, heart block, Hypotension, tachyhdysrhythmias, hyperkalemia	Supportive care, digoxin-specific Fab fragments	Digoxin assay may cross-react but results should be interpreted with caution
Nicotinic: tobacco, lobelia, poison hemlock	Early: nausea, vomiting, tachycardia, hypertension Late: bradycardia, hypotension, seizures	Supportive care Atropine may be useful for late symptoms Benzodiazepines for seizures	Cigarette ingestion is the most common exposure in children
Anticholinergics: nightshade, jimsonweed	Agitation, hallucinations, dry warm skin, decreased bowel sounds, urinary setention	Benzodiazepines for agitation	Physostigmine is not routinely recommended due to the risk of seizures and cardiac arrhythmias
Irritants: philodendron, dumb cane	Pain and swelling at the site of exposure	No specific treatment	Oropharyngeal swelling may potentially compromise the airway
Water hemlock	Status epilepticus	Benzodiazepines are first-line treatment, but anticipate the need for other agents	Responsible for most plant deaths

ingly rare. Table 147.2 lists some common toxic plants along with their clinical effect and management strategies. A comprehensive list is beyond the scope of this chapter. As with all poisonings, supportive care is paramount. A regional poison control center should be contacted immediately to aid in identification and specific treatments when necessary.

Mushrooms

Mushroom hunting is commonplace in some cultures and is very popular in the United States. Although expert mushroom hunters are capable of finding rare delicacies without making a mistake, many novices will attempt to hunt and follow long-held mushroom myths and make terrible mistakes. Such faulty tests of safety include mushrooms that peel easily are harmless to consume; insects found on the mushroom mean it is edible; and boiling them or soaking them in salt will neutralize any possible toxins. Some wild mushrooms ingestions can incur serious morbidity and even mortality. On old saying goes, "There are old mushroom hunters, and there are bold mushroom hunters; but there are no bold, old mushroom hunters." This section will broadly discuss the topic of mushroom toxicity and basic principles of management.

Obtaining as detailed a history as possible is vital in the management of mushroom poisoning. Time, effort, and resources are well spent in this area because a positive and reliable identification of the mushroom will help guide subsequent management. A high index of suspicion must be maintained because in some case there is a prolonged delay between ingestion and symptom onset. If a history of mushroom ingestion is obtained, the amount and variety of different types should be ascertained. If specimens are available for examination, they should be obtained if at all possible. Samples should be stored in the refrigerator until they can be thoroughly examined. Spore prints may also help in the identification process. This technique involves putting the cap of the mushroom with gills facing downward on a sheet of white paper. This cap should be covered in order to prevent drafts from spreading the pores which will settle and become visible on the piece of paper. The spores seen may help identify the mushroom species. Light microscopy of these spores may also provide information. Ideally, the help of a skilled mycologist should be sought to help positively identify the mushroom by its structure and spore print if available.

If a specimen is not available, the patient should be asked for as much descriptive detail as possible about the color, stem, cap, and bulb. Asking the patient to draw the mushroom may help. If the patient has been vomiting and gastric contents are available, the may be filtered through cheesecloth and then centrifuged to obtain spores for microscopic examination.

There are other key parts of the history to obtain. The timeline from ingestion to first symptoms is essential. Nausea and vomiting are the initial symptoms many toxic mushrooms. If

TABLE 147.3

TOXIC MUSHROOMS

Mushroom type and examples	Signs and symptoms

Cyclopeptides
  Aminita phalloides
  Galerina autumnalis
  Lepiota helveola
  Conocybe filaris
	Nausea, vomiting, abdominal pain, diarrhea, encephalopathy, coma, hepatic failure, renal failure, cardiomyopathy

Monomethylhydrazine
  Gyromitra esculenta
  Gyromitra fastigiata
  Helvella lacunose
	Nausea, vomiting, diarrhea, abdominal pain, weakness, headache, seizures, coma

Disulfarim-like toxins
  Coprinus atramentarius
  Clitocybe claviceps
	With ethanol consumption:flushing, metallic taste, headache, hypotension, tachycardia, palpitations

Orellanine
  Aminita smithiana
  Cortinarius orellanus
  Cortinarius splendens
	Nausea, vomiting, diarrhea, decreased urine output, delayed (2–21 days after ingestion) acute renal failure

Muscarine
  Inocybe fastigiata
  Inocybe geophylla
  Clitocybe dealbata
	Miosis, sweating, sialorrhea, diarrhea, abdominal pain, bronchorrhea, tearing, bronchospasm, bradycardia

Isoxazoles
  Aminita muscaria
  Aminita pantheria
  Panaeolus campanulatus
	Fluctuating neurologic status between coma and agitation; mydriasis, euphoria, ataxia, confusion, delirium, nausea, vomiting

Indoles
  Psilocybe cubensis
  Panaeolus foenisecii
  Conocybe cyanopus
  Gymnophilus spectabilis
	Visual hallucinations, confusion, euphoria, bizarre behavior, unintelligible speech, synesthesia; fever and seizures possible in young children

more than 6 hours have passed before the onset of nausea and vomiting, dangerous mushrooms (e.g., *Amanita phalloides*, which can produce severe hepatotoxicty) are a true concern. Symptoms beginning within 6 hours are generally a reassuring sign. However, if a mixture of mushrooms is ingested (as is often the case), this rule will not apply. If the symptoms began after the consumption of alcohol, then mushrooms that convey a disulfiram-like effect (e.g., *Coprinus atramentarius* or "inky caps") should be suspected. As some mycotoxins are heat labile, the preparation method may be useful to know. It is useful to know if multiple people are sick and if they all ate the mushrooms.

Extensive discussion of the presentation and management of individual mushroom poisonings is beyond the scope of this chapter. Table 147.3 summarizes some of the basic features of key poisonous mushroom groups. Some of these poisonings (*e.g. Amanita phalloides*) are potentially life-threatening, and though no perfect antidotes exist, some medical therapies have been investigated. Supportive care should be given as needed. If there are no contraindications, administration of activated charcoal may be helpful. It is encouraged that once a positive identification or clinical suspicion exists for mushroom toxicity, a regional poison center be contacted for consultation and recommendations as to observation time and precise medical therapies.

References

1. Lifshitz M, Shahak E, Sofer S. Carbamate and organophosphate poisoning in young children. *Pediatr Emerg Care* 1999;15:102–103.
2. de Jong AL, Macdonald R, Ein S, et al. Corrosive esophagitis in children: a 30-year review. *Int J Pediatr Otorhinolaryngol* 2001;57:203–211.

Suggested Readings

Abbruzzi G, Stork CM. Pediatric toxicologic concerns. *Emerg Med Clin North Am* 2002;20:223–247.

Berger KJ, Guss DA. Mycotoxins revisited: part I. *J Emerg Med* 2005;28:53–62.

Berger KJ, Guss DA. Mycotoxins revisited: part II. *J Emerg Med* 2005; 28:175–183.

Centers for Disease Control and Prevention. *Managing elevated blood lead levels among young children: recommendations from the advisory committee on childhood lead poisoning and prevention.* Atlanta: CDC; 2002.

Dyer S. Plant exposures: wilderness medicine. *Emerg Med Clin North Am* 2004;22:299–313, vii.

Gold BS, Barish RA, Dart RC. North American snake envenomation: diagnosis, treatment, and management. *Emerg Med Clin North Am* 2004;22:423–443, ix.

Gordon RA, Roberts G, Amin Z, et al. Aggressive approach in the treatment of acute lead encephalopathy with an extraordinarily high concentration of lead. *Arch Pediatr Adolesc Med* 1998;152:1100–1104.

Holstege CP, Kirk M, Sidell FR. Chemical warfare. Nerve agent poisoning. *Crit Care Clin* 1997;13:923–942.

Kales SN, Christiani DC. Acute chemical emergencies. *N Engl J Med* 2004;350:800–808.

Kao LW, Nanagas KA. Carbon monoxide poisoning. *Med Clin North Am* 2005;89:1161–1194.

Kirk MA. Managing patients with hazardous chemical contamination. In: Ford M, Delaney K, Ling L, et al., eds. *Clinical toxicology.* Philadelphia: Saunders; 2001: 115–126.

Lead exposure in children: prevention, detection, and management. *Pediatrics* 2005;116:1036–1046.

Pelclova D, Navratil T. Do corticosteroids prevent oesophageal stricture after corrosive ingestion? *Toxicol Rev* 2005;24:125–129.

Saucier JR. Arachnid envenomation. American Academy of Pediatrics Committee on Environmental Health. *Emerg Med Clin North Am* 2004;22: 405–422, ix.

Singletary EM, Rochman AS, Bodmer JC, et al. Envenomations. *Med Clin North Am* 2005;89:1195–1224.

Truemper E, Reyes de la Rocha S, Atkinson SD. Clinical characteristics, pathophysiology, and management of hydrocarbon ingestion: case report and review of the literature. *Pediatr Emerg Care* 1987;3:187–193.

Victoria MS, Nangia BS. Hydrocarbon poisoning: a review. *Pediatr Emerg Care* 1987;3:184–186.

CHAPTER 148A ■ CARDIOPULMONARY RESUSCITATION

EMILY FONTANE

The 2005 American Heart Association (AHA) guidelines for cardiopulmonary resuscitation (CPR) are based on the most extensive evidence review of CPR published to date and have been streamlined to clarify the most important skills that rescuers need to perform. The AHA believes that children have the best chance for survival when prevention, early basic life support, prompt access to emergency medical services, and timely advanced life support are all optimally ensured. This is the four-link pediatric chain of survival philosophy of the AHA. The delivery of effective CPR requires basic and advanced life support skills. The hospital health care professional caring for the child requiring life support incorporates the skills of both the basic and advanced rescuer. Compressions and ventilations are essential components of CPR. Most out-of-hospital pediatric arrests are due to respiratory failure, sudden infant death syndrome (SIDS), sepsis, neurologic diseases, and injuries. Most in-hospital arrests are due to respiratory failure and shock. Although cardiac arrhythmias amenable to electrical therapy (shocks) are not a common cause of pediatric cardiopulmonary arrest, pediatric basic and advanced life support skills include the ability to deliver shock treatment in the event of a pediatric arrest due to an arrhythmia. The pediatric CPR guidelines are designed for the infant (less than 1 year old, not a neonate) and the child (1 year old to 12 to 14 years old). The act of delivering life support to a patient is called *cardiopulmonary resuscitation*, or *code* in hospital parlance. A code is usually initiated by the individual who has identified a patient who is experiencing a life-threatening event. The stepwise ABCDE (airway, breathing, circulation, disability, exposure) approach taught by the AHA helps students of CPR master the skills and gain the knowledge needed to perform optimally in a code, but in reality many steps are done simultaneously.

NEW GUIDELINES FOR PEDIATRIC AND NEONATAL EMERGENCY CARDIOVASCULAR CARE

An update of previous guidelines for emergency cardiovascular care (ECC) of the pediatric patient as well as cardiopulmonary resuscitation (CPR) and ECC of neonates has been issued. The American Heart Association and the American Academy of Pediatrics published the updates in the May 2006 issue of *Pediatrics*.

The authors emphasize that the "new recommendations do not imply that care involving the use of earlier guidelines is unsafe." Nonetheless, several changes were made on the basis of newly emerging evidence.

The major pediatric advanced life support (PALS) changes and neonatal resuscitation changes are summarized in about 20 key bulleted points at the beginning of the multipart report (Table 148.1).

For the pediatric population, the focus of this chapter, the authors urge caution with the use of endotracheal tubes and emphasize their correct placement. Also, after correct placement of an endotracheal tube, a change from the use of cycles of CPR to continuous compressions "at a rate of 100/minute without pauses for ventilation" is made.

The report also recommends changes in ways to perform and assess ventilation attempts, to administer intravenous epinephrine, and to withhold and discontinue resuscitative efforts.

These recommendations "confirm the safety and effectiveness of many approaches, acknowledge that other approaches may not be optimal, and recommend new treatments that have undergone evidence evaluation," the authors note.

They also point out that the guidelines "will not apply to all rescuers and all victims in all situations. The leader of a resuscitation attempt may need to adapt application of the guidelines to unique circumstances."

PREVENTION

Injury is the leading cause of death in children. It is responsible for more childhood deaths than all causes of death combined. Vehicular-related injuries account for approximately one-half of all pediatric deaths in the United States. Failure to place children in appropriate pediatric car seats and improper use of pediatric car seats and restraints increase the risk of childhood death due to motor vehicle collision. The practice of putting children less than 12 years old in the front passenger seat of cars with airbags is associated with increased risk of child trauma during motor vehicle collisions. Bicycle helmets reduce the severity of head injury after bicycle collisions by approximately 80%. Functional smoke and carbon monoxide detectors are the most effective way to prevent death and injury due to house fires and carbon monoxide poisoning, respectively. Placing an infant on his back to sleep instead of his abdomen or side has been associated with a decrease in the incidence of sudden infant death syndrome. Swimming instruction should emphasize safety as well as skill. Although death due to firearms has decreased since 1995, firearm homicide remains the leading cause of death among African American adolescents. Proper disposition of medical and surgical patients in the hospital (monitored bed versus unmonitored bed) improves patient care and facilitates early identification of patient deterioration. Pediatric pharmacist-assisted drug dosing of medications in children may help limit accidental medication overdosing in pediatric patients.

TABLE 148.1

NEW GUIDELINES FOR PEDIATRIC EMERGENCY CARDIOVASCULAR CARE

BLS HIGHLIGHTS

- Steps for unresponsive infants (<1 year) and children (1 year to puberty): open airway; give 2 breaths if not breathing; begin compressions if no pulse; activate EMS system, use automated external defibrillator (AED) after 5 cycles of CPR in children; if rhythm shockable, give 1 shock and resume CPR for 5 cycles; if rhythm not shockable, resume CPR and check rhythm every 5 cycles until response or PALS providers intercede.
- For sudden collapse in child, activate EMS and get AED before CPR.
- Barrier devices do not reduce infection risk and might increase resistance to air flow.
- Bag-mask ventilation is as effective as endotracheal intubation for short periods; use 100% oxygen until more information known.
- If definite pulse, give 12 to 20 breaths/minute (1 breath every 3–5 seconds) and check pulse every 2 minutes; if no pulse or if pulse ≤60 beats/minute with poor perfusion, begin chest compressions at 100 per minute.
- Cycle consists of 30 compressions (1 rescuer) or 15 compressions (2 rescuers) per 2 breaths. Ideal ratio unknown, but previously recommended 5:1 ratio resulted in less than 60 compressions/minute.
- If rescuer unable to ventilate patient, chest compressions alone are recommended vs no resuscitation.
- Changing rescuer every 2 minutes will maintain good compressions (forceful, fast, full chest recoil, minimal interruptions).
- For severe foreign body airway obstruction, perform subdiaphragmatic abdominal thrusts (child) or 5 back blows alternating with 5 chest thrusts (infant).
- For drowning victims, ventilation, but not compressions, can be started in the water if it does not prolong removal from water.

PALS REVISIONS

- Laryngeal mask airways can be used with caution.
- Cuffed endotracheal tubes can be used if inflation pressure <20 cm.
- Verify endotracheal tube placement.
- When advanced airway in place, perform 100 compressions/minute and 8 to 10 breaths/minute (1 breath every 6–8 seconds) continuously instead of cycles.
- During pulseless arrest, timing of 1 shock, CPR, and drug treatment is same as in advanced cardiac life support.
- Epinephrine is recommended in standard dose, not routine high dose.
- Lidocaine can be used for ventricular fibrillation or pulseless ventricular tachycardia if amiodarone not available.
- Consider induced hypothermia if persistent coma.
- Inodilators can enhance postresuscitation cardiac output.
- Family members prefer to be present during resuscitation.
- Guidelines for resuscitation termination are unreliable as patients can survive prolonged efforts; witnessed collapse, bystander CPR, and early professional treatment are associated with successful resuscitation.

RESPIRATORY FAILURE AND SHOCK

Children are more likely to experience an asphyxial arrest than a cardiac arrest. An asphyxial arrest is the terminal event of progressive respiratory failure or shock. Respiratory failure is associated with an increased respiratory rate and effort, or inadequate respiratory drive, which ultimately impairs ventilation and oxygenation. Shock occurs when blood flow and oxygen delivery fail to support tissue metabolism. Shock may be compensated (early) or uncompensated (late) in children. Central pulses (i.e., femoral pulse and carotid pulse) are usually detectable in compensated shock, and weak or barely detectable in uncompensated shock. Inadequate end-organ perfusion in uncompensated shock is marked by a depressed mental status. Shock in the sick child is confirmed by looking for and identifying multiple signs consistent with shock as opposed to any one sign alone. Capillary refill greater than 2 seconds, decreased urine output, absent tears, dry mucous membranes, ill appearance, tachycardia or bradycardia, and bounding or weak pulses together suggest shock. In children, the most common cause of shock is hypovolemia due to dehydration. Hypovolemia due to hemorrhage is seen in severe multisystem trauma. Before compensatory mechanisms are exhausted in the child in early shock the blood pressure is maintained in the normal range. Systolic blood pressure that is below the 5th percentile of normal for age is associated with decompensated shock. Hypotension in children is defined by the following:

- <60 mm Hg in term neonates (0–28 days)
- <70 mm Hg in infants (1–12 months)
- <70 mm Hg + (2 × age in years) in children 1 to 10 years of age
- <90 mm Hg in children 10 years of age and older

BASIC AND ADVANCED LIFE SUPPORT

In order to deliver quality CPR, a health care professional must be able to rapidly assess and identify cardiopulmonary failure and/or arrest and be prepared to deliver basic and advanced life support in an expedient and skillful manner. Preparation includes receiving instruction and frequent practice in CPR skills including rapid-sequence intubation (RSI) and endotracheal tube placement, keeping abreast of updates in resuscitation guidelines, placing well-stocked pediatric resuscitation carts in strategic locations, and assigning roles to the members of an easily assembled team of rescuers.

Touch the patient and make a loud verbal attempt to rouse the patient. If the child is unresponsive (i.e., she does not move or speak), announce a code to mobilize resuscitation team members and equipment and start CPR. CPR starts with a rapid assessment of the patient's airway and breathing. The head-tilt chin-lift and jaw thrust maneuvers open the mouth, align the upper airway axis, and move the tongue away from the posterior pharynx. The tongue may be the only cause of obstruction in an unconscious patient. Current AHA guidelines for CPR in children recommend the use of the head-tilt chin-lift maneuver in all pediatric patients including trauma patients if the jaw thrust maneuver fails to achieve optimal airway results. Clear the airway of accumulated saliva or blood, vomit, and any visible foreign bodies with a semirigid pharyngeal suction device. Suction forces greater than 120 mm Hg may be needed for use with semirigid device. Forces less than 120 mm Hg should be used when suctioning through an endotracheal tube.

Look, listen, and feel for breaths. Limit the check for breaths to 10 seconds. The chest should visibly rise and fall regularly at a rate consistent with age without the use of accessory muscles in a patient who has normal respiratory function. Agonal gasps are a sign of respiratory failure. In the event of no breathing or agonal gasps, administer two breaths with a manual resuscitator, also called a bag-mask ventilation apparatus. The patient's airway may need to be repositioned and the mask may need to be readjusted a number of times before effective breaths can be delivered. An effective rescue breath will make the patient's chest rise.

Bag-mask ventilation is as effective as ventilation through a properly placed endotracheal tube. Like endotracheal intubation (ETI), bag-mask ventilation requires training and practice for successful implementation; unlike ETI, it is generally safe when used by all rescuers. Self-inflating bags of at least 450 to 500 mL are required to deliver effective tidal volumes to children. Supplemental oxygen is delivered when a self-inflating bag with reservoir is attached to at least 10 L/min oxygen inflow. Adult setups used for pediatric patients require 15 L/min oxygen inflow. In order to avoid hyperventilation and gastric distention, use only the force and tidal volume necessary to make the patient's chest rise and give each breath over 1 second. It is common for health care professionals to deliver excessive ventilation, especially when an advanced airway is in place. Excessive ventilation should be avoided because it impedes venous return to the heart by increasing intrathoracic pressure, it may cause barotrauma in patients with small airway obstruction, it may reduce cerebral blood flow, and it increases the risk of gastric distention, which impedes lung expansion and increases the risk of regurgitation/aspiration. Gastric inflation is minimized by ventilating slowly, and may be minimized by application of cricoid pressure. Cricoid pressure (gentle pressure applied to the neck over the cricothyroid cartilage) indirectly causes esophageal collapse. However, over-aggressive pressure must be avoided because it will collapse the compliant infant trachea and interfere with ventilation.

Cricoid pressure should only be attempted in the unconscious patient. Health care professionals should use 100% humidified oxygen during pediatric resuscitation until better resuscitation science is available regarding the complications, if any, of high-concentration oxygen therapy. Pulse oximetry and serial arterial blood gas determinations should guide oxygen therapy after return of spontaneous circulation in children. Patients with poor lung compliance and/or high airway resistance (respiratory distress syndrome or severe asthma) require high pressures to overcome small airway obstruction. Disabling the pressure-relief valve will allow high pressures to be given. It may be difficult to maintain a tight mask seal in patients with craniofacial abnormalities (congenital or due to trauma) without the coordinated effort of two resuscitation team members. Ventilation delivered by two team members, one to secure the mask to the face and another to compress the bag apparatus, can increase success rates for these patients.

After 2 rescue breaths the team should take no longer than 10 seconds to check for a brachial pulse in an infant and a carotid or femoral pulse in a child. Patient pulses can be difficult to palpate and are commonly overcalled during resuscitations. Therefore, if after 10 seconds no pulse is detected or uncertainty exists, compressions should be initiated in the unresponsive patient. An intravenous or intraosseous line should be placed at this point if one does not already exist.

Chest compressions should be initiated if the pediatric patient's pulse is less than 60 beats per minute and perfusion is poor despite optimal oxygenation and ventilation. Bradycardia associated with poor perfusion (unresponsiveness) despite oxygen therapy is an indication for chest compressions because this combination of findings frequently precedes cardiac arrest. Cardiac output in the young pediatric patient is more dependent on heart rate than stroke volume. If the pulse is equal to or greater than 60 but the infant or young child has no spontaneous breathing, rescue breaths are delivered without compressions. In these cases the pulse should be reassessed for no more than 10 seconds every 2 minutes.

Coordinate compressions (15) with ventilations (2) when ventilating a patient with a bag-mask device. Compressions and ventilations may be administered simultaneously to children older than the neonate after an advanced airway (endotracheal tube [ETT] or laryngeal mask airway [LMA]) is successfully placed. In the hospital setting, a cuffed tube is as safe as an uncuffed tube for infants and children beyond the newborn period. Rapid-sequence intubation facilitates ETI and decreases the incidence of complications. An LMA may be used in the case of a failed ETT attempt. A length-based resuscitation tape provides ETT size and medication doses for children up to 36 kg. Length-based resuscitation tapes are more reliable than formulas.

At a 15 to 2 ventilation–compression ratio, 100 compressions and 8 to 10 breaths are delivered in a minute. Quality and rate of compressions is ensured when compressor fatigue is avoided. Therefore, resuscitation team members assigned to deliver compressions should alternate about every 2 minutes. Chest compressions in children are delivered by using one or two hands over the lower sternum, making sure to avoid excessive pressure over the ribs, xiphoid, and upper abdomen. There is evidence that shows that complete chest recoil after compression improves blood flow to the heart, and that complete recoil is ensured when the compressor's hands are lifted slightly off the chest at the end of each compression. Push hard, push fast, release completely, and minimize interruptions is the chest compression motto emphasized in the 2005 guidelines. Chest compressions in infants may be delivered in two ways: the two thumbs-encircling hands technique and the two-finger technique. Compressions are applied in both techniques just below the intermammary line. The AHA recommends that the two thumbs technique be employed, if possible, during the resuscitation of a child because it produces higher coronary artery perfusion pressures. Effective compressions will compress the child's chest one-third to one-half of the anterior–posterior depth of the chest. The ideal compression-to-ventilation ratio in children is unknown, but studies show that even during ideal conditions, a 5 to 1 compression ventilation ratio delivered fewer than 60 compressions per minute in pediatric manikins. Interruptions to provide ventilation, check for a pulse, and attach a monitor dropped coronary perfusion pressure. Interruptions have also been associated with decreased rate of return of spontaneous circulation in patients. Perfusion pressures are maintained only by uninterrupted, rapid, effective delivery of chest compressions. Cardiac output and subsequent pulmonary blood flow produced by even the most effective chest compressions during resuscitation is low. Therefore, a lower than normal minute ventilation, which translates to fewer rescue breaths during resuscitation, will maintain an adequate ventilation perfusion ratio. It is this deduction, and the dismal results of CPR in patients with cardiopulmonary arrest using the past guidelines, that has spurred the emphasis to administer more effective and rapid compressions and slower, more deliberate ventilations. In fact, a universal (for all ages except neonates) lay rescuer compression ventilation ratio of 30 to 2 has been adopted by the AHA in the hopes that more laypersons will learn CPR (easier to remember one ratio for all) and more compressions will be delivered during lay rescuer CPR. Delivery of CPR is best done while the child is supine on a firm surface. At this time, there are insufficient data to recommend the use of mechanical compression devices in infants and children.

CPR SEQUENCE FOR HOSPITALIZED PATIENTS

The patient is evaluated for unresponsiveness and breathing simultaneously. The unresponsive patient with inadequate or absent respiratory effort is given two 1-second bag-mask ventilations that make the chest rise and allow for recoil after optimal positioning of the airway while a code is announced and the resuscitation team/equipment/defibrillator are assembled. Ideally, no patient should be too far away from a code cart stocked with a length-based measuring tape, appropriately sized equipment, medications, and a well-functioning defibrillator. If no response is noted and no pulse is detected after a 10-second central pulse check, then chest compressions and ventilations are initiated at a 15 to 2 ratio while intravenous (IV) or intraosseous (IO) access is secured (if not already placed). It is important to avoid simultaneous delivery of compressions and ventilations until an advanced airway is secured. The current guidelines emphasize the administration of effective compressions, the avoidance of interruptions of chest compressions, and the avoidance of excessive ventilation. The goal is to deliver 2 minutes of compressions and ventilations at (approximately 100 compressions per minute or 6 cycles per minute) before reevaluating a pulse and applying the defibrillator pads. Team members assigned to deliver compressions should alternate every 2 minutes to avoid rescuer fatigue. Switches in compressor role should not take longer than 5 seconds. Subsequent interventions are guided by patient pulse assessment every 2 minutes, and the cardiac rhythm is noted on the defibrillator monitor. Pulse assessment should be limited to 10 seconds before resuming CPR starting with compressions first.

Optimally, the patient's airway, breathing, circulation (pulse or heart rate), and neurologic status are assessed at the onset and after every 2 minutes of interventions until return of spontaneous circulation. The decision to intubate a patient to secure her airway during a code and allow for uncoordinated compressions and ventilations should be made early. Patients that do not respond to initial breaths after optimal positioning and clearing of the airway will likely benefit from an advanced airway. Health care providers of PALS must be skilled at bag-mask ventilations and should be skilled at ETT placement and ventilation. Bag-mask ventilations have been shown to be as effective as ETT ventilations, especially in situations where a health care provider skilled in ETT placement is not available.

Tracheal intubation is verified by the seeing the tube enter the trachea through the vocal cords, using a carbon dioxide detector, listening for equal breath sounds in the apices and axillae, using an esophageal detector device (in children who weigh more than 20 kg), observing chest rise and fall, observing increases in pulse oximetry, and checking a chest x-ray. Intubated patients may deteriorate due to worsening condition and equipment failure. Consider the DOPE acronym: Displacement of tube, Obstruction of the tube with secretions, Pneumothorax due to barotrauma if high pressures were given, and Equipment failure.

Although lipid-soluble drugs (LEAN acronym: Lidocaine, Epinephrine, Atropine, and Naloxone) may be administered through the endotracheal tube, drug delivery and pharmacologic effect is unpredictable by this route. IV or IO administration of medications is preferred.

RESUSCITATION MEDICATIONS (TABLE 148.2)

Epinephrine is the resuscitation medication of choice in ventricular fibrillation, pulseless ventricular tachycardia, asystole, pulseless electrical activity, and bradycardia because it increases coronary perfusion pressure. Lidocaine and amiodarone are used to treat VF refractory to shocks and epinephrine. Neither has been associated with improved survival to hospital discharge. Calcium has not been shown to improve outcome in pediatric cardiac arrest. There are few data to support the use of procainamide in children. There is not enough evidence to support or refute the use of vasopressin in pediatric resuscitation. Sodium bicarbonate may be used after prolonged arrest, but adequate oxygenation and ventilation should be ensured prior to its use.

RHYTHM ALGORITHMS

Asystole and Pulseless Electrical Activity (Fig. 148.1)

If the monitor shows asystole in two leads or pulseless electrical activity (any rhythm without a pulse not consistent with pulseless ventricular tachycardia or ventricular fibrillation), CPR is continued while 0.01 mg/kg epinephrine is given IV/IO every 3 to 5 minutes until change in rhythm or return of spontaneous circulation.

Pulseless Ventricular Tachycardia and Ventricular Fibrillation (Fig. 148.2)

If the monitor shows pulseless ventricular tachycardia or ventricular fibrillation during a brief pulse-rhythm check after 2 minutes of CPR, CPR is briefly interrupted for electrical therapy starting with 2 J/kg followed by 2 minutes of CPR; 4 J/kg (followed by 2 minutes of CPR) is used for all subsequent shocks as long as the rhythm monitor shows PVT or VF. Epinephrine is given every 3 to 5 minutes during CPR starting

TABLE 148.2

MEDICATIONS FOR PEDIATRIC RESUSCITATION AND ARRHYTHMIAS

Medication	Dose	Remarks
Adenosine	0.1 mg/kg (max 6 mg)	Rapid IV/IO bolus, monitor ECG
Amiodarone	5 mg/kg IV/IO, may be repeated up to 15 mg/kg Maximum: 300 mg	Monitor BP/ECG, prolongs QT Adjust rate (give slowly when pulse present
Atropine	0.02 mg/kg IV/IO, may repeat Minimum dose 0.1 mg Maximum single dose: Child 0.5 mg Adolescent 1 mg	High doses may be needed for organophosphate poisoning
Calcium chloride (10%)	20 mg/kg IV/IO (0.2 mL/kg)	Give slowly, adult dose 5–10 mL
Epinephrine	0.01 mg/kg IV/IO (max 1 mg) 0.1 mg/kg ET (max 10 mg)	May repeat q 3–5 min
Glucose	0.5–1 g/kg IV/IO	$D_{10}W$: 5–10 mL/kg $D_{25}W$: 2–4 mL/kg $D_{50}W$: 1–2 mL/kg
Lidocaine	1 mg/kg IV/IO (max 100 mg) Infusion 20–50 ug/kg/min	
Magnesium sulfate	25–50 mg/kg IV/IO (max 2 g)	Give faster in torsades
Naloxone	<5 yr or <20 kg: 0.1 mg/kg IV/IO/ET >5 yr or >20 kg: 2 mg/dose IV/IO/ET	Use lower dose to reverse therapeutic opioid administration
Procainamide	15 mg/kg IV/IO over 30–60 min Adult: 20 mg/min up to 17 mg/kg	Monitor BP/ECG, prolongs QT
Sodium bicarbonate	1 mEq/kg IV/IO per dose	Give slowly after adequate ventilation

after the second shock until change in rhythm or return of spontaneous circulation. Although the data showing improvement in outcome with the use of antiarrhythmics and magnesium are limited, a trial of amiodorone or lidocaine may be given, especially for ventricular tachycardia, and magnesium may be given for torsades de pointes usually noted in arrests due to hyperkalemia or other electrolyte disorders.

Bradycardia and Tachycardia

Treatment of bradycardia (Fig. 148.3) depends on the hemodynamic status of the patient. If the rate is equal to or greater than 60 beats per minute, ensure adequate oxygenation and ventilation and monitor the patient closely for deterioration or improvement. If bradycardia less than 60 beats per minute exists despite optimal oxygenation and ventilation, start chest compressions. Continue to support the airway and breathing and give an epinephrine bolus. If bradycardia only transiently improves or persists, start an epinephrine or isoproterenol infusion. Treat vagal-induced bradycardia with atropine. Transcutaneous pacing is particularly useful in patients with bradycardia due to heart block or sinus node dysfunction unresponsive to CPR efforts and resuscitation medications, particularly if the arrhythmia is associated with congenital or acquired heart disease. Pacing is not useful in patients with asystole or bradycardia due to hypoxic myocardial insult or respiratory failure.

A narrow-complex tachycardia (Fig. 148.3) may be sinus tachycardia or supraventricular tachycardia (SVT). The evalu-

ation of an electrocardiogram and patient clinical status should help differentiate the two. Consider SVT in young children with heart rates greater than 180 and infants with heart rates greater than 220, without variability. Vagal maneuvers should be attempted in stable children with SVT. Ice is applied to the face of an infant. Massage the carotid artery in the older child. Rapid administration of adenosine is usually effective, especially after a second dose. An unstable patient should be cardioverted with 0.5 to 1 J/kg without delay. If readily available, sedation should be administered prior to cardioversion. Increase to 2 J/kg if SVT is refractory. Consider using amiodorone prior to a third electrical cardioversion attempt. Identify and treat any contributing conditions such as hypovolemia, hypoxia, and hypoglycemia. Ventricular tachycardia (VT) with a detectable pulse is a wide-complex regular tachycardia that should be treated immediately because it can quickly cause patient decompensation. An infusion of amiodorone may be used in the stable patient. Treat unstable VT with synchronized cardioversion in the same doses used for SVT.

FOREIGN BODY AIRWAY OBSTRUCTION (FBAO)

Children less than 5 years old, particularly infants, are at greatest risk for death due to foreign body aspiration. Infants most commonly choke on liquids. Children most commonly choke on small

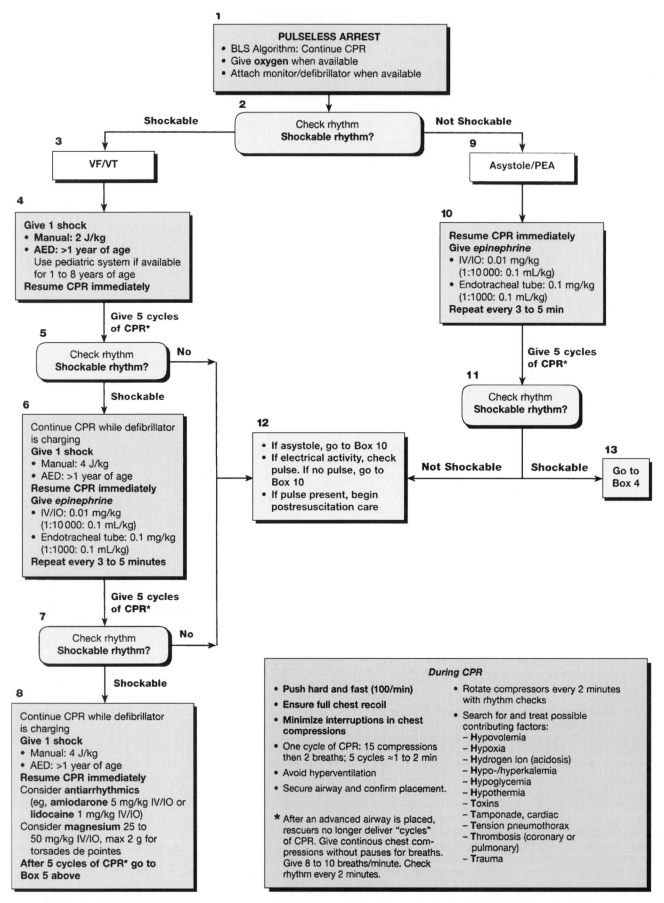

FIGURE 148.1. Pulseless arrest.

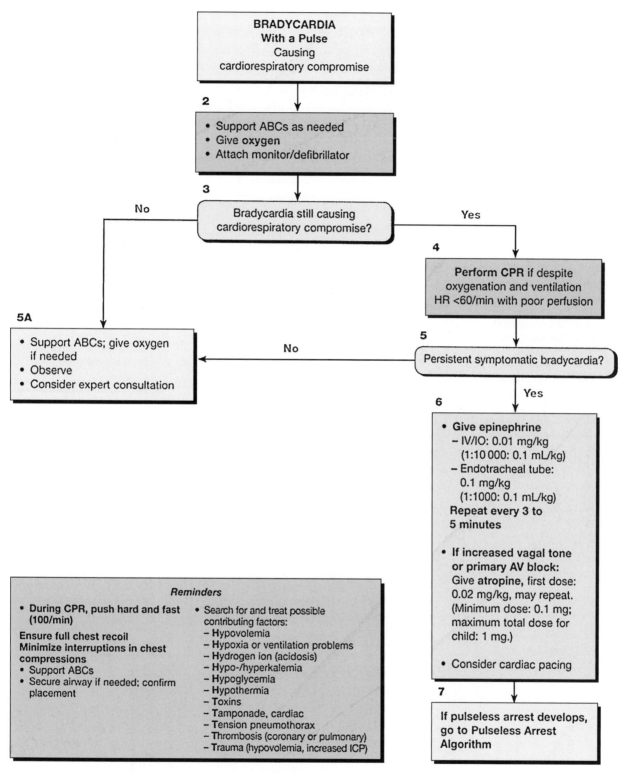

FIGURE 148.2. Tachycardia.

objects such as balloon parts, grapes, nuts, and hot dog pieces. Sudden onset respiratory distress in a child suggests foreign body airway obstruction. Signs include coughing, gagging, stridor, and wheezing. Important differential diagnoses include spasmodic croup and anaphylaxis. Mild airway obstruction will allow a child to cough and make sounds. A child is unable to make any sounds when the airway is completely obstructed. It is this severe obstruction that requires immediate intervention. Infants are given 5 back blows followed by 5 chest thrusts, and children are given subdiaphragmatic abdominal thrusts, also known as the Heimlich maneuver, until the foreign object is expelled or the patient becomes unresponsive. If the infant or child becomes unresponsive CPR, is started. In cases of FBAO, rescuers should look into the patient's mouth before delivering breaths so that the foreign body may be removed if seen. Health care professionals should not attempt blind finger sweeps. Children with mild FBAO should be allowed to cough until the foreign body is expelled while being monitored for complete or severe airway obstruction.

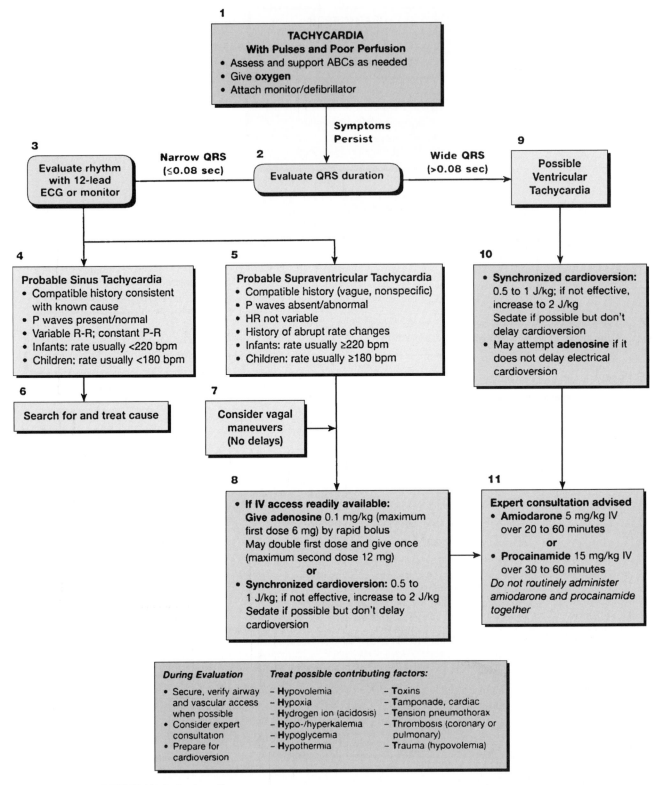

FIGURE 148.3. Bradycardia.

THE TRAUMA PATIENT

Resuscitation principles are the same for the pediatric trauma patient and the pediatric medical emergency patient. Improper resuscitation is a major cause of poor outcome and death in the pediatric trauma patient. Failure to open and maintain an airway and failure to recognize internal bleeding, are common errors. Remember the following when resuscitating a pediatric trauma patient. The pediatric trauma patient's airway should be carefully suctioned, because obstruction may be due to dental fragments or blood. Cervical spine immobilization during airway assessment and interventions prevents secondary spinal cord injury. The jaw thrust maneuver is the recommended approach to open the airway in trauma patients; however, if it is unsuccessful, the head tilt-chin lift maneuver should be attempted while neck and head movement is minimized. Neutral neck position (not flexed, extended, or rotated) in the infant and young child with a large occiput is achieved by elevating the torso with a sheet or towel wedge prior to immobilization. All external bleeding sites should be compressed. Once stabilized, a pediatric multisystem trauma patient should be transferred to a trauma center with pediatric expertise.

PROGNOSIS

For a child in cardiopulmonary arrest to have return of spontaneous circulation and neurologically intact survival, cardiopulmonary resuscitation must be timely and effective. Respiratory arrest is associated with good outcome. More than 70% of children in respiratory arrest survive without neurologic sequelae. Bradycardia is associated with better outcome than asystole and pulseless electrical activity. Prolonged CPR is generally associated with poor outcome except in cases of poisoning (e.g., tricyclic antidepressant toxicity), hypothermia (e.g., drowning in icy water), and arrhythmias amenable to shock therapy (e.g., VF or pulseless VT). Only 2% to 10% of children who progress to cardiac arrest from respiratory failure survive. Most of these survivors are neurologically impaired.

FAMILY PRESENCE

Studies have shown that family presence during resuscitation is beneficial to family members. If the resuscitation team decides to allow family to be present during a code, a team member should be assigned to provide comfort and answer questions.

Suggested Readings

Brown L. Pediatric out-of-hospital cardiopulmonary arrest and public access defibrillation programs for children. *Pediatr Emerg Med Prac* 2005; 2: 1–20.

Hachimi-Idrissi S, Biarent D, Huyghens L. Cardiopulmonary resuscitation in infants and children: new guidelines. *Eur J Emerg Med* 2002;9:287–297.

2005 American Heart Association Guidelines for Cardiopulmonary Resuscitation and Energy Cardiovascular Care. Neonatal Resuscitation Guidelines. *Circulation* 2005;112: Part 13:IV-188–IV-195.

2005 American Heart Association Guidelines for Cardiopulmonary Resuscitation and Energy Cardiovascular Care. Pediatric Advanced Life Support. *Circulation* 2005;112: Part 12:IV-167–IV-187.

2005 American Heart Association Guidelines for Cardiopulmonary Resuscitation and Energy Cardiovascular Care. Pediatric Basic Life Support. *Circulation* 2005;112: Part 11:IV-156–IV-166.

Perondi MM, Reis AG, Paiva EF, et al. A comparison of high-dose and standard-dose epinephrine in children with cardiac arrest. *N Engl J Med* 2004; 350:1722–1730.

Tang W, Weil MH, Jorgenson D, et al. Fixed-energy biphasic waveform defibrillation in a pediatric model of cardiac arrest and resuscitation. *Crit Care Med* 2002;30:2736–2741.

CHAPTER 148B ■ NEONATAL RESUSCITATION

JAMES J. CUMMINGS

Approximately 10% of infants born in the United States require some degree of resuscitation in the delivery room. Positive-pressure ventilation is used in about half of these cases. Most of these infants are considered high risk because of prenatal indicators, but up to one-third are unanticipated. Therefore, persons trained in neonatal resuscitation must be in attendance at *all* deliveries. Recognizing this need, the American Heart Association and the American Academy of Pediatrics collaborated to develop the Neonatal Resuscitation Program (NRP) in the 1980s. A major revision of the NRP based on current, evidence-based consensus recommendations of international experts was released in November 2005. It is considered the "gold standard" reference for neonatal resuscitation.

CONSIDERATIONS UNIQUE TO NEONATAL RESUSCITATION

The sudden separation of the infant from the maternal environment presents challenges not routinely encountered in other resuscitation scenarios.

■ Temperature and fluid regulation
■ Lung inflation and establishment of tidal ventilation
■ Circulatory adaptation, including a 10-fold increase in pulmonary blood flow
■ Metabolic regulation, including glucose homeostasis and acid–base balance

KEY POINTS

Although successful resuscitation involves complex integration of multiple factors, the procedure itself can be simplified by focusing on a few basic principles.

■ *Temperature support*, by warming and drying the newborn, is the *first* step of neonatal resuscitation (except with meconium staining—see below).
■ *Adequate ventilation* is of the utmost importance. Very few depressed neonates require chest compressions or medications, and failure of the infant to respond is most likely due to inadequate ventilation.
■ Resuscitation decisions should be made quickly based on *simultaneous assessment* of breathing, heart rate, and color.

ANTICIPATION AND PREPARATION

Every delivery should be attended by at least one person skilled in neonatal resuscitation. However, certain risk factors may indicate the need for additional personnel with special skills (e.g., endotracheal intubation in deliveries with meconium-stained amniotic fluid). Routine advance preparations include:

■ Screening for maternal risk factors (Table 148.3).
■ Preparation of a warm, clean, well-lit environment.

TABLE 148.3

CONDITIONS ASSOCIATED WITH RISK TO NEWBORNS

Antepartum	Intrapartum
Maternal diabetes	Emergency cesarean section
Pregnancy-induced hypertension	Forceps or vacuum-assisted delivery
Chronic hypertension	Breech or other abnormal presentation
Chronic maternal illness	Premature labor
Cardiovascular	Precipitous labor
Thyroid	Chorioamnionitis
Neurologic	Prolonged rupture of membranes
Pulmonary	(>18 hr. before delivery)
Renal	Prolonged labor (>24 hr.)
Anemia or isoimmunization	Prolonged second stage of labor (>2 hr.)
Previous fetal or neonatal death	Fetal bradycardia
Bleeding in second or third trimester	Non-reassuring fetal heart rate patterns
Maternal infection	Use of general anesthesia
Polyhydramnios	Uterine tetany
Oligohydramnios	Narcotics administered to mother within
Premature rupture of membranes	4 hr. of delivery
Post-term gestation	Meconium-stained amniotic fluid
Multiple gestation	Prolapsed cord
Size–dates discrepancy	Abruptio placentae
Drug therapy	Placenta previa
Lithium carbonate	
Magnesium	
Adrenergic-blocking drugs	
Maternal substance abuse	
Fetal malformation	
Diminished fetal activity	
No prenatal care	
Age <16 or >35 yr.	

- Availability of resuscitation equipment, supplies, and medications (Table 148.4).
- Suction, oxygen source, radiant heater, and laryngoscope should be checked periodically and before each delivery.

RESUSCITATION PROCEDURE

For an algorithm of the resuscitation procedure, refer to Figure 148.4 (see below for altered sequence with meconium staining).

Initial Steps

- Prevent hypothermia—place infant on preheated radiant warmer, dry infant, then rewrap in warm, dry blankets. Polyethylene (food grade) bags may help maintain body temperature of very-low-birthweight infants.
- Position—place the infant in a supine position with the head slightly extended ("sniffing position"); a small roll placed under the shoulders may be helpful.
- Airway—if there are copious secretions compromising the airway, suction the mouth first and then the nose using either a suction bulb or 8F or 10F suction catheter; avoid prolonged and deep suctioning. *Negative pressure should not exceed 100 mm Hg.*
- Tactile stimulation—if the infant remains apneic after drying, positioning, and suctioning, *further tactile stimulation is unlikely to help*; brief, gentle back rubbing or flicking the soles of feet, may be tried, but these efforts should not delay onset of positive-pressure ventilation.

Oxygen Administration

Free-flow 100% oxygen (at least 5 L/min) should be provided to any infant who has central cyanosis, pending further intervention(s). If positive-pressure ventilation (PPV) is begun, 100% supplemental oxygen is recommended. To reduce potential harm from excessive tissue oxygenation in preterm infants, the use of an oxygen blender and pulse oximetry is recommended in order to titrate supplemental oxygen delivery, maintaining oyxgen saturations between 90% and 95%. In any infant, if the heart rate does not respond by increasing to >100 beats per minute, 100% oxygen should be given.

Bag/Mask Ventilation

- Indications—apnea or gasping; heart rate less than 100 beats per minute; central cyanosis despite free-flow oxygen.
- Technique—proper mask size and shape, tight seal between mask and face, proper head position, clear airway, and adequate inflation pressure, ventilation rate of 40 to 60 breaths per minute. If ventilation pressure is being monitored, PPV with an initial inflation pressure of 20 cm H_2O may be effective, but ≥30 to 40 cm H_2O may be required in some term babies without spontaneous ventilation.
- Assessment—increasing heart rate is the primary sign of effective ventilation. Also look for improving color, spontaneous respirations, and improving muscle tone. If the heart rate is not improving, chest wall movement should be assessed and sufficient ventilating pressure should be used to move the chest wall with each breath.

TABLE 148.4

NEONATAL RESUSCITATION SUPPLIES AND EQUIPMENT

Supplies and equipment by category

Suction equipment
  Bulb syringe
  Mechanical suction and tubing
  Suction catheters, 5F or 6F, 8F, and 10F or 12F
  8F feeding tube and 20-mL syringe
  Meconium aspiration device
Bag-and-mask equipment
  Neonatal resuscitation bag with a pressure-release valve
    or pressure manometer (the bag must be capable of
    delivering 90–100% oxygen)
  Face masks, newborn and premature sizes (cushioned
    rim preferred)
  Oxygen with flow meter (flow rate up to 10 L/min) and
    tubing (including portable oxygen cylinders)
Intubation equipment
  Laryngoscope with straight (Miller) blades, no. 0
    (preterm) and no. 1 (term)
  Extra bulbs and batteries for laryngoscope
  Endotracheal tubes: 2.5, 3.0, 3.5, and 4.0 mm internal
    diameter
  Stylet (optional)
  Scissors
  Tape or securing device for tracheal tube
  Alcohol sponges
  CO_2 detector (optional)
  Laryngeal mask airway (optional)
Medication
  Epinephrine 1:10,000 (0.1 mg/mL) 3-mL or 10-mL ampules
  Isotonic crystalloid (normal saline or Ringer's lactate) for
    volume expansion 100 or 250 mL

Sodium bicarbonate 4.2% (5 mEq/10 mL) 10-mL ampules
Naloxone hydrochloride 0.4 mg/mL 1-mL ampules or
    1.0 mg/mL 2-mL ampules
Normal saline, 30 mL
Dextrose 10%, 250 mL
Normal saline "fish" or "bullet" (optional)
Feeding tube, 5F (optional)
Umbilical vessel catheterization supplies
  Sterile gloves
  Scalpel or scissors
  Povidone-iodine solution
  Umbilical tape
  Umbilical catheters, 3.5F, 5F
  Three-way stopcock
Syringes, 1, 3, 5, 10, 20, and 50 mL
Needles, 25-, 21-, and 18-gauge, or puncture device for
  needdleless system
Miscellaneous
  Gloves and appropriate personal protection
  Radiant warmer or other heat source
  Firm, padded resuscitation surface
  Clock (timer optional)
  Warmed linens
  Stethoscope
  Tape, 1/2 or 3/4 inch
  Cardiac monitor and electrodes and/or pulse oximeter
    with probe (optional for delivery room)
  Oropharyngeal airways

■ Gastric decompression—if bag/mask ventilation is prolonged, an 8F orogastric tube should be inserted, aspirated, and left open as a vent to prevent gastric distension.

■ Special note: Flow-controlled pressure-limited mechanical devices (e.g., T-piece resuscitators) are recognized as an acceptable method of administering positive-pressure ventilation during newborn resuscitation; however, self-inflating and flow-inflating bags remain the preferred method for prolonged resuscitation.

Endotracheal Tube (ET) Ventilation

See also "Endotracheal Intubation in Neonates" later in the chapter.

■ Indications—failure to achieve adequate ventilation with bag/mask; prolonged resuscitation (especially if chest compressions are needed); very-low-birthweight infant; need for ventilation in a patient with contraindication to bag/mask ventilation (e.g., diaphragmatic hernia or abdominal wall defect).

■ Technique—ET tube size and length rules of thumb: ET size in mm (internal diameter) = estimated gestational age divided by 10; length in cm to insert ET ("tip to lip") = estimated weight in kg + 6; if less than 750 g, insert to 6 cm (Table 148.5). Ventilation rate is 40 to 60 breaths per minute, or 30 breaths per minute if chest compressions are being given.

■ Assessment—increasing heart rate is the primary sign of effective ventilation. Also look for improving color, spontaneous respirations, and improving muscle tone. Use of a CO_2 detector may facilitate confirmation of ET tube placement. If the heart rate is not improving, chest wall movement should be assessed and sufficient ventilating pressure should be used to move the chest wall with each breath. Also, check for equal breath sounds bilaterally (if absent, suspect intubation of the right mainstem bronchus).

Chest Compressions

■ Note: *Hypoventilation and hypoxia are by far the most common causes of bradycardia in newly born infants*, so almost all depressed infants can be revived by ventilation with oxygen.

■ Indication—heart rate less than 60 beats per minute after 30 seconds of *adequate* ventilation (good chest wall movement and breath sounds).

■ Technique—two-thumb, encircling-hands method is preferred if the infant's size permits; the depth of compression is one-third the anterior–posterior dimension of chest (should produce a palpable pulse).

■ Coordination with ventilations—3:1 ratio (i.e., 3 compressions followed by 1 ventilation) for a total of 120 "events" per minute (90 compressions and 30 ventilations).

Epinephrine

■ Indications—heart rate less than 60 beats per minute despite adequate ventilation and chest compressions for at least 30 seconds (earlier if no detectable heart rate).

■ Dose—IV: 0.1 to 0.3 mL/kg of 1:10,000 solution, drawn up in a 1-mL syringe. Endotracheal: 0.3 to 1.0 mL/kg of a

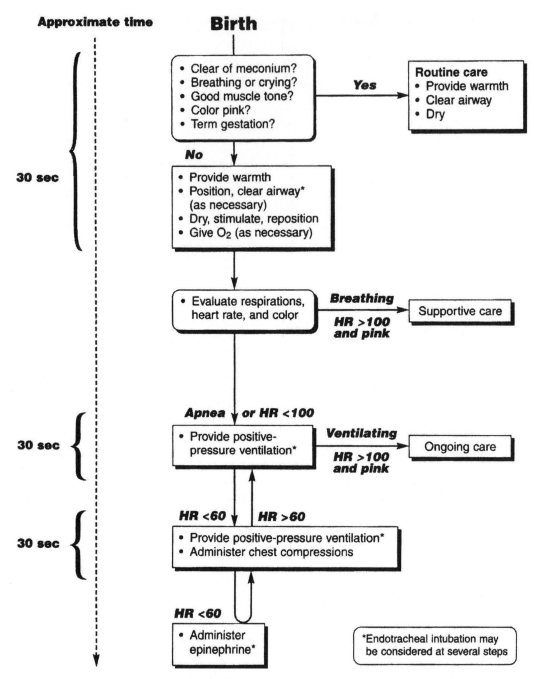

FIGURE 148.4. Algorithm for resuscitation of the newly born infant. (From American Academy of Pediatrics. *Textbook of neonatal resuscitation.* 4th ed. American Academy of Pediatrics and American Heart Association, The American Academy of Pediatrics, Elk Grove Village, Illinois 2000, with permission.)

1:10,000 solution, drawn up in a 3- or 5-mL syringe. Doses may be repeated every 3 to 5 minutes if heart rate is less than 60 beats per minute.
■ Route—initial dose or two may be given via the ET tube; subsequent doses, if needed, should be given IV. (See "Umbilical Vein Catheterization" later in the chapter.)

Volume Expanders

■ Indications—poor response to resuscitation; known or suspected acute blood loss; signs of shock (pallor, poor pulses, perfusion).
■ Dose—10 mL/kg of normal saline or Ringer solution over 5 to 10 minutes IV.

■ O-negative red blood cells if large-volume blood loss.
■ Repeat volume bolus may be indicated, but caution against inappropriate volume expansion especially in small, preterm infant.

Naloxone Hydrochloride

■ Not indicated during the initial steps of resuscitation, but may be given if there is continued respiratory depression *after* positive-pressure ventilation has restored a normal heart rate and color, *and* there is a history of maternal narcotic administration within the past 4 hours.
■ Dose—0.1 mg/kg with either the 0.4 mg/mL or 1.0 mg/mL solution.

- Route—IV preferred; can also be given IM but onset of action will be delayed.
- Patients who respond to naloxone hydrochloride must be monitored for recurrence of apnea (duration of action may be shorter than that of the depressant narcotic).
- Avoid in patients whose mothers are suspected of recent narcotic abuse (may precipitate acute withdrawal).

Bicarbonate

- *Not indicated* in routine neonatal resuscitation.
- May be detrimental because of hyperosmolarity and CO_2 production.
- Possible indication—prolonged resuscitation with *documented* metabolic acidosis after establishment of adequate ventilation and circulation.
- Dose is 1 to 2 mEq/kg of an 0.5-mEq/mL solution infused over at least 2 minutes.

MECONIUM-STAINED AMNIOTIC FLUID

If there is meconium staining of the amniotic fluid, the initial steps of resuscitation may be altered. Once the infant is delivered, the first priority becomes the determination of the need for endotracheal intubation and tracheal suctioning. This depends on whether or not the infant is vigorous. The vigorous infant is defined by NRP as one with good respiratory effort, good muscle tone, and heart rate greater than 100 beats per minute.

Vigorous meconium-stained infants do not require tracheal suctioning. These infants should be placed on radiant warmers and observed without drying or stimulation. Tracheal suctioning should be performed on these infants prior to positive-pressure ventilation if they subsequently develop apnea or respiratory distress.

Nonvigorous infants (i.e., those with poor respiratory effort, decreased muscle tone, or heart rate less than 100 beats per minute) should be intubated immediately. Suction should be applied directly to the ET, which is then slowly withdrawn to suction both the trachea and hypopharynx. Repeat the intubation-suction-withdrawal cycle until little or no meconium-stained secretions are obtained or until further resuscitation (i.e., PPV) is mandated by the infant's condition (e.g., heart rate less than 60 beats per minute). Once meconium is cleared, proceed with usual steps of resuscitation. After stabilization, an 8F orogastric tube may be inserted into the stomach to remove swallowed meconium.

SPECIAL CONSIDERATIONS

Certain congenital anomalies or conditions, often detected antenatally, may require a special approach at the time of delivery to achieve optimal response and minimize further compromise.

- Conditions associated with ventilatory compromise because of mass effect of fluid on the lung (e.g., hydrops, ascites) may require drainage of pleural and/or peritoneal fluid.
- Conditions associated with increased fluid losses and/or potential tissue injury (e.g., omphalocele, gastroschisis, meningomyelocele) require careful handling to protect vascular supply of extruded organs and sterile covering to minimize evaporative fluid and heat losses and decrease the risk of infection.
- Conditions in which bag/mask ventilation is contraindicated because it may result in gastrointestinal distension (e.g., diaphragmatic hernia, gastroschisis, omphalocele); *if*

ventilation is needed in these patients, endotracheal intubation should be performed immediately.
- Conditions in which bag/mask ventilation is likely to be ineffective(e.g., choanal atresia suggested by inability to pass a catheter through the nares)—*if ventilation is needed in these patients, endotracheal intubation should be performed immediately.*

EMERGENCY PROCEDURES

Umbilical Vein Catheterization

Placement of an umbilical venous catheter (UVC) is usually the quickest way to secure venous access. This may be necessary during the resuscitation procedure to give volume expanders or epinephrine.

- Identify the single umbilical vein on the cut surface of the umbilical cord (larger-caliber, thin-walled, and more flattened vessel compared with the two umbilical arteries).
- Fill a 3.5F or 5F single-lumen umbilical catheter with flush solution.
- Insert catheter tip just below skin level until blood returns easily with aspiration.
- Care must be taken to avoid air embolization.
- Remove UVC after the patient is stabilized and alternative vascular access is obtained.

Endotracheal Intubation in Neonates

Endotracheal intubation is most commonly indicated for tracheal suctioning of meconium-stained infants and for prolonged or difficult resuscitations when bag/mask PPV is inadequate. Additionally, intubation may be the preferred method of providing PPV, depending on the skill of the individual and the patient's circumstances (e.g., extremely low birthweight).

- Laryngoscope with a straight blade (Miller size 0 or 1).
- With the tip of the blade in the vallecula, gentle elevation reveals the glottic opening (gentle cricoid pressure may faciliate visualization).
- The tip of the appropriate size ET tube (Table 148.5) should be inserted 1 to 2 cm beyond the vocal cords.
- The appropriate depth of insertion of the ET tube from the level of the upper lip can be estimated by adding 6 cm to the infant's estimated weight in kilograms.
- After passing the ET tube, it should be held securely at the mouth while confirming proper placement by hearing breath sounds bilaterally in the axillae, not hearing breath sounds over the abdomen, and observing good chest wall movement with PPV.
- Tape to the skin above the upper lip.

FAILURE TO RESPOND TO RESUSCITATION

If the infant is not responding well, the following should be considered:

- Pneumothorax—confirm by transillumination if possible; can be relieved by needle aspiration or placement of a chest tube.
- Hemorrhagic shock—aggressive fluid resuscitation needed, possibly with "emergency release" (i.e., non–cross-matched) O-negative red blood cells.
- Error(s) in technique—insufficient ventilatory pressure, malposition of the facemask or ET tube, chest compressions too shallow.

TABLE 148.5

SUGGESTED ENDOTRACHEAL TUBE SIZE AND DEPTH OF INSERTION
ACCORDING TO WEIGHT AND GESTATIONAL AGE

Weight (g)	Gestational age (wks)	Tube size (mm) (ID)[a]	Depth of insertion from upper lip (cm)
<1,000	<28	2.5	6.5–7
1,000–2,000	28–34	3.0	7–8
2,000–3,000	34–38	3.0–3.5	8–9
<3,000	>38	3.5–4.0	>9

[a]ID indicates inner diameter.

■ Some infants cannot be resuscitated (e.g., pre-viable fetuses, lethal anomalies, prolonged severe intrauterine asphyxia)—see next section.

WHEN TO STOP, OR WHEN NOT TO START

■ Both mortality and serious morbidity rates are significantly increased in infants who remain asystolic after 10 minutes of resuscitation. The International Liaison Committee on Resuscitation (ILCOR) and the NRP therefore note that *after 10 minutes of continuous and adequate resuscitative efforts, discontinuation may be justified if there is no heartbeat and no respiratory effort.*

■ Certain conditions, often diagnosed antenatally or obvious postnatally, are either incompatible with survival or associated with extremely poor neurodevelopmental outcome. *Resuscitation may be considered futile therapy in infants with certain conditions* such as anencephaly, trisomy 13, trisomy 18, and extreme prematurity (generally defined as <23 weeks gestation or birthweight <400 g).

■ Some conditions are associated with uncertain prognosis, but borderline survival and high morbidity, and the anticipated burden to the child is high. Examples include prematurity <25 weeks gestation, hypoplastic left heart, diaphragmatic hernia, specific skeletal dysplasias, and holopros-encephaly. In such cases, ILCOR and NRP recommend that *parental desires concerning initiation of resuscitation should be supported.*

■ Finally, it is generally agreed that noninitiation of resuscitation and discontinuation of life-sustaining treatment during or after resuscitation are ethically equivalent. Put another way, initiation of resuscitation does not legally or ethically mandate continued support. Therefore, ILCOR

and NRP recommend that *clinicians should not hesitate to withdraw support when functional survival is highly unlikely.* This is particularly relevant in cases of questionable viability (e.g., extreme prematurity, severe lung hypoplasia). In such cases, additional information may be obtained by assessing the response to resuscitation or after the initial resuscitation (e.g., weighing an infant or obtaining blood gas analysis), which may confirm the suspicion of nonviability.

OUTCOME

■ More than 95% of term infants with a 5-minute Apgar score of 3 or less are developmentally normal.

■ Although the need for cardiac compressions and/or epinephrine in preterm infants is associated with a high mortality, it does not preclude a good neurodevelopmental outcome in survivors.

■ Overall, over 90% of newborns that require resuscitation in the delivery room can be expected to have normal outcomes.

Suggested Readings

American Academy of Pediatrics and the American Heart Association. *Neonatal resuscitation guidelines. Circulation* 2005;112:188–195.

Additional Resources

Neonatal Resuscitation Program (NRP) website at *www.aap.org/nrp. Textbook of neonatal resuscitation.* 5th ed. with DVD-ROM edited by K Tegtmeyer, DA Braner, LP Halamek, et al. Published by American Academy of Pediatrics Elk Grove Village, Illinois 2006 edited by J Kattwinkel.

CHAPTER 149 ■ IDENTIFICATION OF COMMON PSYCHOSOCIAL PROBLEMS AND MENTAL DISORDERS IN AN ACUTE HOSPITAL SETTING

RONALD M. PERKIN

Psychosocial dysfunction in children, first recognized more than 20 years ago as the "new morbidity" in pediatric practice, is now a leading cause of disability in children and adolescents (1). It is estimated that one of every five children and adolescents in the United States has a mental disorder; left untreated these disorders are often debilitating (2). However, the shortage of mental health providers, stigma attached to receiving mental health services, chronic underfunding of the public mental health system, decreased reimbursement to mental health providers, and disparate insurance benefits have contributed to the fact that only 2% of these children are seen by mental health specialists (3). In contrast, approximately 75% of children with psychiatric disturbances are seen in primary care settings, and half of pediatric office visits involve behavioral, psychosocial, or educational concerns.

Despite the growing prevalence of psychiatric illness in children, four out of five children with diagnosable behavioral and emotional problems are not identified by their pediatricians. Furthermore, children are more likely to be recognized and treated if their behavior upsets or annoys adults than if their psychiatric symptoms lead to school failure and poor functioning at home. Poor children are among the least likely to receive adequate mental health attention (2). Numerous studies have shown that untreated mental health problems result in high rates of medical services and place children at high risk for chronic psychosocial morbidity, including antisocial and self-injurious behavior.

There are compelling reasons to encourage an expanding role for pediatricians in the behavioral health care of their patients. All pediatricians and family physicians will have some role in recognizing and responding to mental health concerns that present in their offices or as patients in the acute care hospital (Table 149.1). Pediatric providers' early treatment of behavioral health disorders decreases the risk of long-term disability for children and adolescents (3,4).

Some obstacles to recognition by pediatricians are long-standing. Parents may be reluctant to raise psychosocial concerns, pediatricians may wish to avoid stigmatizing labels, pediatric training underemphasizes mental health and behavioral problems, and reimbursement for psychosocial services is low or unavailable for pediatricians.

Commitment to confronting the new morbidities of psychosocial problems is intrinsic to a pediatric hospitalist's identity. This section describes common psychiatric conditions that may present in an acute hospital admission and discusses approaches to identification, assessment of severity, and treatment planning. Within treatment planning are highlighted guidelines for consulting a pediatric psychopharmacologist, because medication is often an important feature of a comprehensive treatment plan.

TABLE 149.1

ROLE OF THE HOSPITALIST IN MANAGING MENTAL ILLNESS

- Maintain a high index of suspicion.
- Recognize signs of mental health problems.
- Undertake initial assessment.
- Determine diagnosis.
- Educate both patient and family.
- Provide initial management plan (or referral).
- Recognize the need for emergent intervention or urgent referral.
- Facilitate non-urgent referral when needed.
- Ensure short-term follow-up and coordination of care.
- Address family issues that result from the patient's illness, diagnosis, and treatment.

References

1. Cassidy LJ, Jellinek MS. Approaches to recognition and management of childhood psychiatric disorders in pediatric primary care. *Pediatr Clin North Am* 1998;45:1037–1051.
2. Kataoka SH, Zhang L, Wells KB. Unmet need for mental health care among U.S. children: variation by ethnicity and insurance status. *Am J Psychiatry* 2002;159:1548–1555.
3. Williams J, Klinepeter K, Palmes G, et al. Diagnosis and treatment of behavioral health disorders in pediatric practice. *Pediatrics* 2004;114:601–606.
4. Costello EJ, Patino T. The new morbidity: who should treat it? *J Dev Behav Pediatr* 1987;8:288–291.

CHAPTER 150 ■ ASSESSING PSYCHOSOCIAL RISK FOR CHILDREN AND FAMILIES DURING HOSPITAL ADMISSION

MICHAEL E. REICHEL

Pediatric admissions provide clinicians and hospital staff unique opportunities for diagnosis, treatment, and compassionate care, to be integrated with discharge and follow-up by a designated medical home. Much information is generated during typically limited or brief lengths of stay, both by data collection and observation.

Astute clinicians and staff often glimpse dramatic and powerful portraits of family function, psychosocial stressors, the presence or absence of support networks, and elements of ongoing health or psychosocial risk. Databases unique to nursing, social work, and child life services further enhance our understanding and should be effectively shared rather than merely compartmentalized in the chart or electronic medical record.

The experience of inpatient care, when linked to psychosocial information provided or needed by the medical home, can foster better integration of care during the hospital stay and at and beyond discharge.

This applies to each and every hospitalization, whether for an acute or chronic illness. It is an essential feature of family-centered care, in which the context of the admission must be connected to the unique features of each child and family served.

This chapter emphasizes an approach to recognizing psychosocial factors in the inpatient setting, factors that impact both risk and resilience in children and families, factors that may go undetected in other circumstances. It echoes statements by the American Academy of Pediatrics Committee on Psychosocial Aspects of Child and Family Health, that recognition of such factors can and should guide us in all pediatric care.

Key features of psychosocial risk assessment will be reviewed briefly. Some protective factors will be mentioned also, although much needs to be learned, because the traditional attention of clinicians and researchers emphasized the diagnosis and management of pathologies or deficits. There is a rich emerging literature on resilience that can only be referenced in this chapter.

PSYCHOSOCIAL PERSPECTIVES

Erik Erikson first proposed that psychosocial development occurs across the life cycle, with particular stages defining tasks for mastery by infants, toddlers, older children, and adolescents. Drs. Robert J. Haggerty, Stanford B. Friedman, Morris M. Green, T. Berry Brazelton, William B. Carey, Melvin D. Levine, and William Lord Coleman made major contributions in pediatrics by incorporating psychosocial perspectives into the very framework of pediatric care. Wildman and Stancin, in a recent text, have synthesized important work on treating psychosocial problems in primary care, with particular emphasis on barriers to identification and to collaboration between disciplines.

Our understanding of psychosocial development continues to evolve, shaped by contributions from Stanley Greenspan (functional emotional capacities), Allan Schore, Daniel Siegel, and others who have marshaled the explosion of knowledge generated by advances in genetics and neurobiology.

The term *psychosocial* is used to refer to the psychological and social factors that influence mental and physical health. In childhood, healthy psychosocial development encompasses how a child experiences, collects, and integrates their caregiving, attachment, and relationship experiences into behaviors that foster connectedness to others, emotional self-regulation, healthy adaptation and self-care, a sense of personal identity, and the successful emergence of learning and social skills.

PSYCHOSOCIAL PROBLEMS: "THE NEW MORBIDITY"

Since Haggerty first coined this term, a broad range of emotional, cognitive, and behavioral problems that emerge in childhood are now addressed by pediatric and mental health professionals. There is a growing trend for such professionals to be co-located or to work collaboratively; such teamwork may be needed during or beyond specific hospitalizations in which psychosocial problems are identified as causing extreme stress or impairment. Perhaps 20 percent of children in the United States experience such problems, including child maltreatment, substance abuse, attention deficit hyperactivity disorder, mood and anxiety disorders, various learning and behavior problems, and the many stresses that can be associated with adaptation to chronic illness.

Many of these problems often go unrecognized in primary care settings, and because diagnosable mental disorders can emerge from combinations of risk factors and stressors, it is important to use the hospital experience as an opportunity to identify and begin to address these issues. For those families in which risks are already identified, the admission can reinforce coping skills and perhaps even enhance existing support networks.

PSYCHOSOCIAL RISK FACTORS

Commonly accepted risk factors are listed in Table 150.1. The presence of one or more of these factors, however, although

TABLE 150.1

PSYCHOSOCIAL RISK FACTORS

Parental psychopathology or absence
Family conflict, including domestic violence
Premature birth
Prenatal drug and alcohol exposure
Parental substance abuse
Poverty
Child maltreatment, including neglect and emotional abuse
Unstable caretaking
Change in family circumstance, including parental separation, divorce, unemployment or
    homelessness
The presence of chronic illness in one or more family members or important caregivers
Death of an important attachment figure or caregiver
Genetic factors that may predispose to illness or to emotional, cognitive, or behavioral difficulties

enhancing risk of a psychosocial disorder, does not inevitably lead to the development of a specific condition.

All of these categories of risk factors may function as stressful life events, resulting in adversity and maladaptive or disruptive behaviors, and over time may result in or further intensify psychosocial problems, leading to the emergence of childhood emotional or behavioral disorders.

PROTECTIVE FACTORS

Fortunately, many children and families benefit from a variety of protective factors, which seem to foster healthier adaptation and promote resilience. These are resources, whether individual or environmental, that appear to minimize the impact of risk by acting as a "buffering agent to risk exposure." Protective factors are listed in Table 150.2.

USING THE HOSPITAL ADMISSION TO ASSESS FOR PSYCHOSOCIAL RISK

The hospitalization of any infant, child, or adolescent, whether for an acute or chronic illness, is a major stressor for any patient and family. Pediatrics has devoted much thought, energy, and effort into minimizing these stresses over many decades, especially in collaboration with other hospital-based professionals and services.

Valuable opportunities to understand and to aid individual children and their families also exist if organized attention to psychosocial function and risk are addressed during each admission as well.

In primary care settings, many clinical tools are currently used to screen children for developmental progress or identify

TABLE 150.2

PROTECTIVE FACTORS

PROTECTIVE ENVIRONMENTAL FACTORS
    Opportunities for education, employment, and other prosocial activities
    Caring relationships with adults or extended family members
    Social supports from non-family members

PROTECTIVE INTERPERSONAL AND SOCIAL FACTORS
    Attachment to parents
    Caring relationships with siblings
    Low parental conflict
    High levels of commitment to school
    Involvement in conventional activities
    Belief in pro-social norms and values

PROTECTIVE INDIVIDUAL FACTORS
    Social and problem-solving skills
    Positive attitude
    Temperament
    High intelligence
    Low childhood stress

From Jenson JM, Fraser MW. *Social policy for children and families: a risk and resilience perspective.* p. 9.
Copyright 2006 by Sage Publications. Reprinted by Permission of Sage Publications, Inc.

delays, learning or behavior problems, or affective disorders. In a demanding inpatient setting, selective use of brief screening instruments, such as PEDS, the PSC 17 (Pediatric Symptom Checklist), and Family Psychosocial Screening, could be incorporated into an admission database.

Using approaches advocated by Bright Futures or Healthy Steps, it is possible to emphasize the use of open-ended questions and supportive interviewing techniques at some time during the inpatient stay, based on refining the information taken during a standard admission history. Wissow, among others, has studied how residents communicate and encourage or discourage caregivers from seeking help about psychosocial issues.

If such approaches are incorporated into inpatient routines, valuable opportunities for addressing psychosocial concerns can be adopted and linked to the medical home. Variations of this approach usually dominate the care of children who are followed by specialty teams for chronic conditions.

It is time to recognize how generalists, hospitalists, primary care attendings, and residents can emphasize these important aspects of psychosocial care in a more opportunistic way during pediatric inpatient care.

FRAMING YOUR QUESTIONS

Using open-ended questions facilitates more reflective parental (and child) answers; rather than itemizing information only in a "yes" or "no" format, begin as many questions with "why," "how," or "what."

Try to gauge how the family has experienced any recent changes in circumstances over time, by targeting functioning before the illness/admission: "How are things going at home?" "Tell me about any major changes or stresses in your family." Extend this line of inquiry into the past few weeks, and then months, and then perhaps into recent years if needed.

Use affirming questions first, which allow the respondent to tell you how well they feel about a child or themselves: "What makes you most proud of Joey?" "How does Sheila tell you how she feels?"

Barry and Pamela Zuckerman provide a useful list of questions for parental self-reflection, based on the excellent work of Daniel Siegel. Perhaps some of these questions can be used during an admission, especially if there is an ongoing relationship between the clinician and family. An example: "How has your childhood shaped the ways in which you relate to your children?"

It is important to look for evidence of possible protective factors, which may foster resilience, self-esteem, and problem solving in the family. The presence of at least one caring adult who demonstrates acceptance, support, and (ideally) unconditional love for a particular child or family unit is a very positive influence unfortunately lacking in many families. Although kinship care by one or more grandparents is increasingly prevalent, some three-generational households that include adolescent mothers may in fact be associated with less successful coping, if the young mother in essence is allowed to abdicate her parenting responsibilities completely.

CONCLUSIONS

Much outpatient care remains fragmented despite advances in management and care offered in medical homes. When a child is hospitalized, the recognition of such fragmentation, or even of the absence of a fully functioning medical home, is a responsibility the inpatient staff should address with every bit as much dedication as they devote to detailed medical management. Although the stresses and demands of inpatient care extend to attendings, residents, and other hospital staff, an important opportunity exists during inpatient care to redirect attention to comprehensive strategies necessary to provide family-focused care in all settings.

By refining databases to incorporate psychosocial risk assessment, those who provide inpatient hospital care will generate quality service commitments to children and families that can and should extend far beyond a particular hospital admission.

SCREENING TOOLS

Parents' Evaluation of Developmental Status (PEDS) 1997 Birth–9 years (www.pedstest.com)	10 items/ 2 minutes	$30.00
Pediatric Symptom Checklist: *PSC 17* 1999 5 years–adolescence www.ocs.ccri.ws/PS-17.asp	17 items/ 5 minutes	No cost
Family Psychosocial Screening 1996 www.pedstest.com	2 pages 15 minutes (if with interview)	Cost/test $4.40

Online Resources

www.brightfutures.org (Pocket Guide, xiv–xviii, examples of Framing Questions; Mental Health Toolkit)

Suggested Readings

American Academy of Pediatrics Committee on Psychosocial Aspects of Child and Family Health. The new morbidity revisited: a renewed commitment to the psychosocial aspects of pediatric care. *Pediatrics* 2001;108;1227–1230. (*www.pediatrics.org/cgi/content/full/108/5/1227*)

Black MM, Papas MA, Hussey JM, et al. Behavior and development of preschool children born to adolescent mothers: risk and 3-generation households. *Pediatrics* 2002;109;573–580.

Borowsky IW, Mozoyeny S, Ireland M. Brief psychosocial screening at health supervision and acute care visits. *Pediatrics* 2003;112:129–133.

Greenspan SI, Wieder S. *Infant and early childhood mental health.* Arlington, VA: American Psychiatric Publishing; 2006.

Haggerty RJ, Sherrod LR, Garmezy N, et al. *Stress, risk, and resilience in children and adolescents: process, mechanisms, and interventions.* Cambridge, UK: Cambridge University Press; 1996.

Parker S, Zuckerman B, Augustyn M. *Developmental and behavioral pediatrics: a handbook for primary care.* 2nd ed. Philadelphia: Lippincott Williams & Wilkins; 2005.

Schore AN. *Affect regulation and the origin of the self. The neurobiology of emotional development.* Hillsdale, NJ: Erlbaum; 1994.

Siegel DJ. *The developing mind.* New York: Guilford Press; 1999.

Wildman BG, Stancin T. *Treating children's psychosocial problems in primary care.* Greenwich, CT: Information Age Publishing; 2004.

Wissow LS, Larson S, Anderson J, et al. Pediatric residents' responses that discourage discussion of psychosocial problems in primary care. *Pediatrics* 2005;115:1569–1578.

CHAPTER 151A ■ AGITATION/ AGGRESSION/DELIRIUM

RONALD M. PERKIN

AGITATION AND AGGRESSION

Agitation and aggression are not diagnostic terms but rather describe specific sets of symptoms or behaviors associated with myriad psychiatric and medical conditions. *Agitation* is a state of increased mental and motor activity that may present as loud and angry speech, pacing, increased muscle tension, increased autonomic arousal such as diaphoresis and tachycardia, or hostile/irritable affect (1). *Aggression* is defined as any behavior with physical and/or verbal components in which physical harm to others, self, or property would result if the behavior were carried to its completion (1). Aggression has also been defined as a domineering, forceful, or assaultive verbal or physical action toward another person or the motor component of the affects of anger, hostility, or rage.

Behavioral instability may occur in patients with an organic psychiatric disorder, medical illness, as an adverse effect of a medication, or as a result of sensory/communication difficulty. Agitation and aggression may occur separately or in combination. When aggression occurs alone, it is usually considered by medical and nursing staff as a *volitional act* in response to physical, verbal, or psychological stimuli. In fact, such behaviors are often not volitional or intended acts to threaten or cause harm. Aggressive behaviors or responses may occur in patients with preexisting psychiatric conditions, specifically in conduct disorder, oppositional defiant disorder, attention-deficit/hyperactivity disorder, depression, bipolar disorder, psychotic disorders, and pervasive developmental disorders; or they may occur in patients with no premorbid psychiatric history. There are many instances in which agitation and/or aggressive behavior is unrelated to a previous psychiatric condition but rather is a result of an acute medical or physical insult (e.g., brain injury, metabolic or toxic delirium). Therefore, it would follow that the combination of underlying psychiatric condition and medical factors would lead to considerably higher rates of agitation and aggression in medically ill pediatric patients.

The most critical step in treating agitation or aggression is determining the cause of the underlying behavioral symptoms. This is best accomplished with medical, nursing, and psychiatric staff in collaboration and includes review of psychiatric history, assessment of pain, evaluation of substance intoxication or withdrawal, medication interactions or side effects, metabolic abnormalities, sleep deprivation, hypoxia, sepsis, and response to trauma or an acute or chronic medical illness. All such factors may be associated with behavioral instability in medically ill patients and must be fully explored to determine effective intervention.

Initial treatment strategies include treating any underlying psychiatric conditions and medical symptoms associated with the primary disease state. Creating a safe, calming, and nonthreatening environment is essential. Explanation to family members of the cause and treatments for these behaviors may help alleviate their anxiety, ultimately calming the patient. It may be helpful or necessary to have someone to deal with the patient one-to-one during very difficult periods. Providing frequent reassurance, continually reorienting the disoriented patient, and taking measures to maintain normal sleep–wake cycles all may help prevent or minimize behaviorally instability.

In some cases, physical restraints may be required, particularly in cases of delirium. There are strict guidelines and state regulations mandating the manner in which physical restraints may be used (2).

Restraints have been broadly defined as any methods or devices used to restrict a person's freedom of movement, physical activity, or normal access to his body. In the clinical setting, the term *physical restraint* refers to a variety of methods of limiting a patient's movement by holding the patient, either manually or with a variety of devices that restrict the patient physically. These devices include cloth cuffs binding the wrists and/or ankles to a gurney, torso restraints, and in some cases, in older or infirm patients, bedrails. The term "physical restraint" does not apply to mechanisms that are customarily used during transport or during diagnostic or surgical procedures. *Chemical restraint* is the term applied when a medication that is not a standard treatment for the patient's medical or psychiatric condition is used to control behavior or to restrict the patient's freedom of movement. Thus, chemical restraint does not apply to the administration of a psychoactive drug to treat a patient for mental illness, only to the emergency use of a drug to control a patient's behavior.

Several drug classes need to be considered when treating aggression in children and adolescents. These include mood stabilizers, stimulants, beta-blockers, α-antagonists, antihistamines, benzodiazepines, and typical and atypical antipsychotic. Although there is a robust literature on the use of these agents in the adult population, far less evidence-based literature exists for children and adolescents.

Although the mood stabilizers, stimulants, beta-blockers, and α-antagonists may be effective in the treatment of aggression due to underlying psychiatric conditions, they have little use in the acute treatment of behavioral instability associated with acute medical disorders because they do not achieve the primary goal of rapid behavioral stabilization with minimal interference in patient autonomy, cognitive functioning, and underlying medical condition. The primary agents to achieve this balance include antihistamines, benzodiazepines, and antipsychotic agents.

Diphenhydramine and hydroxyzine are frequently used in the treatment of acute agitation in children and adolescents in psychiatric inpatient units. Their flexible route of administration (oral, intravenous, intramuscular) rapid sedative effects, and generally low side-effect profile make them an appropriate choice for treatment of behavioral instability in medically ill pediatric patients. The major potential problems with their use in medically ill children involve significant anticholinergic effects. Constipation, exacerbation of delirium, diminished cognition, cardiac conduction abnormalities, and exacerbation of reactive airway disease are potential side effects that should be considered when choosing these agents.

Benzodiazepines are used in many medical and psychiatric conditions including mood stabilization, treatment of anxiety, sedation, and treatment of withdrawal from alcohol or benzodiazepines in individuals dependent on them. Choice of agent is typically made based on rapidity of onset, length of half-life, and method of metabolism to achieve clinical effect while minimizing side effects.

Although these agents are generally safe, several clinical caveats should be kept in mind with their use. Paradoxical agitation has been described in some children treated with benzodiazepines (1). When used for longer durations, habituation to and physiologic dependence on any of the benzodiazepines may occur. Signs and symptoms of benzodiazepine withdrawal include elevated temperature, increased heart rate and blood pressure, tremor, agitation, delirium, and seizure. It is therefore vital to minimize the potential for withdrawal, particularly in medically ill patients in whom these symptoms may hinder treatment or be confused with symptoms from the primary medical condition. To minimize withdrawal effects, gradual tapering by 10% to 25% every 7 days is recommended when benzodiazepines are used for 2 or more weeks (3). It should be noted that midazolam, a very short-acting benzodiazepine used for conscious sedation, has been associated with paradoxical agitation and withdrawal. Diazepam, although available in intramuscular form, is absorbed erratically from the muscle belly, resulting in unpredictable blood levels and should not be given by this method. Although respiratory failure is unlikely when benzodiazepines are used alone, even in overdose, profound respiratory compromise can occur in conjunction with other sedatives or in patients with preexisting respiratory conditions such as reactive airway disease or sleep apnea (3).

Antipsychotics generally are the mainstay of treatment for behavior instability in both medical and psychiatric emergency settings. As with all pharmacologic interventions, the agent of choice depends on clinical effectiveness, side-effect profile, and flexibility of dosing route. There is often some hesitancy to use antipsychotic agents in children without psychotic symptoms. Families and physicians are often resistant when the use of such medications is suggested. The simple reassurance to family members and medical staff that these are safe and effective agents used for many reasons other than psychosis, and that using them does not imply that a child is "crazy," can facilitate appropriate medical care.

All agents may have potential short-term side effects including extrapryamidal symptoms, neuroleptic malignant syndrome, and lowering of seizure threshold. There is also considerable concern associated with potential prolongation of the QTc interval with resulting cardiac arrhythmias including torsade de pointes. Most antipsychotics, typical and atypical, can prolong the QTc interval.

Dystonic reactions occur acutely in 2% to 10% of patients receiving antipsychotic medication. Dystonia is a neurologic condition characterized by slow, tonic, sustained muscle contractions. It commonly involves the tongue, eyes, jaws, neck, and occasionally the entire body. It is more common with the high-potency typical agents (e.g., haloperidol); however, it has been described with all antipsychotics, typical and atypical. This condition is experienced as both painful and frightening to patients and, in the case of laryngeal dystonia, can be potentially life threatening. A dystonic reaction can be treated acutely with diphenhydramine.

Chlorpromazine was the first antipsychotic developed. Because of its history, there is some stigma associated with its use, particularly in children. However, given its longevity, there is significant clinical experience with this agent. It is indicated for the treatment of psychosis, nausea and vomiting, presurgical anxiety and apprehension, intractable hiccups, and behavioral disturbance and aggression in children as young as 1 year old.

Haloperidol is a commonly used agent in all settings for acute agitation and/or aggression. It has a rapid onset, flexible dosing routes (oral, intramuscular, and intravenous), and a relatively low side-effect profile. There is some concern with the presence of increased risk of torsades de pointes with the use of haloperidol intravenously, but this is extremely uncommon. Of the atypical antipsychotics available, only risperidone has a clinical history of use in children with agitation, aggression, or delirium. It is available in an orally dissolvable form as well as a liquid concentrate.

DELIRIUM

Delirium is primarily a disturbance of consciousness. It is characterized by a reduced awareness of the environment with a reduced ability to focus, sustain, and shift attention. Changes in cognition, such as memory deficits, disorientation, and language disturbance, and hallucinations and delusions may also be present (4). In addition, abnormalities of psychomotor behavior may be a core symptom of delirium. Delirium is characterized by an acute onset and fluctuating course (5).

The clinical signs of delirium show considerable variation in children and adults. Although the presentation in older children may be the same as that seen in adults, in young children, the child's age and developmental stage may influence the clinical picture. Formal psychiatric assessment, including the assessment of orientation in time and place, memory deficits, and language difficulties, may not be possible in young children, and for this reason, observed behavior and caretaker information are important. Psychomotor retardation or agitation, anxiety, difficulty getting the child's attention, and regression with loss of previously acquired skills may be evidence of delirium. An acute onset of symptoms and the fact that the child may be inconsolable support the diagnosis of delirium. The caretakers' opinion is important because caretakers may more readily recognize abnormal behavior in the child.

Delirium appears as a consequence of an illness or its treatment (5). Therefore, delirium as a syndrome may have many etiologies. In children, infections and medication use are the most frequent causes. Pediatric patients are also especially vulnerable to toxic, metabolic, or traumatic central nervous system insults and are at greater risk of delirium with fever regardless of the etiology.

It is wise, however, to realize that often not one single factor but multiple factors contribute to the etiology, such as somatic disorder(s), prescribed medication, and/or medication withdrawal effects. The differential diagnosis of delirium includes regressive states and oppositional behavior due to acute stress, adjustment disorder, dissociative and/or conversion disorder with or without regression, and childhood psychosis.

The diagnosis of delirium in severely ill children, especially in a PICU setting, is usually obvious, although it may be difficult to differentiate delirium from a primary psychiatric diagnosis. Generally, an acute serious general medical condition takes precedence over a primary psychiatric condition. Moreover, one explanation for multiple simultaneous disorders is more likely than simultaneous multiple explanations. Thus, in young children, delirium is more likely to be a consequence of somatic disease than due to the simultaneous occurrence of an unrelated primary psychiatric disorder. More specifically, it has been suggested that the presence of subtle higher cortical disturbances occurring during regression, such as dyspraxia or dysphasia, is more likely to be due to organic disease than due to acute emotional distress. Also, the acute onset of incoherent speech is usually organic in origin. Disorders of consciousness are always suggestive of an organic origin, especially when there are simultaneous higher cortical dysfunctions or other neurologic signs and symptoms.

Medical staff members may interpret the distress with delirium as an indication of inadequate analgesic coverage. The patient is frequently given a variety of medications, including opioids and benzodiazepines, in efforts to comfort them. These drugs, however, may be inappropriate treatment for a misdiagnosis of delirium (5). In addition, doses of these drugs are increased when there is already evidence that the patient is overmedicated and the patient's mental status is deteriorating.

Delirium is aggravated by many factors common to the hospital environment: social isolation, immobilization, unfamiliar surroundings, excessive noise, constant monotonous sensory stimulation, and the lack of diurnal light variation.

Sleep deprivation, including a reduction in rapid eye movement sleep, may be a consequence of a stay in the ICU and lead to cognitive and perceptual changes including disorientation, poor concentration, and visual hallucinations. When determining the etiology of delirium, however, nothing is more important than the medical diagnosis and the severity of the illness.

The occurrence of acute psychiatric symptoms and behavioral disturbances in severely ill young children should be considered due to delirium until proven otherwise. Delirium should be considered if there is regression to earlier stages of development, chaotic behavior, anxiety, and moaning in severely ill children.

Delirium in children should be treated actively and not conservatively for several reasons. First, it is important to control psychomotor agitation to prevent the child from harming herself, for example, by extubating herself, disconnecting lines, and falling out of bed. Moreover, reducing the stress associated with delirium improves recovery from the somatic disorder. The prognostic impact of delirium in children is not known, but one study suggests that delirium is related to a longer hospital stay and a higher mortality (6). Last, because delirium is a disturbing and frightening experience for both the child and caretakers, treating delirium restores quality of life and may reduce the incidence of posttraumatic stress.

Treatment of delirium in young children consists of both psychosocial and pharmacologic interventions. Psychosocial interventions are directed at restoring orientation and comfort. For example, psychoeducation for the family, the presence of a family member, bringing in favorite toys and picture of the home and family, and restoration of the usual day and night rhythm.

Many authors consider haloperidol as the pharmacologic treatment of choice (5). Resperidone has also been suggested for use in children older than 4 years. There are no prospective or retrospective studies on the administration of neuroleptics for the treatment of delirium in children or adolescents, and the U.S. Food and Drug Administration did not identify these or any other medications as appropriate treatments for delirium (5). However, there is wide clinical experience with haloperidol use in children and low doses are not associated with extrapyramidal or other side effects (4). Suggested dosages for children younger than 4 years of age are 0.25 mg slowly intravenously over 30 to 45 minutes as a loading dose and 0.05 to 0.5 mg/kg/ 24 hr intravenously as a continuing dose.

Because of the serious impact of delirium on prognosis as well as the disruptive nature of the delirium, it should be considered a child psychiatric emergency and treated accordingly. This child psychiatric emergency often goes unrecognized and is undertreated; the complex combination of a serious illness and polypharmacy in a young child often results in reluctance and a delayed decision to add yet another medication to treat the delirium.

CHAPTER 151B ■ PSYCHOSIS

JENIFER L. POWELL AND ROBERT R. SHELTON

The term *psychosis* refers not to a particular mental health disorder, but rather to the presence of any of a set of symptoms, which generally include perceptual experiences or beliefs that are not based in reality and grossly disorganized thought, speech, or behavior (7,8). Psychotic symptoms are relatively rare among children and adolescents when compared either to other mental health symptoms displayed by children and adolescents or to rates of psychotic symptoms seen among adults. Within the acute medical hospital setting, psychotic symptoms displayed by children and adolescents can be particularly upsetting both for families and hospital staff. Familiarity with these symptoms and with the wide variety of factors that can potentially contribute to their development is important for appropriate identification, assessment, consultation, and management.

PSYCHOTIC SYMPTOMS AMONG CHILDREN AND ADOLESCENTS

Hallucinations

Hallucinations are sensory perceptions that are not based in reality or associated with observable environmental stimuli (9–11). In general, hallucinations among children younger than 6 or 7 are considered very rare, with frequency increasing over the course of child and adolescent development (9). As with adults, children and adolescents may experience auditory, visual, tactile, or olfactory hallucinations (8–13). Hallucinations must be differentiated from a variety of normative developmental phenomena, including pretend play, imaginary companions, fantasy, and vivid sensory imagery (8,11). Hallucinations that occur solely when awakening (hypnopompic hallucinations) or when falling asleep (hypnagogic hallucinations), are not considered psychotic symptoms because they are relatively common among normal children and adolescents, particularly under conditions of sleep deprivation (7,14).

The presence of hallucinations among infants and toddlers is extremely difficult to establish given developmental limitations in their expressive language (8). At best, hallucinations could be hypothesized from observations of strange or unusual behaviors in which the child appears to be responding to something in the environment but in which no actual external stimuli can be identified.

When assessing preschool and younger school-age children, differentiation of hallucinations from normative developmental phenomena and internal experiences, such as dreams and thoughts, can be particularly challenging (8).

Pretend play, fantasy characters, personified objects, and imaginary companions all are quite common among younger children. Also, normative limitations in cognitive and expressive language skills can make it difficult for adults to clearly determine the nature of a younger child's experience (8,15). Hallucinations reported among children in this age group are most often visual or tactile (8,10).

In comparison to younger children, school-age children are better able to verbally describe the nature of their experiences. They may describe auditory hallucinations in addition to those in other sensory modalities. In comparison to adolescents or adults, school-age children tend to report hallucinations that are more concrete and that often reflect themes of interest or concern at their developmental level, such as monsters, fantasy figures, family members, pets, animals, and toys (8,9,16). Visual hallucinations described by children of this age often include monsters, ghosts, menacing animals or figures, and more general shapes, scenes, or people (9,12). Auditory hallucinations occasionally are reported as sounds, but most often are reported to be one or more voices. These voices may be heard either inside or outside the child's head, but typically are identified as someone else's voice (17). Similar to adults, a school-age child's auditory hallucinations may include mumbling voices, voices conversing with each other, voices commenting on her activities, voices that criticize, threaten, or tease her (i.e., persecutory hallucinations), or voices telling her to hurt herself, harm others, or to do other "bad things" (i.e., command hallucinations) (8,9,17). Occasionally, children have reported benign, positive, or protective voices (9,17). In comparison to adolescents and adults, the messages from voices heard by school-age children tend to be more simple and vague, often including only brief phrases or sentences (12).

The hallucinations described by adolescents are generally quite similar to those reported by adults (8). In comparison to younger children, adolescents tend to report hallucinations that are less concrete, more complex, more detailed, and more vivid (9,16). Content of hallucinations is generally less tied to childhood interests.

Delusions

Delusions are false or bizarre beliefs or belief systems held with complete conviction and resistant to change in the face of logic or contradictory experience or evidence (7,9). These beliefs are not consistent with the beliefs of others with similar social, cultural, or religious backgrounds. Delusions usually are not described among children younger than school age (8). The expressive language limitations of younger children would likely impede clear communication of delusions. Also, delusions would be difficult to distinguish from normative preschool cognitive processes, such as magical thinking, problems with perspective-taking, attribution of life and intentions to inanimate objects, and difficulties distinguishing between appearances and reality (8).

Delusional beliefs among school-age children can involve many themes similar to those seen among adolescents and adults, including delusions that are persecutory, somatic, grandiose, religious, referential, or bizarre (9,12,16). Children with persecutory delusions may believe that others are spying on them, tricking them, or have some other malicious intent toward them. Somatic delusions have themes involving sensations or functions of the body. A child with grandiose delusions may believe that he has a great, unrecognized talent or special purpose. Religious delusions focus on themes such as having a special religious purpose or message from a deity. Referential delusions or "ideas of reference" are those in which children believe that things in the environment such as certain gestures, media messages, or random events have special meaning and are specifically directed towards them. Bizarre delusions are those that are judged to be impossible, such as having one's thoughts or actions controlled by an outside force (7).

Compared to adolescents and adults, school-age children tend to have delusions that are simpler, more concrete, and less organized (8,9,16). As with hallucinations, the delusions of school-age children often have content focused on themes of interest or concern to them, including parents, monsters, animals, fantasy figures, or aspects of identity (8,12,16). Adolescents tend to have delusions that are more systematic, elaborate, and abstract than those of younger children but less detailed, complex, and systematic than those of adults (8,9,12).

Formal Thought Disorder/ Disorganized Speech

Formal thought disorder refers to abnormalities in the manner of presentation, organization, control, or processing of thoughts (9). Rather than emphasizing all of the possible signs of disordered thought, the DSM-IV-TR focuses primarily on a few aspects of *disorganized speech* as characteristic of psychotic thinking, noting that these features are the most easily defined and observed (7). These aspects of disorganized speech include (1) *derailment* or *loose associations*, patterns of speech in which the speaker changes the "track" of the topic under discussion, switches to another topic that may be vaguely related or unrelated, does not prepare the listener for the change, and may not return to the original topic; (2) *tangentiality*, answering a question with information that is unrelated or only distantly related; and (3) *incoherence*, a pattern of speech that is so disorganized that it is sometimes incomprehensible (7). The DSM-IV-TR emphasizes that speech disorganization must significantly impede effective communication in order to be considered psychotic (7). Researchers who study formal thought disorder in children often use definitions that include illogical thinking in addition to the aspects of disorganized speech included in the DSM-IV-TR definition (9).

Disorganized speech or formal thought disorder usually cannot be distinguished from the normal cognitive and communication processes of preschool and early school-age children (8,9). However, by age 7, frequencies of loose associations decrease significantly, and rates of illogical thinking decrease somewhat in the speech of typically developing children (8,9). Thus, in older children, formal thought disorder usually can be reliably distinguished from normal cognitive processes and speech by the presence of incoherence, loose associations, or high rates of illogical thinking (9,16). Signs of formal thought disorder or disorganized speech typically are similar among psychotic adolescents and adults (8).

Grossly Disorganized Behavior

Grossly disorganized behavior may include a variety of maladaptive behaviors that are qualitatively different from those of typical children or adolescents of that age and developmental level from similar social, religious, or cultural backgrounds. Grossly disorganized behavior can include severe problems in goal-directed behavior, significant difficulties participating in age-appropriate activities of daily living, extreme and unpredictable agitation, and catatonic behaviors (7). Catatonic symptoms include an extreme decrease in responsiveness to the environment, assuming rigid and unmovable or bizarre and inappropriate body postures, or displaying very high levels of purposeless motor activity (7). Even among children and adolescents with primary psychotic disorders, rates of catatonic behaviors appear to be fairly low (14).

ETIOLOGY/DIFFERENTIAL DIAGNOSIS

Psychotic symptoms among children and adolescents are not indicative, in and of themselves, of a particular psychiatric or organic disorder. Instead, a wide variety of potential etiologic factors should be considered. Experts generally recommend investigating and ruling out potential organic etiologies of psychotic symptoms, including general medical conditions, substance abuse, and effects associated with medications (8,10,12,13,15,16,18). The pediatric hospitalist should have particularly strong suspicion of an organic etiology if psychotic symptoms emerge for the first time during an admission for treatment of a general medical condition. Because presentation of primary psychotic disorders before later adolescence is atypical, younger age alone is a reason to weigh potential organic etiologies more strongly within the differential diagnosis (7,19). Children and adolescents who experience visual or tactile hallucinations also are more likely to have an organic source for their symptoms, particularly if they are not also experiencing auditory hallucinations. Organic etiologies also should be strongly considered for children and adolescents with unremarkable psychosocial histories and previously normal development. Although evaluating the most dangerous potential organic etiologies is a priority, the pediatric hospitalist and appropriate consultants often can simultaneously begin the process of exploring potential nonorganic sources of psychotic symptoms.

General Medical Conditions

Table 151.1 summarizes medical conditions that have been associated with the development of psychotic symptoms among children and adolescents (7,10,12,13,15,19). Acute emergence of psychotic symptoms without identifiable precipitants often signals the possibility of an underlying general medical condition (19). Close temporal associations between

---

TABLE 151.1

GENERAL MEDICAL CONDITIONS OR SYMPTOMS THAT CAN BE ASSOCIATED WITH THE DEVELOPMENT OF PSYCHOTIC SYMPTOMS AMONG CHILDREN AND ADOLESCENTS

HIGH FEVER SECONDARY TO A WIDE VARIETY OF MEDICAL CONDITIONS

NEUROLOGIC
Auditory or visual nerve injuries or disease
Cerebrovascular lesions or disease
Congenital CNS malformations
Epilepsy, especially temporal lobe epilepsy, simple or complex partial seizures, frontal lobe epilepsy
Migraine
Neoplasms, especially brain tumors, other neoplasms with CNS involvement
Traumatic brain injuries, primary focal or diffuse

NEURODEGENERATIVE DISEASES
Huntington's disease
Lipid storage disorders
Metachromatic leukodystrophy
Multiple sclerosis

INFECTIOUS DISEASE/CNS INFECTIONS
Encephalitis
Herpes encephalitis
HIV infection
Lyme disease
Meningitis
Neurosyphilis

AUTOIMMUNE DISORDERS WITH CNS INVOLVEMENT, ESPECIALLY SYSTEMIC LUPUS ERYTHEMATOSUS

METABOLIC/ENDOCRINE
Hyper- or hypo-adrenocorticism
Hyper- or hypo-parathyroidism
Hyper- or hypo-thyroidism
Hypoglycemia
Porphyrias
Wilson disease

RENAL OR HEPATIC FAILURE

ELECTROLYTE OR FLUID IMBALANCES

VITAMIN DEFICIENCIES, ESPECIALLY NIACIN, VITAMIN B$_{12}$

DEVELOPMENTAL DISORDERS, ESPECIALLY 22q11 DELETION (VELOCARDIOFACIAL SYNDROME, DIGEORGE SYNDROME)

the onset, exacerbation, or remission of a general medical condition and the course of psychotic symptoms also provide support for a causal relation (7,19). Most experts recommend close attention to any signs of abnormal neurologic functioning that may co-occur with psychotic symptoms, as these signs may provide direction for further workup and investigation. Careful screening for signs of other broad categories of general medical conditions that can be associated with psychotic symptoms may also assist in determining the need for further procedures or tests. For example, co-occurrence of psychotic symptoms with tremors, dystonia, ataxia, and/or progressive loss of skills would suggest suspicion of a neurodegenerative disorder and would merit further workup in that direction (15).

Caplan and Tanguay identified several features of psychotic symptoms that have been associated with general medical conditions (9). The severity of formal thought disorder symptoms generally is consistent with the degree of overall cognitive impairment if symptoms result from a general medical condition. Formal thought disorder symptoms are more likely to persist, rather than fluctuate, when secondary to a general medical condition. Also, severely incoherent or fragmented speech often is related to a general medical condition. Hallucinations that result from a general medical condition are more likely to be fixed, in contrast to the more variable form and content typical of hallucinations associated with psychiatric disorders (9).

Substances/Medications

Table 151.2 lists substances and medications that have been associated with the development of psychotic symptoms among children and adolescents (7,9,10,12,13,15,19–22). As seen in the table, psychotic symptoms have been associated with a wide variety of substances and several medication classes. Psychotic symptoms among children and adolescents have been observed secondary to medication side effects, withdrawal from medications, ingestion of toxins, and intoxication or withdrawal from substances of abuse. The acute emergence of psychotic symptoms among young children warrants careful investigation for possible accidental toxic ingestions, because oral exploration of materials and substances in the environment is common in early childhood (10). Evaluation of possible substance abuse is warranted for adolescents, because drug use and exploration is relatively frequent in this age group (9,15). Clues that psychotic symptoms may be secondary to a substance or medication can be found in associations between the acute onset of psychotic symptoms and the timing of potential exposure to a toxin, substance use, abstinence from a substance after frequent use, or starting, stopping, or changing the dose of a medication. For example, medication side effects would be suspected for a child who develops persecutory delusions within a few days of starting high-dose corticosteroids as part of a chemotherapy regimen.

Even when drug use is confirmed through laboratory results, the pediatric hospitalist should keep in mind that comorbidity of substance abuse is high among adolescents with psychiatric disorders (13,15). Usually, psychotic symptoms secondary only to drug intoxication are relatively time-limited, typically resolving within a few days of abstinence (15). However, psychotic symptoms can persist for longer periods after cessation of drugs with longer half-lives or drugs that can be associated with "flashback" experiences with chronic use (e.g., LSD, cannabis) (15).

ICU "Psychosis"/Delirium

ICU psychosis and *intensive-care syndrome* are terms that are commonly used to refer to a cluster of symptoms sometimes observed among severely ill children and adolescents being cared for in pediatric intensive-care units (PICUs). This cluster

TABLE 151.2

SUBSTANCES AND MEDICATIONS THAT CAN BE ASSOCIATED WITH THE DEVELOPMENT OF PSYCHOTIC SYMPTOMS AMONG CHILDREN AND ADOLESCENTS

TOXIC INGESTIONS
Environmental toxins
Heavy metals (e.g., lead, aluminum)
Solvents

SUBSTANCE INTOXICATION/SUBSTANCE ABUSE
Alcohol
Amphetamines and related substances
Cannabis
Cocaine
Hallucinogens (e.g., LSD, ecstasy)
Inhalants
Phencyclidine (PCP)
Sedatives, anxiolytics, hypnotics (e.g., barbituates, benzodiazepines)

MEDICATION SIDE EFFECTS
Anesthetic agents (e.g., ketamine, isoflurane)
Antiarrhythmic agents
Antibiotics (e.g., amoxicillan, clarithromycin)
Anticholinergic agents
Antiepileptic drugs
Corticosteroids
Decongestants (e.g., pseudoephedrine, triprolidine)
Inotropes
Opiate analgesics
Promethazine hydrochloride
Stimulants (e.g., methylphenidate, dextroamphetamine)

SUBSTANCE/MEDICATION WITHDRAWAL
Alcohol
Sedatives, anxiolytics, hypnotics (e.g., barbituates, benzodiazepines, other sedatives)

of symptoms typically includes several of the following: hallucinations and other perceptual disturbances (e.g., misperceptions, illusions); delusions; thought and speech disturbances; disorientation; confusion; labile affect; irritability; anxiety; reduced awareness of or responsiveness to environmental stimuli; decreased attention and concentration; insomnia; and psychomotor apathy, restlessness, or agitation (22,23). The focus on psychotic symptoms within the term "ICU psychosis" can be misleading, because the symptom cluster referred to is actually consistent with delirium (see also Chapter 151A). When psychotic symptoms occur exclusively during the course of a delirium, the delirium diagnosis takes precedence over other possible diagnoses (7). Delirium usually has an acute onset and the intensity of symptoms tends to fluctuate over the course of the day and over the course of the delirium (7,23). Symptoms often are more intense at night.

A combination of multiple factors may contribute to the development of delirium among children and adolescents in the PICU (7,19,22–25). Although limited in number, available studies suggest that infections and medications are the most common causes of delirium among children and adolescents (23,24). Multiple other serious medical conditions and withdrawal from medications also can be causal factors. Sleep deprivation or severe alterations in sleep–wake cycles frequently occur among children and adolescents in the PICU and can contribute to the development of delirium. Factors often associated with the PICU environment and care also have been implicated in the development or exacerbation of delirium. The PICU environment often is characterized by sources of unpleasant overstimulation, including pain, discomfort, frequent medical care or procedures, noise from ventilators, alarms, and surrounding conversation, and constant or high levels of light. In addition, multiple sources of sensory deprivation have been identified within the PICU environment, including relative social isolation, limited mobility, reduced direct communication, less frequent day/night cues, reduced physical contact outside of medical care, and remaining primarily in one room. Extreme limitations in control over self and environment also have been identified as stressful aspects of PICU care. Prolonged serious illness and extended exposure to these PICU conditions may increase vulnerability to the development of delirium (7,19, 22–25).

A greater focus on psychotic symptoms in "ICU psychosis," along with the fluctuating course typical of delirium, may contribute to the fact that delirium in children and adolescents is often unrecognized or misdiagnosed by physicians (23–25). Even when recognized, physicians may underestimate the seriousness of delirium and may not fully consider, investigate, or treat all of the potential factors that may lead to or exacerbate delirium among severely ill children and adolescents (23–25). However, delirium in children and adolescents has been associated with high rates of mortality, likely due to the severity of the medical conditions of children who are most likely to develop a delirium (23). Response to delirium as a sign of medical and psychiatric emergency may be most appropriate (23,24).

Psychiatric Disorders

Among children and adolescents, psychotic symptoms are not diagnostically specific to a particular psychiatric disorder or group of disorders. The pediatric hospitalist is less likely to encounter the presentation of active psychotic symptoms secondary to psychiatric disorders in comparison to other etiologic factors discussed above. In the absence of concurrent acute medical symptoms, children and adolescents with active psychotic symptoms may be more likely to be evaluated and cared for in other settings (e.g., outpatient mental health practices, inpatient psychiatric units, or emergency departments). However, the pediatric hospitalist may care for children and adolescents who are admitted to the acute medical setting solely for a thorough workup of possible etiologies of new-onset psychotic symptoms, including both organic and nonorganic factors. Children or adolescents who are admitted for treatment of injuries following a traumatic event also could present with psychotic symptoms. In addition, the pediatric hospitalist may treat children and adolescents who have histories of psychotic symptoms secondary to a psychiatric disorder, but who are admitted to the acute hospital for treatment of an unrelated medical condition.

Table 151.3 lists psychiatric disorders or conditions that have been associated with psychotic symptoms among children and adolescents (7–13,15–17). These disorders and conditions vary considerably in terms of the prominence, frequency, and duration of psychotic symptoms and in terms of other symptoms that may be present concurrently.

Psychotic symptoms are prominent and necessary features of the primary psychotic disorders that may be seen among children and adolescents (7). These disorders differ in the number of required psychotic symptoms, the duration of psychotic symptoms, the degree of required functional impairment, and the presence of other associated symptoms (7). Children and adolescents with schizophrenia and related disorders (schizophreniform, schizoaffective) typically have chronic psychiatric problems, including periods with prominent psychotic symptoms. The presence of "negative symptoms" before, during, or after periods of active psychotic symptoms is also common among children and adolescents with schizophrenia or related disorders (7,15). "Negative symptoms" may include flattened affect (reduced emotional expressiveness, poor eye contact, limited facial mobility, and decreased nonverbal cues), avolition (severely reduced initiation or pursuit of goal-directed activity), alogia (speech characterized by few words, very brief responses, and limited meaningful content), anhedonia (lack of pleasure or interest in activities once considered enjoyable), and social withdrawal (7). Insidious, rather than acute, onset of psychotic symptoms, histories of nonspecific, premorbid developmental delays and impairments across multiple areas of functioning, and family histories of psychosis are also common for children with schizophrenia and related disorders (8,12, 13,15,16). The duration criteria of schizophrenia and related disorders make it unlikely that a clear diagnosis of one of these disorders will be made during an acute medical hospitalization, particularly if the onset of active psychotic symptoms is close to or during the time of admission. *Brief psychotic disorder* is defined by the acute onset of at least one prominent psychotic symptom that has a duration of at least 1 day but less than 1 month and by complete recovery to the level of premorbid functioning by the end of 1 month (7). Brief psychotic disorder may occur without any identifiable precipitants, within 4 weeks postpartum, or in response to one or more severe stressors (formerly known as brief reactive psychosis) (7).

Psychotic disorder not otherwise specified (NOS) may be the most likely diagnosis for a child or adolescent presenting with psychotic symptoms to receive during an acute medical admission unless she was admitted with a preexisting psychiatric diagnosis or unless a clear organic etiology was identified during the admission. Children and adolescents often receive this diagnosis in the period soon after onset of psychotic symptoms, while a variety of etiologies are being considered and evaluated.

Children and adolescents also can experience psychotic symptoms as associated features of severe mood disorders, including major depressive disorder and bipolar disorder (7). A primary mood disorder is most likely to be diagnosed when hallucinations and delusions occur only during the course of a mood episode or when affective symptoms are more prominent and prolonged than psychotic symptoms (7,8,15,16). Children and adolescents who experience psychotic symptoms secondary to a primary mood disorder often, but not always, have hallucinations or delusions that are congruent with the predominant affective state of the mood episode (e.g., delusions of guilt or hearing critical voices during a depressive episode) (7). When a primary mood disorder is the source of symptoms, psychotic symptoms tend to have an acute onset, and family histories often include mood disorders but not primary psychotic disorders (8,15).

Psychotic symptoms also have been occasionally reported in association with a variety of other disorders, such as posttraumatic stress disorder, other anxiety disorders, or adjustment disorders (see Table 151.3). When psychotic symptoms occur in association with these disorders, the child or adolescent often has recently experienced one or more major life stressors such as the death of a loved one, physical or sexual abuse, exposure to family violence, or other traumatic experiences (8,11,17). In these cases, the characteristic symptoms of the associated disorder are typically more prominent than psychotic symptoms.

TABLE 151.3

PSYCHIATRIC DISORDERS OR CONDITIONS THAT CAN BE ASSOCIATED WITH
PSYCHOTIC SYMPTOMS IN CHILDREN AND ADOLESCENTS

**DISORDERS FOR WHICH PSYCHOTIC SYMPTOMS ARE ESSENTIAL FEATURES:
PRIMARY PSYCHOTIC DISORDERS**
Schizophrenia
Schizophreniform disorder
Schizoaffective disorder
Brief psychotic disorder
Psychotic disorder not otherwise specified

**DISORDERS FOR WHICH PSYCHOTIC SYMPTOMS CAN BE ASSOCIATED FEATURES:
PRIMARY MOOD DISORDERS**
Major depressive disorder, severe with psychotic features
Bipolar disorder, severe with psychotic features

**DISORDERS OR CONDITIONS FOR WHICH ASSOCIATED PSYCHOTIC SYMPTOMS
HAVE BEEN REPORTED**
Posttraumatic stress disorder
Acute stress disorder
Generalized anxiety disorder
Anxiety disorder not otherwise specified
Bereavement
Adjustment disorders
Physical or sexual abuse
Exposure to family violence
Visual, tactile, and phobic hallucinations/benign phobic hallucinosis
Tourette's disorder

**DISORDERS WITH SYMPTOMS THAT MAY RESEMBLE PSYCHOTIC SYMPTOMS
AND/OR IN WHICH TRANSIENT OR SUBTHRESHOLD PSYCHOTIC SYMPTOMS
MAY BE OBSERVED**
Disorders or conditions listed in the category immediately above
Obsessive-compulsive disorder
Autistic disorder
Asperger's disorder
Childhood disintegrative disorder
Pervasive developmental disorder not otherwise specified
Communication disorders
Dissociative disorders
Factitious disorders (including by proxy)
Conduct disorder
Schizotypal personality disorder
Schizoid personality disorder
Borderline personality disorder
Paranoid personality disorder

Visual and tactile hallucinations that appear to be phobic in nature have been reported among very young children, ranging from about 2 to 7 years of age (8,10–13). The hallucinations usually have an acute onset and continued prominence at night (10,13). These hallucinations are considered fairly benign because they usually resolve spontaneously or with supportive care within a few days to a few weeks (10,11).

Table 151.3 lists several other disorders that have symptoms that may be difficult to distinguish from psychotic symptoms or in which transient and/or subthreshold psychotic symptoms may be experienced by children and adolescents. For example, children may have difficulty clearly distinguishing between psychotic symptoms and symptoms of posttraumatic stress disorder, such as flashbacks, intrusive thoughts, nightmares, and dissociative symptoms (13). Children and

adolescents with obsessive-compulsive disorder may report persistent illogical thoughts and strange ideas associated with ritualistic behaviors that can resemble delusions (7,9,13). Children and adolescents with autistic disorder or other pervasive developmental disorders may exhibit strange beliefs, odd behaviors, and atypical sensory experiences and may experience transient delusions or hallucinations (13,15).

ASSESSMENT

Assessment of new-onset psychotic symptoms among children or adolescents should include a comprehensive history, medical examination, and psychiatric evaluation (8,12,13,15,16,18). Detailed information should be collected about developmental history, history of academic and social functioning, medical history, potential for toxic exposures, substance abuse history, prior psychological functioning, previous mental health treatment, family medical and psychiatric history, and history of psychosocial stressors (8,10,12,16,18).

Medical evaluation should include a thorough physical exam and review of systems and a neurologic history and exam (8,10,12,13,15,16,18). Current and recent medications should be reviewed, with special attention to any recent changes in medications. Initial laboratory tests often suggested include a full blood count, ESR, and biochemistries, a urinalysis, urine and/or blood toxicology screens, and other studies to screen for endocrine, metabolic, renal, hepatic, or infectious origins of symptoms (13,15,18). Obtaining an EEG and a MRI and consulting a pediatric neurologist are also often recommended (10,12,15,16,18). Genetic evaluation may be valuable if dysmorphic features are observed (13,15,16). Additional tests and/or consultation with other pediatric specialists may be indicated by the results of initial exams and laboratory tests or by the clinical course.

Psychiatric assessment should include evaluation of mental status, with particular attention to possible signs of delirium, such as disorientation and altered or fluctuating levels of consciousness (8,12,13,15,16,18). To the degree possible, the child or adolescent should be evaluated for suicidal ideation, homicidal ideation, and dangerous or impulsive behaviors (12). Information should be collected about the child or adolescent's premorbid functioning, including changes or deterioration in functioning before the onset of psychotic symptoms (8,12,18). The nature, onset, timing, severity, and course of psychotic symptoms should be investigated (8,12,16,18). In addition, history of and/or concurrent presence of mood, anxiety, or "negative" symptoms should be assessed (8,12,13,15,16). The pediatric hospitalist should consider consultation with a mental health professional, such as a psychiatrist and/or psychologist with experience in working with children and adolescents, for assistance in conducting the psychiatric assessment and with obtaining other history.

Within the acute medical hospital, the nature of assessment of psychotic symptoms among children and adolescents will depend, in part, on the context in which the symptoms developed. For example, if a child develops psychotic symptoms during the course of an admission for treatment of a general medical condition and is known to have a fairly normal developmental, psychosocial, and psychiatric history, the assessment is likely to focus most strongly on evaluation of general medical conditions and medications. The assessment may be curtailed if a fairly obvious source of symptoms, such as a fever or medication withdrawal, is quickly identified. A child who is admitted solely for assessment of new-onset psychotic symptoms will likely have an assessment that includes all the components discussed above. However, a complete assessment of the source of psychotic symptoms may be quite prolonged and may require information from multiple sources and observation of symptoms and response to treatment across several months (8,12,13). If possible organic etiologies are largely ruled out during an acute medical admission, further assessment most likely will be carried out in a mental health setting. Assessment of an adolescent with a preexisting psychiatric diagnosis with associated psychotic features may largely involve collecting information about assessment and treatment that has already taken place, including contacting mental health and medical professionals who have been caring for that adolescent on an outpatient basis.

TREATMENT

The pediatric hospitalist, mental health consultants, and other hospital staff should view safety as the first priority of treatment (8,12). If assessment indicates that a child or adolescent with psychotic symptoms may be dangerous to himself or to others, a range of safety measures including the following should be considered: (1) removal of as many potentially harmful materials as possible from the room (e.g., sharp objects, cords, etc.); (2) frequent observation; (3) constant, one-to-one supervision; and/or (4) physical or chemical restraints. If available within the hospital, transfer of the child or adolescent to an inpatient psychiatric unit while acute medical assessment and treatment continue also can be considered. The severity of assessed risk and the child or adolescent's level of behavioral control are guides to which safety measures should be implemented.

Treatment of psychotic symptoms among children and adolescents will vary according to etiology of the symptoms. Beginning treatment of underlying conditions, if identified, often will be the most effective treatment. For example, psychotic symptoms may resolve as an underlying general medical condition is treated, as medications with psychotic side effects are stopped or changed, or as withdrawal symptoms are addressed by tapering a medication more slowly or by starting a medication to treat withdrawal. Psychotic symptoms that are secondary to a psychiatric disorder may start to improve with interventions such as starting psychotropic medications and/or psychotherapeutic interventions.

Psychopharmacologic treatment, if indicated, may be started within the acute medical setting. A consulting child and adolescent psychiatrist may provide the pediatric hospitalist with valuable assistance in managing psychopharmacologic interventions. "Typical" and "atypical" antipsychotic medications are the most common psychopharmacologic agents used to directly treat active psychotic symptoms among children and adolescents (8,12,13,15,16; see also Chapter 152). "Typical" or "conventional" antipsychotic medications include haloperidol, chlorpromazine, thioridazine, thiothixene, fluphenazine, and trifluoperazine (12,13,15). "Atypical" antipsychotic medications include clozapine, risperidone, olanzapine, quetiapine, zotepine, amisulpiride, and ziprazidone (12,13,15). Research studies investigating the use of these medications with children and adolescents are fairly limited in number and scientific rigor (12,13,15). There is no clear consensus on whether treatment with typical or atypical antipsychotics is preferable among children and adolescents (8,12,13,15).

Available studies generally suggest that typical antipsychotics are at least somewhat better than placebos in reducing hallucinations, delusions, and thought disorder but usually have more limited effects on negative symptoms (12,13,15). Several weeks may be required for the onset of a therapeutic effect for some children and adolescents, and treatment resistance is not uncommon (8,15). Careful monitoring for serious side effects, including acute dystonia, extrapyramidal side effects, oversedation, cognitive blunting, tardive dyskinesia, and neuroleptic malignant syndrome, is important when typical antipsychotic medications are used to treat children and adolescents (8,12,13,15; see also Chapter 152).

A few studies of children and adolescents suggest that some atypical antipsychotics may result in greater improvement in hallucinations and delusions in comparison to typical antipsychotics (15). In addition, atypical antipsychotics seem to have the added benefits of treating negative symptoms more effectively, lower rates of treatment resistance, and lower rates of extrapyramidal side effects, tardive dyskinesia, and neuroleptic malignant syndrome (13,15). Common side effects of atypical antipsychotics among children and adolescents include sedation, excessive weight gain, and anticholinergic side effects. Some less common, but serious, side effects also have been seem among children and adolescents treated with atypical antipsychotics, including hematologic abnormalities, seizures, hyperglycemia, and diabetes (13,15,16; see also Chapter 152). Due to the risk of serious symptoms, monitoring for serious side effects through routine blood testing is recommended when atypical antipsychotics are prescribed (15).

Antipsychotic medications are most likely to be used for longer-term periods with children and adolescents if psychotic symptoms are believed to be secondary to a primary psychotic disorder. However, they may be used in the short-term to decrease active psychotic symptoms while other underlying conditions are being treated (e.g., a mood disorder, delirium, or organic factors). When nonpsychotic psychiatric disorders are believed to be the source of psychotic symptoms, other psychotropic medications, such as antidepressants, lithium, or anxiolytics, may be used instead of or in addition to antipsychotic medications. In other cases, psychotic symptoms may resolve without the use of any psychotropic medications. Examples include hallucinations that resolve after treatment of an infection with antibiotics, after psychotherapy for an anxiety disorder, or after recovery from substance intoxication (11,17). If any psychotropic medications used during an acute medical admission will be continued after discharge, the pediatric hospitalist needs to arrange for close outpatient follow-up of these medications by a psychiatrist or primary care provider who is knowledgeable about and comfortable with the management of these medications among children and adolescents.

During an acute medical admission, a variety of psychosocial interventions can also be beneficial for children and adolescents experiencing active psychotic symptoms and for their families. Comfort items from home (e.g., stuffed animals, pictures, favorite music) and the presence of familiar caregivers can be helpful for children and adolescents who are frightened or disturbed by psychotic symptoms. Although staff and family can provide information that their own perceptions or beliefs are different, they should not argue about the content of delusions or hallucinations, because these symptoms are experienced as real to the child or adolescent at that time. Instead, staff and family members can be encouraged to provide frequent support and reassurance, to respond empathetically to emotions expressed in relation to psychotic symptoms, and to avoid prolonged participation in the hallucinations or delusions. Emotional support, education about psychotic symptoms, and regular information and updates about assessment results and treatment plans are usually helpful for family members. Mental health consultants, such as psychiatrists or psychologists experienced in working with children and adolescents, may provide the pediatric hospitalist with valuable assistance in these aspects of treatment and in educating and supporting other staff members interacting with these patients and their families.

A combination of psychopharmacologic and psychosocial interventions has been recommended for children and adolescents suffering from delirium or "ICU Psychosis," because multiple factors often contribute to or exacerbate delirium (22–25). Some clinicians have found short-term use of antipsychotic medications (often, haloperidol) to be effective in relieving some of the symptoms associated with delirium, including psychotic symptoms (23,24). In addition to the psychosocial interventions described above, children and adolescents with delirium often benefit from frequent reorientation, increased direct communication, developmentally appropriate explanations of procedures and medical care, good pain management, increased day/night cues and other sleep hygiene techniques, consistent caregivers, and encouragement of visitation and therapeutic touch by family members (22–25). Although not always possible given the child or adolescent's medical needs, other efforts to reduce sources of unpleasant overstimulation and to increase positive sensory stimulation may include interventions such as positioning for comfort, silencing alarms quickly, moving equipment to increase open space around the bed, playing familiar music, increasing availability of toys or leisure activities, taking trips out of the room, and increasing opportunities for mobility and control (22–25).

Children and adolescents who experience psychotic symptoms secondary to substance abuse and other psychiatric disorders will likely need treatment beyond that which can be provided during an acute medical admission. Mental health consultants often can assist the pediatric hospitalist in identifying the level and nature of further assessment or treatment that may be indicated for a particular child or adolescent and in making appropriate referrals. Referral to inpatient or outpatient substance abuse treatment should be considered for adolescents who have experienced psychotic symptoms secondary to substance abuse. Once organic factors have been ruled out, transfer to an inpatient psychiatric unit for further assessment and stabilization may be appropriate for children and adolescents who continue to experience active psychotic symptoms or who are judged to be at high risk of harming themselves or others (8,12).

A variety of outpatient follow-up services may be appropriate for other children and adolescents who have experienced psychotic symptoms secondary to a psychiatric disorder but who are relatively stable by the end of an acute medical admission. The nature of services needed after discharge will vary depending on diagnoses that remain within the differential diagnosis and on the severity of symptoms and functional impairments that remain at the time of discharge. For example, outpatient monitoring and supportive therapy by a mental health professional may be appropriate for preschoolers who have experienced visual and tactile phobic hallucinations (10). Referral for regular outpatient psychotherapy may be appropriate for some children and adolescents who experienced psychotic symptoms in relation to conditions such as an anxiety disorder, traumatic experiences, or bereavement (11,17). Children with more severe mood or anxiety disorders may require more intensive outpatient services, such as intensive in-home therapy and/or case management, in addition to outpatient psychotherapy and medication management. Children and adolescents believed to have schizophrenia or a related disorder will likely require long-term, multimodal outpatient treatment services, which may include medication management, supportive individual and/or group therapy, social skills training, behavior modification, family therapy, educational and supportive services for family members, case management, in-home therapeutic services, special education services, therapeutic recreation, and vocational rehabilitation (8,12, 13,15,16). Residential or group home placement eventually may be considered for some children and adolescents who need more intensive treatment services than can be provided on an outpatient basis, but who do not currently need inpatient psychiatric placement. Because approval for placement in residential treatment is usually a prolonged process, it would be unusual for initial placement to be arranged from the acute medical hospital. However, children or adolescents with known histories of serious psychiatric disorders often may return to residential treatment after discharge from an acute medical admission.

CASE STUDY

A 7 yr old girl experienced serious toxic side effects of chemotherapy. Treatment required surgical intervention and a prolonged PICU stay. After extubation and weaning of paralytic and most sedative medications, she began to experience new-onset psychotic symptoms. Although she had experienced some emotional adjustment symptoms in relation to her cancer diagnosis and treatment, the child otherwise had a normal psychiatric and developmental history. A pediatric psychologist had been working with the child and her family since the time of her initial cancer diagnosis as part of the standard care of her oncology team.

Psychotic symptoms initially began at night, with the child displaying fearful and agitated behavior and reporting hallucinations. Symptoms fluctuated over the course of the day, but they generally progressed in severity and frequency over the next few days. The child sometimes seemed more responsive to the external environment and more connected to reality when she was taken out of her PICU room. She began to experience more frequent hallucinations throughout the day and night, including reporting that stuffed animals were talking to her, participating in conversations with siblings who were not present, and reporting that she was seeing and hearing characters from familiar movies or TV programs. The child also began to respond fearfully to physicians during exams, reporting that she thought they were trying to hurt her. As symptoms progressed, her speech sometimes approached incoherence. In addition to psychotic symptoms, the child displayed distractibility, emotional lability, extreme insomnia, and increasing confusion and disorientation. Disorientation eventually progressed to the point that the child often did not recognize her parents or respond to her own name.

Thorough medical evaluation during this period suggested that the child's overall medical condition was improving rather than worsening. No signs of infection were identified.

Careful review of records revealed that initial symptoms had begun a few hours after complete discontinuation of a benzodiazepine that had been tapered. However, little to no improvement in symptoms was observed when another benzodiazepine was administered. As symptoms progressed, many staff members began to characterize the child's symptoms as "ICU psychosis." However, symptoms of delirium continued to worsen after the child was transferred from the PICU to a step-down unit that provided more normal sensory stimulation and was more familiar to her.

A number of psychosocial interventions were implemented by staff members, including providing comfort, reassurance, and support to the child, providing education and emotional support to family members, attempting to correct sources of overstimulation and sensory deprivation, increasing day/night cues and routines, and providing frequent re-orientation. The pediatric psychologist recommended consultation with child and adolescent psychiatry when symptoms worsened in spite of psychosocial interventions. The consulting child and adolescent psychiatrist agreed with the diagnosis of delirium and recommended a trial of an antipsychotic medication and continuation of psychosocial interventions.

The child displayed marked improvement of many of her symptoms after one to two doses of the antipsychotic medication, with complete resolution of psychotic symptoms within 2 days and resolution of other delirium symptoms within a week. Antipsychotic medication was discontinued after the psychotic symptoms resolved.

CHAPTER 151C ■ DEPRESSION

ROBERT R. SHELTON AND JENIFER L. POWELL

Children and adolescents can experience a wide range of depressed mood and depressive symptoms. Depression has the capacity to cause significant distress for patients and their families, as well as to interfere with the ability of children and adolescents to benefit fully from the treatment they receive in acute care settings. Pediatric hospitalists can respond to depressive symptoms quickly and effectively with appropriate assessment, consultation, and interventions in order to prevent or minimize the impact of a depressive episode.

Major depressive disorder (MDD) is the most severe of the depressive disorders described by the DSM-IV-TR (26). It is often a recurring condition that children or adolescents may struggle with into adulthood. MDD can have serious implications for academic, vocational, and social functioning, as well as utilization of health services. Accurate diagnosis and effective treatment are crucial for helping the child and family learn strategies to cope with this disorder. MDD consists of one or more major depressive episodes. The essential feature of such an episode is at least a 2-week period of pervasive depressed mood or loss of interest or pleasure in nearly all activities. DSM-IV-TR specifies that mood may be irritable rather than sad for children and adolescents. At least four other symptoms must also be present from a longer list of symptoms, including primarily somatic complaints and primarily cognitive complaints. Possible somatic symptoms of a major depressive episode include marked increases or decreases in appetite and significant weight loss or weight gain. Children may fail to gain weight at expected rates. Disturbed sleep, often insomnia, is another of the somatic symptoms. Psychomotor agitation (e.g., difficulty sitting still, pacing, picking at the skin, clothing, or other objects) or psychomotor retardation (e.g., slowed speech and body movements) that is significant enough to be noted by others may occur. Another somatic symptom that is frequently reported during a major depressive episode is pervasive fatigue or markedly decreased energy (26).

Symptoms that are more cognitive in nature include a sense of worthlessness or unrealistic guilt. Children or adolescents with this symptom may blame themselves for a multitude of negative events or harshly evaluate their perceived failings. This excessive guilt can reach delusional proportions for some individuals. Those experiencing a major depressive episode often exhibit persistent difficulties with concentrating, thinking, and making decisions. Children and adolescents may experience a drop in school performance secondary to these cognitive difficulties. A major depressive episode also may include frequent thoughts of death or suicidal ideation. Morbid or suicidal thoughts of children and adolescents can range in severity from passive escape wishes, to thoughts that no one would care if they died, to a sense that the lives of others would be improved if the child or adolescent died, to thoughts of killing themselves, to formulating possible plans to kill themselves. At the most severe end of this spectrum, thoughts of death or suicide may progress to the child or adolescent attempting suicide (26).

To qualify as a major depressive episode, the child or adolescent must either experience clinically significant distress or exhibit functional disturbances in social, academic, or other important domains. "Clinically significant distress" refers both to the individual's subjective experience and to the clinician's judgment of the seriousness of the distress. In addition, the depressive symptoms are not secondary to the direct physiologic effects of a substance (e.g., a drug of abuse or a prescribed medication) or a general medical condition (e.g., diabetes). Also, to be considered a major depressive episode, bereavement does not better account for the symptoms (26).

In addition to requiring one or more major depressive episodes for a diagnosis of major depressive disorder, the DSM-IV-TR specifies that one of the bipolar disorders should be diagnosed instead of MDD if the child or adolescent has ever experienced a manic episode, a hypomanic episode, or a mixed episode (which includes both manic and depressive symptoms). Furthermore, MDD should not be diagnosed if the symptoms are better accounted for by schizoaffective disorder (a psychotic disorder with a significant mood component) or if the depressive symptoms are superimposed on schizophrenia, schizophreniform disorder (similar to schizophrenia but of shorter duration), delusional disorder, or psychotic disorder not otherwise specified (26).

As noted above, the DSM-IV-TR describes a few modifications to the diagnostic criteria when applied to children and adolescents (e.g., that mood may be irritable rather than depressed). However, because the criteria were developed primarily for adults, their application to children can be challenging.

When gauging the type and severity of depressive symptoms that a child or adolescent is experiencing, several other psychiatric disorders should be considered within the differential diagnosis. Dysthymic disorder differs from MDD in its chronic nature (at least 1 year for children and adolescents), in its relatively less severe depressive symptoms (e.g., the absence of suicidal ideation), and in the fewer number of depressive symptoms required for diagnosis. The criteria for dysthymic disorder specify that symptom-free intervals have lasted less than 1 month, and that symptoms have not met criteria for a major depressive episode during the 1-year period (26).

Children or adolescents may also exhibit depressive symptoms during the course of an adjustment disorder. These disorders are characterized by a psychological response to an identifiable stressor or stressors that result in clinically significant emotional or behavioral symptoms. The clinical significance of the symptoms is defined by marked distress or impairment in social, academic, or vocational functioning. According to DSM-IV-TR, an adjustment disorder must resolve within 6 months after the occurrence of a discrete stressor. However, the symptoms may persist for a prolonged period if the stressor is chronic (e.g., a chronic, disabling medical condition). Adjustment disorders described by the DSM-IV-TR that may include depressive symptoms are adjustment disorder with depressed mood, adjustment disorder with mixed anxiety and depressed mood, and adjustment disorder with mixed disturbance of emotions and conduct (26).

Depressive disorder not otherwise specified may be diagnosed if depressive symptoms represent a significant component of the presentation but do not meet criteria for a specific depressive disorder. Examples include episodes lasting at least 2 weeks in which depressive symptoms are present but are fewer than required for a diagnosis of MDD, and situations in which depressive symptoms are present concurrently with a general medical condition, and the clinician is unable to determine whether the depression is primary or secondary to the medical condition (26).

Children and adolescents experiencing bereavement may exhibit symptoms indistinguishable from those of MDD. The DSM-IV-TR specifies that MDD should not be diagnosed for a bereaved child or adolescent unless the symptoms persist longer than 2 months after the death of the loved one (26). If the depressive symptoms result in marked impairment or include psychomotor retardation, psychotic symptoms, suicidal ideation, or morbid preoccupations with worthlessness or guilt, the diagnosis of MDD may be made during the first 2 months after the loss (26). However, it should be noted that bereaved children and adolescents often experience intermittent sadness and other grief symptoms for periods much longer than 2 months.

The pediatric hospitalist may encounter children and adolescents who are experiencing multiple traumatic stressors. For example, after a motor vehicle accident with a fatality, an injured child may be struggling to cope with the stressful hospital environment, with his own injuries, and with the loss of a loved one. Children's understanding of and reaction to death varies depending on their level of cognitive development. Children younger than 6 typically do not have a full understanding of the irreversibility and universality of death or of the fact that all life functions cease at death (27). Children older than 6 typically begin to grasp these key elements, with comprehension approaching adult levels during adolescence. Although younger children may exhibit less anxiety about death than older children, they are at greater risk for more adverse reactions over the long term (27). The pediatric hospitalist needs to ensure that bereaved children and adolescents have adequate family and social support, as well as support from available staff, such as chaplains, child life specialists, and mental health professionals. The child's family may benefit from education on signs to monitor (e.g., significant or prolonged behavioral and emotional changes) that would indicate a need for future professional treatment.

During crisis times, children and adolescents may also demonstrate sadness, depressed mood, or withdrawal that does not represent a psychiatric condition. For example, many children and adolescents exhibit short-term, but significant, distress in response to separation from parents or friends, newly diagnosed medical conditions, invasive procedures, or traumatic injuries. In addition, most children and adolescents are strongly affected by their parents' distress, even when parents are making efforts to shield their children from these emotions. At times, support and clear information provided to parents may be the most effective way to help a child in distress, as this will better enable them to be present for their child.

It should be noted that sadness is part of the normal range of human experience, along with joy, fear, and anger. Any hospitalized child who is subjected to unwanted, uncomfortable, or frightening medical procedures may feel unhappy and irritable. The clinician may bear the brunt of the child's moodiness because she is the one who ordered the procedures. Before concluding that the child is depressed, it will be important for the hospitalist and/or mental health consultants to question the patient, parents or guardians, and other staff about the child's affect and behavior at other times. Is the child interested in typical activities? Does he exhibit a normal mood at other times? Do the parents or guardians believe their child is significantly "different" in terms of behavior and mood? How does the child describe his mood? What other symptoms besides sad, irritable, or withdrawn affect does the child report or display? It should be noted that patients, family members, and staff members sometimes used the term "depressed" in a colloquial sense, referring to significant sadness without necessarily meaning to imply other depressive symptoms. This colloquial use of "depressed" or "depression" may or may not be associated with the symptoms of MDD or other disorders with depressive symptoms.

The pediatric hospitalist will often encounter children with chronic medical conditions, such as asthma, cancer, diabetes, juvenile rheumatoid arthritis, and sickle-cell disease. Researchers have investigated the incidence of psychiatric conditions among populations of chronically ill or disabled children and adolescents and have concluded that although these young people are more vulnerable to psychiatric conditions than the general population, psychological maladjustment is not necessarily a predictable outcome (28). Instead, many chronically ill or disabled children or adolescents are remarkably resilient. Adjustment disorders are the most commonly diagnosed condition among these pediatric populations. Psychiatric problems seem to be most pronounced for children or adolescents who have sensory or neurologic deficits (29). The clinician should be cautious about assuming that a child or teen is depressed simply because she has a chronic medical condition or disability. Subjective and objective symptoms of depression should also be present. Risk factors for adjustment problems among children and adolescents with chronic illnesses or disabilities include child experiences of high stress levels and low self-esteem, family environments lacking in cohesion and supportiveness, family relationships high in conflict, and maternal distress (28).

DEVELOPMENTAL CONSIDERATIONS

Depressive symptoms can manifest differently depending on the age of the patient (30). The existence of depression in children from birth to age 2 is controversial. Because many depressive symptoms are cognitive, some argue that children so young are incapable of depression in the same sense as older children and adolescents. Nevertheless, infants and toddlers who experience severe deprivation or maltreatment often exhibit symptoms that resemble depression. Infants who have been deprived of emotional contact with a major attachment figure in the first year of life may exhibit "anaclitic depression," which is characterized by whining, withdrawal, weight loss, slowed growth, lowered immune system, dazed or immobile facial expression, and intellectual decline (30).

From ages 3 to 5, sadness, weight loss, and psychomotor retardation may be seen. Depressed preschoolers frequently may appear tired, angry, and apathetic. Irritability and social withdrawal may also be observed. Some depressed preschoolers may express suicidal ideation, but attempts are very rare in this age group. Some young children may display a sense of guilt and increased responsibility for events over which they have no control. Furthermore, they may have unrealistic beliefs about their ability to change another person's situation (31).

Depressive symptoms of school-age children (6 to 12 years) more closely begin to resemble adult symptoms. School-age children may exhibit all of the symptoms of a major depressive episode. As children's cognitive abilities develop, their capacity to experience the cognitive symptoms of depression increases. School-age children more clearly exhibit a depressed mood, and they may be able to speak about their depressed cognitions and affect. However, verbalizations may be limited by lack of vocabulary. For example, school-age children may describe depressive symptoms with complaints of feeling bored or stupid. Lack of pleasure, apathy, and lowered self-esteem may be evident. Parents or guardians first may become aware of depressive symptoms due to declining performance in school, sports, or chores. School-age children experiencing depressive symptoms may report a sense of being disliked or rejected by peers. Although depressed children may be more likely to have negative attributions about benign interactions

with peers, they may also experience genuine shunning, since depressive symptoms can have a serious impact on a child's desirability as a companion (30).

From ages 12 to 18, the full gamut of affective, cognitive, and somatic symptoms characteristic of major depressive episodes may be seen. In addition, depressive symptoms may be accompanied by more acting-out behaviors during this developmental period. Adolescents may exhibit volatile mood, rage, poor school performance, delinquency, substance abuse, and sexual acting out in association with depressive symptoms. This acting-out must be differentiated from the emotional and behavioral turmoil that has become somewhat normative for adolescents in western culture. Adolescents encounter significant developmental tasks (e.g., increasing independence, identity exploration, beginning to form romantic relationships) that expose them to increased opportunities for stress, disappointment, and failure. Many adolescents experience transient unhappiness and dissatisfaction, which can be distinguished from the symptoms of clinical depression by severity and uniqueness (30).

SUICIDE

As indicated above, children and adolescents with MDD are at increased risk for suicidal ideation. The pediatric hospitalist is likely to encounter young people in the acute medical setting who have attempted suicide (see also Chapter 151E). If a child or adolescent is considered to be depressed, suicidality should always be assessed.

Completed suicide is rare in prepubertal children, and on average, is less common among adolescents than among adults (32). In 2000, 3,877 youths in the United States between ages 15 and 24 committed suicide, resulting in a suicide rate of 10.1 per 100,000 for this age group (32). In the same year, 297 children and adolescents between ages 5 and 14 committed suicide for a rate of 0.7 per 100,000 for their age group. Suicide is the third leading cause of death in young people from ages 15 to 24, after accidents and homicides (33). Rates of suicidal ideation reported by young people in large surveys have ranged from 14.5% to 24.9% for girls and from 3.3% to 13.7% for boys. Rates of reported suicide attempts have ranged from 7.1% to 10.9% for girls and from 2.4% to 5.7% for boys (33). In one study, approximately 2.6% of attempts resulted in injury or the need for medical attention. Children who report suicidal ideation are more likely to attempt suicide as adolescents. Reports from children and adolescents about suicidal thoughts must be taken seriously and attended to. Although most often thought of as a depressive symptom, suicidal behavior is often seen among children and adolescents with other psychiatric disorders, including anxiety, conduct, substance abuse, developmental, and personality disorders.

Acute medical settings should have a policy regarding management of children and adolescents who have attempted suicide or who report suicidal ideation while in the hospital. This policy should include evaluation by a mental health professional (psychiatrist or psychologist) if available. The policy should also include guidance for other hospital staff to ensure the child's safety while in the acute setting. Such guidance may include statements about limiting access to potentially harmful objects (e.g., belts, shoelaces) and about the level(s) of staff observation that a suicidal patient requires. A challenge faced by the mental health consultant is that prediction of attempted or completed suicide is a very inexact science. There are a variety of predictors that have been associated with increased risk of attempting or completing suicide (e.g., sense of hopelessness, past attempts, impulsiveness, conduct problems, family history of attempts), but none of these predict very accurately.

Depending on the severity of the situation, the child or adolescent who has attempted suicide may require inpatient psychiatric hospitalization once he is medically stable. At a minimum, the mental health consultant will probably arrange some type of outpatient psychiatric or psychotherapeutic aftercare as soon after discharge as possible.

ASSESSMENT

When should the pediatric hospitalist become concerned about the possibility of depression? Assessment of potential depressive symptoms is warranted for children or adolescents in the acute hospital who frequently appear sad or who are socially withdrawn. Markedly decreased or lack of interest in preferred activities, apathy, high levels of irritability, and overall moodiness are also warning signs. Involving mental health staff (psychologist or psychiatrist experienced in working with children and adolescents) early when concerns arise may be useful for assistance with assessment and differential diagnosis.

Given the potential that depressive symptoms have for negatively affecting a child or adolescent's ability to function for an extended period, attending to complaints of sadness, unhappiness, or boredom is important. The pediatric hospitalist and appropriate consultants should interview the parents or guardians directly about their perceptions of the child's mood. Information regarding the symptoms of a major depressive episode should be gathered from the parents and, as developmentally appropriate, from the child or adolescent. Younger children should be observed over extended periods to assess the quality of their interactions with family, friends, and typical play materials. Children older than 5 years may be questioned directly about feeling sad, down, or unhappy over a period of time. They should be asked directly, with developmentally appropriate language, about suicidal ideation. Interviews with parents/guardians and with the patient should be conducted separately, if possible. Older children and adolescents may be willing to discuss their feelings, concerns, and experiences more openly without family present. Nurses and therapeutic staff (e.g., occupational therapists, physical therapists, speech therapists, recreation therapists, child life specialists) can provide information about how the child or adolescent is interacting with others and participating in treatment. It is important to be aware, however, that correlations often are not very high between children's or adolescents' self-report of their mood and activities and the reports of parents or other observers.

The assessment of potential depressive symptoms also should include gathering information about the patient's school and social functioning, the patient's history of past mental health treatment or mood disturbance, and family history of mood disturbances and mental health treatment. In addition, the pediatric hospitalist and/or mental health consultants should gather information about the home setting, family stressors (e.g., financial, recent deaths, divorces), and the quality of family relationships (e.g., cohesive, supportive, low conflict versus chaotic, high conflict, low support). Older children and adolescents should be questioned about their use of alcohol or other drugs.

The pediatric hospitalist must be especially concerned about differentiating depressive symptoms secondary to a psychiatric disorder from those secondary to a general medical condition. O'Brien and associates offer guidance for distinguishing between depression as a psychiatric condition and medical conditions that produce depressive symptoms (9). They recommend consultation with a psychiatrist or psychologist who is experienced in working with children and adolescents in medical settings for assistance in differential diagnosis. They note that cognitive symptoms (e.g., sense of worthlessness or thoughts of death) should be emphasized over somatic complaints, because cognitive symptoms are more typical of primary depressive disorders, while somatic symptoms are frequent both for primary depressive disorders and general medical conditions. Family history of psychiatric illness and treatment also may lend support to a psychiatric etiology of symptoms. Clues that a medical condition may be causing depressive symptoms include: (1) sudden onset of depressive symptoms that have no or barely recognized precipitants, (2) temporal association between onset, worsening, and remission of symptoms with the course of the medical condition, and (3) presence of atypical features, such as otherwise mild depressive symptoms accompanied by severe weight loss. A thorough neurologic examination may assist in identifying or ruling out potential neurologic abnormalities that could cause symptoms that resemble a depressive disorder. When a patient does not respond to standard care for the presumed etiology, O'Brien and colleagues recommend that a thorough search be conducted for psychiatric and medical symptoms that may previously have been overlooked. Furthermore, they highlight the important points that psychiatric diagnoses require the presence of symptoms and not merely the exclusion of medical conditions, and that co-morbid psychiatric and medical conditions are not uncommon (34).

Table 151.4 lists medical conditions with symptoms that can resemble those of a depressive disorder (35). Tests the hospitalist may consider to screen for these medical conditions include a complete blood cell count with differential, electrolyte concentrations, liver function tests, thyroid function tests, blood urea nitrogen and creatinine levels, urinalysis, and electrocardiogram. Electroencephalography and CT or MRI may be clinically indicated to assess for seizure activity or other organicity (36).

INTERVENTIONS

If depressive symptoms are mild and appear to be a response to factors related to hospitalization, children and adolescents in the acute medical setting may respond well to environmental changes. Such changes may include instituting a regular schedule, including wakeup times, out of bed times (if appropriate), activity times, homework times (if school is in session), and scheduled times for therapies or other regular aspects of care. Many children and teens respond positively to such structure, which often provides them with increased senses of predictability and control. Ensuring adequate family involvement also may be a helpful intervention if obstacles are preventing family members from being present at the hospital as often as they would like or as the child needs. Hospital social workers may be able to assist in overcoming potential obstacles to family involvement (e.g., transportation, accommodations). Child Life staff often can provide invaluable assistance in ensuring that the child has access to a variety of age-appropriate toys, games, and activities and in helping children better understand and cope with medical procedures. Psychologists or psychiatrists may provide assistance in identifying and coordinating potentially helpful environmental interventions and in educating the patient, family, and staff about why these changes may be beneficial.

For more serious depression, mental health consultants may recommend a variety of therapeutic interventions, depending in part on the age of the child. For younger children, family therapy and play therapy may be beneficial. Family therapy attempts to activate the existing family as a resource to improve the child's mood and level of functioning. Play therapy utilizes the children's natural medium of expression and communication as a means of increasing their sense of control

TABLE 151.4

CONDITIONS MIMICKING DEPRESSION IN CHILDREN AND ADOLESCENTS

INFECTIONS
Infectious mononucleosis
Influenza
Encephalitis
Subacute bacterial endocarditis
Pneumonia
Tuberculosis
Hepatitis
Syphilis (CNS)
AIDS

NEUROLOGIC DISORDERS/TUMORS
Epilepsy
Postconcussion
Subarachnoid hemorrhage
Cerebrovascular accident
Multiple sclerosis
Huntington's disease

ENDOCRINE
Diabetes
Cushing's disease
Addison's disease
Hypothyroidism
Hyperthyroidism
Hypoparathyroidism
Hyperparathyroidism
Hypopituitarism

MEDICATIONS
Antihypertensives
Barbituates
Benzodiazepines
Corticosteriods
Oral contraceptives
Cimetidine
Aminophylline
Anticonvulsants
Clonidine
Digitalis
Thiozide diuretics

OTHERS
Alcohol abuse
Drug abuse and withdrawal
    Cocaine
    Amphetamine
    Opiates
Electrolyte abnormality
    Hypokalemia
    Hyponatremia
Failure to thrive
Anemia
Lupus
Wilson disease
Porphyria
Uremia

Reprinted from Weller EB, Weller RA, Rowan AB, et al. Depressive disorders in children and adolescents. In: Lewis M, ed. *Child and adolescent psychiatry: a comprehensive textbook.* 3rd ed. Philadelphia: Lippincott Williams & Wilkins; 2002: 773, with permission.

and of providing a safe way to vent feelings such as anger, fear, and sadness.

Older children and adolescents with significant depressive symptoms may benefit from family therapy, interpersonal therapy, or cognitive-behavioral therapy. Interpersonal therapy focuses on the development of a therapeutic relationship and the use of that relationship to help the child or adolescent learn more adaptive means of coping. Cognitive-behavioral therapy focuses on identifying and modifying cognitions or behaviors the children or adolescents typically have (though are often unaware of) that tend to lead to or sustain depression. Examples include thoughts such as "I never get things right" or "things always go wrong for me," or behaviors such as remaining in bed when feeling down even though physically capable of getting out of bed. Through discussion and example, the therapist helps the child or adolescent learn and use more adaptive cognitions and behaviors. There is a growing consensus that a therapeutic approach that integrates the best of the above therapies and of psychodynamic therapy has good potential to ameliorate the depressive symptoms of children and adolescents (12).

Therapeutic interventions in an acute hospital setting frequently will be brief and time-limited given the typical length of an acute admission. Often the goals will be to enable the child or adolescent to tolerate the hospitalization and to provide a positive therapeutic experience so further inpatient or outpatient treatment of depressive symptoms will be more acceptable to him. Therapeutic interventions within the acute hospital may be more intensive and of longer duration for children who experience frequent or prolonged hospital admissions.

In some cases, depressive symptoms are so severe that mental health consultants may recommend psychopharmacologic treatment. The American Academy of Child and Adolescent Psychiatry has issued a practice parameter for the treatment of major depression and dysthymia (37). According to this practice parameter, antidepressant medications are indicated for children and adolescents with non-rapid-cycling bipolar disorder or MDD with psychotic features, for those with depressive symptoms that are severe enough to prevent effective psychotherapy, for those whose depressive symptoms fail to respond to an adequate trial of psychotherapy, and for those with chronic or recurrent depression. Many antidepressants require a week or longer to have a therapeutic effect, and most have potential side effects that should be monitored. For this reason, many mental health consultants may recommend referral to an outpatient psychiatrist or other physician who can assess and treat the depression in an ongoing fashion. For those children or adolescents whose symptoms warrant transfer to an inpatient psychiatric unit after medical stabilization (i.e., those who are considered at high risk of harming themselves or others), medication trials are usually delayed until after transfer unless chemical restraint for safety is needed within the acute setting. A depressed child or adolescent who must be in the acute hospital for an extended period or who will have frequent admissions due to the chronic nature of her medical condition may benefit from starting antidepressant medications while in the acute hospital. If psychotropic medications are indicated during the acute admission, the pediatric hospitalist may find consultation with a child and adolescent psychiatrist helpful in selecting medications most appropriate for the needs of a particular patient.

Antidepressant medications that commonly may be recommended include the SSRIs, or selective serotonin reuptake inhibitors (e.g., fluoxetine, paroxetine). There have been few double-blind, controlled studies related to the use of SSRIs in children and adolescents. Initial reports indicate that these agents may be beneficial for treatment of depression and should be maintained for at least 8 to 10 weeks (36). Tricyclic antidepressants (TCAs) were frequently the drug of choice for child and adolescent depression in the past. However, the advent of SSRIs, apparent lower risks associated with the use of SSRIs (e.g., less dangerous in conditions of overdose), and reports of sudden deaths associated with the use of TCAs as prescribed, have limited the use of TCAs for treating children and adolescents.

In 2004, the FDA issued warnings related to the use of antidepressants with children and adolescents (38). This was due to a concern about an increased risk of suicidal thoughts in children or adolescents taking antidepressant medications. The American Psychiatric Association and the American Academy of Child and Adolescent Psychiatry protested these warnings (39). In an information pamphlet for parents, the APA and AACAP stressed the fact that no suicides actually occurred in the 23 studies the FDA reviewed. The two organizations also criticized the FDA's methodology in conducting the review and supported the ongoing use of antidepressants for children and adolescents who meet the criteria for such treatment.

CASE STUDY

A 16-year-old female with a long history of type I diabetes mellitus was admitted to an acute medical hospital for 4 days for treatment of diabetic ketoacidosis (DKA). She had a history of several past admissions for DKA. As with past admissions, her blood work suggested chronic hyperglycemia. The teen admitted to intermittent nonadherence to many aspects of her home diabetes regimen, though the degree and details of reported nonadherence varied in conversations with different staff members. The teen's attending physician requested a pediatric psychology consult to explore potential psychological factors that might be negatively impacting adherence. From the clinical interview and the patient's responses on a standardized self-report questionnaire about depressive symptoms, the psychologist learned that the teen had been experiencing pervasive sadness, hopelessness, and decreased interest in activities and peer relationships for several months. She also had several other symptoms consistent with a major depressive episode. Although several of the somatic symptoms the teen reported (e.g., increased appetite, sleep problems, fatigue) might also have been affected by her chronic hyperglycemia, she also reported several cognitive symptoms of depression, including excessive guilt, high levels of self-criticism, and feelings of worthlessness. She denied current or past active suicidal plans, intent, or attempts. However, of particular concern, she shared that her motivation to follow her diabetes regimen was very low, since she often passively wished for escape from the stresses of her life and frequently thought that her family members would be happier if she died. The teen also described experiencing several significant personal and family stressors. She had participated in outpatient counseling for depressive symptoms in the past but had not received any treatment for several months. After ruling out other possible psychiatric disorders through interview and history, the psychologist arrived at a working diagnosis of MDD and of psychological disorder (MDD) affecting general medical condition (diabetes). As part of discharge planning, the psychologist recommended and assisted in arranging outpatient appointments with a therapist for psychotherapy and with a child and adolescent psychiatrist for consideration of possible psychopharmacologic intervention.

CHAPTER 151D ■ POSTTRAUMATIC STRESS DISORDER

RONALD M. PERKIN

Since the introduction of posttraumatic stress disorder (PTSD) as a diagnostic category in DSM-III in 1980, there has been a growing awareness that children and adolescents as well as adults can experience this disorder (40).

PTSD refers to the development of a characteristic triad of symptoms following exposure to a particularly severe stressor. The diagnostic criteria for this disorder have undergone revisions from those originally proposed in DSM-III. The definition of *traumatic stressor* in DSM-IV (1994) does not require that the event be outside the realm of normal human experiences as suggested by DSM-III. This revision occurred in response to recognition that some stressors known to result in PTSD symptoms are not rare (such as rape, child abuse, and exposure to domestic violence, community violence, or conditions of war). The stressor must, however, be "extreme"; that is, it must involve either experiencing or witnessing an event capable of causing death, injury, or threat to physical integrity to oneself or another person; or learning about a significant other being exposed to such an event. This exposure constitutes the first criterion for PTSD. The child's reaction must include intense fear, horror, helplessness, or disorganized or agitated behavior. Children's initial response to trauma is often characterized by physiologic and behavioral hyperarousal, and when the trauma is ongoing, the response may become complicated by dissociation (41). DSM-IV includes a partial list of several events that may fit the definition of an extreme traumatic stressor but gives the clinician latitude in making this determination depending on the specifics of the situation.

To meet criteria for PTSD, the child's response must include a specific number of symptoms from each of three broad categories: reexperiencing, avoidance/numbing, and increased arousal (Table 151.5). There have been revisions in DMS-III-R (1987) and *DSM-IV* regarding the specific symptoms included under each of these categories, with progressively

TABLE 151.5

DIAGNOSTIC CRITERIA FOR POSTTRAUMATIC STRESS DISORDER

A. The person has been exposed to a traumatic event in which both of the following were present:
   (1) The person experienced, witnessed, or was confronted with an event or events that involved actual or threatened death or serious injury, or a threat to the physical integrity of self or others.
   (2) The person's response involved intense fear, helplessness, or horror.
   Note: In children, this may be expressed instead by disorganized or agitated behavior.

B. The traumatic event is persistently reexperienced in one (or more) of the following ways:
   (1) Recurrent and intrusive distressing recollections of the event, including images, thoughts, or perceptions.
   Note: In young children, repetitive play may occur in which themes or aspects of the trauma are expressed.
   (2) Recurrent distressing dreams of the event.
   Note: In children, there may be frightening dreams without recognizable content.
   (3) Acting or feeling as if the traumatic event were recurring (includes a sense of reliving the experience, illusions, hallucinations, and dissociative flashback episodes, including those that occur on awakening or when intoxicated).
   Note: In young children, trauma-specific reenactment may occur.
   (4) Intense psychological distress at exposure to internal or external cues that symbolize or resemble an aspect of the traumatic event.
   (5) Physiological reactivity on exposure to internal or external cues that symbolize or resemble an aspect of the traumatic event.

C. Persistent avoidance of stimuli associated with the trauma and numbing of general responsiveness (not present before the trauma), as indicated by 3 (or more) of the following:
   (1) Efforts to avoid thoughts, feelings, or conversations associated with the trauma
   (2) Efforts to avoid activities, places, or people that arouse recollections of the trauma
   (3) Inability to recall an important aspect of the trauma
   (4) Markedly diminished interest or participation in significant activities
   (5) Feeling of detachment or estrangement from others
   (6) Restricted range of affect (eg., unable to have loving feelings)
   (7) Sense of foreshortened future (eg., does not expect to have career, marriage, children, or a normal life span)

D. Persistent symptoms of increased arousal (not present before the trauma), as indicated by 2 (or more) of the following:
   (1) Difficulty falling or staying asleep
   (2) Irritability or outbursts of anger
   (3) Difficulty concentrating
   (4) Hypervigilance
   (5) Exaggerated startle response

E. Duration of the disturbance (symptoms in criteria B, C, and D) is more than 1 month.

F. The disturbance causes clinically significant distress or impairment in social, occupational, or other important areas of functioning.

From American Psychiatric Association. Posttraumatic stress disorder. In: *Diagnostic and statistical manual of mental disorders.* 4th ed, text revision (DSM-IV-TR). Washington (DC): American Psychiatric Association; 2000: 467–468.

more attention given in each revision to alternative ways in which children may manifest these symptoms. There also have been changes and ongoing debate on whether the required number of symptoms in each category is appropriate for children (40). The current requirements are that the child must exhibit at least one reexperiencing symptom, three avoidance/numbing symptoms, and two increased arousal symptoms to receive a *DSM-IV* PTSD diagnosis. These requirements are based on current diagnostic criteria for adult PTSD, which may require amendment for younger children.

Reexperiencing symptoms include recurrent and intrusive distressing memories of the event, which in young children may be manifested by repetitive play with traumatic themes; recurrent distressing dreams about the trauma or frightening dreams without recognizable content; acting or feeling as if the trauma were recurring, including trauma-specific reenactment (for example, reenacting sexual acts the child experienced during sexual abuse); intense distress at exposure to cues that symbolize or resemble an aspect of the trauma; and physiologic reactivity at exposure to such cues.

Avoidance of stimuli associated with the event and numbing of general responsiveness must not have been present before the trauma and may be manifested by efforts to avoid thoughts, feelings, or conversations associated with the trauma; efforts to avoid reminders of the trauma; amnesia for an important aspect of the trauma; diminished interest or participation in normal activities; feelings detached or estranged from others; restricted affective range; and a sense of a foreshortened future (e.g., believing one will not live a normal life span).

Persistent symptoms of increased arousal must be newly occurring since the trauma and include sleep difficulties, irritability, or angry outbursts; difficulty concentrating; hypervigilance; and exaggerated startle response. The symptoms must be present for at least 1 month and must cause clinically significant distress or impairment in functioning.

The course of PTSD is quite variable. Some individuals develop symptoms immediately following the trauma. In the first month after a traumatic event, the diagnosis applied is acute stress disorder (ASD). The symptoms of ASD are similar to those of PTSD, although somewhat milder. Moreover, with ASD there is a greater emphasis on the symptom of dissociation. After a month, the diagnosis becomes PTSD. However, some trauma survivors may not develop symptoms of PTSD for months or even years after exposure to a trauma (42).

Once someone develops PTSD, it can become a lifetime illness. Many persons with PTSD experience multiple traumas over the course of their lives. For them, the symptoms of PTSD can continue for decades (42).

CLINICAL PRESENTATION

PTSD can present with a wide variety of clinical features. Developmental factors clearly play a strong role in these variations (42).

In general, as children mature, they are more likely to exhibit adult-like PTSD symptoms. Thus adolescents with PTSD may meet strict DSM-IV criteria with reexperiencing symptoms such as intrusive thoughts and nightmares, avoidance of discussion of the traumatic event and places or people psychologically associated with the event, amnesia for an important aspect of the trauma, withdrawal from friends or usual activities, detachment from others and sense of foreshortened future, and hyperarousal such as sleep difficulties, hypervigilance, and increased startle response. Adolescents with chronic PTSD who have experienced prolonged or repeated stressors may present with predominantly dissociative features, including derealization, depersonalization, self-injurious behavior, substance abuse, and intermittent angry or aggressive outbursts.

Clinical reports have suggested that some elementary school-age children may not experience amnesia for aspects of the trauma and with acute PTSD may not have avoidant or numbing symptoms. They also may or may not have visual flashbacks (41). Children in this developmental stage may show frequent posttraumatic reenactment of the trauma in play, drawings, or verbalizations. They also may have skewed sense of time during the traumatic event. Sleep disturbances may be especially common in prepubertal children.

Very young traumatized children may present with relatively few DSM-IV PTSD symptoms. In part this may be because 8 out of 18 DSM-IV criteria require verbal descriptions from patients of their experiences and internal states (40). The limited cognitive and expressive language skills in young children make inferring their thoughts and feelings difficult. Infants, toddlers, and preschool children, therefore, may present with generalized anxiety symptoms (separation fears, stranger anxiety, fears of monsters or animals), avoidance of situations that may or may not have an obvious link to the original trauma, sleep disturbances, and preoccupation with certain words or symbols that may or may not have an apparent connection to the traumatic event, rather than with more typical DSM-IV manifestations. Scheering and associates proposed an alternative checklist to DSM-IV criteria for detecting PTSD in young children (43). These authors differentiate between posttraumatic play (which is compulsively repetitive, represents part of the trauma, and fails to relieve anxiety) and play reenactment (which also represents part of the trauma but is less repetitive and more like the child's pretrauma play). Either of these may fulfill the reexperiencing criteria, as can nonplay recollections of the trauma (which are not necessarily distressing) or nightmares. Scheering and colleagues also suggested that in the avoidance/numbing category, only one of the following be required: constriction of play (with or without posttraumatic play), social withdrawal, restricted range of affect, or loss of acquired developmental skills (43). These authors further suggested that only one symptom of increased arousal be required to diagnose PTSD in very young children, but they suggested requiring at least one item from an added category, new fears and/or aggression. Thus, there is no clear consensus about the "typical" clinical presentation of PTSD in very young children.

Many recent studies suggest that PTSD is a significant outcome for many different forms of childhood trauma (44–49).

ASSESSMENT

The assessment of PTSD in children depends first and foremost on careful and direct clinical interviews with the child and the parents. If a parent is the alleged perpetrator of the child abuse or domestic violence that is the identified traumatic event, the nonoffending parent or another caretaker should be interviewed. Briefly, both parents and child should be asked directly about the traumatic event and about PTSD symptoms in detail. Specific questions related to reexperiencing and avoidant and hyperarousal symptoms as described in DSM-IV should be asked. Particular attention should be given to the use of developmentally appropriate language when asking the child about these PTSD symptoms. The clinician should be aware of developmental variations in the presentation of PTSD symptoms, particularly with preschool children, and should include questions about developmentally specific symptoms when interviewing young children.

There are many unanswered questions regarding how to assess children for the presence of PTSD. Although several questionnaires and semistructured interviews purport to measure this disorder, there is no single instrument accepted as a "gold standard" for making this diagnosis or monitoring its symptom course.

CLINICAL IMPLICATIONS

Identification of children who have responded to an event (trauma, medical condition, medical procedure) with posttraumatic stress is not purely of academic interest. There is a growing body of literature that suggests PTSD can have a cascading negative effect on children's development and functioning (45,46).

Experiencing traumatic events can have significant behavioral and psychological consequences. These include increased propensity to anger, aggression, suicidal ideation, substance dependence, health care use, learning problems, and engaging in criminal acts (50). The psychological consequences of childhood victimization can also include developmental delays, increased anxiety and depressive symptoms, and sexually inappropriate and regressive behaviors (50).

Recent investigation documents that childhood traumatic stress exposure and posttraumatic symptomatic distress make significant independent contributions to the explanation of childhood health problems over and above the contributions of key demographic, family, and maternal characteristics (e.g. child sex, family income, maternal substance abuse) (51).

Clinical efforts must be made to prevent the development of posttraumatic stress responses in medical settings through "trauma-aware" care, which focuses on decreasing the helplessness and fear that transforms a stressful procedure or event into a traumatic one (46). Dr. Rennick and colleagues have highlighted the significant risk of PTSD and the possible association of invasive procedures as a potential contributor to PTSD in pediatric intensive-care survivors (52).

TREATMENT

Despite the paucity of empirical treatment outcome studies, strong clinical consensus among experts in the field suggests essential components of treatment for children with PTSD, including direct exploration of the trauma, use of specific stress management techniques, exploration and correction of inaccurate attributions regarding the trauma, and inclusion of parents in treatment (40).

Direct exploration with the child of the traumatic event and its impact makes intuitive sense if PTSD is conceptualized as a direct response to that event. However, some clinicians avoid directly discussing the event for fear of transiently increasing the child's symptoms or because of their own need to avoid the negative affect associated with such discussion. There is a powerful adult desire to "let sleeping dogs lie" in children, even if PTSD symptoms suggest that the impact of the trauma is not dormant. The child's own avoidance of talking about the trauma also is often a reason therapists hesitate to discuss it directly. Many therapists have been discouraged from directly discussing certain traumatic events (e.g., child abuse) for fear of tainting the child's potential testimony in subsequent legal proceedings. This concern has arisen from recent controversy about the suggestibility of children's memories and the idea that repeated suggestive questioning may change a child's memory of the factual aspects of an event. However, even if this premise is accepted, and empirical evidence is quite contradictory on this score, direct exploration of the traumatic experience and its meaning to the child as used in psychotherapy does not involve repeated suggestive attempts to alter the child's description of what occurred. Rather, it involves encouraging a child, through relaxation and desensitization procedures, to describe the event with diminished hyperarousal and negative affect.

Another element common to most interventions for traumatized children involves evaluation and reconsideration of cognitive assumptions the child has made with regard to the traumatic event. Faulty attributions regarding the trauma (e.g., "it was my fault," "nothing is safe anymore") should be explored and challenged, beyond mere reassurances. Challenging most often is accomplished through step-by-step logical analysis of the child's cognitive distortions within therapy sessions. Other issues, such as survivor guilt and omen formation, also should be challenged.

Expert consensus also indicates that inclusion of parents and/or supportive others in treatment is important for resolution of PTSD symptoms. Parental emotional reaction to the traumatic event and parental support of the child are powerful mediators of the child's PTSD symptoms. Including parents in treatment helps them monitor the child's symptoms and learn appropriate behavior management techniques, both in the intervals between treatment sessions and after therapy is terminated. In addition, helping parents resolve their emotional distress related to the trauma, to which the parent usually has had either direct or vicarious exposure, can help the parent be more perceptive of and responsive to the child's emotional needs.

Review of current studies suggests that structured treatment focusing on PTSD and trauma symptoms can ameliorate the effects of child and adolescent trauma (50). This suggests that there may be value in increasing the skills of front-line, child-serving professionals, and in particular pediatricians, to directly conduct brief psychosocial supportive treatment for children exposed to trauma.

PSYCHOPHARMACOLOGY

A few studies have indicated that some children with PTSD exhibit physiologic abnormalities similar to those seen in adults with PTSD. Although findings are preliminary, these reports have led clinicians to prescribe a variety of medications for children with PTSD, despite a lack of randomized trials supporting efficacy. Looff and associates reported that carbamazepine resulted in complete remission of symptoms in 22 of 28 children with PTSD (53). These findings were complicated by the fact that several of the children were concurrently taking methylphenidate, clonidine, selective serotonin reuptake inhibitors (SSRIs), or tricyclic antidepressants. Famularo and co-workers demonstrated significant decreases in PTSD symptoms in 11 sexually and/or physically abused children following a 5-week course of propranolol (54). Neither study used a control group or randomization of treatment. Harmon and Riggs reported a decrease in at least some PTSD symptoms in all 7 children included in an uncontrolled clinical trial using clonidine patches (55). Brent and associates suggested that antidepressants may be helpful for some children with PTSD, particularly those with a predominance of depressive or panic disorder symptoms (56). To date, there have been no empirical studies of antidepressants for PTSD in children.

At this time there is inadequate empirical support for the use of any particular medication to treat PTSD in children. Drawing from the adult literature, it seems that the use of conventional psychotropic medication for PTSD is at most mildly effective (40). Because of the lack of adequate empirical data, clinicians must rely on judgment to determine the appropriateness of psychopharmacologic interventions in children with PTSD who have prominent depressive, anxiety, panic, and/or ADHD symptoms. Medication should be selected on the basis of established practice in treating the co-morbid condition (e.g., antidepressants for children with prominent depressive symptoms). Because of their favorable side-effect profile and evidence supporting effectiveness in treating both depressive and anxiety disorders, SSRIs often are the first psychotropic medication chosen for treating pediatric PTSD. Imipramine also is used frequently in children with co-morbid panic symptoms.

CHAPTER 151E ■ SUICIDALITY

THOMAS G. IRONS

Suicide is the third leading cause of death in young Americans between the ages of 10 and 19, behind accidents and homicide. Boys are at 5 to 7 times greater risk for suicide than girls, although girls attempt it more frequently. Between 1992 and 2001, the overall rate in this age group declined slightly, but age distribution and suicide method changed significantly. Suicides by firearm decreased by an average of 8.8% annually, while suicides by suffocation increased by an average of 5.1% annually. Beginning in 1997, suicides by suffocation in the 10 to 14 age group exceeded those by firearm, such that by 2001 suffocation was almost twice as likely as firearm death. Suicides by poisoning also declined in both the 10 to 14 and 15 to 19 age groups, but overall accounted for only about 1 suicide in 9. Although data on suicide attempts are much less reliable, it is reasonable to assume that attempts by poisoning are far more frequent than those by hanging or firearm, simply because of the lethality of the latter (57).

Risk factors for suicide attempt include somatic symptoms; same-sex romantic attraction (boys only); exposure to violence, violence perpetration, or violent victimization; alcohol and marijuana use; school problems; a history of mental health treatment; and of course, depression (58). Although the link with depression is stronger than with all other factors, it is never suspected in over half of suicides. Further, it is very difficult if not impossible to ascertain whether the treatment of depression reduces suicide risk. Nevertheless, because it is the most frequently identified preexisting condition in successful suicide, it is reasonable to treat with a selective serotonin reuptake inhibitor (SSRI), along with counseling, under the assumption that treatment affords some protection. The superior effectiveness of the SSRIs in adolescents, with or without counseling, has been clearly documented (59). New concerns about increased suicidal ideation in children and youth treated with these agents require that patients and families be fully informed about this potential risk and be alerted to signs that such ideation is present (60). This will be discussed in more detail later in this chapter.

WHEN TO HOSPITALIZE

Patients hospitalized on pediatric units after suicide attempts are most likely to have used prescription or nonprescription medications, illegal drugs, or poisons. Some may have attempted suicide by self-mutilation, such as cutting of the wrists, and others by more lethal methods that have been aborted or failed. Others may present to the outpatient clinic or emergency department with somatic symptoms or other complaints. Ascertaining the presence or absence of suicidal thoughts is extremely important, and can be difficult in less communicative patients. A direct, open, and compassionate approach is most likely to be effective. Many pediatricians, including this author, ask directly "Have you thought about, or are you thinking about, taking your own life?" when there is any indication of suicide risk. Horowitz and associates at Boston Children's Hospital in 2001 evaluated a 14-item suicidality screening instrument designed for use by non-mental health professionals in the emergency department. The subjects were 144 children and adolescents, mean age 13.6 years (61). In their study, there were two minimally different combinations of 4 questions that were as highly sensitive as the entire questionnaire, and with an acceptable specificity of about 40%. The most sensitive combination was the following:

1. "Are you here because you tried to hurt yourself?"
2. "In the past week, have you ever thought about killing yourself?"
3. "Have you ever tried to hurt yourself in the past other than this time?"
4. "Has something very stressful happened to you in the past few weeks?"

The second-most sensitive combination substituted this similar question for item three: "Did you ever seriously consider killing yourself in the past?" Until this instrument or a similar one is proven effective in a larger sample, it is prudent to make a similar question set routine where suicidality is suspected.

DIAGNOSTIC WORKUP AND MANAGEMENT

Where hospitalization is dictated by a medical condition such as overdose, suicide precaution policies should be followed. In the case of failed attempts using more lethal methods, such as shooting or suffocation, the first priority is to address the immediate medical and surgical needs. As recovery progresses, however, it is critically important to involve a mental health professional to work with both patient and family. At times, a decision to hospitalize an older child or teen is indicated strictly because of suicide risk, despite the absence of evidence that it is protective against completed suicide. Most of these hospitalizations are in psychiatric units, which are best equipped to handle the unique needs of these patients. However, a pediatric inpatient unit may be all that is available when the need arises. When this is the case, the pediatrician, mental health professional, social worker, and nursing staff should develop a plan aimed at protecting the patient from self-harm, assessing degree of suicidality, and evaluating and, when indicated, beginning treatment for depression. In addition to the standard admission history, questions should be asked about family history of suicide and mental illness, especially major depression and bipolar disorder. The patient should also be queried about completed suicide by peers or friends. The family, school, and social situation should be thoroughly assessed. Specific risk factors such as exposure to physical or sexual violence, same-sex orientation, alcohol and marijuana use, major life stresses, and treatment for mental disorders should be explored directly and non-judgmentally.

A thorough physical examination is important, though often unproductive. One should be careful to look for scars indicative of self-mutilation, other evidence of trauma, signs consistent with marijuana use such as conjunctival erythema and dry mouth, or systemic illness that might cause depression. Laboratory workup should include complete blood count with differential, renal function, and liver function tests. Other studies are generally indicated only when specific signs and symptoms are present. An exception is a thyroid panel, which is indicated if there is any concern about hypothyroidism. Some recommend that thyroid function be checked routinely in all patients. Where drug use is suspected, a drug screen is also useful.

A written plan for ongoing treatment and follow-up should be generated and reviewed with the patient and family prior to discharge. These hospitalizations may be very brief, so it is imperative that a clear plan be in place and that steps are taken to assure compliance. Specific co-morbidities should be directly addressed. In the case of hypothyroidism, treatment of the underlying disorder may be all that is necessary. This is not usually the case, however, when depression accompanies another chronic disease. Depression usually requires a separate, but integrated management strategy. The combination of an SSRI and cognitive-behavioral therapy has been shown to be more effective than either treatment alone, and is recommended. When these agents have been prescribed, as mentioned earlier, the patient and family should be fully informed about the possible risk of a transient increase in suicidal thoughts, and a monitoring program put in place. This can usually be accomplished by telephone. The care team might arrange for twice-weekly calls for the first 2 weeks, followed by weekly calls 1 week apart. The family should have 24-hour number to call if concerns about increased suicidality arise. With older teens, it is ideal for the patient to talk directly with the pediatrician or other designated team member. Parents should be counseled to remove all firearms from the home and property if at all possible and, if not, to place them in a locked cabinet with ammunition locked elsewhere. Similarly, potentially toxic medications and other poisons should be locked away, though the risk of completed suicide using these agents is quite small. Until the situation has stabilized, the family should be especially cautious about leaving the child alone at home during the school day or when parents and siblings are involved in school, faith organization, or community activities. Above all, the hospital care team should try to assure that a strong community-based support structure is available for both the patient and family, and that every possible step is taken to assure that the family can access the services they need.

Suggested Readings

AAP Committee on Adolescence. Suicide and suicide attempts in adolescents. *Pediatrics* 2000;105;871–874.

Adler RS, Jellinek MS. After teen suicide: issues for pediatricians who are asked to consult to schools. *Pediatrics* 1990;86;982–987.

Gould MS, Marrocco FA, Kleinman M, et al. Evaluating iatrogenic risk of youth suicide: a randomized controlled trial. *JAMA* 2005;293;1635–1643.

Keith CR. Adolescent suicide: perspectives on a clinical quandary. *JAMA* 2001;286;3126–3127.

Weissman MM, Wold S, Goldstein RB, et al. Depressed adolescents grown up. *JAMA* 1999;281;1707–1713.

Zametkin AJ, Alter MR, Yemini T. Suicide in teenagers: assessment, management, and prevention. *JAMA* 2001;286;3120–3125.

CHAPTER 151F ■ CONVERSION DISORDER

ROBERT R. SHELTON AND JENIFER L. POWELL

Conversion disorder is classified by DSM-IV-TR as part of the more general category of somatoform disorders. These disorders all are characterized by reported physical symptoms that are suggestive of a general medical condition but that are not fully accounted for by a medical condition, the effects of a substance, or other psychiatric disorders. The physical symptoms must cause marked distress or significantly impaired functioning. Patients with somatoform disorders do not voluntarily produce their physical symptoms. In contrast, patients with a factitious disorder or malingering intentionally manufacture or feign symptoms of a medical condition (62).

The other somatoform disorders include somatization disorder, which is a chronic disorder characterized by a combination of pain, gastrointestinal, sexual, and pseudoneurological symptoms. Undifferentiated somatoform disorder is similar to somatization disorder but requires fewer unexplained physical symptoms and a relatively shorter duration (i.e., months rather than years). Psychological factors are believed to play a strong role in the timing, maintenance, or exacerbation of the severe pain experienced by patients with pain disorder. Hypochondriasis is characterized by the misinterpretation of bodily sensations or symptoms and associated preoccupation with fears of having a serious disease. Patients with body dysmorphic disorder are preoccupied with an imagined or exaggerated defect in appearance. Somatoform disorder not otherwise specified describes unexplained physical symptoms that do not fully meet the criteria for one of the other somatoform disorders (62).

DIAGNOSIS

Conversion disorder is characterized by symptoms or deficits involving voluntary motor control or sensory functions. These deficits are suggestive of a neurologic or other general medical condition. Psychological factors and psychosocial stressors are considered to be associated with the onset and/or increase in severity of the symptoms or deficits. As noted above for somatoform disorders in general, the symptoms are not considered voluntary or intentional. A diagnosis of conversion disorder is excluded if the symptoms are consistent with culturally sanctioned experiences or if deficits can be fully explained by a medical condition or the effects of a substance. The physical symptoms must be severe enough to require medical evaluation, to cause significant distress, and/or to result in impairment in social, academic, vocational, or other major areas of functioning. Finally, pain or sexual dysfunction is not the sole deficit, and the deficit does not occur only in the presence of somatization disorder, and another mental disorder does not better account for the deficit (62).

It should be kept in mind that the diagnostic criteria for conversion disorder were developed from clinical work and research with adults rather than with children and adolescents. The incidence in adults ranges from 1% to 3%. Conversion symptoms seem to be very rare in children younger than 6 years of age. The incidence in older children and adolescents remains relatively rare but increases in frequency across this period of development (63). Incidence of conversion disorder appears to be higher among girls than among boys (63). Higher rates of conversion disorder have also been reported for children living in rural areas or in developing nations (62,63). Research has tentatively suggested that conversion symptoms in childhood or adolescence may be more common in families with lower socioeconomic status, lower levels of parent education, and less sophisticated understanding of or knowledge about physiologic and psychological functioning (62,63). Pediatric neurologists and pediatric hospitalists in tertiary care settings appear to encounter higher rates of conversion symptoms in comparison to practitioners in general pediatric community settings (63).

Motor symptoms of conversion disorder can include impaired coordination or balance, paralysis or localized weakness, hoarseness, aphonia, or coughing. Sensory symptoms can include loss of touch or pain sensation, deafness, and disturbances in vision, including blindness. Nonepileptic seizures, jerking movements, and convulsions may also be seen. Among children and adolescents, pseudoseizures, gait disturbances, paresthesia, localized weakness, fainting, and unprecipitated falls are more commonly exhibited symptoms (63). Gait disturbances and pseudoseizures are the most common presentations among children under 10 years of age (63). Symptoms often do not follow known physiologic or neural pathways, but instead reflect the patient's understanding of how the body works. The more naïve a child or adolescent is, the more implausible the presenting symptoms may be. More sophisticated patients who have greater familiarity with medical conditions may present with subtle deficits that are more difficult to distinguish from the genuine article (63).

ASSESSMENT AND DIFFERENTIAL DIAGNOSIS

As noted above, symptoms that are not *fully* accounted for by a medical condition are key to the diagnosis of conversion disorder. Potential underlying medical conditions must be ruled out before a diagnosis can be confidently made. Therefore, thorough medical and neurologic evaluations are vitally

TABLE 151.6

DISTINCTIVE PHYSICAL EXAMINATION FINDINGS IN CONVERSION DISORDER

Condition	Test	Conversion findings
Anesthesia	Map dermatomes	Sensory loss does not conform to recognized pattern of distribution.
Hemianesthesia	Check midline	Strict half-body split
Astasia-abasia	Walking, dancing	With suggestion, those who cannot walk may still be able to dance, alteration of sensory and motor findings with suggestion
Paralysis, paresis	Drop paralyzed hand onto face	Hand falls next to face, not on it
	Hoover test	Pressure noted in examiner's hand under paralyzed leg when attempting straight leg raising
	Check motor strength	Give-away weakness
Coma	Examiner attempts to open eyes	Resists opening; gaze preference is away from doctor
	Ocular cephalic maneuver	Eyes stare straight ahead, do not move from side to side
Aphonia	Request a cough	Essentially normal coughing sound indicates cords are closing
Intractable sneezing	Observe	Short nasal grunts with little or no sneezing on inspiratory phase; little or not aerolo solization of secretions; minimal facial expression; eyes open; stops when asleep; abates when alone
Syncope	Head-up tilt test	Magnitude of changes in vital signs and venous pooling do not explain continuing symptoms
Tunnel vision	Visual fields	Changing pattern on multiple examinations
Profound monocular blindness	Swinging flashlight sign (Marcus–Gunn)	Absence of relative afferent papillary defect
	Binocular visual fields	Sufficient vision in "bad eye" precludes plotting normal physiologic blind spot in good eye
Severe bilateral blindness	"Wiggle your fingers, I'm just testing coordination"	Patient may begin to mimic new movements before realizing the slip.
	Sudden flash of bright light	Patient flinches.
	"Look at your hand"	Patient does not look there
	"Touch your index fingers"	Even blind patients can do this by proprioception

From Sadock BJ, Sadock VA. *Synopsis of psychiatry: behavioral sciences/clinical psychiatry.* 9th ed. Philadelphia: Lippincott Williams & Wilkins; 2003:650.

important for establishing a conversion disorder diagnosis. Table 151.6 lists findings from the physical examination that can assist in differentiating symptoms of conversion disorder from those of a general medical condition (64).

A legitimate concern is prematurely diagnosing conversion disorder when there is actually an underlying medical condition that has not yet been identified. Data on rates of misdiagnosis of conversion disorder in children and adolescents are limited. A systematic review of misdiagnosis in adults over the past five decades found that misdiagnosis has declined considerably (65). In the 1950s, the mean rate of misdiagnosis of conversion disorder among adults was 29%. However, by the 1990s, this rate had declined to an average misdiagnosis rate of 4%, perhaps due to improved diagnostic tests and better case definitions.

Depending on the presentation, consultation of pediatric specialists may be valuable for evaluation of the presence or absence of medical conditions within their areas of expertise (e.g., neurology, infectious disease). The pediatric hospitalist and involved consultants should keep in mind that conversion disorder frequently is comorbid with a medical condition. For instance, a patient with a genuine seizure disorder can present with pseudoseizures.

Coexisting psychiatric conditions also are not uncommon among children and adolescents with conversion disorder. Depressive disorders, anxiety disorders, and other somatoform disorders are often comorbid conditions. Histrionic or dependent personality characteristics are sometimes seen as well. The possibility of intentional production of symptoms should be assessed. Malingering should be considered if there is an identifiable external incentive for manufacturing symptoms. Factitious disorder would be indicated if the motivation for symptom production is to assume a sick role. Factitious disorder by proxy occurs when symptoms are intentionally produced in the child by another person (e.g., a parent injecting a diabetic child with extra insulin). However, conversion disorder can and does occur in the absence of any other preexisting or co-occurring psychiatric diagnoses. A psychologist or psychiatrist who is experienced in working with children and adolescents in a hospital setting can provide assistance with assessment when conversion disorder is being considered with the differential diagnosis, including obtaining information about potential psychosocial stressors and assessing for other psychiatric disorders that might co-occur or better explain the presenting symptoms.

ASSOCIATED FEATURES AND ETIOLOGIC FACTORS

Primary Gain

From a traditional psychoanalytic perspective, internal conflicts are kept from entering conscious awareness by "converting" the tension associated with these conflicts into physical symptoms. From this viewpoint, the "gain" is avoidance of the conflict, and the symptom has some sort of symbolic value. However, the symbolic value is frequently not very clear in the presenting symptoms. Therefore, primary gain may not always be clearly understood (64).

Secondary Gain

Children and adolescents may gain advantages from being sick that reinforce illness behaviors, so that physical symptoms begin to have a functional purpose or value. From an operational conditioning perspective, the child may have had earlier experiences of sickness that allowed her to escape a negative situation (i.e., negative reinforcement) or to obtain perceived benefits (i.e., positive reinforcement). When stressors arise later, the child reverts to this learned mechanism. From this viewpoint, it is likely that the illness behaviors will persist as long as the reinforcing events continue. Examples of possible reinforcers include avoidance of school and increased positive attention and nurturing from parents, extended family members, teachers, and/or peers (62,64).

Role Model

The patient frequently has a role model of serious or chronic illness or injury in the immediate family system. Some case series studies have found that 25% to 50% of children with conversion disorder had presenting symptoms that resembled those of a close friend or relative (63). From a social learning viewpoint, the child has witnessed a significant other (often a parent or caregiver) obtain benefits from a period of infirmity. This observation vicariously reinforces the child's own illness behaviors. It should be noted that these behavioral models do not imply a conscious effort on the child to learn and reproduce these behaviors or an intentionally provided model. This type of learning occurs outside the level of awareness (66).

La Belle Indifference

The child or adolescent may appear to have an air of indifference or a lack or concern towards his illness or disability. Parents and physicians may appear to be much more distressed or bothered by symptoms or deficits in comparison to the child who is actually experiencing the symptoms. However, this feature is not always present. In some cases, the patient may be extremely worried about the condition (63,64).

Stressors

By definition, some type of stressor(s) or conflict(s) should be identified in association with a diagnosis of conversion disorder. Stressors may be acute and traumatic or chronic. However, the level of stress experienced by a child with conversion disorder often is not unusual or extreme when compared with children who develop other psychiatric conditions. Examples of potential stressors include family chaos, family conflict, financial problems, school difficulties, child abuse, serious illness or disability of family members, a family preoccupation with disease, or the death of a loved one. The child and family may not be aware of or may underestimate the degree of stress the child has experienced. When compared to healthy peers, some children and adolescents with conversion disorder seem to experience higher levels of stress in response to fairly normal or everyday events and interpersonal interactions (66).

Family System

For younger children, the child's family of origin constitutes the world in which they live. For children of any age, their family of origin has taught them how to experience their bodies, the world, and other people. The child develops his capacity for coping with stressful situations from within this learning environment. The families of children with conversion disorder may appear superficially stable but on closer examination may be experiencing an inordinate amount of stress. Tension and anger often may be denied rather than dealt with directly. The family may appear to invest a great deal of energy in the child's illness. From a family systems perspective, the focus of attention and energy on the child's symptoms may allow the family to avoid dealing with other problems (66,69).

Ultimately, as with so many behavioral health issues, the nature of conversion disorder may best be understood as multifactorial.

MANAGEMENT

Once a diagnosis of conversion disorder has been proposed, a primary concern is the response of staff. The temptation on the part of the medical team may be to confront the patient and family with what appear to be manufactured symptoms. Not surprisingly, medical personnel are sometimes frustrated by such a symptom presentation and may feel manipulated. The pediatric hospitalist is in a position to educate staff about conversion disorder and to coach the most appropriate and helpful responses. Confronting the child and the family often results in defensiveness and anger and sometimes leads to an AMA discharge and/or a prolonged period of seeking multiple opinions at several different medical institutions. Unfortunately, in this scenario, it is unlikely that the child will experience improvement in the presenting symptoms.

Considering the possible contributory factors discussed above, the pediatric hospitalist can encourage staff to view the symptoms not as a deliberate manipulation but rather as the only mechanism the child currently possesses to cope with stress and/or to obtain increased nurturing from her environment. This approach allows the medical team and other staff to tailor discussions of impressions and to develop interventions in a manner that helps the child and family feel more confident that the child's symptoms are being appropriately evaluated and addressed and that facilitates their participation in the treatment plan. For example, the child who has a gait disturbance is not told there is nothing wrong with him and immediately expected to skip and run. If he presents with a gait disturbance, treatment begins with that gait disturbance. The primary goal of treatment is complete restoration of functioning. A secondary goal is improvement on the part of the child (and family) in managing stress.

Psychologists or psychiatrists experienced in working with children and adolescents may provide helpful consultation in developing how to best approach the patient and family and what to tell them. The child's developmental level and the degree of sophistication of the child and family in coping with explanations of a psychological nature will affect how to best communicate with the patient and family about the conceptualization of symptoms. Most families benefit from reassurance that the major serious conditions or illnesses that can produce similar physical symptoms have been ruled out. Speed suggests informing the patient and family that all tests have come back within normal ranges (if that is the case), and that functioning can be restored (68). In the case of presenting motor disturbances, the added explanation may be given that messages from the brain have not been transmitted to the muscles in a normal fashion, but that physical and/or occupational therapies will reestablish a normal flow of these messages. Parents and older children with less severe deficits may benefit from a discussion of mind–body connections and the possible relation of stress to presenting symptoms.

A number of consultants may assist the pediatric hospitalist with management and discharge planning. A child and adolescent psychiatrist may provide recommendations for psychopharmacological interventions if significant co-morbid mood or behavior disturbances accompany the presentation of conversion disorder. Depending on the level of social stress the patient and family experience, consultation with social work staff may also be useful. Social workers may also provide valuable assistance in reporting child abuse and communicating with child protective services if child abuse is identified as a family stressor or if evidence begins to suggest factitious disorder by proxy instead of conversion disorder.

Child and adolescent psychologists or psychiatrists can provide recommendations for ongoing treatment after discharge from the acute hospital. The nature of recommended treatment will depend in part on the type and severity of functional deficits. For example, outpatient treatment with an emphasis on individual psychotherapy and possibly family therapy may be recommended for children and adolescents presenting with pseudoseizures. A referral for inpatient rehabilitation may be considered if the child has a gait disturbance or paralysis that creates severe functional impairments, since children with these deficits often benefit from the intensive therapies available in inpatient rehabilitation programs. Physical medicine and rehabilitation consultants, if available, may assist in determining if inpatient or outpatient rehabilitation therapies might be appropriate for a child or adolescent displaying severe motor deficits.

Communication among treatment providers is vital. Good communication is more easily accomplished in inpatient rehabilitation programs, in which intervening professionals are already functioning as a unified team. If the child is not transferred to inpatient rehabilitation, she may be separately involved with a physical therapist, an occupational therapist, a psychologist, and the referring physician. If this team is able to regularly and effectively communicate regarding diagnosis and treatment expectations, success will be enhanced.

If inpatient or outpatient rehabilitation is necessary, several authors recommend a "restrained" approach (67,68). Clearly defined rehabilitation goals are established, and the patient progresses in a stepwise fashion from goals of lower to higher difficulty and complexity. This approach is restrained in the sense that a patient is not allowed to move ahead to favored physical activities until all rehabilitation goals at lower levels are met. Hope for and expectation of improvement are incorporated in all exchanges with the patient and family. Working toward and achieving goals is positively reinforced with frequent praise and sometimes with concrete rewards or privileges.

The child or adolescent ideally should participate in psychotherapy concurrently with rehabilitation therapies. Younger children may benefit from a combination of play therapy and family therapy. Older children and adolescents can benefit from cognitive-behavioral therapy as well as family therapy. Because it is possible that these children label their emotional states as physiologic experiences, one goal of therapy is to assist the child in identifying various feeling states. Other therapy goals often include identification of sources of stress and teaching more adaptive coping strategies (66). Family therapy can help identify patterns of interaction that may reinforce the illness behaviors and can help change these interactions. In addition, family therapy can reduce the overall stress level the child experiences by increasing open and clear communication within the family (66,69).

PROGNOSIS

The majority of children and adolescents with conversion disorder improve within a month. Sudden onset, easily identifiable stressors, good premorbid adjustment, and an absence of comorbid psychiatric or medical conditions are associated with better prognosis. The long-term outcome worsens when conversion symptoms are present for longer periods. A Turkish study of 40 children and adolescents diagnosed with conversion disorder found that 85% (34) of the patients fully recovered within 4 years, with nearly half of those 34 displaying improvement within the first month (70). Patients whose recovery takes longer are at risk for ongoing psychiatric problems, especially mood disorders (64).

Case Study

An 8-year-old boy presented to the hospital emergency department with an 11-day history of lower extremity weakness. He recently had been diagnosed by his pediatrician with otitis media and had been treated with amoxicilin. He complained of his head spinning, of headaches, and of weakness and pain in his lower extremities that made it impossible for him to walk. In the ED, he was given Rocephin. He was admitted to the acute hospital, and he underwent a full array of diagnostic tests. His head CT was negative, and his lumbar puncture was unremarkable. Neurology was consulted, and all recommended tests came back negative. Blood and CSF cultures were all negative. White blood cell counts were within normal limits, and his ESR was reassuring. A psychology consultation did not find co-morbid mood disorders but revealed a history of a learning disability, which might affect the level of stress experienced at school. The psychologist learned that the child's father had been injured in a fall 2 years earlier, which resulted in a permanent limp and an inability to return to his former job. The family lived with a grandparent, and the patient's mother alluded to tension at home, although she would not discuss this openly. The patient also had a younger sibling who was noted to be very active and to demand much of the parents' attention.

After a 6-day stay in the acute hospital, the patient was transferred to inpatient rehabilitation. During his 2-week rehabilitation stay, the nature of his condition was repeatedly demonstrated through inconsistent performance in therapies, observations of moving without difficulty when distracted (e.g., when playing games), and observations of exaggerated effort and uneconomic postures. In addition, the child was observed to exhibit qualitatively worse functioning when certain family members were present. Due to limited sophistication displayed by family members during family conferences, the medical team, in consultation with psychology, made the decision not to use the label "conversion disorder" with the family. The child's course of treatment was reviewed with them, emphasizing that any prior infectious process was now resolved, and that recovery was expected to be complete after a course of rehabilitation therapies.

The child continued to deny awareness of any stressors. The psychologist focused on educating family members about potential reinforcers for his illness behavior as well as possible sources of stress. A child life specialist/recreation therapist developed a poster of a "goal mountain" that portrayed gradual, concrete goals for the patient to meet with input from physical and occupational therapists. Challenges in treating this patient included his father's ongoing focus on a physiologic reason for the symptoms. His mother's observations of her son's variable presentation as she remained with him during the rehabilitation admission likely contributed to her increasing comfort with the possibility that her son's symptoms were at least partially psychogenic in nature. Another challenge was adequately educating the treating staff and ensuring that they were "on the same page" regarding the patient's treatment plan. Some staff seemed overly focused on "proving" that the child was faking symptoms. Ultimately, the patient was discharged having made substantial improvements, although some minor gait disturbance was still noted. Discharge planning included arrangement of outpatient physical therapy and outpatient psychological services, with a focus on family therapy.

CHAPTER 151G ■ EATING DISORDERS

THOMAS G. IRONS

Eating disorders most commonly have their onset during adolescence. The fourth edition of the *Diagnostic and Statistical Manual of Mental Disorders* (71) identifies two primary categories: anorexia nervosa (AN) and bulimia nervosa (BN). A third category, identified as "eating disorder, not otherwise specified (ED-NOS)," reflects the diversity of presentations of these disorders, which not uncommonly occur, over time, in the same patient. Some patients included in the ED-NOS category are likely to be those whose symptoms have not progressed to the point where a definitive diagnosis is possible. Proof is lacking, but it is quite possible that aggressive treatment of these patients before they have progressed to a definitive diagnosis may significantly improve outcomes.

Although disordered eating presents primarily in adolescent females, specialists in the field have identified a growing number of early school-age girls who already are obsessively concerned with dieting, exercise, and weight loss. And the number of male teens with eating disorders, now about 10% of all those diagnosed, appears to be also growing.

Outside the developed world, these diagnoses are rare. They appear to primarily occur in societies where "food is plentiful and where thinness for women is correlated with attractiveness" (72). It is well known that in anorexic patients whose treatment begins in adulthood, the prognosis is much less favorable than in those treated during adolescence. In the United States, their prevalence on college and university campuses is such that most student health services have defined programs aimed at prevention, symptom identification, and treatment. The common factor among all the diagnostic categories is dieting. It is not surprising that in this affluent society where dieting is pervasive, these disorders are far more common than they were a few decades ago. There is also a strong link with so-called "visual sports" such as ballet, gymnastics, and modeling. Although it is clear that social, cultural, and economic conditions play an important role, uncertainty about the underlying etiology still exists. Psychiatrists have traditionally associated this group of disorders with certain family dynamics, using such descriptive phrases as "enmeshed mother, distant father" or "enmeshed, controlling family." It is far from clear, however, that these dynamics play a causative role. They are usually identified at the time the diagnosis is made, when symptoms may have been present for months. It can be speculated that these dynamics evolve along with the disease process, as the family unit responds to the child's symptoms. Whatever the role of these dynamics, it is unwise and perhaps harmful to approach the family from this angle rather than from the perspective of helping the child and family deal with the symptoms and their relationships more successfully.

ANOREXIA NERVOSA: HISTORY, DIAGNOSIS, AND MANAGEMENT

Anorexia usually begins in adolescence. Perfectionism appears to be a strongly predisposing personality trait. The disorder is characterized by severe distortion of body image, refusal to maintain body weight above a minimally acceptable level relative to height, obsession with diet and exercise, irrational fear of weight gain, and in post-menarchal females, amenorrhea. The DSM-IV criteria (71) specify a weight below 85% of the expected weight and amenorrhea (assuming the absence of hormone therapy) for 3 months. Two types are defined. In the restricting type, the patient is not regularly engaged in bingeing or purging (with vomiting, laxatives, or diuretics), while in the bingeing and purging type she is.

Patients almost never seek help for this condition from peers, nonparent adults, parents, or health professionals. Patients may present because of an entirely different problem, but more often are brought in by concerned parents, often after prolonged family struggles and increasing conflict. If a parent says to the pediatrician that he suspects an eating disorder, the odds that such is present are high. The cognitive distortions and eating and weight loss patterns are so distinctive as to make it difficult to confuse these patients with thin, otherwise healthy people, those with inflammatory bowel disease, or those with primary endocrine disorders.

In the outpatient setting, they are managed by a team led by the primary care physician, with the close partnership of mental health and nutrition professionals. Treatment is weight-focused, with weight goals carefully monitored in the office setting. A gradual increase in calorie intake, which is often less than 700 kcal/day, is required, so that the patient reaches an intake level sufficient for a weight gain of 0.5 to 0.9 kg or 1 to 2 lbs/week. In the United States, patients and families think of weight almost exclusively in pounds. Patients must be weighed at a consistent time, wearing only underpants and gown, and after voiding. They are at best passive about treatment and more often actively resistant. It is important that the team set firm goals and stick to them, remaining as positive as possible but always holding out the possibility of hospitalization should the patient fail to meet these goals. Medical and nutritional management are complemented by cognitive-behavioral therapy (CBT) delivered by a mental health professional experienced in the care of these patients. This therapy is aimed at helping the patient recognize intrusive, irrational thoughts and develop strategies for dealing with them. Ideally, families also receive therapeutic interventions, ranging from family therapy to support groups. Oral contraceptives may be used to restore menstruation, but are ineffective at reducing the osteopenia associated with this disorder.

Hospitalization

The effects that lead to hospitalization are largely related to starvation, though concomitant mental disorders, such as depression and suicidality, may of themselves demand inpatient care. Patients with more advanced disease, or those who are progressing despite intensive, team-based outpatient therapy, should whenever possible be hospitalized where defined, team-based eating disorder care is available. Teams are comprised, at a minimum, of a primary care physician, mental health professional, nutritionist, and nurses. All must have sufficient background knowledge and training sufficient to care for these very challenging patients and families. For more severely affected patients, eating disorder centers are an ideal choice. These may be based in psychiatric or pediatric adolescent facilities, often depending upon the specialty training of the program director. Wherever the program is based, a strong partnership between mental health, pediatric, nursing, and nutrition professionals is extremely important.

Hospitalization should be seriously considered for any patient whose weight is below 75% of ideal weight for height. Even if the weight is at 85% of ideal weight but the patient is not meeting preset weight gain goals or continuing to lose weight, hospitalization is required. Occasionally, early psychiatric hospitalization may be required because of a psychiatric co-morbidity such as suicidality. The obsessions associated with this disorder are powerful and strengthened continually as weight loss continues. Patients who are in serious physical danger may strongly resist hospitalization. Although it is important to be both compassionate and supportive, goals must be reinforced with firmness and resolve. Other indications for immediate hospitalization include orthostatic hypotension, prolonged QT interval on ECG, pulse < 50, electrolyte imbalance (usually related to purging), or any intercurrent illness that increases the risk of a major adverse event.

Physical Findings and Diagnostic Studies

On physical examination, aside from an often-striking apathy, the findings are consistent with starvation. Despite the flat affect and denial, these patients are in pain and acutely sensitive to their interactions with the health care team. The Something Fishy website (www.something-fishy.org) uses quotes from actual provider–patient interactions to illustrate this. The blood pressure and body temperature are low. Among the commonly observed findings are dry skin with lanugo hair, atrophic breasts, bradycardia, scaphoid abdomen with palpable stool, peripheral edema, and decreased deep tendon reflexes. Those with the bingeing and purging type may have loss of tooth enamel, especially on lingual surfaces; enlarged, tender parotids; knuckle calluses; and a tender epigastrium. Laboratory studies should include complete blood count, urinalysis, serum electrolytes, calcium, phosphorus, magnesium, creatinine, fasting glucose, and thyrotropin. An electrocardiogram is indicated for any patient whose weight is below 75% of that expected, bradycardia less than 50, or orthostatic hypotension resulting in a pulse drop < 20 or BP drop < 10 mm Hg.

Refeeding

Most refeeding regimens set the initial daily caloric intake at 1,200 to 1,500 calories. The nutritionist should work with the patient and family to negotiate food choices within the daily minimum. In the first few days, most centers use total liquid nutrition. Solid foods are added gradually as weight gain commences. The calories are generally increased in 500-kcal increments about every 4 days. The target intake most often recommended is 3,500 kcal for females and 4,000 kcal for males. Supplemental night-time tube feeding is generally not helpful and may increase resistance of the patient to treatment. Units expecting to hospitalize these patients should have written protocols for inpatient management. Review of the excellent clinical pathway developed and published by clinicians at Stanford (73) will be helpful in protocol development.

Close monitoring is required. Balancing the requirement for such monitoring with the patient's need to preserve some autonomy is difficult, but very important. In addition to daily weights, on the same scale, in the morning, after voiding, and in only gown and underpants, vital signs must be monitored, as should electrolytes, phosphorus, and magnesium. Orthostatic vital signs should be taken every 8 hours until hypotension has resolved. Supplementation is required when indicated, as are daily multivitamin-mineral combinations. Calcium supplementation is standard, and daily zinc sulfate is often given. Patients should be observed very frequently, if not continuously, during and for an hour after feeding. Monitoring during bathroom use is necessary to prevent secretive purging

and/or exercise. During refeeding, patients are especially vulnerable to hypophosphatemia and hypokalemia. Those who are more severely affected, especially those who present with abnormalities on ECG other than bradycardia, require continuous cardiac monitoring. A prolonged QT interval is particularly ominous because of the risk of arrhythmia. Hypothermia, especially during sleep, may be sufficiently severe as to require a warming blanket. Kohn and associates have described a refeeding syndrome in more severely affected patients, the manifestations of which include pedal edema (common) and much more serious complications including QT interval prolongation, hypophosphatemia, weakness, and confusion (74). These are very unusual in patients fed orally according to the previously described standard protocols. When the patient has reached the target weight, usually at least 75% of ideal body weight, is able to demonstrate reasonable independence in maintaining appropriate caloric intake, and physiologic indicators have stabilized, discharge is appropriate. Early discharge is likely to result in clinical deterioration and rehospitalization. A written plan for team-based follow-up, treatment, and monitoring should be in place at the time of discharge, and the patient and family should be able to accurately outline it. Long-term concerns include osteopenia, menstrual irregularities, cerebral atrophy, and psychological co-morbidities. Hospitalization is only one component of a comprehensive management plan that may be in place for years, even in those who fully recover. Such patients often use descriptive phrases like "It never really leaves you. . . you just learn to live with it."

BULIMIA NERVOSA

Bulimia nervosa is a disorder in which symptoms are similar to those of the bingeing-purging type of anorexia, but where weight loss may be minimal or not have progressed to the level consistent with anorexia. When that weight is reached, the primary diagnosis becomes AN, no matter what the previous course has been. Although some suggest that the entities are points along a continuum, and some bulimics transiently or permanently progress to anorexia, there are certain characteristics that are unique to each diagnostic group. On the whole, bulimics have a somewhat later age of onset, often are of normal weight, and have less serious body image distortion and exercise obsession. Of possible therapeutic value is the fact that patients with bulimia are generally less resistant to admitting to the problem and accepting help. It can be said, though it is certainly not universal, that bulimics "hate" their disease. The aforementioned Something Fishy website posts many poignant comments about this aspect of the disease.

Bulimics are more likely to abuse alcohol and to act out sexually. There is a strong association with depression. Uniquely, they are more likely to improve (in terms of symptoms of bulimia) with treatment using serotonin reuptake inhibitors, such as fluoxetine, whether or not the diagnostic criteria for depression are met. A response is most likely when the dose is at a relatively high level, usually about 60 mg/day, with the maximum dosage being achieved over a 7- to14-day period. This is almost always accomplished in the outpatient setting. It is of course important to warn patients and families of the potential for increased suicidal thinking whenever using these agents, and to monitor patients closely, especially in the early days and weeks of treatment.

Pediatric hospitalization for bulimics might occasionally be required as a result of complications or co-morbidities. A suicide attempt is almost always a cause for hospitalization (see Chapter 151E). Occasionally these patients will suffer esophageal tears or even a ruptured viscus as a result of prolonged, forceful gagging and vomiting. Electrolyte disturbances such as hypochloremic alkalosis may occur, but this is far more likely to happen in those with anorexia of the bingeing-purging type. There are case reports of sudden death due to hypokalemia. Psychiatric hospitalization, which is not within the scope of this volume, is frequently required at some point in the course of this disease. As in anorexia, a team-based management approach is important. Although weight monitoring is not usually necessary, periodic physical exams and counseling by the primary care physician are essential. Likewise, the nutritionist must work with the patient over a long period, at least several months, to help her acquire healthy, sustainable eating habits.

PEARLS

- The cornerstone of management of eating disorders is team-based therapy in or out of the hospital. All members of the team, physicians, mental health professionals, nutritionists, and nurses, should have adequate knowledge and training in the management of these patients.
- Most patients with AN have severe cognitive distortions and deny the seriousness of their disease. Bulimics are much more accepting of both the diagnosis and treatment.
- Clinical units where eating disorders are treated should have written treatment protocols.
- Refeeding is a slow and sometimes tedious process. Patience is important.
- The most serious potential complications to which one should be alert are metabolic disturbances and cardiac arrhythmias.
- Anorexics rarely benefit (in terms of symptoms of AN) from antidepressant therapy, while bulimics often do. A dosage at the high end of the therapeutic range is usually required.
- At the time of discharge, every patient and family should have a written plan that applies to all components of management, and should be able to clearly outline that plan.

Suggested Readings

American Academy of Pediatrics. Policy statement: Committee on Adolescence. Identifying and treating eating disorders. *Pediatrics* 2003;111:204–211.
American Psychiatric Association work group on eating disorders. Practice guideline for the treatment of patients with eating disorders (revision). *Am J Psychiatry* 2000;157(suppl):1–39.
Elliott DL, Goldberg L, Moe EL, et al. Preventing substance use and disordered eating. *Arch Pediatr Adolesc Med* 2004;158:1043–1049.
Le Grange D, Loeb KL, Orman SV, et al. Bulimia nervosa in adolescents. *Arch Pediatr Adolesc Med* 2004;158:478–482.
Marítnez-González MA, Gual P, Lahortiga F, et al. Parental factors, mass media influences, and the onset of eating disorders in a prospective population-based cohort. *Pediatrics* 2003;111:315–320.
Mehler PS. Bulimia nervosa. *N Engl J Med* 2003;349:875–881.
Rome ES, Ammerman S, Rosen DS, et al. Children and adolescents with eating disorders: the state of the art. *Pediatrics* 2003;111:e98–e108.
Yager J, Andersen AE. Anorexia nervosa. *N Engl J Med* 2005;353:1481–1488.

References

1. Cummings MR, Miller BD. Pharmacologic management of behavioral instability in medically ill pediatric patients. *Curr Opin Pediatr* 2004;16:516–522.
2. Dorfman DH, Mehta SD. Restraint use for psychiatric patients in the pediatric emergency department. *Pediatr Emerg Care* 2006;22:7–12.
3. Riddle M, Bernstein G, Cook E, et al. Anxiolytics, adrenergic agents, and naltrexone. *J Am Acad Child Adolesc Psychiatry* 1999;38:546–556.
4. Schieudd JNM, Lecentjans AFG. Delirium in severely ill young children in the psychiatric intensive care unit. *J Am Acad Child Adolesc Psychiatry* 2005; 44:392–394.
5. Martini DR. Commentary: The diagnosis of delirium in pediatric patients. *J Am Acad Child Adolesc Psychiatry* 2005;44:395–397.
6. Turkel SB, Travarc CJ. Delirium in children and adolescents. *J Neuropsychiatry Clin Neurosci* 2003;15:431–435.
7. American Psychiatric Association. *Diagnostic and statistical manual of mental disorders.* 4th ed., text revision (DSM-IV-TR). Washington, DC: American Psychiatric Association; 2000.
8. Volkmar FR. Childhood and adolescent psychosis: a review of the past 10 years. *J Am Acad Child Adolesc Psychiatry* 1996;35:843–851.
9. Caplan R, Tanguay P. Development of psychotic thinking in children. In: Lewis M, ed. *Child and adolescent psychiatry: a comprehensive textbook.* 3rd ed. Philadelphia: Lippincott Williams & Wilkins; 2002:359–366.
10. Pao M, Lohman C, Gracey D, et al. Visual, tactile, and phobic hallucinations: recognition and management in the emergency department. *Pediatr Emerg Care* 2004;20:30–34.
11. Schreier HA. Hallucinations in nonpsychotic children: more common than we think? *J Am Acad Child Adolesc Psychiatry* 1999;38:623–625.
12. Sorter M. Psychotic disorders. In: Klykylo WM, Kay J, Rube D, eds. *Clinical child psychiatry.* Philadelphia: Saunders; 1998:397–409.
13. Tsai L, Champine DJ. Schizophrenia and other psychotic disorders. In: Wiener JM, Dulcan MK, eds. *Textbook of child and adolescent psychiatry.* 3rd ed. Washington, DC: American Psychiatric Publishing; 2004:379–409.
14. Wills L, Garcia J. Parasomnias: epidemiology and management. *CNS Drugs* 2002;16:803–810.
15. Hollis C. Schizophrenia and allied disorders. In: Rutter M, Taylor E, eds. *Child and adolescent psychiatry.* 4th ed. Oxford: Blackwell; 2002:612–635.
16. Volkmar FR, Tsatsanis KD. Childhood schizophrenia. In: Lewis M, ed. *Child and adolescent psychiatry: a comprehensive textbook.* 3rd ed. Philadelphia: Lippincott Williams & Wilkins; 2002:745–754.
17. Mertin P, Hartwig S. Auditory hallucinations in nonpsychotic children: diagnostic considerations. *Child Adolesc Mental Health* 2004;9:9–14.
18. Bailey A. Physical Examination and medical investigations. In: Rutter M, Taylor E, eds. *Child and adolescent psychiatry.* 4th ed. Oxford: Blackwell; 2002:141–160.
19. O'Brien RF, Kifuji K. Summergrad P. Medical conditions with psychiatric manifestations. *Adolesc Med* 2006;17:49–77.
20. Cherland E, Fitzpatrick R. Psychotic side effects of psychostimulants: a 5-year review. *Can J Psychiatry* 1999;44:811–813.
21. Przybylo HJ, Przybylo J, Davis T, et al. Acute psychosis after anesthesia: the case for antibiomania. *Pediatr Anesth* 2005;15:703–705.
22. Baker C. Preventing ICU syndrome in children. *Paediatr Nurs* 2004;16:32–35.
23. Turkel SB, Tavare CJ. Delirium in children and adolescents. *J Neuropsychiatry Clin Neurosci* 2003;15:431–435.
24. Schieveld JN, Leentjens AF. Delirium in severely ill young children in the pediatric intensive care unit (PICU). *J Am Acad Child Adolesc Psychiatry* 2005; 44:392–394.
25. Martini DR. Commentary: the diagnosis of delirium in pediatric patients. *J Am Acad Child Adolesc Psychiatry* 2005;44:395–398.
26. American Psychiatric Association. *Diagnostic and statistical manual of mental disorders.* 4th ed., text revision (DSM-IV-TR). Washington, DC: American Psychiatric Association; 2000.
27. Schroeder CS, Gordon BN. *Assessment and treatment of childhood problems: a clinician's guide.* New York: Guilford Press; 1991.
28. Wallander JL, Thompson RJ Jr., Alriksson-Schmidt A. Psychosocial adjustment of children with chronic physical conditions. In: Roberts MC, ed. *Handbook of pediatric psychology.* 3rd ed. New York: Guildford Press; 2003:141–158.
29. LeBlanc LA, Goldsmith T, Patel DR. Behavioral aspects of chronic illness in children and adolescents. *Pediatr Clin North Am* 2003;50:859–878.
30. Kronenberger WG, Meyer RG. *The child clinician's handbook.* Boston: Allyn & Bacon; 1996.
31. Goodyer IM. Symptoms of depression. In: Lewis M, ed. *Child and adolescent psychiatry: a comprehensive textbook.* Philadelphia: Lippincott Williams & Wilkins; 2002:352–358.
32. Shaffer D, Gutstein J. Suicide and attempted suicide. In: Rutter M, Taylor E, eds. *Child and adolescent psychiatry.* 4th ed. Oxford: Blackwell; 2002:529–554.
33. Pfeffer CR. Suicide and suicidality. In: Wiener JM, Dulcan MK, eds. *Textbook of child and adolescent psychiatry.* 3rd ed. Washington, DC: American Psychiatric Publishing; 2004:891–902.
34. O'Brien RF, Kifuji K, Summergrad P. Medical conditions with psychiatric manifestations. *Adolesc Med* 2006;17:49–77.
35. Weller EB, Weller RA, Rowan AB, et al. Depressive disorders in children and adolescents In: Lewis M, ed. *Child and adolescent psychiatry: a comprehensive textbook.* 3rd ed. Philadelphia: Lippincott Williams & Wilkins; 2002:767–781.
36. Weller EB, Weller RA, Danielyan AK. Mood disorders in adolescents. In: Wiener JM, Dulcan, MK, eds. *Textbook of child and adolescent psychiatry.* 3rd ed. Washington, DC: American Psychiatric Publishing; 2004:437–481.
37. American Academy of Child and Adolescent Psychiatry. Practice parameters for the assessment and treatment of children and adolescents with depressive disorders. *J Am Acad Child Adolesc Psychiatry* 1998;37(suppl). 1234–1238.
38. United States Food and Drug Administration. FDA launches a multi-pronged strategy to strengthen safeguards for children treated with antidepressant medications. Press release, October 15, 2004. Downloaded from www.fda.gov.
39. American Psychiatric Association and American Academy of Child and Adolescent Psychiatry. The use of medication in treating childhood and

adolescent depression: information for patients and families. Downloaded from www.apa.org.

40. American Academy of Child and Adolescent Psychiatry. Practice parameters for the assessment and treatment of children and adolescents with posttraumatic stress disorder. *J Am Acad Child Adolesc Psychiatry* 1998;37(suppl): 4S–26 S.

41. Carrium VG, Weems CF, Ray R, et al. Toward an empirical definition of pediatric PTSD: the phenomenology of PTSD symptoms in youth. *J Am Acad Child Adolesc Psychiatry* 2002;4:166–173.

42. Brown EJ. Efficacious treatment of posttraumatic stress disorder in children and adolescents. *Pediatr Ann* 2005;34:139–146.

43. Scheering MS, Zeanah CH, Drill MJ, et al. Two approaches to diagnosing posttraumatic stress disorder in infancy and early childhood. *J Am Acad Child Adolesc Psychiatry* 1995;34:191–200.

44. Connolly D, McCloug S, Hayman L, et al. Posttraumatic stress disorder in children after cardiac surgery. *J Pediatr* 2004;114:480–484.

45. Lonigan CJ, Phillips BM, Richey JA. Posttraumatic stress disorder in children: diagnosis, assessmemt, and associated features. *Child Adolesc Psychiatr Clin* 2003;12:171–194.

46. Mintzer LL, Stuber ML, Secord D, et al. Traumatic stress symptoms in adolescent organ transplant recipients. *Pediatrics* 2005; 15:1640–1644.

47. Peters V, Sottiaux M, Appelboom J, et al. Posttraumatic stress disorder after dog bites in children. *J Pediatr* 2004;144:121–122.

48. Stuber ML, Shemesh E, Saye GN. Posttraumatic stress responses in children with life-threatening illnesses. *Child Adolesc Psychiatric Clinics North Am* 2003;12:195–209.

49. Hobbie WL, Stuber M, Meeske K, et al. Symptoms of posttraumatic stress in young adult survivors of childhood cancer. *J Clin Oncol* 2000;18:4060–4066.

50. Taylor TL, Chemtob CM. Efficacy of treatment for children and adolescent traumatic stress. *Arch Pediatr Adolesc Med* 2004;158:786–791.

51. Grupp-Phelan J, Zatzick D. Post-traumatic stress and its effect on health outcomes in children. *J Pediatr* 2005;146:309–310.

52. Rennick JE, Morin I, Kim D, et al. Identifying children at high risk for psychological sequelae after pediatric intensive care unit hospitalization. *Pediatr Crit Care Med* 2004;5:358–363.

53. Looff D, Grimley P, Kuiler F, et al. Carbamazepine for posttraumatic stress disorder. *J Am Acad Child Adolesc Psychiatry* 1995;34:703–704.

54. Famularo R, Kinscheiff R, Fenton T. Propranolol treatment for childhood posttraumatic stress disorder. *Am J Dis Child* 1988;142:1244–1247.

55. Harmon RJ, Riggs PD. Clinical perspectives: clonidine for posttraumatic stress disorder in preschool children. *J Am Acad Child Adolesc Psychiatry* 1996;35:247–1249.

56. Brent DA, Perper JA, Mariez G, et al. Posttraumatic stress disorder in peers of adolescent suicide victims. *J Am Acad Child Adolesc Psychiatry* 1995;34: 209–215.

57. Department of Health and Human Services, Centers for Disease Control and Prevention. Methods of suicide among persons aged 10–19—United States, 1992–2001. *MMWR* 2004;53:471–478.

58. Borowsky IW, Ireland M, Resnick MD. Adolescent suicide attempts: risks and protectors. *Pediatrics* 2001;107:485–493.

59. Treatment for adolescents with depression study team. Fluoxetine, cognitive-behavioral therapy, and their combination for adolescents with depression. *JAMA* 2004;292;807–820.

60. Newman TB. A black-box warning for antidepressants in children? *N Engl J Med* 2004;351;1595–1598.

61. Horowitz LM, Wang PS, Koocher GP, et al. Detecting suicide risk in a pediatric emergency department: development of a brief screening tool. *Pediatrics* 2001;107;1133–1137.

62. American Psychiatric Association. *Diagnostic and statistical manual of mental disorders*. 4th ed., text revision (DSM-IV-TR). Washington, DC: American Psychiatric Association; 2000.

63. Fritz GK, Campo JV. Somatoform disorders. In: Lewis M, ed. *Child and adolescent psychiatry: a comprehensive textbook*. 3rd ed. Philadelphia: Lippincott Williams & Wilkins; 2002:847–858.

64. Sadock BJ, Sadock VA. *Synopsis of psychiatry: behavioral sciences/clinical psychiatry*. 9th ed. Philadelphia: Lippincott Williams & Wilkins; 2003: 643–659.

65. Stone J, Smyth R, Carson A, et al. Systematic review of misdiagnosis of conversion symptoms and "hysteria." *BMJ*, doi:10.1136/bmj.38628.466898.55 (published 13 October 2005).

66. Kronenberger WG, Meyer RG. *The child clinician's handbook*. Boston: Allyn & Bacon; 1996.

67. Speed J. Behavioral management of conversion disorder: retrospective study. *Arch Phys Med Rehab* 1999;77:147–154.

68. Calvert P, Jureidini J. Restrained rehabilitation: an approach to children and adolescents with unexplained signs and symptoms. *Arch Dis Child* 2006,88: 399–402.

69. Griffith JL, Polles A, Griffith ME. Pseudoseizures, families, and unspeakable dilemmas. *Psychosomatics* 1998;39:144–153.

70. Pehlivanturk B, Unal F. Conversion disorder in children and adolescents: a 4-year follow-up study. *J Psychosom Res* 2002;52:187–191.

71. American Psychiatric Association. *Diagnostic and statistical manual of mental disorders*. 4th ed (DSMIV-TR). Washington, DC: American Psychiatric Association; 1994.

72. Rome ES, Ammerman S, Rosen DS, et al. Children and adolescents with eating disorders: the state of the art. *Pediatrics* 2003;111:e98–e108.

73. Lock J. How clinical pathways can be useful: an example of a clinical pathway for the treatment of anorexia nervosa in adolescents. *Clin Child Psychol Psychiatry* 1999;4:331–340.

74. Kohn MR, Golden NH, Shenker IR, et al. Cardiac arrest and delirium: presentations of the refeeding syndrome in severely malnourished adolescents with anorexia nervosa. *J Adolesc Health* 1998;22:239–243.

CHAPTER 152A ■ GENERAL PRINCIPLES OF PHARMACOLOGIC TREATMENTS IN MENTAL DISORDERS

RONALD M. PERKIN

ROLE OF PHARMACOLOGIC TREATMENT IN CHILD PSYCHIATRY

Drug treatment represents a powerful way of altering the behavior and mental states of children. There are large differences in prescribing practices between countries, and current usage includes drugs that may be ineffective or even hazardous. In the United States, the use of medication tends to exceed what has been validated by objective evidence for safety and efficacy (1).

Since the early 1990s, the use of psychotropic medication in children has increased. This includes, to differing degrees, several classes of drugs: stimulants, antidepressants (especially selective serotonin reuptake inhibitors [SSRIs]), antianxiety agents, and antipsychotics. Evidence of increasing use among children of various ages has been mounting for years. Previous studies have demonstrated higher rates of psychoactive prescription use in adolescents, preschoolers, and those in between (2). These medications have been prescribed for attention-deficit/ hyperactivity disorder (ADHD), conduct disorder, depression, and various other behavioral, mental, or learning disorders.

There is an understandable worry about medication in children, particularly in terms of possible long-term side effects, yet there are few data on whether children really are more vulnerable to side effects. Some children are denied treatment with medication, either because of ideological opposition to this form of therapy, or lack of knowledge. Medication has an important place in child psychiatric treatment, and expertise in the theoretical and practical aspects of drug use should be available in all child mental health services.

In almost every case, pharmacologic treatment for children with psychiatric disorders should be just one part of a package of psychological, social, and educational intervention. Even in conditions where drug treatment plays a significant part—and there are many where it does not—drug treatment will nearly always only be a component of a multimodal treatment plan (Table 152.1).

MAIN CLASSES OF DRUGS USED IN CHILD PSYCHIATRY (TABLES 152.2 AND 152.3)

Stimulants

Basic Pharmacology and Mechanism of Action

Stimulant drugs, including methylphenidate and dexamphetamine, are widely used and effective in the treatment of ADHD.

Stimulants act by releasing monoamines from nerve terminals in the brain. Noradrenaline and dopamine are the most important mediators, but serotonin release also occurs. They increase intrasynaptic concentrations of dopamine by blocking the dopamine transporter, and by displacement of monoamines from synaptic vesicles.

Side Effects and Toxicity

Although the stimulants are safe, dose-dependent side effects may occur, and are similar for all stimulants. The most common side effects are delay of sleep onset, reduced appetite, stomachache, headache, jitteriness, and dysphoria. They often wear off spontaneously, or may be reduced by lowering the dose.

Antipsychotic Drugs

Basic Pharmacology and Mechanism of Action

The antipsychotic drugs are all dopamine receptor antagonists, although many of them also act on other targets, such as serotonin, noradrenaline, and glutamate receptors. The main categories of antipsychotic drugs are the *classical* or *typical* antipsychotics, and the newer drugs, which are often called *atypical*. The classical group includes chlorpromazine, haloperidol, and thioridazine. Relatively new drugs in this group include pimozide and sulpiride. The atypical or newer antipsychotics have different pharmacologic profiles (serotonin-dopamine antagonism), generally have fewer extrapyramidal side effects, and may be effective in groups of patients resistant to treatment with the classical antipsychotics. Clozapine was the first atypical antipsychotic agent introduced and remains the only one to be therapeutically superior to other antipsychotics in efficacy (in resistant schizophrenia). The other atypical antipsychotics include risperidone, olanzapine, amisulpride, quetiapine, and ziprasidone. The behavioral effects of all antipsychotics are similar, but their side effects differ.

Side Effects and Toxicity

Antipsychotic drugs have the potential to produce significant side effects, in particular extrapyramidal side effects (including acute dystonias, akathisia, parkinsonism, and dyskinesias), sedation, and rarely, neuroleptic malignant syndrome (3). The dyskinesias are the most serious of these, and the prevalence in children ranges from 8% to 51%. This includes both tardive dyskinesia and withdrawal dyskinesia. Withdrawal dyskinesia may occur with either gradual or sudden cessation of antipsychotic agents, with one-third or more of children developing these movements when the drug is abruptly withdrawn. Withdrawal dyskinesia is

TABLE 152.1

SUMMARY OF CHILD PSYCHIATRIC DISORDERS IN WHICH DRUG TREATMENT PLAYS A SIGNIFICANT ROLE

Disorder	First-line drugs	Second-line drugs
Psychosis	Atypical antipsychotics Risperidone Olanzapine Amisulpride	Typical antipsychotics Haloperidol Chlorpromazine Clozapine
Hyperactivity	Stimulants Methylphenidate Dexamphetamine	Imipramine Clonidine Venlafaxine
Obsessive-compulsive disorder	SSRIs Sertraline Fluoxetine Paroxetine Fluvoxamine Citalopram	Clomipramine
Depression	SSRIs Sertraline Fluoxetine Paroxetine Citalopram Fluroxamine	Tricyclic antidepressants Imipramine Amitriptyline Clomipramine Atypical antidepressants

Modified from Heyman I, Santosh P. Pharmacological and other physical treatments. In: Rutter M, Taylor E, eds. *Child and adolescent psychiatry*. 4th ed. Oxford: Blackwell; 2002: 998–1018.

TABLE 152.2

SUMMARY TABLE OF DRUGS AND THEIR INDICATIONS

Drug class (specific examples)	Main indications
STIMULANTS	
Methylphenidate Dexamphetamine	ADHD, narcolepsy
ANTIPSYCHOTIC AND ANTIMANIC DRUGS	
Chlorpromazine, thioridazine, trifluoperazine, and other phenothiazines	Schizophrenia, acute aggression
Haloperidol, droperidol, pimozide, sulpiride	Schizophrenia, acute aggression
Atypical antipsychotics: clozapine, olanzapine, amisulpride, risperidone	Schizophrenia, acute aggression
Lithium	Mania, bipolar disorder
Carbamazepine	Mania, bipolar disorder
Sodium valproate	Mania, bipolar disorder
ANTIDEPRESSANTS	
Tricyclic and related antidepressants: amitriptyline, clomipramine, imipramine, trimipramine, dothiepin	ADHD (especially those with anxiety and/or tics), enuresis
SSRIs and related antidepressants: fluoxetine, fluvoxamine, paroxetine, sertraline, citalopram, venlafaxine	OCD, depression, panic disorder
MAOIs	Resistant depression
ANXIOLYTICS, SEDATIVES AND MISCELLANEOUS DRUGS	
Benzodiazepines	Sedation, acute aggression
Antihistamines	Sedation, acute aggression
Clonidine	ADHD, tics, sleep problems

ADHD, attention deficit hyperactivity disorder; MAOI, monoamine oxidase inhibitor; SSRI, selective serotonin reuptake inhibitor; OCD, obsessive compulsive disorder.
Modified from Heyman I, Santosh P. Pharmacological and other physical treatments. In: Rutter M, Taylor E, eds. *Child and adolescent psychiatry*. 4th ed. Oxford: Blackwell; 2002: 998–1018.

TABLE 152.3

DOSAGE RANGE OF PSYCHOTROPIC MEDICATION
USED IN CHILDREN AND ADOLESCENTS

Drug	Dose range
STIMULANTS	
Methylphenidate	5–60 mg/day
Dexamphetamine	2.5–40 mg/day
ANTIDEPRESSANTS	
Tricyclic antidepressants	10–20 mg/day in <6 year olds
Imipramine, desipramine	10–75 mg/day in >6 years (prepubertal)
Clomipramine	50–150 mg/day postpubertal
Selective serotonin reuptake inhibitors (SRIs)	10–200 mg/day
Fluoxetine	10–60 mg/day
Fluvoxamine	50–300 mg/day
Sertraline	25–150 mg/day
Paroxetine	10–60 mg/day
Citalopram	10–60 mg/day
ANTIPSYCHOTICS	
Haloperidol	0.5–8 mg/day (prepubertal)
Sulpiride	1–16 mg/day (postpubertal)
Clozapine	25–500 mg/day
Pimozide	50–600 mg/day
Olanzapine	1–12 mg/day
Risperidone	2.5–20 mg/day
Amisulpride	0.25–6 mg/day
Sertindole	25–1000 mg/day
Ziprasidone	2–16 mg/day
Quetiapine	40–120 mg/day
Others	25–500 mg/day
Lithium carbonate	0.4–1.0 mEq/L (serum level)
Clonidine	0.05–0.25 mg/day
Buspirone	10–45 mg/day
Naltrexone	12.5–50 mg/day

Modified from Heyman I, Santosh P. Pharmacological and other physical treatments. In, Rutter M, Taylor E, eds. *Child and adolescent psychiatry.* 4th ed. Oxford: Blackwell; 2002: 998–1018.

usually reversible, whereas tardive dyskinesia may persist even if the antipsychotic agent is discontinued.

The atypical antipsychotics are less likely to cause extrapyramidal side effects, although there are case reports of risperidone-induced dyskinesias in children.

Main Indications for Antipsychotic Drugs

Antipsychotic medication continues to be the only specific treatment of documented efficacy for psychosis, although most of the evidence for efficacy in children is an extrapolation from the adult literature. The antipsychotic drugs are also widely used in a range of behavioral emergencies.

Antidepressant Drugs

Basic Pharmacology and Mechanisms of Action

Antidepressant drugs comprise a diverse group, and new agents frequently appear on the market, reflecting the recognized shortcomings of those that are currently available. The main shortcomings (see below) are limited clinical efficacy, delayed onset of action, and prevalence of side effects.

The pharmacologic rationale for these drugs rests mainly on the monoamine theory of depression, which holds that depression results from a functional deficit of monoamine transmitters, particularly noradrenaline and serotonin. Currently, the main types of antidepressant drugs are the following:

- Tricyclic antidepressants (TCAs—e.g., imipramine, amitriptyline, clomipramine, desipramine).
- Selective serotonin reuptake inhibitors (SSRIs—e.g. fluoxetine, fluvoxamine, paroxetine, sertraline, citalopram). These widely used drugs appear to be as efficacious as TCAs (and possibly more so in children, see below), with fewer side effects.
- Monoamine oxidase inhibitors (MAOIs—e.g., phenelzine, tranylcypromine, moclobemide).
- Atypical antidepressants (e.g., maprotiline, bupropion, venlafaxine, trazodone, nefazodone, mianserin, mirtazapine). This is a heterogeneous group. Maprotiline inhibits noradrenaline uptake, and resembles the TCAs, although its chemical structure and side effects are different. Venlafaxine inhibits both serotonin and noradrenaline reuptake, and has weaker receptor-blocking actions than TCAs. The mechanism of action of bupropion is unclear. The others act mainly as antagonists of various monoamine receptors, including presynaptic adrenoceptors and serotonin receptors.

Side Effects and Toxicity

TCAs. TCSs and drugs classified as atypical antidepressants are active as antagonists at several different monoamine receptors, notably muscarinic cholinoceptors, histamine (H_1) receptors, and noradrenaline (α_1) receptors, as well as various different serotonin receptors, and these actions account for many of these side effects:

- Sedation (mainly amitriptyline, trazodone, clomipramine, maprotiline; uncommon with bupropion).
- Anticholinergic side effects (dry mouth, blurred vision, constipation, urinary retention).
- Postural hypotension (mainly TCAs, maprotiline, trazodone); paradoxically, hypertension at rest sometimes occurs, particularly with imipramine.
- Weight gain (mainly TCAs).
- Seizures (especially bupropion, but also reported with TCAs).
- Cardiotoxicity, evident as a slowing of conduction and tachycardia, which can progress to ventricular dysrhythmias, is the most serious adverse effect of TCAs, and sudden deaths have been reported in children. Other antidepressants are much safer in this respect.

SSRIs. The side effects appear to be associated with the primary mechanism of action of these drugs, and there is little evidence that individual SSRIs differ significantly from each other; venlafaxine has a similar profile:

- Agitation and insomnia
- Headache
- Nausea and vomiting, mainly at the beginning of treatment

Sexual dysfunction, a major problem associated with SSRIs in adults, is inconsequential in young children but may be important in adolescents.

MAOIs. The serious side effects of first-generation MAOIs, especially hypertensive crisis ("cheese reaction"), greatly limited their clinical utility, particularly in children.

Clinical Uses and Efficacy

A depressive disorder starting in childhood or adolescence is a serious psychiatric condition that may become a chronic illness. The prevalence of major depressive disorder and dysthymia increases dramatically in adolescents, reaching close to adult levels in late teenage years. Treatment of depression includes effective resolution of the current episode and effective prophylaxis to prevent further episodes or to reduce their morbidity if they do occur. Medication should be used in conjunction with interventions designed to improve interpersonal, social, and academic functioning.

There is increasing evidence that SSRIs are effective in child and adolescent depression, and should generally be the first choice of medication (4). Commonly used SSRIs include fluoxetine and paroxetine, with accumulating experience with sertraline and fluvoxamine.

Lithium

Basic Pharmacology and Mechanism of Action

The psychotropic effects of lithium were discovered in 1949 by Cade, and this inorganic cation is still a mainstay in the prophylaxis of manic-depressive (bipolar) illness in adults. Its mechanism of action is uncertain, although it is known to interfere with two important second messenger systems, and thus to have widespread and complex effects on neurotransmitter function.

Side Effects and Toxicity

Lithium is generally well tolerated in children and adolescents, although younger children with neurologic problems may be more vulnerable to side effects. Common side effects in chil-

dren are nausea, tremor, polyuria, and enuresis. Other potential side effects documented in adults include weight gain, acne, hypothyroidism, and impaired renal function. In younger children (aged 4–6 years), more neurologic side effects have been reported, including tremor, drowsiness, ataxia, and confusion, especially at the beginning of treatment, suggesting that a strong clinical indication would be needed to justify lithium use in such young children. Lithium has a narrow therapeutic index, and monitoring of the plasma concentration is an essential part of treatment (5). Acute lithium toxicity can cause coma, convulsions, and death, and may need treatment with plasmapheresis.

Main Indications, Including Trial Data or Other Evidence of Efficacy

The main indication for lithium use in young people, as in adults, is for the prophylaxis of bipolar disorder, and the treatment of acute mania. There have been very few good studies in children, and in general use of lithium in children is based on evidence from adult studies. There is some evidence for efficacy in the treatment of aggression, and little evidence for efficacy in the treatment of ADHD and conduct disorder.

CHAPTER 152B ■ ATYPICAL ANTIPSYCHOTIC MEDICATIONS: THERAPEUTIC CONCERNS AND OVERDOSE

DAVID L. ELDRIDGE AND ADAM K. ROWDEN

There are growing mental health concerns in the pediatric population. These problems cover a wide spectrum ranging from uniquely pediatric problems like pervasive developmental disorders that may have aggressive behavior as a component (e.g., autism) to more adult-like psychiatric disorders like schizophrenia and bipolar disorders. Behavioral therapy and psychiatric counseling remain the key to the management of these problems. In attempt to better serve these patients and their families, different medical therapies are currently being explored. One such group of medications is the *atypical antipsychotics* (Table 152.4). Though none of these are currently approved by the Food and Drug Administration (FDA) for use in children,

their use in children is becoming increasingly prevalent. The pediatric hospitalist may find her patients taking these medications for a number of currently "off-label" indications (Table 152.5). The purpose of this chapter is to familiarize the pediatric hospitalist with these medications in terms of basic pharmacology, side effects, and adverse events that occur even at therapeutic doses. It is strongly recommended that initiation and dose titration of these medications be left to those with more extensive experience with these medications, that is, child psychiatrists and developmental pediatricians.

TABLE 152.4

THE ATYPICAL ANTIPSYCHOTICS

Trade name	Generic name
Abilify	Aripiprazole
Clozaril	Clozapine
Riserdal	Risperidone
Seroquel	Quetiapine
Zyprexa	Olanzapine
Geodon	Ziprasidone

TABLE 152.5

PEDIATRIC DISORDERS WHERE ATYPICAL ANTIPSYCHOTICS ARE CURRENTLY BEING STUDIED/USED

- Aggressive or disruptive behavior secondary to developmental disorders
- Bipolar disorder
- Conduct disorder
- Eating disorders
- Obsessive compulsive disorder
- Schizophrenia
- Tic disorders

PHARMACOLOGY

The pharmacology of the first ("typical") generation of antipsychotics, such as haloperidol, involved blockade of certain neurologic dopamine receptors (specifically D_2 receptors). Although this blockade does seem to provide the desired mental health benefits of these drugs, it also seems responsible for their undesired side effects. These present in a collection of movement orders known as *extrapyramidal symptoms* (EPS) and tardive dyskinesia (TD).

In an attempt to lower the risk of these side effects, a new generation of antipsychotics was produced and is now used prominently. They differ from the typical antipsychotics by their therapeutic mechanism (Table 152.6). Though they still maintain some D_2 receptor antagonism, they do not bind as tightly as typical antipsychotics do. Instead, they exert much of their activity through serotonin receptor blockade (particularly $5-HT_{2A}$ receptors). Depending on the agent, these drugs also exert blockade on histamine, acetylcholine (muscarinic), and α_1-adrenergic receptors. These other properties help to explain many of the side effects seen with these drugs both at therapeutic dosing and in overdose. The advantage of atypical antipsychotics over the older agents is that they have similar efficacy with an improved side effect profile in regard to movement disorders.

DOSING

Therapeutic dosing of atypical antipsychotics in children has no FDA approval at this time. Currently, therefore, all uses are "off-label." The authors, again, strongly encourage that the treating physician discuss these medications carefully with a physician well-versed in their use before initiating them or titrating their dose.

There are some data in adults to suggest doses at which additional clinical benefit may not occur with further dosing increases (Table 152.7). At these doses, the risk of adverse events may very well outweigh any potential benefits. If encountering patients on doses higher than these amounts, it seems reasonable to scrutinize these doses, particularly in children.

SIDE EFFECTS OF ATYPICAL ANTIPSYCHOTICS

Though the second generation of antipsychotics does seem to have an overall decreased risk of the movement disorder that made the older class so worrisome, they are not without side effects (Table 152.8). Besides those known side effects, there is concern that these drugs, which have never been studied long term in developing children, may have unknown, long-term effects yet to be discovered.

Some of these side effects are chronic problems and are unlikely to be of acute significance in the hospital setting. This

TABLE 152.7

PROPOSED ATYPICAL ANTIPSYCHOTIC DOSES FOR NEAR-MAXIMAL THERAPEUTIC BENEFIT

Drug	Near-maximal effective dose (per day)
Aripiprazole	10 mg
Clozapine	400 mg[a]
Quetiapine	150–600 mg
Olanzapine	16 mg[a]
Risperidone	4 mg
Ziprasidone	120–160 mg (acute)
	80–160 (maintenance)

[a]Higher doses may be beneficial.
Data from Davis JM, Chen N. Dose response and dose equivalence of antipsychotics. *J Clin Psychopharmacol* 2004;24:192–208.

includes w*eight gain* and *hyperlipidemia*—problems reported with each of these medications and requiring periodic monitoring. Along these same lines of chronic health concerns, *diabetes* also now appears to be strongly associated with the use of these drugs. *Hyperprolactinemia* has been seen primarily with risperidone and can lead to gynecomastia, galactorrhea, menstrual irregularities, and sexual dysfunction. *Anticholinergic* side effects (dry mouth, constipation, tachycardia, sedation, and urinary retention) are most common with those drugs that have significant muscarinic blockade (olanzapine and clozapine). *Orthostatic hypotension* also is commonly reported, especially when using those medications with α_1-adrenergic blockade. Some degree of *sedation* is reported with all of these drugs. Other therapeutic side effects may have more acute significance. The *agranulocytosis* reported with clozapine is well known and feared. It occurs in approximately 1% of patients who use it and generally occurs within the first 2 to 3 months of use. Another rare but possibly fatal consequence of clozapine use is *myocarditis*.

Prolongation of the QTc interval has probably received the most attention and concern with these medications. Increases in this electrocardiographic interval can progress to torsades de pointes and then to ventricular tachycardia, ventricular fibrillation, and death. Although ziprasidone produces the most significant increase in the QTc interval, most of the others have this effect as well. Interestingly, aripiprazole has actually been reported to shorten it. The pediatric hospitalist needs to be keenly aware of this phenomenon both in therapeutic dosing and in overdoses involving these medications. Furthermore, caution should be used when combing these drugs with any others that have reported to prolong the QTc interval.

TABLE 152.6

RECEPTOR BLOCKADE BY ATYPICAL ANTIPSYCHOTICS

Serotonin
Dopamine
Histamine
α_1-Adrenergic
Acetylcholine (muscarinic)

TABLE 152.8

SIDE EFFECTS WITH ATYPICAL ANTIPSYCHOTIC USE

Anticholinergic (e.g., dry mouth)
Diabetes
Hyperlipidemia
Hyperprolactinemia
Orthostatic hypotension
Sedation
Weight gain
Clozapine only:
   Agranulocytosis
   Myocarditis

MOVEMENT DISORDERS

A distinct clinical advantage of atypical antipsychotics over their predecessors is the decreased risk of movement disorders. However, these phenomena continue to be reported with the new drugs as well.

Extrapyramidal Symptoms

Extrapyramidal symptoms (EPS) are a collection of adverse effects related to antipsychotic use. "Extrapyramidal" refers to areas of the brain's motor system other than the pyramidal (corticospinal) tract that are effected by the dopamine receptor blockade provided from these drugs (e.g., the basal ganglia). This side effect of these drugs gives rise to this unique set of motor disturbances. Although similar in some ways, each has some distinguishing features (Table 152.8).

Acute dystonia refers to sustained, involuntary muscle contractions that are typically focal and occur very soon after an antipsychotic is initiated. The timeline of symptom onset is generally acute and will range anywhere from within hours of the first dose to the first week of beginning the drug. Facial and oropharyngeal muscles (e.g., tongue and throat) are often involved, as are the neck muscles. Involvement of the trunk, eyes, and extremities has also been reported. Mental status is usually clear during these events, with the patient being significantly distressed by the concurrent pain and discomfort. Treatment for an acute dystonic reaction is intravenous or intramuscular administration of an anticholinergic agent, typically diphenhydramine. Due to the long half-lives of antipsychotics, if a response is seen with the initial dose of diphenhydramine, it is recommended to continue regular oral dosing for the next 2 to 3 days to prevent recurrence.

Akathisia is a particularly disturbing phenomenon for patients that provides them with a great deal of anxiety and unease. It is a more subjective movement disorder described best as a perceived inner motor restlessness. Onset may occur within hours, but generally starts within days to weeks of starting the medication. Some will report that they feel this restlessness throughout their body, but others may report that it is limited to their legs. Patients will present very anxious or tense with psychomotor agitation that may be channeled through pacing, rocking back and forth, or other forms of constant movement. Beta-blockers are recommended by some in this situation, although decreasing the antipsychotic dose will likely be an effective intervention in many cases.

Antipsychotic medication use can also lead to a drug-induced *parkinsonism* that resembles true Parkinson disease. The patient will exhibit similar features: tremor, bradykinesia, masked facies, shuffling gait, and bradykinesia. These symptoms usually take a few weeks to develop. Treatment may include anti-parkinsonian, anticholinergic medications. However, decreasing the dose of antipsychotic in question often leads to improvement.

Tardive Dyskinesia

Despite the concern about the EPS syndromes discussed above, *tardive dyskinesia* is the most feared movement disorder secondary to antipsychotic use because it does not respond well to therapy and may be permanent. Usually a patient has been taking antipsychotic medication for some time (months to years of therapy) before this develops. Because pediatric patients are being started on these drugs very early in life, it is reasonable to be concerned that they will be on them for years to come and be vulnerable to this syndrome. Fortunately, this is thought to be a very rare occurrence with the atypical antipsychotics.

The features of TD may be very subtle at first. Family members are often the first to notice these symptoms and report them to a physician. The patient will often start with involuntary twitching of orofacial muscles. This can initially be as understated as excessive eye blinking or slight involuntary movements of the tongue. Early movements may also include repetitive strumming or tapping movements of the fingers and toes. These relatively benign actions may give way to much more disturbing movements. Facial and jaw muscle involvement can progress to involuntary chewing, biting, grimacing, and lip smacking and puckering. Choreoathetoid movement of the extremities (typically distal) also occurs. All in all, these movements are socially stigmatizing and difficult for the patient to suppress.

Prevention is the key to TD. One of the first precautions is generally to use an atypical antipsychotic preferentially over first-generation (e.g., haloperidol) drugs. Using the lowest dose clinically possible for as brief a time as possible is also recommended. Regular follow-up visits with the patient's primary physician managing the patient's antipsychotic medications are a requirement. Early recognition of these symptoms should be the goal of the pediatric hospitalist. Once diagnosed, there is no one treatment that has been found to be successful in all cases. Reviewing each proposed medication for the treatment of TD is beyond the scope of this chapter. It is strongly advised that if TD is suspected during a hospital admission, consultation with a child psychiatrist or another physician well-versed in these medications be obtained.

ATYPICAL ANTIPYSCHOTICS IN OVERDOSE

In overdose, it is useful to consider the atypical antipsychotics as a group. Although each individual member of this class has specific receptor activity, this specificity is often lost in overdose. As a result, any atypical agent is capable of causing the clinical findings below.

Clinical Presentation

Much like some of the side effects in therapeutic dosing, many of the clinical effects seen in overdoses involving the atypical antipsychotics can best be understood if their pharmacology is considered. The various receptor blockades imparted by these medications lead to the symptoms seen in overdose.

The predominant neurologic finding in antipsychotic overdose is *sedation*. This is likely at least partially mediated by histamine receptors. Depending on the dose ingested, this CNS depression can be subtle or profound. Although confusion, lethargy, and slurred speech lie on the mild end of this spectrum, coma and respiratory depressions are common. The sedation caused by large ingestions of atypical antipsychotics can be prolonged (at times lasting days). Though CNS depression is the main neurologic finding, others are possible. The complete reverse may be seen and the patient may be agitated and delirious. Increased muscle tone and hyperreflexia are also noted in some cases. Seizures are also possible in antipsychotic overdose but appear more common with the older typical agents. The seizures are not typically difficult to control. Cardiovascular findings are mediated by adrenergic blockade, which contributes to orthostatic hypotension and dizziness at therapeutic levels, and are more pronounced in overdose. This blockade causes vasodilation and can lead to hypotension with reflex tachycardia. The hypotension seen is usually not profound and typically responds to intravenous fluid administration.

The common ocular finding in atypical overdose is miosis. This miosis is mediated by α_1-adrenergic blockade. The finding of miosis is a very helpful clinical clue if the nature of the ingestion is unknown because relatively few ingested substances cause this finding (e.g., opioids, clonidine, organophosphate pesticides). Small pupils and depressed mental status can sometimes be mistaken for opioid toxicity. In this situation, the clinician may be tempted to administer naloxone. Although not harmful, naloxone in the setting of antipsychotic overdose will not offer any benefit.

Anticholinergic symptoms, due to muscarinic receptor blockade, may also be seen. In this case, the patient may have physical exam findings such as dry mucous membranes, urinary retention, flushing, decreased bowel sounds, and dry skin. Large pupils (mydriasis) may also be seen for this reason.

Prolonged QTc interval is commonly seen with antipsychotic overdose. The mechanism is interference with potassium efflux from the repolarizing cardiac myocyte, which manifests as lengthening of the QT interval on the ECG. Prolonging of the QTc interval is a risk factor for cardiac dysrhythmias, particularly torsades de pointes. The initial assessment for antipsychotic poisoning should include an ECG and cardiac monitoring for QTc prolongation while the patient remains symptomatic. If the QTc interval is prolonged, electrolytes should be monitored closely with special attention to calcium, potassium, and magnesium.

Treatment

Close monitoring of the ABCs (airway, breathing, and circulation) with appropriate supportive care is the first priority. As coma is possible and the patient may be "found down" for an unknown amount of time, the existence of complications possible with such overdoses should be excluded (e.g., aspiration and rhabdomyolysis). Endotracheal intubation may be required for airway protection or if respiratory depression is evident. Close, continued monitoring of the poisoned patient is also warranted as sedation can worsen over time.

Intravenous fluid boluses of isotonic fluid usually are sufficient to correct hypotension and its accompanying reflex tachycardia. If hypotension persists after an adequate fluid challenge, vasopressor therapy may be necessary. As the main reason for this hypotension is α_1-adrenergic receptor blockade, first choices to correct this should be drugs with α-agonist activity. Phenylephrine and norepinephrine have both been recommended for this reason.

The finding of QTc prolongation on ECG requires continued cardiac monitoring. Although relatively rare with antipsychotics, torsades de pointes is a concern in this setting. Intravenous magnesium sulfate (50 mg/kg up to 1–2 g maximum) can be given for prolonged QTc. Overdrive pacing may also have a role in torsades de pointes. However, if torsades de pointes is unstable, it should be treated with cardioversion.

If seizures occur, benzodiazepines are a first-line agent. Phenobarbital is the next choice if needed. As with most drug-induced seizures, phenytoin offers little benefit and may, in some cases, be harmful.

Suggested Readings

Bebarta VS, Kostic MA, Gonzalez MG. Managing adverse reactions to psychotropic medications. *Pediatr Ann* 2005;34:947–954.

Dubois D. Toxicology and overdose of atypical antipsychotic medications in children: does newer necessarily mean safer? *Curr Opin Pediatr* 2005;17:227–233.

Findling RL, Steiner H, Weller EB. Use of antipsychotics in children and adolescents. *J Clin Psychiatry* 2005;66(suppl 7):29–40.

Gomez-Criado MS, Bernardo M, Florez T, et al. Ziprasidone overdose: cases recorded in the database of Pfizer-Spain and literature review. *Pharmacotherapy* 2005;25:1660–1665.

Kao LW, Furbee RB. Drug-induced Q-T prolongation. *Med Clin North Am* 2005;89:1125–1144, x.

Marken PA, Pies RW. Emerging treatments for bipolar disorder: safety and adverse effect profiles. *Ann Pharmacother* 2006;40:276–285.

Patel NC, Crismon ML, Hoagwood K, et al. Unanswered questions regarding atypical antipsychotic use in aggressive children and adolescents. *J Child Adolesc Psychopharmacol* 2005;15:270–284.

Rashid JF, Rosner, F. Tardive dyskinesia: clues to the diagnosis and treatment. *Resid Staff Physician* 2005;51:33–38.

Tandon R. Safety and tolerability: how do newer generation "atypical" antipsychotics compare? *Psychiatr Q* 2002;73:297–311.

Wills B, Erickson T. Drug- and toxin-associated seizures. *Med Clin North Am* 2005;89:1297–1321.

CHAPTER 152C ■ NEUROLEPTIC MALIGNANT SYNDROME AND SEROTONIN SYNDROME

ADAM K. ROWDEN AND DAVID L. ELDRIDGE

The use of psychotropic medications, such as antidepressant and antipsychotic medications, for the treatment of a wide spectrum of pediatric behavioral and psychiatric disorders has become increasingly more common in the pediatric population. Although these drugs often have a proven track record in the adult world, their use in the pediatric population is more often done in an "off-label" fashion. Unlike their colleagues in the world of adult medicine, pediatricians are generally less familiar with the typical indications, clinical pharmacology, and possible adverse effects of these drugs. Two such serious effects are serotonin syndrome (SS) and neuroleptic malignant syndrome (NMS). Each syndrome can occur secondary to a regimen of one or more psychotropic medications. Reaching either diagnosis requires both an indicative medical history and physical exam while at the same time excluding other serious disease processes that can cause similar clinical pictures. Both may lead to serious morbidity and even mortality—though this is generally a far greater concern with NMS. If either NMS or SS are suspected, appropriate supportive care should be initiated, and certain specific clinical interventions begun. With increased utilization of psychotropic drugs in the pediatric population, the pediatric hospitalist will need to become familiar with these clinical entities so optimal care can be started as early as possible.

DRUG-INDUCED HYPERTHERMIAS

NMS and SS share fever as a common clinical symptom. Though this chapter will discuss them specifically in detail, it is appropriate to briefly discuss other instances where drugs may induce fever. Other examples of drug-induced hyperthermia include sympathomimetic toxicity, anticholinergic toxicity, and malignant hyperthermia (MH). One axiom in the management of each of the conditions discussed here (including NMS and SS) is the lack of a role for antipyretic medications in their treatment.

Although this chapter deals with SS specifically, *sympathomimetic toxicity* and SS share many common features, and may be a continuum of the same pathophysiologic process. Classically, sympathomimetic toxicity has been attributed to a host of stimulants (e.g., cocaine, amphetamines, methamphetamines), and ecstasy (methylenedioxymethamphetamines or MDMA). Other potential causes are listed in Table 152.9. Sympathomimetic toxicity is typically characterized by agitation, hypertension, tachycardia, dilated pupils, and diaphoresis. *Anticholinergic toxicity* can result from any toxin or drug which decreases acetylcholine levels in the nerve synapse. Common agents causing anticholinergic toxicity are listed in Table 152.10. This syndrome is characterized by agitation, confusion, visual hallucinations, tachycardia, mild hyperthermia, dry skin and mucous membranes, decreased gut motility, dilated pupils, and urinary retention. Although this anticholinergic toxicity shares many clinical characteristics with the sympathomimetic toxidrome, it can be reliably differentiated by the presence of urinary retention and decreased bowel sounds on exam, which is not typical of sympathomimetics. Dry mucous membranes and skin also is more indicative of anticholinergic poisoning.

Malignant hyperthermia results from a genetic defect in calcium release from the sarcoplasmic reticulum of skeletal muscle in response to inhalational anesthetics and some medications used to induce a depolarizing neuromuscular blockade. It is characterized by hyperthermia, muscle rigidity, and autonomic instability after exposure to the above drugs.

NEUROLEPTIC MALIGNANT SYNDROME

Neuroleptic malignant syndrome (NMS) is a feared adverse event associated primarily with the use of neuroleptic (antipsychotic) medications. It is also reported with the abrupt cessation of dopaminergic receptor agonists (such as those used in the treatment of Parkinson disease). Generally, NMS is thought to be more common with the use of the older, original, "typical" (high-potency) classes of antipsychotic medications, such as haloperidol. With these older neuroleptics, the incidence of NMS occurrence is reported to be 0.07% to 2.2%. However, this syndrome is reported even with the use of

TABLE 152.9

COMMON SYMPATHOMIMETIC AGENTS

Amphetamines
Methamphetamines
MDMA (ecstasy)
Cocaine
Ephedrine
Pseudoephedrine
Caffeine
Ma Huang (herbal supplement)
Ephedra

TABLE 152.10

COMMON ANTICHOLINERGIC AGENTS

ANTIHISTAMINES	OTHERS
Chlorpheniramine	Amantadine
Diphenhydramine	Atropine
Doxylamine	Benztropine
Hydroxyzine	Glycopyrrolate
	Hyoscyamine
MUSCLE RELAXANTS	Meclizine
Carisoprodol	Phenothiazines
Cyclobenzaprine	Quinidine
	Quinine
PLANTS	Scopolamine
Jimsonweed	Tricyclic antidepressants
Nightshade	

newer, "atypical" (low-potency) antipsychotic medications, such as risperidone. As the use of these newer medications is expanding in the pediatric population, the pediatric hospitalist is increasingly likely to encounter this syndrome. Because it is associated with a significant risk of both morbidity and mortality, it is imperative that NMS be in the differential diagnosis of any patient who presents with suggestive clinical symptoms and is taking any of the medications linked with this illness. Appropriate care can then be initiated.

Clinical Presentation

Although the exact criteria for the diagnosis of NMS varies depending on the source, the clinical quartet of *hyperthermia, motor dysfunction* (most commonly muscular rigidity), *altered mental status, and autonomic dysfunction* are generally held as the keystones of diagnosis. These core clinical features, which vary in precise presentation and severity (Table 152.11), may present at different times in a given course. In contrast to the acute onset of serotonin syndrome, the symptoms of NMS generally evolve more slowly over the course of 24 to 72 hours. Some have suggested this progression of symptoms typically begins with altered mental status and gradually will include the other classic symptoms, but this is not consistent. Even with appropriate therapy, the clinical course of NMS may be as long as 2 to 3 weeks.

A fever of 38°C or greater is generally seen, and temperatures in excess of 41°C have been reported. The muscle rigidity of NMS is most commonly described as a generalized "lead-pipe rigidity"—increased tone with noticeable resistance to passive movement. Though rigidity is the classic muscular

TABLE 152.11

CLINICAL SYMPTOMS DESCRIBED IN NEUROLEPTIC MALIGNANT SYNDROME

HYPERTHERMIA	Opisthotonos
ALTERED MENTAL STATUS	Chorea
Coma	Trismus
Agitation	Dysphagia
Confusion	
	AUTONOMIC INSTABILITY
MOTOR DYSFUNCTION	Altered blood pressure
Muscle rigidity	(usually hypertension)
("lead-pipe")	Diaphoresis
Decreased chest wall	Tachycardia
compliance	Tachypnea
Dystonia	Mutism

finding of NMS, other motor findings have also been described with NMS (Table 152.11). One major clinical concern regarding this rigidity is that it may herald the onset of significant rhabdomyolysis. The patient may develop decreased chest-wall compliance with compromise of respiratory function. The autonomic dysfunction seen in NMS is variable, with blood pressure swings to either extreme (though hypertension predominates). Other signs of autonomic dysfunction include tachycardia, diaphoresis, and respiratory disturbances. Mental status changes reported with NMS range from severe agitation at one end of the spectrum to stupor or coma at the other.

Diagnosis

NMS is a diagnosis of exclusion. In any patient presenting with fever and altered mental status, there are other life-threatening and treatable disease processes that must be considered in the differential diagnosis (Table 152.12). Therefore, diagnostic testing may not confirm NMS but will help eliminate other equally serious illnesses. For example, even though the information provided by a lumbar puncture will not help in the diagnosis of NMS, it will often be needed to help exclude CNS infections. Though imaging of the CNS does not directly aid in the diagnoses of NMS, it is often performed to help eliminate other concerning disease processes.

For the diagnosis of NMS to be entertained, the patient must first have a history of using a medication associated with this diagnosis (Table 152.13). Even if a patient is on an atypical antipsychotic, the diagnosis should be entertained. Analysis of cases reported in the literature has lead to the identification of some risk factors that, if placed in the context of a suggestive clinical picture, may elevate the pediatrician's clinical suspicion (Table 152.14).

Although no laboratory test clinches the diagnosis of NMS, there are two abnormalities that are fairly consistently seen.

TABLE 152.12

DIFFERENTIAL DIAGNOSIS FOR NEUROLEPTIC MALIGNANT SYNDROME AND SEROTONIN SYNDROME

DRUG-INDUCED HYPERTHERMIAS
Malignant hyperthermia
Anticholinergic toxidrome
Sympathomimetic toxidrome

DRUG OVERDOSES
Salicylates
Monoamine oxidase inhibitors (MAOIs)

DRUG WITHDRAWAL
Benzodiazepines
Barbiturates
Ethanol

INFECTIOUS
Sepsis
Encephalitis
Meningitis

OTHERS
Heat stroke
Strychnine
Tetanus
Thyrotoxicosis

TABLE 152.13

MEDICATIONS ASSOCIATED WITH NEUROLEPTIC MALIGNANT SYNDROME

WITHDRAWAL OF ANTIPARKINSONIAN DRUGS
Amantadine
Levodopa-carbidopa

USE OF ANTIPSYCHOTIC MEDICATIONS
Typical antipsychotics (high-potency at central dopamine receptors)
Chlorpromazine
Fluphenazine
Haloperidol
Loxapine
Thioridazine
Thiothixene
Atypical antipsychotics
Clozapine
Olanzapine
Quetiapine
Risperidone
Ziprasidone

Along with the clinical finding of muscle rigidity, an elevated creatine phosphokinase (CPK) level is often seen and serves as an indicator of rhabdomyolysis. It is not uncommon for CPK to be extremely elevated in NMS and for myoglobinuria to be present as well. The second common laboratory abnormality is leukocytosis, with an increase in the band count as well. Depending on the severity of the presentation, metabolic acidosis, elevated transaminases, and coagulation abnormalities indicative of disseminated intravascular coagulation may also be found.

Treatment

Neuroleptic malignant syndrome and its complications (Table 152.15) carry a great risk of morbidity and mortality (estimated from 10%–30%). The treatment for NMS begins with the immediate withdrawal of the suspected trigger medication (or the reinstating of the dopaminergic agent that has recently been withdrawn) and appropriate supportive care. Often these patients will require close monitoring in an intensive-care setting. If NMS is suspected, initial stabilization of the patient and transfer to such a setting should be strongly considered. The primary directive of maintaining airway, breathing, and circulation is critical. As these patients often present with a decreased level of consciousness and risk of aspiration, intubation may be needed in order to protect their airway. From a cardiovascular standpoint, autonomic dysfunction can produce hypotension or hypertension requiring medical intervention. To compound this

---

TABLE 152.14

POSSIBLE RISK FACTORS FOR DEVELOPMENT OF NEUROLEPTIC MALIGNANT SYNDROME

Previous brain injury
Dehydration
Malnutrition
Antipsychotic dosing patterns
High doses
Rapid increase of dose over short time period
Use of two or more antipsychotics at once
Concomitant use with lithium

TABLE 152.15

POSSIBLE COMPLICATIONS OF NEUROLEPTIC
MALIGNANT SYNDROME

Rhabdomyolysis
Hepatic failure
Renal failure
Sepsis
Aspiration pneumonia
Cardiac arrhythmia
Cardiopulmonary arrest
Pulmonary embolism
Seizures
Disseminated intravascular coagulation

problem, hyperthermia and diaphoresis may lead to hypovolemia. Therefore, close monitoring of fluid input and output with appropriate intravenous fluid supplementation is important. Continuous cardiac monitoring is recommended as cardiac arrhythmias are also reported.

Hyperthermia may be profound and should be addressed with direct cooling methods (e.g., fans, cooling blankets, ice). There is no role for antipyretic medication in the management of the hyperthermia of NMS. Renal dysfunction secondary to rhabdomyolysis is a serious concern. If an elevated CPK level or myoglobinuria is discovered, appropriate intravenous fluid support to preserve renal function should be initiated. The clinical symptoms of NMS may predispose to deep vein thrombosis and pulmonary embolism. Compressive stockings and kinetic nursing beds are often used. Anticoagulation therapy should be considered.

Management with a variety of drug therapies has been advocated by some experts and minimized by others. Some of this discord stems from disagreement on the true pathophysiology of NMS. As NMS is both rare and solely a clinical diagnosis, there is a lack of good, prospective clinical trials for any particular drug therapy. Much of the research with any medical therapy is limited to case reports. Reported success with any proposed medication is widely variable. However, because NMS has a relatively high risk of mortality, if supportive care has been maximized, it seems prudent to utilize these medical therapies that may be potentially advantageous. The most commonly examined and utilized, *bromocriptine* and *dantrolene*, will be discussed here. They have both been used separately and together for the treatment of NMS.

Bromocriptine, a dopaminergic agonist, has often been utilized in the treatment of NMS. Some studies report both a shortening of the course of NMS and a decreased risk of mortality with its use. It is solely an oral medication and therefore may have to be given via a nasogastric tube. Some reports describe decreased temperature and rigidity as well as improved blood pressure. The generally recommended dosing of bromocriptine varies from 2.5 mg to 10 mg four times a day. Hypotension is a commonly reported side effect. Nausea, and in some cases psychosis, can also be seen.

Dantrolene, a muscle relaxant that blocks intracellular calcium release from the sarcoplasmic reticulum, has long been considered the drug of choice for malignant hyperthermia. Its use in NMS is also common. Its desired effects are muscle relaxation and decreased heat production. Dosage range of dantrolene has been suggested at 1 to 10 mg/kg/day (oral 50–200 mg/day). The most concerning possible side effect of dantrolene is hepatotoxicity.

One concern is the issue of recurrence of NMS upon restarting antipsychotic therapy. Rather then restarting with "high-potency" typical antipsychotics, an attempt is made to switch to one of the newer, "low-potency" atypical antipsychotics. Many experts advocate waiting at least 2 weeks after NMS symptoms have completely resolved and having the patient in a state of good physical health before restarting any antipsychotic medication. At this point, one may gradually increase the medication dose as needed over time while monitoring carefully for any symptoms concerning for a recurrence of NMS.

SEROTONIN SYNDROME

Serotonin syndrome (SS) was first reported in 1955 from an interaction between meperidine and a monoamine oxidase inhibitor (MAOI). The most infamous suspected case of SS involved the death of Libby Zion. Her death served as a catalyst to changes in resident work hours. SS now is recognized to occur in association with drugs such as selective serotonin reuptake inhibitors (SSRIs), which increase serotonin receptor agonism. Since these first initial cases, extensive study has occurred in an effort to prevent, diagnose, and treat this serious drug-induced syndrome. SS may be mild, requiring only removal of the offending agent, or may be a life-threatening medical emergency requiring aggressive therapy to prevent mortality.

Clinical Presentation

The patient with SS typically presents with a symptoms in three general categories: *neurocognitive dysfunction, autonomic dysfunction,* and *neuromotor dysfunction.* Although one may predominate, usually there are findings in all three areas (Table 152.16). Clinical findings usually begin shortly, typically within hours, after a dosing change or addition of new medications or substances that result in increased serotonin activity. Although most cases are mild and self-limited, deaths have been reported.

TABLE 152.16

CLINICAL SYMPTOMS DESCRIBED IN SEROTONIN
SYMDROME

NEUROCOGNITIVE DYSFUNCTION
  Altered mental status
  Confusion
  Coma
  CNS depression
  CNS stimulation
  Agitation
  Seizures

AUTONOMIC DYSFUNCTION
  Hypertension
  Tachycardia
  Diaphoresis
  Diarrhea
  Hypotension
  Fever
  Dilated Pupils

NEUROMOTOR DYSFUNCTION
  Increased muscle tone (especially in lower extremities)
  Myclonus
  Tremor
  Ataxia
  Hyperreflexia
  Nystagmus
  Bruxism

Neurocognitive dysfunction in SS is usually typified by altered mental status. This altered mental status may vary wildly from CNS depression to stimulation. Although agitation is most commonly seen in mild cases, the behavioral changes may manifest simply as confusion. Coma is also possible especially in the late stages of SS. Seizures are occasionally reported and may be refractory in the setting of severe serotonin syndrome.

The second feature of SS is autonomic dysfunction with hypertension and tachycardia being the most common symptoms in this category. Although typically not severe, disturbances in cardiovascular stability can be dramatic and lead to arrhythmias and ischemic complications. In later stages, hypotension is possible and is a poor prognostic sign. Diaphoresis, dilated pupils, and diarrhea are common findings also linked to this autonomic dysfunction. Hyperthermia, which can be profound, is a grave finding and indicates a critically ill patient in need of aggressive therapy.

The third class of symptoms in SS is neuromotor dysfunction. This most common form of this is increased muscle tone that is frequently more pronounced in the lower extremities. Inducible myoclonus and hyperreflexia are common in even mild cases. Sustained myclonus and muscle rigidity are signs of more severe disease and should prompt the clinician to suspect rhabdomyolysis. Ataxia, nystagmus, and bruxism are also reported.

The critically ill patient with serotonin syndrome will typically present with extreme agitation, hypertension, tachycardia, lower extremity myclonus, and hyperreflexia. Without appropriate, early treatment, the clinical picture may progress to include general muscle rigidity, hyperthermia, hypotension, coma, and seizures.

Diagnosis

Like NMS, SS is defined by observed clinical symptoms alone and is a diagnosis of exclusion. It is generally agreed that the symptoms seen will fall into three general categories: *neurocognitive dysfunction, autonomic dysfunction,* and *neuromotor dysfunction* (Table 152.16). Because there are no laboratory tests to confirm the diagnosis, it is important for clinicians to maintain a high index of suspicion for serotonin syndrome while considering other possible diagnoses (Table 152.12). Other disease processes should be explored thoughtfully, utilizing all necessary laboratory tests and other studies to eliminate other, similar potentially life-threatening disease processes.

Besides identifying possible clinical findings, a pertinent history compatible with SS must be obtained. The most important component of the medical history is exposure to serotonergic agents (Table 152.17), which is key to the diagnosis. SS typically occurs soon after a change in the dosage of a serotonergic drug, or after the addition of another drug with serotonergic activity. Single agents, particularly some drugs of abuse, are capable of inducing serotonin syndrome by themselves. Although a wide variety of prescription antidepressants are well known to most physicians to have serotonergic activity, the clinician should also inquire into some common over-the-counter (OTC) agents that also may lead to SS (Table 152.17). Two notable examples are the antitussive dextromethorphan and the herbal product St. John's wort. The importance of history cannot be overemphasized, because identifying and withdrawing the offending agent is essential to treatment.

If the patient is also taking antipsychotic medications, choosing between the diagnoses of SS and NMS can be challenging. These clinical syndromes have many overlapping symptoms, such as fever and altered mental status, and are often confused. However, if a patient's medication list necessitates consideration of both diagnoses, there are some clinical

TABLE 152.17

DRUGS IMPLICATED IN SEROTONIN SYNDROME

L-tryptophan
Monoamine oxidase inhibitors
Amphetamines
Methamphetamines
MDMA (ecstasy)
Cocaine
Tricyclic antidepressants
Selective serotonin reuptake inhibitors (SSRIs)
Venlafaxine
Dextromethorphan
Meperidine
Tramadol
Linezolid
Reserpine
Fenfluramine
Lithium
Nefazodone
Sumatriptan
St. John's wort
Bupropion

differences that may allow the pediatric hospitalist to discriminate between the two (Table 152.18).

Treatment

The treatment of serotonin syndrome hinges on recognizing the disease so that the offending agent or agents can be withdrawn. Equally important is good supportive care and anticipation of complications (Table 152.19). As with any patient, airway, breathing, and circulation should be addressed and managed appropriately. A variety of pharmacotherapies have been proposed in the treatment of SS, but should be utilized with caution as the clinical evidence supporting them is largely anecdotal. Severe cases of SS will likely require an intensive-care setting for management. Finally, if SS is suspected, phone consultation with a medical toxicologist can be sought from a regional poison control center for specific treatment recommendations.

Benzodiazepines are considered first-line agents in most cases of SS. Their pharmacology makes them a logical choice

TABLE 152.18

CLINICAL CONTRASTS OF NEUROLEPTIC MALIGNANT SYNDROME AND SEROTONIN SYNDROME

	NMS	SS
Time of onset	Symptoms typically evolve over days	Symptoms typically evolve over minutes to hours
Myoclonus	Less common	More common
Muscle rigidity	More common	Less common
Increased CPK	More common	Less common
Leukocytosis	More common	Less common
Metabolic acidosis	More common	Less common
Time of symptom resolution	Typically over days	Typically over 24 hours

TABLE 152.19

COMPLICATIONS OF SEROTONIN SYNDROME

Hyperthermia
Seizures
Rhabdomyolysis
Disseminated intravascular coagulation
Cardiovascular collapse
Coma
Stroke

to counteract the clinical symptoms seen with SS. Benzodiazepines exert their effect on the central nervous system by facilitating the activity of the neurotransmitter gamma-aminobutyric acid (GABA), the major inhibitory neurotransmitter of the central nervous system. This general inhibitory action by benzodiazepines has several benefits: (1) calming the agitated patient, (2) decreasing the CNS-mediated release of catecholamines to help counter the hypertension and tachycardia usually encountered in SS, (3) serving as a muscle relaxant to relieve rigidity, and (4) if seizures are suspected, serving as an anticonvulsant. In addition to these benefits, most pediatricians are very familiar with these drugs, which are widely available, can be given IV, have a wide margin of safety, and can be titrated carefully to effect. Despite their wide use in clinical practice, the evidence for their effectiveness is not rigorous and is largely based on case reports. There are no large-scale clinical trials to support their use in SS.

More profound symptoms may require more aggressive therapy. If muscle rigidity is severe and does not respond readily to benzodiazepines, other therapies may be considered. Dantrolene, commonly used in the treatment of MH, has also been proposed as a treatment for SS. Though available data show mixed results with no clear benefit, in the face of refractory muscle rigidity, dantrolene may be warranted. Severe muscle rigidity should also prompt the pediatrician to obtain a CPK level and urine myoglobin to look for signs of rhabdomyolysis. If rhabdomyolysis is a concern, appropriate intravenous fluid should be used to help prevent renal failure. In the hyperthermic patient direct, active cooling should be utilized when necessary. Antipyretics have no role in the hyperthermia induced by serotonin syndrome. Hypertension and tachycardia rarely require specific interventions and usually respond well to benzodiazepines. Antidotal therapy aimed at antagonizing the serotonin receptor has been used in some cases. The drug most commonly utilized is cyproheptadine. The evidence for its use is largely based on case reports of some success with this medication. Animal models have shown some evidence of potential benefit, but only when pretreated with dosages that far exceed what is typically used in humans. Until further evidence exists, this agent should be thought of as adjutant to supportive care.

References

1. Heyman I, Santosh P. Pharmacological and other physical treatments. In: Rutter M, Taylor E, eds. *Child and adolescent psychiatry*. 4th ed. Oxford: Blackwell; 2002:998–1018.
2. Conrad P. Prescribing more psychotropic medications for children. *Arch Pediatr Adolesc Med* 2004;158:829–830.
3. Campbell M, Rapoport JL, Simpson GM. Antipsychotics in children and adolescents. *J Am Acad Child Adolesc Psychiatry* 1999;38:537–545.
4. Emslic GJ, Walters JT, Pliszka SR, et al. Nontricyclic antidepressants: current trends in children and adolescents. *J Am Acad Child Adolesc Psychiatry* 1999;38:517–528.
5. Tueth MJ, Murphy TK, Evan DL. Special considerations: use of lithium in children, adolescents, and elderly populations. *J Child Psychol Psychiatry* 1998;59:66–73.

Suggested Readings

Adnet P, Lestavel P, Krivosic-Huber R, et al. Neuroleptic malignant syndrome. *Br J Anaesth* 2000;85:129–135.
Asch DA, Parker RM. The Libby Zion case. One step forward or two steps backward? *N Engl J Med* 1988;318:771–775.
Bhanushali MJ, Tuite PJ. The evaluation and management of patients with neuroleptic malignant syndrome. *Neurol Clin* 2004;22:389–411.
Boyer EW, Shannon M. The serotonin syndrome. *N Engl J Med* 2005;352:1112–1120.
Chandran GJ, Mikler JR, Keegan DL, et al. Neuroleptic malignant syndrome: case report and discussion. *CMAJ* 2003;169:439–442.
Farver DK. Neuroleptic malignant syndrome induced by atypical antipsychotics. *Expert Opin Drug Saf* 2003;2:21–35.
Graudins A, Stearman A, Chan B. Treatment of the serotonin syndrome with cyproheptadine. *J Emerg Med* 1998;16:615–619.
Gupta S, Nihalani ND. Neuroleptic malignant syndrome: a primary care perspective. Primary care companion to the Journal of Clinical Psychiatry (Prim Care Companion J clin Psychiatry) *J Clin Psychiatry* 2004;6:191–194.
Halloran LL, Bernard DW. Management of drug-induced hyperthermia. *Curr Opin Pediatr* 2004;16:211–215.
Mills KC. Serotonin syndrome. A clinical update. *Crit Care Clin* 1997;13:763–783.
Radomski JW, Dursun SM, Reveley MA, et al. An exploratory approach to the serotonin syndrome: an update of clinical phenomenology and revised diagnostic criteria. *Med Hypotheses* 2000;55:218–224.
Rusyniak DE, Sprague JE. Toxin-induced hyperthermic syndromes. *Med Clin North Am* 2005;89:1277–1296.
Susman VL. Clinical management of neuroleptic malignant syndrome. *Psychiatr Q* 2001;72:325–336.
Thomas CR, Rosenberg M, Blythe V, et al. Serotonin syndrome and linezolid. *J Am Acad Child Adolesc Psychiatry* 2004;43:790.
Ty EB, Rothner AD. Neuroleptic malignant syndrome in children and adolescents. *J Child Neurol* 2001;16:157–163.

Page numbers followed by *f* refer to illustrations; page numbers followed by *t* refer to tables.